PHARMACOLOGIC ASPECTS *of* NURSING

PHARMACOLOGIC ASPECTS *of* NURSING

EDITED BY

ANN M. PAGLIARO, R.N., B.S.N., M.S.N.

Associate Professor of Nursing,
Faculty of Nursing,
University of Alberta,
Edmonton, Alberta

LOUIS A. PAGLIARO, M.S., Pharm.D., Ph.D.

Associate Professor and Coordinator, Master of Pharmacy Program,
Faculty of Pharmacy and Pharmaceutical Sciences,
University of Alberta,
Edmonton, Alberta

with 335 illustrations

The C. V. Mosby Company

St. Louis · Toronto · Princeton   1986

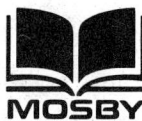

MOSBY

A TRADITION OF PUBLISHING EXCELLENCE

Project Editor: Teri Merchant
Manuscript Editors: Kathy Brown, Jeff Friedman, Nelle Garrecht, Dale Woolery
Production: Barbara Merritt, Teresa Breckwoldt, Kathleen L. Teal
Design: Nancy Steinmeyer

The C.V. Mosby Company

11830 Westline Industrial Drive, St. Louis, Missouri 63146

Library of Congress Cataloging in Publication Data

Main entry under title:

Pharmacologic aspects of nursing.

Includes bibliographies and index.
1. Pharmacology. 2. Drugs. 3. Nursing.
I. Pagliaro, Ann M. II. Pagliaro, Louis A.
[DNLM: 1. Drug Therapy—nurses' instruction.
2. Pharmacology—nurses' instruction.   QV 4 P5345]
RM300.P49 1986   615'.1   85-31739
ISBN 0-8016-3747-3

GW/VH/VH 9 8 7 6 5 4 3 2 1   03/D/318

Contributors

Jon Auricchio, Pharm.D.
Assistant Director, Internal Medicine Residency Program;
Assistant Professor of Clinical Pharmacy, Washington State
University, Spokane, Washington

Leslie Z. Benet, Ph.D.
Professor and Chairman, Department of Pharmacy, School
of Pharmacy, University of California, San Francisco, San
Francisco, California

Larry Bettesworth, B.S.
Clinical Instructor, College of Pharmacy, Washington State
University, Spokane, Washington

David F. Biggs, Ph.D.
Professor, Faculty of Pharmacy and Pharmaceutical
Sciences, University of Alberta, Edmonton, Alberta

Steven H. Butler, M.D.
Assistant Professor of Anesthesiology, Attending Physician
in Pain Clinics, School of Medicine, University of
Washington, Seattle, Washington

**Ronald T. Coutts, Ph.D., D.Sc., F.C.I.C., F.R.I.C., F.P.S.,
F.R.S.C.**
University Professor and Professor of Medicinal Chemistry,
Faculty of Pharmacy and Pharmaceutical Sciences,
University of Alberta, Edmonton, Alberta

**William G. Dewhurst, M.A., B.M., B.Ch., M.R.C.P.,
D.P.M., F.R.C.P.(C.), F.A.C.Psych., F.R.C.Psych.**
Chairman and Professor, Department of Psychiatry, Faculty
of Medicine, University of Alberta, Edmonton, Alberta

John B. Dossetor, B.M., B.Ch., Ph.D., F.R.C.P., F.A.C.P.
Professor, Faculty of Medicine, University of Alberta,
Edmonton, Alberta

David M. Fawcett, B.Sc., M.D., M.Sc., Ph.D.
Professor, Faculty of Medicine, University of Alberta;
Medical Biochemist, Department of Laboratory Medicine,
University of Alberta Hospital, Edmonton, Alberta

Abram J.D. Friesen, B.S., M.A., Ph.D.
Associate Professor, Faculty of Pharmacy and
Pharmaceutical Sciences, University of Alberta, Edmonton,
Alberta

Gerald R. Greene, M.D., M.P.H.
Associate Adjunct Professor, Director, Pediatrics Inpatient
Service, Department of Pediatrics, School of Medicine,
University of California, Irvine, Irvine, California

Sharon M. Hall, Ph.D.
Associate Professor in Residence, Medical Psychology,
Langley Porter Psychiatric Institute, University of
California, San Francisco, San Francisco, California

Philip D. Hansten, Pharm.D.
Professor, College of Pharmacy, Washington State
University, Pullman, Washington

Donna R. Helmer, M.A.
University of Evansville, Evansville, Indiana

Betty-ann Hoener, Ph.D.
Vice Chairwoman and Associate Professor, Department of
Pharmacy, School of Pharmacy, University of California,
San Francisco, San Francisco, California

Debbie L. Huie, Pharm.D.
Drug Information Service, Department of Pharmacy
Services, Stanford University Hospital, Stanford, California

Richard L. Jones, B.S., M.S., Ph.D.
Associate Professor, Faculty of Medicine, University of
Alberta, Edmonton, Alberta

John F. Kittel, B.S.Pharm., Pharm.D.
Chief, Pharmacy Services, Veteran's Administration Medical
Center, Spokane, Washington

Loren W. Kline, B.Sc., M.Sc., Ph.D.
Professor, Faculty of Dentistry, Department of Oral Biology,
University of Alberta, Edmonton, Alberta

**Thavisakdi Kovithavongs, M.D., Ph.D., F.A.C.P.,
F.R.C.P.(C.)**
Associate Professor of Medicine, Faculty of Medicine,
University of Alberta, Edmonton, Alberta

Don Leach, Pharm.D.
Director of Pharmacy, Cascade Valley Hospital, Arlington,
Washington

Donald R. McLean, M.D., F.R.C.P.(C.)
Director and Professor of Neurology, Division of Neurology,
Faculty of Medicine, University of Alberta, Edmonton,
Alberta

Philip K. Ng, B.Pharm., Pharm.D., M.D.
Honorary Assistant Professor, Pediatrics, Faculty of
Medicine, University of Alberta, Edmonton, Alberta

Sharon D. Ow-Wing, Pharm.D.
Staff Pharmacist, Pediatric Satellite Pharmacy, Department of Pharmacy Services, Stanford University Hospital, Stanford, California

Ann M. Pagliaro, R.N., B.S.N., M.S.N.
Associate Professor of Nursing, Faculty of Nursing, University of Alberta, Edmonton, Alberta

Louis A. Pagliaro, M.S., Pharm.D., Ph.D.
Associate Professor and Coordinator, Master of Pharmacy Program, Faculty of Pharmacy and Pharmaceutical Sciences, University of Alberta, Edmonton, Alberta

Lynn M. Paulsen, Pharm.D.
Associate Professor, College of Pharmacy, Washington State University, Spokane, Washington

Shirley C. Peeke, Ph.D.
Associate Adjunct Professor, Medical Psychology, Langley Porter Neuropsychological Institute, University of California, San Francisco, San Francisco, California

Margaret A. Peterson, B.Sc.Pharm., M.Sc., Ph.D.
Assistant Professor, Faculty of Pharmacy, University of Manitoba, Winnipeg, Manitoba

Frederick G. Pfeiffer, M.S., Pharm.D.
Attending Clinical Pharmacist, Family Medical Center, Clinical Assistant Professor, University of Iowa, Iowa City, Iowa

Randall A. Prince, Pharm.D.
Associate Professor, College of Pharmacy, University of Iowa, Iowa City, Iowa

Stuart A. Ross, M.B., Ch.B., F.R.A.C.P.
Director of Diabetic Daycare Centre, Foothills Provincial Hospital; Assistant Professor, Faculty of Medicine, University of Calgary, Calgary, Alberta

Sheldon H. Roth, B.Sc., M.Sc., Ph.D.
Professor, Departments of Anesthesia and Pharmacology and Therapeutics, Faculty of Medicine, University of Calgary, Calgary, Alberta

Eric Schloss, M.D., F.R.C.P.(C.)
Associate Clinical Professor, Pathology and Dermatology, Faculty of Medicine, University of Alberta, Edmonton, Alberta

Alec Shysh, B.Sc., M.Sc., Ph.D.
Professor, Faculty of Pharmacy and Pharmaceutical Sciences, University of Alberta, Edmonton, Alberta

Branimir Ivan Sikic, B.S., M.D.
Assistant Professor, Department of Medicine (Oncology and Clinical Pharmacology), Stanford University, Stanford, California

William D. Snively, Jr., M.D., F.A.C.P.
Professor Emeritus of Life Sciences, University of Evansville, Evansville, Indiana

George C. Stone, Ph.D.
Professor of Medical Psychology, Director of Graduate Academic Programs, Department of Psychiatry, University of California, San Francisco, San Francisco, California

David S. Tatro, Pharm.D.
Assistant Clinical Professor, School of Pharmacy, University of California, San Francisco; Assistant Director of Pharmacy for Drug Information and Educational Services, Stanford University Hospital, Stanford University Medical Center, Stanford, California

Norman R. Thomas, B.D.S., B.Sc., Ph.D.
Professor, Department of Oral Biology, Faculty of Dentistry, University of Alberta, Edmonton, Alberta

Elliot S. Vesell, M.D.
Professor and Chairman, Department of Pharmacology, College of Medicine, The Pennsylvania State University, Hershey, Pennsylvania

Leonard I. Wiebe, B.S.P., M.Sc., Ph.D.
Professor and Assistant Dean (Research), Faculty of Pharmacy and Pharmaceutical Sciences, University of Alberta, Edmonton, Alberta

D. George Wyse, B.S.P., M.Sc., M.D., Ph.D., F.R.C.P.(C.), F.A.C.P., F.A.C.C.
Director, Foothills Hospital Pacemaker and Clinical Electrophysiology Center; Associate Professor, Faculty of Medicine, University of Calgary, Calgary, Alberta

Walter W. Yakimets, M.D., F.R.C.S.(C.), F.A.C.S.
Professor, Faculty of Medicine, University of Alberta, Edmonton, Alberta

Karin E. Zenk, Pharm.D.
Pharmacist-Specialist in Pediatrics, University of California Irvine Medical Center; Assistant Adjunct Professor of Pediatrics, University of California, Irvine; Assistant Clinical Professor of Pharmacy, University of California, San Francisco, San Francisco, California

Nursing Advisory Committee

Marjorie C. Anderson, R.N., B.Sc., M.N.
Assistant Professor, Faculty of Nursing, University of Alberta, Edmonton, Alberta

Audrey L. Barlock, R.N.
Oncology Nurse Consultant, Silver Spring, Maryland

Frances Fothergill Bourbonnais, R.N., B.Sc.N., M.N.
Assistant Professor, School of Nursing, University of Ottawa, Ottawa, Ontario

Muriel Burry, R.N.
Head Nurse of Neurology and Neurosurgery, Health Sciences Centre, Winnipeg, Manitoba

Anne L. Cavanaugh, R.N.
Director, Patient Respresentative Program, The Bryn Mawr Hospital, Bryn Mawr, Pennsylvania

Marcia A. Cohen, C.N.A, R.N., B.S., C.M.H.N.P.
Director of Nursing, Council for Jewish Elderly, Lieberman Geriatric Health Centre, Skokie, Illinois

Margaret Cotterell, R.N., M.A., A.N.P.
Clinical Instructor, Geriatric
Nurse Practitioner Program, New York Hospital School of Continuing Education for Nurses, New York Hospital–Cornell Medical Center, New York, New York

Carolyn D. Davis, R.N., B.S.N., M.S. Admin. Med.
Hypertension Practitioner, William S. Middleton Memorial Veteran's Hospital, Madison, Wisconsin

Teresa M. Davis, R.N., B.N., M.Ed., Ph.D.
Associate Professor of Nursing, Faculty of Nursing, University of Alberta, Edmonton, Alberta

Rene A. Day, R.N., B.Sc., M.Sc. (Nursing)
Associate Professor of Nursing, Faculty of Nursing, University of Alberta, Edmonton, Alberta

Kathleen A. Dier, R.N., B.Sc., M.Sc. (Nursing)
Associate Professor of Nursing, Faculty of Nursing, University of Alberta, Edmonton, Alberta

Charlotte E. Eliopoulos, R.N., M.P.H.
Vice President for Clinical Services, Levindale Hebrew Geriatric Center and Hospital, Baltimore, Maryland

Gail Federspiel, R.N., M.Ed.
Faculty of Nursing, University of Alberta, Edmonton, Alberta

Janis W. Fink, R.N., M.S.N.
Formerly Nurse Educator, National High Blood Pressure Education Program, Kappa Systems, Inc., Bethesda, Maryland

Patricia E. Greene, R.N., M.S.N., F.A.A.N.
Assistant Vice President for Cancer Nursing, American Cancer Society National Office, New York, New York

Shirley M. Gullo, R.N.
Chemotherapy Coordinator, Cleveland Clinic Foundation, Cleveland, Ohio

Patricia Turk Horvath, R.N., M.S.N.
Assistant Professor and Coordinator, Cardiovascular Specialty, Medical-Surgical Nursing Program, School of Nursing, Yale University; Clinical Nurse Specialist, Cardiac Surgery, Yale–New Haven Hospital, New Haven, Connecticut

Susan M. Hubbard, R.N., B.S.
Director International Cancer Information Center, Office of International Affairs, National Cancer Institute, Bethesda, Maryland

Virginia H. Kemp, R.N., Ph.D.
Assistant Professor, Parent-Child Nursing, Medical College of Georgia, School of Nursing, Augusta, Georgia

Margaret King-Collier, R.N., B.Sc.N., M.N.
Nurse Epidemiologist, University of Alberta, Edmonton, Alberta

Sharon Krumm, R.N., M.S.N.
Director of Nursing, Ellis Fischel State Cancer Center, Columbia, Missouri

Angela Ladyshewsky, R.N.
Neuroscience Unit, St. Boniface General Hospital, Winnipeg, Manitoba

Laura Jean Looper, R.N., M.A.
Professor, Department of Nursing, College of Marin, Kentfield, California

Mildred L. Matthes, R.N., M.A.
Director, Diabetic Day Care, Maricopa Medical Center, Maricopa County Department of Health Services, Phoenix, Arizona

Constance W. McAdams, R.N., M.S.N., Ph.D.
Assistant Professor of Nursing, School of Nursing, University of California at Los Angeles, Los Angeles, California

Margo McCaffery, R.N., M.S., F.A.A.N.
Consultant in the Nursing Care of People with Pain, Santa Monica, California

Mary Ann Mikulic, R.N., M.N.
Rehabilitation Clinical Nurse Specialist, Veterans Administration Medical Center, Seattle, Washington

Susan E. Norman, R.N., M.S.N.
Clinical Nurse Specialist, Sleep Disorders/Pulmonary Medicine, Mount Sinai Medical Center, Miami Beach, Florida

Kathleen Oberle, R.N., M.N.
Assistant Director of Nursing, University of Alberta Hospitals, Edmonton, Alberta

Maureen Osis, R.N., B.Sc.N.
Nursing Consultant, Osis Consulting Services, Ltd., Calgary, Alberta

Yechiam Ostchega, R.N., B.S.N., M.S.N.
Clinical Nurse Specialist (Research), Cancer Nursing and Medicine Branch, National Cancer Institute, Bethesda, Maryland

Anne Griffin Perry, R.N., M.S.N.
Associate Professor of Nursing, School of Nursing, St. Louis University Medical Center, St. Louis, Missouri

Sharon C. Posey, R.N., M.S.N., M.S.Ed.
Associate Professor, School of Nursing, Purdue University, West Lafayette, Indiana

Roberta Ronayne, R.N., B.Sc.N., M.Sc.[A.]
Lecturer, Faculty of Health Sciences, School of Nursing, University of Ottawa, Ottawa, Ontario

Janice Selekman, R.N., M.S.N., D.N.S.
Associate Professor, Thomas Jefferson University, Philadelphia, Pennsylvania

Maxine Soules, R.N., M.S., E.T.
Enterostomal Clinical Specialist, St. Luke's Hospital, San Francisco, California

Janet L. Stanford, R.N., B.S.N.
Cardiovascular Research Nurse, Emory University School of Medicine, Atlanta, Georgia

June L. Stark, R.N., B.S.N., C.C.R.N.
Critical Care Instructor, Staff Education, Renal Consultant, New England Medical Center Hospital, Boston, Massachusetts

Claudette G. Varricchio, R.N., D.N.S.
Assistant Professor, Medical-Surgical Nursing, Niehoff School of Nursing, Loyola University of Chicago, Chicago, Illinois

Emalou R. Vaterlaus, R.N., B.S.N.
Craven-Hagan Clinic, Williston, North Dakota

Lynne Vear, R.N.
Evening Co-Ordinator, Psoriasis Education and Research Centre, Toronto, Ontario

Marilyn A. Wales, R.N., B.Sc.N., M.S.N.
Assistant Professor, Faculty of Nursing, University of Alberta, Edmonton, Alberta

Mary E. Walesky, R.N.
Metabolic Research Nurse, Division of Endocrinology, School of Medicine, Yale University, New Haven, Connecticut

Anne West, R.N., M.S.N., C.C.R.N.
Adult Nurse Practitioner, Bristol, Tennessee

Marge J. White, R.N.
Screening and Advice Nurse of Pittsburg Health Center, Contra Costa County Medical Services, Martinez, California

Jane Wilson, R.N., B.A.
Ottawa, Ontario

To our mothers,
Grace M. Webb and Mary J. Pagliaro,
and to the memory of our fathers,
Donald D. Webb and James A. Pagliaro

At no other time has the understanding of drugs, how they work, and their place in therapeutic practice been more important than today. The number of agents continues to increase; the sometimes startling effects of interactions can be frightening to clinicians and patients alike. The complexity of drug therapy related to diverse social and economic factors, age groups, and illnesses requires that students and practitioners are provided the best possible sources of information.

We are confident that *Pharmacologic Aspects of Nursing* is the most accurate, up-to-date, and comprehensive text available. This book took over 6 years to develop and write. All drugs and dosages were painstakingly cross-referenced by computer data base to pharmacologic standards and industry data. Incredible detail went into cross-referencing material and providing easy access to information through thorough indexes. A drug handbook is even combined right into the text in the *Nursing Drug Digest*—it's like getting two books in one.

Take a moment to read and compare. I think you will find *Pharmacologic Aspects of Nursing* the best drug resource and text available. It is accurate, comprehensive, and a real value.

THE PUBLISHER

Preface

The administration of medications and the monitoring of their effects in the patient comprise some of the most important and complex aspects of nursing. A great need exists, therefore, for an authoritative pharmacology text and reference book written with a specific and contemporary nursing focus. The purpose of this book is to present a comprehensive and readily accessible compilation of pharmacologic and related clinical data concerning the use and effect of drugs in the patient, together with the consequent general implications for nursing care.

The text is organized into 15 sections. The first section concerns the role of the professional nurse in drug therapy and includes a historical overview and an indepth discussion of the preparation and administration of medications and the monitoring of their effects. The second section deals with the general basic principles that influence the selection and efficacy of drug therapy. The remaining sections, arranged according to pharmacologic classification, contain detailed information about specific drugs. This information is presented in narrative form to facilitate learning or review of material, and in tabular form to facilitate retrieval of needed information. These sections also contain chapters that review the basic anatomy, physiology, and assessment of the major organ systems to help the user understand the use and mechanism of action of drugs in specific organs or body systems and recognize and monitor therapeutic and toxic effects.

The contributing authors of the various chapters have been carefully chosen for their demonstrated clinical experience, expertise, and interest in specific areas of pharmacology and drug therapy. The varied backgrounds of this prestigious group of clinicians and educators provide this text with an added depth and dimension that have been significantly missing from other nursing pharmacology texts and should help establish this book as the standard pharmacology text and reference for nurses.

The nursing advisory committee, composed of a distinguished group of nurses actively involved in a variety of nursing areas including service, research, and education, further contributes to the depth and scope of this text and has helped to ensure its nursing focus. This committee represents the rich and varied interests of nurses and reflects the diversified needs that this text has addressed.

The drugs discussed in this text are referred to by their nonproprietary (generic) USAN names; however, nurses who use trade or brand names may gain access to the information they seek by consulting the General Index. A comprehensive listing of brand names can be found in L. A. Pagliaro and A.M. Pagliaro, *Drug Reference Guide to Brand Names and Active Ingredients*, St. Louis: The C.V. Mosby Co., 1986. This reference guide alphabetically lists drug trade names for both single and multiple active ingredient products and gives the nonproprietary names of the active ingredients for both prescription and nonprescription medications that are available in either Canada or the United States.

All doses included in this text are average doses and are therefore approximate. In all cases, variability in patient response because of genetic, physiologic, or environmental differences may necessitate alterations in the dosages or dosage regimens (see Section II of this text, General Principles of Pharmacology, for further information and examples). Accepted guidelines for the use of each drug, including drug information centers, patient package inserts, or other authoritative references, should be consulted whenever there is further question about a particular use or dose of a drug. When additional age-specific information regarding drug therapy is required in relation to the care of either children or the elderly, the nurse is referred to L. A. Pagliaro and A.M. Pagliaro (Eds.), *Problems in Pediatric Drug Therapy* (2nd ed.), Hamilton, Ill.: Drug Intelligence Publications, 1986, or L. A. Pagliaro and A.M. Pagliaro (Eds.), *Pharmacologic Aspects of Aging*, St. Louis: The C.V. Mosby Co., 1983, respectively.

It is hoped that by using the information presented in this text nursing students and nurse clinicians will be better able to provide patients with maximum benefits of drug therapy with a minimum of adverse effects.

Ann M. Pagliaro
Louis A. Pagliaro

Introduction

The role of the professional nurse in drug therapy is complex and requires expert knowledge and skills. This role is one of increasing responsibility and accountability. Nurses today require increased knowledge regarding pharmacology and related nursing care so that individual drug therapy regimens can be planned in collaboration with patients and other health team members so that patients can obtain the optimum benefits of drug therapy with a minimum of adverse effects.

The role of nurses is often blurred and is not explicit. Nurses today must make explicit the domain of nursing, particularly as it relates to drug therapy. The basic philosophy used in this text is that drug therapy is an integral part of the domain of nursing. Nursing has an overlapping domain in regard to drug therapy with other health professions, particularly pharmacy and medicine, but also a unique domain as well.

SECTION I—THE ROLE OF THE PROFESSIONAL NURSE IN DRUG THERAPY

Section I of this text describes the role of the professional nurse in drug therapy. Nurses are often not cognizant of their rich history or the contributions that many nurses have made, particularly during the last decades, to the development of nursing science in relation to drug therapy and nursing practice, education, and research. These contributions must continue to be built upon to further develop nursing as both an art and a science. The evolving and expanding role of nurses in relation to drug therapy is presented in Chapter 1, "Pharmacologic Aspects of Nursing: A Historical Overview."

Preparation, administration, and monitoring of medications are important aspects of the nurse's role in drug therapy. The safe and accurate preparation and administration of medications are essential parts of nursing practice. Research has shown that nursing errors in drug therapy are generally caused not only by a lack of knowledge regarding pharmacology, but also by inattention to fundamental techniques and procedures developed to ensure patient safety. The correct nursing techniques for the preparation and administration of medications and the monitoring of their effects are discussed in Chapter 2, "Preparation, Administration, and Monitoring of Medications."

SECTION II—GENERAL PRINCIPLES OF PHARMACOLOGY

To help nurses prepare drug dosage forms, select routes of administration, and monitor patient response, knowledge and understanding of the general principles of pharmacology are required, including the mechanisms of drug action, factors affecting drug availability and distribution, metabolism and elimination, pharmacokinetics, age-dependent drug selection and response, psychologic and genetic factors affecting drug response, drug interactions, drug toxicity, and drug abuse and addiction. These principles are presented in Section II, General Principles of Pharmacology, and serve as a basis for the material presented in subsequent chapters of this text. The following overview of the individual chapters in Section II identifies the importance and relevance of these principles and their application to nursing practice.

Mechanisms of drug action

A knowledge of the general mechanisms of drug action (see Chapter 3) will enable nurses to understand how and why drugs work in the human body and appreciate each drug's distinct mechanism of action. With this knowledge nurses can plan nonpharmacologic nursing measures to promote drug action, make decisions or recommendations about drug therapy, and discuss drug therapy knowledgeably with patients and other health team members. This knowledge will also help nurses understand the mechanisms of drug interactions and adverse side effects.

Drug availability and distribution

For a drug to have a systemic effect in the body it must be made available for absorption and distribution. This is discussed in Chapter 4, "Drug Availability and Distribution." An understanding of the physical and physiologic processes involved in transporting a drug from its site of administration via the systemic circulation to its specific site of action will enable nurses to appreciate that (1) not all drugs are equally available to the systemic circulation, and (2) various factors (e.g., dosage form, route of administration, timing of oral drug administration in relation to meals) can significantly affect drug availability. Knowledge regarding drug availability and distribution will help nurses make decisions regarding the selection or recommendation of dosage forms and routes of administration.

Drug metabolism and elimination

Once a drug has been absorbed and distributed, it must be metabolized and eliminated from the body for its action to cease. Hepatic and renal dysfunction can affect drug metabolism and elimination and may require that a drug be administered at a lower dose or at less frequent dosing intervals. An understanding of the basic mechanisms by which medications are inactivated and eliminated from the body can enable nurses to appreciate how changes in physiologic factors can significantly affect drug metabolism and elimination and necessitate a change in drug therapy. These principles will also help nurses understand and anticipate antagonistic (e.g., coumadin and phenobarbital) and synergistic (e.g., penicillin and probenecid) drug interactions that are mediated by the processes of metabolism and elimination.

Pharmacokinetic considerations in drug response

Pharmacokinetics is the study of the absorption, distribution, metabolism, and elimination of drugs from the body and the mathematical modeling that represents these events. An understanding of pharmacokinetic principles and the use of drug blood level monitoring will enable nurses to appreciate the scientific and physiologic basis for dosage scheduling. An understanding of the use of drug blood levels in monitoring for therapeutic drug effects and adverse side effects will enable nurses to plan appropriate drug administration schedules and make decisions or recommendations regarding the need for drug therapy modifications. Pharmacokinetic considerations are discussed in Chapter 6, and therapeutic blood levels for selected agents are presented in Appendix VII.

Age-dependent drug selection and response

Drug selection and patient response are significantly affected by the age of the patient. Generally, children and the elderly react differently to certain drugs or classifications of drugs than do young or middle-aged adults. Children are particularly at risk for problems in drug therapy because of the immaturity of their body systems and thus they cannot be dosed simply as "little" adults. The older person, be-cause of the changes that occur as a result of the normal aging process such as diminished renal and hepatic function, commonly require special alterations in drug therapy. The specific age-related factors that must be taken into consideration when planning to meet the drug therapy needs of these special patient groups are presented in Chapter 7, "Age-dependent Drug Selection and Response."

Psychologic factors in drug response

Increasing attention is being given to the psychologic effects that influence drug response. The placebo response and other psychologic effects have received much attention. Psychologic effects play a significant role in relation to both the success of drug therapy and the incidence of adverse side effects. Nurses have an integral role to play in this regard as discussed in Chapter 8, "Psychologic Factors in Drug Response."

Genetic factors affecting drug response

Genetic factors significantly affect drug therapy and help identify and account for some of the uniqueness that is observed in individual patient response to drug therapy. Specific genetic conditions that particularly affect drug therapy are identified and discussed in Chapter 9, "Genetic Factors Affecting Drug Response." An understanding of these genetic factors will help nurses recognize and meet individual patient needs in relation to drug therapy.

Drug interactions

To provide optimum care, nurses must have a general understanding of drug interactions, including their frequency and severity. Nurses should be aware of which drugs can interact with each other or with foods so that undesirable interactions can be anticipated and avoided. With an understanding of drug interactions, nurses can often prevent common interactions by avoiding concurrent or concomitant dosing of interacting drugs. Nurses can also identify if an observed interaction necessitates a change in drug therapy, and, if so, select or recommend a drug or dosage form that can be safely and appropriately substituted. For example, a patient may safely and effectively take both oral tetracycline and antacids (two drugs that significantly interact when coadministered) *providing* that the two drugs are dosed sufficiently apart from each other to avoid binding together in the stomach. Some drugs can interfere with certain laboratory tests, and attention to these possible interactions is also essential, particularly when scheduling and interpreting laboratory tests and planning drug administration schedules. Basic principles of drug interactions are discussed in Chapter 10, "Drug Interactions."

Drug toxicity

Chapter 11, "Drug Toxicity," presents a basic overview of the various types and principal mechanisms of drug toxicity. With this information, nurses should be able to anticipate potential drug toxicities and plan to prevent these toxicities when possible or minimize them when they are unavoidable. Generally, nurses spend more time with patients than any other health care professional and thus are in a unique position to monitor patients for drug toxicity. This is particularly important when drugs are dosed to their toxic levels or when patients are receiving drugs that have potentially irreversible toxic effects.

Drug abuse and addiction

Drug abuse and addiction are major problems in North America affecting both children and adults in all socioeconomic and cultural groups. Drug addiction has been a concern of nurses in planning pain management regimens and in relation to the misuse and abuse of available over-the-counter preparations commonly indicated for such conditions as simple constipation or coughs and colds. The misuse and abuse of illicit and social drugs are increasing concerns. These areas are discussed in Chapter 12, "Drug Abuse and Addiction." A knowledge of the principal drugs and substances of abuse will enable nurses to more effectively recognize and deal with both patients and colleagues who have drug abuse problems.

DRUG CHAPTERS

Sections III, IV, V, VI, VII, VIII, and XII present drugs classified according to their actions on specific body systems, including the central and peripheral nervous systems, respiratory system, cardiovascular system, gastrointestinal system, renal system, and cutaneous system. A general chapter reviewing the anatomy, physiology, and assessment of the associated major organ system is included in each of these sections. This material should help nurses learn or review the anatomy, physiology, and assessment of these systems particularly as they relate to drug therapy and pharmacologic principles.

Section IX, Antiparasitic Medications; Section X, Antibacterial, Antifungal, and Antiviral Medications; Section XI, Antineoplastic Medications; Section XIII, Antiinflammatory Medications; Section XIV, Hormones and Hormone Antagonists; and Section XV, Miscellaneous Therapeutic and Diagnostic Agents, are classified according to major drug classes because the agents in these chapters have effects on many organ systems. The anatomy, physiology and assessment content has been integrated as appropriate to these chapters.

The chapters in Sections III through XV have been written using the individual styles and emphasis of the respective authors. These chapters generally discuss drug use, pharmacokinetics, pharmacodynamics, dosing, and recent therapeutic developments as they pertain to the specific drug classification. For consistency, and to facilitate use of this text, each chapter includes the common Adverse/Side Effects of the drugs discussed in the chapter, Clinically Significant Drug Interactions, General Nursing Implications, General Instructions for Discharge/Outpatients, and a Nursing Drug Digest.

Adverse/Side Effects lists alphabetically, according to body system, the most common adverse side effects associated with the specific drugs discussed in each chapter. A body system format readily adaptable to physical assessment approaches has been used to facilitate the identification and the monitoring of adverse side effects.

Clinically Significant Drug Interactions lists the drugs discussed in the chapter in alphabetical order together with the corresponding interacting drugs, the possible effects, and the probable mechanisms of the interaction when these have been established.

The effects are listed as "possible" because interactions depend on dose, duration of therapy, and individual patient variables (e.g., hepatic or renal function, genetic predisposition, health state) and thus rarely occur with 100% frequency.

The probable mechanisms of the interactions are identified to provide nurses with insight into how and why the interactions occur and provide the necessary information for the nurse to plan to minimize interactions. For example, if under probable mechanisms it is noted that one drug inhibits the gastrointestinal absorption of another drug by binding with it in the stomach, the nurse can plan to space the dose of the two interacting drugs apart, thus avoiding the interaction and allowing the patient to continue to receive both drugs.

Only those drug interactions that have been assessed as clinically significant have been included in these tables.

General Nursing Implications presents a conceptualized approach to help nurses care for patients who require a specific classification of drug and has been organized so that it can be used by nurses regardless of which conceptual model or nursing theoretical framework they may use in practice.

Important areas that should be considered when

assessing patients and planning therapy or when collaborating with the prescriber and other health care team members include Assessment, Sensitivity, Contraindications, Cautions, Drug Interactions, Administration, Monitoring Patient Response, and Patient Education. These areas are outlined in the General Nursing Implications of each drug chapter and are discussed briefly as follows.

Assessment. As with other aspects of nursing, drug therapy should not be implemented until the patient's requirements for drug therapy and nursing assistance or care have been assessed and a plan has been developed to help patients and families meet these requirements. Evaluation criteria must be established so that therapy can be revised as needed. Assessment must take into consideration sensitivity, contraindications, cautions, and possible drug interactions.

Administration. After assessment is completed, drug therapy regimens can be planned and implemented. Because drug administration can vary in relation to the drug, types of dosage forms available, and individual patient factors, points for planning drug administration are presented in the administration section.

Sensitivity. Virtually all drugs have the ability to cause a hypersensitivity reaction in susceptible individuals. This section identifies those drugs that are most likely to cause such a reaction, and, when possible, identifies patients who are at particular risk.

Contraindications. The contraindications section identifies the general types or groups of patients who should not receive the category of drug being discussed, even though they may have an indication for its use. For example, mild to moderate hypertension is an accepted indication for the use of propranolol; however, use of propranolol in a patient with asthma who has moderate hypertension would be contraindicated because of its negative or deleterious effect on the asthmatic condition.

Cautions. This section includes information on those conditions that do not contraindicate the use of the particular drug classification, but rather indicate that increased monitoring or a modification of dosage may be required. For example, if a drug is eliminated from the body primarily in unchanged form in the urine, then impaired renal function may necessitate a reduction in dose or change in the dosing interval.

Drug interactions. This section identifies interactions that occur with the class of compounds (e.g., barbiturates and narcotic analgesics causing increased CNS depression) and, where applicable, offers suggestions for dealing with these interactions. Specific drug interactions involving individual agents are listed in Clinically Significant Drug Interactions.

Monitoring. Monitoring patient response to drug therapy in relation to the occurrence of desired therapeutic drug effects and adverse side effects is essential for optimum drug therapy. Nurses in acute care settings are generally with patients more than any other health care team members and thus have an excellent opportunity to monitor patient response to drug therapy. Community health nurses working with patients in various community settings likewise have an excellent opportunity to monitor drug therapy.

Monitoring the patient's therapeutic response to drug therapy is particularly important so that patient drug regimens can be appropriately modified when the desired response does not occur as, or when, expected. Some drugs may take weeks to months to provide maximum therapeutic effects and other drugs, particularly those with a narrow therapeutic index, require careful monitoring to avoid potentially serious or irreversible toxic effects.

Since adverse effects often necessitate discontinuation of drug therapy, another increasingly important nursing consideration is monitoring patients for adverse side effects. Specific information related to the monitoring of patients for therapeutic drug effects and for adverse side effects for each classification of medications is outlined. Nursing measures that can be used to maximize therapeutic effects and to prevent or minimize adverse side effects are also included.

Patient education. Patient education in relation to drug therapy is an increasingly important aspect of the nurse's role in drug therapy. All patients whenever possible should have a clear understanding of their drug therapy so that they can make informed decisions about their therapy. Generally, patients should have a clear understanding of the planned drug regimen including the reasons for drug therapy, the exact name of their medication, its basic action, dosage, contraindications, and cautions. They should know how to administer their medication and should be able to monitor for therapeutic effects. Patients should be aware of what adverse side effects can occur and how to prevent or minimize these effects when possible. Patients and families as indicated should know what signs indicate that the nurse or other health care provider should be notified so that a change in the drug therapy regimen can be made. This information and other related patient education information are outlined under Patient Education.

General Instructions For Discharge/Outpatients outlines in lay language and terminology the general medication instructions for discharged or out-

patients who require the particular medication. These instructions can be modified and individualized by nurses to promote drug therapy according to the individual patient's abilities and needs. These instructions can be used during in-hospital patient education sessions as well as by patients when at home to refer to as needed to increase their understanding of the use of the medications and compliance.

Nursing Drug Digest, included at the end of each drug chapter, contains an alphabetical listing, by generic name, of all drugs discussed in the chapter that are currently available for use in either Canada or the United States. Most drugs are available in both countries. When a drug is generally available in only Canada, its entry is preceeded by a maple leaf; when available only in the United States, its entry is preceded by a star. Some experimentally available drugs are also included when it was felt that these agents may be more generally available in the near future.

An alphabetical listing of trade or brand names can be found under the generic name of each drug. When the trade or brand name product contains an additional active ingredient, it is identified by an asterisk. For a comprehensive listing of brand names and a complete listing of all active ingredients see L.A. Pagliaro and A.M. Pagliaro, *Drug Reference Guide to Brand Names and Active Ingredients*, St. Louis: The C.V. Mosby Co., 1986.

The second and third columns of the Nursing Drug Digest contain a list of indications for the use of the drug and the corresponding usual dosages together with the route of, and recommendations for, administration. The remaining columns contain specific detailed information for each drug concerning its Preparation and Storage; Contraindications, Cautions, and Comments; and Monitoring.

The Nursing Drug Digest is included in each drug chapter to facilitate retrieval of information needed by nurses to properly prepare, administer, and monitor drug therapy. When additional details or information are needed, nurses are referred to the text and other tables in the chapter, as well as to Sections I and II of this text.

APPENDICES

Various appendices have been included to facilitate the use of this text. These include Appendix I, an alphabetized glossary of terms used in each chapter. The terms listed in the glossary are generally italicized when they first appear in the text. Appendix II consists of a comprehensive list of abbreviations used throughout the text. Because of the various errors that have occurred because of confusion with drug names, Appendix III lists pairs of drugs whose names look or sound alike. A chart of intravenous incompatibilities, which lists the most commonly used admixtures, is presented in Appendix IV for quick reference. Poisoning treatment is presented in Appendix V. Appendix VI presents a list of drugs lacking adequate evidence of effectiveness, and Appendix VII lists the therapeutic blood levels of selected therapeutic agents.

INDEXES

A comprehensive cross-referenced General Index has been compiled and included at the end of this text to facilitate retrieval of needed information. In addition, two additional indexes, the Adverse Drug Effects Index and the Drug Interaction Index, have been included to further help nurses gain quick and complete access to the information they may require in assessing, planning, implementing, and monitoring drug therapy.

SUMMARY

This text provides comprehensive and accurate information regarding drugs and drug therapy that is required by today's professional nurses. This information should help nurses meet their expanding roles and responsibilities in relation to drug therapy and thus significantly contribute to optimizing patient care.

Preface

The administration of medications and the monitoring of their effects in the patient comprise some of the most important and complex aspects of nursing. A great need exists, therefore, for an authoritative pharmacology text and reference book written with a specific and contemporary nursing focus. The purpose of this book is to present a comprehensive and readily accessible compilation of pharmacologic and related clinical data concerning the use and effect of drugs in the patient, together with the consequent general implications for nursing care.

The text is organized into 15 sections. The first section concerns the role of the professional nurse in drug therapy and includes a historical overview and an in-depth discussion of the preparation and administration of medications and the monitoring of their effects. The second section deals with the general basic principles that influence the selection and efficacy of drug therapy. The remaining sections, arranged according to pharmacologic classification, contain detailed information about specific drugs. This information is presented in narrative form to facilitate learning or review of material, and in tabular form to facilitate retrieval of needed information. These sections also contain chapters that review the basic anatomy, physiology, and assessment of the major organ systems to help the user understand the use and mechanism of action of drugs in specific organs or body systems and recognize and monitor therapeutic and toxic effects.

The contributing authors of the various chapters have been carefully chosen for their demonstrated clinical experience, expertise, and interest in specific areas of pharmacology and drug therapy. The varied backgrounds of this prestigious group of clinicians and educators provide this text with an added depth and dimension that have been significantly missing from other nursing pharmacology texts and should help establish this book as the standard pharmacology text and reference for nurses.

The nursing advisory committee, composed of a distinguished group of nurses actively involved in a variety of nursing areas including service, research, and education, further contributes to the depth and scope of this text and has helped to ensure its nursing focus. This committee represents the rich and varied interests of nurses and reflects the diversified needs that this text has addressed.

The drugs discussed in this text are referred to by their nonproprietary (generic) USAN names; however, nurses who use trade or brand names may gain access to the information they seek by consulting the General Index. A comprehensive listing of brand names can be found in L. A. Pagliaro and A.M. Pagliaro, *Drug Reference Guide to Brand Names and Active Ingredients*, St. Louis: The C.V. Mosby Co., 1986. This reference guide alphabetically lists drug trade names for both single and multiple active ingredient products and gives the nonproprietary names of the active ingredients for both prescription and nonprescription medications that are available in either Canada or the United States.

All doses included in this text are average doses and are therefore approximate. In all cases, variability in patient response because of genetic, physiologic, or environmental differences may necessitate alterations in the dosages or dosage regimens (see Section II of this text, General Principles of Pharmacology, for further information and examples). Accepted guidelines for the use of each drug, including drug information centers, patient package inserts, or other authoritative references, should be consulted whenever there is further question about a particular use or dose of a drug. When additional age-specific information regarding drug therapy is required in relation to the care of either children or the elderly, the nurse is referred to L. A. Pagliaro and A.M. Pagliaro (Eds.), *Problems in Pediatric Drug Therapy* (2nd ed.), Hamilton, Ill.: Drug Intelligence Publications, 1986, or L. A. Pagliaro and A.M. Pagliaro (Eds.), *Pharmacologic Aspects of Aging*, St. Louis: The C.V. Mosby Co., 1983, respectively.

It is hoped that by using the information presented in this text nursing students and nurse clinicians will be better able to provide patients with maximum benefits of drug therapy with a minimum of adverse effects.

Ann M. Pagliaro
Louis A. Pagliaro

Preface

The administration of medications and the monitoring of their effects in the patient comprise some of the most important and complex aspects of nursing. A great need exists, therefore, for an authoritative pharmacology text and reference book written with a specific and contemporary nursing focus. The purpose of this book is to present a comprehensive and readily accessible compilation of pharmacologic and related clinical data concerning the use and effect of drugs in the patient, together with the consequent general implications for nursing care.

The text is organized into 15 sections. The first section concerns the role of the professional nurse in drug therapy and includes a historical overview and an in-depth discussion of the preparation and administration of medications and the monitoring of their effects. The second section deals with the general basic principles that influence the selection and efficacy of drug therapy. The remaining sections, arranged according to pharmacologic classification, contain detailed information about specific drugs. This information is presented in narrative form to facilitate learning or review of material, and in tabular form to facilitate retrieval of needed information. These sections also contain chapters that review the basic anatomy, physiology, and assessment of the major organ systems to help the user understand the use and mechanism of action of drugs in specific organs or body systems and recognize and monitor therapeutic and toxic effects.

The contributing authors of the various chapters have been carefully chosen for their demonstrated clinical experience, expertise, and interest in specific areas of pharmacology and drug therapy. The varied backgrounds of this prestigious group of clinicians and educators provide this text with an added depth and dimension that have been significantly missing from other nursing pharmacology texts and should help establish this book as the standard pharmacology text and reference for nurses.

The nursing advisory committee, composed of a distinguished group of nurses actively involved in a variety of nursing areas including service, research, and education, further contributes to the depth and scope of this text and has helped to ensure its nursing focus. This committee represents the rich and varied interests of nurses and reflects the diversified needs that this text has addressed.

The drugs discussed in this text are referred to by their nonproprietary (generic) USAN names; however, nurses who use trade or brand names may gain access to the information they seek by consulting the General Index. A comprehensive listing of brand names can be found in L. A. Pagliaro and A.M. Pagliaro, *Drug Reference Guide to Brand Names and Active Ingredients*, St. Louis: The C.V. Mosby Co., 1986. This reference guide alphabetically lists drug trade names for both single and multiple active ingredient products and gives the nonproprietary names of the active ingredients for both prescription and nonprescription medications that are available in either Canada or the United States.

All doses included in this text are average doses and are therefore approximate. In all cases, variability in patient response because of genetic, physiologic, or environmental differences may necessitate alterations in the dosages or dosage regimens (see Section II of this text, General Principles of Pharmacology, for further information and examples). Accepted guidelines for the use of each drug, including drug information centers, patient package inserts, or other authoritative references, should be consulted whenever there is further question about a particular use or dose of a drug. When additional age-specific information regarding drug therapy is required in relation to the care of either children or the elderly, the nurse is referred to L. A. Pagliaro and A.M. Pagliaro (Eds.), *Problems in Pediatric Drug Therapy* (2nd ed.), Hamilton, Ill.: Drug Intelligence Publications, 1986, or L. A. Pagliaro and A.M. Pagliaro (Eds.), *Pharmacologic Aspects of Aging*, St. Louis: The C.V. Mosby Co., 1983, respectively.

It is hoped that by using the information presented in this text nursing students and nurse clinicians will be better able to provide patients with maximum benefits of drug therapy with a minimum of adverse effects.

Ann M. Pagliaro
Louis A. Pagliaro

Introduction

The role of the professional nurse in drug therapy is complex and requires expert knowledge and skills. This role is one of increasing responsibility and accountability. Nurses today require increased knowledge regarding pharmacology and related nursing care so that individual drug therapy regimens can be planned in collaboration with patients and other health team members so that patients can obtain the optimum benefits of drug therapy with a minimum of adverse effects.

The role of nurses is often blurred and is not explicit. Nurses today must make explicit the domain of nursing, particularly as it relates to drug therapy. The basic philosophy used in this text is that drug therapy is an integral part of the domain of nursing. Nursing has an overlapping domain in regard to drug therapy with other health professions, particularly pharmacy and medicine, but also a unique domain as well.

SECTION I—THE ROLE OF THE PROFESSIONAL NURSE IN DRUG THERAPY

Section I of this text describes the role of the professional nurse in drug therapy. Nurses are often not cognizant of their rich history or the contributions that many nurses have made, particularly during the last decades, to the development of nursing science in relation to drug therapy and nursing practice, education, and research. These contributions must continue to be built upon to further develop nursing as both an art and a science. The evolving and expanding role of nurses in relation to drug therapy is presented in Chapter 1, "Pharmacologic Aspects of Nursing: A Historical Overview."

Preparation, administration, and monitoring of medications are important aspects of the nurse's role in drug therapy. The safe and accurate preparation and administration of medications are essential parts of nursing practice. Research has shown that nursing errors in drug therapy are generally caused not only by a lack of knowledge regarding pharmacology, but also by inattention to fundamental techniques and procedures developed to ensure patient safety. The correct nursing techniques for the preparation and administration of medications and the monitoring of

their effects are discussed in Chapter 2, "Preparation, Administration, and Monitoring of Medications."

SECTION II—GENERAL PRINCIPLES OF PHARMACOLOGY

To help nurses prepare drug dosage forms, select routes of administration, and monitor patient response, knowledge and understanding of the general principles of pharmacology are required, including the mechanisms of drug action, factors affecting drug availability and distribution, metabolism and elimination, pharmacokinetics, age-dependent drug selection and response, psychologic and genetic factors affecting drug response, drug interactions, drug toxicity, and drug abuse and addiction. These principles are presented in Section II, General Principles of Pharmacology, and serve as a basis for the material presented in subsequent chapters of this text. The following overview of the individual chapters in Section II identifies the importance and relevance of these principles and their application to nursing practice.

Mechanisms of drug action

A knowledge of the general mechanisms of drug action (see Chapter 3) will enable nurses to understand how and why drugs work in the human body and appreciate each drug's distinct mechanism of action. With this knowledge nurses can plan nonpharmacologic nursing measures to promote drug action, make decisions or recommendations about drug therapy, and discuss drug therapy knowledgeably with patients and other health team members. This knowledge will also help nurses understand the mechanisms of drug interactions and adverse side effects.

Drug availability and distribution

For a drug to have a systemic effect in the body it must be made available for absorption and distribution. This is discussed in Chapter 4, "Drug Availability and Distribution." An understanding of the physical and physiologic processes involved in transporting a drug from its site of administration via the systemic circulation to its specific site of action will enable nurses to appreciate that (1) not all drugs are equally available to the systemic circulation, and (2) various factors (e.g., dosage form, route of administration, timing of oral drug administration in relation to meals) can significantly affect drug availability. Knowledge regarding drug availability and distribution will help nurses make decisions regarding the selection or recommendation of dosage forms and routes of administration.

Drug metabolism and elimination

Once a drug has been absorbed and distributed, it must be metabolized and eliminated from the body for its action to cease. Hepatic and renal dysfunction can affect drug metabolism and elimination and may require that a drug be administered at a lower dose or at less frequent dosing intervals. An understanding of the basic mechanisms by which medications are inactivated and eliminated from the body can enable nurses to appreciate how changes in physiologic factors can significantly affect drug metabolism and elimination and necessitate a change in drug therapy. These principles will also help nurses understand and anticipate antagonistic (e.g., coumadin and phenobarbital) and synergistic (e.g., penicillin and probenecid) drug interactions that are mediated by the processes of metabolism and elimination.

Pharmacokinetic considerations in drug response

Pharmacokinetics is the study of the absorption, distribution, metabolism, and elimination of drugs from the body and the mathematical modeling that represents these events. An understanding of pharmacokinetic principles and the use of drug blood level monitoring will enable nurses to appreciate the scientific and physiologic basis for dosage scheduling. An understanding of the use of drug blood levels in monitoring for therapeutic drug effects and adverse side effects will enable nurses to plan appropriate drug administration schedules and make decisions or recommendations regarding the need for drug therapy modifications. Pharmacokinetic considerations are discussed in Chapter 6, and therapeutic blood levels for selected agents are presented in Appendix VII.

Age-dependent drug selection and response

Drug selection and patient response are significantly affected by the age of the patient. Generally, children and the elderly react differently to certain drugs or classifications of drugs than do young or middle-aged adults. Children are particularly at risk for problems in drug therapy because of the immaturity of their body systems and thus they cannot be dosed simply as "little" adults. The older person, be-

cause of the changes that occur as a result of the normal aging process such as diminished renal and hepatic function, commonly require special alterations in drug therapy. The specific age-related factors that must be taken into consideration when planning to meet the drug therapy needs of these special patient groups are presented in Chapter 7, "Age-dependent Drug Selection and Response."

Psychologic factors in drug response

Increasing attention is being given to the psychologic effects that influence drug response. The placebo response and other psychologic effects have received much attention. Psychologic effects play a significant role in relation to both the success of drug therapy and the incidence of adverse side effects. Nurses have an integral role to play in this regard as discussed in Chapter 8, "Psychologic Factors in Drug Response."

Genetic factors affecting drug response

Genetic factors significantly affect drug therapy and help identify and account for some of the uniqueness that is observed in individual patient response to drug therapy. Specific genetic conditions that particularly affect drug therapy are identified and discussed in Chapter 9, "Genetic Factors Affecting Drug Response." An understanding of these genetic factors will help nurses recognize and meet individual patient needs in relation to drug therapy.

Drug interactions

To provide optimum care, nurses must have a general understanding of drug interactions, including their frequency and severity. Nurses should be aware of which drugs can interact with each other or with foods so that undesirable interactions can be anticipated and avoided. With an understanding of drug interactions, nurses can often prevent common interactions by avoiding concurrent or concomitant dosing of interacting drugs. Nurses can also identify if an observed interaction necessitates a change in drug therapy, and, if so, select or recommend a drug or dosage form that can be safely and appropriately substituted. For example, a patient may safely and effectively take both oral tetracycline and antacids (two drugs that significantly interact when coadministered) *providing* that the two drugs are dosed sufficiently apart from each other to avoid binding together in the stomach. Some drugs can interfere with certain laboratory tests, and attention to these possible interactions is also essential, particularly when scheduling and interpreting laboratory tests and planning drug administration schedules. Basic principles of drug in-assessing patients and planning therapy or when collaborating with the prescriber and other health care team members include Assessment, Sensitivity, Contraindications, Cautions, Drug Interactions, Administration, Monitoring Patient Response, and Patient Education. These areas are outlined in the General Nursing Implications of each drug chapter and are discussed briefly as follows.

Assessment. As with other aspects of nursing, drug therapy should not be implemented until the patient's requirements for drug therapy and nursing assistance or care have been assessed and a plan has been developed to help patients and families meet these requirements. Evaluation criteria must be established so that therapy can be revised as needed. Assessment must take into consideration sensitivity, contraindications, cautions, and possible drug interactions.

Administration. After assessment is completed, drug therapy regimens can be planned and implemented. Because drug administration can vary in relation to the drug, types of dosage forms available, and individual patient factors, points for planning drug administration are presented in the administration section.

Sensitivity. Virtually all drugs have the ability to cause a hypersensitivity reaction in susceptible individuals. This section identifies those drugs that are most likely to cause such a reaction, and, when possible, identifies patients who are at particular risk.

Contraindications. The contraindications section identifies the general types or groups of patients who should not receive the category of drug being discussed, even though they may have an indication for its use. For example, mild to moderate hypertension is an accepted indication for the use of propranolol; however, use of propranolol in a patient with asthma who has moderate hypertension would be contraindicated because of its negative or deleterious effect on the asthmatic condition.

Cautions. This section includes information on those conditions that do not contraindicate the use of the particular drug classification, but rather indicate that increased monitoring or a modification of dosage may be required. For example, if a drug is eliminated from the body primarily in unchanged form in the urine, then impaired renal function may necessitate a reduction in dose or change in the dosing interval.

Drug interactions. This section identifies interactions that occur with the class of compounds (e.g., barbiturates and narcotic analgesics causing increased CNS depression) and, where applicable, offers suggestions for dealing with these interactions. Specific drug interactions involving individual agents are listed in Clinically Significant Drug Interactions.

Monitoring. Monitoring patient response to drug therapy in relation to the occurrence of desired therapeutic drug effects and adverse side effects is essential for optimum drug therapy. Nurses in acute care settings are generally with patients more than any other health care team members and thus have an excellent opportunity to monitor patient response to drug therapy. Community health nurses working with patients in various community settings likewise have an excellent opportunity to monitor drug therapy.

Monitoring the patient's therapeutic response to drug therapy is particularly important so that patient drug regimens can be appropriately modified when the desired response does not occur as, or when, expected. Some drugs may take weeks to months to provide maximum therapeutic effects and other drugs, particularly those with a narrow therapeutic index, require careful monitoring to avoid potentially serious or irreversible toxic effects.

Since adverse effects often necessitate discontinuation of drug therapy, another increasingly important nursing consideration is monitoring patients for adverse side effects. Specific information related to the monitoring of patients for therapeutic drug effects and for adverse side effects for each classification of medications is outlined. Nursing measures that can be used to maximize therapeutic effects and to prevent or minimize adverse side effects are also included.

Patient education. Patient education in relation to drug therapy is an increasingly important aspect of the nurse's role in drug therapy. All patients whenever possible should have a clear understanding of their drug therapy so that they can make informed decisions about their therapy. Generally, patients should have a clear understanding of the planned drug regimen including the reasons for drug therapy, the exact name of their medication, its basic action, dosage, contraindications, and cautions. They should know how to administer their medication and should be able to monitor for therapeutic effects. Patients should be aware of what adverse side effects can occur and how to prevent or minimize these effects when possible. Patients and families as indicated should know what signs indicate that the nurse or other health care provider should be notified so that a change in the drug therapy regimen can be made. This information and other related patient education information are outlined under Patient Education.

General Instructions For Discharge/Outpatients outlines in lay language and terminology the general medication instructions for discharged or out-

teractions are discussed in Chapter 10, "Drug Interactions."

Drug toxicity

Chapter 11, "Drug Toxicity," presents a basic overview of the various types and principal mechanisms of drug toxicity. With this information, nurses should be able to anticipate potential drug toxicities and plan to prevent these toxicities when possible or minimize them when they are unavoidable. Generally, nurses spend more time with patients than any other health care professional and thus are in a unique position to monitor patients for drug toxicity. This is particularly important when drugs are dosed to their toxic levels or when patients are receiving drugs that have potentially irreversible toxic effects.

Drug abuse and addiction

Drug abuse and addiction are major problems in North America affecting both children and adults in all socioeconomic and cultural groups. Drug addiction has been a concern of nurses in planning pain management regimens and in relation to the misuse and abuse of available over-the-counter preparations commonly indicated for such conditions as simple constipation or coughs and colds. The misuse and abuse of illicit and social drugs are increasing concerns. These areas are discussed in Chapter 12, "Drug Abuse and Addiction." A knowledge of the principal drugs and substances of abuse will enable nurses to more effectively recognize and deal with both patients and colleagues who have drug abuse problems.

DRUG CHAPTERS

Sections III, IV, V, VI, VII, VIII, and XII present drugs classified according to their actions on specific body systems, including the central and peripheral nervous systems, respiratory system, cardiovascular system, gastrointestinal system, renal system, and cutaneous system. A general chapter reviewing the anatomy, physiology, and assessment of the associated major organ system is included in each of these sections. This material should help nurses learn or review the anatomy, physiology, and assessment of these systems particularly as they relate to drug therapy and pharmacologic principles.

Section IX, Antiparasitic Medications; Section X, Antibacterial, Antifungal, and Antiviral Medications; Section XI, Antineoplastic Medications; Section XIII, Antiinflammatory Medications; Section XIV, Hormones and Hormone Antagonists; and Section XV, Miscellaneous Therapeutic and Diagnostic Agents, are classified according to major drug classes because the agents in these chapters have effects on many organ systems. The anatomy, physiology and assessment content has been integrated as appropriate to these chapters.

The chapters in Sections III through XV have been written using the individual styles and emphasis of the respective authors. These chapters generally discuss drug use, pharmacokinetics, pharmacodynamics, dosing, and recent therapeutic developments as they pertain to the specific drug classification. For consistency, and to facilitate use of this text, each chapter includes the common Adverse/Side Effects of the drugs discussed in the chapter, Clinically Significant Drug Interactions, General Nursing Implications, General Instructions for Discharge/Outpatients, and a Nursing Drug Digest.

Adverse/Side Effects lists alphabetically, according to body system, the most common adverse side effects associated with the specific drugs discussed in each chapter. A body system format readily adaptable to physical assessment approaches has been used to facilitate the identification and the monitoring of adverse side effects.

Clinically Significant Drug Interactions lists the drugs discussed in the chapter in alphabetical order together with the corresponding interacting drugs, the possible effects, and the probable mechanisms of the interaction when these have been established.

The effects are listed as "possible" because interactions depend on dose, duration of therapy, and individual patient variables (e.g., hepatic or renal function, genetic predisposition, health state) and thus rarely occur with 100% frequency.

The probable mechanisms of the interactions are identified to provide nurses with insight into how and why the interactions occur and provide the necessary information for the nurse to plan to minimize interactions. For example, if under probable mechanisms it is noted that one drug inhibits the gastrointestinal absorption of another drug by binding with it in the stomach, the nurse can plan to space the dose of the two interacting drugs apart, thus avoiding the interaction and allowing the patient to continue to receive both drugs.

Only those drug interactions that have been assessed as clinically significant have been included in these tables.

General Nursing Implications presents a conceptualized approach to help nurses care for patients who require a specific classification of drug and has been organized so that it can be used by nurses regardless of which conceptual model or nursing theoretical framework they may use in practice.

Important areas that should be considered when

Contents

SECTION III

CENTRAL NERVOUS SYSTEM MEDICATIONS

SECTION IV

PERIPHERAL NERVOUS SYSTEM MEDICATIONS

SECTION XI

ANTINEOPLASTIC MEDICATIONS

SECTION XII

DERMATOLOGIC MEDICATIONS

SECTION XIII

ANTIINFLAMMATORY MEDICATIONS

SECTION XIV

HORMONES AND HORMONE ANTAGONISTS

SECTION XV

MISCELLANEOUS THERAPEUTIC AND DIAGNOSTIC AGENTS

APPENDICES

INDEXES

INDEXES

PHARMACOLOGIC ASPECTS *of* NURSING

THE ROLE OF THE PROFESSIONAL NURSE IN DRUG THERAPY

Pharmacologic Aspects of Nursing

A HISTORICAL OVERVIEW

Ann M. Pagliaro

Nursing's integral involvement with drug therapy is not often recognized, and many nurses view pharmacology as being primarily a medical discipline. However, the role of the professional nurse has traditionally incorporated various aspects of drug therapy, including the preparation and administration of medications and the monitoring of their effects, which required nurses to have specific pharmacology knowledge and skills. In early nursing this knowledge and skills were obtained empirically.

As the role of the nurse has expanded into modern concepts of primary care and independent nursing practice, the nurse's role in relation to drug therapy has also expanded. This role will continue to expand as models of advanced nursing practice develop and as increasing technologic advances require expert nursing knowledge and skills based on research and scientific principles. This historical perspective is presented to illustrate the basic association of the discipline of pharmacology with nursing practice, aspects of which are an integral part of the domain of nursing.

EARLY NURSING PRACTICE

Although the professions of medicine and pharmacy have extensive records dating from the earliest civilizations that document their knowledge and practice, nursing's early records are scant and almost nonexistent. It is known that nursing existed in relation to the roles of mother, wet nurse, and midwife from the earliest times, but it is only in the records of the ancient Hindus (2000-250 BC) that we find actual reference to the nurse figure and descriptions of nursing knowledge and practice, including the nurse's role in relation to drug therapy.

Ancient Hindu nurses were probably young men or in special cases elderly women. They were to be clever, pure in mind and body, and devoted to their patients. In addition to being "skilled in every kind of service that a patient might require" (Dock & Stewart, 1931, pp. 25-26), they were to have "knowledge of the man-

ner in which drugs were prepared and compounded for administration" (Nutting & Dock, Vol. 1, 1907, p. 32).

The earliest continuous records of nursing, other than those of the ancient Hindus, came in the first centuries of the Christian Church. Nursing was greatly influenced by concepts of Christianity. Both men and women sacrificed wealth and worldly possessions to serve Christ by nursing the poor and sick, for nursing was seen as direct service to God as well as penance for sins or solace for unhappy lives.

The great monastic movement began in the fourth and fifth centuries AD after the disintegration of the Holy Roman Empire and continued through the Middle Ages. Nursing was one of a number of activities carried out by the monks and nuns in the early monasteries that spread throughout the Western World preserving culture and learning while offering places of refuge. Medicinal gardens were cultivated, music and languages were studied, poetry and drama were written, and ancient knowledge was preserved by the copying of manuscripts. As time progressed, several monastic orders were founded whose sole aim was the alleviation of sickness and suffering.

The duties of the nursing brothers at the monastery at Monte Cassino (529 AD), the most famous of the Benedictine monasteries, included changing beds, bathing patients, dressing wounds, and providing food, drink, and warmth, as well as preparing and administering medications. The brothers were never to be angry or hasty in their care because under the rule of St. Benedict, "before all things and above all things care must be taken of the sick," as if indeed Christ was being directly served (Nutting and Dock, Vol. 1, 1907, p. 154).

Another of the early monastery hospitals was St. Gall (720 AD) in Switzerland, also a Benedictine monastery. At St. Gall, a hospital plan was conceived that provided for separate wards for the seriously ill, for those who had been bled, for a pharmaceutical dispensary, for a bathroom, kitchen, lavatories, and for

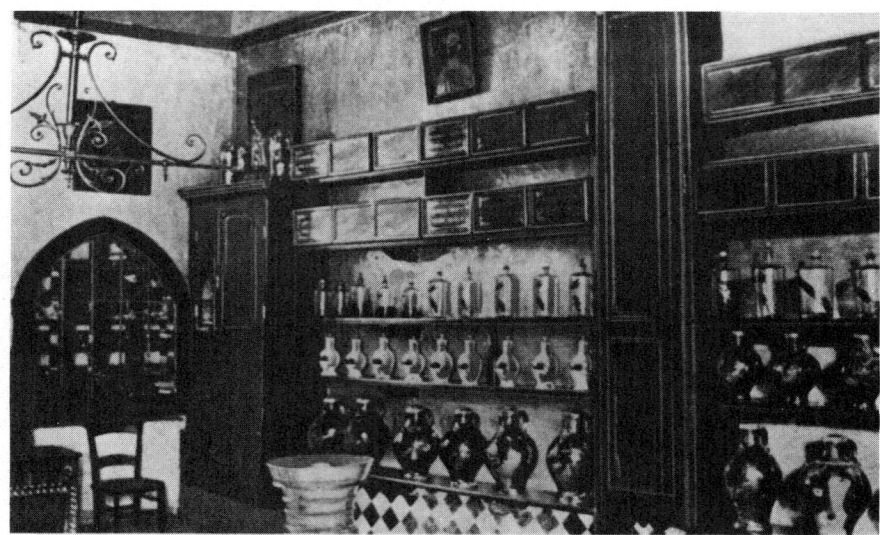

FIGURE 1-1. **The drug room of a nursing sisterhood, St. John's Hospital, Bruges. (From Dock, L.L., and Nutting, M.A.** *A history of nursing,* **Vol. 1. New York: G.P. Putnam's Sons, 1907.)**

staff rooms, all looking out on a garden where the most common medicinal herbs were grown by the nursing monks.

Of the three medieval hospitals built outside monastery walls, the most famous is the Hôtel Dieu, Paris (650 AD). This hospital was staffed by one of the earliest purely nursing orders, the Augustinian Sisters.

The Augustinian Sisters admitted the sick, homeless, and aged to their hospital and provided for their warmth, sustenance, and cleanliness. They dressed wounds and ulcers with herbal medications and prepared the dead for Christian burial. The nursing sisters also administered medications that during the Middle Ages were usually derived from medicinal herbs often combined with offensive substances such as insects, urine, animal excreta, powdered earthworms, or the "ground skull of an 'unburied' man."

The drug department in the hospital had an old nursing sister in charge. A younger nursing sister and a boy helped carry the drugs to the wards. The young sister also did the cleaning of the drug rooms. Eventually, the charge of the drug room was transferred from the sisters to a licensed apothecary, because reports indicate that drugs were sold to outsiders. Records in the late 1700s indicate that the sisters often countermanded orders for medications and diet, infuriating physicians who requested that their orders be followed exactly.

In an effort to regain the Holy Land from the Moslems, seven Crusades were launched between 1096 and 1291. The crusaders learned much from the Arabs in relation to medical knowledge and the establishment of hospitals. Several military nursing orders developed during the Crusades with half-knights, or knights themselves, nursing the sick and wounded between battles.

The best-known and purely military nursing order was that of the Knights Hospitalers of St. John of Jerusalem who organized hospitals and cared for the sick. Part of their nursing duties included drug administration.

The Beguines, a group of lay nurses originated in Liege, Flanders, about 1170, devoted themselves to the care of the widows and orphans of the crusaders and established hospitals eventually staffed by the Sisters of St. Martha of Burgundy. Two of their hospitals were at Beaune and Chalon-sur-Saone where there were beautifully decorated and immaculately kept drug rooms (Figure 1-1) from which the nursing sisters did the dispensing.

In 1534, Henry VIII (1491-1547) made himself the head of the Church of England. To demonstrate his independence from Rome he dissolved the monasteries and suppressed the religious nursing orders that served the hospitals. Thus hospitals became staffed by secular and less devoted staff and often became places of horror.

In France, the Catholic Reformation fostered the ideals of individuals such as St. Vincent de Paul (1576-1660). He founded many charitable organizations and eventually a secular nursing order, the Sisters of Charity.

In relation to drug therapy, the Sisters of Charity were to act with great respect for the doctors. They were never to condemn them or contradict their orders. The Sisters were to follow the physician's orders exactly without ever presuming to prepare the medicines according to their own way of thinking. They were to follow punctually what was prescribed, both "with regard to the quantity of the dose and the ingredients of which it was composed, because upon this fidelity and exactness depends nothing less, perhaps than the life of the patient." However, St. Vincent also encouraged them to observe and remember the methods of the physicians for treating the sick so that when they were in the villages where there was no physician they could bleed their patients and apply cupping glasses correctly. The Sisters were also to learn the different remedies used for the treatment of various diseases and the proper time and manner for administering them (Nutting & Dock, Vol. 1, 1907, pp. 424-425).

EARLY AMERICAN AND CANADIAN NURSING

Although great numbers of early colonists in America suffered from smallpox, scurvy, and yellow fever, an organized system of nursing was not brought to the American colonies. In the United States, nursing was done by family members or certain skilled individuals who also practiced as midwives. Formal nursing was, however, brought to the colonies of New France by the publication of the Jesuit *Relations* in 1633, in which the Jesuit Fathers pleaded for Sisters to care for the Indians.

The Duchesse d'Aiguillon, a niece of Cardinal Richelieu, read the Jesuit *Relations* and provided the financial support for building the first hospital on the shores of the St. Lawrence, the Hôtel Dieu at Quebec in 1639. She arranged for three Augustinian Sisters to staff the early hospital, and they suffered many hardships as they nursed colonists and Indians during severe winters, Indian wars, and epidemics of typhus and smallpox. In 1 year they treated more than 150 patients, including Indians, who would go to their hospital to be purged or bled or to ask for medicines. The Sisters dispensed over 450 medicines and exhausted their supply of drugs.

The second hospital in New France was the Hôtel Dieu at Montreal, which was founded by Canada's first lay nurse, Jeanne Mance (1606-1673). At first her hospital was little more than a dispensary constructed within the fort itself. Because of increasing numbers of patients from Indian attacks, a separate hospital building was constructed for her in 1645. Jeanne dressed wounds of all kinds and compounded her own medicines using a mortar and scales she had brought from France. She also had a syringe with an ivory tube as well as razors and lances and experience in bloodletting. Jeanne was later assisted in her work by Sisters of the Order of St. Joseph de la Flêche whom she brought to Montreal.

One of the sisters, Judith de Brésoles, had special training in nursing and in the preparation of drugs. On arriving in Montreal, she was placed in charge of the nursing at the hospital. She took the pharmacy under her care and later cultivated her own wild herbs. She "invented and prepared remedies which gained a high reputation throughout all the colony" (Nutting & Dock, Vol. 1, 1907, p. 395).

DARK AGE OF NURSING

The 1700s to the mid 1800s was a period of revolution, political strife, and pestilence. Nursing as a profession sank to its lowest level. Nurses were recruited from the lowest social ranks, for nursing was considered a type of domestic service. They worked long hours in hospitals and homes for poor pay and usually under terrible working conditions. Nurses were usually illiterate and were unable to read the labels on the medicines they were to give. They were well known for their drunkeness and abuse of patients. Charles Dickens (1844) portrayed this class of nurse in the characters of Sairey Gamp and Betsey Prig in his book, *The Life and Adventures of Martin Chuzzlewit*. People dreaded and avoided both hospitals and hired nurses, preferring to treat themselves with homemade remedies.

In the country areas, people often sought the help of self-taught nurses or "old women," who had special experience in healing and often dealt with herbs, spells and witchcraft. It was such a self-taught nurse in Shropshire, England, who cured dropsy (generalized edema) with an herbal remedy made with foxglove when the standard remedies of the day failed. Later, Dr. William Withering (1741-1799) extracted and identified the cardiac glycoside, digitalis, from her guarded recipe that contained up to 20 herbs.

In Canada after the American Revolution pioneer loyalists also depended on home remedies and self-taught nurses. One such pioneer nurse was Jane Pushie, the wife of a trumpeter in Washington's army. She was the only dispenser of medicine, practical nurse, and midwife in Antigonish, Nova Scotia. At her death at the age of 103, she had delivered approximately 1000 babies.

The self-taught Loyalist nurses concocted many common remedies that were used for all kinds of problems. Many of these "folk remedies" were used until relatively recent times. "Goose grease was always applied for a sore throat, and coughs were cured with a syrup made of onions and molasses boiled together." Frost-bites were cured with strawberry jam. In addition, roots, barks, leaves, seeds, and fruits were gathered for their desired medicinal properties. (Gibbon & Mathewson, 1947, p. 64).

NURSING IN THE EARLY 1800s

During the first half of the nineteenth century nursing was done according to individual ideas and knowledge picked up from practice or from assisting individual physicians. Nursing was a hazardous occupation at this time because many contagious diseases were brought to North America on ships, such as cholera, typhus, and smallpox. Patients were visited and nursed in the home, and nurses kept many guarded recipes of their treatments. One recipe for weak joints was a plaster that contained rosin, sulfur, beeswax, castile soap, and lard boiled in half a pint of good spirits until thick enough for spreading. "Beeves" galls, camphor, oil, and turpentine mixed with a pint of Jamaica rum was recommended for the treatment of rheumatism. This recipe, however, did not specify if the concoction was taken by mouth or applied at the site of the problem (Gibbon & Mathewson, 1947, p. 69).

Surgery during this period was not done under aseptic conditions. Patients kept most of their clothes on and Jamaican rum was used instead of anesthetics. During the 1840s the use of ether for surgical operations was being explored in the United States, and nitrous oxide was being used in the extraction of teeth. The year 1848 marked the gradual introduction of anesthetics into the surgical wards of Canadian hospitals—the use of ether coming from Boston and chloroform from Edinburgh. The use of anesthesia in surgical operations resulted not only in a great increase in the number of recoveries from casualties and major operations, but also in a greater demand for nurses to carry out the instructions for later care from surgeons as well as to administer the anesthetic.

In spite of the advances in surgery, calomel, castor oil, and bleeding were the treatments of choice for medical conditions.

In addition to self-taught nurses, nursing of quality was performed by the religious nursing orders in Canada and the United States.

The Grey Nuns brought nursing west across Canada and by 1850 were established in St. Boniface treating measles, dysentery, and smallpox with medicines they brought from Montreal. They also learned the uses of the herbs that grew in the country.

Knowledge of the medicinal use of plants was a highly developed art, not only among the native Indians but also among the white people. Nearly every plant that grew on the prairie had a special purpose. "Wild mint, goldenrod, gentian, plaintain, bloodroot, pumpkin seeds, rose-berries, wild strawberries, corn tassels, rhubarb, dandelions, black currants, milkweed, cherry bark, and spruce sap and a host of other things were made into poultices, ointments, and tasty concoctions each for a specific ailment" (Gibbon & Mathewson, 1947, p. 89). Most of the Sisters were skilled in the preparation of these medications and provided their nursing primarily in the homes of the sick.

At St. Luke's hospital in New York City, founded in 1858, the Sisters were instructed to prepare and administer all medications rather than have the patients be responsible for taking their own medications as was common in the early 19th century hospitals:

Patients cannot be trusted with their own medicine. They cannot be made to understand the fallacy of the argument, that if a teaspoonful of anything will cure a man slowly, the whole bottle will do it immediately (Dolan, 1978, p. 146).

In addition, it was not uncommon for patients to rub oral medication into the injured limb or to orally take the topical medication by the teaspoonful faithfully after meals. Thus, it was felt that the nurse should administer the medications to prevent such "gross mistakes." To perform this duty the nursing sisters were required to understand the nature of the medication, its usual dose, and expected effect. Any mistakes that might occur were to be honestly and immediately reported.

FLORENCE NIGHTINGALE

Although there are other nurses who may be considered to be leaders in nursing during the mid-1800s, it is generally felt that it is with the contributions of Florence Nightingale (1820-1910) that nursing became recognized as a profession requiring specific training, knowledge, and skills and moved into its modern period.

Nightingale's own formal nursing preparation was scant. Because nursing was being done by the servant class and was amid its darkest period in England, most of her knowledge was gained through reading all the health reports and related materials she could find.

In 1850 and again in 1851, she briefly visited the renowned school of nursing at Kaiserswerth, Germany, that the Pastor Fliedner and his wife had instituted in 1836. There the nurse deaconesses were given instruction in nursing techniques as well as in medicine and pharmacy by members of the respective professions so that they would know something about these related areas. Nightingale's early nursing preparation was followed by a brief visit to the Hôtel Dieu in Paris where she observed the nursing of the Sisters of Charity.

In 1853, Nightingale took her first nursing position as the superintendant of The Institution for the Care of Sick Gentlewomen in Distressed Circumstances. Later she was asked to become the superintendant of nurses at King's College Hospital and had just begun her work there when England and France declared war on Russia and sent their armies to the Crimea. Nightingale's work in the Crimea is well known and she received numerous honors for her services there.

After the war, Nightingale published many papers and books including *Notes On Nursing: What It Is and What It Is Not.* In *Notes,* she uses the term *nurse* indiscriminately for lay and professional nurses alike, because she believed that all women needed knowledge of the laws of health and the care of the sick in the home. Although she felt that cure and medication per se were "doctor's subjects" and preferred not to enter deeply into them, she did discuss the importance of "sound and ready observation" and the accurate measurement of medications.

To Nightingale, the ability to make accurate observations was one of the most important lessons to be given to nurses so that they could distinguish individual reactions to disease, treatments, and medications. Careful and accurate observation was especially important in relation to drug action and effects:

The same remark applies to the action of narcotics, of aperients [a very mild laxative, for example, magnesium oxide], which, in the one, take effect directly, in the other not perhaps for twenty-four hours.... The experienced nurse can always tell that a person has taken a narcotic the night before by the patchiness of the colour about the face, when the reaction of depression has set in; that very colour which the inexperienced will point to as a proof of health (Nightingale, 1860, pp. 115-117).

In relation to the measurement of medication she states:

I have known several of our real old-fashioned hospital "sisters," who could, as accurately as a measuring glass, measure out all their patients' wine and medicine by the eye, and never be wrong. I do not recommend this, one must be very sure of oneself to do it (Nightingale, 1860, p. 113).

The inexperienced administration of medicines was another area she spoke to, for this appeared to

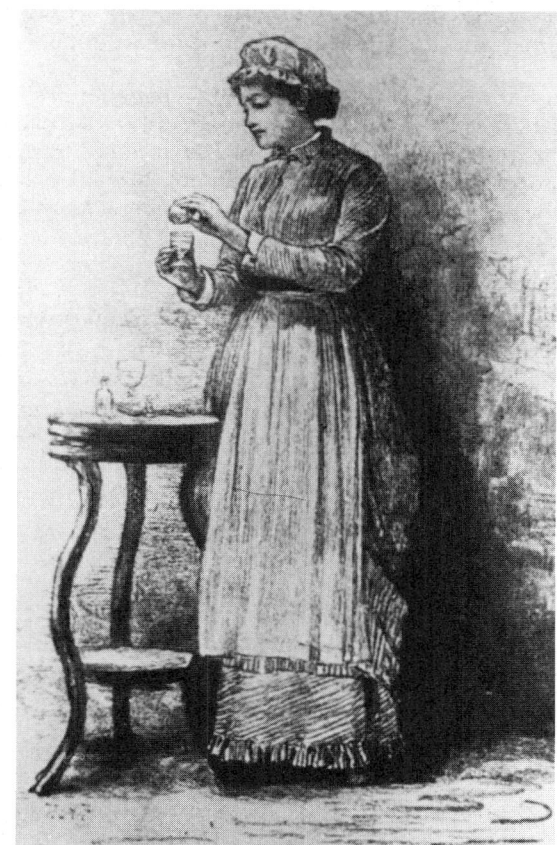

FIGURE 1-2. **Trained nurse preparing medications. Isabel A. Hampton (Robb), Bellevue, 1882. (From Dock, L.L., and Nutting, M.A.** *A history of nursing,* **Vol. 1. New York: G.P. Putnam's Sons, 1907.)**

be a problem in the mid 1800s. She knew that some ladies shared their medications with friends and poorer neighbors and recommended that instead of giving medicine, of which they did not know "the exact and proper application, nor all its consequences," it would be better

to persuade and help your poorer neighbors to remove the dung hill from before the door, to put in a window which opens, or an Arnott's ventilator, or to cleanse and limewash the cottages? Of these things the benefits are sure. The benefits of the inexperienced administration of medicines are by no means so sure (Nightingale, 1860, p. 131).

She especially warned against the giving of alcohol, narcotics, or dangerous soothing syrups to infants. If lay women were to give medicines, however, she felt that they should give a homeopathic medicine. "It won't do any harm" (Nightingale, 1860, p. 132).

However, to Nightingale, nursing was more than the administration of medications and treatments:

I use the word nursing for want of a better. It has been limited to signify little more than the administration of medicines and the application of poultices. It ought to signify the proper use of fresh air, light, warmth, cleanliness, quiet, and the proper selection and administration of diet—all at the least expense of vital power to the patient (Nightingale, 1860, p. 8).

Having recognized the need for specially prepared and educated nurses to provide care to the sick, Florence Nightingale founded the Nightingale Training School for Nurses at St. Thomas' Hospital in London in 1860. Before she died, she saw the initiation of thousands of schools for nurses based on her plan in Europe, the United States, and Canada as well as in other parts of the world. The dark age of nursing was now over (Figure 1-2).

EARLY SCHOOLS OF NURSING

By 1892, approximately 148 schools of nursing were established across the United States and by the early 1900s more than 70 training schools sprang up all across Canada. The schools were organized by both lay hospitals and religious sisterhoods. Instruction at these training schools was in the art of nursing, the care of wards and sick rooms, the cleaning and disinfection of equipment, and the observation of the sick in regards to pulse, breathing, skin condition, sleep, appetite, effect of diet, and the effects of stimulants and medicines (Figure 1-3). Students received lectures in chemistry, sanitary science, physiology, anatomy, hygiene, various medical conditions, and materia medica (drugs).

Most of the early training schools were associated with hospitals, and students soon became a source of inexpensive labor for the hospitals. At the World's Fair Congress on Hospitals, Dispensaries, and Nursing in 1893 nursing leaders were addressing this issue as well as other nursing problems of the day.

NURSING AT THE TURN OF THE CENTURY

In 1906, Isabel Hampton Robb (1860-1910), one of the first graduates of the New York Training School for Nurses at the Bellevue Hospital and a famous nursing leader who had been at the World's Fair Conference, completed her third "revised and enlarged" edition of *Nursing: Its Principles and Practices*. This reference was directed for hospital and private use and outlined a 3-year curriculum plan for training schools. She felt that shorter programs were ineffective because of the increasing amount of knowledge nurses required and because nursing students, being used for labor, were too tired to make good use of their lectures.

The program included a 6-month preliminary course in which the domestic duties of the probationer, who was not to do any actual nursing, were outlined. Included in her book is a chapter outlining the method of administration of drugs, dosage, weights and measures, care of medicine closets, and the use of medicine lists. Nursing techniques and responsibilities were also described as well as routes of administration, care of equipment, and the observation of the patient's individual reaction to medication.

The administration of medicines was a duty that began early in the first year of a nurse's instruction, and there were rules that students learned were never to be disobeyed in relation to the safe administration of medications. It is often surprising how many of these rules are still practiced today. The medicine label and dose were to be read twice before giving any drug, once before it was measured out, and just before it was given to the patient. Nurses were never to give a medicine from a bottle or box that was not properly labeled, and nurses were never to record that a medicine had been given before the patient actually had taken it.

Although Robb's book was published more than 75 years ago, it is interesting and informative to note the nurse's role in relation to the preparation, administration, and monitoring of drug therapy. Let us look at the nurse's role in relation to drug administration at this time.

Oral route of administration

The oral route was the most common route for drug administration. Drugs given by mouth were given in solution or in the form of powders, pills, capsules, triturates, and wafers.

Liquid dosage forms. Many drugs in solutions as well as oil preparations were given for various conditions. Many of these were bad tasting. To increase palatability and "lessen the sensibility of the nerves of taste and render the flavor of the dose less noticeable" a nurse gave a small piece of ice to the patient to hold in his mouth just before the medicine was given. The nurse also mixed medicines with crushed ice or seltzer water to make them more palatable. In addition to these techniques, it was recommended that the nurse have the patient hold brandy, whiskey, or hot water in the mouth for a few minutes, or hold the nose while the dose was given. Immediately afterward, the nurse should also provide her patient with a little cold water

DATE, May 20, 1892.   PLATE VI.

Hour.	Temp	Pulse.	Sleep.	Urine	Stool.	Medicine.	Stimulant.	Nourishment.	Remarks.
A. M.									
1	...	...	...	{ Per cath 200 c. c, }	...	...	...	Enema { Pep. milk, ℥iij / Brandy, ℥j. }	Retained enema. Has had much pain.
2	...	...	...	...	...	Tr. capsici, gtt. iij	...		
3	...	...	1 hour.	...	...	...	...		
4	98.6	72	...	...	...	...	...		Vomited greenish clear fluid, ℥ijss
5	...	...	...	...	...	...	...	Enema { Pep. milk, ℥iij / Brandy, ℥j. }	Retained enema. [night.
6	...	...	...	...	...	...	...		Has been noisy the latter part of
7	...	...	...	...	...	...	...		
8	99.6	80	...	{ Per cath 170 c. c }					
9	...	...	½ hour.	...				{ By mouth: Milk and lime-water, ℥j.
10	...	...	½ hour.	...			Brandy, ♏xxx	{ Milk and lime-water, ℥ij.
11	...	...	...	...				{ Milk and lime-water, ℥ij,
12 **P. M.**	99.8	76	...	...					Headache. No other pain.
1	...	...	¾ hour.	...				{ Milk and lime-water, ℥iij.
2	...	...	...	{ Voided 100 c. c }			Brandy, ♏xxx	
3	...	...	...	...				{ Milk and lime-water, ℥iij.
4	100	78	...	...					Enema, { Oil, ℥ij : / Turpentine, ℥ss.
5	...	...	...	...				{ Milk and lime-water, ℥iij. }	Enema, { Soapsuds, Oj ; / Rochelle salts, ℥ss.
6	...	...	½ hour.	...			Brandy, ♏xxx		Enema expelled ; partially-formed stool, moderate amount.
7	...	...	...	...	1			{ Milk and lime-water, ℥iv.	
8	99.6	82	...	...	...	Tr. capsici, gtt. iij		{ Milk and lime-water, ℥iv.	
9	...	...	1 hour.	...				{ Milk and lime-water, ℥iv.	Rectal tube inserted. Flatus expelled.
10	...	...	...	...			Brandy, ♏xxx		
11	...	{ 45 min.	Voided 300 c. c }					{ Milk and lime-water, ℥iv. }	Comfortable. No pain.
12	99.8	72							

SUMMARY: Sleep, 5 hrs. Urine, 770 c. c. Tr. capsici, gtt. vj. Stimulant, brandy, ℥ij. Nourishment, milk and lime-water, ℥ij. by mouth ; milk by enema, ℥vj ; brandy by enema, ℥ij. Purgative enemata, ij. Stool, 1.

FIGURE 1-3. A bedside record of nursing care including medications administered (1892). (From Robb, I.H. *Nursing: Its principles and practice* (3rd ed.). Toronto: The J.F. Hartz Co., Ltd., 1906.)

or seltzer to rinse the mouth and to take away the taste. For administering oils:

> two drachms of sherry may be placed in a medicine-glass, the rim and sides being moistened with it, and the oil then poured carefully into the center; lastly, another drachm of sherry is poured on the top, and the whole is taken in one swallow (Robb, 1910, pp. 220-221).

When giving oil to children, the nurse emulsified it by shaking it with a little milk and sugar to prevent vomiting. Castor oil was best given at bedtime, and for the "obstinate child" Robb (1910) recommended that the nose "be held firmly enough to oblige the little patient to open his mouth in order to breathe." At just the right moment, the nurse could then insert the spoon, press the back of the tongue gently down with it, and slowly empty the medicine (pp. 221-222).

Solid dosage forms. Tasteless powders were mixed with a little water. "Effervescing" powders were always given in 1/2 to 2/3 glass of cold water and taken during effervescence. Insoluble powders, including calomel or acetanilid, were placed directly on the tongue and washed down with a drink of water.

For convenience in giving some medicines, triturates or tablets were used. Triturates were prepared by adding certain proportions of milk sugar or "sulfite of soda" to the solid drug and triturating (i.e., grinding and rubbing until thoroughly pulverized). The powder was mixed into a paste with weak alcohol that evaporated, leaving a freshly made pill. The nurse was to be sure that her pills were freshly made up because they would become hard and dry if allowed to stand too long and would not dissolve when given to the patient, passing through the alimentary canal without producing the desired effect. When giving a pill, especially to a patient who had difficulty swallowing, the nurse placed it far back on the tongue and followed it quickly with a drink of water.

If the patient was ill or if it was "difficult to get him to take his medicine," an admixture made of the medication and a little milk or glycerin would facilitate swallowing.

Wafers were also used by the nurse, especially when giving unpleasant tasting powders. Quinine-containing preparations were wrapped in wafers of rice paper or enclosed in capsules of gelatin, which rapidly dissolved in the stomach. If wafers were not available, thin pieces of tissue paper were used.

When pills were given to children, the pill was concealed in a small piece of bread or in a small amount of jelly. If this did not work, it was crushed and given as a powder. The nurse was never to use force when giving a pill to a child, for there was "danger of pushing it into the larynx."

Rectal route of administration

Various rectal medications were given for therapeutic purposes, as were numerous kinds of enemas.

Rectal medications. The rectal site of administration of medication was selected when local effects were desired, when the stomach was unable to retain anything, or if it "must have its work lessened." Because it was believed that the mucous membrane of the large intestine did not absorb quickly, requiring twice as long as the stomach, medicines that were given for a stimulating effect were administered in solution and injected "as high up as possible" (10 inches) in the same manner as enemas (Robb, 1910, p. 227).

Sedative medicines were sometimes given by the rectal route. Bromides and chloral hydrate were administered for their systemic sedating effects, and it was recommended that these drugs always be given with the tube inserted at least 6 inches. Opium in some form, usually a suppository, was administered for localized pain.

Enemas. There were many types of enemas, or enemata, used at the turn of the century. Simple, laxative, and purgative enemas were common, and there were many others that had to be prepared and administered by the nurse to treat various conditions.

The nurse's role in the administration of enemas included the actual preparation of the enema solutions, which often contained several different medications and other ingredients; preparation of the patient; administration of the enema; the care of the equipment afterward; and the recording of the treatment and results.

When one reviews the nursing literature, it is often surprising how accurate the rationale given for the nursing measures was and how many of the principles are still in use today.

The patient was positioned on the left side with the knees flexed because "the sigmoid flexure of the colon lies in the left iliac fossa, and the fluid will thus be more easily retained". The bed was protected with a rubber sheet and towel, with the bedpan in near readiness and always "comfortably warm." For serious constipation the knee-chest position was ordered; however, this was considered to be rarely necessary. The basin of water was placed on the rubber sheet and the "enema administered under cover" with a bulb syringe (Robb, 1910, p. 157).

Suppositories. Suppositories were used in the same manner as they are today. The most common suppositories of this time were those that contained some preparation of opium, which was used as a "local sedative." When administering a suppository, the nurse first oiled it and then "slipped [it] in without force" with the patient lying on the left side. The nurse was careful that the suppository was placed beyond the internal sphincter muscle, pressing the anus with a towel if necessary until any desire to expel the suppository passed (Robb, 1910, p. 227).

Parenteral route of administration

Hypodermic medications. Hypodermic medication meant the administration of drugs by injecting them under the skin. The correctly held belief was that the chief advantages of this route was the rapidity in which absorption of the drug occured and the avoidance of gastric disturbance. In the early 1900s, drugs such as morphine or solutions of the active principles of drugs were often given hypodermically in dosage ranges from 1 to 15 minims (1 minim ≈ 1 drop). In the case of "stimulants" such as whiskey, brandy and ether, a "syringeful" was given at one time when "rapid stimulation" was required (Robb, 1910, pp. 223-224).

The principle drugs used hypodermically were made up in the form of compressed tablets (hypodermic tablets) that were dissolved in a teaspoon of distilled or boiled water. This greatly helped the nurse make up fresh solutions for administration at a moment's notice.

Injections were given in a fine syringe to which a hollow needle was attached. The nurse was taught that risk could be reduced to a minimum if proper care and technique were used.

To prepare the needle for a hypodermic injection, the nurse passed it through an alcohol flame just before insertion. Because this technique was said to blunt the needle and therefore cause the injection to be painful for the patient, a preferred method, performed before the syringe was loaded, was to boil the needle for a few minutes in a tablespoonful of water or 1% soda solution over an alcohol or gas flame (Figure 1-4). It was then attached to the syringe with a clean piece of sterilized gauze.

The nurse was to be sure that the syringe and solution were "perfectly aseptic" so that "virulent germs" would not be introduced into the surrounding tissues, resulting in inflammation and "abscess-formation." The skin was well prepared with absolute alcohol, the nurse selecting the "outer side of the arms, thighs, hips, or the abdomen." A "fair-sized" fold of skin was pinched up between the thumb and finger of the left

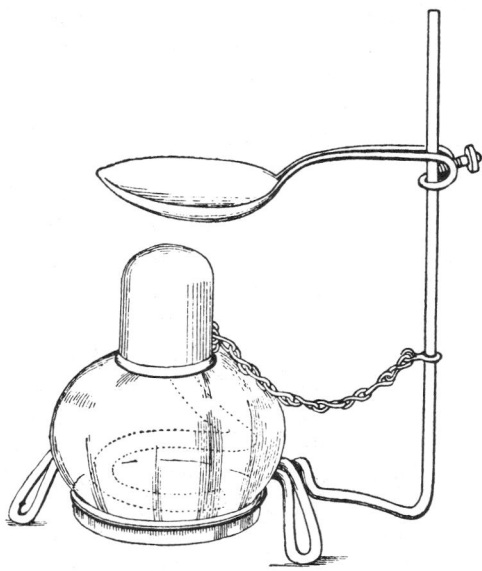

FIGURE 1-4. **Alcohol lamp and spoon-shaped pan for sterilizing hypodermic needles. (From Pope, A.E. *Pope's manual of nursing procedure.* New York: G.P. Putnam's Sons, 1919.)**

hand, and the needle inserted quickly in a slanting direction into the tissues for at least half an inch; it was then withdrawn slightly so that the nurse could be sure that the injection only penetrated the fleshy part of the body, since it was believed that injection into a vein would cause the drug to be "carried directly to the heart and may reach the nerve-centres in concentration in a few seconds, producing alarming symptoms." She was also careful to avoid penetrating nerves and injecting the medication over a bony prominence, for this was believed to injure the bone. The medication was injected slowly and the needle quickly withdrawn. A clean pad was pressed lightly over the site to "prevent fluid from escaping," and the area was rubbed gently in an upward fashion to assist in the absorption of the drug. However, if the rubbing was at all painful to the patient, it was not to be done (Robb, 1910, pp. 223-224).

Injections of normal salt (saline) solution. In the early 1900s, the administration of "injections of normal salt solution" had been well established as a therapeutic agent. Subcutaneous infusion into the tissues was the procedure most often used, although intravenous infusion was also used at this time. Supplies of normal salt solution were kept on hand in the general hospitals. The apparatus included a graduated jar that had a glass nipple projecting from the side near the bottom and 6 feet of sterile rubber tubing with a "moderate-sized" aspirating needle attached.

Other routes of administration

Douches. Vaginal, nasal, and aural douches were also given for cleanliness, for their stimulating effects, or to relieve inflammation. A fountain spout and bag apparatus were used and given in much the same way as enemas.

Tampons. Nurses also made tampons of lamb's wool for the application of antiseptics, powders, and soothing drugs in inflammatory conditions of the vagina. The tampon was inserted with a speculum and long dressing forceps and removed after 24 hours, followed by a vaginal douche per order.

Inunction. The administration of medications by "inunction" or the "rubbing in" of various substances, was rare in the early 1900s. However, mercurial inunctions were often used at this time for the treatment of syphilis. In addition, tuberculosis, in cases in which there was much emaciation, was treated with cod liver oil in this way.

The areas generally used for inunction were the axillary spaces, inner surfaces of the thighs, chest, and abdomen. Before an inunction was given, the circulation of the skin was increased by a warm bath and then the ointment was rubbed in well by the nurse.

Inhalation. To obtain absorption of medications via the lungs, atomizers or "insufflators" were used at the turn of the century. The spray from an atomizer was most commonly used; however, the inhalation of vapor was also a favorite method. The drug was mixed in hot water in a small teakettle that was heated over a lighted gas or alcohol lamp with a flame just large enough to allow a small stream of steam to pass constantly through the spout. The patient held his mouth over this stream at a comfortable distance.

Volatile drugs such as ammonia, eucalyptus, chloroform, and ether were poured on sponges or small pieces of cloth and held near the nostrils. "Nitrite of amyl is best inhaled from a small piece of fine linen or handkerchief," and was the treatment of choice for angina. The nurse was to be especially careful when using irritating substances with unconscious patients, being careful to hold the cloth far enough away to prevent injury (Robb, 1910, p. 228).

Anesthetics. Nurses in the early training schools at the turn of the century were often called on in private practice to administer an anesthetic (Figure 1-5). Nurses gained competence in this by taking every opportunity to watch the administration of anesthesia in the hospital, to ask questions when a "fitting occasion" arose, and to practice the technique whenever possible. The nurse was to make herself familiar with the principles and methods involved and the dangers to be watched for and how to prevent them (Robb, 1910, p. 417).

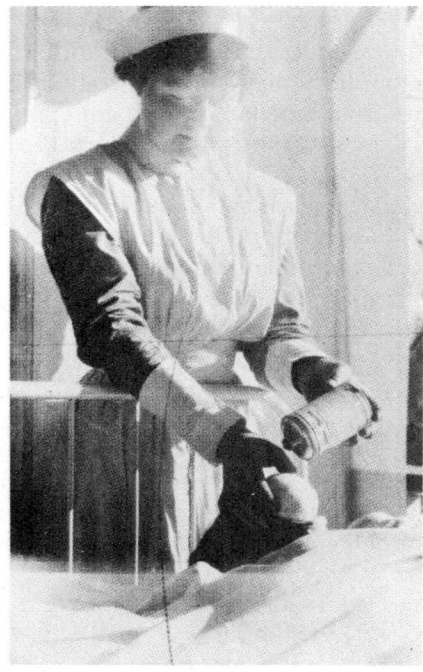

FIGURE 1-5. **Student nurse administering ether to a patient. (From Archivos, Archer Memorial Hospital of Lamont)**

Anesthetics were administered in the form of a vapor or gas to produce a general effect and were administered in liquid form by subcutaneous injection into the tissues or applied externally to obtain a local effect. Ether, administered in an ether cone, and chloroform were used most in surgery and obstetrics. Nitrous oxide had been used before the introduction of ether and chloroform, but was now used mainly in dentistry.

Nursing responsibilities. By the turn of the century, it was the responsibility of the head nurse in the hospital to write out accurate lists with patient names, medicines, doses, and hours of administration. One nurse was set apart and held responsible for the "prompt and correct administration" of the medications (i.e., a "medication" nurse). However, a nurse "under no circumstances" was to "take upon herself the responsibility of suggesting or prescribing a medicine. If consulted as to what it would be best to give, she should always refer the consultant to the physician in charge" (Robb, 1910, p. 232).

Drug monitoring. The nurse during the early 1900s not only received training in the administration of drugs, but also was required to understand the effects of the drugs in common use and to recognize the ordinary indications for their discontinuance. Nurses were also to be aware of the maximum and minimum doses of drugs and the symptoms of overdose. It was expected that the nurse recognize that the nature of the disease, the patient's age, temperament, and habits, and the time of administration could affect individual patient drug response and the action of the medications.

It was recognized that children required "much smaller doses than adults," and that the elderly had "less resisting powers than the middle-aged person for depressing drugs" (Robb, 1910, p. 229). The most generally accepted rule, at this time, for calculating the doses for children under 12 years of age was to make a fraction, the numerator of which, represented the age of the child in years and the denominator, the age of the child with twelve added. This gave the part of the adult dose that was required. Thus a 4-year-old child would receive one fourth of the adult dose according to the general rule: $\frac{4}{(4 + 12)} = \frac{1}{4}$.

Generally for patients between 12 and 21 years of age, the recommended dose was half of the full dose. There were exceptions to be remembered to the rule, however. For example, purgatives like calomel or castor oil were given to children in half of the adult dose; with opium, "since children are very susceptible to this drug," a smaller dose than the rule was given. On the other hand, children being "very tolerant of belladonna," the dose was adjusted accordingly (Robb, 1910, pp. 229-230).

It was up to the nurse to recognize not only the therapeutic response of the prescribed drug, but also other results that may follow its use, since it was known that the drug may not act in the same way with everyone. Certain individuals, such as those with "nervous temperaments," would be affected by certain medication in "some peculiar way that would not ordinarily be expected," and thus the nurse was to be very careful to note the symptoms following the first dose of a medicine. If any peculiar symptoms were observed, they were to be "reported to the physician" and the dose "not be repeated without further instructions" (Robb, 1910, p. 230). Thus it was imperative that the nurse should understand the symptoms that may follow the use of the various drugs because "often only through her can such occurrences be detected" (Robb, 1910, p. 231)."

It was also recognized that some drugs, when given over a long period of time, could gradually accumulate in the system, resulting in "marked symptoms of poisoning." This was especially true of drugs such as strychnine. In addition to watching for this "accumulative" effect, the nurse was to observe for reactions to drugs that might show that the system had become "accustomed" to them, resulting in the need for an increase in the dose to obtain the desired result. The possibility of patient addiction was another problem that the nurse was to be alert to: . . . "the patient thinks he cannot do without it, as is so frequently seen with opium, and its alkaloid morphine" (Robb, 1910, p. 230).

Addiction. Addiction had been a recognized problem since the Civil War when morphine was widely administered by syringe to the wounded soldiers to relieve pain. Addiction became so widespread in the veterans that it became known as the "army disease."

By the early 1900s, there were over 100,000 narcotic addicts in the United States. Opiates were often found in patent medications such as pain killers, cough mixtures, and other preparations. Morphine sulfate and opium were mixed with molasses or sassafras for flavor and were sold widely. In addition, opiates were widely prescribed along with whiskey and brandy by physicians of the late 1800s and early 1900s for diarrhea, dysentery, and other illnesses.

Heroin was introduced as a remedy for the treatment of coughs and was considered to be "the most powerful and most reliable drug at our command" (Schleif, 1902). In relation to the use of this new drug, nurses were to be alert to "after effects" including constipation, nausea, drowsiness, and itching. In addition, stupor, giddiness, or severe headaches could also be noted.

Heroin was used successfully, according to the literature of the day, as a cure for opium (i.e., morphine) addiction. In addition, it was often substituted for morphine injections because it was thought to have the properties of an opiate without the problem of addiction. Thus, it was widely used alone and in pharmaceutical preparations in Europe and the Americas for a few decades.

Because of the continued problems related to addiction, Congress passed the Federal Pure Food and Drug Act in 1906. By 1914, the Harrison Narcotic Act was passed.

Often, when a habit was becoming apparent, a placebo was substituted by the nurse in order to "quiet the mind of the patient" and to not further contribute to the addiction. However, Robb (1910) felt this was "to be deprecated from a moral standpoint and no nurse should resort to hypodermics of water or salt solution or any of the various substitutes without the direct orders from the physician" (p. 231).

Timing of drug administration. The timing of drug administration in relation to its absorption was also considered to be required nursing knowledge at this time. It was known that absorption was more rapid when the stomach was empty and that the medication was not to be given when the stomach was full of food if rapid action was desired. Fast-acting purgatives were given 1 hour before breakfast and more slowly acting cathartics were given at bedtime. Alkaline tonics were given before meals, and to decrease gastrointestinal upset, irritating or acid substances were given when food was in the stomach. Narcotics were given after patients were prepared for the night and nothing was to be done to arouse or disturb them once the drugs had been given.

Drug interactions. It was also a nursing responsibility to know what foods certain medicines were incompatible with. For example, nurses were required to know that milk and acids being given together would cause the milk to be rejected or cause gastric pain. In addition, nurses were required to know that some drugs were physiologically or chemically incompatible with others. For example, corrosive sublimate, being incompatible with all albuminous bodies (i.e. eggs, milk, blood), was to be given alone.

Storage of medications. Medicines were kept in stock on the wards in small quantities to ensure freshness, and in locked immaculately kept medicine closets. All unused medications were returned to the hospital pharmacy, thus cutting down on expenses. For safety, all extracts, active principles, and "powerful drugs" were kept in small quantities in bottles holding no more than 2 ounces supplied with two labels. One label specified the name of the drug and the strength of the preparation. The other label, bright red as a precaution, was marked "poison". External applications were stored in colored glass bottles with rough surfaces so that the moment the nurse's fingers touched it, she would recognize that it was a poisonous substance. The nurse always poured the medication away from the label so it would not be damaged or rubbed off, and a small damp cloth was used to wipe the bottle before returning it to the shelf after it was "carefully corked to prevent evaporation" (Robb, 1910, p. 233).

THE WAR YEARS (1914-1918)

During the war years, the fifth edition of Lavinia Dock's *Materia Medica for Nurses* was copyrighted; it had previously been published in 1890, 1897, 1901, and 1905. Compelled by many years of experience, she reminded nurses of the subtle dangers of many potent remedies with which they were entrusted and encouraged them to never lose sight of the dreadful possibility of falling under the influence of certain drug habits "unfortunately but too easily acquired in accession to the relief offered by drugs in moments of fatigue or of nerve exhaustion." The nurse was encouraged "not to prop her failing strength by stimulating drugs" (Dock, 1915, p. IV). Thus it seems drug abuse among trained nurses by 1915 may have been a problem.

Recognizing that the study of materia medica was part of the course of study in all nursing training schools, Dock prepared her textbook along the then current curriculum models. She felt that books written for the use of the medical profession were not appropriate for nurses because the application of medicine to disease was not part of a nurse's study, and these books contained not only what the nurse needed to know but what she did not need to know. It was her goal to collect from all available sources the scattered points that concerned a nurse, and to give them simply and directly, including the source and composition of drugs, their physiologic actions, signs indicating their favorable or unfavorable results, and symptoms of poisons with their antidotes, and practical points on drug administration.

In addition, this nursing pharmacology reference reflected the newest teaching of the period and encouraged a philosophy of less and less drug giving, for it was thought that "the patient who takes a medicine must recover twice—once from the disease and once from the medicine." Dock (1915) emphasized:

> The use of drugs to produce emesis is not so prevalent as it was years ago, and if it becomes necessary to cause vomiting, the simpler means (such as drinking large draughts of tepid water and putting one's finger down the throat) should be tried whenever possible (p. 275).

Inorganic materia medica (i.e., alkalies, metals, nonmetal elements, inorganic acids, and carbon compounds) and organic materia medica (i.e., vegetable and animal matter) were included in the text, as well as poisons and their treatments, emetics, hypodermics, serum therapy, electrotherapeutics, and radiology. She also included synthetic remedies but made no attempt to present a full list of the "innumerable drugs" that were then available.

Individual patient peculiarities continued to be emphasized, as previously discussed. She encouraged the nursing student to be aware that:

> The more highly strung nervous organizations respond more quickly, as a rule, to the actions of drugs than do those of coarser fibre, and more quickly show evidence of overdosing and mild poisoning....With frequent repetition comes "toleration," when the system accommodates itself to the drug, and larger doses can be taken with relatively less effect. Beyond this point comes "habit," when the system not only tolerates but craves the drug in ever increasing quantities . . . as is most strikingly shown in the ascendency of alcohol and opium over the individual (Dock, 1915, p. 3).

Drug "accumulation" and the "cumulative action" of drugs were other things for which the nurse was responsible, as well as giving "strong drugs" carefully to children and the aged. In relation to prescribing, Dock (1915) noted that:

> It is never necessary to tell a good nurse not to prescribe for others—she scorns an act which is not only unprofessional, but in the worst possible taste (Dock, 1915, p. iv).

Drug forms

By 1915, drug preparations varied and included tablets; "collapsubes"—collapsible tubes containing ointments and creams; solubes, which were substances put up in soluble coverings for local application as lotions; sterules—glass capsules of sterile solutions for ophthalmic or general use; vescettes—compressed effervescent salts that were dissolved in water before being administered; cachets—hollowed disks, two of which were used to enclose powdered medications; and lamellae—small gelatin disks containing drugs that were inserted between the lower lid and the eyeball.

As in the early 1900s, the making of solutions continued to be a phase of nursing procedure that necessitated exact knowledge and careful technique. It was recommended that this be taught in the hospital drug room by the pharmacist, "since here only is to be found the requisite combination of expert knowledge and suitable equipment which makes for efficient teaching. By actually handling drugs, and by observation under expert supervision of exact methods of weighing and measuring, the nurse will more readily grasp the underlying principles and realize the necessity for caution and accuracy" (Dock, 1915, p. 13).

The nurse was always to know what she was giving, as well as the usual doses of the different classes of drugs. Thus, it was essential that she recognize the most important ingredients contained in prescriptions and to find out "by arithmetic process" the exact amount of each ingredient. For example, it was often necessary for nurses to administer a fractional dose of a drug when the preparation on hand was in a solution whose strength was indicated in terms of percentage:

> Strychnine gr. 1/50 is called for,
> the solution on hand has a strength
> of 1%
> Since ♏100 [100 minims] contains gr. i.
> ∴ ♏ I [1 minim]   "   " 1/100.
> ∴ gr. 1/50 will be contained in as many minims as
> grain 1/100 is contained in gr. 1/50.
> $$1/50 \div 1/100 = 1/50 \times 100/1 = 2.$$
> Minims 2 of the stock solution represents
>   the amount called for, viz., gr. 1/50.
> (Dock, 1915, p. 16).

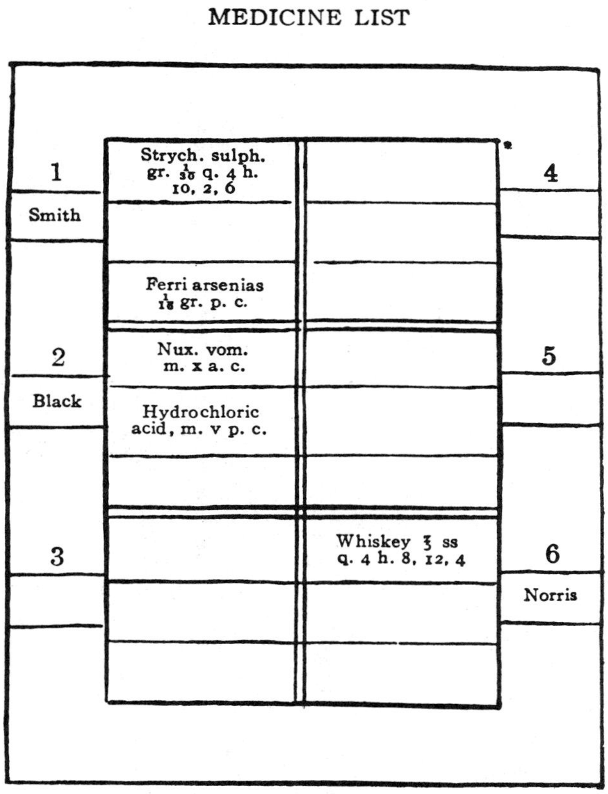

MEDICINE LIST

1	Strych. sulph. gr. ₃₀ q. 4 h. 10, 2, 6		4
Smith			
	Ferri arsenias ⅛ gr. p. c.		
2	Nux. vom. m. x a. c.		5
Black	Hydrochloric acid, m. v p. c.		
3		Whiskey ℥ ss q. 4 h. 8, 12, 4	6
			Norris

FIGURE 1-6. **A medicine list used after World War I. (From Pope, A.E.** *Pope's manual of nursing procedure.* **New York: G.P. Putnam's Sons, 1919.)**

Hypodermic and intramuscular injections

The hypodermic administration of drugs was growing steadily in favor by this time. The best location for the injection being considered the extensor surfaces of the extremities, as well as the back, chest, or abdomen, avoiding the region of large blood vessels and nerves. The dose given was usually half the amount given by mouth.

The nurse was to be familiar with the various forms and sizes of hypodermic syringes in use and their care and sterilization. Two methods of making the injections were now identified as superficial and deep. Morphine and strychnine were usually injected superficially "about the fleshy part of the shoulder," although they could be "put in lower down on the arm or in other parts of the body."

Deep, or intramuscular, injections were used for irritating drugs and were given with the same precautions as superficial injections. Mercury, in the form of the bichloride salt or "gray oil," was injected deep into the buttocks. Ether, camphor, ammonia, alcohol, and caffeine were also injected into the muscles in order to obtain their rapid stimulating effects. Digitaline, ergotine, and arsenic, in the form of atoxyl, were likewise "put in deep."

A new technique incorporated into the nurse's rep-

ertoire was that of the administration of serums. The nurse was to have an understanding of the action and immunity of sera, of which two kinds were identified: antitoxic, such as antitetanus, antidiphtheritic, and anticellular; and antibacterial, such as antipneumococcic, antityphoid, and antiplague (Dock, 1910, p. 282). Antitoxin was usually administered deeply into the tissues of the back, buttocks, or thigh, between the shoulder blades, or in the lumbar muscles, the preferred sites at that time.

Injections of normal salt solution

By 1915, a salt solution apparatus was kept on hand, including a graduated bottle, a rubber tube, a needle, and sterilized normal salt solution (0.9%). When used, it was still heated, as it was in the earlier part of the century, to a temperature of 110° F and maintained at that point during infusion. The bottle was suspended 3 to 6 feet above the patient, and the fluid was injected into the tissues behind the breast or into the thigh. The nurse was not to become alarmed if a large swelling occurred because persistent kneading of the tissues around the site would reduce it. The infusion rate was 500 ml over 20 to 30 minutes.

POSTWAR YEARS (1919 through the 1920s)

During the postwar years nursing still included such things as the application of poultices, the use of counterirritants, bloodletting, cupping, and the use of leeches. In addition, there were numerous points of special importance to be remembered regarding the care, measuring, and administration of medicines.

Care of medicines

Nurses were to keep medicine cupboards locked and were not to leave the key where patients could get it. To expedite the giving of medicines, it was recommended that medicine lists (Figure 1-6) be used and that medicines be kept in alphabetical order, keeping those intended for external use and stronger poisons separate from others. Oils were kept in a cool place. Poisons continued to be placed in colored bottles with rough exteriors marked carefully with "poison" or "for external use only." Nurses were never to have medicines in unmarked bottles nor were they to use a dose of medicine that had been left in an unmarked glass. Nurses were instructed never to order a large amount of a medicine at a time because there were few drugs that did not deteriorate with age, and for the same reason any drug that had an unusual appearance was not to be used.

Measuring

Medicines were to be given on time, and while measuring medicines, the nurse was "never [to] think of anything but the work at hand and never speak to anyone nor allow anyone to speak to you." In addition, patients were never to be allowed to carry medicine to another patient because "innumerable mistakes have been thus made" (Pope, 1919, pp. 409-411).

Medication administration

When giving medications to the patients, the nurse carried a small tray, a pitcher of fresh cold water, a glass rod for stirring, a dropper, glass tubes to be used as straws for the administration of medication mixtures that could injure the teeth, and plenty of graduated medicine glasses so that each patient would be given medicine in a clean glass. After the medicine was given, each glass was carefully washed. Glasses used for oils were washed separately from the others in hot soapy water. This washing was never to be entrusted to any patient.

Increased attention was given to the safe administration of medications and the need for written orders from physicians:

In order to prevent mistakes in receiving and carrying out physicians' orders and to protect nurses from unjust accusations, it was a common practice in hospitals for each ward or floor to be provided with a "prescription book." Nurses, except in emergencies, were not allowed to give medicines or treatments until the order was written in the book by the physician or, if he authorized a nurse to write it, signed by him. If the order was given by telephone or for any other reason it was impossible for the doctor to write or sign it, the nurse receiving the order was required to write it in the book and sign her name (Pope, 1919, pp. 406-407).

In addition, nurses were encouraged to practice reading prescriptions and were responsible for understanding their component parts.

Nursing curricula at this time correlated the practical work of nursing with theory. To facilitate teaching, many techniques were demonstrated to students in the classroom before they were expected to perform them in the clinical area with actual patients. Many

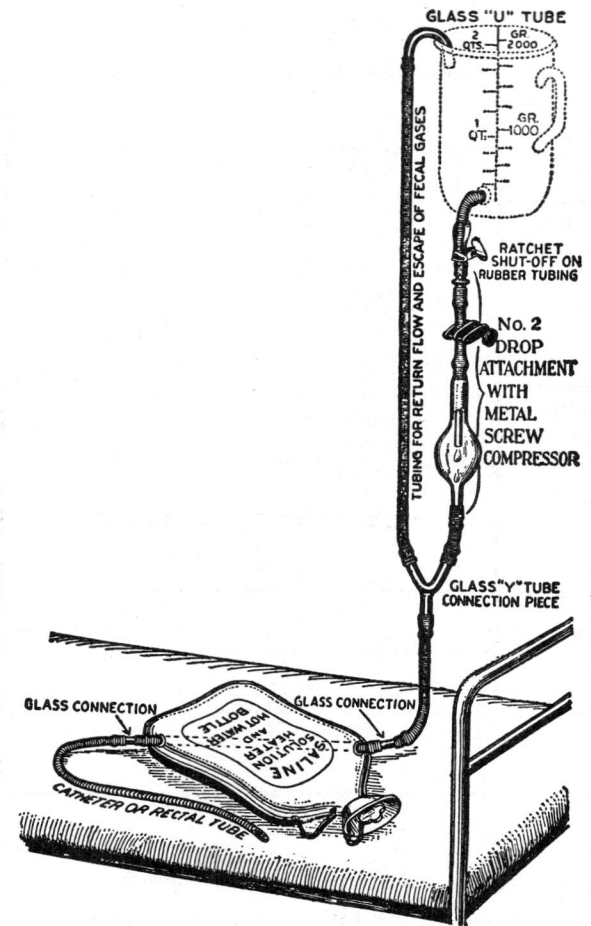

FIGURE 1-7. **Proctoclysis apparatus. (From Pope, A.E. *Pope's manual of nursing procedure.* New York: G.P. Putnam's Sons, 1919.)**

of the demonstrations included aspects of medication administration such as subcutaneous injections.

As a rule, subcutaneous injections were the only injections demonstrated in class, and it was highly recommended that the students give each other hypodermic injections "for nurses should know what they feel like." Sterile water instead of a drug was used during student practice (Pope, 1919, p. 462).

Dangers that nurses were alert to in relation to injectable therapy were causing abscesses, breaking the needle in the flesh, and injecting the drug into a vein.

During the postwar years, proctoclysis, enteroclysis, hypodermoclysis, and intravenous infusion were primarily to supply the body with fluid.

The nursing technique of proctoclysis consisted of the slow introduction of fluid into the intestine in amounts that could be readily absorbed but not irritate the bowel. The flow was regulated by height of the reservoir or by the use of an apparatus that regulated the flow so that the solution would enter the rectum drop by drop, which some nurses found easier to regulate (Figure 1-7).

Enteroclysis, injecting fluid into the colon in a steady stream under low pressure, was used to cleanse the bowel of inflammatory products such as mucus, to remove irritating substances, or to destroy microorganisms such as the ameba that caused amebic dysentery.

Hypodermoclysis, injection of fluid into the cellular tissue, was used when protoclysis was not advisable. The nurse gathered the necessary equipment and prepared the patient. She was especially alert to monitoring the patient's pulse so that she would be able to tell if it was improved by the treatment. She cleaned and disinfected her hand and the site for the infusion: in women the loose tissue at the base of the breasts and in men the loose tissue of the flanks just below the axilla or at the base of the scapula. She connected the apparatus, being careful to handle the needles only at their "sockets" and prepared the solution at the correct temperature, being sure that the air was expelled from the tubing. The physician usually injected an anesthetic before inserting the needles, "but the treatment was sometimes given by senior and graduate nurses for, though it is very important to carry out the technique most carefully, to do so does not require knowledge that cannot be gained by frequently seeing the treatment given" (Pope, 1919, 394-395).

Nurses were careful to maintain strict asepsis and to regulate the infusion with the rate of absorption. At the conclusion of the treatment, the nurse removed the needles, placed a sterile sponge over each puncture, and gently massaged the surrounding parts until the fluid ceased to "ooze from the holes." These were then sealed with collodion and when dried, covered with sterile sponges strapped in place with narrow strips of adhesive plaster.

Intravenous infusion, the injection of fluid directly into the vein, was used when an immediate result was required, such as for conditions of shock or hemorrhage. Either adrenaline or pituitrin was added to the solution at this time to help establish blood pressure.

The most common solutions for intravenous infusion according to Pope (1919) included normal saline (0.9% sodium chloride), Lock's solution (sodium chloride 0.9 gm, potassium chloride, 0.042 gm, calcium chloride 0.0024 gm, sodium bicarbonate 0.03 gm, dextrose 0.1 gm, and sufficient distilled water to make 100 ml), Ringer-Lock solution (same as Lock solution minus the dextrose), and Dawson's solution (0.8% sodium chloride and 0.5% of sodium bicarbonate). Drugs such as salvarsan (i.e., arsphenamine) and certain sera were also given intravenously.

For substances to be injected into the vein, it was recognized that they had to be sterile, isotonic with the blood, and free from any substance that affected its "coaguable property." It was also recognized that air or other substances if admitted into a vein could cause "destruction of blood platelets and so initiate the formation of a thrombus, which, under the influence of the treatment will almost surely be followed by embolism."

The nurse was responsible for the preparation of equipment, and usually two nurses were involved to maintain asepsis in the handling of sterile and unsterile materials. The infusion was always given by the physician; however, the nurse was expected to have a knowledge of the nature of the procedure so that she could give efficient assistance. The nurse was also responsible for maintaining the temperature of the solution as well as for the amount infused. She was also to keep track of the patient's radial pulse and to observe for air bubbles that might gain entrance into the tubing. After the procedure, the nurse stayed with the patient 20 to 30 minutes, especially if normal saline solution was used because this caused the patient to have a chill. The cause of the chill was not definitely known at this time. The nurse reassured the patient, however, and kept hot water "bags" in the bed until the chill ceased.

Inhalation

Many drugs continued to be given by inhalation including amylnitrite, which came by now in a "Pearl," a small capsule of thin glass that could be crushed in some gauze. Five drops were placed on a clean gauze and held a short distance from the patient's nose and mouth. It was kept in place until the symptoms were relieved or until the drug had evaporated. The nurse was warned to be alert not to inhale the drug herself because it caused dilation of the arteries and when not required, headache, dizziness, and faintness.

Stramonium and belladonna were sometimes given by inhalation to relieve asthmatic spasms "because they are absorbed by the mucous membranes with which they come in contact and, by depressing the secretory and bronchial motor nerve endings, they lessen the secretion of mucus and the contraction of the bronchial muscles" (Pope, 1919, pp. 416-417). When drugs were given by inhalation, "leaves containing them were burned and the smoke inhaled." The leaves could also be bought in the form of cigarettes and were smoked in the same manner as tobacco. The

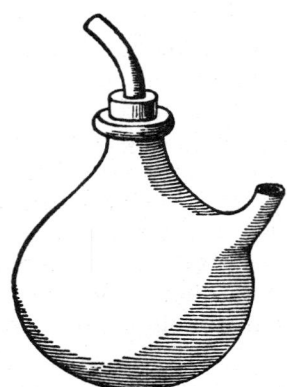

FIGURE 1-8. **Maw's inhaler. (From Pope, A.E. *Pope's manual of nursing procedure*. New York: G.P. Putnam's Sons, 1919.)**

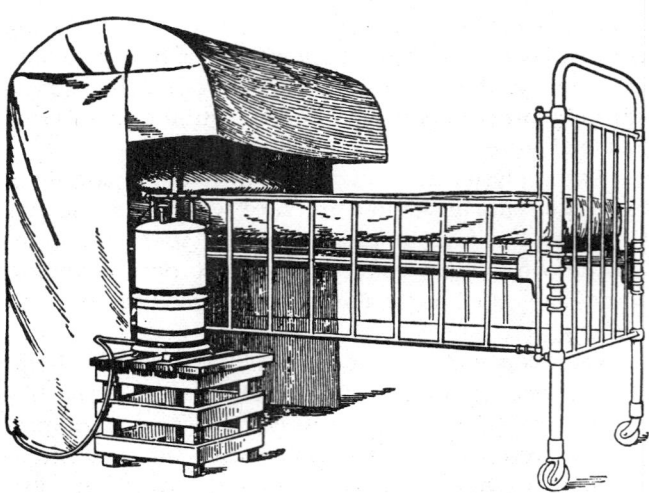

FIGURE 1-9. **Croup tent. (From Pope, A.E. *Pope's manual of nursing procedure*. New York: G.P. Putnam's Sons, 1919.)**

patient was to be "instructed to inhale as much of the smoke as possible" (Pope, 1919, p. 417).

In addition to various drugs, gases were used therapeutically as well. Oxygen inhalations were used to counteract conditions of cyanosis and were administered from a steel container. The gas was bubbled through water to prevent the drying of mucous membranes. A Maw's inhaler (Figure 1-8) was often used for the administration of steam, as were a croup kettle and a croup tent (Figure 1-9).

THE RIGHT PATIENT, THE RIGHT DRUG, AND THE RIGHT TIME IN THE 30s

The nurse in the 30s was not to be ignorant, disinterested, or mechanical in the administration of drugs. Her responsibilities included seeing "that the medication was received by the patient accurately, promptly, and in such a way as to give the best results" (Harmer, 1931, p. 448). In order to do this "intelligently," she needed to consider the nature of the drug, its action, dosage range, the desired effect, and symptoms of overdose.

By this time, it was recommended that the label be read "thrice," as it is today: before the medication was taken from the shelf, and before and after pouring out the drug (Figure 1-10). Liquid medicines that had sediments or were not perfectly clear were to be shaken. To avoid defacing the label while pouring, the bottle was held so that the label was on the upper side and the nurse was not to let her hand come in contact with it. Before replacing the bottle on the shelf, the rim was wiped with a piece of clean gauze. A nurse was not to alter or change a label because this was to be done by the pharmacist only. Medicines that

changed color when mixed together or formed precipitates were not to be given without speaking to the physician, and some foods were not to be given near the time certain medicines were administered. For example, milk and eggs were not to be given near a dose of calomel, the protein of which would combine with the mercury to form an albuminate of mercury. The nurse was referred to the current *Materia Medica* for drugs and foods that should not be given at the same time.

In the early 1930s the nurse was to ensure that the "right patient is given the right medicine at the right time," and each hospital had developed its own system or procedure to ensure this. Two-inch colored tickets were used to identify medications when they were prepared and taken to patients in order to prevent errors in distribution. In some areas index carding systems were used as well. Colors were used for the number of doses per day or to identify the route of administration. If medication tickets or cards were used instead of a medicine list, the patient's name was read before the medicine was given.

By the early 1930s, it was emphasized that nurses be familiar with habit-forming drugs and the necessity for and the means of restricting their use. By 1933, the first antibiotics were introduced, and by 1935 the sulfonamides were available. It should be noted that during this time intramuscular injections were usually given by the physician.

Oxygen therapy was being increasingly used, and nurses were interested in enhancing their practice in relation to nursing care of patients in oxygen tents.

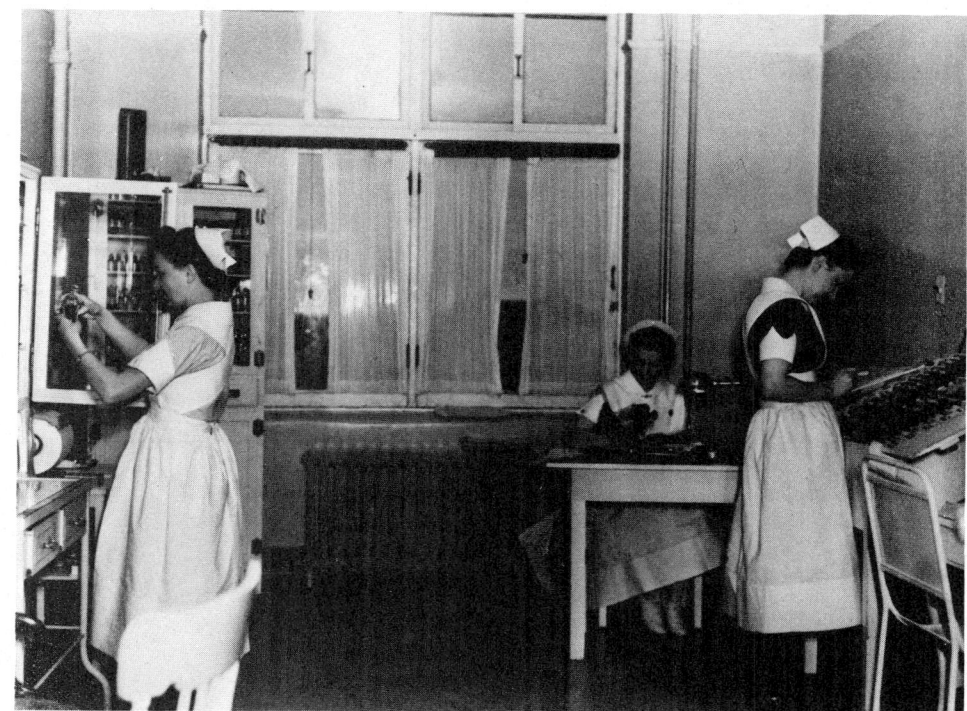

FIGURE 1-10. **Nurse and students preparing medications and recording medication administration in the hospital drug room. (From the University of Alberta Archives, The University of Alberta Hospital, 1939.)**

Some of the current issues involved the use of rubber mattress covers to prevent the escape of oxygen, the danger of giving alcohol rubs to patients where high oxygen concentrations were being used, and how to provide necessary nursing care while maintaining oxygen concentration in the tent. An interesting study was completed by Hawthorne, Henderson, Montag, and Warfield in 1938 to answer some of these questions and to guide nursing practice. They found that by manipulating the tent so that care of the face was given initially, the canopy could then be moved to cover only the head and the remainder of nursing care could be satisfactorily provided. In their summary they recommended that "nurses become sufficiently familiar with methods of testing the tent oxygen concentration to enable them to regulate the oxygen flow effectively."

NURSING IN THE 40s

By 1940 the "wonder drugs" significantly changed health care. People no longer had to be nursed through long and often fatal infections such as pneumonia. Hospitals continued to grow in sophistication and complexity, requiring highly skilled nurses to monitor and closely observe patients as procedures

traditionally done in the doctors office were now performed more safely in the hospital.

In the late 1930s and early 1940s, "physician's sheets" were kept in large notebooks at the nurses station and used routinely to prevent mistakes in receiving and carrying out medication orders as well as to provide more efficient nursing service and a permanent record of therapy.

All orders were written by the attending physician or intern on the order sheet. Nurses were not permitted to carry out verbal orders, and telephone orders were taken only by interns or the head nurse, who was responsible for transcribing them on the order sheet. The physician's name was signed and initialed by the nurse. In addition, all prescription orders were marked in red ink and initialed when sent to the pharmacy.

By this time, all narcotics and other drugs listed under the Harrison Narcotic Act were kept in locked drawers and recorded on specific sheets.

Nurses in the 40s used medication cards (Figure 1-11) more at this time when administering medications and were responsible for selecting appropriate vehicles for giving them. Cards were kept in index card boxes to ensure accuracy of medication administra-

Mrs. J. Jones R 437
Rx 26548
Elixir Sodium Bromide
dr. i = gr. x
Dr. i (gr. x) T.I.D.a.c.

Mr. L. Brown R 329
Rx 35679
Tr. Digitalis
7 cc. = 1 cat unit
1 cat unit (7 cc.) O.D.

Mrs. L. Smith R 462
Rx 27654
capsule
Codeine Sulf. gr. ss
Aspirin gr. x
1 capsule Q 4 H

Mr. G. James R 318
Rx 25695
Aminophyllin
1 cc. = gr. ii3/4
1 cc. (gr. ii3/4) I.V. B.I.D.

FIGURE 1-11. **Medication cards. (From Day, M.A.C. *Basic sciences in nursing arts* (2nd ed.). St. Louis: The C.V. Mosby Co., 1947.)**

tion and to prevent loss (Figure 1-12). A drug was never to be given without careful consideration of the dosage, the purpose for which it was given, the condition of the patient, and the expected results. As in the early 1930s, the nurse was to ensure that the "right patient was given the right medicine at the right time."

Students in the 40s gave medications, but not before the dosage was worked out on paper and checked by the supervisor with the student "always remembering" that medications could never be given without a written order from the physician. In addition, she was never to give a medication that had been prepared by another, and when in the least doubt about a medication dosage, "a drug should under no circumstances be administered" (Day, 1947, p. 419). The nurse was to address the patient by name when administering the medication and was to stay with him until the medication had been taken.

Medications were carefully arranged on trays (Figure 1-13) and often delivered to patients arranged on medication carts (Figure 1-14). After the medication was given, the nurse was responsible for recording the name of the drug, time administered, the amount, the route or method of administration, and the results obtained, as well as any unusual reactions.

More attention was directed at the nurse's professional role and to the psychologic aspects of drug therapy. For example, the nurse, especially when giving suppositories, was to be careful to explain the procedure adequately to the patient and to screen and drape the patient. It was preferable for the nurse to insert the suppository rather than to permit the patient to do so. The nurse's attitude was to be "impersonal and strictly professional, in order to spare the patient all possible embarrassment and to eliminate undesirable psychologic and physiologic reactions" (Day, 1947, p. 426).

Hypodermic medications were also given. Whether a specific drug was to be given by subcutaneous or intramuscular injection was designated by the physician. Successive injections were not to be given in the same site and by now, drugs such as morphine and codeine came in solution in glass ampules. Medications also came in multidose vials with rubber caps that required the insertion of air to withdraw the medication.

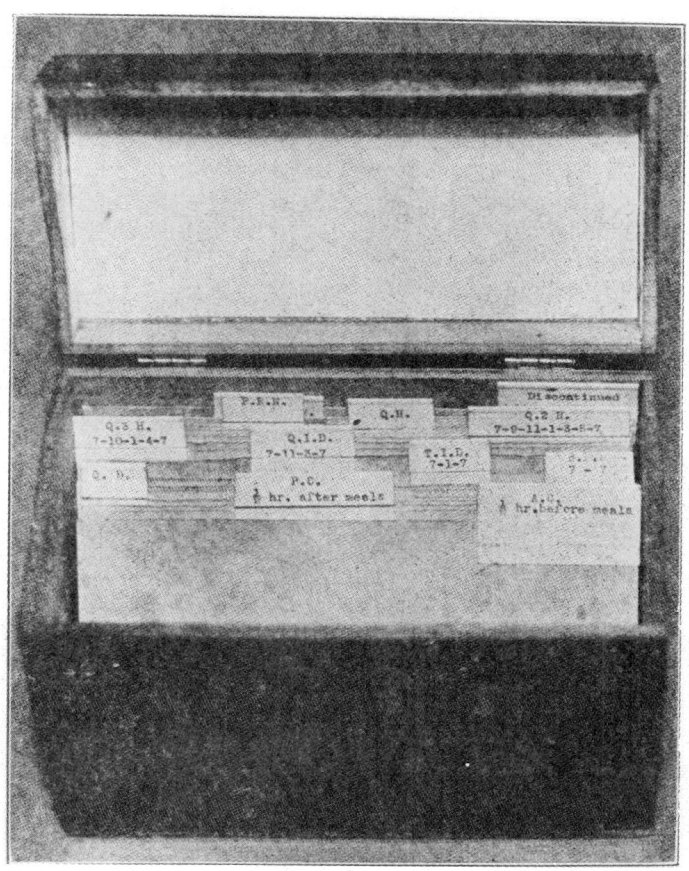

FIGURE 1-12. **Index file system for medication administration cards. Cards are removed from their respective pockets when medicines are to be administered. (From Day, M.A.C.** *Basic sciences in nursing arts* **(2nd ed.). St. Louis: The C.V. Mosby Co., 1947.)**

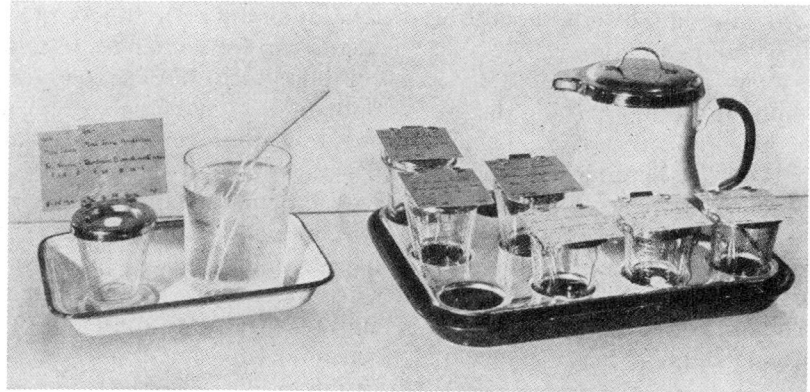

FIGURE 1-13. **Medications and trays:** *(left)* **tray to be used when medications are given individually;** *(right)* **a convenient setup for group technique in giving medicines. (From Day, M.A.C.** *Basic sciences in nursing arts* **(2nd ed.). St. Louis: The C.V. Mosby Co., 1947.)**

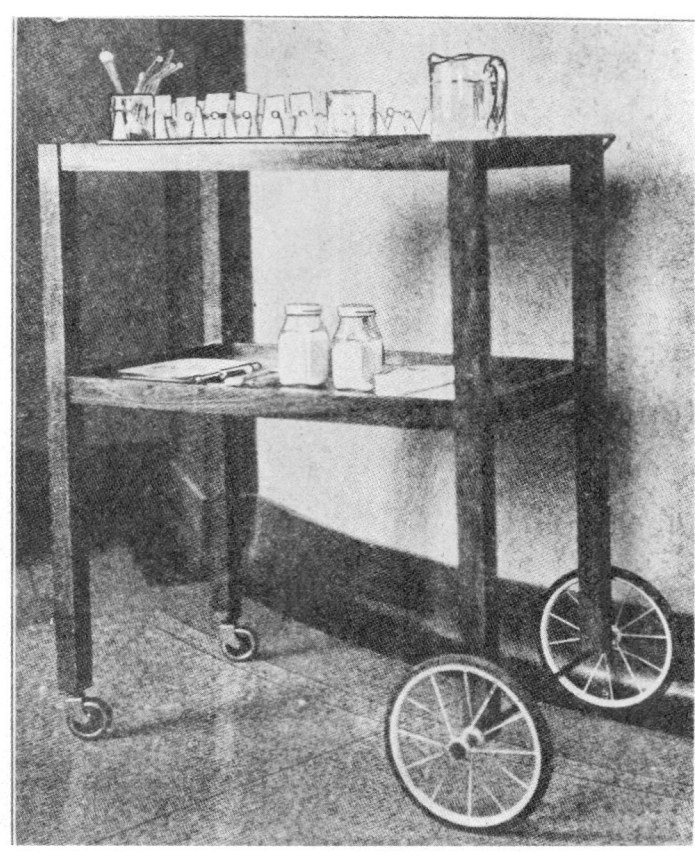

FIGURE 1-14. **Medication cart and tray for administering numerous medications. (From Day, M.A.C. *Basic sciences in nursing arts* (2nd ed.). St. Louis: The C.V. Mosby Co., 1947.)**

When intramuscular injections were given, it was now recommended that the deltoid muscle of the arm be "gently yet firmly grasped with one hand, and the tissues tightly squeezed and lifted simultaneously, pulling the muscle away from the bone." "The skin under tension" would allow more ready insertion of the needle, decrease pain, and minimize the danger of striking the bone especially in thin patients. The needle was inserted at a 45-degree angle for subcutaneous injections and at right angles for intramuscular injections. The plunger was pulled back slightly to ascertain whether the needle was in a blood vessel. After the injection was given, the site was massaged until the fluid was "completely absorbed and no lumps [could] be felt beneath the skin" (Day, 1947, p. 424).

By the 1940s the intravenous route (Figure 1-15) was recognized as the most practical route of administering parenteral therapy, although hypodermoclysis was still common and used, especially with infants. There

was less emphasis on the maintainance of a specific temperature of the solutions because it was recognized that reactions more often resulted from too rapid administration of fluid and improper care of equipment than from changes in temperature. In addition, solutions were now prepared by reputable chemical houses and were labeled "pyrogen free."

Intravenous infusions were started by the intern or the nurse under strict aseptic technique. The patient was to be made comfortable and was never to be left for more than a few minutes at a time so that the nurse could observe for any reaction. After the infusion, the nurse recorded the time the infusion was started, by whom, the amount and type of solution, the time completed, and any immediate or delayed reactions.

A common continuous intravenous infusion used at this time for the treatment of syphilis was Mapharsen (oxophenarsine) therapy, which was administered over 5 days. Patients were admitted to the hos-

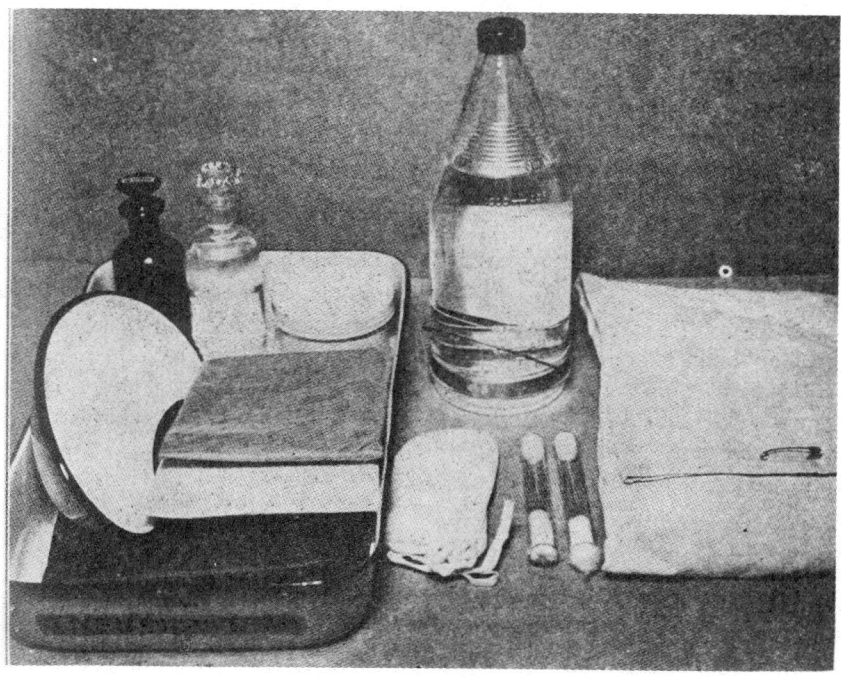

FIGURE 1-15. **Intravenous fluid apparatus. (From Day, M.A.C. *Basic sciences in nursing arts* (2nd ed.). St. Louis: The C.V. Mosby Co., 1947.)**

pital for the treatment and put into an isolation room to protect other patients and staff. Nursing responsibilities included explaining the procedure to the patient, providing understanding and support, and preparing the Mapharsen. This consisted of mixing 60 mg of Mapharsen in 5 ml of distilled water, drawing the solution into a syringe and injecting it into the flask of an intravenous set containing 600 ml of 5% glucose in distilled water. The rate of the drip was regulated so that 200 ml of solution would infuse per hour. This was repeated 4 times during each of the 5 days. When the patient had received the required daily dose, the needle was removed from the vein, and alternate arms were used daily. The nurse was to observe for signs of toxic reactions, including elevated temperature, nausea and vomiting, and early signs of hemorrhagic encephalitis, which included dizziness or personality change.

In the early 40s, State Board Examinations reflected the advances in nursing education at the time. Knowledge of the action of drugs, the active principles of drugs, types of pharmaceutical preparations, apothecary, household, wine, and metric measurement equivalents, and drug classifications was required. For example, questions related to pharmacology and therapeutics included the following questions and the corresponding answers:

What must a nurse know about drugs in order to administer them safely?

She must know the range of dosage of all preparations in common use and know how to prepare prescribed doses of drugs from pure drugs, tablets, and stock solutions.

She must know what action to expect of each drug in order that she may detect idiosyncrasies and recognize early toxic symptoms.

She must know the physical and chemical characteristics of drugs and what standards determine purity and quality in pharmaceutical preparations.

She must know the therapeutic uses of drugs to be able to administer them intelligently (Foote, 1942, pp. 301-302).

If you find a pulse of a patient receiving digitalis to be 60, what should you do?

This is the most important symptom of digitalis poisoning and should always be reported to the physician. The treatment usually is to discontinue the drug and keep the patient quiet in bed (Foote, 1942, p. 322).

Effects of World War II

World War II broke out in 1939, and as the war went on, more and more nurses were required to care for the wounded. Blood, plasma, and penicillin were available now, and these helped save many lives. Nurses were involved in working at blood banks and overseas.

Amphetamines were used by armed forces of the United States, Great Britain, Germany, and Japan to help counteract fatigue, increase endurance and vigilance, and heighten mood. Aircraft crews on long bombing runs had them available to combat sleep and fatigue. After the war, amphetamine derivatives became widely available in inhalers. This liquid form of amphetamines was soon abused, especially for intravenous injection. In addition, amphetamines, because of their central nervous system stimulant effects (increased activity level and appetite suppression), were commonly prescribed for weight control and for depression. With its widespread use through availability in inhalers and medical uses, amphetamines became a source of common abuse in the 1950s. Later, amphetamines became heavily used by truck drivers and students. During this period nurses and other health care professionals became involved in drug abuse prevention and treatment programs.

Interest in mental health nursing increased by the end of the second World War. Advances in such treatments as insulin shock and electroconvulsive therapy required careful nursing attention, and the demands for specially trained nurses increased. The postwar period also saw the development of antipsychotic tranquilizers, which decreased the need for physical restraint, and nurses became more oriented toward treatment as custodial care was less emphasized.

Civilian hospitals were depleted during the war, and this continued as nurses who returned either left nursing for marriage or preferred the more independent role of the public health nurse. Nursing aide, orderly, and vocational or practical nurse programs were started as a result during the postwar years. This led to the evolution of the nursing team concept, which resulted in the Registered Nurse relinquishing some of her direct patient care responsibilities to others as she concentrated more and more on the giving of treatments, on the administration of medications, and on ward management.

RESEARCH AND TEACHING IN THE 50s

During much of the modern period, nurses have been dependent on others for research. Since World War II, there has been an increased growth in nursing research in relation to the functions, status, problems, viewpoints, and education of nurses, as illustrated since 1952 in the journal *Nursing Research* and other nursing journals. Interestingly, there were also studies completed on aspects of the nurse's role in preparing medications for administration such as, "Are organisms introduced into vials containing medication when air is injected?" (Baer, et al., 1953).

By the mid 50s, patient centered models of nursing practice as well as the health team concept were emphasized. Types of orders varied in relation to drug administration including standing orders, single orders, and stat orders. A written physician's order was required before a nurse could administer medications or gases as "legal implications for administering them without a written order were serious." The written order greatly decreased errors caused by misunderstandings. Of course, the nurse was responsible for questioning any order that in her judgment was incorrect or unsafe.

The nurse was to have a sound knowledge of the "therapeutic agents" that she administered. This was important because of the number of drugs that were then becoming available on the market. Many were ordered that did not have sufficient information available to the nurse, who was also often confronted with similarity of drug names. It was recommended that new drugs not be given without first checking the spelling and information about the drug action and possible untoward effects. Any errors in drug administration were to be reported immediately to the physician, and an "accident" or "medication error report" was to be filled out in detail so that periodic reviews could be completed in order to identify weaknesses in procedures and increase safety.

Polyethylene tubing and hypospray, the administration of a drug through the skin without a needle, became available. Medications given directly into the vein were given by physicians, and nurses were to follow the policies in the area they worked. By now, patient identification bands were widely used in order to increase safety in medication administration (Figure 1-16).

The use of nursing care plans was increasingly being encouraged and used in practice, and because it was felt that the nurse was "afforded an excellent teaching opportunity when administering therapeutic agents," the nurse by the mid 50s was including a more specific teaching role in her care plan as it related to drug therapy. In addition, it was generally thought:

While it is the physician who is usually responsible for telling the patient what he is receiving, the practice of refusing to tell patients the nature of what they are receiving is fast disappearing. In fact, now it is considered far more reassuring to a patient to be well informed about his therapy, and often it is the nurse who is responsible for the teaching (Fuerst & Wolff, 1959, p. 437).

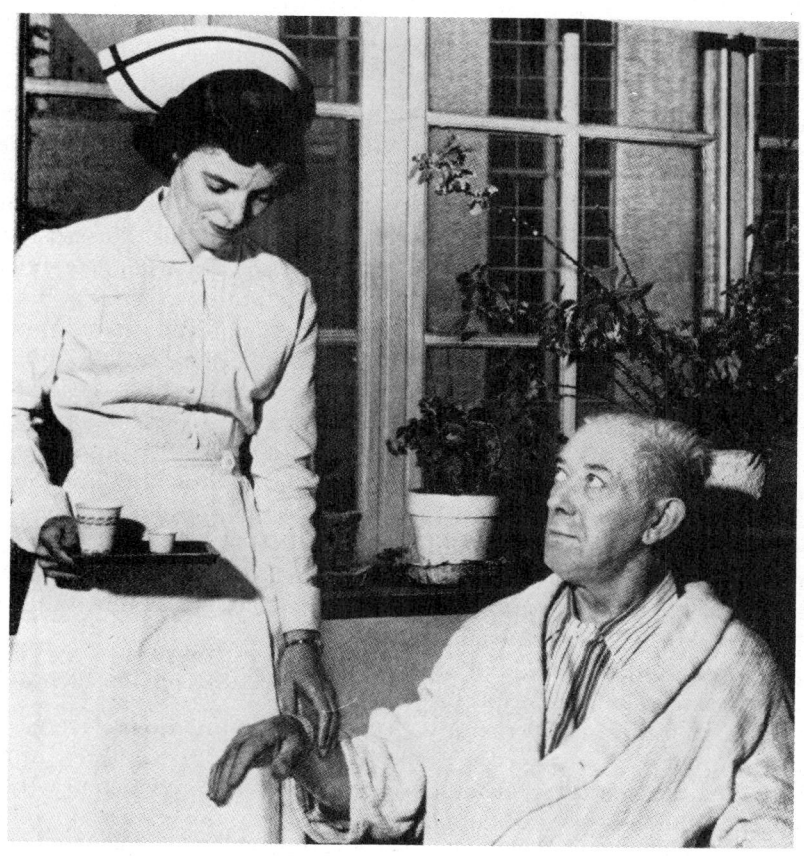

FIGURE 1-16. **Nurse checking the patient identification band to ensure giving the medication to the "right" patient. (From Fuerst, V.V., and Wolff, L.V. *Fundamentals of nursing* (2nd ed.). Philadelphia: J.B. Lippincott Co., 1959.)**

There was no rule as to what patients should be told or taught. This was usually up to the physician. However, it was recognized that the nurse played "an important part in assisting the patient to understand the dangers of practicing self-medication and the careless use of habit-forming drugs." The nurse's teaching responsibilities included teaching the patient how to prepare and take drugs, explaining results, such as that belladonna may cause a dry mouth, bismuth may cause dark stools, or oxytetracycline may cause diarrhea. Patients were warned to watch closely for "toxic signs" such as "a reduction in urine with sulfa drugs or headache and skin eruptions from bromides." Instruction also included demonstrations and supervised practice in the measurement and administration of drugs. "It is as much the nurse's function to teach the patient how to take medications as to give them to him" (Harmer & Henderson, 1955, pp. 695-696).

By the late 1950s Associate Degree programs had developed, and there was more emphasis on nursing practice and research at the master's level. The great advances in knowledge required that nurses be further prepared in all areas of nursing including drug therapy.

EXPANDING ROLES AND ADVANCES IN DRUG DELIVERY SYSTEMS IN THE 60s AND 70s

The 60s and 70s have seen the evolution of the centralized unit dose medication systems, which influenced nursing roles in relation to drug therapy in both the United States and Canada.

The main reason for the development of these systems was to prevent medication errors that statistics had indicated were becoming too frequent in all aspects of health care, to decrease cost of health care by decreasing drug waste, and to increase nursing efficiency and to allow the nurse to focus more attention on the nursing functions of medication administration and assessment of patient responses to drug therapy (Stewart, et al., 1976).

Medications were individually prepared and packaged by the pharmacist for each ward or station, and nurses compared the dose with the order and administered it according to the correct patient, time, and route.

By the mid 70s, drug companies began individual packaging and uniform labeling for unit dose systems, and pharmacists began preparing intravenous additive orders that were delivered to the ward refrigerators. Increasing numbers of nursing homes and acute care hospitals began using these systems.

By the late 60s and early 70s, Master's preparation in nursing was gaining in recognition, and clinical nurse specialists were evolving with expanded knowledge in specific areas such as maternal and child health nursing, perinatal nursing, mental health nursing, public health nursing, and acute care, and geriatric nursing. This expanded specialized knowledge included drug therapy as well, and hundreds of articles describing advanced responsibilities in preparation, administration, and monitoring of drug therapy appeared in the nursing journals.

In the United States, nurse practitioners, registered nurses with additional preparation and skills obtained in Nursing Board specified programs, began to define a more independent nursing practice role during the 1970s. Maternity nurse practitioners, pediatric nurse practitioners, psychiatric nurse practitioners, and other nurse practitioners demonstrated their ability to function in expanded roles, which necessitated greater understanding of drug therapy and clinical therapeutics. To facilitate nursing's expanding role, over 30 states revised their nurse practice acts during the 70s. Prescription became legal for nurses at this time in over half of these states. However, most acts were revised or rewritten to allow only indirect prescribing by nurses. In these states, nurses had to prescribe in accordance with written protocols or through a physician or pharmacy.

The 70s also saw a growing trend toward self-care and health promotion. Conceptual frameworks for nursing evolved to guide practice in this area. Nurses began to more formally see their role as promoting wellness. This concept involved all areas of nursing practice including drug therapy. Individuals and families were encouraged to become more actively involved in decisions about drug therapy. In order that the client might make a more informed decision about care, the nurse increasingly became involved in teaching aspects of individual drug therapy, self-medication, and monitoring.

By the late 70s there was increased emphasis on nurses' accountability for practice and their role in decision making and nursing diagnosis. Attention was increasingly given to patient assessment, including data collection from nursing histories and physical examination or health assessment. The importance of diagnosis by nurses of drug-related problems was recognized, but it was felt that both in nursing education and practice, drug-related problems were given little attention. LeSage (1979) identified one reason for this: the conceptual process for making such diagnosis was not well defined in relation to drug therapy. Emphasizing that diagnosis and intervention related to the outcome of drug therapy were the domain of both nurses and physicians, she proposed a conceptual process for diagnosing drug incompatibility. The conceptual framework did not define the domain of nursing practice, but could be used in its development.

INCREASED ACCOUNTABILITY IN THE 80s

Although unit dose systems in the 80s are becoming more and more common, nurses have shared their concerns and anxieties in working with the new systems. Many nurses are uncomfortable not using the traditional medication cards to identify their medications. Other nurses find the unit dose carts that carry a 24-hour or more supply of regularly dispensed medications with a backup dose of each drug for each patient as well as controlled prn and stock drugs heavy and cumbersome in ward areas and noisy at night. The design of carts has also received complaint; so has the packaging of the drugs—they are often difficult to open. However, this system has many advantages, including safe drug administration for patients because both nurses and pharmacists are involved in interpretation of orders. Six-day patient profiles are kept on each patient, assessing their concurrent drug usage, adverse drug reactions, allergies, and antibiotic treatment problems. With this system medications are not misplaced in front of medication cards, medicines are no longer poured into unidentified medication cups, and medication errors are usually caught within 24 hours and not days.

The use of these systems has also opened some additional areas of legal concern. For example, a case has occurred in which a nurse left her cart unlocked and unattended and a confused patient unfortunately took medications and died. Nurses also borrow drugs from other patients when missing drugs occur, and this practice is illegal; so is changing labels when doses and frequency of drug administration is altered by the prescriber.

In order to look at the role of the nurse in relation to such drug delivery systems, nurses must take an active role in planning for and evaluating these systems in relation to their practice. An interesting pilot study conducted by Long (1982) examined the interaction between "frequency of medication errors reported by nursing units, administering medications through various combinations of nursing care (functional, team, total, primary) and medication delivery systems (unit dose, complete floor stock, individual prescription)." The study found that the effects of medication delivery systems on monitoring medication errors were influenced by the nursing care system used.

Nurses must not lose sight of changing aspects of their role in relation to drug preparation, administration, and monitoring. As these systems come into practice, the nurse's role will change, and nurses will be required to be more knowledgeable and skilled in aspects of drug preparation, administration, and monitoring as well as in patient preparation for drug therapy and teaching.

Research, such as that completed by Markowitz (1981) and her research group, has reported that nurses are the least knowledgeable when compared with physicians and pharmacists in relation to knowledge of hazards of medication. This lack of pharmacology knowledge represents a major risk to public health and safety. Nurses because of their direct contact with patients are in a prime position to effectively contribute to better drug therapy by recognizing and attending to adverse drug reactions. Since the 70s adverse drug reactions—"any unintended, undesirable reaction experienced by a patient as a consequence of the administration of medication"—have become the most common form of iatrogenic disease in North America. Several hundred thousand adverse reactions occur each year, resulting in extended hospital stays, unnecessary pain, disability, increased cost and demand for health resources, and death.

Another question for the 80s is the manner in which basic pharmacology should be taught to nurses. Over the last few decades, pharmacology has not usually been taught as a separate course, but has been integrated into nursing curricula. To date no standards have been set regarding required drug knowledge. Markowitz (1981) suggests that drug knowledge is less than adequate and that drug knowledge be monitored through examination and quality assurance programs as well as through peer review. In addition, it is felt that further research should be completed and that rigorous monitoring systems be developed to guide nursing practice in relation to drug therapy.

Nurse practitioners began defining their roles and moving toward independent nurse practice in many states and some provinces in the 70s and 80s. In defining their roles they are moving toward the prescription of drugs. For example, in 1981 nurse practitioners were prescribing medications under special pilot projects in Utah.* Nurse practitioners "working in collaboration with any participating physician" could administer local anesthetics and prescribe drugs or medicines according to protocols jointly developed by the nurse practitioner and the physician. The Utah law does not specify or limit the kind of drugs to be prescribed. However, in other states, such as Oregon, nurse practitioners must have been practicing for 1 year and have obtained credit in 30 hours of pharmacology obtained through continuing education before they can prescribe medications. In addition, Oregon nurses can only prescribe drugs that are listed in an official formulary.

Nurse practitioners state that they are actually performing the same role that they had been in these states, but are now able to base their practice on a firmer legal base. They do not have to resort to presigned prescription pads, calling in procedures, or appending the physician's name to their own signatures—practices that were sometimes illegal. Many states and provinces must still address this issue and with the revision of Nurse Practice Acts more nurses will be legally sanctioned to perform in this expanded role.

By the end of this century, we will see significant changes in laws as these relate to nursing practice and the prescription, preparation, administration and monitoring of drug therapy.

The problem of diagnosis and prescribing in nursing is not primarily a legal one, but a professional one. Whenever a nurse diagnoses, or prescribes, she must be sure that she is competent to do so. Competency is not created by law. The law, as always, follows rather than precedes; it merely recognizes and formalizes the authority which competence bestows. (Clark, 1978, p. 488)

We will also see the further development and use of conceptual models and nursing theories. Conceptual models are currently being used to guide nursing curricula, research, and practice. Harper (1984) con-

---

*Many different and worthwhile pilot prescribing projects have been carried out by nurses in different parts of North America.

ducted a research study applying Dorothea Orem's theoretical constructs to self-medication behaviors in the elderly. Her findings will be added to those of other nurse researchers of the 1980s such as Nichols, Barstow, and Cooper (1983), McGuire (1984), and Vanbree, Hollerbach, and Brooks (1984).

Nichols' group studied the incidence of phlebitis and frequency of changing intravenous tubing and percutaneous site. McGuire studied the measurement of clinical pain, the results of which can be used by nurses to evaluate pharmacologic and other interventions. Vanbree, Hollerbach, and Brooks investigated the effect of three techniques for administering subcutaneous low-dose heparin.

Studies such as these will help further delineate the role of the professional nurse in drug therapy, particularly how it relates to the preparation and administration of medications and the monitoring of their effects. These studies and others will also further enable nurses to assist patients with decisions regarding drug therapy, self-medication, minimizing adverse side effects, and effects on self-care practices or activities of daily living.

SUMMARY

Since nursing's earliest recorded history aspects of pharmacology have been an integral part of the domain of nursing. Although the emphasis placed on the various aspects of preparation, administration, and monitoring of drug therapy has waxed and waned through nursing history, nurses have always been responsible for elements of these aspects of drug therapy in their nursing practice. Even prescription of medication, which many nurses and other health professionals think of as "new" or not a "true" nursing function, was widely and competently practiced by early American and Canadian nurses.

Today, more so than at any other time in history, nurses throughout the world are involved in every aspect of drug therapy. Pharmacology as a discipline or science is an integral component of the domain of nursing. Nurses today thus have an increased responsibility to fully integrate the pharmacologic aspects of nursing into their own concept of nursing practice.

BIBLIOGRAPHY

Baer, M.H., et al. Are organisms introduced into vials containing medication when air is injected? *Nursing Research*, 1953, *2*, 23-32.

Baker, N. Prescriptive authority for nurse practitioners. *Geriatric Nursing*, 1981, *2*, 420-421.

Clark, J. Should nurses diagnose and prescribe? *Journal of Advanced Nursing*, 1978, *3*, 485-488.

Day, M.A.C. *Basic sciences in nursing arts* (2nd ed.). St. Louis: The C.V. Mosby Co., 1947.

Dickens, C. *The life and adventures of Martin Chuzzlewit.* Paris: Baudry's European Library, 1844.

Dock, L.L. *Materia medica for nurses* (5th ed.). New York: G.P. Putnam's Sons, 1915.

Dock, L.L., & Stewart, I.M. *A short history of nursing: From the earliest times to the present day* (3rd ed.). New York: G.P. Putnam's Sons, 1931.

Dolan, J.A. *Nursing in society: A historical perspective* (14th ed.). Philadelphia: W.B. Saunders Co., 1978.

Faddis, M.O. Eliminating errors in medication. *American Journal of Nursing*, 1939, *3*, 1217-1223.

Foote, J.A. *State board questions and answers for nurses.* Philadelphia: J.B. Lippincott Co., 1942.

Fuerst, E.V., & Wolff, L.V. *Fundamentals of nursing: The humanities and the sciences in nursing* (2nd ed.). Philadelphia: J.B. Lippincott Co., 1959.

Gibbon, J.M., & Mathewson, M.S. *Three centuries of Canadian nursing.* Toronto: The Macmillan Co. of Canada Ltd., 1947.

Hampton, I.A. *Nursing of the sick, 1893.* New York: McGraw-Hill Book Co., 1949.

Hansen, H.F. *A review of nursing with outlines of subjects, questions, and answers* (5th ed.). Philadelphia: W.B. Saunders Co., 1937.

Harmer, B. *Text-book of the principles and practice of nursing* (2nd ed.). New York: The Macmillan Co., 1931.

Harmer, B. & Henderson, V. *Text-book of the principles and practice of nursing* (4th ed.). New York: The Macmillan Co., 1939.

Harmer, B., & Henderson, V. *Textbook of the principles and practice of nursing* (5th ed.). New York: The Macmillan Co., 1955.

Harper, D.C. Application of Orem's theoretical constructs to self-care medication behaviors in the elderly. *Advances in Nursing Science*, 1984, *6* (3), 29-46.

Hawthorne, M.J., et al. Oxygen therapy. *American Journal of Nursing*, 1938, *38*, 1203-1216.

Krantz, J. *Historical medical classics involving new drugs.* Baltimore: Williams & Wilkins, 1974.

Leitch, C.J., & Mitchell, E.S. A state by state report: the legal accomodation of nurses' practicing expanded roles. *Nurse Practitioner*, 1977, *2*, 19-22, 30.

LeSage, J., Beck, C., & Johnson, M. Nursing diagnosis of drug incompatibility: a conceptual process. *Advances in Nursing Science*, 1979, *1*, 63-67.

Long, G. The effect of medication distribution systems on medication errors. *Nursing Research*, 1982, *31*, 182-184.

Markowitz, J.S., et al. Nurses, physicians, and pharmacists: their knowledge of hazards of medications. *Nursing Research*, 1981, *30*, 366-370.

Mayers, M.H. Legal guidelines. *Geriatric Nursing*, 1981, *2*, 417-421.

McGuire, D.B. The measurement of clinical pain. *Nursing Research*, 1984, *33* (3), 152-156.

Milby, J.B. *Addictive behavior and its treatment.* New York: Springer Publishing Co., 1981.

Nichols, E.G., Barstow, R.E., & Cooper, D. Relationship between incidence of phlebitis and frequency of changing IV tubing and percutaneous site. *Nursing Research, 1983, 32* (4), 247-252.

Nightingale, F. *Notes on nursing: what it is, and what it is not.* New York: D. Appleton & Co., 1860.

Nutting, M.A., & Dock, L.L. *A history of nursing* (Vols. 1 and 2). New York: G.P. Putnam's Sons, 1907.

Pagliaro, A.M. *History of nursing* (five parts). Edmonton: CFRN Television, 1982.

Palmer, D.A. Unit dose. *American Journal of Nursing, 1980 80,* 2062-2063.

Pope, A.E. *Pope's manual of nursing procedure.* New York: G.P. Putnam's Sons, 1919.

Robb, I.H. *Nursing: Its principles and practice for hospital and private use.* Toronto: The J.F. Hartz Co., Ltd., 1910.

Sarsfield, M. The five day treatment for syphilis. *American Journal of Nursing,* 1941, *41,* 1045-1046.

Seymer, L.R. *A general history of nursing.* New York: Macmillan Publishing Co., 1933.

Smith, L.L. Fun and frolic with unit dose. *RN,* 1981, *44,* 99-100.

Spalding, E.K., & Notter, L.E. *Professional nursing: foundations, perspectives, and relationships.* Philadelphia: J.B. Lippincott Co., 1962.

Stewart, I.M., & Austin, A.L. *A history of nursing from ancient to modern times: A world view* (5th ed.). New York: G.P. Putnam's Sons, 1962.

Stewart, D.Y., Kelly, J., & Dinel, B.A. Unit dose medication: a nursing perspective. *American Journal of Nursing,* 1976, *76,* 1308-1310.

Talbot, C.H. *Medicine in medieval England.* London: Oldbourne Book Co., Ltd., 1967.

Trandel-Korenchuk, D.M., & Trandel-Korenchuk, K.M. Current legal issues facing nursing practice. *Nursing Administration Quarterly,* 1980, *5,* 37-55.

Vanbree, N.S., Hollerbach, A.D., & Brooks, G.P. Clinical evaluation of three techniques for administering low-dose heparin. *Nursing Research,* 1984, *33* (1), 15-19.

Preparation, Administration, and Monitoring of Medications

Ann M. Pagliaro

The pharmacologic aspects of nursing involve, in some cases, the selection and prescription of drug therapy. However, today in most areas of practice, the role of the registered nurse primarily involves the preparation, administration, and monitoring of drug therapy as ordered by a prescriber. In addition, nurses have an extremely important role in relation to patient assessment and the planning, implementation, and evaluation of nursing care as they relate to drug therapy. The role of the nurse is not dependent, but interdependent, one that requires specialized knowledge and skills.

Nurses today are legally accountable for the safe preparation, administration, and monitoring of medications. They are responsible for recognizing safe dosage ranges, computing and measuring dosages correctly, administering medication dosage forms skillfully, and monitoring the effects of drug therapy (including individual patient response) accurately. These are essential in providing optimum drug therapy.

The nurse requires a sound knowledge of dosage forms, drug incompatibilities or interactions (i.e., drug-drug, drug-food, drug-patient), and the care and storage of the medications with which she is entrusted. She also requires a sound knowledge of the therapeutic ranges of drugs, which can vary in relation to an individual's age, weight, body surface area, hepatic or renal function, and in relation to various other factors (see Section II of this text for details). If medication orders are not within recommended ranges (according to the nurse's knowledge or resources) in relation to these individual patient factors, she is required by law to consult with the prescriber *before* the medication is given. In this regard, nurses share full responsibility for any drug they administer. Nurses legally, professionally, and morally are responsible for all of their nursing actions, which must be based on current nursing knowledge and expert skill.

Nurses are also responsible for the provision of individualized drug therapy. Patients and their families should be involved as much as possible in decisions about their therapy. They require knowledge about the names of their medications, their dosages, desired actions, precautions, and how the drug may effect their everyday activities.

The patient's right to know what medication he is receiving and why is a continuing problem perplexing nursing practice that still needs to be formally addressed. Murchison et al. (1982) describe the importance of the professional and legal responsibility of the nurse to inform patients of the benefits and risks associated with medications, especially in relation to manufacturer's warnings and side effects.

In fact, it is the duty of professional nurses to incorporate into their patient teaching any known risks associated with the drug being administered, in a manner consistent with the medical requirements of disclosure . . . nurses must consider what their role should be in relation to reinforcing or initiating disclosure relative to drug therapy (Murchison, et al., 1982, pp. 91-92).

Patients may also require teaching about the preparation, administration, and monitoring of medications that they require. Some hospital policies allow certain medications, such as antacids, birth control pills, and nitroglycerin, to be kept at the bedside by the patient. The nurse must be sure that the patient understands the use of these medications and that the medication and any cups or other necessary equipment are available for the patient's use. Other hospitals are exploring self-medication programs in which adult patients are responsible for specific self-medication regimens, including deciding when medications such as analgesics are required and actually charting and recording their medication use. These regimens may follow those that the patient was on at home, or else they may be implemented or revised in the hospital so that the patient can continue them after discharge. In addition, the nurse should be alert to recording the self-medication abilities of the patient and to monitoring the effects of drug and related therapy.

The nurse is increasingly becoming responsible for the provision of expert drug therapy as related to her nursing care. Thus, nurses today must understand factors that affect individual response to drug therapy, including mechanisms of drug action, drug availability and distribution, drug metabolism and elimination, pharmacokinetic factors, age-dependent drug selection and response, psychologic factors in drug response, genetic factors affecting drug response, drug interactions, drug toxicity, and drug abuse and addiction. These factors are individually addressed and discussed in the chapters of the following section of this text.

NURSING ASSESSMENT AND DIAGNOSIS

Nursing assessment includes the gathering of relevant data. In relation to drug therapy, this includes individual patient factors: biographic data, the patient's knowledge and skills in self-medication, information about the patient's health and disease state, and specific drug-related information. The nurse obtains the necessary data by using a nursing history, finding other relevant data sources, and employing physical assessment, from which patient problems can be diagnosed and the delivery of nursing care planned.

Careful drug histories should be completed on all patients as an important part of the nursing history. Drug histories should be completed whenever the patient enters the health care system. In acute or general hospitals it is usually completed on admission or within 24 to 48 hours. The drug history should record both prescription and nonprescription medications, including illicit and social drugs, taken by the patient as well as any medication allergies the patient may have.

When a history of allergic response to medications is obtained, the actual response to the drug should be explored, because many reports of drug allergies are not accurate. In addition, the complete history should include not only the medications taken, but also how they are taken. Self-medication can be assessed, and nursing assistance in relation to increasing the patient's knowledge and ability to self-medicate is included in the plan of care as indicated. Home remedies should also be assessed in relation to prescribed therapy.

PLANNING

Planning nursing care in relation to drug therapy should involve the patient and family as indicated. Individualized objectives should be identified with the patient and family and specific evaluation criteria formulated to measure goal attainment. Planning should include such areas as route selection; timing of doses in relation to therapeutic effects or unavoidable adverse effects of drugs; modifications in daily activities; patient education including the name of the medication, purpose, dosage, adverse side effects, and how these can be prevented or minimized; and the promotion of self-medication, particularly if the patient will be responsible for taking medications on a discharge/outpatient basis. Nursing actions or orders should be clearly specified in relation to helping patients achieve their objectives as related to drug therapy. The roles of the nurse, patient, and family as indicated should be clearly specified. The plan should be kept current and revised as needed. Collaboration with the prescriber in planning may be indicated.

IMPLEMENTATION

The implementation of the care plan includes preparation of the patient and equipment as related to the prescribed drug therapy. The actual role of the nurse or patient in relation to the preparation, administration, and monitoring of drug therapy can be shared. Nursing actions and patient reactions are recorded and communicated to other health care members.

EVALUATION

The evaluation of the care plan is completed in relation to the achievement of objectives. It is systematic and ongoing. If the objectives are not met, the plan is revised. Monitoring is particularly important in the process of evaluation because it is only through monitoring that the nurse can ascertain whether the objectives in relation to drug therapy have been met.

ORAL MEDICATIONS

Oral medications are available in the form of liquids, tablets, and capsules and are taken by mouth and swallowed. The major advantages of oral medications are convenience and economy. There are, however, some disadvantages to this method of drug administration. Nausea and vomiting are problems often associated with oral medications that irritate the gastric mucosa, and some medicines because of their unpleasant taste, are refused or not taken.

Absorption of oral medications is influenced by the dosage form and by the nature of the drug itself (i.e., acidity or alkalinity, lipid solubility, molecular size). Drugs given orally usually require more time for absorption as compared with other methods of administration, and their absorption can be incomplete and unpredictable. For example, absorption can be slowed by the presence of food in the stomach or can be influenced by the actions of certain medications, such as anticholinergics, which slow gastrointestinal motility, and parasympathomimetics, which increase gastrointestinal motility (see Chapter 4, "Drug Availability and Distribution," for additional details).

Liquids. Numerous oral medications are prepared for administration in liquid form, including solutions, syrups, elixirs, suspensions, and oils. Liquid preparations are more readily absorbed than capsules or tablets because they do not have to go through the disintegration and the dissolution processes.

Solutions are preparations in which one or more drugs are dissolved in water. Syrups contain drugs in a homogeneous solution in a sugar base and are clear. Some syrups, such as cough preparations, are given for soothing effects and thus should not be given with water. Because of their high sugar content syrups should be given with caution to diabetics.

Suspensions are preparations in which fine particles of the drug are suspended in a liquid base and are thus cloudy. Suspensions must be shaken well before the medication is given because of the tendency for the drug to settle to the bottom of the container when stored. For this reason, suspensions should be given as soon as possible after they are poured. Some medications also come in liquid form because they can be more easily formulated in this manner. For example, drugs that are soluble in alcohol can often be more readily made into elixirs than into solid dosage forms. Elixirs, because they contain various percentages of alcohol, should *not* be administered to patients for whom alcohol is contraindicated, such as those receiving disulfiram therapy for the treatment of alcoholism.

Oil preparations such as castor oil or mineral oil are given carefully in order to prevent aspiration of the oil into the respiratory tract, which could result in lipid pneumonia. Patients often find oil preparations unpleasant to take, and they are often given over ice or in fruit juice to help make them more palatable.

Liquid preparations are usually prescribed for individuals, especially children under 5 years of age and some elderly, who have difficulty swallowing tablets and capsules. Pharmaceutical companies prepare drugs in liquid form with various flavorings, including chocolate, lemon, and cherry, that can be used for both children and adults in relation to their individual preferences to make oral medications more palatable.

It is important to check expiration dates on liquid preparations and to be sure that the medication is stored correctly. Most liquid preparations should be stored in a cool dark area. All outdated medications should be returned to the pharmacy. Because of their sugar content, many of these preparations can cause the lid of the bottle to become stuck and the label sticky and illegible. Liquid medications should be carefully poured away from the label, and the lip of the bottle should be carefully wiped before it is returned to the shelf or medication refrigerator.

Tablets. Tablets are solid oral dosage forms that contain drugs mixed with a binder that sticks the ingredients of the tablet together, a disintegrator that usually absorbs fluid and helps the tablet break apart in the gastrointestinal tract, a lubricant for manufacturing purposes, and various other excipients (fillers) to make the tablet size convenient and appearance aesthetic. Tablets are the most widely used dosage form because of their convenience, economy, accuracy of dosage, compactness, ease of administration, and portability. Various forms of tablets are made. The color, size, shape, and dose of these tablets varies according to the drug manufacturer.

Many tablets are prepared with sugar or film coatings to help prevent them from breaking apart or flaking when they are shaken or knocked together in their containers. The coating also prevents them from dissolving in the mouth before they are swallowed.

Some tablets are protected by an enteric coating so that they will be dissolved in the alkaline secretions of the duodenum and not in the stomach where the medication may be destroyed by the acidic pH. These tablets should not be chewed, nor should the nurse crush them to facilitate administration because the medication would be destroyed by the stomach acid. Some medications, such as bisacodyl, are enteric coated to protect the stomach from the irritating effect of the drug, and some liquids, such as milk, can destroy the protective coating of enteric-coated medications and should not be used when they are given.

When it is desired that the drug be gradually released in the gastrointestinal tract, it is often embedded in sustained-release tablet form. Sustained-release tablets offer sustained blood levels of medication over a longer period of time and can therefore be given less frequently. These tablets likewise would not work as desired if crushed.

Tablets also come in chewable form. It is especially important that the nurse explain to the patient that these tablets must be thoroughly chewed before swallowing if they are to be properly absorbed. Some of these tablets (e.g., antacids) may be sucked and dissolved in the mouth instead of chewed. They should *not* be swallowed whole, however, because they may fail to dissolve and an intestinal obstruction may result.

Capsules. Capsules are small gelatin cases that are used to enclose medications. Various powdered, granular, and liquid forms of drugs are prepared in capsules that vary in color, size, and shape depending on the manufacturer. Because they are formulated of gelatin, capsules should be stored in a cool area. Capsules that crack or stick together should be discarded or returned to the pharmacy.

Empty gelatin capsules are also available and come in various sizes. These may be used to give unpleasant or bitter medications. For example, a codeine (1 grain, 60 mg) tablet can be placed in an empty gelatin capsule and administered more pleasantly.

Capsules usually dissolve in the stomach after being swallowed with water. If the patient has difficulty swallowing, many capsules can be taken apart and the medication administered as a powder or liquid in an appropriate vehicle to disguise the taste.

Some capsules contain time-released particles. These can also be opened and given in an appropriate vehicle because each particle is individually coated and protected; however, the patient must be cautioned against chewing the particles.

Although the oral route is the most convenient route for medication administration and has many advantages, it is *contraindicated* when the patient is vomiting, has gastric suction, is unconscious and unable to swallow or is unable to take foods or fluids by mouth because of other conditions (e.g., tests or surgery).

Preparation

Except for when unit dose systems are being used, oral medications are usually prepared in the medication or drug room area by the nurse. Because the oral cavity is not sterile, preparation is carried out using a "clean technique."

A tablet or capsule is poured from the container into its cap and then into a paper souffle cup for delivery to the patient (Figure 2-1). There are numerous medication measuring cups, spoons, and droppers available for use when preparing liquid medications. The 30 ml plastic medication cup is usually used for measuring liquid medications for both adults and children because it is calibrated in 5 ml measurements as well as in drams and ounces. The most

accurate measurement of liquid medications is made with the syringe, since it is calibrated in tenths of a milliliter and it expels all of the medication that is drawn up. The syringe should be used when liquid medications are measured, especially those with low therapeutic index such as anticonvulsants. The standard household teaspoon should not be used because it has been found to hold from 2.5 ml to 9.7 ml, depending on the viscosity of the medication, and can even deliver between 3 ml and 7 ml of the same liquid when measurement is completed by different individuals. Some medications, such as pediatric digoxin elixir, are supplied with their own calibrated droppers. In controlled studies these have been found to be accurate; however, they should be used *only* with the particular medication they have been supplied with because the viscosities of various liquid preparations may differ and affect the accuracy of the calibration.

When preparing oral medications, the nurse must consider individual preferences as well as the patient's ability to take the various dosage forms. For example, before administering medications in tablet or capsule form, the nurse must assess the patient's ability to take tablets or capsules. This ability is especially important in relation to children, individuals with hemiparesis, the frail elderly, and others who have difficulty swallowing.

If a patient has difficulty swallowing, certain medications in tablet form can be crushed to facilitate administration, and many capsules can be taken apart. The medication can then be mixed in a small amount of fluid or food.

When crushing tablets, the nurse must be careful that the medication is not lost and the dose thus altered. It is recommended that the tablet be placed in a souffle cup and another cup inserted on top of it. The tablet can then be crushed with the small end of a pestle without popping out.

When mixing crushed tablets or drugs from opened capsules with fluid and foods, the nurse must be alert to incompatibilities or drug-food interactions as well as to the individual preferences of the patient. For infants and young children applesauce or other puréed fruits are often used because these are some of the first foods introduced to the infant, and allergies are rare. These foods offer a consistency that is easily handled in administration; however, cultural variations need to be considered because all infants may not be familiar with these foods. The medication can also be mixed with a little water and administered in a syringe with the needle *removed*. The problem with mixing medications with foods is that often an aver-

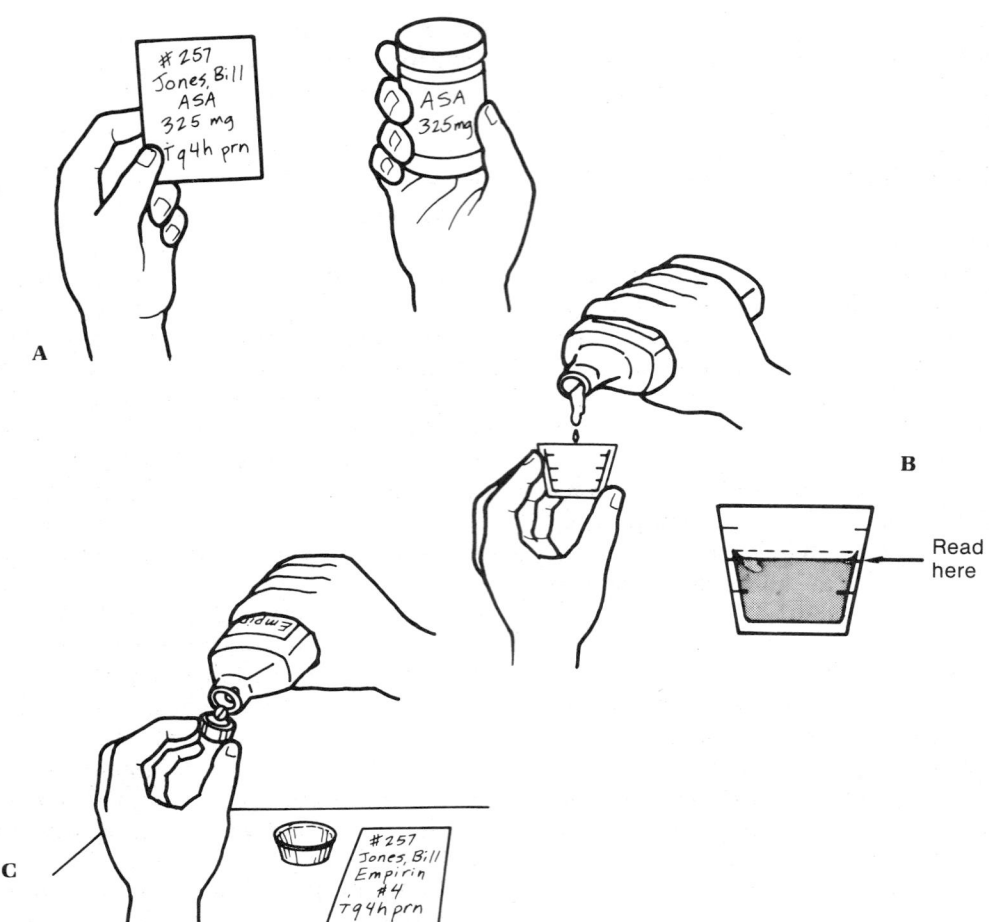

FIGURE 2-1. **The preparation of oral medications. The accurate preparation of oral and other medications is essential. A, Medication cards should be carefully checked with prescriber's orders. Before pouring the medication, the nurse should compare the label to the medication card. All medication labels should be read three times to ensure the correct medication is given: (1) when the container is taken from the shelf, (2) when compared with the medication card before pouring, and (3) when it is returned. B, Liquid medications are poured away from the label and are measured at eye level on a flat surface. Before returning to the shelf or refrigerator, the nurse should wipe the lip to prevent the lid from sticking or the label from being damaged. C, Tablets and capsules are poured from their containers into the cap and then into a paper souffle cup for delivery to the patient. Capsules and tablets should not be handled by the hands. It is also recommended that tablets and capsules be poured into individual cups even if they are for the same patient so that medications can be administered more accurately.**

sion to the food can result. Thus, essential foods should *never* be used to mix medications especially for infants and young children. Medication should never be put into a full bottle of formula or milk. The smallest amount of liquid or food possible, to ensure that the patient will take the entire amount of medicine, should be used.

Some tablets are scored and can be halved with a lance. However, if the medication is supplied in unscored tablets that must be halved or if any tablet must be quartered to obtain the correct dosage, the nurse should consult with the pharmacist because the dosage will not be accurate if the tablet is broken into smaller pieces.

Administration

The nurse must establish a positive relationship with infants and children and should give medications in such a way as to maintain trust and cooperation. Medication administration should never be seen as punishment. The child should be praised for taking medicine but should also be allowed to express fears and dislikes. Even young children can be given simple, honest explanations of why the medication is necessary.

Many children will take unpleasant tasting medications if they are made more palatable. For example, ampicillin comes in vanilla-pineapple, fruit, and cherry flavors. Liquid preparations of amoxicillin come in strawberry, banana, and bubble gum flavors. Erythromycin is supplied in orange and cherry-cinnamon flavors, and penicillin V comes in many flavors, such as coconut-custard and cinnamon root-beer. The nurse should be alert to the availability of different flavors of preparations and should consult the pharmacist when faced with a child on regular medications who "just does not like the taste." It is also helpful if the nurse actually knows what the preparations taste like.

Sometimes firmness is required in administering medications to children. The nurse must be consistent in her approach, and reinforce positive behavior. Negative behavior should be ignored. A crying child should not be given oral medication because it can be easily aspirated.

Providing the child a choice he can make often helps in increasing his control over his care and increases cooperation. For example, the child does not have a choice regarding taking medications, but he does have a choice in relation to taking it from a cup, syringe, in another oral form, or with a certain drink. The manner of administration will have to be planned individually with the child and parent in relation to the medications he is receiving. The child may also respond to being given a choice as to where he would like to take the medicine—in the nurse's lap or in the chair. Depending on the child's age, he may or may not prefer the parent to give it.

Parents should be involved as much as possible in the administration of oral medications in order to promote their abilities in administering medication to the child and to decrease the probability of medication error once the child is sent home. When involving the parent in the care of the child, the nurse must be sure to check hospital policy in relation to philosophy and liability.

When medications are administered, the patient is called by name, and his identification band is checked

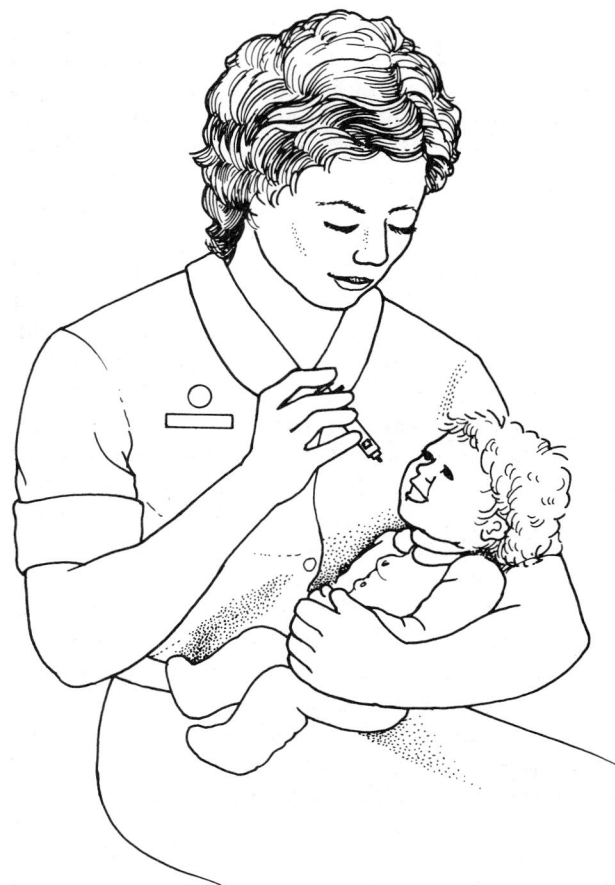

FIGURE 2-2. **The administration of oral medications to children involves a positive approach. Toddlers and preschoolers can be held in the lap and gently restrained if necessary, with the near arm behind the nurse and the other arm held with the nurse's free hand. The child should be in a sitting position to prevent aspiration. Liquid forms of medication are usually given to infants and young children, and can be given in a plastic cup or needleless syringe.**

for safety with the medication card, which has been carefully checked against the prescriber's order. When unit dose systems are used, the label on the prepared medication is checked with the patient's identification band.

The young infant is held as for feeding, and liquid oral medications are given through a nipple that the infant will suck readily, since the sucking reflex is strong. The medication may be taken more readily if the child is hungry. If the infant refuses the nipple, the medication can be given by a *needleless* syringe (Figure 2-2). The medication can be injected in small amounts (0.5 to 1.0 ml) into the infant's cheek at the gums toward the back of the mouth because the infant can choke or drool if too large a volume of medication is given at one time. The infant should be allowed to swallow between each injection, and should *not* be returned to the crib until the medication has been completely swallowed.

Toddlers and preschoolers can also be held and the medication can be given with a plastic medicine cup or a needleless syringe. The child can be gently restrained when held in the nurse's lap with the near arm behind the nurse and the other arm held with the nurse's free hand if necessary. Children over 5 years of age and adults should be in a sitting position to enhance swallowing and to prevent aspiration. Liquid medications can be taken directly from the plastic cup. For solid dosage forms, the patient should be told to place the tablet or capsule on the back of the tongue and to swallow the medication with water or juice if this is not contraindicated. Some medications, such as sulfonamides, are to be taken with a full glass of water to ensure adequate dissolution and to minimize the occurence of crystalluria. The nurse should stay with the patient until the medication is swallowed.

Cases of drug-induced esophagitis associated with delayed passage of capsules or tablets even without obvious GI abnormalities or dysphagia have been reported as well as cases resulting in death. Esophageal transit time of capsules and tablets is affected by both the position of the patient and the amount of fluids taken with the medication. It is recommended that, unless contraindicated, patients should stand or sit up while swallowing capsules or tablets and should take them with at least 100 ml liquid. This will prevent local irritation from prolonged drug contact with esophageal mucosa if the tablet or capsule adheres to the wall and disintegrates there. This is particularly important with medications such as potassium chloride, tetracycline, doxycycline, fluorouracil, and clindamycin. If these measures are contraindicated, liquid preparations should be used. Patients should likewise be monitored for sensations of a lump in the throat or difficulty swallowing.

Many children and adults who have been on regular medication therapy take numerous tablets or capsules at one time without difficulty; however, to prevent aspiration, they should usually be taken one at a time.

When giving medications to the elderly adult, the nurse must also incorporate a wide range of communication skills. In addition, normal sensory changes that can occur with aging should be considered. For example, because of yellowing of the lenses, patients may not be able to see a white pill in a white souffle medication cup or differentiate between different colored tablets (e.g., white and yellow, green and blue) during teaching sessions related to self-medication. The patient, because of auditory changes that may occur with aging, may not hear explanations and instructions regarding the taking of oral medications. Thus, an oral medication that should be chewed might be swallowed. When administering medications, the nurse should remember to give the aged time, to avoid background noise, and to use quiet areas for medication instruction. The nurse should not shout at the elderly. The tone should be kept low, but normal, and not exaggerated, and the nurse should speak slowly and distinctly. The patient should be asked to repeat the instructions to ensure that he has heard and interpreted them correctly. Clearly printed instructions should also be provided. This is especially important if the patient will be discharged with medications.

A confused elderly person often presents a challenge to the nurse in relation to the administration of oral medications. Medications are usually administered in crushed form in a small amount of food because tablets may be refused and there is also danger of aspiration. The patient should be positioned for feeding and the medication given from a spoon in a small amount of food so that the nurse can be sure that the total dose is taken. Liquid medications may also be used.

It is especially important that the nurse be alert to drug-food interactions. Because of alterations in taste caused by aging, sweet-tasting preparations are usually taken more readily. When liquid forms of medication are being given, the nurse must be alert to mixing them in small amounts of compatible liquids. For example, perphenazine oral concentrate can be mixed with milk or orange juice but not with coffee, tea, or apple juice because a precipitate will form.

Psychiatric patients may also need special nursing considerations in relation to the administration of medications. These measures are dealt within Chapter 18, "Drugs Used to Treat Psychotic Disorders," and Chapter 19, "Drugs Used to Treat Affective Disorders."

When giving oral medications to patients with nasogastric tubes, the nurse must consider if the medications can be given with tube feedings or not. It is also important to note that only liquid forms of medication can be given by this route. The patient should be positioned in a semi-Fowler's or high Fowler's position and the medication administered according to tube feeding after it has been ascertained that the tube is properly placed. The tubing is clamped off and a syringe that has had the barrel removed is attached. The correct amount of medication is poured into the syringe and the tubing unclamped so that the medication can flow in by gravity. Force should not be used. The procedure should be stopped immediately if the patient shows signs of distress or discomfort. The flow rate can be regulated by lowering or raising the syringe or by clamping the tube. The tubing should be flushed with 30 to 50 ml of water (20 to 25 ml for children) before the medication empties out. This prevents the medication from remaining on the sides of the tubing and prevents clogging of the tubing. The syringe is then removed and the tubing clamped. The patient should remain in an upright position or on the right side for 30 minutes.

Monitoring

The nurse must be especially alert to monitoring the infant, child, or adult after oral administration of medications. Many medications, such as elixir of phenobarbital, potassium chloride solution, theophylline elixir, and phenylbutazone, are irritating to the gastric mucosa and can cause nausea or vomiting. In addition, other medications taken orally, such as ampicillin, can also cause diarrhea. Diluting the drug or giving it with meals, if not contraindicated, is sometimes helpful in reducing the nausea and vomiting. If vomiting occurs soon after a medication is given, the vomitus should be examined for undissolved drug. The dose should not be repeated unless ordered. For such side effects, other oral dosage forms or alternate routes of administration may be required. In some hospitals, nurses can alternate dosage forms or routes of administration using their own judgment. In some areas of practice, the prescriber will have to be consulted. It is up to the nurse to be aware of the parameters of her practice in the context in which she practices. If the nurse can make judgments about alternative routes, it is important to recognize that drug dose may vary because of differences in bioavailability (see Chapter 4, "Drug Availability and Distribution").

The therapeutic effects and the adverse side effects of specific oral medications must also be monitored in relation to individual patient response. These are outlined in the General Nursing Implications and the Nursing Drug Digest of each medication chapter in Sections III through XV of this textbook.

RECTAL MEDICATIONS

Drugs are administered rectally when the oral route is contraindicated, such as when patients are unconscious or are vomiting. The rectal route may also be used when patients are receiving gastric suction or when local effects are desired. Rectal medications are usually given in the form of suppositories.

Suppositories are conical-shaped preparations in which the drug is combined with a cocoa butter, polyethylene glycol, or a glycerinated gelatin base that melts at body temperature, thus releasing the drug for local effect or absorption by the capillaries of the rectal mucosa for systemic effect. The rectal administration of medications is contraindicated in conditions where the bowel is inflamed or irritated, if diarrhea is present, or if the patient is prone to rectal abscesses.

Suppositories are manufactured and supplied in various sizes and shapes. The action of medications administered rectally in suppository form is affected by the placement of the suppository and the presence of fecal matter in the rectum, which can prevent its contact with the bowel wall. Suppositories given for local effects (e.g., bisacodyl) often act within 30 minutes. However, absorption of suppositories given for systemic effects (e.g., aminophylline) is unpredictable and erratic in both children and adults. When giving suppositories, the nurse should use the intact dosage form. Suppositories should not be split or halved; because of their irregular shapes, this does not guarantee an accurate dose. In addition, because the amount of medication may not be evenly distributed in the suppository, the nurse should consult the pharmacist for appropriate doses of suppositories as needed.

The medication should be stored in the refrigerator or in a cool place until used.

Preparation

Both adults and children must be prepared for the procedure with adequate explanation of the reason for the suppository, the procedure, and the results expected. The administration of medications rectally can be especially upsetting to the preschool child because it can be seen as an "attack from behind" because of castration and body integrity fears that are common with this age group. Thus great care and careful preparation are required in administration of medications by this route.

Administration

The nurse should wear a disposable examination glove to administer the suppository. Infants, children, and adults are positioned on the left side with the upper leg flexed (Figure 2-3). Adequate draping is required to provide privacy and to relieve anxiety. After the foil wrapper is removed, the suppository is lubricated with a water-soluble lubricant or water. The child or adult is told to take a deep breath to distract him as well as to relax the external sphincter muscle. The external anal sphincter is gently dilated with the fifth digit for infants and children 1 to 3 years of age.

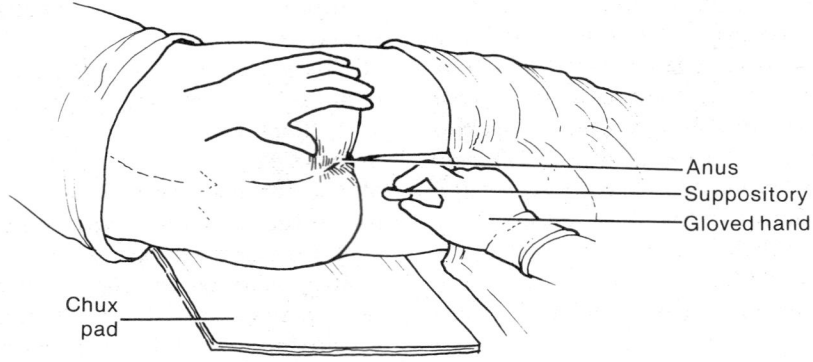

FIGURE 2-3. **The rectal administration of medications. Medications are usually administered rectally in suppository form. Before inserting the suppository, the nurse should carefully remove the foil and roll the suppository gently in the gloved hand, to smooth the ridges that are formed when it is made. Insertion will be more comfortable for the patient. The patient is positioned on his side and carefully draped. The buttocks are separated and the anal sphincter dilated. The suppository is then inserted with the rounded end first. Lubrication of the suppository with a water-soluble lubricant or water facilitates insertion and patient comfort.**

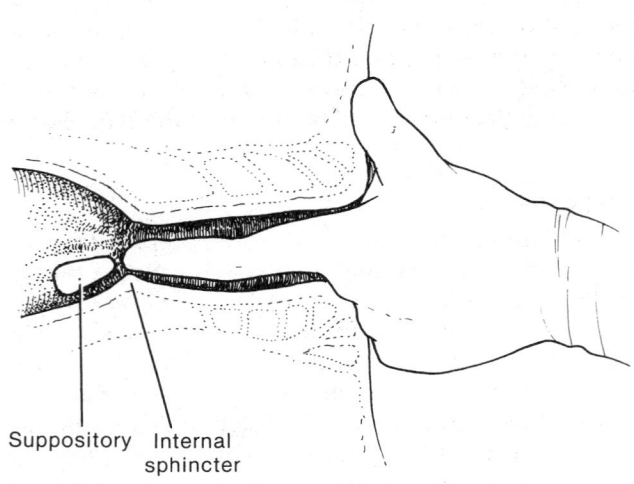

FIGURE 2-4. **When inserting the suppository into the rectum, the nurse should not insert it into feces. It should be inserted against the bowel wall beyond the internal sphincter.**

The index finger is used for children over 3 years of age and adults. Once the nurse feels the external sphincter relax around her finger, the suppository is introduced, rounded end first—the length of her finger at an angle toward the umbilicus to be sure it is correctly placed in contact with the bowel wall (Figure 2-4). The finger is withdrawn and the buttocks are held together until the desire to expel the suppository passes.

Monitoring

The nurse must be sure that the suppository is retained and not expelled after insertion before it has had a chance to elicit its local effect or to be absorbed. The patient's response to the medication must also be monitored. If the suppository was given for systemic effects and was expelled within 30 minutes, the prescriber should be notified. If the suppository was given for laxative purposes, the stool characteristics and results must be charted. The nurse must also be alert to any untoward signs, such as cramping or discomfort as well as lack of results by a specified time, depending on the indication for the medication.

VAGINAL MEDICATIONS

Vaginal medications are available in the forms of creams, foams, jellies, ointments, suppositories, and tablets. These medications are used to treat local irritation or infections or for contraception. An interesting development is the intrauterine polymer reservoir system, which can deliver a constant daily dose of a medication (i.e., progesterone) for more than 1 year. Vaginal medications are used infrequently in infants and children; however, preadolescent and adolescent girls and adult women may require their use for various conditions. Aged adult women may, in addition, require medications such as hormonal preparations by this route. Douches or irrigations are also available, but generally not recommended because of the associated danger of peritonitis.

Preparation

Toddlers and preschoolers, because of their developmental levels, require careful preparation to reduce psychologic trauma. An individual approach to children is essential, and explanation and reassurance at their level must be completed; sometimes role playing with dolls is helpful to the preschooler.

School-aged children and adolescents can understand explanations and reasons for the treatment. They will require information about the vaginal area and its functions, as well as what to expect in relation to the administration of the medication, and individual sexuality must be explored. Parental involvement is also important.

Adults should also receive careful explanation of the purpose for the procedure and proper instruction regarding the specific procedure. Adolescents and adults can usually be instructed to administer their own vaginal medications and to care for their equipment.

Administration

The patient should be asked to void before the procedure. She is positioned on her back comfortably with the knees and hips flexed and the thighs abducted and rotated externally. If desired, the hips can be slightly elevated on a pillow. Good visualization is essential, especially in children, to prevent trauma because the vaginal area is small.

Vaginal creams, foams, suppositories, and tablets are usually administered with their own specially designed applicators so that the medication can be inserted in the upper vaginal vault to ensure maximum effect. Each patient should have her own equipment, which is carefully washed after use. Sterile technique is not required unless open lesions are present, however, clean technique should be routinely followed. The nurse should use gloved hands and spread the labia gently so that the vaginal orifice can be seen. Using the other hand, the nurse should insert the medication gently with the appropriate applicator about 3 inches (7.5 cm) along the posterior fornix or posterior wall of the vagina in the adult. The plunger is pushed to insert the medication, and the applicator is gently removed. The patient should remain in a recumbent position to prevent the medication from leaking from the vaginal orifice. Because many vaginal medications can stain underclothing, a perineal pad should be used. It is not recommended that tampons be used because they tend to absorb the medication.

Monitoring

The patient should be assessed for comfort and effects of drug therapy. In addition, self-medication abilities and understanding of the purpose for the therapy should be observed. Unusual discharge or odor should be noted as well as pruritus or other discomfort especially if antibiotic therapy is being used because this may indicate overgrowth of nonsusceptible organisms.

OPHTHALMIC MEDICATIONS

There are numerous ophthalmic medications used for a variety of conditions of the eye, including infection and inflammation. There are also ophthalmic preparations used for diagnostic purposes and for the treatment of glaucoma. Most ophthalmic preparations are available in solution, suspension, or ointment forms. Although some liquid preparations are supplied in bottles with droppers, most are supplied in plastic squeeze bottles that release one drop of medication at a time. Ointments are supplied in tubes. A newer development is the polymer reservoir system, which is inserted into the conjunctival sac where the drug (e.g., pilocarpine) is continuously released for 1 week.

Preparation

Ophthalmic preparations are often stored under refrigeration, but should be warmed to room temperature when administered, to decrease blinking and local irritation. Before administering ophthalmic medications, the nurse should inspect the container for the date of expiration, and solution preparations should be examined for cloudiness, which may indicate contamination or drug deterioration. Any liquid or ointment that is questionable should be discarded or returned to the pharmacy. Suspensions should be thoroughly shaken before use.

Infants, children, and adults may find the administration of eye drops or ointments uncomfortable and even frightening. The child can be positioned on his parent's or the nurse's lap with the head back, or he can lie supine on the bed or treatment table. A pillow can be placed under the shoulders so that the child's head is lower than the body because gravity will help disperse the medication over the cornea. The child will usually cooperate if he is told the reason for the medication and if he is given directions. It is important that the nurse have the cooperation of the child because struggling can result in injury, and crying results in the medication being rinsed out of the eye, thereby decreasing or nullifying the drug's effect. The infant or child may need to be gently restrained.

The adult can lie supine, with a pillow under the shoulders to extend the neck, or can tilt the head back while in a sitting position, if preferred. The dropper should be introduced from the side, and the patient should be asked to look up to decrease the corneal reflex and blinking or moving that might occur when the dropper is directed toward the eye.

Before drops or ointments are administered into the eye, the eye should be gently wiped from the inner to the outer canthus with a sterile gauze sponge moistened with normal saline solution, so that the eye and lashes are free from exudate. A separate sponge should be used for each eye.

The bottle label should be carefully checked to ensure that the medication is for ophthalmic use and the exact concentration noted.

Administration

The eye is not sterile; however, when instilling ophthalmic medications, a sterile technique is essential to prevent the introduction of pathogens into the eye. The dropper or tip of the ointment tube should never come in contact with the patient's eye or eyelashes because this may cause bacterial contamination of the solution or ointment. Ophthalmic preparations should be individually dispensed for each eye to prevent cross infection and should *not* be used for any other person.

It is important to note that because the normal volume of tears if 7 μl, the nonblinking eye can accommodate up to 30 μl, but blinking keeps the maximum at 10. Any excess is rapidly drained from the eye. The usual drop size of drug solution is 25 to 50 μl, and thus any volume greater than one drop is lost. As volume increases, the rate of absorption increases. The ideal volume is 5 to 10 μl to decrease loss of drug and systemic absorption. This has implications for multiple drop therapy, because much of the first drop will be lost when the second medication is given.

If multiple drop therapy must be used, the interval between drops should be about 5 minutes to permit therapeutic effect and to prevent loss through the nasolacrimal duct.

For both children and adults, the nurse should stand at the patient's left, if right-handed and retract the lower lid gently with the nondominant hand and administer the drops as ordered into the conjunctival sac of the appropriate eye (Figure 2-5). The lower lid can also be grasped below the lashes and pulled out to form a pouch in which ophthalmic medication can be administered. The dropper should be placed as close as possible to the eye without touching it in order to decrease both splattering of the medication and patient discomfort. The nurse may need to use

the thumb and index fingers to gently separate the lids. The nurse should rest her hand on the patient's forehead when instilling the drops so that if he or she moves, the eye will not be injured by the dropper because the nurse's hand moves with the patient. The skin is released to its normal position, and the patient is asked to gently close the eye. The patient should also be asked to move the eye back and forth from side to side under the closed lid to evenly distribute the medication, and should remain in a recumbent position for a few minutes and avoid blinking (at least 30 seconds) so that the medication will have maximum contact with the eye. A tissue should be provided so that any medication that runs out of the eye can be gently blotted.

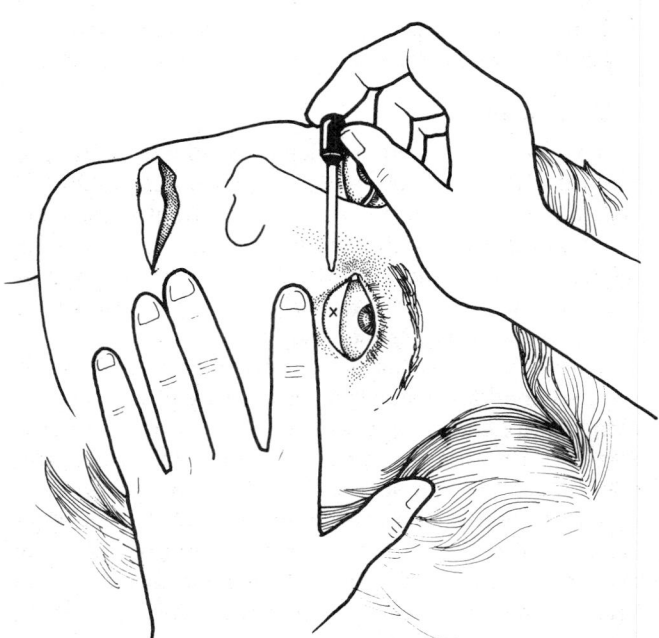

FIGURE 2-5. **The administration of ophthalmic drops. When instilling ophthalmic drops, the nurse's hand should be stabilized on the patient's forehead to prevent injury to the eye if the patient moves unexpectedly. (If the nurse is right-handed, she should stand at the patient's left side; if left-handed, at the patient's right.) The patient should be asked to look up so that the corneal reflex is diminished, and the dropper should be introduced from the side. The lower lid is gently retracted, and the ordered number of drops are instilled into the conjunctival sac of the correct eye. Drops should not be dropped directly onto the cornea because this can result in pain and damage to the eye. After the drops are instilled, the lid is gently released to its normal position.**

To prevent undesired systemic effects from some medications (e.g., epinephrine) and to prevent loss of medication, the nasolacrimal duct should be gently blocked by applying digital pressure at the inner canthus for 2 minutes. This increases corneal contact time and prevents medication from entering the duct and resultant absorption into the general circulation. After 2 minutes excess medication can be wiped away with a clean tissue.

Eye ointment. The administration of ointment into the eye is completed much like drops (Figure 2-6). To facilitate flow of ointment, the tube can be held for a few minutes in the hand to warm it before use. A small amount of ointment (½ in, 1.3 cm) is squeezed in a line along the conjunctival sac of the lower lid, rotating the tube with a twisting motion to stop the flow. The lid margin should be gently released, and the child or adult should remain in position with his eyes closed for a few minutes. If desired and not contraindicated, the lid can be gently massaged to evenly distribute the medication. A small amount of ointment should be squeezed onto a sterile gauze sponge and discarded to ensure that the tube maintains asepsis. The tip should be wiped with a sterile gauze sponge and the cap replaced. If a second type of ointment is required, it should not be administered within 10 minutes of the first one.

Monitoring

The nurse should chart individual reactions to the medication and make specific observations related to

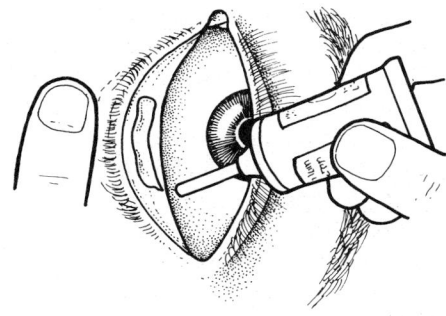

FIGURE 2-6. **The administration of ointment into the eye. Eye ointment is administered in much the same way as eye drops. The lower lid is retracted gently, and a small amount of ointment is squeezed along the conjunctival sac of the lower lid of the correct eye. The lid is gently released, and the patient is asked to gently close the eye. The patient should remain in the recumbent position or with the head back for a few minutes to allow the medication to have maximum contact with the eye.**

the action of the drug as well as to the details of administration. She should include observations that indicate therapeutic response or reactions such as swelling, itching, stinging, inflammation, or discharge. For example, patients receiving mydriatic medications before eye examinations or surgery should be observed for pupil dilation and cautioned regarding temporary blurring of vision or photophobia. Safety precautions and assistance with daily activities may be required. Sunglasses may diminish glare. When miotic drugs are administered, patients should be monitored for complaints of headache, blurred vision, pain or spasms in the treated eye. In addition, patients should be monitored for systemic absorption of eye preparations including facial flushing, dry mouth, and tachycardia with mydriatics or nausea, vomiting, bradycardia, or diaphoresis with miotics. See individual drugs for other aspects of monitoring patient response. To prevent infection or irritation, children and adults should be encouraged not to rub the eye after the medication has been administered.

OTIC MEDICATIONS

Ear instillations are used for their local effects and to treat infections, inflammation, and other disorders of the internal and external ear. Often, softening agents are instilled into the external auditory canal so that ear wax can be removed, particularly in elderly patients. Otic medication comes in liquid form and is instilled into the external auditory canal with a soft plastic dropper. Sterile technique is not used because the ear canal is not sterile; however, "clean" technique should be observed. If the tympanic membrane is ruptured or if there is any drainage from the canal, a sterile technique should be used. Otic medications are dispensed for each patient and should be used only for individual patients as specified.

Preparation

Before otic drops are instilled, the medication should be examined for sediment or discoloration. The bottle should be shaken if indicated and a small amount of the medication drawn up into the dropper. This can be held against a light source for inspection. If the medication is discolored, has sediment, or looks different than usual, it should be discarded and not used. The infant or child is restrained and placed on the side, or in a supine position, if preferred, with the affected ear exposed for the administration of the medication. The older child and adult will cooperate with appropriate preparation and explanation of the pro-

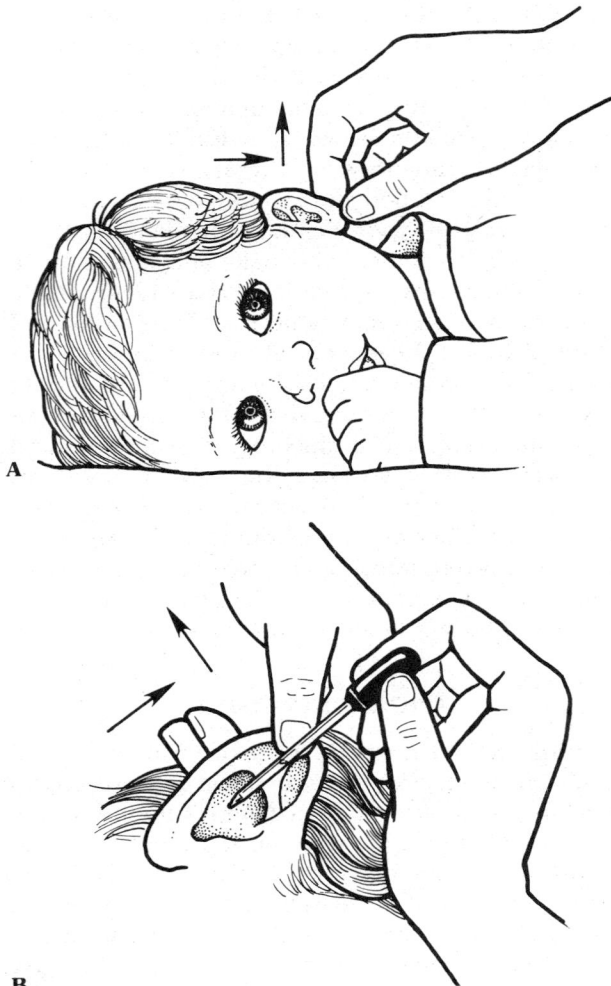

FIGURE 2-7. **The administration of otic medications. The infant, child, or adult is positioned on the unaffected ear. A, The nurse pulls the pinna down and back to administer ear drops to infants and children under 3 years of age. B, When administering ear drops to children older than 3 years and adults, the nurse gently pulls the pinna up and back. The nurse should stabilize her hand on the patient's head for safety and instill the prescribed number of drops. The drops are directed towards the ear canal to avoid hitting the tympanic membrane, which can cause pain. The patient should remain in the position for 5 to 10 minutes. Otic drops should be warmed before they are instilled to prevent nausea or vertigo.**

cedure. The adult is positioned on the unaffected side. The external auditory meatus is wiped with a sterile cotton-tipped applicator. If there is much exudate, this may be removed with sterile sponges and sterile normal saline.

In a child under 3 years of age the external auditory canal is cartilaginous and straight. To separate the walls of the canal for instillation, the auricle or pinna is pulled gently downward and back. In children over 3 years of age and adults, the ear canal has more ossification, and the canal angles slightly so that the pinna should be gently pulled up and back to straighten it.

Administration

The dropper is filled with the required amount of medication and is carefully inserted into the external ear canal so that it does not touch the canal, which may be sensitive or become irritated (Figure 2-7). The nurse's hand should rest on the patient's head when instilling the drops to stabilize the hand as well as to prevent injury if the patient should move unexpectedly. The drops should be directed toward the ear canal because drops that hit the tympanic membrane directly may cause pain. If the drops are cold, they may induce nausea or vertigo and should thus be warmed before administration. This can be done by rolling the bottle in the hands for a few minutes. The prescribed drops are instilled and the tragus of the ear is massaged gently or pressed two to three times to assist movement of the drops into the ear canal. The patient should remain in a side-lying position for approximately 5 to 10 minutes. A sterile cotton ball can be placed gently into the external ear canal to absorb any medication that may flow out when the patient sits up.

Monitoring

The patient should be observed for specific reactions to the medication, including subjective complaints of itching, burning, or pain. The infant and young child should be observed for rubbing or tugging at the ear, which may indicate pain or discomfort. The nurse should also monitor for drug effectiveness. For example, if the drops are given for an infection, the ear should be inspected for exudate, odor, and temperature. These observations, as well as the charting of the procedure specifying the drug, number of drops, and ear instilled, should be recorded.

NASAL MEDICATIONS

Nasal medications are often used to relieve nasal congestion or to treat allergic or inflammatory conditions of the nasal passages. The medication usually comes in a dropper or a spray bottle, both of which are individually dispensed and should not be used for other patients. The instillation of medication into the nares is a clean but not a sterile procedure. Because the nares drain into the back of the mouth and the throat, the instillation of medication may cause a tickling in the throat or a difficulty in breathing. In addition, the patient may be able to taste the medication after instillation, which some find unpleasant. With careful positioning this can be prevented.

Preparation

The nares may need to be cleansed of excess mucus before administration of the medication, and this can be easily accomplished with a gauze sponge and normal saline. In addition, it is helpful to have older children and adults gently blow their nose if not contraindicated before the administration of the nasal medication. Careful preparation and instruction should be completed before nasal medications are instilled.

Infants often react negatively to having drops placed into the nose because they are nose breathers. The older child may also protest. Proper explanation and restraint of the child are important factors in preventing injury. The older child and adult will cooperate with adequate explanation of the procedure. They should be warned that they may be able to taste the medication after it is given.

Administration

The infant is positioned with a pillow under the shoulders, and his head is allowed to fall back over the edge of the pillow onto the nurse's arm. Her hand can be used to restrain the infant's arms if necessary. The drops can then be administered with the free hand. If preferred, the infant can be held in the lap (Figure 2-8). Older children and adults can be positioned on the bed with a pillow under the shoulders to extend the neck.

Nose drops. The drops are administered with the dropper just inside the nares (½ in, 1.3 cm). The prescribed number of drops are directed toward the midline of the superior concha of the ethmoid bone so that they will not run down the throat. To avoid injuring the tissues and contaminating the dropper, the nurse should not touch the mucous membranes of the nostrils. The patient should be encouraged to relax and to breathe through the mouth, maintaining the position for 1 to 5 minutes to permit the medication to be absorbed by the nasal mucosa.

Nasal sprays. Older children and adults can assume a sitting position with the head slightly tilted back. The opposite nostril should be held closed by the patient, and he should be told to breathe in through the nostril being sprayed. The spray should

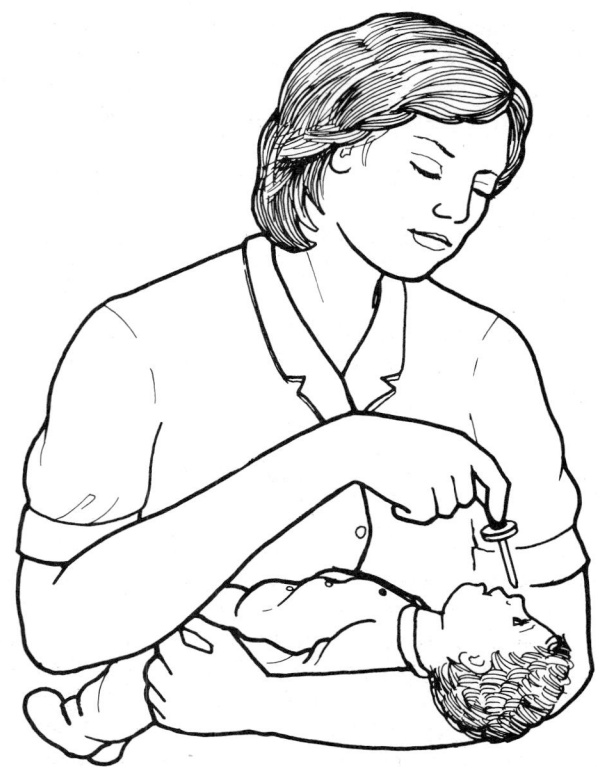

FIGURE 2-8. **The administration of nose drops. When administering nose drops to infants and young children, the nurse positions them with a pillow under the shoulders, and the head is allowed to fall back onto the nurse's arm. The nurse's hand can be used to restrain the child's arm if necessary. The drops are instilled with a soft dropper just inside the nares. The dropper should not be allowed to touch the mucous membranes. The child should be maintained in the position for 1 to 5 minutes. Nose drops should be given about 20 minutes before feedings. Because infants are nose breathers, they may squirm when the nose drops are administered. With this position, the nurse can stabilize the infant's head between her arm and body. If necessary, a mummy restraint can be used or the child held by another nurse.**

be directed toward the midline of the superior concha of the ethmoid bone for optimum effect. The bottle should be squeezed the prescribed number of times.

Monitoring

The patient's response to the medication is noted, as are observations related to the patient's condition, including exudate from the nose and subjective complaints. The medication, number of drops, and position of the patient are also recorded. Although nose drops are used primarily for their local effects, nasal products can be systemically absorbed though the nasal mucosa and elicit systemic effects. For example, ephedrine or epinephrine in nasal products can cause tachycardia as well as nervousness in sensitive individuals.

The infant, child, and adult should be closely observed for choking or vomiting during or following nasal instillation. In addition, if nasal decongestants are used routinely, the nurse should be alert to monitoring for rebound nasal congestion as well as for signs of dependence, particularly in adolescents.

Patient education regarding misuse or abuse is essential.

TOPICAL MEDICATIONS

There are numerous forms of topical medication including emollients, lotions, powders, ointments, pastes, creams, solutions, soaps, and shampoos. Topical medications are administered for their local effect on the skin or mucous membrane at the site of application. Diaper rash, wounds, burns, dermatitis, and other skin conditions, as well as external parasitic conditions, are treated with topical medications. They also are used to decrease pruritus or to treat local bacterial or fungal infections (see Section XII, "Dermatologic Medications" for further discussion of the use and administration of specific topical preparations).

Preparation

Before topical medications are applied, a careful assessment of the skin should be completed and charted as a point of reference. With this baseline documentation, therapeutic results as well as untoward effects can be properly assessed and evaluated. The young child and adult will require adequate explanation of the procedure, which will vary in relation to the patient's condition and the treatment selected.

Administration

The topical medication is applied to a clean skin surface from the inner to the outer aspects using "clean" technique. If lesions are present, sterile technique should be used. The lotion or emollient can be poured onto a sterile gauze and gently applied to the affected area. It is *not* patted or rubbed on because this may cause irritation or injury to the area being treated. When large areas are treated, long, smooth strokes should be used and the medication applied in the direction of hair growth to prevent folliculitis. When applying powders, the nurse must be careful not to inhale them or to cause the infant, child, or

adult to inhale them because they may be irritating to the respiratory tract.

Cream preparations are removed from the jar with a sterile tongue blade and placed onto a sterile gauze. The cap is immediately replaced after the required amount of cream is removed. Creams may also be supplied in tubes. Ointments are usually supplied in tubes, and these are squeezed onto a sterile tongue blade or gauze and the cap replaced. Creams and ointments are *not* squeezed directly from the tube onto the site to prevent contamination. Ointments and creams are usually applied evenly with gloved hands or applied with sterile tongue blades in a thin coat, unless otherwise directed. This is especially important to prevent the medication from being absorbed through the nurse's skin, which can cause unwanted effects. It should be noted that some research has indicated that generally patients prefer to be touched with nongloved hands. If not contraindicated (for the nurse) because of local absorption, irritation, or allergy, the hands can be used to apply the topical preparation. The nurse should be sure to wash her hands carefully after application of the medication.

If open lesions are present or if burns are being treated, strict sterile technique is used.

Monitoring

Observation of the lesion being treated, as well as individual reaction to the treatment, must be documented. The area treated must be carefully assessed for rashes, inflammation, or other local irritation that might be caused by the medication. If such reactions are noted, they should be reported to the prescriber immediately and the medication stopped until further direction is obtained.

Whenever applying topical preparations to the skin, the nurse must always be aware of not only local effects of the medication, but also potential systemic effects. This awareness is especially important when topical preparations are being applied over large areas, particulary with infants, as well as whenever topical preparations are applied to abraded or denuded areas of skin, which allow greater absorption. Use of occlusive dressings may also increase the systemic absorption of topically applied medications.

Itching may also be a problem for patients requiring topical medications, and they may need to be cautioned against scratching or rubbing treated sites. Nails should be trimmed short, and restraints may be indicated to prevent disruption of the healing process as well as secondary infection. Restraints are often necessary, especially with infants and young children.

It may also be necessary to administer drugs that relieve itching (e.g., diphenhydramine), and this should be discussed with the prescriber.

PARENTERAL MEDICATIONS

Parenteral medications are medications not taken via the digestive system and commonly refer to all medications given by injection. Although medications can be injected by way of intraarterial, intracardiac, intradermal, intraarticular, and intralesion routes for local effects, the major routes utilized for the administration of parenteral medications for systemic effects are subcutaneous (SC), intramuscular (IM), and intravenous (IV). The physical and chemical properties of the drug, including lipid solubility and tissue-irritating qualities, influence the selection of the route of administration. Thus, all parenteral medications cannot be given by all parenteral routes. This is discussed in more detail in Chapter 4, "Drug Availability and Distribution."

Medications administered parenterally usually have a more rapid onset of action than most orally administered medications and a higher extent of absorption. The major disadvantage, however, is that the administration of these medications involves penetration of the protective skin layer, and thus, strict aseptic technique is required in their preparation and administration in order to prevent infection.

Subcutaneous route. The subcutaneous route is used when a predictable and sustained effect is desired because drugs are usually absorbed slowly and completely from the subcutaneous tissues. However, any factor that influences subcutaneous blood flow (e.g., edema, shock, burns, exercise) will affect the medication's rate of absorption. Research has also shown that absorption from various subcutaneous sites (e.g., anterior thigh or lateral aspect of the upper arm) can vary significantly.

Drugs in aqueous solution are rapidly absorbed subcutaneously; however, some drugs, because of their desired effects, are formulated so that their absorption is intentionally prolonged (e.g., protamine insulin). Irritating medications are not to be administered by this route because pain, necrosis, and sloughing of the tissues can result. Concentrated drug solutions are also not to be given subcutaneously because they can cause the formation of sterile abscesses.

Intramuscular route. The intramuscular route is used for drugs that are concentrated or that cause irritation and cannot be given subcutaneously or intravenously. Generally, absorption from this route is more rapid than subcutaneous absorption because muscular tissue is more vascularized. However, the rate of absorption from intramuscular sites (e.g., deltoid, dorsogluteal) can vary.

As with some subcutaneous medications, some intramuscular medications are prepared so that they will be absorbed more slowly and their action sustained, for example, aqueous suspensions (e.g., penicillin G benzathine) and solutions in oils (e.g., progesterone). These preparations are *not* to be given intravenously. The intramuscular route is not recommended for use when patients are receiving anticoagulants (e.g., heparin, warfarin) because of the dangers of bleeding and resultant tissue sloughing.

Intravenous route. Medications are administered by the intravenous route when immediate or rapid action is desired or when medications, because of their chemical characteristics or action, cannot be given subcutaneously or intramuscularly. For example, some medications (e.g., diazepam and phenytoin) are manufactured with propylene glycol or alcohol solvents. These preparations are not usually administered by the intramuscular route because the solvents are rapidly diluted by the interstitial fluid, resulting in the drug precipitating at the injection site, followed by slow and erratic absorption.

The major advantage of the intravenous route is that therapeutic blood levels of medications can be obtained quickly and predictably. It is the common route for the administration of antibiotics and antidysrhythmics to hospitalized patients and is used for administering drugs in emergencies. Many irritating drugs can be diluted and administered by this route. The intravenous route is also used to maintain fluid and electrolyte balance, especially for patients who cannot take fluids by mouth, for various reasons, and to replace fluid and electrolytes lost through surgery, vomiting, diarrhea, suctioning, or wound drainage (see Chapter 67, "Fluids and Electrolytes").

Equipment for parenteral administration

Parenteral medications are usually supplied in sterile glass ampules and vials.

Ampules. Ampules are designed to hold a single dose of liquid medication. Today, most ampules are prescored so the stem can be easily broken off and the medication withdrawn. To ensure withdrawing the accurate volume of medication, the nurse must be sure that all of the medication is in the base of the ampule before breaking it open. To bring the medication down, the nurse can gently flick the stem with the finger.

If the ampule is not prescored, it should be placed on its side on a counter and gently scored around the neck with a file. The base of the ampule is grasped with one hand and the stem with the other. The tips of the thumbs should be facing each other. A piece of sterile gauze or a wrapped sterile alcohol swab is placed around the stem to protect the fingers, and the stem is broken off. The ampule should be broken away from the nurse so glass particles will not fly into the eyes.

To withdraw the medication, the nurse inserts the needle, and the required amount of drug is withdrawn into the syringe. Air is not injected into the ampule because it is an open system. To prevent contamination of the needle, it should not be allowed to touch the edges of the ampule where it was broken. It is recommended that a filter needle be used to withdraw the medication to avoid drawing up glass particles that may be tracked through or deposited in the tissues when the injection is given. Medication can also be withdrawn with the ampule inverted. This technique is used when shorter needles are used to withdraw medication. The needle must be kept in the solution so that the capillary pressure will be maintained or the drug will dribble out. Keeping the vial upright when withdrawing the medication encourages glass particles to stay at the bottom of the ampule. The medication should be withdrawn quickly since the system is open, and airborne contamination can result. The needle should be changed before the injection is given.

Vials. Medications for parenteral use are also supplied in single or multidose vials. Vials are small sterilized glass bottles sealed with rubber stoppers. They are supplied in various sizes and usually hold from 0.5 ml to 50 ml of solution or powdered medication ready for reconstitution.

To protect the rubber stopper, vials are usually packaged with a plastic cover that can be snapped off with the thumb or a soft metal cap that can be lifted off with a file. The rubber stopper should be cleansed with a sterile alcohol swab before the medication is withdrawn. Because a vial is a closed system, the needle is inserted, and an amount of air equal to the volume of medication to be withdrawn is introduced. To decrease the possibility of introducing rubber cores into the medication, it is recommended that the nurse insert the needle, bevel side up, with slight pressure exerted laterally (Figure 2-9). The drug is drawn into the syringe at eye level, with the bevel kept below the surface of the solution.

Sterile water for injection or sterile normal saline is usually used to reconstitute powdered medications. The manufacturer's directions on the label or package insert regarding the type and the amount of diluent to use should be followed exactly (see General Nursing Implications and the Nursing Drug Digest of the medication chapters in Sections III through XV for information regarding the reconstitution of specific agents). To dissolve the powder, the nurse should shake the vial or (if this is contraindicated because of the possibility of frothing) roll it gently in the hands for a few minutes. The vial should be examined carefully for any undissolved drug before the medication is withdrawn. After reconstitution, multidose vials must be stored according to the manufacturer's directions and must be labeled with the date and time of reconstitution, type and amount of diluent used for mixing, date of reconstitution, and the name or initials of the nurse who reconstituted it. With some preparations, such as

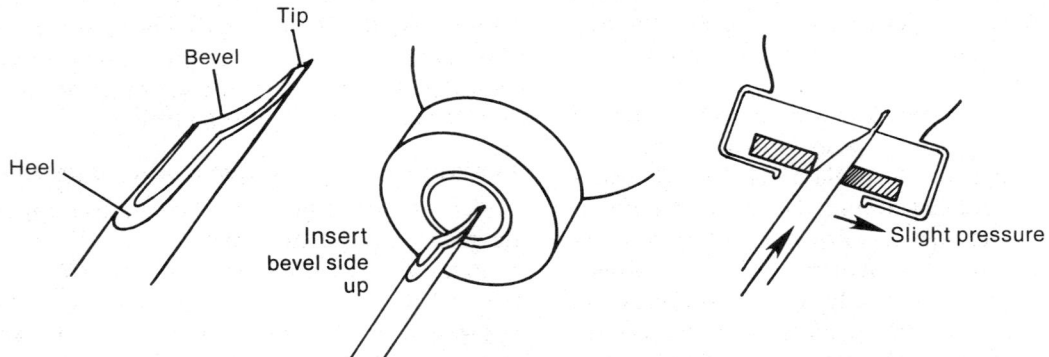

FIGURE 2-9. **Preparing medication in vials. The injection of diluent or air, as well as the withdrawal of medication from vials, often causes the introduction of rubber cores into the medication by the needle. To prevent this, it is recommended that the needle be inserted, bevel side up, with slight pressure exerted laterally as the needle is pushed in.**

Solu-Cortef, a special diluent is supplied with the powder in a double-stopper vial. The cap is removed and the vial is placed on a flat surface. A slight pressure is necessary to press down the stopper even with the lip of the vial. This pressure forces the inner stopper into the lower base of the vial, releasing the diluent to mix with the powdered medication. The medication readily dissolves with gentle shaking.

In addition to ampules and vials, parenteral medications are also supplied in prefilled cartridges, such as the Tubex system, that screw into a reusable syringe holder or Carpuject sterile cartridge-needle units. The cartridges are disposed of once the prescribed medication is administered.

Needles. Needles used for injection have three parts, the hub, which attaches to the syringe; the stem, or shaft; and the bevel (Figure 2-10)

When preparing medications for injection, the nurse must select the length, gauge, and bevel of the needle in relation to the volume and viscosity of the medication and route of administration. She also must determine individual patient factors, including the amount of subcutaneous fat or size of the muscle to be injected.

Shorter, finer-gauge needles are used for subcutaneous injections, and longer needles are used for intramuscular injections, depending on the size of the patient.

Most needles are made of stainless steel. In addition to being supplied in individual sterile packages, for convenience as well as to preserve asepsis, they are disposable. Needles, for the administration of medication, are available in various gauge numbers ranging from 18 to 27. The smaller the diameter of the needle, the larger is its gauge number. When giving injections, the nurse should use the largest gauge needle number (i.e., the smallest diameter) possible, considering the medication and site, in order to minimize the pain of injection. Viscous medications usually require small-numbered gauge needles (i.e., larger diameter needles), although, more watery or thin medications may be given in larger-gauge (i.e., smaller diameter) needles.

The bevel of the needle will vary in relation to its intended use. It makes a narrow opening that, after the injection is made, readily closes to prevent leakage of medication or serum and to decrease bleeding. The longer the bevel, the sharper the needle. Regular bevels are used for subcutaneous and intramuscular injections (Figure 2-11). Shorter, less sharp bevels are used for intravenous needles so that the needle can penetrate the vein when inserted, but will not easily penetrate the opposite vein wall, resulting in infiltration (Figure 2-12).

Syringes. Most syringes used for the preparation and administration of parenteral medications today are made of disposable plastic and are individually packaged for sterility and convenience.

Syringes are usually available in 2, 3, and 5 ml sizes

FIGURE 2-10. **Needles and syringes are available in various sizes and are selected in relation to the route of administration, type of medication to be injected, and specific patient factors.**

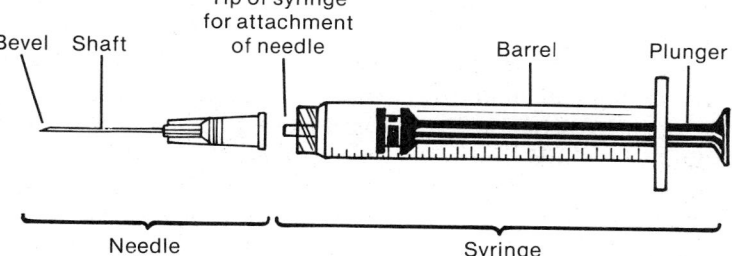

FIGURE 2-11. **Regular bevel. Regular bevels are used for intramuscular and subcutaneous injections. Because bevels can be dulled when inserted through rubber vial stoppers, the needle should be changed before the injection is given. Changing needles before giving an injection also prevents the tracking of medication through tissues, which can result in pain or irritation in some cases.**

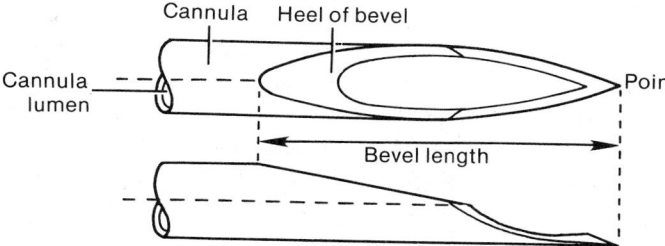

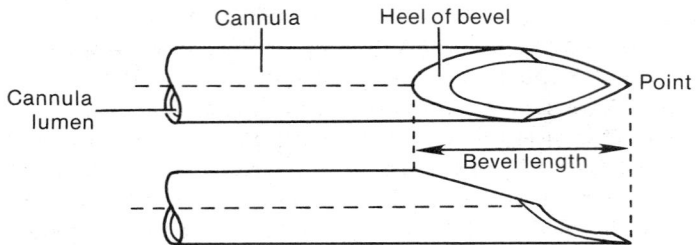

FIGURE 2-12. **Short bevel. The short bevel is used for intravenous injections. Because it is not as sharp as the regular bevel, there is less of a tendency for it to penetrate the opposite vein wall, which would result in extravasation. It is recommended by some that the butterfly needle be inserted bevel down to further decrease the chance of the penetration of the opposite vein wall. It is also recommended that the syringe be rotated after a needle is inserted intravenously with the bevel up so that the needle is positioned bevel down before the injection is made.**

and are calibrated in cubic centimeters. Larger syringes are also available. Most commonly used syringes for injection are supplied with detachable needles for convenience. There are also 1 ml insulin and tuberculin syringes.

Before I proceed, a note of explanation about the notation used for volumes of parenteral medications is in order. A cubic centimeter (cc) is the basic unit of measure for the volume of a gas, and milliliter (ml) is the basic unit of measure for the volume of a liquid. However, because of custom and the fact that these two measures are virtually equal in capacity, the nurse will find that the two terms, *cc* and *ml*, are used interchangeably in the literature, on packaged equipment, and when parenteral therapy is ordered by the prescriber. However, milliliter (ml) is the correct term for liquid volume and should be used by nurses as consistently as possible.

The selection of the syringe depends on the kind and amount of medication to be prepared and the route by which it will be administered. The barrel should be marked in units appropriate to the medication ordered. The syringe should be handled carefully to prevent contamination of the barrel, plunger, or tip.

The tuberculin syringe was designed for use with the tuberculin skin test and is calibrated in tenths and hundredths of a milliliter. This syringe is often used for the administration of small dosages of drugs and thus is especially useful when drugs are given to children.

Insulin syringes are calibrated in 100-unit scales for use with U100 insulin, which has largely replaced the previously used U40 and U80 insulins and syringes in order to decrease dosage error. A "lo-dose" 0.5 ml insulin syringe is also available for giving 50 units or less

of U100 insulin. This syringe is supplied with a "microfine" 27.5 gauge, ½ inch (12.7 mm) needle.

When syringes are selected and medications are prepared, it is important that syringe deadspace be considered. Deadspace is the volume of fluid left in the syringe after the plunger is pushed to the needle end of the barrel. When a needle is attached, this volume is increased. Consideration of deadspace is especially important when small volumes of drugs with narrow margins of safety are given, because dosage can be significantly altered. The ratio of deadspace to syringe volumes is greatest for the 1 ml syringe. Thus, great care should be made when drawing up small volumes of medications in this syringe. It is recommended that the amount of deadspace be calculated and an air bubble slightly greater than this volume be drawn into the syringe to ensure delivery of the total amount of medication. When possible, syringes with negligible deadspace should be used.

Syringes and needles should be disposed of carefully according to hospital procedure. It is important to note that it is no longer recommended that needles be snipped or syringes destroyed because of the danger of infection associated with airborne transmission of organisms. In addition, because of the risk of needle exposure to nurses when recapping needles after performing injections, some recommend that needles not be recapped, but disposed of readily in appropriate and accessible containers. This is particularly important in relation to caring for patients who are at risk for or who have been diagnosed with hepatitis or AIDS or at high risk (e.g., intravenous drug abusers, homosexual or bisexual men). Further attention should be given to care of injection equipment after use to prevent needlestick exposure to infected blood or blood products.

Major parenteral routes

Subcutaneous injections

Preparation of equipment. Subcutaneous injections are usually given with 24 to 27 gauge needles, ½ to ⅝ inch long (1.3 to 1.6 cm). The length of the needle is selected in relation to the amount of subcutaneous fat. For obese patients, a ⅝ inch or 1 inch needle is used and inserted at a 90-degree angle. Because only small volumes of medication are given, 1 ml to 3 ml syringes are often used for convenience. Insulin is administered in the appropriate insulin syringe. Depending on the health of the tissue, the nurse should inject from 0.5 to 1.5 ml of medication. Various medications, including heparin, insulins, narcotics, and vaccines, can be given by this route.

Preparation of the patient. Injections are frightening as well as painful, and infants, young children, and even adults, may need to be restrained gently but firmly to prevent them from moving unexpectedly which can result in the injection being given in the wrong site or in the needle being withdrawn prematurely. A sudden movement can cause the needle to break or scratch the patient.

The administration of injections can be particularly upsetting to children who have body integrity fears; preparing them carefully for injections is essential in relation to promoting mastery and trust. Therapeutic play, including needle play, can be used before and after injections. Timing of therapeutic play and explanations must be directed at the child's level of development and must be carefully individualized. Often the nurse can introduce another nurse to help the child keep still during the injection. The child should be allowed to cry "ouch," close his eyes, wiggle his toes, or squeeze a hand, but he must keep the site still. A combative child should not be restrained by numerous individuals because this is psychologically traumatic. Time should be taken for adequate preparation. If the injection has been upsetting, the nurse should spend time after the injection to work with the child as this child will have difficulty developing trust in the staff as well as have difficulty coping with future injections. Colorful stickers and Band-Aids can be used to make the experience more positive to the child.

Parents should be involved when possible because it helps them understand their child's care. They are usually placed at the child's head to provide support and reassurance. If they cannot handle the situation, an extra nurse should stand in for them. Evans (1981) recommends that a parent not be involved in restraining the child for injections or other painful procedures because the child may find it confusing and distress-ing that the parent is not protecting them from the painful procedure. Parents will need assistance on how to help their child cope with unpleasant or painful procedures and how to support their child for future injections.

Subcutaneous injection sites. Subcutaneous injections for both children and adults are given beneath the epidermal layers of the skin into the subcutaneous fat layers. The preferred sites are the anterior thighs, buttocks, upper arms, and abdomen. Sites on the upper back below the scapulae are also used. The site must be free from hematomas, rashes, lesions, excoriations, exudate, and drainage.

Administration. After carefully preparing the patient and explaining the purpose of the medication and procedure, the nurse cleanses the site in a circular fashion, from the center out with an alcohol or povidone-iodine swab to prevent the introduction of microorganisms. If the patient has an allergy to iodine, the site should be cleansed with alcohol. When giving a subcutaneous injection, the nurse inserts the needle, with the bevel up, at a 45-degree angle to the skin surface as the skin is held taut (Figure 2-13). If preferred, the tissue can be gently pinched up and the needle inserted at a 90-degree angle in the pocket formed. To prevent pain, the nurse should insert the needle quickly and advance it smoothly into the tissue. The tissue should be released, and the syringe gently aspirated to ensure that the needle is not in a blood vessel. The medication is then slowly injected if no blood appears in the syringe. Releasing the tissue prevents painful stimulation of the subcutaneous nerve endings that can occur if the medication is injected into compressed tissue. Releasing the tissue also allows the medication to distribute more readily into the tissues. If blood appears in the syringe, the needle should be withdrawn and slight pressure should be applied to the site with an alcohol or povidone-iodine swab or sterile gauze. The medication should be disposed of as per hospital policy, and a new injection should be prepared. (For further information regarding the administration of heparin and insulin see Chapters 34 and 60, respectively.)

After the medication is injected, the needle is quickly withdrawn at the same angle it was inserted. An antiseptic swab should be held at the site as the needle is withdrawn. The swab can then be used to apply pressure to the site and to massage it to increase absorption of the medication unless this is contraindicated, such as when heparin is given.

Monitoring. For patients receiving numerous injections, the rotation of sites is essential to prevent tissue damage (Figure 2-14). This is particularly important

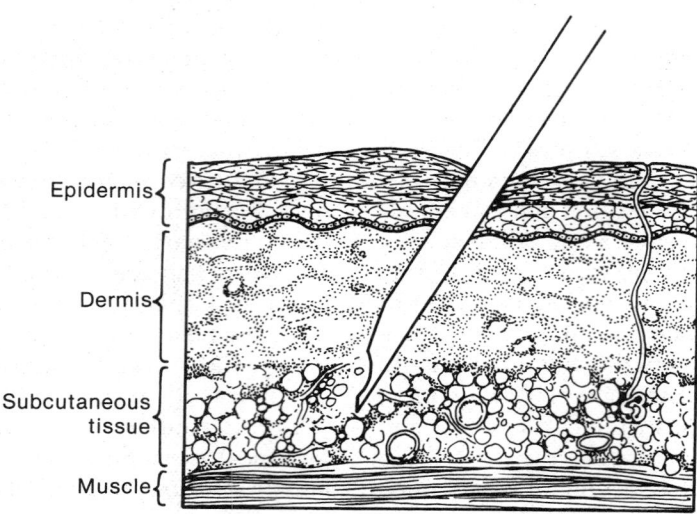

Epidermis

Dermis

Subcutaneous
tissue

Muscle

FIGURE 2-13. **Subcutaneous injections. Subcutaneous injections are given with ½-to ⅝-inch (1.3 to 1.6 cm) needles depending on the amount of subcutaneous tissue; 24- to 27-gauge needles are used. The length of the needle can be determined by gently grasping the skin and measuring the width of the skin fold from the top to the bottom. The length of needle closest to this measurement should be selected. There are various techniques for administering subcutaneous injections, and recommendations are often conflicting. Both heparin and insulin, commonly given by this route, also can be injected with variations of the technique (see Chapters 34 and 60, respectively). McConnell (1982) recommends that a 90-degree angle be used with ½-inch (1.3 cm) needles and that ⅝-inch (1.6 cm) needles be inserted at 45-degree angles to the skin surface. The skin is grasped to elevate the subcutaneous tissue and to prevent the needle from entering the wrong skin layer, and is released once the needle is inserted. McConnell also recommends that an air-lock of 0.2 to 0.3 cc of air be drawn into the syringe before the injection is given to help seal the medication into the subcutaneous tissue.**

when heparin or insulin is administered. Heparin has been associated with bleeding at the injection site, resulting in ecchymotic areas in the subcutaneous tissue. Lipodystrophy and hypertrophy have often been problems associated with the frequent administration of insulin. Although these have become less of a problem with the newer purified insulin preparations, it is still recommended that no area 1 inch (2.5 cm) in diameter be used more than once every 3 to 4 weeks (see Chapter 34, "Vasodilators, Antilipemics, Anticoagulants, and Platelet Aggregation Inhibitors," and Chapter 60, "Insulin and Related Medications," for more detail).

Intramuscular injections. Giving intramuscular injections requires careful site selection and adequate preparation of the infant, child, or adult. The nurse must take into consideration the patient's age, the type of drug, the dosage and volume of medication, the number of injections to be given, and the patient's general condition and preference when selecting sites and equipment.

Preparation of equipment. Intramuscular injections require the use of a 1 to 3 inch (2.5 to 7.5 cm) needle, depending on the amount of subcutaneous fat over the injection site (Figure 2-15), to ensure penetration of the muscle tissue. For infants, children, thin adults or, frail elderly patients, a 1 inch (2.5 cm) or smaller needle can be used. A 19 to 23 gauge needle is usually used depending on the viscosity of the medication to be given. For example, procaine penicillin G, because of its viscosity, is administered with a 19 or 21 gauge needle. If the needle appears bent in any way, it should *not* be used because it could break at the weakened point. The drug is drawn up as for a subcutaneous injection. To prevent the medication from leaking out before or during the injection, 0.2 ml of air should be drawn into the syringe. The bubble will rise to the plunger end when the injection is given and the syringe is inverted. It is harmless and reduces leakage along the needle injection path after the injection is made.

Preparation of patient. As with subcutaneous injec-

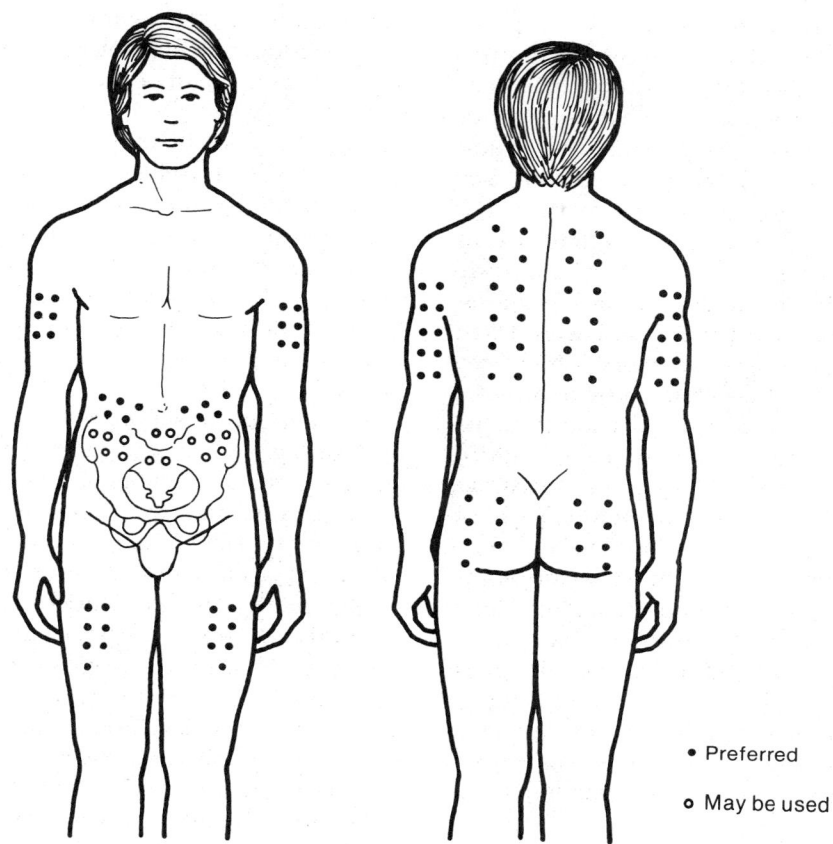

FIGURE 2-14. **Subcutaneous injection sites.**

• Preferred

o May be used

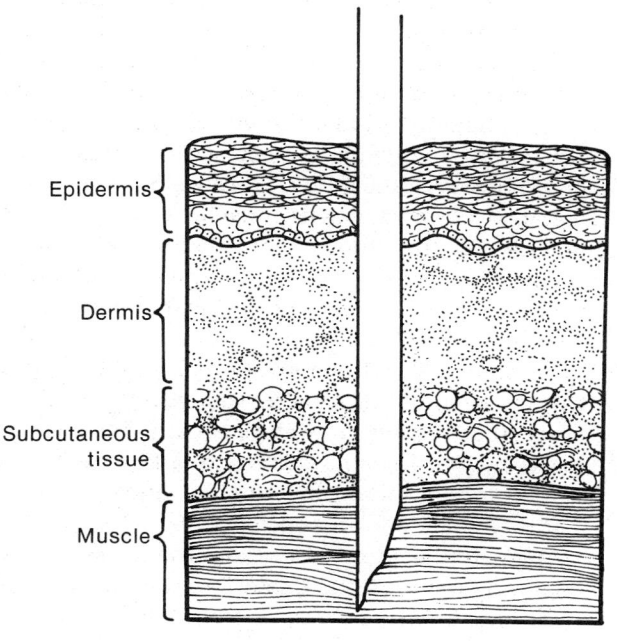

Epidermis

Dermis

Subcutaneous tissue

Muscle

FIGURE 2-15. **Intramuscular injections. Intramuscular injections are given with 1 to 3 inch (2.5 to 7.5 cm) needles depending on the amount of subcutaneous fat present over the muscle site; 19- to 25-gauge needles are usually used and are selected in relation to the viscosity of the medication to be injected. To minimize the pain of injections, the nurse should use the largest number gauge needle possible (i.e., smallest diameter). Intramuscular injection needles must be carefully selected so that the medication will be delivered to the muscle and not the subcutaneous tissues because irritation and severe sloughing with some medications can occur.**

tions, adults and children can move during the injection. Infants and small children should be restrained firmly but gently. The older child and adult may need assistance with the restraining of the extremity to be injected. For intramuscular injections, the nurse should tell the patient to relax the muscle being used because this will decrease pain. A positive attitude is important with children. Distraction is often helpful. The injection should never be introduced as punishment, and therapeutic needle play is important, especially for preschoolers and young children. Older children should be encouraged to express their feelings. It is helpful to the older child to be allowed to talk about fears, anger, or other feelings about the injection. The nurse can talk to the adult while giving the injection to distract him. Many approaches can be used, and parents or other family members can be involved (see section on subcutaneous injections).

Intramuscular injection sites. Site selection is important in administering intramuscular injections. Medications should not be delivered to subcutaneous tissue but to muscle mass. Muscles contain more blood vessels and have fewer sensory nerve endings than other sites; however, the potential for puncturing blood vessels, which may result in bleeding or the inadvertent administration of the medication intravenously, is great.

Only healthy muscle that is well vascularized is selected. It should not be painful to touch or have evidence of hardened masses. Necrotic areas, abscesses, and sloughing tissue must be avoided. After the site is selected, the muscle should be rolled between the fingers and assessed for twitching. Extrasensitive areas will twitch when the muscle mass is rolled under the fingers. Injection into this area can cause referred or sharp pain as if a nerve had been hit.

Intramuscular injections can also cause nerve and bone damage resulting in pain and perhaps permanent disability, including paralysis and periostitis. Because of these dangers, it is important that the nurse visualize and palpate landmarks and boundaries carefully in a good light. Although she should ensure patient privacy, the site must be sufficiently exposed for accurate site location.

A number of sites can be used for the administration of intramuscular injections. The usual sites used are the deltoid muscles of the upper arms, the gluteal muscles of the buttocks, and the rectus femoris and vastus lateralis muscles of the quadriceps muscle group of the thighs. The site selected depends on the age of the patient, the size of the muscle and its condition, the medication being injected, and the number of injections to be given.

DELTOID SITE. The deltoid muscle is *seldom* used now for intramuscular injections because of its small size. However, it can be used for some immunizations or when rotation of sites is necessary for extensive therapy. Only small amounts of medication should be given at this site. To locate the densest area of muscle and to avoid the radial nerve and major blood vessels, the nurse should identify a point on the lateral aspect of the upper arm, about 1 to 2 inches (2.5 to 5 cm) inferior to the lower edge of the acromion process in line with the axilla (Figure 2-16). The needle is inserted at a right angle or pointed slightly toward the acromial process.

The deltoid muscle is *not* recommended for children under 1½ years of age because of its small size and the position of nerves and vessels. Immunizations, however, are routinely given in this site because of its accessibility. For children under 15 years of age, 0.5 ml can be given. Those 15 years and older can receive 0.5 to 2 ml. It is recommended however, that this site be used *only* when necessary and for small volumes (0.5 ml or less) of medication. For some elderly and for others in wheelchairs who are self-propelling, the deltoid is better developed than other sites because of its use and offers an alternate intramuscular site.

DORSOGLUTEAL SITE. The dorsogluteal site is *not* recommended for use in infants less than 18 months of age because the muscle mass is not well developed until the child has begun walking for at least a year. Up to 1 ml can be administered to the 2½- to 3-year-old child, although great care must be taken in correct site identification, because of the proximity of the sciatic nerve. The 3- to 6-year-old can receive up to 1.5 ml of medication by this route and the 6- to 15-year-old 1.5 to 2 ml. Those older than 15 can receive 2 to 4 ml comfortably if the muscle mass is healthy. In active healthy adults, the gluteal muscles are the most commonly used muscles for intramuscular injection. However, the gluteal muscles have the slowest drug absorption rate. This muscle is likely to be degenerated in the elderly, nonwalking, or emaciated patient. The nurse must be accurate in identifying landmarks to avoid injuring the sciatic nerve and superior gluteal arteries.

The patient should be positioned on the abdomen with the femurs internally rotated. Research has shown that toeing in reduces pain and bleeding caused by the injection. The patient is made comfortable and draped; however, the dorsogluteal site must be available for mapping.

To locate the site for injection, the nurse draws an imaginary line from the posterior superior iliac spine to the greater trochanter of the femur. This line is

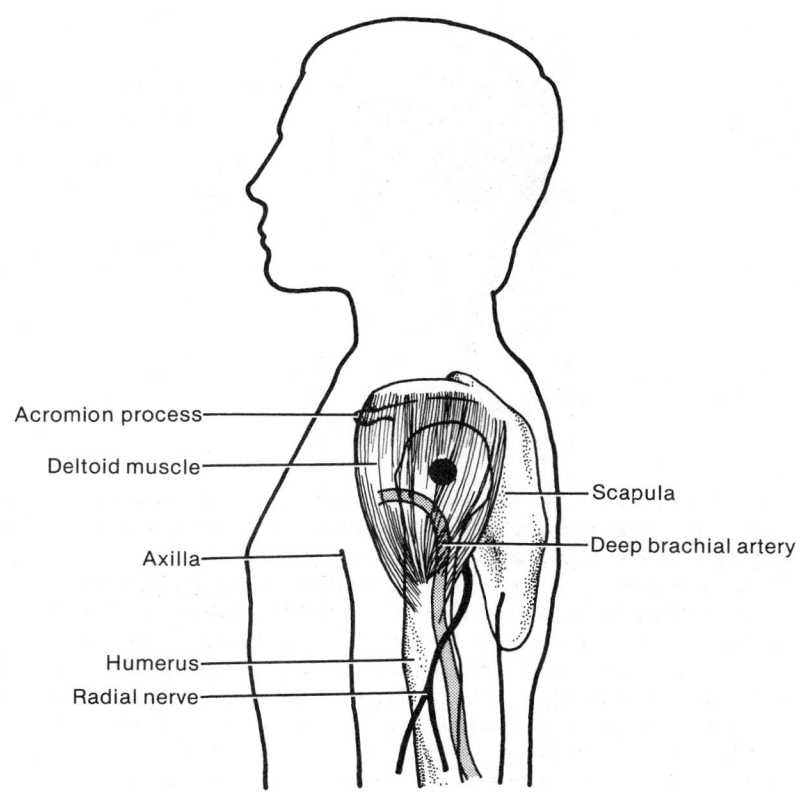

FIGURE 2-16. **Deltoid site for intramuscular injection. To locate the densest area of muscle and to avoid the radial nerve and deep brachial artery, the nurse should identify a point on the lateral upper arm, 1 to 2 inches (2.5 to 5 cm) inferior to the lower edge of the acromion process in line with the axilla. The needle is inserted at a right angle or pointed slightly toward the acromion process. Because of the small size of this muscle and the proximity of major nerves and blood vessels, this site should only be used when necessary and for small volumes of medication (0.5 ml).**

lateral to and parallel to the sciatic nerve and thus a site selected laterally and superiorly to this line will be away from the sciatic nerve as well as from the major blood vessels (Figure 2-17). The gluteal muscle can also be injected with the patient standing with toes in or lying on his side. To relax the muscle when the patient is on his side, the nurse should position the patient with the knee and hip of the upper leg flexed and anterior to the lower leg.

The child must be prone on a flat surface and the injection given at right angles to the surface on which he is lying.

This site can be selected for injecting irritating drugs using the Z-track method of administration (a discussion of this method follows later in this chapter).

VENTROGLUTEAL SITE. The ventrogluteal site uses the gluteus medius and gluteus minimus muscles. This site has a larger muscle mass and less subcutaneous tissue than the dorsogluteal site. It is accessible from supine, prone, standing, and lateral recumbent positions. Since this site is relatively free from major nerves and vessels, it is recommended for children over 3 years who have been walking; however, care must be taken that the injection is not made into a bone or a joint. This site is not generally recommended for children under 3, although it can be used for children older than 18 months, if other sites are not available. An injection of up to 1 ml can be given. For preschool children 1.5 ml can be given and for school age children up to 2 ml. Adolescents and adults can be given up to 2 to 2.5 ml. This site is also commonly used in elderly, nonwalking, and emaciated patients because the muscle mass of the gluteus medius and vastus lateralis are likely to be degenerated.

To locate this site, the nurse locates the greater trochanter of the femur with the heel of the hand, with

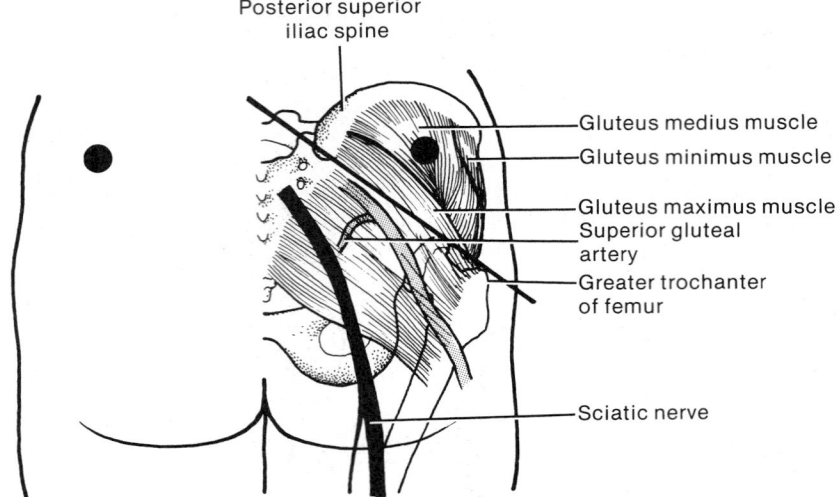

Posterior superior
iliac spine

Gluteus medius muscle

Gluteus minimus muscle

Gluteus maximus muscle

Superior gluteal
artery

Greater trochanter
of femur

Sciatic nerve

FIGURE 2-17. **Dorsogluteal site for intramuscular injection. To locate the site for injection, the nurse should draw an imaginary line from the posterior superior iliac spine to the greater trochanter of the femur. Because this line is lateral to and parallel to the sciatic nerve, a site selected laterally and superiorly will be away from the nerve as well as the superior gluteal artery. The injection is made into the gluteus medius muscle. To relax the muscle for injection and to reduce pain, the patient should toe-in. The needle should be inserted at right angles to the surface on which the patient is lying. The dorsogluteal site is *not* recommended for use in infants less than 18 months of age because the muscle mass is not well developed until the child has been walking for at least a year. Great care must be taken in mapping this site because of the proximity of the sciatic nerve and major vessels.**

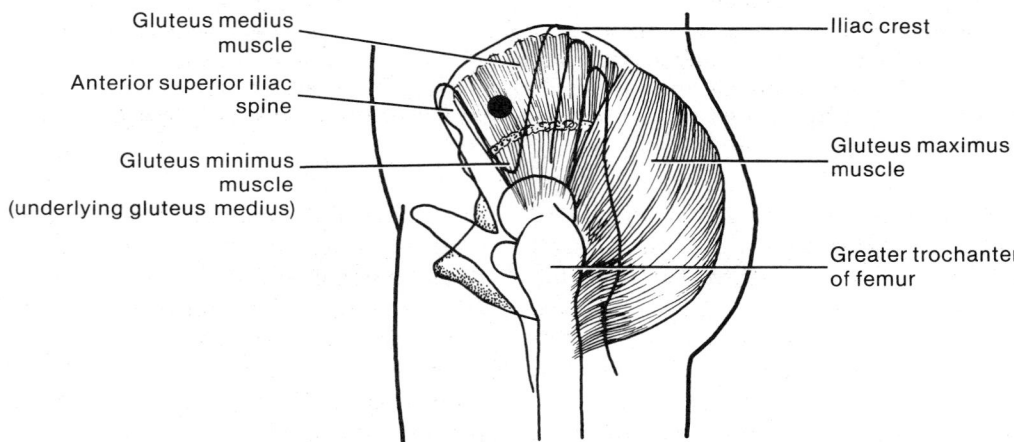

Gluteus medius
muscle

Anterior superior iliac
spine

Gluteus minimus
muscle
(underlying gluteus medius)

Iliac crest

Gluteus maximus
muscle

Greater trochanter
of femur

FIGURE 2-18. **Ventrogluteal site for intramuscular injection. To locate this site, the nurse palpates the greater trochanter of the femur with the heel of the hand. The index and middle fingers are spread to form a V from the anterior superior iliac spine to just below the iliac crest. The triangle formed between the index finger, the middle finger, and the crest of the ilium is the injection site. The injection is made in the center area of the triangle with the needle directed slightly toward the iliac crest or at a right angle to the muscle. This site is relatively free from major nerves and vessels and has a larger muscle mass and less subcutaneous tissue than the dorsogluteal site. It is recommended for adults and children over 3 years of age who have been walking.**

the fingers pointing toward the patient's head. The right hand is used for palpating the left hip, and the left hand is used for palpating the right hip. The index and middle fingers are spread to form a V from the anterior superior iliac spine to just below the iliac crest. The triangle formed between the index finger, the third finger, and the crest of the ilium is the injection site (Figure 2-18). Injections are made in center of the triangle with the needle directed slightly toward the iliac crest or at a right angle to the muscle.

The drug can be administered at this site with the patient lying on the back or side. A prone position with the toes pointed inward or a sidelying position with the top knee flexed and in front of the lower leg is recommended to relax the muscle.

For adults, a 20 to 23 gauge, 1½ to 3 inch (3.8 to 7.6 cm) needle is used, and 1 to 5 ml can be injected.

VASTUS LATERALIS SITE. The vastus lateralis can be used for deep IM and Z-track injections because the site is free from major nerves and vessels. It is the preferred intramuscular injection site for children. The muscle is well developed at birth.

In the child, the medial outer aspect in the center one-third portion of the thigh is selected. The belly of the muscle is one third the distance between the greater trochanter and the knee. The muscle mass is gently lifted away from the bone for injection. The needle should not be longer than 1 inch in the child. Up to 0.5 to 1 ml can be administered per injection to infants less than 18 months, and toddlers can receive 1 ml comfortably. Preschoolers can receive up to 1.5 ml and the school age child to 15 years can receive 1.5 to 2 ml.

The vastus lateralis site is recommended for giving larger volumes of medication for these reasons: the muscle is large in healthy active adults, has only a thin covering of fat, is away from major blood vessels and nerves, and tolerates up to 5 ml well.

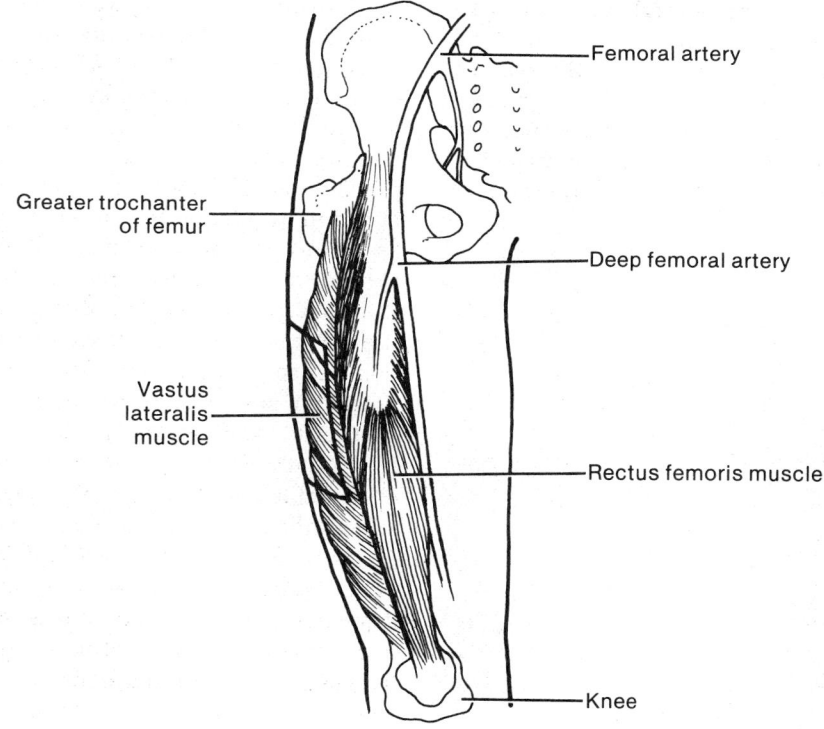

FIGURE 2-19. **Vastus lateralis site for intramuscular injection. The vastus lateralis site is located on the medial outer aspect in the center third portion of the thigh in children. The belly of the muscle is one-third the distance between the greater trochanter and the knee. It is the preferred site in children as it is well developed at birth. It is also recommended for adults because the muscle is large and can take up to 5 ml of medication per single injection. In the adult the site for injection is from one hand's breadth below the greater trochanter to a hand's breath above the knee. The injection should be given at a right angle to the muscle or on an angle slightly toward the knee.**

In the adult the vastus lateralis is located on the anterolateral aspect of the thigh from a hand's breadth below the greater trochanter to a hand's breadth above the knee (Figure 2-19). The patient can be positioned on the back or in a sitting position. The needle should be inserted on an angle slightly toward the knee or at right angles to the muscle.

The muscle is likely to be degenerated in the elderly, nonwalking, and emaciated patient, and should *not* be used.

RECTUS FEMORIS SITE. The rectus femoris muscle is located on the anterior aspect of the thigh (Figure 2-20). It is recommended for use in infants and children because it is better developed and is an alternate site for the vastus lateralis. It is also used by patients for self-injection because of its accessibility. Injections can be given when the patient is sitting or lying flat.

For adults, it is recommended that a 22 to 25 gauge, ½ to 1 inch (1.3 to 2.5 cm) needle be used, and 1 to 3 ml can be injected into this site.

Administration. The amount of medication that can be injected into a site varies, but usually 1 to 5 ml is considered to be the maximum range in the average adult. The maximum in infants, frail elderly, or emaciated patients is 1 to 2 ml. The nurse must use her judgment in determining the amount of the injection, based on assessment of the patient in relation to health state, size and health of muscle, adequacy of blood supply, and individual preferences.

To decrease the pain associated with giving the injection, it is recommended that a plastic glove of ice be held at the selected site for a few minutes to numb it. The site is prepared with ethyl alcohol or povidone-iodine to prevent the introduction of microorganisms. Before using iodine preparations, the nurse should find out if the patient has an allergy to iodine. The site is cleansed in a circular fashion from the center out for approximately 2 inches (5 cm). The syringe is held at a 90-degree angle, unless otherwise specified, and quickly inserted with a darting action to minimize pain. The tissue is released, and the plunger is gently aspirated so that it can be determined if the needle is in a blood vessel. If no blood is withdrawn into the syringe, the medication is slowly injected to allow it to spread into the tissue under less pressure. If blood appears in the syringe with aspiration, the needle should be withdrawn, and the injection prepared again using sterile equipment. A sterile antiseptic swab is held at the site. The needle is withdrawn quickly and smoothly and the area is wiped with an antiseptic swab. The relaxed muscle may be massaged to distribute the medication and to increase absorption unless this is contraindicated. A Band-Aid can be placed over the site if desired. This is especially important to children in relation to maintaining body integrity and as a reward. Exercise of the limb will also increase absorption and reduce pain.

Z-TRACK INJECTION. The Z-track injection is used for the administration of thick irritating drugs such as iron dextran to avoid subcutaneous irritation and discoloration or staining of the subcutaneous tissues (Figure 2-21). A 19- to 20-gauge, 2 to 3 inch (5 to 7.5 cm) needle is used to draw up the medication. The needle is changed to avoid tracking the medication through the subcutaneous tissue, and 0.2 to 0.5 ml of air is drawn up into the syringe to prevent leakage of the medication into the subcutaneous tissues after injection. After the site is selected, at least a 4-inch (10 cm) area is cleansed with an alcohol or povidone-iodine swab. The skin, and subcutaneous fat are retracted laterally down and medially, at least 1 inch with the ulnar side

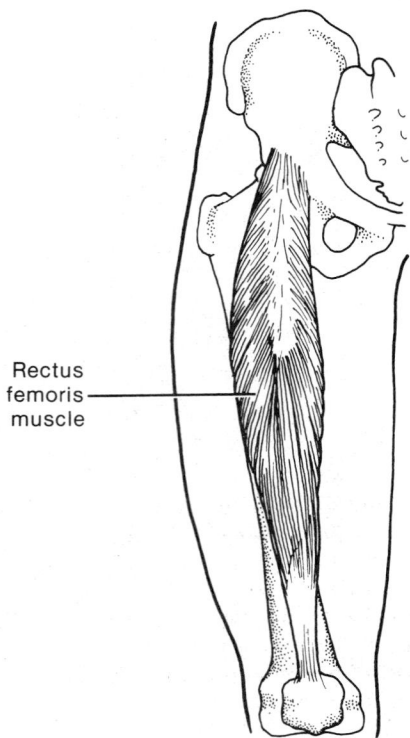

Rectus
femoris
muscle

FIGURE 2-20. **Rectus femoris site for intramuscular injection. The rectus femoris is located on the anterior aspect of the thigh and is recommended as an alternate site for the vastus lateralis in infants and children. The site can also be used for adults.**

of the nondominant hand at the injection site before the needle is inserted at a 90-degree angle. It is important to note that although the skin and subcutaneous layers are retracted, the muscle remains at the original landmarked site. The plunger is gently aspirated and if no blood appears, the medication is injected slowly. The skin is held continuously in the retracted position for 10 seconds before the needle is withdrawn. The needle is quickly and smoothly removed straight out, and the tissues are allowed to return to their normal position. Pressure is applied at the site. The site should *not* be rubbed or massaged. No more than 2 ml of iron dextran should be administered into one site. The dorsal gluteal and vastus lateralis muscles, because of their size, should be selected. The tissue should be retracted down and medially when the dorsal gluteal site is used. For courses of therapy in which more than one or two injections are required, intravenous therapy with an appropriate injectable form of iron should be considered. The prescriber and hospital policy will need to be consulted.

This method of injection has been recommended as an alternative method of administering other intramuscular medications at the gluteal and vastus lateralis sites.

Monitoring. The absorption rate of intramuscular and subcutaneous medications depends on the blood flow to the injection site.

When a patient is receiving numerous intramuscular injections, rotation of the injection sites is important. Drug absorption is thus enhanced and pain is decreased.

Serum creatine phosphokinase (CPK) levels can rise after IM injections of various medications because of trauma and destruction of muscle tissue. The nurse should consider this when monitoring patients for CPK levels. Intramuscular injections should *not* be used when patients are being treated with anticoagulants (i.e., heparin or warfarin) or when patients have severe platelet depression because deep bleeding in the muscles can result and cause tissue sloughing.

Various lesions, including nodular masses, indurated areas, deposits of unabsorbed or precipitated drug, hematomas, and abscesses, have been identified following intramuscular injections. In addition, deformities such as quadriceps contracture can result, particularly in children, from multiple intramuscular injections because of extensive fibrosis of the quadriceps femoris muscles caused by the injections. Careful monitoring and palpation of intramuscular injection sites is thus important.

Follow-up care may be indicated, especially in relation to quadriceps contracture because damage is not usually seen until after infants or children are discharged. Parents may report that their child has difficulty crawling and climbing stairs, or a stiffness of

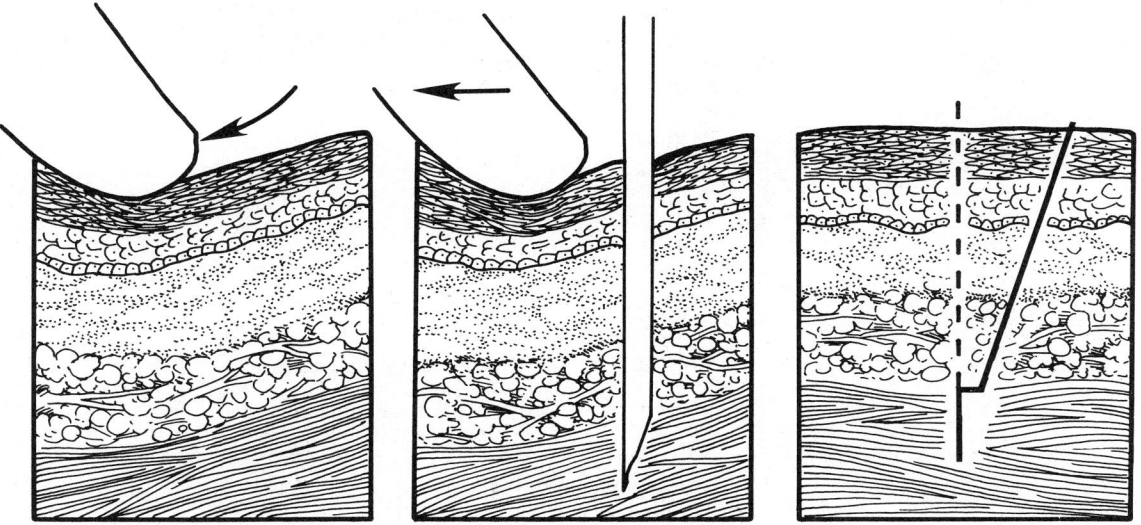

FIGURE 2-21. **Z-track technique for intramuscular injections. The skin and subcutaneous fat are retracted laterally at the injection site before the needle is inserted at a 90-degree angle. The plunger is gently aspirated, and if no blood appears, the nurse injects the medication slowly. The skin is held continuously in the retracted position for 10 seconds. The needle is removed smoothly, and the tissues are returned to their normal position.**

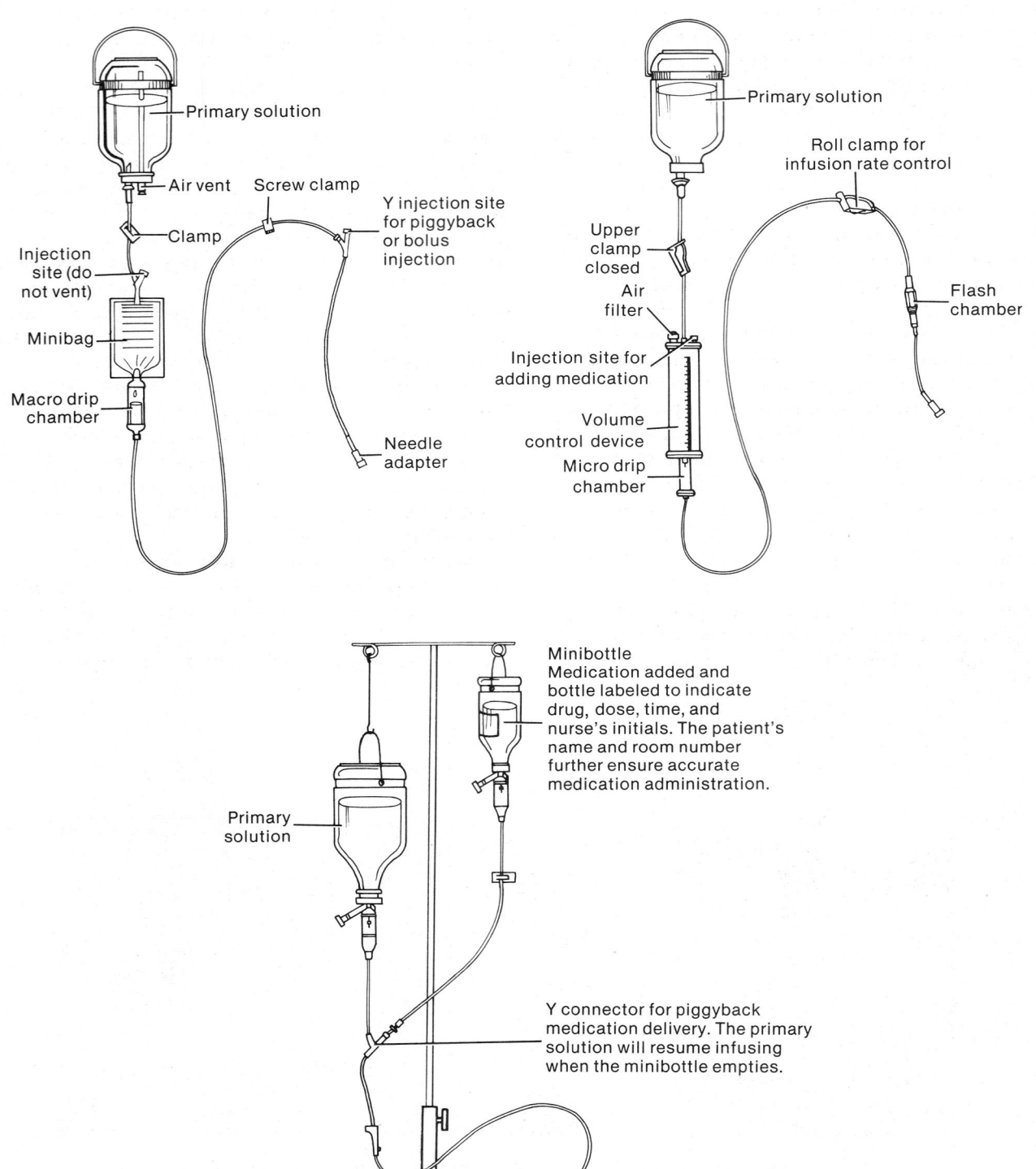

FIGURE 2-22. **Various delivery systems are available for the administration of intravenous medications.**

the knee from 4 weeks to 1 year after intramuscular injections have been given. Because of the severity of this condition, the development of which is contributed to by volume and frequency of injections, it is recommended that careful records of site rotation be kept at the patient's bedside and that the nurse follow up on children receiving large numbers of IM injections. The neonate and infant, because of the limited sites for injection, are at particular risk. Monitoring of the child is essential for early recognition of knee stiffness. It is also recommended that simple, regular, passive range-of-motion knee exercises, as well as the application of warm soaks and massage, be completed after each injection to stretch the tissue and to prevent shortening and extension contracture at the knee. Continued research in the administration of intramuscular medications is essential.

Intravenous medications. The intravenous route is used for the administration of medications (e.g., trimethaphan) when immediate drug action is required. It is also the route of choice for patients who have compromised peripheral circulation (e.g., shock, congestive heart failure) because it does not depend on blood flow to different tissues for absorption. This method of drug administration is used when volumes greater than 5 ml of a medication must be given frequently to prevent the pain and damage caused by frequent intramuscular injections. Many medications can be administered intravenously; however, because of the danger of emboli formation, aqueous suspensions and drugs prepared in oil should *not* be given by this route.

Nurses are guided by state or provincial regulations and hospital policy with regard to which medications they are allowed to administer intravenously, including those infused in various volumes of solution as well as those injected in small volumes directly into the vein. Because exaggerated or unusual pharmacologic effects can occur immediately with intravenous administration, there is little margin for error. As a safeguard in most hospitals intravenous drugs are diluted in 50 to 100 ml of solution and when possible, infused slowly rather than given as a bolus. Thus, if an undesired reaction occurs, the nurse can stop the infusion before the patient receives the total dose of medication.

When reconstituting medications for intravenous administration, the nurse must be alert to the type of diluent to add, the amount of diluent required, and how long and under what conditions the drug can be safely stored or infused once it is reconstituted or diluted.

Preparation of equipment. The equipment for establishing intravenous therapy for drug administration

varies according to the manufacturer and the therapy to be given (Figure 2-22). Various solutions (e.g., normal saline [NS], 5% dextrose in water [D$_5$W], Ringer's lactate) are supplied in sterile vacuum-sealed glass bottles or plastic bags for intravenous use. They are available in various sizes including 250, 500, and 1000 ml. Minibags, minibottles, and partial-fill bottles (i.e., 50 ml, 100 ml) are also available for intravenous medication administration.

Solution bottles are fitted with rubber stoppers and sealed with metal caps or collars. They should be examined carefully to be sure that the seal is intact before use. The bottle should not be used if the cap or metal collar is not intact. Bags should be inspected for puncture marks and leaks, especially at the additive port. Both bags and bottles should be held up to the light and rotated carefully as they are inspected for hairline cracks and cloudiness or particulate matter. The nurse should ensure that the expiration date on the solution container is current. The label, as with other medications, should be read three times to ensure accuracy in selecting solutions. Some bottles have indwelling vents, and others do not and will require vented tubing to permit air to enter the vacuum and displace the solution. Bags compress as they empty, and nonvented tubing can be used.

Intravenous tubing is supplied in sterile packages by various manufacturers and is designed for specific intravenous therapy uses. There are also various filters available that are used to decrease the risk of contamination and the amount of particulate matter that may be delivered into the bloodstream. These range from 0.22 to 5 microns.

Drip chambers are available in macrodrip or microdrip systems. The number of drops delivered per milliliter for macrodrip systems can vary according to the manufacturer. The number of drops in 1 ml is indicated on the box that the drip chamber and tubing are supplied in. It is important that the nurse know the amount delivered in each drop in order to be able to calculate the rate of infusion. For example, micro-

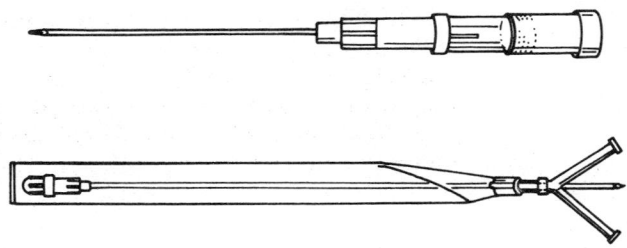

FIGURE 2-23. **Various catheters are also available for intravenous therapy.**

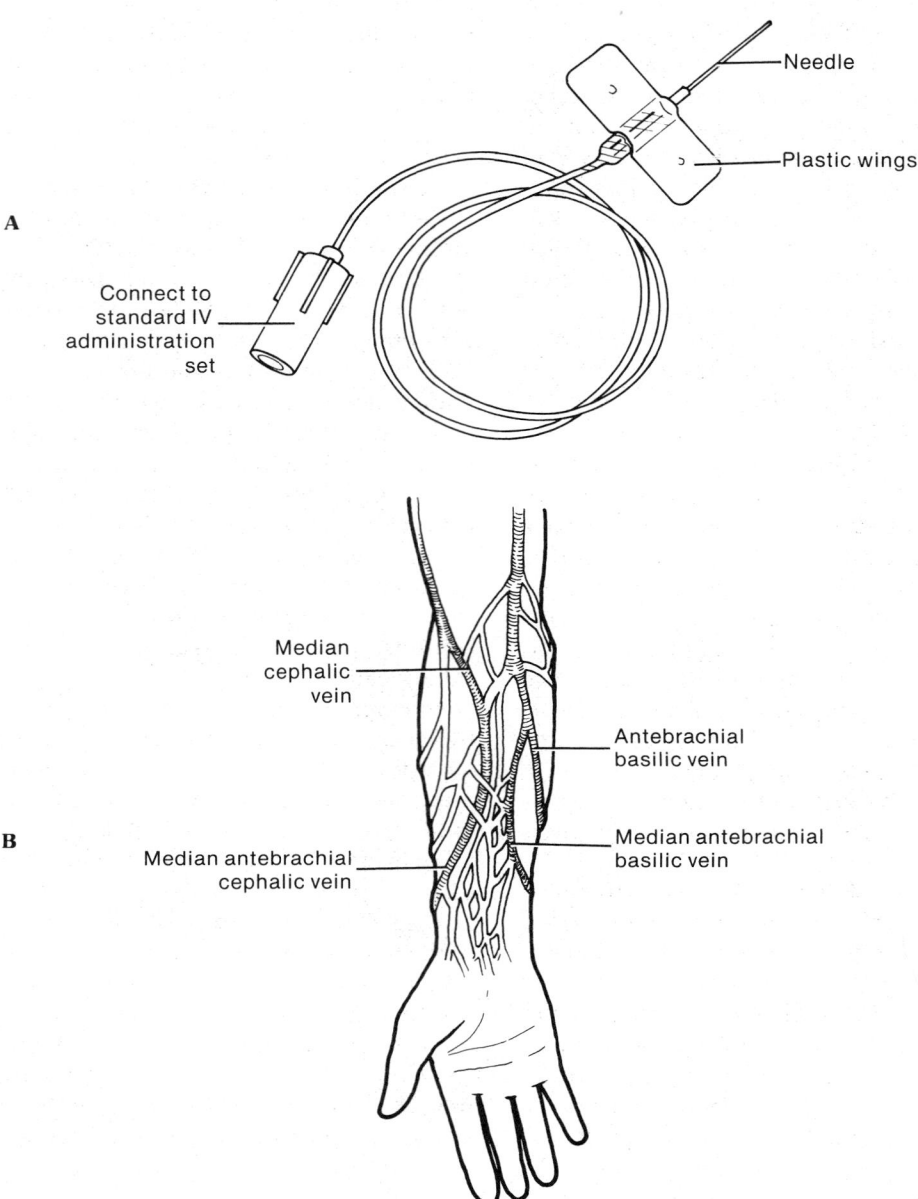

FIGURE 2-24. *A,* **The winged-tip, or butterfly, needle for intravenous injection. But-terfly needles are the most commonly used needles for intravenous injection and are available in ½ to 1¼ inch (1.3 to 3.2 cm), 18- to 25-gauge. The tubing length can vary from 3 to 12 inches (7.5 to 30 cm).** *B,* **Sites for intravenous injection. The superficial ventral basilic and cephalic veins are used, selecting distal sites first in children and adults.**

drip systems that are identified with a small needle projection at the top of the chamber deliver 60 drops per milliliter, whereas average macrodrip chambers deliver 10 to 20 drops per milliliter.

Intravenous needles and catheters (cannulas) (Figure 2-23) come in various sizes in individual sterile packages. They are coated with silicone to decrease clotting and to facilitate insertion. Over-the-needle catheters as well as inside-the-needle catheters, usually made of Teflon, are also available. They range in size from 1¼ inch (3.2 cm) to 5½ inch (14 cm) with a 12- to 22-gauge diameter. The most commonly used intravenous needles, however, are metal winged-tip or butterfly needles (Figure 2-24), which are supplied in ½ to 1¼ inch (1.3 to 3.2 cm), 18- to 25-gauge with short bevels to prevent puncture of the opposite vein wall after placement. The tubing extending from the needle may be 3 to 12 inches (7.5 to 30 cm) in length.

The age of the patient, size and condition of the vein, and the type of infusion determines the needle

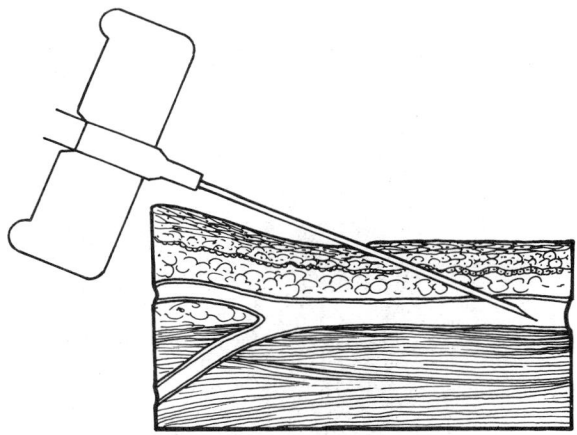

FIGURE 2-25. **Venipuncture. The vein is selected, and the site is prepared with an antiseptic as per hospital policy. A tourniquet is applied above the site, and the patient is asked to make a fist, clenching and unclenching the hand to distend the veins. The arm is grasped and the thumb is placed about 1 inch below the site to anchor the vein by gently pulling skin and vein (at bifurcation) toward the hand. The needle is inserted next to the vein at a 15-degree angle and gently advanced through the vein wall. Blood return indicates correct placement. The needle or catheter is taped securely, and the tourniquet released before injection of medication or infusion of solution. The needle should be inserted with the bevel up to facilitate insertion. If the tourniquet is not readily removed, a hematoma can result, and if the infusion is started, the vein can be damaged and the site lost.**

or cannula selected. Butterfly or winged-tip needles are generally used; however, for long-term therapy and depending on individual hospital policy, cannulas may also be used. The smallest diameter (i.e., largest gauge number needle and cannula possible should be used to minimize vein damage and to increase the amount of blood flow at the tip. Needles and catheters should be carefully inspected for defects and inaccuracies in packaging before use. The ½ inch (1.3 cm), 25-gauge scalp vein wing-tipped needle is used for infants and children; 21- to 23-gauge needles are used for older children and adults. The selection of equipment often depends on the nurse's personal preference (i.e., some nurses prefer butterfly needles and others prefer cannulas) as well as on hospital policy. The butterfly may be selected because it is easily used; however, it is not as stable after insertion as the cannula and can more easily damage the vein and cause infiltration. The cannula allows the patient more mobility and is usually selected for long-term therapy. The site, however, must be carefully assessed for infection and phlebitis, problems that tend to occur more often than with wing-tipped needles. More research is required on how medications, various needles and cannulas, the length of time the site is used, and site dressing procedures influence infiltration, inflammation, or infection rates.

Preparation of patient. In many areas of practice, the venipuncture and establishment of the intravenous site (Figure 2-25) for the delivery of intravenous fluids or medications by various systems is the responsibility of the nurse. In other areas of practice, this responsibility is shared with the physician or IV team. Before intravenous therapy is initiated, however, the patient must be carefully prepared for the procedure. Both adults and children should have an understanding of the reasons for the medications they are to receive and how these will be administered. The patient must also understand how the intravenous therapy will affect his mobility and other activities of daily living. The patient, and family as indicated, should know how to maintain the intravenous site and what to watch for in relation to its care and to any complications that might occur. With the recognition that intravenous therapy can cause fear and anxiety, the nurse must prepare patients carefully and at the patient's level of understanding. The patient should be positioned comfortably, the site prepared for the desired intravenous therapy as per hospital policy, and the venipuncture completed.

Intravenous injection sites. The site for venipuncture is selected in relation to the patient's age, purpose of infusion, state of health, duration of therapy, medication to be infused or injected, and individual patient preference (i.e., dominant or nondominant hand). Many hospitals have policies as to the sites nurses may use or not use. For example, nurses usually cannot start IV infusions in scalp or foot veins, but can start IVs below the elbow (Figure 2-24, *B*). When selecting a vein in the respective site, the nurse should select any visibly prominent vein with adequate blood flow and good elasticity.

Generally, the smallest-gauge device should be used as well as the largest possible vein to decrease phlebitis by allowing increased blood to dilute medication as it enters the vein and to reduce irritation of the vein walls by the device.

The infant and young child have small and fragile veins. Thus the venipuncture must be completed carefully. The scalp veins are large in infants proportionately, and these are usually used (Figure 2-26). The hair is shaved, and this may cause distress for parents who need to be reassured that the hair will grow out. It is essential that sites be maintained carefully so that frequent and unnecessary venipunctures are avoided.

In older children and adults the basilic and cephalic veins on the dorsal aspect of the hand are most often used for IV injections and infusions (Figure 2-27). Distal sites should be selected first and then more proximal sites selected as needed. It is preferred that the needle be inserted away from a movable joint to prevent extravasation of the needle once it is in place. Thus the antecubital fossa is usually *not* used except to draw blood or for one-time injections.

Patients requiring long-term therapy may need frequent site changes to avoid phlebitis or other complications. Sites on alternate arms should be selected to allow healing between punctures.

The infant, young child, and confused adult require restraint while the IV is started. Once the IV is started, it is carefully secured with tape and covered with a transparent dressing so that the tubing is free from kinks and the site is easily observed. An arm-board may be used to immobilize the site. Even young children learn to be careful with their IVs, and soft restraints are often not required although the young infant must be restrained when not held or supervised so that the tubing is not inadvertently pulled and the IV dislodged. Plastic cups are often cut in half and taped over the site to prevent dislodgement of the needle. In many pediatric areas, a controlled volume device (100 to 150 ml) is attached to the primary solution bottle to limit the amount of fluid that can be infused. This ensures the delivery of accurate volumes and prevents the possibility of the child receiving a large quantity directly from the bottle in a short time.

Administration. Some drugs (e.g., furosemide), because of their desired pharmacologic effect, are ad-

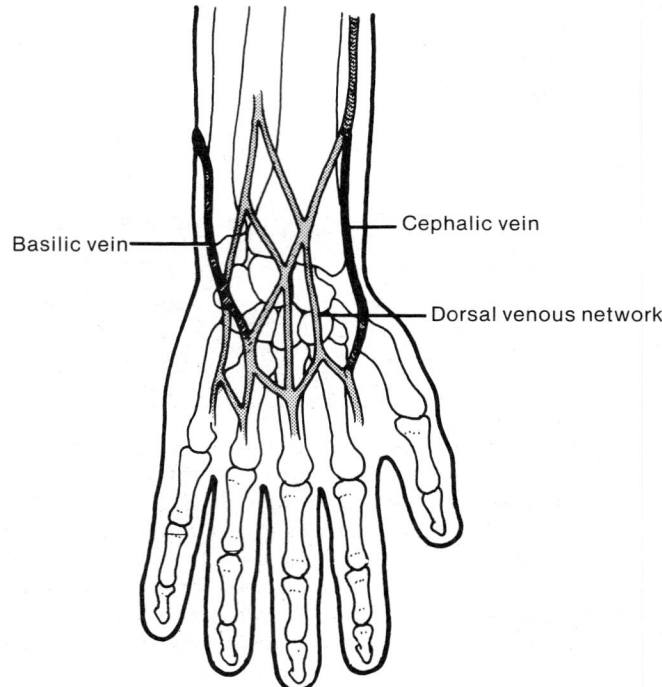

FIGURE 2-27. **Sites for intravenous injection. The basilic and cephalic veins on the dorsal aspect of the hand are the most often used sites for intravenous injections and infusions. To prevent extravasation, the nurse should not use the needle sites near movable joints, except as needed for one-time injections.**

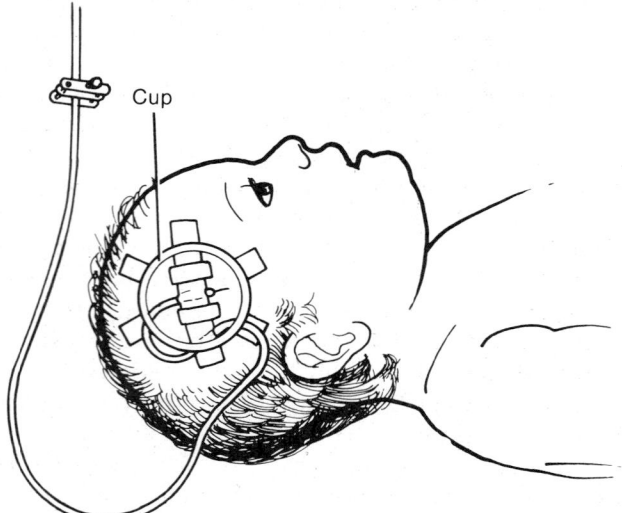

FIGURE 2-26. **Scalp vein infusion for infants.**

ministered all at once or by slow IV push. Medications that cannot be diluted because of the possibility of incompatibility (e.g., diazepam and phenytoin) are likewise administered by IV push or bolus injections. Other intravenous medications, usually because of their toxicity, are administered as continuous intravenous infusions (e.g., amphotericin B, corticotropin, multivitamins, polymyxin B, and potassium chloride) and are slowly infused, usually over 8 hours or longer. Others (e.g., amikacin, gentamicin, miconazole) are administered by intermittent intravenous infusion over 30 to 60 minutes in piggyback or volume-control devices (e.g., Buretrol, Metriset, Soluset, and Vol-U-Trol).

There are several important points for the nurse to consider when preparing and administering medications intravenously by any of these methods. The nurse must consider not only the properties of each drug, the desired action, untoward effects, and individual patient variables, but also the type and amount of drug diluent, rate of administration, the length of time the reconstituted drug can be stored, and drug incompatibility.

After the nurse prepares the medication and determines the dilution required and the rate at which to infuse the medication, she is ready to administer it. Medications can be infused slowly and continuously in primary solutions as admixtures, they can be given intermittently, or they can be given by IV bolus directly into a patent line, a heparin lock, or vein.

ADMINISTRATION OF INTRAVENOUS MEDICATIONS IN PRIMARY SOLUTIONS. Many medications are added to primary IV solutions for slow continuous infusion. When adding medications to primary solutions, the nurse must be especially alert to incompatibilities that may be caused by acid-base or chemical reactions resulting in the destruction of the drug administered (see Appendix IV, "Intravenous Incompatibilities"). When mixing admixtures, the nurse must be observant to color changes and cloudiness, which often indicate incompatibilities. It is recommended that the most concentrated drug be added first and mixed thoroughly before other drugs are added. Colored additives should be added last because they may mask possible precipitates or cloudiness. Liquid medications for intravenous use can be added directly to the primary solution with sterile technique. Others can be added after reconstitution. A filter should be used when drawing up the medication so that particulate matter can be removed. The filter should be removed before the medication is injected into the solution.

When adding medications to a bottle that has already been superimposed with vented tubing, the nurse carefully removes the air vent and injects the medication into the air vent port. For vented bottles, the medication is injected into the triangle area on the rubber stopper after it is carefully wiped with an alcohol swab. When adding medication to a bag, the nurse wipes the medication port with an alcohol swab and injects the medication.

To prevent delivering the drug all at once to the patient, the nurse should close the flow clamp before injection of the medication and gently rotate the bottle or bag to mix the medication after it is injected. The clamp is then opened, and the flow rate adjusted accordingly. A label indicating the medication added, the dose, time, date, and initials of the nurse is attached to the bag or bottle and the medication and any other pertinent observations are recorded.

Because of the complexity of admixture preparation, as well as the risk of contamination, the pharmacy departments at some hospitals are completing the procedure with the use of laminar air flow hoods. Prepared IV additives are supplied to the nurse in partial-fill bottles or minibags. In addition, some drugs in bulk vials can be frozen by the pharmacist after reconstitution, thus preventing loss of stability during prolonged storage.

INTERMITTENT ADMINISTRATION OF INTRAVENOUS MEDICATIONS. IV additive sets or volume-control devices are used for intermittent administration of medications. Intermittent infusion therapy is used when a patient needs an IV drug regularly but does not need additional fluid or activity restrictions imposed by a continuous IV. The use of additive sets enables the nurse to administer different drugs at different times and can be used when the drug is not compatible with the primary solution.

Medication is added under sterile technique to partial-fill bottles, minibottles, or minibags that are superimposed into primary intravenous lines or into heparin locks. The medication can be infused simultaneously with the primary solution, or if it is incompatible, it can be infused alone. Medication is also delivered in intermittent infusion devices (i.e., volume-control devices), which are available in various models (e.g., Buretrol, Metriset) with membrane or floating valve filters. The operation of various devices can differ, and the nurse should refer to the directions on the package or seek hospital in-service instruction.

When the drug is incompatible with an infusing solution, the tubing must be cleared with a compatible solution before the medication can be introduced. After the medication is infused, the tubing will have to be cleared with compatible solution again before the primary solution is allowed to infuse again. A common example is the incompatibility of antibiotics with solutions of multiple vitamins, which can diminish the potency of the antibiotics.

BOLUS OR PUSH ADMINISTRATION OF INTRAVENOUS MEDICATIONS. Some IV medications are delivered by "push" directly into the vein, IV tubing of a continuous IV, or heparin lock. For example, diazoxide must be delivered intravenously over 5 minutes because it is highly protein bound. Other medications may be delivered in less than 5 minutes, such as atropine, sodium bicarbonate, or vincristine. The rate of administration varies among drugs.

Generally, medications that are injected directly into the vein should be given slowly and in not less than 1 minute because the blood from a peripheral vein can reach the heart and brain in 15 seconds under normal circulatory conditions. Blood flow through the entire circulatory system is completed in approximately 1 minute. If medications are administered too rapidly, speed shock can occur, in which the drug may reach the heart or brain in high concentrations resulting in headache, tightness in the chest, shock, or cardiac arrest. When the medication is given slowly, it has a chance to mix with the blood before delivery to the heart and brain. Recommended rates of infusion are indicated by manufacturers, and these guidelines should be carefully followed because intravenous absorption is instantaneous. Emergency equipment and medications should be on hand in case of reactions, especially for the first dose of medications. The rate of bolus intravenous administration can be computed by dividing the total amount of medication to be injected by the recommended time. No drug should ordinarily be administered by IV push in less than 1 minute.

When administering compatible medications into the IV tubing of a primary line by IV push, the nurse swabs the injection port with an antiseptic and inserts the needle into the center area indicated on the rubber port. The tubing behind the point of insertion is pinched or, if preferred, clamped with the roller or screw clamp. The syringe plunger is gently pulled back to check for blood return. If the needle or cannula is patent, the medication is injected at the prescribed rate. The patient should be observed for at least 15 seconds after the medication is first introduced for side effects or untoward reactions. The clamp is opened and the solution allowed to run through the tubing to clear the medication and to decrease irritation of the vein. Then the flow rate is adjusted. The administration of the medication and other pertinent information is recorded.

HEPARIN LOCKS. Heparin locks are increasingly being used for both intermittent and bolus intravenous injections because they allow more freedom for the patient and prevent the need for repeated needle injections. They are used for both children and adults.

The heparin lock is a needle or catheter that is placed into the vein, filled with heparin solution to prevent back flow and clotting of blood, and capped with a special rubber cap. The heparin lock is maintained with heparinized solutions of 10 to 100 units of heparin per milliliter of saline. The cap can be taped to prevent it from inadvertently coming apart, and the child as well as the adult should be cautioned against tampering with it. As with the IV butterfly or cannula, if it should be inadvertently pulled out, the patient and family should have knowledge about applying pressure to the site to stop bleeding and to notify the nurse. All patients on any type of heparin therapy should be monitored for blood coagulation problems before and during treatment. The nurse should observe the site for hemorrhage, discoloration, or other signs of prolonged clotting time.

Strict aseptic technique is used as with all other intravenous therapy. The heparin lock is wiped with an alcohol swab, the site is checked for patency, and the medication is injected with a 1 inch (2.5 cm) needle according to the required rate of administration. The syringe is withdrawn and normal saline is injected to flush the medication through the tubing followed by the heparinized solution (e.g., 1 ml dilute heparin solution 100 units/ml) to prevent coagulation and to keep the tubing patent until the medication is administered again.

When medications are given continuously by intravenous infusion, it is important that the rate be maintained accurately. Thus it becomes necessary, especially with potent medications, that an electronic infusion-control system such as a gravity controller or an infusion pump be used.

There are many models of electronic infusion control devices (ICD); however, there are basically two main types: the gravity controller and the infusion pump (e.g., syringe, peristaltic, or cassette pump). Both types are available in volumetric or nonvolumetric models that deliver fluid at a constant volume or at a constant drop rate, respectively. Drugs such as dopamine, nitroglycerin, sodium nitroprusside, or oxytocin are best infused with a nonvolumetric ICD; whereas total parenteral nutrition (TPN) could be infused with a volumetric ICD. These could also be used in providing therapy to patients requiring accurate fluid volume regulation such as neonates or patients with renal dysfunction or severe congestive heart failure. Because the viscosity of a solution can affect drop size, the volumetric ICD is more accurate than the nonvolumetric ICD. Although an alarm will indicate a malfunction in these systems, infusion pumps will continue to deliver fluid even if the needle is in an interstitial space. This can result in severe tissue infiltration especially if irritating or vesicant drugs are infused. There are some electronic monitoring devices to prevent this; however, the nurse is still required to monitor therapy carefully. ICDs are not infallible in relation to dry chambers, air in the tubing, occluded lines, and improper rates; thus they should be calibrated by the nurse for safety. There are also battery-powered pumps that can be used, allowing the patient more freedom. The nurse must be sure that batteries are charged and that the ICD is functioning correctly.

Monitoring. The nurse must be alert to and monitor for several complications that are associated with intravenous therapy. These include fluid overload, infection, sensitivity reactions, infiltration, phlebitis, and embolism or thrombus formation.

Circulatory overload is a problem with intravenous therapy, especially in relation to compromised patients, the elderly, those with congestive heart failure or renal disease, and infants and young children. The infusion of IV fluid and medication thus requires close monitoring in the infant, child, and critically ill adult. Because of the possibilities of fluid overload, careful regulation of the rate of infusion is essential. IV drip rates should be monitored every 15 to 30 minutes and the hourly amounts administered recorded. ICDs should be used as indicated.

Because the vein is penetrated, the intravenous administration of medications poses the everpresent risk of infection. The nurse should be alert to not only the signs of local infection, but also to the signs indicating systemic infection, which can result from contaminated equipment or solutions, poor patient instruction on site care, or poor nursing technique.

When medications are administered intravenously, the nurse must also be alert to signs of drug sensitivity. Since effects are immediate, especially with bolus injections, the patient needs close monitoring. Patients should be asked to report any unusual effects including chills, nausea, local pain, burning, or itching. If these occur, the infusion should be stopped immediately and the prescriber notified. The nurse should observe the patient's behavior toward the IV and ability to perform activities of daily living, including ambulation and movement in bed. She should also be alert to the flow rate, patency of the line, and the level of fluid in the bottle, especially if a small amount of fluid is used for medication administration. The nurse must be certain that the medication has infused completely and that the patient is not experiencing any untoward

effects from the drug. In addition, infusion bottles must be regularly checked so that they do not run dry and result in the site being lost.

The most common local complications of intravenous drug therapy are infiltration and phlebitis. Infiltration is infusion of the solution into the subcutaneous tissue spaces which results when the needle is not in the vein. Swelling around the site of the needle or cannula can be observed, and the patient may complain of pain. The involved extremity should be compared with the opposite extremity. An early sign the nurse should be alert to is a sluggish or slowed rate of infusion. Infiltration can occur when the IV bottle is hung excessively high—the higher the bottle is hung, the greater the gravitational force, the faster the flow and the greater the risk of phlebitis and infiltration. All other things being equal (i.e., patient's position, patency of tubing, placement of needle) simply raising the IV bottle from 3 feet (91 cm) to 6 feet (183 cm) above the patient would cause the flow rate to increase 400%. Lowering the bottle slows the flow rate the same degree. The infusion of intravenous fluids thus requires constant monitoring in relation to position, clamp regulation, movement and stretching of the line. The effect on flow rate when an IV infusion container is raised or lowered can be calculated as follows:

$$\frac{(\text{present height})^2}{(\text{previous height})^2} \times 100\% \text{ of original flow rate}$$

To reduce the possibility of infiltration, the nurse must avoid placing the IV needle near a movable joint and use a heparin lock if the patient requires frequent IV medications but does not require continuous fluids.

Because many medications are extremely irritating to tissues, it is imperative that the nurse be sure of the patency of the infusion line before medications are administered in order to prevent extravasation. Severe sloughing of tissue has resulted, especially with medications such as antineoplastics, from needles improperly positioned outside of the vein.

Another important side effect of administering medications by the IV route is phlebitis, which results from trauma of the vein caused by the needle, the cannula, or the medication. Some drugs, such as potassium chloride and cephalothin, are irritating, and when patients are receiving these medications, the skin should be observed for redness and increased skin temperature over the course of the vein. Patient complaints of burning pain along the vein should be heeded. If these are observed, the infusion is to be stopped and restarted in an alternate site before the medication is readministered. Further use of the vein is to be avoided. It is important that the infusion site not be taped over or covered so that it can be observed carefully at the beginning of drug infusion and when it is finished. The use of collodion dressings is recommended.

To check for developing phlebitis, the nurse can pinch the IV line just behind the venipuncture and gently compress the flash chamber. This dilates the vein at the entry site, which causes pain if the vein is inflamed.

Research regarding the development of phlebitis secondary to IV infusion has found that the rates of phlebitis were decreased with more frequent tubing changes, thus, it is recommended that IV tubing be changed at least every 24 hours.

The amount of air required for fatal embolism has not been determined and is often a concern of patients. When infusing medications, the nurse must be careful not to inadvertently administer air when a bottle or Vol-U-Trol is allowed to run out. The amount of air in the tubing is approximately 10 ml, but blood usually backs up into the line, occluding the needle, and the line is lost and needs to be restablished. This may result in thrombus formation at the needle end. Under no circumstances should the site be irrigated with a syringe because the thrombus can be detached, resulting in severe complications (e.g., pulmonary embolus).

Thus, monitoring and appropriate nursing action in response to observed complications of intravenous drug therapy play an extremely important role in providing the patient with optimum drug therapy.

SUMMARY

Nursing responsibilities are expanding in relation to the increased complexity of drug therapy. In order to provide optimum drug therapy to patients, nurses must apply unique nursing knowledge and skills in preparing, administering, and monitoring medications.

The preparation, administration, and monitoring of oral, rectal, vaginal, ophthalmic, otic, nasal, topical, and parenteral medications has been discussed. The administration of inhalants is discussed in Section V, "Respiratory and Related Medications." Additional information in relation to specific drugs can be found in the medication chapters of Sections III to XV of this text.

BIBLIOGRAPHY

Akers, M.J. Ocular bioavailability of topically applied ophthalmic drugs. *American Pharmacy*, NS23, *1*, 1983, 33-36.

Amonsen, S., & Gren, J.E. Relationship between length of time and contamination in open intravenous solutions. *Nursing Research*, 1978, *27*, 372-374.

Bell, S.K. Guidelines for taking a complete drug history, *Nursing 80*, 1980, (March), 10-11.

Bruning, W.C. & Setaro, J. Oral solid dosage forms: be sure before you crush them. *Pharmacy Times*, 1983, Nov., 28-30.

Chapin, G., Shull, H., & Welk, P.C. Potential for error using textbook technique for intramuscular administration. *Am. J. Hosp. Pharm.*, 1983, *40*, 385.

Cockshott, W., et al. Intramuscular or intralipomatous injections? *New England Journal of Medicine*, 1982, *307*, 356.

Cohen, M.R. Medication errors, *Nursing 80*, 1980, June, 12.

Coyle, N. Analgesics at the bedside. *American Journal of Nursing*, 1979, *79*, 1554-1557.

Drehobl, P. Quadriceps contracture. *American Journal of Nursing*, 1980, *80*, 1650-1651.

Erickson, R. Tube talk: principles of fluid flow in tubes. *Nursing '82*, 1982, July, 55-62.

Evans, M.L., & Hansen, B.D. Administering injections to different-aged children. *Maternal Child Nursing*, 1981, *6*, 194-199.

Geolot, D.H., & McKinney, N.P. Administering parenteral drugs. *American Journal of Nursing*, 1975, *75*, 788-793.

Giving medication through a nasogastric tube. *Nursing '80*, 1980, May, 71-73.

Hayter, J. Why response to medication changes with age. *Geriatric Nursing*, 1981, *2*, 411-416.

Huey, F.L. Setting up and troubleshooting. *American Journal of Nursing*, 1983, *83*, 1026-1028.

Hurd, P.D., & Blevins, J. Aging and the color of pills. (Letter to the editor) *The New England Journal of Medicine*, Jan. 19, 1984, p. 202.

Jerrett, M.D. Taking the ouch out of Injections, *The Canadian Nurse*, 1983, *79* (1), 24-27.

Kim, K.K. & Grier, M.R. Pacing effects of medication instruction for the elderly. *Journal of Gerontological Nursing*, 1981, *7*, 464-468.

Kimminau, M. Spoons provide potential for dosing errors. *American Pharmacy*, 1979, *NS19*, 25-27.

Koszuta, L.E. Choosing the right infusion control device for your patient, *Nursing '84*, 1984, March, 54-56.

Kruszewski, A.Z., Lang, S.H., & Johnson, J.E. Effect of positioning on discomfort from intramuscular injections in the dorsogluteal site. *Nursing Research*, 1979, *28*, 103-105.

Lang, S.H., Zawacki, A.M. & Johnson, J.E. Reducing discomfort from IM injections. *American Journal of Nursing*, 1976, *76*, 800-801.

Lenz, C.L. Make your needle selection right to the point, *Nursing '84*, 1984.

Lundin, D.V. You *can* inject heparin subcutaneously, *RN*, 1978, *41* (12), 51-54.

MacLaughlin, J.E. Intravenous containers - variability in measurement. *The Canadian Nurse*, 1981, Sept., 28-30.

MacCara, M.E. & Gillis, M.C. Children's therapy compliance is a matter of taste. *Canadian Pharmaceutical Journal*, 1982, *115*, 274-276.

MacCara, M.E. Extravasation: a hazard of intravenous therapy, *Drug Intelligence and Clinical Pharmacy*, 1983, *17*, 713-717.

Mar, D.D. Intravenous admixtures. *American Journal of Nursing*, 1981, *81*, 574-575.

Masoorlie, S.T. Toward impeccable IV technique-trouble free IV starts, *RN*, 1981, Feb., 21-27.

Mayers, M.H. Legal guidelines. *Geriatric Nursing*, 1981, (Dec.), 417-441.

McCloskey, J.R. & Chung, S.M. Quadriceps contracture as a result of multiple intramuscular injection. *American Journal of Diseases in Children*, 1977, *131*, 416-417.

McConnell, E.A. The subtle art of really good injections. *RN*, 1982, *45*, 25-34.

Meguerdichian, D. Improving self-medication in an HRF, *Geriatric Nursing*, 1983, (Jan./Feb.), 30-34.

Millam, D.A. Tips for improving your venipuncture techniques. *Nursing '83*, 1983, (Aug.), 40-43.

Murchison, I., Nichols, T.S. & Hanson, R.S. Legal accountability in the nursing process (2nd ed.). St. Louis, The C.V. Mosby Co., 1982.

Mynick, A. Instituting a postpartum self-medication program. *Maternal Child Nursing*, 1981, *6*, 422-424.

Newton, D.W., & Newton, M. Route, site, and technique: three key decisions in giving parenteral medication. *Nursing '79*, 1979, *9*, 18-25.

Newton, M., Gilbert, J.P., & Newton, D.W. Parenteral antibiotics: the hazards to watch for. *RN*, 1981, *44*, 44-51.

Nichols, E.G., Barstow, R.E., & Cooper, D. Relationship between incidence of phlebitis and frequency of changing IV tubing and percutaneous site. *Nursing Research*, 1983, *32*, 247-252.

Nurses Drug Alert. What's in a spoon? *Nurses Drug Alert*, 1980, *4*, 71.

Ormond, E.A.R., & Caulfield, C. A practical guide to giving oral medications to young children. *Maternal Child Nursing*, 1976, *1*, 320-325.

Parker, W.A. Canadian oral solid dosage forms that should not be crushed. *Canadian Pharmaceutical Journal*, 1983, Nov., 465-474.

Petrillo, M., & Sanger, S. Emotional care of hospitalized children (ed. 2), Philadelphia, J.B. Lippincott Co., 1980.

Pontious, S.L. Practical Piaget: helping children understand. *American Journal of Nursing*, 1982, *83* (1), 114-117.

Rapp, P.R., Elgert, J.F., & Piecoro, J.J. Guidelines for the administration of commonly used intravenous drugs. *Drug Intelligence and Clinical Pharmacy*, 1980, *14*, 193-208.

Rimar, J.M. Guidelines for the intravenous administration of medications used in pediatrics. *Maternal Child Nursing*, 1982, *7*, 184-197.

Schilder, E. Insulin injection sites. *The Nurse Practitioner*, 1981, *6* (3), 43.

Shepherd, M.J. & Swearington, P.L. Z-track injections: a step-by-step how-to for an underused IM technique. *American Journal of Nursing*, 1984, *84* (6), 746-747.

Sklar, C. Nursing negligence in the administration of medication . . . could it happen to you? *The Canadian Nurse*, 1979, *75*, 51-53.

Tanner, S. Toward impeccable IV technique IV bolus leaves no room for errors. *RN*, 1981, *44*, 54-55.

Todd, B. What does a good drug history include? *Geriatric Nursing*, 1981, (Jan-Feb), 63-64.

Todd, B. Drugs and the elderly. Using eye drops and ointments safely. *Geriatric Nursing*, 1983, (Jan-Feb), 53-57.

Vanbree, N.S., Hollerbach, A.D., & Brooks, G.P. Clinical evaluation of three techniques for administering low-dose heparin. *Nursing Research*, 1984, *33* (1), 15-19.

Weeks, H.F. Administering medication to children. *Maternal Child Nursing*, 1980, *5*, 63-64.

Welk, D.S. Preventing insulin induced lipodystrophies. *Nursing 79*, 1979, *9*, 42-45.

Wertsching, J.H. Reconstituting parenteral antibiotics for children. *Maternal Child Nursing*, 1982, *7*, 128-133.

Wittig, P. & Semmler-Bertanzi, D.J. Pumps and controllers: a nurse's assessment guide. *American Journal of Nursing*, 1983, *83*, 1022-1025.

Wong, D.L. Significance of dead space in syringes. *American Journal of Nursing*, 1982, *82*, 1237.

Wormser, G.P., Joline, C., & Duncanson, F. Needle-stick injuries during the care of patients with AIDS. (Letter to the editor). *The New England Journal of Medicine*, 1984, *310* (22), 1461-1462.

Zimmerman, T.J. et al. Improving the therapeutic index of topically applied ocular drugs. *Arch. Ophthalmol.* 1984, *102*, 551-553.

GENERAL PRINCIPLES OF PHARMACOLOGY

CHAPTER 3

Mechanisms of Drug Action

Louis A. Pagliaro

Nurses are concerned with the response patients have to a particular drug. An understanding of the basic mechanisms of drug action at the molecular or primary level is necessary for the nurse to appreciate patient response and to understand how a variety of factors influence drug action.

Structure-activity relationship. Understanding a drug's primary mechanism of action will enable the nurse to appreciate how slight chemical modifications of the structure of a drug molecule can give rise to a new drug in the same class or family with different properties. This concept is known as "structure-activity relationship." An example is found in the group of drugs known collectively as the penicillins (see Chapter 45).

Penicillin G, the prototype or original member of the penicillin family, is not effective against *Haemophilus influenzae* or penicillinase-producing bacteria, such as *Staphylococcus aureus*. However, other penicillins with slight molecular modifications are effective against these organisms. For example, ampicillin is effective against *Haemophilus influenzae,* and methicillin is effective against *Staphylococcus aureus.*

Pharmacodynamics. Before we proceed to examine the individual mechanisms of action, it is important to briefly examine the relationship between the dose of a medication administered to a patient (or group of patients) and the observed pharmacologic effect(s). The relationship between drug concentration over time and observed pharmacologic effect is often referred to as the "pharmacodynamics" of the drug.

Dose-response curve. The pharmacodynamic relationship of drug level to effect is probably best conceptualized by examining the dose-response curve (Figure 3-1). For most drugs, if the log of the dose* administered is plotted against the percent of observed pharmacologic response in a single subject,

one typically obtains an S-shaped, or sigmoidal, curve. The curve indicates that a graded response is obtained from differing doses of drug. The upper and lower ends of the curve usually are reciprocal of each other, although the lower end of the curve may be absent or difficult to observe in some cases (e.g., in the presence of dose-dependent kinetics—see Chapter 5, "Drug Metabolism and Elimination"). Figure 3-1 is an example of a typical sigmoidal dose-response curve. It should be noted, however, that the slope of the curve (i.e., whether the **S** is flattened or stretched) depends on which drug and which pharmacologic effect are plotted.

The curve in Figure 3-1 is divided into three portions, *A*, *B*, and *C*. Examination of the lower portion of the curve *(A)* indicates that a minimal or theshold dose of drug (i.e., a pharmacologic or therapeutic quantity) must be administered before a pharmacologic effect is observed.

The middle or linear portion of the curve *(B)* is the part that is most often encountered in clinical practice. This portion of the curve is responsible for the *law of conservation of dose.* Basically, this law states that dose is directly proportional to plasma concentration and thus effect. Under this law, if one were to increase or decrease the dose of a medication, the expected effect should proportionately increase or decrease. This law accounts for the empirical modification of dose based on the patient's response. Examination of Figure 3-1, however, reveals that the law clearly does not apply when the dose and response are at either extreme end of the curve (i.e., *A* or *C*). In addition, the law does not apply for certain drugs (e.g., aspirin, phenytoin) that exhibit what is known as capacity limited, or dose-dependent kinetics (see Chapter 5, "Drug Metabolism and Elimination").

Examination of the upper portion of the dose-response curve *(C)* indicates that, as 100% pharmacologic response is approached, the curve tapers off or becomes more horizontal and a ceiling effect is obtained. In other words, once a maximal effect

---

*The same type of curve is obtained if dose is plotted against response. Use of the log of the dose, however, creates a more standardized S-shaped curve with a steeper slope.

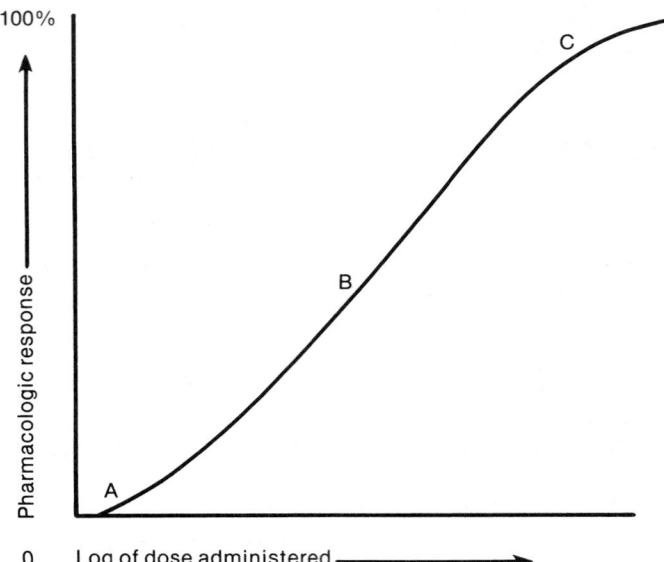

FIGURE 3-1. **Dose-response curve illustrating the typical relationship between dose and response.**

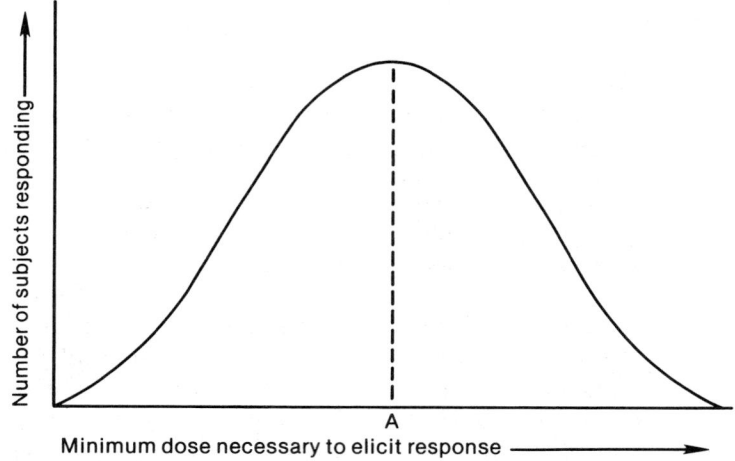

FIGURE 3-2. **Normal distribution of subjects pharmacologically responding to a minimum effective dose of drug.**

is reached, increasing the dose will not increase the effect, but may increase adverse or toxic effects, which have not yet reached their maximum, or ceiling.

A curve that may help conceptualize the variability of drug response in a population of patients is shown in Figure 3-2. When one plots the minimum dose necessary to achieve a certain pharmacologic effect against the number of individuals who respond to that particular dose, a bell-shaped, or normal distribution, curve is obtained. This curve indicates the wide range of variability in response that can be expected when a certain dose of medication is administered to a number of different patients.*

Most individuals elicit the desired pharmacologic response when administered the average dose (A), but for some individuals (approximately 15%) at either extreme of the curve shown in Figure 3-2, the average dose or ED_{50} (minimum dose effective for 50% of the population) will be either too small or too large. The average dose is calculated to produce a pharmacologic effect with a relatively low incidence of adverse effects in the average patient. It is thus used as a starting dose and as such is found effective in most patients.

The safety of the average dose varies from drug to drug, as nurses are well aware. The margin of safety can be defined as the difference between the *maximum* therapeutic dose and the *minimum* toxic dose.† Some drugs such as the penicillins have a large margin of safety, and extremely large doses can usually be given safely. Other drugs such as the antidysrhythmics have a small margin of safety, and the difference between the therapeutic and toxic dose may be only a few micrograms. The nurse must keep these considerations in mind and, by careful observation of the patient, recommend increasing or decreasing the dose when appropriate.

With this brief introduction let us now examine the specific primary mechanisms by which drugs elicit their pharmacologic effects.

MECHANISMS OF DRUG ACTION

Drugs act through a variety of mechanisms to elicit their pharmacologic effects. These mechanisms have been divided into five categories: (1) binding at a receptor site, (2) chemical reaction, (3) physical effect, (4) functional disruption, and (5) psychologic effect.

Before proceeding, it should be noted that the mechanisms of action discussed in this chapter apply to *all* pharmacologic effects, desired and undesired. For example, allergic reactions to penicillins are caused by the chemical binding of a penicillin and a hapten, which results in an antigen-antibody response.

---

*Individual variability in drug response can be explained for the most part by age (see Chapter 7), psychologic status (see Chapter 8), and genetic makeup (see Chapter 9).

†Toxicity in this context is defined differently for different drugs, depending on the use of the drug, the availability of alternatives, and societal values. Thus, the minimum toxic dose may refer to the dose at which side effects of any type are first noted, the dose at which major side effects are noted, or the minimum lethal dose.

Binding at a receptor site

Because of the selectivity and specificity of drug action it is believed that most drugs work at a molecular level by binding (attaching) to specific macromolecules in the body, known as drug receptors.* According to the receptor theory of drug mechanism of action, a drug must be attracted to and bind to a receptor for a biologic response to be obtained. This binding starts a series of biochemical and physiologic reactions (changes) that ultimately result in the observed pharmacologic effect of the drug. An interesting corollary of this mechanism of drug action is that a drug cannot create a new action or function in the organism, but simply starts or regulates an endogenous function.† Another corollary of this mechanism of action is that only the free (unbound) portion of a drug dose, and *not* the protein-bound (or complexed) portion, can interact with a drug receptor and cause a pharmacologic effect.

The concept of receptors dates back to Paul Ehrlich, who introduced the term *receptor* in 1905. Receptors or receptor sites have since been established for several drugs (e.g., acetylcholine, estrogen, insulin, morphine, nicotine); however, for most drugs this mechanism is still a hypothesis. This mechanism of action was originally thought of in terms of a lock-and-key model. Although this representation is not entirely accurate, it may help conceptualize the interaction between drug and receptor site.

The three-dimensional structure of the receptor, which determines its spatial relationship (compatibility) with the drug, and its physiochemical properties (i.e., polarity or charge), which determine the affinity (binding or attraction) toward the drug, work in unison to determine if the drug will cause a certain effect (i.e., activity or efficacy) and how strong the effect will be in relation to a specific dose (i.e., potency or intrinsic activity).

Figure 3-3 is a stylized illustration of the drug-receptor model. Note the various types of attracting forces (bonds) that function to hold the two components, drug and receptor, in place. Note also how the chemical structure of the drug is compatible with the physical characteristics or structure (i.e., cavities and flat surfaces) of the receptor. This compatibility allows the drug to get close enough to the receptor to bind and thus elicit a pharmacologic response. Of course,

---

*How the drug gets to the receptor site is discussed in Chapter 4, "Drug Availability and Distribution."

†See the "functional disruption" section of this chapter for a noted exception to this corollary.

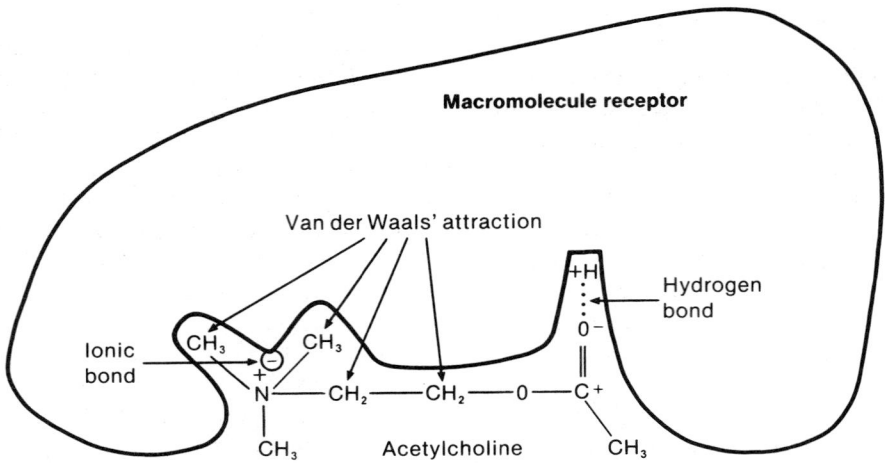

FIGURE 3-3. **Stylized illustration of acetylcholine interacting at its receptor site.**

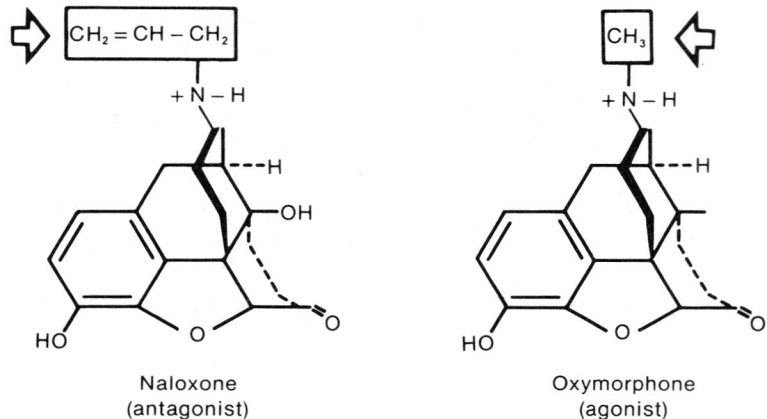

FIGURE 3-4. **Structural similarity between antagonist (naloxone) and agonist (oxymorphone). Note that the only chemical and structural difference is in the attachment to the nitrogen (N) atom, indicated above by a box and arrow.**

other factors such as the number of functioning receptors and drug dose also play a major role in determining drug response.

It should be noted that for most drugs, binding to a receptor site is a reversible process. Thus, primary drug action may be terminated by unbinding the drug and the receptor. This process allows interactions involving competition for binding sites to occur between drugs (see Chapter 10, "Drug Interactions").

Study of drug-receptor binding and interactions has given rise to two terms, *agonist* and *antagonist*, which are widely used in relation to pharmacologic effects. An agonist is a drug that binds to the receptor site and causes a direct effect by activating the receptor

(e.g., oxymorphone). An antagonist is a drug that binds to the receptor site but produces no direct pharmacologic response (e.g., naloxone). However, an antagonist produces an indirect effect in the presence of an agonist by competing for (and thus reducing) the agonist's available binding sites. Thus, if naloxone is administered alone, it displays almost no pharmacologic effect; however, if administered with oxymorphone (or other narcotics), it effectively antagonizes (blocks) the pharmacologic effects of the narcotic. Obviously, the chemical structure of agonists and antagonists must be closely related (Figure 3-4). Because of this, one often finds antagonists (e.g., nalorphine) that possess some agonist properties (i.e., *partial* agonist-antagonist). In fact some drugs work as either agonist or antagonist as a function of dose. Figure 3-4 compares the chemical structures of oxymorphone (an agonist) and naloxone (an antagonist).

Chemical reaction

Chemical reactions involved in drug mechanism of action typically involve the binding or recombining of two ions or groups, one positively charged and one negatively charged. This can be easily conceptualized by the following representative equation:

$$X^{(+)} + Y^{(-)} \rightleftharpoons XY$$

It should be noted that some prefer to think of one of these elements (e.g., X) as the drug and the other element (e.g., Y) as the receptor and would thus include chemical reactions under the rubric of "binding at a receptor site." Either classification is acceptable; however, it is felt that a clearer understanding of drug mechanisms is provided by using a separate classification for chemical reaction. Examples of drugs that elicit their effect by way of chemical reactions include antacids, many antidotes, and acid-base regulators.

Antacids (Chapter 39) neutralize hydrochloric acid, which is secreted into the stomach. This is accomplished by a simple chemical reaction in which antacids, which are basic compounds, combine with hydrochloric acid to form carbon dioxide, water, and a chloride salt (e.g., calcium chloride if the antacid contains calcium, such as calcium carbonate, or sodium chloride if the antacid contains sodium, such as sodium bicarbonate).

Many antidotes, such as the metal chelating (binding) agent edetate calcium disodium (Chapter 71) and the heparin antidote protamine sulfate (Chapter 34), also elicit their pharmacologic effects by chemically binding with, and thus neutralizing, their counterpart agents. Edetate calcium disodium has a high affinity for (attraction to) lead. Thus, the calcium in the molecule is readily displaced by lead. The lead, which is no longer in a free (active) form, is subsequently excreted as the soluble lead-edetate complex. Protamine sulfate (a strong base) combines with heparin (a strong acid) to form a physiologically inert complex and thus elicits its effect as an antidote for heparin overdosage. Antitoxins (Chapter 69) provide passive immunity by binding to specific toxins and thereby neutralizing their effects.*

---

*This mechanism of action can also be thought of as a false receptor, for the antitoxin binds with the toxin and thereby prevents the toxin from binding with its physiologic receptor.

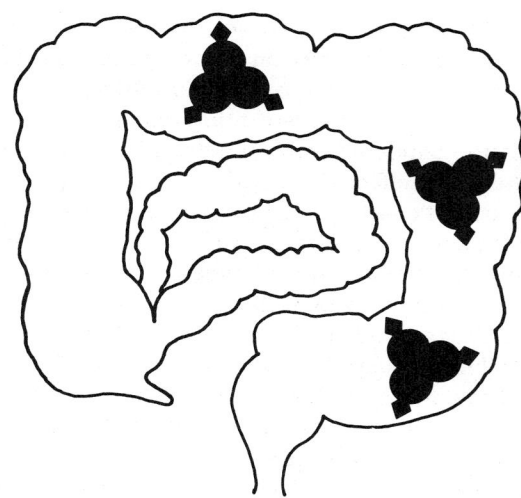

FIGURE 3-5. **Schematic representation of bulk-forming laxatives placing direct physical pressure on the receptors in the wall of the colon, thereby eliciting their pharmacologic effect.**

Acidifiers (e.g., ammonium chloride) increase free hydrogren ion concentration, and alkalinizers (e.g., sodium bicarbonate) decrease free hydrogen ion concentration and thus lower or raise, respectively, the pH of the blood or urine (see Chapter 67, "Fluids and Electrolytes").

Another way in which drugs act by way of chemical reactions can be demonstrated by observing the mechanism of action of vitamins (Chapter 66). The B vitamins (i.e., nicotinic acid, pyridoxine, thiamine) act as coenzymes to permit or enhance the efficiency of various chemical (metabolic) reactions in the body.

Physical effect

Some drugs exert their pharmacologic effect by means of a direct physical effect. A common example of this mechanism of drug action is found in the bulk-forming and lubricant laxatives (see Chapter 41). Bulk-forming laxatives (such as methylcellulose and plantago seed) absorb fluid from the gastrointestinal tract to increase their bulk and facilitate peristalsis of the colon by direct physical pressure on the receptors (Figure 3-5). Lubricant laxatives, such as mineral oil, form a barrier between the wall of the colon and feces to prevent reabsorption of water and thereby facilitate formation and passage of the feces.

Osmotic diuretics (e.g., mannitol and urea—see Chapter 36) increase urine volume by a simple physical mechanism of action. By their presence in the renal tubules, they cause the concentration of the tubular solution to increase. Water then passes through the membrane of the proximal convoluted tubules of the nephron from a region of lower concentration to a region of higher concentration in an attempt to equalize the concentration on both sides of the membrane (osmotic effect). The end result is an increased rate of urine flow. Certain laxatives (e.g., magnesium sulfate [Epsom salt]) work by the same osmotic principle, except that instead of drawing water into the renal tubules they draw water into the colon.

Some drugs elicit their direct physical effect on the exterior skin surface. These include drugs such as zinc oxide which, when applied as a paste, forms a physical barrier to protect the skin from both the irritating effects of overexposure to the sun (when it is used as a sunscreen applied to the face) and the irritating effects of urine (when it is used on infants to prevent diaper rash). Fibrinolysin is an enzyme that cleanses wounds by dissolution of protein matter. Rapidly evaporating solutions (e.g., isopropyl alcohol) cool the skin simply by means of evaporation.

Another interesting physical mechanism of action involves the use of petroleum jelly (petrolatum) to treat infestation of pediculi on the eyelashes. When applied to the eyelashes, petroleum jelly physically suffocates the pediculi without causing irritation to the eye.

Functional disruption

The mechanism of drug action mediated by means of functional disruption can occur on several different levels, including molecular, cellular, and organ. Disruption, or alteration of the genetic material (i.e., DNA), caused by some of these drugs may result in the creation of *new* function(s) for the affected cells. This is a noted exception to the corollary stated in the receptor-mechanism section of this chapter.

At the molecular level agents such as the anticancer drugs (e.g., cisplatin, mitomycin [Chapter 53]) elicit their effect by directly cross-linking or binding together deoxyribonucleic acid (DNA) strands or chains (Figure 3-6), which in turn results in improper DNA replication and cell death. The antineoplastic antimetabolites (see Chapter 52) also work at the molecular level. Methotrexate, for example, binds to the enzyme dihydrofolate reductase, thereby preventing the reduction of folic acid to tetrahydrofolate (a precursor compound necessary for DNA synthesis in the cell). Azathioprine inhibits the synthesis of the amino acid purine, which is necessary for DNA synthesis.

Griseofulvin (Chapter 51) binds with the microtubule protein of fungal cells, disrupting the mitotic spindle, thereby preventing cell division and growth of the fungus.

In bacteria, paraaminobenzoic acid (PABA) is chemically converted to folic acid and then further to tetrahydrofolic acid, which is an enzyme necessary for cell growth. Sulfonamides (Chapter 49) have a chemical structure similar to PABA and thus act to inhibit the incorporation of PABA into folic acid, thereby preventing the production of tetrahydrofolic acid and inhibiting bacterial cell growth. Humans use preformed folic acid and are therefore not affected by this effect of the sulfonamides.

Psychologic effect

This mechanism is mediated through the brain and central nervous system. One can think of this mech-

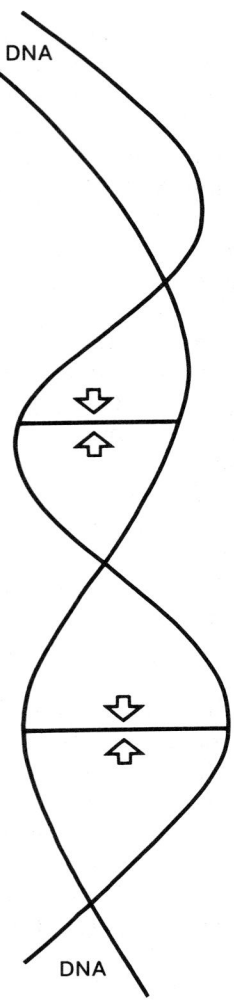

FIGURE 3-6. **Disruption of DNA function by the inappropriate binding together (cross-linking) of the DNA strands** (arrows) **caused by anticancer agents such as cisplatin and mitomycin.**

anism as working on the principle of mind over matter. The mind can activate body systems to actually cause physical effects* and can also make one think that the drug is causing an effect that it is not. Common examples of psychologic drug effects include habituation, or psychologic dependence to drugs, and the placebo effect.

A placebo is a pharmacologically inert substance that is usually administered, therapeutically or experimentally, for its psychologic effect. Although many clinicians associate the placebo effect with the use of placebos (e.g., injections of normal saline, sugar pills), it should be noted that any drug is capable of eliciting a placebo response or effect.

The placebo effect can be defined as any effect that has no direct relationship to the drug being used. In other words, the drug objectively does not have specific activity that would cause the observed effect. In this regard one might say that the discussion of placebo response should not be included here because it does not involve a direct drug action. However, it does involve at least an indirect action, for if the drug had not been administered, the effect would not have been observed.

The placebo effect is initiated in a psychologic mechanism. Because of this, the effect may be modified not only by the patient's self-perceived expectations, but also by the suggestion and expectation of the clinician who recommends and administers the medication. This effect, induced by the clinician's attitude, applies to all medications, whether directly pharmacologically active or placebo. A common example of the placebo response is observed when one takes one or two aspirin tablets for a simple tension headache and obtains almost immediate relief, even though the aspirin has not yet been substantially absorbed from the gastrointestinal tract and has not yet achieved a "pharmacologically" significant blood level.†

---

*These effects can be either positive or negative. They can result in healing, such as disappearance of warts or alleviation of headache, but they can also cause side effects, such as nausea or vomiting.
†For more details on drug absorption and the relationship of blood levels to effect, see Chapter 4, "Drug Availability and Distribution," and Chapter 6, "Pharmacokinetic Considerations in Drug Response."

Psychologic effects of drug therapy, including placebo and psychosomatic response, are dealt with in more detail in Chapter 8, "Psychologic Factors in Drug Response."

SUMMARY

The exact mechanism of action for most medications remains unknown. However, several specific types of mechanisms of action have been identified and discussed in this chapter. An awareness of a drug's mechanism of action enables the nurse to better understand why different drugs in the same pharmacologic class have similar actions. The nurse will more fully appreciate that because of slight chemical or structural modifications, related drugs may be more (or less) potent and may have more (or fewer) side effects. Knowledge of drug mechanisms of action also frequently enables one to predict drug interactions, to more fully appreciate their significance, and to rationally deal with them by substituting a similar type of drug with a different mechanism of action. Further information on the specific mechanisms of action for various classes of drugs can be found in the following sections of this text.

BIBLIOGRAPHY

Ariens, E.J. Drug levels in the target tissue and effect. *Clinical Pharmacology and Therapeutics*, 1974, *16*, 155-175.

Ariens, E.J., & Simons, A.M. Receptors and receptor mechanisms. In Saxena, P.R., & Forsyth, R.P. (Eds.). *Beta-adrenoceptor blocking agents.* Amsterdam: North Holland Publishing Co., 1976.

Furchgott, R.F. Pharmacological characterization of receptors. *Federation Proceedings*, 1978, *37*, 115-120.

Synder, S.H. Opiate receptors in the brain. *New England Journal of Medicine*, 1977, *296*, 266-271.

Vrhovac, B. Placebo and its importance in medicine. *International Journal of Clinical Pharmacology*, 1977, *15*, 161-165.

Wertheimer, A.I. The placebo effect. *Pharmacy International*, 1980, *1*, 12-13.

CHAPTER 4

Drug Availability and Distribution

Betty-ann Hoener

This chapter examines how a drug gets from its dosage form to its site of action in the body. Dosage forms (e.g., tablets, capsules, suppositories, and injectables) will be referred to as *drug delivery systems*, since they are intended to deliver the drug(s) they contain to the patient. The place in the body where the drug acts, its site of action, will be defined as the *biophase*. The study of all the controllable variables that can be manipulated in order to input a drug to its biophase is known as *biopharmaceutics*. The variables can be divided into two categories: pharmaceutical variables, and patient variables. Table 4-1 presents a summary of these variables.

AVAILABILITY

Pharmaceutical variables

Pharmaceutical variables depend on the physical and chemical properties of the drug and its dosage form. These properties are determined by the structure of the drug and of any inert ingredients added to make the dosage form. Added ingredients are called inert because they exert (at least in the amount[s] present) no pharmacologic effects of their own. They can, however, influence the delivery of the drug from the dosage form. The pharmaceutical variables also include the manufacturing processes: how a pharmaceutical manufacturer chooses to make its dosage forms, the inert ingredients selected, the order of mixing, and the machinery used. Thus, although all aspirin is chemically alike, not all aspirin tablets will be alike, nor will they all necessarily act alike in the body.

Patient variables

The second category of variables is the patient variables. These include both the anatomic and physiologic characteristics of the patient. Hence, we may anticipate that the sex, age, and state of health of our patients could modify drug delivery. In addition, patients may modify drug delivery by taking their dosage forms with or without food, just before or after strenuous exercise, or with other drugs. These patient and pharmaceutical variables may also interact. For example, they may work together to either increase or decrease drug delivery, or they may work against each other.

Blood level versus time curve

In order to find out if these controllable variables have been successfully manipulated in order to maximize drug delivery, we will need a tool to determine whether the drug has gotten out of its dosage form and into the biophase. The tool typically used is the blood level versus time curve (C_b versus t). We will be looking at the concentration of the drug in the blood, plasma, or serum over an extended period of time. The blood can be called the sample compartment, since it is the part of the body that is sampled (by drawing out some blood and measuring the concentration of drug in the sample). We will assume that the drug in the blood is in equilibrium with the drug in the biophase. Thus if the concentration of the drug in blood increases or decreases, there will be a proportionate change of drug in the biophase. The blood is sampled because it is, usually, more accessible than the biophase. Consider how difficult it would be to measure one drug molecule sitting on one pain receptor in the central nervous system. The amount of drug or drug metabolites excreted in the urine can also be used to describe how effectively the drug was delivered to the body.

We will be looking at some blood level curves of drugs to determine how much of the administered dose of a drug actually got out of its dosage form and into the general circulation of a patient. We will also look at how fast this process occurs. This is what we call *bioavailability*—the rate and extent of delivery of a drug to the general circulation. Pharmacokineticists attempt to mathematically describe these blood level versus time curves. That is, they study the kinetics of the absorption, distribution, metabolism, and excretion (ADME) of drugs and construct models to account for their observations (see Chapter 6, "Pharmacokinetic Considerations in Drug Response"). We will attempt to describe, in a nonmathematical way, the bioavailability of a drug by looking at its blood level versus time curve.

Let us begin by looking at what happens when a single intravenous bolus dose of a drug is administered. In Figure 4-1 we see that the concentration of drug is highest at time = 0 hours. This is because all of the drug has been administered directly into the sample compartment, the general circulation. Then, as the drug is eliminated from the body, by metabolism or excretion, the concentration declines until at some later time (i.e., time = infinity) it is once again zero. The time it takes to completely eliminate the drug depends, of course, on both the drug and the patient. Drugs eliminated by renal excretion will be more slowly eliminated by patients with decreased renal function. Likewise, some, but not all, liver diseases slow

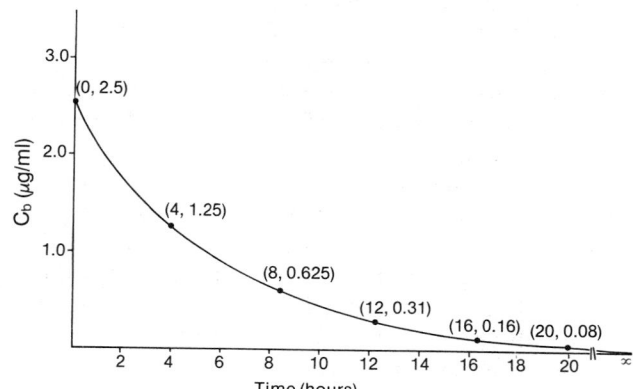

FIGURE 4-1. **The blood level versus time curve of an intravenous bolus dose of 50 mg of a drug. The time it takes to eliminate one half of the drug in the body is the biologic half-life. The $T_{1/2}$ = 4 hours for this drug.**

TABLE 4-1

Factors influencing drug availability

Pharmaceutical variables	Patient variables
Drug	
Chemical structure	Sex
Purity	Age
Water solubility	State of health
Lipid solubility	Physical activity
pKa	Emotions
Crystal form	Timing of dose relative to meals‡
Salt form	Route of administration
Degree of hydration	Fluids available to solubilize the drug
Particle size	pH of environment
Chemical stability (to water, light and oxygen)	Size of dose that can be delivered
Physical stability (vapor pressure, melting or boiling point)	Potential for first-pass metabolism
Dosage form	Blood flow to site of administration
Inert ingredients*	Other drugs and diet taken concurrently
Suspensions†	Willingness to comply with therapy
Viscosity	
Ease of shaking	
Pourability	
Topical preparations†	
Spreadability	
Solid dosage forms†	
Order of mixing, method and size of granulation	
Compression pressure or packing density	
Special coatings including their water solubility and the pH dependence of solubility	

*The same factors found above under Drug also apply to each inert ingredient found in the preparation.
†Only those factors distinctive for the particular dosage form are listed. For each dosage form all items listed under inert ingredients apply.
‡These factors are detailed in Table 4-3.

the elimination of drugs metabolized by the liver. In general, we can indicate how rapidly or slowly a drug is eliminated from the body by giving its biologic half-life. This half-life is the time it takes for one half of the drug in the body to be eliminated.

Intravenous. We are interested, in this chapter, in both how much of and how fast the drug gets into the general circulation. For an IV bolus, how fast we push on the syringe determines the rate at which the drug is delivered to the bloodstream. Once administered, it is considered to be instantaneously mixed and distributed throughout the body by the general circulation. The few minutes it takes to do so should not significantly alter the blood level curve. Thus, for an IV bolus dose neither the rate nor the extent of availability is a consideration. Since the drug is administered directly into the general circulation, the answer to the question, "How much?" is "All of it." Thus, the fraction available, F, is one for an IV dose (i.e., $F_{IV} = 1$), by definition.

We can use this same blood level (C_b) versus time (t) curve to illustrate a method that will allow us to compare the relative extents of availability of the same drug given under different conditions. To do so we look at the area under the blood level curve (AUC). This is the area calculated from time zero to time infinity. The shaded portion of the curve in Figure 4-2 is the AUC for a 50 mg dose of drug. What would the curve look like if we administered a 100 mg IV bolus dose? What would happen to the AUC? The AUC will exactly double, yielding a curve with every concentration twice as high as the 50 mg dose. Thus at t = 0, C_b = 5 μg/ml, at t = 2 hr, C_b = 3.5 μg/ml; and at t = 4 hr, C_b = 2.5 μg/ml, and so on. The area is twice as large because the dose is twice as large. Pharmacologically this is known as the *rule of normalization* and applies to all commonly encountered drugs except those (e.g., aspirin, phenytoin) that display what is known as zero order or dose-dependent kinetics (see Chapter 5, "Drug Metabolism and Elimination"). The AUC can be used to compare the relative extents of availability if an adjustment for any differences in the dose administered is made. (NOTE: we can compare the AUCs for the same drug given under different conditions or at different doses but we *cannot* compare the AUCs for *different* drugs under any conditions.)

Nonintravenous. Let us now look at some blood level curves of a drug given by a nonintravenous route of administration. The curves we will be looking at could be for any route in which the drug is not injected directly into the general circulation. These routes include intramuscular, intrathecal, subcutaneous, oral, buccal, sublingual, nasal, vaginal, rectal, inhalation, in-

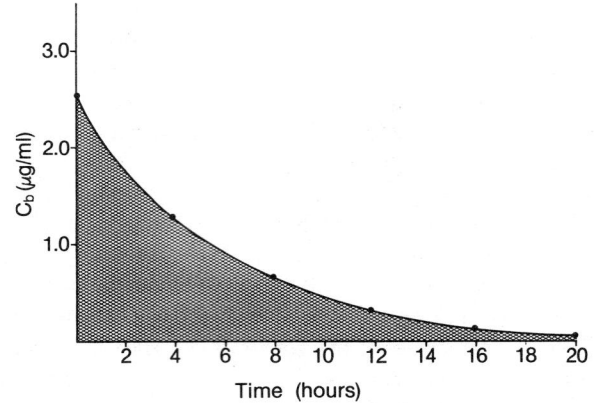

FIGURE 4-2. **The same IV dose of 50 mg as in Figure 4-1 with the area under the curve (AUC) shaded in. The AUC is 14.4 μg/ml · hr.**

tradermal, topical, ophthalmic, and otic. At t = 0, there will be no drug in the sample compartment. Likewise, there will be no drug at time = infinity. We now have two points for our curve in Figure 4-3. It seems reasonable to assume that the blood levels will rise as the drug is released from its dosage form and is absorbed into the general circulation. The drug that reaches the general circulation will be eliminated, but drug will still be entering so we can expect the curve to continue rising. Then, as the amount of unabsorbed drug becomes small we might expect that absorption will contribute less and less to the curve while elimination will become the dominant factor. Hence, the blood levels will decline until all of the drug is eliminated. We now have the entire blood level versus time curve of Figure 4-3.

MEC, MTC, T_{peak}. Note the line labeled MEC. This is the *minimum effective concentration*. At drug levels above the MEC we will see a pharmacologic effect. Below this level there will be no effect. The line labeled MTC *(minimum toxic concentration)* is the concentration above which toxic effects would begin to be seen. The time at which the blood level curve rises above the MEC is the *onset of action*. In Figure 4-3 this time is 0.9 hours. The length of time the concentration stays above the MEC is the *duration of action*. In Figure 4-3 this is 5.3 hours.

There is one other time of particular interest in Figure 4-3. That is the time at which the blood level is at its maximum, its t_{peak}. It can be shown mathematically that t_{peak} is directly related to the rate at which the drug reaches the general circulation. (NOTE: we can use t_{peak} to compare the rate of absorption of the *same* drug administered under different conditions. However, we must assume that the *clearance*

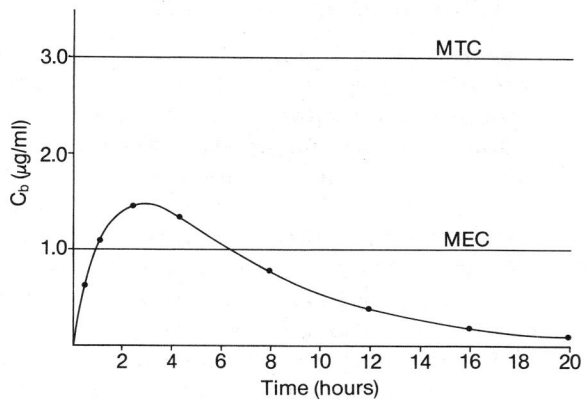

FIGURE 4-3. **A 50 mg dose of the same drug has been given by a nonintravenous route. The minimum effective concentration (MEC) is 1 μg/ml. The minimum toxic concentration (MTC) is 3 μg/ml. The time to reach the peak (t_{peak}) is 2.7 hours. The AUC is 13 μg/ml · hr.**

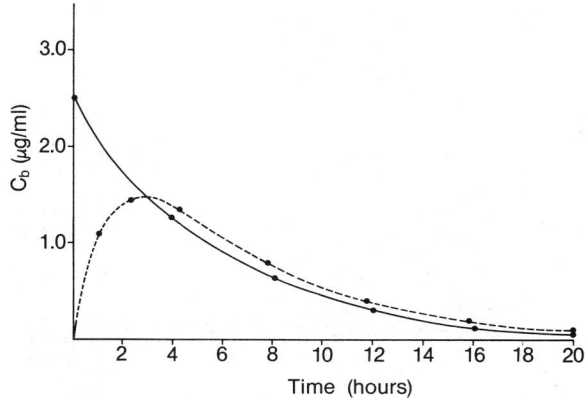

FIGURE 4-4. **The 50 mg IV (—) dose and the 50 mg non-IV (---) dose are plotted.**

[elimination] of the drug is *constant* under these different conditions). Now ask yourself, "What would happen to the C_b versus t curve if the patient took twice the dose of this drug?" Stop and think what that would do to each concentration, to the t_{peak}, to the onset, to the duration, and to the AUC. Note that each blood level is twice as high, the onset is sooner, and the duration longer. The concentrations are much closer to the MTC. However, the t_{peak} is the same. The AUC should be twice as big (since the dose was twice as big). Now, if we were to compare $AUC_{50\ mg}^{nonIV}$ to $AUC_{100\ mg}^{nonIV}$, we would find the relative availability equals one. The extent is the same.

$$\frac{AUC_{50\ mg}^{nonIV}}{50\ mg} \bigg/ \frac{AUC_{100\ mg}^{nonIV}}{100\ mg} = 1$$

Let us compare the 50 mg non-IV dose with the 50 mg IV dose of this drug (Figure 4-4). The t_{Peak}^{IV} occurs at t = 0 hours. Thus, the drug is much more rapidly available to the general circulation than is the same drug given by the non-IV route. Now let us compare the AUCs. $AUC_{50\ mg}^{nonIV}/AUC_{50\ mg}^{IV}$ = 0.9. We know, by definition, that F_{IV} = 1. Therefore the absolute availability of the non-IV dose is 0.9.

$$\frac{AUC^{nonIV}}{AUC^{IV}} = \frac{F^{nonIV}}{F^{IV}} = F^{nonIV}$$

What happened to the other 0.1 (or 10%) fraction of the drug? It is not available to the general circulation of the patient. It might not have gotten out of its dosage form. If it were an oral tablet, it might not have dissolved completely (e.g., some enteric-coated aspirin tablets). Some of the drug might have been destroyed

by the stomach acid (e.g., erythromycin stearate or penicillin G). Some of it may have complexed with food or other drugs in the GI tract (e.g., tetracycline and antacids) and passed out into the feces. There are many possibilities. The blood level curve tells us only that the drug did not reach the sample compartment. It cannot tell us where it did go.

Now, let us compare two non-IV dosage forms of our drug. We will use the 50 mg dose of Figure 4-3. Let us suppose that it was an oral solution. Now let us administer a 50 mg tablet of the same drug to the same patient. Since it is the same drug we can assume that clearance (elimination) is a constant. We anticipate, however, that the rate and extent of availability could be different. In Figure 4-5 we have drawn the blood level curves to indicate a difference. Is this difference in the rate (compare the t_{peak} of each) or in the extent (compare the AUCs)? Notice that the "eyeball" method of determining t_{peak} and AUCs gives you a reasonably accurate indication of what is happening. The t_{peak} of the solution is 2.7 hours, but the t_{peak} of the tablet is 4.5 hours. Thus, the rate of availability of the two dosage forms is different. However, the AUCs appear to be the same. Certainly the common, shaded portion under the curves is equal. It remains for us to decide if the two other portions are equal.

Finally, see that changing the rate or the extent of availability dramatically changes the shape of the blood level curve. These changes effect the onset and duration of the pharmacologic effect. They also determine if toxic concentrations are reached. Thus, bioavailability studies can provide information that will enable us to administer a drug in a dosage form or by a route of administration that will maximize the therapeutic benefits of drug therapy while minimizing side effects.

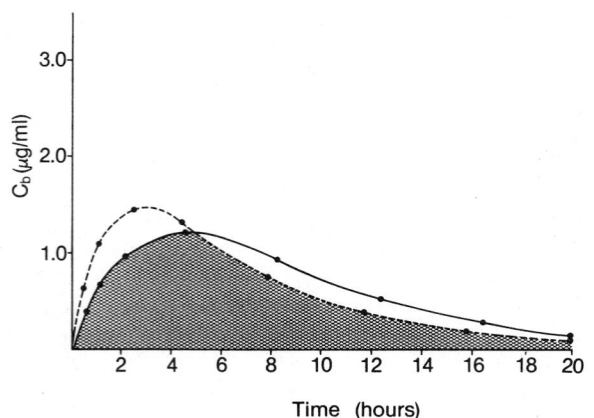

FIGURE 4-5. **A 50 mg dose of the drug as an oral solution (---) and a 50 mg dose as an oral tablet (—). Each t_{peak} is different, but the AUCs are the same.**

ROUTES OF ADMINISTRATION*

We will now turn our attention to biopharmaceutics in order to learn something about those variables that can be controlled to optimize the amount of drug reaching the general circulation. We will begin by looking at the various routes of administration and the patient and pharmaceutical variables of each. These routes, illustrated in Figure 4-6, can be divided into three categories: (1) direct injection into the general circulation (e.g., intravenous and intraarterial), (2) absorption across a membrane barrier (e.g., oral, buccal, sublingual, intramuscular, subcutaneous, intradermal, vaginal, rectal, nasal, inhalation, ophthalmic), and (3) absorption across the skin (i.e., topical).

---

*For information on the preparation, administration, and monitoring of drugs in relation to route of administration, see Chapter 2.

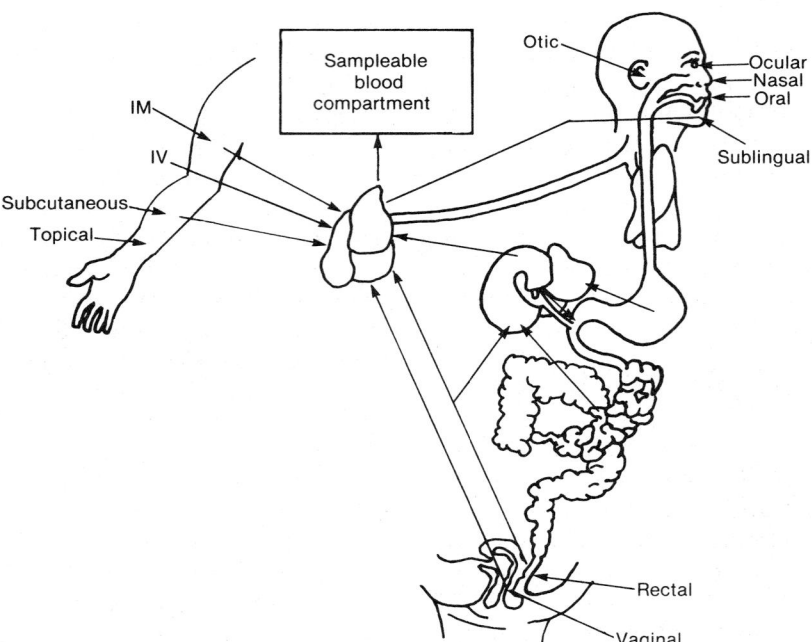

FIGURE 4-6. **Various pathways by which a drug may be delivered to the general circulation. The diagram has been drawn to emphasize the organs that the blood leaving a site of absorption must pass through before reaching the general circulation. This figure shows that a drug may be metabolized on its first-pass through the liver following oral or rectal administration. In addition, the lungs may also eliminate the drug before it reaches the general circulation. This first-pass lung effect might be observed for all of the routes illustrated. (From Benet, L.Z. In F. McMahon (Ed.).** *Principles and techniques of human research and therapeutics* **(Vol. 3), New York: Futura Publishing, 1974.)**

In our discussion about blood level versus time curves we have covered intravenous injection. So we begin with the intraarterial route.

Direct injection into the systemic circulation

Intraarterial route. This route is used infrequently. Radiopaque materials may be injected for diagnostic purposes. Therapeutically, some antineoplastic drugs such as carmustine may be injected intraarterially. This route may be used to deliver the drug directly into the general circulation. Both the liver and lung are avoided on the first pass of the drug through the body. We will discuss the advantage of bypassing these organs. On occasion it may be desirable to inject a drug into a specific organ or tumor. Then injection into the principal artery leading to the tissue may be attempted. In general, these injections are an attempt to deliver the drug directly to its site of action. The subsequent dilution by the blood entering and leaving the target tissue is, in this case, a side effect that cannot be avoided.

Absorption across a membrane barrier

Oral route. Among those routes involving membrane transport, the oral route, at least as far as number of dosage forms administered, is by far the most important. It is estimated that at least 70% to 80% of all dosage forms taken are oral capsules or tablets. If we add in the oral solutions and suspensions, we can easily assume that up to 90% of all medications are taken orally. We can divide the process by which drugs taken orally reach the general circulation into four steps: (1) getting the drug to its site of absorption, (2) getting the drug into solution, (3) getting the drug through the membrane, and (4) carrying the drug away to the general circulation. The order of the first two steps is interchangeable. That is, a drug may get into solution and then get to the site, or it may reach the site and then get into solution. It must however, be in solution before it can be absorbed.

Getting the drug to its site of absorption. The principal site of absorption for most drugs is the small intestine. The main reason for this is the large surface area of the small intestine relative to the rest of the GI tract. Although absorption may begin in the stomach, even alcohol is primarily absorbed in the small intestine. Thus, anything that affects the rate of stomach emptying will potentially affect the rate at which a drug gets to its absorption site and may, therefore, affect its rate of absorption.

Those factors that can affect stomach emptying are numerous. Strenuous exercise will delay emptying. On the other hand, the chronically inactive will have slower gastric emptying. Light physical activity will stimulate gastric emptying. If a patient is lying on the right side, emptying of the stomach contents will be facilitated, whereas if the patient is lying on the left side, the stomach contents will have to move uphill, and emptying may be delayed. The emotional state of the patient may either increase or decrease stomach emptying. Other drugs may affect the stomach emptying rate by altering GI motility.

The stomach protects the intestine from extreme conditions. Therefore, if the stomach contents differ significantly with respect to pH, temperature, osmolarity, or viscosity from those conditions normally encountered in the intestine, emptying will be delayed until those conditions approach normal. Food, by altering these factors, will effect gastric emptying. Thus, the timing of meals relative to the timing of an oral dose can influence the rate and possibly the extent of drug availability.

Drugs known to be affected by food are listed in Table 4-2. Other factors affecting availability are summarized in Table 4-3. Remember, most of these factors may affect the rate of availability. They may or may not also affect the extent of availability. We shall see that the rate as well as the extent of availability may increase, decrease, or not change. Thus, there are nine possible outcomes including no effect on either the rate or extent of availability. We will look at several of these possibilities. As you examine the figures, remember to look at the t_{peak} to determine the relative rates of availability and at the AUC to measure the relative extents of availability.

Figure 4-7 shows the average serum level curves obtained after oral administration of a 500 mg capsule of cephradine, an antibiotic. Each subject received the capsule once on an empty stomach and once with a meal. Note the change in t_{peak}. It is about 1 hour when the subjects are fasting and a little over 2 hours when they are eating. Thus food, by delaying stomach emptying, has delayed the rate of availability of cephradine. It appears, however, that the AUCs are not different. We conclude that food does not affect the extent of availability of cephradine. This information can be used to maximize therapy. If we wish a rapid onset, cephradine should be administered 1 hour before or 2 hours after a meal. If we wish a longer duration and are not concerned about a rapid onset, we may wish to administer cephradine with food.

Often it is recommended that drugs be taken with food to minimize possible GI distress. Such recommendations may also alter the shape of the blood level

TABLE 4-2

Effect of food on the bioavailability of drugs*

Decreased rate	Decreased extent	Increased extent	Not affected
Acetaminophen	Alcohol	Canrenone	Ampicillin (suspension)
Alclofenac	Ampicillin (capsules)	Carbamazepine	Amoxicillin
Amoxicillin	Amoxicillin (capsules)	Diazepam	Aspirin (coated granules in
Aspirin (effervescent tablets,	Aspirin (enteric-coated tab-	Dicumarol	capsule)
tablets)	lets, tablets)	Diftalone	Bendroflumethiazide
Cefaclor	Aspirin (Ca^{++})	Erythromycin estolate (cap-	Chlorpropamide
Cephalexin	Demeclocycline	sules)	Digoxin (elixir)
Cephradine	Doxycycline	Erythromycin ethyl succi-	Erythromycin ethyl car-
Cimetidine	Erythromycin (coated tablets,	nate (coated tablets, sus-	bonate (suspension)
Digoxin (tablets)	tablets)	pension)	Erythromycin estolate (sus-
Erythromycin (coated tab-	Erythromycin estolate (cap-	Erythromycin stearate	pension)
lets, tablets)	sules)	Griseofulvin	Erythromycin stearate
Furosemide	Erythromycin stearate (coat-	Hetacillin	(suspension)
Indoprofen	ed tablets)	Hydralazine	Glipizide
Nitrofurantoin	Isoniazid	Hydrochlorothiazide	Glyburide
Phenobarbital	Levodopa	Lithium citrate	Indoprofen
Potassium	Methacycline	Metoprolol	Metronidazole
Sulfadiazine	Nafcillin	Nitrofurantoin	Oxazepam
Sulfadiazine (Na$^+$)	Oxytetracycline	Phenytoin	Penicillin V (tablets)
Sulfanilamide	Penicillin G	Propoxyphene	Prednisone
Sulfadimethoxine	Penicillin V (suspension, tab-	Propranolol	Propylthiouracil
Sulfasymazine	lets)	Riboflavin	Tolbutamide
Sulfisoxazole	Penicillin V (Ca^{++})	Spironolactone	
	Penicillin V (K$^+$)		
	Phenethicillin		
	Pivampicillin		
	Propantheline		
	Rifampin		
	Tetracycline		
	Theophylline		

Compiled from Melander, A. *Clinical Pharmacokinetics*, 1981, *3*, 333-351; Toothaker, R.D., and Welling, P.G. *Annual Review of Pharmacology and Toxicology*, 1980, *20*, 173-199; and Welling, P.G. *Journal of Pharmacokinetics and Biopharmaceutics*, 1977, *5*, 291-334.
*For those drugs that appear in more than one category the dosage and salt forms have been listed. On occasion, however, the same drug with the same dosage and salt forms may appear in more than one category (e.g., erythromycin estolate, capsules). For these drugs variability in study design and subject population may account for the apparent discrepancy.

TABLE 4-3

Physiologic factors influencing drug absorption

GASTRIC EMPTYING	
Factor	*Effect on gastric emptying*
Volume of ingested material	As volume increases, there initially is an increase followed by a decrease in rate of emptying; bulky material tends to empty more slowly than liquids
Type of meal	
Fats	Decrease rate of emptying
Carbohydrates	Decrease rate of emptying
Temperature of ingested material	As temperature increases to body temperature, rate of emptying increases
Viscosity of ingested material	As viscosity increases, rate of emptying decreases
Osmotic pressure of ingested material	As osmotic pressure increases, rate of emptying decreases
Body positioning	When a person lies on the left side, rate of emptying decreases
Psychologic state	Aggressive emotional states appear to increase rate of emptying; depressive states tend to decrease rate of emptying
Drugs	
Anticholinergics (e.g., atropine)	Decrease rate of emptying
Narcotic analgesics (e.g., morphine, meperidine)	Decrease rate of emptying
Analgesics (e.g., acetaminophen, aspirin)	Decrease rate of emptying
Disease states	
Stomach neoplasm	Decreases rate of emptying
Gastric ulcer	No effect
Ulcer of pyloric antrum or associated with duodenal ulcer	Decreases rate of emptying
Uncomplicated duodenal ulcer	Increases rate of emptying
Diabetic diarrhea	Decreases rate of emptying
Miscellaneous factors:	
Acidification (e.g., HCl, H_2SO_4, tartaric acid, citric acid)	Decreases rate of emptying
KCl	Decreases rate of emptying
NaCl, $NaHCO_3$, urea, glycerol	Increase rate of emptying up to a maximum concentration, and thereafter decrease rate of emptying
$NaHCO_3$, 1 hour after a meal	Decreases rate of emptying
Bile salts	Decrease rate of emptying
Alcohol before a meal	Decreases rate of emptying

INTESTINAL MOTILITY AND INTESTINAL TRANSIT TIME	
Factor	*Effect on intestinal motility and/or intestinal transit time*
Food	Retards transit
Increased viscosity	Tends to retard transit rate; decreases diffusion as well as decreasing dissolution rate, and thus decreases absorption
Disease states	
Constipation	Decreases rate of transit
Diarrhea	Increases rate of transit
Lack of digestive juices	Decreases rate of transit
Insulin, hypoglycemia	Increases intestinal motility and probably increases rate of transit
Lack of thyroxine secretion	Decreases transit rate

From Mayersohn, M.A. *Canadian Pharmaceutical Journal*, 1971, *6*, 164-169.

Continued.

TABLE 4-3—cont'd

Physiologic factors influencing drug absorption

INTESTINAL MOTILITY AND INTESTINAL TRANSIT TIME—cont'd	
Factor	*Effect on intestinal motility and/or intestinal transit time*
Drugs	
Anticholinergics (e.g., atropine)	Reduce the motor activity of the GI tract and as a result will decrease intestinal transit rate
Various other drugs that have an action antagonistic to anticholinergics (e.g., parasympathomimetics, anticholinesterases, ganglionic stimulants)	Increase intestinal muscle tone and increase intestinal transit rate
Morphine	Increases the tone of the intestinal musculature and thus enhances motility
Tricyclic antidepressants	Possess anticholinergic activity and may thus decrease transit rate
Miscellaneous factors	
Pregnancy	Transit rate decreases probably because of smooth muscle relaxation
Bile secretion	Increases transit rate

GASTROINTESTINAL BLOOD FLOW	
Factor	*Effect on gastrointestinal blood flow*
Food	Blood flow to the gastrointestinal tract increases
Physical exercise	Appears to decrease blood circulation to the gastrointestinal tract
Hypotensive conditions and syncope	Reduce blood flow to the gastrointestinal tract

INTERACTION OF DRUGS WITH FOOD	
Factor	*Effect*
Food in the gastrointestinal tract	In addition to altering gastric emptying rate, may provide substances to which the drug can bind; such binding, particularly if an insoluble complex is formed, will decrease the amount of drug that can be absorbed (e.g., binding of tetracycline antibiotics by calcium [cheese, milk] and aluminum salts [antacids]).

DRUG INTERACTION WITH GASTROINTESTINAL COMPONENTS	
Factor	*Effect*
Gastrointestinal membrane (membrane is lined by a mucous material, which is viscous)	This material is able to bind certain drugs and reduce their absorption (e.g., quaternary ammonium compounds form a nonabsorbable complex with mucous, and in vitro studies have shown that streptomycin and dihydrostreptomycin bind to mucus)
Intestinal enzymes	Metabolic alterations of drugs; pancreatin and trypsin can deacetylate *N*-acetylated compounds (e.g., several sulfonamides); intestinal esterases act on the acetoxymethylester of benzylpenicillin
Bile	
Various components of bile (e.g., bile salts, lecithin) have surface activity	Surface active agents may increase the wetting of solid particles and enhance drug dissolution rate
Bile	Several drugs (e.g., neomycin and kanamycin) form insoluble complexes with bile salts, thus decreasing absorption of these compounds. Other antibiotics (e.g., nystatin, polymyxin, and vancomycin) are inactivated by bile salts.
Intestinal fluid pH	May increase degradation and reduce absorption of certain compounds that are unstable in acid

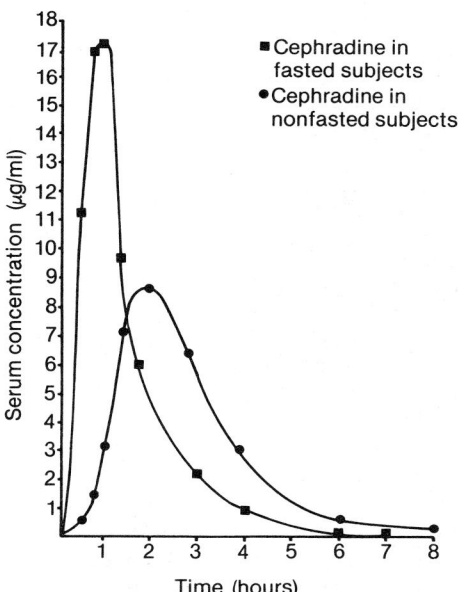

FIGURE 4-7. **Average serum concentrations of cephradine following oral administration of a 500 mg dose to fasting or nonfasting subjects. (From Mischler, T.W., et al. *Journal of Clinical Pharmacology*, 1974, 4, 604-611.)**

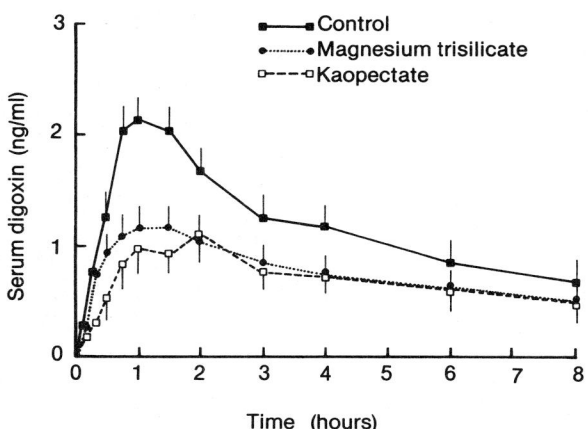

FIGURE 4-8. **Average (± SE) serum concentrations of digoxin following oral administration of 0.75 mg to 10 healthy adults. The tablets were given alone (control) and with magnesium trisilicate or Kaopectate. (From Brown, D.D., and Juhl, R.P. *New England Journal of Medicine*, 1976, 295, 1034-1037.)**

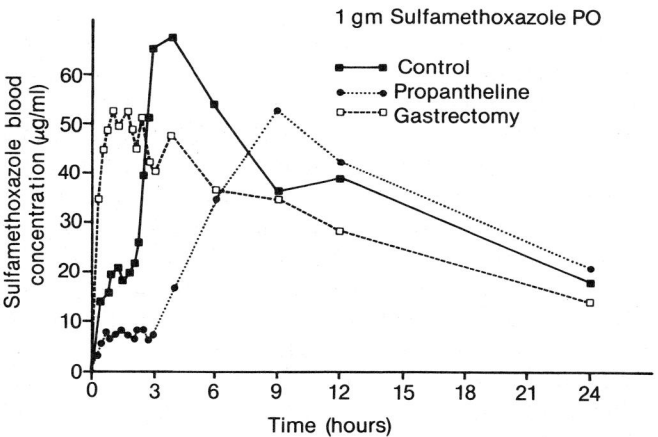

FIGURE 4-9. **Average blood levels of nonmetabolized sulfamethoxazole following oral administration of two 0.5 gm tablets, under three different conditions. (From Antonioli, J.A., et al. *International Journal of Clinical Pharmacology*, 1971, 5, 212-215.**

versus time curves. What is important is that we are aware of these possibilities. Once a patient's dosing regimen has been established, it is important that the timing of the dosing schedule relative to meals is kept constant. Otherwise, the patient will be shifting from one curve to the other and risking either dropping below the effective concentration or rising above the minimum toxic level.

Figure 4-8 shows the effect of an antacid and an antidiarrheal on the availability of digoxin. Digoxin is a particularly troublesome drug, since there is little difference between its therapeutic and its toxic concentrations (i.e., it has a low therapeutic index). Volunteer subjects took a 0.75 mg oral dose of digoxin alone or with the antacid magnesium trisilicate or the antidiarrheal Kaopectate. Notice that the t_{peak} of each is the same, but both the magnesium trisilicate and the Kaopectate decrease the extent of availability. Once again, if a patient were routinely taking only digoxin, that patient's dosage could be adjusted to give therapeutic but not toxic levels.

Suppose, however, the patient developed an ulcer and an antacid was prescribed. Now the patient might drop below a therapeutic level. It is important to realize that in addition to treating the patient's ulcer, we must also monitor the digoxin. On the other hand, what would happen if the patient had

been taking an antacid while the initial dosing regimen of digoxin was established, and then stopped taking the antacid? The patient's digoxin levels might rise above the MTC.

In Figure 4-9 we see the effect of propantheline (a drug that slows GI motility) on the absorption of the antibiotic sulfamethoxazole. Propantheline decreases both the rate and extent of availability. We might have predicted the effect on the rate, but the decrease in

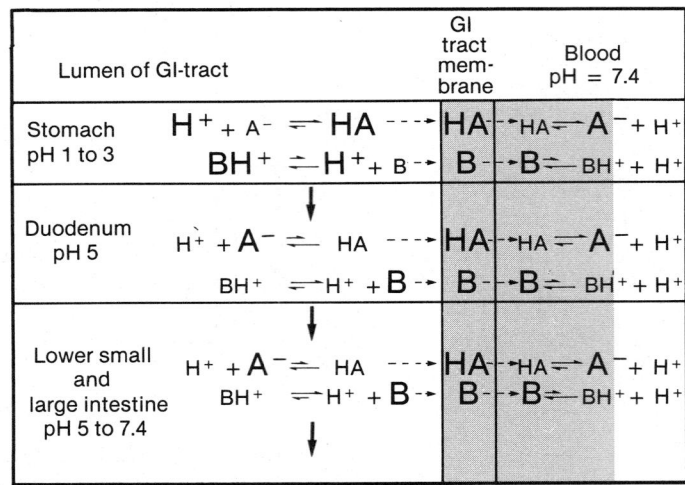

FIGURE 4-10. **The effect of the changing pH along the GI tract on the ionization of acidic and basic drugs.** *HA,* **acidic drug (a drug that can donate a proton);** *B,* **basic drug (a drug that can accept a proton). The relative sizes of H$^+$, HA, A$^-$, B, and BH$^+$ are proportional to their concentration.**

extent is more difficult to rationalize. We might speculate that since it stayed in the stomach acid longer, some of the sulfamethoxazole was degraded. One other interesting effect is shown in Figure 4-9. If stomach emptying controls the rate at which a drug reaches its site of absorption, then we might predict that in a patient who has undergone a partial or total gastrectomy the drug would arrive directly at its site of absorption. Hence, in Figure 4-9, the gastrectomy patient has the fastest rate of availability of sulfamethoxazole.

Ask yourself how an intestinal bypass or resectioning would effect the bioavailability of a drug. Would the length of the bypassed section be important? Would its location (i.e., ileostomy versus colostomy) be significant? We might expect that for a drug well absorbed high up in the GI tract that there would be little or no effect. Likewise, the shorter the bypassed section and the further it is down the GI tract, the less likely it will interfere with drug availability. However, extensive resectioning may markedly decrease the extent of availability of a drug.

Dissolution. The second step in the process of oral absorption is getting the drug into solution. This step will be affected not only by the solubility of the drug itself but also by the kind(s) and amount(s) of inert ingredients in the dosage form. The dissolution rate will also depend on the fluids of the GI tract. Most drugs are either weak acids or weak bases. Hence their solubility will depend on the relative acidity/basicity of the fluids in the GI tract. The relatively low (acidic)

pH (1 to 3) of the stomach contrasts with the higher (more basic) pH (5 to 7) of the duodenum, and the still higher pH (7.4) in the ileum and colon.

The left hand side of Figure 4-10 illustrates the degree of ionization for acidic and basic drugs as they move down the GI tract. An acidic drug will be more soluble in the aqueous fluids of the GI tract when it is ionized. Acids will become increasingly ionized as the pH increases (i.e., as the pH becomes more basic). Thus, they become more ionized and more water soluble as they move down the GI tract. Bases, on the other hand, are ionized at low pH, and thus will be more soluble higher up in the GI tract.

Antacids that raise the stomach pH might, therefore, decrease the dissolution rate of basic drugs taken concurrently but increase the dissolution rate of acidic drugs. Patients who are deficient in stomach acid, achlorhydric, might also be expected to have abnormal blood level curves of some drugs.

In addition, both acidic and basic drugs can be given in their salt forms. With rare exception, these salts are more soluble than the parent acids or bases. Some drugs are available for oral use as both the parent and various salt forms—for example, penicillin G and penicillin G sodium, tetracycline and tetracycline hydrochloride or tetracycline phosphate. Others are available only as the parent compound (e.g., diazepam), or only as the salt (e.g., procainamide hydrochloride). Often the choice is made by the manufacturers. Their decision might be based on bioavailability studies but is more likely based on physical and chemical stability, the ease of handling, and cost.

Inert ingredients may also dramatically effect the dissolution rate of the active ingredients. Disintegrants, (e.g., starch) may hasten the breaking apart of a tablet or capsule into many fine particles that will dissolve more rapidly than one large one. On the other hand, binders (e.g., gelatin) are usually added to hold the particles together so that a tablet will not fall apart before the patient has a chance to swallow it. These inert ingredients will vary from manufacturer to manufacturer. Two tablets made by two different manufacturers may, even if they contain the same amount of the same active ingredient, have different blood level versus time curves because they dissolve at different rates. Thus, getting the drug into solution depends on both patient variables (e.g., composition of the GI fluids) and pharmaceutical variables (e.g., solubility of the drug and the inert ingredients).

Membrane transport. The third step in absorption, membrane transport, also depends on both patient and pharmaceutical variables. The body has special active transport systems for absorbing some nutrients. Drugs that have chemical structures similar to these nutrients can also be absorbed by active transport. We will, however, consider only drugs absorbed by passive diffusion.

Biologic membranes typically act as lipid barriers. This lipid membrane barrier will be permeable to drugs with at least some degree of lipid solubility. For an acidic or basic drug the nonionized form is more lipid soluble than the ionized form. Acids will be more nonionized at a low (acidic) pH, and bases will be more nonionized at a high (basic) pH. The right side of Figure 4-10 illustrates these concepts. Thus acids are more rapidly transported through this barrier in the stomach and bases, in the small intestine. However, no acidic or basic drug will be 100% ionized or nonionized anywhere along the GI tract. There will be an equilibrium between the ionized and nonionized form. Once one nonionized molecule gets through the lipid barrier, the equilibrium will shift and another nonionized molecule will be available. This process may be slow and may cause the drug to be slowly absorbed. On the other hand, many acidic drugs (e.g., aspirin) are well absorbed from the small intestine, even though they are extensively ionized, because of the high surface area of the small intestine relative to the stomach.

If you compare this discussion with the section on dissolution, you will notice that we predicted that bases will dissolve most rapidly in the stomach and acids in the intestine, whereas membrane transport for bases and acids (because of the surface area) will be most rapid in the intestine. Which then will be the predominant effect? The answer is, "It depends." It depends on which one is the slowest step. In any rate process with more than one step, it is the slowest step that determines the rate at which the task gets done. This is also known as the *rate limiting step.* In our case, the task is to get the drug to the general circulation. Whether stomach emptying, dissolution, or membrane transport is the rate limiting or determining step depends on which of the steps is (for a particular drug in a given dosage form, taken under certain circumstances by an individual patient), the slowest. Can we predict which step will be slowest? In some cases, as in Figure 4-9 with propantheline, the answer is "probably." Usually, however, we must examine the results of a well-designed bioavailability study for determination of both the rate and extent of absorption and then draw our own conclusions. For some drugs these studies have been done. For many they have not. Pharmacists are the members of your health care team who have the most extensive training in how these studies should be performed and their results interpreted. You should consult with them. Even if they cannot immediately answer your question, they should be able to find out if the information is available.

Blood flow to the general circulation. The final step in absorption involves carrying the drug away from the site and into the general circulation. For the oral route this step will depend on the rate of blood flow to the GI tract. It is possible that this could be the slowest step in oral dosing. However, there are, as yet, no known cases where it is. There is, however, another important consideration. As the blood carrying the drug leaves the small intestine, it travels through the liver and to the heart, then from the heart to the lungs and then back to the heart before it reaches the general circulation (see Figure 4-6). If the drug (e.g., nitroglycerin) is both rapidly and extensively metabolized on its first pass through the liver, then it will not be available to the general circulation. It is true that the drug did get out of the intestine and into the blood, but not all of it gets to the general circulation intact. We call this the first-pass effect. What other routes will show a first-pass effect? The rectal route is estimated to have a potential first-pass effect of up to 50%. The blood from the other tissues will reach the liver after the general circulation. If the drug is also rapidly and extensively metabolized in the lung, which routes will show a first-pass lung effect? For all the routes shown in Figure 4-6 the blood leaving the tissue goes through the lung before reaching the general circulation. Can you think of any route that would avoid this first-pass

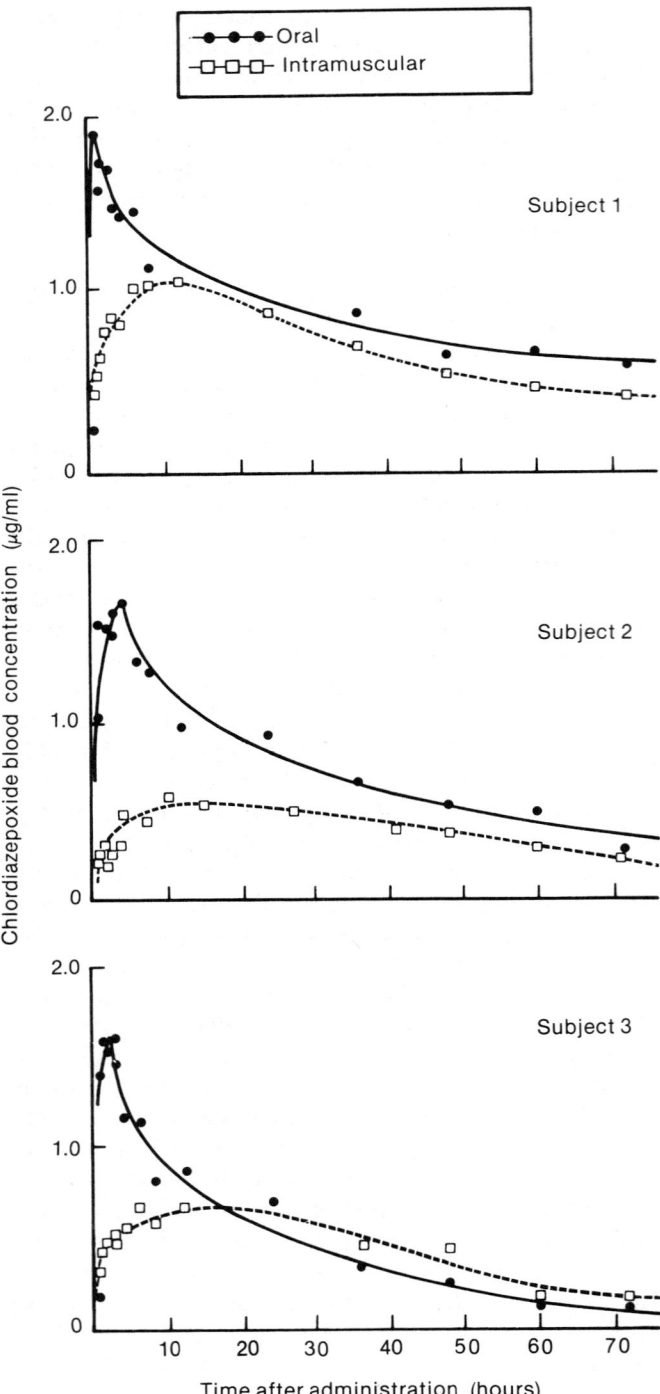

FIGURE 4-11. **Blood levels of chloridiazepoxide following a 50 mg dose given orally (●—●) (two 25 mg capsules) or intramuscularly (□---□) (50 mg/2 ml). (From Greenblatt, D.J., et al. *New England Journal of Medicine*, 1974, *291*, 1116-1118.)**

lung effect? Only the intraarterial route would allow drugs to avoid the first-pass lung effect and be delivered to the general circulation. For drugs administered directly to the site of action (e.g., intrathecal) neither lung nor liver metabolism on the first pass will be important.

In all of the remaining routes of administration involving membrane transport, the drugs are applied directly to the site of absorption. Thus, we need consider only three steps—dissolution, membrane transport, and blood flow to the general circulation.

Buccal and sublingual routes. Some drugs that are extensively metabolized on their first pass through the liver (e.g., nitroglycerin or testosterone) may be administered in sublingual or buccal tablets. These tablets are held under the tongue or in the cheek pouch. In general, sublingual tablets are designed to dissolve rapidly whereas buccal tablets dissolve slowly. Since the buccal membranes are well perfused, absorption can be rapid and complete. Unfortunately, some of the dissolved drug may be swallowed with the saliva or the patient may mistakenly swallow the entire tablet, thus defeating the purpose of using these routes.

Intramuscular and subcutaneous routes. The notion that because a needle and syringe are used to inject a drug (either a solution or suspension), either intramuscularly or subcutaneously, it will be instantaneously available is not necessarily true. Dissolution and blood flow to the area may be significant problems. Even if we inject a solution, the drug may precipitate in the muscle mass or in the subcutaneous fat. Phenytoin crystals have actually been seen in the muscle tissue following IM injection (*against* the manufacturer's advice). Phenytoin is not very water soluble. The miniscule volume and pH 7.4 fluids of the muscle cause the phenytoin to precipitate from the injection solution. These crystals dissolve slowly and unpredictably to give low blood levels. The directions accompanying the phenytoin solution, therefore, recommend a slow (50 mg/min) IV push.

An IM injection of a drug may actually be less rapidly available than an oral capsule form of the same drug because of such solubility problems. The blood level curve obtained after an IM or oral dose of chlordiazepoxide is shown in Figure 4-11. Which is the more rapidly absorbed? Which has the greatest extent of availability? The answer to both of these questions is the oral route. It has an earlier t_{peak} and larger AUC.

Consider the problem of blood flow to the site of injection. The area of the absorbing membrane is small at the site of injection. Thus we must rely on the blood to carry away the absorbed molecules so that those

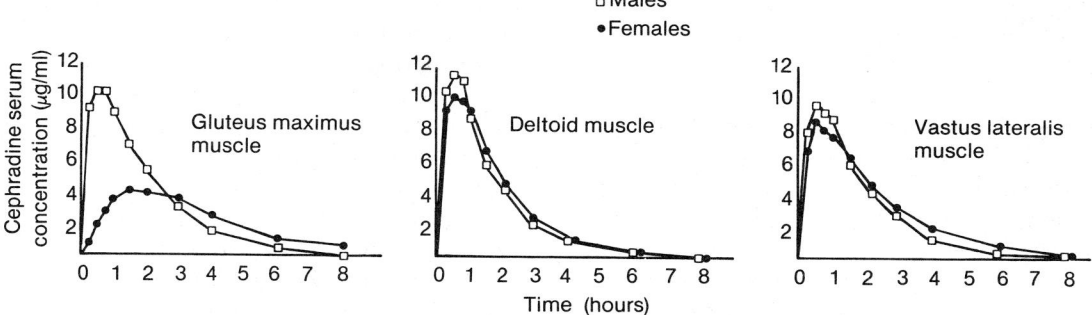

FIGURE 4-12. **Average cephradine serum concentrations following intramuscular injection of a 475 mg dose at different sites in men (□) or women (●). (From Vukovitch, R.A., et al. *Clinical Pharmacology and Therapeutics*, 1975, *18*, 215-220.)**

remaining to be absorbed can be passively transported. However, the circulation to the area can be low or variable. Consider insulin. Studies have shown that joggers who inject insulin experience an undesirably precipitous drop in blood sugar after a SC injection into the thigh but not if the injection is into the arm or abdomen. Running markedly increases the blood flow to the leg area. The dose of insulin is rapidly carried into the general circulation, and the blood glucose level drops immediately. Blood flow to the arm or abdomen does not change so dramatically, so absorption is slow but steady. Likewise, the blood glucose level drops slowly to the desired level.

Another interesting patient variable is illustrated in Figure 4-12 with the IM administration of cephradine. There is no difference in bioavailability for male and female subjects when the injection is into the deltoid or vastus lateralis muscle. There is a marked difference, however, in rate for the injection into the gluteus maximus. This has been attributed to the different distribution of subcutaneous fat around the musculature in men and women. Since fat is less well perfused, we would expect that if blood flow were the rate-determining step in absorption, then women will have a later t_{peak}.

Intradermal route. Intradermal injections are made directly below the superficial layer of the skin. This route is used for diagnostic tests (e.g., TB, allergy) or for vaccination (e.g., smallpox). Absorption into the general circulation will be slow and is considered to be a side effect.

Intrathecal route. Many drugs do not readily penetrate the central nervous system. Some drugs (e.g., antibiotics for spinal meningitis) must, therefore, be injected directly into the fluid in the spinal canal (i.e., intrathecally). This is an injection directly into the bio-

phase and thus bioavailability is not usually considered to be a problem. In fact, the drug that does reach the general circulation is *no* longer available to the target tissue.

Vaginal route. This route of administration is most often used for local effects. Antibiotic (e.g., metronidazole), contraceptive (e.g., progestin), and hormonal (e.g., conjugated estrogens) medications can be administered by this route for their local effects. The vagina is well perfused and could, in theory, be used as a route for systemic drug delivery. It has not, however, and thus bioavailability, in terms of getting the drug to the general circulation, is generally considered to be an undesirable side effect for this route of administration.

Rectal route. Rectal suppositories and solutions (e.g., microenemas) can be used for both local and systemic effects. This route is often a viable alternative for patients with nausea and vomiting. It also has the advantage of at least partially avoiding any first-pass liver metabolism, since only about 50% of the blood leaving the rectal tissues goes through the liver before reaching the general circulation. Bioavailability following rectal administration can be rapid and complete if the suppository has been properly formulated, inserted, and placed correctly, and is retained by the patient. A major disadvantage is poor patient acceptability, and therefore, poor compliance. No dosage form is bioavailable if the patient refuses or neglects to take it.

Ophthalmic route. Solutions, suspensions, and ointments can be administered ophthalmically. In general, the drops or ointment are placed in the conjunctival sac between the lower lid and the cornea. The volume of the dose administered is accordingly small. In addition, much will be washed away by tears.

Hence, most ophthalmic preparations are used for their local effects. Again, as with the vaginal route, delivery of the drug to the general circulation is usually considered to be a side effect.

Nasal route. Nasal solutions (or rarely gels) can be used for both local (e.g., treatment of congestion) and systemic (e.g., treatment of diabetes insipidus) effects. The nasal membranes are well perfused with blood. Absorption can be rapid. A disadvantage is that only a small volume can be delivered. In addition, much of the dose may get into the pharynx, where it will be swallowed and made available by the oral route. It is difficult, therefore, to perform and interpret bioavailability studies using the nasal route.

Inhalation route. Inhalation therapy can be effective both locally and systemically. Certainly antiasthmatic drugs (e.g., isoproterenol) and anesthetic gases (e.g., nitrous oxide) are rapidly and extensively available to the general circulation through the membranes of the lung. The rate of availability may approach that of IV administration. There are, however, few controlled studies examining this potential.

Absorption across the skin

Topical route. When dosage forms (e.g., solutions, suspension, lotions, creams, or ointments) are applied topically, the drug must first get out of the dosage form, then partition into the epidermis, diffuse through the epidermis partition into the dermis, and then go into the capillary beds where it will be picked up by the blood and delivered to the general circulation.

The epidermis is a dense, highly keratinized layer of dead cells (see Chapter 54, "Review of the Anatomy, Physiology, and Assessment of the Cutaneous System"). It is a formidable barrier. One of its major functions is to protect the body from the external environment. In doing so, it also prevents the absorption of most drugs. Topical applications are, thus, usually not used for their systemic effects. The drug is usually so slowly absorbed that no measurable blood levels will be achieved. Most drugs are applied topically for their effects on the epidermis or dermis.

Penetration of a drug can be maximized by chemical modification to produce an increased solubility in the epidermal barrier. Selection of the correct vehicle (e.g., ointment or cream) can also increase penetration. Solvents such as DMSO will enhance penetration of many drugs by physically altering the barrier layer. None have, however, been approved for clinical use. Finally, using an occlusive dressing (e.g., plastic wrap) can cause hydration of the skin. The hydrated skin will be less dense and more permeable to drugs. Whenever modifications are made that increase drug penetration of the skin, systemic absorption and resultant systemic toxicity can occur and should be monitored for. Patient noncompliance is often significant because messy, greasy, smelly ointments are not well tolerated by many patients. In addition, the most aesthetic topical preparations are often rubbed off or washed off by perspiration before releasing all their drug. (See Section XII, "Dermatologic Medications," for further details on topical medications.)

Otic route. The external ear canal is lined with keratinized epithelial cells. Therefore, systemic absorption is highly improbable. Otic drops can be used for local infections of the external canal or to soften ear wax. Infections of the middle ear, however, must be treated systemically.

DOSAGE FORMS THAT ATTEMPT TO CONTROL THE RATE OF DRUG RELEASE

We have considered the four steps in getting a drug into the general circulation and therefore to its site of action. At each step we have considered how the pharmaceutical and patient variables may interact and affect the rate or extent of drug availability. There is considerable interest in designing dosage forms that will reliably deliver, at a fixed rate, their active ingredients. Recall that the slowest step in any rate process is the rate-determining step. Therefore, the pharmaceutical designers must slow the release of drug from its dosage form, since they cannot alter the patient. The usual approach has been to attempt to design dosage forms with known release rates. The intent is to achieve a blood level just above the minimum effective concentration and then sustain that level.

Sustained-release capsules and tablets have been manufactured (e.g., Spansules, Lontabs, Extentabs). These usually contain the drug inside a special coating or matrix. The coating dissolves in the GI tract to release the drug, or the drug is leached out of the matrix. Both require action by the GI fluids, which are a patient variable. Furthermore, food in the GI tract and GI transit time can significantly affect these dosage forms. Some are more or less successful, but none are totally controlled. In addition, they are usually more expensive than a therapeutically equivalent amount of drug in a conventional dosage form (e.g., Measurin versus generic aspirin).

There are, however, some interesting and successful control-release dosage forms available. A brief list would include a contraceptive intrauterine device (i.e., Progestasert) that steadily releases a low-dose progestin over the period of 1 year. Ocuserts, small pliable disks containing pilocarpine, are inserted in the conjunctival sac between the lower eyelid and the cornea. They can be worn for 7 days to treat glaucoma. They slowly release the pilocarpine to produce a low level of drug. Patients are spared the inconvenience of three to four daily applications of the ophthalmic drops. They also avoid the blurred vision caused by the high levels of pilocarpine when they first apply the drops. There is also a small flexible patch containing scopolamine. Applied behind the ear, it releases sufficient drug to the systemic circulation to protect the wearer from motion sickness. Other products are currently being designed and tested. Certainly the goal of controlling the rate and extent of delivery of a drug to its site of action is a desirable one. Considering, however, the degree of interpatient variability and the multiplicity of disease states, it is not likely to be a universally achievable one.

DISTRIBUTION

So far we have been concerned with getting a drug out of its dosage form and into the general circulation. This is the absorption step of pharmacokinetics. The next steps are distribution, metabolism, and excretion. The latter two topics are discussed in Chapter 5. Our remaining subject is distribution. Now that the drug has gotten into the general circulation, it will be distributed to all those places in the body that the blood goes. In short, everywhere. It is unlikely, however, that the drug will be uniformly distributed throughout the body. The amount of the drug and its time course in each tissue or organ will depend on several factors: (1) the size of the organ or tissue into which the drug distributes, (2) the partition coefficient of the drug between the tissue or organ and the circulating blood, (3) the blood flow to the area, and (4) the extent of protein binding of the drug in the blood and the tissue or organ.

Notice that these factors depend on the drug's physical/chemical properties and the patient's physiology. They are relatively beyond our control. It is true that blood flow to different areas may vary. For example, as we saw previously with insulin, strenuous physical activity will increase blood flow to the muscles being exercised. Likewise, blood flow to the GI tract is greatest during and just after a meal. Nevertheless, well-perfused organs (e.g., the liver) are more likely to see more of the drug. However, a drug may, because of its solubility characteristics, partition into less well perfused areas (e.g., muscle). Lipid-soluble drugs (e.g., phenobarbital) are more likely to accumulate in the fat than are drugs with poor lipid solubility (e.g., aspirin). On the other hand, for drugs with low lipid solubility, we often calculate the dose for obese patients using not their actual weight but their desired weight. Since the drug does not distribute into their fat, a dose per kilogram of real weight would generally result in an overdose.

The extent of protein binding of drug in the blood versus the tissues can be a critical factor. We usually assume that it is the free (unbound) drug in blood that is available to the site of action (See Chapter 3, "Mechanisms of Drug Action"). We further assume that the unbound drug in blood is in equilibrium with the unbound drug in the tissues. Other drugs or endogenous compounds may compete with and displace or be displaced by a drug (e.g., free fatty acids and aspirin). Binding may also be altered in disease states (e.g., phenytoin in cirrhosis). Thus, the free and bound concentrations of drug in the blood and tissues may be altered. Such changes in free drug may affect the blood level versus time curve and modify the availability to the site of action. Whether there is a need to modify drug therapy is a complex and difficult decision. It is a decision often recognized retrospectively. In Chapter 10, "Drug Interactions," drugs altering the protein binding of other drugs are further discussed.

SUMMARY

We have used blood level curves to determine the bioavailability of drugs. We have discussed the patient and pharmaceutical variables that will affect both the rate and extent of availability of a drug from its dosage form. We have used the intravenous route of administration as our reference point. Our emphasis has, however, been on the oral and intramuscular routes of administration. We have also very briefly considered the factors that determine the distribution of a drug throughout the body. Our discussions have been necessarily brief and nonmathematical. You will, however, be using these concepts when you learn about the pharmacologic activity of the specific drugs in the following chapters.

BIBLIOGRAPHY

Antonioli, J.A., Schelling, J.L., Steininger, E. & Borel, G.A. Effects of gastrectomy and of an anticholinergic drug on gastrointestinal absorption of a sulfonamide in man. *International Journal of Clinical Pharmacology*, 1971, *5*, 212-215.

Ballard, B.E. Prolonged-action pharmaceuticals. In A. Osol (Ed.), *Remington's pharmaceutical sciences*. Easton, PA: Mack, 1980.

Benet, L.Z. Input factors as determinants of drug activity: route, dose, dosage regimen, and drug delivery system. In

F. Gilbert McMahon (Ed.), *Principles and techniques of human research and therapeutics* (Vol. 3). New York: Futura, 1974.

Benet, L.Z. The effect of route of administration and distribution on drug action. In G.S. Banker & C.R. Rhodes (Eds.), *Modern Pharmaceutics*. New York: Marcel Dekker, 1979.

Brown, D.D., & Juhl, R.P. Decreased bioavailability of digoxin due to antacids and kaolin-pectin. *New England Journal of Medicine*, 1976, *295*, 1034-1037.

Greenblatt, D.J., Shader, R.I. & Koch-Weser, J. Slow absorption of intramuscular chlordiazepoxide. *New England Journal of Medicine*, 1974, *291*, 1116-1118.

Hersey, J.A. Depot Medication. In G.S. Banker & C.T. Rhodes (Eds.), *Modern Pharmaceutics*. New York: Marcel Dekker, 1979.

Hoener, B. & Benet, L.Z. Factors influencing drug absorption and drug availability. In G.S. Banker & C.T. Rhodes (Eds.), *Modern Pharmaceutics*. New York: Marcel Dekker, 1979.

Kolvisto, V.A., & Felig, P. Effects of leg exercise on insulin absorption in diabetic patients. *New England Journal of Medicine*, 1978, *298*, 79-83.

Mayersohn, M. Pharmacologic factors influencing drug absorption. *Canadian Pharmaceutical Journal*, 1971, *6*, 164-169.

Melander, A. Influence of food on the bioavailability of drugs. *Clinical Pharmacokinetics*, 1981, *3*, 337-351.

Mischler, T.W., Sugerman, A., Willard, D.A., Brannick, L.J., Neiss, E.S. Influence of probenecid and food on the bioavailability of cephradine in normal male subjects. *Journal of Clinical Pharmacology*, 1974, *14*, 604-611.

Shaw, J.E., & Chandrasekaran, K. Controlled topic delivery of drugs for systemic action. *Drug Metabolism Review*, 1978, *8*, 223-233.

Toothaker, R.D., & Welling, P.G. The effect of food on drug bioavailability. *Annual Review of Pharmacology and Toxicology*, 1980, *20*, 173-199.

Welling, P.G. Influence of food and diet on gastrointestinal drug absorption: a review. *Journal of Pharmacokinetics and Biopharmaceutics*, 1977, *5*, 291-334.

Welling, P.G., & Craig, W.A. Pharmacokinetics in disease states modifying renal function. In L.Z. Benet (Ed.), *The effect of disease states on drug pharmacokinetics*. Washington, D.C.: American Pharmaceutical Association, 1976.

Williams, R.L., & Benet, L.Z. Drug pharmacokinetics in cardiac and hepatic disease. *Annual Review of Pharmacology and Toxicology*, 1980, *20*, 389-413.

Vukovitch, R.A., Brannick, L.J., Sugerman, A.A., & Neiss, E.S. Sex differences in the intramuscular absorption and bioavailability of cephradine. *Clinical Pharmacology and Therapeutics*, 1975, *18*, 215-220.

CHAPTER 5

Drug Metabolism and Elimination

Ronald T. Coutts

DRUG METABOLISM

Drug metabolism may be defined as the chemical modification of a drug in a biologic environment. The procedure is also commonly referred to as drug biotransformation or drug detoxification. Most drugs undergo metabolic modification in the body; only a few (e.g., acetazolamide, barbital, decamethonium, hexamethonium, penicillin G) are excreted almost quantitatively in unchanged form. Drugs that are metabolized (e.g., phenothiazines) may be converted to many products or may form only one major metabolite (e.g., metabolic conjugation of benzoic acid to hippuric acid). Normally drug metabolism is enzymatically controlled via oxidases, reductases, esterases, and enzymes involved in conjugation reactions, but sometimes nonenzymatic reactions occur in the body. Nitroso compounds, for example, may be oxidized to nitro compounds in the presence of oxygen but without the involvement of an enzyme. The process of drug metabolism produces metabolites.

Purposes of drug metabolism

Drug metabolism in the organism has two *principal* functions:

1. To convert drugs to products (metabolites) that are less pharmacologically active. Otherwise a pharmacologic reaction would continue indefinitely.

2. To convert drugs to products that are much more water soluble (i.e., more polar or ionized) than the parent drug and therefore more readily and rapidly excreted. Because of their polarity, most metabolites do not undergo tubular reabsorption in the kidney to any great extent, and are thus excreted in the urine.

Although it is true that most metabolites are less active pharmacologically and more polar than the parent drug, there are exceptions to this generalization. Some products are referred to as "active metabolites" because they possess a pharmacologic activity equal to, greater than, or different from, the parent drug itself; some may have appreciable activity. Occasionally, a metabolite is more lipophilic than the drug from which it was formed. Some sulfonamides, for example, are metabolically converted to lipophilic N-acetylated metabolites (see Metabolic Activation section later in this chapter).

Sites of drug metabolism

Drug metabolism occurs mainly in the liver and to a lesser extent in the kidney, blood, brain, lungs, gastrointestinal tract, skin, and other tissues.

The most important metabolic reaction is drug oxidation (discussed later) and this occurs mainly in the liver. The liver contains various cells including heptocytes where metabolic oxidation occurs. In the cytoplasm of the liver cell there are various structures (Figure 5-1), including a network of channels called *smooth endoplasmic reticulum,* which contain the oxidase enzymes and the *granular,* or *rough, endoplasmic reticulum.* The granular endoplasmic reticulum, however, is not involved in drug metabolism. Its main function is protein synthesis. Metabolic reductions also occur in the liver. The most common ones are the reverse of known oxidative mechanisms (e.g.,

$$\underset{/}{\overset{\backslash}{C}} = O \leftrightharpoons \underset{/}{\overset{\backslash}{C}}HOH)$$

and require the same enzyme system. Actually many enzymatic reactions are reversible, but usually the reaction equilibrium favors one direction.

Metabolism of drugs is also carried out by microorganisms of the gastrointestinal tract, which tend to cause reductions rather than oxidations, and also to catalyze the hydrolysis of esters and amides.

Metabolic pathways

Drug metabolism reactions are classified as phase 1 or phase 2 reactions (see Metabolic Pathways on following pages). A phase 1 metabolic reaction is one in which a new chemical group is introduced into a drug molecule, especially by oxidative, reductive, and hydrolytic methods. A phase 2 metabolic reaction is one in which a drug or phase 1 metabolite is conju-

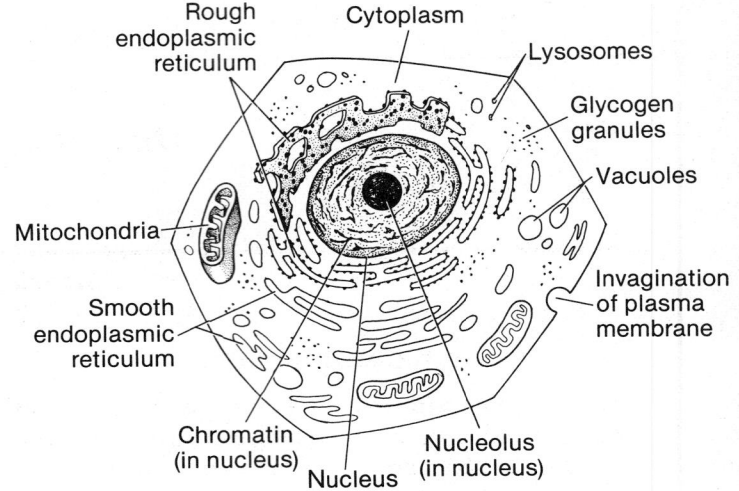

FIGURE 5-1. **Stylized drawing of parenchymal liver cell (hepatocyte).**

Metabolic pathways

Phase 1 reactions
Oxidation

1. Primary alcohols; aldehydes.
   These are oxidized to acids.

   EXAMPLE
   $$CH_3CH_2OH \rightarrow CH_3CHO \rightarrow CH_3COOH$$
   Alcohol   Acetaldehyde   Acetic acid

2. Secondary alcohols.
   These are oxidized to ketones.

   EXAMPLE
   $$CH_3CH_2CHOHCH_3 \rightleftharpoons CH_3CH_2COCH_3$$
   2-Butanol   2-Butanone

3. Aliphatic carbon atoms.
   These are oxidized to alcohols.

   EXAMPLES

   a. $C_4H_9NHCONHSO_2$—⟨ ⟩—CH_3 Tolbutamide

   $\downarrow$

   $C_4H_9NHCONHSO_2$—⟨ ⟩—CH_2OH Alcohol metabolite

   The alcohol metabolite undergoes further metabolic oxidation to the corresponding acid (cf. reaction 1).

Metabolic pathways—cont'd

Phase 1 reactions—cont'd
Oxidation—cont'd

b.

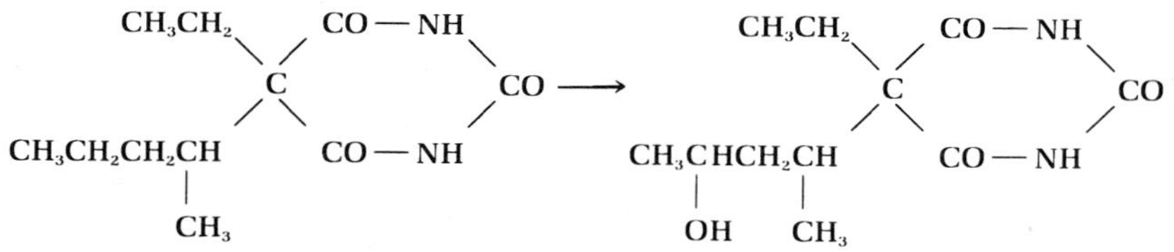

$$CH_3CH_2\text{, } CH_3CH_2CH_2CH(CH_3)\text{—}C(CO\text{—}NH)(CO\text{—}NH)\text{—}CO \longrightarrow CH_3CH_2\text{, } CH_3CHCH_2CH(OH)(CH_3)\text{—}C(CO\text{—}NH)(CO\text{—}NH)\text{—}CO$$

Pentobarbital   Pentobarbital alcohol

4. Aromatic carbon atoms

These are often oxidized in the *para* (p) position to phenols.

EXAMPLES

a. ⟨benzene⟩—$CH_2CH(CH_3)NH_2 \longrightarrow$ HO—⟨benzene⟩—$CH_2CH(CH_3)NH_2$

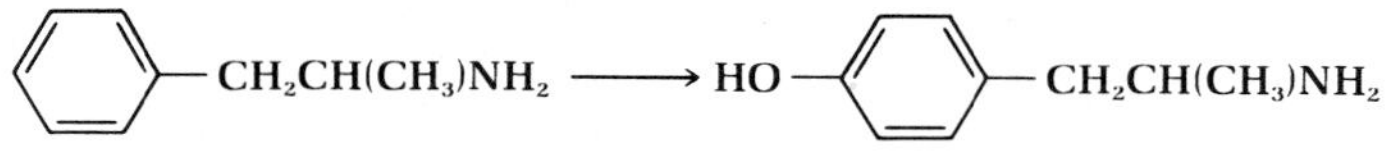

   Amphetamine   *p*-Hydroxyamphetamine

b. CH_3CH_2—⟨benzene⟩—C(CO—NH)(CO—NH)—CO $\longrightarrow$ HO—⟨benzene⟩—CH_3CH_2—C(CO—NH)(CO—NH)—CO

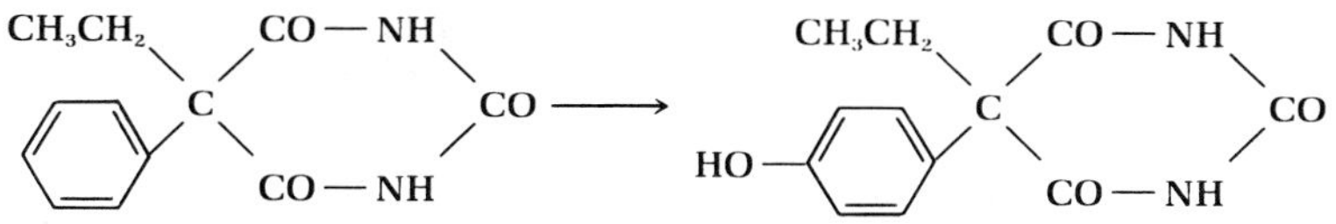

   Phenobarbital   *p*-Hydroxyphenobarbital

5. Dealkylation

N-Alkyl, O-alkyl, and S-alkyl compounds are metabolically dealkylated.
This is an oxidation reaction, and a general reaction can be drawn:

$$R^1\text{—}X\text{—}CH_2R^2 \rightarrow [R^1\text{—}X\text{—}CHOHR^2] \rightarrow R^1\text{—}XH + R^2CHO$$

Dealkylated
product

X = NH, N-alkyl, N-aryl, O, S.

EXAMPLES

a. CH_3CH_2O—⟨benzene⟩—$NHCOCH_3 \longrightarrow$ HO—⟨benzene⟩—$NHCOCH_3$

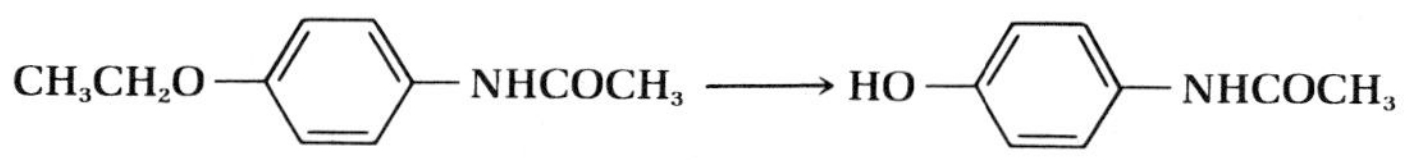

   Phenacetin   *p*-Hydroxyacetanilide
                        (acetaminophen)

b. ⟨benzene⟩—$CHOHCH(CH_3)NHCH_3 \longrightarrow$ ⟨benzene⟩—$CHOHCH(CH_3)NH_2$

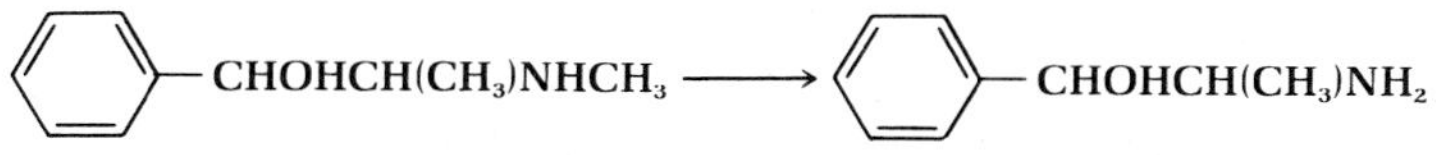

   Ephedrine   Norephedrine

Continued.

Metabolic pathways—cont'd

Phase 1 reactions—cont'd
Oxidation—cont'd

6. Deamination

Amines undergo the following oxidative reaction. A general reaction can be drawn:

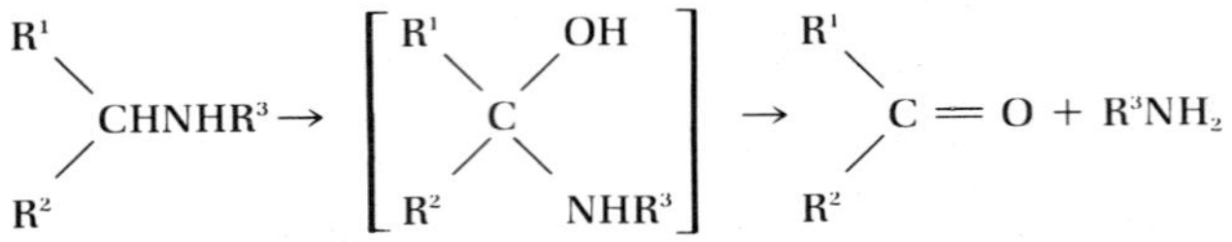

$$\underset{R^2}{\overset{R^1}{\diagdown}}CHNHR^3 \rightarrow \left[\underset{R^2}{\overset{R^1}{\diagdown}}\underset{NHR^3}{\overset{OH}{C}}\right] \rightarrow \underset{R^2}{\overset{R^1}{\diagdown}}C = O + R^3NH_2$$

The mechanism is the same as that observed in dealkylation; the initial product is the result of oxidation at the carbon atom adjacent to the nitrogen atom.

EXAMPLE

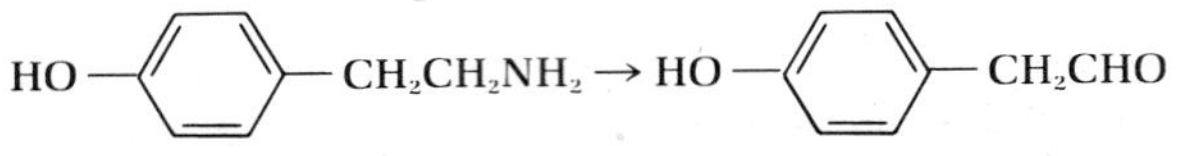

$$HO-\langle\ \rangle-CH_2CH_2NH_2 \rightarrow HO-\langle\ \rangle-CH_2CHO$$

p-Tyramine   *p*-Hydroxyphenylacetaldehyde

The metabolite is oxidized further to *p*-hydroxyphenylacetic acid (cf. reaction 1).

7. *N*-Oxidation

This reaction is observed mainly with tertiary amines that are converted into tertiary amine *N*-oxides. A few primary and secondary amines have been observed to undergo metabolic *N*-oxidation. The products are hydroxylamines and are toxic.

EXAMPLE

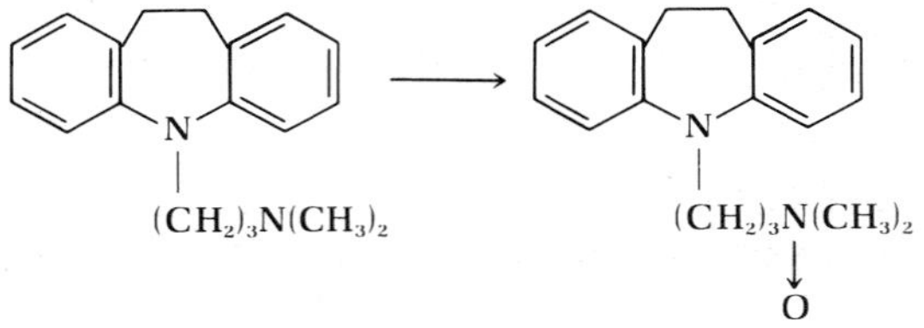

$(CH_2)_3N(CH_3)_2$ $(CH_2)_3N(CH_3)_2$
$\downarrow$
O

Imipramine   Imipramine *N*-oxide

8. *S*-Oxidation

This has been observed mainly with phenothiazine drugs.

EXAMPLE

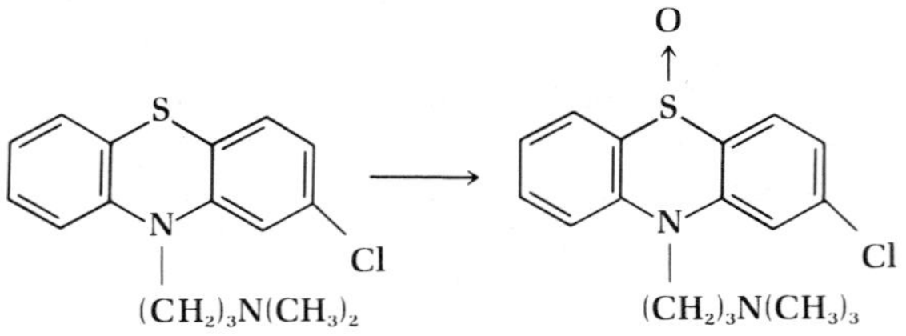

O
$\uparrow$
S

$(CH_2)_3N(CH_3)_2$ — Cl $(CH_2)_3N(CH_3)_3$ — Cl

Chlorpromazine   Chlorpromazine *S*-oxide

Chlorpromazine is also metabolically *N*-oxidized (cf. reaction 7), *N*-dealkylated (cf. reaction 5); deaminated (cf. reaction 6), and ring hydroxylated (cf. reaction 4).

Metabolic pathways—cont'd

Phase 1 reactions—cont'd
Reduction

1. Aldehydes and ketones

   They are reduced to primary and secondary alcohols respectively. Secondary alcohols produced in this way will be optically active.

   EXAMPLE

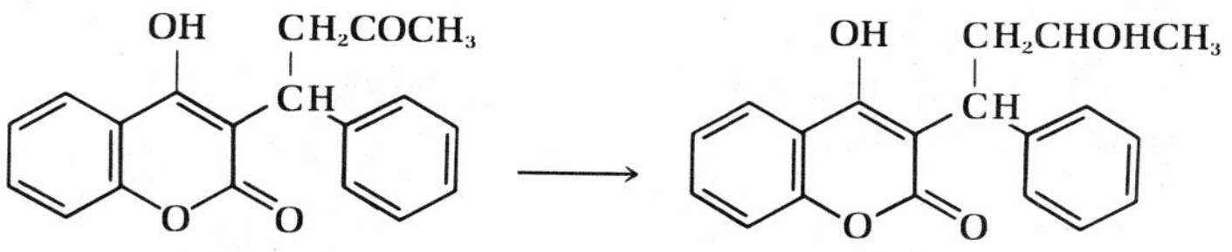

   Warfarin   Warfarin alcohol

2. Aromatic nitro compounds

   They are reduced to primary amines and also to intermediate reduced forms (nitroso compounds and hydroxylamines). A general reaction can be drawn:

   $$R-NO_2 \rightarrow R-N=O \rightarrow R-NHOH \rightarrow R-NH_2$$

   EXAMPLE

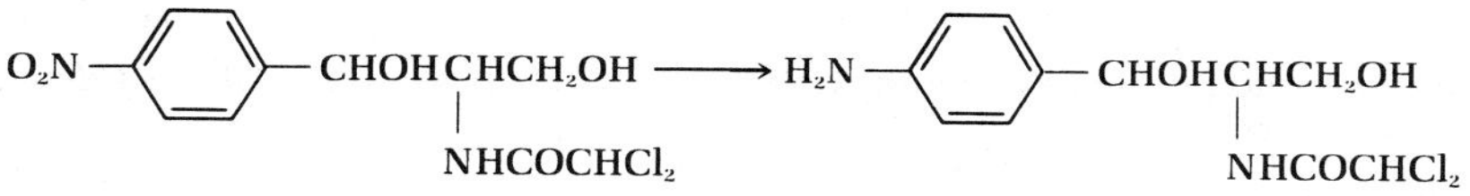

   Chloramphenicol   Reduced chloramphenicol

3. Miscellaneous reductions

   Alkenes may be reduced to alkanes; azo compounds are reduced to hydrazo derivatives; then to primary amines (e.g., prontosil → sulfanilamide); disulfides are reduced to thiols (e.g., disulfiram → dithiocarbamic acid); and sulfoxides may be reduced to sulfides.

Hydrolysis

1. Esters

   They are hydrolyzed by esterases to the corresponding acid.

   EXAMPLES

   a.

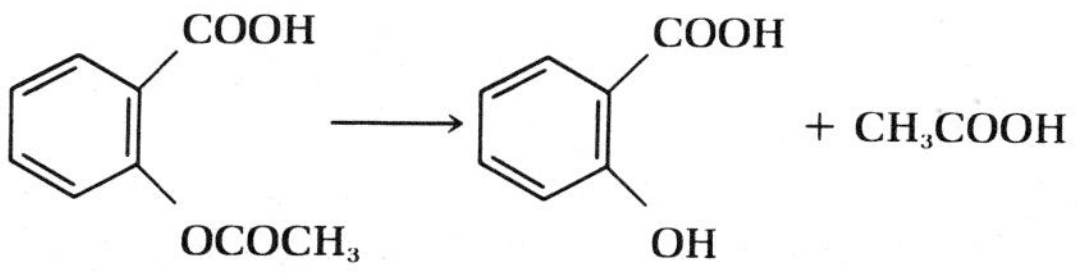

   $+ CH_3COOH$

   Acetylsalicylic acid   Salicylic acid
   (aspirin)

   b.

   $+ CH_3CH_2OH$

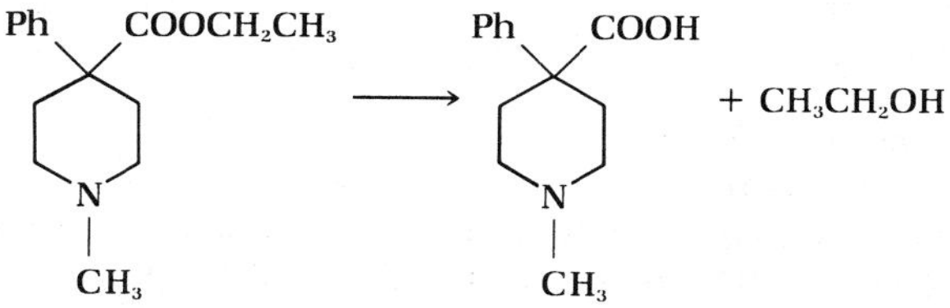

   Meperidine   Meperidinic acid

Continued.

Metabolic pathways—cont'd

Phase 1 reactions—cont'd
Hydrolysis—cont'd

2. Amides

Metabolic hydrolysis of amides is generally of little significance in humans. Most amide drugs undergo alternative metabolic reactions; a few are extensively hydrolyzed.

EXAMPLE

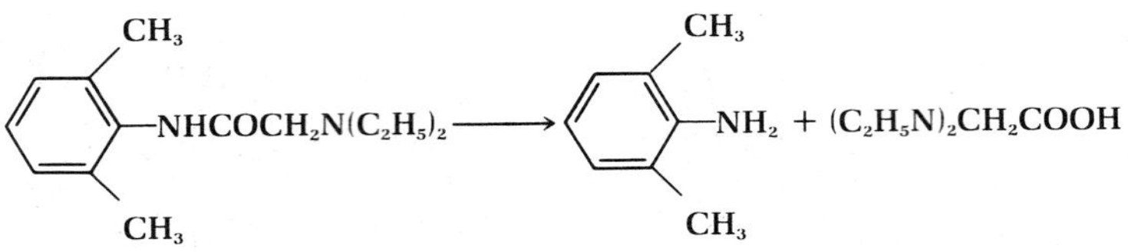

Lidocaine → 2,6-Xylidine

Phase 2 reactions
Glucuronide formation

REQUIRES

UDPGA (Uridine diphosphate α-D-glucuronic acid) and a UDP-glucuronyl-transferase (occurs mainly in the liver but also in other tissues such as the kidney, gut, skin).

SUBSTRATES

Numerous compounds containing one or more of the groups $-OH$, $-COOH$, $-NH_2$, $-NHR$, $-SH$.

REACTION

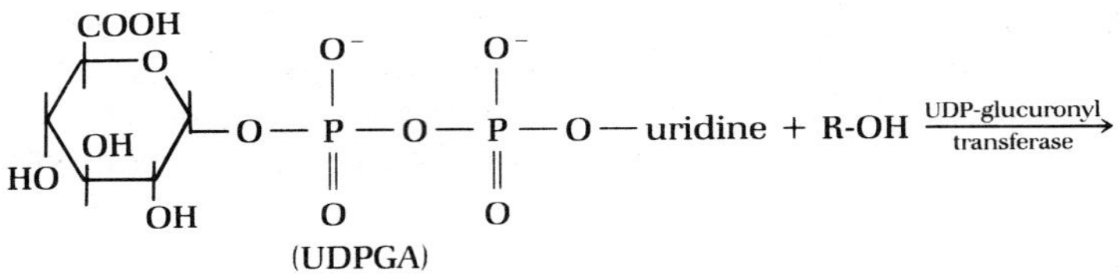

(UDPGA)

EXAMPLE

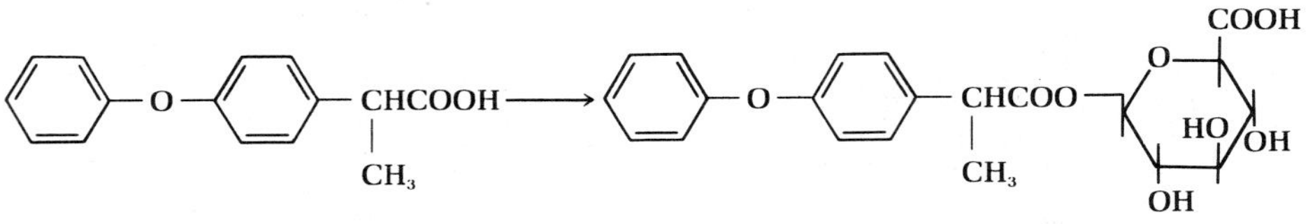

Fenoprofen → Fenoprofen glucuronide

NOTES

1. This is a most important metabolic pathway in mammals.
2. Inversion occurs during the reaction.
3. Amines form N-glucuronides (unstable); thiols form S-glucuronides.
4. When administered orally, morphine forms a glucuronide in the epithelial cells of the intestine.

Metabolic pathways—cont'd

Phase 2 reactions—cont'd
Glucuronide formation—cont'd

PROPERTIES

Glucuronides are water soluble. Phenols (which are common products of metabolism), for example, are commonly converted to glucuronides. Most phenols are ionized to less than 1% at physiologic pH 7.4 and are only slightly soluble in biologic fluids. At pH 7.4, glucuronides are 99.99% ionized (pk$_a$ $\simeq$ 3.5), and are so polar that they do not enter cells and are efficiently removed by the kidney (i.e., glomerular and tubular secretion) from the bloodstream and do not undergo tubular reabsorption.

If a glucuronide is formed in the liver and if the molecular weight of the glucuronide is in excess of 400 to 500, it is likely to be excreted into the small intestine in the bile (i.e., biliary excretion), and excreted in the feces. It may also be hydrolyzed in the gut by β-glucuronidase present there, and the aglycone may be reabsorbed.

Sulfate formation

REQUIRES

PAPS (3'-phosphoadenosine-5'-phosphosulfate) and a sulfotransferase (occurs in the soluble fraction of liver; also present in the kidney, gut).

SUBSTRATES

Phenols, some alcohols and aromatic amines, N-hydroxy compounds.

REACTION

PAPS

PAP

EXAMPLE

Phenol   Phenol sulfate

NOTES

1. O-sulfates are much more common than N-sulfates.
2. In humans, the sulfate conjugation system can be quickly exhausted. If so, glucuronidation takes over.
3. Sulfate formation of some drugs (e.g., isoproterenol, terbutaline, rimiterol, isoetharine) may occur in the columnar epithelial cells of the intestine.

Continued.

Phase 2 reactions—cont'd

Acetate formation

REQUIRES

Acetyl coenzyme A (CH_3CO-S-CoA) and an N-acetyltransferase (present in liver-mitochondrial enzyme; also present in other tissues).

SUBSTRATES

Compounds with a primary amino group (i.e., aromatic and some aliphatic amines, amino acids, hydrazines, hydrazides). Only of importance with sulfonamides, isoniazid (a hydrazide), and histamine.

REACTION

$$CH_3CO-S-CoA + R-NH_2 \xrightarrow[\text{transferase}]{\text{N-acetyl-}} R-NHCOCH_3 + HS-CoA$$

Acetyl coenzyme A   Drug   Acetylated drug   Coenzyme A

EXAMPLE

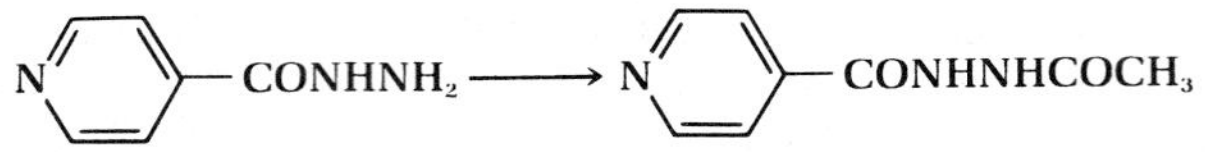

Isoniazid   Acetylisoniazid

NOTE

1. Metabolism of isoniazid in humans shows a bimodal distribution with both rapid and slow acetylators (see Chapter 9, "Genetic Factors Affecting Drug Response").

Conjugation with glycine

REQUIRES

ATP (adenosine triphosphate), CoA-SH (coenzyme A), an acylthiokinase, glycine (H_2NCH_2COOH), N-acyltransferase (present in liver and kidney).

SUBSTRATES

Only carboxylic acids with an aromatic ring (aryl and arylaliphatic acids), especially benzoic acid and related compounds.

REACTION

$$R-COOH \xrightarrow[\text{acylthiokinase}]{\text{ATP, CoA}} R-CO-S-CoA \xrightarrow[\text{N-acyltransferase}]{\text{H}_2\text{NCH}_2\text{COOH}} RCONHCH_2COOH + CoA-SH$$

EXAMPLE

$$C_6H_5COOH \longrightarrow C_6H_5CONHCH_2COOH$$
Benzoic acid   Hippuric acid

NOTE

This is a Phase 2 reaction that is often *not* preceded by a Phase 1 reaction.

Methylation

REQUIRES

S-Adenosylmethionine and a methyltransferase (present in liver and other tissues such as brain).

SUBSTRATES

Mainly endogenous compounds (e.g., epinephrine, histamine) and analogous exogenous compounds.

REACTION

$$\text{Adenosine}-\overset{\overset{\textstyle R}{\textstyle |}}{\underset{+}{S}}-CH_3 + R'-XH \xrightarrow[\text{transferase}]{\text{methyl}} R'-XCH_3 + \text{Adenosine}-\overset{\overset{\textstyle R}{\textstyle |}}{S} + H^+$$

$$[R = CH_2CH_2CH(NH_2)COOH]$$

Phase 2 reactions—cont'd
Methylation—cont'd

EXAMPLE

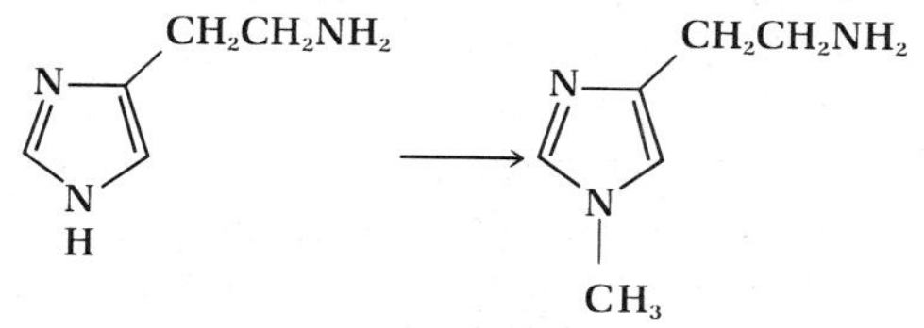

Histamine → tele-Methylhistamine

NOTES

1. In humans metabolic *O*-, *N*-, and *S*-methylation is observed.
2. Catecholamines are major substrates:

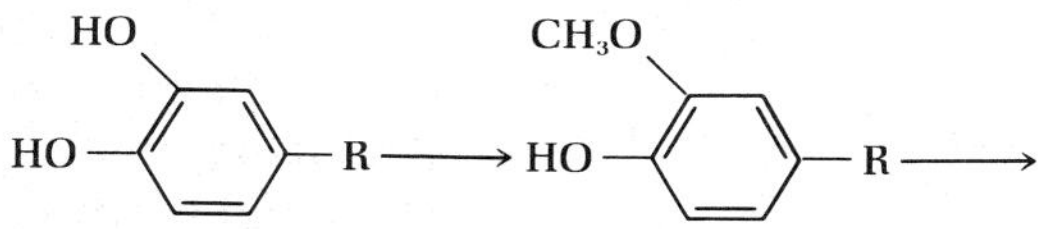

(where R = an amino side chain—e.g., $CHOHCH_2NH_2$ in norepinephrine)

3. Few drugs undergo metabolic methylation. In those that do (e.g., estradiol), it is often a minor metabolic pathway.

Conjugation with glutathione and mercapturic acid formation

REQUIRES

Glutathione and glutathione-S-aryltransferase (present in liver).

SUBSTRATES

Aromatic hydrocarbons, some halogenated and nitro derivatives, and other miscellaneous compounds.

EXAMPLE

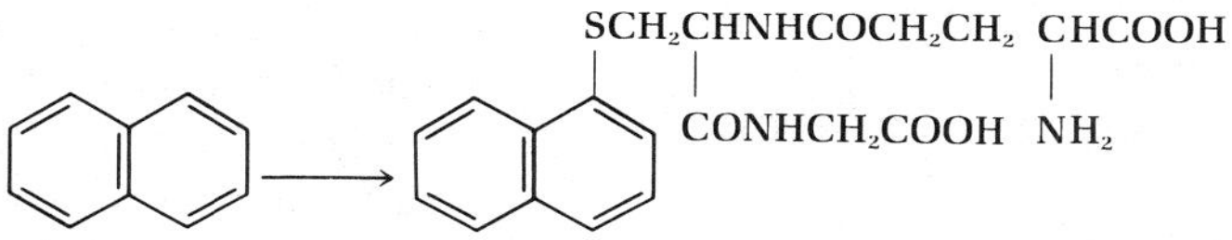

Naphthalene → Naphthalene glutathione conjugate 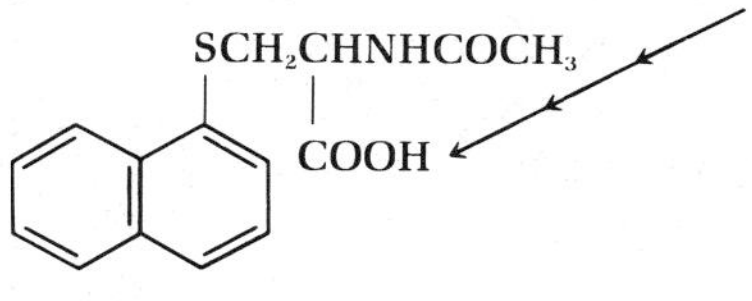 → Mercapturic acid conjugate

NOTES

1. The conversion of the glutathione conjugate to the mercapturic acid conjugate is a complex reaction.
2. Many species, including humans, form glutathione conjugates.
3. Humans are sometimes deficient in enzymes that are required for mercapturic acid conjugate formation.
4. *N*-Hydroxyacetaminophen is a minor metabolite of acetaminophen, and it is normally inactivated by liver glutathione. When toxic quantities of acetaminophen are ingested, larger quantities of *N*-hydroxyacetaminophen are produced. Glutathione stores are depleted and the excess *N*-hydroxymetabolite reacts with vital liver cell constituents, causing cell necrosis.

gated by an enzymatic process with a small endogenous molecule. Glucuronide and sulfate formation are excellent examples.

Numerous examples of phase 1 metabolic reactions have been observed; many are oxidative reactions. The primary mechanism by which oxygen is introduced into a molecule is complex. The reaction is catalyzed by the mixed function oxidases of the endoplasmic reticulum of the liver and other tissues. This has been referred to as the P-450 system (i.e., cytochrome P-450, cytochrome P-450 reductase, cytochrome C reductase), which requires molecular oxygen and NADPH (or NADH) for the introduction of one atom of oxygen into the drug. The overall reaction can be depicted as follows:

$$R\text{-}H + O_2 + NADPH + H^+ \xrightarrow[\text{system}]{P\text{-}450} R\text{-}OH + NADP^+ + H_2O$$
(drug)   (oxidized drug)

The phase 1 metabolic reactions depicted in Metabolic Pathways on the preceding pages are representative. Phase 2 metabolic reactions are conjugation reactions of drugs and drug metabolites of general formula R-XH, where X = NH, NR^1, O, or S. Most examples involve compounds of structure R-OH. Metabolic conjugation reactions that have been observed follow:

1. Conjugation with glucuronic acid
2. Sulfate formation
3. Acetate formation
4. Conjugation with glycine
5. Methylation
6. Conjugation with glutamine
7. Conjugation with glutathione → mercapturic acid formation
8. Other conjugation reactions

Of these reactions, conjugation with glucuronic acid (which yields a glucuronide) is the most important in humans. Reactions 2 through 5 are observed in humans, but are of less importance. The other conjugation reactions are relatively unimportant in humans.

Rate of metabolism

When most drugs that undergo metabolism are administered at therapeutic dose levels, the rate of metabolism (and hence the rate of drug elimination from the plasma) is directly proportional to the plasma concentration of the drug. The rate of metabolism therefore decreases with a decrease in plasma drug concentration. If the rate of metabolism $\propto C_p$, equation 1 applies.

$$\text{Rate of metabolism} = k_m C_p \tag{1}$$

where C_p = plasma concentration of drug (e.g., in μg/ml) and k_m = metabolic rate constant in reciprocal time units (e.g., hr^{-1}). Thus if $k_m = 2 \times 10^{-4} \ min^{-1}$ and $C_p = 5 \ \mu g/ml$, the rate of metabolism = $2 \times 10^{-4} \times 5 \times 1000 = 1 \ ng \ ml^{-1} \ min^{-1}$. NOTE: $k_m = \dfrac{V_{max}}{K_m}$.

Plots of typical data will often appear as illustrated (Figure 5-2).

Equation 1, however, is a simplified form of a more complex relationship (equation 2), which describes rate of metabolism more accurately:

$$\text{Rate of metabolism} = \frac{V_{max} C_p}{K_m + C_p} \tag{2}$$

in which V_{max} is the maximum possible rate of metabolism of a drug and depends on the amount of metabolizing enzyme available, and K_m is a Michaelis constant and represents the drug concentration at which the rate of metabolism is half that of the maximum rate. At therapeutic dose levels of most drugs, the value of C_p is much less than that of K_m, and the enzyme system is never exhausted. Thus the value of $K_m + C_p$ approximates that of K_m alone.

$$\text{Rate of metabolism} = \frac{V_{max} C_p}{K_m} = k_m C_p \tag{1}$$

The rate of metabolism of most drugs, therefore, obeys first order kinetics, and the elimination from the plasma of most drugs that undergo first order metabolism is also first order. In other words, regardless of dose, a certain percent of the drug in the body is eliminated per unit time interval (i.e., x % hr^{-1}).

The rates of metabolism of some drugs, however, including salicylates, phenytoin, and others are *dose dependent.* These drugs obey zero order or Michaelis-

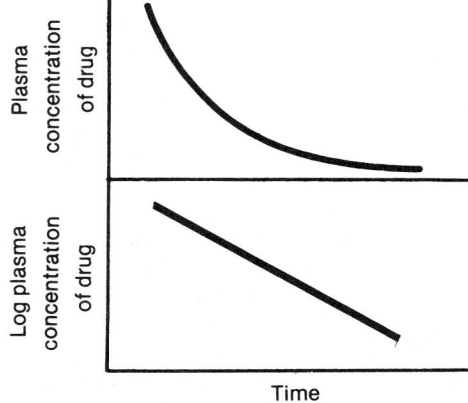

FIGURE 5-2. **Plots of plasma concentrations as a function of time for intravenous administration of a single bolus dose.**

Menten kinetics and eliminate a certain *amount* (as opposed to percent) of drug from the body per unit time (i.e., x mg hr^{-1}). If plasma concentrations of these drugs are high (such as in acute overdose) then equation 2 must be applied. At high plasma concentrations of drugs, metabolism is not a first order process, and observed rates of metabolism and drug elimination from plasma are slower than when plasma concentrations of drug are in the therapeutic range. Since both K_m and C_p in equation 2 are increased at high plasma drug concentrations, the half-life (i.e., the time it takes a drug to fall to one half of its plasma concentration) (Figure 5-3) of these drugs also increases. The combination of a high plasma concentration and a slower rate of metabolism often results in a toxic situation. Some properties of zero and first order metabolic processes are listed in Table 5-1. (Further discussion of half-life can be found in Chapter 6, "Pharmacokinetic Considerations in Drug Response.")

METABOLIC FACTORS AFFECTING THE SYSTEMIC AVAILABILITY* OF A DRUG

Intestinal metabolism

If a drug is administered orally, it may be metabolized during absorption by an enzyme system present in the gastrointestinal epithelium, so that significant quantities of an inactive metabolite and a much re-

---

*See Chapter 4, "Drug Availability and Distribution" for further details.

TABLE 5-1

Comparison of some properties of zero and first order metabolism

Zero order	First order
$T_{1/2}$ *depends* on dose	$T_{1/2}$ is *independent* of dose
Metabolic pattern may be influenced by dosage form	Metabolic characteristics are independent of dosage form
Drug decline in the body is *nonexponential* (i.e., decline is at a constant rate, x mg hr^{-1})	Drug decline in the body is *exponential* (i.e., percent decline is constant, X % hr^{-1})
Percent of dose recovered as a particular metabolite *changes* with respect to dose	Percent of dose recovered as a particular metabolite is *constant* for an individual
Competitive inhibition of metabolism is *present*	Competitive inhibition of metabolism is *absent*
An *abnormal* dose-response relationship may be observed:	A *normal* dose-response relationship is observed:

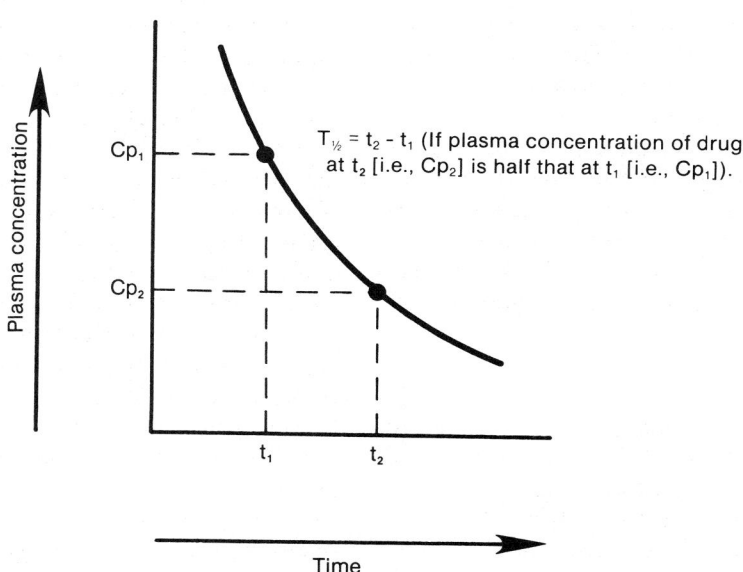

FIGURE 5-3. **Graphical representation and determination of half-life ($T_{1/2}$).**

duced amount of the drug are absorbed. Sulfate formation is of particular importance. Some drugs are conjugated with sulfate in significant amounts in the intestinal wall. The sulfate conjugate is absorbed but quickly eliminated in the urine. This explains why larger amounts of certain drugs (including the bronchodilators isoproterenol and isoetharine) are excreted as pharmacologically inactive sulfate conjugates when the drugs are given orally than when the drugs are given by intravenous infusion. These drugs are therefore less effective orally than when given by injection. A list of drugs that form conjugates in the intestine follows.

Drugs that are metabolically conjugated in the intestine

Chlorpromazine	Levodopa	Rimiterol
Diethylstilbestrol	Methyldopa	Salicylamide
Isoetharine	Morphine	Testosterone
Isoproterenol	Progesterone	Terbutaline

Intestinal sulfate formation can be reduced significantly if another substance that is sulfated is given concomitantly with the drug. Vitamin C, for example, is sulfated in the GI tract and is therefore a competitive inhibitor of intestinal drug sulfation.

Other conjugation reactions also occur in the intestinal mucosa. Morphine, for example, is believed to be conjugated, to a significant extent, with glucuronic acid during absorption. This explains why plasma levels of morphine after oral administration are lower than those observed when comparable doses of the drug are administered intravenously. Significant amounts of various esterases, decarboxylases, and digestive enzymes are also present in the GI tract and are involved in biotransformations.

Gastrointestinal organisms also contribute to metabolic processes. Enzymes present in these organisms are capable of catalyzing many reactions, including hydrolysis of amides, esters, glucuronides, glycosides, sulfates, and conjugates; dehydroxylation; decarboxylation; dealkylation; reduction; aromatization; and dehalogenation.

First-pass effect

A drug may be absorbed intact from the GI tract. It will then be transported to the liver *via* the portal vein having to pass through the liver to reach the systemic circulation. During its passage through the liver the drug may be extensively metabolized (occasionally completely metabolized) to pharmacologically inactive products. Thus significantly reduced amounts of the active drug reach the systemic circulation for transportation to the site of action. This process is called the *first-pass effect* (i.e., the effect of the first pass of the drug through the liver) and is one of the explanations for differences in the fraction of drug available to the systemic circulation when the same amount of drug is given orally and by intravenous injection. Drugs subject to extensive first-pass metabolism in humans include lidocaine, phenacetin, and propranolol.

The best way to completely avoid the first-pass effect is to administer the drug intravenously. Drugs that are administered rectally also significantly avoid the hepatic first-pass effect. Efforts are being made to improve products (e.g., suppositories, creams) that will permit more efficient rectal absorption of drugs that could be self-administered by the patient and that would avoid to a great extent the first-pass effect.

ELIMINATION OF DRUGS AND METABOLITES

Drugs and metabolites are excreted from the systemic circulation by different pathways (e.g., in urine, bile, feces, saliva, sweat, expired air, and breast milk—Table 5-2). Of these pathways, excretion into the urine is by far the most important.

Renal excretion

The kidneys are implicated in the elimination of virtually all drugs or drug metabolites in humans. Four distinct processes may be involved in renal excretion: glomerular filtration, active tubular secretion, and active and passive reabsorption. These processes are illustrated in Figure 5-4. (See Chapter 35, "Review of the Anatomy, Physiology, and Assessment of the Renal System" for further details.)

Arterial blood flows into the glomerulus of the kidney through an afferent arteriole. In the glomerulus, plasma water and low molecular weight molecules are filtered from the blood. Blood cells and large molecules (i.e., those with a molecular weight in excess of 50,000) are not filtered in the normal, undamaged glomerulus. Thus, the urine is virtually protein free and only free drugs (i.e., drugs *not* bound to plasma protein) can be filtered. The total glomerular filtration in a healthy adult approaches 200 L of fluid per day, but about 99% of this fluid is reabsorbed in the tubular portion of the kidney. The remainder, approximately 1.5 L (or 1 ml/min), is excreted as urine. This fluid reabsorption procedure results in high urinary concentrations of solutes, including drugs and metabolites that are less efficiently reabsorbed.

Some drugs and metabolites undergo tubular se-

TABLE 5-2

Drug excretion

Excretion pathway	Mechanism	Examples
Urine	Glomerular filtration and active tubular secretion (Figure 5-4)	Virtually all non-protein-bound ("free") drugs are filtered. "Bound" drugs may undergo tubular secretion (e.g., dicloxacillin—see text)
Bile	Active transport and passive diffusion from blood into the bile in the bile ductular region	Organic carboxylic and sulfonic acids, other acids (e.g., chlorothiazide), quaternary bases, ouabain, cardiac glycosides (e.g., digoxin), numerous glucuronides
Feces	Biliary excretion	Drugs that are excreted into the bile, drugs excreted into the saliva
Saliva	Active and passive secretory processes	Numerous drugs including penicillins and tetracyclines
Sweat	Probably passive diffusion	Numerous drugs including urea, medicinal sulfonamides, and benzoic acid
Expired air	Passive diffusion	Drugs and metabolites with high vapor pressures (e.g., guaiacol), gaseous metabolites (e.g., carbon dioxide)
Breast milk	Active and passive diffusion	Numerous acidic and basic drugs. See Chapter 7, "Age-Dependent Drug Selection and Response."

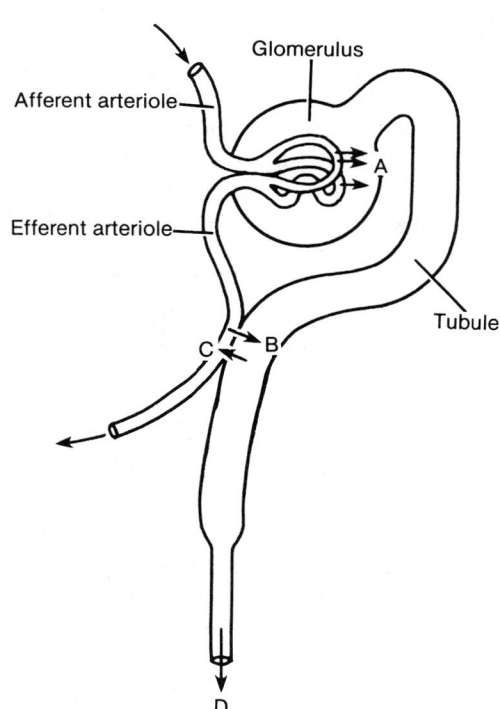

FIGURE 5-4. **Diagrammatic illustration of drug excretion by the kidneys. The represented functional and structural unit of the kidney composed of the glomerulus and the tubule is known as a nephron.** *A,* Glomerular filtration; *B,* active secretion; *C,* active or passive reabsorption; *D,* urinary excretion.

cretion. This is termed an active transport process, whereby the drug diffuses with the aid of a carrier transport system against a concentration gradient from efferent arterioles through the tubular membrane into the kidney tubule. Plasma protein binding does not interfere with tubular secretion. Dicloxacillin and other drugs are known to bind extensively with plasma protein, and yet these drugs are excreted mainly in the urine. This is believed to be the result of rapid tubular transport of the unbound drug, and subsequent rapid dissociation of the drug-protein complex in an attempt to maintain free drug–bound drug equilibrium.

Active and passive reabsorption of drugs and metabolites also occurs in the renal tubules. The former process requires a carrier transport system, whereas passive reabsorption depends on the principles of diffusion: concentration gradient between the concentrated urine and blood, pH of urine, pK_a of drug or metabolite, and lipid solubility of the drug or metabolite. Lipid soluble drugs are efficiently reabsorbed passively. Compounds that are not lipid soluble or that are ionized in the urine are poorly reabsorbed.

Urine pH. The renal clearance of weak acids and bases is greatly influenced by urinary pH. The renal clearance of weak acids (e.g., barbiturates, nalidixic acid, probenecid, salicylic acid) is increased if the urine is made alkaline, because more of the drug will be in ionized form in alkaline urine than in neutral urine. Similarly the renal clearance of weak acids is decreased in acidic urine because more drug will then be in nonionized form. The converse is true of weak bases (e.g., amphetamine, codeine, imipramine, meperidine, morphine); renal clearance will be increased in acidic urine and lowered in alkaline urine. Common procedures used to alter urinary pH follow.

MANIPULATION OF URINARY pH

To render the urine acidic, administer one of the following compounds:
  Ammonium chloride
  Ascorbic acid
  Amino acid hydrochloride (HCl) salts (e.g., arginine HCl, lysine HCl)
To render the urine basic, administer one of the following compounds:
  Acetazolamide
  Antacids (e.g., calcium carbonate, sodium bicarbonate)
  Sodium glutamate
  Thiazide diuretics

Renal clearance. The renal clearance of a drug is defined as the volume of blood that is cleared of the drug by the kidneys per minute.

$$CL_R = \frac{C_u V}{(1 - p)C_p t} \text{ ml/min}$$

CL_R = renal clearance
C_u = concentration of drug in urine (mg/ml)
C_p = concentration of drug in plasma (mg/ml)
p = fraction of drug bound to protein (fraction of 1)
V = volume of urine excreted (ml)
t = duration of urine collection (min)

In healthy individuals the renal clearance of glucose is zero (i.e., complete tubular reabsorption occurs), and the renal clearance of aminohippuric acid is approximately equal to renal plasma flow (i.e., 650 ml/min), indicating that aminohippuric acid is so efficiently excreted by the renal tubules that it is essentially cleared from the plasma in a single pass through the kidney. The best biologic estimate of glomerular filtration rate, and thus renal clearance without tubular secretion or reabsorption, is given by creatinine clearance, which ranges from 80 to 120 ml/min in the normal adult without renal impairment. If the renal clearance value of a drug or metabolite exceeds 130 ml/min, then tubular secretion is probably occurring; renal clearance values that fall below 130 ml/min in a normal, healthy adult are generally indicative of the occurrence of tubular reabsorption. Estimates of renal clearance can, therefore, provide information on excretion mechanisms.

Biliary excretion

The liver continually produces bile fluid, which is transported by the bile duct to the gall bladder where it is stored. Up to 1 L of bile is produced and emptied daily into the duodenum. During the passage of the bile through the bile duct, free exchange of drugs and metabolites to and from the blood occurs. Thus the bile can be a pathway of excretion of some drugs and metabolites. These drugs and metabolites enter the small intestine and are either excreted in the feces or are reabsorbed into the systemic circulation. The latter situation is referred to as enterohepatic reabsorption or recycling (Figure 5-5). Enterohepatic recycling may continue until metabolism, renal excretion, and fecal excretion eventually eliminate the drug from the body. Thus drugs that exhibit enterohepatic reabsorption may persist in the body for lengthy periods of time. In humans, various drugs including thyroxine, estrone, estradiol, testosterone, norethynodrel, eryth-

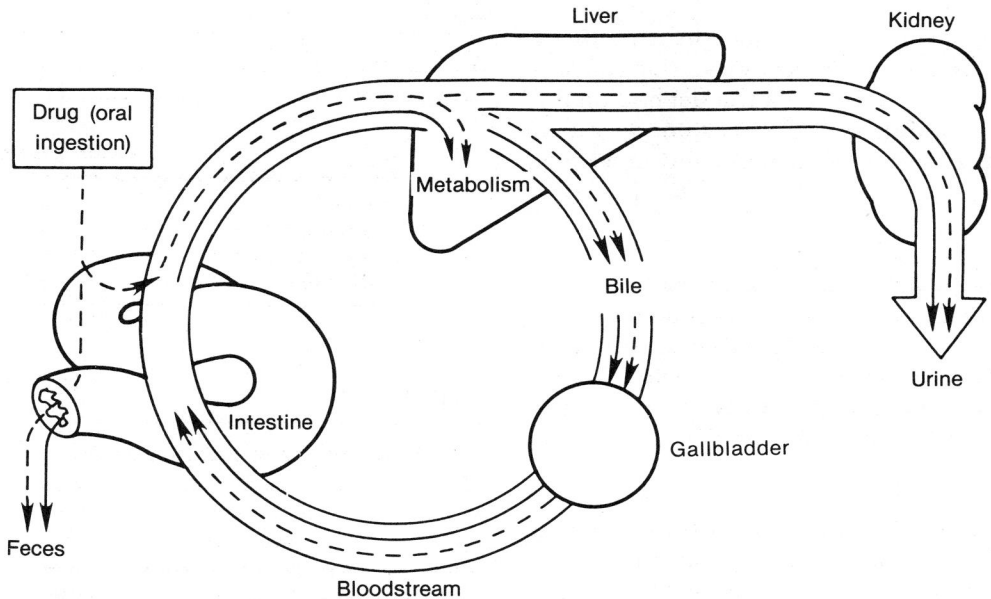

FIGURE 5-5. **Enterohepatic recycling. (Commencing at *Drug* and following the arrows represent diagrammatically the likely fate of a drug (--→) and a metabolite (→) in the body. The cycle—liver ⇒ bile ⇒ gallbladder ⇒ intestine ⇒ bloodstream ⇒ liver— illustrates enterohepatic recycling.**

romycin, and chloramphenicol may undergo significant enterohepatic recycling.

Biliary excretion is an important elimination procedure for compounds that are polar and possess molecular weights greater than 400. Above this threshold molecular weight, biliary excretion increases at the expense of renal excretion. Both unchanged drugs and metabolites are excreted in the bile. Appreciable quantities of erythromycin, penicillin, and digitoxin, for example, have been isolated from bile in unchanged form. Many drugs are excreted as conjugates in the bile. Examples are indomethacin, morphine, and estradiol.

Salivary excretion

This is not an important route of excretion, since most drugs present in saliva will pass to the GI tract and be reabsorbed or excreted in the feces. Examples of drugs that are excreted in the saliva are the penicillins and the tetracyclines.

Saliva/plasma drug concentration ratios for some drugs (e.g., lithium, phenytoin, theophylline) are relatively constant, and in these instances drug concentrations in saliva can be used to estimate plasma concentration. Saliva/plasma ratios have been determined for numerous drugs. Drugs with ratios in excess of 0.1 are identified in Table 5-3.

TABLE 5-3

Drugs excreted in the saliva

Drug	*Saliva/plasma ratio*
Acetaminophen	1.40
Aminopyrine	0.79
Amobarbital	0.35
Antipyrine	0.92
Caffeine	0.55
Carbamazepine	0.26
Digoxin	0.66
Ethosuximide	1.04
Isoniazid	1.02
Lidocaine	1.78
Lithium	2.85
Pentobarbital	0.42
Phenacetin	0.60
Phenobarbital	0.32
Phenytoin	0.11
Primidone	0.97
Procainamide	3.50
Quinidine	0.51
Streptomycin	0.15
Sulfacetamide	0.92
Sulfadiazine	0.31
Sulfadimidine	0.72
Sulfamerazine	0.32
Sulfanilamide	0.87
Sulfapyridine	0.81
Sulfathiazole	0.23
Theophylline	0.75

Mammary excretion

Almost all drugs that are present in a mother's blood will also be present in her milk. The concentrations of these drugs in the milk will depend on the lipid solubility of the drug, concentration, degree of protein binding, degree of ionization, and molecular weight.

Sweat excretion

Numerous drugs and other substances have been detected in sweat. Examples are *p*-aminohippuric acid, antipyrine, arsenic, benzoic acid, boron, bromine, iodine, iron, lead, mercury, salicylic acid, sulfonamides, thiamine, and urea. Sweat/plasma ratios have been determined for some sulfonamides (Table 5-4).

Lung excretion

A few volatile drugs and metabolites are excreted into expired air. Gaseous drugs (e.g., gaseous anesthetics) and metabolites such as carbon dioxide are obvious examples, but other drugs are also excreted in this way:

Drugs excreted in expired air

Alcohol	Gaseous anesthetics
Ammonium chloride	Guaiacol
Camphor	Iodides
Coumarin	Paraldehyde

FACTORS THAT INFLUENCE DRUG METABOLISM AND ELIMINATION

Various factors can affect the absorption, distribution, biotransformation, and elimination of a drug. Factors that affect drug metabolism and elimination are now considered.

Age*

In general, plasma half-lives are shortest in infants, children, and adults; longer in elderly subjects; and longest in the newborn.

Newborn. Compared with adults, neonates have a low drug-metabolizing capacity. They have a low ability to form glucuronide and glycine conjugates. Thus in the newborn an inability to conjugate chloramphenicol can lead to severe chloramphenicol toxicity (i.e., gray baby syndrome), and an inability to conjugate bilirubin causes kernicterus. The reduced rate of excretion of salicylate in the newborn has also been attributed to an inability to form glucuronides.

---

*See Chapter 7, "Age-dependent Drug Selection and Response," for further details.

TABLE 5-4

Sulfonamides excreted in sweat

Drug	Sweat/plasma ratio
Sulfadiazine	0.11
Sulfanilamide	0.69
Sulfapyridine	0.58
Sulfathiazole	0.13

TABLE 5-5

Development of metabolic processes

Age	Process
Birth	Sulfation, some oxidation and acetylation
1-2 Weeks	Oxidation, reduction
1 Month	Acetylation
2 Months	Glucuronidation
3 Months	Conjugation with glycine
	Conjugation with glutathione
	Other conjugations

In contrast, however, the newborn does possess a reasonably efficient acetylation enzyme system and is able to conjugate drugs with sulfate, but this latter pathway quickly becomes saturated, and there is no glucuronidation system to take over. Rates of metabolic oxidation are also greatly reduced in the newborn. A comparison of amobarbital half-lives in a mother (16 hours) and her newborn (40 hours) illustrates this.

The ability to metabolically oxidize and acetylate drugs develops rapidly after birth, and conjugation reactions proceed efficiently after the third month. The development of metabolic processes in the newborn is summarized in Table 5-5.

Infants and children. Rates of drug metabolism in this group are similar to, and sometimes even faster than, rates observed in adults. An excellent example of the latter situation is provided by theophylline, the average half-life of which is 5.5 hours in adults and 3.7 hours in children. Efficient enzyme systems involved in drug metabolism rapidly develop in children.

Elderly. The general decline in organ function, including the liver and kidney, that results with aging causes a decrease in the rates of all drug metabolism processes and hence a longer plasma half-life for most drugs. Propranolol, when given in the same dose to young adults and to elderly patients, for example, results in much higher (i.e., greater than fourfold) mean plasma propranolol levels in the elderly patients. Elderly patients also have a reduced ability to form conjugates.

Genetic factors*

Intersubject variations in plasma drug levels in comparable patients given the same dose of a drug are often caused by differences in rates of drug metabolism. That these rates are genetically controlled is attestable by the following observations:

1. Identical (i.e., monozygotic) twins metabolize drugs (phase 1 and phase 2 reactions) at identical rates, whereas fraternal (i.e., dizygotic) twins do not.

2. Some drugs (e.g., isoniazid and debrisoquin) show bimodal distributions of drug metabolism rates. With such drugs, "fast metabolizers" and "slow metabolizers" can be identified. In Figure 5-6, a typical graphic illustration of bimodal metabolism rates is presented.

With isoniazid, fast and slow acetylators can be identified:

$$N \diagdown \text{—CONHNH}_2 \longrightarrow N \diagdown \text{—CONHNHCOCH}_3$$

Isoniazid

and with debrisoquin, fast and slow C-oxidizers are recognized:

Debrisoquin

It is of significance that slow acetylators of isoniazid are also slow acetylators of other drugs (e.g., sulfonamides). Although debrisoquin undergoes alicyclic metabolic C-oxidation, there is evidence that slow oxidizers of debrisoquin are also slow oxidizers of drugs that are metabolically C-oxidized in aromatic rings and aliphatic side chains. Since slow metabolizers will have increased plasma concentrations of unmetabolized drug, excessive amounts will accumulate in the plasma if the dose administered is the same as that

*See Chapter 9, "Genetic Factors Affecting Drug Response," for further details.

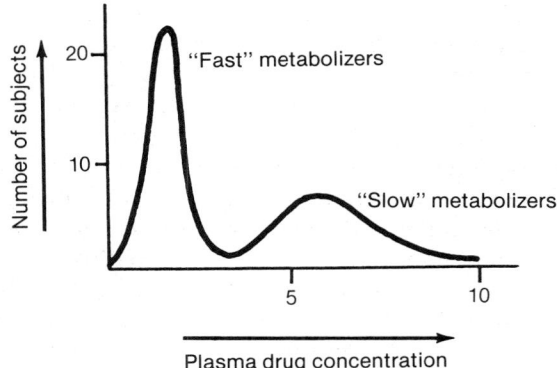

FIGURE 5-6. **Drug concentrations in plasma—a fixed time interval after administration of the same dose of drug, calculated on a weight per kilogram basis, to a large patient sample.**

given to the fast metabolizer. It has been advocated, therefore, that before isoniazid, debrisoquin, and other similar drugs are routinely administered to patients that it be determined whether they are fast or slow metabolizers. Dosages of these drugs could then be adjusted accordingly. (See Chapter 9 for a more complete discussion of genetic effects).

Disease

Liver disease. Since most drug metabolism occurs in the liver, it may be expected that liver dysfunction would result in an altered rate of drug metabolism. In practice, however, liver disease must be particularly severe before drug metabolism is altered significantly. Some studies show no differences in drug metabolism between patients with known liver impairment and those with normal liver function.

Studies with antipyrine are informative. Antipyrine is used to assess liver function, since it is virtually completely oxidized metabolically in patients with normal liver function. Thus the plasma half-life of antipyrine is a sensitive indicator of liver function. The antipyrine half-life in adult men and women under the age of 33 years is approximately 12 hours. Most persons with *acute reversible liver disease* have similar antipyrine half-lives (i.e., 12 hours). In contrast, persons suffering from *chronic severe liver disease* (e.g., alcoholic hepatic cirrhosis, chronic hepatitis) have elevated antipyrine half-lives, usually in the 26- to 34-hour range.

If antipyrine half-lives are increased, then drug metabolism rates are reduced. Similar effects can be expected with other drugs that are metabolically oxidized. Such is the case with diazepam, lidocaine, and meperidine, whose rates of metabolism are reduced in patients with *alcoholic hepatic cirrhosis.*

Contradictory results have been observed in patients with *acute viral hepatitis.* Plasma half-lives of hexobarbital, diazepam, meperidine, and antipyrine were prolonged, but returned to near-normal when liver function improved. In contrast, plasma half-lives of phenobarbital and phenytoin are not significantly altered in patients with acute viral hepatitis.

In summary, acute liver dysfunction (i.e., viral hepatitis) often has little clinical significance, and it is difficult to say whether drug dosage should be modified in patients who have acute liver disease. Generally, doses should be kept as low as possible, consistent with the desired therapeutic effect. It is recommended, however, that particular care should be taken when sedative-hypnotics, analgesics, and antidepressant drugs are administered.

Hepatic dysfunction can be induced with drugs. Acetaminophen, for example, is hepatotoxic at elevated doses. Acute hepatic necrosis can occur. If it does, the rates of metabolism of many drugs, such as acetaminophen itself, antipyrine, phenytoin, and phenobarbital, are reduced significantly. Many drugs in clinical use produce hepatic damage, though few, such as chloroform and carbon tetrachloride, are true hepatotoxins. Most drugs that adversely affect the liver appear to act as liver sensitizing agents. The following drugs can produce hepatic damage in susceptible individuals.

Major hepatotoxic drugs

Acetaminophen	Mercaptopurine
Allopurinol	Methyldopa
Aminosalicylic acid	Methotrexate
Barbiturates	Nitrofurantoin
Chlorambucil	Nitroglycerin
Chloramphenicol	Oxytetracycline
Chlorpromazine	Penicillin
Chlorpropamide	Perphenazine
Chlortetracycline	Phenelzine
Contraceptives, oral	Phenylbutazone
Cortisone	Phenytoin
Diazepam	Prochlorperazine
Digoxin	Promazine
Furosemide	Sulfonamides
Hydralazine	Tetracycline
Indomethacin	Thioridazine
Iproniazid	Trifluoperazine
Isocarboxazid	Zoxazolamine
Isoniazid (in combination with aminosalicylic acid)	

Renal disease. Patients with impaired renal function eliminate drugs *via* the urine at a slower rate than do healthy patients. One would expect, however, that rates of drug metabolism should not be significantly affected, since few drugs are metabolized to any great extent in the kidneys. Drug metabolites, of course, would accumulate in the plasma, but in most instances, metabolites are not pharmacologically active. In those instances when pharmacologically active metabolites are formed (e.g., primidone → phenobarbital; aromatic amines → aromatic hydroxylamines), their accumulation in the blood could result in toxicity. Quinidine toxicity is observed in patients with renal insufficiency; accumulation of active metabolites in the blood is thought to be the reason.

Rates of acetylation of various drugs (e.g., isoniazid, hydralazine, sulfisoxazole), the rate of hydrolysis of procainamide, and the rate of metabolic reduction of cortisol are altered in renal failure. None of these drugs is metabolized in the kidney; nevertheless, impairment of renal function somehow alters the normal metabolic rates.

Relatively few studies have been conducted on the nephrotoxicity of therapeutic agents. Those drugs that are recognized as being nephrotoxic in susceptible individuals are listed below.

Nephrotoxic drugs

Antibiotics	Antibiotics—cont'd
Amikacin	Tetracyclines
Amphotericin B	Vancomycin
Bacitracin	Analgesics
Cephaloridine	Acetaminophen
Colistin	Phenacetin
Gentamicin	Salicylates
Kanamycin	Other drugs
Neomycin	Aminosalicylic acid
Penicillins	Paradione
Polymyxin B	Phenylbutazone
Streptomycin	Trimethadione
Sulfonamides	

Congestive heart failure. This disease condition can affect the rate of elimination of drugs and metabolites. An active metabolite of lidocaine (monoethylglycinexylidide), for example, accumulates in the plasma of patients with congestive heart failure and causes CNS toxicity (see also Chapter 6, "Pharmacokinetic Considerations in Drug Response").

Hormone imbalance—thyroid disease. Normal hepatic drug elimination depends on a body hormone balance. In thyroid disease, hormone balance is upset, and drug metabolism is affected. Extensive studies have been carried out on antipyrine. Hypothyroidism is associated with an increased antipyrine plasma half-life (i.e., decreased rate of metabolic C-oxidation), whereas hyperthyroidism results in a decreased antipyrine half-life (i.e., increased rate of metabolism).

Similar effects are observed with digoxin, methimazole, and propylthiouracil.

Pregnancy

Phase 2 conjugation reactions that take place in the liver, especially glucuronidation, occur with endogenous compounds and exogenous materials (e.g., organic chemicals in food, drugs, environment chemicals). Especially during late pregnancy, a strain is placed on the liver to conjugate the large number of organic endogenous compounds that pass through it. Rates of phase 2 conjugation reactions are therefore decreased, and sometimes drug-induced liver damage can result. Cases of death from liver damage following administration of tetracycline during pregnancy have been reported. During pregnancy, increased blood levels of progesterone and pregnanediol are also observed. Normally pregnanediol is efficiently excreted as a glucuronide.

Drug interactions*

Enzyme induction. Some drugs and other organic compounds, when administered in therapeutic doses daily for a short period (i.e., 2 to 4 weeks), can cause (1) increased liver weight and liver blood flow; (2) an increase in total liver protein (including microsomal protein) per unit weight of liver; (3) an increased amount of smooth endoplasmic reticulum (which can be seen on electron microscopy); and (4) an increase in the P-450 system (i.e., cytochrome P-450, P-450 reductase, cytochrome C reductase), which is involved in metabolic oxidation reactions. The clinical result of inducing the production of increased amounts of the cytochrome P-450 system is a dramatic increase in the rate of metabolism of other drugs, or the inducer itself, if the drugs are metabolized by an oxidative process (i.e., a decrease in the efficacy of the drug is usually observed unless, of course, an active metabolite, which is not further metabolized, is produced).

There are hundreds of compounds that have been observed to induce the production of increased amounts of the P-450 system in the liver, but only a few are important clinically, especially phenobarbital and other barbiturates, phenytoin, rifampin, and chronic alcohol ingestion (Table 5-6). An excellent and often quoted example of enzyme induction, which has clinical significance, is the concomitant administration of phenobarbital and warfarin (or other oral anticoagulants), since the differences in dosages of anticoagulant that are ineffective and those that are likely to produce dangerous hemorrhage are small. For ex-

ample, the desired mean prothrombin time of warfarin (about 20 seconds) is reduced if phenobarbital is given for 2 weeks concomitantly, and an increase of warfarin dosage by 30% to 50% may be required to maintain this prothrombin time. Dangerous overdosage of warfarin would thus likely result if the phenobarbital was withdrawn without a concomitant decrease in warfarin dosage.

In many instances, drugs that stimulate hepatic microsomal enzyme production may also stimulate their own metabolism (i.e., self-induction). This partially explains the development of tolerance when some drugs are given chronically.

Drugs that induce their own metabolism

Carbamazepine	Nitroglycerin
Chlorcyclizine	Phenobarbital
Diazepam	Phenylbutazone
Glutethimide	Phenytoin
Hexobarbital	Probenecid
Meprobamate	Tolbutamide

Many environmental chemicals also stimulate drug metabolism. Exposure to insecticides (e.g., DDT, lindane) decreases the half-lives of numerous drugs, whereas exposure to polycyclic hydrocarbons, which are found in cigarette smoke and industrial effluents, induces the metabolism of many drugs. This explains why cigarette smokers often develop lower plasma levels of drugs than nonsmokers when both are given comparable doses.

Enzyme inhibition. Some drugs, when given concomitantly with another drug, have been found to inhibit the metabolism of the other drug, thus prolonging its pharmacologic effect. This is often the result of substrate competition for metabolic enzyme(s). Many drugs are metabolized by the cytochrome P-450 enzyme system. If two concomitantly administered drugs are both metabolically oxidized by this system, the one will act as a competitive inhibitor of the metabolism of the other. Typical examples of this competitive inhibition include monoamine oxidase inhibitors and sympathomimetic amines, disulfiram and alcohol, and chloramphenicol and phenytoin. Clinically important examples of microsomal enzyme inhibitors are identified in Table 5-7. (See Chapter 10 for further discussion of drug interactions.)

METABOLIC ACTIVATION

Some drugs are metabolized to other products that retain the pharmacologic actions of the parent drugs. It may be that in many instances it is the metabolite that is the pharmacologically active species. In some

---

*See Chapter 10, "Drug Interactions," for further information.

TABLE 5-6

Inducers of microsomal enzymes

Drug whose metabolism is induced	Inducer	Effect

Antidepressants, tricyclic
  Amitriptyline
  Desipramine
  Doxepin
  Imipramine
  Nortriptyline
  Protriptyline
	Barbiturates	Decreased antidepressant effect

Barbiturates	Rifampin	Decreased barbiturate effect
Bishydroxycoumarin and other oral anticoagulants	Alcohol—chronic abuse Barbiturates Glutethimide Griseofulvin Rifampin	Decreased anticoagulation
Contraceptives, oral	Rifampin	Decreased contraception
Corticosteroids	Barbiturates Phenytoin Rifampin	Decreased corticosteroid effect (phenytoin interacts especially with dexamethasone)
Digitoxin	Barbiturates Rifampin	Decreased digitoxin effect
Doxycycline	Barbiturates Carbamazepine	Decreased antibiotic effect
Isoniazid	Rifampin	Increased isoniazid toxicity
Meprobamate	Alcohol-chronic abuse	Decreased sedation
Methadone	Rifampin	Methadone withdrawal symptoms

Phenothiazines
  Acetophenazine
  Butaperazine
  Carphenazine
  Chlorpromazine
  Fluphenazine
  Mesoridazine
  Perphenazine
  Piperacetazine
  Prochlorperazine
  Promazine
  Thioridazine
  Trifluoperazine
  Triflupromazine
	Barbiturates	Decreased phenothiazine effect

Phenytoin	Alcohol—chronic abuse	Decreased sedation
Quinidine	Barbiturates Phenytoin	Decreased quinidine effect
Tolbutamide	Alcohol—chronic abuse Rifampin	Decreased hypoglycemia

TABLE 5-7

Inhibitors of microsomal enzymes

Drug whose metabolism is inhibited	*Inhibitor*	*Effect*
Alcohol	Disulfiram Metronidazole	Accumulation of acetaldehyde in blood and tissues
β-adrenergic blockers	Cimetidine	Increased blood levels of β-adrenergic blockers with resultant toxicity

Bishydroxycoumarin and other oral anticoagulants	Alcohol—acute intoxication
	Allopurinol
	Chloramphenicol
	Cimetidine
	Disulfiram
	Hypoglycemics, oral
	   Acetohexamide
	   Chlorpropamide
	   Tolazamide
	Metronidazole
	Oxyphenbutazone
	Phenylbutazone
		Increased anticoagulant effect

Carbamazepine	Propoxyphene Troleandomycin	Increased carbamazepine effects

Hypoglycemics, oral
  Acetohexamide
  Chlorpropamide
  Tolazamide
	Bishydroxycoumarin and other oral anticoagulants
	Chloramphenicol
	Phenylbutazone
		Increased hypoglycemia

Phenytoin	Alcohol—acute intoxication	Increased anticonvulsant effect leading to acute phenytoin toxicity
	Bishydroxycoumarin and other oral anticoagulants Chloramphenicol Cimetidine Disulfiram Isoniazid	Increased phenytoin toxicity

Tyramine (present in some foods, beer, wine)	Monoamine oxidase inhibitors
	   Furazolidone
	   Isocarboxazid
	   Pargyline
	   Phenelzine
	   Procarbazine
	   Tranylcypromine
		Inhibition of tyramine metabolism, which results in an increased central and peripheral release of norepinephrine and resultant physiologic effects (e.g., hypertensive crisis)

TABLE 5-8

Metabolic activation

Drug	Active metabolite(s)	Pharmacologic action(s) and comments
Acetohexamide	Hydroxyhexamide	Hypoglycemic; uricosuric
Allopurinol	Oxipurinol	Uricosuric
Amitriptyline	Nortriptyline	Antidepressant
Aspirin	Salicylic acid	Analgesic; antipyretic; antiinflammatory
Chloral hydrate	Trichloroethanol	Hypnotic
Chlordiazepoxide	Desmethylchlordiazepoxide	Antianxiety agent
Chlorpromazine	7-Hydroxychlorpromazine	Antipsychotic
Codeine	Morphine	Analgesic
Cortisone	Cortisol	Corticosteroid; metabolic activation mandatory
Daunorubicin	Daunorubicinol	Antibiotic; cytotoxic agent
Diazepam	N-Desmethyldiazepam	Antianxiety; sedative
Digitoxin	Digoxin	Cardiotonic; metabolic activation mandatory
Diphenoxylate	Hydrolyzed drug	Antidiarrheal; metabolite is 1-(3-cyano-3,3-diphenylpropyl)-4-phenylpiperidine-4-carboxylic acid
Dopamine	Norepinephrine	Endogenous amine
Fenfluramine	Norfenfluramine	Anorexiant
Flurazepam	Desethyl- and didesethyl-flurazepam	Hypnotic; other metabolites may also be active
Glutethimide	4-Hydroxyglutethimide	Hypnotic
Imipramine	Desipramine	Antidepressant
Meperidine	Normeperidine	Narcotic analgesic
Mephobarbital	Phenobarbital	Sedative; anticonvulsant
Methamphetamine	Amphetamine	CNS stimulant; anorexiant
Methsuximide	N-Desmethylsuximide	Anticonvulsant
Phenacetin	Acetaminophen	Analgesic; antipyretic
Phenylbutazone	Oxyphenylbutazone and 3-hydroxy-analog of phenylbutazone	Uricosuric
Phendimetrazine	Phenmetrazine	CNS stimulant; anorexiant
Prednisone	Prednisolone	Corticosteroid
Propranolol	4-Hydroxypropranolol	Antidysrhythmic; antihypertensive
Primidone	Phenobarbital	Anticonvulsant; sedative
Procainamide	N-Acetylprocainamide	Antidysrhythmic
Rifampin	Deacetylated rifampin	Antibacterial
Thioridazine	Mesoridazine	Antipsychotic
Trimethadione	Dimethadione	Anticonvulsant
Vitamin D	1,25-Dihydroxycholecalciferol	Antirachitic vitamin; metabolic activation mandatory

instances (e.g., cortisone, vitamin D) a metabolic activation reaction is mandatory. In Table 5-8, typical examples of drugs that are metabolized to pharmacologically active products in humans are listed.

TOXIGENESIS

Some drugs are metabolized in humans to products that are extremely toxic. A few examples are worthy of comment.

Acetaminophen (III) is normally excreted mainly as the glucuronide (IV) and sulfate (V). N-Hydroxyacetaminophen (VI) is a minor metabolite that dehydrates to the quinonoid compound (VII) in the body. This reactive product is normally inactivated as VIII by reacting with liver glutathione. When excessive amounts of acetaminophen are ingested, glutathione stores become depleted, and the intermediate (VII) then reacts with vital liver cell constituents, resulting in cell necrosis.

Metabolism of acetaminophen in humans. Glutathione is represented by RCH_2SH, in which

$$R = HOOCCH_2NHCOCH- \quad \begin{array}{c} COOH \\ | \\ NHCOCH_2CH_2CHNH_2 \end{array}$$

A similar metabolic reaction has been suggested to explain the chronic nephrotoxic properties of phenacetin (IX). The N-hydroxylated metabolite (X) is believed to be implicated.

Patients receiving the monoamine oxidase inhibitor, pargyline (XI), develop severe nausea after ingesting alcoholic beverages because of elevated blood acetaldehyde levels. A metabolite of pargyline is responsible. Pargyline is metabolized to N-methylbenzylamine, N-benzylpropargyline, and benzylamine as expected. Also produced is propiolaldehyde (XII). Found to be an irreversible inhibitor of mitochondrial aldehyde dehydrogenase, it thus prevents the further metabolic oxidation of the acetyldehyde derived from alcohol (cf. Table 5-1; oxidation example 1).

SUMMARY

A basic overview of the principles and mechanisms of drug metabolism and elimination has been presented. Factors that influence drug metabolism and elimination, including concurrently administered medications and disease states, were discussed to provide insight into some of the reasons for individual variability in drug action and patient response. Although metabolism functions primarily to detoxify or deactivate chemicals and drugs that are in the body, some drugs are metabolized to active, and sometimes toxic, metabolites. Just as some chemicals and drugs stimulate the systems responsible for drug metabolism, others have the ability to inhibit these same systems. An understanding and appreciation of these concepts should enable the nurse to anticipate and monitor pharmacologic effects that may be affected by changes in drug metabolism and elimination.

BIBLIOGRAPHY

Adverse interactions of drugs. *The Medical Letter,* 1979, *21*(2), 5-12.

Coutts, R.T., & Beckett, A.H. Metabolic N-oxidation of primary and secondary aliphatic medicinal amines. In F.J. Di Carlo, (Ed.), *Drug Metabolism Reviews* (vol. 6). New York: Marcel Dekker, 1977.

Drayer, D.E. Pharmacologically active drug metabolites: therapeutic and toxic activities, plasma and urine data in man, accumulation in renal failure. *Clinical Pharmacokinetics,* 1976, *1,* 426-443.

Gorrod, J.W. (Ed.). *Biological oxidation of nitrogen.* New York: Elsevier/North-Holland, 1978.

Gorrod, J.W., & Beckett, A.H. (Eds.). *Drug metabolism in man.* London: Taylor & Francis, 1978.

Parke, D.V., & Smith R.L. (Eds.) *Drug metabolism from microbe to man.* London: Taylor & Francis, 1976.

Shirota, F.N., DeMaster, E.G., Elberling, J.A., & Nagasawa, H.T. Metabolic depropargylation and its relationship to aldehyde dehydrogenase inhibition *in vivo. Journal of Medicinal Chemistry,* 1980, *23,* 669-673.

Testa, B., & Jenner, P. *Drug metabolism: chemical and biochemical aspects.* New York: Marcel Dekker, 1976.

Pharmacokinetic Considerations in Drug Response

Leslie Z. Benet
Louis A. Pagliaro

When a nurse administers a dose of a drug to a patient, the ultimate concern is with the efficacy of that drug product in treating a particular condition or disease state. As depicted in Figure 6-1, a number of steps may be interposed between administration of the dose and its therapeutic efficacy. The three steps at the top of the figure—input, distribution, and loss—represent the pharmacokinetic characteristics of the drug. In most cases the drug will be administered by the most convenient route, usually orally, that will result in therapeutic drug concentrations in the blood. The pattern of the concentration-time curve for the drug will be a function of the input, distribution, and loss characteristics. For example, if the elimination of a drug from the body is rapid, then input must be rapid if the clinician expects to achieve reasonable blood levels over any time period.

In most cases, the concentration of drug in the general circulation will be related to a concentration of drug at the site of action. The presence of the drug at the site of action will then elicit a number of pharmacologic effects: the clinical effect desired, a toxic effect, and in some cases an effect completely unrelated to efficacy or toxicity of the drug. The clinician then must balance the toxicity potential of a particular dose of a drug with its efficacy in order to determine the therapeutic utility.

Pharmacokinetics plays its role in the dose-efficacy scheme by attempting to provide a more quantitative relationship between efficacy and dose by interposing measurements of drug concentrations in various biologic fluids. The importance of pharmacokinetics in patient care will depend on the improvement in efficacy, which can be attained and predicted as a result of the measurement of drug levels in the general circulation rather than relating efficacy directly to dose of the drug. This allows the clinician to take into account the various pathologic (i.e., disease states) and physiologic (i.e., age, genetic characteristics) features in the particular patient that makes him or her different from the normal individual given the usual dose. See Chapter 9 for a discussion of the genetic factors affecting drug response.

Pharmacokinetics may be defined as the study of the kinetics of the absorption, distribution, metabolism, and excretion of drugs and the corresponding pharmacologic, therapeutic, or toxic response in humans. Before 1970, the majority of research work in pharmacokinetics was concentrated on those drugs that could be analyzed easily, using simple (and often imprecise and nonspecific) spectrophotometric and microbiologic techniques. In this pre-1970 stage a great deal of effort was directed toward the development of sophisticated mathematic models that, at times, were much more complex than was needed to describe the limited data available. Initiates to the field often indicated that they believed that the mathematic modeling techniques had far outstripped the meager amount of good data describing the time course of drugs or metabolites measured using a specific assay.

During the past decade, the analytic capabilities for measuring drug and metabolite levels have improved considerably. More and more drug studies are being reported in which specific analytic techniques have been developed so that drug concentrations may be measured accurately at levels seen following the usual drug dosing regimen.

Surprisingly, as our analytic techniques began to improve, we found that the sophisticated mathematic models previously developed were not adequate. It became increasingly difficult to delineate which of the many pharmacokinetic parameters should be used in comparing drug absorption and disposition with pharmacologic response data in normal subjects. This uncertainty became particularly acute when investigators began to study drug kinetics in the patient as opposed to the healthy volunteer. In addition, if one wishes to apply pharmacokinetics in patient care, it is necessary to use models that may adequately and simply be related to physiologic parameters in the

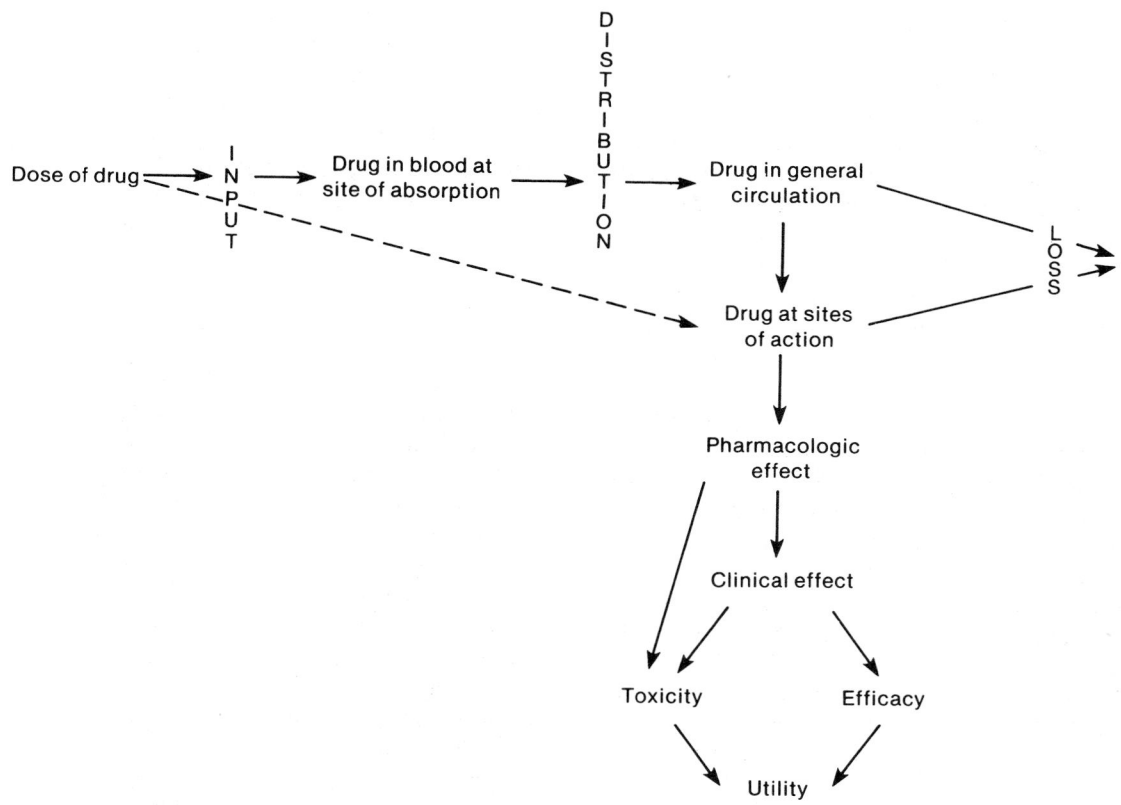

FIGURE 6-1. **A schematic representation of the dose-efficacy relationship for a drug.**

body whereby the clinician can rationally make a judgment as to drug dosing in the disease state.

KINETIC MEASUREMENTS

The need to apply pharmacokinetic parameters to patient care has led to a consideration of three basic types of kinetic measurements: (1) volume of distribution, (2)(elimination half-life, and (3) clearance. The first, a volume of distribution (Vd), relates a given measured concentration in the body to a given amount of drug in the body (i.e., when the amount of drug is divided by the distribution volume, the measured concentration is obtained). The second term is the most generally used parameter, the half-life ($T_{1/2}$) of elimination for the drug. The elimination half-life may be simply defined as the amount of time it takes a drug to "fall" to one half of its initial or current serum or plasma level (Figure 6-2). It should be noted that the discussion here, and throughout the remainder of this chapter, may *not* always apply to drugs that display dose-dependent or capacity-limited kinetics. For a

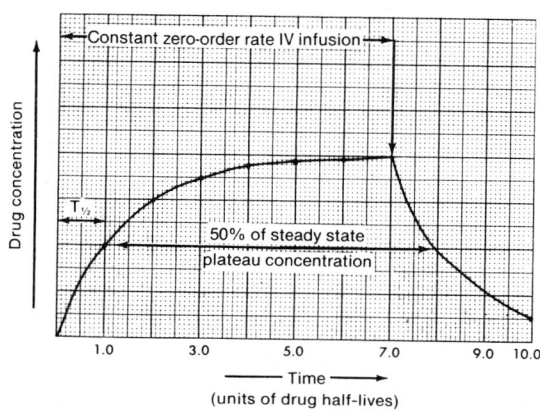

FIGURE 6-2. **Relationship between $T_{1/2}$ and time to drug concentration plateau.**

brief description and discussion of these exceptions, the reader is referred to Chapter 5, "Drug Metabolism and Elimination."

Although knowledge of half-life is necessary in developing multiple-dose drug regimens, we have begun to realize during the past few years that the change in half-life is often not a good measure of changes in blood concentration and response in relation to changes in the pathologic state of a patient. For example, it has been demonstrated with a number of drugs that in patients with congestive heart failure, the half-life of elimination of an administered drug may remain unchanged, but the volume of distribution decreases. Consequently, the serum concentration of the drug increases in proportion to the decrease in volume of distribution unless the dose is appropriately decreased. In fact, a clearance term has been found to be more useful in this respect.

Clearance essentially represents the product of the volume of distribution and the rate constant of elimination, where the rate constant of elimination may be defined as 0.693 (i.e., the natural logarithm of 2) divided by the half-life. Changes in clearance and volume of distribution appear to be the independent variables in the above relation that may be correlated to specific physiologic and pathologic conditions in the body, whereas the rate constant or half-life change appears to depend on the changes of the other two parameters. This is discussed in more detail later in this chapter. Let us first consider the volume of distribution.

VOLUME OF DISTRIBUTION

It is well known that the plasma volume of a "normal" 70 kg man is approximately 3 L, the blood volume is about 5.5 L, and the total body water is approximately 42 L. Consider then the fact that in a normal 70 kg individual when 600 μg of digoxin is administered intravenously, a plasma concentration of approximately 1 ng/ml is observed. Dividing the amount of drug in the body by the plasma concentration yields a volume of distribution for digoxin of approximately 600 L. This value is certainly much greater than the 42 L total body water and is actually 9 times as great as the total body volume of a 70 kg man. This example serves to emphasize the fact that the volume of distribution does *not* represent a real volume, but rather must be considered as the "apparent" size of a pool of body fluids, *assuming* that the drug is equally distributed throughout all portions of the body. It is thus often referred to as an "apparent" volume of distribution. For example, digoxin, which is relatively hydrophobic, distributes into muscle and adipose tissue readily; thus the amount of drug remaining in the plasma is relatively small, and this in turn results in the high apparent volume of distribution.

Depending on a number of factors, including the acid dissociation constant (pK_a) of the drug, the degree of plasma protein binding, the partition coefficient of the drug into fatty tissues, and the degree of binding to other tissues, the volume of distribution may vary widely. For example, in a normal 70 kg man furosemide yields a volume of distribution of 7 L, gentamicin 14 L, antipyrine 33 L, lidocaine 77 L, procainamide 130 L, and quinacrine as high as 40,000 L.

CLEARANCE

Whereas the volume of distribution is a constant representing an apparent space, which may not be readily comparable to the size of an individual, clearance is a measure that is much more clearly related to actual physiologic processes. Figure 6-3 depicts either a plasma or blood volume, depending on where concentrations are measured, as well as on equations relating renal and total clearance (i.e., CL_R and CL_T). Assume that we are dealing with a drug in which concentrations are measured in plasma. The renal clearance for this drug approximates the glomerular filtration rate (GFR) and is approximately 100 ml/min. In essence, we are saying that in every minute the kidney has the ability to completely remove the drug from 100 ml of plasma (i.e., the dotted area in Figure 6-3).

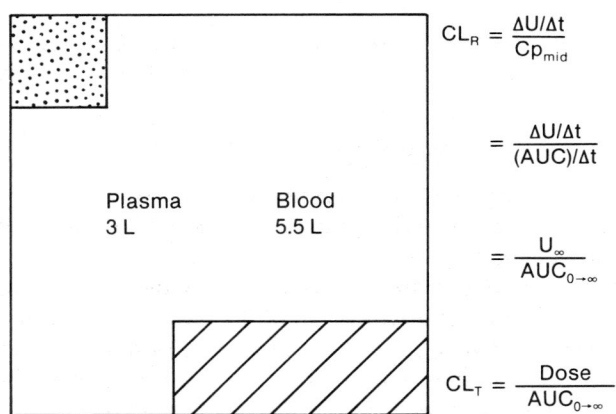

$$CL_R = \frac{\Delta U/\Delta t}{Cp_{mid}}$$

$$= \frac{\Delta U/\Delta t}{(AUC)/\Delta t}$$

$$= \frac{U_\infty}{AUC_{0\to\infty}}$$

$$CL_T = \frac{Dose}{AUC_{0\to\infty}}$$

Plasma 3 L   Blood 5.5 L

FIGURE 6-3. **Hypothetical plasma or blood volume where dotted area represents fraction of volume cleared of drug per minute by renal mechanisms (e.g., 100 ml/min for renal clearance measured with respect to drug concentrations in plasma), and the area containing diagonal lines represents fraction of volume cleared of drug per minute by all elimination mechanisms (e.g., 300 ml/min). Equations demonstrate relationship between renal and total body clearances.**

Renal clearance. Renal clearance (CL_R) is usually calculated by the top equation in Figure 6-3; that is, the rate of drug elimination in the urine, $\Delta U/\Delta t$ (i.e., the amount excreted unchanged in the urine over any given time period), divided by the midpoint plasma concentration (Cp_{mid}) during that time period. This midpoint plasma concentration is, in fact, supposed to represent the average plasma concentration during the time of drug elimination. The average plasma concentration may be more accurately represented as the area under the plasma concentration time curve, AUC (i.e., the amount of drug available to the systemic circulation), during the time interval divided by the time interval (Δt), as represented in the second equation in Figure 6-3. Eliminating the change in time (i.e., Δt) from the numerator and denominator of the second equation yields the result that the renal clearance is in fact the amount of drug eliminated over any time period divided by the area under the plasma concentration time curve during that time period. The third equation in Figure 6-3 allows the time period discussed to be the entire time necessary to describe the course of drug disposition; that is, the total amount of drug eliminated unchanged in the urine (U_∞) divided by the total area under the plasma concentration time curve ($AUC_{0 \to \infty}$).

Total plasma clearance. Whereas renal clearance represents that fraction of the total plasma or blood pool that is cleared by the kidney per unit time, the total plasma or blood clearance represents the volume of the plasma or blood pool that is cleared per unit time by all elimination mechanisms. Thus it may readily be seen that total clearance (CL_T) differs from renal clearance (CL_R) only in that the total dose appears in the numerator of the equation rather than simply the amount eliminated by the renal route.

Relationship between clearance and physiologic processes. In Figure 6-3, the total plasma clearance is 300 ml/min (i.e., the portion of the figure represented by diagonal lines). In this example, renal clearance would represent 100 ml/min while other mechanisms of elimination, most likely the hepatic route, would be responsible for 200 ml/min. Now it is possible to see that clearance measurements, unlike volumes of distribution, will have some real limitations related to physiologic parameters.

Hepatic clearance could never be any faster than blood flow to the liver, since the drug must be delivered to the liver before it can be eliminated. Thus if one were measuring blood levels, the maximum hepatic clearance would be approximately 1.5 L/min. Likewise, the maximum renal clearance would be approximately 1.2 L/min, the blood flow to the kidney. For a drug that is eliminated by kidney filtration only, the maximum clearance would be equal to the glomerular filtration rate (i.e., approximately 120 ml/min).

When we discuss actual physiologic clearances and attempt to relate them to body processes, it is important to deal with *blood* clearances. Plasma clearances may be converted to blood clearances when one knows the hematocrit as well as the partition of the drug between the red blood cells and the plasma.

Table 6-1 presents plasma clearance values broken down into the hepatic and renal route for five representative drugs. Lidocaine and antipyrine represent drugs that are cleared almost exclusively by the hepatic route. However, there is a large difference in their clearance values that, in fact, represents different mechanisms. The plasma clearance of lidocaine, 700 ml/min, approaches the maximum clearance possible (i.e., lidocaine clearance is a function of plasma flow to the liver), whereas antipyrine clearance at 38 ml/

TABLE 6-1

Selected hepatic, renal, and total plasma clearances and half-lives for five representative drugs in a healthy 70 kg man

Drug	Hepatic clearance (ml/min)	Renal clearance (ml/min)	Total plasma clearance (ml/min)	Half-life	References
Antipyrine	38	Negligible	38	10.0 hours	Branch, et al., 1976
Digoxin	40	140	180	1.8 days	Koup, et al., 1976
Gentamicin	3	77	80	2.0 hours	Gyselynck, et al., 1974; Lockwood & Bower, 1973
Lidocaine	700	Negligible	700	1.8 hours	Thomson, et al., 1973
Procainamide	500	330	830	3.0 hours	Galeazzi, et al., 1976

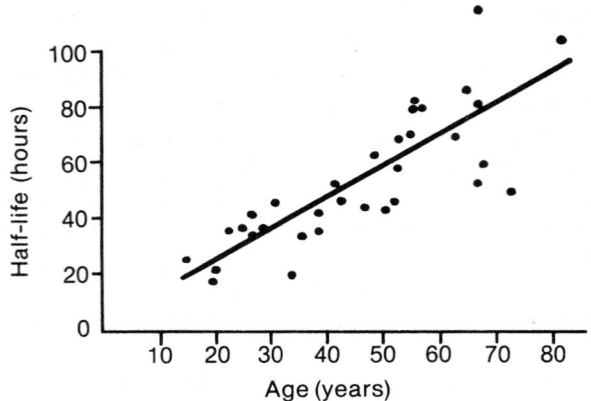

FIGURE 6-4. **Correlation of diazepam half-life and age in 33 normal individuals as described by Klotz, U., et al.** *Journal of Clinical Investigation,* **1975,** *55,* 347-359.

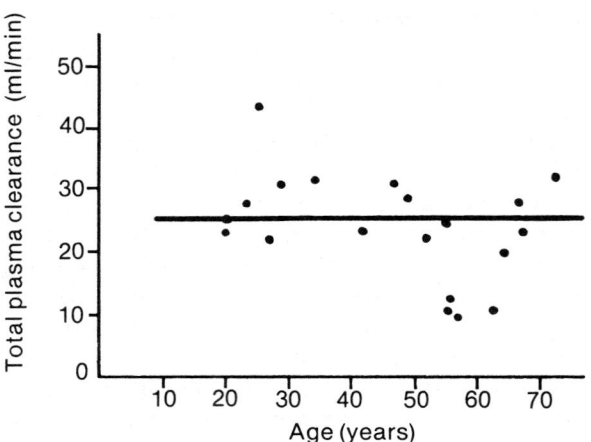

FIGURE 6-5. **Correlation of total plasma clearance of diazepam with age for 20 normal individuals as described by Klotz, U., et al.** *Journal of Clinical Investigation,* **1975,** *55,* 347-359.

min would probably be independent of plasma flow and is generally designated as a drug showing capacity-limited metabolism (see Chapter 5, "Drug Metabolism and Elimination"). One would expect that changes in metabolic enzymes either through induction or competition would lead to changes in antipyrine clearance but not necessarily to changes in lidocaine clearance. That is, the capacity of the liver to metabolize lidocaine is large, and induction would not have an affect on drug metabolism, since apparently lidocaine clearance is limited by blood flow rate. However, changes in blood flow as in a disease state such as congestive heart failure may lead to changes in lidocaine clearance but not changes in antipyrine clearance. In contrast, digoxin and gentamicin are two drugs cleared predominately by the renal route. Thus changes in renal function should have a marked affect on drug clearance. Procainamide is intermediate, with approximately half of its clearance by metabolic and half of its clearance by renal routes.

Relationship between clearance and half-life. It should be noted that half-lives would *not* be good predictors of clearance. Digoxin and gentamicin have total clearances (i.e., 180 and 80 ml/min) that differ by a factor of two, yet their half-lives (i.e., 1.8 days and 2 hours) differ by twentyfold. This is because of the marked differences in the volume of distribution for the two compounds (i.e., 640 L and 14 L). In the case of digoxin the kidney is essentially able to clear plasma at the glomerular filtration rate (GFR). However, since little drug is in the plasma (i.e., large volume of distribution), the half-life of drug in the body is long.

It is important to understand the differences between clearance and half-life when one is attempting to define the underlying mechanisms for the effect of a disease state on drug disposition. For example, in Figure 6-4 Klotz and co-workers (1975) found that the half-life of diazepam increased with the age of the patient. One could speculate that the ability of the liver to metabolize this drug therefore decreases as a function of age. However, when clearance is plotted versus age for 20 normal individuals (Figure 6-5), it is readily apparent that there is no change with age (as denoted by the virtually horizontal line through the data points). That is, the increased half-lives actually result from changes with age in the volume of distribution, and the metabolic processes responsible for eliminating the drug are fairly constant.

APPLICATION

Following this brief overview of pharmacokinetic concepts, we may now discuss how these concepts may be used in treating patients. As stated earlier, most early pharmacokinetic treatments and models were so complicated that it was impossible to use them in a clinical situation. However, most pharmacokinetic adjustment of doses in a patient can be made using one simple relationship; that is, rate in equals rate out. When this is applied to the clinical situation in a particular patient in whom the clinician wishes to maintain a certain average plasma level, $\overline{C}_p$, the rate in equals rate out equation may be converted to equation 2.

Calculations at steady state

$$\text{Rate in} = \text{Rate out} \qquad (1)$$

$$\frac{F \times \text{Dose}}{\tau} = \text{Clearance} \times \overline{C}_p \qquad (2)$$

For Drug "X":

assume desired C_p
= 8 μg/ml

Clearance = 60 ml/min

$$\frac{(F \times \text{Dose})}{\tau} = 60 \text{ ml/min} \times 8 \text{ μg/ml}$$

$$= 480 \text{ μg/min} = 28.8 \text{ mg/hr}$$

$$\approx 30 \text{ mg/hr}, 120 \text{ mg/4hr}, 240$$
$$\text{mg/8 hr}$$

WHERE:

F (availability) is the fraction of a dose available to the systemic circulation. For example, F would be equivalent to 1.0 for a drug administered by the IV route; and F would be equivalent to some fraction less than or equal to 1.0 depending on: the amount absorbed from the gastrointestinal tract for a drug administered by the oral route (see Chapter 4, "Drug Availability and Distribution").

τ (tau) is the dosing interval
$\overline{C}_p$ is the average desired plasma drug concentration

The example calculation given in equation 2 might be for a patient with normal renal function, a situation where the clinician wishes to maintain an average Drug "X" plasma level of 8 μg/ml. The rate in will equal clearance times this steady-state level; that is, 480 μg/min, or 28.8 mg/hr. Since the availability, F, of parenteral Drug "X" is approximately 1, the clinician then may choose the dosing scheme at multiples of approximately 30 mg/hr. The clinician may choose to dose the drug six times a day and therefore would give 120 mg every 4 hours or may choose to dose the drug three times a day, giving 240 mg every 8 hours.

Although these equations are most useful in reaching a given average level, it is important to realize that the change in the dosing interval will cause the plasma level time curve to have different maximum and minimum values depending on the dosing interval even though the average level will always be 8 μg/ml. If the clinician chose to infuse Drug "X" at a continuous rate of 480 μg/min then the level of 8 μg/ml will be maintained continuously. However, if one of the other dosing schemes suggested (e.g., 4- or 8-hour intervals) was chosen, then the maximum and minimum levels would differ.

A simplified way of calculating these maximum $(C_p^{ss}{}_{max})$ and minimum $C_p^{ss}{}_{min}$ values is given in equations 3 and 4. These equations *assume* that absorption

is much faster than elimination and that the system comes quickly into distribution equilibrium.

Maximum and minimum levels at steady state (assuming absorption is much faster than elimination)

$$C_{p_{max}}^{ss} = \frac{F \times \text{Dose}/V_d}{\text{Fraction lost in a dosing interval}} =$$

$$\frac{240 \text{ mg/14 L}}{0.94} = 18.3 \text{ μg/ml} \qquad (3)$$

$$C_{p_{min}}^{ss} = C_{p_{max}}^{ss} \times \text{Fraction remaining after dosing interval} =$$

$$18.3 \text{ μg/ml} \times 0.06 = 1.1 \text{ μg/ml} \qquad (4)$$

The denominator of equation 3, the fraction lost in a dosing interval, may be easily calculated when one knows the half-life. For example, an 8-hour dosing interval was chosen for Drug "X"; assuming a half-life of 2 hours, 50% of the amount of drug in the body would be lost in the first 2 hours after the last dose was given, 75% in 4 hours, 88% in 6 hours, 94% in 8 hours and 97% in 10 hours. Correspondingly, only 6% would remain at the end of the 8-hour dosing interval. Thus with this dosing regimen a maximum level of 18.3 μg/ml and a minimum level of 1.1 μg/ml would be achieved. This would probably not be a good dosing scheme in this patient, since high, potentially toxic levels would be maintained for over 1 hour, and levels possibly below the minimum effective concentration would be expected over 4 hours during each 8-hour dosing interval. A possibly better choice would be 120 mg every 4 hours, where the fraction lost in a dosing interval would be 0.75, and maximum and minimum levels at steady state would be 11.4 and 2.9 μg/ml, respectively. However, in either case, the average level would still be 8 μg/ml.

In this example, the fraction of drug eliminated from the body was derived from the simple algorithm, which states that 50% of the amount of drug *remaining* to be eliminated is eliminated within the time frame of each successive half-life. Thus, it takes five half-lives after the cessation of therapy for a drug to be virtually entirely (i.e., 97%) eliminated from the body. It is interesting to note that the same algorithm also applies to drug accumulation within the body toward a plateau that occurs with multiple dosing and constant rates of IV infusion (see Figure 6-2).

Figure 6-6 graphically illustrates the relationship between frequency of dosing and minimum/maximum plasma concentrations. In this figure, it is noted that after five half-lives of the drug have passed, all three curves (i.e., dosing regimens) yield the same average plasma concentration (i.e., the steady-state plasma concentration). However, they differ significantly

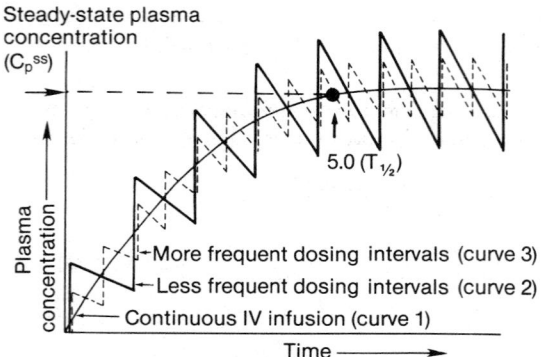

FIGURE 6-6. **Relationship between frequency of dosing interval (T) and minimum/maximum plasma concentrations.**

from one another in relation to their observed minimum and maximum plasma concentrations.

The constant IV infusion provides constant plasma concentration once the steady-state level has been achieved. Less frequent dosing intervals (i.e., curve 3) have the greatest variability in minimum and maximum plasma concentrations. As dosing intervals become more frequent (i.e., curve 2) this variability decreases geometrically. For example, if the dosing interval for curve 2 is half of that for curve 3 (i.e., 120 mg every 4 hours versus 240 mg every 8 hours in the Drug "X" example given earlier) then the average minimum and maximum plasma concentrations will be closer to the actual steady-state concentration.

As noted, it generally takes approximately 5 half-lives to reach steady-state drug concentration. When, however, full, rapid pharmacologic effect is necessary, as is often the case for digitalization and antidysrhythmic therapy, a "loading" dose can be given to rapidly achieve steady-state levels.

TARGET LEVEL CONCEPT

With the simple equations presented above, the nurse should be able to suggest an appropriate drug dosing regimen using the target level concept (i.e., a specific steady-state concentration that is believed to be effective would be the objective of the dosage regimen suggested). Sheiner and Tozer (1977) have discussed under what criteria the target level concept is applicable.

First, the target level concept is applied best when there is marked interindividual (i.e., between different patients) variability in dose to plasma level, with much less intraindividual (i.e., within the same patient) vari-

ability. That is, in Figure 6-1, the concentration of drug in the general circulation should correlate much better with efficacy than dose, since the interindividual differences in input, distribution, and loss can be eliminated when levels are measured and compared with effect.

Second, the target level concept is most useful when evaluation of the target effect is not possible. For example, for the antidysrhythmics, such as quinidine, lidocaine, and procainamide, toxicity may actually resemble lack of efficacy. That is, for these drugs, a dysrhythmia may result from toxic levels of the drug. Thus an effect measurement is not an adequate means of predicting whether the dose should be increased or decreased. A second situation where the target effect is not measurable occurs when the drug is used for prophylaxis of a dangerous event. For example, antiepileptic drugs are dosed to levels so that seizures are prevented. Measurement of an effect would mean that an inadequate dose had been given, but then the damage would have been done. Measurement of target effects are not possible for compounds where efficacy is delayed or difficult to measure, such as with the digitalis glycosides, and a target effect is probably not a good measure when there is no flattening of the dose-response curve, such as for the bronchodilator theophylline (Figure 6-7).

A third important criteria for use of the target level concept is that the drug has a small therapeutic index (TI) and that toxicity from overdosing of the drug is serious. Therapeutic index in this sense is defined as the ratio of the minimum toxic dose to the minimum effective dose. The digitalis glycosides serve as a good example for this criteria. In many cases the therapeutic index is two or less, and toxicity from overdosing the drug can lead to death. The use of the target level concept is best if drug levels are *directly* related to effects and if a constant effect is desired. Then a constant blood level can be maintained that should elicit the required response.

Koch-Weser (1972) has listed 10 drugs that appear to meet the target level criteria, as presented in Table 6-2, with their usual therapeutic ranges. This table does not include any antibiotics where a number of compounds, especially the aminoglycosides, fit the above criteria. More recently, Benet and Sheiner (1980) have compiled effective and toxic concentrations for about 100 drugs, from which pharmacokinetic data may be used in making dosage regimen decisions.

Sheiner and co-workers (1975) have shown that the target level criteria can be used successfully with the cardiac glycoside, digoxin. Using the best information

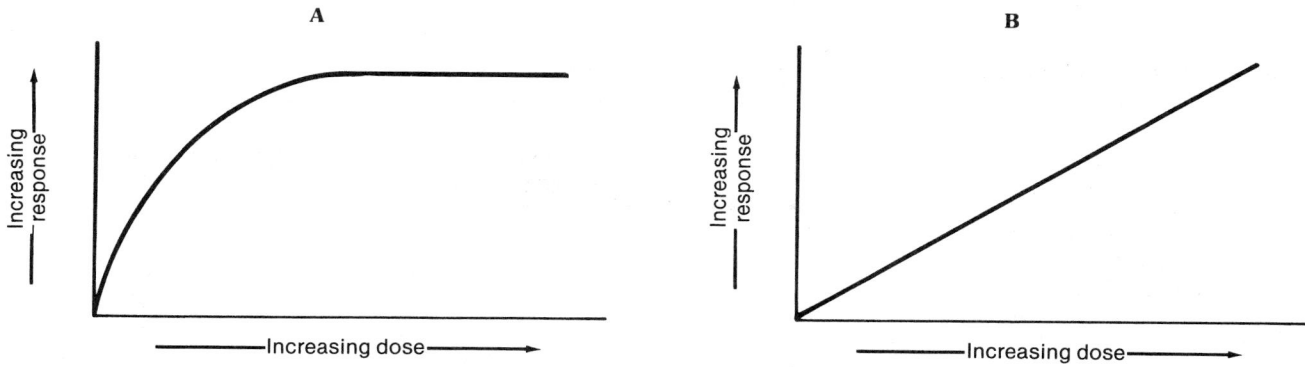

FIGURE 6-7. *A,* **Normal dose-response curve. Note the plateauing of the response.**
***B,* Abnormal dose-response curve. Note the lack of response plateau.**

TABLE 6-2

Usual range of therapeutic plasma concentrations for 11 drugs that appear to meet the target level criteria

Drug	Therapeutic plasma concentration range*
Digitoxin	10-22 ng/ml
Digoxin	0.5-2 ng/ml
Lidocaine	1.2-6 μg/ml
Lithium	0.5-1.5 mEq/L
Nortriptyline	50-140 ng/ml
Phenytoin	10-20 μg/ml
Procainamide	4-9 μg/ml
Propranolol	20-100 ng/ml
Quinidine	2-6 μg/ml
Salicylates	100-250 μg/ml
Theophylline	10-20 μg/ml

*Data from Koch-Weser, J. *New England Journal of Medicine,* 1972, *287,* 227-231; and Benet, L.Z., & Sheiner, L.B. Design and optimization of dosage regimens: pharmacokinetic data. In A.G. Gilman, L.S. Goodman, & A. Gilman (Eds.), *Goodman and Gilman's The pharmacological basis of therapeutics* (6th ed.). New York: Macmillan, 1980.

available as to the patient's weight, sex, renal function, and degree of heart failure, these workers were able to use pharmacokinetics to predict dosage regimens that would maintain blood levels in the 0.5 to 2.0 ng/ml concentration range. However, essentially 8% of the population treated would have a toxic response while 8% would have levels that would be ineffective using predictions based on these patient variables alone. Sheiner et al. (1975) pointed out, however, that if two

drug measurements of digoxin in plasma were taken, then it was possible, using the target level concept and the pharmacokinetic principles presented here, to decrease the patients exhibiting toxic and ineffective levels to 2% in each case. Similarly, Koch-Weser et al. (1974), in a survey of adverse reactions to digoxin in eight hospitals, as presented in Table 6-3, showed that the incidence of toxic reactions to digoxin could be reduced from 13.9% to 5.9% when blood levels were measured in patients at the Massachusetts General Hospital.

EFFECT OF DISEASE STATES

Within the last few years, studies in pharmacokinetics have been concerned with the changes brought about in drug absorption and disposition in patients with a particular disease. The book *The Effect of Disease States on Drug Pharmacokinetics* was one of the first texts that attempted to bring together our knowledge of this particular field (Benet, 1976). One of the initial well-controlled studies in this area was carried out by Thomson and co-workers (1973), who studied the disposition of lidocaine in normal individuals, patients with congestive heart failure, patients in renal failure, and patients with alcoholic cirrhosis. Figure 6-8 depicts the plasma concentration time curves for lidocaine (Thomson, et al., 1971) following 50 mg intravenous bolus doses injected into seven patients with heart failure as compared with the average values found in normal subjects. It is obvious that the levels in the heart failure patients are significantly greater than those found in the normal subjects. Table 6-4 lists some of the representative values found by Thomson

TABLE 6-3

Frequency of adverse reactions to digoxin in eight hospitals

	Number of patients receiving digoxin	Percent with adverse reactions
Boston V.A. Hospital	330	15.2
Boston City Hospital	273	16.2
Hadassah Hospital (Israel)	128	13.1
Lemuel Shattuck Hospital (Boston)	485	19.4
Peter Bent Brigham Hospital (Boston)	736	16.9
Roger Williams General Hospital (Providence, R.I.)	336	14.3
St. Joseph's Hospital (London, Ontario)	137	16.8
TOTAL	2425	AVERAGE 16.0
Massachusetts General Hospital (Boston) 1966-1968	459	13.9
Massachusetts General Hospital (Boston) 1970-1972	253	5.9

From Koch-Weser, J., Duhme, D.W., & Greenblatt, D.J. *Clinical Pharmacology and Therapeutics*, 1974, *16*, 284-287.

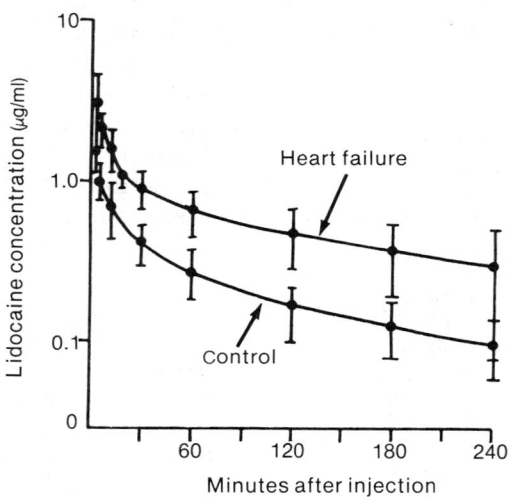

FIGURE 6-8. **Arithmetic mean values ± SD for plasma concentrations of lidocaine in seven subjects with heart failure following a 50 mg IV bolus, illustrating that plasma concentrations in heart failure subjects were elevated throughout the period of observation. (From Thomson, P.D., et al. *Annals of Internal Medicine* 1973, *78*, 499-508).**

et al. (1973) in the four classes of patients. As indicated, clearance is decreased in both the heart failure patients and those with alcoholic cirrhosis. In addition, however, the volume of distribution in the heart failure patients is also significantly less than that found in the normal subjects. Both of these effects are probably related to the decreased cardiac output seen in heart

failure patients. That is, the drug distributes less readily to remote portions of the body when the cardiac output is decreased, thereby decreasing the volume available for drug disposition.

It is important to realize that when the volume of distribution decreases by approximately 40%, as in this case, the blood levels will increase by that per-

TABLE 6-4

Lidocaine pharmacokinetic parameters found in four groups of patients

Patient group	Number	Half-life terminal phase (min)	Volume of distribution steady-state (L/kg)	Plasma clearance (ml/min/kg)
Normal subjects	10	107.8	1.32	10.0
Heart failure	8	11.5	0.88 (p<0.05)*	6.3 (p<0.05)
Renal disease	6	77.4	1.20	13.7
Liver disease	8	296 (p<0.05)	2.31 (p<0.05)	6.0 (p<0.05)

From Thomson, P.D., et al. *Annals of Internal Medicine*, 1973, *78*, 499-508.
*Statistical significance calculated in comparison with normal subjects.

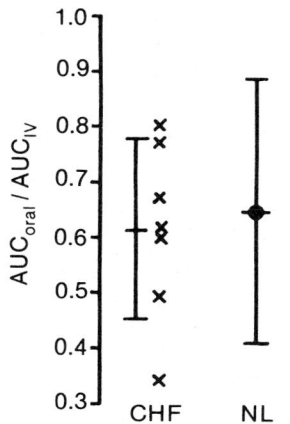

Furosemide availability

FIGURE 6-9. **Comparisons of the mean and range for the extent of oral availability found in seven patients with congestive heart failure (CHF) by Benet and co-workers as compared with the range found in normal patients (NL) by Kelly et al. (From Benet, L.Z., et al. Gastrointestinal absorption of drugs in patients with cardiac failure. In L.Z. Benet (Ed.).** *The effect of disease states on drug pharmacokinetics*, **Washington D.C.: APhA Academy of Pharmaceutical Sciences, 1976; and Kelly, M.R., et al.** *Clinical Pharmacology and Therapeutics*, **1974,** *15*, **177-186.)**

trast, the volume of distribution for the cirrhotic alcoholics is greater than that found in normal patients. However, in spite of the increased volume, clearance still decreases, probably because of decrease in the ability of the liver to eliminate the drug. Although there is an increase in volume, the decrease in clearance is more substantial, and thus the half-life increases for lidocaine in these liver failure patients.

The decrease in volume of distribution for lidocaine in heart failure has also been noted for procainamide and apparently for quinidine, as reviewed by Benet, et al. (1976). However, Greither and co-workers (1979) found that the volume of distribution for furosemide, a highly protein bound acidic drug, was not different when heart failure and normal patients were compared. These workers were interested in determining whether the decreased cardiac output in congestive heart failure caused a decreased gastrointestinal absorption of furosemide. A compilation of the availability results are presented in Figure 6-9. These workers found that there was a marked variation in the oral availability of furosemide in heart failure patients ranging from 33% to 80%. However, this variation in drug availability was similar to that found in normal patients by Kelly and co-workers (1974). Thus it appears that absorption of furosemide in heart failure patients may be erratic and unpredictable, but this unpredictability is similar to that found in normal individuals.

Table 6-5 compiled by Sheiner (1976) presents examples of pathologic conditions that may affect the relationship of dosage regimens to the effects seen with particular cardiovascular drugs. Awareness of the changes found in the disease states listed will give the nurse the ability to make predictions on the basis of clearance concepts as to what dosage regimens should be used to attain the target blood levels listed previously in Table 6-2.

centage. In addition, the clearance of the drug is decreased because the blood flow to the clearing organ, the liver, is decreased in heart failure for this drug, which apparently approaches blood flow rate, limiting clearance conditions. The decrease in volume of distribution and the decrease in clearance appear to counteract each other for this particular drug so that the apparent half-life of lidocaine is the same in both the normal patients and heart failure patients. In con-

TABLE 6-5

Examples of pathophysiologic conditions that may affect the relationship of dosage regimen to effect for some cardiovascular drugs*

Drug	Renal failure (uremia)	Hepatic failure— cirrhosis	Hypoalbuminemia (e.g., nephrotic syndrome)	Congestive heart failure	Malabsorption
		Condition			
Digitoxin	? ↓ Clearance ↓ Protein binding	? ↓ Clearance	↓ Protein binding		
Digoxin	↓ ↓ Clearance ↓ Volume of distribution	? ↓ Clearance		? ↓ Clearance	↓ Oral bioavailability
Procainamide	↓ Clearance ↑ Active metabolites			↓ Clearance, ↓ Volume of distribution ↓ Oral bioavailability	
Phenytoin	↓ ↓ Protein binding ↑ Volume of distribution ↑ ↑ Clearance	↓ Clearance	↓ ↓ Protein binding ↑ Volume of distribution ↑ ↑ Clearance		
Lidocaine	↑ Active metabolites	↓ Clearance		↓ Clearance, ↓ Volume of distribution	
Quinidine	↑ Active metabolites		↓ Protein binding	? ↓ Volume of distribution	
Propranolol		? ↓ Clearance	↓ ↓ Protein binding	↓ Clearance	

Adapted from Sheiner, L.B. *Practical Cardiology*, 1976, *2*, 35-41.

*This table is not meant to be exhaustive but, rather, illustrative. Other conditions may cause variability in the kinetics of the drugs listed, and the effects of the conditions listed are not necessarily restricted to those indicated. *One arrow*, moderate changes in direction indicated; *two arrows*, major changes in direction indicated; *question mark*, inconsistency in noted effect.

SUMMARY

A simplified explanation of the mathematics of pharmacokinetics has been presented using the clearance concept. Realizing that a target blood level can be maintained if the rate of drug administration matches the rate of drug elimination, the clinician may readily select the appropriate dosage regimen for a particular drug. Using the principles presented here, with a knowledge of the changes in the physiologic processes affecting drug clearance as a function of disease states, the clinician will be able to make the appropriate dosage regimen corrections that will allow the maintenance of the patient at a target blood level appropriate for the particular disease state being treated.

BIBLIOGRAPHY

Benet, L.Z. (Ed.). The *effect of disease states on drug pharmacokinetics*. Washington, D.C.: APhA Academy of Pharmaceutical Sciences, 1976.

Benet, L.Z., Greither, A., & Meister, W. Gastrointestinal absorption of drugs in patients with cardiac failure. In L.Z. Benet (Ed.), *The effect of disease states on drug pharmacokinetics*. Washington, D.C.: APhA Academy of Pharmaceutical Sciences, 1976.

Benet, L.Z., & Sheiner, L.B. Design and optimization of dosage regimens: pharmacokinetic data. In A.G. Gilman, L.S. Goodman, & A. Gilman (Eds.), *Goodman and Gilman's The pharmacological basis of therapeutics* (6th ed.). New York: The Macmillan Co., 1980.

Branch, R.A., James, J.A., & Read, A.E. The clearance of antipyrine and indocyanine green in normal subjects and in patients with chronic liver disease. *Clinical Pharmacology and Therapeutics*, 1976, *20*, 81-89.

Galeazzi, R.L., Benet, L.Z., & Sheiner, L.B. Relationship between the pharmacokinetics and pharmacodynamics of procainamide. *Clinical Pharmacology and Therapeutics*, 1976, *20*, 278-289.

Goldstein, A., Aronow, L., & Kalman, S.M. *Principles of drug action* (2nd ed.). Toronto: John Wiley & Sons, 1974.

Greither, A., Goldman, S., Edelen, J.S., Benet, L.Z., & Cohn, K. Pharmacokinetics of furosemide in patients with congestive heart failure. *Pharmacology*, 1979, *19*, 121-131.

Gyselynck, A.M., Forrey, A., & Cutler, R. Pharmacokinetics of gentamicin: distribution and plasma and renal clearance. *Journal of Infectious Diseases*, 1971, *124 Supp.*, S70-S76.

Kelly, M.R., Cutler, R.E., Forrey, A.W., & Kimpel, B.M. Pharmacokinetics of orally administered furosemide. *Clinical Pharmacology and Therapeutics*, 1974, *15*, 178-186.

Klotz, U., Avant, G.R., Hoyumpa, A., Schenker, S., & Wilkinson, G.R. The effects of age and liver disease on the disposition and elimination of diazepam in adult man. *Journal of Clinical Investigation*, 1975, *55*, 347-359.

Koch-Weser, J. Serum drug concentrations as therapeutic guides. *New England Journal of Medicine*, 1972, *287*, 227-231.

Koch-Weser, J., Duhme, D.W., & Greenblatt, D.J. Influence of serum digoxin concentration measurements on frequency of digitoxicity. *Clinical Pharmacology and Therapeutics*, 1974, *16*, 284-287.

Koup, J.R., Greenblatt, D.J., Jusko, W.J., Smith, T.W., & Koch-Weser, J. Pharmacokinetics of digoxin in normal subjects after intravenous bolus and infusion doses. *Journal of Pharmacokinetics and Biopharmaceutics*, 1975, *3*, 181-192.

Lockwood, W.R., & Bower, J.D. Tobramycin and gentamicin concentrations in the serum of normal and anephric patients. *Antimicrobial Agents and Chemotherapy*, 1973, *3*, 125-129.

Michelson, P.A., Miller, W.A., Warner, J.F., Ayers, L.W., & Boxenbaum, H.G. Multiple dose pharmacokinetics of gentamicin in man: evaluation of the Jelliffe nomogram and the adjustment of dosage in patients with renal impairment. In L.Z. Benet (Ed.), *The effect of disease states on drug pharmacokinetics.* Washington, D.C.: APhA Academy of Pharmaceutical Sciences, 1976.

Pagliaro, L.A., & Benet, L.Z. Critical compilation of terminal half-lives, percent excreted unchanged, and changes of half-life in renal and hepatic dysfunction for studies in humans with references. *Journal of Pharmacokinetics and Biopharmaceutics*, 1975, *3*, 333-383.

Sheiner, L.B. Clinical application of plasma drug concentrations in cardiovascular therapy. *Practical Cardiology*, 1976, *2*, 35-41.

Sheiner, L.B., Halkin, H., Peck, C., Rosenberg, B., & Melmon, K.L. Improved computer assisted digoxin therapy: a method using feedback of measured serum digoxin concentrations. *Annals of Internal Medicine*, 1975, *82*, 619-627.

Sheiner, L.B., Benet, L.Z., & Pagliaro, L.A. A standard approach to compiling clinical pharmacokinetic data. *Journal of Pharmacokinetics and Biopharmaceutics*, 1981, *9*, 59-127.

Sheiner, L.B., & Tozer, T.N. Clinical pharmacokinetics: the use of plasma concentrations of drugs. In K.L. Melmon & H.F. Morrelli (Eds.), *Clinical pharmacology* (2nd ed.). New York: The MacMillan Co., 1977.

Smith, D.E., Lin, E.T., & Benet, L.Z. Absorption and disposition of furosemide in healthy volunteers, measured with a metabolite-specific assay. *Drug Metabolism and Disposition*, 1980, *8*, 337-342.

Thomson, P.D., Melmon, K.L., Richardson, J.A., Cohn, K., Steinbrunn, W., Cudihee, R., & Rowland, M. Lidocaine pharmacokinetics in advanced heart failure, liver disease and renal failure in humans. *Annals of Internal Medicine*, 1973, *78*, 499-508.

Thomson, P.D., Rowland, M., & Melmon, K.L. The influence of heart failure, liver disease, and renal failure on the disposition of lidocaine in man. *American Heart Journal*, 1971, *82*, 417-421.

CHAPTER 7

Age-dependent Drug Selection and Response

Louis A. Pagliaro

Ann M. Pagliaro

Drug therapy must be tailored to meet the individual needs of each patient, taking into consideration such unique variables as general state of health, concurrent diseases or conditions, psychologic status, past medical history, genetic predisposition, current physical condition (including vital organ function), known allergies, and other prescription and nonprescription medications the patient is currently taking. The clinician uses this information to devise a drug regimen that will provide the patient with optimal therapeutic benefits with minimal adverse effects.

Whereas drug therapy must be individualized to the needs of all patients, it is well recognized that two groups in particular, the very young and the very elderly, require special attention in relation to drug selection and dosage.

One can readily observe the many similarities in the manner in which the young and the elderly respond to medications. For example, decreased renal function in both of these groups increases the half-life of elimination for drugs that are eliminated primarily unchanged in the urine. In general, however, as in the case of decreased renal function, the reason for the similarities in handling drugs is quite different. In the young, immature body systems are still developing to their full capacity, whereas in the elderly, aging body systems, in response to the normal physiologic process of aging, are losing their functional capacity.

Nurses have recognized for some time the special needs of these two populations and have established specialized programs for pediatric and geriatric nurses. It is important, however, for all nurses to appreciate the special needs in relation to drug therapy for the very young and the very old.

SPECIAL DRUG CONSIDERATIONS IN THE YOUNG

Because of the variety of factors involved in human physiologic development, drug therapy must be spe-cially tailored and monitored in the young. This process begins before birth, because of the teratogenic potential of many drugs, and it continues through adolescence when the young complete physiologic maturation and become adults.

Teratogenesis

Special considerations for drug therapy in the young must begin before birth to minimize the risk of a teratogenic drug insult. A teratogen may be defined as an agent or factor that causes the production of physical or developmental abnormalities in the developing embryo or fetus. Birth defects caused by drugs that the mother consumes have been fairly well documented and could be prevented if the health care professional working with the mother is aware of their occurrences and effectively educates her.

Because of the sequence of human development (Figure 7-1), the developing embryo or fetus is most susceptible to a teratogenic drug during the first trimester of pregnancy. Following this period the next most troublesome period is usually at birth, when the drug may exhibit its pharmacologic effect in the neonate. For example, heroin-addicted mothers may deliver neonates suffering from heroin withdrawal symptoms, and mothers treated with thiopental during labor may have neonates who exhibit neurobehavioral depression. Fortunately, the adverse effects noted at birth that are an extension of the normal or expected pharmacologic effect of a particular medication are usually reversible with proper recognition and care. Birth defects such as cleft lip, congenital heart disease, and other multiple congenital anomalies are not as easily or as successfully dealt with. For these other more serious effects the best "treatment" is education and prevention.

The placenta, which in the past had often been referred to as the *placental barrier,* is physiologically like a sieve that allows the passage of most substances. The major mechanisms by which drugs cross the pla-

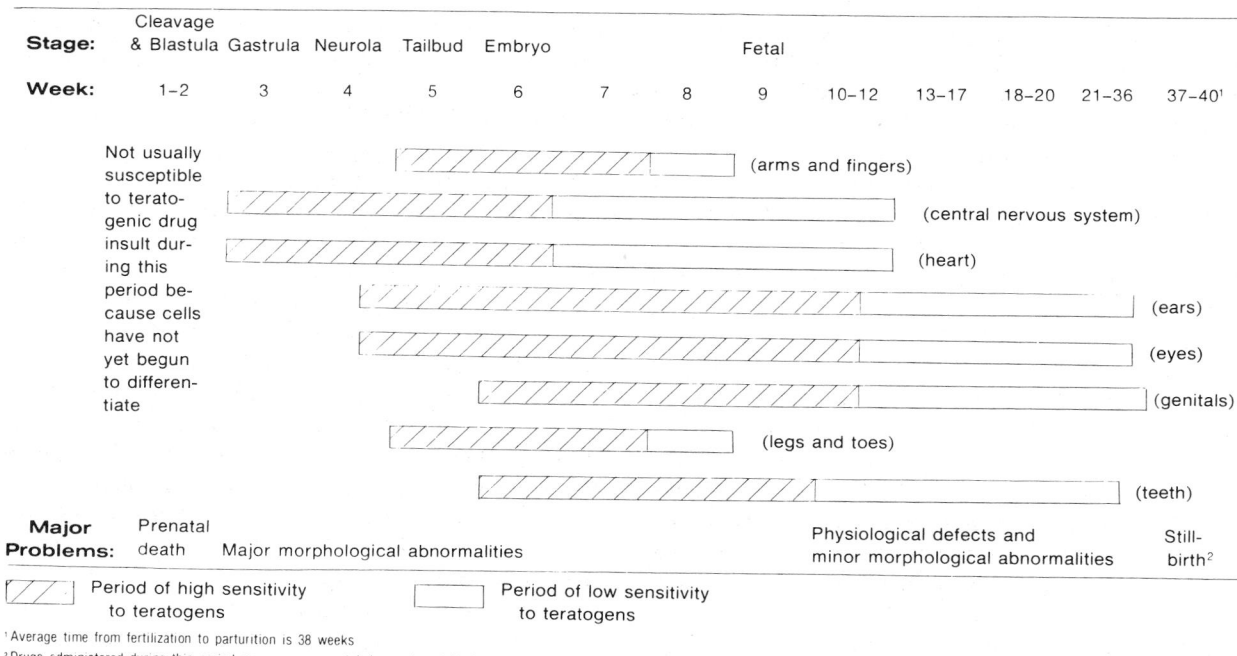

FIGURE 7-1. **Overview of human development with particular reference to timing of potential teratogenic drug insult. (From Pagliaro, L.A., & Levin, R.H. Teratogenesis. In L.A. Pagliaro & R.H. Levin (Eds.).** *Problems in pediatric drug therapy.* **Hamilton, Ill.: Drug Intelligence Publications, 1979, p. 41.)**

centa are active transport, breaks in the placental villi, facilitated diffusion, pinocytosis, simple diffusion, and ultrafiltration. Drug transfer across the placenta is governed by the concentration gradient between the maternal and fetal sides, as well as by the characteristics of the drug including degree of ionization, lipid solubility, and molecular weight (i.e., size of the molecules). In general, nonionized drugs, which are lipid soluble and have a low molecular weight, have the best chance of crossing the placenta to the fetus. Drug transfer and the relationship between a drug bound to tissue or plasma protein are illustrated in Figure 7-2.

Most drugs can cross the placenta, but not all are dangerous or harmful to the fetus. Those most likely to cause a teratogenic effect and that should always be *avoided* in pregnant women include alcohol, aminopterin, chlorpropamide, diazepam, diethylstilbestrol, ethinyltestosterone, heroin, iodide, lithium, mepivacaine, mercury, methadone, methyltestosterone, methylthiouracil, norethindrone, phenytoin, propranolol, propylthiouracil, secobarbital, tetracycline, thalidomide, trimethadione, and warfarin.

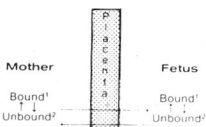

[1] The portion of drug bound to serum protein or ionized which does not cross the placenta
[2] The portion of unionized or unbound drug which crosses the placenta

FIGURE 7-2. **Schematic representation of drug transfer across the human placenta. (From Pagliaro, L.A., & Levin, R.H. Teratogenesis. In L.A. Pagliaro & R.H. Levin (Eds.).** *Problems in pediatric drug therapy.* **Hamilton, Ill.: Drug Intelligence Publications, 1979, p. 41.)**

Drugs excreted in breast milk

Unless information to the contrary exists for a particular drug, it can be assumed that any drug taken by a nursing mother will be excreted in her breast milk. For the vast majority of drugs, however, the concentration in the milk will be insufficient to cause any pharmacologic effect or elicit any clinical symptoms in the nursing infant.

The excretion of drugs into breast milk depends on many factors, including the maternal blood concentration of the drug, the physiochemical properties of the drug (e.g., molecular weight, lipid solubility, and degree of ionization), composition of the milk, and the nursing behavior of the infant (i.e., time and amount of feeding). It is in relation to nursing behavior in particular that the nurse should educate the patient. If a mother must consume a medication the best time in relation to breast feeding would be about 15 minutes after nursing or 3 to 4 hours before the next feeding, because this schedule would minimize the amount of medication excreted in the breast milk. It should be noted, however, that this is a general rule and will *not* apply to all drugs (e.g., the milk concentration of salicylate is maximal 4 hours after maternal administration).

Although most drugs do not cause a problem for the nursing infant, the nurse should be alert to the drugs that may cause associated pharmacologic effects in nursing infants. These drugs include bromide, cascara sagrada, chloral hydrate, chloramphenicol, cyclophosphamide, diazepam, ergot alkaloids, gallium citrate, heroin, iodide, lithium, methadone, methotrexate, phenindione, phenytoin, propylthiouracil, radioactive iodine, tetracycline, and thiouracil. If these or other medications present a problem for the nursing infant and the mother is not able to discontinue the medication, then breast feeding should be stopped.

Pediatric poisonings

Accidental pediatric poisoning is a major health problem. As soon as an infant can crawl (about 6 months of age) an accidental poisoning can occur. However, it is usually in children between 2 and 5 years of age that the majority of poisonings with medications occur. This is because of the child's curiosity, a tendency to put most objects in the mouth, greater mobility (starting with the toddler stage), and lack of sufficient cognitive development to appreciate danger.

The majority of accidental poisoning deaths related to medication ingestion result from ingesting analgesics (particularly aspirin), antipsychotics, iron preparations, and sedative-hypnotics.

To minimize accidental poisoning with medications, parents and others caring for young children should be informed about the seriousness of the problem and advised to have all of their medications in containers with childproof caps and to store these in a locked medicine cabinet. It should be stressed that nonprescription medications, such as aspirin and iron tablets, are just as hazardous to young children as prescription medications. A list of specific antidotes for some specific types of poisons can be found in Appendix V of this text.

Adverse drug reactions

Children, because of their immature mechanisms of metabolism, excretion, and drug receptors, are particularly sensitive to some medications even if adjustments in dosage are made on the basis of body surface area. Examples of drugs that may cause specific adverse effects in children include: corticosteroids, which when administered to children may inhibit both normal epiphyseal development and growth hormone effects resulting in growth suppression; the possible association between aspirin use in children with chickenpox or influenza and Reye's syndrome; chloramphenicol, which when administered to newborn infants may cause the gray syndrome because of an immature metabolic pathway (e.g., glucuronide conjugation) present during the first few days of life; hexachlorophene, which when applied as a soap to the scalps of neonates can be significantly absorbed and cause neurotoxicity; succinylcholine, which when administered to children may cause myoglobinemia significantly more often than when administered to adults; and tetracycline, which if administered to children under 8 years of age may become incorporated in developing teeth and cause permanent staining and enamel hypoplasia.

Renal function

Renal blood flow is lower in the neonate and the glomerular filtration rate of the infant is approximately 50% of the normal adult rate. The renal system matures relatively rapidly, however, and by the sixth to twelfth month of life should reach the adult rate. Until this time, however, drugs that are primarily excreted unchanged in the urine (e.g., digoxin, gentamicin, penicillin) will have a much longer half-life of elimination than one would normally expect, and their dose or dosage regimens must be adjusted accordingly (see Chapter 6, "Pharmacokinetic Considerations in Drug Response," and Chapter 35, "Review of the Anatomy, Physiology, and Assessment of the Renal System").

Hepatic function

Hepatic function is not fully developed at birth, so some enzymes produced in the liver and responsible for drug metabolism (e.g., glucuronyl transferase, which is needed to conjugate chloramphenicol) are not available in the neonate and administering even pediatric doses of some medications may cause severe unexpected reactions, such as the gray syndrome. Several medications, including amphetamines, diazepam, nalidixic acid, phenacetin, phenytoin, and phenylbutazone, are more slowly metabolized in the neonate and therefore have a longer half-life of elimination, which must be considered in devising a dosing regimen. Fortunately, by the end of the neonatal period most drug metabolizing enzymes are fully functioning.

Another important factor in relation to pediatric hepatic function is protein binding. Protein binding of drugs is important in determining their volume of distribution and pharmacologic effect.* The major serum protein to which drugs bind is albumin, which is produced by the liver. Until a child is about 2 years of age, the mechanism for producing albumin is not fully developed, so younger children may have a higher percentage of free (active) drug circulating in their blood from a given dose of medication. This may occur even though the dosage was reduced according to the weight, age, or body surface area of the child.

Volume of distribution

Fluid constitutes approximately 80% of the body weight of an infant. This percentage gradually decreases to the adult percentage of body weight (55%) by 2 years of age.

Because of the differences in percentage of total body water and its associated fluid spaces (i.e., intracellular and extracellular) the volume of distribution of some drugs (e.g., digoxin, gentamicin), which are highly water soluble, will be expected to be larger in neonates and infants as opposed to adults. Thus, alterations in dose or dosage regimen may need to be made to reflect the altered volume of distribution.

Drug receptors

Health care professionals have observed for some time that some drugs demonstrate either a remarkably strong (e.g., atropine, curare, kanamycin) or weak (e.g., halothane, succinylcholine) effect when administered to children.† Although most of these effects can be explained by the factors previously discussed, some have postulated that some drug receptors may not be fully developed in children.

Altered or "immature" receptors may also account for the majority of seemingly paradoxical drug effects (e.g., the calming effect of the stimulant methylphenidate) in children.

---

*Recall that it is only the free drug (not the protein-bound drug) which elicits a pharmacologic effect (see Chapter 3, "Mechanisms of Drug Action").

†Some authors refer to this phenomenon as children being particularly sensitive or resistant to the effects of certain medications.

Pediatric dosing and administration

Several dosing formulae (e.g., Clark's rule, Fried's rule, Young's rule) have been developed to estimate pediatric dosage as a fraction of the normal adult dose. Body surface area, which uses two measures—height and weight—(Figure 7-3), is generally believed to provide better estimates for pediatric dosing than the formulae based on age or weight. In some cases the pediatric dose calculated may exceed the maximal recommended adult dose; however, one should *never* administer a dose to children exceeding the maximal recommended adult dose, except in rare cases where the dosage guidelines specifically recommend this. A specific case involves theophylline. Because of its shorter half-life of elimination in children its dosage may at times exceed the normal adult dose.

It should be emphasized that formulae or nomograms are used to calculate approximate pediatric doses. Because of the influence of the factors previously discussed, however, it is only by means of careful titration and adjustment that the optimal dosage will be arrived at for each individual pediatric patient.

When administering medications to a young child nurses should try to administer the entire dose in one spoonful, avoid administering drugs with important foods because the child may begin to associate the unpleasant drug taste with the food, avoid making medications so flavorful or treated in such a manner that they may later be sought out as candy, advise parents and others responsible for the care of young children always to keep all medications (prescription and nonprescription) in child-resistant containers and out of children's reach, and remember that administering medications to young infants and small children always requires tact and skill.* For more details or information in relation to drug administration see Chapter 2, "Preparation, Administration, and Monitoring of Medications."

Pediatric dosages have been specified whenever possible in the Nursing Drug Digest of each medication chapter in Sections III through XV of this text. If the nurse needs more detailed information on pediatric drug therapy (e.g., the affect of prematurity on drug dosing, neonatal drug dosing) he or she should refer to the comprehensive pediatric drug therapy reference by Pagliaro and Levin listed in the Bibliography of this chapter.

---

*For an interesting anecdote by Robb on pediatric drug administration, see Chapter 1, "Pharmacologic Aspects of Nursing: A Historical Overview."

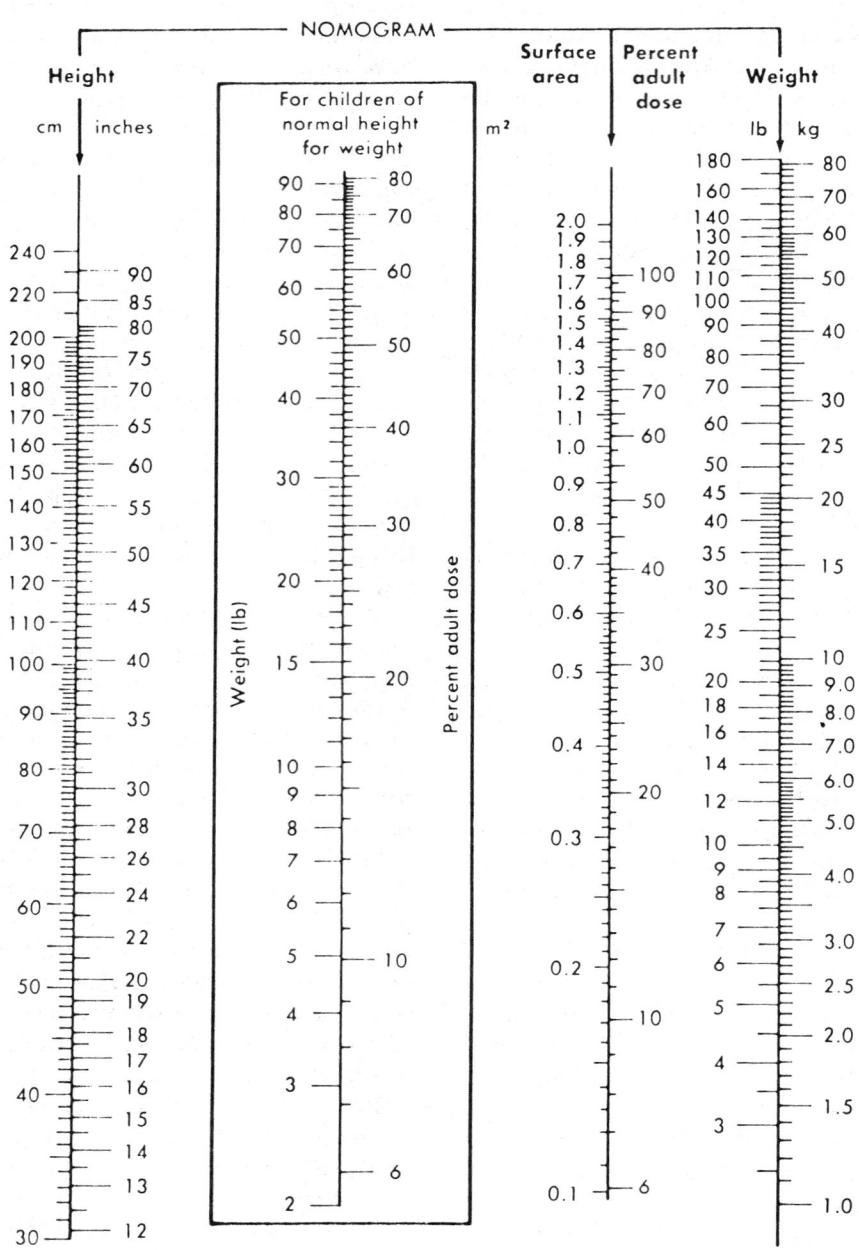

FIGURE 7-3. West's nomogram for the calculation of body surface area. (From Kegel, S.M., & Singer, M.I. Critical care of infants and children after the neonatal period. In D.A. Zschoche (Ed.). *Mosby's comprehensive review of critical care.* St. Louis: The C.V. Mosby Co., 1976. Modified from Nelson, W.E. *Textbook of pediatrics* (8th ed.). Philadelphia: W.B. Saunders, 1964.)

SPECIAL DRUG CONSIDERATIONS IN THE ELDERLY

The elderly suffer 2 to 5 times the frequency of adverse effects from drug therapy than the younger adult, and from 5% to 30% of geriatric admissions to hospitals may be associated with inappropriate drug therapy.

Clinicians are often not adequately aware of the problems in geriatric drug therapy because of the following factors: a low level of suspicion, ascribing symptoms to old age, more than one clinician prescribing for the client, a failure to inquire about nonprescription drug use, atypical presentation of symptoms in the elderly (e.g., higher pain threshold, more referred pain), a difficulty in communication (e.g., poor vision and hearing), and a lack of time necessary to adequately work up a geriatric patient. In addition, physiologic changes that are a natural result of aging profoundly influence drug therapy in the elderly even in the absence of disease.

Before proceeding, so as not to inadvertently contribute to the stereotype of ageism, it should be noted that the physiologic changes noted below occur in the *average* elderly patient (i.e., aging is a unique and individual process that occurs at different rates in different individuals). However, whereas the occasional elderly individual may be found who is in better shape than a person one half of his or her age, for the vast majority of individuals the physiologic changes noted here are accurate.

Renal function

Renal blood flow and the dependent mechanisms of glomerular filtration and tubular secretion are decreased in the elderly. There is also a reduction in the number of functioning nephrons. Consequently, drugs that are eliminated predominantly in unchanged form via the kidneys (e.g., digoxin, gentamicin, kanamycin, lithium, penicillin, sulfamethizole) will stay in the body longer and will have a longer half-life of elimination.* If dosages are not reduced, overdosing will result at an increased frequency, as will the severity of adverse and side effects.

Composition of body mass

Several changes occur in the composition of the body mass as a natural consequence of aging. These include increased fat (as opposed to lean) body tissue that can cause delayed onset followed by accumula-

---

*See Chapter 6, "Pharmacokinetic Considerations in Drug Response," for more details concerning the effect of renal function on pharmacokinetics.

tion on repeated dosing with fat soluble drugs (e.g., barbiturates, diazepam, lidocaine), and reduction of heart, kidney, and muscle mass that can cause toxic blood or tissue levels of a drug when a normal adult dose is administered. Total body fluid also decreases as a percentage of total body weight, from 55% in the younger adult to 45% in the elderly adult.

Volume of distribution

In patients who have congestive heart failure the volume of distribution of many drugs (e.g., digoxin, furosemide, lidocaine) is reduced so that a normal adult dose may result in toxic blood levels (see Chapter 6, "Pharmacokinetic Considerations in Drug Response," for further details).

Another factor affecting the volume of distribution in the elderly is a significantly reduced albumin concentration. Thus, as noted previously for young children, the concentration of a free (active) drug can be significantly higher than expected if a normal adult dose of a highly protein-bound drug (e.g., meperidine, phenytoin, phenylbutazone, warfarin) is administered to an elderly patient. Greater competition of drugs for protein-binding sites also exists in the elderly and the potential for drug interactions mediated via a protein-binding mechanism is significantly increased.

Hepatic function

The rate of some forms of hepatic metabolism (i.e., hydroxylation and conjugation reactions—see Chapter 5, "Drug Metabolism and Elimination") for several drugs (e.g., acetaminophen, antipyrine) has been demonstrated to be significantly decreased (on average) in the elderly. This decrease is associated with longer half-lives of elimination for these drugs in the elderly. These findings are not generalizable to all other drugs, and it appears that most drugs are normally metabolized in the elderly. However, it should be noted that the elderly may be more susceptible to drug-induced liver toxicity (e.g., hepatitis caused by isoniazid) than are younger adults.

Drug receptors

As was the case for pediatrics, health care professionals have observed for some time that the elderly appear to be particularly susceptible or resistant to the effects of certain drugs (e.g., barbiturates). Most of these effects can be explained by the geriatric factors previously discussed; however, it has been postulated that these effects may be the result, at least in part, of decreased numbers of drug receptors in the elderly or of the decreased responsiveness of some drug receptors in the elderly.

Aging body systems

Because of the decreased functional reserve in a variety of body systems (e.g., cardiovascular, nervous, renal) and the resultant lack of a safety margin with which to cope with drug effects, the elderly may experience more seemingly paradoxic drug responses and side effects than individuals in other age groups. These effects may also be the result of age-related changes in the structure, number, or sensitivity of drug receptors in the elderly.

Interactions with multiple disease states

Multiple disease states and pathologic disease states caused by polypharmacy involving prescription, as well as nonprescription, medications are very common in the elderly. Therefore, drug–drug and drug–disease state interactions are much more frequently observed in this age group.

Interactions involving psychotherapeutic agents that additively or synergistically depress the sensorium are especially troublesome in the elderly. They contribute to poor self-esteem in the elderly patient and to the significant number of elderly who are inappropriately classified as suffering from senile dementia.

Geriatric dosing and administration

Because of the factors previously discussed, special consideration for dosing and monitoring the effects of medications in the elderly are particularly important. Because these factors are relatively newly discovered and have not previously been given wide attention, dosing in the elderly is not as exact as in the young. In the young specific dosages and general formulae have been extensively worked out; however, only for a very few drugs has an exact dosage been identified for the elderly, and because of the multitude of factors affecting drug therapy in the elderly, the only equations that have been devised are as yet necessarily complex and laborious to use.

Geriatric dosages have been included whenever possible in the Nursing Drug Digest of each medication chapter in Sections III through XV of this text. If the nurse needs more detailed geriatric drug therapy knowledge he or she should refer to the comprehensive geriatric drug therapy reference by Pagliaro and Pagliaro in the Bibliography at the end of this chapter.

Principles of geriatric drug therapy

Nurses should be aware of the following principles in relation to geriatric drug therapy. The major factors that necessitate special considerations in geriatric drug therapy are (1) polypharmacy, (2) multiple coex-

istent disease states, and (3) the natural physiologic changes of aging. In dealing with these factors the nurse must keep the following points in mind: (1) Is drug therapy necessary?; (2) What is the therapeutic endpoint of therapy?; (3) Is the drug correct?; (4) Is the dosage correct?; (5) Is the dosage form correct?; (6) What adverse or side effects may occur?; (7) What drug interactions may occur?; (8) Is the drug correctly labeled and packaged?; (9) Who is responsible for drug administration?; (10) Is the patient compliant?; and (11) Can any of the patient's other medications be discontinued?

Because specific drug therapy regimens have not been generally developed for the elderly, each of these principles will be briefly commented on and examples that may make the rationale for the principle more apparent will be presented.

Is drug therapy required? Often, drug therapy is not the therapy of choice.* This is particularly true for the elderly, who because of the natural consequences of aging are more likely to have multiple medical conditions, each of which necessitates some form of therapy.

In this regard nurses must use their knowledge and skills to determine if an alternate therapy may be used to treat the patient's problem. Can a sedative–hypnotic drug be avoided if the patient receives increased physical activity, avoids caffeinated beverages in the evening, avoids large volumes of fluids near bedtime, or drinks a warm glass of milk at bedtime?† Another example might be that an antidepressant drug can be avoided if voluntary visiting is arranged to decrease the patient's loneliness or if the medications causing the depression (e.g., reserpine) are stopped. However, old age should not be used as a criterion to withhold rationally formulated drug therapy that may improve the quality and dignity of life for the elderly.

What is the therapeutic endpoint of therapy? Rational drug therapy should always be associated with a general goal (e.g., curing a condition, relieving symptoms, prolonging life) and a predefined endpoint that can indicate whether the goal has been (or is being) achieved. Quantitative measures (e.g., blood pressure equal to 130/90) should be established to serve as indicators of the success or failure of drug therapy. Other measures may also serve as indicators that the drug therapy should be reevaluated, or a

---

*For an interesting anecdote see Nightingale's comments on drug therapy in Chapter 1, "Pharmacologic Aspects of Nursing: A Historical Overview."

†It should be noted that milk contains the amino acid tryptophan, which may have a sedating effect on the central nervous system.

timeframe (e.g., every 6 months) may be associated with this variable. Drug therapy should *never* be prn for an indefinite period without a definite timeframe for reevaluation.

Is the drug correct? Misdiagnosis is particularly common when dealing with the elderly. Ideally, as more educational programs are designed to meet this need and as more geriatric clinicians begin practice the problem of choosing the correct drug will decrease. Commonly misdiagnosed and misprescribed conditions in the elderly involve: using a cardiac glycoside in elderly patients with dependent edema without congestive heart failure; using cardiac glycosides in elderly patients who had temporary congestive heart failure perhaps caused by anemia or a severe respiratory infection, but which resolved itself when the primary condition was treated; and using antipsychotic drugs in the elderly when their confusion is the result of other medications they are taking.

Similar types of problems commonly seen in the elderly also include prescribing a drug that is the drug of choice for the particular disease state in a younger adult, but is contraindicated in the elderly patient because of the physiologic factors noted earlier. Also to be considered is whether the disease can be treated by a different drug with fewer or less severe side effects.

Is the dosage correct? As previously noted, specific dosages have not yet been generally determined for the elderly. However, in general we know that loading doses are often not needed and that smaller than normal adult doses are usually required to prevent toxicity because of the physiologic changes (e.g., decreased renal function, decreased volume of distribution) that occur as a natural consequence of aging. Some medications (e.g., antibiotics, diuretics) may need to be administered in higher than normal doses if the desired therapeutic response is not obtained. In general, therefore, the elderly often initially require more follow-up to adjust and titrate properly the drug dosage to their individual needs.

Is the dosage form correct? Some elderly patients find liquid dosage forms easier to swallow than capsules or tablets, and changing to liquid forms may significantly increase compliance. Sometimes suppositories may be preferred. One must check that the bioavailability (see Chapter 4, "Drug Availability and Distribution") is not significantly changed by changing the dosage form, and if it does to adjust the dose accordingly.

What adverse or side effects may occur? The nurse should not only know which adverse or side effects to look for, but should also see that the patient is properly educated about adverse and side effects. This should be done so the patient will be aware of what minor effects to expect (and thus increase compliance), as well as be aware of what adverse effects should alert one to stop taking the medication and to inform the health care provider.

Orthostatic hypotension is a particularly troublesome side effect for the elderly. It may cause a fall that often leads to a fractured femur and hospitalization. Any antihypertensive drug (Chapter 33), including the thiazide diuretics, may cause this effect. The nurse should caution the patient about the problem of orthostatic hypotension and provide instruction in measures that may minimize its occurrence.

What drug interactions may occur? Because of a variety of factors, including polypharmacy and decreased albumin concentration, the elderly are at a particular risk of experiencing a drug interaction. In addition, because of their decreased functional reserve (as previously noted), the probability of the interaction having an adverse effect is significantly increased in the elderly.

It is always necessary to be aware of possible drug interactions and of their potential severity (e.g., does the interaction necessitate a change in therapy, and if so, which drug can be safely substituted?). The patient must also be carefully informed about which drugs and foods may interact with the drug and should thus be avoided (see Chapter 10, "Drug Interactions").

Is the drug correctly labeled and packaged? In addition to the usually required information (i.e., name of medication, strength, quantity, dosage, name of patient, and name of prescriber) and auxillary information (i.e., major potential side effects, activities, foods, and drugs to avoid) the elderly patient often has other special drug labeling and packaging needs. Is the print on the labels large enough for the patient to read? Does the patient read English? If not, are directions available in his or her foreign language or is a responsible family member available who reads English and can assist? Can the elderly patient open childproof containers?

Who is responsible for administering the drug? Can the patient administer his or her own medication or is he or she blind or too disabled with arthritis to administer a parenteral medication (i.e., insulin)? Can the patient follow complicated multidrug regimens or is he or she too confused or forgetful to comply? Possible solutions to this problem are having a family member administer the medications, or developing memory aids (e.g., dosing cards, calendars, or containers) to assist the patient to remember when the medications should be taken. The community or public health nurse can also assist with administering medications in the home for the elderly. Finally, patients and nurses may find it helpful to use dosing regimens or longer-acting dosage forms that need to be administered only once daily (e.g., phenothiazines), once weekly (e.g., large doses of vitamin D for osteomalacia), or once monthly (e.g., fluphenazine decanoate).

Is the patient compliant? Estimates of noncompliance in the elderly range from 20% to 80%. If nurses use the principles presented here in their practice the major reasons for noncompliance will have been effectively dealt with. In addition, nurses should ensure that the patient has been provided with both verbal and written instructions in relation to drug therapy and explain to the patient the importance of compliance. The patient should be asked to repeat the instructions in his or her own words to assess comprehension of the directions (i.e., the appropriate directions may have been correctly given, but this does not ensure that the patient understood them).

Nurses should also foster in the elderly patient, according to his or her abilities, the concept of self-care. Provided with proper education, patients should be assisted in assuming as much of the responsibility for their own self-care in relation to drug therapy as possible.

Can any of the patient's other medications be discontinued? Take advantage of the opportunity whenever evaluating a patient for new medications to reevaluate thoroughly the previous therapeutic regimen and to discontinue those medications (both prescription and nonprescription) no longer needed. Not only will this save the patient the time, money, and trouble of taking an unnecessary medication, but this may also improve the patient's quality of life by perhaps eliminating an unnecessary side effect (e.g., mental confusion), as well as decrease the presence of potential adverse drug interactions.

Whenever a medication is removed from a drug regimen the nurse should ascertain if a change in dosage of the remaining drugs is necessary. For example, if a medication that enhances drug metabolism* (e.g., phenobarbital) is discontinued, then the dosage of another drug the patient is taking (e.g., warfarin) may need to be decreased to prevent toxicity, because it will not continue to be metabolized at the same rate. This same procedure should be followed whenever any medication is added to a drug regimen. For example, if a medication that enhances drug me-

---

*See Chapter 5, "Drug Metabolism and Elimination," for examples and a discussion of drugs that stimulate metabolism.

tabolism (e.g., phenobarbital) is started, then the dosage of another drug the patient is taking (e.g., warfarin) may need to be increased to obtain the same pharmacologic effect.

SUMMARY

This chapter has focused on two special groups of patients, the very young and the very old, who have special needs and considerations in relation to drug therapy. Special mechanisms responsible for altered pharmacologic response in pediatric and geriatric groups have been summarized. The pharmacologic principles for effectively dealing with these mechanisms to optimize therapeutic drug response in these patient populations have also been presented. The nurse should keep in mind that many of the principles presented in this chapter can also be generalized to assist in developing optimal drug therapy regimens for other patient groups.

BIBLIOGRAPHY

Coleman, J.H., & Dorevitch, A.P. Rational use of psychoactive drugs in the geriatric patient. *Drug Intelligence and Clinical Pharmacy,* 1981, *15,* 940-944.

Dietsche, L.M., & Pollmann, J.N. Alzheimer's disease: advances in clinical nursing. *Journal of Gerontological Nursing,* 1982, *8,* 97-100.

Garcia, C.A., Reding, M.J., & Blass, J.P. Overdiagnosis of dementia. *Journal of the American Geriatrics Society,* 1981, *29,* 407-410.

Goldberg, R.J. Drug excretion into human milk. *Pharmacy Times,* 1982, *48,* 60-67.

Gossel, T.A., & Wuest, J.R. The right first aid for poisoning. *RN,* 1981, *44,* 73-75.

Greenblatt, D.J., Sellers, E.M., & Shader, R.I. Drug disposition in old age. *New England Journal of Medicine,* 1982, *306,* 1081-1088.

Hastreiter, A.R., Simonton, R.L., van der Horst, R.L., Benawra, R., Mangurten, H., Lam, G., & Chiou, W. Digoxin pharmacokinetics in premature infants. *Pediatric Pharmacology,* 1982, *2,* 23-31.

Hayes, M.H., Langman, M.J., & Short, A.H. Changes in drug metabolism with increasing age: warfarin binding and plasma proteins. *British Journal of Clinical Pharmacology,* 1975, *2,* 69-72.

Hayter, J. Why response to medication changes with age. *Geriatric Nursing,* 1981, *2,* 411-416.

Lamy, P.P. Special features of geriatric prescribing. *Geriatrics,* 1981, *36,* 42-52.

Lenhart, D.G. The use of medications in the elderly population. *Nursing Clinics of North America,* 1976, *11,* 135-143.

Lerner, R. Sleep loss in the aged: implications for nursing practice. *Journal of Gerontological Nursing,* 1982, *8,* 323-326.

Lovejoy, F.H., & Berenberg, W. Poisoning in children under age 5. *Postgraduate Medicine,* 1978, *63,* 79-89.

Mullen, E.M., & Granholm, M. Drugs and the elderly patient. *Journal of Gerontological Nursing,* 1981, *7,* 108-113.

Pagliaro, L.A., & Levin, R.H. (Eds.). *Problems in pediatric drug therapy.* Hamilton, Ill.: Drug Intelligence Publications, 1979.

Pagliaro, L.A., & Pagliaro, A.M. (Eds.). *Pharmacologic aspects of aging.* St. Louis: The C.V. Mosby Co., 1983.

Pagliaro, L.A., and Pagliaro, A.M. (Eds.). *Problems in pediatric drug therapy* (2nd ed.). Hamilton, Ill.: Drug Intelligence Publications (in press).

Playfer, J.R., Baty, J.D., Lamb, J., Powell, C., & Price-Evans, D.A. Age related differences in the disposition of acetanilide. *British Journal of Clinical Pharmacology,* 1978, *6,* 529-533.

Ritschel, W.A. Pharmacokinetics approach to drug dosing in the aged. *Journal of the American Geritatrics Society,* 1976, *24,* 344-354.

Sloan, R.W. How to minimize side effects of psychoactive drugs. *Geriatrics,* 1982, *37,* 51-64.

Steinberg, S. Drug therapy in the elderly—problems and recommendations. *On Continuing Practice,* 1981, *8,* 15-19.

CHAPTER 8

Psychologic Factors in Drug Response

George C. Stone
Shirley C. Peeke

Psychologic factors are important in pharmacotherapeutics in several distinct but overlapping ways. Every individual's behavior with respect to drugs and even the physiologic response to drug therapy can be modified by the individual's unique experiences, beliefs, understandings, and feelings present when the therapeutic regimen is prescribed. These factors influence (1) the schedule on which the drugs are taken, (2) the psychophysiologic state that will prevail in the body, and (3) the psychologic reactions to the effects the drugs will produce in the body.

To enhance the nurse's understanding of the complexity of the psychologic factors that influence the individual patient's unique response to drug therapy, the following four areas will be discussed: (1) somatopsychic effects of drugs, (2) expectation and other nonspecific factors, (3) personality factors, and (4) communication.

SOMATOPSYCHIC EFFECTS OF DRUGS

Somatopsychic effects of drugs include the changes in psychologic functioning that result from the administration of drugs. There are many different kinds of psychologic side effects of drugs, ranging from alterations of sensory and motor capacities and alterations of mood to hallucinations or paranoid psychoses.

Drugs that have been studied with the aid of many behavioral and psychologic tests are mostly those that are prescribed with the intent to change such functions (e.g., the psychotropic drugs;* such as the stimulants, sedative-hypnotics, antidepressants, and antipsychotics) and drugs that are self-administered for recreational purposes (e.g., alcohol, barbiturates, caffeine, cannabis, and nicotine). Psychologic effects of other kinds of drugs or drug combinations are usually noticed only when they are very marked, and they are then usually described with such imprecise terms as "confusion," "memory disturbances," or "fatigue." We will provide a sampling of some of the more specific available information, but before doing so we want to point out a secondary kind of psychologic effect that can occur, the reaction to a primary drug effect based on the individual's interpretation of that effect.

A drug such as chlorpromazine or methyldopa that may reduce sexual potency can have a very profound effect on a young, sexually active male who is unaware of the source of his difficulties, but may have no psychologic effect at all on another person with different sexual behavior patterns and concerns. Similarly, a person who is already concerned with possible losses of mental capacity because of advancing age may be very much disturbed by a drug that impairs memory or sensory capacity, whereas a younger person might pay little or no attention to the same effect.

Thus, there are two levels at which drugs can create psychologic effects: (1) primary psychologic effects that actually change the functioning of the nervous system and other physiologic systems that directly influence behavior and experience, and (2) secondary psychologic effects that may through *any* detectable or perceived change in bodily function give rise to behavior mediated by the meaning attributed to the change noted.

Primary psychologic effects

Primary psychologic effects may give rise to misinterpretations by the nurse, who may attribute the effects to the personality characteristics or mental limitations of patients. To avoid such distortions, it is important to know about the kinds of primary psychologic effects drugs can produce. Identifying and describing such effects has not progressed very far as yet. It is probably appropriate to consider the possibility that any kind of unusual behavior on the part of

---

*See Section III, "Central Nervous System Medications," for the detailed pharmacology of these agents.

a patient who is taking a drug may be influenced to some degree by the action of the drug.

Idiosyncrasies of individual metabolism and complexities of interactions between drugs and the circumstances under which they are taken support this idea. For example, increasingly convincing evidence exists that some children whose activity level is high enough and whose capacity to attend to a particular activity is low enough to produce marked disturbances around them (e.g., some of the so-called hyperactive children) may be stimulated to this socially unaccepted behavior by a kind of allergic response to dyes or other chemical substances added to foods. An example of the influence of circumstances on response to drugs is found in the interaction between the overall arousal level of the individual (i.e., the tonic state of the ascending reticular activating system and associated parts of the nervous system) and the individual's susceptibility to depressant drugs.

Secondary psychologic effects

Secondary psychologic effects can be as various and as complex as are people themselves. They can greatly increase the difficulty of working with patients, but they can usually be greatly reduced if patients are encouraged to express their concerns explicitly and if those concerns are then included in the total set of problems that need to be handled in planning treatment or nursing care. Sometimes, simply explaining that a particular side effect is common and reversible will suffice. Other times, it may be appropriate to consider whether some different treatment ought to be selected for a particular patient. In providing reassurance about some side effect, the nurse will want to keep in mind the most unfortunate examples of side effects that were once thought to be reversible, but which turned out not to be, such as the tardive dyskinesias associated with the use of antipsychotic medications (see Chapter 18, "Drugs Used to Treat Psychotic Disorders").

The secondary psychologic effects of drugs are based on interpretations made by patients, and can often be treated by nurses' skillful communication.

With these general principles introduced, we turn to examples of some of the kinds of direct impact on the psychologic functioning of patients that drugs have been found to produce. Our review is organized in terms of the complexity of the observed behavior to change as a result of the drug's action, starting with the simplest input and output functions and progressing to the most complex verbal interpretations of inner experience.

Sensorimotor capacities

We begin with sensorimotor capacities because our information about what an organism, human or otherwise, can do with information and what it is experiencing is derived almost entirely from the movements we observe, or from their consequences (e.g., speech production). Skilled and complex movements require the integrity of large parts of the nervous system, and sensitive tests for impairments of central nervous system (CNS) functions by depressants and other drugs have been based on measures of such movements. The time that a rat or mouse can remain balanced on a rotating rod, how long it takes a rat to climb a short piece of vertically suspended rope, and the percentage of time that a human can keep a stylus in contact with a moving target (i.e., pursuit rotor test) or walk a straight line are examples of this kind of test. Slurred speech is a common indicator of CNS impairment that is readily detected, although not easily quantified.

Fortunately for our purposes of assessing other psychologic functions, it is possible to arrange for the output of a variety of tasks to be coded so that reliance on the ability to perform the motor function can be reduced to a minimum in the measurement of those other functions. We can train an animal or instruct a human to close a simple switch when and only when certain conditions prevail, and thereby assess the capacity to appraise conditions. This very simple response provides us with the ability to measure thresholds for stimuli, recognize differences between stimuli, recognize subtly displayed emotional states, and discover analogic relationships that tap some of the highest intellectual functions. Of course, we are usually interested in behavioral toxicities much less pronounced than those that would seriously disrupt speech, so we can also investigate processes of memory storage and retrieval, mood state, and social judgment by asking people questions to which they respond verbally.

Sensory capacities are impaired by CNS depressants such as the barbiturates. A careful analysis of this effect, using a sophisticated experimental procedure that can isolate different components of the process, permitted Rundele, Williams, and Boyd (1978) to determine that secobarbital affects primarily the intake of information in a visual stimulus, whereas alcohol, in the same task, affects the selection of one response from among a small set, but not the preprocessing of the stimulus. Other investigators, using measures of the electric responses of the brain, have been able to show that alcohol slows the processing of the auditory pathway from the midbrain to the thalamus.

The effects of drugs on sensory systems are determined in considerable part by the neurochemistry of those systems. The retina apparently uses dopamine as its primary neurotransmitter, and therefore such dopamine antagonists as the antipsychotic drugs may affect retinal function. The pattern of electric activity of the retina has been demonstrated to be slowed down by administering one such drug, thioridazine. This observation might possibly be related to an earlier report that chlorpromazine, another drug with dopamine-blocking actions, slowed the disappearance of the very brief (about one half second), imaged memory for a visual stimulus, whereas neither scopolamine, an anticholinergic, nor pentobarbital, a sedative–hypnotic, had such an effect.

Increased sensitivity to stimuli has been reported following the administration of the opiate antagonist naloxone. The most likely way for this kind of effect to show itself is as hyperalgesia (i.e., excessive sensitivity to pain). The difficulty of making unambiguous statements about these effects is highlighted by a report that, in a group of normal young adults, those who initially had low sensitivity to pain showed an increased pain response to a test stimulus after receiving naloxone, whereas those who were initially pain sensitive showed reduced pain.

Most studies of the effects of drugs on sensorimotor performance have not attempted to isolate the particular aspect of the task that is the source of the difficulty. However, by collecting many well-controlled studies of nonpatients performing psychomotor tasks that make differential demands on input and output functions, Wittenborn (1978) was able to discern some general patterns. Hypnotic and depressant drugs led to significant impairment in over one half of the comparisons with the placebo condition, with the most pronounced effects occurring in the tasks that required more complex processing of information (e.g., card sorting, digit-symbol substitution).

Drugs prescribed primarily for anxiety, such as diazepam, were not so often studied with these tasks, but when studied they uniformly showed impairment. These anxiolytics also produced impairment of eye-hand coordination with greater frequency than did the barbiturate sedative–hypnotics, but were less likely to impair tapping speed, a more purely motor output task. Altogether, the anxiolytics produced significant improvement of performance in 4 of 49 tasks (8%).

Antipsychotic drugs, stimulants, and antidepressants were studied much less frequently, so that trends among tasks could not be assessed. These classes of drugs rarely produced impairment of psychomotor function; the antipsychotics produced impairment in only 2 of 13 comparisons, and the antidepressants in only 2 of 8. Stimulants led to significant impairment in only 1 of 13 studied (eye-hand coordination) and significant improvement in 6 of the 13.

Effects on processes of attention. Our sensory receptors are constantly bombarded by far more information than our brains can possibly cope with. Out of this enormous flow of information, we select what our previous experience has shown to be most likely to be important for our survival and adaptation to environmental circumstances. The processes by which this selection is accomplished are collectively known as the mechanisms of selective attention (Figure 8-1).

Like most other psychologic processes, attention is complex and by no means completely understood. We can organize much of what is known about one aspect of attention with the aid of a simple metaphor. Imagine oneself in a dark place with a search light that has a limited capacity to illuminate. To see what is around one, one can adjust the beam so it is very broad, and casts a dim light on much of the space around one, or one can narrow it to play a bright light on a small region. A substantially separate set of mechanisms allows us to predetermine certain kinds of signals that we want to be sure to detect if they occur, and to sensitize them so that even a dim light will let us recognize them. Most of what we know about the effects of drugs on attention is related to the first of these mechanisms. Generally speaking, depressants impair the capacity of the beam to be narrowed; amphetamine-like drugs keep it narrowed even when it might be advantageous to have a broader beam. Our capacity to keep the beam fixed on a particular part of the world is often labeled concentration in everyday language.

There appears to be some correlation between how often the fixation is changed and how narrow the beam is, but the relationship is not simple. At moderate doses, drugs that focus attention may produce rapid shifting, hence a kind of distractability. At high doses, however, the effect is sometimes a pathologic fixation that appears obsessive. In animal studies, this effect often takes the form of ceaseless repetition of some very stereotyped behavior, which may even lead to serious tissue damage from stereotyped licking or biting. Inability to focus attention may be interpreted by the health care provider as disorientation or confusion. These signs are often interpreted as having serious importance, but could be no more than a reflection of a hyperstimulation.

Effects on storage and retrieval of information. The processes of learning and the storage and retrieval

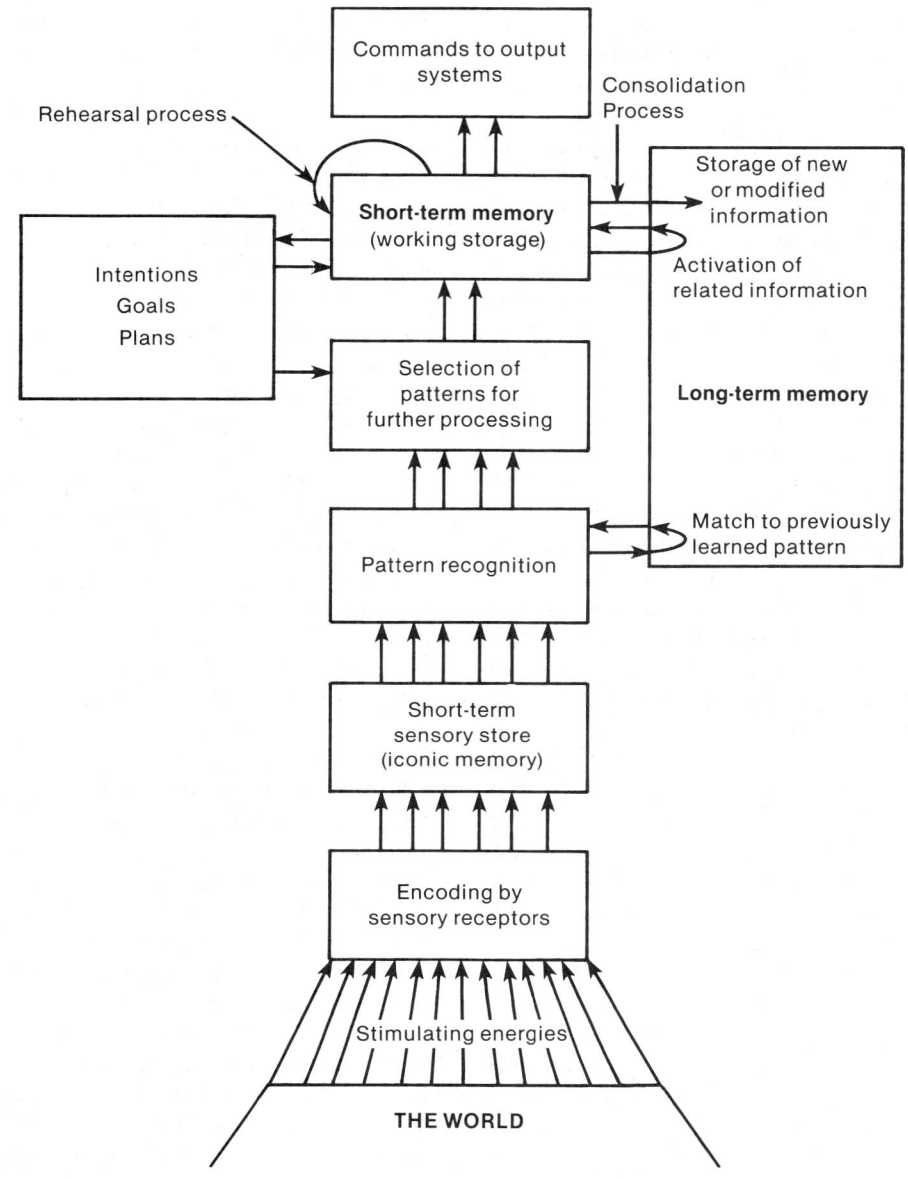

FIGURE 8-1. **Current conceptions of the relationships among sensorimotor input–output systems and the brain's information-processing systems.**

of information are not well understood. It is exceedingly difficult to separate the influences of the underlying physiologic process of information use from the motivating factors that regulate using such processes. In humans, at least, the picture is further complicated by the more or less conscious use of such deliberate strategies as rehearsal, imaging, and memory search, which can profoundly affect the level of performance. Thus, if we observe a drug effect, it will be very difficult to know how it is produced. Furthermore, we can expect that any drug that affects mood, arousal, motivation, attention, or body sensations will be capable of altering the way in which a person handles information or learns.

According to current conceptions, human memory is based on distinctively different processes for storing information and for retrieving information that has been previously stored. Furthermore, in addition to the very brief sensory memory referred to previously, there appear to be at least two different types of memory, usually referred to as short-term memory (STM) and long-term memory (LTM). STM is limited in the number of items it can retain, and depends on continued attention to those items. It is the process used when one looks up a telephone number and then remembers it long enough to dial. LTM appears to be virtually unlimited in the amount of information that can be retained, and requires no attention for maintenance of the information once it has been stored. Activating a memory stored in LTM so that it can influence current behavior occurs as a result of a certain degree of correspondence between present circumstances and those that prevailed when the memory was stored.

The process of entering information into LTM takes minutes to hours. This process, called consolidation, is enhanced by many CNS stimulants (e.g., amphetamines, strychnine, picrotoxin) and retarded by depressants (e.g., barbiturates). Cholinergic drugs also improve storage and retrieval in LTM, and do not affect STM. Drug effects on STM appear to occur mostly through modifying the attention mechanisms. There are also indications that the mechanism of STM may relate to the sodium pump. The pharmacologic implications of this possibility have yet to be tested. Tetrahydrocannabinol (THC), the most active principle in marijuana, appears to be particularly disruptive of the storage of new information into LTM from STM.

People learn to remember by creating enriched stimuli in STM so that the item to be stored in LTM has more associated cues that can be used later for retrieval. One kind of enrichment is the result of visualizing some image involving the stimuli, especially meaningless stimuli such as lists of words. Another is achieved by sorting the words to be remembered into meaningful categories so that remembering one word in a category provides cues for others. These active processes of memorizing require effort. The impairment of the learning process by alcohol and other CNS depressants is probably in part the result of the person's inability or disinclination to put forth the necessary effort.

Many, perhaps most, drugs give rise to body sensations (e.g., taste, changes in heart rate, changes in skin temperature) that can be detected by the person who has taken the drug. Even though people rarely separate the effect of one of their drugs from all the other sensations associated with their illness, one particular effect can still become part of the complex of cues associated with memories established during the time when the drug was active in the body.

Then, when retrieval of the information would be useful (as in remembering instructions), if the drug cues are not present, it may be harder for the person to recall. This phenomenon, known as state dependent learning, is associated not just with cues produced by drugs, but by any kind of internal stimuli, such as those produced by emotional states or by sensations produced by disease processes. It can give rise to apparent fluctuations in memory, so that a patient may remember things at some times and not at others. All of us are subject to this phenomenon all of the time, but it may be more pronounced in patients whose internal states are subject to wide variations from time to time.

Effects on mood. The term *mood* refers to a kind of bias toward remaining in or returning to a particular emotional state. Psychologists have been able to isolate at least six relatively pure emotions: fear, anger, sorrow, disgust, surprise, and happiness (actual emotions are often blends of these). Corresponding to four of these emotions, mood states can be recognized: (1) anxiety, although complex, is related to fear; (2) irritability is the disposition to anger; (3) depression is also complex, but related to sorrow; and (4) euphoria is the name most frequently used for the disposition to be happy. In our culture, at least, there are not well-recognized moods associated with surprise or disgust.

For many years, the pharmacology of moods was largely that of the monoamines of the CNS (e.g., epinephrine, norepinephrine, dopamine, and serotonin). Substantial evidence exists that norepinephrine can produce irritability and anger, and epinephrine is associated with fear. Insufficiency of serotonin and dopamine seems to be more involved with the state of depression, although norepinephrine may also play a role. All three of the monoamines widely found in the brain (epinephrine is not) seem to have an energizing effect on behavior, so that in excess they produce states that are described as elevated mood, progressing to euphoria and mania. When they are insufficient, the result is depression.

More recently, the brain peptides, including the enkephalins and vasopressin, are being studied for their possible direct effect on mood. In particular, the enkephalins that have been called endorphins, because of the similarity of their actions to those of morphine and the opiates, appear to be involved in the mediation of pleasure and the resistance to pain. The well-known euphoriant effect of the opiates may be caused by their mimicking these endogenous substances. The morphine antagonist naloxone also antagonizes the endorphins, and is thus a powerful tool for exploring their pharmacology.

Moods are always present, even though we name them usually only in their more extreme forms. They are central states that integrate the influences of all of the nervous and hormonal systems on the emotional substrate. Thus, fluctuations of moods are likely to be one of the most noticeable results of both the primary and secondary effects of drugs. The host of feedback links within the neuroendocrine systems and the impact of cognitive appraisal on emotional responses create a situation in which any drug can influence mood, but very few drugs will affect them consistently and predictably.

Effects on intellectual function. In our society, we usually think of the processes of judgment, decision making, analysis, and the creative synthesis of ideas as the highest functions of the brain. They depend critically on the integrity of the cerebral cortex for their performance, but they also depend on the subcortical systems to provide the information, the attentional states, and the output systems as the context for these intellectual functions (Figure 8-2).

Perhaps because of the complexity of the various aspects of intellectual function, much less attention has been paid to them by psychopharmacologists than to the simpler forms of behavior. Few comprehensive reviews exist of the work that has been done on those

effects of drugs. In general, it has not been possible to demonstrate conclusively the long-term effects of even those drugs that have been suspected of altering mental function, with the notable exception of the memory deficit found in the Wernicke-Korsakoff syndrome, which is associated with chronic, severe alcoholism. LSD, for example, in spite of its dramatic hallucinatory effects, has not been shown to lead to the systematic impairment of intellectual function. Methodologic difficulties in such research are, however, severe (e.g., how can one tell whether any disturbed judgment that might be found in a long-time user of a drug is the result or the cause of the drug abuse?).

Drugs that impair the simpler functions will, on acute administration, usually have an even greater effect on the more complex functions. However, this is not always the case, as they may reduce patients' anxiety and thereby permit an improvement in performance under some conditions.

When the psychedelic drugs first became the subject of laboratory studies there were many anecdotal reports of their capacity to enhance creativity. Marijuana for many years enjoyed a reputation for enhancing the performance of jazz musicians. However,

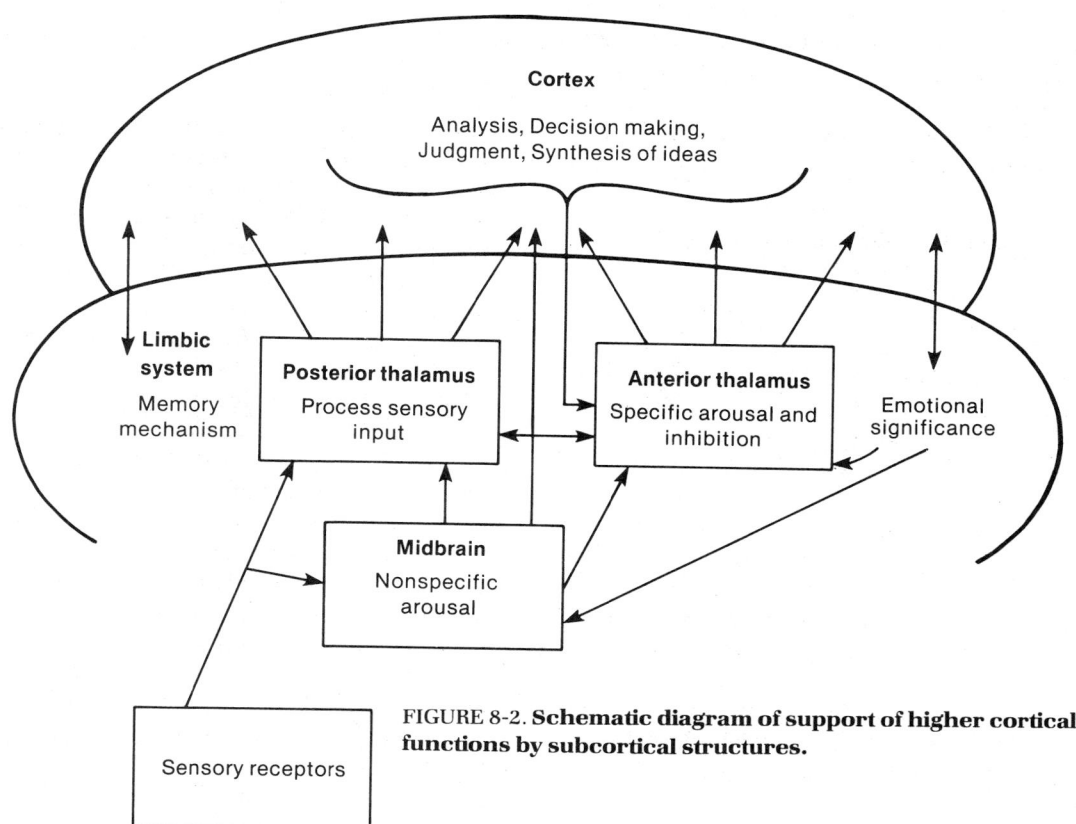

FIGURE 8-2. **Schematic diagram of support of higher cortical functions by subcortical structures.**

careful studies that have attempted to document such enhancement have usually found impairment instead. Weckowicz, Fedora, Mason, Radstack, Bay, and Yonge (1975) found some indication of greater word fluency and higher divergent production scores at low doses of marijuana but impairment at high doses. Some question remains whether the conditions of the tests were sufficiently similar to those in which the enhanced performances were observed, because many of the effects of the recreational drugs are very susceptible to social influences.

It is fitting to conclude this section on the effects of drugs on psychologic measures with the warning that many of the generalizations we have offered may before long be qualified by the demonstration of differences among different subject groups and in different circumstances. We have already mentioned the differing effects of naloxone in patients according to their sensitivity to pain in the absence of the drug. As another example we can cite a study by Jones and Jones (1976), which showed that females reach a higher blood level of alcohol than do males, when given the same dose per kilogram of body weight, that this difference is enhanced in the premenstrual period, and that the resulting cognitive deficit is greater in the afternoon than in the morning. As future research further clarifies the influence of internal hormonal effects, and as more and more of the body's endogenous chemicals are found to have psychologic effects, we can expect first to observe and then to understand many such complex patterns.

EXPECTATION AND OTHER NONSPECIFIC FACTORS

Until recent years little attention has been paid to the role of set and expectation in the patient's response to a drug. The term "nonspecific drug factors" is often used to refer to all nonpharmacologic factors that can influence reactions to drugs. The importance of these nonspecific factors is becoming more apparent as more research is directed toward their investigation. In addition to attitude and expectations of the patient, other nonspecific factors include variables of age, race, sex, duration and severity of present symptoms, history of previous occurrence of the illness (including prior hospitalizations and prior medications), and the success of previous treatments. Equally important are the attitudes and the expectations of the health care providers regarding treatment, and the characteristics of the setting in which the treatment is carried out.

Placebo effect

One of the most pervasive examples of nonspecific drug factors is the placebo response, an effect that functions primarily through psychologic mechanisms. The placebo effect is any effect of a medical intervention that cannot be attributed to the specific action of a drug or treatment. The definition can include not only drug effects but also any kind of medical or therapeutic intervention including hospitalization, psychotherapy, and rehabilitative treatments.

Placebo effects have a negative connotation. In research, placebo effects are viewed as artifacts and tend to be controlled or ignored rather than studied directly. This is true even though until relatively recently almost all medications prescribed were largely ineffective and the majority of improvement in patients' conditions was the result of a placebo effect. Today there is a trend toward using research designs that attempt to differentiate specific drug effects from placebo effects and recognizing that all treatments consist of a combination of the two.

To the extent that all drug treatment consists of a combination of specific drug effects and placebo effects, much can be learned about the role of expectation through the study of placebos. A placebo may be an inert substance or a pharmacologically active substance for which there is no known basis for the drug's effectiveness in the particular illness being treated. Although a placebo effect is attributed to suggestion or expectation, it may still show such characteristics as a time-effect curve, cumulative effects, tolerance, and side effects. Placebos have been shown to be addictive, to mimic the effects of active drugs, to reverse the action of potent drugs, and to have direct effects on body organs and on organic illnesses.

Negative placebo effects have also been reported. These consist of side effects and a worsening of symptoms. Side effects may be similar to those that would be found with the active medication or may be the symptoms of the original disease. They may represent heightened sensitivity to body sensations or may signify unfulfilled expectations about the drug. Although objective changes such as dermatitis and changes in gastric mucosa have been attributed to placebo use, most side effects are related to changes in mood and emotion. Negative placebo effects are more often reported by clinic patients than by private patients.

The efficacy of a placebo is influenced by color, taste (i.e., bitter or highly flavored pills are more effective), size (i.e., large pills are more effective), and whether administration is oral or by injection (i.e., injections are more effective). An element of mysticism and a certain amount of discomfort contribute to placebo efficacy.

Patient variables. The question of the extent of effectiveness of placebos has often been raised. The number of persons showing a placebo effect may range from 0% to 100% depending on the population being tested, nature of the illness, type of treatment, and whether the setting is an experimental test or a clinical application. Beecher (1969) reviewed 15 experiments in which placebos were used in the clinical study of pain. The placebo was reported to relieve pain satisfactorily in 35% of the patients. However, the placebo response is quite unreliable. A patient showing a placebo response on one occasion may not respond on another occasion or to a different drug. Lasagna, et al (1954) reported that fewer than 50% of the patients who received more than a single treatment with placebos responded consistently. Thus, no data exist to support the idea that certain individuals are consistent placebo responders.

Sex, age, education, IQ, race, and social class have not shown any systematic relation to placebo effects. However, certain personality traits may predispose some persons to react to placebos. McNair et al. (1968) divided patients into acquiescers (i.e., those who tend to agree uncritically with authoritatively stated generalizations or clichés) and nonacquiescers. Patients were treated with diazepam or a placebo for 2 weeks. Nonacquiescers showed substantially greater symptom reduction on the active drug than on the placebo; acquiescers showed marked improvement on the placebo that equaled or exceeded the improvement on the active drug. There was some evidence that acquiescers were nondiscriminating in assessing their symptoms and more unreliable in their verbal reports. They also may have responded adversely to the somatic cues of the active drug. Shapiro and Morris (1978) report on a number of other studies and reach the conclusion that a weak relationship exists between placebo reaction and suggestibility, acquiesence, and compliance.

Prescriber and staff variables. The attitude of the prescriber or treatment staff members is very important in influencing the response to a drug treatment. When the attitude toward the patient is one of friendly personal interest, warmth, and sympathy, the response to the drug will be more favorable than when the attitude consists of lack of interest or rejection. The attitude of treatment staff members to the particular drug is also influential.

A study by Wheatley (1968) in which prescribers' attitudes were classified as optimistic, indifferent, or pessimistic with respect to the expected outcome of treatment of anxiety by chlordiazepoxide and amobarbital showed that the greatest improvement in anxiety symptoms was obtained with optimistic prescribers, less improvement with indifferent prescribers, and the least improvement with pessimistic prescribers. However, in treating neurotic depression by imipramine and phenobarbital, prescribers' attitudes had no differential effect on symptom reduction.

Usually, in the absence of specific information to the contrary, one can assume that attitudes of belief, enthusiasm, conviction, and optimism result in a more effective response than do skepticism, disbelief, and pessimism; although there is a danger of a clinician overselling a treatment and raising patient expectations unrealistically high.

Social and situational variables. Social and situational variables also affect responses to a drug or a placebo. A harmonious, supportive therapeutic milieu has a positive influence on placebo effectiveness to the extent that in one study when patients were informed they were being given sugar pills, they continued to improve in spite of the disclosure. A connection between social setting and pharmacologic action can occur through an effect of social setting on physiologic processes, as well as on perceptions of body sensations such as pain (e.g., endocrine levels are related to social status variables such as dominance).

Barchas and Barchas (1977) describe a study in which endocrine levels of subjects were altered by changes in their social status in a group setting. A change in base level complicates the interpretation of subsequent drug effects. Another example of the contribution of social setting to the effectiveness of pharmacologic agents is a study by Schacter and Singer (1962). They gave subjects Adrenalin or a placebo under varying conditions of information about the drug. Those who received Adrenalin with no information used social cues provided by the experimental setting to give meaning to their aroused condition. Others have also reported that normal responses to active drugs were not found when patients were not told the nature of the drug they were administered.

Other examples of social influence on drug response are the opinions and reactions of relatives, friends, and other patients; the influence of group pressure to comply with treatment; the impact of stress and life events; the cost of treatment; the clinician's reputation; and the use of aids such as written directions and information sheets.

Possible mechanisms of placebo effects. The mechanism by which placebos exert their influence has not been established. Among the mechanisms that have been proposed are social influence and expectance. Suggestibility is the type of social influence most often cited, and attempts have been made to relate susceptibility to hypnotic suggestion with the placebo response. The research indicates that whereas tests of suggestibility successfully predict hypnotic responders, they fail to predict placebo responders. Other types of social influence that might underlie placebo effects are persuasion (the power of the clinician's arguments in favor of the treatment), transference (the patient's feelings of love and trust or hatred and distrust stemming from past relationships are transferred to the patient-clinician relationship and influence the drug response), and role demands (the positive drug response is thought to reflect the patient's attempt to be a good patient).

Many types of expectancy mechanisms have been used to account for placebo effects. One type is the health care team's expectations and the patient's preconceived ideas derived from prior experience with the drug or information about it. Another mechanism is classical conditioning (exemplified by Pavlov's studies in which dogs who had received many pairings of a bell ringing and meat powder came to salivate when the bell alone rang). Via this mechanism, the patient who has previously experienced physical reactions to a drug may have the same reactions when about to receive the drug again or when given a placebo.

Another sign of a classically conditioned drug response is when the physiologic reaction to the drug occurs more quickly than it should if it were induced only by the pharmacologic mechanism of the drug (e.g., when headache relief is obtained immediately after taking an aspirin tablet). Another expectancy mechanism is cognitive dissonance, which refers to the tendency of people to resolve conflicting reactions by modifying the reaction that offers the least resistance to change. If the expectation of a drug's effect and the physiologic reaction to that drug are in conflict, and if the expectation is very strongly held, it may be the physiologic reaction to the drug that yields in order to comply with expectations.

Another possible explanation of placebo effects has to do with the manner in which the effectiveness of a drug is evaluated and the objectivity of the evaluation. If the evaluator is biased in favor of the drug, then a change in the patient's condition may be attributed to the drug when it is actually caused by some other factor. There is also the issue of response artifact, (i.e., the persistent tendency of a person to respond similarly in a variety of situations). A given patient might be predisposed to give the benefit of the doubt to any

treatment or to do the opposite. Most patients are also uncomfortable with any change in the body state that cannot be explained or labeled. A patient's label for an ambiguous body state might be determined by having just received a drug treatment. Thus, many symptoms may be attributed to the drug that are not related but are conveniently explained by it.

It is apparent that placebo effects are an important and neglected aspect of the total response to a drug. However, there is a tendency for the placebo effect to be a kind of wastebasket concept, a convenient label for any unexplained drug effect. Such an attitude impedes the effort to separate specific from nonspecific drug effects. Fisher (1970) cautions against overusing the concept of the placebo effect when a drug's efficacy cannot be explained. What is considered a placebo effect may, in some cases, actually be a conventional pharmacologic effect that is overlooked because of incomplete understanding of the drug or because of a lack of knowledge regarding the interaction of the drug and the CNS.

Fisher discusses two conceptual models for determining the respective contributions of pharmacologic and nonspecific factors in responses to a drug: the additive model and the interactional model. In the additive model, the effects of a placebo can be directly subtracted from the effects of the active drug to yield an estimate of drug effect uninfluenced by the placebo. In the interactional model the two effects are not additive but vary in their respective contribution to the total reaction as a function of other variables. The interactional model seems to be applicable in most studies of human subjects. Fisher has derived some general principles regarding the relative importance of drug and nonspecific factors in any given situation. Among them is the principle that the more the cortical processes such as awareness, consciousness, and feelings are involved, the greater the role of nonspecific factors will be. Also, the more potent the drug is, the less sensitive it will be to nonspecific factors. Fisher suggests that a maximal drug response can be obtained by administering it in the presence of the most favorable placebogenic factors.

The discovery of the endorphins, mentioned earlier, poses new problems for our understanding of placebo effects. Are these substances the principal physiologic mediators of all of the social and psychologic effects that have been discussed in this section, or are there other mechanisms as yet unknown? Dissociation between the effects on the experimental pain of acupuncture, which is blocked by naloxone, and hypnotism, which is not, suggest that more than one mechanism may be involved.

PERSONALITY FACTORS IN DRUG RESPONSE

The personality factors and individual reactions that tend to complicate responses to drug treatments are also present in all medical and nursing procedures. These personality factors determine the patient's reaction to the stress of illness, vulnerability to pain, the presence of a psychosomatic component in the illness, and the meaning of the illness in terms of secondary gain (i.e., the benefits of being ill). These reactions will help to determine the patient's compliance with the drug regimen and the total effectiveness of the drug in treating the illness. These personality factors create special problems for the health care providers. Thus, the ability to predict and anticipate these adverse or complicating responses permits more effective treatment and may prevent staff members' frustration.

The process of illness or hospitalization is highly stressful for all patients. It strains the coping abilities of the well-adjusted, as well as the neurotic, patient in terms of the threat to independence and self-sufficiency, the requirement for trust in strangers, and fears of loss of competency, love, and respect. The patient invariably responds to the stress of illness with loss of self-esteem plus varying degrees of depression, anxiety, shame, guilt, and feelings of helplessness, and may cope through using inappropriate or unrealistic mechanisms.

Patients differ greatly in their vulnerability to the stress of illness. Certain personality types experience particular problems. Ruesch and Bowman (1953) studied cases in which recovery from illness was slower than expected given the nature of the illness. They found that one personality constellation tended to have greater susceptibility to disease and accident, to have a poorer chance for recovery, and a slower convalescence. These were patients who had excessive needs for dependence, who persistently tried to obtain affection and approval by subordinating themselves, by accepting excessive responsibilities, or by striving for unusual achievements. They tended to show a lack of adaptive behavior and to have unsatisfactory techniques for meeting social changes, so that in times of stress their ability to cope effectively broke down.

Hypochondriasis. Another personality type that creates special problems for nurses is the patient for whom the illness itself fills a need or is a means of coping with life's conflicts. The hypochondriac patient is dominated by a preoccupation with body functions and has an unshakeable belief that a physical illness is present. The somatic complaints are vague and shifting and tend to be exaggerated in relation to physical findings.

Symptoms are not relieved by traditional medical treatment and there is usually a long history of unsuccessful medical treatments for a variety of symptoms. The onset of symptoms is often related to a loss in the patient's life. It is important to recognize that the hypochondriac patient is not consciously trying to deceive anyone. The patient may be a dependent, clinging person who is unable to meet life's challenges. The dependency, and the anger associated with it, get expressed through the hypochondriasis. For some patients, the sickness may be a form of self-sacrifice through which the patient maintains equilibrium as a person whose life is based on self-sacrifice. This patient has a low sense of self-esteem and a sense of hopelessness with few relationships or interests outside of the hospital or clinic. The patient's belief in the illness protects and enhances self-esteem and the illness thus becomes necessary to keep coping defenses intact.

Treatment or management of the hypochondriac patient is particularly frustrating for the health care staff, and their emotional reserves can become quickly exhausted by this patient. The patient makes persistent demands for care, but the symptoms do not respond to treatment. If these demands are dismissed as being psychologically based, the patient becomes more hostile. If referred to a psychiatrist, the hypochondriac patient rarely will follow through with the appointment.

Altman (1975) has suggested that the appropriate attitude is to be supportive and sustaining rather than to insist on insight or reason with the patient to induce the surrender of symptoms. Reassurance that nothing is wrong will not work nor will making a positive diagnosis followed by treatment. Altman suggests that the staff members listen to the patient's symptoms without challenging them or making a diagnosis; if a diagnosis is given it should imply a chronic but benign disease is present. The patient will react poorly to drug treatment unless allowed to help in deciding which drug to use, but probably no improvement will occur in the patient's condition. Treatment sessions should be short, with a brief physical examination. The health care professionals' role should be fairly passive, with sympathetic listening as the primary function. An increased demand for treatment probably indicates that something negative has happened in the patient's life. It should be noted that many patients are temporary hypochondriacs and develop symptoms of this type only occasionally and when under stress or when suffering a severe loss.

Obviously, neurotic personality disorders such as hypochondriasis create problems in drug treatment, but personality differences in nonneurotic patients also result in diverse reactions to drugs. Klerman, DiMascio, Greenblatt, and Rinkel (1959) have identified two clusters of personality characteristics that react in opposite ways to certain drugs. One type, labeled "intellectually-oriented" and characterized by a passive relationship to the environment and aesthetic interests, reacted in the expected way to drugs with sedative effects (i.e., secobarbital and chlorpromazine). They became more calm, experienced no negative feelings, showed an increase in rapport, and improved on tests of intellectual functioning after receiving these drugs. The other type, labeled "athletically-oriented" and characterized by extraversion, high ego strength, a high level of psychomotor activity, and an acting-out relationship with the environment, reacted in a paradoxic way to the sedatives. They expressed irritability, apprehension, increased anger, became more agitated, and showed thought confusion and impaired learning. It may be that the motor-inhibiting characteristic of the sedatives was ego threatening to the athletic-type patients because of a disruption of their basic pattern of personality organization.

Paradoxic reactions to benzodiazepines and antidepressants have also been reported for nonneurotic subjects. When subjects whose scores on an anxiety scale indicated they were very low in anxiety were given diazepam and chlordiazepoxide, they reported an increase rather than a decrease in anxiety. Subjects who had an unusually low score for depressive traits on a personality inventory reacted paradoxically to imipramine by reporting increased depression. An explanation of these effects is not readily available, but a differential degree of side effects was ruled out as an explanation.

Another way in which personality may be related to illness is through psychosomatic disease. In psychosomatic disease, psychologic factors play a necessary role in the predisposition and onset of the disease. One prominent idea has been that specific personality factors are associated with particular illnesses.

Writing from a psychoanalytic point of view, Alexander (1950) suggested that it was not specific personality factors but rather specific underlying, unresolved neurotic conflicts that were associated with specific illnesses. He also emphasized that some constitutional organ vulnerability was also necessary. According to Alexander's formulations, peptic ulcer was found in patients who were in severe conflict between their strivings for oral dependency and their ego ideal of independence. These frustrated oral strivings were discharged through autonomic pathways to the stomach with excessive acid secretion and eventual ulceration. Similar formulations were made for ulcerative colitis, rheumatoid arthritis, bronchial asthma, essential hypertension, Graves' disease, and neurodermatitis.

Although much effort has gone into attempts to demonstrate scientifically that a neurotic conflict can result in disease, so far the control problems have been insurmountable and there is little convincing evidence for this view. For example, some diseases are slow and insidious in their onset but can themselves shape personality development. The attempt to determine causality through retrospective studies has not been successful and the use of prospective studies is rare. One exception is the type A personality constellation that seems to be associated with coronary artery disease. The type A individual is highly ambitious and hard driving, and has an excessive urgency about deadlines. Type A individuals are impatient with treatment and their compliance tends to be poor.

More recently the focus has shifted from personality traits to studies of the relationship between life stress and the onset of disease. Individuals who have recently suffered a severe loss or have changed an important facet of their lives appear to be more likely to fall ill, whether it be with a common cold, a heart attack, or cancer. But personality variables are also present in this line of research because certain personality types may tend toward living a more stressful life than others. It is probable that in most cases of psychosomatic disease, personality type, life stress, and physiologic predisposition combine interactively.

Compliance. The issue of compliance with drug regimens is very important and receives surprisingly little attention, considering the waste of time and money that occurs when extensive diagnostic procedures are negated by patients' failing to follow through with treatment. Health care personnel tend to overestimate compliance rates, perhaps because it is uncomfortable to believe that one's efforts are often wasted.

We mentioned earlier that specific personality types (e.g., the type A personality) tend toward noncompliance, but the problem is more pervasive. It is estimated that 30% to 75% of patients do not adequately follow instructions for taking medication. Lundin (1983) and others have noted a number of factors in noncompliance. Perhaps the most important is the patient's failure to understand the purpose of the treatment and the consequences of noncompliance. The role of effective communication in increasing compliance will be discussed later. An important factor is the patient's concerns and fears regarding the action of the medication and the possible side effects. The patient's attitudes and values are also important in compliance. An attitude of denial or complacency regarding the disease or values (including religious) against drug taking are difficult to detect and deal with. For some patients, resistance to authority leads to noncompliance, whereas for others noncompliance results from a failure to have an action-oriented approach to the control of life events, including illness.

Individual responses to pain. One of the most common and perplexing problems for health care personnel is the individuality of responses to pain and pain-reducing medication. Pain constitutes a major stress itself and compounds the intensity of the other forms of stress experienced during illness. In some patients, pain fosters regression and may produce a childlike feeling that leads to a demand for immediate relief through medication. Other patients may be overly stoic and their tendency to ignore pain may have life-threatening consequences (e.g., a woman suffering from an acute appendicitis attack insisted on finishing cleaning house before going to the hospital). Pain threshold varies enormously and seems to be lowest in anxious and hypochondriac patients. Pain threshold is partially biologically determined and is also related to the patient's emotional state (i.e., whether depressed, angry, or anxious), to the level of attention, and to the body part affected. Just as some patients demand relief from even minor pain, others seem to be unable to ask for help, even including medication, for severe pain.

Pain is the most common presenting problem that brings patients to the health care system and is usually taken as evidence of the presence of disease. But pain can have a psychogenic, as well as a physiologic, basis and even pain with a physiologic origin is complicated by the psychologic reaction of the patient and the special meaning the pain might have. Melzack (1974) points out that pain is not a simple function of tissue damage but rather a complex of psychologic processes, including suggestion and prior learning. Pain may serve as a solution to a psychologic conflict, as when pain is needed by the patient or when pain serves the purpose of secondary gain. Pain may also be a substitute for an underlying depression.

Differential diagnosis of psychogenic from physiologic pain is a major problem—clinicians often assume that when pain resists drug treatment it must have a psychogenic basis, but this is an unjustified conclusion. The important role of information and expectations in the experience of pain is indicated in a study by Egbert, et al (1964). In their study, a group of patients who were scheduled to have abdominal surgery all received preoperative visits by the anesthesiologist. For one half of the patients he provided information about the recovery room, the pain to be expected, and the medication that would be available to them. For the remaining patients he did not provide this information. After surgery those patients who received the information left the recovery room sooner and required less medication for pain than those who had not been given the information.

Chronic pain (i.e., pain that is a persistent and daily experience for at least 6 months) produces special problems for treatment. This pain may have physical findings related to it but is not associated with a specific underlying disease process that can be alleviated by known treatments. One model of chronic pain views it as a symptom involving self-inflicted punishment that serves to ease feelings of guilt. Such a person may present himself or herself as a martyr tolerating pain and therefore deserving comfort. Another model views chronic pain as a form of learned behavior governed by rewarding consequences in the patient's environment and recommends withdrawing the positive results that are the consequence of the pain complaints. Another view is that chronic pain is a form of communication and interpersonal manipulation between a patient and a clinician. Some patients appear to be at a high risk for chronic pain, but specific personality characteristics have not been established yet (pain is also discussed in Chapter 17, "Analgesics and Narcotic Antagonists").

COMMUNICATING WITH PATIENTS ABOUT DRUGS

To ensure that patients get the greatest possible value from the drugs that are prescribed or recommended for them, it is essential that they have appropriate expectations regarding drug effects and that they take them according to the appropriate schedule. It is necessary to discover all of the drugs a person is taking, both those that were prescribed and those that were obtained by over-the-counter purchase, to identify incompatibilities and drug interactions (see Chapter 10, "Drug Interactions"). People need to be informed about the possible side effects of the drugs, and special issues that arise out of cultural or religious backgrounds need to be explored so that they can be explained and put into appropriate perspective. All of these tasks and others like them depend on effective communication for their accomplishment.

This chapter cannot undertake any extensive discussion of the principles and skills that lead to effective communication. Most nursing curricula provide extensive instruction in communications skills. Here, we wish only to outline briefly an approach particularly compatible with the special issues that arise in communicating about the use of drugs.

Communication consists of an exchange of information between two or more persons so that each accomplishes some purpose that has been activated in the process. Each person's communication is guided by active intentions or goals. In some cases, these goals will have to do with giving or receiving information about drugs. In other circumstances, purposes may be to protect one's self-esteem, to look professional, or to end an uncomfortable situation. Clearly, the more such secondary agenda items encroach on the communication, the more difficult it will be to accomplish the business about drugs.

Another kind of difficulty can arise because of differences between the nurse and the patient in vocabulary and in understanding the actions of drugs on the body. Studies of noncompliance have often identified patients' lack of comprehension of the instructions they received as a major factor in their failure to follow instructions.

A third common obstacle to effective communication occurs when patients are in an abnormal physiologic state, either as a result of drugs already taken, of the disease process, or because of a highly emotional state accompanying their illness or its treatment. Receiving and storing information so it can be used at a later time, and retrieving information previously stored to serve present purposes are both very complex psychologic processes that are quite easily disrupted. Such disruption usually is seen as the patient forgetting the instructions about the drug regimens. The problem can be greatly reduced, in some circumstances, by providing clear, written instructions to the patient.

The principal recommendation we can offer to avoid the possible problems in communication that can arise from the three sources just listed is that the nurse should have a clear intention to communicate fully and to accept patients as they are without making judgments about whether they are right or wrong, responsible or irresponsible, appealing or unappealing. Whereas it is definitely possible to improve one's skills in detecting psychologic states from facial expressions and body posture (almost everyone has learned in the course of growing up to recognize when others are experiencing discomfort, irritation, puzzlement, or inattention), what is called for to produce effective communication is to accept these psychologic states without becoming defensive, to acknowl-

edge them to the patient in a way that makes it clear it is all right to feel that way, and to explore the reasons for the presence of the indication that all is not well with the communication. If the patient looks irritated, the nurse's statement, "You seem upset by what I am telling (or asking) you," may permit the patient to reveal a perceived slight, a lack of comprehension of some word or phrase, or a practical obstacle to following the prescribed regimen in the patient's life circumstances. Or, the patient might admit to an inability to pay attention to complicated questions or instructions while preoccupied with the implication for the future of the real or fantasized health problem that is being confronted.

It is usually a good idea to ask patients to restate in their own words the main points of the instructions to be followed. Not only may patients fail to admit they have not understood all of the directions, but they may actually say that they understand when they do not. If the communication is carried on in an atmosphere of mutual respect, patients usually appreciate the opportunity to check their grasp of what they have been advised to do.

The value of a written recapitulation of instructions has already been mentioned. In one recent experiment, patients were pleased to be given tape recordings of the portion of their interactions with their clinician that included the instructions for their treatment. However, without specific verification of understanding there may still be slip-ups. Patients have been found, for example, to take medications anywhere from 1 hour before to 1 hour after a meal in response to the written instruction, "Take with meals." Such variation can have important effects on the absorption of the drug or on the gastric irritation experienced, and can in other ways influence responses to the drug.

When general principles of effective communication are followed, there may still remain special problems in which patients' responses to drugs are influenced by communication processes. One of these has already been introduced in our discussion of the influence of expectations. We know that what people expect influences what they experience, but we are nevertheless faced with the necessity to provide and gather information about side effects. Everyday experience suggests that telling patients they may experience nausea, loss of sexual potency, or blurred vision will increase the likelihood that some patients will experience such effects. Not much empirical evidence exists regarding this question. Laboratory studies, including some of those cited in the section on expectations, show clearly that responses can be influenced by suggestion. In reviewing studies of the impact of package inserts, however, Morris and Halperin (1979) found only two reports on the impact of written information about side effects, and in neither case was there any effect. Another study that provided a combination of written and oral consultation did find an increased willingness of patients to report the adverse effects they experienced. Because full disclosure of potential side effects is now the ethical norm, it is important to learn more about how such information can be communicated for the maximal benefit of the patient.

Another special problem in communicating with patients about drugs arises when there are substantial cultural differences between health care providers and patients. People with different ethnic, religious, or social class backgrounds have different beliefs about illness, different ways of reacting to pain, and different ways of expressing health complaints. Topics that can be talked about freely in some subcultures are totally taboo in others. Thus, people who experience the identical physical effects of a drug (if there were some way to establish that) may make very different reports, may respond to questioning in very different ways, and may have different inner experiences. Health care providers need to recognize that these differences cannot be approached from a position that considers the patient's views erroneous and their own views as correct. With regard to physiologic and health care facts the professionally trained person is more expert, but with regard to subjective, inner experiences, and beliefs about what topics may be discussed with a stranger—even a professionally trained stranger—it is not possible to establish right and wrong views. What is needed is a respectful and nonevaluative exploration of patients' views that assists patients to be as clear as possible about how their health can best be promoted, maintained, or restored.

The views presented here are not intended to suggest that the nurse should fail to confront patients with what appears to be nonadaptive behavior. The point is that the confrontation should convey respect and inspire trust.

We can conclude this section on the impact of communication processes on response to drugs by pointing to some common, human tendencies of health care providers. Four deficiencies in therapeutic behavior stem from an unreadiness of the health care provider to deal with interpersonal discomfort. Each of these deficiencies can result in significant or serious problems in the patient's drug response: (1) the health care provider may assume greater adherence to the prescribed regimen than is actually the case; (2) the

health care provider may prescribe an unnecessary medication as a means of ending an unsatisfying or uncomfortable visit; (3) the prescriber may yield to explicit or implicit demands arising from the patient's belief that no adequate medical care has been given unless some medication is prescribed; and (4) nurses, pharmacists, and other health care providers who generally do not have primary responsibility for prescribing drugs may be insensitive to or simply ignore errors of the kinds just listed, or actual errors in prescription rather than confront the displeasure of a prescriber whose error is pointed out.

To reduce the impact of these tendencies, two things are required. First, the health care provider must have a personal knowledge that these tendencies exist. Reading about their existence is the first step, but full acceptance will come about only when one observes them operating in the health care provider's own segment of the health care system. Second, the health care provider needs to form a clear intention to overcome these tendencies in practice. Education in interpersonal relations, such as is often found in courses and workshops on communication, can provide a safe environment in which to experiment with confronting the discomfort that people typically experience when they contemplate direct and honest communication about sensitive topics. Many people find the mastery of new modes of communication to be very rewarding.

SUMMARY

Psychologic factors influence the ways in which people take drugs, the state of the body into which the drugs are taken, and the response of the body to the drugs. Many drugs have a direct influence on behavioral capacities and psychologic experience.

Psychologic reactions to these direct effects create an enormous range of possible responses. Primary effects include alterations of sensorimotor capacities, alteration of attentional processes that select from sensory input and relate it to ongoing processes, alteration of the processes of storage and retrieval of information from memory, and of emotional states and moods. All of these processes combine to support intellectual and affective functioning.

These direct effects can be modified or mimicked by the influence of people's beliefs and expectations about their bodies and about the drugs they are taking. A dramatic and important kind of nonspecific drug response is the placebo effect, whereby pharmacologically inert substances can have a powerful impact on the body. Placebo effects are influenced not only by the psychologic characteristics of the person who takes them, but by the attitudes of the health care team and by the social and situational variables of the environment in which the placebo is taken. Research suggests that some placebo effects may be mediated through a neurohumoral system involving peptides of the brain (the endorphins).

Many less specific aspects of the patient's personality affect reactions to the stress of illness and the therapeutic regimens that are advised to deal with them. People vary in their ability to cope with stress. Some become very dependent on health care personnel. Others may find short-run relief of life's pressures in their illness, and may be reluctant to give it up, or they may attribute deep symbolic meanings to symptoms or to the illness that can greatly complicate their treatment. Some theorists have proposed that psychologic symbolism contributes to the development of specific patterns of psychosomatic diseases (e.g., asthma, rheumatoid arthritis, and stomach ulcer). It is now clear that the way one lives, the pace one sets, the stresses one is exposed to, and one's ways of dealing with such stresses have a major impact on health, sickness, and responses to drugs.

How the patient behaves in relation to the stresses of illness and of therapeutic regimens is an important aspect of the health care picture. Whether prescriptions are filled and taken, how the patient deals with pain and distress, the forms of patients' complaints, and communication with health care personnel all affect treatment. These forms of patient behavior are, like all behavior, complexly determined by individual, social, and cultural factors.

The primary means at the nurse's disposal for dealing with the psychologic factors in drug responses are to understand them and to communicate effectively with patients about them. The basis for effective communication is the intention to make oneself understood and a willingness to press past barriers of discomfort that can arise in confronting sensitive issues. An approach that views communication in health transactions as a joint problem-solving activity can aid in identifying and overcoming barriers to the effective delivery and use of health care.

BIBLIOGRAPHY

Alexander, F. Psychosomatic medicine. New York: W.W. Norton and Company, Inc., 1950.

Altman, N. Hypochondriasis. In J.J. Strain & S. Grossman (Eds.), Psychological care of the medically ill: a primer in liaison psychiatry. New York: Appleton-Century-Crofts, 1975.

Baldessarini, R.J., & Tarsy, D. Tardive dyskinesia. In M.A. Lipton, A. DiMascio, & K.F. Killam (Eds.), Psychopharmacology: a generation of progress. New York: Raven Press, 1978.

Barchas, P.R., & Barchas, J.D. Sociopharmacology. In J.D. Barchas, P.A. Berger, R.D. Ciaranello, & G.R. Elliott (Eds.), Psychopharmacology. New York: Oxford University Press, 1977.

Barrett, J.E., & DiMascio, A. Comparative response to "minor tranquilizers" in "high" and "low" anxious student volunteers. Diseases of the Nervous System, 1966, 27, 483-486.

Beecher, H.K. Measurement of subjective responses: quantitative effects of drugs. New York: Oxford University Press, 1969.

Bertakis, K.D. The communication of information from physician to patient: a method for increasing patient retention and satisfaction. The Journal of Family Practice, 1977, 5, 217-222.

Birnbaum, I.M., Parker, E.S., Hartley, J.T., & Noble, E.P. Alcohol and memory: retrieval process. Journal of Verbal Learning and Verbal Behavior, 1978, 17, 325-335.

Buchsbaum, M.S., Davis, G.C., & Bunney, W.E. Naloxone alters pain perception and somatosensory evoked potentials in normal subjects. Nature, 1977, 270 (5638), 620-622.

Butt, H.F. A method for better physician-patient communication. Annals of Internal Medicine, 1977, 86, 478-480.

Davis, G.C., Buchsbaum, M.S., & Bunney, W.E. Naloxone decreases diurnal variation in pain sensitivity and somatosensory evoked potentials. Life Sciences, 1978, 23, 1449-1460.

Davis, K.L. Psychological effects of nonpsychiatric drugs. In J.D. Barchas, P.A. Berger, R.D. Ciaranello, & G.R. Elliott (Eds.), Psychopharmacology: from theory to practice. New York: Oxford University Press, 1977.

Davis, K.L., Mohs, R.C., Tinkelberg, J.R., Pfefferbaum, A., Hollister, L.E., & Kopell, B.S. Physostigmine: improvement of long-term memory process in normal humans. Science, 1978, 201, 272-274.

DiMascio, A., Meyer, R.E., & Stiffler, L. Effects of imipramine on individuals varying in level of depression. American Journal of Psychiatry, 1968, 124, 55-58.

Dornbush, R.L. Marijuana and memory: Effects of smoking on storage. Annals of the New York Academy of Science, 1974, 234, 94-100.

Dunn, A.J. Neurochemistry of learning and memory: an evaluation of recent data. Annual Review of Psychology, 1980, 31, 343-390.

Egbert, L.D., Batit, G.E., Welch, C.E., & Bartlett, M.K. Reduction of post-operative pain by encouragement and instruction to patient. New England Journal of Medicine, 1964, 270, 825.

Ekman, P., & Friesen, W. Unmasking the face. Englewood Cliffs, N.J.: Prentice Hall, 1975.

Filip, V., & Balik, J. Possible indication of dopaminergic blockade in man by electroretinography. International Pharmacopsychiatry, 1978, 13, 151-156.

Fisher, S. Nonspecific factors as determinants of behavioral response to drugs. In A. DiMascio, & R.I. Shader (Eds.), *Clinical handbook of psychopharmacology*. New York: Science House, 1970.

Friedman, M., & Rosenman, R.H. Type A behavior pattern: its association with coronary heart disease. *Annals of Clinical Research*, 1971, *3*, 300-312.

Gordis, L. Conceptual and methodologic problems in measuring patient compliance. In R.B. Haynes, D.W. Taylor, & D.L. Sackett (Eds.), *Compliance in health care*. Baltimore: Johns Hopkins University Press, 1979.

Groves, P.M., & Rebec, G.V. Biochemistry and behavior: some central actions of amphetamine and antipsychotic drugs. *Annual Review of Psychology*, 1976, *27*, 91-127.

Hayes-Bautista, D.E. Modifying the treatment: patient compliance, patient control and medical care. *Social Science and Medicine*, 1976, *10*, 233-238.

Ho, B.T., Richards, D.W., & Chute, D.L. (Eds.). *Drug discrimination and state dependent learning*. New York: Academic, 1978.

Jenkins, C.D. Cultural differences in concepts of disease and how these affect health behavior. In I. Barofsky (Ed.), *Medication compliance*. Thorofare, N.J.: Charles B. Slack, Inc., 1977.

Jones, B.M., & Jones, M.K. Alcohol effects in women during the menstrual cycle. *Annals of the New York Academy of Sciences*, 1976, *273*, 576-587.

Jones, B.M., & Jones, M.K. States of consciousness and alcohol: relationship to the blood alcohol, curve, time of day, and the menstrual cycle. *Alcohol, Health and Research World*, 1976, *1*, 10-15.

Klerman, G.L., DiMascio, A., Greenblatt, M., & Rinkel, M. The influence of specific personality patterns on the reactions of phrenotropic agents. In J. Masserman (Ed.), *Biological psychiatry*. New York: Grune & Stratton, Inc., 1959.

Lasagna, L., Laties, V.G., & Dohan, J.L. Further studies on the "pharmacology" of placebo administration. *Journal of Clinical Investigation*, 1958, *37*, 533-537.

Lasagna, L., Mosteller, F., von Felsinger, J.M., & Beecher, H.K. A study of the placebo response. *The American Journal of Medicine*, 1954, *16*, 770-779.

Levine, J.D., Gordon, N.C., & Fields, H.L. The mechanism of placebo analgesia. *Lancet*, 1978, *ii*, 654-657.

Lundin, D. Medication taking behavior and compliance in the elderly. In L.A. Pagliaro & A.M. Pagliaro (Eds.), *Pharmacologic aspects of aging*. St. Louis: The C.V. Mosby Co. 1983.

Mayer, D.J., Price, D.D., & Rafii, A. Antagonism of acupuncture analgesia in man by the narcotic antagonist naloxone. *Brain Research*, 1977, *121*, 368-372.

Mazzulo, J.M., Lasagna, L., & Griner, P.F. Variation in interpretation of prescription instructions. *Journal of the American Medical Association*, 1974, *227*, 929-931.

McCreary, C., & Jamison, K. The chronic-pain patient. In R.O. Pasnau (Ed.), *Consultation-liaison psychiatry*. New York: Grune & Stratton, Inc., 1975.

McGeer, P.L., & McGeer, E.G. Chemistry of mood and emotion. *Annual Review of Psychology*, 1980, *31*, 273-307.

McNair, D.M., Kahn, R.J., Dropplenian, L.F., & Fisher, S. Patient acquiescence and drug effects. In K. Rickels (Ed.), *Non-specific factors in drug therapy*. Springfield, Ill.: Charles C Thomas, Publisher, 1968.

Melzack, R. Psychological concepts and methods for the control of pain. In J.J. Bonica (Ed.), *Advances in neurology, vol. 4. International symposium on pain*. New York: Raven Press, 1974.

Morris, L.A., & Halperin, J.A. Effects of written drug information on patient knowledge and compliance. *American Journal of Public Health*, 1979, *69*, 47-52.

Nakano, S., & Hollister, L.F. Early clinical testing of antianxiety drugs: an experimental model. *Progress in Neuropsychopharmacology*, 1978, *2*, 101-105.

Nash, H., & Stone, G.C. Psychological effect of drugs: a factor analytic approach. *Journal of Nervous and Mental Disease*, 1974, *159*, 444-448.

Rahe, R.H., Fløistad, I., Bergan, T., Ringdal, R., Gerhardt, R., Gunderson, E.K., & Arthur, R.J. A model for life changes and illness research. *Archives of General Psychiatry*, 1974, *31*, 172-177.

Rank, S.G., & Jacobson, C.K. Hospital nurses' compliance with medication overdose orders: a failure to replicate. *Journal of Health and Social Behavior*, 1977, *18*, 188-193.

Rapp, D.J. Does diet affect hyperactivity? *Journal of Learning Disabilities*, 1978, *11*, 383-389.

Ruesch, J., & Bowman, K.M. Personality and chronic illness. In A. Weider (Ed.), *Contributions toward medical psychology* (vol. 1), New York: Ronald Press, 1953.

Rundele, O.H., Williams, H.L., & Boyd, B.K. Secobarbital and information processing. *Perceptual and Motor Skills*, 1978, *46*, 1255-1264.

Schacter, S., & Singer, J.E. Cognitive, social and physiological determinants of emotional state. *Psychological Review*, 1962, *69*, 379-399.

Shapiro, A.K., & Morris, L.A. The placebo effect in medical and psychological therapies. In S.L. Garfield & A.E. Bergin, (Eds.), *Handbook of psychotherapy and behavior change* (2nd ed.). New York: John Wiley & Sons, Inc., 1978.

Squieres, K.C., Chu, N., & Starr, A. Acute effects of alcohol on auditory brain stem potentials in humans. *Science*, 1978, *20*, 174-176.

Stimson, G.V. Obeying doctors' orders: a view from the other side. *Social Science and Medicine*, 1974, *8*, 97-104.

Stone, G.C. Patient compliance and the role of the expert. *Journal of Social Issues*, 1979, *35*(1), 34-59.

Stone, G.C., Callaway, E.C., Jones, R.T., & Gentry, T. Chlorpromazine slows decay of visual short term memory. *Psychonomic Science*, 1969, *16*, 229-230.

Swanson, J.M., & Kinsbourne, M. Food dyes impair performance of hyperactive children on a laboratory learning test. *Science*, 1980, *207*, 1485-1487.

Weckowicz, T.E., Fedora, O., Mason, J., Radstaak, D., Bay, K.S., & Yonge, K.A. Effect of marijuana on divergent and convergent production cognitive tests. *Journal of Abnormal Psychology*, 1975, *84*, 386-398.

Wittenborn, J.R. Behavioral toxicity in normal humans as a model for assessing behavioral toxicity. In M.A. Lipton, A. DiMascio, & K.F. Killam (Eds.), *Psychopharmacology: a generation of progress*. New York: Raven Press, 1978.

Wheatley, D. Effects of doctors' and patients' attitudes and other factors on respone to drugs. In K. Rickels (Ed.), *Nonspecific factors in drug therapy*. Springfield, Ill.: Charles C Thomas, Publisher, 1968.

CHAPTER 9

Genetic Factors Affecting Drug Response

Elliot S. Vesell

Most courses and texts in pharmacology imply that many drugs can be administered in a single fixed dose that will be satisfactory for all patients regardless of the patient's age, sex, diet, disease, or genetic constitution. In practice the concept of the single ideal patient who can represent all other patients with respect to response to many drugs is false. Yet this misconception has deep roots in pharmacology and arose in part because of the common pharmacologic practice of ignoring individual pharmacokinetic and pharmacodynamic values by ostensibly eliminating these differences through the device of averaging all values to derive a single mean value such as the dose of a drug that is lethal in 50% of animals (LD_{50}) or the dose of a drug that is pharmacologically effective in 50% of animals or humans (ED_{50}).

The true picture is the reverse: patients vary extensively in their response to drugs because patients differ in many important ways, each of which can profoundly influence drug disposition and response. Thus, in practice health care providers deal not with single abstract values, such as an ED_{50} or an ideal universally applicable dose of a drug, but rather with patients who often exhibit large differences in rates of drug elimination. Some of the critical variables that affect drug disposition and response, that produce these large variations in drug elimination among patients, and that differ markedly from patient to patient are identified in Figure 9-1. Probably many other, as yet unidentified, similar factors exist. The next few years should witness their identification because clinicians are now becoming aware of the influence of such factors on drug disposition and response and are beginning to search more diligently for them. Accordingly, clinicians have become more alert recently to the existence of large variations among patients' drug responses and consequently now individualize the dosage of many more drugs than they did previously.

Several reasons can be offered for this recent salutary change in prescribing habits. Many studies published in the last few years in leading health care jour-

nals have advocated individualizing drug therapy both because of the large magnitude of interindividual variation in drug response that can range up to fortyfold, depending on both the drug and the population, and the recent trend among pharmaceutic houses to produce new drugs with higher maximal effects and lower therapeutic indices.

The purpose of this chapter is to acquaint nurses with several host factors that can dramatically alter drug response. For purposes of convenience in presentation these host factors will be divided into (1) those involving the genetic constitution of the host and (2) those impinging on the host as a result of the external or internal environment. In practice, these genetic and environmental factors should not be considered as though they were separate and independent, but conceptually they should be recognized to interact continuously and dynamically. For that reason the environmental factors in Figure 9-1 (outer circle) are connected to each other and are also connected by wavy arrows to the inner circle representing the effects on drug disposition exerted by the genetic constitution. Most important, in disease states the relative effects produced by each of the factors can change from hour to hour and day to day, depending on the fluctuating course and severity of the disease in the particular patient, including the medications administered and the changing functional status of critical organs (e.g., heart, liver, kidney). In a given patient this changing relationship among the factors shown in Figure 9-1 means that the therapeutic dose of a particular drug at one time may become toxic even for the same patient at another time or ineffective on a third occasion. These facts show why patients must be monitored closely when drugs with low therapeutic indices are used, such as drugs in which the margin between the minimal effective and the minimal toxic dose is small (e.g., digoxin and the antidysrhythmics). Close observation is necessary to assure that each patient derives the maximal therapeutic benefit from the dose selected rather than suffer toxicity or ineffective-

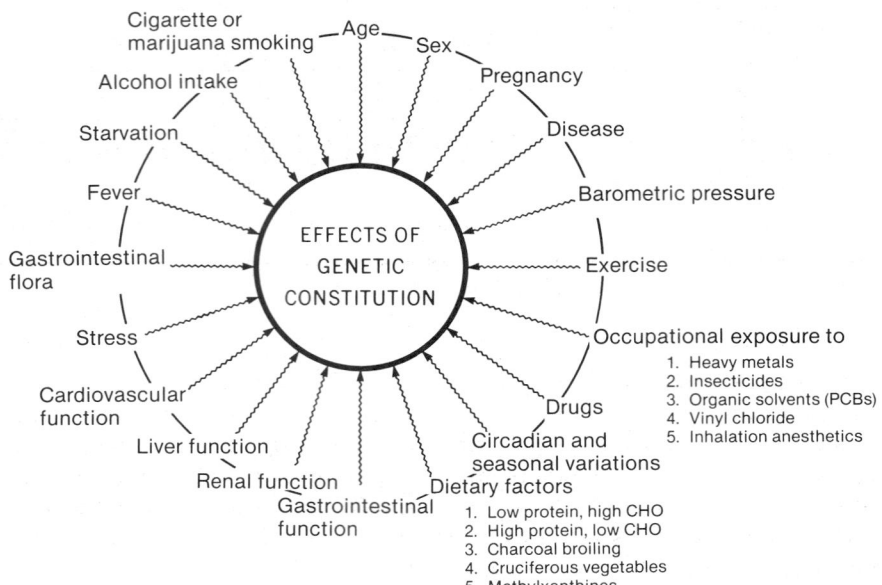

FIGURE 9-1. **This figure shows established or suspected environmental factors that can alter genetically controlled rates of drug elimination. Lines from each environmental factor are wavy to suggest that modification of genetically controlled rates can occur at multiple levels. Such environmental effects need not occur directly at the genetic level. A line joins environmental factors to suggest that several are associated and interdependent, rather than independent.**

ness that could be avoided simply by changing the dose.

Pharmacogenetics deals with the genetic causes of variation among patients in response to drugs. Response to drugs includes the five processes of drug (1) absorption, (2) distribution, (3) biotransformation, (4) interaction with receptor sites, and (5) excretion.

Each of these five processes is generally controlled by different genes, hence by different proteins, and is often located in different tissues of the body. Genetic as well as environmental factors shown in Figure 9-1 can operate simultaneously on several of these processes. The net effect of these simultaneously operating factors exerted on these five different processes may be either to cancel out different influences (if they operate in opposing directions) or to be additive (if they operate in the same direction). In other words, measuring the rate of elimination of a drug indirectly reflects the effects that take place separately and individually at the sites of drug absorption, distribution, biotransformation, action, and excretion.

Epidemiologic studies reveal that about 1 patient in 5 enters a hospital in the United States for treatment for an adverse drug reaction. Further, 15% to 30% of all hospitalized patients have at least one such reaction. Although wide disparity in patients' responses

to drugs is only one of many causes of adverse reactions, it nevertheless constitutes a significant contribution to this major health care problem because it demands individualizing dosages.

Multiple factors have been systematically investigated and identified as contributing to wide interindividual variations in drug disposition and response (Figure 9-1). They include age, sex, time of day or season of drug administration, disease, hormonal and nutritional status, stress, and exposure to inducers or inhibitors of the hepatic microsomal drug-metabolizing enzymes, including chronic administration of any one of several hundred drugs (see Chapter 5, "Drug Metabolism and Elimination," and Chapter 7, "Age Dependent Drug Selection and Response," for additional details in relation to metabolism and age).

MONOGENIC, PHARMACOGENETIC CONDITIONS DIRECTLY AFFECTING DRUG RESPONSE

Table 9-1 presents a partial list of genetically transmitted conditions affecting drug disposition and action at various sites in the body. These conditions may all be regarded as special forms of an inborn error of metabolism in which the substrate happens to be a

TABLE 9-1

Pharmacogenetic conditions with putative aberrant enzymes, mode of inheritance, frequency, and drugs that can elicit the signs and symptoms of the disorder

GENETIC CONDITIONS PROBABLY TRANSMITTED AS SINGLE FACTORS ALTERING THE WAY *THE BODY ACTS ON DRUGS*

Name of condition	Aberrant enzyme and location	Mode of inheritance	Frequency	Drugs that produce the abnormal response
Acatalasia	Catalase in erythrocytes	Autosomal recessive	Mainly in Japan and Switzerland, reaching 1% in certain small areas of Japan	Hydrogen peroxide
Slow inactivation of isoniazid	Isoniazid acetylase in liver	Autosomal recessive	Approximately 50% of U.S.A. population	Isoniazid, sulfamethazine, phenelzine, dapsone, hydralazine
Suxamethonium sensitivity or atypical pseudocholinesterase	Pseudocholinesterase in plasma	Autosomal recessive	Several aberrant alleles; most common disorder occurs 1 in 2500	Suxamethonium or succinylcholine
Phenytoin toxicity caused by deficient parahydroxylation	? Mixed function oxidase in liver microsomes that parahydroxylates phenytoin	Autosomal or X-linked dominant	Only 1 small pedigree	Phenytoin
Dicumarol sensitivity	? Mixed function oxidase in liver microsomes that hydroxylates dicumarol	Unknown	Only 1 small pedigree	Dicumarol
Phenacetin-induced methemoglobinemia	? Mixed function oxidase in liver microsomes that deethylates phenacetin	Autosomal recessive	Only 1 small pedigree	Phenacetin
Deficient N-glucosidation of amobarbital	? Mixed function oxidase in liver microsomes that N-glucosidates amobarbital	Autosomal recessive	Only 1 pedigree: screening of over 100 unrelated, normal volunteers revealed that approximately 2% were homozygous affected	Amobarbital
Polymorphic hydroxylation of debrisoquin in man	? Mixed function oxidase in liver microsomes that 4-hydroxylates debrisoquin	Autosomal recessive	94 volunteers and 3 families with a frequency of homozygous affected individuals of approximately 3%	Debrisoquin

Continued.

TABLE 9-1—cont'd

Pharmacogenetic conditions with putative aberrant enzymes, mode of inheritance, frequency, and drugs that can elicit the signs and symptoms of the disorder

Name of condition	*Aberrant enzyme and location*	*Mode of inheritance*	*Frequency*	*Drugs that produce the abnormal response*
GENETIC CONDITIONS PROBABLY TRANSMITTED AS SINGLE FACTORS ALTERING THE WAY *DRUGS ACT ON THE BODY*				
Warfarin resistance	? Altered receptor or enzyme in liver with increased affinity for vitamin K	Autosomal dominant	2 large pedigrees	Warfarin
Glucose-6-phosphate dehydrogenase deficiency, favism or drug-induced hemolytic anemia	Glucose-6-phosphate dehydrogenase	X-linked incomplete codominant	Approximately 100,000,000 affected in world; occurs in high frequency where malaria is endemic; 80 biochemically distinct mutations	Many different drugs (e.g., aspirin, primaquine, sulfonamides, vitamin K)
Drug-sensitive hemoglobins Hemoglobin Zurich	Arginine substitution for histidine at the 63rd position of the β-chain of hemoglobin	Autosomal dominant	2 small pedigrees	Sulfonamides
Hemoglobin H	Hemoglobin composed of 4 β-chains			Many different drugs
Inability to taste phenylthiourea or phenylthiocarbamide	Unknown	Autosomal recessive	Approximately 30% of Caucasians	Drugs containing N-C-S group such as phenylthiourmethyl and propylthiouracil
Malignant hyperthermia with muscular rigidity	Unknown	Autosomal dominant	Approximately 1 in 20,000 anesthetized patients	Various anesthetics, especially halothane

drug. With respect to metabolism, pharmacogenetic errors arising from an aberrant enzyme decrease production of product, and accumulation of parent drug occur, as in other inborn errors. This accumulation of parent drug can lead to toxicity.

Thus, pharmacogenetics may be regarded as a specialized topic in toxicology in which very specific genetic differences among patients render particular individuals extremely sensitive to what would generally be considered normal doses of a drug. Obviously, in these sensitive patients, the dose is not normal, but toxic. Individuals bearing pharmacogenetic aberrations are generally normal medically until they receive a dose of a particular drug to which they are sensitive. This dose, when given chronically, can produce toxicity that can lead to the identification of the aberrant enzyme. Once the discovery of the aberrant enzyme is made, thereby revealing the cause of the drug toxicity, a major aim in pharmacogenetics is to identify similar individuals in the same family and also in the general population who possess this aberrant enzyme before they also develop severe toxicity caused by the chronic administration of the drug(s) to which they are sensitive. For this reason, it is important for health care providers to recognize that pharmacogenetic conditions exist, some in high frequency, that render certain patients particularly susceptible to drug toxicity, by virtue of their genetic constitution. If health care providers are alert to this possibility, they will be able to avoid or discontinue the drug before serious toxicity occurs.

Terminology of genetic transmission of traits

Familiarity with several terms related to the modes of genetic transmission of characteristics or traits is necessary to follow the rest of this chapter. A brief review will be presented for the convenience of the reader.

Genetic disorders are primarily transmitted by one of the following modes: (1) autosomal recessive, (2) autosomal dominant, (3) sex-linked recessive, and (4) sex-linked dominant. Autosomal indicates that the characteristic is transmitted by a chromosome other than a sex chromosome. Conversely, sex-linked means that the characteristic or trait is transmitted via (or located on) either the X or Y sex chromosome.

Dominant characteristics are transmitted to the offspring if either one or both of the parents possess the characteristic dominant gene(s). Recessive characteristics, however, are transmitted only if both parents possess the characteristic recessive gene(s). There are also several variant combinations of transmissions (hy-

brids) intermediate between dominant and recessive, as well as carrier states, which occur.

Homozygous means having the same gene at specific loci (sites) on homologous chromosomes, whereas heterozygous means having different genes at specific loci on homologous chromosomes.

An allele is one of two or more alternate forms of a gene, each of which contains specific inheritable characteristics.

Monogenic means that a characteristic is controlled entirely by genes at a single locus on a chromosome, whereas polygenic means that more than one locus on a chromosome is involved.

Pharmacogenetic categories and associated conditions

Pharmacogenetic conditions may be divided into two general categories: (1) genetic conditions probably transmitted as single factors altering the way the body acts on drugs and (2) genetic conditions probably transmitted as single factors altering the way drugs act on the body.

Genetic conditions probably transmitted as single factors altering the way the body acts on drugs. Eight major conditions are associated with the genetic conditions probably transmitted as single factors altering the way the body acts on drugs: (1) acatalasia, (2) slow inactivation of isoniazid and other acetylated drugs, (3) succinylcholine sensitivity, (4) deficient parahydroxylation of phenytoin, (5) dicumarol sensitivity, (6) phenacetin-induced methemoglobinemia, (7) deficient N-glucosidation of amobarbital, and (8) polymorphic hydroxylation of debrisoquin.

Acatalasia. In 1946, the Japanese otorhinolaryngologist Takahara discovered acatalasia in an 11-year-old Japanese girl. In a series of classic studies he demonstrated that the defect was transmitted as an autosomal recessive trait. Takahara's original patient lacked catalase activity in her oral mucosa and erythrocytes, as did three of her five siblings. The patient's parents were second cousins: consanguinity is a hallmark of the inheritance of rare autosomal recessive conditions.

Mild, moderate, and severe cases of acatalasia have been described. The mild form is characterized by ulcers of the dental alveoli, in the moderate form alveolar gangrene and atrophy occur, and in the severe form recession of alveolar bone develops with exposure of the necks and eventual loss of the teeth. The enzyme is deficient in tissues such as mucous membranes, skin, liver, muscle, and bone marrow. Trace levels of catalase activity occur in some patients, and the term "severe hypocatalasia" seems more appropriate than does acatalasia. Heterozygotes who usually have values of catalase activity between those of affected and unaffected persons would be classified as having intermediate hypocatalasia. In certain Japanese kindreds, some heterozygotes do not exhibit intermediate levels of catalase activity, but rather have values that overlap the normal range, suggesting heterogeneity.

In 1959, a Korean patient was reported with acatalasia, the first non-Japanese subject to be described. Two years later Aebi and associates found three affected individuals by screening 73,661 blood samples from Swiss Army recruits. All three were healthy and showed none of the dental defects typical of the Japanese cases. The Swiss acatalasic patients, unlike the Japanese ones, exhibited residual catalase activity, possibly protecting them against the hydrogen peroxide formed by certain microorganisms thought to be responsible for the oral lesions. The catalase from the Swiss patients also differed from that of unaffected persons in electrophoretic mobility, pH, heat stabilities, and sensitivity to certain inhibitors. These facts suggest that in Swiss families acatalasia is a structural gene mutation.

Slow inactivation of isoniazid and other acetylated drugs. Although isoniazid (INH) was synthesized in 1921, its bacteriostatic effect was not discovered until 1952. Soon great differences among subjects were reported in the metabolism of INH, but each patient maintained an unchanged pattern of excretion during long-term therapy. Slow inactivators show reduced activity of acetyl transferase, the soluble hepatic enzyme responsible for the metabolism of INH and of sulfamethazine, as well as other monosubstituted hydrazines, such as phenelzine and hydralazine. Toxic effects of these drugs occur chiefly in slow acetylators. Acetylation (see Chapter 5, "Drug Metabolism and Elimination") of procainamide is polymorphic (i.e., occurs in more than one form) and thus the effect of this antidysrhythmic agent varies appreciably according to the genotype of the patient to whom it is administered. Toxicity caused by chronic INH administration takes the form of polyneuritis as a result of a vitamin B_6 (pyridoxine) deficiency; this potential deficiency of pyridoxine to which slow acetylators are particularly susceptible can be easily overcome by giving this vitamin with INH whenever INH is administered for long periods.

Another form of toxicity to which slow acetylators appear to be more disposed than rapid acetylators is both the drug-induced and spontaneous forms of disseminated lupus erythematosus. Thus, susceptibility to certain diseases may be linked to genetic differences among patients in their capacity to biotransform drugs and other compounds that do not apparently bear any direct pathogenetic relationship to the diseases.

The sedative nitrazepam also shows a similar variation in response. Acetylation of other drugs, such as aminosalicylic acid and sulfanilamide, is accomplished by a different acetylase and no genetic differences among patients occur in the metabolism of these drugs. Interestingly, neither the slow nor the rapid acetylase genotype is more liable to resistance to tubercle bacilli or reversion. The half-life of INH ranges from 45 to 80 minutes in the plasma of rapid inactivators, whereas the half-life extends from 140 to 200 minutes in slow inactivators. Although slow acetylators excrete approximately 70% of a dose in the urine as metabolites, rapid acetylators excrete 97% of a dose as metabolites, thereby being exposed to higher concentrations of potentially toxic reactive metabolites. Such toxic intermediates have been implicated as the cause of the severe hepatic necrosis and hepatitis that occur in approximately 1% of the patients receiving INH chronically for prophylactic purposes. However, the transient elevation of serum transaminases caused by liver damage in approximately 10% to 20% of patients receiving isoniazid or isoniazid plus rifampin chronically seems to occur predominantly in slow acetylators.

Slow inactivation of INH is inherited as an autosomal recessive trait. The best evidence suggests that the different phenotypes result from a structural gene mutation. Diverse geographic and racial distributions of the gene are documented. Most uncommon in Canadian Eskimos (5%), slow inactivation is only slightly more frequent in Far Eastern populations, where it occurs in approximately 10% of Japanese people. Slow inactivation is common among Blacks and European populations, in nearly 80% of whom the aberrant gene is present whether in the homozygous or the heterozygous state. Approximately one half of the United States population are slow acetylators.

Succinylcholine sensitivity. Shortly after the muscle relaxant succinylcholine was introduced in 1952 and its use became widespread, patients occasionally were found to be extraordinarily sensitive to it; indeed, several deaths associated with its use were reported. Normally the action of the drug is short (i.e., 2 to 3 minutes); this brevity is caused by the exceedingly rapid hydrolysis of succinylcholine by plasma pseudocholinesterase, which catalyzes the sequential removal of choline radicals. Serum pseudocholinesterase activity was reduced in the initially published reports of prolonged apnea. This difficulty can be reversed by transfusing with either normal plasma or a highly purified preparation of human enzyme. The abnormality is the result of a structurally altered enzyme with kinetic properties much different from those of the usual enzyme. The abnormal enzyme exerts no measurable effect on succinylcholine at concentrations of the drug usually present during anesthesia, whereas the normal enzyme shows marked hydrolytic activity.

The atypical enzyme is more resistant than the normal one to many pseudocholinesterase inhibitors (e.g., both fluoride and organophosphorus compounds inhibit the typical and atypical enzyme differentially). Dibucaine, also a differential inhibitor of typical and atypical pseudocholinesterases, can distinguish three phenotypes: homozygous normals, heterozygotes, and affected individuals who could not be satisfactorily separated simply by measuring the pseudocholinesterase activity of their plasma. The percentage of inhibition of pseudocholinesterase activity produced by a 10^{-5} molar solution of dibucaine was designated the dibucaine number (DN). Whereas atypical pseudocholinesterase is inhibited only 20%, the normal enzyme is inhibited about 80%, and heterozygotes exhibit a 50% to 70% inhibition. Tetracaine, unlike other previously studied compounds, is hydrolyzed faster by atypical pseudocholinesterase than by normal pseudocholinesterase, and an even larger separation of phenotypes apparently can be achieved with the procaine–tetracaine ratio than with the DN. The discovery of additional genetic variants resulted from using sodium fluoride as an inhibitor.

In some families, the DNs do not follow the typical pattern of inheritance. These persons are thought to be heterozygous for a rare, so-called silent gene. Heterozygotes for this gene exhibit two thirds of the normal serum cholinesterase activity; they widely overlap normal values. A few rare individuals are presumably homozygous for the silent allele, reflecting a complete absence of serum and liver pseudocholinesterase activity. Apparently normal otherwise, these persons lack all four of the usual isozymes of serum pseudocholinesterase; the absence of antigenically cross-reacting material was revealed by immunodiffusion and immunoelectrophoretic studies.

This silent mutation may affect the controlling element of the gene, thereby completely disrupting protein production. Alternatively, a single structural mutation may affect both the active site and the antigenic determinants. Another silent allele has been described in which there is some (about 2%) residual enzymatic activity, indicating further heterogeneity.

Family studies suggest that the inheritance of various types of atypical pseudocholinesterase occurs through allelic codominant or recessive genes at a single locus. Symptoms may occur after treatment with succinylcholine in persons homozygous for any of the variant alleles and in some mixed heterozygotes. At least four alleles have been definitely identified with the ten resultant genotypes: $E_1^u E_1^u$, $E_1^u E_1^a$, $E_1^a E_1^a$, $E_1^s E_1^u$, $E_1^s E_1^s$, $E_1^s E_1^a$, $E_1^f E_1^u$, $E_1^f E_1^f$, $E_1^f E_1^a$, and $E_1^f E_1^s$, where E_1 signifies the pseudocholinesterase genetic locus and u, a, s, and f indicate the usual, atypical, silent, and fluoride sensitive alleles, respectively. A new allele (E_1^j) has been described that apparently causes reduction of the usual (E_1^u) molecules by about 60%.

The incidence of atypical pseudocholinesterase remains comparatively constant in different geographic areas. Persons who are homozygous recessive for the atypical allele number about 1 in 2500. An exceptionally high incidence of the silent mutation was discovered in a population of southern Eskimos. Before this survey in Alaska, only 10 individuals homozygous for the silent gene had been described. The gene frequency of 0.12 in this locality, extending from Hooper Bay to Unalakleet and centered on the lower Yukon River, suggested that 1.5% of this Alaskan population was sensitive to succinylcholine. The isolation and consequent inbreeding of these natives may have resulted in the high frequency of the rare silent gene in this region of Alaska, although only 2 of the 11 Eskimo families are known to be related.

Deficient parahydroxylation of phenytoin. Since its introduction, phenytoin has become one of the most popular anticonvulsants. However, it can cause multiple toxic reactions, including nystagmus, ataxia, dysarthria, and drowsiness reactions that are clearly dose related. The drug is metabolized in humans mainly by parahydroxylation of one of the phenyl groups to yield 5-phenyl-5'-para-hydroxyphenylhydantoin (PPHP), which is conjugated with glucuronic acid and then eliminated in the urine.

Many lipid-soluble drugs, such as phenytoin, are rendered more water soluble, and hence more excretable, through metabolism by the oxidative microsomal enzyme systems in the liver. The earliest published example of a genetic defect of hepatic mixed function oxidases in humans was a deficient hydroxylation of phenytoin, although only one affected family was described. Several additional cases of such a deficiency have been published subsequently. The true incidence is unknown because populations have not been screened systematically for the condition. However, if it is associated with a deficient 4-hydroxylation of debrisoquin, as seems to be the case (see the section on the polymorphic hydroxylation of debrisoquin), then the incidence of deficient parahydroxylation of phenytoin may be very high in certain populations, as high or higher than 7%.

A study of two generations of the affected family in the earliest case described revealed two affected and three unaffected members, suggesting that the low activity of phenytoin hydroxylase may exhibit a dominant transmission. Toxic symptoms developed in the proband (i.e., the initial individual whose condition led to the study of the genetically transmitted condition) on a commonly used dosage of 4.0 mg/kg, but not on a dose of 1.4 mg/kg. Abnormally low urine levels of the metabolite PPHP occurred in combination with prolonged high blood levels of unchanged phenytoin. Apparently phenylalanine and such drugs as phenobarbital are parahydroxylated by enzymes different from those hydroxylating phenytoin, because the proband's capacity to parahydroxylate these compounds was normal.

Recently, slow inactivation of isoniazid has been identified as a more important cause of phenytoin intoxication than an inheritable deficiency of parahydroxylase activity. In 29 patients receiving phenytoin and isoniazid, all five patients who developed symptoms of phenytoin toxicity were slow isoniazid inactivators. Both isoniazid and aminosalicylic acid interfered with phenytoin parahydroxylation in microsomal fractions isolated from rat livers. This example shows how genetic constitution can influence the clinical severity of a drug interaction.

Dicumarol sensitivity. Dicumarol sensitivity occurred in a patient receiving the drug for an acute myocardial infarction. On a dose of 150 mg the patient's plasma dicumarol half-life was 82 hours compared to normal values of 27 ± 5 hours. The patient's mother suffered a spinal cord hematoma, causing permanent paraplegia, while she was receiving a small weekly dose of 2.5 to 5 mg of warfarin. Although familial studies were not performed because of lack of cooperation, this unfortunate event in the treatment of the patient's mother suggests the possibility of hereditary transmission of dicumarol sensitivity.

Warfarin and dicumarol are extensively hydroxylated in the rat. Genetic factors influence responsiveness to anticoagulants in rabbits, as they do in rats, in which resistance to warfarin as a rodenticide is transmitted as an autosomal dominant trait. The metabolites in humans are not fully characterized, but the patient with dicumarol sensitivity just described, and his mother, may have a metabolic defect involving a deficiency of a hepatic microsomal hydroxylase.

Increased sensitivity to coumarin anticoagulants also can result from acquired conditions, including vitamin K deficiency, increased turnover of plasma proteins, and numerous forms of liver disease that impair a patient's capacity to produce vitamin K-dependent clotting factors. Various drugs can increase the prothrombinopenic response to coumarin anticoagulants. Cinchophen may damage liver cells; phenothiazines may produce cholestasis, thereby diminishing the absorption of vitamin K; phenylbutazone increases sensitivity by displacing warfarin from plasma albumin; and phenyramidol inhibits the hepatic microsomal enzymes responsible for the metabolism of coumarin drugs. Resistance to warfarin derivatives also has been reported.

Phenacetin-induced methemoglobinemia. Severe methemoglobinemia and hemolysis occurred in a 17-year-old girl after she had taken phenacetin. Multiple studies excluded inheritable erythrocytic disorders, including hemoglobinopathies, and extracorpuscular compounds seemed to be causing hemolysis. As much as one half of the patient's hemoglobin was occasionally in the form of methemoglobin. After administering phenacetin, large amounts of 2-hydroxyphenetidin and 2-hydroxyphenacetin derivatives were discovered in her urine. In unaffected persons more than 70% of a 2 gm dose of phenacetin appears in the urine as N-acetyl-para-aminophenol with only minute amounts of the hydroxylated products that were so prevalent in the reported patient's urine. One sister, a brother, and both parents of the patient had normal responses to phenacetin, but another sister likewise responded abnormally.

These observations suggest an autosomal recessive inheritance of a defect in which the patient's hepatic microsomal mixed function oxidases were deficient in deethylating capacity. Instead of being deethylated as in unaffected persons, phenacetin, in the patient and in her 38-year-old sister, was hydroxylated.

The toxicity observed after phenacetin administration was probably produced by these hydroxylated products, because the induction of the hepatic microsomal phenacetin hydroxylating enzymes before administering phenacetin by phenobarbital exacerbated the condition (i.e., severe neurologic symptoms, including bilateral positive Babinski's responses, and profound methemoglobinemia developed). After the same pretreatment, an unaffected volunteer developed neither methemoglobinemia nor neurologic changes.

Deficient N-glucosidation of amobarbital. Pursuing their initial observations based on a twin study that showed large interindividual variations in elimination rates of amobarbital to be predominantly under genetic control, Kalow, et al (1977) investigated the family of one set of twins with a deficiency in N-hydroxylation, but not C-hydroxylation, of amobarbital. The family study of these twins disclosed that this deficiency was most likely produced through autosomal recessive transmission, although only urinary ratios of these metabolites were measured. Later, Kalow, et al reported that the urinary metabolite was mistakenly identified as an N-hydroxylamobarbital and that the actual metabolite was instead N-β-D-glucopyranosyl amobarbital.

This metabolite showed great variability in the urine of 129 volunteers studied after a single oral dose of amobarbital: one volunteer completely lacked the metabolite, whereas 14 had it as the primary form. Of these 14, 4 were of Chinese origin, suggesting possible racial differences in the pattern and pathway of metabolite formation. These studies on amobarbital illustrate the utility of searching whenever possible for a monogenic origin of pharmacogenetic conditions, the necessity for performing genetic analyses in families, and the need, whenever more than a single metabolite is produced from the parent drug, to measure rates of metabolite formation, rather than measuring only the disappearance of the parent drug.

Polymorphic hydroxylation of debrisoquin. The antihypertensive drug debrisoquin is used in both England and Canada, but is not yet approved by the FDA in the United States. It was observed that patients receiving debrisoquin vary widely in their hypotensive response to the adrenergic-blocking action of the drug, and that a close correlation exists between debrisoquin plasma concentrations and the resultant decline in blood pressure. In 94 unrelated volunteers the urinary ratio of the parent drug to the primary metabolite, 4-hydroxy-debrisoquin, was measured after a single oral dose of 10 mg debrisoquin. In 3 of these 94 volunteers the ratio was high, suggesting a possible hepatic microsomal enzyme deficiency of *N*-hydroxylation of debrisoquin. Furthermore, family studies of the three volunteers with abnormally high ratios of debrisoquin to 4-hydroxy-debrisoquin in the 8-hour urinary collection suggested the transmission of the metabolic deficiency as an autosomal recessive trait.

Most side effects, as well as most pronounced antihypertensive activity, of debrisoquin occurred in the slow metabolizers (those individuals with the highest urinary ratio of parent drug to metabolite). This result, which could have been predicted given that the main metabolite is devoid of antihypertensive action, illustrates both the direct clinical and toxicologic consequences of pharmacogenetic conditions, and also the need for health care providers observing an unusual drug response in a patient to consider genetic factors as a potential cause.

A fascinating development in this commonly occurring, genetically controlled variation is that patients who metabolize debrisoquin slowly also have a similar reduction in the capacity to eliminate several other drugs (e.g., patients who 4-hydroxylate debrisoquin slowly also exhibit reduced rates of para-hydroxylation of phenytoin and of O-deethylation of phenacetin).

Genetic conditions probably transmitted as single factors altering the way drugs act on the body. Five major conditions are associated with genetic conditions probably transmitted as single factors altering the way drugs act on the body: (1) warfarin resistance, (2) glucose-6-phosphate dehydrogenase (G-6-PD) deficiency, (3) drug-sensitive hemoglobins, (4) phenylthiocarbamide tasting ability, and (5) malignant hyperthermia and muscular rigidity.

Warfarin resistance. Genetically controlled resistance to warfarin was found in a 71-year-old patient receiving anticoagulants for a myocardial infarction. Physical and laboratory examination showed no abnormalities other than a reproducible reduction in the one-state prothrombin concentration to about 60% of normal. Anticoagulants were initially withheld because of the patient's low prothrombin time. They were administered after 1 month, at which time the patient proved to be resistant, rather than sensitive, to dicumarol. A daily dose of 145 mg was required to reduce the prothrombin concentration to therapeutic levels (i.e., nearly 50 standard deviations above the mean).

Detailed studies showed that the drug was absorbed normally from the gastrointestinal tract. Kinetic and binding studies were also normal. Even after administration of very high doses, warfarin was not excreted unchanged in the urine or stools, and amounts of a metabolite of warfarin similar to those recovered from the urine of unaffected persons who were given equivalent amounts of the drug were recovered from the patient's urine. The patient also showed resistance to dicumarol and the indandione anticoagulant phenindione, but not to heparin.

An enzyme or receptor site with an altered affinity for vitamin K or for anticoagulant drugs was postulated as the mechanism responsible for resistance to warfarin in this patient. Five other members of both sexes of the patient's family over three generations were also resistant to warfarin, suggesting an autosomal dominant transmission of the trait. A second large kindred of 18 patients with warfarin resistance in two generations has been reported.

Various environmental conditions lead to resistance to coumarin anticoagulants as phenocopies of the genetic defect. Most commonly the resistance is related to the simultaneous administration of inducing agents (e.g., barbiturates, glutethimide, chloral hydrate, and griseofulvin—see Chapter 5, "Drug Metabolism and Elimination") that reduce the blood concentration of anticoagulant drugs by stimulating their metabolism.

Glucose-6-phosphate dehydrogenase (G-6-PD) deficiency. Formerly called primiquine sensitivity, or favism, glucose-6-phosphate dehydrogenase (G-6-PD) deficiency is the most common hereditary enzymatic abnormality in humans and is transmitted as a sex-linked (X chromosome) recessive disorder. More than 80 physicochemically discrete molecular variants are described, each being associated with slightly different clinical features. Ordinarily only the male homozygote shows significant drug-related hemolysis. Female patients may be affected mildly, as would be predicted from the Lyon hypothesis (which states that only one of the two X chromosomes in females is functional, the other having become inactive early in development), or more severely, as in populations wherein the gene frequency is high enough that homozygosity is appreciable. A mild, usually self-limited anemia is associated with the common variant of G-6-PD found in blacks, in whom drugs can be given repeatedly without danger, because only the susceptible, older RBCs are removed from the circulation by hemolysis; they are rapidly replaced by resistant younger cells.

In numerous Mediterranean G-6-PD variants, hemolysis affects a larger proportion of the total erythrocyte population and occurs more rapidly after the administration of smaller doses of drugs. The severity of the hemolysis depends not only on the total activity of the mutant G-6-PD but also on its other properties, including stability. Several properties in addition to symptomatic severity can characterize the variants, including the total erythrocyte G-6-PD activity, enzymatic electrophoretic mobility, and various kinetic measurements. The specific amino acid substitution in G-6-PD A^+ and in G-6-PD Hektoen has been elucidated by microfingerprinting techniques. Hemolytic anemia in the newborn can be particularly severe in the Mediterranean area in babies with G-6-PD deficiency.

Hemolysis apparently may occur spontaneously or during infection in certain G-6-PD variants. Obviously, enough stress can be placed on the metabolism of G-6-PD-deficient erythrocytes to cause hemolysis by several environmental alterations in addition to those produced by drug administration.

Drug-sensitive hemoglobins. A life-threatening hemolytic anemia developed in a 2-year-old Swiss girl and her father after they received sulfa drugs. Both patients registered an abnormal hemoglobin content, the electrophoretic mobility being between that of hemoglobins A and S. Further studies showed an abnormality in the beta chain, with arginine taking the place of the usual histidine residue at the sixty-third position, where the heme group is attached. Of the 65 relatives examined, 15 showed the abnormal hemoglobin feature, designated hemoglobin Zürich, a defect transmitted as an autosomal dominant trait. In another family, discovered in Maryland, with the same substitution the severity of the hemolytic episodes was less than in the Swiss cases.

Another drug-sensitive hemoglobin, hemoglobin H, is a special form of α-thalassemia. Composed of four beta chains, hemoglobin H is sensitive to the oxidant drugs described under the G-6-PD deficiency. In certain regions, such as Thailand, the frequency of homozygous hemoglobin H is high (i.e., 1 in 300 individuals).

Phenylthiocarbamide tasting ability. The ability to taste phenylthiocarbamide (PTC) is transmitted as an autosomal dominant trait, and tasters may be either heterozygous or homozygous. This polymorphism was discovered in 1932 when Fox, who synthesized the compound, noted that he could not detect a bitter taste from the dust of the compound arising as it was poured into a container, whereas a colleague in the same room complained of the bitter taste.

Although this polymorphism seems to be benign, some researchers have related the ability to taste PTC to thyroid disease. Administration of PTC can, for example, produce goiter in the rat. Compounds related to PTC by possessing the $N-C=S$ group, such as the antithyroid drugs methylthiouracil and propylthiouracil, also have the same bimodality in taste perception exhibited by patients to PTC. Of 134 patients with nodulant goiter, 41% were nontasters, an observation confirmed in 447 patients who underwent thyroidectomy for various reasons. In male patients with multiple thyroid adenomas, a marked increase in nontasting frequency was also noted. Nontasters seem to be more susceptible to athyreotic cretinism and to adenomatous goiter. These data suggest to some investigators that nontasters may be more susceptible than tasters to environmental goitrogens. The physicochemical basis for the difference in taste perception in affected individuals is unknown.

Malignant hyperthermia and muscular rigidity. In 1962 hyperthermia was reported to be the cause of death in 10 of 38 family members who had received anesthesia for various surgical procedures. This was the first indication that the rare, hitherto seemingly sporadic, malignant hyperthermia afflicting persons exposed to various anesthetic agents might be genetically transmitted. More than 200 cases of malignant hyperthermia have been identified and shown to have a hereditary basis. The condition is associated with muscular rigidity and appears to be transmitted as an autosomal dominant trait. It develops during anesthesia with nitrous oxide, methoxyflurane, halothane, ether, cyclopropane, or combinations thereof, and is more common in association with the use of succinylcholine as a preanesthetic agent. During anesthesia the body temperature rises rapidly, occasionally reaching 46° C.

The incidence of malignant hyperthermia is in the range of 1 in 20,000 cases of general anesthesia and exhibits no sex preference, but occurs more in younger than in older anesthetized patients. Approximately two thirds of the patients die, usually from cardiac arrest. The degree of rigidity is variable, differing from patient to patient and sometimes being absent. This variability may indicate that the term "malignant hyperthermia" refers to several discrete diseases.

Occasionally, rigidity is so marked that the body literally becomes as stiff as a board, progressing without interruption into rigor mortis. Intravenous administration dantrolene, procaine, or procainamide is reported to alleviate the rigidity and fever in certain cases. Curare is ineffective. Interestingly, a limb under tourniquet does not become rigid, suggesting a peripheral rather than a central lesion. Animal models have been produced in dogs and in Landrace pigs treated with halothane and dinitrophenol.

GENETIC FACTORS AFFECTING THE DISPOSITION OF COMMONLY USED DRUGS

Because most of the conditions just described are rare and produce toxicity with only a few drugs, they probably contribute only a small extent to the current major health care problem of adverse drug reactions. However, another development in pharmacogenetics suggests that genetic differences among patients that directly affect drug disposition play a prominent role in commonly encountered forms of drug toxicity. This idea was suggested by a series of experiments that examined rates at which healthy, adult, identical and fraternal twins cleared commonly used drugs administered to them in single doses (Figure 9-2). These twins were in a basal state with respect to most of the factors shown in Figure 9-1. This means they were nonmedicated, living in different households, but not exposed at work or at home to such inducing agents as alcohol or chronic cigarette smoking.

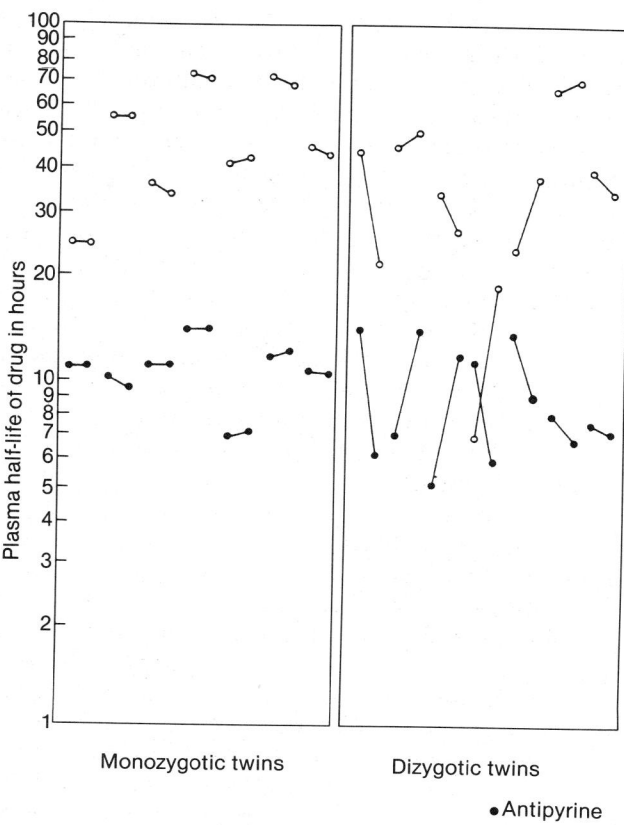

FIGURE 9-2. **Plasma half-lives of dicumarol and antipyrine were measured separately at an interval of more than 6 months in healthy monozygotic (identical) and dizygotic (fraternal) twins. A solid line joins the values for each set of twins for each drug. Note that intratwin differences in the plasma half-life of both dicumarol and antipyrine are smaller in monozygotic than in most dizygotic twins.**

Twins are of two types: identical twins have identical heredities because they arise from a single fertilized egg and are accordingly termed monozygotic, whereas fraternal twins arise from two fertilized eggs, are called dizygotic, and are no more alike genetically than siblings except that they are born at the same time. After administration of alcohol, antipyrine, dicumarol, halothane, nortriptyline, phenylbutazone, phenytoin, or salicylate, large interindividual variations that existed among unrelated people vanished within sets of identical twins but were preserved in most, but not all, sets of fraternal twins (Figure 9-2). The magnitude of interindividual variations in rates of drug elimination among unrelated people was thirtyfold for nortriptyline, tenfold for dicumarol, fourfold for phenylbutazone and antipyrine, threefold for halothane, and twofold for alcohol. Family studies on three of these drugs substantiated observations made in twins; in families, predominantly polygenic mechanisms appeared to control large interindividual variations in the disposition of the tested drugs. More studies have to be done using twins and families in which rates of production of metabolites are examined both in blood and in urine, rather than simply examining the disappearance of the parent drug.

Precise determination of the mode of inheritance is usually quite easy with single-gene traits, especially if they are rare. Family studies are invaluable; alleles segregate during gamete formation and rejoin in the offspring to form gene combinations that can be detected by their phenotypic expression.

Polygenic inheritance produces a different picture. Instead of alleles at only a single gene locus, alleles at several sites on a chromosome or chromosomes contribute to the formation of the phenotype. The effect of each gene is not as profound as it is with single-gene inheritance; instead, the final expression is a combination of genetic plus environmental effects.

The possibility remains that the long-sustained influence of certain environmental factors could be responsible in some measure for the particular rate of drug disposition of a patient who might otherwise appear to be in a basal state. To explore this possibility, a careful inquiry into the patient's exposure at home and at work to these factors is necessary. The existence and operation of numerous environmental factors (Figure 9-1), each with different capabilities of altering the near basal, genetically controlled rate of drug disposition, make it exceedingly difficult to attribute quantitatively different portions of the total interindividual variation to specific single environmental factors. The task of partitioning the total interindividual variation in drug elimination of large heterogeneous populations into component parts is further complicated because such seemingly pure environmental factors as smoking and diet are closely associated with other environmental factors, as well as with genetic factors.

Extrapolation to a large population of the precise contribution of a particular trait, such as vegetarianism, to interindividual variations in the rate of drug elimination observed in a selected, small study population can be hazardous. Such extrapolations should be accompanied by a demonstration that the frequency of the particular trait in the study group is similar to its frequency in the larger population. Without such a demonstration, the quantitative contribution of the trait cannot legitimately be extrapolated from the small study group to the large population.

The simultaneous contributions of multiple genetic and environmental factors to the particular drug-metabolizing activity of a given individual, as well as the change in relative importance of these different factors with time and condition, such as during aging, fever, disease, dietary change, drug administration, and acute or chronic exposure to environmental chemicals, make it exceedingly difficult to quantify the relative influence of the numerous factors involved at any given time, other than in a transient, relatively basal state. Also, for these reasons, carefully controlled studies are required.

SUMMARY

Pharmacogenetics deals with the genetic causes of variability among patients in response to drug therapy. Pharmacogenetic conditions may be divided into two general categories: (1) genetic conditions probably transmitted as single factors altering the way the *body acts on drugs*, and (2) genetic conditions probably transmitted as single factors altering the way *drugs act on the body*. Pharmacogenetics helps explain, at least in part, what often has been previously referred to as an idiosyncratic response by an individual to a particular medication. Specific genetic conditions can significantly influence the outcome of drug therapy and warrant special consideration. Familiarity with the concepts of pharmacogenetics will enable the nurse to more effectively plan nursing care for patients in whom genetic makeup predisposes an idiosyncratic response to drug therapy.

BIBLIOGRAPHY

Alexanderson, B., Price Evans, D.A., & Sjoqvist, F. Steady-state plasma levels of nortriptyline in twins: influence of genetic factors and drug therapy. *British Medical Journal*, 1969, *4*, 764-768.

Andreasen, P.B., Frøland, A., Skøvsted, L., Andersen, S.A., & Hauge, M. Diphenylhydantoin half-life in man and its inhibition by phenylbutazone: the role of genetic factors. *Acta Medica Scandinavica*, 1973, *193*, 561-564.

Cascorbi, H.F., Vesell, E.S., Blake, D.A., & Helrich, M. Genetic and environmental control of halothane metabolism in twins. *Clinical Pharmacology and Therapeutics*, 1971, *12*, 50-55.

Endrenyi, L., Inaba, T., & Kalow, W. Genetic study of amobarbital elimination based on its kinetics in twins. *Clinical Pharmacology and Therapeutics*, 1976, *20*, 701-714.

Kalow, W., Kadar, D., Inaba, T., & Tang, B.K. A case of deficiency of N-hydroxylation of amobarbital. *Clinical Pharmacology and Therapeutics*, 1977, *21*, 530-535.

Kopun, M., & Propping, P. The kinetics of ethanol absorption and elimination in twins and supplementary repetitive experiments in singleton subjects. *European Journal of Clinical Pharmacology*, 1977, *11*, 337-344.

O'Reilly, R.A. The second reported kindred with hereditary resistance to oral anticoagulant drugs. *New England Journal of Medicine*, 1970, *282*, 1448-1451.

O'Reilly, R.A., Aggeler, P.M., Hoag, M.S., Leong, L.S., & Kropatkin, M.L. Hereditary transmission of exceptional resistance to coumarin anticoagulant drugs: first reported kindred. *New England Journal of Medicine*, 1964, *271*, 809-815.

Vesell, E.S. Factors altering the responsiveness of mice to hexobarbital. *Pharmacology*, 1968, *1*, 81-97.

Vesell, E.S. Advances in pharmacogenetics. *Progress in Medical Genetics*, 1973, *9*, 291-367.

Vesell, E.S. Genetic and environmental factors affecting drug disposition in man. *Clinical Pharmacology and Therapeutics*, 1977, *22*, 659-679.

Vesell, E.S. Twin studies in pharmacogenetics. *Human Genetics*, 1978, *S1*, 19-30.

Vesell, E.S. Pharmacogenetics: multiple interactions between genes and environment as determinants of drug response. *American Journal of Medicine*, 1979, *66*, 183-187.

Vesell, E.S. Intraspecies differences in frequency of genes directly affecting drug disposition: the individual factor in drug response. *Pharmacological Reviews*, 1979, *30*, 555-563.

Vesell, E.S., & Page, J.G. Genetic control of drug levels in man: phenylbutazone. *Science*, 1968a, *159*, 1479-1480.

Vesell, E.S., & Page, J.G. Genetic control of drug levels in man: antipyrine. *Science*, 1968b, *161*, 72-73.

Vesell, E.S., & Page, J.G. Genetic control of dicumarol levels in man. *Journal of Clinical Investigation*, 1968c, *47*, 2657-2663.

Vesell, E.S., Page, J.G., & Passananti, G.T. Genetic and environmental factors affecting ethanol metabolism in man. *Clinical Pharmacology and Therapeutics*, 1971, *12*, 192-201.

Drug Interactions

Philip D. Hansten

Over the past two decades, there has been increasing awareness that certain drug combinations can produce adverse effects or the inhibition of a desired drug response. In many health care settings nurses have the first opportunity to observe the unwanted effects of drug interactions; thus it is important that they have a basic understanding of how drugs interact. This chapter will explore the fundamental principles of drug interactions, many of which have a direct application to the practical management of drug interaction problems in specific patients. Note that many chapters throughout this book contain tables (i.e., Clinically Significant Drug Interactions in the medication chapters of Sections III through XV) describing specific interactions of the drugs discussed in those chapters. Incompatibilities of drugs in intravenous solutions are discussed in Appendix IV of this text and will not be considered here.

CLINICAL IMPORTANCE OF DRUG INTERACTIONS

The impact of drug-drug interactions on public health is still a matter of some debate. Epidemiologic studies of drug interactions have been conducted, but the results have been highly variable and have not allowed accurate estimates of the incidence of adverse drug interactions. However, several patterns have emerged from these reports. First, it has been found that many patients receive *potentially* interacting drugs, whether these patients are hospitalized, ambulatory, or in a nursing home. Second, relatively few of the patients who receive potentially interacting drugs actually develop significant adverse effects. Third, it has become obvious that the adverse effects of drug-drug interactions that do occur are infrequently recognized as such by the health care professionals caring for the patient. This is unfortunate because it is clear that some individual patients develop serious difficulties when the interactive potential of certain drug combinations is not recognized.

CLINICAL CHARACTERISTICS OF DRUG INTERACTIONS

For the nurse to deal effectively with potential drug interaction problems in specific patients, it is necessary to appreciate some of the general characteristics of drug interactions.

1. *It is rarely necessary to avoid giving interacting drug combinations.* Very few drug interactions constitute absolute contraindications. The adverse consequences of drug interactions can nearly always be prevented by adjusting drug dosage, by changing dosing times to minimize mixing in the gastrointestinal (GI) tract, or by monitoring the patient more carefully for evidence of the interaction.
2. *Few interactions cause immediate reactions.* The adverse effects of drug interactions usually occur gradually over several days to 1 week or more. There are some interactions that do occur acutely within 15 or 20 minutes of administration, but such reactions are rare.
3. *Large interpatient variability.* A striking feature of most drug interactions is the enormous variation in response from patient to patient. It is usually difficult to predict whether a given patient will manifest an interaction and, if so, to what degree.

MECHANISMS OF DRUG INTERACTIONS

Most drug interaction mechanisms fall into one of two broad categories: pharmacokinetic or pharmacodynamic. Pharmacokinetic interactions include those in which one drug affects the absorption, distribution, metabolism, or excretion of another drug. Pharmacodynamic interactions result from the combined pharmacologic effects of two or more drugs, usually resulting in additive, potentiated, or antagonistic effects. It should be noted that some drug interactions involve multiple mechanisms, and some interactions involve mechanisms that are poorly under-

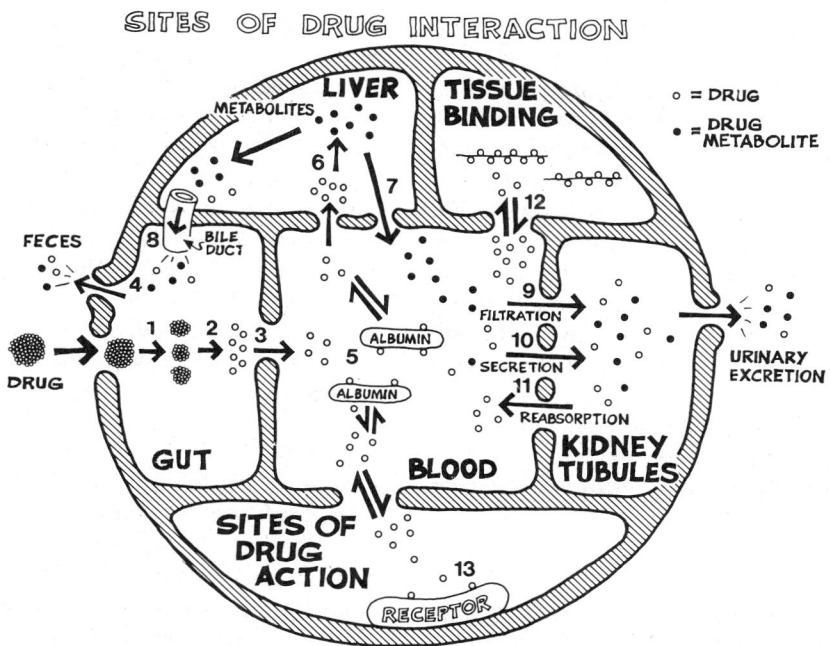

SITES OF DRUG INTERACTION

FIGURE 10-1. **Drugs may interact at a variety of sites within the body. The process of gastrointestinal absorption is represented by disintegration (1), dissolution (2), and absorption across the gut wall (3). Elimination of drug or metabolites in the feces is represented in 4. Some drugs may interact at sites of binding to serum albumin (5). Hepatic metabolism of some drugs (6) may be enhanced or inhibited by concurrent drug therapy. Metabolites formed in the liver may return to the blood (7) or undergo biliary excretion (8). Several drug disposition processes in the kidney are susceptible to drug interaction, including glomerular filtration (9), active tubular secretion (10), and passive tubular reabsorption (11). Tissue binding of one drug may be affected by another (12). Finally, drugs may have additive or antagonistic pharmacologic effects through action on receptors (13).**

stood. Using Figure 10-1 as a model, specific drug interaction mechanisms are described.

Absorption

When a solid dosage form, such as a tablet, arrives in the GI tract, disintegration takes place, resulting in smaller particles (Figure 10-1, *1*), followed by dissolution into individual molecules (Figure 10-1, *2*). It is only after the drug is in solution that it can be absorbed into the blood (Figure 10-1, *3*). The proportion of the drug that is not absorbed is subsequently excreted in the feces (Figure 10-1, *4*). Few clinically significant drug interactions seem to occur through interference with drug disintegration or dissolution. Instead, absorption interactions usually occur when the dissolved drug is adsorbed on a drug with a very large surface area such as antacids, kaolin-pectin, charcoal, or attapulgite (found in some antidiarrheal mixtures). Alteration in GI motility by a drug may also alter the absorption of other drugs. A drug that slows gut motility, such as

an anticholinergic, may *increase* absorption of a drug that is not very soluble by simply giving the poorly soluble drug more time to dissolve. For example, the absorption of the poorly soluble drug nitrofurantoin may be increased if given in the presence of an anticholinergic such as propantheline.

In summary, the majority of clinically significant absorption drug interactions occur with the use of high-surface-area drugs such as antacids and kaolin-pectin. When possible, one should administer these adsorbing agents in such a way as to minimize their contact with other drugs in the GI tract. This usually can be accomplished by spacing the doses of the interacting drugs.

Protein binding

After gaining access to the blood, most drugs are bound to a greater or lesser extent to plasma proteins (Figure 10-1, *5*). The drug thus bound does not exert a pharmacologic effect, nor is it as easily excreted by the kidneys or metabolized by the liver. Hence, the protein binding of drugs in the plasma is much like a reservoir, with the release of the drug from binding sites occurring as the concentration of unbound (free) drug in the plasma decreases because of metabolism, renal excretion, or tissue binding. The potential for drug interaction occurs when two drugs compete for plasma protein binding sites. When this occurs, the free plasma level of one or both drugs increases and can result in more of the drug being available to interact with receptors, resulting in an increased pharmacologic (or toxic) effect. However, in such cases liver metabolism and kidney excretion also tend to be increased, and the enhanced pharmacologic effect usually returns to normal after several days to 1 week or more, even if the interacting drugs continue to be given in the same dose.

Metabolism

The primary site of drug metabolism is the liver, where drug molecules are generally made more water soluble and thus are more easily excreted by the kidneys (Figure 10-1, 6, 7). Some drugs can stimulate the production of hepatic drug-metabolizing enzymes, especially those enzymes involved in the oxidative metabolism of drugs. Such enzyme stimulators are called enzyme inducers. Examples of enzyme-inducing drugs follow.

Examples of enzyme-inducing drugs

Barbiturates	Phenytoin
Carbamazepine	Primidone
Glutethimide	Rifampin

The pharmacologic effect of certain other drugs may be substantially reduced by the concurrent use of an enzyme-inducing drug. Examples would include the reduction in the anticoagulant response to oral anticoagulants with the concurrent use of a barbiturate, and reduction in the effect of corticosteroids in the presence of phenytoin therapy. It should be noted that enzyme induction takes place gradually and usually requires 7 to 10 days for the maximal effects to be seen. Similarly, it generally takes 1 to 2 weeks for the effects of enzyme induction to dissipate fully.

Whereas some drugs are able to stimulate drug metabolism by the liver, others tend to inhibit these processes. Examples of enzyme-inhibiting drugs follow.

Examples of enzyme-inhibiting drugs

Chloramphenicol	Methyldopa
Cimetidine	Metronidazole
Disulfiram	Phenylbutazone
Isoniazid	Sulfonamides

When one of these inhibitors is used concurrently with a drug susceptible to enzyme inhibition, the blood level and pharmacologic effect of the latter drug may be increased (e.g., phenytoin intoxication may occur if an enzyme inhibitor such as chloramphenicol is concurrently taken). Unlike enzyme induction, which develops slowly over 1 week or more, enzyme inhibition generally occurs much more quickly. In some cases, clinical evidence of an interaction involving the inhibition of drug metabolism may be seen within 1 to 2 days of starting the inhibiting drug (see Chapter 5, "Drug Metabolism and Elimination," for additional details on drug metabolism).

Renal excretion

As previously stated, the kidney is the primary route of excretion of the more water-soluble drug metabolites formed in the liver. For some drugs, excretion by the kidneys without prior hepatic metabolism is an important route of disposition. Such drugs arrive in the kidney tubules via glomerular filtration (Figure 10-1, 9), active tubular secretion (Figure 10-1, 10), or by both processes. Because serum albumin does not normally cross the glomerulus, the drug bound to albumin tends to remain in the blood. However, competition for plasma protein binding between two drugs can increase the amount of free drug available for glomerular filtration. Only certain drugs are actively secreted into the renal tubules. Examples of drugs that may interact via active tubular secretion follow.

Examples of drugs that may interact via active tubular secretion

Cephalosporins	Probenecid
Methotrexate	Salicylates
Penicillins	Sulfinpyrazone
Phenylbutazone	Thiazide diuretics

When two or more of these drugs are given concurrently, there may be interference with the secretory process, resulting in higher blood levels of one or both drugs.

Another potential site of drug interaction in the kidney involves the process of reabsorption from the renal tubules back into the blood (Figure 10-1, 11). Because the reabsorption process involves passing through lipid membranes, a more lipid-soluble drug would tend to be reabsorbed more readily. For certain drugs that are weak bases, a more alkaline urine would increase the proportion of the drug in the nonionized (i.e., more lipid soluble) form and would tend to promote reabsorption with resultant elevated blood levels. Conversely, a more acid urine would result in more of the weak base being in the ionized (i.e., more water soluble) form and reabsorption would decrease, resulting in lowered blood levels. Examples of weak base drugs that have been shown to be affected by changes in urinary pH include amphetamines, methadone, and quinidine. A patient on quinidine, for example, may develop quinidine toxicity if given another drug that increases the alkalinity of the urine. The behavior of certain weak acids susceptible to reabsorption interactions is the opposite. With weak acids, an alkaline urine would tend to reduce reabsorption back into the blood, resulting in a reduction in blood levels (e.g., a patient receiving large doses of aspirin for arthritis may develop reduced blood salicylate levels with the administration of a drug that alkalinizes the urine).

Tissue binding

Most drugs are bound, to a greater or lesser extent, to the various tissues of the body (Figure 10-1, *12*). The concurrent use of other drugs may alter this binding (e.g., one of the mechanisms by which quinidine is able to substantially increase blood levels of digoxin is by reducing the binding of digoxin to peripheral tissues such as skeletal muscle). However, there are relatively few proven clinical examples of tissue-binding interactions.

Pharmacologic interactions

When two or more drugs with similar pharmacologic effects are given concurrently, one would expect to see an increase in the intensity of the pharmacologic response. Such interactions may or may not involve an action by more than one drug on the same receptor. Conversely, the concurrent use of drugs with opposing pharmacologic activity may result in an antagonism of the pharmacologic effect. When pharmacologic interactions are considered, it is important to consider the secondary and the primary pharmacologic effect(s) for which the drug was given (e.g., the concurrent use of several drugs with secondary anticholinergic effects may result in intestinal ileus, urinary retention, and blurred vision). Pharmacologic drug interactions are relatively common in clinical practice. If they are anticipated and proper precautions are taken, they may be innocuous or even beneficial. If not anticipated, or at least quickly diagnosed, they can occasionally result in a serious adverse drug interaction.

NURSING IMPLICATIONS OF DRUG INTERACTIONS

With an understanding of the processes involved in drug interactions, the nurse can be involved in both the prevention and the early detection of adverse drug interactions in specific patients.

Prevention

If the nurse is aware that a potentially interacting drug combination has been prescribed, he or she may be in a position to inform the prescriber before the interacting combination is administered. As mentioned previously, it is usually not necessary to avoid the concurrent use of interacting drugs. However, some other measures such as a dosage adjustment or closer laboratory or clinical monitoring may reduce the likelihood of untoward effects. Another situation in which the nurse may be involved in preventing drug interactions is in GI absorption interactions. By separating the dosing times of the interacting drugs, the nurse may be able to minimize the importance of many of these interactions.

Detection

For many adverse drug interactions, early identification of the problem is important to reduce the likelihood of serious effects. Some of the more serious drug interactions reported in the literature involved those patients where the interaction was misdiagnosed. In many situations the nurse is the first health care professional to observe the adverse results of a drug interaction. Thus, a working knowledge of drug interactions is useful to any nurse directly involved in patient care.

IMPORTANT INTERACTING DRUGS

Certain drugs are more likely than others to be involved in adverse drug interactions. This is largely because of the intrinsic properties of these drugs that tend to promote interactions. The following discussion covers specific drugs and drug classes that have a high interactive potential and includes a description of those properties that tend to promote interactions with these drugs. Specific examples of important interactions involving these drugs will also be given.

Alcohol

Alcohol has variable effects on drug metabolism, depending on the amount and duration of alcohol intake. Chronic ingestion of large amounts of alcohol tends to stimulate hepatic microsomal drug metabolism. However, any person who is acutely intoxicated will tend to metabolize concurrently administered drugs *less* rapidly. Also, chronic alcoholics with serious associated liver disease may not be able to me-

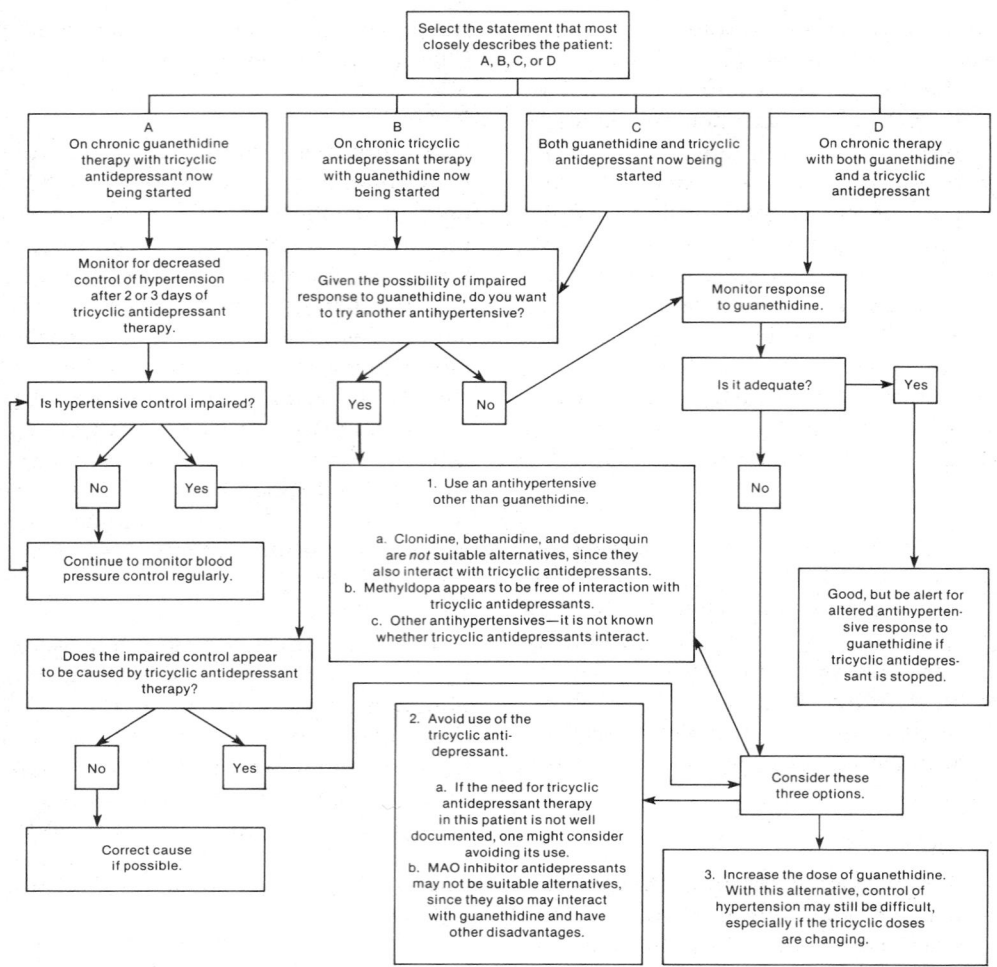

FIGURE 10-2. Evaluation of drug interactions in specific patients. Once it has been determined that a patient is receiving a potentially harmful interacting drug combination, one must address two important questions. First, can the interaction be essentially disregarded because the situation for this patient is such that the risk of adverse effects is minimal? Second, if the interaction cannot be disregarded, what is the appropriate course of action to minimize the likelihood of adverse consequences? The algorithm for the interaction between guanethidine and tricyclic antidepressants demonstrates the process of assessing risk and determining a course of action. Note that the algorithm addresses factors such as sequence of administration, drug dosage, patient monitoring, and use of alternative noninteracting drugs.

tabolize drugs normally. Because alcohol is a central nervous system (CNS) depressant, it may exhibit additive effects with other agents that depress the CNS. Finally, some drugs are capable of sensitizing the patient to alcohol, resulting in a disulfiram-like (Antabuse) reaction with findings such as flushing, tachycardia, nausea, and dyspnea.

Alcohol interactions	Result
CNS depressants	Additive CNS depression
Sensitizing agents	Disulfiram-like symptoms
Chloral hydrate	
Chlorpropamide	
Disulfiram	
Metronidazole (possibly)	

Antacids

Antacids have a large surface area on which concomitantly administered drugs may be adsorbed, decreasing absorption from the GI tract.

Antacid interactions	Result
Digoxin	Possibly reduced GI absorption of digoxin
Tetracyclines	Reduced GI absorption of tetracyclines (except for doxycycline)

Anticholinergics

Anticholinergics tend to reduce GI motility, which may increase the bioavailability of poorly soluble drugs (e.g., nitrofurantoin) and reduce the bioavailability of drugs degraded within the GI tract (e.g., levodopa). In addition, the combined use of more than one drug with anticholinergic properties may result in adverse reactions such as urinary retention, paralytic ileus, tachycardia, and blurred vision.

Anticholinergic interactions	Result
Combined anticholinergics	Excessive anticholinergic effect (e.g., paralytic ileus, urinary retention)
Levodopa	Reduced absorption of intact levodopa

Barbiturates

Barbiturates are enzyme inducers and can stimulate the hepatic microsomal metabolism of several other drugs. One may also see additive effects when barbiturates are given with other CNS depressants.

Barbiturate interactions	Result
Increased metabolism of: Anticoagulants (oral) Antidepressants (tricyclic) Beta-adrenergic blockers Contraceptives (oral) Corticosteroids Doxycycline Phenothiazines Quinidine	Reduced effect of drug given with barbiturate
Valproic acid	Increased barbiturate effect

Beta-adrenergic blockers

Nonspecific beta-adrenergic blockers such as propranolol may alter the response to concurrently administered sympathomimetics such as epinephrine. More specific beta-adrenergic blockers such as metoprolol seem less likely to do so. Also, when given orally, some beta-adrenergic blockers undergo extensive metabolism in the first pass through the liver. Thus, their rate of metabolism may be altered by other drugs that can increase or decrease first-pass metabolism. Finally, beta-adrenergic blockers may alter glucose homeostasis, resulting in inhibition of the return of blood glucose to normal following hypoglycemia.

Beta-adrenergic blocker interactions	Result
Antidiabetic agents	Hypoglycemic episodes prolonged; inhibition of signs of hypoglycemia; hypertension during hypoglycemia
Barbiturates	Decreased beta-adrenergic blocker effect
Furosemide	Increased propranolol effect
Indomethacin	Decreased antihypertensive effect of beta-adrenergic blocker
Sympathomimetics (especially epinephrine)	Hypertension, especially with nonspecific beta-adrenergic blockers

Cholestyramine and colestipol

Cholestyramine and colestipol are designed to bind with bile acids in the GI tract, but may also bind with drugs that are present in the gut at the same time. Although orally administered drugs would be expected to be most likely to interact, parenterally administered drugs that undergo enterohepatic circulation (e.g., warfarin) may also be bound in the gut by cholestyramine or colestipol.

Cholestyramine and colestipol interactions	Result
Coumarin anticoagulants	Decreased anticoagulant response
Dextrothyroxine	Decreased dextrothyroxine effect
Digitoxin	Decreased digitoxin effect
Levothyroxine	Decreased levothyroxine absorption

Cimetidine

Cimetidine is capable of inhibiting the hepatic metabolism of several other drugs. It has also been proposed that cimetidine may have an additive effect with other drugs (e.g., carmustine, phenytoin), which may cause bone marrow depression.

Cimetidine interactions	Result
Benzodiazepines (chlordiazepoxide and diazepam, but not lorazepam or oxazepam)	Enhanced benzodiazepine effect
Coumarin anticoagulants	Increased anticoagulant response
Phenytoin	Increased phenytoin effect
Propranolol	Increased propranolol effect
Theophylline	Increased theophylline effect

Corticosteroids

Corticosteroids are susceptible to enzyme induction. Thus, a patient with a disease controlled by corticosteroid therapy may develop an exacerbation of that disease if an enzyme inducer is given. Some corticosteroids can also promote renal potassium excretion, thus adding to the hypokalemic effect of other drugs. The diabetogenic effect of corticosteroids may affect antidiabetic drug requirements.

Corticosteroid interactions	Result
Antidiabetic agents	Increased requirements for antidiabetic drugs

Enzyme inducers
  Barbiturates
  Phenytoin
  Rifampin
	Decreased corticosteroid effect

Potassium-losing diuretics	Hypokalemia

Contraceptives (oral)

Oral contraceptives that reduce the circulating level of estrogenic hormones may result in menstrual irregularities such as breakthrough bleeding and, more importantly, may result in unwanted pregnancy. Enzyme inducers may stimulate the metabolism of oral contraceptives. Another site of interaction is the GI tract. An important pathway for the disposition of estrogens is conjugation in the liver and excretion into the intestine via the bile. Intestinal bacteria then hydrolyze the conjugated estrogen, leaving free drug to be reabsorbed, thus maintaining the serum level of estrogen. Antibiotics, which reduce the population of these bacteria, may interfere with this enterohepatic circulation of estrogen, resulting in lower serum estrogen levels. Oral contraceptives with a low hormonal content are probably more susceptible to both enzyme inducers and antibiotics.

Oral contraceptive interactions	Result

Antibiotics
  Ampicillin (probably)
  Neomycin (theoretically)
  Tetracycline (possibly)
	Menstrual irregularities; unplanned pregnancies

Enzyme inducers
  Barbiturates
  Phenytoin
  Rifampin
	Menstrual irregularities; unplanned pregnancies

Coumarin anticoagulants

Coumarin anticoagulants are metabolized by hepatic microsomal enzymes and are susceptible to both enzyme induction and enzyme inhibition. They are also extensively bound to plasma proteins and may be displaced by other highly bound drugs. Further, alteration in the effect of coumarin anticoagulants may have serious consequences because an enhanced response may produce bleeding and a reduced response may produce a thrombotic episode.

Coumarin anticoagulant interactions	Result

Inhibiting agents
  Barbiturates
  Carbamazepine
  Cholestyramine
  Gluthethimide
  Griseofulvin
  Rifampin
	Increased risk of thrombosis; possible bleeding if inhibitor discontinued without reducing anticoagulant dose

Potentiating agents
  Anabolic steroids
  Cimetidine
  Clofibrate
  Disulfiram
  Metronidazole
  Phenylbutazone
  Salicylates
  Sulfinpyrazone
  Thyroid hormones
	Enhanced anticoagulation, possible bleeding

Digitalis glycosides

A drug-induced electrolyte imbalance (e.g., hypokalemia) may increase the likelihood of digitalis toxicity. Also, digoxin is susceptible to inhibition of GI absorption by various other drugs. Because the tissue binding and renal excretion of digoxin may be reduced by quinidine, the possibility must be considered that other drugs may have a similar effect on digoxin. Hepatic metabolism is more important for the disposition of digitoxin than it is for digoxin; thus, enzyme inducers may stimulate digitoxin metabolism.

Digitalis interactions	Result

Absorption inhibitors
  Antacids (oral)
  Cholestyramine
  Colestipol
  Kaolin-pectin
  Sulfasalazine
	Reduced digoxin effect in some patients

Potassium depleting agents
  Amphotericin B
  Corticosteroids
  Potassium-losing diuretics
	Increased likelihood of digitalis toxicity

Quinidine	Increased digoxin serum levels; possible digoxin toxicity

Hypoglycemics (oral)

Sulfonylurea hypoglycemics seem to be susceptible to inhibitors of hepatic microsomal enzymes such as phenylbutazone and sulfonamides. Also, some sulfonylureas may be displaced from plasma protein-binding sites by other highly bound drugs. Finally, the dosage requirement for oral hypoglycemics may be altered by drugs with intrinsic hyperglycemic or hypoglycemic effects.

Oral hypoglycemic interactions	*Result*
Chloramphenicol	Enhanced hypoglycemia with chlorpropamide and tolbutamide
Clofibrate	Enhanced hypoglycemic effect
Hyperglycemic agents Corticosteroids Diazoxide Estrogens Nicotinic acid (large doses) Thiazide diuretics	Increased dosage requirement of antidiabetic drug
Hypoglycemic agents Alcohol (large doses) Anabolic steroids Guanethidine Monoamine oxidase (MAO) inhibitors Propranolol Salicylates (large doses)	Decreased dosage requirement of antidiabetic drug
Phenylbutazone	Enhanced hypoglycemia with acetazolamide, chlorpropamide, and tolbutamide
Sulfonamides	Enhanced hypoglycemic effect with some sulfonamides

Indomethacin

The ability of indomethacin to reduce prostaglandin activity may be responsible for its interaction with diuretics, beta-adrenergic blockers, lithium, and sympathomimetics.

Indomethacin interactions	*Result*
Beta-adrenergic blockers	Reduced antihypertensive effects
Diuretics Furosemide Thiazides	Reduced natriuretic and antihypertensive effects
Lithium carbonate	Increased serum lithium levels; possible lithium toxicity
Sympathomimetics	Hypertensive reaction with phenylpropanolamine; possibly with other sympathomimetics

Kaolin-pectin

Because of its large surface area and adsorbing properties, kaolin-pectin may adsorb drugs administered orally concomitantly. Thus, doses of other drugs should be spaced so that mixing with kaolin-pectin in the GI tract is minimized.

Kaolin-pectin interactions	*Result*
Digoxin	Reduced digoxin serum levels and effect
Lincomycin	Reduced lincomycin effect

Levodopa

Some of the orally administered levodopa appears to be degraded within the gut before it reaches sites of absorption. Thus, agents that slow GI motility may increase intraluminal degradation and thereby reduce serum levels of levodopa. Further, some drugs such as phenytoin, papaverine, and the phenothiazines may directly antagonize the antiparkinsonism effects of levodopa. The addition of carbidopa to levodopa therapy effectively prevents the inhibition of levodopa by pyridoxine and prevents the hypertensive reaction that occurs with the concurrent use of levodopa and MAO inhibitors.

Levodopa interactions	*Result*
Anticholinergics	Reduced levodopa absorption
Antagonists of CNS effects of levodopa Clonidine Papaverine Phenytoin Phenothiazines	Reduced antiparkinsonism effect

Lithium carbonate

Agents that deplete sodium such as diuretics may result in lithium carbonate retention with elevated serum lithium levels and possibly toxicity. Other drugs may produce signs of lithium intoxication in the absence of any change in the serum lithium level; this probably results from combined effects on the CNS.

Lithium interactions	*Result*
Indomethacin	Lithium intoxication
Methyldopa	CNS lithium toxicity (serum lithium may not be elevated)
Sodium-depleting diuretics	Lithium intoxication

MAO inhibitors

Because MAO inhibitors increase adrenergic neuron stores of norepinephrine, administration of indirect acting sympathomimetics such as amphetamines and phenylpropanolamine may release large amounts of norepinephrine, resulting in a hypertensive crisis. Tyramine found in foods may have a similar effect. Direct-acting sympathomimetics such as epinephrine and norepinephrine appear to be less dangerous than indirect-acting agents in the presence of MAO inhibitors. MAO inhibitors may also exhibit intrinsic hypoglycemic effects, thus affecting dosage requirements for antidiabetic drugs.

MAO inhibitor interactions	Result
Antidiabetic agents	Enhanced hypoglycemia
Direct-acting sympathomimetics	
Epinephrine	Little or no interaction
Levarterenol	Little or no interaction
Phenylephrine	Hypertensive crisis
Indirect-acting sympathomimetics	Hypertensive crisis
Amphetamines	
Ephedrine	
Metaraminol	
Phenylpropanolamine	
Pseudoephedrine	
Levodopa	Hypertensive crisis (but not if patient is also receiving carbidopa)
Meperidine	Hypertension, excitation, rigidity

Phenylbutazone

Phenylbutazone can interact by a variety of different mechanisms. It can inhibit the metabolism of other drugs such as warfarin and phenytoin. Paradoxically, phenylbutazone also seems capable of *stimulating* drug metabolism; one may see reduced serum digitoxin levels in the presence of phenylbutazone. Phenylbutazone can also interact at the level of the kidney by altering the renal excretion of some other drugs such as acetohexamide and possibly methotrexate. Phenylbutazone is also extensively bound to plasma albumin and may be involved in plasma protein-binding drug interactions. Finally, the ability of phenylbutazone to inhibit platelet function may increase the likelihood of bleeding if the patient is also receiving other drugs that impair hemostasis.

Phenylbutazone interactions	Result
Anticoagulants (oral)	Marked increase in hypoprothrombinemic response; bleeding
Digitoxin	Reduced digitoxin effect
Hypoglycemics (oral)	Enhanced hypoglycemic effect
Methotrexate	Possible methotrexate toxicity
Phenytoin	Increased phenytoin serum levels; possible phenytoin toxicity

Quinidine

The elimination of quinidine involves both hepatic metabolism and the excretion of unchanged drug in the urine. Drug interactions can affect both of these processes. Enzyme inducers stimulate the hepatic metabolism of quinidine, thus lowering serum quinidine levels. Also, the renal excretion of quinidine is pH dependent; a more alkaline urine promotes reabsorption of quinidine from renal tubules, thus increasing serum quinidine levels. Finally, quinidine

has been shown to displace digoxin from tissue-binding sites and also to reduce the excretion of digoxin. Thus, it seems possible that quinidine might affect other drugs similarly.

Quinidine interactions	Result
Digoxin	Increased digoxin serum levels; possible toxicity
Enzyme inducers	Reduced quinidine effect
Barbiturates	
Phenytoin	
Rifampin	
Urinary alkalinizers	Increased quinidine serum levels; possible toxicity
Acetazolamide	
Sodium bicarbonate	

Salicylates

When salicylates are given in larger doses (i.e., over 3 to 4 gm daily), two of their hepatic metabolic pathways become saturated, thus increasing the proportion of salicylate excreted unchanged in the urine. When this occurs, the pH of the urine becomes an important determinant of the rate of renal salicylate excretion. Thus, alkalinization of the urine tends to increase renal salicylate excretion, resulting in lower serum levels. Salicylates also may interact with drugs that are involved in active renal tubular secretion, such as methotrexate, probenecid, and phenylbutazone. The ability of aspirin (but not most other salicylates) to impair platelet function may increase the likelihood of bleeding if the patient is also receiving other drugs that impair hemostasis. Larger doses (i.e., over 3 to 4 gm a day) of aspirin or other salicylates may exhibit a hypoprothrombinemic effect. Aspirin has been shown to reduce the GI absorption of various other drugs (e.g., indomethacin), although the magnitude of the reduction is usually minor. Although aspirin has a reputation for displacing other drugs from plasma protein-binding sites, this mechanism seems seldom to cause clinically significant problems. Finally, the known adverse effects of aspirin on the GI tract may add to the effect of other drugs with similar properties (e.g., alcohol, corticosteroids).

Salicylate interactions	Result
Alcohol	Increased GI irritation
Anticoagulants (oral)	Increased bleeding tendency
Antidiabetic agents	Increased hypoglycemic effects in some patients
Heparin	Increased bleeding tendency
Methotrexate	Reduced methotrexate excretion; possible methotrexate toxicity
Probenecid	Reduced uricosuric effect of probenecid, particularly with arthritic doses of salicylates

SUMMARY

Most drug interaction mechanisms fall into one of two broad categories: (1) pharmacokinetic, and (2) pharmacodynamic. *Pharmacokinetic* interactions include those in which one drug affects the absorption, distribution, metabolism, or excretion of another drug. *Pharmacodynamic* interactions result from the combined pharmacologic effects of two or more drugs, usually resulting in additive, potentiated, or antagonistic effects. Although some drug interactions involve multiple mechanisms, the majority of interactions encountered in clinical practice involve the pharmacodynamic mechanism. Several general clinical characteristics of drug interactions have been noted: (1) it is rarely necessary to avoid giving interacting drug combinations (i.e., appropriate countermeasures can minimize the likelihood of adverse effects); (2) few interactions cause immediate reactions (i.e., most reactions from drug interactions occur over several days or more); and (3) large interpatient variability is noted (i.e., it is difficult to predict accurately whether a specific drug interaction will occur in a specific patient). In many situations, the nurse is the first health care professional to observe the adverse results of a drug interaction. With an understanding of the processes involved in drug interactions, the nurse can prevent and more readily detect adverse drug interactions.

BIBLIOGRAPHY

Drug interaction update. *The Medical Letter,* 1984, *26,* 11-14.

Gelehrter, T.D. Enzyme induction (part I). *New England Journal Medicine,* 1976, *294,* 522-526.

Gelehrter, T.D. Enzyme induction (part II). *New England Journal of Medicine,* 1976, *294,* 589-595.

Gelehrter, T.D. Enzyme induction (part III). *New England Journal of Medicine,* 1976, *294,* 646-651.

Hansten, P.D. *Drug interactions* (5th ed.). Philadelphia: Lea & Febiger, 1985.

Jinks, M.J., Hansten, P.D., & Hirschman, J.L. Drug interaction population. *American Journal of Hospital Pharmacy,* 1979, *36,* 923-927.

Jusko W.J., & Gretch, M. Plasma and tissue protein binding of drugs in pharmacokinetics. *Drug Metabolism Reviews,* 1976, *5,* 43-140.

LeSage, J., Beck, C., & Johnson, M. Nursing diagnosis of drug incompatibility: a conceptual approach. *Advances in Nursing Science,* 1979, *1,* 63-77.

May F.E., Stewart R.B., & Cluff L.E. Drug interactions and multiple drug administration. *Clinical Pharmacology and Therapeutics,* 1977, *22,* 322-328.

McElnay, J.D., & D'Arcy, P.F. Sites and mechanisms of drug interactions. I. In vitro, intestinal and metabolic interactions. *International Journal of Pharmaceutics,* 1980, *5,* 167-185.

Mitchell, G.W., Stanaszek, W.F., & Nichols, N.B. *American Journal of Hospital Pharmacy,* 1979, *36,* 653-657.

Simborg, D.W. Medication prescribing on a university medical service—the incidence of drug combinations with potential adverse interactions. *Johns Hopkins Medical Journal,* 1976, *139,* 23-26.

Wightman, E.R. Medicine interactions observed in a year of ward pharmacy. *Journal of Clinical Pharmacology,* 1978, *3,* 183-188.

CHAPTER 11

Drug Toxicity

David S. Tatro
Sharon D. Ow-Wing
Debbie L. Huie

In general, when drug therapy is indicated, the expected benefits should outweigh the potential risks. The exact frequency with which adverse drug reactions accompany drug therapy is not known. However, numerous studies and extrapolations have cast some light on the magnitude of the adverse drug reaction problem.

To date, the most meaningful statistics associated with the incidence of adverse drug reactions come from the Boston Collaborative Drug Surveillance Program (Jick, 1974). The findings from this group are based on data from patients admitted to a general medical service and are summarized as follows.

1. During their hospital stay, 30% of general medical patients experience at least one adverse drug reaction.
2. Of all hospital admissions to general medical services, 3% are the result of adverse drug reactions.
3. Deaths caused by adverse drug reactions occur in nearly 0.3% of hospitalized general medical patients.

Adverse drug effects reportedly occur with the highest incidence in females, in the elderly, and in patients with impaired renal function. Drugs most frequently implicated in causing hospital admission include antibiotics, anticoagulants, aspirin, corticosteroids, digoxin, and diuretics. Digoxin and cytotoxic agents are most frequently named in association with drug reactions during a patient's hospital stay in a medical ward.

ADVERSE DRUG REACTIONS

There is no commonly agreed on definition of an adverse drug reaction. In this chapter, an adverse drug reaction is considered to be any drug effect that is not intended when the agent is used for diagnosis, treatment, or prophylaxis. Thus, illicit use of drugs will not be discussed (see Chapter 12, "Drug Abuse and Addiction"). A clinically significant adverse reaction is any unexpected or unintended response to a drug requiring an alteration in therapy, such as discontinuation of the drug or administration of an antidote.

Over the years, adverse drug reactions have been receiving an increasing amount of attention. Because nurses are frequently the first to observe an adverse drug reaction, it is essential for them to be familiar with potential types of drug-induced diseases. Adverse drug reactions will be discussed according to the following classifications.

1. Side effects
2. Overdosage
3. Drug interactions
4. Laboratory test interferences

SIDE EFFECTS OF DRUGS

Three general subgroups of drug side effects will be considered: pharmacologic, idiosyncratic, and allergic.

Pharmacologic side effects. Pharmacologic side effects are dose-related actions of the drug and can occur in all patients, provided sufficient quantity of the drug is ingested. Most adverse pharmacologic drug reactions conform to a sigmoid or S-type response curve (Figure 11-1). Thus, a small number of patients will show an adverse reaction to low doses of a drug, and, as the dose is increased, the number of patients reacting increases. An example of this type of side effect is the troublesome drowsiness following administration of the antihistamine diphenhydramine. This side effect of sedation is frequently used clinically. It should be noted that some side effects, such as drowsiness following amitriptyline administration, subside with continued therapy.

Idiosyncratic side effects. Idiosyncratic reactions are usually considered to be a catchall category for

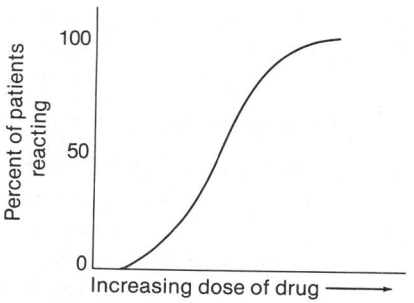

FIGURE 11-1. **Dose-response curve for pharmacologic side effects.**

inadequately understood side effects. As more clinical information becomes available, many drugs in this group may be reclassified based on the observed mechanism of action. Idiosyncratic reactions tend not to be dose-related, affect only a small portion of the total patient population, and are usually associated with genetic defects (see Chapter 9, "Genetic Factors Affecting Drug Response"). These genetic defects, frequently caused by excesses or deficiencies in specific enzymes, can lead patients to respond adversely to drugs. Patients vary in the rate at which they metabolize procainamide. For example, patients with decreased amounts of N-acetyltransferase, the liver enzyme responsible for inactivating procainamide, metabolize this drug more slowly. If slow metabolizers and rapid metabolizers receive the same dose of procainamide, toxic levels may accumulate more quickly in the slow metabolizer group. Indeed, patients who are slow acetylators of procainamide develop systemic lupus erythematosus more frequently than do patients who are rapid acetylators. Because each idiosyncratic reaction is genetically determined, a full understanding of the mechanism of a specific reaction requires information about both the genotypic and the phenotypic characteristics of the patient.

Allergic side effects. All allergic drug reactions are the result of an immune (antigen-antibody) response and do not occur with the first exposure to the agent. In general, allergic reactions involve the body's response to foreign or exogenous proteins (antigens). Because drugs are not usually protein, they do not, by themselves, act as antigens. However, following metabolism, drugs may combine with endogenous proteins to form reactive compounds, against which the body may produce antibodies. Following the initial sensitizing contact to the drug, subsequent exposure may produce an allergic hypersensitivity. This group of side effects is not pharmacologic and, therefore,

reactions are not dose-related and involve only a small portion of the total number of patients receiving the drug.

Allergic drug reactions manifest themselves in a wide variety of forms affecting different organs and tissues. For example, a drug allergy affecting the blood may produce agranulocytosis (e.g., chlorpromazine), thrombocytopenia (e.g., quinidine), or hemolysis (e.g., cephalothin). Based on their immunologic mechanism, allergic drug reactions may be classified into type I, type II, type III, and type IV.

Type I, anaphylactic reactions, are acute, life-threatening reactions, occurring within 30 minutes of drug exposure. Anaphylaxis may occur with all routes of administration, but is most frequently seen following parenteral use. Signs and symptoms may include hypotension, urticaria, bronchospasm, laryngeal edema, and increased gastrointestinal (GI) contractility. The reaction results from an antigen reacting with an antibody that is fixed to the surface of mast cells or basophils. Anaphylactic reactions are most frequently associated with penicillin. Drug treatment usually involves subcutaneous administration of epinephrine, intramuscular or intravenous diphenhydramine, and intravenous aminophylline. Following adequate volume replacement, administration of vasopressors may be indicated for profound and persistent hypotension.

Type II reactions are cytotoxic reactions in which the antigen (drug-protein combination) attaches to a cell surface. Circulating antibodies may then react with the antigen and destroy the cells. These drug reactions frequently result in damage to individual organs, such as the liver, kidney, and blood. This reaction is illustrated by thrombocytopenia induced by meprobamate and transfusion reactions.

Type III reactions involve circulating antigen-antibody complexes that may destroy various tissue. The best known example of this type of allergic reaction is serum sickness, which may be caused by such drugs as penicillin, phenytoin, and streptomycin. Symptoms may include rash, fever, nephritis, arthritis, and lymphadenopathy.

Type IV reactions are the delayed or tuberculin type in which the antigenic material produces tissue inflammation after interacting with antibodies that are attached to lymphocytes. Tuberculin skin reactions are an example of Type IV reactions.

In types II through IV reactions, the mainstay of treatment is to discontinue the offending agent and to treat the accompanying symptoms. Inflammatory reactions can be treated with salicylates or corticosteroids, whereas urticaria may be treated with antihistamines or epinephrine.

Allergic drug reactions are difficult to predict and difficult to prevent. A careful and complete drug history will allow one to avoid administering a medication to a patient reporting prior allergic symptoms to the drug.

Clinical considerations

Drug side effects can mimic almost any naturally occurring illness; therefore, distinguishing between a nondrug disease and a drug-induced illness may be extremely difficult. Constant awareness, careful patient interviews, and close monitoring of patients will enable the rapid detection of side effects. Diagnosis is facilitated by accurate patient, historical, physical, and laboratory information. Knowledge of certain factors aid in making an association between a drug and an adverse event. When considering a potential adverse drug reaction, one must assess if there is a reasonable temporal association between administration of the drug and occurrence of the reaction (i.e., was the medication given before the onset of the reaction?). In addition, other factors, which could contribute to the patient's reaction, such as the patient's clinical status, should be evaluated. Also, the results of a dechallenge should be observed (i.e., if the drug is discontinued, does the patient's condition improve?).

OVERDOSAGE

A drug overdosage, which is usually associated with elevated blood levels of the drug, can occur by various means. Frequently this will be the result of the deliberate ingestion of toxic amounts such as occurs with suicide attempts, accidental ingestion by children, or drug abuse. In other instances overdosage may result from impaired drug metabolism or excretion, allowing toxic amounts of the agent to accumulate in the body. Thus, patients with impaired renal function may show signs of gentamicin toxicity (e.g., ototoxicity), if the usual therapeutic dosages are administered. Careful monitoring of renal function and proper adjustment in dosage can easily circumvent these potential adverse reactions.

The signs and symptoms of overdosage generally manifest themselves as an exacerbation of the desired pharmacologic action of the drug (e.g., the severe and prolonged bleeding following excessive doses of the anticoagulant warfarin).

Clinical considerations

There are relatively few specific antidotes for treating overdosage (see Appendix V of this text for listings). Supportive therapy is the most important aspect of treatment. Care for the patient starts with supporting the cardiovascular and respiratory systems, as well as discontinuing the offending agent. Following these initial steps, attempts should be made to decrease the systemic availability of the drug by the most appropriate means: inducing vomiting, decreasing absorption, increasing elimination, or administering a pharmacologic antidote.

DRUG INTERACTIONS

Whenever a patient receives more than one medication, the possibility of a drug-drug interaction exists. Drug interactions occur by numerous mechanisms. The most common interactions involve cumulative or antagonistic effects resulting from multiple drug therapy (e.g., excessive sedation seen in a patient receiving flurazepam for sleep, narcotics for pain, diazepam for tension, and diphenhydramine for an allergy). Drugs may also interact pharmacokinetically to influence the absorption, metabolism, distribution, and elimination of one another. The mechanisms involved in these interactions are often complex and poorly understood (see Chapter 10, "Drug Interactions").

Interactions may result in either increases or decreases in the amount or rate of drug absorption. Thus, a drug that is absorbed very slowly may never achieve therapeutic levels. Oral administration of ferrous sulfate interferes with the GI absorption of tetracycline. This will lead to decreased serum levels of the antibiotic. Patients should not receive tetracycline and iron (or other divalent and trivalent cations) within 2 hours of each other.

The effects of one drug on the metabolism of a second are well documented. The concurrent administration of two drugs may lead to an interaction causing a decrease or an increase in the rate of metabolism. Decreased liver metabolism may be caused by reversible competition for the same enzyme system or an irreversible inhibition of the enzyme. Chloramphenicol decreases the metabolism of tolbutamide, resulting in an increase in the pharmacologic half-life of tolbutamide and the potential for prolonged and protracted hypoglycemia. Conversely, administration of one drug may increase the amount of liver enzymes available for metabolizing a second drug. To circumvent these interactions, it may be necessary to decrease the dosing interval, to increase the dosage, or to seek a suitable alternative agent. Hepatic enzyme induction is a reversible occurrence and once the enzyme stimulator is discontinued, the metabolism will revert to the predrug rate. Alcohol increases the rate of metabolism of tolbutamide, producing potentially decreased therapeutic effects of tolbutamide.

Many drugs are reversibly bound to plasma proteins. Concurrent administration of more than one drug bound to the same protein fraction may displace one or the other agent from its binding site. Drugs bound to plasma proteins are inactive pharmacologically; in addition, the bound form is not available for metabolism or excretion. That one drug displaces another from its binding site is insufficient to predict the pharmacologic outcome of an interaction. Not only will more amounts of the drug be free to exert its pharmacologic action, but additional amounts of the drug will also be available for metabolism, excretion, and redistribution to other tissues. For example, phenylbutazone displaces warfarin from its protein-binding site, which may produce severe bleeding.

Altered renal excretion is another means by which drugs may interact. Significant drug interactions involving interference with elimination have been reported. This may involve either enhancement or inhibition of excretion. Triamterene inhibits the renal elimination of potassium chloride, which may result in hyperkalemia. When possible, concomitant use of these two drugs should be avoided. However, if both drugs are administered, serum potassium levels should be monitored very carefully.

Clinical considerations

Whereas the concurrent administration of multiple drugs in the treatment of patients creates an environment in which drug interactions may occur, these interactions are seldom a contraindication to the use of either drug. Most potentially interacting drug combinations can be administered concomitantly if the patients are monitored and appropriate adjustments are made in the dose, dosing interval, or route of administration. Knowledge of the mechanism by which a drug interaction may occur will frequently enable one to circumvent clinically significant problems. (See Chapter 10, "Drug Interactions," for further details).

LABORATORY TEST INTERFERENCES

Many pharmaceutical products are capable of altering clinical laboratory tests. The adverse effects of drugs on laboratory tests are generally considered to occur by two mechanisms: (1) pharmacologic properties of the drug or (2) interference with the testing procedure. The former involves actual changes in laboratory tests, frequently resulting from a drug side effect, such as elevated serum glutamic oxaloacetic transaminase (SGOT) resulting from isoniazid hepatotoxicity, whereas interference with the testing procedure usually involves direct alterations in the obtained laboratory test value or interference with the laboratory test measurement by the drug or its metabolite(s). Thus, cephalothin may produce a black-brown or green-brown color with the use of Clinitest tablets, which could be misinterpreted as a positive test for glucose.

Clinical considerations

Altered laboratory tests may indicate the development of a drug side effect. A drug-induced cause should be considered in the differential diagnosis when unexpected or unexplained abnormal laboratory measurements, such as in renal and hepatic function tests, are present. Laboratory test alterations seldom result in invalid conclusions in general medical service patients. Routine monitoring of all patients for potential drug-induced alterations in any laboratory test is not warranted; however, routine monitoring of certain laboratory tests when patients are receiving specific drugs may be appropriate. Thus, periodic assessment of renal function is in order for patients receiving gentamicin therapy.

SPECIFIC ORGAN TOXICITY

Because drug reactions can mimic most naturally occurring diseases, making diagnosis difficult, awareness and identification of potential causative agents and modification of therapy is of prime importance. In this section, adverse effects of drugs on specific organ systems are discussed. Special attention has been given to those drugs implicated in causing organ toxicity.

The following categories of adverse drug reactions are considered.

1. Cutaneous
2. Fever
3. Hematologic
4. Hepatic
5. Ocular
6. Otic
7. Pulmonary
8. Renal
9. Sexual

Gastrointestinal and central nervous system toxicities have not been included because nearly all drugs have been implicated in causing nausea, vomiting, diarrhea, or drowsiness.

For comprehensive information regarding specific types of reactions occurring with a particular drug, the reader is referred to the Adverse Side Effects and Nursing Drug Digest of the medication chapters found in Sections III through XV of this text.

Cutaneous toxicity

Skin eruptions may be produced by almost any drug and, in many instances, a single drug may produce a variety of dermatoses, frequently making diagnosis difficult by mimicking common dermatologic diseases. Immediate identification of the offending agent, and modification of therapy, is of prime concern. The drug-induced cutaneous eruptions reviewed in this section are photosensitivity, acneform eruptions, alopecia, fixed drug reactions, toxic epidermal necrolysis, and erythema multiforme.

Photosensitivity. Drug-induced photosensitivity reactions require the presence of both the drug and a light source for the cutaneous eruptions to occur. When considering drug-induced photosensitivity reactions, it is important to differentiate between photoallergic and phototoxic mechanisms.

Photoallergic reactions: (1) are preceded by an initial sensitizing exposure; (2) are not related to the dose of the medication administered; (3) exhibit cross-sensitivity between chemically related compounds; (4) usually involve a light spectrum of longer wavelengths than phototoxic reactions; (5) may occur at distant dermatologic sites from those previously exposed to the offending agent; (6) take a wide variety of morphologic forms including sunburn-like reactions, urticarial lesions, erythematous papules or nodules, and bullous eruptions; and (7) occur within 2 days of exposure to the drug.

In contrast, phototoxic reactions: (1) may occur with the first exposure to the drug, usually within 6 hours; (2) occur at wavelengths close to the absorption peak of the drug; (3) are dose related; (4) do not exhibit cross-reactivity; and (5) are sunburn-type reactions, occurring only on the light-exposed areas of the skin.

Patients taking known photosensitizing drugs should be cautioned to avoid exposure to sunlight by wearing protective clothing and using chemical sunscreening agents.

Acneform eruptions. Although acneform eruptions resemble true acne, the drug-induced reactions are characterized by their sudden onset, absence of comedones, and involvement of unusual sites.

Alopecia. Hair loss induced by drugs may affect any portion of the body. However, because 90% of the scalp hairs are in the active phase of growth (anagen), it is here that the adverse effect is most notable.

Fixed eruptions. Fixed drug eruptions represent a hypersensitivity reaction in which repeated exposure to the causative agent produces lesions at the same, or almost identical, sites, as previously affected. Fixed eruptions are often characterized by erythematous, bullous, urticarial, or pruritic plaques. When the drug is discontinued, hyperpigmented areas may remain.

Toxic epidermal necrolysis. Toxic epidermal necrolysis is a life-threatening reaction, which in the early stages is characterized by skin eruptions of an erythematous and tender nature. This is followed by large flaccid bullae that easily rupture and peel. These lesions are predominantly in the epidermis, with little or no dermal involvement, and heal within 2 weeks, without residual scarring unless complicated by infection. When death occurs, it is frequently a result of a secondary infection. Toxic epidermal necrolysis is a hypersensitivity reaction. In addition to drugs, other etiologic factors that have been implicated as a cause of this reaction include bacterial metabolites and foods. However, irrespective of cause, the pathogenesis is the same.

Erythema multiforme. As implied by its name, erythema multiforme can involve variable skin lesions. Lesions involve the skin and mucous membranes, and include urticarial, macular, papular, vesicular, or purpuric eruptions. These reactions are most common in children and young adults. The duration of the reactions is 2 to 6 weeks. Stevens-Johnson syndrome is a fatal variant of erythema multiforme. Death is estimated to occur in 5% to 18% of patients. Etiologic factors include drugs, foods, infections, deep radiograph therapy, and neoplasms.

Fever

The precise mechanism by which drug-induced fever occurs is incompletely understood. However, for clinical application, five types of drug fever have been described.

The most common type of drug fever involves an immunologic mechanism that may become manifest alone or with accompanying signs and symptoms such as rash, urticaria, and eosinophilia. On subsequent administration of an offending agent, fever will often ensue within hours.

Idiosyncrasy is a second mechanism by which drugs have been implicated to induce temperature elevation. Such a reaction occurs when certain individuals with abnormal muscle metabolism receive depolarizing skeletal muscle relaxants.

Febrile reactions may also occur as a direct result of a drug's pharmacologic action, such as the release of endotoxins, resulting from the bactericidal effect of antibiotics on sensitive microorganisms (e.g., Jarisch-Herxheimer reaction).

Drugs may elevate temperature by a direct effect on the physiologic mechanisms involved with temperature regulation. The mechanisms by which drugs have been implicated include interference with the dissipation of heat (e.g., atropine), increases in metabolism (e.g., thyroxine), and alterations in the thermoregulatory center (e.g., phenothiazines).

A final mechanism for drug-induced febrile reactions results from administering impurities or pyrogens while administering the drug parenterally. Although this is not truly caused by the drug, it is an important source of unexplained fever.

Whenever drug fever is suspected, the best therapy is to discontinue the offending agent. If administration of the drug is essential, concurrent use of corticosteroids, unless contraindicated, often suppresses the fever and accompanying manifestations.

Hematologic complications

Numerous drugs have been implicated as causing untoward effects on the cells of the hemopoietic system. Hematologic drug reactions usually destroy peripheral blood cells or inhibit bone marrow cell development. Blood cells disappear more rapidly in the former instance than in the latter. Four categories of drug-induced blood dyscrasias are presented here: (1) agranulocytosis, (2) aplastic anemia, (3) hemolytic anemia, and (4) thrombocytopenia.

Agranulocytosis. Agranulocytosis is characterized by a decrease in white blood cells or leukocytes to less than 3000 mm³ of blood. Signs and symptoms include chills, fever, necrosis of the mucous membranes of the mouth, throat, rectum, and vagina, as well as prostration. Red blood cells and platelets are not usually affected. Recovery is frequently complete, occurring within 2 weeks of discontinuing the offending agent. However, if the reaction is complicated by infection, death may result.

Aplastic anemia. Aplastic anemia is characterized by bone marrow that has few, if any, hemopoietic cells and a preponderance of fatty spaces. This reaction is the most severe, but least frequent, of the drug-induced blood dyscrasias. Death frequently occurs and is associated with infection and hemorrhage.

Hemolytic anemia. Drug-induced hemolytic anemia is associated with a rapid fall in erythrocytes (i.e., hemolysis of red blood cells) and normoblastic hyperplasia of the bone marrow.

Thrombocytopenia. A fall in platelets characterizes drug-induced thrombocytopenia. Thus, the major symptom is hemorrhaging from skin and mucous membranes, but internal bleeding may also be present. Recovery is rapid once the causative drug is discontinued.

Hepatotoxicity

As with other drug reactions, drug-induced liver disease may occur as a result of toxicity, hypersensitivity, or idiosyncrasy. Signs and symptoms, as well as mortality, are dependent on the type of injury produced. In general, hepatotoxicity takes the form of cholestatic, cytotoxic, or mixed injury. The latter involves a combination of both cholestatic and cytotoxic forms. Mortality is highest with cytotoxic reactions.

Cholestatic hepatitis may be canalicular (i.e., without portal inflammation) or hepatocanalicular (i.e., with portal inflammation). Canalicular hepatitis is characterized clinically by a normal or slightly elevated alkaline phosphatase. In hepatocanalicular hepatitis, alkaline phosphatase levels are relatively high (i.e., more than three times normal) and cholesterol levels may also be markedly elevated. Both canalicular and hepatocanalicular hepatitis are associated with modest elevations in transaminase levels. Jaundice and pruritis predominate. Death rarely occurs.

Cytotoxic reactions include necrosis or steatosis; both involve overt parenchymal damage and show a moderate elevation in alkaline phosphatase. Necrotic lesions resemble viral hepatitis. Here serum glutamic pyruvic transaminase (SGPT) and SGOT are markedly elevated.

Ocular complications

Ocular complications of drugs may occur following both systemic and topical administration. A wide variety of drugs may adversely affect almost any portion of the eye. Because one cannot predict when this will occur, initial and subsequent examinations should be performed on patients receiving any drug with known adverse ocular effects.

Ototoxicity

Side effects of drugs on hearing may range from an annoying ringing in the ear (i.e., tinnitus) to total and irreversible deafness. Reactions are usually associated with hearing loss (auditory toxicity) or dysfunction of the vestibular apparatus. Frequently these disturbances may be traced to alterations in the neural structures of the inner ear and the eighth cranial nerve. The inner ear contains all the receptors for hearing (cochlea) and equilibrium (utricle for static equilibrium and semicircular canals for dynamic equilibrium). Thus drugs often produce ototoxicity by damaging the inner ear. Kanamycin and neomycin exert their toxicity on the cochlear portion of the labyrinth, whereas gentamicin and streptomycin effects are mainly on the vestibular portion.

Renal complications

Drug-induced renal disease may include signs and symptoms associated with renal disease of other causes, including (1) acute renal failure, (2) chronic renal failure, (3) the acute nephrotic syndrome, (4) the chronic nephrotic syndrome, (5) renal colic, (6) hematuria, (7) tubular defects, and (8) obstructive nephropathy.

Therefore, in any patient with renal disease, it is imperative to obtain a thorough drug history and to carefully monitor renal function tests. When a drug is suspected of causing renal damage, it should be discontinued. The mechanisms by which drug-induced renal disease occurs are incompletely understood.

Pulmonary complications

Drug-induced pulmonary disease is not common; however, when a patient is seen with a respiratory disorder of unknown etiology, drugs should be considered in the differential diagnosis. As with drug-induced renal disease, the exact mechanisms by which drugs cause pulmonary disease are ill-defined. As the mechanisms become better understood, recognition of drugs as a cause may increase. The pulmonary disorders frequently associated with drugs include (1) asthma, (2) interstitial pulmonary fibrosis, and (3) pulmonary eosinophilia (infiltrates).

Sexual dysfunction

Information describing drug-induced sexual dysfunction is sparse. The classes of drugs that significantly interfere with sexual function are the antihypertensives, the antipsychotics, and the anticholinergics. The mechanisms by which drugs produce sexual dysfunction are poorly understood; however, these mechanisms probably involve the autonomic and central nervous systems, as well as hormonal balance. The effects of drugs on sexual dysfunction include decreased libido, erectile problems, and impaired ejaculation.

SUMMARY

The subject of adverse drug reactions is complex and varied. An understanding of the different classes of adverse drug reactions, as well as the mechanism by which they occur, frequently makes it possible for those attending the patient to anticipate potential adversities and to take the appropriate actions (e.g., monitor laboratory tests, conduct a thorough drug history) necessary to prevent, detect, or treat adverse drug reactions.

BIBLIOGRAPHY

Batist, G., & Andrews, J.L., Jr. Pulmonary toxicity of antineoplastic drugs. *Journal of the American Medical Association*, 1981, *246*, 1449-1453.

Bennett, W.M., Plamp, C., & Porter, G.A. Drug-related syndromes in clinical nephrology. *Annals of Internal Medicine*, 1977, *87*, 582-590.

Bernheim, J.L., & Korzets, Z. Indomethacin-induced renal failure. *Annals of Internal Medicine*, 1979, *91*, 792.

Carlstedt, B.C. The clinical lab CBC and diff red blood cells. *US Pharmacist*, 1978, *3*, 14-17.

Carlstedt, B.C. The clinical lab complete blood count: white blood cells and differential. *US Pharmacist*, 1978, *3*, 26-33, 92.

Cole, N.J. Drugs causing sexual problems. *Pharmacy International*, 1981, *2*, 63-67.

Cripps, G.W., Martinez, D.R., Gilliam, A., & Caldwell, T.J. Significance of drug-altered laboratory test values. *American Journal of Hospital Pharmacy*, 1973, *30*, 603-608.

Curtis, J.R. Drug-induced renal disease. *Drugs*, 1979, *18*, 377-391.

Drug-induced bullous eruptions. *British Medical Journal*, 1971, *282*, 421-422.

Drury, P.L., Asirdas, L.G., & Bulger, G.V. Mefenamic acid nephropathy: further evidence. *British Medical Journal*, 1981, *282*, 865-866.

Ettinger, B., Mandel, N.S., & Darling, S. Triamterene-induced nephrolithiasis. *Annals of Internal Medicine*, 1979, *91*, 745.

Evaluations of drug interactions (2nd ed.). Washington, D.C.: American Pharmaceutical Association, 1976.

Filipek, W.J. Drug-induced pulmonary disease. *Postgraduate Medicine*, 1979, *65*, 131-140.

Fisher, A.A. Drug-induced skin eruptions: typical treatments for topical problems. *Geriatrics*, 1979, *34*, 45-64.

Fleckenstein, L. Adverse effects of drugs on the liver-update. *Alta Bates Hospital Drug Information Service Newsletter*, 1975, *7*, 23-38.

Fraunfelder, F.T. Interim report: national registry of possible drug-induced ocular side effects. *Ophthalmology*, 1979, *86*, 126-130.

Friedlander, I.R. Ototoxic drugs and the detection of ototoxicity. *New England Journal of Medicine*, 1979, *301*, 213-214.

Grant, I.W.B. Drug-induced diseases: drug-induced respiratory disease. *British Medical Journal*, 1979, *1*, 1070-1077.

Hansten, P.D. Drug-induced pulmonary disease. *Alta Bates Hospital Drug Information Service Newsletter*, 1970, *2*, 14-16.

Hansten, P.D. *Drug interactions* (4th ed.). Philadelphia: Lea & Febiger, 1979.

Irey, N.S. Diagnostic problems in drug-induced illness. *Annals of Clinical and Laboratory Science*, 1976, *6*, 272-277.

Jick, H. Drugs—remarkably nontoxic. *New England Journal of Medicine*, 1974, *291*, 824-828.

Jick, H., Walker, A.M., & Porter, J. Drug-induced liver disease. *Journal of Clinical Pharmacology*, 1981, *21*, 359-364.

Koetting, J.F. Ocular and visual side effects of drugs—a reconsideration. *Journal of the American Pharmaceutical Association*, 1975, *15*, 558-597, 600.

Lee, G.L. Drug-induced sexual dysfunction. *Pharmacy and Therapeutics Forum of the University of California, San Francisco*, 1981, *29*, 1-4.

Lee, H.A. Drug-induced diseases: drug-related disease and the kidney. *British Medical Journal*, 1979, *2*, 104-107.

Lien, E. & Lien, L. Structure side-effect sorting of drugs III: hepatotoxicities. *California Pharmacist*, 1978, *26*, 34-44.

Linton, A.L., Clark, W.F., Driedger, A.A., Turnbull, D.I., & Lindsay, R.M. Acute interstitial nephritis due to drugs. *Annals of Internal Medicine*, 1980, *93*, 735-747.

Maddrey, W.C., & Boitnott, J.K. Drug-induced chronic hepatitis and cirrhosis. *Progress in Liver Diseases*, 1979, *7*, 595-603.

Miller, R.R. Hospital admissions due to adverse drug reactions. *Archives of Internal Medicine*, 1974, *134*, 219-223.

Mitchell, J.R., McMurtry, R.J., Statham, C.N. & Nelson, S.D. Molecular basis for several drug-induced nephropathies. *American Journal of Medicine*, 1977, *62*, 518-526.

Ockner, R.K. Drug-induced liver disease. *Western Journal of Medicine*, 1979, *131*, 36-45.

Paxes, G.E. Eye irritation and lithium carbonate. *Archives of Ophthalmology*, 1980, *98*, 930.

Petz, L.D., & Garratty, G. Drug-induced haemolytic anemia. *Clinics in Haemotology*, 1975, *4*, 181-197.

Photosensitivity from drugs, perfumes and cosmetics. *Medical Letter*, 1980, *22*, 64.

Pisciotta, A.V. Drug-induced agranulocytosis. *Drugs*, 1978, *15*, 132-143.

Pisciotta, A.V. Idiosyncratic hematologic reactions to drugs. *Postgraduate Medicine*, 1974, *55*, 105-113.

Raymond, G.G., Saenz, R.V., & Chandler, C., Jr. Drug induced skin manifestations. *US Pharmacist*, 1970, *3*, 44-61.

Rosenstein, S. & Lamy, P.P. Drug-induced disease: blood dyscrasias. *Hospital Form Management*, 1970, *5*, 13-18.

Schiff, G. Adverse drug reactions: recognition of the problem. *Facts and Comparisons Drug Newsletter*, 1984, *3*, 49-51.

Schwinghammer, T.L., & Britton, H.L. Adverse effects of drugs on the eye. *US Pharmacist*, 1979, *4*, 49-60.

Shinn, A.F. Drugs and ototoxicity. *US Pharmacist*, 1978, *3*, 54-64.

Stauffer, J.L. Drug-induced lung disease: the price of progress. *California Medicine*, 1973, *119*, 48-56.

Stohs, S.J. Drugs and sexual function. *US Pharmacist*, 1978, *3*, 51-66.

Stuurman, A. Drugs affecting sex. *Pharmacy International*, 1981, *2*, III.

Sullivan D., Dsuka, M.E., & Blanchard, B. Erythromycin ethylsuccinate hepatotoxicity. *Journal of the American Medical Association*, 1980, *243*, 1074.

Swanson, M. Drugs, chemicals and hemolysis. *Drug Intelligence and Clinical Pharmacy*, 1973, *7*, 6-24.

Tarpey, C.A. Drug-induced liver injury—update, 1981. *Alta Bates Hospital Drug Information Service Newsletter*, 1981, *11*, 1-8.

Tatro, D.S. Drug-induced cutaneous eruptions: part I. *Alta Bates Hospital Drug Information Service Newsletter*, 1970, *2*, 36-42.

Tatro, D.S. Drug-induced cutaneous eruptions: part II. *Alta Bates Hospital Drug Information Service Newsletter*, 1970, *2*, 48-55.

Tatro, D.S. Drug-induced cutaneous eruptions: part III. *Alta Bates Hospital Drug Information Service Newsletter*, 1970, *2*, 56-62.

Villeneuve, J.P., & Warner, H.A. Cimetidine hepatitis. *Gastroenterology*, 1979, *77*, 143-144.

Walshe, J.J., & Venuto, R.C. Acute oliguric renal failure induced by indomethacin: possible mechanism. *Annals of Internal Medicine*, 1979, *91*, 47-49.

Zanowiak, P. Contact dermatitis caused by drugs and cosmetics. *Journal of the American Pharmaceutical Association*, 1977, *17*, 626-628.

Zimmerman, H.J. Drug-induced liver disease. *Drugs*, 1978, *16*, 25-45.

CHAPTER 12

Drug Abuse and Addiction

Sharon M. Hall

Drug addiction is a physiologic condition marked by an increased tolerance for a drug and a withdrawal syndrome when the drug is withdrawn. *Tolerance* occurs when successively greater doses of the drug are required to obtain a comparable effect from it, or conversely, when the initial dose of the drug no longer produces a noticeable effect. The *withdrawal syndrome* is a constellation of physiologic symptoms that occur when the amount of drug administered is decreased, or when it is removed entirely.

Physiologic addiction may exist concurrently with *psychologic dependence*, the habitual use of a drug, usually across a variety of situations. On removing the drug, a sense of loss or craving for the drug may be felt without other, more specific physiologic symptoms. Physical addiction and psychologic dependence are not two separate entities but represent the endpoints of the biologic-psychologic continuum, with many symptoms, such as anxiety and craving, quite plausibly linked to either somatic or environmental determinants (e.g., whereas some theorists assume craving for alcohol to be a sign of a tissue need, others interpret reports of craving as expectancy of pleasant drug effects).

Drug abuse may not entail either addiction or dependency, but is usually assumed to occur when drug use interferes with the health and personal or social functioning of the individual. Usually, either addiction or dependency are involved to some degree. But the term "drug abuse" is sufficiently encompassing that it may refer to the drug-taking behavior of the addicted heroin user, the drinker who uses alcohol only twice a year but becomes violent on these occasions, and the cigarette smoker who continues to smoke despite early signs of chronic pulmonary disease.

In practice, lines between drug abuse and acceptable drug use are often not clear cut, and the demarcation line frequently reflects a multitude of factors, including the values, health, and life requirements of the individual and the norms and values of the society in which he or she exists. Among these is the social evaluation of the implications of use of the drug, an evaluation that rests heavily on the time and place in which the drug use occurs. Heavy drinking may be considered acceptable, and is socially encouraged, among some segments of society (e.g., midwestern male factory workers) and unhealthy and undesirable in other segments of the same society (e.g., upper-middle-class women).

A more subtle point, but one that ultimately has great influence on the life and treatment of the user, is the severity with which particular cultures view *addiction*, per se, to a particular drug. Perhaps the most striking example of the effects of societal views of addiction to a particular substance is offered by Brecher (1972), who describes the metamorphosis in attitudes towards the use of opiates, which was from one of mingled disapproval and tolerance at the turn of the century to one of near hysteric fear in the early 1970s.

In the late nineteenth and early twentieth centuries, patent elixirs, containing opiates, were over-the-counter drugs, advertised as effective for a variety of common disorders, and were used by more or less respectable segments of the population. Several forces, both moralistic ones and ones related to increasing tax revenue, resulted in the passage of the Harrison Narcotics Act in 1914. This act, later related acts, and the ways in which the courts interpreted them resulted in tight controls over the dispensation of narcotic drugs, particularly with respect to prescribing narcotics for a known addict.

Before passage of the Harrison Narcotics Act, physicians had been able to prescribe narcotics to individuals who were already addicted; after its passage, it became impossible for an addict to obtain legal drugs via medical prescriptions. Criminals took control of the drug market, and the addict became a criminal.

Use of the pure drug had few physical consequences other than addiction. Illegal narcotics, the contaminants used to dilute them, and the conditions of their use, resulted in serious illness, including bacterial endocarditis, abscesses, and diseases related to malnutrition. The mild disapproval directed toward early drug use mushroomed into the near hysteric fear of the early 1970s, when the addict was seen as a doomed, diseased, and crazed criminal, and this perversion was solely the result of the use of a particular substance, heroin. Whereas it is true that the change in attitude followed a change in the character of the addict, the change in the addict was initially the result of the social evaluation of the seriousness of drug addiction, and of resulting legal attempts to control it.

Thus, despite the descriptive simplicity with which we may offer definitions of addiction, abuse, tolerance, and withdrawal, the actual implications of these occurrences for the drug abuser vary tremendously depending on the time, place, and resulting social context of addiction.

THEORIES OF ADDICTION

Independent of the particular substance studied, theories of the etiology and treatment of drug abuse and addiction can be grouped into three general categories: (1) somatic theories, including metabolic–biochemical and genetic transmission theories; (2) intrapsychic theories, most of which posit the existence of an addictive personality predisposing one to drug use; and (3) conditioning theories, which assume that addiction reflects the past experience of the individual, experience with both the drug and the particular social context in which the individual lives.

Somatic theories

One variant of somatic theories is the metabolic deficiency model, which suggests that drug abuse develops because the drug abuser has a particular biologic deficiency satisfied by the drug. Whereas many individuals may experiment with a drug, only those who possess the particular deficiency will, according to this theory, ultimately become addicted. A typical example of such a theory is that of Dole and Nyswander (1980), who suggest that experimentation with heroin occurs more or less because of simple adolescent curiosity. Most individuals who use the drug once or twice have either mixed positive and negative effects, or predominantly negative effects, and terminate use. However, some individuals continue to use the drug to the point of addiction, perhaps because their physiologic makeup is such that initial experiences are predominantly pleasurable. Once use occurs, especially repeated use, the nervous system is changed irrevocably, according to this theory. Precisely how it is changed, or what characterizes individuals who

continue drug use versus those who do not is not known, but the assumption is that these changes lead to physical dependence, characterized by discomfort in withdrawal. This discomfort, then, impels the addict to continue to seek drugs and can continue in subtle forms long after detoxification.

Dole and Nyswander's theory evolved from their pioneering work using methadone to maintain heroin addicts. They found that substituting methadone for heroin resulted in the ability of patients to abstain from heroin, and ultimately, for most of the patients, in rehabilitation. Because their patients were able to resume well-functioning lives without a great deal of psychotherapy, they assumed that the deficiency was the result almost entirely of a metabolic dysfunction rather than of either environmental or intrapsychic factors.

Nationwide experience with thousands of patients on methadone maintenance produced generally favorable outcomes, but outcomes that are considerably less impressive than those of Dole and Nyswander's initial sample. In retrospect, it would seem that much of Dole and Nyswander's success reflected the novelty and enthusiasm of a new treatment, and of a fairly select patient population. Methadone alone, without provision of adequate rehabilitation services, does not seem to result in major rehabilitative changes; in fact, some writers have suggested that the primary purpose of methadone is simply to attract addicts to clinics where they can gradually become involved in activities related to mainstream society (Bourne, 1974). Dole and Nyswander (1980) argue that such failures should not reflect on methadone per se, or on the metabolic theory of addiction, but may indicate the failure of the rehabilitative therapies provided. Although this may be the case, these failures simply point out the limited scope of a model that does not include them, and suggest that metabolic models are, at best, partial ones.

Some somatic models focus on genetics. Such models are not mutually exclusive of metabolic deficiency models (e.g., a certain genetic makeup may predispose one to developing a metabolic deficiency), but their focus differs. Shuckit (1980) has reviewed the major theories and research related to genetic mechanisms causing a predisposition to drug use, and concluded that good evidence exists, from divergent methods, that indicates genetic predispositions are a contributory factor in alcoholism. Whereas some investigations have been completed linking a genetic predisposition to the use of other drugs, the evidence is limited, and not nearly so compelling as is the case with alcoholism. Shuckit suggests that a complicated polygenic model that considers interaction with the environment may be the most useful one (i.e., probably a combination of genes predispose a person to drug abuse, and some might act to protect a person from drug abuse; these will interact with environmental events that either facilitate or discourage drug abuse).

Whatever the role of underlying somatic aberrations concerning drug abuse, they provide at best a partial model, especially with respect to rehabilitation, where the importance of social and personal factors appear preeminent. Somatic theories may ultimately lead to preventing the development of addictions. Such an occurrence is probably far in the future, however, and it seems unrealistic to expect that they will provide a magic bullet to cure addiction via amelioration of a biochemical abnormality.

Intrapsychic theories

The original intrapsychic theories were psychoanalytic ones, which constructed an elaborate psychologic picture of the character of the addicted individual. Typical are the theories of Rado (1933), who saw all addictions as representative of personal immaturity, and the desire to return to an infantile, narcissistic state. A more recent analytic perspective has been provided by Ausabel (1961), who proposed the existence of specific personality types most susceptible to addiction. These included the inadequate personality, which he characterized as irresponsible, passive, and unable to delay gratification, and the anxious, depressed individual. In later elaboration of the theory, Ausabel (1980) suggested that for a small proportion of psychopathic addicts, drug use may simply provide a means of acting out. Finally, Ausabel suggests that under extreme conditions even mature individuals may use drugs for a limited time to dull feelings of hopelessness.

Later variants of intrapsychic theories have been more limited and have suggested that drug use reflects one or more fairly specific emotional states. One of the most widely researched of these is the anxiety-reduction model, and the related tension-reduction hypothesis, which has been most widely applied to alcohol, although variants of it have been proposed to apply to cigarette smoking and opiate abuse. The tension-reduction hypothesis assumes that the primary purpose of drug use is to reduce anxiety, and implies that the experience of stress will increase the probability of drug use. According to the model, the drug user need not necessarily be higher in trait anxiety than nonusers. However, many writers, when discussing the tension-reduction hypothesis, assume this to be the case. Despite the popularity of this model,

and its intuitive appeal, the research available does not consistently support either the assumption that drug consumption reduces stress or that increases in stress consistently increase the probability of drug use.

The older, more general versions of the intrapsychic model have rather gloomy implications for treatment. Because the disorder is assumed to stem from enduring personality characteristics, and because massive characterologic modifications are difficult at best, the probability of any more than a temporary superficial change in drug abuse is slight. Of course, although many may care to argue with this particular view, there is little to disprove it at this point.

Research on personality similarities among addicts proposed by intrapsychic theories has not generally supported the assumption that certain personality types would be found among abusers of particular substances. No matter what the substance studied, constellations of particular traits appearing vary from study to study, and frequently several different constellations are found within a sample. It can also be argued that any similarities in personality ascribed to addicts can be just as easily explained by the pressures of addiction and the lifestyle it entails; of course, this is an especially compelling argument with illegal drugs.

The anxiety-reduction model suggests that more specific treatments designed to ameliorate anxiety should be of value in treating drug abuse. However, neither psychologic treatments designed to reduce anxiety, nor pharmacologic agents with anxiety-reducing properties, if used alone, are effective in producing either the termination of cigarette smoking or excessive drinking. It thus appears that whereas these treatments may be of value as ancillaries in drug treatment, the problems involved are too complex to yield to such a simple, single-factor solution.

Conditioning theories

Perhaps one of the most widely cited theories of addiction is Wikler's (1973) conditioning theory. Wikler proposed that withdrawal symptoms and other responses, primarily internal responses preceding drug use, become classically conditioned to the environmental stimuli associated with them (i.e., the environment in which withdrawal occurs gradually comes to evoke some aspects of it; most notably, craving). Recurrence of these environmental stimuli cause a conditioned abstinence syndrome that is suggested to be causally related to relapse. The model proposes that the conditioned abstinence syndrome can be extinguished (eliminated) by repeated pairings of the environmental stimuli with the absence of the euphoric or withdrawal effect. This theory has been extended to alcohol abuse and has been proposed as useful in understanding substance misuse in general.

Empirical evidence for the usefulness of the model, however, is weak. The influence of craving and withdrawal symptoms on relapse is questionable. On a clinical level, trials with naltrexone, a narcotic antagonist, which blocks drug receptor interaction and therefore precipitates withdrawal effects, indicates that, contrary to predictions, extinction of drug use does not occur during an antagonist administration, for when administration is terminated, drug use resumes.

A second conditioning theory of some consequence is the opponent process theory, which suggests that within the brain there exists a system that functions to decrease emotional arousal (e.g., whereas initially the response of the heroin addict to an opiate injection may be euphoria and a rush, with time the response can best be described as relief; this diminution in intensity reflects the operation of the opponent process).

The opponent process model proposes two states following drug administration. The first, (the A state) is the extreme pleasure following drug use. In the second state (the B state), craving and irritating withdrawal symptoms occur. Once the A state occurs, the B state must also occur. The A state and the B state describe what happens during the first few stimulations. During later stimulations, the intensity of the A state is automatically decreased by the operation of the opponent process, whereas the intensity of the B state automatically increases (e.g., in later stimulations, the heroin addict experiences only relief instead of the euphoric rush, and craving and abstinence anxiety are increased).

According to this model, then, opiate, alcohol, barbiturate, amphetamine, or nicotine addiction occur because the B state lasts a long time and is aversive and becomes more so with continued daily use. Also, because reelicitation of the A state removes the B state, the user employs the drug to elicit the A state to get rid of the B state. Solomon and Corbit (1973) suggest that a major therapeutic task is to weaken the B state, because this is the state that mediates the strongest escape and avoidance behavior. These behaviors, which are drug use behaviors, repeatedly arouse the A state and thereby actually strengthen the B state.

The opponent process theory appeals to many because it suggests a basic mechanism with which to explain all addictions. However, if one looks closely at the treatment recommendations that result from the opponent process theory, the result is rather disappointing because they generally do not suggest new intervention strategies over and above simple conditioning theories.

Conditioning theories tend to be undeveloped with respect to social learning and interpersonal reinforcement for drug use, and often fail to mention, or adequately discuss, the cognitions that may mediate drug use. Still, they have led to some innovative drug abuse intervention strategies; these are discussed later. These conditioning models are also incomplete because they focus purely on interactions between the drug and the individual, rather than considering the broader social context in which addiction occurs. Factors that must be considered are the role models for the addicted individual, the value the addict places on the addict's role as opposed to the nonaddict's role, interpersonal, social, and vocational skills available to the addict other than those attached to the addict's role, and all of the reinforcers accruing to the use of the substance.

SUBSTANCES OF ABUSE

The range of substances abused by human beings is truly a testimony to the versatility of humanity. This list includes narcotics, stimulants, depressants, inhalants, hallucinogens, marijuana, caffeine, nicotine, and alcohol.

Rates of use of drugs of abuse rise and fall in popularity because of socioeconomic factors, such as availability, publicity, and price. In spite of such fluctuations, three classes of abused drugs have been consistently related to major health and social problems in the United States and Canada. Two of these, alcohol and tobacco, are legal, relatively inexpensive, easily attainable, and are used by large numbers of people. Together they account for more than 25% of drug-linked premature deaths, and about 25% of total deaths in North America. A third drug, heroin, is neither legal, easily obtainable, nor cheap, and its use affects a much smaller segment of the population. However, the effects of heroin addiction in our society are so devastating that heroin is worth considering in depth.

Opiates

Opiates are a class of drugs employed primarily for analgesia, but they also have other uses (see Chapter 17, "Analgesics and Narcotic Antagonists"). Known and used several hundred years before the birth of Christ, the opiate predominantly used until relatively modern times was opium, derived from the juice of the poppy, *Papaver somniferum*. Frequently abused drugs falling into this class include morphine, codeine, as well as the synthetic opiates of heroin, methadone, meperidine, and pentazocine. The most common drug abused is heroin, made from morphine by acetylation.

Incidence and prevalence of heroin addiction. In 1975, there were 550,000 heroin addicts in the United States; by 1977 the number had decreased to 450,000. Whereas this decline is encouraging, two sobering facts must be taken into account. First, the prevalence in 1977 was about double that known in the mid-1960s. Also, reports of increases in heroin production via increased production of opium from Iran and other Mideastern countries during 1979 and 1980 may ultimately result in another increase in the number of addicted individuals. Groups at high risk include residents of ghettos and other low-income areas, where heroin is easily available, individuals exposed to large supplies of heroin in foreign countries, and health practitioners, especially physicians and nurses.

Accurate estimates of the numbers of occasional heroin users are virtually impossible to obtain. The occasional user both fears legal sanctions and has no need of a treatment system that might reveal his or her existence.

Psychologic effects of heroin addiction. Psychologic effects of heroin addiction are well known: the drug produces euphoria, analgesia, drowsiness, and relaxation. It may also produce nausea and vomiting, which addicts describe as unimportant in comparison to the euphoria produced by the drug. With continued use the euphoric and other pleasant effects of heroin injection appear to vanish as tolerance develops, and heroin may only alleviate the withdrawal symptoms and make the addict feel normal.

Health consequences of heroin use. Acute overdose of the opiates causes central nervous system (CNS) and respiratory depression, which can result in death. In general, however, opiate use per se appears to have no long-term permanent effect on the human body. Temporary effects include decreased sexual potency and libido, cessation of menses, and decreased likelihood of pregnancy. Other effects are constriction of the pupils, constipation, and excessive sweating. A potentially dangerous effect is analgesia, which results in the addict failing to feel and recognize pain, potentially postponing seeking medical care in the presence of serious diseases.

In contrast to the relatively benign effects of the use of pure opiates, heroin addiction has devastating effects on health. Complications of heroin use include bacterial endocarditis, viral hepatitis, skin lesions, and renal disease. Pulmonary impairment, including pulmonary infections and emboli caused by the presence of inert substances in heroin preparation, are common. All of these disorders can be traced to the addict lifestyle and using contaminated or adulterated drugs, rather than to the opiate itself.

Babies born to addicted mothers tend to show a variety of signs that are generally thought to be withdrawal symptoms. However, whether this is the result of general immaturity, reflected specifically in the maturity of the nervous system, or other actual withdrawal symptoms is not clear. The former is a clear possibility because many infants born to heroin addicts suffer low birth weights and other signs of immaturity. Special programs to treat the pregnant addict are becoming increasingly common. Such programs attend to the mothers' health, special problems occurring during delivery (such as use of analgesics), and the care of the newborn.

Withdrawal symptoms of heroin addiction. Termination of heroin use results in typical withdrawal symptoms, which may range from mild to severe. In peak severity, they may include lacrimation, diarrhea, severe anxiety, sweating, shakes, and gooseflesh. In the mild form, they may resemble the common cold, with lacrimation and rhinorrhea being the prevalent symptoms. Addicts undergoing withdrawal and displaying few physical withdrawal symptoms may report severe anxiety.

Treatment modalities for heroin addiction. There are four widely used treatment modalities for heroin addiction in the United States and Canada: (1) outpatient detoxification, (2) therapeutic communities, (3) drug-free outpatient treatments, and (4) methadone maintenance.

Outpatient detoxification. Outpatient detoxification from heroin usually involves using gradually decreasing doses of methadone as a substitute narcotic. In the period from 1977 to 1980, 17% of all admissions to federally funded drug abuse programs went to outpatient detoxification. Detoxification is not only a treatment in its own right, but it is also an essential adjunct to all treatments for heroin addiction except methadone maintenance. Treatment facilities offering detoxification generally have as goals the termination of heroin use and entrance into longer term rehabilitation treatment. However, few clients (3% to 20%) terminate heroin use during detoxification. Treatment completion rates from 0% to 69% have been reported, but are generally less than 40%, and only rarely do clients enter into more intensive rehabilitation following detoxification.

In general, then, outpatient detoxification, despite its popularity, has not been a notably successful procedure. In spite of this, its relative inexpensiveness and its presence as an alternative to more restrictive treatments, such as methadone maintenance and therapeutic communities, have encouraged continuing its use.

Some attempts have been made to improve the efficacy of detoxification, including innovations using self-regulation of dose and rapid detoxification schedules. Other innovations include using antihypertensives as detoxification adjuncts; Washington, Resnick, and Rawton (1979) have reported that clonidine reduces opiate withdrawal symptoms during detoxification. However, whether symptom reduction is related to reduced heroin use or to better rehabilitative outcomes has not yet been determined.

Therapeutic communities. Therapeutic communities are residential programs. The therapeutic community treatment modality centers on confrontative encounter therapy, usually modeled after the Synanon Game. The aim is to destroy the personal illusions of the addict while providing support for new identities and behaviors. The therapeutic communities also rely on nonprofessional health care providers to a greater extent than most other drug abuse treatment modalities. Primary staff members are usually former addicts and drug abusers who have been rehabilitated themselves in therapeutic communities. Therapeutic communities vary widely in other respects, including their emphasis on planning for reentry into the community, their acceptance of professionals as service providers, and their willingness to accept research on the outcome of the treatment as meaningful.

In part because of the general disdain of many therapeutic communities for research, and in part because of methodologic difficulties, it is difficult to draw clear conclusions about the effectiveness of this modality. However, available data indicate dropout rates are high. Somewhere between 40% and 90% of the individuals who enter therapeutic communities do not complete treatment (i.e., leave before staff think treatment has been completed). Because therapeutic communities frequently require extended time commitments (e.g., 12 to 18 months), it should be noted that even dropouts receive some treatment. Also, even when dropouts are included in data analyses it appears that the therapeutic community experience does result in patients using fewer opiates and other drugs, lower arrest rates, less additional treatment, and higher employment rates during follow-ups, ranging from 1 to 5 years posttreatment, than observed before the treatment.

It is difficult to estimate the efficacy of therapeutic communities, in part because of the high dropout rate. Until outcomes of therapeutic communities are compared with outcomes for similarly motivated individuals who have not received treatment, or who received less restrictive treatment, one cannot accurately assess the benefit of the therapeutic community treatment relative to other treatments available. The high dropout rates do suggest that therapeutic communities are either too ambitious in their treatment goals or that they are of value only to a proportionately small number of drug abusers.

Outpatient drug-free treatment. Almost as many heroin abusers participate in drug-free treatment as in methadone maintenance, which is somewhat surprising considering the relative amounts of attention given to the modalities by both the scientific community and the media; these two treatment modalities each consistently account for approximately 20% of all drug treatment clients.

Treatment modalities used vary from program to program, ranging from storefront rap centers to behavior therapy and family therapy. Most programs emphasize traditional supportive counseling and referral to other community agencies for health, educational, legal, and other services. It is difficult to compare the effectiveness of outpatient treatment to other treatment approaches, in part because the modality tends to attract specific subgroups of patients: young patients, patients recently released from prison, and patients who need posttreatment support. Outcomes reported are mixed; this is not surprising when one considers the diversity of the programs offered and the wide variance in the types of patients who use them. None of the evaluations reported to date have been controlled, random assignment studies, and most do not involve comparable patients across modalities, so little can be said with any certainty about the efficacy of drug-free treatment. There seems to be an impression, however, that drug-free treatment is less likely to retain patients than most other drug treatment programs, especially methadone maintenance.

Methadone maintenance. Methadone maintenance therapy consists of substituting a synthetic opiate, methadone, for heroin. Pioneered by Nyswander and Dole in the 1960s, methadone maintenance is designed to eliminate illegal opiate use by substituting a similar, but longer acting, narcotic. By eliminating the need constantly to hustle for drugs on the street, it attempts to provide the addict with the opportunity to redirect energies to personal, social, and vocational rehabilitation. Most methadone maintenance programs offer a variety of adjunctive therapies, including family, individual, and vocational counseling, and support education groups in topics such as parenting and general health care. Both the extent and quality of such services vary greatly from program to program.

Methadone maintenance results have been more widely studied than other treatment modalities. Overall, it appears to be moderately effective according to the three most commonly used indices of success: program retention, criminal behavior, and employment and educational status.

A major concern with methadone maintenance has been the difficulty of detoxifying a patient from methadone (i.e., to become free of methadone addiction). Clinic reports indicate that a zero dose is reached only by a minority of those who attempt to detoxify (25% to 40%). Similarly, relapse to opiate use after detoxification is frequent. Reported posttreatment abstinence rates varied from a low of 8% at 42 months to 79% at 9 months. Further, the use of other drugs, most notably alcohol, following detoxification is frequently reported. Again, promising innovations in treatment have been reported (e.g., evidence exists that small decrements in dose may facilitate detoxification). Similarly, other research indicates that providing psychologic support, such as group therapy and relaxation training, may be of value in detoxification.

Tobacco

Of the several hundred compounds generated by the burning of tobacco, most attention has been paid to nicotine, which has long been thought to be the primary CNS-active component of cigarette smoke. Of the forms of ingestion possible, by far the most common is smoking the dried leaf of the tobacco plant.

Incidence and prevalence of tobacco smoking. American males began smoking cigarettes at the beginning of the twentieth century, especially during World War I. By 1925, approximately 50% of adult males smoked. Smoking among females lagged behind that of males by 25 to 30 years. The proportion of adult females smoking cigarettes did not exceed one quarter of the population until the onset of World War II. However, following the Surgeon General's Report on Smoking and Health (1964), cigarette smoking began to decline, more notably among males than among females. From 1965 to 1978, the proportion of adult male cigarette smokers declined from 51% to 37%. In a roughly comparable time period (1965 to 1976) the proportion of adult female smokers remained virtually unchanged at 32% to 33%; however, from 1976 to 1980 the proportion of female smokers declined to below 30%. The overall smoking prevalence of 32.3% of both sexes in 1978 represented the lowest recorded value in 45 years, although it appears that smoking has since increased, particularly among teenage girls.

Smoking usually begins during adolescence. Several studies have indicated that a higher risk of smoking initiation occurs if the adolescent comes from a home where one or both parents smoke, or where an older sibling or peer group member smokes. Smokers are generally prone to be less achievement motivated and have lower rates of aspiration than nonsmokers in high school populations. They are also less frequently involved in extracurricular school activities and have high rates of absenteeism. Some writers have conceptualized smoking as a response to stress, and general feelings of unattractiveness, incompetency, lack of efficacy, and limited opportunities for growth.

Psychologic effects of tobacco smoking. Psychologically, tobacco appears to have multiple effects, although these are just beginning to be studied. Nicotine, which is the principal CNS-active component of tobacco, affects the CNS in a variety of ways. The drug produces an altered pattern in electroencephalograms (EEG) and in reported behavioral arousal. It appears to have a paradoxic effect in that some smokers reported increases in level of arousal, whereas others reported that it had a relaxing effect.

The sociopsychologic effects of cigarette smoking are also multiple. For some individuals smoking is simply something to do with one's hands. For others it is a social gesture, a way of controlling unpleasant emotions, or a way of putting distance between oneself and others.

Health effects of tobacco smoking. In addition to nicotine, the cigarette smoker ingests several hundred different compounds, including carbon monoxide, methyl alcohol, ammonia, formaldehyde, phenols, creosote, tars, anthracin, arsenic, and benzopyrene. Shuman (1971) noted that diseases related to, though not necessarily caused by, tobacco smoking contribute to 37% of the total deaths in the United States, and that for smokers between the ages of 35 to 60 years of age, approximately one third of all deaths would not have occurred had they had the same death rate as nonsmokers.

With respect to the cardiovascular system, smoking is known to cause an increased incidence of atherosclerosis and is correlated with an increased risk of heart disease, especially in relatively young men. Smoking also increases the incidence of angina.

Cigarette smoking appears to be the main cause of two major chronic obstructive lung diseases, chronic bronchitis and pulmonary emphysema. It is generally known that cigarette smoking is causally related to lung cancer, but smoking is also causally related to cancer of the mouth, pharynx, and larynx. The risk of developing such cancers is greater among tobacco smokers who are also heavy drinkers. Whereas the existence of a causal relationship is open to question, smoking has also been shown to be related to retarded fetal growth in children born to smoking mothers, and to a significantly higher infant mortality rate resulting from stillbirths and neonatal deaths.

Withdrawal symptoms of tobacco smoking. Some authorities have questioned the existence of a withdrawal syndrome for tobacco smoking. It is now generally accepted that the syndrome does occur, but its manifestations are variable. Among the many changes that occur during tobacco withdrawal are decreases in the heart rate and in the diastolic blood pressure, and metabolic changes, including decreasing excretion of epinephrine and norepinephrine. Also reported are changes in alertness, with some studies indicating that alertness decreases on smoking cessation, and others indicating that it increases. Another well-documented result of withdrawal is weight gain. The cause of the gain, however, is not clear. Although it may reflect only increased food intake, some researchers suggest that it may be the result of slowed metabolic processes. Changes in mood as a result of smoking cessation are extremely variable, with many smokers reporting increased irritability, hostility, anxiety, and craving. Some evidence exists that the worst of the subjective withdrawal symptoms subside within 10 days after termination of cigarette smoking. Shiffman's work (1979) indicates that gradual withdrawal may result in levels of withdrawal symptoms that do not differ greatly from abstinence, suggesting that a treatment that attempts gradually to withdraw individuals from cigarettes may simply succeed in perpetuating the abstinence syndrome.

Treatment modalities for tobacco smoking

Self-care methods. It is estimated that 95% of exsmokers who have stopped have done so on their own. Self-care methods include any method not requiring outside assistance: going cold turkey, devising one's own programs or techniques, or using aids such as a manual or a book. The printed aids are varied, with several books and pamphlets available describing ways to quit. Book content ranges from material designed to provide insight into reasons for smoking to descriptions of specific behavioral techniques. Also, at least two systems of commercial filters that gradually reduce tar and nicotine levels are available. In general, outcome data on self-help methods are lacking.

Educational methods. Perhaps the second level of effort to self-treatment is using rational, educational approaches that rely on providing information about the effects of smoking on health. Until recently, most of these campaigns have been conducted in high

schools and colleges and have generally met with limited success. Because most of these campaigns were health oriented and because adolescents generally do not feel vulnerable to health problems, the focus may well have been inappropriate.

Clinical methods. Clinical methods include individual counseling, support groups, medications, hypnosis, aversive conditioning, and developing self-control skills (e.g., self-monitoring and self-reward programs). In general, most result in long-term abstinence rates of 20% to 25% by 1 year posttreatment. The single exception to this may be aversive satiation therapy. In aversive satiation (or rapid smoking, as it is sometimes called), the smoker puffs and inhales at a very rapid rate (i.e., usually every 6 seconds) until reaching a point of nausea. Small-scale studies using this technique with motivated smokers has resulted in an abstinence rate of up to 60% at the end of 1 year.

Research suggests that there are some pharmacologic determinants to smoking. Nicotine is the most likely candidate for such a determinant. Trials in both North America and Europe have indicated that nicotine replacement by nicotine gum may be a useful treatment modality for a dependent smoker. The gum is available as a prescription drug in the United States and Canada (see Chapter 26, "Ganglionic Stimulants and Blockers and Neuromuscular Blocking Agents").

Widely available public and commercial programs. Formal programs for smoking cessation range from programs provided for with a minimal or no fee through the American Cancer Society, the American Heart Association, and the American Lung Association, to SmokeEnders, Schick Laboratories, and St. Helena programs that charge several hundred dollars for a course of treatment. Content is as variable as price. Nonprofit programs, such as those offered by health-related societies, frequently use volunteer staff members to provide tips, group support, and positive reinforcement. On the other end of the continuum, the St. Helena Hospital and Health Center in Deer Park, California offers a 5-day inpatient program, which includes individual and group counseling, lectures, films, physical therapy, and exercise.

Again, outcome data are not available on most of these programs, so it is difficult to evaluate their basic cost-benefit effectiveness. An exception to this is the SmokeEnders program, which has allowed some research into its effectiveness. Kanzler, Jaffe, and Zeidenberg (1976) reported a 70% cessation rate immediately posttreatment, with follow-up rates of 57% for men and 30% for women. These figures are probably an overestimation of efficacy, because a substantial proportion of participants could not be contacted.

Alcohol*

Problems of definition. Most experts consider it practical to distinguish between alcoholism and problem drinking, because many alcohol-related problems involve excessive use but do not involve addiction to alcohol per se. Many definitions of alcoholism have been advanced. In general, they all have in common the following elements: high alcohol consumption is almost always present; some type of addiction occurs; cessation or reduction of the usual drinking pattern results in withdrawal symptoms; and drinking has resulted in some type of impairment to physical health or to social or psychologic functioning.

Other than these general criteria, there is considerable disagreement on how alcoholism should be defined. Usually, differing definitions reflect differences in the etiologic models underlying the definitions. Some models such as Jellinek's (1960) seek to identify the alcoholic via both physiologic addiction and by a loss of control whenever drinking is initiated. Other definitions, which assume a similar etiology, also imply that an inability to return to normal drinking is a hallmark of the alcoholic.

In contrast to these physical disease models, other models have classified alcoholism as a coping strategy for adapting to conflicting needs (e.g., the World Health Organization, 1976).

Problem drinking, on the other hand, is used as a catchall term to describe a variety of drinking patterns that have resulted in harmful consequences, but that do not represent alcoholism per se. Problem drinkers are considered to include individuals who drink very heavily, but who function adequately and do not experience physical symptoms. Others may drink infrequently, but when they do they cause accidents or become aggressive.

Incidence and prevalence of alcoholism. Estimating the number of alcoholics and problem drinkers in the United States and Canada is difficult, in part because of these differing definitions, and also in part because of the stigma involved in being an alcoholic. In 1978, the National Institute on Alcoholism and Alcohol Abuse (NIAAA) estimated that there were somewhere between 9.3 and 10 million problem drinkers in the United States. At the time this was 10% of the men in the country, and 3% of the women. However, many experts feel these statistics with respect to women are inaccurate, because alcoholism may take dif-

---

*Much of the information presented in this section is summarized from E. P. Noble (Ed.). *Third special report to the U.S. Congress on alcohol and health.* Washington, D.C.: Department of Health, Education, and Welfare, 1978.

ferent undiagnosed forms in women. There were marked increases in alcohol consumption in the United States during the decade of 1960 to 1970. Alcohol consumption in the period from 1971 to 1976 was fairly constant. However, during that 6-year period an increase in alcohol consumption for women was noted, the result primarily of the women who moved into the moderate drinking (7 to 20 drinks a week) category. Some interpretations of these data suggest that this increase in modest drinking in women is caused by increased numbers of women entering into the workforce, because employment for women is generally correlated with alcohol consumption whereas being a homemaker is not. However, in general, the relationship between changes in women's roles and increases in drinking are not clear.

Problem drinking is not confined to adults: it is estimated that there are 3.3 million problem drinkers among youths 14 to 17 years of age and this figure constitutes 19% of that age group. This is a particularly disturbing statistic because many young people are unable to handle even moderate or light doses of alcohol, and become impulsive, aggressive, or to engage in tasks they should avoid, such as driving a car while drunk.

As is the case with many drugs, there is some evidence that alcohol abuse is especially a problem among ethnic groups who are denied access to more satisfying means of fulfillment. There is some evidence that problem drinking tends to be greater in the Spanish-speaking American community than in the general population. Within the black American culture, little adequate data are available; however, alcohol use patterns do not seem to differ markedly from those of Caucasians, except that black women are more likely to be either abstainers or heavy drinkers than are Caucasian women. However, impressionistic and observational data suggest that heavy alcohol consumption and alcohol abuse are some of the central social and mental health problems of the black community. It is not known if it is a relatively greater problem than in other segments of society.

Among all of the special population groups in the United States, the highest frequency of problems associated with drinking has been attributed to Native Americans. However, there is little evidence to indicate that rates of alcohol abuse among Native Americans are actually higher than those of other ethnic groups. Further, although it has long been assumed that Native Americans are genetically predisposed to pathologic responses to alcohol, no evidence exists to support this assumption.

Psychologic effects of alcoholism. Alcohol is a

CNS depressant; among the psychologic effects of the drug are relaxation, euphoria, and drowsiness. Along with these subjectively pleasant effects, the other effects of alcoholism as a CNS depressant include impaired judgment, decreased reaction and coordination, and loss of emotional control.

Health consequences of alcoholism. Excessive use of alcohol results in a plethora of aversive health consequences, including damage to the esophagus, stomach, lower intestine, and pancreas. These effects are the result primarily of chronic inflammation and irritation caused by the alcohol. Alcoholism has been found to be related to cirrhosis of the liver and to hepatitis. Excessive alcohol ingestion clearly results in decreased intellectual functioning, which reflects underlying damage to the brain. Further, excessive alcohol use has been associated with heart disease. Major coronary diseases are significantly higher in moderate to heavy drinkers.

There is also evidence that alcohol is related to cancer. Heavy drinkers have been regularly found to show high mortality rates from cancer of the mouth, pharynx, larynx, esophagus, liver, and lungs. If levels of cigarette smoking are controlled for, the correlation between alcohol ingestion and lung cancer disappears. However, there is some suggestion that alcohol and tobacco interact synergistically to increase rates of cancer of the mouth, pharynx, larynx, and esophagus. The relationship to stomach cancer is questionable.

A final health-related risk of alcohol consumption is that to the unborn child. Fetal alcohol syndrome (FAS) is considered the third leading cause of birth defects in the United States, and is the only one that is now preventable. The unborn child is at risk of developing the syndrome if its mother drinks 1 ounce of absolute alcohol (i.e., approximately 2 drinks) or more per day during her pregnancy. The features of the syndrome include growth deficiencies, unique facial features, heart defects, brain abnormality, and intellectual deficits.

Withdrawal symptoms of alcoholism. Withdrawal symptoms of alcoholism range from disturbed sleep, nausea, weakness, anxiety, and mild tremors to cramps, vomiting, and tremors so severe that the patient cannot even lift a glass. In extreme cases, patients may hallucinate, experience grand mal seizures, and become confused, disoriented, and agitated. Death because of cardiovascular collapse may occur.

Treatment modalities for alcoholism

Alcoholics Anonymous. Alcoholics Anonymous (AA) is an organization, a fellowship to its members, of alcoholics. The members offer each other support, understanding, and a coherent philosophy by which to lead abstinent lives. Alcoholics Anonymous very likely treats more alcoholics than any other modality. From 1935, when AA was founded by two alcoholics, to 1975, this group has expanded to 7500 chapters, which hold a total of 10,000 meetings per year in the United States, District of Columbia, Canal Zone, Canada, and Puerto Rico. Estimates of membership generally exceed 250,000. Alcoholics Anonymous is frequently criticized by professionals because of the organization's general disdain for data, outcome, and professional intervention. The success rate of AA is estimated at 30 to 35%.

Pharmacologic agents. Disulfiram produces adverse effects when alcohol is consumed. It increases heart and respiratory rates, and results in a cold sweat. Administration of disulfiram was once thought to be a panacea for alcoholism, but it is very questionable how many alcoholics prescribed disulfiram actually continue to take it for any length of time. It is contraindicated for individuals with arteriosclerosis, heart disease, cirrhosis, kidney disease, diabetes mellitus, and some other chronic disorders. It may cause hepatitis, acute brain syndrome, and convulsions. Although it may be of value to some alcoholics, especially highly motivated ones, its use *without* adjunctive therapy aimed at the cause of the alcoholism is discouraged.

Behavioral treatments. Behavioral treatments are based on a learning etiology (i.e., they are based on the idea that alcoholism is not a disease, but an overlearned drinking pattern). It assumes that relearning experiences can result in a decrease in excessive drinking. Early attempts to treat alcoholism behaviorally relied almost entirely on aversive conditioning. Early reports came from Kantorovich (1930), who used electric shock as the aversive stimulus. He reported a 70% abstinence rate at 3 to 20 months follow-up; however, controlled attempts to replicate these results produced questionable outcomes. Other clinicians have used chemical aversion, most notably emetine, to produce abstinence in alcoholics. Lemere and Voegtlin (1950) reported 60% abstinence in 1 year; however, when the effects of aversive conditioning are considered in controlled studies, whether the aversive stimulus be a chemical or electric shock, the results are not at all definitive. It appears that many of the clinical effects noted are the result of anticipation and other nonspecific factors.

A controversy in the study of alcoholism is whether alcoholics and alcohol abusers can be taught to drink moderately, rather than insisting on total abstinence. Several outcome studies have been reported that compare training in moderate drinking strategies with various controls, including regular hospital treatment and bibliotherapy. The outcome usually has favored the moderate drinking training and has indicated that a sizeable proportion of patients do maintain controlled levels of drinking. However, no controlled comparisons between abstinence and moderate drinking strategies are available, so an answer to the controversy is not available. It would seem that if moderate drinking is a possible and desirable outcome for some alcohol abusers, it will be a somewhat limited number, probably those who drink heavily but who have not suffered severe physical, psychologic, or social damage as a result of their drinking.

Even with respect to abstinence, behavioral approaches are generally moving away from aversion to a broader perspective. Innovations include assertiveness training for alcoholics who are unable to express themselves appropriately in certain demanding situations and training in marital interaction and interpersonal communication.

Other treatments. Many therapeutic communities that deal primarily with drug abusers also treat alcoholics. Because such communities differentiate very little between the drug addict and the alcoholic, treatment for the alcoholic is essentially the same as for the drug addict.

Additionally, many hospitals are developing or have developed inpatient programs for alcoholics. The usual program includes detoxification, physical rehabilitation, counseling, group therapy, and AA sessions. Other programs have techniques as diverse as hypnosis, LSD, psychovitamin therapy, sensitivity groups, psychodrama, acupuncture, behavior modification, biofeedback, and controlled drinking training. So far, there are no general statistics available about outcomes from these programs. However, it should be noted that inpatient programs do treat many alcoholics. In the decade from 1962 to 1972 the percentage of alcoholics admitted to state and county facilities increased from 15% to 26.1%; the percentage admitted to Veteran's hospitals increased four times to 30%.

OTHER COMMONLY ABUSED DRUGS

Phencyclidine

Phencyclidine (PCP) was first introduced by Parke, Davis, and Company as an anesthetic for humans. It was withdrawn from human use because of severe psychologic and behavioral effects. However, it is still marketed for use as an animal tranquilizer. It first made its appearance on the streets in capsule form around 1965. However, in this form users found it dif-

ficult to titrate, and bad effects were extremely common. The drug rapidly developed a bad reputation on the street and its use practically disappeared. It was reintroduced on the street about 1972. However, the principal mode of administration at that time was to sprinkle PCP in dust form on leaf material such as parsley, marijuana, or tobacco and smoke it. In the NIDA Drug Abuse Survey of 1976, 3% of 12 to 17 year olds said they had used the drug at least once. Of the 18 to 25 year olds surveyed, 9.5% said they had used PCP at least once. It appeared that PCP use was increasing rather rapidly, for in 1977 5.8% of the 12 to 17 year olds and 13.9% of the 18 to 25 year olds had used the drug.

There is some question about why PCP gained popularity, because the effects emphasized in both the media and in clinical reports are negative. The reports are of perceptual disturbances, restlessness, disorientation, anxiety, paranoia, irritability, psychosis, and violent behavior. However, surveys indicate some users occasionally find great enjoyment in the drug and many, but not all, users report positive effects occuring during PCP use although negative effects may also be present. Positive effects include heightened sensitivity to outside stimuli, mood elevation, inebriation, relaxation, and tranquility.

The drug has numerous CNS, autonomic nervous system, and cardiovascular effects. Small doses do lead to a drunken state, whereas higher doses can lead to analgesia and anesthesia. Sensory impulses seem to be blocked from reaching the cortex or reach there only in distorted forms. Cataleptic motor responses and convulsions have been reported. The drug also increases the heart rate and blood pressure. Clinical reports indicate that tolerance is possible, but withdrawal symptoms have not been reported other than craving.

Luisada (1978) describes the existence of a schizophrenic-like reaction to PCP characterized by an initial state of violent psychotic paranoid behavior, which gradually decreases over the course of about 10 days, but that seems to be reactivated by other incidences of PCP use. There is some evidence that schizophrenia is linked to this form of PCP sensitivity. Luisada (1978) reports gradual amelioration of the psychosis using chlorpromazine. Other authors suggest using diazepam or haloperidol in the treatment of PCP toxicity.

Marijuana

Marijuana, or cannabis, the dried top of the hemp plant, is generally smoked, although it is sometimes eaten, either baked into other foods or sprinkled on top of them. Some users drink the tea-like infusion.

The psychoactive substance in *Cannabis sativa*, the plant from which marijuana is derived, is delta-9-tetrahydrocannabinol (THC). The proportion of THC in marijuana and hashish may vary considerably: from 1% to 8% for a marijuana cigarette (i.e., joint or reefer); up to 15% for the resin (i.e., hashish or ganja); and up to 60% for the extract (i.e., hashish oil or weed oil).

Marijuana use is common, and is increasingly becoming a socially acceptable drug for a broad spectrum of Americans. In 1977, 42 million Americans had used it at least once and 16 million considered themselves current users. Whereas daily use is generally believed to be uncommon, in the 3 years from 1975 to 1978 the percentage of high school seniors reporting daily use almost doubled, rising from 6% to 11%.

Further, marijuana use began at an earlier age in 1979 than it did a decade before. For example, from 1976 to 1977, the percentage of those between 12 and 17 years of age who had ever used marijuana increased 25%, and the number who had used it in the month preceding the survey increased 30%. By contrast, use in the over 18-year-old group did not change significantly. This statistic is a cause for some concern because evidence also exists that many of the effects of marijuana (discussed later in detail) lead to impaired classroom learning.

The effects of marijuana are varied, and depend to a great extent on the dose, the expectation users have about the drug, and the environment in which they consume it. Users' reports of increased well-being, relaxation, euphoria, spontaneous laughter, and increased perceptual sensitivity explain the popularity of the drug. On the other hand, at high doses, or among inexperienced users, transient mild paranoia and anxiety are common. Some evidence exists that marijuana use may lead to an exacerbation of psychotic symptoms in patients in partial remission from schizophrenia.

Marijuana's acute effects appear to be detrimental to individuals in learning situations (i.e., youngsters in school). Particularly relevant are impaired concept formation, reading comprehension, and short-term memory.

Marijuana may have other effects to be considered, especially with chronic use. Many authorities suggest that daily use of the drug may result in lung damage not different than that found in heavy smokers, but as yet the data are indirect, especially with respect to humans, because heavy marijuana users are often heavy cigarette smokers.

Even more controversial is the effect of marijuana on the reproductive system, although authorities agree that use during pregnancy is unwise. Although research on the effect of marijuana on the immune response, on chromosomal abnormalities, and on brain damage continues, the data remain inconclusive. The drug does perpetuate chest pain in those with already impaired functions, and its use in the presence of coronary disease is not recommended.

Most authorities agree that tolerance to marijuana use occurs and that both the magnitude and the rapidity with which it develops depends on the size and frequency of repeated dose. However, whether tolerance is related to drug-seeking behavior is unclear.

Because marijuana users rarely perceive its use as a problem and do not often present themselves for treatment, no specific treatment modalities are available. Like alcohol, however, excessive marijuana use may be part of the adjustment problems noted particularly in adolescents, and referrals to supportive counseling, psychotherapy, or family therapy may be appropriate. A growing concern involves driving while under the influence of marijuana. Marijuana, even when used at social levels, can significantly impair driving skills and may be a major contributing factor to highway traffic accidents and death.

There is evidence also that marijuana is becoming increasingly involved in emergency room admissions. During a 1-year period beginning May 1976 and ending April 1977, marijuana ranked thirteenth among drugs mentioned in emergency room contacts. By 1978, however, marijuana had risen to sixth place. The cause of this increase is not easily discernable, and may reflect either increased use, less concern about revealing use, or increased potency of the drug.

Cocaine and amphetamines

Over 2 million Americans have tried cocaine. In spite of the cost, as of 1977, it seemed clear that cocaine use is increasing. In 1976, 9% of the 18 to 25 year olds reported having used cocaine. In 1977, 19% of the individuals in that age group reported prior use.

The CNS effects of cocaine include euphoria, increased confidence, increased energy, and increases in heart rate, blood pressure, body temperature, and metabolic rate. Use of the drug also results in dilated pupils and a constriction of blood vessels. Tolerance to cocaine apparently does occur, but a withdrawal syndrome has not been reported. Cocaine is *not* physically addicting, but has an extremely high potential to reinforce severe psychologic dependence. With chronic use symptoms such as irritability and difficulty in concentration are seen. Some individuals show serious psychologic dependence, spending vast amounts of money to maintain their cocaine habit.

The other class of commonly abused stimulant drugs are amphetamines. Subjectively, their effects seem to differ little from cocaine. Amphetamines are often used to dilute (i.e., cut) cocaine in the illicit market to increase profits. Use of amphetamines, however, at least intravenously, has decreased sharply in the United States from the late 1960s to the late 1970s.

Nonmedical use of prescription drugs

Nonmedical use of prescription drugs has become a problem of increasing concern, in part because it is difficult to determine the extent to which this exists, and to what extent the prescribing clinicians are involved. For all age groups except the 18 to 25 year olds, the use of prescription drugs from 1972 to 1977 stayed fairly constant, and fairly low. For example, the percentage of adults over 25 years of age who reported nonmedical use of sedatives was 4% in 1972; in 1977 it was 6%. However, in the short time period from 1976 to 1977 the percentage of 18 to 25 year olds reporting nonmedical use of prescription drugs increased markedly from 12% to 18%, and this trend appears to be continuing to date.

The psychopharmacology of these drugs are discussed elsewhere in this book (see Chapters 15, "Sedative-Hypnotics," and 17, "Analgesics and Narcotic Antagonists"). To appreciate the enormity of the problem of the nonmedical use of prescription drugs one must only consider the informed estimates stating that up to 30% of the barbiturates currently *legally* manufactured in the United States and Canada are diverted to the black market.

Of all the prescription drugs that are commonly abused, barbiturates are not only among the most common, but are also the most dangerous, and therefore deserve special mention.

With respect to lethality, between May 1977 and April 1978 barbiturates accounted for 20% of the drugs mentioned in connection with deaths reported by emergency rooms to the Drug Abuse Warning Network (DAWN). Some authorities have suggested that there are as many as 500,000 barbiturate abusers in the United States alone. How many individuals are actually addicted to barbiturates is unknown.

Most authorities assume there is a good deal of variability in the characteristics of barbiturate-dependent individuals. They may range from older middle-class individuals who overdose themselves, often secretly using medication prescribed for dysphoric states, to the younger, street-wise individuals who acquire the drug through peers, and use it in social settings.

The effects of barbiturate intoxication are qualitatively similar to intoxification with alcohol. Users report elevated mood; decreased self-criticism, anxiety, and guilt; and increased energy and self-confidence. However, sadness, mood lability, hypochondriac concerns, and agitation are also experienced.

Jaffee et al. (1980), among others, note that there are marked similarities in the withdrawal syndromes seen with barbiturates and those seen with methaqualone, glutethimide, meprobamate, benzodiaze-pines, and related sedative-hypnotics. In its mildest form, this general depressant syndrome may consist of only an increase in anxiety and insomnia. Sudden cessation or marked decrease in high-dosage self-medication of sedative-hypnotics results in a characteristic abstinence syndrome (i.e., withdrawal), which includes anxiety, nausea, vomiting, hyperactive reflexes, generalized convulsions, delirium, desensitization, and psychosis. Barbiturate withdrawal is much more severe than heroin withdrawal, is potentially fatal, and is best carried out on an inpatient basis, where longer-acting barbiturates (e.g., phenobarbital) are substituted for the shorter-acting substances of addiction, and the dosage is gradually reduced over a period of several days to weeks.

Hallucinogens

With the exception of PCP, the use of hallucinogens seems to be declining rapidly. This category includes many drugs, however, the most widely researched of these drugs is lysergic acid diethylamide (LSD). Psilocybin, dimethyltryptamine (DMT) and diethyltryptamine (DET), mescaline, and 2, 5-demethoxy-4 methyl amphetamine (DOM), are also included in this category.

Drugs of this type can produce illusions (i.e., false interpretations of a real sensory image), hallucinations (i.e., false perceptions not based in reality), pseudo-hallucinations (i.e., voluntarily induced hallucinations), and marked changes in mood. Loss of body boundaries, and feelings of calmness and oneness with the universe have been reported; on the other hand, under different conditions with different individuals these same drugs can produce severe anxiety, feelings of depersonalization, and a fear of the fragmentation of self.

Most authorities agree that chronic use of hallucinogens is not common, and that most individuals who use them chronically for a time soon tire of them. Both acute panic reactions to drug effects and anxiety aroused by flashbacks, (i.e., spontaneous recurrence of the drug's effects after a normal nonuse period) have been reported as therapeutic problems. Most authorities suggest a calm environment and reassurance as central to treatment, with adjunctive use of diazepam or chlorpromazine if the reassurance fails.

Attempts have been made to use LSD to facilitate psychotherapeutic changes in alcoholics, and in opiate addiction, but the potentially adverse side effects of the drugs, as well as their uncontrollability, has led to a decrease in interest in them. These same factors probably influenced their decline in street usage, although legal strictures no doubt also contributed to this effect.

SUMMARY

Drug abuse and addiction are endemic in society. The causes are variant and multifactorial. The various theories that have been proposed to account for addiction have been examined and briefly discussed in this chapter. These include the somatic, intrapsychic, and learning theories. Common illicit and prescription substances of abuse were also presented along with various approaches to dealing with problems of abuse. With a knowledge and understanding of the complexities of drug and substance abuse, nurses can work towards preventing this increasingly growing problem. In addition, they can better recognize signs of drug abuse and assist patients with problems associated with addiction.

BIBLIOGRAPHY

Abruzzi, W. Drug-induced psychosis. *International Journal of the Addictions*, 1977, *121*, 183-193.

Ausabel, D.P. Causes and types of narcotic addiction: a psychosocial view. *Psychiatric Quarterly*, 1961, *35*, 523-531.

Ausabel, D.P. An interactional approach to narcotic addiction. In D.J. Lettieri, M. Sayers, & H.W. Pearson (Eds.). *Theories on drug abuse: selected contemporary perspectives*. NIDA Research Monograph, 1980, *30* (GPO No. not available).

Babor, T.F., Meyer, R.E., Mirin, S.M., McNamee, H.B., & Davies, M. Behavioral and social effects of heroin self-administration. *Archives of General Psychiatry*, 1976, *33*, 363-367.

Balster, R.L., & Chait, L.D. The behavioral pharmacology of phencyclidine. *Clinical Toxicology*, 1976, *9*, 513-528.

Bourne, P.G. Issues in addiction. In P.G. Bourne (Ed.). *Addiction*. New York: Academic Press, 1974.

Brecher, E.M., & the Editors of Consumer Reports. *Licit and illicit drugs*. Boston: Little, Brown and Co., 1972.

Danaher, B.G., & Lichtenstein, E. *Become an ex-smoker*. Englewood Cliffs, N.J.: Prentice-Hall, Inc., 1978.

DeAngeles, G.G., & Goldstein, E. Long-term treatment of adolescent PCP abuse. In R.C. Peterson & R.C. Stillman (Eds.). *Phencyclidine (PCP) abuse: an appraisal*. NIDA Research Monograph, 1978, *21* (GPO No. 017-024-00785-4).

DeLeon, G., & Rosenthal, M.S. Therapeutic communities. In R.I. Dupont, A. Goldstein, and J. O'Donnell (Eds.). *Handbook on drug abuse*. NIDA Research Monograph, 1979, *27*, (GPO No. 017-024-00981-4).

Dole, V.P., & Nyswander, M.E. Methadone maintenance: a theoretical perspective. In D.J. Lettieri, M. Sayers, & H.W. Pearson (Eds.). *Theories on drug abuse: selected contemporary perspectives*. NIDA Research Monograph, 1980, *30* (GPO No. not available).

Dutta, S.N. Sedative hypnotics. In S.N. Pradhan & S.N. Dutta (Eds.). *Drug abuse: clinical and basic aspects*. St. Louis: The C.V. Mosby Co., 1977.

Foy, D.W., Miller, P.M., Eisler, R.M., & O'Toole, D.H. Social skills training to teach alcoholics to refuse drinks effectively. *Quarterly Journal of Studies in Alcohol*, 1976, *37*, 1340-1345.

Fulwiler, R.L., Hargreaves, W.A., & Bortman, R. Detoxification from heroin using self vs. physician regulation of methadone dose. *International Journal of the Addictions*, 1979, *14*, 289-298.

Gay, G.R., & Inaba, D.S. Acute and chronic toxicology of cocaine abuse: current sociology treatment and rehabilitation. In S.J. Mule (Ed.). *Cocaine: chemicals, biological, clinical, social, and treatment aspects*. Cleveland, Ohio: CRC Press, 1976.

Gilbert, D.G. Paradoxical tranquility and emotion reducing effects of nicotine. *Psychological Bulletin*, 1979, *86*, 643-661.

Gold, M.S., Redmond, D.E., & Kleber, H.D. Nora adrenergic hyperactivity in opiate withdrawal supported by clonidine reversal of opiate withdrawal. *American Journal of Psychiatry*, 1979, *136*, 100-102.

Grinspoon, L., & Bakalar, J.B. Cocaine. In R.I. Dupont, A. Goldstein, & J. O'Donnell (Eds.). *Handbook on drug abuse*. NIDA Research Monograph, 1979, *27* (GPO No. not available).

Gritz, E.R., Brunswick, A., & Bierman, K.L. Psychosocial and behavioral aspects of smoking in women. In J.S. Pinney (Ed.). *Health consequences of smoking for women: a report of the Surgeon General*. Bethesda, Office on Smoking and Health, 1980.

Hall, R.G., Sachs, D.P.L., & Hall, S.M. Medical safety of rapid smoking. *Behavior Therapy*, 1979, *10*, 249-259.

Hall, S.M. The abstinence phobia. In N.A. Krasneger (Ed.). *Behavioral analysis and treatment of substance abuse*. NIDA Research Monograph Number, 1979, *25* (GPO No. 017-024-00939-3).

Hall, S.M., Bass, A., Hargreaves, W.A., & Loeb, P.L. Contingency management and information feedback in outpatient heroin detoxification. *Behavior Therapy*, 1979, *10*, 443-451.

Ikard, F.F., & Tompkins, S. The experience of affect as a determinant of smoking behavior: a series of validity tests. *Journal of Abnormal Psychology*, 1973, *81*, 172-181.

Jaffe, J.H., & Martin, W.R. Opiod analgesics and antagonists. In A.G. Gilman, L.S. Goodman, and A. Gilman (Eds.). *The *pharmacological basis of therapeutics.* New York: Macmillan, Inc., 1980.

Jellinek, E.M. *The disease concept of alcoholism.* New Haven: College and University Press and Hillhouse Press, 1960.

Jones, R.T. Human effects: an overview. In R.C. Peterson (Ed.). *Marijuana research findings: 1980.* NIDA Research Monograph, 1980, *31* (GPO No. not available).

Jones, R.T., & Benowitz, N. The 30-day trip-clinical studies of cannabis tolerance and dependence. In M.C. Branda & S. Szara (Eds.). *Pharmacology of marijuana.* New York: Raven Press, 1976.

Jones, R.T., Benowitz, N., & Bachman, J. Clinical studies of cannabis tolerance and dependence. *Annals of the New York Academy of Science,* 1976, *282,* 221-239.

Kantorovich, N.V. An attempt at associative reflex therapy in alcoholism. *Psychological Abstracts,* 1930, *1,* 493.

Kanzler, M., Jaffee, J., & Zeidenberg, P. Long and short-term effectiveness of a large scale-proprietary smoking cessation program—a 4 year follow-up of SmokeEnders participants. *Journal of Clinical Psychology,* 1976, *32,* 551-569.

Kleber, H.D. Detoxification from methadone maintenance: the state of the art. *International Journal of the Addictions,* 1977, *12,* 870-880.

Kleber, H.D., & Slobetz, F. Outpatient drug-free treatment. In R.I. Dupont, A. Goldstein, and J. O'Donnell (Eds.). *Handbook on drug abuse.* NIDA Research Monograph, 1979, *27* (GPO No. not available).

Lemere, F. Normal drinking in recovery alcohol addicts: further comment on the articles by D.L. Davies. *Quarterly Journal of Studies in Alcohol,* 1978, *24,* 727-728.

Lemere, F., & Voegtlin, W.L. An evaluation of the aversion treatment of alcoholism. *Quarterly Journal of Studies in Alcohol,* 1950, *11,* 199-204.

Lerner, S., & Burns, R.S. Phencyclidine use among youth: history, epidemiology and acute and chronic intoxification. In R.C. Peterson & R.C. Stillman (Eds.). *Phencyclidine (PCP) abuse: an appraisal.* NIDA Research Monograph, 1978, *21* (GPO No. 017-024-00785-4).

Luisada, P.V. The phencyclidine psychosis: phenomenology and treatment. In R.C. Peterson & R.C. Stillman (Eds.). *Phencyclidine (PCP) abuse: an appraisal.* NIDA Research Monograph, 1978, *21* (GPO No. 017-024-00785-4).

Marlatt, G.A. Craving for alcohol, loss of control and relapse: a cognitive-behavioral analysis. In P.E. Nathan, G.A. Marlatt, & T. Loberg (Eds.). *Alcoholism: new directions in behavioral research and treatment.* New York: Plenum Press, 1978.

Marlatt, G.A. Alcohol, stress and cognitive control. In I.G. Sarason & C.D. Speilberger (Eds.). *Stress and anxiety.* Washington, D.C.: Hemisphere Publishing Corp., 1976.

Marlatt, G.A., and Gordon, J.R. Determinants of relapse: implications for the maintenance of behavior change. In P.O. Davidson & S.M. Davidson (Eds.). *Behavioral medicine: changing health lifestyles.* New York: Bruner/Mazel, Inc., 1980.

McAllister, A., Puska, P., Koskela, K., Pallonen, U., & Maccoby, N. Mass communication and community organization for public health education. *American Psychologist,* 1980, *35,* 375-379.

Miller, P.M., & Eisler, R.M. Assertive behavior of alcoholics. *Behavior Therapy,* 1977, *8,* 146-149.

Misra, R.K. Achievement, anxiety and addiction. In D.J. Lettieri, M. Sayers, & H.W. Pearson (Eds.). *Theories on drug abuse: selected contemporary perspectives.* NIDA Research Monograph, 1980, *30* (GPO No. not available).

Nathan, P.E. Alcoholism. In H. Leitenberg (Ed.). *Handbook of behavior modification and behavior therapy.* Englewood Cliffs, N.J.: Prentice-Hall, Inc., 1976.

Noble, E.P. (Ed.). *Third special report to the U.S. Congress on alcohol and health.* Washington, D.C.: Department of Health, Education and Welfare, 1978.

Nowlan, K., & Cohen, S. Tolerance to marijuana: heart rate and subjective "high." *Clinical Pharmacology and Therapeutics,* 1977, *22,* 550-556.

Pehacek, T.F. An overview of smoking behavior and its modification. In N.A. Krasnegor (Ed.). *Behavioral analysis and treatment of substance abuse.* NIDA Research Monograph, 1979, *25* (GPO No. 017-024-00939-3).

Peterson, R.C. Marijuana and health: 1980. In R.C. Peterson (Ed.). *Marijuana research findings: 1980.* NIDA Research Monograph, 1980, *31* (GPO No. not available).

Peterson, R.C., & Stillman, K.C. Phencyclidine: an overview. In R.C. Peterson & R.C. Stillman (Eds.). *Phencyclidine (PCP) abuse: an appraisal.* NIDA Research Monograph, 1978, *21* (GPO No. 017-024-00785-4).

Pittel, S., & Oppendahl, M.C. The enigma of PCP. In R.I. Dupont, A. Goldstein, & J. O'Donnell (Eds.). *Handbook on drug abuse.* NIDA Research Monograph, 1979, *27* (GPO No. not available).

Platt, J., & L'abate, C. *Heroin addiction: theory, research and treatment.* New York: John Wiley & Sons, Inc., 1976.

Pomerleau, O.F. Commonalities in the treatment and understanding of smoking and other self-management disorders. In N.A. Krasnegor (Ed.). *Behavioral analysis and treatment of substance abuse.* NIDA Research Monograph, 1979, *30* (GPO No. 017-024-00939-3).

Pomerleau, O.F., & Pomerleau, C.S. *Break the smoking habit.* Champaign, Ill.: Research Press, 1977.

Pradhan, S.N., & Hollister, L.E. Abuse of LSD and other hallucinogenic drugs. In S.N. Pradhan & S.N. Dutta (Eds.). *Drug abuse: clinical and basic aspects.* St. Louis: The C.V. Mosby Co., 1977.

Rado, S. The psychoanalysis of pharmacothymia (drug addiction). *Psychoanalytic Quarterly,* 1933, *2,* 22.

Report of the National Research Council Committee on Clinical Evaluation of Narcotic Antagonists. Clinical evaluation of naltrexone treatment of opiate dependent individuals. *Archives of General Psychiatry,* 1978, *35,* 335-340.

Schwartz, J.L. Smoking cures: ways to kick an unhealthy habit. In M.E. Jarvik, J.W. Cullen, E.K. Gritz, T.M. Vogt, & L.S. West (Eds.). *Research on smoking behavior.* NIDA Research Monograph, 1977, *17* (GPO No. 017-024-00694-7).

Senay, E., Dorus, W., Goldberg, F., & Thornton, W. Withdrawal from methadone maintenance. *Archives of General Psychiatry,* 1977, *34,* 361-367.

Sheffet, A., Quinones, M., Lavanhar, M.E., Doyle, K., & Praeger, C. An evaluation of detoxification as an initial step in the treatment of heroin addiction. *American Journal of Psychiatry,* 1976, *133,* 270-274.

Shiffman, S.M. The tobacco withdrawal syndrome. In N.A. Krasnegor (Ed.). *Cigarette smoking as a dependence process.* NIDA Research Monograph, 1979, *23* (GPO No. 017-024-0895-8).

Shiffman, S.M., & Jarvik, M.E. Smoking withdrawal symptoms in two weeks of abstinence. *Psychopharmacology,* 1976, *50,* 35-39.

Showalter, C.V., & Thornton, W.E. Clinical pharmacology on phencyclidine toxicity. *American Journal of Psychiatry,* 1977, *134,* 1234-1238.

Shuckit, M.A. A theory of alcohol and drug abuse: a genetic approach. In D.J. Lettier, M. Sayers, & H.W. Pearson (Eds.). *Theories on drug abuse: selected contemporary perspectives.* NIDA Research Monograph, 1980, *30* (GPO No. not available).

Shuman, L.M. The benefits of the cessation of smoking. *Chest,* 1971, *59,* 421-427.

Siegal, R.K. Phencyclidine and ketamine intoxication: a study of the four populations of recreational users. In R.C. Peterson & R.C. Stillman (Eds.). *Phencyclidine (PCP) abuse: an appraisal.* NIDA Research Monograph, 1978, *21* (GPO No. 017-024-00785-4).

Smith, D.E., Wesson, D.R., & Seymour, R.B. The abuse of barbiturates and other sedative hypnotics. In R.I. Dupont, A. Goldstein, & J. O'Donnell (Eds.). *Handbook on drug abuse.* Washington, D.C.: National Institute on Drug Abuse, 1979.

Smith, E.C., Wesson, D.R., Buxton, M.E., Seymour, R., & Kramer, H.M. The diagnosis and treatment of the PCP abuse syndrome. In R.C. Peterson & R.C. Stillman (Eds.). *Phencyclidine (PCP) abuse: an appraisal.* NIDA Research Monograph, 1978, *21* (GPO No. 017-024-00785-4).

Solomon, R.L., & Corbit, J.D. An opponent-process theory of motivation II: cigarette addiction. *Journal of Abnormal Psychology,* 1973, *81,* 158-171.

Tennant, F.S. Outpatient treatment and outcome of prescription drug abuse. In L.S. Harris (Ed.). *Problems of drug dependence.* NIDA Research Monograph, 1979, *27* (GPO No. 017-024-00981-4).

U.S. Department of Health, Education and Welfare, Public Health Service. *Smoking and health.* Washington, D.C.: U.S. Government Printing Office, 1964.

VanLancker, J. Smoking and disease. In M.E. Jarvik, J.W. Cullen, E.R. Gritz, T.M. Vogt, & L.J. West (Eds.). *Research on smoking behavior.* NIDA Research Monograph, 1977, *17* (GPO No. 017-024-00694-7).

Vischi, T.R., Jones, K.R., Shank, E.L., & Lima, L.H. *The alcohol drug abuse and mental health national data book.* NIDA Research Monograph, 1980, (GPO No. not available).

Vogler, R.E., Lunde, S.E., Johnson, G.R., & Martin, P.L. Electrical aversion conditioning with chronic alcoholics. *Journal of Consulting and Clinical Psychology,* 1970, *34,* 302-307.

Washington, A.M., Resnick, R.B., & Rawson, R.A. Clonodine hydrochloride: a nonopiate treatment for opiate withdrawal. In L.S. Harris (Ed.). *Problems of drug dependence,* NIDA Research Monograph, 1979, *27* (GPO No. 017-024-00981-4).

Wikler, A. Dynamics of drug dependence: implications of a conditioning theory for research and treatment. *Archives of General Psychiatry,* 1973, *28,* 611-616.

World Health Organization. *Alcohol related problems in the disability perspective.* Geneva: World Health Organization, 1976.

CENTRAL NERVOUS SYSTEM MEDICATIONS

Medications discussed in this section

CHAPTER 18

Acetophenazine
Butaperazine
Carphenazine
Chlorpromazine
Chlorprothixene
Droperidol
Fluphenazine
Haloperidol
Loxapine
Mesoridazine
Methotrimeprazine
Molindone
Perphenazine
Pimozide
Piperacetazine
Prochlorperazine
Promazine
Thiopropazate
Thioridazine
Thiothixene
Trifluoperazine
Triflupromazine

CHAPTER 19

Amitriptyline
Amoxapine
Clomipramine
Desipramine
Doxepin
Imipramine
Isocarboxazid
Liothyronine
Lithium carbonate
Maprotiline
Nomifensine
Nortriptyline
Phenelzine
Protriptyline
Pyridoxine
Tranylcypromine
Trazodone
Trimipramine

CHAPTER 20

Amantadine
Amphetamine
Benzphetamine
Benztropine
Biperiden
Bromocriptine
Caffeine
Caramiphen
Chlorphenoxamine
Chlorphentermine
Clortermine
Cycrimine
Deanol acetamidobenzoate
Dextroamphetamine
Diethylpropion
Diphenhydramine
Doxapram
Ethamivan
Ethopropazine
Fenfluramine
Levodopa
Levodopa-benserazide
Levodopa-carbidopa
Mazindol
Methamphetamine
Methylphenidate
Nikethamide
Orphenadrine
Pemoline
Pentylenetetrazol
Phendimetrazine
Phenmetrazine
Phentermine
Pipradol
Procyclidine
Trihexyphenidyl

CHAPTER 21

Acetazolamide
Amobarbital
Bromide
Carbamazepine
Clonazepam
Corticotropin
Diazepam
Ethosuximide
Ethotoin
Magnesium sulfate
Mephenytoin
Mephobartital
Metharbital
Methsuximide
Paraldehyde
Paramethadione
Pentobarbital
Phenacemide
Phenobarbital
Phensuximide
Phenytoin
Primidone
Thiopental
Trimethadione
Valproic acid

CHAPTER 13

Review of the Anatomy, Physiology, and Assessment of the Central Nervous System

Norman R. Thomas

The purpose of this chapter is to provide an overview of the structure and function of the central nervous system to enable the student and practitioner to achieve a better understanding of the mechanism of action of drugs on the central nervous system. Awareness of one's environment results from the integrative and correlative functioning of the nervous system.

The nervous system consists of a group of tissues made up of highly specialized cells possessing properties of excitability and conductivity. The nervous system proper is divided into central and peripheral components (Figure 13-1). (See Section IV for a discussion of the peripheral nervous system and related medications.) The central nervous system consists of the brain contained within the skull and the spinal cord lying in the vertebral canal. The peripheral nervous system is composed of 43 pairs of nerves that leave the central nervous system and pass to various parts of the body. Two kinds of conducting fibers are present in the peripheral system (Figure 13-2). One group, termed the afferent or sensory fiber system, carries information from the periphery to the central nervous system, and the second, the efferent or motor fiber system, conveys impulses from the central system to muscles, glands, and other organs.

The nervous system may also be considered as divided into two anatomic and functionally distinct components: the somatic and autonomic systems. Both the somatic and autonomic systems have central and peripheral components. The somatic nervous system is concerned with the registering of changes that occur in the environment and those voluntary responses that the organism makes to those stimuli. The autonomic or vegetative nervous system controls the visceral functions of the body, and for the most part these occur at a subconscious or involuntary level.

TYPES OF NERVE CELLS

The nervous system contains two major types of cells: neuroglia, which are the supporting elements of the nervous system, and neurons, the basic functional conducting element of the nervous system.

Neuroglia

The nonnervous element consists of supporting connective tissue and blood vessels and is known collectively as the neuroglia. Morphologically four different cell types are observed in the neuroglia component of the nervous system. These are the astrocytes, so called because of their star-shaped morphology; the oligodendroglia cells, which have few and short processes; the microglia, small cells with a limited number of processes; and the ependyma, a specialized neuroglia cell that lines the cavities or ventricles of the brain and spinal cord (Figure 13-3).

Neurons

The basic functional unit of the nervous system is the neuron (Figure 13-4). These cells have the property of conducting electrical impulses from one part of the body to another. The neuron is made up of a cell body and various cellular extensions or processes. The cell body is composed of a granular cytoplasm, the perikaryon, in which can be observed mitochondria, Nissl substance, neurofibrils, Golgi apparatus, and a centrally placed nucleus. Axons and dendrites are processes that extend from the cell body and have complementary functions. The axon is a cytoplasmic extension that is responsible for conducting nerve impulses away from the cell body, whereas the dendrites conduct impulses toward the cell body. The axon consists of an axis cylinder, a myelin sheath, a neurilemma, and a Schwann cell. The myelin sheath

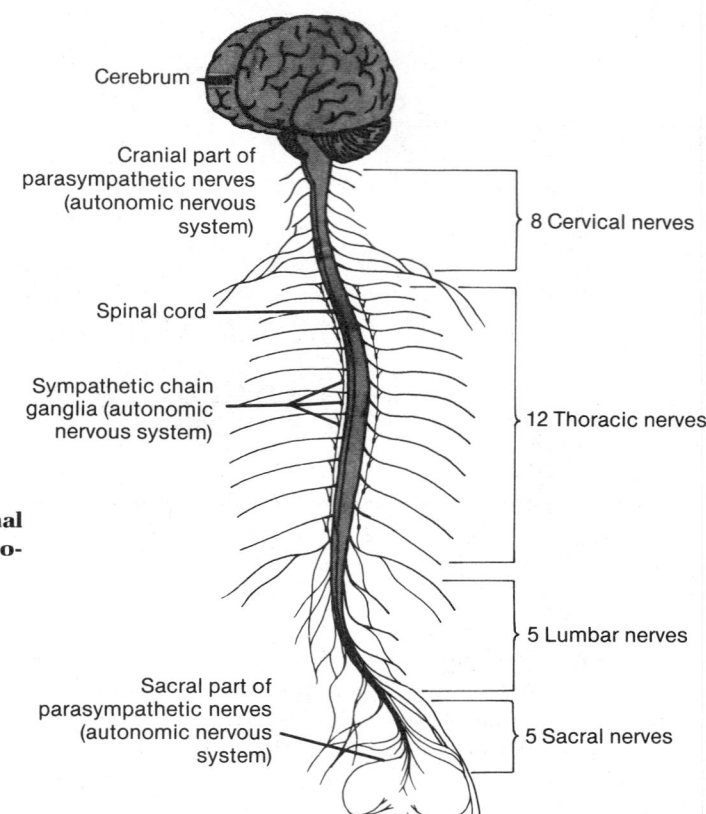

Cerebrum

Cranial part of
parasympathetic nerves
(autonomic nervous
system)

Spinal cord

Sympathetic chain
ganglia (autonomic
nervous system)

Sacral part of
parasympathetic nerves
(autonomic nervous
system)

8 Cervical nerves

12 Thoracic nerves

5 Lumbar nerves

5 Sacral nerves

FIGURE 13-1. **The central nervous system. The proximal portions of the peripheral nervous system and autonomic nervous system.**

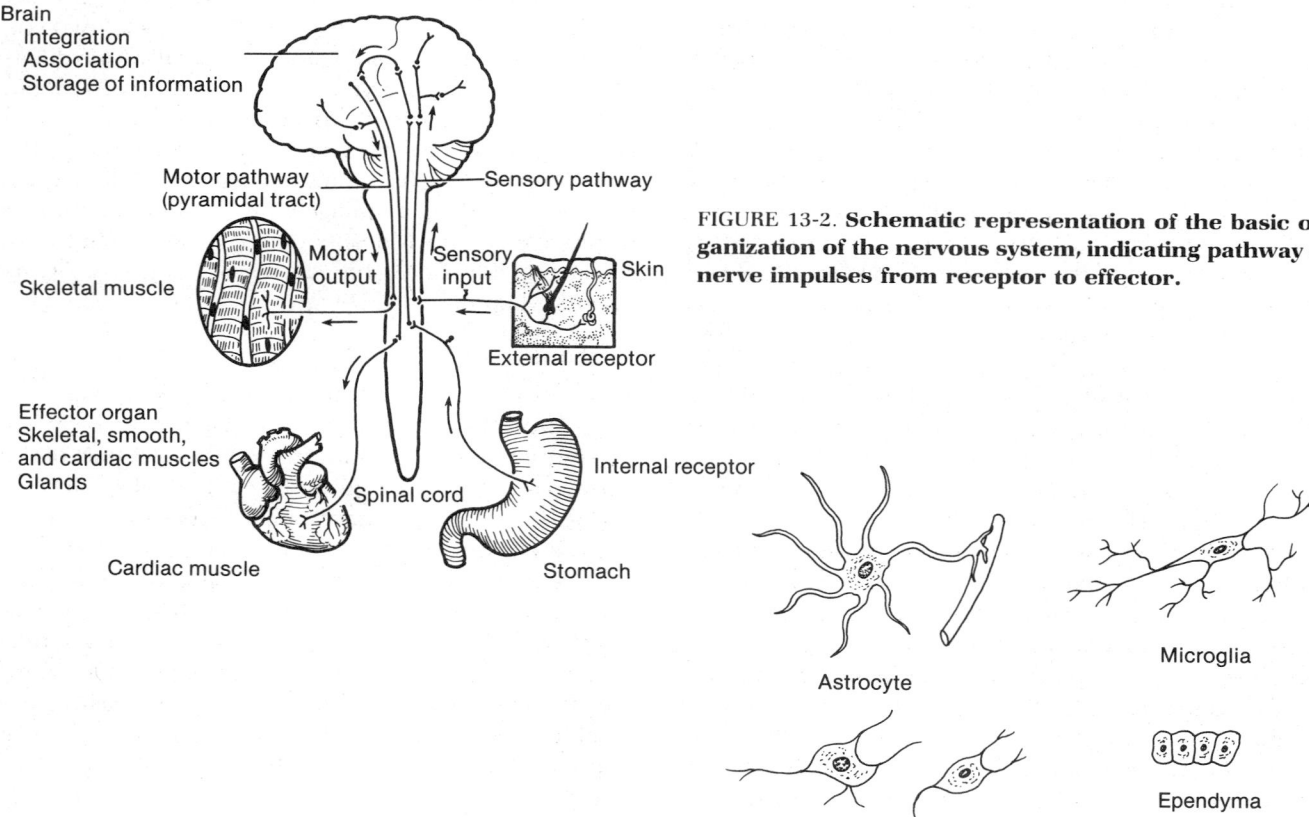

Brain
Integration
Association
Storage of information

Motor pathway
(pyramidal tract)

Sensory pathway

Motor
output

Sensory
input

Skin

Skeletal muscle

External receptor

Effector organ
Skeletal, smooth,
and cardiac muscles
Glands

Spinal cord

Internal receptor

Cardiac muscle

Stomach

FIGURE 13-2. **Schematic representation of the basic organization of the nervous system, indicating pathway of nerve impulses from receptor to effector.**

Astrocyte

Microglia

Ependyma

Oligodendroglia

FIGURE 13-3. **Neuroglia of central nervous system.**

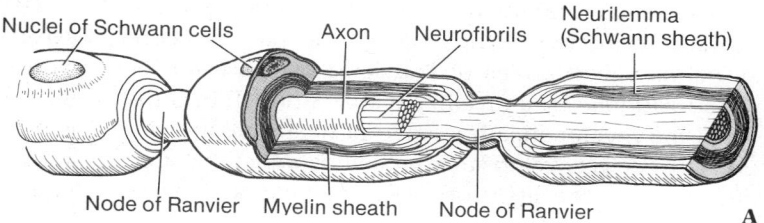

FIGURE 13-4. *A,* **General structure of nerve fiber;** *B,* **Types of neurons.** 1, **Bipolar.** 2, **Unipolar.** 3, **Multipolar.**

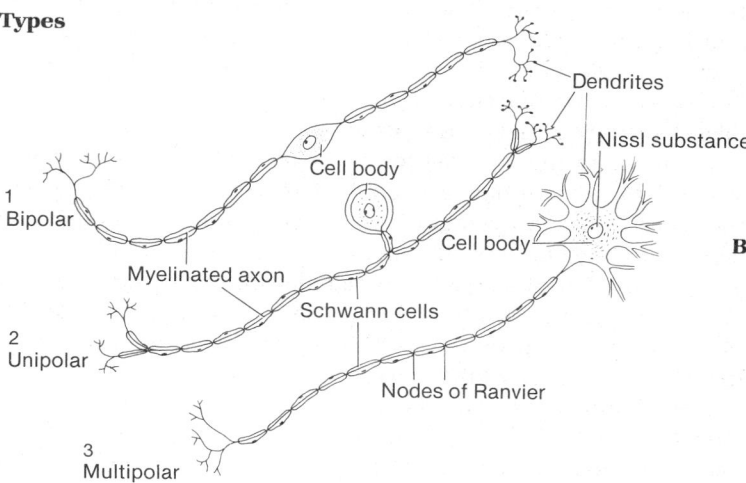

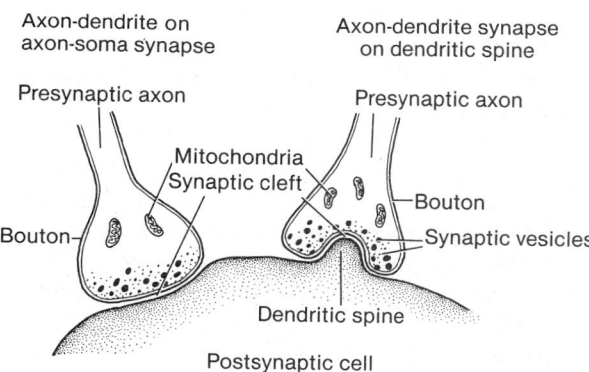

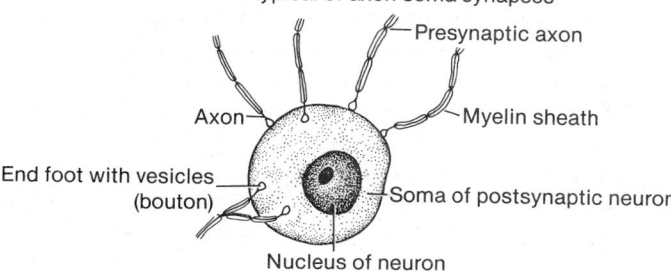

FIGURE 13-5. **Various forms of synaptic junctions.**

wraps itself around the nerve fiber except for a portion at the termination of the axon and at periodic constrictions called nodes of Ranvier. Peripheral nerves are surrounded by a myelin sheath, although in some cases the myelin sheath instead of wrapping individual nerve cells envelops a group of fibers that are often described in the literature as nonmyelinated nerve fibers.

The neurilemma is a thin membrane that surrounds the nerve fiber, forming an outer covering. Within the neurilemma is found a group of cells known as Schwann cells. Fibers in the brain and spinal cord do not possess neurilemma or Schwann cells and the oligodendrocytes take the place of Schwann cells. Nerve fibers in the gray matter of the central nervous system do not contain a sheath of myelin and are therefore true nonmyelinated fibers. The larger fibers containing myelin sheaths conduct impulses at a greater rate than the smaller so-called nonmyelinated fibers because the conducted impulse must jump action potential from one node to the next because of the high resistance of the intervening myelin sheath. The Nissl substance consists of nucleoproteins and is found throughout the cell and the cytoplasm of the dendrites. Nissl substance tends to be clear at the point where the axon leaves the neuron termed the axon hillock. Nissl substance serves as a catalyst for oxidation and also functions in the reaction of the nerve to injury.

Injury to a nerve results in Wallerian degeneration of the processes distal to the site of injury. That portion of the nerve still attached to the cell body will undergo proliferation in an attempt to reestablish communication between the nerve fiber and the innervated receptor via the distal remnants of the myelin tube. Nerve cells devoid of a neurilemmal sheath, such as those of the spinal tracts, cannot repair themselves, since the protective neurilemma sheath is not able to assist this process.

Neurons fall into three groups: unipolar, bipolar, and multipolar, depending on the number of processes that the cell body develops (Figure 13-4). A unipolar neuron has only a single process in its axon. Unipolar cells are rare in a mature individual, but are commonly seen in embryonic tissue. Bipolar neurons such as those found in the retina have a single dendrite and single axon. Although multipolar neurons have a single axon, they may have many dendrites. Most of the cells of the nervous system are multipolar. In addition to the afferent and efferent fibers described, internuncial neurons conduct impulses from one nerve cell to another, thereby forming links within the central nervous system.

Two mechanisms of nerve transmission are observed in the human nervous system. The transmission of an impulse along a single nerve fiber is an electrical process. The transmission of an impulse across a synapse (Figure 13-5) from one neuron to another is a chemical process caused by the liberation of a neurotransmitter from the presynaptic cell that acts upon the cell membrane of the postsynaptic cell to set up another electrical impulse that will travel along the postsynaptic nerve.

ORIGIN OF THE RESTING POTENTIAL

It can be shown that during rest the interior of nerve cells is negatively charged with respect to the outside. This negative charge is known as the resting potential. It can be demonstrated by using the Nernst equation in association with experiments involving differential ion concentrations that the electronegativity of the inside is caused by differences in potassium ion concentration across the cell membrane (Figure 13-6). A number of factors contribute to this differential potassium ion concentration gradient. The membrane that surrounds the nerve is a relatively impermeable membrane. However, potassium ions can diffuse easily through the membrane, whereas sodium ions can only do so with considerable difficulty because of their larger size. In addition to this a sodium pump present within the cell membrane augments the differential diffusion rates of sodium and potassium by extruding any sodium that passes across the cell membrane to gain entrance to the cell interior. The sodium pump does this by exchanging potassium ions for any sodium ions that are extruded.

The internal components of a cell are largely protein, and under the existing physiologic pH conditions the protein is negatively charged. This negatively charged protein cannot diffuse out of the cell because of the impermeability or relative impermeability of the cell membrane. Thus the negatively charged protein material within the cell tends to bind the potassium ions that can diffuse easily across the cell membrane. The increased concentration of potassium ions within the cell with respect to the outside gives rise to a concentration gradient. Thus potassium ions continually leak to the outside despite the function of the sodium-potassium pump until an equilibrium potential develops—the resting potential. The physiologic value for the resting electrical potential across the cell membrane, inside/outside is about -80 mV and the concentration of potassium ions inside the nerve cell attains a level of 140 mEq/L in contrast to only 5 mEq/L in the extracellular compartment.

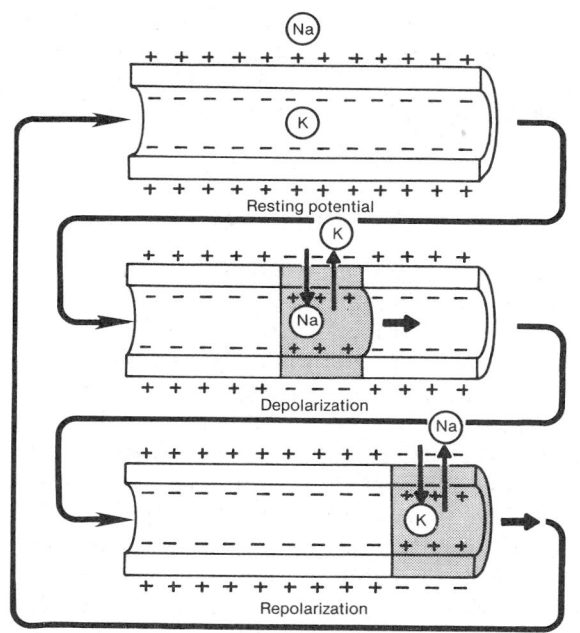

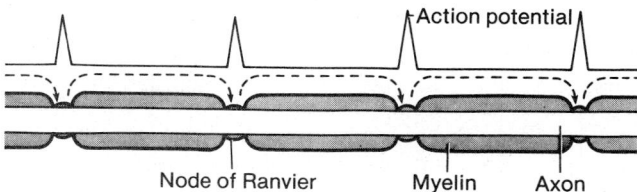

FIGURE 13-7. **In myelinated neurons, action potentials occur at nodes of Ranvier, and a nerve impulse "jumps" along the neuron from node to node.**

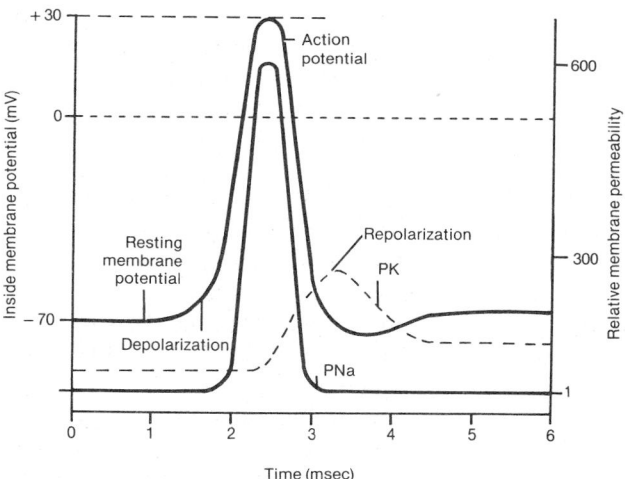

FIGURE 13-6. **Resting and action potentials.**

DEPOLARIZATION, REPOLARIZATION AND THE ACTION POTENTIAL

As long as the membrane of the nerve fiber is undisturbed, the resting potential remains approximately -80 mV. Any factor that suddenly increases the permeability of the membrane elicits a change in the membrane potential known as depolarization. This is achieved under physiologic conditions by the development of a receptor potential that occurs in response to an adequate stimulus.

If the stimulus is strong enough to evoke a response,

an action potential or nerve impulse occurs. Once that impulse has been initiated, it will rise to constant and maximum magnitude independent of any further increase or intensity of the stimulus. This phenomenon is accorded the term *all or none process.*

The change in permeability of the cell membrane and the subsequent development of an action potential occurs in two separate stages called depolarization and repolarization. During stimulation the permeability of the nerve membrane to sodium ions suddenly increases such that sodium ions rush to the inside of the fiber carrying enough positive charges to the inside to cause a disappearance of the normal resting potential and the development of a positive state inside the nerve fiber called the reversal potential. Almost immediately after depolarization the pores of the membrane once again become totally impermeable to the sodium ions. The reversal potential inside the fiber therefore disappears and the normal resting potential returns. This is called repolarization.

The exact cause of the increased permeability to sodium is not entirely understood. It has been postulated however that the sodium *channels* are lined by positive calcium ions that prevent sodium ions from moving down the channels toward the interior of the cell. During stimulation it is thought that the structure of the protein in the cell membrane undergoes configuration changes so as to release calcium, permitting an increasing rate of sodium diffusions from the outside of the cell membrane to the inside. The concentration of sodium ions outside the cell membrane attains a level of about 142 mEq/L, whereas the concentration of sodium ions within the cell under resting conditions is only 10 mEq/L.

An action potential elicited at any one point on the excitable nerve membrane usually excites adjacent portions of the membrane resulting in propagation of the action potential or wave of negativity along the nerve membrane surface (Figure 13-7). It is known that local anesthetics act by stabilizing the nerve membrane against increased permeability to sodium and hence the action potential. It therefore appears that local anesthetics must bind to the calcium binding sites so that they stabilize the membrane during physical or chemical stimulation, thereby preventing changes in sodium permeability and the setting up of an action potential. A variety of other pharmacologic agents are also known to act in a similar manner, such as antihistamines and aspirin, although their binding properties are clearly not as successful as those of the classical local anesthetics. An action potential lasts only a fraction of a second, and the fiber then becomes ready to transmit new impulses. However, during the period of repolarization of the cell membrane following the passage of an action potential the nerve is for a period of time refractory to further stimulation. The refractory period is composed of absolute refractory and relative refractory phases. During an absolute refractory period the nerve is entirely unresponsive. During the relative refractory period it is possible to set up a response, but the stimulus required is greater than that necessary to stimulate a resting nerve.

TRANSMISSION OF THE IMPULSE AT SYNAPTIC AND MYONEURAL JUNCTION

A nerve fiber terminates in knoblike bodies known as boutons (see Figure 13-5) that are closely associated with the dendrites or body of another cell to form a synapse. When the nerve impulse in the presynaptic nerve reaches the synapse, a neurotransmitter agent is released from the boutons to diffuse across the synapse toward the second cell or postsynaptic surface. Thus, transmission at the synapse is a chemical process. An excitatory or an inhibitory agent may be produced by the bouton. In the case of an excitatory agent, usually acetylcholine, the agent diffuses the synapse to act on the postsynaptic cell membrane to increase its permeability to sodium ions, setting up a wave of depolarization in the postsynaptic nerve. In about 2 msec the destruction of acetylcholine by the enzyme cholinesterase permits reestablishment of the resting potential in the postsynaptic nerve.

Acetylcholine is also produced at the junction between a nerve and muscle fiber—the myoneural junction. The increased sodium permeability of the sarcolemma or muscle membrane induced by acetylcholine evokes an action potential that travels along the muscle fiber at a rate of about 5 m/sec. This action potential passing into the substance of the muscle results in the liberation of calcium ions from the endoplasmic reticulum to cooperate with ATP in the interaction of actin and myosin in contraction of the muscle fiber. In myasthenia gravis weakness of muscle contraction occurs because of the inhibition of transmission at the myoneural junction. Myasthenia gravis is commonly treated by drugs that inhibit the action of cholinesterase (see Chapter 25, "Anticholinesterases and Cholinesterase Reactivators").

PHYSIOLOGY OF THE SPINAL REFLEX

The reflex arc is the nerve chain between the receptor and its effector organ (Figure 13-8). The afferent neuron conveys information to the central nervous system, whereas the efferent nerve leaves the cord to activate the effector organ, muscle, or gland. Between these two neurons may be found the so-called internuncial or intercalated neuron. The reflex arc constitutes the functional unit of the central nervous system. Paralysis of the muscles or failure of the gland to secrete can be caused by cutting efferent fibers that pass toward the effector organ. Cutting of the afferent root would bring about a loss of sensation, touch, pain, and heat sensitivity from that part of the body giving rise to the afferent nerve.

A reflex reaction serves to protect or warn the body of impending danger. An example of a reflex action is that produced when the patella tendon in the knee is tapped. Tension on the tendon stimulates the receptor, which in this case is the muscle spindle. An electrical potential induced in the muscle spindle results in depolarization of the supplying afferent nerve, which if it reaches threshold level results in an action potential that passes toward the central nervous system. In the case of the knee tap (myotatic reflex) the afferent fiber synapses directly with the efferent fiber. This is called a monosynaptic reflex (Figure 13-9). Other reflexes, such as the withdrawal of the leg when the toe is noxiously stimulated (flexion reflex), and internuncial neurons become intercalated between the afferent and efferent nerves. Superficial reflexes follow cutaneous stimulation; deep reflexes involve stimulation of deep structures such as muscle tendons. Damage or injury to any component of the reflex arc including alteration in inhibitory or facilitatory influences will cause a pathologic reflex (e.g., a transection of the spinal cord will abolish reflexes at the level of transection). Below the point of injury to the spinal cord, the deep reflexes will be increased, since the inhibitory influences from the higher centers are removed. Above the level of the injury the deep reflexes are unchanged.

CENTRAL SYNAPTIC TRANSMISSION

An action potential in an axon will cause the discharge of a neurotransmitter from the presynaptic terminals. A synaptic delay of approximately 0.5 msec in

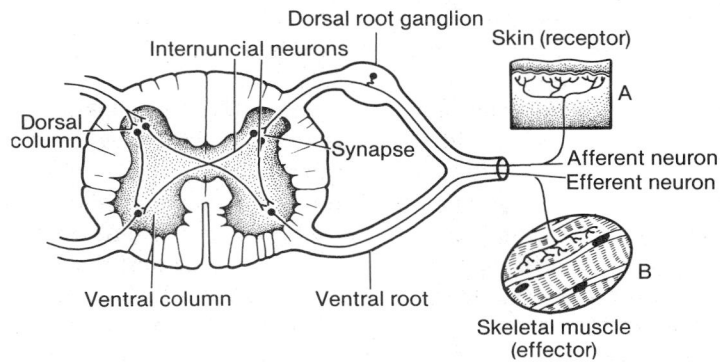

FIGURE 13-8. **Reflex arc between the receptor** (A) **and its effector organ** (B).

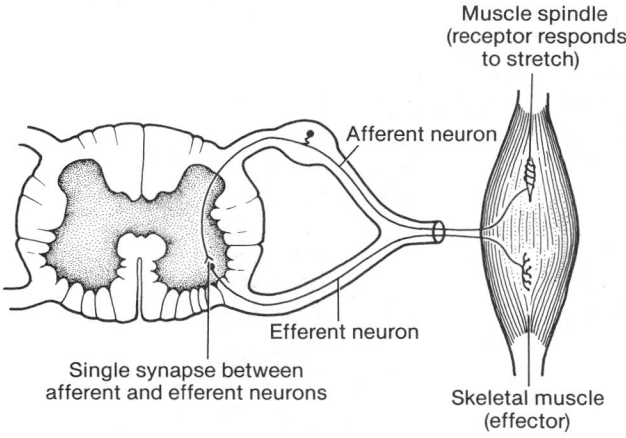

FIGURE 13-9. **Monosynaptic reflex (myotatic reflex).**

the central nervous system is the result of the time required for diffusion of the neurotransmitter across the synapse. Facilitatory impulses bring about a local graded depolarization of the postsynaptic membrane known as the excitatory postsynaptic potential (EPSP). The EPSP is a transient potential lasting a few milliseconds. Gradation of the EPSP is a consequence of the convergence of many presynaptic terminals from afferent fibers on the postsynaptic cell; that is to say, each presynaptic fiber produces a neurotransmitter at the synapse that gives increments in the depolarization level of the postsynaptic cell. In short, the neurotransmitter algebraically summates with other neurotransmitters that are liberated within a short period. When the threshold level of depolarization—which is about 10 mV below that of the resting potential—is reached, the postsynaptic cell generates a propagated action potential. The EPSP is of longer duration than the action potential. Only rarely can an impulse in a single presynaptic fiber bring the EPSP to threshold

level. Thus threshold may be accomplished by a train of action potentials in a single presynaptic fiber (temporal summation) or by single action potentials in many presynaptic fibers (spatial summation). Temporal summation is caused by the residual effects of previous action potentials, whereas spatial summation is achieved by synchronous trains of impulses in several converging afferent fibers.

Inhibition at a synapse can be achieved by two distinct processes: postsynaptic inhibition and presynaptic inhibition. Postsynaptic inhibition results from the release of a transmitter that increases or hyperpolarizes the synaptic membrane; that is, the interior of the cell becomes even more negative than that obtained under resting condition. The potential change is called the inhibitory postsynaptic potential (IPSP). Inhibitory transmitters exert their hyperpolarizing effects by altering membrane permeability to potassium and chloride ions, but not to sodium ions. Presynaptic inhibition results from the activation of internuncial neurons, which synapse on the presynaptic terminals of another afferent fiber. These inhibitory interneurons partially depolarize the presynaptic terminals; consequently impulses in these presynaptic fibers are reduced in magnitude or blocked and are therefore less effective in releasing their excitatory neuron transmitter from their terminals. Presynaptic inhibition is of long duration, probably because of repetitive firing of the internuncial neuron.

TRANSMITTERS OF THE CENTRAL NERVOUS SYSTEM

Two common neurotransmitters are acetylcholine and norepinephrine, and they are generally found throughout the central nervous system as well as in the peripheral nervous system. Those synapses liberating acetylcholine are known as cholinergic synapses, and those that use norepinephrine are defined as adrenergic synapses. The enzymes used in the synthesis and degradation of acetylcholine are choline acetylase and acetylcholinesterase respectively. Cholinergic synapses are in high concentrations in the hypothalamus, the cranial nerve nuclei, and the fiber tracts that descend in the spinal cord to innervate the cells of the preganglionic sympathetic nervous system. The enzymes of synthesis of norepinephrine are tyrosine hydroxylase, dopa decarboxylase, and β-hydroxylase. The degradation enzymes for norepinephrine are monoamine oxidase and catechol-O-methyltransferase. Many of the adrenergic synapses are inhibitory, although there are some that are not. Other compounds with neurotransmitter action are serotonin, dopamine, GABA, and glutamate. Some pharmacologic agents act on the central nervous system by altering nerve membrane permeabilities (e.g., local anesthetics); others act by inhibiting or facilitating synaptic transmission (e.g., monoamine oxidase inhibitors).

BRAIN

The three developmental divisions of the brain are the forebrain (prosencephalon), midbrain (mesencephalon), and hindbrain (rhombencephalon) (Figure 13-10). The forebrain is subdivided into the cerebrum and diencephalon. The cerebrum consists of the covering cerebral cortex, which is composed of gray matter, and an underlying white core. The diencephalon consists of the thalamus and the hypothalamus. The forebrain is supported by the midbrain, which separates it from the hindbrain, or rhombencephalon. The midbrain consists of the cerebral peduncles and corpora quadrigemina. The hindbrain is subdivided into the pons, the medulla oblongata, and the cerebellum.

Cerebrum

It is in the nerve centers of the cerebrum that sensory and motor activities are located. Perception, memory, and intelligence are further functional components of the cerebrum. During development the cerebral cortex expands out of proportion to the rest of the brain, causing the gray matter of the cerebral cortex to roll and fold upon itself such that a bulge called a gyrus is formed; the groove between the bulges is known as a sulcus, or fissure (Figure 13-11). The longitudinal fissure separates the right and the left hemispheres of the brain (Figure 13-12). These cerebral hemispheres are mirror images of each other and possess a full set of centers for the sensory and motor activities of the body. Thus, the right side of the brain controls the left side of the body, and the left side of the brain controls the right side of the body.

The two cerebral cortices are connected by the corpus callosum (Figure 13-13), which is composed of a series of connecting fibers that allows the integration

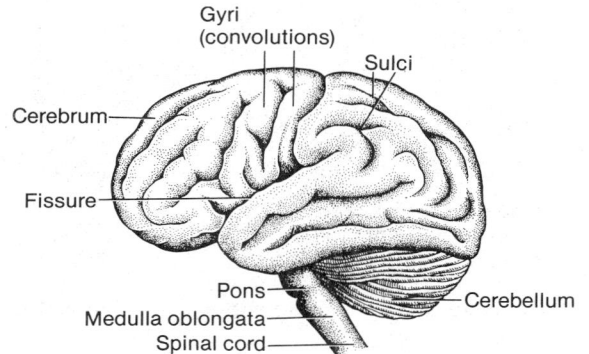

FIGURE 13-11. **Lateral view of the surface of the brain. The surface of the cerebral hemispheres has numerous convolutions that are separated by either sulci or fissures.**

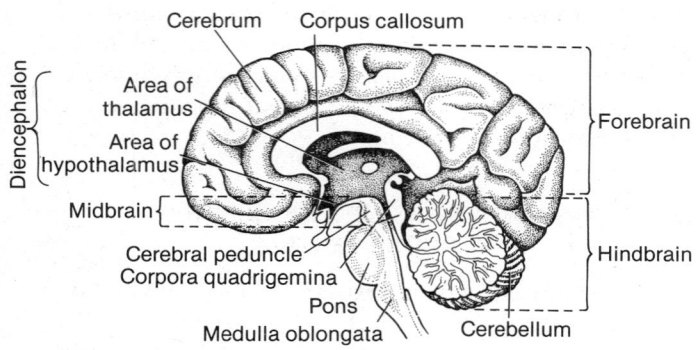

FIGURE 13-10. **Midsagittal section of the brain and brainstem.**

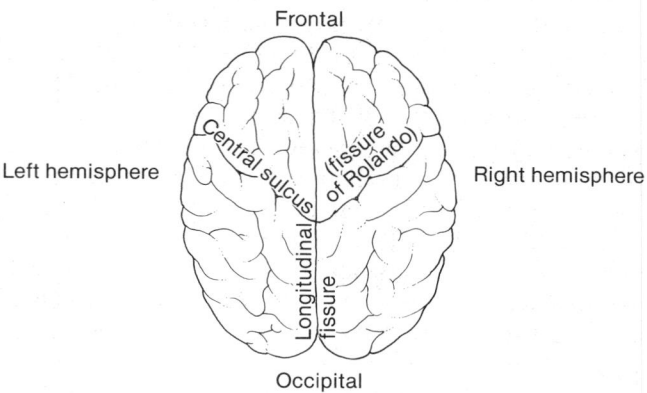

FIGURE 13-12. **Major fissures of the brain, superior view.**

of their functions. The lateral sulcus, or fissure of Sylvius, cuts horizontally and posteriorly over the temporal lobe of the brain (Figure 13-14). It is above and below the lateral sulcus that centers for speech and hearing are found, respectively. The central sulcus, otherwise known as the fissure of Rolando, starts at the middle of the superior border of the cortex and extends downward toward the lateral sulcus, separating the rostral cerebral cortex into frontal and parietal lobes. The precentral gyrus anterior to the central sulcus—the primary motor area—is concerned with the motor activities of the body, whereas the postcentral gyrus posterior to the sulcus is concerned with sensory functions and is known as the primary sensory area (Figure 13-15). On the medial aspect of the cerebral hemisphere is found a sulcus running parallel to the corpus callosum. This is known as the cingulate sulcus (Figure 13-13), and the cortex surrounding the sulcus is concerned with emotion and olfaction.

A wedge-shaped region in the posterior pole of the cerebral cortex, the occipital lobe, is superiorly delineated on the medial surface by the calcarine sulcus (Figure 13-13); this region comprises the visual cortex and association areas. The region of the cerebral cortex anterior to the central sulcus and superior to the lateral sulcus is called the frontal lobe and is responsible for higher intellectual psychic functions and drive. That region posterior to the central sulcus excluding the wedge posteriorly of the visual cortex is known as the parietal lobe. The parietal lobe extends inferiorly to the lateral sulcus and includes hand skills and speech and sensory function (Figure 13-15). Inferior to the lateral sulcus is the temporal lobe, which is concerned with auditory perception and memory. Thus, damage to the parietal lobe results in aphasia, which includes inability to speak or understand language. Auditory perception, occurs in the temporal lobe, but since auditory impulses pass through both hemispheres, damage or injury to one temporal lobe

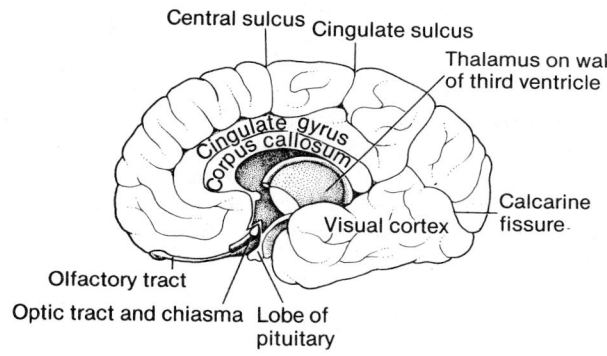

FIGURE 13-13. **Medial surface, right hemisphere.**

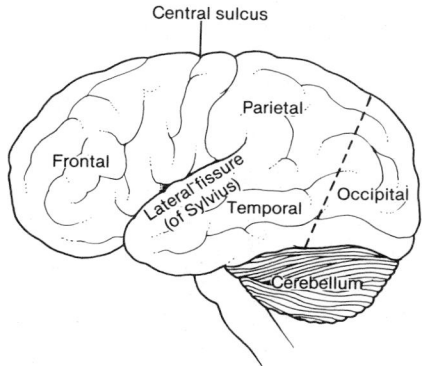

FIGURE 13-14. **Lateral surface, left hemisphere.**

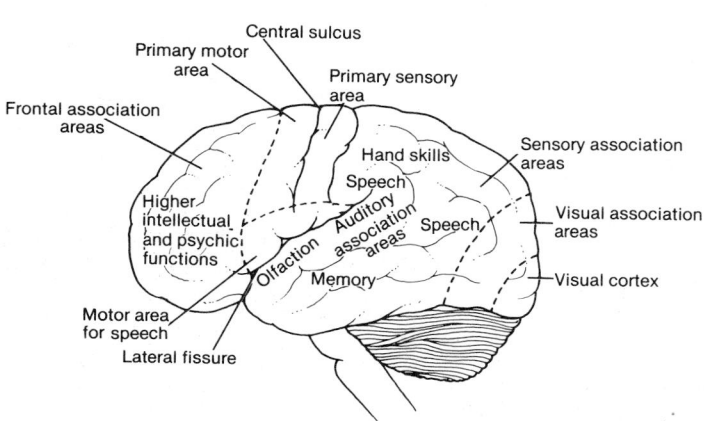

FIGURE 13-15. **General functional areas of the left cerebral cortex, lateral aspect.**

does not usually result in disturbances in audition. This, however, does not apply to speech comprehension, because one or the other hemisphere, usually the left, becomes dominant in respect to this modality. Therefore, damage to the relevant parts of the language centers of the dominant hemisphere results in inability to understand the spoken or written word (receptive aphasia). The motor cortex lying anterior to the central fissure is concerned with the voluntary control of movement; specific areas control specific parts of one side of the body. The control of the head region, for example, is found in the inferior part of the motor cortex, whereas the feet and toes are found in the superior aspect of the motor cortex. Thus motor aphasia, or inability to speak, is associated with damage to the inferior motor cortex of the dominant hemisphere. A similar somatopic localization occurs in the sensory cortex posterior to the central sulcus (Figure 13-16).

The sensory and motor cortices are sometimes known as projection areas, since fibers pass to and from these regions, respectively. Motor fibers project to the lower motor neurons via the pyramidal tract (Figure 13-2). The pyramidal tract crosses to the opposite side of the brainstem and exercises voluntary control over movement. Sensory information is transmitted to the sensory cortex from lower sensory neurons (see Figure 13-2). A large part of the cerebral cortex is composed of so-called association areas, since fibers pass between these areas and into the sensory, motor, and visual cortices. Thus, association fibers passing between the visual cortex found in the posterior pole of the brain and the motor cortex associated with movements of the lips and tongue permit a visual experience to be correlated with motor function and speech. An individual, for example, vocalizing a particular word by command from the motor cortex is able through the relevant association fibers to visualize the object verbalized.

Embedded in the white matter beneath the gray covering of the cerebral cortex are found masses of gray material known as the basal ganglia. The basal ganglia form part of the extrapyramidal system and include the caudate and lentiform nuclei. These nuclei together with the adjacent white matter comprise the corpus striatum of the internal capsule (Figure 13-17).

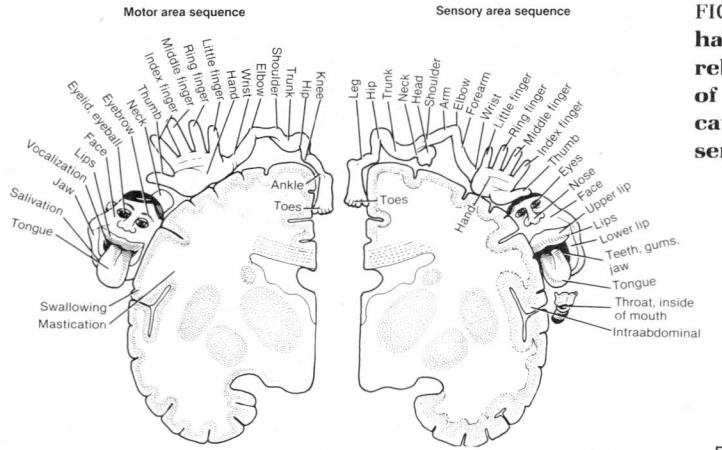

FIGURE 13-16. **Frontal section of the cerebrum. The left half indicates the locations of neurons within the cerebral cortex that control voluntary motor movement of specific structures. The right half indicates the locations of regions of the cerebral cortex that receive sensory nerve impulses from specific body structures.**

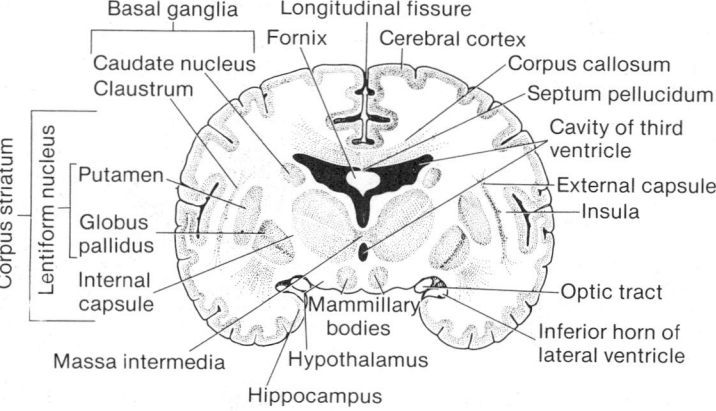

FIGURE 13-17. **Frontal section of the cerebrum and the diencephalon showing the cerebral cortex (gray matter) surrounding the white matter and the basal ganglia deep within the white matter.**

The interconnections between the basal ganglia are complex and appear to be important for smoothing and refining body movements.

Effects of injury to the cerebral cortex. Damage to the corpus striatum can produce variable degrees of paralysis if the white fibers are involved; the white fibers are really projecting from the motor cortex to the lower motor neurons. If the gray material of the basal ganglia is involved, then extrapyramidal effects develop, such as tremor, and rigidity and disturbance of movement, gait, and posture. Damage to the motor cortex itself may result in hemiplegia or paralysis of the opposite side of the body. Scar formation in the precentral gyrus gives rise to epileptiform discharges, which are seizures occurring in specific parts of the body, depending on the part of the motor cortex involved.

Injury to the prefrontal lobes lying anterior to the motor cortex results in the loss of an individual's drive and moral judgment. Prefrontal lobotomy, in which the association fibers passing to the frontal lobes are severed, is a surgical procedure once used to relieve anxiety and compulsion neuroses in mentally ill patients. Relief of the compulsion neurosis is exchanged for alterations in the personality of the individual. Damage to the temporal lobe results in auditory aphasia and uncinate fits that are accompanied by olfactory hallucinations and other mental aberrations. Damage to the occipital lobe may result in blindness of the nasal half of one visual field and the temporal half of the other.

Diencephalon

The diencephalon of each hemisphere is composed of the thalamus and hypothalamus (Figures 13-13 and 13-17). The thalami are bilateral gray nuclei found within the white core of the cerebrum inferior to the corpus callosum and third ventricle. A relay center for sensory information passing from the periphery to the cerebral cortex, the *thalamus* acts as an integrative center for pain and other sensory information. Through the activity of the thalamus the sensation of muscle and joint movements is first received by the individual. Stereognosis and sensory discrimination also are controlled within the thalamus. In addition to its sensory functions, the thalamus is also concerned with the facilitation or inhibition of motor commands passing from the cerebral cortex to lower motor centers. Information passing from the hypothalamus to the frontal lobes of the cerebral cortex is also relayed through the thalamus, which serves a function in the integration and correlation of emotional behavior.

The hypothalamus is found on the ventral surface of the thalamus (Figure 13-13). It is concerned with the control of the autonomic nervous system. Thus, many of the body's functions that occur at subconscious levels are controlled through the activity of the hypothalamus. Water balance, temperature control, and sexual behavior, as well as stress reactions are coordinated both directly through the action of the hypothalamus and indirectly by its control over the endocrine system by way of the pituitary gland. The hypothalamus exerts its control over the pituitary by the release of certain releasing factors that stimulate the liberation of anterior pituitary hormones. The supraoptic and parahypophyseal nuclei of the hypothalamus control the release of posterior pituitary hormones (i.e., antidiuretic hormone and vasopressin).

Midbrain

Figure 13-10 shows that the midbrain is found between the forebrain and the hindbrain. On the dorsal

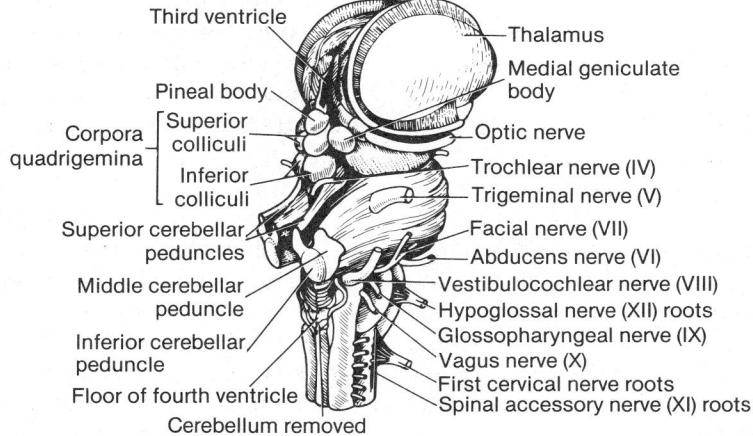

FIGURE 13-18. **A dorsolateral view of the brainstem.**

aspect of the midbrain are found four elevations known as the corpora quadrigemina. The upper two, or superior, colliculi are concerned with visual reflexes, whereas the lower two, or inferior, colliculi are associated with hearing. On the ventral aspect of the midbrain are found the cerebral peduncles, which contain the main motor pathway, or pyramidal tract, that passes from the motor cortex to lower motor neurons. Deep within the structure of the midbrain is the tegmentum, which contains important afferent and efferent pathways as well as the red nucleus, which is important in motor movement and postural reflex mechanisms (Figure 13-18).

Hindbrain

The hindbrain consists of the cerebellum, pons, and medulla oblongata (Figure 13-10).

Cerebellum. The cerebellum consists of two lateral hemispheres and a central vermis that attaches to the dorsal aspect of the brainstem beneath the mesencephalon. The outer covering of the cerebellum is composed of gray matter and is set into folds and fissures such that in cross section the cerebellum resembles a tree, giving it the name of arbor vitae. The cerebellum is concerned with movement and equilibrium and is connected by incoming and outgoing fibers with all parts of the central nervous system. Incoming fibers inform the cerebellum of the muscular activity of the organism as well as bringing information from the eyes, the ears, touch receptors, and organ of balance in the middle ear. In cooperation with the cerebrum the efferent supply from the cerebellum refines and coordinates the movements of the body, and it also helps maintain the posture of the individual. Cerebellar function is assessed by numerous cerebellar tests including Romberg, rhythmic patting, heel to shin, heel-to-toe walking, shallow knee bend, and observation of posture, balance, arm swing, and leg movement.

Pons. The pons is found on the ventral aspect of the brainstem and consists of white fiber tracts passing to and from various parts of the brain and brainstem. It also contains several important cranial nerve nuclei.

Medulla oblongata. The medulla oblongata is the upward continuation of the spinal cord and connects superiorly with the pons and cerebellum. The dorsal aspect of the medulla oblongata forms the floor of the fourth ventricle, lying beneath the cerebellum. The ventral surface of the medulla is formed by the pyramids, which are the motor tracts passing caudally through the brainstem from the motor cortex. Many of the cranial nerve nuclei are found in the floor of the fourth ventricle, whereas afferent and efferent tracts form the white matter of the medulla oblongata. The centers for cardiovascular and respiratory control are found in the substance of the medulla.

Reticular activating system. Throughout the midbrain, pons, and medulla oblongata are scattered large star-shaped cells giving rise to the reticular formation of the brainstem. Some of these large cells are collected into reticular nuclei, but have as their function the modification of reflex activity of the spinal neurons. The reticular activating system also has the property of alerting the brain or inhibiting it during sleep. The reticular activating system plays an important part in the extrapyramidal influence on voluntary movements.

CRANIAL NERVES

There are twelve pairs of cranial nerves. They include the olfactory, optic, oculomotor, trochlear, trigeminal, abducens, facial, vestibulocochlear, glossopharyngeal, vagus, accessory, and hypoglossal nerves (Figure 13-19).

The *olfactory nerve*, the first cranial nerve, is formed by filaments that lead from the olfactory mucous membrane of the nasal cavity passing superiorly through the cribriform plate to join the olfactory bulb. The olfactory tract runs posteriorly from the bulb to the lateral and medial olfactory gyri. The first cranial nerves are responsible for the sensation of smell and, during testing, each nostril should be closed to permit examination of the presence of smell for each olfactory nerve. Complete absence of smell is known as anosmia.

The *optic nerve*, the second cranial nerve, is responsible for vision. Receptors for the optic nerve are found in the retina of the eye. These receptors are known as rods and cones; the rods subserve night vision and the cones day vision. The nerve cells arising from these receptors pass backward to form the optic nerves, which pass into the cranial cavity to join with the nerves of the opposite side to form the optic chiasma. The fibers pass from the nasal aspect of the retina on each side across to the opposite side to form the optic tract. The optic tract terminates in the lateral geniculate body of the thalamus and superior colliculus. Fibers arising in the lateral geniculate body pass posteriorly toward the occipital lobe via the optic radiations. Assessment of this nerve involves testing visual acuity and testing the visual fields. This nerve is also involved in pupillary reaction to light. The Snellen chart is used for assessing visual acuity, although gross assessment can be made by asking the patient to read from a newspaper or other written material. Peripheral

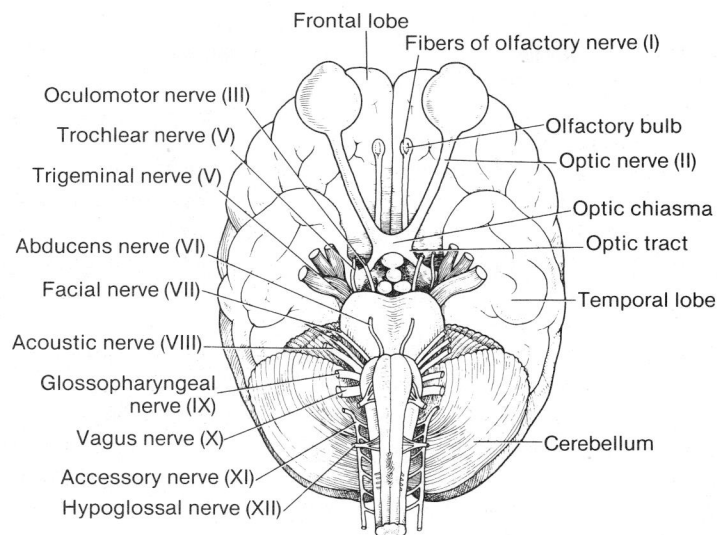

FIGURE 13-19. **The ventral surface of the brain showing the cranial nerves.**

vision can be grossly assessed using the visual field confrontation test or the perimeter or tangent screen tests.

The oculomotor nerve, the third cranial nerve, supplies four of the six external muscles that move the eye, namely: (1) the superior and (2) inferior recti, which turn the eye superiorly and inferiorly, respectively; (3) the medial rectus, which turns the eye in toward the nose; and (4) the levator palpebrae superioris muscle, which raises the upper eyelid. Direct and consensual pupillary reaction to light and accommodation are used in testing oculomotor function. Screening of the six cardinal fields is also used in oculomotor assessment as well as in assessing trochlear and abducens nerve function.

The *trochlear nerve*, which is the fourth cranial nerve, supplies the superior oblique muscle of the eye, turning the eye downward and laterally. The convergence test is used to test trochlear as well as oculomotor function.

The *trigeminal nerve*, or fifth cranial nerve, is the largest of the cranial nerves and supplies sensory information to the face, the nose, the mouth, the forehead, and the top of the head as well as the motor supply to the muscles of mastication. The trigeminal nerve is divided into three divisions: (1) the ophthalmic, which supplies the forehead and internal parts of the orbit of the eye; (2) the maxillary, which supplies the upper face; and (3) the mandibular division, which supplies the lower face and lower jaw. The trigeminal nerve also supplies the mucous membrane of the nose via the nasal branches of the maxillary nerve as well

as sensation to the anterior two thirds of the tongue by the lingual branch of the mandibular division of the trigeminal nerve. Integrity of the trigeminal nerve is diagnosed by testing sensory stimulation to forehead, face, and lower jaw regions. Testing of corneal reflex is also used. Weakness in the motor division is tested by asking the patient to clench the teeth. Contraction of the elevator muscles is substantiated by palpation of the relevant musculature.

The *abducens nerve*, or sixth cranial nerve, supplies the lateral rectus muscle of the eye and is responsible for moving the eye outward.

The *facial nerve*, the seventh cranial nerve, is composed of fibers that supply the muscles of the face and scalp, the muscles of facial expression. It also contains parasympathetic fibers to the lacrimal, submandibular, and sublingual glands. It also includes afferent sensory fibers from the mucous membranes of the anterior two thirds of the tongue responsible for gustation, or taste, via the chorda tympani branch. Damage to the facial nerve results in paralysis of the muscles of the face. This may be elucidated by asking the patient to wrinkle the forehead, to frown, or to laugh. Loss of sensory function to the tongue may be tested by applying sweet substance, salt, or bitter substance such as quinine to the tongue to check for taste.

The *vestibulocochlear*, acoustic or eighth cranial nerve, subserves the function of hearing and balance. This nerve consists of two parts, the auditory (cochlear), which is responsible for hearing, and the vestibular portion, which is responsible for balance or equilibrium. Injury to the auditory nerve results in deafness.

Injury to the vestibular portion produces symptoms of either loss of balance or vertigo and nystagmus, a rapid staccato movement of the eyes usually in a horizontal direction. Audition may be grossly tested by whispering in each ear. The Weber and Rinné tests are also used in hearing assessment. More precise examination of the hearing may be evaluated by using an audiometer. Damage to the vestibular nerve may simply be tested by asking the patient to close the eyes and to point at an object that he or she has previously visualized or simply to observe the patient's state of balance during closure of the eyes. Nystagmus may also be observed in a patient who has suffered damage to the vestibular nerve.

The *glossopharyngeal*, or ninth nerve, is responsible for the function of general sensation and taste for the posterior third of the tongue. It also receives information from the carotid sinus that indicates to the brain the blood pressure level, and from the carotid body, which monitors the carbon dioxide concentration of the blood. The secretory parasympathetic fibers of the glossopharyngeal nerve are distributed to the parotid gland and the mucous membrane of the pharynx. The motor component of the glossopharyngeal nerve supplies the stylopharyngeus muscle, which aids in movements of the pharynx. Screening is completed by assessing swallowing and the gag reflex. Loss of sensory function to the tongue may be tested by applying sweet, salty, or sour substances to assess taste.

The *vagus nerve*, the tenth cranial nerve, innervates the pharyngeal, laryngeal and smooth muscles of the esophagus, stomach, and intestine. It also contains nerves that depress cardiac action and produce constriction of the terminal bronchioles of the airway. The integrity of the vagus nerve is tested by observing pharyngeal muscles during function. The common test here is to ask the patient to say "ahh," during which movements of the soft palate and uvula are examined.

The *accessory nerve*, the eleventh nerve, supplies motor fibers to the trapezius and sternocleidomastoid muscles. Thus, the integrity of the accessory nerve is tested by asking the patient to raise the shoulders against resistance. This will indicate the state of nerve supply to the trapezius muscle. Weakness in the sternocleidomastoid muscle is evaluated by asking the patient to turn the head to the left or to the right against the resistance of the examiner's hand.

The *hypoglossal nerve*, or twelfth nerve, innervates the muscles to the tongue. Integrity of the hypoglossal nerve can be tested by observing speech or by asking the patient to protrude and wag the tongue. Deviation of the tongue toward one side or the other indicates injury to the hypoglossal nerve.

SPINAL NERVES

There are 31 pairs of spinal nerves named for the vertebrae anterior to their emergence. There are eight pairs of cervical, twelve thoracic, five lumbar, five sacral, and one coccygeal spinal nerve (Figure 13-20). The spinal nerves are grouped into small fascicles, each surrounded by a perineurium (Figure 13-21). From the fibrous perineurium, strands of connective tissue pass into the spaces between the individual nerve fibers. This is known as the endoneurium. The epineurium forms an overall covering for the entire nerve unit. As seen in Figure 13-22 the spinal nerves are formed by union between a dorsal and ventral root. Along the dorsal root is found an expansion, the dorsal

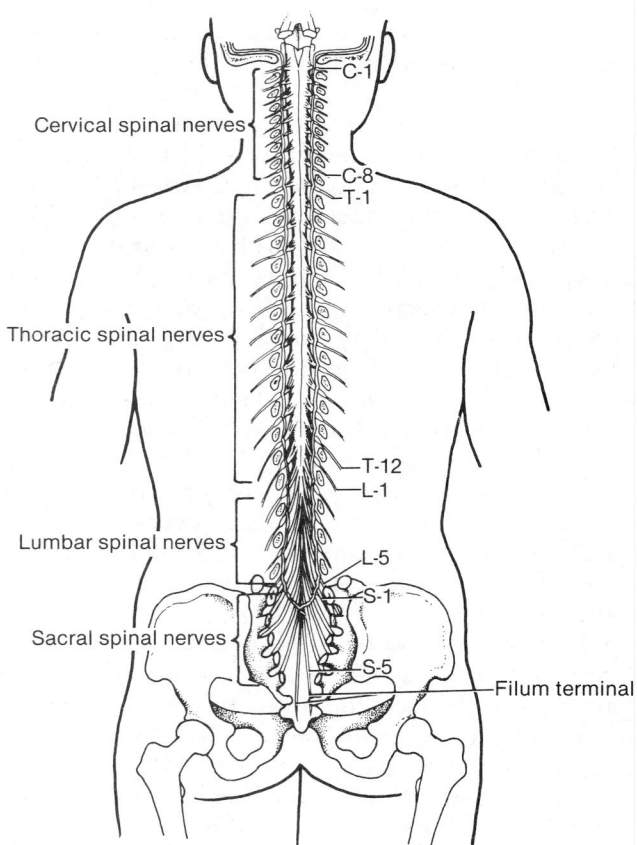

FIGURE 13-20. **The spinal cord and the proximal portions of the spinal nerves. The letters indicate specific spinal nerves: C, cervical, T, thoracic, L, lumbar, S, sacral.**

root ganglion. This contains the first order neurons of the sensory or afferent nerve fibers in the root. After union between the dorsal and ventral roots, the nerves emerge from the bony spinal canal or vertebral canal. On its emergence from the spinal canal a meningeal branch is given off to supply the meninges of the spinal cord. The dorsal ramus conveys nerve fibers serving the muscles and skin of the back of the head, neck, and trunk. The ventral part of the trunk is supplied by the ventral ramus.

Communicating fibers are received from and sent to the sympathetic chain of the autonomic nervous system. These communicating fibers are known as the gray and white rami communicantes, respectively. The latter are fibers that pass to and from the bilateral autonomic ganglia of the autonomic chains that provide sympathetic innervations to the viscera, blood vessels, and glands. The strip of skin supplied by the afferent portion of the spinal nerves is known as the sensory dermatome. The pattern of distribution or loss of sensation in the sensory dermatomes is important to the diagnosis and location of spinal nerve compression and injury. A coronal section through the spinal cord reveals a central gray matter shaped like an H, which contains the nerve cell bodies of the spinal cord (Figure 13-22). The white matter of the cord consists of the nerve fibers passing through the spinal segment, which have ascending and descending tracts as well as local communicating fibers that form the basis of the spinal reflex. (See Chapter 22, "Review of the Anatomy, Physiology, and Assessment of the Peripheral Nervous System," for further information.)

SUMMARY

Many drugs affect the central nervous system directly and indirectly. Those drugs that directly affect this system are discussed in the following chapters in this section. The brief overview presented in this chapter describing the anatomy, physiology, and assessment of the central nervous system should assist the nurse in better understanding the mechanisms of action and the effects of these agents, as well as the central nervous system side effects and toxicity associated with drugs discussed in other sections of this text.

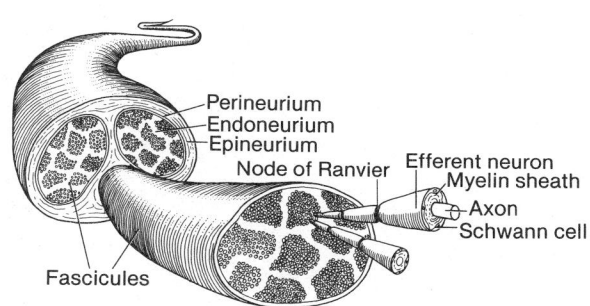

FIGURE 13-21. **Diagram showing components of a peripheral nerve and neuron.**

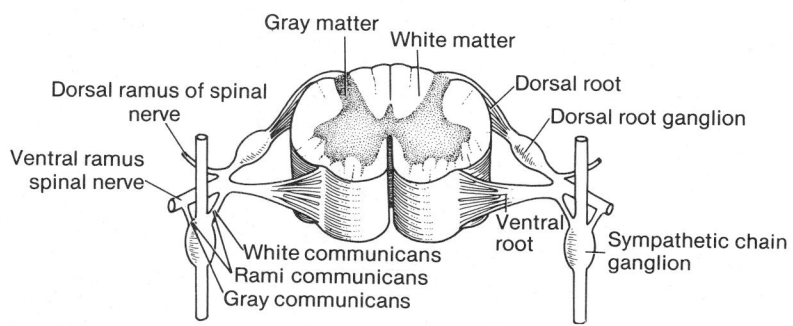

FIGURE 13-22. **A segment of the spinal cord showing the formation of a pair of spinal nerves from dorsal and ventral roots.**

BIBLIOGRAPHY

Brobeck, J.R. *Best and Taylor's physiological basis of medical practice* (10th ed.). Baltimore: The Williams & Wilkins Co., 1979.

Fox, S.I. *Human physiology.* Iowa: Wm. C. Brown Publishers, 1984.

Francis, C.C. *Introduction to human anatomy* (5th ed.). St. Louis: The C.V. Mosby Co., 1968.

Gatz, A.J. *Manter's essentials of clinical neuroanatomy and neurophysiology* (3rd ed.). Philadelphia: F.A. Davis Company, 1966.

Malasanos, L., Barkauskas,, V., Moss, M., & Holtenberg-Allen, K. *Health assessment* (2nd ed.). St. Louis: The C.V. Mosby Co., 1981.

Mason, E.B. *Human Physiology.* Menlo Park, Calif.: Benjamin/Cummings Publishing Co., Inc., 1983.

Mountcastle, V.B. *Human physiology* (vols. 1 and 2) (14th ed.). St. Louis: The C.V. Mosby Co., 1980.

Ruch, T.C., & Patton, H.D. *Physiology and biophysics* (19th ed.). Philadelphia: W.B. Saunders Co., 1966.

Somjen, G. *Neurophysiology: the essentials.* Baltimore: Williams & Wilkins Co., 1983.

General Anesthetics

Sheldon H. Roth

Medications discussed in this chapter

Inhalation anesthetics
  Gases
    Cyclopropane
    Ethylene
    Nitrous oxide
  Volatile liquids
    Chloroform
    Ether
    Enflurane
    Halothane
    Isoflurane
    Methoxyflurane

Intravenous anesthetics
  Etomidate
  Fentanyl and droperidol
  Ketamine
  Methohexital
  Thiamylal
  Thiopental

Anesthesia began in antiquity. Humans searched for various means to conquer the pains of surgery and trauma, and centuries ago, discovered that certain plants and herbs possessed the powers within that freed the patient from anguish and suffering. The Chinese prescribed hashish as an anesthetic and an analgesic, and the Egyptians used opium, belladonna alkaloids, and alcohol. Physical methods of alleviating pain were also practiced. The Romans used intense cold and nerve compression, and the Assyrians and Italians practiced strangulation and cerebral concussion. Such methods as concussion did provide relief from pain of surgery but added greatly to the risk; reversible unconsciousness was predicted if "the wooden bowl placed on the head of the patient were struck with sufficient force to crack the shell of an almond, but not the skull!" Most often, however, the patient was simply restrained by sheer physical force by the surgeon's assistants.

The introduction of ether and nitrous oxide in the 1840s began the age of modern surgical anesthesia. It is interesting to note that the analgesic properties of these agents were known long before their use in surgery; the primary interest in their effects reserved for entertainment at carnivals and "ether frolics." It was mainly the determination of dentists who observed pain routinely in their practice that convinced physicians that pain during surgical procedures could be abolished.

HISTORY

In 1842, Dr. Crawford Long administered ether to his patient, James Venable, and then removed a cyst from the patient's neck. Crawford failed to document his experience until 1849, 3 years after Dr. William T.G. Morton presented the famous demonstration of ether anesthesia at the Massachusetts General Hospital in Boston, October 18, 1846. Dr. Morton was credited as the "inventor and revealor of anesthetic inhalation." Three hundred years before this demonstration, Paracelsus had described the pain-relieving properties of ether in 1540, the year the substance was synthesized by Valerius Corud.

Nitrous oxide would have been the first anesthetic introduced for surgery in 1845 if Dr. Horace Wells, a dentist, had not failed in his attempt to demonstrate the effects of this gas at the same hospital where Morton had succeeded. Nitrous oxide was synthesized in 1776 by Priestley. In the late 1790s, he and Humphrey Davy commented on its anesthetic properties and suggested its use during surgical operations. Faraday, in the early 1800s reported that the effects of nitrous oxide were similar to those of ether. Colton, not a physician, reintroduced the use of nitrous oxide, and in 1868 the gas was readily available in cylinders in combination with oxygen.

In 1831, chloroform was independently discovered by Guthrie in the United States, Soubeiran in France, and Von Liebig in Germany. Dr. James Simpson, a Scottish obstetrician, was the first to use chloroform in humans in 1847. The major highlight for acceptance of chloroform was the administration by John Snow to Queen Victoria in 1853 during the birth of Prince Leopold. Snow became known as the first anesthesiologist.

Nitrous oxide, diethyl ether, and chloroform were the major anesthetics used well into the twentieth century. In 1929, cyclopropane was discovered by accident when the impurities in propylene were being studied. After clinical trials, cyclopropane was introduced into practice in 1934 and remained the agent of choice for nearly 20 years. The explosive property of this anesthetic became an important factor because of the increased use of electrical equipment in the operating room. Therefore, development of a nonexplosive substance was pursued.

The development of fluorinated compounds during World War II led to the synthesis of nonexplosive volatile anesthetics such as halothane by the British group at Imperial Chemical Industries. Introduced into clinical practice in 1956, halothane became the most widely used anesthetic agent. The introduction of other halogenated volatile anesthetics into clinical anesthesia continued from the late 1950s up to the present.

Intravenous agents have not played a major role in general anesthesia. Since the introduction of hexobarbital and thiopental in the mid 1930s, few other agents have been successful in clinical trials. Of the many agents tested, a few remaining steroids, narcotic combinations, and dissociative agents are useful in special procedures or as adjuvants to ensure that *hypnosis*, *analgesia*, relaxation, or visceral reflexes are controlled.

GENERAL ANESTHETICS

There are a large number of substances that could be regarded as general anesthetics. These include a wide variety of structurally unrelated compounds. These agents share the common property of being lipid soluble and capable of reversibly depressing excitable or nervous tissue, thus producing the physiologic phenomenon known as *narcosis*. Narcosis is defined as stupor or loss of consciousness. As a result of nonspecific actions on many different tissues and the problems associated with profound adverse effects and toxicity, few have remained acceptable for clinical use.

There are basically two classes of general anesthetics: (1) inhalation anesthetics, which include gases (nitrous oxide, cyclopropane) and volatile liquids (ether, halothane); and (2) intravenous agents such as barbiturates (thiopental, methohexital), narcotics (In-

TABLE 14-1

Medications associated with general anesthetics

Pharmacologic classification	Drug
Anticholinergics (see Chapter 23)	Atropine Scopolamine
Sedative-hypnotics (see Chapter 15)	Chlordiazepoxide Diazepam Flurazepam Lorazepam Nitrazepam Oxazepam Pentobarbital Secobarbital
Narcotic analgesics (see Chapter 17)	Fentanyl Meperidine Morphine
Neuroleptic agents (see Chapter 18)	Droperidol Promazine Promethazine Triflupromazine
Neuromuscular blockers (see Chapter 26)	Alcuronium Fazadinium Gallamine Pancuronium Succinylcholine Tubocurarine
Neuromuscular block antagonists (anticholinesterases) (see Chapter 25)	Neostigmine Physostigmine

novar, fentanyl) and "dissociative" agents (ketamine).

In the course of general anesthesia, many other drugs or adjuvants are often administered for various purposes. Some of these agents are discussed in the following sections; others are discussed in other chapters (Table 14-1).

GENERAL ANESTHESIA

Anesthesia can be defined as a reversible drug-induced disturbance of neuronal behavior. General anesthesia is associated with a loss of perception of sensation, including touch, sight, taste, hearing, smell, pain, and awareness of environment, and usually involves unconsciousness. Local anesthesia is the inhibition of perception of certain senses in a specific region of the body in conscious and otherwise completely aware patients.

The state of anesthesia is unquestionably complex. It is not simply a loss of sensation and unconsciousness; it also results in varied degrees of *amnesia*, analgesia, hyporeflexia, and skeletal muscle relaxation. It is associated with many alterations of the psyche as well as certain body functions.

Anesthesia consists of progressive stages of excitation and depression. It is difficult to define precisely without a clear understanding of consciousness. Most likely, a single state does not exist, but rather many states forming a continuous spectrum, which may differ for each anesthetic agent.

There are many risks associated with general anesthesia. These agents are potentially lethal; however, death from anesthesia is rare.

BALANCED ANESTHESIA

The purpose of general anesthesia is to produce a state consisting of analgesia and relaxation as well as a lack of awareness that is required to perform the surgical procedures (i.e., a balance between the effects of drugs and surgical stimuli). Balanced anesthesia implies that all aspects of discomfort be controlled or modified, which extends the concept of abolishing only pain or rendering the patient asleep. Balanced anesthesia is the result of a balanced pharmacologic approach. A single drug, such as an anesthetic, cannot produce all the desirable effects. The objectives of balanced anesthesia follow.

1. Analgesia—loss of pain, sensory perception
2. Relaxation—prevention of reflex activity; skeletal muscle relaxation; prevention of movement
3. Unconsciousness—loss of awareness (sleep)
4. Amnesia—loss of memory

COURSE OF CLINICAL ANESTHESIA

The course of anesthesia is divided into six parts: premedication, induction, maintenance, reversal, recovery, and postoperative period. Each part has its own specific definition, purpose, and related pharmacology. Combined, a balanced anesthesia is achieved, as is a smooth, safe, and comfortable recovery.

Premedication

Premedication provides the patient relief from anxiety and pain; promotes sedation and amnesia, and prevents parasympathetic effects of the anesthetic, such as secretions, emesis, and bradycardia. This stage facilitates the induction of anesthesia.

The drugs used in this stage include narcotic analgesics, antianxiety agents, anticholinergics, neuroleptics, and sedatives (see Table 14-1).

Before premedications are given, the patient should be encouraged to void, and vital signs should be taken to serve as baseline data. Premedications are usually given 30 to 60 minutes before surgery. After administration, the patient should be positioned comfortably with the bedside rails in place. Nursing measures to decrease stimulation and to promote relaxation should be used.

Induction

The principal objective of induction is to induce a chemical hypnosis or sleep, not to produce anesthesia. Usually, short-acting, rapid-onset intravenous anesthetic agents are administered. The drugs used to induce anesthesia and together with the premedicants are often termed preanesthetic agents.

Maintenance

Maintenance is the period following induction during which the surgical procedure is conducted. The drugs used in this period include all the general anesthetic agents that are described in detail later in this chapter.

Reversal

The removal or reduction of an inhalation anesthetic and continuation of oxygen will lead to reversal and recovery from anesthesia. Rapid reversal is possible because most inhalation anesthetics are eliminated primarily by the lungs.

Recovery

The recovery period can be divided into an early and late phase. During early recovery oxygen may be continued and cholinesterase inhibitors, analgesics, and antiemetics may be administered. The role of the nurse is extremely important during this and the later period of recovery.

Postoperative period

Various procedures such as coughing, deep breathing, and frequent turning by or of the patient may be necessary. See General Nursing Implications.

IDEAL ANESTHETIC

There are a number of criteria for the "perfect," or ideal anesthetic. Some of the newer volatile anesthetics fulfill many of the requirements for an ideal agent;

however, an anesthetic has not been developed, to date, that can be termed *ideal*. The properties that are desired of such an inhalation anesthetic are listed in the box below.

SIGNS AND STAGES OF ANESTHESIA

Between 1847 and 1858 John Snow attempted to determine the depth of anesthesia of his patients under chloroform or ether. He described certain signs during the anesthesia that were related to the senses known at that time, such as seeing, feeling, breathing (pattern), movement and reflexes of the eyes, pulse, and condition of skin (wet or dry). In 1920 Guedel presented the classic description of the stages of anesthesia. Extending Snow's descriptions, Guedel divided anesthesia into four stages. The third (surgical) stage was further divided into three planes. Guedel used ether, the ideal agent for this exercise because of its slow onset and distinguishable progressive effects. In 1943 Gillespie refined Guedel's classification by including certain reflexes and responses to surgical

stimulus (incision). In 1954 Artusio subdivided stage 1 into three planes describing the progressive changes in memory and analgesia. It is not possible to distinguish all the stages and planes with the modern anesthetics, and it must be noted that preanesthetic agents can alter the many signs of depth of anesthesia. The classification of Guedel is of historical interest and demonstrates only the pattern of anesthetic effects that may occur in various tissues (Table 14-2).

UPTAKE AND DISTRIBUTION

Volatile and gaseous anesthetics are administered via inhalation. The principles of uptake and distribution for inhalation anesthetics are different from intravenous drugs. A knowledge of these principles will provide a better understanding of the manner in which these agents are administered.

To produce anesthesia, it is necessary to achieve a certain partial pressure of anesthetic in the brain. The transfer of an anesthetic gas from one phase to another (e.g., lung to blood, blood to tissue) depends on the

---

Properties of an ideal inhalation anesthetic

Physical

Gas that is easily liquified for storage, or a liquid that is reasonably volatile

High vapor pressure

Boiling point above room temperature and below 70° C

Low blood/gas solubility ratio (provides high partial pressure in alveoli)

Moderate oil/water solubility ratio (relates to potency and fat storage)

Low water solubility

Chemical

Nonflammable, nonexplosive

Stable (should neither decompose on exposure to moisture, light, heat, or air nor corrode or react with rubber, plastic, or metal)

Compatible with carbon dioxide absorber

Easily manufactured from readily available raw material

Simple and accurate analysis of blood and alveolar concentrations

Pharmacologic

Potent, smooth, rapid induction and elimination

Nonirritating

Pleasant odor and taste

Good muscle relaxation

Minimal respiratory and cardiovascular effects

Good analgesia

Minimal postanesthetic effects (e.g., nausea, vomiting)

Does not provoke allergic reactions

Compatible with all drugs used during anesthesia

Adequate oxygenation possible (at least 50%)

Inert—no metabolites; eliminated unchanged via lungs

Nontoxic to all organs

Wide margin of safety

Does not cross placental barrier

difference in partial pressure between the phases (partial pressure gradient). The partial pressure in the brain is determined by the partial pressure in the blood, which is determined by the partial pressure in the alveolar gas. The partial pressure in the alveoli depends on the concentration in the inhaled gas mixture. Henry's law states that the concentration of a gas (anesthetic) in a liquid is directly proportional to the partial pressure of the gas. At equilibrium, the partial pressure in the liquid phase (e.g., blood) is *equal* to the partial pressure in the gaseous phase. However, the concentrations may *not* be equal. Concentration in tissue or blood is equal to the partial pressure times the solubility.

The rate of induction of anesthesia depends on the rate of increase of partial pressure in the brain. The factors that affect this rate are the concentration of gaseous mixture, alveolar concentration, and uptake by blood and by tissues.

The concentration of gas mixture is determined at the source by metered devices or controlled vaporization.

Alveolar concentration is determined by
1. Inspired anesthetic concentration
2. Alveolar ventilation
3. Residual lung volume (functional residual capacity)
4. Uptake by blood

Uptake by blood is determined by
1. Diffusion across alveolar membrane
2. Blood/gas solubility ratio, which is equivalent to the Ostwald solubility coefficient
3. Cardiac output
4. Pulmonary blood flow

Uptake by tissue is determined by
1. Regional blood flow, for example, richly perfused (brain) versus poorly perfused (fat)
2. Tissue/blood solubility ratio

TABLE 14-2

Signs and stages of ether anesthesia (modified Guedel's classification)

Stage	Respiration	Cardiovascular		Eye		Loss of reflex	Description
		Heart rate	Blood pressure	Pupils	Movement		
Stage I: analgesia	Slight increase			React to light			Consciousness, amnesia, analgesia, euphoria, slight distortion of smell, vision, hearing, speech
Stage II: delirium	Rapid, irregular	Increase	Increase	Wide dilation	Increase		Loss of consciousness, hyperreaction to stimuli, involuntary activity
Stage III: Plane 1 surgical anesthesia	Regular	Decrease	Normal	Constriction	Marked increase	Eyelid, "gag"	Sleep
Plane 2	Expirations longer		Normal	Slight dilation	None	Eyelid, corneal, laryngeal	Sensory loss
Plane 3	Diaphragm		Decrease	Dilation	None	Eyelid, corneal, cough	Muscle tone loss
Plane 4	Decrease	Decrease	Decrease	Wide dilation	None	Eyelid, corneal, cough	Intercostal paralysis
Stage IV: medullary paralysis	Complete paralysis	Failure	Decrease	Maximum dilation	None	Eyelid, corneal	Diaphragm paralysis

228

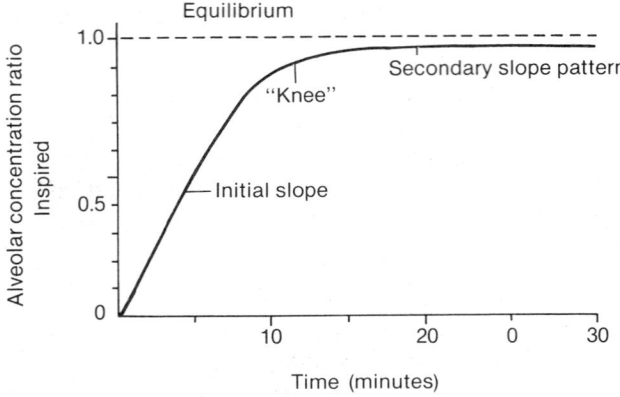

FIGURE 14-1. **Representation of an equilibrium curve for an inhalation anesthetic agent. The relationship (ratio) between the alveolar concentration and inspired concentration is exponential with time. Equilibrium is equal to a ratio of 1.0.**

It is important to note that any of these factors may be altered by disease or pregnancy, which will affect the uptake and consequently the rate of induction of anesthesia. For example, in pregnancy the functional residual capacity (residual lung volume) is reduced, but it is increased in emphysema. In shock the cardiac output is decreased.

The rate of uptake for most anesthetics is exponential with time. If the ratio of the alveolar partial pressure to inspired partial pressure is plotted against time, then an equilibrium curve is generated (Figure 14-1). The equilibrium curve consists of an initial steep slope, a knee (bend), and a secondary slope (plateau) that approaches equilibrium (ratio, 1.0).

The lower the solubility, the faster the "knee" is reached; therefore many factors will alter the shape of this curve, including the type of anesthetic, concentration of inspired anesthetic, cardiac output, and to a lesser degree metabolism and diffusion into body cavities and through skin.

Other factors will affect the uptake and distribution of anesthetics.

Concentration effects

A high concentration of anesthetic in the inspired mixture will create a high concentration in the alveoli. Removal of this anesthetic from the alveoli by pulmonary blood will effectively lower the gas pressure (or volume) in the alveoli and create a "suction" effect, which will effectively increase alveolar ventilation. The opposite effect can occur when the administration of the anesthetic is discontinued: large volumes of gas move from blood to alveoli, thereby reducing the "vol-ume" of oxygen, creating an apparent *diffusion hypoxia.*

Second gas effect

The uptake of a large volume of a primary gas (e.g., nitrous oxide) can accelerate the rate of rise of alveolar partial pressure of a second gas (e.g., halothane) contained in the mixture in a lower concentration, by the same mechanism as described for the concentration effect.

INHALATION ANESTHETICS

Administration

The physical properties of the gaseous and volatile anesthetics are such that they possess perfect characteristics for administration via the respiratory system. A certain concentration of anesthetic "gas" can be delivered with oxygen to the patient, and thus a desired partial pressure in the central nervous system can be achieved that produces anesthesia. In addition, a combination of anesthetic gases (e.g., halothane plus nitrous oxide) can be administered simultaneously. This method of delivery affords rapid induction and elimination, continuous control of concentration, a source of oxygen, and a method of ventilation.

The gaseous anesthetics (nitrous oxide, cyclopropane) are administered with oxygen using a system of flow meters and mixing apparatus. The liquid volatile anesthetics must be vaporized. This can be accomplished simply by the open drop method or using specialized vaporizers (Copper Kettles).

Open drop method. This method of administration is performed by dripping the anesthetic onto a gauze mask placed on the patient's mouth and nose (Figure 14-2). Ether is most commonly applied in this manner. Another form of the open drop method is dripping the anesthetic into a stream of gas (oxygen). The advantages of the open drop method are portability and simplicity; however, there are a number of disadvantages, for example, lack of control of concentration, loss of anesthetic to the atmosphere (waste and pollution), and loss of heat during vaporization, which lowers temperature within the gauze and diminishes vaporization.

Vaporizers. The volatile liquid anesthetics in use at present are vaporized using specilized vaporizers (Copper Kettle). The modern vaporizer is designed to deliver a precise concentration of anesthetic with a constant flow of oxygen (approximately 5 L/min). The vaporizer is incorporated into a breathing system or circuit.

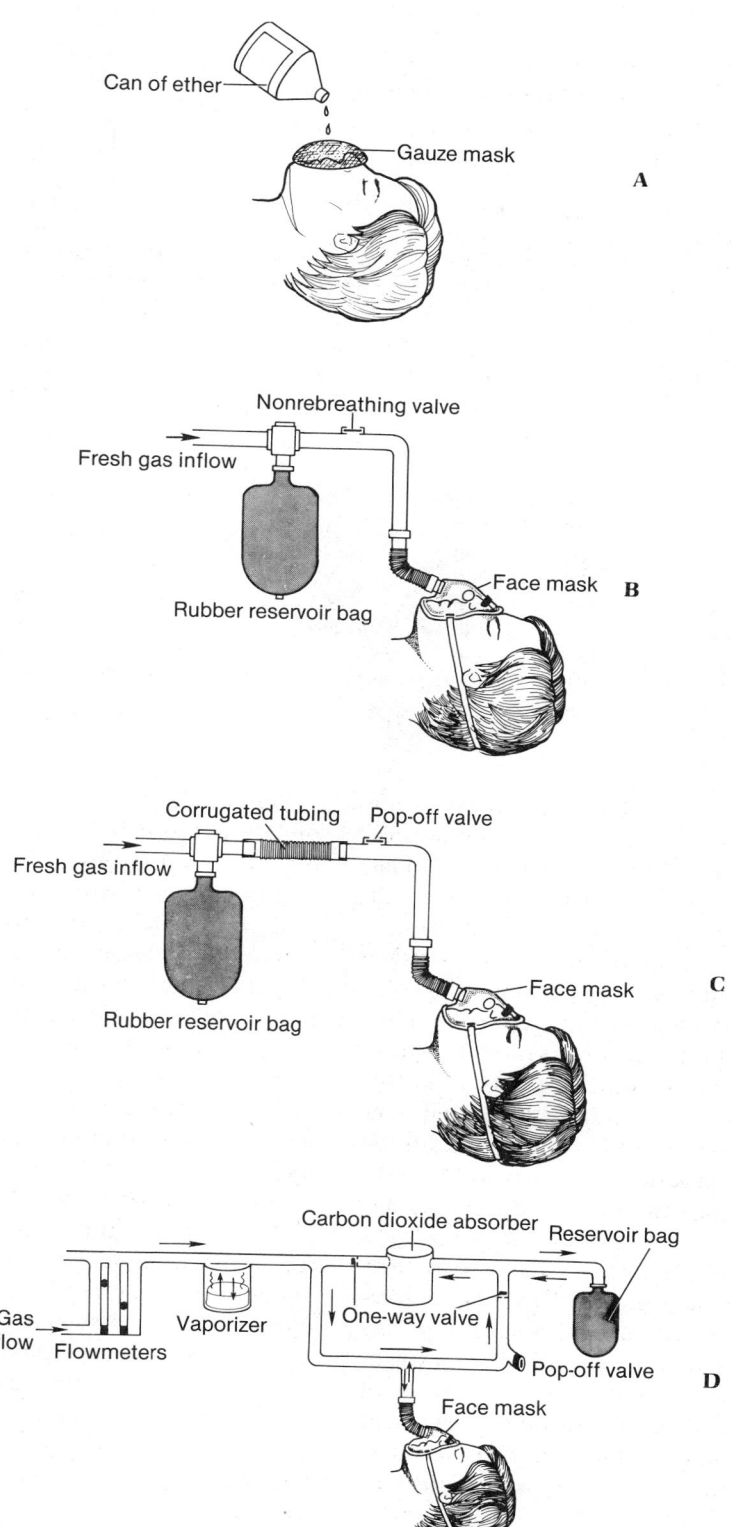

FIGURE 14-2. **Schematic diagrams of different breathing circuits (systems) used to administer inhalation anesthetic agents.** *A,* **Open drop method.** *B,* **Semiopen system.** *C,* **Mapleson, or Magill, system.** *D,* **Circle (semiclosed) system.**

TABLE 14-3

Some physical properties of inhalation anesthetic agents

Agent	Molecular weight	Boiling point (°C)	Vapor pressure mm Hg (20° C)	Flammable	Explosive	Partition coefficients (37° C)		
						Blood/gas	Brain/blood	Oil/gas
GASES								
Nitrous oxide	44.02	−89.0	gas	No	No	0.47	—	1.4
Cyclopropane	42.08	−33.0	gas	Yes	Yes	0.42	1.3	11.2
Ethylene	28.06	−103.0	gas	Yes	Yes	0.14	1.2	1.3
VOLATILE LIQUIDS								
Diethyl ether	74.12	34.6	442	Yes	Yes	12.1	1.14	65
Divinyl ether	70.09	28.3	553	Yes	Yes	2.8	1.14	54.6
Chloroform	119.38	61.2	160	No	No	10.3	1.0	265
Halothane	197.4	50.2	242	No	No	2.5	—	224
Methoxyflurane	164.97	104.7	20	No	No	13.0	2.5	825
Enflurane	184.0	56.5	180	No	No	1.91	—	98.5
Isoflurane	184.5	48.5	250	No	No	1.4	—	99.0

Vaporization. Most liquid anesthetics have vapor pressures that favor vaporization at room temperature (Table 14-3). Vaporization requires energy; heat is lost during the process. A decrease in temperature will decrease the vapor pressure, thus reducing vaporization. For this reason, vaporizers or Copper Kettles are constructed of substances that are good heat conductors to prevent a significant decrease in temperature of the liquid. The temperature at which the vapor pressure is equal to the atmospheric pressure is the *boiling point.* The critical temperature is the temperature above which a gas cannot be liquified at atmospheric pressure. Modern vaporizers are usually made for one specific agent; for example, the Fluotec is designed for halothane.

Breathing circuits. The systems used to deliver volatile gaseous anesthetics consist of a source of oxygen and often nitrous oxide (tanks), a source of anesthetic (vaporizer or tank), a method of removal of exhaled carbon dioxide (carbon dioxide absorber of free exhaust), reservoir for gases (reservoir bag), and mechanisms for adequate ventilation. The circuit is connected to the patient by means of a face mask or endotracheal tube.

The basic purpose of the breathing circuit is to provide an input of fresh oxygen plus a certain concentration of anesthetic gas and an effective method of removal of the exhaled carbon dioxide.

One method of removing carbon dioxide is to simply allow the exhaled gases to be released to the atmosphere. This type of system (open or semiopen) requires an excessive supply of fresh gas inflow.

Carbon dioxide may also be removed by chemical reaction with an alkaline substance. A carbon dioxide absorber contains granules of sodium and calcium hydroxide, and the reactions that occur are

$$CO_2 + NaOH \longrightarrow H_2O + Na_2CO_3 + heat$$
$$Na_2CO_3 + Ca(OH)_2 \longrightarrow 2\ NaOH + CaCO_3$$

The heat produced warms the container and is a good indicator of a functioning absorber. A colorimetric pH indicator is also included, which indicates exhaustion of the hydroxide material.

There are a number of different designs for breathing circuits. They can be classified generally as open, semiopen, semiclosed, or closed systems. The semiclosed or closed systems provide the most efficient and perhaps safest systems but are complicated in design. The basic characteristics are described.

Nonbreathing systems (open and semiopen). These systems are relatively simple and efficient with spontaneously breathing patients. Unidirectional valves may or may not be incorporated into the systems; therefore, there is usually little resistance to flow of gases. Exhaled gases are released into the atmosphere. Examples of open systems include open-drip method, insufflation, and simple T-piece. Examples of semiopen systems include the Mapleson or Magill system and the Bain system (a modification of the Magill system, it warms gas inflow).

Partial rebreathing systems (semiclosed). The circle system is the most popular. The system is complex, involving unidirectional valves, which produce an increase in resistance to gas flow. A reservoir bag is incorporated into the system. Carbon dioxide and water vapor may accumulate. A high concentration of anesthetic vapor is provided.

Rebreathing system (closed system). The gas mixture (fresh inflow and expired gases) are rebreathed. The system contains a reservoir bag and a carbon dioxide and moisture absorber. The fresh gas inflow is required only to provide the necessary oxygen that was consumed and the amount of anesthetic taken up. It is the most economical system because it conserves heat, moisture, and anesthetic. It also reduces the hazard of explosion and pollution. Regulation of respiration is possible by means of the breathing bag.

Effective dose and potency of inhalation anesthetics

To establish a desired depth of anesthesia, it is necessary to achieve a certain partial pressure of anesthetic at the active site (brain). It is essential to determine the concentration of anesthetics administered because there is always the danger of delivering a potentially lethal dose. The therapeutic index (TI) for most anesthetics is small; that is, there is only a twofold to fourfold difference between the dose (concentration) that produces respiratory and cardiovascular arrest and the dose that produces the desired effect.

The concentration of an anesthetic in the brain cannot be practically measured. At a steady state, the partial pressure in the alveoli is equal to the partial pressure in the brain, and there is rapid equilibration between the alveoli (blood) and the brain. Therefore, the concentration in the alveoli is a relatively accurate measure of the concentration in brain. The minimal alveolar concentration (MAC) of anesthetics has been accepted as a measure of the effective "dose" of general anesthetics. MAC is the minimum concentration of anesthetic in the alveoli at equilibrium that is sufficient to just prevent mobility as a result of a standard noxious or surgical stimulus in one half (50%) of the patient population. Measurements are made at 1 atmosphere. This is a measure of anesthetic *potency.* Potency is regarded as the activity per unit weight of substance and is usually expressed as a concentration in the blood or other fluid. Since a "fixed" dose of anesthetic is not administered, but rather a continuous (and variable) concentration of gaseous mixture,

the concept of alveolar concentration as a measure of potency for inhalation anesthetics is suitable. Potency is equal to the reciprocal of the partial pressure required to give a desired anesthetic effect; it is different from *efficacy,* which is a measure of each substance's inherent activity. Each anesthetic has a different MAC value (Table 14-4) and also will produce an effect different in magnitude.

The dose response curves for most general anesthetics are steep. MAC represents only a single point on the curve, and the slope cannot be predicted from this value. The variation in MAC is small; more than 99% of the population responds at 1.1 MAC (the working range is 0.9 to 1.1 MAC). Only a few physiologic factors affect MAC.

FACTORS THAT AFFECT MAC

1. Age (decreases with increasing age)
2. Body temperature (hypothermia reduces MAC)
3. Thyroid function (hyperthyroidism raises MAC)
4. Drugs (narcotics, anxiolytics, methyldopa decrease MAC)
5. Hepatic function (decreased hepatic function usually decreases MAC)

FACTORS THAT DO NOT AFFECT MAC

1. Duration of anesthesia
2. Circadian rhythms
3. Hypothyroidism
4. Changes in arterial oxygen (Pao_2)
5. Changes in arterial pressure
6. Changes in carbon dioxide ($Paco_2$)
7. Anemia
8. Changes in metabolic acidosis/alkalosis

Effects of general anesthetics

Inhalation gaseous and volatile anesthetics are often classified as nonspecific drugs, for they are capable of affecting all excitable tissues. They do not appear to have a specific structural requirement for activity; rather the potency is best related to lipid solubility. The effects of general anesthetics are concentration (dose) dependent. Although the effects on various organ systems appear to be similar, there are significant differences between the agents that warrant individual description.

It is generally accepted that the major effect of anesthetics is depression of the central nervous system. Principal sites of action are proposed to be the ascending reticular activating system (RAS) and certain synaptic pathways in the spinal cord. The precise central "site" is unknown.

Respiration is usually depressed, most likely a result

TABLE 14-4

Effective concentrations of inhalation anesthetic agents

| Agent | Inspired concentrations | | Anesthesia (maintenance) | MAC* volume % | Current status |
| | Volume % | | | | |
	Induction	Analgesia			
GASES					
Nitrous oxide	75	50-70		105	Commonly used
Cyclopropane	25-50	3-5	10-20	9.2	Rarely used
Ethylene	90	20-50	80-90	—	Rarely used
VOLATILE LIQUIDS					
Diethyl ether	10-30	1.5-3.0	5-15	1.92	Obsolete
Divinyl ether		0.2	2-4	0.5	Obsolete
Chloroform	1-2	0.2-1	0.75-1.5	0.5	Rarely used
Halothane	1-4		0.5-2.0	0.75	Used
Methoxyflurane	2-3	0.3-0.8	0.25-1.0	0.16	Disappearing
Enflurane	2-5	—	1.5-3.0	1.68	Used
Isoflurane	1-4	—	0.8-2.0	1.40	Used

*MAC = minimum alveolar concentration

of (1) depression of the central respiratory center and RAS and (2) reduction of sensitivity to carbon dioxide. Certain agents such as ether may stimulate respiration or produce tachypnea.

Heart rate, blood pressure and cardiac output are commonly decreased. These effects may be reflexly antagonized by a sympathetic stimulation of the autonomic nervous system. Cardiac dysrhythmias are common. Certain agents such as cyclopropane, ether, and fluroxene may enhance cardiac output.

The general effects on muscle relaxation and analgesia are variable. Splanchnic blood flow is decreased, as are certain kidney functions, including glomerular filtration rate, renal blood flow, and urine volume.

GASEOUS ANESTHETICS

Nitrous oxide

Physical properties. Nitrous oxide is a colorless inorganic gas, heavier than air, with a slight odor and taste. It is nonexplosive and nonflammable, but at high concentrations will support combustion. Nitrous oxide is commonly called "laughing gas."

Actions. Nitrous oxide is a gaseous anesthetic of low potency (MAC = 105%), but in combination with oxygen will produce excellent analgesia. Its major uses are in dental procedures and as a component of bal-

anced anesthesia. Inhalation of pure nitrous oxide produces effects similar to other intoxicants: dizziness, loss of inhibition, confusion, and often dreams and hallucinations. The gas does not irritate the respiratory tract and has little effect on respiratory, cardiovascular, kidney, and liver functions. It must be administered with at least 20% oxygen, for there is the potential danger of producing hypoxia when attempting to produce satisfactory surgical anesthesia. Nitrous oxide has all the properties for creating a concentration, or second gas effect. Emergence from anesthesia using nitrous oxide must be accompanied with sufficient oxygen in order to avoid diffusional hypoxia. Muscle relaxation does not occur; in fact, tone may be increased. Therefore a neuromuscular blocker must be used. Although the depression produced by a clinical dose of nitrous oxide (70% in oxygen) is subtle, the MAC values of potent inhalation anesthetics are reduced.

Side effects. Nitrous oxide produces virtually no effect on the gastrointestinal, hepatic, renal, cardiovascular, and respiratory systems. Approximately 15% of patients will have postoperative nausea and vomiting.

Metabolism. No significant metabolic transformation has been reported for nitrous oxide.

Toxicity. There is no significant evidence of toxicity.

Preparation/administration. Nitrous oxide is

stored compressed as liquid in steel cylinders in equilibrium with its gas phase; it is usually administered in closed systems.

Cyclopropane

Physical properties. Cyclopropane is a stable, colorless, heavier than air gas, with a mild pungent odor. It is explosive and flammable in air or oxygen. It may be used with a carbon dioxide absorber.

Actions. Cyclopropane is a potent anesthetic, producing analgesia at 3% to 5% and anesthesia at 25%. Induction (approximately 50%) is rapid (1 to 2 min), and the gas does not irritate the respiratory tract. The anesthetic produces a descending depression of central nervous system centers, initially affecting the respiratory center, which may lead to acidosis. The vasomotor center is not significantly affected. Dysrhythmias may develop, and peripheral resistance may be increased. The myocardium can be depressed. Sympathetic stimulated release of catecholamines may account for some of the cardiovascular effects and may induce dysrhythmias. Adequate skeletal muscular relaxation is produced, but the smooth muscle of the uterus and the intestine is not affected.

Side effects. In addition to the effects described above, cyclopropane produces little effect on the kidney and liver. At deep anesthetic levels dysrhythmias may be produced and marked respiratory depression may occur. Postoperative "cyclopropane shock" may occur with a resultant decrease in blood pressure. This is probably the result of accumulation of carbon dioxide and may be avoided with adequate ventilation during emergence. Postanesthetic delirium has been known to occur.

Metabolism. Approximately 0.5% of the inhaled drug is metabolized to carbon dioxide and water.

Toxicity. There is no evidence of hepatotoxicity.

Preparation/administration. Compressed gas is stored in steel containers. Cyclopropane is administered using a closed system and carbon dioxide absorber.

Status. It is rapidly disappearing or obsolete because of its explosive nature.

Ethylene

Physical properties. Ethylene is a highly volatile gas that is lighter than air. It is colorless, slightly sweet, and has an unpleasant odor. It is explosive and flammable in oxygen.

Actions. At concentrations of 20% to 50%, ethylene produces analgesia, at concentrations of 80% to 90%, anesthesia. Induction is smooth and rapid (2 to 5 minutes) and has effects similar to nitrous oxide, but slightly more potent. It does not irritate the respiratory tract and produces no change in respiration or cardiovascular functions. Muscle relaxation is absent.

Side effects. Ethylene produces moderate postoperative nausea and vomiting but no significant effects on the kidney or liver.

Metabolism. Approximately 10% of ethylene is metabolized.

Toxicity. No toxicity has been established.

Preparation/administration. Ethylene is stored under pressure in steel cylinders and administered with oxygen in closed systems.

Status. Ethylene is obsolete because of its explosive nature.

VOLATILE LIQUIDS

Ether

Physical properties. Ether is a highly volatile, flammable, colorless liquid. It is explosive in mixtures of air or oxygen. It is not a stable substance and decomposes on exposure to light, air, and moisture.

Actions. Ether presents the classic signs and stages described by Guedel of irregular descending depression of the central nervous system. Induction at a concentration of 10% to 12% will cause an increase of pulse rate and blood pressure that will return to normal during maintenance. Peripheral vasodilation and depression of the myocardium are usually reversed as a result of stimulation of sympathetic activity.

Bronchial secretions are increased, and respiration is reflex stimulated as a result of irritation of the respiratory mucosa.

Ether relaxes skeletal muscles by blocking the neuromuscular junction. Uterine smooth muscle contractions may be decreased and slowed. Intestinal muscle tone and peristalsis are also depressed. Urinary output, glomerular filtration rate, and renal plasma flow are decreased. The anesthetic crosses the placental barrier in 15 to 20 minutes.

Side effects. Postoperative nausea and vomiting are common. This may be caused by gastric mucosa irritation. Recovery from ether anesthesia is slow, similar to the induction, and stages of excitation and analgesia can be experienced.

Metabolism. Approximately 5% to 10% of the anesthetic is converted to acetaldehyde, which is then metabolized to water and carbon dioxide.

Toxicity. Respiratory arrest may occur during the induction phase. Prolonged exposure to ether may result in respiratory failure and depression of the cardiovascular system. It is possible for the patient, during emergence, to aspirate mucus or vomitus.

Preparation/administration. Ether is kept in tightly sealed metal containers, and contents from a previously opened container should *not* be used. It can be administered in a variety of ways, such as open drop or closed systems. A concentration of 1% will produce analgesia, 3% unconsciousness, and 3% to 5% anesthesia. An inhaled concentration of 6% to 8% may produce respiratory arrest.

Status. Although regarded as a relatively safe anesthetic, its irritant properties, explosive and flammable nature, slow induction and recovery, and high incidence of postoperative nausea and vomiting have resulted in ether being used mainly as a solvent for fats and oils rather than a general anesthetic.

Divinyl ether

Physical properties. Divinyl ether is similar to ether but more volatile; it is also explosive and flammable.

Actions. Its actions are similar to those of ether, but divinyl ether has a more rapid induction and recovery. It produces a progressive rhythmic twitching, and ultimately may cause convulsions by stimulating the motor centers. It will also depress the respiratory center with little irritation of the mucosa.

The most characteristic effect on the cardiovascular system is sinus tachycardia. Skeletal muscles are relaxed, as well as bronchial smooth muscle. Analgesia is produced at 0.2% and anesthesia at 2% to 4% concentrations.

Side effects. Divinyl ether has fewer side effects than ether.

Metabolism. The metabolism is unknown.

Toxicity. Hepatotoxicity as a result of hypoxia can occur after exposure periods of ½ hour or more; kidney damage and convulsions are commonly produced in children.

Preparation/administration. It is available in dropper bottles and administered by open drop, semiclosed, or closed systems.

Status. It is rarely used.

Chloroform

Physical properties. Chloroform is a clear and colorless liquid with a characteristic sweet odor and taste. It is neither flammable nor explosive.

Actions. Chloroform produces a rapid induction and emergence. Analgesia can be produced at concentrations of 0.2% or more, and anesthesia at 1% to 2%. It does not irritate the respiratory tract but will increase rate and decrease minute volume of respiration.

It has a direct depressant action on the myocardium and is prone to produce dysrhythmias. Uterine and vascular smooth muscle and skeletal muscle are relaxed.

Side effects. Nausea and vomiting may occur postoperatively but can be controlled by antiemetic agents. The slowing of heart rate is a stimulated vagal reflex and may be antagonized by atropine.

Metabolism. About 5% to 8% of the drug can be dechlorinated, but most is excreted via the lungs unchanged.

Toxicity. Chloroform has been reported to be lethal in many cases, probably a result of hypoventilation or severe liver damage. Kidney toxicity has also been suggested.

Preparation/administration. Chloroform is stored in amber bottles and administered in a variety of ways.

Status. Chloroform is seldom used today, although there have been many suggestions to reintroduce this agent, since its toxicity can be significantly reduced using modern techniques of ventilation and carbon dioxide removal.

Ethyl chloride

Physical properties. Ethyl chloride is a highly volatile, colorless liquid that is flammable and explosive.

Actions. Ethyl chloride is a potent anesthetic producing analgesia at concentrations of 1.5% and anesthesia at 3% to 5%. It depresses the myocardium and respiration and has a narrow margin of safety; respiratory arrest occurs at about 5% concentration. It produces minimal muscle relaxation.

Metabolism. The metabolism of ethyl chloride has been suggested but not defined.

Toxicity. It is hepatotoxic.

Preparation/administration. Ethyl chloride evaporates so quickly that it will freeze tissues on contact and thus is useful as a local anesthetic.

Status. The lack of control of depth of general anesthesia with ethyl chloride and possible cardiac arrest make it unsuitable for clinical use.

Halothane

Physical properties. Halothane is a nonirritating, clear, colorless, volatile liquid with a pleasant odor. It is neither flammable nor explosive. Slight decomposition can occur on exposure to light, but this is prevented by the use of a stabilizer (0.01% thymol).

Actions. Halothane is used for a wide variety of surgical procedures. Induction and emergence are smooth and rapid. Anesthesia can be maintained with gaseous concentrations of 1% to 3% (10 to 20 mg/dl in blood). When it is vaporized in a mixture of oxygen and 65% nitrous oxide, the effective concentration is reduced to 0.08%.

Halothane depresses airway secretions and pharyngeal, laryngeal, and bronchial reflexes. The respiratory rate is initially enhanced and then depressed with an increase in depth of anesthesia.

Unconsciousness can be achieved in 5 to 10 minutes and, emergence is complete in 20 to 30 minutes. Relaxation of skeletal muscle is minimal; therefore, muscle relaxants may be required. Bronchial and uterine smooth muscle are relaxed. Intracranial pressure may increase. Contractile force, stroke volume, and thus cardiac output are diminished; peripheral blood vessels are dilated. The net result is hypotension. The decrease in heart rate and blood pressure may be reversed with administration of atropine. The myocardium is sensitized to catecholamines. Effects on the gastrointestinal system are minimal.

Side effects. The hypotensive effects caused by alterations of cardiac rate and rhythm and the depression of respiration are commonly encountered but can be controlled. Since the uterine muscle is significantly relaxed, contractions during labor may cease; therefore, halothane is not recommended for obstetric anesthesia.

Metabolism. Halothane is metabolized to the extent of 20% to 35% by microsomal enzymes. The major metabolites excreted in urine are bromides, chlorine, and trifluoracetic acid. There is also a small quantity of free fluorine produced.

Toxicity. There is no clear indication of kidney damage, although a few cases of renal failure following halothane anesthesia have been reported; decreases in urine excretion and renal blood flow are short lived. There is a conflict regarding the possibility of hepatic necrosis. The National Halothane Study by the Committee on Anesthesia, National Academy of Sciences, National Research Council in 1966 concluded that the occurrence of halothane-induced hepatic necrosis could not be ruled out, but was rare. Since then more halothane-induced hepatitis case reports have appeared in the literature. It is accepted that repeated exposure may increase the risk of liver damage; therefore, this must be seriously considered in certain patients. If possible, its use should be avoided in patients with known hepatic or biliary disease.

Halothane is a potent volatile anesthetic with a small therapeutic index; however, since it can be administered with adequate oxygen it has proved to be a "safe" anesthetic. Caution is recommended with administration of catecholamines.

Preparation/administration. Halothane is supplied in amber bottles and can be used in all types of circuits; however, a completely closed circuit is not recommended. The use of a calibrated vaporizer is necessary to control concentrations, adequate ventilation must be maintained, and vital signs should be monitored frequently. Halothane can be used with a carbon dioxide absorber.

Methoxyflurane

Physical properties. A stable, colorless liquid with a high boiling point, methoxyflurane is neither flammable nor explosive and has a fruity odor.

Actions. Methoxyflurane is a potent substance, but induction and emergence are slow. It possesses analgesic potency, and provides good muscle relaxation. There is little effect on uterine activity, and most vital functions are well sustained. The myocardium is sensitized to catecholamines, but there is relative safety in the presence of epinephrine. In combination with 50% nitrous oxide, concentrations of methoxyflurane can be reduced by half. Analgesia occurs at concentrations of 0.3% to 0.8%.

Metabolism. The metabolism of methoxyflurane causes production of free fluoride.

Toxicity. Methoxyflurane produces a dose-related nephrotoxicity (renal tubule damage) because of the fluoride metabolite.

Preparation/administration. Methoxyflurane is supplied in glass bottles containing 0.01% butylated hydroxytoluene as an antioxidant. It can be administered using a variety of methods of open and closed systems.

Status. Its use in clinical anesthesia is disappearing.

Enflurane

Physical properties. Enflurane is one of the many fluorinated methyl ethyl ethers introduced in the 1970s. It is a stable, nonflammable, nonexplosive, volatile liquid. The blood/gas solubility ratio is low, which provides rapid induction (less than 10 minutes) and rapid elimination.

Actions. The clinical effects of enflurane are similar to halothane; however, its potency is approximately half that of halothane. It produces a unique EEG response, with high-frequency waves associated with light anesthesia, and slow waves superimposed on the high-frequency waves at deeper levels of anesthesia.

Enflurane does not irritate the respiratory tract, and it produces direct bronchodilation, slight secretions, and pronounced respiratory depression.

The myocardium is sensitized to epinephrine; decreased blood pressure (hypotension) usually occurs only with overdose.

There is marked relaxation of skeletal muscles, and the effects of nondepolarizing neuromuscular blockers such as tubocurarine, gallamine, and pancuronium are potentiated.

Side effects. The side effects are minimal, which suggests that enflurane is superior to halothane and is useful for all types of surgical procedures in patients even with cardiorespiratory diseases, allergic disorders, neuromuscular disease, pheochromocytoma, and endocrine disorders.

Metabolism. A minimal amount of drug is biotransformed (about 2.5%); the metabolites include both organic and free fluoride ion.

Toxicity. This drug has not been associated directly with hepatotoxicity to date, and no effects on the kidney have been demonstrated. There are a few reports that repeated exposure to enflurane may be associated with hepatic necrosis.

Isoflurane

Physical properties. Isoflurane is an isomer of enflurane, but it is more stable and does not require antioxidants or stabilizers.

Actions. The effective concentrations of isoflurane are between halothane and enflurane. It appears that there are a number of advantages with isoflurane, such as absence of cardiac dysrhythmias, greater compatability with epinephrine, greater analgesia and muscle relaxation, and lack of neuromuscular irritation.

Induction and emergence are slightly more rapid than with enflurane. A slight rise in heart rate may occur. Blood pressure may progressively decrease, but circulation remains near normal.

Respiratory depression is greater than with halothane. Smooth muscle of the uterus is relaxed. There is marked potentiation of nondepolarizing muscle relaxants similar to enflurane.

Metabolism. Little of isoflurane is biotransformed (about one tenth of trifluoroacetic acid compared with halothane), although the same amount of fluoride ion is produced.

Toxicity. Isoflurane is currently under clinical investigation. No hepatotoxicity seems to be associated with this drug, and effects on the kidney are minimal. A report of possible neoplasms resulted in the withdrawal of isoflurane from trials for a few years.

Development of new inhalation anesthetic agents

The biotransformation of the inhalation anesthetics presently in clinical use presents major problems associated with the production of active and potentially toxic metabolites. The toxicity and possible teratogenicity of volatile anesthetics has been of great importance recently. It is well recognized that fetal tissues are vulnerable to the effects of many anesthetics and perhaps the metabolites. Although not firmly established, there appears to be a greater than average risk of spontaneous abortion in female operating room personnel. Nephrotoxicity and hepatotoxicity are of great concern and have resulted in the discontinuation of many agents. Many new aliphatic and alicyclic polyhaloalkanes and polyhaloethers are being synthesized and tested; however, only a few appear promising. The ideal anesthetic is yet to be developed.

INTRAVENOUS AGENTS

Barbiturates

Sodium thiopental is a potent barbiturate that is frequently used for induction of anesthesia. The induction is smooth and pleasant, and unconsciousness occurs in one arm-to-brain circulation time (10 to 30 seconds). The duration of action is relatively short (i.e., 20 to 30 minutes) for an average dose because of redistribution of the drug into fat tissue. Prolonged administration will delay the recovery time as a result of saturation of the sites of redistribution.

In general, thiopental and methohexital depress the myocardium, cardiovascular reflexes, and respiration. Relaxation of skeletal muscle is minimal except at high doses. Even deep levels of anesthesia, however, will not relax abdominal muscles adequately.

Barbiturates are metabolized in the liver; this is not involved in the immediate recovery of thiopental, but is important in the duration of action of methohexital.

There are no reports of liver or kidney damage caused by thiopental. One major disadvantage is the possibility of medullary paralysis. The drug is not recommended for use in patients with severe heart disease, hepatic dysfunction, anemia, respiratory disease or porphyria.

Thiopental is available for injection in glass ampules containing sodium carbonate as a buffer. Solutions of 2% to 2.5% have a pH of about 10 to 11. The initial dose (approximately 4 mg/kg) is delivered in about 15 seconds, with subsequent doses repeated every 30 to 60 seconds as required for hypnosis.

Other short-acting barbiturates such as methohexital and thiamylal have few advantages over thiopental.

Onset of action following injection of propanidid is rapid (20 to 25 seconds). Recovery is fast following a short duration (4 minutes) as a result of rapid metabolism. The drug is initially hydrolyzed by plasma pseudocholinesterases and then hepatic microsomal cholinesterases. Dosage should be reduced accordingly in the elderly to avoid increased duration of action.

Propanidid produces a dose-dependent depression of the myocardium, which results in hypotension, often to a greater degree than with barbiturates. Respiration is initially stimulated then depressed. The drug is associated with a greater risk of venous thrombosis at the site of injection than the barbiturates. Since the drug is metabolized by plasma pseudocholinesterase, as is suxamethonium, the action of the latter agent may be prolonged by about 50%.

Ketamine

Ketamine is a cyclohexanone derivative of the psychotomimetic drug, phencyclidine. It produces a state of anesthesia different from other anesthetics: a state described as similar to a cataleptic state (i.e., dissociation from sensation), thus the terminology *dissociative anesthetic.*

The onset of action following intravenous administration is rapid (less than 1 minute), and the duration is between 5 and 10 minutes. Intramuscular administration prolongs the onset to 5 minutes, and the duration to 10 to 25 minutes. The patient appears awake but unresponsive to stimuli. Ketamine produces a marked analgesia that lasts approximately 40 minutes, and a state of amnesia that can last 1 to 2 hours. The eyelids often remain open, and some degree of nystagmus and slight involuntary movement is common. There are occasional violent responses to stimuli.

Ketamine produces little skeletal muscle relaxation and often a hypertonus response. The pharyngeal and laryngeal reflexes are retained, but the cough reflex is suppressed.

Respiration is depressed significantly only with rapidly delivered high doses. Airway resistance is decreased and bronchospasm is usually abolished.

Ketamine increases sympathetic activity; therefore arterial blood pressure, heart rate, and cardiac output are increased. Cerebrospinal fluid pressure is elevated.

The drug is metabolized in the liver, and the metabolites are believed to be active. It readily crosses the placental barrier, but little metabolism occurs in the newborn.

The recovery phase from ketamine anesthesia is associated with excitation, delirium, pleasant or unpleasant dreams, confusion, euphoria, and even hallucinations. Some of these effects can be controlled by the benzodiazepines. These emergent reactions appear to occur most often in the middle adult (over 30 years of age), rather than in children or the elderly. They may last a few hours, and some reports have indicated recurrences up to 24 hours postoperatively. The site of action of ketamine is proposed to be the cortex or limbic system.

Ketamine is not recommended for patients with hypertension or those suffering from emotional disorders. It is useful in children for diagnosis or repeated anesthesia.

Innovar

Innovar is a combination of a short-acting narcotic analgesic and long acting neuroleptic (fentanyl citrate 0.05 mg plus droperidol 2.5 mg per milliliter of solution). This combination produces *neuroleptanalgesia,* which is characterized by a state of quiescence, dissociation, or indifference to painful stimuli, and decreased motor activity. The patient is awake and cooperative but without pain. In combination with 65% nitrous oxide, a state of *neuroleptanesthesia* is produced, which provides an almost perfect state of anesthesia: hypnosis, analgesia, and muscle relaxation.

The actions and side effects of Innovar are related to each component, which are described below separately. The dose is usually 0.5 to 2.0 ml IM, 45 to 60 minutes preoperatively, and often half the preoperative dose is given two to three times postoperatively. The common side effects include hypotension, bradycardia, decreased cerebral blood flow, and intracranial pressure. Marked respiratory depression occurs and may require the use of a ventilator. On recovery, the patient is free of pain, drowsy, arousable, and may be confused and depressed.

Fentanyl

Fentanyl is a narcotic analgesic with activity approximately 100 times that of morphine. The onset of action is faster than morphine (intravenous is 3 to 5 minutes, intramuscular is 5 to 15 minutes) with durations of action 30 to 60 minutes and 1 to 2 hours, respectively.

Preoperative doses of 0.05 to 0.1 mg will produce effective analgesia. Side effects include hypotension, respiratory depression, miosis, nausea, vomiting, euphoria, constipation, and pruritus, which are morphinelike. Narcotic antagonists such as naloxone will reverse the effects. Toxicity can result in respiratory depression and muscle rigidity. All central nervous system depressants will potentiate the sedative and respiratory depressant effects of fentanyl. The drug is metabolized in the liver, and the half-life is in the range of 1 to 4 hours.

Droperidol

Droperidol is a butyrophenone neuroleptic that produces a state of tranquility, reduced motor activity, and indifference to surroundings. The patient remains awake and responsive to commands but may experience considerable drowsiness. Muscle tone and voluntary movements are depressed. Droperidol is also effective in blocking α-adrenergic receptors, producing some hypotension, in addition to the antiemetic, antifibrillatory, and anticonvulsant actions.

Onset occurs in 3 to 10 minutes, and the duration of action is approximately 3 to 6 hours ($T_{1/2} \approx 2$ hours). The drug is metabolized in the liver and excreted in the urine.

Side effects include extrapyramidal symptoms such as tremor, and some reports include dizziness, chills, and restlessness. Droperidol can enhance the effects of other central nervous system depressants. Dosages are in the range of 2.5 to 10 mg administered 30 to 60 minutes before induction.

PREANESTHETIC MEDICATION

The administration of preanesthetic medication (premedication) is an important step in the preparation of a patient to ensure satisfactory anesthesia. The use of premedication was introduced in the 1860s primarily to facilitate induction.

The *purpose* of premedication is to
1. Provide relief from anxiety and pain
2. Provide sedation and encourage amnesia
3. Prevent parasympathetic effects of anesthetics

Calming of the patient can be achieved with a variety of drugs such as barbiturate sedative-hypnotics, neuroleptics, and anxiolytics. In addition, many narcotic analgesics, anxiolytics, and neuroleptics will provide some degree of, or at least encourage, amnesia. Many of the neuroleptics also have potent antiemetic properties that will prevent postoperative nausea and vomiting. Sedatives can also be administered the night before to provide the patient with a restful sleep. Narcotic analgesics are commonly prescribed as the drugs of choice used to alleviate pain and discomfort before and following the anesthetic or surgical procedure.

Exposure to certain anesthetic agents and noxious stimulation (e.g., intubation or injection) may stimulate autonomic reactions primarily of the parasympathetic pathways. These responses include increase in secretion from salivary, mucous, and sweat glands. Accumulation of bronchial secretions, especially in close proximity to the larynx can provoke coughing or laryngospasm. Other parasympathetic effects include spasm of smooth muscle in the intestinal, urinary, biliary, or respiratory tracts and vagus-induced bradycardia. Many autonomic responses can be prevented by administration of anticholinergic agents, which will also act on various exocrine glands, decrease gastric secretions, and produce mydriasis and loss of visual accommodation. Most premedications are given ½ to 2 hours before anesthesia. It is important to be aware of the duration of action of the premedication to avoid possible interaction with anesthetics.

The neuromuscular blocking agents also provide muscle relaxation during anesthesia. These agents are described in detail in Chapter 26.

CLINICAL USE OF GENERAL ANESTHETICS

The pharmacokinetics and pharmacodynamics of anesthetic agents and adjuvants are affected by body weight, age, certain diseases or disorders, alcohol and drug use, and inherited traits.

The effects of age on anesthetic response can be briefly described in relation to children or elderly patients. Neonates and children, in general, require 30% to 50% higher concentrations of anesthetic than adults proportionately based on body weight for desired effect. Higher concentration of other agents such as premedications may also be necessary, but it must be emphasized that there is a greater risk of respiratory depression with administration of other depressants.

An elderly patient may respond with slower onset and longer duration of action to many agents used in anesthesia. Reduction of dose in inhalation anesthetics, induction agents, muscle relaxants, and premedication drugs is usually recommended. The alterations in pharmacokinetics may be a result of decreased metabolic rate and slower circulation times. In addition, the elderly patient may respond with an exaggerated response or even exhibit a hypersensitivity reaction. This may be a reflection of the "aging process" of many functions.

A variety of diseases can present problems or risks with administration of anesthetic agents. For example, cardiovascular disease may increase the risks of hypotension or hypertension, dysrhythmias, fibrillations, or even cardiac arrest. A slower circulation time will produce changes in the pharmacokinetics and may result in possible overdose. Bronchoconstriction, laryngospasm, and increased production of secretions may be aggravated in the presence of respiratory disease. Patients suffering from allergic disorders may respond with a variety of adverse drug reactions or bronchoconstriction. The risk of anesthetic-induced hypoglycemic or hyperglycemic states must be avoided in a diabetic patient.

Renal disease presents complicated problems associated with hypertension; water, electrolyte, and acid-base balance; anemia; and renal failure. In addition, anesthetics can cause potentially fatal kidney damage in kidneys that would be at greater risk in renal disease. Patients suffering from uremia exhibit a sensitivity to barbiturates; therefore, doses must be adjusted accordingly.

Hepatic disease presents similar problems. Hypotension, hypoxia, or hypercapnia as a result of anesthesia must be avoided to prevent further damage.

Epileptics are at risk of convulsions and drug interactions. Individuals with hypothyroidism may exhibit increased sensitivity to depressant drugs. Complications associated with pregnancy affect both mother and fetus.

TOXICITY OF ANESTHETIC AGENTS

A number of studies have demonstrated a variety of toxic effects of anesthetics. Interpretation of the results is often difficult in light of the high concentrations of anesthetics used. Bone marrow depression has been shown to occur after prolonged exposure to nitrous oxide. The risk of impairment and perhaps severe damage to kidney and liver function has been implicated for most inhalation anesthetics, and recent reports emphasize the role of metabolites, which are now known to be produced in significant amounts.

Concern has been expressed of the possibility of trace amounts of inhalation and gaseous anesthetics predisposing operating room personnel to increased risk of malignancy, spontaneous abortion, and congenital defects and mental deficiencies in their offspring. The evidence to date remains controversial, and it is obvious that research in this area is severely lacking. It has only recently been realized that many general anesthetics can be biotransformed to metabolic products that may be potentially reactive and toxic.

MALIGNANT HYPERPYREXIA (MALIGNANT HYPERTHERMIA)

A small portion of the population may be at risk of developing an adverse reaction to anesthetic agents known as malignant hyperpyrexia. This disease is inherited as an autosomal dominant trait with variable expression. It may be caused by a disorder of the binding of calcium to the sarcoplasmic reticulum and sarcolemma. It is most often associated with the administration of halothane and succinylcholine. The clinical symptoms of this myopathy include muscle

contracture, acidosis, and hyperkalemia followed by a fever in which the body temperature rises at a rate of at least 2° C per hour. Many fatalities have been known to occur. It has been recommended that dantrolene 1 mg/kg IV, to a maximum single dose of 10 mg/kg, be administered immediately to treat this life-threatening reaction.

MECHANISM OF ACTION OF GENERAL ANESTHETICS

General anesthesia can be produced by a wide variety of structurally dissimilar chemical substances. The one common property among these agents is lipid solubility. There does not appear to be a specific receptor for the anesthetics; these agents can affect most tissues. No specific chemical antagonist has been found, and a strong correlation between lipid solubility and anesthetic potency exists. The physical interaction of an anesthetic molecule with hydrophobic regions in the membrane of excitable cells provided the basis of a very general "theory" of mechanism: that is, the Unitary Theory of Lipid Solubility Theory of Anesthesia.

The correlation of anesthetic potency and lipid solubility was first noted by Meyer and Overton in 1901, and later extended into a theory of anesthesia by K.H. Meyer in 1935. The original concept stated that anesthesia resulted when a critical concentration of anesthetic was attained in the cell membrane. This "theory" focused on the importance of the hydrophobic interaction (lipid solubility) but did little to provide an explanation of mechanism.

The lipid solubility theory of anesthesia merely expressed a rule of activity for anesthetic agents. Attempts to develop this "rule" into a theory of mechanism were made by a number of investigators. In 1954 L.J. Mullins postulated that the "volume" occupied in the membrane by the anesthetic was the critical factor for potency, and that the shape and size of the molecule would determine its effect. In the early 1970s K.W. Miller and his associates modified Mullins' concept and developed the Critical Volume Hypothesis, which suggested that anesthesia was the result of "expansion" of a hydrophobic region in the membrane beyond a "critical" volume. Expansion of membranes was accounted for by a decrease in resistance to lateral diffusion (motion) of molecular components in the membrane. This was termed fluidization. Thus fluidization provided an explanation for "perturbation," which could then account for the alteration of excitability of neurons (anesthesia).

It is well recognized, however, that all anesthetic

agents do not produce the same effects, and this selectivity of action strongly suggests that a common (unitary) mechanism of action cannot exist.

In clinical anesthesia, a variety of patterns of anesthesia can be observed in the central nervous system as well as in many peripheral systems such as the respiratory and cardiovascular systems. Recently, selectivity of action of anesthetic agents at the cellular level has also been demonstrated.

There appears to be more than one site of action for anesthetics. Lipid solubility is an obvious requirement, but structural configuration may play a role in the potency and effect of an agent.

The precise site(s) within the central nervous system associated with general anesthesia have not been identified. Anesthetics can affect a number of regions in the brain (e.g., cortex, medial thalamus, basal ganglia, hypothalamus, mesencephalic region, hippocampus, or reticular formation). In addition, anesthetic agents are capable of both exciting and depressing various regions of the CNS; the ultimate effect is a disorganization of central activity.

Current concepts do not support a unitary theory of anesthesia. It is more probable that a number of mechanisms account for the production of anesthesia.

Although historically it was generally accepted that anesthetic agents were nonspecific agents, it is now becoming more evident that they possess selective actions.

The mechanisms of action of anesthetic agents still remain unsolved. The difficulty in defining the phenomenon of anesthesia provides further complication to the problem. Research continues to provide more information on the structure and function of the central nervous system, and ultimately general anesthesia and the mechanisms of action of the drugs that produce this effect will be better understood.

SUMMARY

This chapter examines the various types and uses of general anesthetics. With an understanding of the various individual agents, their actions and side effects, as well as the related preanesthetic agents, the nurse will be better able to provide appropriate care to the patient before, during, and following the administration of these agents. Patient education can be enhanced, adverse effects anticipated and monitored for, and clinically significant drug interactions avoided by using the information presented in this chapter.

ADVERSE/SIDE EFFECTS OF GENERAL ANESTHETICS*

ALLERGIC REACTIONS

Histamine release (narcotics)
Hypersensitivity (etomidate)

AUTONOMIC NERVOUS SYSTEM

Catecholamine release stimulated
Parasympathetic stimulation—eye,
  mucous and salivary glands, sweat
  glands, smooth muscle
Vagal stimulation leads to bradycardia

BEHAVIOR

Amnesia
Catalepsy (ketamines)
Convulsions (vinyl ether, enflurane)
Electroencephalogram changes
Hypnosis
Restlessness (phenothiazines)
Vivid dreams, hallucinations (keta-
  mines)

CARDIOVASCULAR SYSTEM

Dysrhythmias
Hypotension
Hypothermia (result of decreased
  peripheral resistance)
Myocardial depression (direct and via
  vagal stimulation)
Peripheral resistance decreased
Sensitization of myocardium to cate-
  cholamines
Thromboembolism—increased risk
  postoperatively in patients taking
  oral contraceptives
Vascular dilation

CENTRAL NERVOUS SYSTEM

Cerebrospinal fluid pressure increase
Descending depression (e.g., respira-
  tory, vasomotor)
Extrapyramidal effects (neuroleptics)
Stimulation of motor centers (divinyl
  ether)

GASTROINTESTINAL SYSTEM

Nausea, vomiting from irritation of
  gastric mucosa (cyclopropane,
  diethyl ether)
Nausea, vomiting from stimulation of
  chemoreceptor trigger zone (narcotics)

HEMATOLOGIC SYSTEM

Anemia

HEPATIC SYSTEM

Hepatotoxicity

METABOLIC and ENDOCRINE SYSTEMS

Carbohydrate metabolism disturbed
  (diethyl ether)
Hyperglycemia (usually less than 5
  mmol/L)
Metabolic acidosis
Lacticacedemia (caused by increased
  glycogenolysis secondary to
  increased sympathetic activity)

NEUROMUSCULAR SYSTEM

Increased tone of gastrointestinal
  tract (narcotics)
Occasional muscle movements
Skeletal muscle relaxation
Relaxation of bronchioles, uterus
Spasms (narcotics)

RENAL SYSTEM

Decreased glomerular filtration rate
Decreased renal blood flow
Decreased urine output
Increased tubular reabsorption of
  water
Renal tubule damage (fluoride metab-
  olite of methoxyflurane)

RESPIRATORY SYSTEM

Bronchial secretions stimulated (via
  parasympathetic nervous system)
Bronchoconstriction
Bronchodilation
Decreased responsiveness to carbon
  dioxide (narcotics)
Irritation of respiratory mucosa
Respiratory depression and stimula-
  tion
Retardation of mucociliary flow

*See Chapter 11, "Drug Toxicity," for an overview of drug toxicity.

CLINICALLY SIGNIFICANT DRUG INTERACTIONS*

Primary drug	Interacting drug	Possible effects(s)	Probable mechanism(s)
General anesthetics	Alcohol(ism)	Abnormal biotransformation	Altered liver function
General anesthetics	Antibiotics (neomycin, amikacin, kanamycin, streptomycin, tobramycin, netilmicin)	Potentiation of neuromuscular blockers (respiratory arrest)	Inhibit neurotransmitter release reduction of EPP
General anesthetics	Reserpine	Hypotension and bradycardia	Potentiation of reserpine effects
General anesthetics	Tricyclic antidepressants	Cardiac dysrhythmias	Potentiation of myocardial depression
Halothane	Ketamine	Decreased cardiac output, heart rate, blood pressure	Blockade of ketamine's cardiovascular stimulating effects
Halothane	Theophylline	Cardiac dysrhythmias	Synergistic effect
Methoxyflurane	Tetracycline	Increased risk of polyuric renal failure	Unknown
Propanidid	Neuromuscular blockers (e.g., pancuronium, succinylcholine)	Prolonged activity of suxamethonium by 50%	Inhibition of plasma pseudocholinesterase
Volatile anesthetics	Antihypertensive agents	Exaggerated myocardial depression	Beta-blockade
Volatile anesthetics	Catecholamines (epinephrine, norepinephrine)	Sensitization of myocardium, dysrhythmias	Possible release of endogenous neurotransmitter

*See Chapter 10, "Drug Interactions," for an overview of drug interactions.

GENERAL NURSING IMPLICATIONS

Nursing of patients requiring anesthetics

PREOPERATIVE ASSESSMENT

A careful drug history should be obtained during the nursing admission history and assessment to identify sensitivity, contraindications, and cautions related to preoperative medications or anesthetics. Numerous medications can interact with anesthetic agents (see Clinically Significant Drug Interactions.

Some medications need to be discontinued several days before surgery, and the use of such medications requires careful verification. If a patient is on regular medication, this needs to be discussed with the surgeon and anesthesiologist in advance so that it may be determined which if any of the medications should be held until after surgery or if the medication should be administered parenterally. Patients receiving corticosteroid therapy may require the corticosteroid parenterally before surgery.

Preoperative laboratory work including hematologic studies (e.g., hemoglobin and hematocrit) serum electrolytes, and urinalysis must be completed and abnormalities immediately reported. Consents, surgical preparations, and other related procedures must also be completed. Depending on the patient's age and condition, absence of food and drink for at least 4 hours before anesthesia should be maintained. Older children and adults are usually fasting from midnight on before the day of the surgery.

Patients are often anxious before surgery and this needs to be assessed. Nursing measures to relieve anxiety should be used. Medication to promote sleep may be indicated the night before surgery. Patient need and response should be carefully assessed and monitored. Preoperative teaching and involving the patient in care can do much to decrease anxiety.

SENSITIVITY

Generally, allergic reactions to the general anesthetics are rare; however, any drug has the potential to cause a hypersensitivity reaction in a susceptible individual. See the Nursing Drug Digest.

CONTRAINDICATIONS

The use of anesthetic agents is contraindicated in hypersensitivity. See the Nursing Drug Digest for contraindications associated with specific individual agents.

CAUTIONS

Administer anesthetics with caution to Severely debilitated patients

GENERAL NURSING IMPLICATIONS—cont'd

Nursing of patients requiring anesthetics—cont'd

CAUTIONS—cont'd

Patients with severe cardiovascular disorders
Patients with severe anemia
Extremely obese patients
Patients with asthma or respiratory obstruction
Elderly patients

Health risks have been associated with anesthetic gas exposure in operating room and recovery room personnel, including

Risks to unborn children of exposed women
Various forms of cancer
Myeloneuropathy (halothane)
Interference with vitamin B_{12} metabolism (nitrous oxide)
Hepatic and renal disease

DRUG INTERACTIONS

Because of the varied chemical structures of the anesthetic agents, drug interactions do not generally occur with all the agents. For specific drug interactions associated with individual anesthetic agents, see Clinically Significant Drug Interactions.

ADMINISTRATION

Administration of anesthetics varies, depending on the chemical structure and grouping of the specific anesthetic. For example, all barbiturate anesthetics (e.g., thiopental) are administered intravenously, whereas other agents (e.g., nitrous oxide, halothane) are administered by inhalation.

Nurses generally do not administer anesthetic agents. This is usually done by the anesthesiologist or nurse anesthetist. Preoperative medication is often given to relieve anxiety and to enhance the effect of the anesthetic, and nurses can do much in relation to this aspect of care.

Premedication

Before administration of the preoperative medication as ordered, the patient must be carefully prepared and gently restrained if necessary to prevent injury. This is especially important when injections are administered to children and apprehensive adults. Before the premedication is given, the pa-

tient should be encouraged to void, the vital signs should be obtained to serve as a baseline, and in some hospitals catheterization and the establishment of intravenous infusion or nasogastric suction may also be indicated. The patient's gown is changed; dentures are removed, or if they are to be removed in surgery because of patient embarrassment, this is indicated on the chart; jewelry is removed, or the wedding ring taped. Most hospitals have preoperative checklists, and these need to be carefully filled out because they are sent with the chart when the patient goes to the operating room and are used by the nurses there in planning their nursing care. Thus, the nursing care plan should also accompany the chart.

After the premedication, the patient should be positioned and made comfortable. Nursing measures to relieve anxiety and to reduce stimuli should be used. The bedside rails should be used and the patient monitored for drug effects. The medication is charted as are the patient's response and general condition and emotional state. Any unusual observations should be readily reported.

MONITORING PATIENT RESPONSE

Therapeutic response

Preoperative

The premedication should relieve pain (if present) and anxiety and provide sedation.

Intraoperative

After administration of the anesthetic, the patient will lose perception of sensation and progress through the stages of anesthesia. Monitor for analgesia, relaxation, and unconsciousness.

Postanesthetic recovery is considered to be an extension of the intraoperative period. Anesthetic effects persist in the immediate postanesthetic period, thus knowledge of the scope of anesthesia and intensive care nursing is essential.

The nurse must be familiar with all aspects of the management of the unconscious patient. The nurse must obtain a complete report of the procedure, premedication, anesthetic

agents, and response to surgery. This information is usually recorded on the patient's chart. However, it is helpful to talk directly to the anesthesiologist and surgeon when the patient is received in order to clarify questions. A plan of individualized care can then be developed using these data.

Careful assessments related to respiratory status, including the presence of an airway; oxygen; excessive secretions, laryngospasms, or edema; bronchospasm; or hypoventilation need to be completed frequently (every 5 minutes).

Circulatory assessment and monitoring of hypotension and shock as well as monitoring for hypertension resulting from hypoxia, hypervolemia, or pain are completed. Cardiac status should also be assessed.

Nausea and vomiting may occur, and positioning and turning should be completed carefully.

Renal status should be monitored. Oliguria is not uncommon in the immediate postsurgery period. A urinary output of less than 30 ml/hour should be reported.

Hypothermia may result, as may shivering as the temperature approaches normal. The patient should be positioned comfortably and warmth maintained. Vasodilation and heat loss must be prevented. The nurse should have a sound knowledge of emergency care, possessing skills in venipuncture, airway maintenance, manual ventilation, and intravenous fluid administration, as well as all aspects of management of the unconscious patient. Disturbances should be avoided during recovery. Auditory sense is the first to recover, although the recovery period varies according to the anesthetic used. During stage II, because the patient is aware of the surroundings and can hear what is said, the environment should be kept quiet and stimuli kept to a minimum to avoid excitement. Restlessness could be indicative of pain or hypoxia. As the patient moves to stage I, the nurse must continue to talk

Continued.

GENERAL NURSING IMPLICATIONS—cont'd

Nursing of patients requiring anesthetics—cont'd

Intraoperative—cont'd

to the patient during assessment and procedures. Pain must be carefully evaluated. Pain medications should be administered as needed per order with caution, and if given, should be carefully recorded. When the patient is transferred back to the nursing unit, this information should be brought to the attention of the nurse in charge of caring for the patient.

The patient should be provided with positive encouragement and orientation to procedures. Family and significant others will also need to be considered, especially if the patient is to remain in recovery for an extensive time. The recovery time should be noted and the postanesthetic recovery score or equivalent recorded.

Postoperative

When monitoring patient response to anesthetics postoperatively, the nurse should know the scope of anesthesia and care in the recovery room. The nurse must also obtain a complete report from the recovery room nurse and anesthesiologist and surgeon as indicated. The chart will have records of the patient's status and response to surgery.

POSTOPERATIVE PROCEDURES

1. Monitor vital functions, pulse, and respiration.
2. Observe color, hue of skin, eyes, reflexes, peripheral perfusion, body temperature, secretions, and drainage.
3. Provide as indicated oxygen therapy, analgesics, antiemetics, and fluids.
4. Prevent incorrect positioning of patient, nerve injuries, pulmonary complications, vomitus aspiration, and injury.

The nurse should monitor for signs of thrombosis or embolisms, hypoxemia, and hypotension.

Vasodilation and heat loss must be prevented.

It is important to be aware of possible postoperative complications, such as hypotension, nausea and vomiting, oliguria, intestinal distention, and hypoventilation.

The nurse must be familiar with possible drug interactions and complications postoperatively that may involve other medications that may be required. For example, when administering a narcotic analgesic postoperatively, the nurse should be aware of which anesthetic has been administered to avoid potential additive respiratory depression such as may occur if the patient has received Innovar, which contains fentanyl (a narcotic) and droperidol.

Adverse side effects

Adverse effects of anesthetics commonly encountered that may pose risk for the patient and should be monitored for include respiratory depression and hypotension. See Adverse/Side Effects of General Anesthetics and the Nursing Drug Digest for specific anesthetic agents.

PATIENT EDUCATION

Preoperative teaching may be completed by unit or operating room staff. Preparation should be individualized, and family and significant others should be involved as indicated. Patients should be encouraged to practice coughing and deep breathing, splinting, leg exercises, turning, and other techniques required postoperatively. A knowledge of what to expect during the preoperative, intraoperative, and postoperative periods is essential including preoperative medications, anesthesia, and postoperative medications.

GENERAL INSTRUCTIONS FOR DISCHARGE/OUTPATIENTS

Follow the after surgery directions given to you for your specific surgery or condition.

If you have any questions or notice any unusual effects, contact your health care provider.

IMPORTANT FOR THE OUTPATIENT

Because of drowsiness do not drive or operate dangerous machinery.

Do not ingest any alcohol or other sedative drugs for 24 hours unless authorized by your nurse or physician.

If you note any irregular heart beats, notify your nurse or physician.

NURSING DRUG DIGEST

Medication (trade name)	Indication	Usual dosage and administration	Dosage forms, preparation, and storage	Contraindications, cautions, and comments	Monitoring
Chloroform	Volatile liquid anesthetic (obsolete)	Analgesia 0.2%-0.7% Anesthesia 1%-2.0%	Liquid in amber bottles	Rapid induction; muscle relaxant; lowers blood pressure; may produce dysrhythmias with sympathomimetics, cardiac paralysis; acidosis on recovery; hepatotoxic; *obsolete*	Monitor cardiac function when used with epinephrine
★ **Cyclopropane**	Anesthetic gas (rarely used)	*Adults:* (vapor concentration) Analgesia 3%-5% Anesthesia 10%-25% Administer in closed system with oxygen	Gas supplied in orange cylinders	Rapid induction; moderate skeletal muscle relaxation; sensitizes myocardium to catecholamines; may produce dysrhythmias, laryngospasms, postanesthesia nausea, vomiting, and headache. *Explosive with oxygen*	Monitor cardiac function when used with epinephrine
★ **Enflurane** Ethrane	General anesthetic Obstetric analgesic for vaginal delivery	*Adults:* (vapor concentration) Induction 2%-4.5% Maintenance 0.5%-3% Use calibrated vaporizer *only* *Adults:* (vapor concentration) 0.25%-1.25%	Liquid: 125 and 250 ml amber bottles	*Contraindicated* in hypersensitivity and seizure disorders. Rapid induction (7-10 min). May produce some motor activity, hypotension, respiratory depression, dysrhythmias and shivering; potentiates nondepolarizing neuromuscular blockers; induction and recovery are rapid. Use avoided in pregnancy; *not* to exceed 3% for maintenance. Use with caution in patients with renal impairment	Monitor cardiac function when used with epinephrine

Continued.

NOTE: For additional details regarding the individual agents listed in this table see the text and other tables in this chapter.
✦ Indicates that the drug is generally available only in Canada.
★ Indicates that the drug is generally available only in the United States.

NURSING DRUG DIGEST—cont'd

Medication (trade name)	Indication	Usual dosage and administration	Dosage forms, preparation, and storage	Contraindications, cautions, and comments	Monitoring
★ **Ether**	Volatile liquid anesthetic (rarely used)	Vapor concentration Analgesia 1.5%-3.0% Anesthesia 3.4%-4.5%	Liquid supplied in metal containers	*Contraindicated* in patients with respiratory disease Slow, unpleasant induction and recovery; irritates respiratory mucosa; postanesthetic nausea and vomiting; muscle relaxant may produce respiratory paralysis *Explosive with oxygen*	Monitor respiration
★ **Ethylene**	Anesthetic gas (rarely used)	Vapor concentration Anesthesia 80%-90% Analgesia 20%-50%	Gas supplied in red cylinders	Primary complication is hypoxia; high (about 80%) concentrations required for anesthesia; short induction; poor muscle relaxant; explosive and flammable	Monitor for hypoxia
★ **Etomidate** Amidate Hypnomidate	General anesthetic (for short operative procedures)	*Adults:* 0.2-0.6 mg/kg IV *Children:* less than 10 years of age—use *not* recommended	Injectable: 2 mg/ml	Cardiovascular and respiratory depression are *low*; myoclonus may develop; commonly causes pain on injection	Monitor for any untoward effects because experience with this agent is still limited
Fentanyl and droperidol combination Innovar	General anesthetic as an adjunct to nitrous oxide and oxygen Anesthetic premedication	Variable depending on intended use and individual patient response Administration is by slow IV infusion or drip *Adults:* 1-2 ml IM 45-60 min preoperatively *Children:* 0.03 ml/kg IM 45-60 min preoperatively	Injectable: 0.05 mg fentanyl and 2.5 mg droperidol per ml Can be diluted with D_5W Protect from light Store at room temperature	*Contraindicated* in hypersensitivity or intolerance to either component Produces a quiescent and analgesic state with reduced motor activity; complete loss of consciousness usually does not occur without the use of an additional agent	Observe for hypoventilation; reduce dosage of narcotic analgesics postoperatively Monitor blood pressure for hypotension

Drug	Category	Dosage	Remarks	Nursing implications
Halothane Fluothane Somnothane	General anesthetic	*Adults:* (vapor concentration) Induction 1%-3% Maintenance 0.5%-1.5% (0.8% with 65% nitrous oxide)	Liquid supplied in 125 and 250 ml amber bottles (0.01% thymol) Do *not* store in contact with rubber or plastic because these may be deteriorated by halothane *Contraindicated* in shock and cardiac dysrhythmia Use caution with certain antibiotics (respiratory arrest) Danger of malignant hyperthermia occurring in genetically susceptible patients; potent anesthetic May produce respiratory depression, myocardial depression, moderate muscle relaxation, hypotension, hypoxia, and acidosis; induction and recovery are rapid Produces little secretions, bronchodilation; sensitizes myocardium to catecholamines May produce dysrhythmias; may cause apnea neonatorum if administered during labor Treat shivering on recovery Use is *not* recommended for obstetric anesthesia	Monitor all vital signs; monitor cardiac function frequently when epinephrine administered
Isoflurane Forane	General anesthetic	*Adults:* (vapor concentration) Induction 2.5%-4.5% (1.5%-3% with 50%-70% nitrous oxide) Maintenance: 1.5%-3.5% (1%-2.5% with 50%-70% nitrous oxide) *Children:* over 2 years of age same as adults	Liquid supplied in 100 ml amber bottles *Contraindicated* in hypersensitivity Absence of cardiac dysrhythmias; depression of respiration; muscle relaxant, marked uterus relaxation, progressive decrease of blood pressure; no irritation of respiratory airways	Monitor respiration
Ketamine Ketaject Ketalar Ketaset	General anesthetic (*not* recommended if skeletal muscle relaxation is required)	*Adults:* Induction 1-4.5 mg/kg IV slowly over 60 sec; or 6.5-13 mg/kg IM Maintenance 50%-100% of full induction dose May need to decrease dose in renal failure	Injectable: 10, 50, and 100 mg/ml Dilute 100 mg/ml concentration with D_5W, NS, or sterile water for injection *before* administration *Contraindicated* in hypertension and hypersensitivity *Contraindicated* in cerebrovascular accident patients	Monitor blood pressure Observe for emergence reactions

Continued.

NURSING DRUG DIGEST—cont'd

Medication (trade name)	Indication	Usual dosage and administration	Dosage forms, preparation, and storage	Contraindications, cautions, and comments	Monitoring
Ketamine—cont'd				Produces a rapid state of "dissociative anesthesia" and analgesia; increases blood pressure Excitement as well as respiratory depression may occur; emergence can be associated with disturbing reactions (ketamine is a potent hallucinogen); may cause neurobehavioral depression in the neonate if administered during labor Do *not* disturb patient on emergence; patient should be placed in a quiet area postoperatively and may require a sedative (diazepam) Ketamine has a high therapeutic index	
Methohexital Brevimytal Natrium Brevital Brietal	General anesthetic (for short surgical procedures)	*Adults:* Induction 50-120 mg IV drip 0.2% (1 drop/sec) Rate of injection of 1% solution approximately 1 ml/5 sec (i.e., 2 mg/sec) Maintenance continuous IV drip of 0.2% solution at a rate of 1 drop/sec	Injectable: 0.5, 2.5 and 5 gm vials or ampules Dilutions must be aseptic To prepare 0.2% drip solution, add 500 mg to 250 ml of sterile water for injection, D_5W, or NS; solution is incompatible with silicone (as on some rubber stoppers) and with acidic solutions (e.g., atropine, succinylcholine) Incompatible with lactated Ringer's solution Do not use diluents that contain bacteriostatics Store at room temperature Discard unused solution after 24 hr	*Contraindicated* in hypersensitivity to the barbiturates *Contraindicated* in porphyria May cause myocardial and respiratory depression, laryngospasm, hypotension, and tachycardia; short duration; administration during labor may cause neurobehavioral depression in the neonate	Monitor for allergic reactions

Methoxyflu-rane Methofane Penthrane	General anesthetic in combination with oxygen and 50% nitrous oxide Analgesic	*Adults:* (vapor concentration) Induction 0.5%-3% Maintenance 0.1%-0.5%	Liquid supplied in 15 and 125 ml bottles Protect from light Do *not* freeze	*Contraindicated* in renal dysfunction Sympathomimetics and nephrotoxic drugs *contraindicated;* recovery prolonged and may require analgesics; may be used in combination with nitrous oxide Complete anesthetic; moderate skeletal muscle relaxation; lowers blood pressure; slow induction may produce respiratory depression *Avoid* deep anesthesia	Monitor urinary output and renal function
★ **Nitrous oxide**	Weak anesthetic gas, anesthetic supplement, analgesic, used in dentistry and second stage labor	Variable; administer with at least 20% oxygen	Compressed gas supplied in blue cylinders	Good analgesia; weak anesthetic; no skeletal muscle relaxation; alters pulse and respiration; may produce cyanosis; *nonexplosive* To avoid hypoxemia, administer with at least 20% oxygen	Monitor pulse and respiration
Thiamylal Surital	General anesthetic (for short surgical procedures)	*Adults:* Induction 1 ml of 2.5% solution every 5 sec Maintenance continuous IV drip of 0.3% solution to maintain anesthesia	Injectable: 1, 5, 10 gm dry powder; a 2.5% solution can be made by dissolving 1 gm in 40 ml of sterile water for injection; may be further diluted with D₅W or NS; Ringer's lactate solutions may cause precipitation; do *not* mix with solutions of atropine; Use *only* clear solutions; if stored at room temperature, discard after 24 hours; if refrigerated, discard after 6 days	*Contraindicated* in porphyria *Contraindicated* in hypersensitivity to the barbiturates May cause myocardial and respiratory depression, laryngospasm, hypotension and tachycardia; short duration; administration during labor may cause neurobehavioral depression in the neonate Extravasation may cause pain and tissue necrosis	Monitor cardiac function and respiration

Continued.

NURSING DRUG DIGEST—cont'd

Medication (trade name)	Indication	Usual dosage and administration	Dosage forms, preparation, and storage	Contraindications, cautions, and comments	Monitoring
Thiopental Pentothal	General anesthetic (for short surgical procedures)	*Adults:* Induction and maintenance 1-3 ml of 2.5% solution (i.e., 25-75 mg) IV at a rate of 0.1 ml/sec; wait 1 min to observe patient response, then repeat at 20-60 sec intervals as required; *or* a continuous IV drip of 0.2%-0.4% solution (diluted in D_5W or NS) at a rate to produce adequate anesthesia	Injectable: 0.5, 1, 5, 10 gm/vial Prepare dilutions aseptically; use sterile water for injection or NS or D_5W; use only fresh solution (discard after 24 hr)	*Contraindicated* in hypersensitivity to the barbiturates May cause myocardial and respiratory depression, laryngospasm, hypotension and tachycardia; short duration; administration during labor may cause neurobehavioral depression in the neonate	Monitor cardiac function and respiration

BIBLIOGRAPHY

Aldrete, J.A., & Britt, B.A. (Eds.). *Malignant hyperthermia.* New York: Grune & Stratton, Inc., 1978.

Britt, B.A. Malignant hyperthermia. *Clinical Anesthesia,* 1975, *11,* 61.

Cohen, D.N. Toxicity of inhalational anesthetic agents. *British Journal of Anaesthesiology,* 1978, *50,* 665.

Dantrolene for malignant hyperthermia during anesthesia. *Medical Letter,* 1980, *22,* 61.

Davie, I.T. Specific drug interactions in anesthesia. *Anesthesia,* 1977, *32,* 1000.

Dienstag, J.L. Halothane hepatitis. *New England Journal of Medicine,* 1980, *303,* 102.

Dobkin, A.B. (Ed.). Development of new volatile inhalation anaesthetics. *Monographs in Anaesthesiology,* Vol. 6, *Exerpta Medica Amsterdam,* 1979.

Dundee, J.W., & McCaughey, W. Drugs in anaesthetic practice. In G.S. Avery (Ed.), *Drug treatment.* New York: Adis Press, 1980.

Eckenhoff, J.E. (Ed.). *Controversy in anesthesiology.* Philadelphia: W.B. Saunders Co., 1979.

Etomidate for induction of anesthesia. *The Medical Letter on Drugs and Therapeutics,* 1983, *25,* 71-72.

Fink, B.R. *Molecular mechanisms of anesthesia. Progress in anesthesiology.* New York: Raven Press, Vol. 1 (1975) Vol. 2 (1980).

Grad, R.K., & Woodside, J. Obstetrical analgesics and anesthesia. *American Journal of Nursing,* 1977, *77,* 242.

Grinblat, J., Lewitus, Z., & Rosenfeld, J. Renal tubular necrosis and liver damage. *Drug Intelligence and Clinical Pharmacy,* 1980, *14,* 431.

Johnston, R.R., Eger, E.I.II, and Wilson, C. A comparative interaction of epinephrine with enflurane, isoflurane and halothane in man. *Anesthesiology and Analgesia,* 1976, *55,* 709.

Lichtiger, M., & Moya, F. (Eds.). *Introduction to the practice of anesthesia.* New York: Harper & Row Publishers, Inc., 1978.

Lunn, J.N. *Lecture notes on anaesthetics.* Oxford: Blackwell Scientific Publications, 1979.

Mattia, M.A. Hazards in the hospital environment. *American Journal of Nursing,* 1983, *83*(1), 72-77.

Rawlings, M.D. Drug interaction and anesthesia. *British Journal of Anaesthesia,* 1978, *50,* 689.

Roth, S.H. Physical mechanisms of anesthesia. *Annual Review of Pharmacology and Toxicology,* 1979, *19,* 159.

Roth, S.H. Mechanisms of anaesthesia: a review. *Canadian Anaesthetists Society Journal,* 1980, *27,* 433.

Sakai, T., and Takaori, M. Biogradation of halothane, enflurane and methoxyflurane. *British Journal of Anaesthesiology,* 1978, *50,* 785.

Smith, T.C., Cooperman, L.H., & Wollman, H. History and principles of anesthesiology. In A.G. Gilman, L.S. Goodman, and A. Gilman (Eds.), *The pharmacological basis of therapeutics.* New York: MacMillan Publishing Co., Inc. 1980.

Strunin, L. *The liver and anaesthesia.* London: W.B. Saunders Co., 1977.

Thornton, J.A., & Levy, C.J. Topics in anesthesia and intensive care. London: Henry Kimpton Publishers, 1979.

CHAPTER 15

Sedative-Hypnotics

John F. Kittel

Medications discussed in this chapter

Benzodiazepines
Alprazolam
Bromazepam
Chlordiazepoxide
Clorazepate
Diazepam
Flurazepam
Halazepam
Lorazepam
Lormetazepam
Nitrazepam
Oxazepam
Prazepam
Temazepam
Triazolam
Barbiturates
Amobarbital
Aprobarbital
Barbital
Butabarbital
Butalbital

Barbiturates—cont'd
Hexobarbital
Mephobarbital
Pentobarbital
Phenobarbital
Secobarbital
Talbutal
Miscellaneous agents
Bromisovalum
Carbromal
Chloral Hydrate
Chlormezanone
Ethchlorvynol
Ethinamate
Glutethimide
Hydroxyzine
Meprobamate
Methaqualone
Methyprylon
Paraldehyde
Triclofos

Sedative-hypnotics are drugs that produce a depression of the central nervous system (CNS) leading to behavioral changes or to a loss of consciousness. The extent to which this CNS depression occurs will determine in large part whether a drug is classified as a sedative or as a hypnotic. Stated another way, the sole difference between a sedative and a hypnotic may well be one of degree, and a higher dose of a "sedative" may indeed produce hypnosis, or sleep. Some authors have noted that sedation, drug-induced sleep, and general anesthesia are all an extension of CNS depression and can, with the exception of the benzodiazepines, be produced by virtually all members of this pharmacologic drug class. The sedative-hypnotics have been divided into three groups for discussion in this chapter: (1) barbiturates, (2) benzodiazepines, and (3) miscellaneous agents.

The modern use of drugs to modify a CNS response dates back to the middle 1800s when bromides were first used. With the introduction of barbital in 1903 and phenobarbital in 1912, the channel was opened for a flood of pharmacologic agents, mostly barbiturate derivatives, which produced a variety of CNS depressant effects. The barbiturates continued as the primary sedative-hypnotic agents until the development of the benzodiazepine class of drugs, specifically chlordiazepoxide, in 1960. Although the barbiturates continue to be widely used as sedative-hypnotics, their use has declined in favor of the benzodiazepines.

Sedative-hypnotics are, as the name implies, most often used to induce a calming effect or to produce sleep. Sedatives have also been used, however, to treat epilepsy (see Chapter 21, "Drugs Used to Treat Epilepsy"), alcohol withdrawal, and skeletal muscle spasms (see Chapter 16, "Muscle Relaxants"). Because a discussion of anxiety and its treatment is included in Chapter 19, "Drugs Used to Treat Affective Disorders," this chapter will focus primarily on the use of drugs to induce sleep.

PHYSIOLOGY OF SLEEP

Natural sleep is composed of two basic stages that occur cyclically: (1) *rapid eye movement* sleep (*REM sleep*), and (2) *non–rapid eye movement* sleep (*non-REM sleep*). During a normal sleep episode, an individual will progress from wakefulness to a non-REM stage, consisting of four phases, and then to a REM stage that is lighter than the non-REM stage and during which dreaming occurs. As the sleep episode continues, the individual will cycle back and forth from REM to non-REM stages until wakefulness is again experienced (Figure 15-1). Each of the sleep stages are associated with other physical changes (e.g., postural changes and dreaming occur during REM sleep, whereas postural immobility and cerebral deactivation

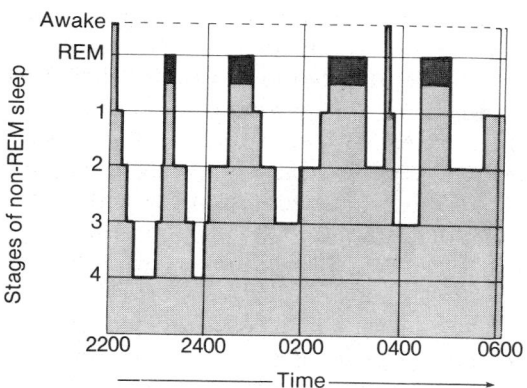

FIGURE 15-1. **In a night's sleep for an adult, the first REM sleep normally occurs after 1 to 2 hours; the cycle of alternating REM and non-REM phases continues through the night, and REM periods lengthen toward morning. In narcolepsy, sleep usually begins with a REM period.**

occur during non-REM sleep). Pathologic changes such as gastric acid secretion or nocturnal angina attacks occur during REM sleep, whereas night terrors and sleepwalking most often originate during non-REM sleep. The physiologic value of each of the sleep stages has not been well defined. However, that definite biologic changes take place during specific sleep stages makes it important for one to note the effect of individual agents on each sleep stage.

POTENTIAL ADVERSE EFFECTS

Inherent in the use of any drug is the possibility of inducing adverse drug effects. The sedative-hypnotic class of drugs is no exception to this dictum and several relative contraindications to their use exist.

Patients with clinical conditions related to sleep

Table 15-1 presents various clinical conditions with sleep-related physiologic changes. Such conditions should be considered before initiating sedative-hypnotic therapy. Patients with duodenal ulcers are often given hypnotic drugs if insomnia also exists. Because gastric acid has been shown to increase during REM sleep, it might at first seem desirable to give the patient a sedative-hypnotic that suppresses REM sleep and thereby avoid excess hydrochloric acid production during sleep. However, the suppression of REM sleep may lead at some later date to a phenomenon known as *REM rebound*, where REM sleep is sharply increased and is often associated with increased dreaming, nightmares, and insomnia. If REM rebound occurs

TABLE 15-1

Clinical disorders related to sleep

Clinical condition	Sleep laboratory finding
MEDICAL DISORDERS	
Coronary arteriosclerosis	Anginal attacks and ECG changes; increase during REM sleep
Duodenal ulcer	Gastric acid secretion is markedly increased during REM sleep
Bronchial asthma	Attacks occur at all sleep stages except stage 4; especially true in children
Hypothyroidism	Stage 4 markedly decreased; substantial increase after treatment when patient has euthyroid condition
Depression	REM sleep is slightly decreased; stage 4 is markedly decreased; with successful treatment, stage 4 sleep increases
SLEEP DISORDERS	
Sleepwalking and night terrors	Virtually all episodes occur out of stage 4 sleep
Enuresis	Most episodes occur out of non-REM sleep
Insomnia	Autonomic activity is at higher levels during sleep as compared to normal sleepers

From Kales, A., & Kales, J. Evaluation, diagnosis and treatment of clinical conditions related to sleep. *Journal of the American Medical Association,* 1970, *213,* 2229.

then the patient with a sleep-related disorder may notice an acute exacerbation of the disease during sleep episodes. REM rebound may occur in any of the following situations: (1) the patient takes a REM suppressant drug for an extended period of time and uses it chronically (such patients may experience REM "breakthrough" where REM sleep occurs even though a REM suppressant drug is being taken); (2) the patient sleeps past the clinical effects of the REM suppressant drug; or (3) the patient naps during the day without taking the REM suppressant drug.

Drug interactions

Several drug interactions may occur when sedative-hypnotics are used, particularly the barbiturates (see

Clinically Significant Drug Interactions). That sedative-hypnotic drugs may be taken intermittently makes predicting clinical effect difficult at best.

History of drug abuse

Because of the CNS depressant activity of this class of drugs, the potential for abuse exists and must be considered before initiating therapy.

In terms of clinical importance, as well as pharmacologic effects, sedative-hypnotics can be divided into three categories: the benzodiazepines, the barbiturates, and other miscellaneous drugs.

BENZODIAZEPINES

Since the introduction of the first benzodiazepine, chlordiazepoxide, in 1960, a plethora of information has been developed concerning these agents. A large number of clinically similar, but sometimes pharmacologically distinct, preparations have been marketed and, whereas dissimilarities do exist among members of the class, enough similar properties are exhibited to permit a discussion of the class as a group.

Mechanism of action

Even though benzodiazepines have been commercially available for over 20 years, the precise site and mechanism of action is not well defined. It appears that benzodiazepines act in concert with gamma-aminobutyric acid (GABA) to cause an inhibition of neurotransmission in parts of the limbic system, the thalamus, and the hypothalamus. A benzodiazepine receptor has been postulated. However, the precise mechanism by which the benzodiazepines exert their effects is unknown.

Drug effects

Central nervous system effects. Like all members of the sedative-hypnotic class of drugs, the benzodiazepines have marked CNS depressant activity. This CNS depression may be manifested by such identifiable characteristics as an attenuation of aggressive behavior, an induction of sleep, a reduction of anxiety as a result of various causes, the prevention of convulsions, and a reduction of muscle spasms.

The benzodiazepines, however, are unlike other members of this class of drugs in that an increase in dose will not cause progressive depression past the lighter stages of sleep from which patients can be easily aroused.

Effects on sleep. The benzodiazepines do not affect normal physiologic sleep stages when given at usual doses. REM stage sleep occurs, as does non-REM sleep in normal phases; REM rebound does not occur following withdrawal of the drug. At higher than normal doses, however, REM *suppression* may occur. Recent work with the newer benzodiazepines has suggested that those drugs with short half-lives (e.g., triazolam, nitrazepam, and flunitrazepam) may cause rebound insomnia, whereas benzodiazepines with longer half-lives (e.g., diazepam and flurazepam) do not appear to cause this effect. These findings have been disputed in other studies and additional work will need to be done to substantiate or disprove this claim.

Tolerance. As with the other CNS active drugs in this class, *tolerance* and physical dependence may develop with the continued chronic use of the benzodiazepines. The potential for such effects, however, is generally regarded as much lower with the benzodiazepine class than with the other sedative-hypnotics.

Respiratory effects. The benzodiazepines cause only a slight degree of respiratory depression even in overdosage and generally do not require supportive measures in such circumstances. An exception to this may be in the case of rapidly injected intravenous diazepam, which has caused *apnea*. However, animal studies have demonstrated similar effects with the solvent for diazepam injection, propylene glycol. Thus it is not clear whether diazepam or propylene glycol is responsible for the cessation of breathing.

Cardiovascular effects. Cardiovascular effects of the benzodiazepines are slight and although hypotension and tachycardia have occurred, they do not appear to be clinically significant for the majority of patients.

Effects of the benzodiazepines on other organ systems appear to be clinically insignificant in most patients.

Adverse effects. The benzodiazepines, when used in recommended doses, are remarkably free from ad-

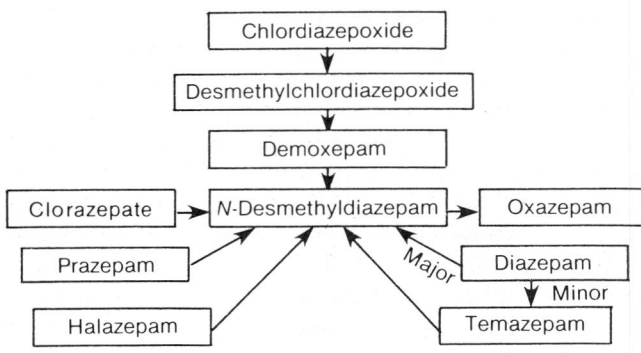

FIGURE 15-2. **Major metabolic pathways of selected benzodiazepines.**

verse effects. Side effects that most commonly occur are an extension of the CNS depressant activity and include oversedation, lethargy, disorientation, and a lack of motor coordination. The incidence of these side effects appears to be higher in elderly patients who have taken moderate to higher doses (e.g., 30 to 60 mg of flurazepam). Other adverse effects infrequently reported with the benzodiazepines include a variety of reactions affecting most organ systems (see Adverse/Side Effects). In addition, the benzodiazepines can cause *psychologic dependence*. Whether they cause physical addiction is currently a controversial issue.

Individual agents

Benzodiazepines, as a drug class, show remarkable structural and metabolic similarities (Figure 15-2). The primary differences among class members exist in (1) the duration of action as determined by the rate of metabolism, and (2) the presence or lack of active metabolites (Table 15-2). It is interesting that, despite the seeming similarities among benzodiazepines, they have been promoted for differing indications. Flurazepam and temazepam are promoted strictly as hypnotics, whereas chlordiazepoxide, clorazepate, diazepam, prazepam, lorazepam, and oxazepam are pro-

TABLE 15-2

Selected pharmacokinetic properties of the benzodiazepines when given orally

Drug	Onset of action	Adult serum half-life (hours)	Duration of action	Active metabolites?
Alprazolam	Rapid	12-15	Intermediate	Yes—alphahydroxy alprazolam
Bromazepam	Rapid	8-19	?	?
Chlordiazepoxide	Rapid	7-20	Intermediate	Yes—desmethylchlordiazepoxide, demoxepam, N-methyldiazepam, (nordiazepam) (desmethyldiazepam)
Clorazepate	Slow	50-99	Long	Yes—N-methyldiazepam (nordiazepam) (desmethyldiazepam)
Diazepam	Rapid	14-90	Long	Yes—N-methyldiazepam (desmethyldiazepam) (nordiazepam) temazepam
Flurazepam	Rapid	30-100	Long	Yes—desalkyl-flurazepam
Halazepam	Rapid	14	Long	Yes—N-methyldiazepam (desmethyldiazepam) (nordiazepam) (3-hydroxy-halazepam)
Ketazolam	Rapid	34-52	Long	?
Lorazepam	Rapid	9-22	Short	No
Lormetazepam	Rapid	11-15	Short	No
Nitrazepam	Rapid	18-34	Long	No
N-methyldiazepam*	Slow	50-99	Long	Yes—oxazepam
Oxazepam	Rapid	6-24	Short	No
Prazepam	Slow	63-70	Long	Yes—N-methyldiazepam (desmethyldiazepam) (nordiazepam) (norprazepam)
Temazepam	Rapid	5-15	Short	No
Triazolam	Rapid	3-5	Short	Yes—7-alphahydroxy-triazolam

*Not available as a separate drug entity.

moted primarily as *anxiolytic* agents. At least one benzodiazepine, clonazepam, is used primarily as an anticonvulsant, whereas another, diazepam, is used in treating status epilepticus (see Chapter 21, "Drugs Used to Treat Epilepsy").

BARBITURATES

The barbiturates are among the oldest sedative-hypnotic agents in use today, dating from the introduction of barbital in 1903. Yet they also represent the entry into the modern era of drug therapy of insomnia and anxiety, because before their introduction the only agents available for this purpose were the bromides, paraldehyde, urethane, sulfonal, and chloral hydrate. They are among the most widely modified group of drugs because over 2500 different barbiturates have been synthesized. Of these, only about 50 have been commercially marketed and of this number approximately 10 are still on the market. That the barbiturates are still widely used is evidenced by the over 12 million prescriptions that were written in 1980 for these agents. This contrasts, however, with 20 million prescriptions written for barbiturates in 1973. The reason for the decline in the use of this drug class is twofold: (1) increased Drug Enforcement Administration (narcotic) controls and (2) the increased replacement in clinical use by benzodiazepines.

Mechanism of action

Barbiturates vary greatly in potency and in pharmacokinetic properties. These differences are ex-plained in part because lipid solubility varies to a great degree among members of this class (Table 15-3). As one might suspect, thiopental (the most lipid soluble) is the most potent in onset of action; barbital (the least lipid soluble) is the least potent. It has been postulated, therefore, that barbiturates penetrate the CNS membrane lipid and alter ion channels or enzymes to cause specific physiologic changes. Pharmacologic actions other than induction of sleep, however, do not correlate well with lipid solubility (e.g., anticonvulsant activity). This would seem to indicate that additional factors may be present.

Drug effects

Central nervous system effects. In general, all barbiturates exhibit some degree of CNS depressant activity and, depending on the drug, dose, and route of administration, a variety of pharmacologic effects may be seen. Useful applications of this effect are induction of sleep and general anesthesia. Potentially lethal extensions of this depression, coma and death, may also occur in overdose. Barbiturates, notably phenobarbital and mephobarbital, are also useful adjuncts in the therapy of epilepsy and have been used as antianxiety agents. There is little evidence, however, to suggest any antianxiety effect other than sedation, and the benzodiazepines remain the anxiolytic agents of choice.

Effects on sleep. The barbiturates have been shown to interfere with the REM stage sleep, as well as stages 3 and 4 of non-REM sleep. Chronic use has led to REM rebound characterized by insomnia, nightmares, or

TABLE 15-3

Selected pharmacokinetic properties of the barbiturates when given orally

Drug	Adult serum half-life (hours)	Duration of action	Relative lipid-solubility	Comments
Amobarbital	8-42	Intermediate	113	
Aprobarbital	14-40	Intermediate	—	
Barbital	—	Long	4	
Butabarbital	34-42	Intermediate	I	
Hexobarbital	3-7	Short	73	
Mephobarbital	12-24	Long	56	75% converted to phenobarbital
Pentobarbital	15-48	Intermediate	106	
Phenobarbital	72-144	Long	34	
Secobarbital	19-34	Intermediate	—	
Talbutal (butalbital)	15	Intermediate	—	
Thiopental	3-8	Short	1000	

more frequent and intense dreams. As mentioned previously, physiologic changes such as angina and exacerbation of ulcers have occurred during such a rebound phenomenon.

Tolerance. Tolerance to the CNS effects of barbiturates, as well as physiologic dependence, may occur depending on the regularity with which the drug is used. With chronic continued use, decreased effectiveness has been demonstrated in sleep laboratories by the second week of drug administration (see Hepatic Effects).

Paradoxic excitation. Barbiturates may produce a paradoxic excitement in children, elderly patients, or debilitated patients. For this reason, barbiturates, particularly phenobarbital and mephobarbital, are best avoided in very young patients, elderly patients, and chronically ill patients.

Respiratory effects. The barbiturates produce a respiratory depression proportional to the dose of drug received (i.e., the larger the dose, the greater the degree of respiratory depression). Lower doses, such as those used for hypnosis, may decrease respirations to the level of normal sleep. Higher doses, however, will cause a decrease in the rate, depth, and volume of respiration and an overdose may cause a respiratory arrest.

Cardiovascular effects. Normal therapeutic doses of the barbiturates have little cardiovascular effect aside from a transient hypotension and a decrease in the heart rate. An overdose, however, may cause a profound hypotension leading to renal shutdown and cardiovascular collapse.

Hepatic effects. Barbiturates do not affect liver tissue pathologically. They are metabolized by the liver, however, and thus patients with liver disease may show an increased sensitivity to the usual barbiturate dose. For this reason, barbiturates are best avoided in patients with liver disease. Barbiturates may also alter the metabolic functions of the liver in that they may stimulate the hepatic microsomal enzyme system. Microsomal enzymes are associated with one of the primary drug metabolizing systems of the body and are discussed at some length in Chapter 5, "Drug Metabolism and Elimination." Barbiturates, as well as some other members of the sedative-hypnotic drug class, stimulate this metabolizing mechanism to the extent that other drugs also metabolized by the liver may be removed from the body at a much faster rate, thereby decreasing their effectiveness. Probably the best known example of this effect is the concurrent administration of barbiturates with oral anticoagulants such as warfarin. If not adjusted, the plasma levels of warfarin may be decreased to the point where the drug

is no longer effective. On the other hand, patients who are taking both barbiturates and warfarin and who stop taking the barbiturate may experience a tremendous increase in the level of anticoagulant activity once the microsomal enzyme response returns to normal.

OTHER MISCELLANEOUS SEDATIVE-HYPNOTICS

Chloral hydrate

Chloral hydrate is the oldest member of the sedative-hypnotic drug class, having been used clinically since 1869. It is most often used as a hypnotic agent, either as chloral hydrate or as the monosodium salt of the phosphate ester of trichloroethanol, triclofos sodium. Once ingested, both forms are quickly converted to the active metabolite, trichloroethanol, which is believed responsible for the pharmacologic actions of the drug.

Drug effects

Central nervous system effects. Like other members of the sedative-hypnotic drug class, chloral hydrate produces CNS depression resulting, at appropriate doses, in induction of sleep. Chloral hydrate also experimentally has some anticonvulsant activity. However, the dose required to produce anticonvulsant effects is too close to the hypnotic dose, rendering it impractical for use in treating convulsive disorders.

Effects on sleep. Unlike the barbiturates, chloral hydrate does not appreciably affect REM-stage sleep, at least in the usual doses of 0.5 to 1 gm. Higher doses have been reported to cause REM suppression on initiation of therapy. A return to normal sleep patterns is usually seen within 2 weeks. REM rebound does not occur after the discontinuation of the drug.

Tolerance. Continued chronic use of chloral hydrate may lead to a tolerance of the physiologic effects, necessitating an increase in dose or conversion to another agent. This may be because the amount of trichloroethanol formed from chloral hydrate decreases as the drug is continuously administered.

Respiratory and cardiovascular effects. Chloral hydrate does not produce a noticeable effect on respiration or the cardiovascular system in normal doses. An overdose, however, produces serious respiratory depression and hypotension. In addition, patients with a preexisting cardiac disease appear to be at risk for developing cardiac complications when given large doses of chloral hydrate.

Adverse effects. Chloral hydrate and, to a lesser extent, triclofos sodium are irritating to the gastric mucosa and may cause various GI side effects, including nausea, stomach pain, and occasional vomiting.

Trichloroethanol appears to displace various drugs from protein-binding sites, thereby subjecting them to increased metabolic degradation and variable clinical effects (e.g., potentiation or antagonism of the action of oral anticoagulants may be seen depending on the dose of each agent and the frequency of dosing).

Other drugs

A number of other nonbarbiturate, nonbenzodiazepine sedative-hypnotics have been developed in the last 20 years. For all practical purposes, these medications have been largely replaced in clinical therapy by the benzodiazepines, both for treating anxiety and for inducing sleep.

Drug effects

Central nervous system effects. Drugs in this subclass of sedative-hypnotics all cause CNS depression to varying degrees. Some, such as chlormezanone, are mildly sedating and therefore are not suitable for hypnosis. Others, such as methyprylon, are rapidly absorbed and metabolized and are therefore not useful for daytime sedation or for treating anxiety.

Effects on sleep. Virtually all drugs in this class cause a decrease in REM sleep, an increase in non-REM sleep, and a REM rebound following the discontinuation of the drug. The two exceptions may be meprobamate, which has been observed to produce an increase in REM sleep, and methaqualone, which increases REM sleep at low doses while suppressing REM sleep at higher doses.

Tolerance. All drugs in this group, with the exception of hydroxyzine, may produce a tolerance to their clinical effects with continued use; physical dependence is also possible. Sudden cessation of the therapy will produce symptoms of withdrawal similar to those seen with the barbiturates.

Adverse effects. As one might suspect, the primary adverse effects seen with this group of drugs are related to their CNS activity. Drug hangover, paradoxic excitement, confusion, mental clouding, or disorientation may occur, especially with continued chronic use. Respiratory depression and hypotensive effects similar to the barbiturates may be seen in overdose.

Whereas drugs of this group show similar pharmacologic actions, some unique differences exist, particularly related to adverse effects. Ethchlorvynol can produce a giddiness and facial numbness, as well as a mintlike aftertaste. Methaqualone may cause transient paresthesias and a peripheral neuropathy that may continue after the drug is discontinued. Metha-

qualone, incidentally, is subject to a high degree of abuse, purportedly because of the mistaken belief that it has aphrodisiac properties. A more likely reason, however, is that in high doses it produces a dissociative high without the sedative effects seen with the barbiturates. Methyprylon, glutethimide, and ethchlorvynol may all stimulate the hepatic microsomal enzymes and thus interfere with the action of other drugs metabolized by the liver.

Paraldehyde is also worthy of note, not because it is a superior sedative-hypnotic, but because its use may lead to severe problems. Paraldehyde is a liquid preparation that, in years past, was administered to patients with alcoholic liver disease who were experiencing delirium tremens. It was given in the mistaken belief that a major portion of the drug was excreted through the lungs and thus would spare the liver from metabolizing an additional pharmacologic agent. It is true that a small percentage of a paraldehyde dose is excreted via the lungs. Between 70% and 80% of the dose, however, is metabolized in the liver to acetaldehyde and then to carbon dioxide and water. A patient with alcoholic liver disease may not be able to handle this increased metabolic demand and may experience toxic effects of the drug that are similar to those seen with chronic alcoholism. Overdose or mismanagement of therapy may thus easily occur. In addition, paraldehyde, once opened and exposed to air, readily decomposes to acetic acid. Cases of acetic acid poisoning from deteriorated paraldehyde are a matter of record.

SUMMARY

A variety of sedative-hypnotic agents are available for the effective induction of sleep or reduction of anxiety. When choosing an individual agent, however, the following ideal qualities should be considered: (1) it should cause effective induction and maintenance of sleep (this effectiveness should not diminish quickly nor necessitate an increased dose); (2) it should have a quick onset of action; (3) it should have little or no interference with REM sleep or other sleep stages; (4) it should not cause a hangover effect (i.e., there should be no drug accumulation with continued use); (5) it should not cause interference with other current drug therapies; and (6) it should be inexpensive.

Whereas the barbiturates are effective CNS depressants, enough adverse effects are possible that their continued widespread use for inducing sleep must be questioned. Respiratory depression, interference with REM sleep, drug interactions, REM rebound phenomenon, decreased effectiveness with continued chronic use, and drug accumulation are all potentially serious enough to dissuade one from using this group of drugs as hypnotic agents. Chloral hydrate, although an older hypnotic agent, is still effective. It does not suppress REM sleep nor cause REM rebound when discontinued. At normal doses, it does not suppress respiration or cause alterations in blood pressure, although an overdose may affect both of these physiologic systems. The drug is metabolized outside of the microsomal enzyme system and therefore may be of some use, particularly for elderly patients.

Since the introduction of the benzodiazepines for the treatment of anxiety and the induction of sleep, other drug entities are approaching obsolescence. That the benzodiazepines are as effective as barbiturates, yet have many fewer side effects, speaks strongly in favor of their use when a sedative-hypnotic is indicated. Additionally, the benzodiazepines do not interfere with REM sleep at normal doses, do not interfere with hepatic metabolic mechanisms to the extent that barbiturates do, do not produce an appreciable tolerance (although physical dependence is possible), and have a very high therapeutic index. Cost remains the most serious objection to their use. However, with time and the institution of generic drug forms, this surely too will be resolved in their favor.

ADVERSE/SIDE EFFECTS OF THE SEDATIVE-HYPNOTICS*

ALLERGIC REACTIONS

Angioneurotic edema (barbiturates)
Asthma
Nonthrombocytopenic purpura
Skin rash (morbilliform, urticarial, and
  maculopapular)

BEHAVIOR

Depression
Disorientation, confusion
Insomnia (particularly following with-
  drawal)
Lethargy
Paradoxic anxiety attacks
Paradoxic excitatory effects (particu-
  larly in children and debilitated
  and elderly patients)

CARDIOVASCULAR SYSTEM

Palpitations
Syncope
Tachycardia or bradycardia
Various dysrhythmias

CENTRAL NERVOUS SYSTEM

Dizziness
Drowsiness
Fatigue and ataxia
Hallucinations, nightmares

HEMATOLOGIC SYSTEM

Agranulocytosis
Aplastic anemia
Megaloblastic anemia (particularly
  with phenobarbital)
Neutropenia
Thrombocytopenia
NOTE: most hematologic effects are
  seen only with continued, high-
  dose usage

GASTROINTESTINAL AND HEPATIC SYSTEMS

Constipation
Jaundice
Nausea (particularly with chloral hydrate and paraldehyde)
Stimulation of microsomal enzyme
  system (by barbiturates, ethchlorvynol, glutethimide, and methyprylon)

OCULAR SYSTEM

Blurred vision
Diplopia
Nystagmus

*See Chapter 11, "Drug Toxicity," for an overview of drug toxicity.

CLINICALLY SIGNIFICANT DRUG INTERACTIONS*

Primary drug	Interacting drug	Possible effect(s)	Probable mechanism(s)
Barbiturates	Alcohol	Increase CNS depression	Additive effects
Barbiturates	Anticoagulants (oral)	Decrease anticoagulant effect	Increased liver metabolism; decreased absorption of dicumarol
Barbiturates	Antidepressants (tricyclic)	Decrease antidepressant serum levels	Increased metabolism of antidepressant
Barbiturates	Beta-adrenergic blockers	Decrease serum level of beta-adrenergic blocker	Increased liver metabolism
Barbiturates	CNS depressants	Increase CNS depression	Additive effect
Barbiturates	Corticosteroids	Decrease clinical effect of corticosteroid	Increased liver metabolism
Barbiturates	Griseofulvin	Decrease serum levels of griseofulvin	Decreased absorption of griseofulvin
Barbiturates	Methoxyflurane	Possible nephrotoxicity	Increased liver metabolism may cause nephrotoxic metabolites
Barbiturates	MAO inhibitors	Increase barbiturate effect	Decreased metabolism of barbiturates
Barbiturates	Oral contraceptives	Decrease contraceptive effect	Increased liver metabolism
Barbiturates	Phenytoin	Decrease phenytoin serum levels	Increased liver metabolism
Barbiturates	Quinidine	Decrease quinidine serum levels	Increased liver metabolism
Barbiturates	Sulfonamides	Increase barbiturate effect	Displacement from protein-binding site
Barbiturates	Tetracyclines	Decrease tetracycline serum levels	Increased liver metabolism
Benzodiazepines	Alcohol	Increase CNS depression	Additive effect
Benzodiazepines	Cimetidine	Increase benzodiazepine effect	Decreased liver metabolism
Benzodiazepines	Levodopa	Decrease levodopa serum levels	Unknown
Chloral derivatives	Alcohol	Increase serum levels of both alcohol and chloral derivative	Decreased alcohol metabolism and increased active metabolites from chloral derivative
Chloral derivatives	Anticoagulants (oral)	Increase risk of bleeding	Displacement from protein-binding site
Ethchlorvynol	Anticoagulants (oral)	Decrease anticoagulant effect	Increased liver metabolism
Glutethimide	Alcohol	Increase CNS depression	Additive effects
Glutethimide	Anticoagulants (oral)	Decrease anticoagulant effect	Increased liver metabolism
Methyprylon	Anticoagulants (oral)	Decrease anticoagulant effect	Increased liver metabolism
Meprobamate	Alcohol	Increase CNS depression	Additive effect
Paraldehyde	Disulfiram	Acute disulfiram reaction	Paraldehyde is metabolized to acetaldehyde

*See Chapter 10, "Drug Interactions," for an overview of drug interactions.

GENERAL NURSING IMPLICATIONS

Nursing of patients requiring sedative-hypnotics

ASSESSMENT

Sleep habits and rest and sleep needs vary greatly among patients. Although insomnia can occur in any patient, it is a frequent complaint of patients hospitalized for the diagnosis or treatment of medical, surgical, or psychologic disorders. Primary insomnia characterized by difficulty falling asleep, numerous awakenings during the night, or early morning or secondary insomnia brought about by a change in sleeping environment, psychologic stress, pain, or physical discomfort are often treated by resolving the causative factors or with sedative-hypnotic medication if the causative factors are unknown or untreatable.

Patients with insomnia or other sleep disorders should be evaluated carefully. Assessment of the patient is especially important so treatment can be directed at the cause of the sleep disturbance and the use of the sedative-hypnotics avoided whenever possible. It is recommended that sedative-hypnotic medication be used only when other methods of promoting sleep have failed and then only for the shortest possible period of time. Assessment should include a general sleep history, psychologic assessment, and a careful drug history. Baseline data gathered during the initial assessment of the patient can assist the nurse in identifying potential sleep and rest problems, as well as assist in planning with the patient to minimize the disruption of established patterns. Because the sedative-hypnotics are often ordered on a prn basis, nursing assessment of the patient's need for medication and monitoring individual response are especially important.

The sleep history should include a description of the patient's usual sleep-wakefullness pattern, including the following: number of hours of sleep each day; usual times for retiring and arising; usual number of awakenings during nights, as well as reasons for awakenings; number, time, and length of daytime naps; usual sleep environment (e.g., type of bed, number of pillows used, sleeps alone or with someone or a significant object, number of blankets, amount of ventilation, and amount of light); sleeping aids used (e.g., bedtime rituals, ingestion of snacks or beverages, bath or shower, use of medication); daily exercise pattern; activities used to rest (e.g., reading, relaxation techniques); worries or concerns including health, work, or family; home responsibilities; dreams; and a description of daily activities, including sexual activity.

Patients should be asked to describe in their own words their pattern of sleep and wakefulness over 24 hours. Special attention should be given to the patient's affective response of the description of the quality of sleep.

The patient's own beliefs about sleep and rest requirements for optimal functioning should be identified so that assistance in meeting sleep requirements can be made.

When a patient has insomnia, the database for assessment should include a description of the patient's sleep latency or inability or difficulty falling asleep, frequency of nocturnal awakenings, early morning awakenings, and total sleep time. Assessment should include signs that indicate a lack of sleep over 1 to 2 days, including irritability, tension, complaints about difficulty resting or sleeping, and subjective feelings of fatigue or tiredness. The assessment of daytime alertness is important in the treatment of insomnia.

Because the sedative-hypnotics are contraindicated in certain medical conditions (e.g., peptic ulcer disease, myocardial infarction, a history of drug abuse), the presence of other medical conditions should be carefully identified. A drug history should also be completed because many medications can affect sleep (e.g., caffeine, amphetamines), and the withdrawal of medications that have been taken for a long time can affect usual sleep patterns. In addition, possible sensitivity, contraindications, cautions, potential drug interactions, and drug-taking patterns should be identified before initiating sedative-hypnotic therapy.

SENSITIVITY

Generally, allergic reactions to the sedative-hypnotics are rare; however, any drug has the potential to cause a hypersensitivity reaction in susceptible individuals.

Barbiturates may produce paradoxic excitement in children and elderly or debilitated patients and should generally be avoided in these patients.

Barbiturates are best avoided in patients with hepatic dysfunction because the drugs are metabolized by the liver and patients with liver disease may show an increased sensitivity to the usual barbiturate dose.

CONTRAINDICATIONS

The use of sedative-hypnotics is contraindicated in patients with the following conditions: a known hypersensitivity to a specific sedative-hypnotic; severe respiratory compromise; acute intermittent porphyria; history of drug or alcohol abuse or suicide attempt by overdose; pain, unless pain control has been accomplished, because discomfort will increase; pregnancy; and oral contraceptive use, because a reduced efficacy and increased incidence of breakthrough bleeding have been reported with the concomitant use of barbiturates and oral contraceptives.

CAUTIONS

These medications have not been safely established for use in pregnancy. Congenital defects have been associated with their use during the first trimester. Use during the third trimester has resulted in a physical dependence by the fetus and neonatal depression. These drugs are also excreted in small amounts in breast milk, which has been associated with lethargy and weight loss in breast-fed infants.

Mental or physical abilities may be impaired. Safety precautions should be implemented and patients warned of these effects. Bed-side rails, restraints, and other measures may be indicated. It is especially important to monitor smoking; one may need to remove the patients cigarettes.

Continued.

Nursing of patients requiring sedative-hypnotics—cont'd

CAUTIONS—cont'd

These drugs may be habit forming and tolerance is seen with barbiturates. Prolonged use can result in psychic dependence; withdrawal symptoms after the chronic use of large doses can cause delirium, convulsions, and death.

DRUG INTERACTIONS

Additive CNS depression effects, including a potential for respiratory depression can occur when sedative-hypnotics are coadministered with each other (e.g., a barbiturate and benzodiazepine) or with other CNS depressant drugs (e.g., narcotic analgesics, phenothiazines, antihistamines, alcohol). In addition, barbiturates, because of their effect on metabolism can effect the metabolism of drugs metabolized by the liver (e.g., warfarin). See Clinically Significant Drug Interactions for further information.

ADMINISTRATION

The sedative-hypnotics are available in various dosage forms for oral, intramuscular, intravenous, and rectal administration. Thus, administration should be individualized to the patient. The recommended dose varies with the individual drug, as well as the patient, and is usually reduced initially in elderly patients (see the Nursing Drug Digest for specific information regarding the administration of specific drugs).

Generally, smaller dosage ranges of the sedative-hypnotics administered 2 or 3 times a day are used for sedation. Hypnotic doses are larger and are administered ½ hour to 1 hour before bedtime for the treatment of insomnia. Medication for preoperative sedation is usually given 1 to 1½ hours before surgery, depending on patient factors and route of administration.

When the sedative-hypnotics are administered, the following activities should be completed to enhance the effect of the medication:

Before administering any sedative-hypnotic explore with the patient the possibility of sensitivity. This is usually obtained during the history, but with the excitement of admission or stress because of the patient's condition, this should be further addressed. Identify conditions that cause symptoms of anxiety or sleeplessness so that non-pharmacologic measures can be explored and used in treating the problem or condition. The administration of sedative-hypnotics must be seen as an adjunctive symptomatic treatment that is not curative, but a means to alleviate distress so the underlying problem can be worked on more effectively.

Use and encourage conservative measures, including listening, providing understanding, teaching relaxation techniques, and other therapeutic measures to create a relaxing atmosphere. Increase daytime activity and promote evening relaxation, as well as decrease caffeine intake during the day to promote sleep at night. A warm bath and warm milk are often helpful in promoting sleep.

Provide comfort measures with the medication, including a back rub and a quiet comfortable environment to enhance the patient's ability to fall asleep. These measures enhance the hypnotic effect of the medication. Bedrails should be raised as a safety precaution for those patients who exhibit deep sleep or have demonstrated sleepwalking. Restraints may also be indicated as an extra safety precaution in some patients, and cigarettes or other smoking materials may need to be removed from the bedside.

Plan with the patient so that usual patterns of daily living are maintained. Unnecessary disruption should be prevented in daily routines and alterations in the patient's usual routines should be minimized. Involve the patient in care planning and explain the need for scheduling diagnostic tests and procedures and explain the rationale for interruptions. This can do much to promote rest and sleep.

Do not awaken patients for unnecessary procedures and allow at least 90 minutes of uninterrupted rest or sleep whenever possible.

Because illness can increase the need for sleep and rest, plan early morning naps as opposed to afternoon naps, which can cause the patient to have difficulty falling asleep at night (afternoon naps are proportionately high in non-REM sleep, whereas morning naps are proportionately high in REM sleep). Substitute restful activities for afternoon naps.

Nursing measures should be used to assist the patient with worry, fear, anxiety, or tension if any of these conditions are the cause for insomnia. Referral to social services for financial assistance may be indicated. Patients should receive counseling, as indicated, to promote coping styles. Pain should be prevented and managed carefully, and physical comfort should be enhanced through positioning, adjustment in room temperature, ventilation, lighting, and other environmental conditions before the sleep period.

MONITORING PATIENT RESPONSE
Therapeutic response

The onset and duration of the sedative-hypnotic effect is largely dependent on the dosage form, route of administration, and on individual patient factors. *Ultrashort-acting* drugs given orally, intramuscularly, or intravenously have an action onset of a few minutes with a duration of 1 hour. *Short-acting* drugs have an onset of action of 10 to 15 minutes with a duration of 3 hours or less after oral or intramuscular administration. *Intermediate-acting* drugs have an onset of action of 10 to 30 minutes, lasting for 3 to 6 hours, and *long-acting* drugs have an onset of 30 to 60 minutes with a duration of action from 6 to more hours after oral or intramuscular administration.

Monitor *sedative* doses for calming, relaxing, or anxiolytic effects.

Monitor *hypnotic* doses for effect. Monitor for reduced sleep latency or time required to fall asleep, decreased number of nocturnal awakenings or early morning awakenings, and increased sleep efficiency or the ratio of time asleep to time in bed. The effect on daytime alertness, performance, mood, and the patient's perception of effectiveness of the medication should also be monitored and documented. It is important to document daytime alertness in patients with insomnia who may otherwise experience daytime drowsiness because of poor quality sleep. Because hypnotics are indicated

Nursing of patients requiring sedative-hypnotics—cont'd

Therapeutic response—cont'd

for the short-term treatment of insomnia, monitoring is especially important.

Adverse side effects

Adverse side effects vary among the sedative-hypnotics. Common adverse effects are outlined in Adverse/Side Effects of the Sedative-hypnotics. The most common effects should be carefully monitored for and nursing measures provided to minimize or prevent these effects.

Monitor for hypersensitivity and observe and report symptoms of blood dyscrasias such as a sore throat or a fever.

Monitor for increased CNS depression, especially with increased doses.

Monitor for signs and symptoms of intoxication (effect similar to alcohol intoxication): slurred speech, ataxia, silliness, dizziness, diplopia, and blurred vision.

Monitor for "next day effects," including hangover, headache, dizziness, dry mouth, and nervousness, especially with patients receiving benzodiazepines, including triazolam.

Monitor for daytime sedation, confusion, or other behavior changes, including paradoxic excitement, hostility, rage, confusion, depersonalization, and hyperactivity (especially with elderly patients).

Monitor for symptoms of REM rebound, particularly with patients with duodenal ulcer, coronary arteriosclerosis, bronchial asthma, hypothyroidism, or depression.

Monitor for tolerance, which can develop within several days. The patient may find that a dose of the drug that relieved symptoms a few days earlier no longer works well and may resort to an increased dose to produce the desired effect. Cross-tolerance can develop, so switching drugs is not often helpful.

Monitor for physical and psychologic dependence that can occur with hypnotic dosages over time.

For barbiturates, monitor for symptoms of withdrawal after physical dependence has developed, if the drug is abruptly discontinued, 24 hours to 2 weeks after the last dose depending on the drug half-life; including the following: insomnia, weakness, muscle tremors, anxiety, sweating, anorexia, fever, nausea, vomiting, headache, incoordination, restlessness. Continued withdrawal symptoms include the following: postural hypotension, tinnitus, delirium, psychosis, convulsions, status epilepticus, cardiovascular collapse, and loss of the temperature-regulating mechanism. Barbiturate withdrawal is considered a medical emergency, because if it is untreated it can result in death. Withdrawal is usually accomplished by substituting a long-acting barbiturate (e.g., phenobarbital) and gradually decreasing the dose over a 2- to 4-week period.

Monitor for toxicity, especially with elderly patients, who experience more toxic reactions because of a diminished hepatic capability to metabolize and eliminate drugs. Increased large doses can lead to coma and death.

PATIENT EDUCATION

The patient and the family, as indicated, should have a clear understanding of the medication regimen, as well as the exact name of the medication, its action, dosage, storage, administration, adverse side effects, and measures that can be used to prevent or minimize these effects. The patient should know how to monitor the therapeutic response and should be able to identify signs that indicate the prescriber or health care provider should be notified. Assisting patients with using the sedative-hypnotics is extremely important. Patient education should also include an overview of normal sleep, as well as self-care measures that can be used to promote sleep and rest.

The patient should recognize that sleep requirements change with age and can be altered by a disruption in usual routines brought about by travel, hospitalization, nervousness, depression, or stress related to work, family, or illness. The patient should recognize common myths about sleep and these should be clarified. Patients should understand the limits of the sedative-hypnotics and should be encouraged to use nonpharmacologic measures to establish and maintain appropriate sleep and wakefulness patterns.

In general, the patient should do the following: use presleep routines, including reading, a warm bath, or shower; establish a sleep and wakefulness pattern; recognize that afternoon naps may decrease the amount of stage 3 and 4 non-REM sleep during the following night; recognize that alcohol in small amounts can increase relaxation and promote sleep but in increased amounts can suppress REM sleep; realize that coffee (caffeinated) decreases sleep time especially during the later half of the night and should be avoided at least 4 to 5 hours before going to bed; and establish an exercise program to meet individual requirements, because a usual pattern of physical exercise several hours before bedtime can promote muscle relaxation and aid sleep. The patient should also recognize that excessive exercise before retiring, especially if the patient is unconditioned, can cause fatigue and make relaxation and sleep more difficult.

In addition to these measures, the patient and the family should be able to identify environmental conditions that may make sleep difficult. They may require assistance in assessing home environments and in making environmental changes to promote sleep.

The patient and the family should understand that the sedative-hypnotics may be effective on a short-term basis and that these drugs can disrupt sleep patterns. Routine use of these preparations can decrease their effectiveness and they should be used only when other measures have failed. Patients should be encouraged to use non-pharmacologic measures to promote the action of the sedative-hypnotics when indicated.

It is especially important for patients who are hospitalized to recognize that difficulty in sleeping may be a problem caused by a change in sleep environment or by stress or anxiety. It is often helpful to use established sleep routines as much as possible and to inform patients that adaptation usually occurs in 1 to 2 days.

GENERAL INSTRUCTIONS FOR DISCHARGE/OUTPATIENTS

This medication is a *sedative-hypnotic* and it is used to help you relax and to fall asleep, as well as to prevent you from awakening frequently during the night and in the early morning. If you have any questions about why you are receiving this medication, ask your nurse or health care provider.

Follow the instructions on the prescription exactly. If you have any questions about how this medication should be used, ask your nurse, pharmacist, or physician.

This medication may cause you to become dizzy, lightheaded, drowsy, or less alert than you would normally be. If taken at bedtime, it may cause you to be drowsy or less alert on arising.

Until you learn how this medication affects you, do not drive, operate dangerous machinery, or put yourself in situations where decreased mental alertness may be dangerous.

This medication will add to the effects of alcohol and other medicines that slow down the nervous system, such as tranquilizers, antihistamines, narcotics, or other prescription pain medicine. Check with your nurse, pharmacist, or physician before taking any of the above.

Along with the desired effects, a medicine may cause some unwanted effects. Although these side effects do not occur very often, when they do occur they may require medical attention. Check with your nurse, pharmacist, or physician if any of the following occur: confusion or depression, shortness of breath or trouble breathing, skin rash, sore throat or fever, unusual behavioral changes, unusually slow heartbeat, yellowing of eyes or skin, or unusual bleeding or bruising.

The following side effects occur more commonly and usually do not require medical attention. However, if any of the following become bothersome to the point where they interfere with daily activities, check with your nurse, pharmacist, or physician: clumsiness or unsteadiness, dizziness or lightheadedness, drowsiness, "hangover" effect, diarrhea, or headache.

This medication has been prescribed especially for you. Do not trade or give this medication to any relatives or friends.

Notify your nurse or physician if you start or stop taking any other medications while taking this medication.

Keep this and all medications out of the reach of children.

NURSING DRUG DIGEST

Medication (trade name*)	Indication	Usual dosage and administration	Dosage forms, preparation, and storage	Contraindications, cautions, and comments	Monitoring
Alprazolam Xanax	Anxiety	*Adults*: 0.5-4 mg PO daily in divided doses *Elderly*: 0.25 mg b.i.d. to t.i.d. Elderly or debilitated patients may be overly sensitive to usual adult doses	Tablets: 0.25, 0.5, 1 mg	*Contraindicated* in acute narrow-angle glaucoma: may be used in patients with open-angle glaucoma who are receiving appropriate treatment Continued use may lead to tolerance or physical dependence May be excreted in the milk of nursing mothers Use with caution in patients with impaired liver or renal function	Observe for oversedation Monitor for other common adverse effects: drowsiness, dizziness, lightheadedness, unsteadiness, ataxia, headache, or depression Monitor for symptoms of tolerance or physical dependence
Amobarbital Amytal	Sedation and anxiety Hypnosis Convulsive seizures	*Adults*: 15-100 mg PO b.i.d. to t.i.d. Should *not* be used in children under 6 years of age *Adults*: 65-200 mg PO q.h.s. *Adults*: 65-500 mg deep IM or 1 ml/min IV (10% solution) (maximal dose is 1 gm) *Children*: 6-12 years of age, 65-500 mg IV (not to exceed 1 ml/min of 10% solution) NOTE: IV injection rate faster than 1 ml/min may cause apnea or hypotension IM injection should be administered deeply into a large muscle; do *not* use more than 5 ml per IM injection site	Tablets: 15, 30, 50, 100 mg Elixir: 8.8 mg/ml (alcohol 34%) Injectable: 125, 250, 500 mg (dry powder) Capsules: 65 and 200 mg Do *not* use cloudy injection solution; use injection within 30 minutes after opening to minimize deterioration *Do not shake* the ampule; rotate it to dissolve contents Reconstitute dry powder with sterile water for injection	*Contraindicated* in patients with severely impaired liver function *Contraindicated* in patients with latent or active porphyria Should be avoided, if possible, in patients taking oral anticoagulants because of difficulty in stabilizing prothrombin times Use cautiously in patients with CNS or respiratory depression, or in patients with liver disease Continued use may lead to tolerance or physical dependence	Observe for oversedation Observe for respiratory depression or hypotension if given parenterally Observe for paradoxic excitement in children or in elderly or debilitated patients

Continued.

NOTE: For additional details regarding the individual agents listed in this table see the text and other tables in this chapter.

*Indicates a multiple active ingredient product. For a complete listing of all active ingredients see the *Drug Reference Guide to Brand Names and Active Ingredients*.

✦ Indicates that the drug is generally available only in Canada.

★ Indicates that the drug is generally available only in the United States.

NURSING DRUG DIGEST—cont'd

Medication (trade name)	Indication	Usual dosage and administration	Dosage forms, preparation, and storage	Contraindications, cautions, and comments	Monitoring
★ **Aprobarbital** Alurate	Sedation Hypnosis	*Adults:* 40 mg (1 tsp) PO t.i.d. *Adults:* 40-160 mg (1-4 tsp) PO q.h.s. *Children:* Should *not* be used in children Elderly or debilitated patients may be overly sensitive to usual adult doses	Elixir: 40 mg/5 ml (alcohol 20%)	*Contraindicated* in patients with severely impaired liver function *Contraindicated* in patients with latent or active porphyria Should be avoided, if possible, in patients taking oral anticoagulants because of difficulty in stabilizing prothrombin times Use cautiously in patients with CNS or respiratory depression or in patients with liver disease Continued use may lead to tolerance or physical dependence	Observe for oversedation Observe for paradoxic excitement in elderly or debilitated patients
★ **Barbital** Embinal Hynodol Medinal Plexonal* Veronal	Hypnosis	*Adults:* 300-600 mg PO q.h.s. *Children:* 75-300 mg PO q.h.s.	Tablet: 300 mg Elixir: 175 mg/5 ml	*Contraindicated* in patients with severely impaired renal function *Contraindicated* in patients with latent or active porphyria Drug is not metabolized in the liver and may be used in the presence of liver disease Rarely used because of newer agents Use cautiously in patients with CNS or respiratory depression Continued use may lead to tolerance or physical dependence	Observe for oversedation Observe for paradoxic excitement in children or in elderly or debilitated patients

Bromazepam
Lectopam

Anxiety

Adults: 6-30 mg/day PO in 2-3 divided doses
Maximum: 60 mg/day
Elderly: 3 mg PO daily in 2 divided doses

Tablets: 3, 6 mg

Contraindicated in acute narrow-angle glaucoma; may be used in patients with open-angle glaucoma who are receiving appropriate treatment
Continued use may lead to tolerance or physical dependence
May be excreted in the milk of nursing mothers
Use with caution in patients with impaired liver or renal function

Observe for oversedation
Other common adverse effects include: drowsiness, light-headedness, unsteadiness, and ataxia
Observe for signs of bromism (e.g., acne, headache, cold extremities, sleepiness, weakness, or decreased libido)

Bromisovalum
Bromural
Isoval

Anxiety
Hypnosis

Adults: 300 mg PO t.i.d. to q.i.d.
Adults: 600 mg PO q.h.s.
Children: Should *not* be used in children
NOTE: Use is *not* generally recommended

Tablet: 300 mg

Low therapeutic index
Overdose may lead to shock lung and intravascular coagulation

Observe for oversedation
Observe for signs of bromism (e.g., acne, headache, cold extremities, sleepiness, weakness, or decreased libido)

Butabarbital
Bubartal
Buta-Barb
Butabell
HMB*
Buticaps
Butigetic
Butiserpazide*
Butisol
Day-Barb
G-2*
G-3*
Intasedol
Mebutal
Minotal*
Nep-Barb
Neurosedine
Phrenilin*
Quibron Plus*

Sedation

Hypnosis

Adults: 15-30 mg PO t.i.d. to q.i.d.
Children: 7.5-30 mg/day PO in divided doses
Adults: 50-100 mg PO q.h.s.
Children: Not established
NOTE: Prolonged therapy (greater than 14 days) is usually not effective and is *not* recommended

Tablets: 15, 30, 50, 100 mg
Elixir: 30 mg/5 ml (alcohol 7%)
Capsules: 15, 30 mg

Contraindicated in patients with severely impaired liver function
Contraindicated in patients with latent or active porphyria
Should be avoided, if possible, in patients taking oral anticoagulants because of difficulty in stabilizing prothrombin times
Use cautiously in patients with CNS or respiratory depression or in patients with liver disease
Continued use may lead to tolerance or physical dependence
Tablets contain tartrazine, which may cause allergic reactions in some patients

Observe for oversedation
Observe for paradoxic excitement in children or in elderly or debilitated patients

Continued.

NURSING DRUG DIGEST—cont'd

Medication (trade name)	Indication	Usual dosage and administration	Dosage forms, preparation, and storage	Contraindications, cautions, and comments	Monitoring
★ **Butalbital** Apectel* Buff-A Comp* Esgic* Florinal with codeine* Fiorinal* Medigesic Plus* Panitol* Plexonal* Rapan* Sandoptal	Hypnosis	Adults: 100 mg PO 15-30 min before bedtime. Children: Not recommended for use in children. NOTE: Use is not generally recommended	Primarily available in a variety of dosages in multiingredient products	Continued use may lead to tolerance or physical dependence. Should be avoided, if possible, in patients taking oral anticoagulants. Use cautiously in patients with CNS or respiratory depression or in patients with liver disease	Observe for oversedation. Observe for paradoxic excitement in elderly or debilitated patients
★ **Carbromal** Adalin Bro-T's* Carbrital* Carbropent* Fydalin Nyctal	Hypnosis	Adults: 1-2 capsules PO q.h.s. Children: Should not be used in children. NOTE: Use is not generally recommended	Capsules: containing pentobarbital, 100 mg, carbromal, 240 mg (Carbropent and Carbrital); bromisovalum, 120 mg and carbromal, 200 mg (Bro-T's)	Contraindicated in patients with severely impaired liver function. Contraindicated in patients with latent or active porphyria. Carbropent and Carbrital should be avoided, if possible, in patients taking oral anticoagulants because of difficulty stabilizing prothrombin times. Use cautiously in patients with CNS or respiratory depression or in patients with liver disease	Observe for oversedation. Observe for paradoxic excitement in elderly or debilitated patients. Observe for signs of bromism (e.g., acne, headache, sleepiness, weakness, cold extremities, or decreased libido)
Chloral hydrate Aquachloral Choralex Choralvan Cohidrate Falsules Lorinal Lycoral Nigracap	Sedation Hypnosis	Adults: 250 mg PO t.i.d., maximum of 2 gm per single dose. Children: 25 mg/kg given in divided doses; maximum of 1 gm per single dose. Adults: 500 mg-1 gm PO q.h.s., maximum dose of 2 gm. Children: 50 mg/kg PO q.h.s.; maximum dose of 1 gm	Capsules: 250, 500 mg. Syrup: 500 mg/5 ml. Suppositories: 500 mg (refrigerate). Store in dark containers	Contraindicated in patients with severe cardiac disease. Contraindicated in patients with severely impaired renal function. Contraindicated in patients with acute pulmonary insufficiency	Observe for oversedation. Observe for GI irritation. Monitor urine output because chloral hydrate may decrease urinary output and uric acid excretion; ensure adequate hydration

Drug (generic and trade names)	Uses	Dosage	Preparations / Administration	Remarks	Nursing implications
Noctec, Novochlorhydrate, Oradrate, Rectules, Somni Sed, Somnos, SK-Chloral Hydrate		Administer with food or milk to decrease GI upset		Should be avoided, if possible, in patients taking oral anticoagulants because of difficulty in stabilizing prothrombin times / Continued use may lead to tolerance or physical dependence / Does not interfere with REM sleep at usual doses / May be excreted in the milk of nursing mothers	
Chlordiazepoxide A-Poxide, C-Tran, Clipoxide*, Corax, Librax*, Librelease, Libritabs, Librium, Lidinium*, Medilium, Nack, Novopoxide, Relaxil, Selium, SK-Lygen, Trilium, Via-Quil	Anxiety and tension / Withdrawal symptoms of acute alcoholism	Adults: 5-25 mg PO t.i.d. to q.i.d. / Children: 5-10 mg PO b.i.d. to q.i.d. / NOTE: Not recommended for use in children under 6 years of age / Elderly: 5 mg PO b.i.d. to q.i.d. / NOTE: Elderly patients may be overly sensitive to usual adult doses / Adults: 50-100 mg PO or IM repeated as needed every 2-4 hr up to 300 mg/day (initial therapy is usually begun with the injectable form) / Elderly: 25-50 mg given as above up to 150 mg/day	Capsules: 5, 10, 25 mg / Tablets: 5, 10, 25 mg / Injectable: 100 mg (refrigerate) / Reconstitute immediately before administration; add diluent supplied with ampule for IM use only / For IV use, dilute 100 mg with 5 ml sterile water for injection or normal saline / Do not use diluent solution if hazy	Contraindicated in acute narrow-angle glaucoma; may be used in patients with open-angle glaucoma who are receiving appropriate treatment / Continued use may lead to tolerance or physical dependence / May be excreted in milk of nursing mothers / Use with caution in patients with severe liver or renal impairment	Observe for oversedation
Chlormezanone Clorilax, Trancopal	Mild anxiety and tension	Adults: 100-200 mg PO t.i.d. to q.i.d. / Children: 5-12 years of age, 50-100 mg PO t.i.d. to q.i.d. / Not recommended for use in children under 5 years of age	Tablets: 100, 200 mg		Observe for oversedation
Clorazepate Azene, Tranxene, Tranxilene	Anxiety	Adults: 15-90 mg PO daily in divided doses / Children: Not recommended for use in patients under 18 years of age / Elderly: 7.5-15 mg PO in divided doses; may increase to 60 mg/day as needed	Tablets: 3.75, 7.5, 15 mg / Capsules: 3.75, 7.5, 15 mg / Sustained-action (SA) tablets: 11.25, 22.5 mg	Contraindicated in acute narrow-angle glaucoma; may be used in patients with open-angle glaucoma who are receiving appropriate therapy	Observe for oversedation

Continued.

NURSING DRUG DIGEST—cont'd

Medication (trade name)	Indication	Usual dosage and administration	Dosage forms, preparation, and storage	Contraindications, cautions, and comments	Monitoring
Clorazepate—cont'd	Adjunct in treatment of partial seizures	Elderly or debilitated patients may be overly sensitive to usual adult doses *Adults:* 7.5 mg PO t.i.d. may increase gradually by 7.5 mg every week to maximum of 90 mg/day *Children:* 9-12 years of age, 7.5 mg PO b.i.d.; increase as above to maximum of 60 mg/day		SA form may be given as single daily dose; should not be used to initiate therapy because of long duration of action May be teratogenic if administered during first trimester of pregnancy Continued use may lead to tolerance or physical dependence May be excreted in the milk of nursing mothers Use with caution in patients with impaired liver or renal function	
Diazepam Apaurin Atensine D-Tran E-Pam Lembrol Meval Neo-Calme Noan Novodipam Paxel Serenack Setonil Stress-Pam Tensium Tranimul Valium Valrelease Vatran Vivol	Anxiety	*Adults:* 2-10 mg PO b.i.d. to q.i.d.; or 2-5 mg IM or IV, repeat in 3-4 hr as necessary NOTE: 15 mg slow-release capsule (Valrelease) administered *once* daily is equivalent to 5 mg tablets administered PO t.i.d. NOTE: IV injection should be given slowly (5 mg/min) because of the risk of apnea and cardiac arrest *Children:* 1-2.5 mg PO t.i.d. to q.i.d. NOTE: Should *not* be used in children under 6 months of age *Elderly:* 2-2.5 mg PO q.d. to b.i.d. Elderly or debilitated patients may be overly sensitive to usual adult doses	Capsule: 15 mg Tablets: 2, 5, 10 mg Injectable: 5 mg/ml Store injectable protected from light Injectable contains propylene glycol (40%) and alcohol (10%) as a vehicle Do *not* mix injectable form with other drugs unless compatibility has been established	*Contraindicated* in acute narrow-angle glaucoma: may be used in patients with open-angle glaucoma who are receiving appropriate therapy Continued use may lead to tolerance or physical dependence May be excreted in the milk of nursing mothers Use with caution in patients with impaired liver or renal function IV use may cause thrombophlebitis Accidental *intraarterial* injection has caused vascular damage and gangrene resulting in amputation Popular street drug known as "V's"	Observe for oversedation Monitor for respiratory depression with IV use particularly with neonates and elderly patients

	Acute alcohol withdrawal	*Adults:* 10 mg PO t.i.d. to q.i.d. during first 24 hr; reduce to 5 mg t.i.d. to q.i.d. as needed; or 10 mg IV or IM, repeat 5-10 mg in 3-4 hr as needed		
	Muscle spasm	*Adults:* 2-10 mg PO t.i.d. to q.i.d.; or 5-10 mg IM or IV initially, then 5-10 mg IM or IV in 3-4 hr		
		Children: 30 days of age to 5 years of age; 1-2 mg IM or IV slowly; repeat every 3-4 hr as necessary		
		Over 5 years of age; 5-10 mg IM or IV slowly repeated every 3-4 hr as needed (respiratory assistance should be available)		
	Status epilepticus	*Adults:* 5-10 mg IV; repeat at 10-15 min intervals up to 30 mg total dose		
		Children: 30 days of age to 5 years of age; 0.2-0.5 mg IV slowly every 2-5 min up to maximum 5 mg		
		Over 5 years of age, 1 mg IV every 2-5 min up to total of 10 mg		
Ethchlorvynol Arvynol Placidyl Serensil	Hypnosis	*Adults:* 500-1000 mg PO q.h.s. *Children:* Should *not* be used in children	Capsules: 100, 200, 500, 750 mg	*Contraindicated* in patients with latent or active porphyria
		Elderly or debilitated patients may be overly sensitive to usual adult doses	750 mg capsules contain tartrazine, which may cause allergic reactions in some patients	Continued use may lead to tolerance or physical dependence
		Administer with food or milk to slow absorption and minimize ataxia and lightheadedness	Store in airtight, light-resistant containers	Abrupt withdrawal may cause severe withdrawal symptoms similar to barbiturate and alcohol withdrawal
				Patients who have demonstrated paradoxic excitement with barbiturates will show the same response with this drug
				Use with extreme caution in patients with mental depression or suicidal tendencies
				Observe for oversedation

Continued.

NURSING DRUG DIGEST—cont'd

Medication (trade name)	Indication	Usual dosage and administration	Dosage forms, preparation, and storage	Contraindications, cautions, and comments	Monitoring
★ **Ethinamate** Valmid Valmidate	Hypnosis	*Adults:* 500-1000 mg PO 20 min before bedtime *Children:* Should *not* be used in children under 15 years of age *Elderly:* 500 mg PO 20 min before bedtime NOTE: Prolonged therapy (i.e., more than 7 days) is usually *not* effective and is *not* recommended	Capsule: 500 mg	Continued use may lead to tolerance or physical dependence	Observe for oversedation
Flurazepam Dalmane Novoflupam	Hypnosis	*Adults:* 15-30 mg PO q.h.s. *Children:* Should *not* be used in children under 15 years of age *Elderly:* 15 mg PO q.h.s. NOTE: Elderly or debilitated patients may be overly sensitive to usual adult doses	Capsules: 15, 30 mg	*Contraindicated* in acute narrow-angle glaucoma; may be used in patients with open-angle glaucoma who are receiving appropriate therapy Continued use may lead to tolerance or physical dependence Does not interfere with REM sleep Hypnotic effect may be more pronounced after second or third dose May be excreted in the milk of nursing mothers Use with caution in patients with impaired liver or renal function	Observe for oversedation
Glutethimide Doriden Eldrodorm Rolathimide Somida	Hypnosis	*Adults:* 250-500 mg PO q.h.s. Maximum: 1 gm/day *Children:* Should *not* be used in children Elderly or debilitated patients may be overly sensitive to usual adult doses	Tablets: 250, 500 mg	*Contraindicated* in active porphyria Reduces intestinal motility Should be avoided, if possible, in patients taking oral anticoagulants because of difficulty in stabilizing prothrombin times	Observe for oversedation Observe for constipation

Generic/Trade Name	Uses	Preparations and Dosages	Contraindications and Precautions	Nursing Considerations
			Abrupt withdrawal may cause severe withdrawal symptoms similar to barbiturate and alcohol withdrawal; Excreted in the milk of nursing mothers; Continued use may lead to tolerance or physical dependence	Observe for drowsiness, which may occur in up to 50% of patients, especially in elderly patients; Observe for oversedation; Observe for paradoxic excitement in elderly or debilitated patients
★ **Halazepam** Paxipam	Anxiety	Tablets: 20, 40 mg *Adults:* 20-40 mg PO t.i.d. to q.i.d. *Children:* Should *not* be used in children under 18 years of age *Elderly:* 20 mg PO q.d. to b.i.d. Elderly or debilitated patients may be overly sensitive to usual adult doses NOTE: Long-term use (i.e., greater than 4 months) has not been established as effective and is *not* recommended	*Contraindicated* in acute narrow-angle glaucoma; may be used in patients with open-angle glaucoma who are receiving appropriate therapy; Continued use may lead to tolerance or physical dependence; May be excreted in the milk of nursing mothers; Use with caution in patients with impaired liver or renal function	
★ **Hexobarbital** Evipal Percobarb* Sombucaps Sombulex Somnalert	Hypnosis	Tablet: 250 mg *Adults:* 250-500 mg PO q.h.s. *Children:* Should *not* be used in children	*Contraindicated* in patients with severely impaired liver function; *Contraindicated* in patients with latent or active porphyria; Should be avoided, if possible, by patients taking oral anticoagulants because of difficulty stabilizing prothrombin times; Use cautiously in patients with CNS or respiratory depression or in patients with liver disease; Continued use may lead to tolerance or physical dependence	

Continued.

NURSING DRUG DIGEST—cont'd

Medication (trade name)	Indication	Usual dosage and administration	Dosage forms, preparation, and storage	Contraindications, cautions, and comments	Monitoring
Hydroxyzine Atarax Ataraxoid* Cartran* Enarax* Equipoise Hy-Pam Marax* Pas Depress Sedaril Vistaril Vistrax*	Anxiety	*Adults:* 50-100 mg PO q.i.d. *Children:* under 6 years of age, *50 mg daily PO* in divided doses; over 6 years of age, 50-100 mg PO daily in divided doses	Tablets: 10, 25, 50, 100 mg Capsules: 25, 50, 100 mg Injectable: 25 mg/ml, 50 mg/ml NOTE: Injectable should be used for IM injection *only* Syrup: 10 mg/5 ml (alcohol 0.5%) Suspension: 25 mg/5 ml	*Contraindicated* in early pregnancy May potentiate narcotics and barbiturates May cause dry mouth, which can be relieved by sucking on hard sugarless candy May be excreted in the milk of nursing mothers May cause pain and necrosis at IM injection site	Observe for oversedation
	Sedation (preoperative)	*Adults:* 50-100 mg IM *Children:* 0.6mg/kg IM			
Lorazepam Ativan Emotival Larpose Lorax Psicopax Tavor Temesta	Anxiety	*Adults:* 1-6 mg/day PO in divided doses NOTE: Most adults respond optimally to a total daily dose of 1-4 mg; increases in dosage should be in increments of 0.5 mg *Children: Not* recommended for use in children under 12 years of age *Elderly:* 0.5-1 mg/day PO in divided doses to initiate therapy; increase as necessary and as tolerated Elderly or debilitated patients may be overly sensitive to usual adult doses	Tablets: 0.5, 1, 2 mg Injectable: 2 mg/ml, 4 mg/ml (refrigerate)	*Contraindicated* in acute narrow-angle glaucoma; may be used in patients with open-angle glaucoma who are receiving appropriate therapy Often causes drowsiness Continued use may lead to tolerance or physical dependence Use with caution in patients with impaired renal function because the drug is excreted primarily via the kidneys May be excreted in the milk of nursing mothers Abrupt withdrawal may induce grand mal seizures Accidental *intraarterial* injection of benzodiazepines has caused vascular damage and gangrene resulting in amputation	Observe for oversedation Observe for withdrawal symptoms on discontinuation of drug, including grand mal seizures

Drug	Use	Dosage	Preparations	Contraindications/Precautions	Nursing Considerations
★ **Lormetazepam** Noctamid	Hypnosis	*Adults:* 0.5-2 mg PO q.h.s. *Children: Not recommended for use in children* Elderly or debilitated patients may be overly sensitive to usual adult doses	Tablet: 1 mg	*Contraindicated* in acute narrow-angle glaucoma; may be used in patients with open-angle glaucoma who are being treated appropriately Continued use may lead to tolerance or physical dependence May be excreted in the milk of nursing mothers Use with caution in patients with impaired renal function because the drug is excreted primarily by the kidneys	Observe for oversedation
Mephobarbital Mebaral Mebroin* Menta-Bal Mephoral Phemitone Prominal	Anxiety Epilepsy	*Adults:* 32-100 mg PO t.i.d. to q.i.d. *Children:* 16-32 mg PO t.i.d. to q.i.d. *Adults:* 400-600 mg/day PO *Children:* Under 5 years of age, 16-32 mg PO t.i.d. to q.i.d.; over 5 years of age, 32-64 mg PO t.i.d. to q.i.d. Elderly or debilitated patients may be overly sensitive to usual adult doses	Tablets: 32, 50, 100, 200 mg	*Contraindicated* in patients with severe liver disease *Contraindicated* in patients with latent or active porphyria Should be avoided, if possible, in patients taking oral anticoagulants because of difficulty in stabilizing prothrombin times Use cautiously in patients with CNS or respiratory depression or in patients with liver disease Continued use may lead to tolerance or physical dependence May be excreted in the milk of nursing mothers Mephobarbital is metabolized to phenobarbital	Observe for oversedation Observe for paradoxic excitement in elderly or debilitated patients

Continued.

NURSING DRUG DIGEST—cont'd

Medication (trade name)	Indication	Usual dosage and administration	Dosage forms, preparation, and storage	Contraindications, cautions, and comments	Monitoring
Meprobamate Aneural, Deprol*, Equagesic*, Equanil, Meditran, Mepavlon, Meprogesic*, Meprospan, Meprotabs, Micrainin*, Milpath*, Miltown, Miltrate*, Pathibamate*, Pensive, Probal, Quietal, Saronil, Tamate, Tranquiline, Trelmar, VioBamate	Anxiety	*Adults:* 1200-1600 mg PO daily in divided doses *Children:* 6-12 years of age, 100-200 mg PO b.i.d. to t.i.d. NOTE: *Not* recommended for use in children under 6 years of age	Tablets: 200, 400, 600 mg	*Contraindicated* in acute intermittent porphyria Continued use may lead to tolerance or physical dependence Concentration in milk of nursing mothers is 2-4 times that of the blood	Observe for oversedation
Methaqualone Hyptor, Mequelon, Mequin, Optinoxan, Parest, Quaalude, Quaalude-300, Rouqualone "300", Sedalone, Somnafac, Sopor, Triador, Tualone-300, Tuazole, Vitalone	Sedation Hypnosis	*Adults:* 75 mg PO q.i.d. *Adults:* 150-300 mg PO q.h.s. *Children: Not* recommended for use in children NOTE: Prolonged therapy (i.e., more than 14 days) is usually not effective and is *not* recommended Elderly or debilitated patients may be overly sensitive to usual adult doses	Tablets: 150, 300 mg	*Contraindicated* in pregnancy or history of porphyria Continued use may lead to tolerance or physical dependence Lower doses (150 mg) do not interfere with REM sleep; higher doses (300 mg) suppress REM sleep Removed from U.S. market in 1983 because of widespread illicit use and overdose	Observe for oversedation
Methyprylon Noludar	Hypnosis	*Adults:* 200-400 mg PO q.h.s. *Children:* Over 12 years of age, 50-200 mg PO q.h.s. NOTE: Should *not* be used in children under 12 years of age	Capsule: 300 mg Tablets: 50, 200 mg	Excreted in the milk of nursing mothers Continued use may lead to tolerance or physical dependence	Observe for oversedation

Drug	Use	Dosage	Dosage forms	Nursing considerations	Observe for
Nitrazepam Megadon Mogadon	Hypnosis	*Adults:* 2.5-10 mg PO q.h.s. *Children: Not* recommended for use in children *Elderly:* 2.5-5 mg PO q.h.s. Elderly or debilitated patients may be overly sensitive to usual adult doses	Tablets: 5, 10 mg	Use cautiously in patients with renal and hepatic dysfunction. Should be avoided, if possible, by patients taking oral anticoagulants because of difficulty in stabilizing prothrombin times. *Contraindicated* in acute narrow-angle glaucoma; may be used in patients with open-angle glaucoma who are receiving appropriate therapy. Continued use may lead to tolerance or physical dependence. Use with caution in patients with impaired liver or kidney function. May be excreted in the milk of nursing mothers. Excessive salivation has been noted in patients given high doses	Observe for oversedation
Oxazepam Adumbran Limbial Praxiten Serax Seranid-D Serapax Seresta	Anxiety	*Adults:* 10-30 mg PO t.i.d. to q.i.d. *Children:* Should *not* be used in children under 6 years of age *Elderly:* 10-15 mg t.i.d. to q.i.d. Elderly or debilitated patients may be overly sensitive to usual adult doses	Capsule: 10, 30 mg Tablet: 15 mg	*Contraindicated* in patients with acute narrow-angle glaucoma; may be used in patients with open-angle glaucoma who are receiving appropriate therapy. Continued use may lead to tolerance or physical dependence. May be excreted in the milk of nursing mothers. Tablets contain tartrazine, which may cause allergic reaction in some patients	Observe for oversedation

Continued.

NURSING DRUG DIGEST—cont'd

Medication (trade name)	Indication	Usual dosage and administration	Dosage forms, preparation, and storage	Contraindications, cautions, and comments	Monitoring
Oxazepam—cont'd				Use with caution in patients with impaired renal function because the drug is excreted primarily via the kidney	
Paraldehyde Paral	Anxiety

Hypnosis | *Adults:* 5-10 ml PO q.i.d. *Children:* 0.15 ml/kg, or 6 ml/m², PO q.4-6 hr. *Adults:* 10-30 ml PO q.h.s. *Children:* 0.3 ml/kg, or 12 ml/m², PO q.h.s. Administer in capsule form or well diluted in milk or fruit juice. NOTE: IV injection is extremely hazardous and should *not* be used. IM injection is also dangerous: special care must be taken to avoid nerve trunks. Do not administer more than 5 ml per IM injection site. NOTE: Use is *not* generally recommended | Capsule: 1 gm. Liquid injection. Caustic liquid; avoid contact with skin. Use *only a glass* syringe because plastic syringes will melt when exposed to the drug. Store in airtight, light-resistant containers. Discard solutions that are discolored, have a vinegar odor, or contain a precipitate. Do *not* leave open bottles in stock because the drug degrades to acetic acid on contact with air. Ventilate patient's room to remove exhaled drug | *Contraindicated* in patients with hepatic insufficiency. *Contraindicated* in patients with acute or chronic respiratory disease. Continued use may lead to tolerance or physical dependence. Avoid use during pregnancy and delivery. IM injection is extremely painful | Observe for oversedation. Observe for GI irritation if given orally. Observe for respiratory depression. Monitor injection site for pain and abscesses |
| **Pentobarbital** Butylone Carbrital* Dorsital Hypnotal Ibatal Nebralin Nembutal Nembutal Sodium Nova-Rectal Pentanca Pentogan WANS* | Sedation

Hypnosis | *Adults:* 30 mg PO t.i.d. to q.i.d. *Children:* 2-4 mg/kg/day PO in divided doses. Maximum: 100 mg. *Adults:* 100 mg PO q.h.s. *Children:* 8-50 mg PO q.h.s. NOTE: Administer IM injection deeply to minimize tissue necrosis. Do *not* administer more than 5 ml per IM injection site. IV route is *not* recommended because of the danger of respiratory arrest. Elderly or debilitated patients may be overly sensitive to usual adult dose | Capsules: 30, 50, 100 mg. Elixir: 20 mg/5 ml (alcohol 18%). Suppositories: 30, 60, 120, 200 mg. Injectable: 100 mg, 1 gm, 2.5 gm. Discard cloudy solutions | *Contraindicated* in patients with severely impaired liver function. *Contraindicated* in patients with active or latent porphyria. Should be avoided, if possible, in patients taking oral anticoagulants because of the difficulty in stabilizing prothrombin times. Use cautiously in patients with CNS or respiratory depression or in patients with liver disease | Observe for oversedation. Observe for respiratory depression. Observe for paradoxic excitement in children or in elderly or debilitated patients |

Continued use may lead to tolerance or physical dependence

Suppresses REM sleep

30 to 100 mg capsules contain tartrazine, which may cause allergic reactions in some patients

Injectable form is very alkaline (pH 9.5)

May predispose patient to laryngospasm if given by IV route

Have facilities for artificial respiration if administered via IV route

May be excreted in the milk of nursing mothers

Popular street drug, known as "yellows" or "yellow jackets"

Drug	Use	Dosage	Preparations	Nursing considerations	Observations
Phenobarbital Amodrine* Antrocol* Atrobarb* Bronkolixir* Cardilate-P* Donnatal* Eskabarb Henotal Hypnolone Liquital Luminal Matropinal* Mudrane* Talpheno	Anxiety Hypnosis	*Adults:* 30-120 mg PO daily in divided doses *Children:* 6 mg/kg, or 180 mg/m², PO daily in divided doses *Adults:* 100-200 mg q.h.s. *Children:* 3-6 mg/kg PO q.h.s. NOTE: Administer IM injection deeply to minimize tissue necrosis IV route *not* recommended because of the danger of severe respiratory depression; if IV route *is* used, do *not* exceed rate of 50 mg/min and have resuscitation equipment at hand	Tablets: 8, 15, 30, 60, 100 mg Capsule: 15 mg Elixir: 20 mg/5 ml Injectable: 120 mg Suppositories: 8, 15, 30, 60, 100, 120 mg Solution for injectable should *not* be used if precipitate is present Reconstitute injectable form with 2 ml sterile water for injection	*Contraindicated* in patients with active or latent porphyria *Contraindicated* in patients with severely impaired liver function Should be avoided, if possible, in patients taking oral anticoagulants because of difficulty stabilizing prothrombin times Use cautiously in patients with CNS or respiratory depression or in patients with liver disease Continued use may lead to tolerance or physical dependence Suppresses REM sleep	Observe for oversedation Observe for paradoxic excitement in children or in elderly or debilitated patients

Continued.

NURSING DRUG DIGEST—cont'd

Medication (trade name)	Indication	Usual dosage and administration	Dosage forms, preparation, and storage	Contraindications, cautions, and comments	Monitoring
★ **Prazepam** Centrax	Anxiety	*Adults:* 20-60 mg PO daily in divided doses *Children:* Should *not* be used in children under 18 years of age *Elderly:* 10-20 mg PO daily in divided doses Elderly or debilitated patients may be overly sensitive to usual adult doses	Capsules: 5, 10, 20 mg	*Contraindicated* in acute narrow-angle glaucoma; may be used in patients with open-angle glaucoma who are receiving appropriate therapy Continued use may lead to tolerance or physical dependence May be excreted in the milk of nursing mothers Use with caution in patients with impaired liver or renal function	Observe for oversedation
Secobarbital Barbosec Bi-Secogen* Duo-Barb*, Hyptran*, Hyptrol Novamo-Secobarb* Secogen Seconal Secotabs Sedonal Natrium Seotal Sodium Seral Tuinal Pulvules* Tuinal* Tuisec Tuo-Barb*	Hypnosis	*Adults:* 100 mg PO q.h.s.; or 120-200 mg PR q.h.s. *Children:* Up to 6 months of age, 15-60 mg PR; 6 months-3 years, 60 mg PR; 3 years and older, 60-100 mg PO or PR NOTE: If given IM, injection should be made deeply to minimize tissue necrosis IV administration is *not* recommended because of the danger of respiratory depression; if the drug *is* given IV do not exceed rate of 50 mg/min If given IV, have facilities available for artificial respiration Prolonged therapy (i.e., more than 14 days) has not been shown to be effective and is *not* recommended	Capsules: 50, 100 mg Suppositories: 30, 60, 100, 120 mg (refrigerate) Sterile secobarbital sodium is compatible with sterile water for injection To reconstitute, rotate ampule; do *not* shake Store aqueous polyethylene glycol solution below 10° C	*Contraindicated* in patients with active or latent porphyria *Contraindicated* in patients with severely impaired liver function Should be avoided, if possible, in patients taking oral anticoagulants because of difficulty in stabilizing prothrombin times Use cautiously in patients with CNS or respiratory depression or in patients with liver disease Continued use may lead to tolerance or physical dependence Suppresses REM sleep May be excreted in the milk of nursing mothers Popular street drug, known as "reds" or "red devils"	Observe for oversedation Observe for paradoxic excitement in children or in elderly or debilitated patients Observe for respiratory depression

Drug	Use	Dosage	Supplied	Cautions	Nursing considerations
★ **Talbutal** Lotusate	Hypnosis	*Adults:* 120 mg PO 15-30 min before bedtime *Children: Not recommended for use in children*	Tablet: 120 mg	*Contraindicated* in patients with severely impaired liver function *Contraindicated* in patients with active or latent porphyria Should be avoided, if possible, in patients taking oral anticoagulants because of difficulty in stabilizing prothrombin times Continued use may lead to tolerance or physical dependence Use cautiously in patients with CNS or respiratory depression or in patients with liver disease Suppresses REM sleep	Observe for oversedation Observe for paradoxic excitement in elderly or debilitated patients
Temazepam Euhynos Forte Restoril	Hypnosis	*Adults:* 15-30 mg PO q.h.s. *Children: Not recommended for use in children* *Elderly:* 15 mg PO q.h.s. Elderly or debilitated patients may be overly sensitive to usual adult doses	Capsules: 15, 30 mg	*Contraindicated* in acute narrow-angle glaucoma; may be used in patients with open-angle glaucoma who are receiving appropriate therapy Continued use may lead to tolerance or physical dependence May be excreted in the milk of nursing mothers Use with caution in patients with impaired renal function because the drug is primarily excreted via the kidneys	Observe for oversedation, particularly in elderly or debilitated patients
Triazolam Halcion	Hypnosis	*Adults:* 0.25-1 mg PO q.h.s. *Children: Not recommended for use in children* *Elderly:* 0.125 mg PO q.h.s. Elderly or debilitated patients may be overly sensitive to usual adult doses	Tablets: 0.25, 0.5, 1 mg	*Contraindicated* in acute narrow-angle glaucoma; may be used in patients with open-angle glaucoma who are receiving appropriate therapy	Observe for oversedation

Continued.

NURSING DRUG DIGEST—cont'd

Medication (trade name)	Indication	Usual dosage and administration	Dosage forms, preparation, and storage	Contraindications, cautions, and comments	Monitoring
		Doses greater than 0.5 mg may produce nonspecific personality changes such as depersonalization, severe anxiety, suicidal ideation, or paranoia		Continued use may lead to tolerance or physical dependence May be excreted in milk of nursing mothers Use with caution in patients with impaired liver or kidney function Does not suppress REM sleep Altered sense of taste or smell has been seen with doses greater than 0.5 mg	
★ **Triclofos** Triclos	Hypnosis	*Adults:* 1500 mg PO q.h.s. *Children:* under 12 yrs of age, 22 mg/kg PO q.h.s. NOTE: Prolonged therapy (i.e., more than 14 days) in persons more than 65 years of age is usually *not* effective and is *not* recommended *Continued* use in children is *not* recommended Administer with food or milk to decrease GI upset	Tablet: 750 mg Liquid: 1.5 gm/15 ml	*Contraindicated* in patients with severe liver or kidney impairment *Contraindicated* in labor or pregnancy because of possible induction of kernicterus in infant Should be avoided, if possible, in patients taking oral anticoagulants because of difficulty in stabilizing prothrombin times Does not suppress REM sleep Continued use may lead to tolerance or physical dependence Abrupt withdrawal may cause precipitation of withdrawal symptoms similar to barbiturate or alcohol withdrawal Instruct patient to swallow tablet whole with a full glass of water (i.e, do not *chew* tablet)	Observe for oversedation

BIBLIOGRAPHY

Costa, E., Guidotte, A., & Mao, C.C. Evidence for involvement of GABA in the actions of benzodiazepines: studies on rat cerebellum. In E. Costa & P. Greengard (Eds.). *Mechanisms of action of benzodiazepines*. New York: Raven Press, 1975.

Cutler, R.W.P. Disorders of sleep (neurology). In *Scientific American medicine* (vol. 2, c. 11). New York: Scientific American, Inc., 1981.

Drugs for psychiatric disorders. *The Medical Letter*, 1983, *25*(635), 45-52.

Greenblatt, D.J., Allen, M.D., & Shader, R.I. Toxicity of high-dose flurazepam in the elderly. *Clinical Pharmacology and Therapeutics*, 1977, *21*, 355-361.

Gustafson, A., Svensson, S.E., & Ugander, L. Cardiac arrhythmias in chloral hydrate poisoning. *Acta Medica Scandanavica*, 1977, *201*, 227-230.

Harris, B. Sedative-hypnotic drugs. *American Journal of Nursing*. 1981, *81*(7), 1329-1334.

Hobson, J.A., Spagna, T., & Malenka, R. Ethology of sleep studied with time-lapse photography: postural immobility and sleep-cycle phase in humans. *Science*, 1978, *201*, 1251-1253.

Hypnotic drugs and treatment of insomnia. *Journal of the American Medical Association*, 1981, *245*, 749.

Kales, A., Scharf, M.B., Kales, J.D., & Soldatos, C.R. Rebound insomnia, a potential hazard following withdrawal of certain benzodiazepines. *Journal of the American Medical Association*, 1979, *241*, 1692-1695.

Killam, E.K., & Suria, A. Antiepileptic drugs: benzodiazepines. In G. H. Glaser, J.K. Penry, & D.M. Woodbury (Eds.). *Antiepileptic drugs: mechanisms of action*. New York: Raven Press, 1980.

Kroboth, P.D., & Juhl, R.P. Triazolam. *Drug Intelligence and Clinical Pharmacy*, 1983, *17*, 495-500.

Nicholson, A.N. The use of short- and long-acting hypnotics in clinical medicine. *British Journal of Clinical Pharmacology*, 1981, *11*, 615-695.

Simon, C. Benzodiazepine hypnotics for insomnia. *American Journal of Nursing*, 1983, *83*(9), 1330-1332.

Young, R.R., & Delwaide, P.J. Drug therapy—spasticity. *New England Journal of Medicine*, 1981, *304*(2), 96-99.

Muscle Relaxants

John F. Kittel

Medications discussed in this chapter

Centrally acting skeletal muscle relaxants
  Baclofen
  Carisoprodol
  Chlorphenesin
  Chlorzoxazone
  Cyclobenzaprine
  Diazepam
  Mephenesin

Centrally acting skeletal muscle relaxants—cont'd
  Metaxalone
  Methocarbamol
  Orphenadrine
Peripherally acting skeletal muscle relaxant
  Dantrolene

The relaxation of skeletal muscle may be achieved by using three pharmacologic categories of drugs: (1) centrally acting muscle relaxants, (2) neuromuscular blocking agents, and (3) peripherally acting muscle relaxants. Each pharmacologic category has generally been used in specific situations (i.e., centrally acting agents, with the exception of baclofen, are most often used to treat acute muscle spasm, neuromuscular blocking agents are most often used in conjunction with anesthesia or surgical procedures, and peripherally acting drugs are usually reserved for treating muscle spasticity caused by neurologic disease).

The discussion of muscle relaxants in this chapter centers primarily on their use to treat two types of muscle reactions: (1) acute muscle spasm resulting from trauma, and (2) muscle spasticity resulting from neurologic disease (for a discussion of the use of muscle relaxants in anesthesia, see Chapter 26, "Ganglionic and Neuromuscular Stimulants and Blockers").

Consideration of the action of muscle relaxants must be prefaced by a definition of pathologic states in which they are used. Acute muscle trauma is, as the name implies, acute injury to skeletal muscle tissue. The cause of the trauma can be varied and may be external, such as a crushing injury or a broken bone, or it may be internal, such as an overextension or a muscle tear. Spasticity is defined as increased tone in a skeletal muscle characterized by exaggerated tendon jerks; it is caused by a pathologic change in nerve tissue rather than the muscle body.

Acute muscle spasms are usually the result of peripheral, localized pathologic conditions, whereas spasticity is usually the result of general, centralized pathologic conditions.

PHYSIOLOGY OF ACUTE MUSCLE SPASMS AND SPASTICITY

Several basic anatomic structures are involved in skeletal muscle function (Figure 16-1). Muscle spindles are structures within the body of the skeletal muscle that are stimulated as the agonist muscle body stretches or contracts. Impulses originating in the muscle spindle travel to the spinal cord via a proprioceptor nerve. The impulse is then transmitted through a synapse to a motor neuron and travels back to the same muscle from whence it came. In addition to this basic reflex arc, at least two modifying influences affect the final muscle response: (1) collateral nerves from the proprioceptor nerve synapse with an interneuron, or internuncial nerve, and then synapse again with the motor neuron; and (2) impulses arising from the muscle spindle of the antagonist muscle body travel to other interneurons that also synapse with the motor neuron.

In summary, activity in a skeletal muscle, such as the biceps, generates an excitatory impulse that travels from the muscle spindle of the agonist muscle (biceps) through a proprioceptor nerve to the spinal cord and back to the same muscle via a motor neuron. This returning excitatory impulse will be modified by at least two inhibitory impulses, one from interneurons stimulated by smaller nerve branches arising from the proprioceptor nerve, and one from interneurons stimulated by nerves from the muscle that normally antagonizes the original muscle (e.g., in the case of the

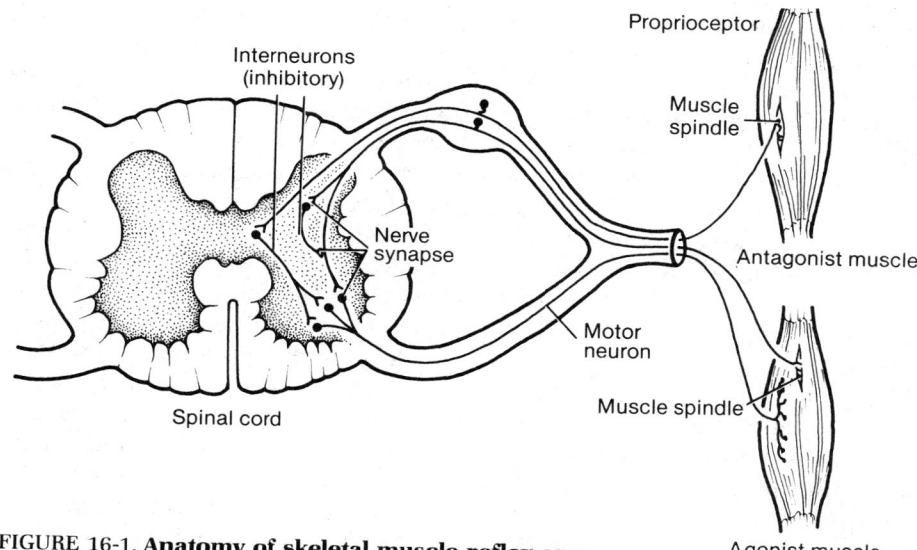

FIGURE 16-1. **Anatomy of skeletal muscle reflex arcs.**

biceps, the antagonist muscle would be the triceps). The summation of these impulses will determine the final response of the muscle.

Acute muscle spasm arises when sensory impulses (such as pain resulting from trauma) are transmitted from the muscle to the spinal cord and back to the muscle, causing a reflex contraction. This reflex contraction stimulates the muscle even more, which in turn causes a stronger spinal cord stimulation, and so on. The net response is a muscle cramp that is caused by a progressively increasing positive spinal cord reflex mechanism as a result of a sensory impulse.

Muscle spasticity, on the other hand, originates in the central nervous system (CNS) and is caused by a lesion that causes an interruption of normal excitatory or inhibitory responses. The result is an abnormal nerve impulse transmission causing sustained contractions, relaxation, or a combination of both. The lesion may occur: (1) in the brain, as in the case of a stroke, head injury, or cerebral palsy; (2) in the spinal cord, as with paraplegia; or (3) in a combination of both the brain and the spinal cord, as with multiple sclerosis or amyotrophic lateral sclerosis (Lou Gehrig's disease).

Drug therapy for either acute muscle spasm or spasticity must be based on a knowledge of the site of action of the various drugs available, as well as of the type of pathologic condition the patient has.

DRUG THERAPY

Using drugs to cause muscle relaxation dates back to a description of the muscle relaxing properties of mephenesin by Berger and Bradley (1946). Following this initial report, investigators reported a number of other compounds (e.g., meprobamate, methocarbamol, and chlorzoxazone) with significant muscle relaxing activity. More sophisticated studies, however, revealed that these compounds, although therapeutically useful, were all dependent on a similar *central* mechanism of action and thus were plagued with a variety of CNS side effects (e.g., drowsiness, dry mouth, ataxia, nervousness). With the introduction of dantrolene in 1974, a new class of muscle relaxants was made available that acted *peripherally* at the muscle fiber. This empirical classification of the muscle relaxants by site of action is a useful tool for further describing the pharmacologic characteristics of these agents.

CENTRALLY ACTING MUSCLE RELAXANTS

Centrally acting muscle relaxants can be represented by three prototype drugs: mephenesin, diazepam, and baclofen. As previously mentioned, mephenesin was the first of the muscle relaxants to be described clinically. Other drugs related to mephenesin include carisoprodol, chlorphenesin, chlorzoxazone, metaxalone, methocarbamol, and orphenadrine. Some of the benzodiazepines, notably diazepam, also have muscle relaxant activity. Finally, baclofen has been found useful in specific cases of spasticity, primarily those caused by spinal cord lesions. It should also be noted that cyclobenzaprine, although structurally related to the tricyclic antidepressant drugs, apparently causes physiologic muscle relaxation qualitatively similar to mephenesin.

Using the centrally acting muscle relaxants to treat acute muscle spasm has long been a subject of controversy. The primary argument has centered on the lack of controlled studies that show these agents to be safe and effective when used to treat acute muscle injury. Because the majority of these injuries are self-limiting and resolve spontaneously within 3 to 4 days, it is very difficult objectively to measure the effectiveness of a given drug. Therefore, most compounds have been studied using various animal models that may or may not accurately reflect responses in humans.

Mechanism of action

Diazepam and cyclobenzaprine appear to act by blocking the transmission of nerve impulses in the internuncial neurons of the spinal cord (Figure 16-2) at a single synapse and are therefore called monosynaptic inhibitors. Baclofen and mephenesin, on the other hand, act at multiple or polysynaptic sites. Of these two, however, the action of baclofen is confined primarily to the spinal cord whereas mephenesin may have higher CNS depressant activity. None of the centrally acting muscle relaxants affect skeletal muscle directly or the nerve-muscle junction, nor do they affect smooth muscle contraction.

Drug effects

Central nervous system effects. Because drugs in this class act centrally, they exhibit many CNS-related effects, including lethargy, ataxia, confusion, weakness, drowsiness, and dizziness. Given that mephenesin and diazepam are less selective in their action, they appear to be more likely to cause CNS side effects than baclofen. This is not to say that baclofen is the preferred drug in all cases of skeletal muscle spasticity. Both spasticity and muscle spasms involve such a complex array of neurologic impulses that therapy often requires some degree of trial and error to find the best drug for a given patient.

Other medications with CNS activity such as alcohol, narcotics, or tranquilizers tend to act additively with centrally acting muscle relaxants. Patients taking one or more CNS-active medications should therefore be cautioned against driving or performing work where decreased mental alertness may cause harm.

Respiratory effects. With the possible exception of diazepam, which may cause depressed respiration in high doses, and baclofen, which may cause nasal stuffiness in normal doses and respiratory depression in acute overdose, the centrally acting muscle relaxants cause no significant respiratory effects.

Cardiovascular effects. Cardiovascular effects are usually not a problem with ordinary doses of this group of drugs. Hypotension (and apnea) has been reported following the IV injection of diazepam, although it is not clear whether this is caused by the active drug or by the solvent, propylene glycol. Also, in view of the cardiotoxic action of the tricyclic antidepressants, cyclobenzaprine should probably be avoided in patients with a known history of cardiac abnormalities.

Adverse effects

As previously mentioned, the primary adverse effects seen with using centrally acting muscle relaxants are a result of an extension of their CNS activity. Elderly or debilitated patients may exhibit increased sensitivity to usual adult doses and should therefore be start-

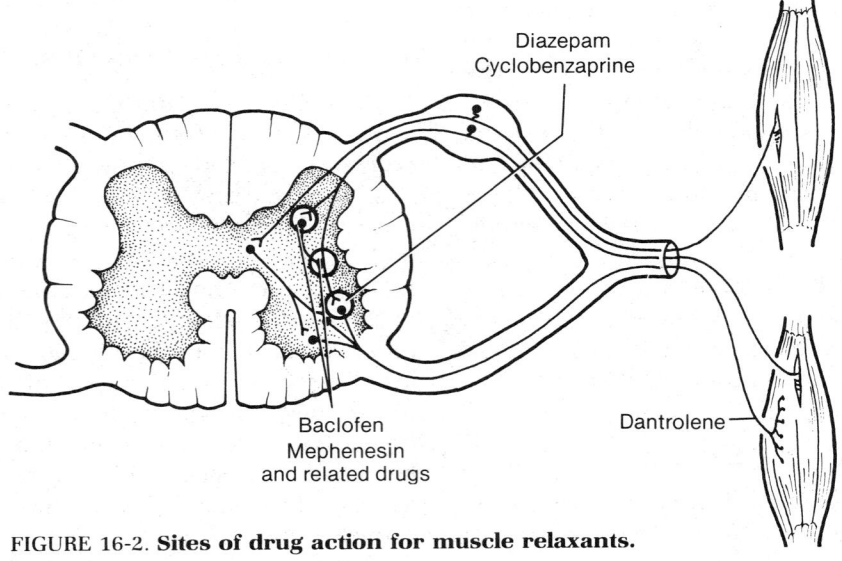

Diazepam
Cyclobenzaprine

Baclofen
Mephenesin
and related drugs

Dantrolene

FIGURE 16-2. **Sites of drug action for muscle relaxants.**

ed with lower doses and observed more closely during the initial phases of therapy.

Patients in whom baclofen therapy is abruptly stopped have been noted to have an increase in the number and severity of muscle spasms; some patients have also had hallucinations. For these reasons, baclofen therapy should be slowly tapered off if discontinued for any reason.

PERIPHERALLY ACTING MUSCLE RELAXANTS

The sole peripherally acting muscle relaxant drug is dantrolene. It is unique in that it acts directly on skeletal muscle without any effect on reflex pathways.

Mechanism of action

Dantrolene weakens the force of contraction of skeletal muscle by interfering with the normal calcium exchange necessary to cause muscle excitation. It does not interfere with nerve impulse transmission like the centrally acting muscle relaxants, and the electromyelogram (EMG) in patients receiving dantrolene will remain unchanged from readings taken before initiating therapy.

Drug effects

Dantrolene usually has little effect on the CNS, although drowsiness and dizziness have been observed. Lethargy, nausea, malaise, diarrhea, and headache have also been reported. Clinical effects on other organ systems are not normally apparent at usual doses.

Dantrolene will not restore normal muscle function in patients who are experiencing muscle spasticity. It can, in fact, cause patients who use their spasticity as an internal bracing mechanism to lose the ability to walk. It should be pointed out, therefore, that not all patients with spasticity need to be treated. Patients in whom therapy should be considered are those in whom spasticity interferes with normal daily activities of living or nursing care.

Parenthetically, dantrolene injection is indicated for treating malignant hyperthermia and may be lifesaving in this medical emergency. Malignant hyperthermia may occur in any age group and is characteristically generated by exposure to certain anesthetic agents such as halothane or succinylcholine. Following exposure to the anesthetic agent, a rapid rise in body temperature may be seen along with tachycardia. Untreated, the patient will exhibit continually deteriorating cardiac function until ventricular fibrillation and death occur. Although all cases of malignant hyperthermia are not uniformly fatal (the mortality rate is

estimated at 60%), the dramatic nature of the symptoms plus the likelihood of some CNS damage from sustained abnormally high body temperature makes rapid treatment a necessity. Dantrolene injection given intravenously will reduce the body temperature to normal levels and stabilize the cardiac rate. On recovery, the patient may complain of muscle pain and tenderness, and some swelling of skeletal muscle may be present, presumably because of sustained contraction.

Adverse effects

The most serious adverse effect seen with dantrolene is drug-induced hepatitis. This idiosyncratic reaction is seen in approximately 0.5% to 1% of the patients receiving dantrolene. An increased risk of hepatitis may be seen in patients in any of the following groups: (1) patients receiving short-term, high-dose therapy; (2) patients receiving more than 300 mg per day for more than 2 months; (3) females; (4) patients over 35 years of age; and (5) patients taking other drugs, especially estrogens. The development of hepatitis is usually preceded by anorexia, nausea, vomiting, abdominal discomfort, or elevation of liver function tests. Before dantrolene therapy is initiated, therefore, baseline liver function tests should be obtained. The patient should also be made aware of prehepatitis symptoms (already noted) to participate in monitoring therapy.

SUMMARY

The skeletal muscle relaxants, both centrally and peripherally acting, are drugs used widely in clinical therapeutics today. Although it is more difficult objectively to prove the usefulness of these agents in treating acute muscle spasm than it is to demonstrate their effectiveness in muscle spasticity, one may expect to see continued use in both types of pathologic conditions.

The centrally acting drugs, such as diazepam, cyclobenzaprine, and mephenesin-related compounds, are generally used to treat acute muscle spasm caused by trauma, whereas baclofen, although classified as centrally acting, is usually reserved for treating muscle spasticity that is spinal cord in origin. CNS side effects such as drowsiness, dizziness, and ataxia may be expected to some degree with all of the agents in this class.

Dantrolene is the only peripherally acting muscle relaxant currently available and is useful as a muscle relaxant in those patients with muscle spasticity caused by a central neurologic disease. It will, in most patients, lessen the force of contraction to the point where limbs are more mobile, although it will not actually restore previously deteriorated function. Patients who use their spasticity as a means of support are not candidates for dantrolene because the drug may interfere with the patient's adaptation to altered muscle tone.

The decision to use any skeletal muscle relaxant must be based on a knowledge of the patient's muscular pathologic conditions, the site of action of the drug, and the goal to which therapy is directed. Consideration of these factors will do much to ensure optimal and rational drug therapy.

ADVERSE/SIDE EFFECTS OF MUSCLE RELAXANTS*

ALLERGIC REACTIONS

Anaphylaxis (IV methocarbamol)
Angioneurotic edema
Asthma
Fever
Photosensitivity
Pleural effusion with pericarditis (dantrolene)
Skin rash

AUTONOMIC NERVOUS SYSTEM

Dry mouth

BEHAVIOR

Confusion
Depression
Insomnia
Irritability

CARDIOVASCULAR SYSTEM

Facial flushing
Hypotension (IV methocarbamol)
Palpitation

Postural hypotension (carisoprodol)
Tachycardia

CENTRAL NERVOUS SYSTEM

Ataxia
Dizziness
Hallucinations (on abrupt withdrawal of baclofen)
Headache
Sedation

GASTROINTESTINAL AND HEPATIC SYSTEMS

Diarrhea
Hepatitis (dantrolene; greater risk in females, patients over 35 years of age, or patients taking other drugs; important to obtain baseline liver function tests before beginning therapy and at regular intervals throughout therapy)
Nausea
Vomiting

GENITOURINARY SYSTEM

Discoloration of urine (chlorzoxazone and methocarbamol)
Urinary frequency or retention

METABOLIC AND ENDOCRINE SYSTEMS

Acneiform rash (dantrolene)
Galactorrhea (cyclobenzaprine, dantrolene)
Gynecomastia (cyclobenzaprine)
Hirsutism (dantrolene)
Hyperhidrosis
Testicular swelling (cyclobenzaprine)

NEUROMUSCULAR SYSTEM

Fatigue
Weakness

OCULAR SYSTEM

Blurred vision

*See Chapter 11, "Drug Toxicity," for an overview of drug toxicity.

CLINICALLY SIGNIFICANT DRUG INTERACTIONS*

Primary drug	*Interacting drug*	*Possible effect(s)*	*Probable mechanism(s)*
Centrally acting muscle relaxants	Alcohol	Increase CNS depression	Additive effect
Cyclobenzaprine	Alcohol	Increase CNS depression	Additive effect
Cyclobenzaprine	Barbiturates	Decrease muscle relaxant effect	Increased liver metabolism
Cyclobenzaprine	Epinephrine	Increase blood pressure	Unknown
Cyclobenzaprine	Levarterenol	Increase blood pressure	Unknown
Diazepam	Alcohol	Increase CNS depression	Additive effect
Diazepam	Cimetidine	Increase benzodiazepine effects	Decreased liver metabolism
Diazepam	Levodopa	Decrease control of parkinsonian symptoms	Unknown

*See Chapter 10, "Drug Interactions," for an overview of drug interactions.

GENERAL NURSING IMPLICATIONS

Nursing of patients requiring centrally or peripherally acting skeletal muscle relaxants

ASSESSMENT

Patients who have acute self-limiting conditions, as well as diagnosed disease conditions of the musculoskeletal system, require careful assessment and evaluation. Assessment is especially important in monitoring therapeutic response. In assessing patients it is important to differentiate between conditions that are a result of lesions of the upper or lower motor neurons. Spasticity and pain associated with lesions of the upper motor neurons should be identified and recorded. Involved muscles, diminished muscle strength, as well as other observations, should be identified. Flaccidity associated with lesions of the lower motor neurons with a loss of muscle tone and atrophy should be noted, as well as the presence of fasciculations and absent or diminished tendon reflexes. In addition to inspection, palpation, and tests for muscle strength and function, diagnostic and laboratory tests including electromyelograms and serum enzyme levels may be indicated to determine the neural adequacy of the muscle or the presence of an intrinsic muscle disease.

A drug history should be completed to identify the patient's drug-taking patterns, possible sensitivity to medications, contraindications, cautions, and potential drug interactions before medication therapy is started.

SENSITIVITY

Patients who are receiving these medications for the first time should be carefully monitored for hypersensitivity reactions such as skin rash, acneform rash, fever, or respiratory difficulty, including asthma.

CONTRAINDICATIONS

The use of these medications is contraindicated with known hypersensitivity.

See the Nursing Drug Digest for specific contraindications to each medication.

CAUTIONS

Other drugs with CNS effects, including alcohol, narcotics, and tranquilizers may have an additive or synergistic effect. Caution patients about activities that require alertness.

Safety precautions should be implemented as indicated, including using bedside rails, restraints, supervision with ambulation, or smoking.

DRUG INTERACTIONS

Additive CNS depression can occur when muscle-relaxants are coadministered with other CNS depressants (e.g., narcotic analgesics, phenothiazines, antihistamines, alcohol).

See Clinically Significant Drug Interactions.

ADMINISTRATION

The specific muscle relaxants are available in various dosage forms for oral, intramuscular, and intravenous administration. Administration and dosage should be individualized. See the Nursing Drug Digest for specific information regarding the administration of these drugs.

MONITORING PATIENT RESPONSE
Therapeutic response

The patient should be carefully monitored for relief of pain associated with muscle spasms and degree of spasticity. It is important to identify sources that may trigger reflex spasms and use the control of these stimuli in promoting drug response. Safety precautions that are required because of spasticity in certain patients should be continued until the response is known.

Depending on the patient's condition and requirements for muscle relaxants, a decrease in painful or recurrent spasms should be noted, as well as changes such as an increased ability to sit, stand, ambulate, or progress in rehabilitation or physiotherapy treatment.

Monitoring is especially important because certain painful spasms not relieved with conservative or pharmacologic treatment may require surgical intervention.

Adverse side effects

Adverse side effects can occur with the various muscle relaxants. See Adverse/Side Effects of Muscle Relaxants. The most common effects should be carefully monitored and nursing measures provided to minimize or prevent these effects.

Monitor vital signs until patient's dosage and physiologic response are stabilized. Children, the elderly, or debilitated patients should be carefully monitored during the initial phases of therapy. Bedside rails should be raised as a safety precaution and ambulation should be supervised.

Monitor for drowsiness because this is one of the most common adverse effects of these drugs. Other CNS-related effects have also been observed, including lethargy, ataxia, confusion, weakness, dizziness, and changes in vision (e.g., complaints of blurred vision and accomodation problems). The nurse should be especially alert to observe and report excessive sedation or other behavioral changes. Although a peripherally acting skeletal muscle relaxant, dantrolene also appears to cause some of these effects.

Continued.

GENERAL NURSING IMPLICATIONS—cont'd

Nursing of patients requiring centrally or peripherally acting skeletal muscle relaxants—cont'd

Adverse side effects—cont'd

Monitor for a balance in intake and output because these drugs can cause urinary retention. An increased urinary output should also be maintained because many of these drugs are excreted by the kidneys. An increased fluid intake is also helpful in preventing constipation, which is also associated with these medications.

Females should be monitored for menstrual irregularities and both males and females should be monitored for breast enlargement (especially those patients taking dantrolene).

Patients taking dantrolene and chlorzoxazone should be monitored carefully for signs of hepatitis, including jaundice, abnormal liver function tests, fever, malaise, weakness, anorexia, nausea, vomiting, and abdominal discomfort.

PATIENT EDUCATION

The patient and the family, as indicated, should have a clear understanding of the medication regimen, the exact name of the medication, its action, dosage, storage, administration, and adverse side effects, as well as measures that can be used to prevent or minimize these effects. The patient's ability to self-medicate requires careful assessment in certain disease conditions (e.g., cerebrovascular accident, multiple sclerosis). The patient and the family should know how to monitor therapeutic response and to be able to identify when the health care provider should be notified. Individualized teaching regarding the preparation and administration of the medication is particularly important in chronic conditions so that increased patient and family participation in care and monitoring can be achieved.

GENERAL INSTRUCTIONS FOR DISCHARGE/OUTPATIENTS

This medication is a muscle relaxant. Follow the instructions on the prescription exactly.

This medication may cause you to become dizzy, lightheaded, drowsy, or less alert than you normally would be. Until you learn how this medication affects you (usually, at least 3 days), do not drive, operate any dangerous machinery, or put yourself in situations where decreased mental alertness may cause danger.

This medication will add to the effects of alcohol and other medicines that slow down the nervous system, such as tranquilizers, antihistamines, narcotics, or other prescription pain medicine. Check with your nurse, pharmacist, or physician before taking any of the above.

Along with the desired effects, a medicine may cause some unwanted effects. Although these side effects do not occur very often, when they do occur they may require medical attention. Check with your nurse, pharmacist, or physician if any of the following occur:
Hallucinations
Bloody or dark urine
Skin rash
Mental confusion or depression
Unusual excitement, nervousness, or irritability
Unusual tiredness or weakness
Yellowing of eyes or skin

The following effects occur more commonly and usually do not require medical attention. However, if they become bothersome to the point where they interfere with daily activities, check with your nurse, pharmacist, or physician:

Blurred vision
Clumsiness or unsteadiness
Diarrhea
Dizziness or lightheadedness
Drowsiness
Headache
Nausea

This medication has been prescribed especially for you. Do not trade or give this medication to any relatives or friends.

Notify your nurse or physician if you stop or start taking any other medications while taking this medication.

Keep this and all medication out of the reach of children.

NURSING DRUG DIGEST

Medication (trade name*)	Indication	Usual dosage and administration	Dosage forms, preparation, and storage	Contraindications, cautions, and comments	Monitoring
Baclofen Lioresal	Spasticity, especially the result of multiple sclerosis or spinal cord injury	*Adults:* titrate to optimal dose as follows 5 mg t.i.d. PO for 3 days, then 10 mg t.i.d. PO for 3 days, then 15 mg t.i.d. PO for 3 days, then 20 mg t.i.d. PO for 3 days Maximum: 80 mg/day *Children: Not* recommended for use in children under 12 years of age Administer with food or milk to decrease GI distress, or administer with a full glass of water to further decrease GI irritation and to help ensure adequate hydration Decrease dosage in renal impairment because baclofen is primarily eliminated via renal excretion	Tablet: 10 mg	*Contraindicated* in early pregnancy Has *not* been shown to benefit stroke patients and is *not* recommended May cause drowsiness Should be used with caution in patients where spasticity is used to sustain upright posture and locomotion or where spasticity is used to obtain increased function (e.g., multiple sclerosis or other CNS injury) Should be used with caution in patients with a history of epilepsy or seizure disorders because deterioration of seizure control and EEG has been reported Drug should be withdrawn slowly if therapy is stopped because hallucinations have occurred with abrupt withdrawal Periodic EEG should be performed	Observe for oversedation and other CNS depressant effects Observe for hypersensitivity (i.e., exaggerated motor response) Laboratory tests (e.g., SGOT, alkaline phosphatase, and blood sugar) may be abnormally high Monitor for signs of overdose: vomiting, blurred vision or any change in vision, muscular hypotonia, hypotension, drowsiness, accommodation disorders, seizures, respiratory depression (assisted respiration may be required)

Continued.

NOTE: For additional details regarding the individual agents listed in this table see the text and other tables in this chapter.

*Indicates a multiple active ingredient product. For a complete listing of all active ingredients see *the Drug Reference Guide to Brand Names and Active Ingredients.*

★Indicates drug is generally available only in the United States.

NURSING DRUG DIGEST—cont'd

Medication (trade name)	Indication	Usual dosage and administration	Dosage forms, preparation, and storage	Contraindications, cautions, and comments	Monitoring
Carisoprodol Carisoma Rela Sanoma Soma Soma Compound with Codeine	Acute, painful musculoskeletal conditions	*Adults:* 350 mg PO t.i.d. and q.h.s. *Children: Not* recommended for use in children under 12 years of age	Tablet: 350 mg	*Contraindicated* in acute intermittent porphyria, hepatic impairment, or renal impairment Excreted in breast milk in 2-4 times maternal plasma levels—may cause sedation and GI upset in nursing infant Mild withdrawal symptoms may occur after abrupt withdrawal from chronic use	Observe for oversedation Observe for idiosyncratic reactions after first dose: extreme weakness, transient quadriplegia, dizziness, ataxia, agitation, confusion, temporary vision loss Observe for signs of respiratory distress
Chlorphenesin carbamate Maolate	Acute, painful musculoskeletal conditions	*Adults:* 400-800 mg PO t.i.d. to q.i.d. *Children:* Should *not* be used in children under 12 years of age NOTE: Should *not* be used for longer than 8 weeks because the drug does not have documented safety and effectiveness for longer periods Administer with food or milk to decrease GI upset	Tablet: 400 mg	*Contraindicated* in hepatic dysfunction	Observe for oversedation Monitor hepatic and renal function Observe for signs of blood dyscrasias: sore throat, weakness, persistent infection
Chlorzoxazone Flexaphen* Myoforte* Paraflex* Parafon Forte* Saroflex* Spasgesic*	Acute, painful musculoskeletal conditions	*Adults:* 250-750 mg PO t.i.d. to q.i.d. *Children:* 125-500 mg PO t.i.d. to q.i.d. Administer with food or milk to decrease GI distress Tablets may be crushed and taken with food or liquid for ease of administration	Tablet: 250 mg	*Contraindicated* in patients with liver disease Has been implicated with hepatitis May color urine orange to reddish	Observe for oversedation Observe for signs of hepatitis: jaundice, abnormal liver tests, malaise

Drug	Uses	Dosage	Contraindications/Precautions	Nursing Implications
Cyclobenza-prine Flexeril	Acute, painful musculoskeletal conditions	Tablet: 10 mg *Adults:* 10 mg PO t.i.d. to q.i.d. (maximum dose is 60 mg q.d.) *Children: Not* recommended for use in children under 15 years of age NOTE: Significant improvement in symptoms has not been demonstrated when used beyond 2-3 weeks; use of the drug for longer periods of time is *not recommended*	*Contraindicated* in hyperthyroidism May produce atropine-like reactions Dry mouth Urinary retention Should be avoided in patients with cardiac abnormalities because this class of drug (tricyclics) has been reported to cause acute exacerbation of cardiac problems Drowsiness is common Use with extreme caution in patients receiving MAO inhibitors or within 14 days after their discontinuation because hyperpyretic crises, severe convulsions, and death have resulted (avoid if possible) Dry mouth can be relieved by sucking on sugarless hard candy	Observe for oversedation Monitor fluid intake and output and for urinary retention Monitor for dry mouth
Dantrolene Dantrium	Spasticity	Capsules: 25, 50, 75, 100 mg Injectable: (protect from light) Each 70 ml vial contains 20 mg dantrolene and sufficient sodium hydroxide to yield a pH of approximately 9.5 when reconstituted with 60 ml of sterile water After adding sterile water, *shake well* until solution is clear *Adults:* 25 mg PO q.d. initially; increase to 25 mg b.i.d., t.i.d. or q.i.d. and then by increments of 25 mg; maintain each dose level for 4-7 days to be certain of maximum effect Maximum: 400 mg/day *Children:* Should *not* be used in children under 5 years of age; over 5 years of age, 0.5 mg/kg PO b.i.d. to q.i.d.; may be gradually increased by 0.5 mg/kg to a maximum dose of 100 mg q.i.d.	*Contraindicated* in acute liver disease *Contraindicated* in chronic obstructive pulmonary disease Chronic pleural effusions and eosinophilia may occur with long-term treatment May cause photosensitivity; patients should be cautioned about exposure to sunlight May cause severe diarrhea	Monitor for edema papules and urticaria if patient is exposed to sunlight because these can occur if sunlight exposure is not avoided Observe for signs of liver toxicity: jaundice, abnormal liver tests, malaise Monitor bowel movements

Continued.

NURSING DRUG DIGEST—cont'd

Medication (trade name)	Indication	Usual dosage and administration	Dosage forms, preparation, and storage	Contraindications, cautions, and comments	Monitoring
Dantrolene—cont'd	Malignant hyperthermia	Therapy should be discontinued if results are not evident in 45 days *Adults:* 1 mg/kg IV push (rapid) *continuing* until symptoms subside or a dose of 10 mg/kg is reached Take special care to avoid extravasation of injection because of alkaline nature of drug (pH 9.5) *Children:* Although *not* recommended for use in children under 5 years of age, risk-benefit determinations may be necessary; dose for children under 5 is the same as adults Administer with food or milk to decrease GI upset or administer with a full glass of water to decrease GI upset and to help ensure adequate hydration Prophylactic administration of 1-2 mg/kg q.i.d. for 1-3 days following IV dose is recommended to prevent recurrence of malignant hyperthermia		Specific therapeutic goal should be decided on before therapy is begun; once goal is achieved, no further increase in dosage is necessary May cause transient drowsiness, weakness, dizziness, malaise, and fatigue Risks of liver toxicity greater in women, patients over 35 years of age, and patients taking other medications of any type, but especially estrogens	Observe for oversedation and weakness as long as therapy is continued Monitor patient's ability to manipulate rehabilitative devices such as crutches and braces
Diazepam Apaurin Atensine D-Tran E-Pam Lemprol Meval Neo-Calme	Anxiety	*Adults:* 2-10 mg PO b.i.d. to q.i.d.; or 2-5 mg IM or IV push; repeat in 3-4 hr if necessary *Children:* 1-2.5 mg PO t.i.d. to q.i.d. NOTE: Should *not* be used in children under 6 months of age	Capsule: 15 mg Tablets: 2, 5, 10 mg Injectable: 5 mg/ml Injectable contains propylene glycol (40%) and alcohol (10%) as a vehicle Protect from light	*Contraindicated* in acute pulmonary insufficiency Continued use may lead to tolerance or physical dependence May cause drowsiness	Observe for oversedation Supervise ambulation and use bedside rails Monitor duration of use and patient response carefully

Noan
Novodipam
Paxel
Serenack
Setonil
Stress-Pam
Tensium
Tranimul
Valium
Valrelease
Vatran
Vivol

Acute alcohol withdrawal

Acute, painful musculoskeletal conditions

Elderly: 2-2.5 mg PO q.d. to b.i.d.

Elderly or debilitated patients may be overly sensitive to usual adult doses

15 mg slow-release capsule (Valrelease) administered q.d. is equivalent to 5 mg tablets administered t.i.d. PO

Absorption from the deltoid IM site is usually rapid and complete, whereas slow and erratic absorption may occur at other IM sites

Do *not* mix with other solutions or drugs in syringe or infusion bottle

NOTE: Do not inject IV at a rate to exceed 5 mg/min because of risk of apnea and cardiac arrest

IV use may cause thrombophlebitis; avoid use of small veins in hands and wrist

Accidental intraarterial injection of diazepam has caused vascular damage and gangrene, resulting in amputation

Adults: 10 mg PO t.i.d. to q.i.d. during first 24 hr; reduce to 5 mg t.i.d. to q.i.d. as needed; or 10 mg IV or IM, repeat 5-10 mg in 3-4 hr as needed

Adults: 2-10 mg PO t.i.d. to q.i.d.; or 5-10 mg IM or IV initially, then 5-10 mg IM or IV in 3-4 hr

Children: 30 days of age to 5 years of age: 1-2 mg IV or IM slowly; repeat q.3-4h. as necessary; over 5 years of age: 5-10 mg IM or IV repeated every q.3-4h. as needed (respiratory assistance should be available)

Do *not* mix injectable form with other medications unless known to be compatible

Abrupt withdrawal following chronic, excessive dosage may produce confusion, toxic psychoses, convulsions, and other symptoms resembling delirium tremens

Administer deep IM and aspirate carefully before injecting medication

Continuous intravenous infusion is not recommended because of the possibility of precipitation in intravenous fluids and adsorption of the medication to the plastic infusion bags or tubing; if diazepam cannot be given by direct IV injection, it should be injected slowly into infusion tubing as close to the patient as possible

Transient retrograde amnesia can result from IV administration

Monitor patients for signs of withdrawal: vomiting, sweating, abdominal cramps, tremor, and convulsions that can persist for several weeks

Continued.

NURSING DRUG DIGEST—cont'd

Medication (trade name)	Indication	Usual dosage and administration	Dosage forms, preparation, and storage	Contraindications, cautions, and comments	Monitoring
Diazepam— cont'd	Status epilepticus	*Adults:* 5-10 mg IV push; repeat at 10- to 15-min intervals, up to 30 mg total dose *Children:* 30 days of age to 5 years of age: 0.2-0.5 mg IV slowly every 2-5 min up to maximum 5 mg; over 5 years of age: 1 mg IV every 2-5 min up to total of 10 mg			Observe for oversedation
★ **Mephenesin** Dioloxol Mephson Oranixon Sinan Tolsaram Tolserol Tolyspaz	Acute, painful, musculoskeletal conditions	*Adults:* 0.5-1 gm PO 1-6 times daily Administer with food or milk to decrease GI upset NOTE: Use is *not* generally recommended	Tablet: 500 mg	Rarely used because newer compounds are available	Observe for oversedation
★ **Metaxalone** Skelaxin	Acute, painful musculoskeletal conditions	*Adults:* 800 mg PO t.i.d. to q.i.d. *Children: Not* recommended for use in children under 12 years of age Administer with food or milk to decrease GI upset *Not* recommended for use longer than 1-2 weeks because of lack of demonstrated effectiveness	Tablet: 400 mg	*Contraindicated* in hepatic and renal dysfunction *Contraindicated* in patients with known tendencies to anemias May cause skin rash	Observe for signs of hepatotoxicity: jaundice, abnormal liver function tests, malaise Observe for signs of blood dyscrasias: sore throat, weakness, persistent infections
Methocarbamol Delaxin Forbaxin Metho-500 Robaxin Robaxisal C-1/4* Robaxisal C-1/8*	Acute, painful musculoskeletal conditions Tetanus	*Adults:* 1-1.5 gm q.i.d. PO; or 1 gm IV t.i.d. up to 3 days *Adults:* 1-2 gm IV stat followed by 1-2 gm as IV drip (3 gm initial dose); repeat q.i.d. until drug can be taken orally; up to 24 gm/day PO can then be given until symptoms subside	Tablets: 500, 750 mg Injectable: 100 mg/ml Store at room temperature Do *not* refrigerate Discard solutions that are discolored or that contain particulate matter	*Contraindicated* in renal dysfunction May color urine green or black on standing	Observe for oversedation Observe for orthostatic hypotension; encourage patient to make position changes slowly; should dangle legs before standing

Drug	Indications	Dosage	Preparations	Side Effects / Contraindications	Nursing Implications
Robaxisal* Spenaxin Tresortil		*Children:* 15 mg/kg IV q.i.d. (tetanus only) *Not* recommended for use in children under 12 years of age NOTE: IM injection may cause tissue sloughing and should not be used IV injection rate *not* to exceed 3 ml/min (may cause thrombophlebitis) Oral therapy should be instituted as soon as possible			Monitor muscle relaxant effects observable within 10 minutes of IV injection Monitor IV site for extravasation because thrombophlebitis, pain, and sloughing can occur Monitor patient for complaints of metallic taste, nausea, nystagmus, diplopia, muscle spasms, incoordination, redness or flushing of face, vertigo, weakness, syncope, bradycardia, and hypotension after IV injection
Orphenadrine Brocasipal Disipal Marflex Mephena-mine Myotrol Norflex Norgesic* Norgesic Forte*	Acute, painful musculoskeletal conditions	*Adults:* 100 mg PO b.i.d.; or 60 mg IV or IM b.i.d. as needed *Children: Not* recommended for use in children Patient should remain in recumbent position for 10-15 min following IV injection Administer IV *slowly* over 5 min	Tablet: 100 mg Injectable: 30 mg/ml	*Contraindicated* in narrow-angle glaucoma, severe renal dysfunction, stenosing peptic ulcers, prostatic hypertrophy, glaucoma, pyloric or duodenal obstruction, bladder neck obstruction, cardiospasm, myasthenia gravis May cause urinary retention	Dryness of the mouth is usually the first adverse effect seen Observe for oversedation, lightheadedness, dizziness, and syncope Monitor fluid intake and output

BIBLIOGRAPHY

Berger, F.M., & Bradley, W. The pharmacological properties of alpha : beta-dehydroxy-gamma-(2-methylphenoxy) propane (MYANESIN). *British Journal of Pharmacological Chemotherapy,* 1946, *1,* 265-272.

Campbell, E.D.R. Muscle relaxant drugs. *Practitioner,* 1979, *223,* 507-509.

Delaney, J.F. Medical treatment of spasticity. *Current Problems in Surgery,* 1980, *17*(4), 245-248.

Jardon, O.M., Wingard, D.W., Barak, A.J., & Connolly, J.F. Malignant hyperthermia. *Journal of Bone and Joint Surgery,* 1979, *61*A(7), 1064-1070.

Knutsson, E. Antispastic medication. *Scandinavian Journal of Rehabilitation Medicine. Supplement,* 1980, *7,* 80-84.

Pinder, R.M., Brogden, R.N., Speight, T.M., & Avery, G.S. Dantrolene sodium: a review of its pharmacological properties and therapeutic efficacy in spasticity. *Drugs,* 1977, *13,* 3-23.

Share, N.N., & McFarland, C.S. Cyclobenzaprine: a novel centrally acting skeletal muscle relaxant. *Neuropharmacology,* 1975, *14,* 675-684.

Young, R.R., & Delwaide, P.J. Spasticity—part I. *New England Journal of Medicine,* 1981, *304*(1), 28-33.

Young, R.R., & Delwaide, P.J. Spasticity—part II. *New England Journal of Medicine,* 1981, *304*(2), 96-99.

CHAPTER 17

Analgesics and Narcotic Antagonists

Steven H. Butler

Medications discussed in this chapter

Narcotic analgesics
  Alphaprodine
  Anileridine
  Brompton's cocktail
  Codeine
  Drocode
  Ethoheptazine
  Fentanyl
  Heroin
  Hydrocodone
  Hydromorphone
  Levorphanol
  Meperidine
  Methadone
  Morphine
  Opium

Narcotic analgesics—cont'd
  Oxycodone
  Oxymorphone
  Propoxyphene
Narcotic agonist/antagonist
  Butorphanol
  Levallorphan
  Nalbuphine
  Pentazocine
Phenothiazine analgesic
  Methotrimeprazine
Narcotic antagonist (pure)
  Naloxone
Nonnarcotic analgesics
  Acetaminophen
  Aspirin

Analgesics, especially the narcotics, have been both a boon and a problem for humanity for centuries. Despite this long association and an increasing sophistication in medical knowledge, problems remain. Prescribing *narcotics* and related drugs is still poorly done by the medical community. There are three main areas of difficulty. The first concerns acute *pain,* such as the case of a postoperative patient, when too often insufficient analgesics are given in terms of unit dose or frequency of administration. This same problem involves many terminal cancer patients suffering from severe pain. In a rather contradictory manner, patients with chronic benign pain are often given high doses of narcotics when there is good evidence that the narcotics have limited usage in long-term pain problems. For these reasons, prescribing practices should be continually audited. The nurse is in a good position to help monitor the analgesics and to encourage appropriate medication use by patients and their supply by prescribers.

An encouraging trend is the recent vast increase in our knowledge about drug activity, especially the narcotics. With the burgeoning research in the field of endorphins and enkephalins, scientists are finding specific sites of action of the opiates in the nervous system. They are unraveling the complex interaction of various nerve pathways that transmit and control pain, and the response of the human organism to the sensations and emotions produced by any stimulus perceived as painful. With this new wealth of information, some of the myths, fears, and confusion about appropriate narcotic use should be dispelled, allowing for more rational and adequate treatment of a wide variety of pain problems.

SITES OF ACTION

The narcotics, both *agonist* and *antagonist,* act in a complex manner in the central nervous system (CNS), the spinal cord, and the gut. Basically, these drugs are (1) chemicals (e.g., opium) naturally produced by plants, (2) a modification of these chemicals (e.g., heroin), or (3) synthesized chemicals (e.g., meperidine) that mimic nervous system transmitter compounds or neuromodulating compounds (endorphins and enkephalins) naturally present in the human body.

In the brain, the action of these transmitter compounds is in the periaqueductal gray area, the medial parts of the thalamus, the amygdala, the frontal cortex, the hypothalamus, and the basal ganglia (see Chapter 13, "Review of the Anatomy, Physiology, and Assessment of the Central Nervous System"). The narcotics *increase* the tone of the system by increasing message transfers. This tends to *lower* the number of *nociceptive* messages received from the peripheral nervous system, perceived in the conscious areas of the brain as pain. Narcotic antagonists (e.g., naloxone) have the opposite effect, because they *decrease* the tone in the pain modulating system and allow *more* nociceptive

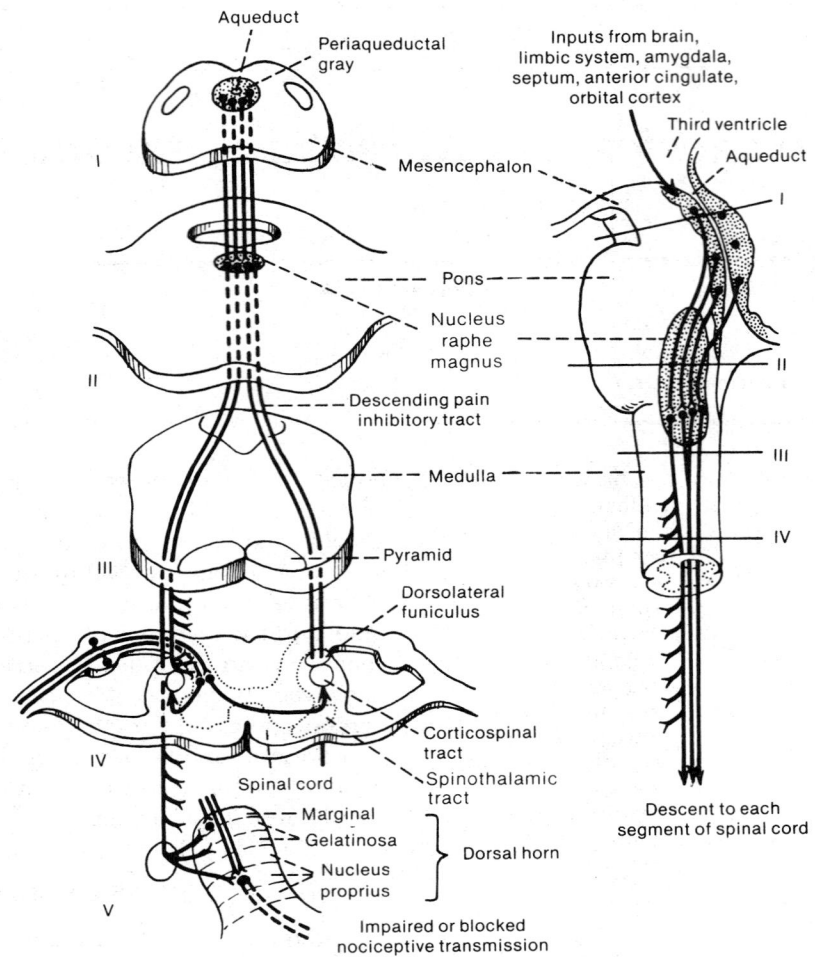

FIGURE 17-1. **This represents the pain transmission and pain modulation systems of the spinal cord and brainstem. The narcotics are active in the spinal cord (marginal and gelatinosa layers of the dorsal horn at the bottom of the figure) blocking pain transmission. They also act in the stippled areas (periaqueductal gray and nucleus raphe magnus) of the brainstem to send pain inhibitory messages to the spinal cord. (From Bonica, J.J.** *The management of pain,* **2nd ed., Philadelphia: Lea & Febiger, In Press.)**

messages to pass through and register pain in the conscious brain. Some compounds act as both agonists and antagonists (e.g., pentazocine). By themselves, they can produce analgesia in the face of nociceptive input, but if given at the same time as a potent narcotic, they will block the effect. Analgesia is not noticed per se unless some nociceptive messages are being sent from the periphery. Rounding out this spectrum of drugs are pure antagonists of opiates and other narcotics (e.g., naloxone). These agents have only blocking properties and *no* stimulating properties.

In the peripheral nervous system, narcotic analgesics and narcotic antagonists act in the dorsal horn (Figure 17-1). Narcotic analgesics can block nociceptive input there and prevent the nervous system messages that are perceived in the consciousness as pain. Narcotic antagonists prevent this blockade and allow more nociceptive neural traffic (i.e., the conscious awareness of more pain).

Narcotic analgesics also act on the gut to slow smooth muscle contraction, causing the constipation seen as a side effect of their administration.

A review of some neurophysiology is essential (see Chapter 13, "Review of the Anatomy, Physiology, and Assessment of the Central Nervous System"). At this point I will discuss, as a way of functionally accounting

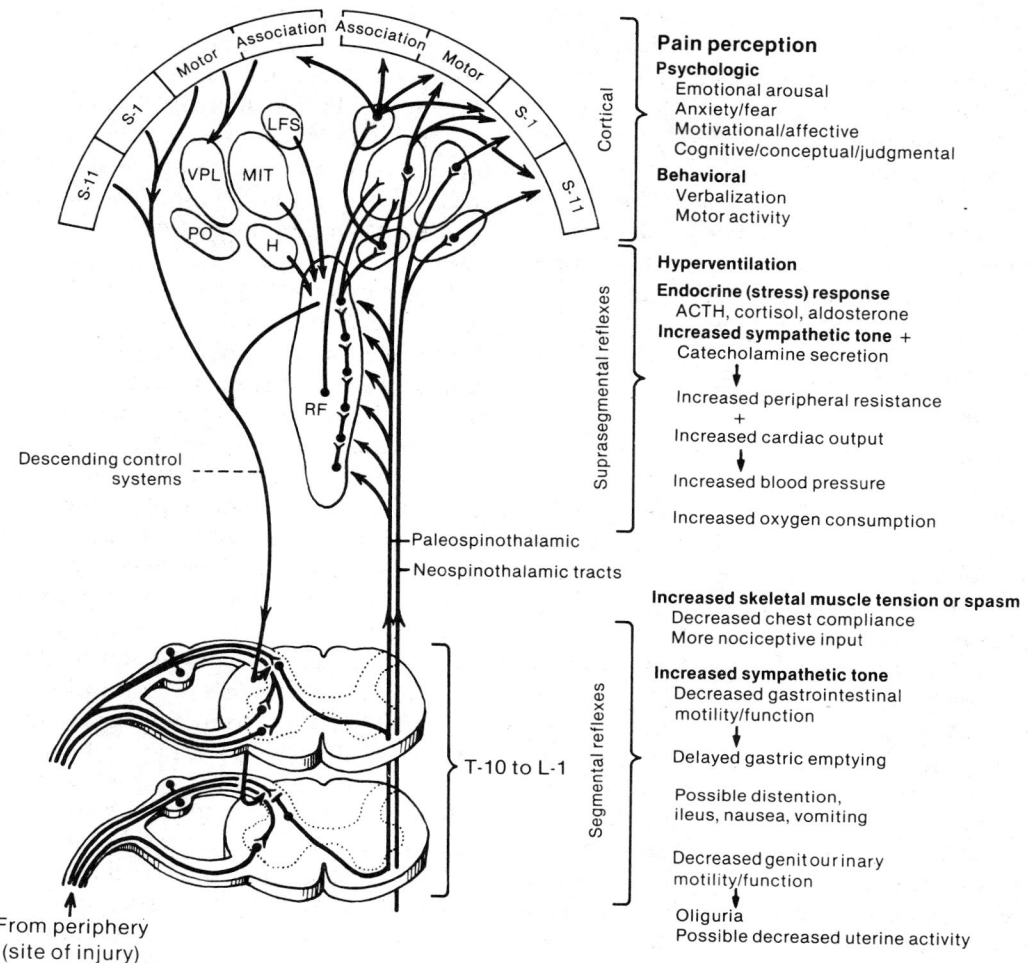

Pain perception
Psychologic
  Emotional arousal
  Anxiety/fear
  Motivational/affective
  Cognitive/conceptual/judgmental
Behavioral
  Verbalization
  Motor activity

Hyperventilation

Endocrine (stress) response
  ACTH, cortisol, aldosterone
Increased sympathetic tone +
  Catecholamine secretion
    ↓
  Increased peripheral resistance
    +
  Increased cardiac output
    ↓
  Increased blood pressure

  Increased oxygen consumption

Increased skeletal muscle tension or spasm
  Decreased chest compliance
  More nociceptive input

Increased sympathetic tone
  Decreased gastrointestinal
  motility/function
    ↓
  Delayed gastric emptying
    ↓
  Possible distention,
  ileus, nausea, vomiting

  Decreased genitourinary
  motility/function
    ↓
  Oliguria
  Possible decreased uterine activity

FIGURE 17-2. **This shows the ascending pain pathways (paleospinothalamic and neo-
spinothalamic tracts) and descending pain inhibitory systems. Besides being active
at spinal and brainstem levels as shown in Figure 17-1, narcotics act in the hypothalamus (H), thalamus (PO, VPL, MIT), amygdala (LFS), and sensory cortex (S-1, S-11).
RF, Reticular formation; H, Hypothalamus; PO, posterior thalamus; VPL, ventral pos-
terolateral thalamus; MIT, medial and intralaminar thalmic nuclei; LFS, limbic forebrain structures; S-1, S-11, somatosensory cortex. (From Bonica, J.J.** *The management of pain,* **2nd ed. Philadelphia: Lea & Febiger, In Press.)**

for the activity of narcotic analgesics, the nervous system and the sites where the enkephalins and endorphins have been found.

First, high concentrations of opiate receptors and
rich enkephalin innervation are found in the dorsal
horn of the spinal cord, the periaqueductal gray area,
and the thalamus. One of the pain systems, the paleospinothalamic tract, connects through these areas
(Figure 17-2). It conducts dull, poorly localized pain
messages such as the ache experienced with a bruise,
not the localized, sharp pain that is felt with the blow

that caused the bruise. Narcotics are believed to decrease pain messages within this system.

High concentrations of opiate receptors and enkephalins are found in the hypothalamus, the amygdala, and the frontal cortex (Figure 17-2). These areas
of the brain are associated with the perception and
expression of emotion. The opiates are felt to decrease
the severity of pain as an emotional, conscious experience through activity here. The euphoria experienced with some narcotics probably is produced here,
as well as psychologic dependence.

Some areas of the brainstem and medulla have high concentrations of *opiate* receptors and enkephalins. Many believe that some of the side effects of narcotics, such as respiratory depression and nausea, are produced here. The desirable suppression of cough also may be caused by activity in this region.

As previously mentioned, the narcotics decrease the transfer of nociceptive information at the spinal cord level so that fewer messages reach the brain. This also decreases the conscious awareness of pain.

CAUTIONS AND COMMENTS

Narcotic analgesics

When narcotic drugs are mentioned, the primary concern for all is addiction or drug dependence (for a more complete discussion of this issue see Chapter 12, "Drug Abuse and Addiction"). This usually refers to a combination of psychologic dependence and physical addiction or tolerance. Psychologic dependence is the desire for the drug because of its euphoric and sedating effects. Physical addiction is the need of the body for the drug to prevent withdrawal symptoms from occurring. With narcotics, these include sweating, nausea, abdominal cramps, diarrhea, and muscle pains. Tolerance is the gradual increase in drug dose required to produce the same physiologic effect.

The fears and concerns of addiction and dependence are overemphasized. Narcotic analgesics should be used primarily for acute, self-limiting pain states where some tolerance may appear but physical addiction is unlikely.* In managing chronic cancer pain, dependence should *not* be a concern if the medications allow a better quality of life for the sufferer, who often has a rather limited life expectancy. It should be noted that patients with severe pain *rarely* become addicted to the narcotic analgesics. Dependence can be a problem in chronic benign pain. It is known that for most chronic pain problems, narcotics do not alter pain levels if given over prolonged periods of time and are seldom appropriate. (In a controlled environment, withdrawal from narcotics of any dose can be easily done in 1 to 2 weeks in terms of physical addiction and tolerance without producing significant physical side effects. Psychologic dependence is more difficult to control, however.) With these thoughts in mind, narcotic analgesics should be tailored to the patient's requirements for acute pain and chronic cancer pain without undue interference from the specter of addiction.

*An exception to this rule is the use of methadone in narcotic addiction maintenance programs (see Chapter 12, "Drug Abuse and Addiction").

Narcotic analgesics should be used with caution in patients with head injuries. The respiratory depression produced leads to an increase in blood carbon dioxide levels that increase blood flow to the brain and intracranial pressure. If intracranial pressure has already been elevated, as is usual, by the head injury itself, then increased brain damage can occur. Vital signs must be monitored extremely closely in these patients.

When narcotic analgesics are given intravenously, they should be given with care. Too rapid infusion can lead to sudden obtundation, airway obstruction, apnea, and hypotension. Therefore, *slow* injection (i.e., over 3 to 5 minutes) is the general rule.

In patients with acute respiratory embarrassment (e.g., asthma, pneumonia, bronchitis), with chronic respiratory disease (e.g., emphysema, bronchitis), or a combination of these conditions, narcotics should be used with caution. Narcotics decrease respiratory drive, predominantly decreasing the rate but also causing an increase in airway resistance by stimulating smooth muscle contraction in the airways. This combination may be fatal in a patient with incipient respiratory failure from the causes just mentioned. Therefore, if narcotics are given to such patients, frequent monitoring of vital signs, especially the respiratory rate, and skin color (for signs of cyanosis), is imperative.

One must also be concerned about hypotension in patients taking narcotics. This is usually orthostatic (i.e., appears when standing) in patients receiving these drugs. It is more common in the elderly and the debilitated patient. One must observe these patients closely, as well as those patients with recent blood or fluid loss.

Because the narcotic analgesics are CNS depressants, any functioning requiring mental concentration and judgment or motor dexterity should be avoided if large doses are administered. This includes such activities as driving and operating or being near mechanical equipment. Both the patient and the family need to be notified about this problem. The tendency for patients to suffer from orthostatic hypotension with the use of large doses of narcotics will also aggravate these functions.

NARCOTIC AGONISTS AND ANTAGONISTS

As listed in the Nursing Drug Digest, most of these agents are used primarily for their agonist or analgesic effects. As such, the previously mentioned precautions for narcotic analgesics also apply to this group. Because these agents have antagonistic properties, they

TABLE 17-1

Relative potency of common stronger narcotics

Drug	Route of administration	Onset (min)	Peak action (hr)	Duration (hr)	Approximate equivalent dose (mg)*
Alphaprodine	SC or IM	5 to 10	within 0.5	1 to 2	40 to 60
Anileridine	SC or IM	within 15	0.5 to 1	2 to 3	30
Codeine	SC or IM	15 to 30	1.0 to 1.5	4 to 6	120
Fentanyl	SC or IM	5 to 15	within 0.5	1 to 2	0.2
Hydromorphone	SC or IM	15 to 30	0.5 to 1.5	4 to 5	1.5
Levorphanol	SC or IM	within 60	1.0 to 1.5	5 to 8	2 to 3
Meperidine	SC or IM	10 to 15	0.5 to 1	2 to 4	75 to 100
Methadone	SC or IM	10 to 15	1 to 2	4 to 8	7.5
Morphine	SC or IM	within 30	0.5 to 1.5	up to 7	10
Opium	PO or PR	within 30	0.5 to 1.0	up to 7	15

*This column lists the doses that should provide approximately the same amount of analgesia (e.g., it would take approximately 120 mg of codeine to provide the same amount of analgesia as 10 mg of morphine).

TABLE 17-2

Relative potency of common weaker analgesics

Drug	Route of administration	Onset (min)	Peak action (hr)	Duration (hr)	Approximate equivalent dose (mg)†
Acetaminophen	PO	10 to 20	0.5 to 1	4 to 6	650
Aspirin	PO	15 to 30	2	4 to 6	650
Codeine*	PO	15 to 30	1.0 to 1.5	4 to 6	32
Pentazocine	PO	15 to 30	1	4	30
Propoxyphene hydrochloride	PO	within 30	2	6 to 12	65
Propoxyphene napsylate	PO	within 30	2	6 to 12	100

*Codeine appears in the previous table and can be used as a comparison between these groups.
†This column lists the doses that should provide approximately the same amount of analgesia (e.g., it would take approximately 650 mg of aspirin to provide the same amount of analgesia as 32 mg of codeine).

are never to be used in conjunction with the pure agonists, because they will block their effect and may prevent or reverse any analgesia produced. When an antagonist is necessary, such as in the case of narcotic overdose, a pure narcotic antagonist (e.g., naloxone) should be used.

For a comparison of the narcotic and weaker analgesics, including the narcotic agonists/antagonists, refer to Tables 17-1, 17-2, and 17-3.

SUMMARY

This chapter has examined the various types and uses of both narcotic and nonnarcotic analgesics, as well as the various narcotic antagonists.* Emphasis has been placed on the sites of action and cautions and comments. Analgesics are one of the most fre-

*See Chapters 12, "Drug Abuse and Addiction," and 58, "Nonsteroidal Antiinflammatory Drugs," for a discussion of related topics.

quently administered classes of medications. With an understanding of the various individual agents, including their actions and side effects, the nurse will be better able to provide optimal care for the patient requiring these medications. Patient education can be enhanced, adverse drug effects anticipated, monitored for, and minimized, and clinically significant drug interactions avoided by using the information presented in this chapter.

TABLE 17-3

Comparison of stronger and weaker analgesics

	Stronger analgesics	*Weaker analgesics*
Indications	Moderate to severe pain of an acute nature (e.g., major surgery, trauma, MI, or renal stones)	Mild to moderate pain. Some chronic pain states (e.g., minor surgery, arthritis, or myalgias)
Contraindications	Chronic pain states with the exception of those associated with some cancers	Severe pain
Action	Primarily central (brain and spinal cord) to decrease nociceptive input and the emotional impact of pain	Primarily peripheral with some central effects. Mostly decreases nociceptive input
Route of administration	Usually parenteral (i.e., SC, IM, or IV)	Usually oral
Adverse effects	Primarily caused by CNS depression with low therapeutic to toxic ratio	Primarily caused by local effects in gut or excretory organs with high therapeutic to toxic ratio
Recipients	Primarily hospitalized patients	Hospitalized and ambulatory patients

ADVERSE/SIDE EFFECTS OF THE ANALGESICS*

ALLERGIC REACTIONS

Pruritus
Rashes
Urticaria (rarely hemorrhagic urticaria)
Wheals and flares may appear over a vein following injection into it

CENTRAL NERVOUS SYSTEM

Agitation
Disorientation and visual disturbances (these are usually related to the size of dose and are seen primarily with rapid intravenous injection)
Dysphoria
Headache

Incoordinated muscle movements
Insomnia
Transient hallucinations
Tremor
Weakness

GASTROINTESTINAL SYSTEM

Anorexia
Biliary tract spasm
Constipation
Dry mouth
Nausea and vomiting

CARDIOVASCULAR SYSTEM

Bradycardia
Faintness

Flushing of the face
Hypotension
Palpitations
Phlebitis (may follow intravenous injection)
Syncope
Tachycardia

GENITOURINARY SYSTEM

Antidiuretic effect
Reduced libido or impotence
Urinary hesitancy or retention

RESPIRATORY SYSTEM

Apnea
Hypoventilation

*See Chapter 11, "Drug Toxicity," for an overview of drug toxicity.

CLINICALLY SIGNIFICANT DRUG INTERACTIONS*

Primary drug	Interacting drug	Possible effect(s)	Probable mechanism(s)
Narcotic analgesics	Alcohol	Increased CNS depression	Additive effect
Narcotic analgesics	Barbiturates	Increased CNS depression	Combined effect CNS; possible increased toxic metabolite of meperidine
Narcotic analgesics	MAO inhibitors	Increased CNS depression Increased duration Hypotension	Potentiation (must be used together with extreme caution; *avoid* MAO inhibitors and meperidine)
Narcotic analgesics	Narcotic antagonists	Acute withdrawal symptoms	Antagonism
Narcotic analgesics	Skeletal muscle relaxants	Increased respiratory depression	Additive effect (use these agents together with extreme caution and careful patient monitoring)
Narcotic analgesics	All CNS depressants (alcohol, barbiturates, phenothiazines, butyrophenones, general anesthetics, benzodiazapines)	Increased CNS depression	Additive effect
Aspirin	Acetazolamide	Inhibition of aspirin effects	Increased urinary excretion
Aspirin	Acidifying agents (urinary)	Potentiation of aspirin effects, which may produce toxicity	Decreased urinary excretion
Aspirin	Alcohol	Increased gastric irritation and GI bleeding	Potentiating of irritating effect of each
Aspirin	Alkalinizing agents (urinary)	Decreased aspirin effects	Urinary excretion
Aspirin	Aminobenzoic acid	Increased aspirin effects	Decreased urinary excretion
Aspirin (simultaneous therapy contraindicated)	Anticoagulants (oral)	Anticoagulation, gastric bleeding	Aspirin decreases prothrombin formation Aspirin causes direct ulceration of the stomach lining Aspirin decreases platelet function
Aspirin	Chlorpropamide	Lowering of blood sugar by chlorpropamide augmented	Unknown
Aspirin	Corticosteroids	Increased chance of peptic ulceration Increased antiinflammatory effects	Additive Additive
Aspirin	Methotrexate	Increased drug activity	Aspirin displaces drug from binding sites
Aspirin (avoid combination)	Phenylbutazone	Increased change of peptic ulceration	Additive
Aspirin	Spironolactone	Aspirin may reverse effects	Unknown
Aspirin	Sulfonamides	Increased antibacterial action and toxicity	Decreased excretion of sulfonamide

*See Chapter 10, "Drug Interactions," for an overview of drug interactions.

GENERAL NURSING IMPLICATIONS

Nursing of patients requiring analgesics

ASSESSMENT

Patients requiring analgesics require a careful assessment of pain. The initial assessment should also include specific data related to the patient's condition, a detailed drug history to identify sensitivity, contraindications, cautions, potential drug interactions, and drug-taking patterns before analgesic therapy is planned and initiated.

Because pain is highly variable, it is helpful to look at assisting patients with analgesics related to acute self-limiting pain, chronic cancer pain, and chronic benign pain. These are outlined in this table following the general overview of analgesics.

SENSITIVITY

Any drug has the potential to cause a hypersensitivity reaction in susceptible individuals, and patients should be questioned carefully regarding known allergies to medications such as codeine or aspirin. Patients receiving analgesics for the first time should be carefully monitored.

CONTRAINDICATIONS

The use of analgesics is contraindicated in patients with hypersensitivity to a specific analgesic, respiratory depression, or respiratory failure.

See the Nursing Drug Digest for specific contraindications to each analgesic.

CAUTIONS

Analgesics should be used cautiously in elderly, sedated, or debilitated patients, and patients with severe renal or hepatic impairment.

The use of narcotic analgesics has the potential to produce both physical and psychologic dependence.

See the Nursing Drug Digest for cautions related to individual agents.

DRUG INTERACTIONS

Analgesics have the potential to interact with numerous drugs, particularly those that can cause CNS depression.

See Clinically Significant Drug interactions.

ADMINISTRATION

Analgesics can be administered orally, rectally, subcutaneously, intramuscularly, or intravenously, depending on the specific drug and dosage form. See the Nursing Drug Digest for specific information regarding the administration of each analgesic. The clinical setting, the patient's self-medication abilities, and type of pain and condition influence the drug therapy regimen and the selection of routes and times of administration. This is further discussed under the three sections: (1) acute self-limiting pain, (2) chronic cancer pain, and, (3) chronic benign pain. One should use adjunctive measures to promote pain reduction and comfort (e.g., positioning, diversional activities).

MONITORING PATIENT RESPONSE
Therapeutic response

The onset and duration of the analgesic effect is dependent on the dosage form, route of administration, and individual patient factors. Monitoring analgesic effects is especially important because if the patient's pain is not relieved, a change in the dosage or the drug, or adding another drug may be indicated so that pain relief can be maintained. See sections on acute self-limiting pain, chronic cancer pain, and chronic benign pain.

Adverse side effects

Adverse side effects vary depending on the chemical family or structure of the particular analgesic. In general, side effects are more common and more severe with the narcotic analgesics (e.g., CNS and respiratory depression, as well as drug abuse and addiction). However, serious adverse side affects can also be associated with the non-prescription analgesics (e.g., using aspirin in children suffering from viral infections has been associated with an increased incidence in Reye's syndrome). See previous section and the Nursing Drug Digest for monitoring adverse side effects for specific agents.

PATIENT EDUCATION

The patient and the family, as indicated, should be fully informed about the nature of the patient's condition, the need for analgesia, and the treatment plan. This information is discussed collaboratively with the physician and others involved in the patient's general care. The patient should be involved in care planning whenever possible and should have a clear understanding of the medication, its exact name, general action, dosage, administration and adverse side effects. The patient should also know how to minimize or prevent side effects whenever possible. The patient should also be informed of the abuse and addiction potential of narcotic analgesics. This should be done without unduly alarming the patient and the family. Instruction concerning the use of narcotics in the home environment is extremely important in preventing abuse and accidental poisoning, which can result in death. Patient education is influenced by the patient's condition and requirements for analgesia. See the following sections on assisting patients with acute self-limiting pain, chronic cancer pain, and chronic benign pain.

GENERAL NURSING IMPLICATIONS—cont'd

Nursing of patients with acute self-limiting pain

Carefully assess the patient's pain, because this is extremely important in individualizing pain management. When a patient complains of pain, do not assume that the pain is related to a patient's trauma (e.g., assuming that a surgical patient is always having surgical pain; the patient may have a headache or a sore back from sleeping on a different bed). Instruct the patient to explain exactly how the pain feels in his or her own words. If this is difficult for the patient, pain assessment tools such as the McGill-Melzack pain questionnaire can be used. Document this information and your assessment on the chart. Include your own observations along with the patient's vital signs; however, these are not considered valid indicators of pain by themselves.

Never administer a pain medication until a note has been made in the patient's chart of when the last medication was given for pain. If pain is not being relieved, this needs to be explored with the patient and the prescriber. Noninvasive nursing measures can be used to increase the effectiveness of the medication. If ineffective, alternate pain management will need to be considered.

Until a postoperative patient is fully recovered from the anesthetic, pain medications, if indicated, must be carefully administered and monitored because they can interact with and potentiate the residual effects of some anesthetics (see Chapter 14, "General Anesthetics").

Before administering a medication to a patient who has not received the medication before, find out if the patient has allergies to the medication. Often during the stress and excitement of admission and even surgery, the patient will forget or possibly not understand what was meant by the question during the nursing history. The patient's response to the medication should be carefully monitored. Observations of any skin rash, localized wheal, flare, generalized urticaria, or other unusual reactions should be reported immediately.

Tell the patient the medication is for pain relief and how long it will take to be effective. Sometimes the patient expects immediate relief. Also, do not forget the importance of using noninvasive nursing measures to alleviate pain and to enhance drug response, including positioning and making the patient more comfortable, washing the patient's face, helping with oral hygiene, helping the patient relax through diversional techniques, and decreasing overstimulation. Monitor the patient's response to the analgesic. Check back with the patient to see if the pain is increased, decreased, or relieved by the medication or other measures. Use bedside rails as a safety precaution for those patients who become somnolent or confused, and always use rails as a precaution when patients are receiving the medication for the first time. Always place the call light in reach. Document your findings.

Schedule activities of daily living, treatments, and postoperative coughing, deep breathing, and leg exercises in relation to peak effects of analgesia. These should not be performed when the patient is in severe pain.

Do not be afraid to awaken the patient at night. When dealing with severe pain problems (e.g., trauma, postoperative pain), care must be taken to deliver analgesics promptly on time, as well as on a pain-contingent basis. This gives the patient confidence and decreases anxiety, which can aggravate pain. It also enables the nurse to monitor responses effectively so that decisions for appropriate changes in dose or schedule can be made to optimize the analgesia. Consultation with the prescriber may be indicated to optimize pain management.

The management of pain in the postoperative patient is directly related to preoperative teaching. Apathy, anger, fear, and tension are common reactions to pain and illness. Preoperative teaching cannot be overemphasized in relation to pain management. Patients with acute trauma also require teaching about tests and procedures, as tolerated.

Narcotic analgesics should be used with caution in the elderly, in debilitated patients, or in patients who have head injuries.

Monitor pulse, blood pressure, and respiratory rate until the patient's dosage and physiologic responses are stabilized. Pay particular attention to the respiratory rate at the time of peak activity of the administered agent.

Report a respiratory rate reduction of 10 or less ventilations per minute, and hold the medication because further respiratory depression can result.

Monitor intake and output and observe for urinary retention, constipation, nausea, or cough suppression.

Individualize teaching for the patient and the family as indicated in relation to observing the effects and side effects of the medication.

Monitor for the development of tolerance of the medication.

Narcotic antagonists should not be administered with potent narcotics, because this will block their effect, unless they are used to treat an overdose.

Continued.

GENERAL NURSING IMPLICATIONS—cont'd

Nursing of patients with chronic cancer pain

Carefully assess the patient's pain and reevaluate it as necessary.

Monitor the effectiveness of the analgesia and tailor it to the patient's individual needs. Reevaluate as necessary.

Dependence should not be a concern if the medication provides a better quality of life.

Administer the analgesic at regular intervals over a 24-hour period, especially through the night, to maintain constant analgesic blood levels. Evaluate the effectiveness of the medication in relation to various periods of the day.

Involve the patient and the family, as indicated, in planning, carrying out, and evaluating programs of pain control.

Plan to minimize drug side effects.

Schedule patient care activities to coincide with the peak action of the analgesic.

Nursing of patients with chronic benign pain

Monitor for signs of physical and psychologic dependence.

Monitor for symptoms of withdrawal that may occur with physical dependence, especially when drug regimens are changed. These include sweating, nausea, abdominal cramps, diarrhea, or muscle pain.

Explore alternative methods of pain relief with the patient and the family, as indicated.

As described by Donovan and Keith (1979), successful management of chronic pain after discharge from the hospital requires careful attention to the equivalent dose of medication when changing from a parenteral to a nonparenteral route. In preparation for the transition from hospital to home medication changes if indicated should be made 48 hours before discharge. This enables the patient to do the following: (1) have an opportunity to experience the change in the route of administration in a controlled environment; (2) evaluate the effectiveness of the medication in relation to individualized goals with assistance, as required; (3) have the dose and interval of administration individualized to the patient's own needs and lifestyle; (4) observe individual reactions to the medication, including adverse side effects; and (5) receive systematic and individualized teaching regarding the preparation, administration, and monitoring of the effects of the medication.

In planning for discharge, the nurse should do the following.

Make sure the patient has written discharge instructions to prevent misunderstandings, even though instructions may have been given verbally. The instruction sheet should be gone over with the patient and the patient's understanding should be assessed. Areas that are not clear or that the patient does not understand should be carefully gone over and reemphasized.

Before discharging the patient from the hospital, establish a time schedule for the pain medications to fit the patient's lifestyle and needs for the analgesic, because the hospital schedule may not be appropriate for the patient's needs when discharged. The patient should understand the importance of an individualized plan.

Emphasize that the medication should not be skipped or doubled in case of an increase in pain or to make up for a missed dose.

Teach the patient to monitor for side effects from the medication.

Provide the patient with teaching cards, specifying the name of the drug, action, and instructions (see General Instructions for Discharge/Outpatients).

GENERAL INSTRUCTIONS FOR DISCHARGE/OUTPATIENTS*

This medication is a *narcotic analgesic* used to treat pain. If you do not understand why you are receiving this medication, consult your health care provider.

Follow the instructions on the prescription exactly.

Do not take alcohol, sleeping medications, tranquilizers, high blood pressure medications, or other pain medications without specific instructions by a nurse, pharmacist or physician who knows you are taking this medication.

Skin rash, lightheadedness, drowsiness, and constipation can occur. If these persist or become extreme notify your nurse, pharmacist, or physician.

This medication can cause drowsiness, which may impair your ability to drive or operate dangerous equipment and can impair mental alertness. If you, a relative, or a fellow employee notices impairment then those situations should be avoided and your nurse or physician should be notified.

This medication has been prescribed specifically for you. Do not sell, trade, or give this medication to relatives, friends, or others.

Keep this and all other medications out of the reach of children.

*These instructions do *not* apply to aspirin or acetaminophen.

NURSING DRUG DIGEST

Medication (trade name*)	Indication	Usual dosage and administration†	Dosage forms, preparation, and storage	Contraindications, cautions, and comments	Monitoring
NARCOTICS **Alphaprodine** Nisentil	Acute pain Dental analgesia Obstetric analgesia	*Adults:* 0.4-0.6 mg/kg IV; or 0.4-1.2 mg/kg SC Maximum: 240 mg/24 hr *Children:* 0.3-0.6 mg/kg SC for dental use *Adults:* 30-60 mg SC, repeat at 2-hr intervals as indicated Do not administer IM	Injectable: 40, 60 mg/ml Discard discolored or cloudy solutions	*Contraindicated* in hypersensitivity Duration of action is 1-2 hr SC and 20-40 min IV; therefore use is limited to short operative procedures such as joint manipulation, suture removal and IV for short anesthetics in combination with other drugs; not appropriate for long-term administration Same adverse effects and drug interactions as all narcotic analgesics	Respiratory depression is the most significant problem of overdose, and respiratory rates less than 10/min indicate significant depression (hold next dose); if used during labor, newborns respirations must be closely monitored (naloxone often given to mother just before delivery)
Anileridine Apodol Leritine	Acute pain Obstetric analgesia	*Adults:* 25-50 mg PO q.4-6h.; or 25-75 mg IM/SC q.4-6h. *Adults:* 50 mg SC, repeat at 3-4 hr intervals as indicated Maximum: 200 mg/24 hr IV use is *not* generally recommended	Injectable: 25 mg/ml Tablets: 25 mg	Duration of action is 2-4 hr; often used as post-operative analgesic for 1-2 days; oral form for outpatient oral surgery; popular as a premedication before surgery	Monitor respiration; if used during labor, newborn's respiration must be closely monitored
Brompton's cocktail	Chronic pain associated with terminal cancer	Dose variable depending on contents and severity of pain; usually administered q.4h. PO around the clock Use has been largely replaced by morphine sulfate solution, which is commercially available	Not available commercially; prepared in hospital pharmacy No uniform formula for this medication; generally contains a narcotic ± cocaine (in the United States a phenothiazine is often included) ± alcohol in a liquid form; narcotic originally was heroin, but morphine is used now	Usually used for pain associated with cancer Precautions are related to varying contents. If you are supervising its use, make yourself familiar with *all* of the ingredients and their effects singly and in combination Brompton's is a potent oral liquid analgesic that can provide a pain-free state *without* the side effects of a clouded sensorium	Monitor respiratory rate

Drug	Indication	Dosage	Preparations	Comments	Nursing considerations
Codeine A.S.A. and Codeine Compound* Bufferin with Codeine No. 3* C3* C4* Empirin with Codeine* Phenaphen with Codeine* Tylenol with Codeine*	Mild acute pain Cough Chronic intermittent pain	*Adults:* 0.5-1 mg/kg q.4-6h. SC/IM/PO *Children:* 0.5 mg/kg q.4-6h. SC/IM/PO *Adults:* 5-10 mg PO q.3-6h. *Children:* 1-1.5 mg/kg/24 hr in 4-6 divided doses Maximum: 60 mg/24 hr *Adults:* 0.5-2 mg/kg PO q.4-6h. *Children:* 0.5-1.0 mg/kg PO q.4-6h. Maximum: 60 mg/24 hr	Tablets: 15, 30, 60 mg Injectable: 15, 30, 60 mg/ml Elixir: 10 mg/5 ml	Studies indicate that cocaine plus morphine offers no analgesic advantage over morphine alone *Contraindicated* in hypersensitivity Duration of action is 4-6 hours by oral or parenteral route; not useful in severe pain states; one of the most constipating of commonly used narcotics; nausea and dizziness are also common side effects; one of the most common narcotics in prescription and nonprescription cough preparations	Be cautious of and monitor for the possibility of patients receiving multiple narcotics simultaneously; patients may receive codeine in a cough preparation, as well as compounded with other agents such as aspirin, acetaminophen, or caffeine in many popular preparations Monitor for abuse and dependence Observe for allergic reaction Monitor for GI distress
★ **Drocode** Compal* Synalgos-DC*	Moderate to severe pain	*Adults:* 0.4-0.5 mg/kg q.4-6h. PO	Tablets: 16, 30 mg Usually found in combination with other active ingredients	Duration of action is 4-6 hr; not a common drug and no real advantage over other agents such as morphine and meperidine This drug has respiratory depressant, circulatory effects, and drug interactions similar to the more common narcotics	Monitor respiration

Continued.

NOTE: For additional details regarding the individual agents listed in this table see the text and other tables in this chapter:

*Indicates a multiple active ingredient product. For a complete listing of all active ingredients see the *Drug Reference Guide to Brand Names and Active Ingredients.*

†No maximum dosages have been provided for the narcotic analgesics. In most individuals, tolerance occurs, which leads to increased dosages needed to provide analgesia. This is *not* usually the case for the elderly, and therefore drug dosages should begin at the lower limit and be increased cautiously. For others, the dose should be titrated to pain relief with somnolence and decreased respiratory rate to 10 or below as an indication of overdosage. These medications should be used with caution in children less than 1 year of age.

✦ Indicates that the drug is generally available only in Canada.

★ Indicates that the drug is generally available only in the United States.

NURSING DRUG DIGEST—cont'd

Medication (trade name)	Indication	Usual dosage and administration	Dosage forms, preparation, and storage	Contraindications, cautions, and comments	Monitoring
★ **Ethoheptazine** Equagesic* Meprogesic* Zactane Zactirin*	Mild acute pain	*Adults:* 75-150 mg PO t.i.d. to q.i.d. To decrease GI upset administer with food or milk	Tablet: 75 mg	Duration of action is 2-4 hr; this drug is little used because it has similar analgesic properties to aspirin or low-dose codeine but shows no other advantage; little respiratory or circulatory depression seen in usual dosages	Observe for GI distress
Fentanyl Innovar* Sublimaze	Adjunct to general anesthetic See also Chapter 14, "General Anesthetics"	*Adults:* 2-20 µg/kg SC/IM No cardiovascular effects even in doses to 0.7 mg/kg IV; duration of action and respiratory depression may be prolonged with higher doses and in the elderly Not to be used in children less than 2 years of age or in pregnant women because of poor knowledge of possible untoward effects	Injectable: 0.05 mg/ml Protect from light Store at room temperature	Duration of action is 20-40 min IV; because of this, it is most often used as an IV analgesic during general anesthesia; it may be used IM as a premedicant (duration 1-2 hr); no real indication otherwise except for short minor surgical procedures without general anesthesia	Close postoperative monitoring of respiratory rate for up to 12 hr following its use in anesthesia may be warranted
Heroin	Rarely used in clinical practice (illegal drug in United States and Canada)	*Adults:* 0.05-0.1 mg/kg SC/IM or IV q.4h.	Not legally available in the United States or Canada	Duration of action 3-4 hr; not available except experimentally in Canada and the United States; some limited use in the United Kingdom for cancer pain, but recent studies have not shown it to be superior to other narcotics for this purpose	Monitor for respiratory depression
Hydrocodone Adatuss D.C. Expectorant* Citra Forte*	Cough suppressant Mild acute pain	*Adults:* 5 mg PO q.4h. *Children:* 2-12 years of age, 1.25-5 mg PO q.4h. *Adults:* 5-10 mg PO q.4-6h. Maximum: 40 mg/24 hr	Tablet: 5 mg Syrup: 2.5, 5 mg/ml	*Contraindicated* in hypersensitivity or respiratory depression	Monitor for abuse and dependence Monitor for respiratory depression

Drug	Use	Dosage forms	Dosage	Remarks
Codone Corutol DH Dicodid Entuss Expectorant Hycodan* Hycomine* Hycotuss* Mercodinone Robidone S-T Forte Tussend Expectorant* Tussend* Tussionex* Vicodin*				Duration of action 4-8 hr; primarily used as a cough suppressant; not superior to codeine As with codeine, the major side effect in long usage to be considered is constipation
Hydromorphone Dilaudid Hymorphan	Moderate to severe acute pain Cough mixture	Tablets: 1, 2, 3, 4 mg Injectable: 1, 2, 3, 4 mg/ml Syrup: 1 mg/5 ml Rectal suppositories: 3 mg	*Adults:* 1-4 mg q.4-6h. PO/SC/IM/IV (IV injections should be administered slowly over 2-3 min); or 3 mg q.6-8h. PR *Adults:* 1 mg q.3-4h. PO	*Contraindicated* in hypersensitivity, increased intracranial pressure, and respiratory depression Duration of action 4-5 hr A good drug for acute severe pain of short duration; the advantage of this medication over others such as morphine or meperidine is its good oral absorption; this drug has a significant abuse potential and is a base for iatrogenic addiction when used inappropriately for chronic pain Similar to morphine because it is a close derivative; equal dosage both orally and parenterally Use with caution in elderly patients	In overdose, monitoring of respiratory rate is important; rates of 10/min or below require treatment with naloxone Monitor for abuse and dependence

Continued.

NURSING DRUG DIGEST—cont'd

Medication (trade name)	Indication	Usual dosage and administration	Dosage forms, preparation, and storage	Contraindications, cautions, and comments	Monitoring
Levorphanol Levo-Dromoran	Moderate to severe acute pain	*Adults:* 1-3 mg q.4-8h. SC/PO Duration of action is about 4-8 hr when given parenterally, but about 6 hr when used orally; for this reason the PO route has been suggested for long-term administration Note difference in *duration* of oral and parenteral forms; dosage timing must be changed, especially when changing from SC to PO because more frequent dosing of PO form can lead to accumulation and toxic effects (e.g., respiratory depression)	Injectable: 2 mg/ml Tablet: 2 mg	Side effects are less than with morphine, and addiction is less of a problem	Monitor for respiratory depression
Meperidine Demer-Idine Demerol Dolantal Dolantin Mefedina Mepergan* Phytadon	Premedication for surgery Intravenous analgesia Acute pain Cancer pain	*Adults:* 1 mg/kg SC/IM 30-90 min before anesthetic *Children:* 1 mg/kg SC/IM 30-90 min before anesthetic *Adults:* 0.5-1 mg/kg IV *Children:* 0.5 mg/kg IV *Adults:* 1 mg/kg SC/IM *Children:* 1 mg/kg SC/IM *Adults:* 1-3 mg/kg PO *Children:* 1-3 mg/kg PO IV dosage should be diluted and administered slowly over 3-5 min with patient in a recumbent position Note difference in dosage between oral and parenteral forms; less drug absorption by the oral route means higher dose levels orally; with IV administration, drug is excreted into the stomach and reabsorbed producing a late increased effect; watch for this especially postoperatively when this has been used as an anesthetic agent; avoid SC injection because this is painful	Elixir: 50 mg/5 ml Injectable: 50, 100 mg/ml vials Ampules: 0.5, 1.0, 1.5, 2.0 mg Tablets: 50, 100 mg Syrup: 50 mg/5 ml Do *not* mix barbiturate and meperidine injectables because they are physically incompatible	*Contraindicated* in patients taking monoamine oxidase inhibitors because patients may have cardiovascular collapse *Contraindicated* in patients with porphyria because it can precipitate an acute attack Duration of action is 2-4 hr when given orally and parenterally; it is a synthetic narcotic with fewer side effects than morphine in terms of smooth muscle spasm, which makes it the drug of choice in renal colic and biliary colic It also causes relaxation of bronchial spasm in asthma and is used as a sedative in acute asthmatic attacks for this reason	Monitor blood pressure

Drug	Use	Dosage	Preparations	Remarks
				Common adverse effects include cardiovascular depression, dizziness, nausea, or vomiting
Methadone Adanon Amidone Athose Dolophine Westadone	Moderate to severe acute pain Cancer pain	*Adults:* 0.1 mg/kg SC/IM *Adults:* 2.5-10 mg PO q3-4h. prn Duration of action is 3-5 hr by parenteral route, 6-8 hr by oral route Note difference in *duration* from parenteral to oral forms; too frequent dosage by the oral route will lead to accumulation of drug and toxicity over a few days (somnolence and respiratory depression are produced) *Reduce dosage in renal impairment* Parenteral route is *not* indicated for more than single dose administration if patients are able to swallow and GI function is intact.	Tablets: 5, 10, 40 mg Injectable: 10 mg/ml Syrup: 5 mg/15 ml Solution: 1 mg/ml (oral)	Because drug has a topical anesthetic effect, oral liquid form (syrup) should be given with a glassful of water. Narcotic antagonist and resuscitation equipment should be immediately available This drug has a low incidence of side effects as compared with morphine; well tolerated for this reason; with long duration of action it is a good drug for treating cancer pain; this plus there is less euphoria than with heroin make it useful for maintenance of narcotic addicts
	Methadone maintenance	*Adults:* 10-120 mg/24 hr PO		
				As with all narcotics, respiratory depression is of particular importance as an indicator of toxicity and must be closely monitored; for morphine and any other narcotic, a respiratory rate of 10/min or less indicates overdose; the next narcotic dose is held; naloxone made available, and continued frequent monitoring of the respiratory
Morphine M.O.S. Syrup RMS Suppositories	Premedication for surgery Intravenous analgesia Acute pain Cancer pain	*Adults:* 0.1-0.2 mg/kg SC/IM 30-90 min before anesthetic *Children:* 0.2 mg/kg SC/IM 30-90 min before anesthetic *Adults:* 0.05-0.1 mg/kg IV *Children:* 0.1 mg/kg IV *Adults:* 0.1-0.2 mg/kg SC/IM *Children:* 0.2 mg/kg SC/IM *Adults:* 0.2-0.4 mg/kg PO, PR q. 4-6h. prn *Children:* 0.2-0.4 mg/kg PO, PR q4-6h. prn Administer IV doses *slowly* NOTE: As a general rule, to switch from parenteral to oral morphine the dose is doubled (e.g., 5 mg IV = 10 mg PO)	Injectable: 2, 4, 8, 10, 15, 30 mg/ml Tablets: 10, 15, 30 mg Syrup: 1 mg/ml (contains 5% alcohol) Solution (oral): 5, 10, 20 mg/5 ml Rectal suppositories: 10, 20 mg	Contraindicated in hypersensitivity; cardiac dysrhythmias, severe hypotension, and severe cirrhosis The prototype of all narcotic analgesics and the yardstick by which they are measured; duration of action is 4-5 hr by the oral or parenteral route; oral absorption is less adequate than with the SC/IM route; side effects include respiratory depression, eu-

Continued.

NURSING DRUG DIGEST—cont'd

Medication (trade name)	Indication	Usual dosage and administration	Dosage forms, preparation, and storage	Contraindications, cautions, and comments	Monitoring
Morphine—cont'd				phoria, nausea, vomiting, constipation, pupillary constriction, or vascular dilatation; decreased cardiac output and cardiac work and oxygen consumption after an MI, but not in the normal heart (this is one reason for it being the drug of choice in MI); it also causes smooth muscle spasm (*not* being the drug of choice in renal or biliary colic); increased sweating and itching are sometimes seen	rate and the level of consciousness is necessary. Monitor for signs of withdrawal, including agitation, pupillary dilatation, GI cramps, or piloerection
Opium alkaloids Pantopon	Acute pain	*Adults:* 20-60 mg/kg SC/IM Maximum: 120 mg/24 hr *Children:* Over 2 years of age, 1 mg/year of age SC/IM	Tablets: 60 mg Injectable: 20 mg/ml Often found in combination (e.g., opium and belladonna)	These are a combination of many drugs both active and inactive; the major active ingredient is morphine (10%-50%), and therefore the comments applicable to morphine should be reviewed	See Morphine
Oxycodone Eudol Mictoben Percobarb* Percocet* Percocet-Demi* Percocet-5* Percodan* Percodan-Demi* Proladone Supeudol Tylox*	Moderate to severe acute pain Cough mixtures	*Adults:* 5 mg PO q.6h. *Children: Not* recommended for use in children *Adults:* 3-5 mg PO q.4-6h.	Solution: 5 mg/5 ml Tablets: 2.5, 5 mg	The duration of action is 4-5 hr; well absorbed orally and a good compound for oral use in moderate to severe pain of short duration; this drug has a high addiction potential and is a frequently abused oral narcotic; *not* to be used for chronic benign pain	Monitor for abuse and dependence

Oxymorphone Numorphan	Moderate to severe acute pain	*Adults:* 1-1.5 mg SC/IM q.4-6h.; or 5 mg PR q.4-6h.	Injectable: 1, 1.5 mg/ml Rectal suppository: 5 mg	Duration of action is 4-5 hr; supposedly with less respiratory depressant activity for equianalgesic effect when compared with morphine Not a high addictive potential A good suppository form available for use when oral route not available and one wishes to avoid IM or SC	Monitor for respiratory depression
Propoxyphene Algodex Darvocet-N* Darvon Darvon with A.S.A.* Darvon-N Darvon-N Compound* Dolene Dolene Compound-65* Doloxene Femadol Levadol Pargesic 65 Progesic Proxagesic	Mild pain	*Adults:* 65 mg (of chloride form) PO q.4h. (maximum 390 mg/24 hr); or 100 mg (of napsylate form) q.4h. (maximum 600 mg/24 hr)	Capsules: 32, 65 mg as chloride salt Tablets: 50, 100 mg as napsylate salt Suspension: 10 mg/ml as napsylate salt	Duration of action is 4-6 hr; except with overdose; no real precautions; despite its reputation as being non-addictive, it is a drug of abuse and frequent requests for repeat prescriptions need investigation; not to be used in severe pain; no real advantage for pain over aspirin or acetaminophen; as effective as low-dose codeine in some studies but without GI side effects; said not to be addictive and without serious side effects, but overdoses have caused death; probably overprescribed presently	Monitor for abuse and dependence
NARCOTIC AGONIST/ANTAGONIST **Butorphanol** Stadol	Acute pain Intravenous analgesia	*Adults:* 1-3 mg IM q.3-4h. *Adults:* 0.5-2 mg IV *Children:* Use is *not* recommended	Injectable: 1, 2 mg/ml Store at room temperature	Duration of action is 3-4 hr; not a widely used drug; perhaps somewhat safer than other narcotics in high doses because it causes less respiratory depression; otherwise,	

Continued.

NURSING DRUG DIGEST—cont'd

Medication (trade name)	Indication	Usual dosage and administration	Dosage forms, preparation, and storage	Contraindications, cautions, and comments	Monitoring
Butorphanol— cont'd				similar to pentazocine; low addiction potential; this drug is more potent than morphine and appears to have a ceiling effect in terms of respiratory depression; this is a theoretical advantage to this drug because a relative overdose should not produce a compromising respiratory depression; this drug is similar in action and side effects to pentazocine, although without pronounced psychotomimetic effects; it causes a significant increase in workload on the heart	
Levallorphan Lorfan	Narcotic overdosage (little used now)	Adults: 1 mg IV followed by 1-2 additional 0.5 mg doses at 15 min intervals Maximum: 3 mg total Children (neonatal): 0.05-0.25 IM/SC or into the umbilical cord vein after delivery NOTE: Use is not generally recommended	Injectable: 1 mg/ml	Since the advent of naloxone, a relatively pure narcotic antagonist, this drug is not as popular, and naloxone, because it is a pure narcotic antagonist, is recommended instead	Monitor for respiratory depression
Nalbuphine Nubain	Acute pain Intravenous analgesia	Adults: 0.2 mg/kg SC/IM q.3-6h. Adults: 0.1-0.2 mg/kg IV q.3-6h. Maximum: 160 mg/24 hr	Injectable: 10, 20 mg/ml Store at room temperature Protect from excessive light	This newer agent needs to age clinically so its true usefullness can be assessed; be aware of its antagonist properties and avoid use in patients on other narcotics to prevent opiate withdrawal symptoms	

Drug	Use	Dosage	Preparations	Remarks	Nursing considerations
				Duration of action is 3-6 hr; another agonist and antagonist drug but with weak antagonist effects	
				About as potent as morphine as an analgesic, but as with butorphanol, there is a ceiling effect to the respiratory depression, which gives it a theoretical advantage over morphine and meperidine; like these drugs, it also lowers the cardiac workload and may be useful for patients in heart failure or following an MI; it can produce an abstinence syndrome if given to people on chronic narcotics; few side effects on low dosage	
Pentazocine Fortalgesic Talwin Talwin Compound* Talwin Nx*	Mild acute pain	*Adults:* 30-60 mg SC/IM/IV q.3-4h.; *or* 50-100 mg PO q.3-4h. Note the difference in dose between oral and parenteral use; SC injection is irritating and should be avoided for long-term administration Pentazocine is about one-fourth to one-third as effective orally as parenterally	Injectable: 30 mg/ml Tablets: 50 mg	Duration of action is 3-4 hr The first useful agonist and antagonist for use as an analgesic; it was synthesized to produce a drug with minimal abuse potential, but it has become a drug of abuse because of its psychotomimetic effects, especially in doses above 60 mg; respiratory depression appears to have a ceiling effect; GI disturbances correspond to equianalgesic doses of morphine at low doses but are less at higher doses	Monitor for abuse and dependence

Continued.

NURSING DRUG DIGEST—cont'd

Medication (trade name)	Indication	Usual dosage and administration	Dosage forms, preparation, and storage	Contraindications, cautions, and comments	Monitoring
Pentazocine—cont'd				Dysphoria, nightmares, and confusion may occur at higher doses; these can be relieved with naloxone Pentazocine can cause withdrawal symptoms in patients on chronic pure narcotic agonists and they should not receive it Because of widespread abuse one formulation (Talwin Nx) contains both pentazocine and naloxone in an attempt to discourage illicit injection of the tablet form of pentazocine	

PHENOTHIAZINE ANALGESIC

Medication (trade name)	Indication	Usual dosage and administration	Dosage forms, preparation, and storage	Contraindications, cautions, and comments	Monitoring
Methotrimeprazine Levoprome Nozinan Veractil	Moderate acute pain Mild chronic pain Premedication for surgery	*Adults:* 0.2-0.3 mg/kg IM q.4-6h. *Adults:* 2-25 mg PO t.i.d. with meals *Adults:* 0.15-0.3 mg/kg IM 45-90 min before anesthetic Must be given *deep IM, not IV* or SC, because of local irritation See also Chapter 18, "Drugs Used to Treat Psychotic Disorders"	Tablets: 2, 5, 25, 50 mg Injectable: 20 mg/ml	Duration of action is 4-6 hr; this is a phenothiazine derivative with tranquilizing and analgesic effects; side effects are orthostatic hypotension (usually clears after a few doses); may produce amnesia, disorientation, drowsiness, slurring of speech, weakness, GI upset, chills, or urinary retention; with continued usage, hepatic dysfunction may be seen Effects may be increased when given with barbiturates, atropine, meprobamate, and antihypertensive agents	

NARCOTIC ANTAGONIST (PURE)

Drug	Indication	Dosage	Comments
Naloxone Narcan	Narcotic overdose	Injectable: 0.4 mg/ml; 0.02 mg/ml (neonatal injection) *Adults:* 0.4-2.0 mg SC/IM/IV q.1-4h. prn for reversal of narcotic effects *Children and neonates:* 0.01 mg/kg IV/IM/SC q.1-4h. prn for reversal of narcotic effects Because of the relatively long duration of action of many narcotics, readminister naloxone at periodic intervals for up to 48 hr	Duration of action is 1-4 hr; this pure narcotic antagonist is the ideal drug for reversal of narcotic side effects, especially respiratory depression; analgesia is also reversed; side effects are minimal with some nausea and occasional vomiting the most common This drug may reverse analgesia and respiratory depression from many nonnarcotic drugs Because of the relatively short duration of action in low doses, careful monitoring of respiratory rates in narcotic overdose is necessary to indicate possible repeat naloxone administration (respiratory rate less than 10 min) Monitor for acute narcotic withdrawal reaction in dependent individuals

NONNARCOTIC ANALGESICS

Drug	Indication	Dosage	Comments
Acetaminophen Acephen Acetamin Aspirin Free Anacin-3* Atasol Bromo-Seltzer* Co Tylenol* Congesprin* Darvocet-N* Datril Datril 500 Daycare* Excedrin* Excedrin P.M.* Femcaps Pamprin* Panadol Percocet* Percocet-5* Percogesic* Tempra Tranquil Tylenol Tylenol with Codeine*	Mild pain, fever	Tablets: 80, 120, 325, 500, 650 mg Elixir: 120, 160 mg/5 ml Syrup: 120 mg/5 ml Drops: 100, 120 mg/ml Capsules: 325, 500 mg NOTE: The drops are approximately 5 times more concentrated than either the elixir or the syrup *Adults:* 300-1000 mg PO q.4-6h. Maximum: 4000 mg/24 hr (short-term use); 2600 mg/24 hr (long-term use) *Children:* 5-15 mg/kg PO q.4-6h. Maximum: 65 mg/kg/24 hr	*Contraindicated* in hypersensitivity and severe hepatic dysfunction Duration of action is 4-6 hr This drug has analgesic and antipyretic effects but no antiinflammatory effects It is the drug of choice in febrile states where aspirin is contraindicated It is not an innocuous drug and with acute overdosage hepatic necrosis, renal tubular necrosis and hypoglycemic coma can occur and be fatal; chronic overdose can produce anemia As with aspirin, this drug should be used only with specific indications, such as mild pain or fever Chronic ingestion can lead to complications and should be discouraged Monitor hepatic function in patients on long-term chronic therapy

Continued.

NURSING DRUG DIGEST—cont'd

Medication (trade name)	Indication	Usual dosage and administration	Dosage forms, preparation, and storage	Contraindications, cautions, and comments	Monitoring
Acetaminophen—cont'd Tylenol Extra Strength Valadol Vanquish Caplet*				Use with caution in presence of impaired hepatic function. Overdose of acetaminophen should be treated with *N*-acetylcysteine 140 mg/kg PO, followed by 70 mg/kg q.4h. for 72 hr	Observe for allergic reaction Monitor for GI distress
Aspirin Acetal Alka-Seltzer Plus* Anacin* Arthritis Pain Formula* Arthritis Strength Bufferin* Aspergum Bayer Aspirin Bayer Children's Aspirin Bayer Timed-Release Aspirin Bufferin with Codeine No.3* Bufferin* Congespirin* Cope* Dolene Compound-65*	Mild pain, especially associated with inflammation (e.g., arthritis); fever. Acute rheumatic fever. Transient (cerebral) ischemic attacks. See also Chapter 58, "Nonsteroidal Antiinflammatory Drugs"	*Adults:* 325-650 mg PO, PR q.4-6h. Maximum: 3.9 gm/24 hr. *Children:* 10-20 mg/kg PO, PR q.6h. Maximum: 3.6 gm/24 hr. NOTE: For treatment of arthritis and rheumatic conditions, a serum salicylate level of 20-30 mg/dl should be maintained. *Adults:* 100 mg/kg/24 hr in divided doses. Maximum: 7.8 gm/24 hr. *Children:* 100 mg/kg/24 hr in divided doses. *Adults* (men): 1300 mg/24 hr PO in 2-4 divided doses	Tablets: 65 to 650 mg. Capsules: 300 mg. Rectal suppositories: 65 to 1300 mg	*Contraindicated* in hypersensitivity, peptic ulcer disease, hemophilia, hemorrhagic states, and acute viral infections in children. Duration of action is 4-6 hr. This is not an innocuous drug; toxic reactions to overdose can be fatal and are too common in children. Avoid in patients with peptic ulcer disease and in those with an allergic history; early signs of toxicity are CNS-related tinnitus; if this is reported, hold the next dose of the drug until the symptoms disappear; review drug interactions	

Empirin Compound*
Empirin with Codeine*
Excedrin P.M.*
Excedrin*
Midol*
Percodan*
St. Joseph Aspirin
Talwin Compound*
Vanquish Caplet*

Use with extreme caution, if at all, in patients receiving anticoagulants

Use should be avoided in children with viral conditions (e.g., influenza, chickenpox) because of the associated higher risk of developing the potentially fatal Reye's syndrome; Reye's syndrome is characterized by vomiting and lethargy, which may progress to delirium and coma in children recovering from viral infections; death occurs in approximately 30% of cases and permanent brain damage in many others

If aspirin has a vinegar odor, discard because it has broken down to acetic acid and is ineffective

BIBLIOGRAPHY

Bonica, J.J. *Management of Pain* (2nd ed.). Philadelphia: Lea & Febiger (in press).

Boyer, M.W. Continuous drip morphine. *American Journal of Nursing*, 1982, *82*(4), 602-604.

Bradberry, J.C., & Raebel, M.A. Continuous infusion of naloxone in the treatment of narcotic overdose. *Drug Intelligence and Clinical Pharmacy*, 1981, *15*, 945-949.

Collins, J.A. "Cocktails" for relief of cancer pain. *Geriatrics*, 1982, *37*(3), 136-143.

Coyle, N. Analgesics at the bedside. *American Journal of Nursing*, 1979, *79*(9), 1554-1557.

DiBlasi, M., & Washburn, C.J. Using analgesics effectively. *American Journal of Nursing*, 1979, *79*(1), 74, 78.

Donovan, C., & Keith, L. Chronic pain management: transition from hospital to home. *Nursing Drug Alert, New York*, 1979, *3*, 16.

Gerbershagen, H. Non-narcotic analgesics. In J. Bonica and V. Ventafridda (Eds.). Advances in pain research and therapy, vol. 2. New York: Raven Press, 1976.

Gever, L.N. Brompton's mixture: how it relieves the pain of terminal cancer. *Nursing 80*, 1980, *10*(5), 57.

Gever, L.N. A new treatment for a new problem—acetaminophen overdose. *Nursing 80*, 1980, *10*(5), 57.

Houde, R.W. Narcotic analgesics. In J. Bonica and V. Ventafridda (Eds.). Advances in pain research and therapy, Vol. 2. New York: Raven Press, 1976.

Jacox, A.K. Assessing pain. *American Journal of Nursing*, 1979, *79*(5), 895-900.

Jaffe, J.N., & Martin, W.R. Opioid analgesics and antagonists. In A.G. Gilman, L.S. Goodman, & A. Gilman (Eds.). The pharmacological basis of therapeutics (6th ed.). New York: MacMillan, Inc., 1980.

Jozwiak, J.S. Acetaminophen overdose a new—and treacherous—care problem. *RN*, 1978, *41*(12), 56-62.

Macy, A.M. Preventing hepatotoxicity in acetaminophen overdose. *American Journal of Nursing*, 1979, *79*(2), 301-303.

Martinson, I.M., Nixon, S., Geis, D., YaDeau, R., Nesbit, M., & Kersey, J. Nursing care in childhood cancer—methadone. *American Journal of Nursing*, 1982, *82*(3), 432-435.

Maxwell, M.B. How to use methadone for the cancer patient's pain. *American Journal of Nursing*, 1980, *80*(9), 1606-1609.

McCaffery, M. *Nursing management of the patient with pain* (2nd ed.). Philadelphia: J.B. Lippincott Co., 1979.

McCaffery, M. Relieve your patient's pain fast and effectively with oral analgesics. *Nursing 80*, 1980, *10*(10), 58.

McCaffery, M. Patients shouldn't have to suffer: how to relieve pain with injectable narcotics. *Nursing 80*, 1980, *10*(10), 34-39.

Meissner, J.E. How can you improve the care of the hospitalized child? McGill-Melzack pain questionnaire. *Nursing 80*, 1980, *10*(10), 50-51.

Mount, B.M., Ajemian, I., & Scott, J.F. Use of the Brompton mixture in treating the chronic pain of malignant disease. *Nursing Digest*, 1977, *5*(2), 49.

Pfeiffer, R.F. Drugs for pain in the elderly. *Geriatrics*, 37(2), 67.

Pierce, P.F. About analgesics and kidney damage. *Nurses' Drug Alert*, 4(12), 89.

Rankin, M.A. Use of drugs for pain with cancer patients. *Cancer Nursing*, 1982, *5*(3), 181-190.

Reilly, M. Lets set the record straight. *Nursing 79*, 1979, *9*(1), 56-61.

Seche, J. Emergency care of an aspirin overdose patient. *RN*, 1978, *41*(10), 83.

Silman, J. The management of pain. *American Journal of Nursing*, 1979, *79*(1), 74.

Vaterlaus, E. A holistic approach to nursing the patient in pain. *The Canadian Nurse*, 1979, *75*(6), 22.

Wachter-Shikora, N., & Perez, S. Unmasking pain. *Geriatric Nursing*, 1982, *3*, 392-393.

West, A. Understanding endorphins: our natural pain relief system. *Nursing 81*, 1981, *11*(2), 50-53.

Wright, Z. From I.V. to P.O. titrating your patient's pain medication. *Nursing 81*, *11*(7), 39-43.

Zimmerman, M. Physiology of nociception. In J. Bonica, J. Liebeskind, & D. Albe-Fessard (Eds.). Advances in pain research and therapy, vol. 3. New York: Raven Press, 1979.

Zola, E.M., & McLeod, D.C. Comparative effects and analgesic efficacy of the agonist-antagonist opioids. *Drug Intelligence and Clinical Pharmacy*, 1983, *17*, 411.

CHAPTER 18

Drugs Used to Treat Psychotic Disorders

Louis A. Pagliaro
Ann M. Pagliaro

Medications discussed in this chapter

Butyrophenones
  Droperidol
  Haloperidol
Dibenzoxazepines
  Loxapine
Dihydroindolones
  Molindone
Diphenylbutylpiperidines
  Pimozide
Phenothiazines
  Acetophenazine
  Butaperazine
  Carphenazine
  Chlorpromazine
  Fluphenazine

Phenothiazines—cont'd
  Mesoridazine
  Methotrimeprazine
  Perphenazine
  Piperacetazine
  Prochlorperazine
  Promazine
  Thiopropazate
  Thioridazine
  Trifluoperazine
  Triflupromazine
Thioxanthenes
  Chlorprothixene
  Thiothixene

Emotional disorders have been defined and grouped in a number of different ways. For convenience, however, they are generally divided into two groups based on their severity and response to drug therapy. These two groups are known as neuroses and *psychoses*.

Neuroses can be defined as emotional disorders caused by an unresolved, unconscious conflict. Several general symptoms usually accompany neuroses, including specific avoidance behavior, change in behavior (e.g., increase or decrease in eating or smoking), lack of interest in the environment, sexual disturbances (e.g., frigidity or impotence), emergency discharges to relieve tension (e.g., shouting), and sleep disturbances. The neuroses are varied in type and include a variety of specific conditions including anxiety neurosis, depersonalization neurosis, hypochondrial neurosis, depressive neurosis, hysteric neurosis, neurasthenic neurosis, obsessive-compulsive neurosis, and phobic neurosis. Drug treatment of the neuroses is dealt with in Chapter 19, "Drugs Used to Treat Affective Disorders."

Psychoses are major mental disorders of physical or psychologic origin in which the individual's ability to think, respond emotionally, and relate to reality are severely impaired. Frequent characteristics of psychoses include regressive behavior, inappropriate mood, diminished impulse control, delusions (e.g., of grandeur or persecution), and hallucinations. Pharmacologic treatment of psychoses is dealt with in this chapter.

Because psychoses usually respond well to treatment with the antipsychotic tranquilizers, whereas neuroses do not, it is important for the nurse to be able to differentiate between these two types of emotional disorders. Typically, the characteristics of these two groups are opposite or converse of each other. Following is a summary of the differentiation between psychoses and neuroses.

Psychoses	*Neuroses*
Hereditary predisposition	*No* hereditary predisposition
May be the result of a biochemical abnormality of the central nervous system	Probably a learned maladaptive response to stress
Severe inability to function in society	Relatively less severe inability to function in society
Often *no* recognizable precipitating stress	Usually a recognizable precipitating stress
Patient usually considers behavior to be normal	Patient often realizes that behavior is abnormal
Often severely out of contact with reality	Usually *no* loss of contact with reality
Psychotherapy usually *not* beneficial	Psychotherapy may be the best treatment
Often responds to treatment with antipsychotic agents and can tolerate large doses well	Antipsychotic agents are usually of *no* benefit and cause similar effects as in normal individuals (e.g., large doses *not* well tolerated)

Before we proceed to a discussion of the drug therapy for the treatment of psychotic disorders, it should be noted that some psychiatric patients will simultaneously display characteristics of both neurotic and psychotic behavior. Mental disorders are no more exclusive than are physical disorders. Just as an individual can concurrently suffer from both hypertension and diabetes, so too can an individual concurrently suffer from more than one type of mental disorder. However, because of the usual absence of physical findings associated with mental disorders, the health care provider must be especially diligent in patient assessment and in monitoring the affects of drug therapy.

ANTIPSYCHOTIC TRANQUILIZERS

The antipyschotic tranquilizers, also known simply as antipsychotics or major tranquilizers, are derived from a number of different chemical families including the butyrophenones, dibenzoxazepines, dihydroindolones, diphenylbutylpiperidines, phenothiazines, and thioxanthenes.

Although chemically diverse, the antipsychotics share several basic pharmacologic characteristics including antipsychotic activity, sedation, potentiation of other CNS depressants, antiemetic activity, adrenergic and cholinergic blocking activity, and production of extrapyramidal symptoms. None of the antipsychotics cause psychologic or physical dependence. The degree of the other effects varies with chemical classification and dosage. See the Nursing Drug Digest for specific information on each individual antipsychotic agent.

The mechanism of action of the antipsychotics is complex and incompletely understood. However, their antipsychotic activity appears to be related to an interaction with dopamine containing neurons, specifically the blockade of dopamine receptors.

The antipsychotics are metabolized in the liver and the metabolites (as well as varying amounts of unchanged drug) are eliminated in the urine and feces. Thus, the dosage must be modified in the presence of hepatic or renal impairment.

Because all of the antipsychotics are efficacious, it should be noted that the choice of an individual agent is typically based on the presence of specific side effects. For example, if a psychotic patient has a heart condition, then an antipsychotic with relatively few cardiac effects should be chosen. Likewise, if a patient is agitated and has difficulty sleeping, an antipsychotic with sedating properties should be chosen.

In all cases, however, the patient's previous response to antipsychotic drug therapy should be used as a guide. If a patient has previously responded favorably to a particular agent, it should generally be used again. Dosage should be gradually increased. In the elderly, who are very susceptible to the adverse effects of the antipsychotics, dosage should be started low and gradually increased. Because most of the antipsychotics have long half-lives (greater than 24 hours), they can frequently be dosed once daily. This is usually done at bedtime to take advantage of any sedative effect and so the patient can often sleep through other minor side effects.

Before proceeding to a discussion of the individual chemical classifications of the antipsychotics, a common misconception should be clarified. Contrary to what has been presented in most other nursing pharmacology texts, the term *minor tranquilizer* is a misnomer and has led to considerable confusion.

Pharmacologically, the only tranquilizers are the major or antipsychotic tranquilizers. The term "minor tranquilizer" was developed as an advertising gimmick by the pharmaceutical manufacturers when the benzodiazepines were introduced to the market place in the early 1960s. However, the benzodiazepines do not possess any tranquilizing activity. They are pharmacologically members of the sedative-hypnotic group of medications and as such are discussed in Chapter 15, "Sedative-Hypnotics."

Following is a brief discussion of the antipsychotics according to chemical family. Familiarity with these groupings should enable the nurse to appreciate the similarities between agents from the same chemical family, as well as to be able to anticipate the action and side effects to be expected from any new agents that may be developed. Because of similarities among agents within a chemical family, it should be readily apparent that administering more than one agent from the same chemical family offers no additional therapeutic benefit and is *not* recommended.

Butyrophenones

Therapeutics. The butyrophenones are similar to phenothiazines; however, they may have a more rapid onset of action. The two members of this class currently approved for use in North America are droperidal and haloperidol, although droperidol is *not* used for its antipsychotic effect.

Adverse effects. Butyrophenones frequently cause extrapyramidal effects including *akathisia* and *dystonia* (especially in children). They may occasionally cause blood dyscrasias, galactorrhea, menstrual changes, postural hypotension, sedation, and *tardive dyskinesias*.

Dibenzoxazepines

Therapeutics. Dibenzoxazepines are similar to the phenothiazines. Loxapine is the only agent in this class that is currently approved for use in North America.

Adverse effects. Loxapine frequently causes extrapyramidal effects, including akathisia. Drowsiness is also common. This agent occasionally causes anticholinergic effects (including blurred vision, dry mouth, decreased gastrointestinal [GI] motility, urinary retention, and tachycardia), convulsions (particularly in epileptic patients), dystonia, hypotension or hypertension, and tardive dyskinesia.

Dihydroindolones

Therapeutics. Molindone is the only agent of the dihydroindolones that is currently approved for use in North America. The anorexia and weight loss associated with molindone may have clinical significance in treating those psychotic patients in whom weight gain is a real or perceived problem.

Adverse effects. Molindone frequently causes extrapyramidal effects, including akathisia. Anticholinergic effects (including blurred vision, dry mouth, decreased GI motility, urinary retention, and tachycardia) are also common. Molindone may occasionally cause anorexia, drowsiness, dystonia, menstrual changes, postural hypotension, and skin rash.

Diphenylbutylpiperidines

Therapeutics. Pimozide is the only agent of the diphenylbutylpiperdines that is currently manufactured and used in North America.

Adverse effects. Pimozide frequently causes *extrapyramidal reactions*, including akathisia, dystonia (especially torticollis), and *parkinsonism*. It may occasionally cause convulsions (particularly in epileptic patients), hypotension, and tachycardia.

Phenothiazines

Because the phenothiazines were the first class of antipsychotics to be synthesized and clinically used in the early 1950s, they are considered to be the prototype antipsychotics against which other agents are compared and contrasted. There are more individual agents in this chemical class than in all the other antipsychotic classes combined.

The phenothiazines are usually well tolerated by psychotic patients. The sedative effects of these drugs are rapidly prominent; however, the full antipsychotic activity may not be apparent for several weeks.

The phenothiazines have been subdivided into three groups (i.e., aliphatic, piperazine, piperidine) according to the chemistry of the phenothiazine sidechain. Because of their chemical similarity, the individual agents within these groups share specific therapeutic and adverse effects.

Aliphatics. The aliphatic phenothiazines include chlorpromazine, methotrimeprazine, promazine, and triflupromazine.

Therapeutics. This group includes the prototype phenothiazine—chlorpromazine. Because of the lower incidence of troublesome extrapyramidal side effects, this group is the widest used of the antipsychotics. The strong sedative effects can be of assistance in treating agitated psychotic patients and in inducing sleep when administered at bedtime.

Adverse effects. Aliphatics frequently cause anticholinergic effects (including blurred vision, dry mouth, decreased GI motility, urinary retention, and tachycardia), drowsiness, and orthostatic hypotension. They may occasionally cause cholestatic jaundice, convulsions (at high doses), electrocardiogram (ECG) changes, extrapyramidal effects including dystonia and tardive dyskinesia (incidence is less than that caused by the piperazine derivatives), menstrual changes, photosensitivity, skin rashes, and weight gain. Long-term, high-dose use may cause lens opacity.

Piperazines. The piperazine phenothiazines include acetophenazine, butaperazine, carphenazine, fluphenazine, perphenazine, prochlorperazine, thiopropazate, and trifluoperazine.

Therapeutics. Piperazines generally have a higher potency on a milligram per milligram basis than the other phenothiazines. They also have a relatively greater antiemetic effect than the other phenothiazines. One of the members of this group, fluphenazine, can be administered as the decanoate or enanthate salt intramuscularly. Administered as such it acts as a depot for the antipsychotic medication, thus assuring compliance over several weeks during long-term maintenance therapy (see the Nursing Drug Digest for further details).

Adverse effects. Piperazines often cause extrapyramidal effects, including akathisia and dystonia. They may occasionally cause anticholinergic effects (including blurred vision, dry mouth, decreased GI motility, urinary retention, and tachycardia), anorexia, drowsiness, galactorrhea, menstrual changes, orthostatic hypotension, photosensitivity, tardive dyskinesia, and weight gain. Long-term, high-dose use may cause lens opacity. They cause *less* sedation and orthostatic hypotension than other phenothiazines.

Piperidines. The piperidine phenothiazines include mesoridazine, piperacetazine, and thioridazine.

Therapeutics. The piperidines are similar to the aliphatic phenothiazines in many regards but have fewer sedative effects.

Adverse effects. Piperidines frequently cause anticholinergic effects (including blurred vision, dry mouth, decreased GI motility, urinary retention, and tachycardia), drowsiness, inhibition of ejaculation in males, orthostatic hypotension, and weight gain. They may occasionally cause extrapyramidal effects including akathisia and tardive dyskinesia, ECG changes, galactorrhea, menstrual changes, and photosensitivity. Long-term high-dose use of these agents may cause *pigmentary retinopathy.*

Thioxanthenes

Therapeutics. Chlorprothixene and thiothixene are the members of the thioxanthenes currently in therapeutic use. They are structurally similar to the phenothiazines, but also possess some antidepressant activity that may be beneficial when treating psychotic patients who have a depressed affect.

Adverse effects. Thioxanthenes frequently cause anticholinergic effects (including blurred vision, dry mouth, decreased GI motility, urinary retention, and tachycardia), drowsiness, extrapyramidal effects including akathisia and dystonia (more common with thiothixene), and orthostatic hypotension (more common with chlorprothixene). They may occasionally cause galactorrhea, menstrual changes, and skin rash. Long-term, high-dose use of thioxanthenes may cause lens opacity.

Miscellaneous

Reserpine and other rauwolfia alkaloids have been used in the past to treat schizophrenia; however, this class of drugs has now been completely replaced by the newer and more efficacious antipsychotics previously discussed. It should be noted that a prominent side effect of reserpine therapy is depression, which is always troublesome, but particularly so in psychiatric patients. Using reserpine for the treatment of psychiatric conditions is obsolete and *not* recommended.

Lithium has been erroneously classified in some texts as an antipsychotic. However, it is used in the treatment of affective disorders, specifically manic-depressive disorders, and as such is discussed in Chapter 19, "Drugs Used to Treat Affective Disorders."

EXTRAPYRAMIDAL EFFECTS

About 30% of patients receiving antipsychotics will develop some sort of extrapyramidal effect. These range in severity from minor effects that abate with a reduction of dosage or continued therapy, to severe tardive dyskinesia (i.e., a late occurring neurologic syndrome characterized by involuntary sucking and smacking of the lips, jaw movements, and darting of the tongue), which in some cases may be irreversible even after discontinuation of the antipsychotic.

The extrapyramidal effects (reactions) include akathisia (i.e., motor restlessness marked by an inability to sit quietly or to sleep), dyskinesia (i.e., impairment of voluntary muscle movements), muscle rigidity, *oculogyric crisis* (i.e., prolonged fixation of eyeballs in one position—usually sideways or upwards), *torticollis*, slurring of speech, hypersalivation, parkinsonism (i.e., a group of neurologic disorders marked by hypokinesia, tremor, and muscle rigidity), and tremors.

These effects can generally be well treated with the antiparkinsonian medications that are discussed in Chapter 23, "Parasympathomimetics and Parasympatholytics," and in Chapter 20, "Antiparkinsonian Medications and Stimulants." Periodic reevaluation and drug holidays have been suggested as a means of minimizing the extrapyramidal effects of the antipsychotics. When antipsychotic and antiparkinsonian medications are discontinued they should be gradually tapered off simultaneously or the antipsychotic tapered off first, over 1 to 2 weeks, with the patient closely monitored.

Tardive dyskinesia, which may be irreversible and untreatable, remains one of the most distressing adverse effects of antipsychotic drug therapy. Various drugs have been used to treat tardive dyskinesia (e.g., baclofen, clonazepam, levodopa, and manganese); however, results have been mixed and their efficacy remains unproven. Because tardive dyskinesia can be caused by any of the antipsychotics, therapy must be aimed at prevention. Recommendations to decrease the incidence of tardive dyskinesia include the following: using the minimum effective antipsychotic dose; reevaluating patient status and incorporating drug holidays (1 month in duration) where the risk–benefit ratio warrants; minimizing, where possible, the chronic use of anticholinergics (e.g., prophylactic use in anticipation of extrapyramidal effects); and finally to monitor the patient closely and to discontinue the antipsychotic at the first sign of tardive dyskinesia whenever possible. Following discontinuation of the antipsychotic, the tardive dyskinesia may initially worsen; however, this is usually only a short-term effect and one can expect that in many cases the disorder will totally and spontaneously remit.

SUMMARY

The antipsychotics have revolutionized the treatment of severe mental disorders since their introduction in the early 1950s. They are clearly not a panacea because approximately 15% of treated patients fail to respond and another 35% respond only marginally, enabling deinstitutionalization, but not providing normality. However, their judicious use, although not usually effecting a cure, has been able to permit the majority of psychotic patients to maintain more normal lives. In addition, their use has enabled the treatment of most psychotic patients on an outpatient basis and freed them from totally institutionalized lives.

ADVERSE/SIDE EFFECTS OF THE ANTIPSYCHOTICS*

ALLERGIC REACTIONS

Asthma
Angioneurotic edema
Contact dermatitis (care should be taken to avoid direct skin contact with solution forms of the antipsychotic medications)
Eczema
Erythema
Itching
Photosensitivity (patient should be instructed to avoid undue prolonged exposure to direct sunlight)

AUTONOMIC NERVOUS SYSTEM

Anticholinergic effects (one of these effects, dry mouth, can be relieved by sucking of sugarless hard candy)
Change in body temperature
Paralytic ileus

BEHAVIOR

Akathisia or uncontrollable restlessness
Impaired function caused by oversedation (most patients will develop tolerance to the sedating effects)
Paradoxic exacerbation of psychoses

CARDIOVASCULAR SYSTEM

Cardiac arrest
ECG abnormalities (shown as an increase in the Q-R interval and a flattened T wave; seen more often with thioridazine)

Postural hypotension (in the event of shock and the possible need for a vasoconstrictor use levarterenol or phenylephrine; *never* use epinephrine because a paradoxic further lowering of blood pressure may result)
Ventricular tachycardia (more likely to occur with sudden large increases in dosage, especially with thioridazine)

CENTRAL NERVOUS SYSTEM

Convulsions (occurs primarily with high doses and with a rapid increase in dosage, especially with chlorpromazine or promazine)
Drowsiness (patients usually develop tolerance to this effect)

HEMATOLOGIC SYSTEM

Agranulocytosis (has a low incidence but is potentially lethal; highest incidence found in elderly caucasian females; discontinue antipsychotic medication)
Anemia
Eosinophilia
Leukopenia

HEPATIC SYSTEM

Cholestatic jaundice (incidence is low but is potentially lethal)

METABOLIC AND ENDOCRINE SYSTEMS

Amenorrhea
Galactorrhea
Gynecomastia
Impaired glucose tolerance
Impotence
Libido change
Weight gain

NEUROMUSCULAR (EXTRAPYRAMIDAL) SYSTEM

NOTE: May be treated by altering dose or coadministering antiparkinsonism agents; persistent severe dyskinesias may necessitate discontinuing the antipsychotic medication
Akathisia
Drug induced parkinsonism
Dystonia
Tardive dyskinesia

OCULAR SYSTEM

Blurred vision
Exacerbation of glaucoma
Mydriasis
Myosis
Pigmentary retinopathy (occurs primarily after long-term administration; most often with patients receiving greater than 1200 mg/24 hr of thioridazine)

*See Chapter 11, "Drug Toxicity," for an overview of drug toxicity.

CLINICALLY SIGNIFICANT DRUG INTERACTIONS*

Primary drug	Interacting drug	Possible effect(s)	Probable mechanism(s)
Phenothiazines	Antacids	Decreased phenothiazine effect	Decreased phenothiazine absorption from GI tract
Phenothiazines	Anticholinergics	Heart failure	Potentiated anticholinergic effect
Phenothiazines	Antidepressants (tricyclic)	Blurred vision, constipation, diplopia, dry mouth, headache, urinary retention	Additive anticholinergic effect
Phenothiazines	Barbiturates†	Drowsiness, lethargy, stupor, respiratory collapse, coma, death	Additive or potentiated CNS depression
Phenothiazines	Alcohol†	Drowsiness, lethargy, stupor, respiratory collapse, coma, death	Additive or potentiated CNS depression
Phenothiazines	Guanethidine	Decreased guanethidine effect	Block drug uptake at adrenergic/dopaminergic neuron
Phenothiazines	Levodopa	Decreased levodopa effects	Block drug uptake at adrenergic/dopaminergic neuron
Phenothiazines	Narcotics	Drowsiness, lethargy, stupor, respiratory collapse, coma, death	Additive or potentiated CNS depression
Thiothixene	Guanethidine	Increased guanethidine effect	Block drug uptake at adrenergic/dopaminergic neuron

*See Chapter 10, "Drug Interactions," for an overview of drug interactions.
†Long-term chronic use may increase the rate of phenothiazine metabolism, thus necessitating an increase in phenothiazine dosage (note: increasing dose may cause the drug interaction listed above).

GENERAL NURSING IMPLICATIONS

Nursing of patients requiring antipsychotics

ASSESSMENT

All patients manifesting symptoms of psychoses require a thorough history and physical examination, including laboratory evaluation of blood and urine, to ensure an accurate diagnosis because many conditions when uncontrolled can resemble psychoses (such as diabetes and hypertension). Viral encephalitis, intracranial tumors, and thyroid disease may also appear with symptoms of psychoses, and a neurologic assessment is often indicated to ensure that the patient's condition is not best treated neurologically.

The initial data base should include a psychiatric history and psychosocial assessment. The psychosocial assessment should include social and psychologic data gathered from interaction with the patient, family, or others, as indicated, including friends or the police, because the patient may be seeking help voluntarily or may be referred by the courts or the police for assessment and care. The source of the data should be identified and recorded.

It is especially important that the patient's perception of the condition be included. The patient's insight and evaluation of the significance of the present situation should be assessed (e.g., whether the patient feels the need for treatment). Data gathered from direct interaction with the patient should include observations of the patient's present psychotic symptoms, including the presence of regressive behavior, agitation, aggressiveness or combativeness, rage or hostility, negativism, thought disorders, delusions (e.g., of grandeur, persecution), paranoia, overactivity related to sensory stimuli, or diminished impulse control.

The patient's general behavior, including posture, appearance, ability to maintain self-care, facial expression, activity level, loudness and coherence of speech, emotional state or mood (including mood changes), hallucinations, compulsions, phobias, fantasies, and daydreams should be carefully assessed and documented.

It should be ascertained if the patient is oriented to time, place, person, and self. The patient's attention span and ability to recall events in the recent and remote past should be assessed along with the patient's general intellectual ability and level of abstract thinking.

A family and personal mental health history should be completed. This is especially important if the patient has responded well to a particular drug in the past, because chances are greater that the patient will again respond well to the same drug. Likewise, if unfavorable reactions have been experienced, that particular drug should generally be avoided.

GENERAL NURSING IMPLICATIONS—cont'd

Nursing of patients requiring antipsychotics—cont'd

ASSESSMENT—cont'd

In addition, the use of alcohol or drugs (including illicit drugs) during the preceding week should be acertained. This is especially important because some drugs, such as amphetamines and cocaine, can cause toxic psychoses. The history should include previous hospitalizations or mental health treatments, past successes with specific medication regimens, history of sensitivity or serious intolerance to medication, or adverse side effects related to previous or present antipsychotic therapy. This is extremely important in planning individualized and optimal therapy.

In addition to these baseline data, psychologic testing, intelligence testing (e.g., use of Stanford-Binet Test), or Rorschach Testing may be indicated. Personality inventories (e.g., the Minnesota Multiphasic Personality Inventory [MMPI] are also often performed. Depending on the patient's condition and history, assessment may require completion over the first days of therapy. Initial assessment should include specific data related to the patient's condition, a detailed drug history to identify sensitivity, contraindications, cautions, potential drug interactions, and drug-taking patterns before antipsychotic drug therapy is initiated.

SENSITIVITY

Generally, allergic reactions to antipsychotics are rare; however, any drug has the potential to cause a hypersensitivity reaction in susceptible individuals. Allergic reactions, including fever and angioneurotic edema, have been observed, particularly with the phenothiazines. The most common allergic response is a pruritic maculopapular rash that usually appears on the face, neck, and chest 2 to 10 weeks after the drug is first administered. No treatment is required for mild rashes because these usually remit on their own. If the rash is severe, however, the medication should be discontinued and a different antipsychotic substituted. It is important to recognize that contact dermatitis can occur with the injectable or liquid concentrate forms of the phe-nothiazines, and direct contact with the skin should be avoided by both the patient and the nurse.

Lower doses of antipsychotics may be tried (e.g., 25 to 50 mg PO or 25 mg IM of chlorpromazine) to test for hypersensitivity or adverse side effects. If no untoward reaction is noted in 1 to 2 hours, then small daily divided doses are administered and then the dose is titrated to clinical improvement with minimal side effects.

CONTRAINDICATIONS

The use of antipsychotics is contraindicated in patients with the following conditions: hypersensitivity; bone marrow depression or a history of blood dyscrasias; liver dysfunction, because these patients may be at increased risk of developing obstructive jaundice and may not be able adequately to detoxify or inactivate the antipsychotics; CNS depression or patients who are in a coma as a result of the use of alcohol, barbiturates, narcotics, or as a result of brain trauma, because synergistic CNS depression can result in respiratory paralysis or circulatory collapse.

CAUTIONS

Whereas psychotic patients can tolerate large doses of antipsychotics, the administration of these medications to nonpsychotic individuals is not well tolerated and can actually precipitate symptoms of psychoses.

Because antipsychotics can cause cardiac effects, patients with a history of cardiac disease should be evaluated by a cardiologist and undergo an ECG when treatment is planned.

Use antipsychotics with caution particularly the butyrophenones in parkinsonism because the increased dopamine blockade may cause a resumption of symptoms even when patients are taking antiparkinsonian medications.

Pregnant women should be treated only when necessary, especially during the first trimester of pregnancy. Although not conclusively teratogenic, many antipsychotics can pass the pla-cental barrier. Use of antipsychotics has resulted in postnatal depression syndrome followed by agitation in the neonate. Antipsychotics are also excreted in breast milk in small quantities. The use of these agents must be weighed against the risk to mother and infant.

Antipsychotics, especially chlorpromazine and thioridazine, should be used cautiously in the elderly because the elderly are more sensitive to the anticholinergic effects of antipsychotics. They experience adverse side effects at lower doses and more quickly develop toxic reactions, including atropine psychoses.

The elderly are prone to have severe sedative effects and orthostatic hypotension, which can result in falls and trauma. Elderly men, especially with prostatic hypertrophy, are prone to urinary hesitancy or retention, and elderly women experience more constipation and bowel obstruction.

When antipsychotics are used in combination with other drugs that have anticholinergic properties (e.g., antiparkinsonian medications), anticholinergic effects can be potentiated. Patients should be carefully monitored for the following: agitation; confusion; disorientation; dry, flushed skin; tachycardia; sluggish, dilated pupils; bowel hypomotility; dysarthria; and memory impairment. If these signs are noted, the antipsychotic should be discontinued. Physostigmine (IM, IV) should be readily available for treatment of severe cases.

DRUG INTERACTIONS

Antipsychotics have the potential to interact with numerous drugs in a variety of mechanisms.

See Clinically Significant Drug Interactions.

ADMINISTRATION

Antipsychotics can be administered orally, rectally, or by intramuscular injection. Dosage requires adjustment when routes of administration are changed because of variability in availability and distribution (see Chapter 4,

Continued.

GENERAL NURSING IMPLICATIONS—cont'd

Nursing of patients requiring antipsychotics—cont'd

ADMINISTRATION—cont'd

"Drug Availability and Distribution"). The clinical setting, the patient's self-medication abilities, and the acute severity of the patient's condition influence the drug therapy regimen and the selection of routes of administration.

Generally, because antipsychotics have a high therapeutic index, they can be given at relatively high doses with minimal risk. Because the dosage of antipsychotics is titrated against symptoms of psychosis and the appearance of adverse side effects, there is wide variation in dose and dosage schedules (see the Nursing Drug Digest for recommended dosage ranges for specific antipsychotics).

Although in some situations patients may be observed for up to 2 weeks or longer in the clinical setting before drug therapy is initiated, patients who are combative or assaultive and in danger of hurting themselves or others require immediate antipsychotic treatment. For the initial treatment of acute agitation or violent behavior, antipsychotic medication is administered intramuscularly for rapid onset of action. Patients may require from 2 to 10 consecutive doses at 30- to 60-minute intervals for sedation or control of symptoms. The patient's blood pressure and pulse rate should be closely monitored in lying and standing positions if possible before each dose to assess hypotensive effects. Mental status should also be monitored carefully and recorded. As behavior is controlled, oral medication (tablet, capsule, or liquid concentrate) should be substituted.

Over the first 5 to 10 days following an acute episode, oral medication is administered in daily divided doses 3 to 4 times a day. Dosing is then gradually changed to twice a day or once a day. Single daily doses are usually given at bedtime to maximize the drug's sedative properties and to minimize experienced adverse side effects, because the patient can sleep through them.

Some patients requiring antipsychotic medications may be agitated or resistant and the nurse may need assistance to administer needed medication. If restraint is indicated, civil liberties must be honored. Involuntary treatment can only be performed according to due process as required by state or provincial mental health laws. Care must be taken to ensure that medication is administered in relation to these laws and to ensure patients' rights.

Patients are generally cooperative when approached by a nurse or other health care provider they know and trust. Building a relationship that establishes trust may take time and patience. The nurse may need to work with other health care team members the patient trusts to gain the patient's cooperation so that medication is accepted as necessary for the improvement of the patient's condition. It is important for the development of self-medication abilities to observe the patients' behavior and to talk to them about the meaning the medication may have to them (e.g., a patient with paranoia may refuse medication because it is thought that the nurse is giving some other substance [i.e., poison] than medication; this type of patient may also refuse suppository medication because it may be seen as an attack from behind).

Suicidal and self-destructive patients may avoid taking medications knowing that this action will be destructive to their physical condition. They may not only refuse antipsychotic medication but other required medication (e.g., antidiabetic or antihypertensive medication) if indicated. Medication may be cheeked or hoarded by patients and they require oral assessment after administration and monitoring for behaviors that may indicate medication stashing (e.g., returning to room or other area where no one is around after taking medication). The nurse should remain with the patient until the medication is swallowed. It is important that trust is established with the patients and they should be approached honestly. The patients should be told the purpose of the medication, as well as the need for supervision until they can be trusted to take their medication.

Patients should understand that the medication is required to control disturbed behavior and to promote their well-being. Approaches should be discussed with health team members involved in the patient's care so that approaches can be consistent. Approaches must be individualized to provide optimal patient care and depend on the nurse's philosophy and model of nursing practice.

Because of the long-term toxic effects of antipsychotics, drug holidays are generally recommended as part of the maintenance program. It is recommended that patients on long-term maintenance come off medications at least every 6 months to monitor response. Patients may receive medication every other day or Monday through Friday, with medication not being taken on the weekends.

Although treatment is highly individualized, patients are usually kept on antipsychotics for 6 months to 1 year following the initial psychotic episode. After maximal clinical improvement, antipsychotics can be gradually tapered off and discontinued. Abrupt withdrawal can cause relapse, withdrawal dyskinesia, or other effects (e.g., chlorpromazine and thioridazine can cause nausea, vomiting, and diarrhea within 48 hours of the drug being withdrawn).

The long-acting parenteral forms of medication can be used for patients who are ambivalent about taking oral medication or who prefer not being totally responsible for self-medication. Fluphenazine enanthate, 12.5 to 50 mg every 3 to 14 days, or fluphenazine decanoate, every 2 to 4 weeks (fewer side effects) can be selected depending on the individual patient's needs, thus eliminating the need to take medication one or more times a day or without supervision.

The medication must be administered by the community health nurse or by family members who have been taught to administer the drug and monitor its effects. It is important that allergy is ruled out. The drug should be admin-

GENERAL NURSING IMPLICATIONS—cont'd

Nursing of patients requiring antipsychotics—cont'd

ADMINISTRATION—cont'd

istered deep intramuscularly, usually in the dorsogluteal site.

Maintenance doses are usually required for sustained improvement. Because there is higher probability of relapse in patients with a history of recurring psychotic episodes, long-term maintenance is often indicated in these patients. After the acute phase, which usually lasts from 4 to 12 weeks, doses can be lowered to a maintenance dose of one half to one fifth of the highest dose used to control acute symptoms. The lowest effective dose should be used.

Self-medication is often required for outpatients on maintenance antipsychotic therapy, and should be planned carefully to ensure as much success as possible. Divided daily doses are often not required, because antipsychotics have a prolonged half-life and dosage regimens can be planned to help the patient maintain self-medication abilities. When antipsychotics can be taken once a day, doses can be remembered and medication does not have to be carried during the day. Because fewer tablets or capsules are required, cost can be reduced, which is important to some patients in maintaining therapy. In addition, antipsychotics with sedative effects can be taken at bedtime so that not only are doses more easily remembered, but sleep is promoted and the patient can sleep through many of the adverse side effects.

MONITORING PATIENT RESPONSE

Therapeutic response

The onset and duration of an antipsychotic effect is largely dependent on the dosage form and the route of administration, as well as on individual patient factors. Antipsychotics are rapidly absorbed after oral or intramuscular administration. Clinical effects can be noted within 30 to 60 minutes after oral administration and within 10 minutes after intramuscular injection. Antipsychotic effects occur from several hours to weeks after the first dose, and after initial effects are observed, weeks to months may be required for full improvement to occur. It is important that patients be made aware of this lag period because they can become discouraged with therapy.

Patients should be closely monitored for improvement in mood, reduced agitation, calming of disturbed behavior without oversedation, emotional quieting, improvement in disordered thought, decreased hallucinations and paranoid ideation, or a decrease in other presenting symptoms.

Monitoring of therapeutic response is especially important. If the patient is unresponsive to one class of antipsychotic drugs, another may be more beneficial in controlling symptoms.

Some patients who do not respond to lower doses of medication do respond to very high doses.

Refractory patients require trial and error doses often at two to four times the usual doses. In some instances, patients have required doses 30 to 60 times the usual dosage ranges with constant monitoring. When patients are not responsive to drug therapy after a full drug trial of 3 to 6 weeks, a second drug may be tried from another drug class or subclass. A third drug trial may be used or an alternate dosage form may be tried (e.g., intramuscular injection may work better because of absorption properties).

Self-medication should be monitored if no effect is noted. Medication-taking behaviors should also be monitored because the drug may be cheeked. Blood level determinations can frequently be used to indicate if the drug is being taken correctly and at sufficient doses to produce therapeutic blood levels and response. Other therapy (e.g., electroconvulsive therapy (ECT) may be indicated.

In monitoring response it is important to keep in mind that antipsychotics are *not* addicting and do *not* produce euphoria or tolerance to antipsychotic effects.

Adverse side effects

Adverse side effects vary widely, depending on the chemical family or structure of the particular antipsychotic agent (see Adverse/Side Effects of the Antipsychotics, as well as the discussion in the text). However, major adverse side effects encountered in patients on antipsychotic therapy include blood dyscrasias and extrapyramidal effects, including drug-induced parkinsonism, akathisias, dystonic reactions, and dyskinesias. The nurse should have an understanding of the occurrence, severity, and symptoms of these effects because they frequently have a rapid onset and require immediate attention. Other common adverse side effects, although less severe or dangerous, are uncomfortable and frightening to patients and require immediate recognition and appropriate treatment to enhance the course of therapy.

It is helpful to keep in mind that many adverse side effects diminish after several days or weeks of treatment, and others can be treated by decreasing the dose of medication. Although tardive dyskinesia is usually not reversible, most other adverse side effects are. Although some antipsychotic drugs have increased risk for specific adverse side effects, any adverse side effect can occur with any of the antipsychotics. Monitoring is important so that if adverse side effects are noted the medication dosage can be decreased or the medication can be stopped or changed. In some instances, the administration of counteractants may be indicated.

The most common adverse side effects are anticholinergic effects, orthostatic hypotension, and sedation. These occur during the first 1 to 2 weeks of therapy but subside with continued therapy. Monitor patients carefully for the following.

Anticholinergic effects

Monitor for dry mouth, nasal congestion or stuffiness, blurred vision, palpitations, constipation, urinary hesitancy or retention, and paralytic ileus (this is rare).

Orthostatic hypotension

Monitor for dizziness, weakness, lightheadedness, and palpitations or tachycardia. Monitor these symptoms es-

Continued.

GENERAL NURSING IMPLICATIONS—cont'd

Nursing of patients requiring antipsychotics—cont'd

Orthostatic hypotension—cont'd
pecially in the morning when the patients get out of bed or after they have been lying down. Because postural hypotension can cause falls and injury, especially in the elderly, monitor for these symptoms carefully. In addition, monitor blood pressure during initial therapy in lying and standing positions before and one half hour after each dose of medication. A fall of 30 mm Hg in blood pressure is significant.

Sedation
Monitor for drowsiness during the day.

Hypersensitivity
Monitor for rashes, pruritus, difficulty in breathing, or other allergic effects.

Agranulocytosis
Monitor for sore throat, fever, malaise, sores in the mouth, and spontaneous bleeding. If these symptoms are noted, a CBC should be drawn because leukopenia confirms this condition. It is an extreme emergency. The drug should be stopped and reverse isolation instituted. If not fatal, the leukocyte count returns to normal within 10 days, with rapid recovery.

Anemia
Monitor for fatigue, pale color, or decreased hematocrit, hemoglobin.

Cholestatic jaundice
Monitor for early signs: malaise, fever, nausea, and abdominal pain. Monitor for later signs (1 week): itching and jaundice. Cholestatic jaundice is treated with bedrest and a high protein and carbohydrate diet. The drug should be stopped (common with chlorpromazine during the first month of treatment). Another drug may be selected if needed.

Metabolic and endocrine
Monitor menstrual cycles for changes in pattern; because amenorrhea may be indicative of pregnancy, this must be ruled out. It is important to note false positive pregnancy tests while patients are on antipsychotics.

Monitor for impaired glucose tolerance. Monitor S & A especially if patient is diabetic because an alteration in insulin and diet requirements may be necessary; may unmask undiagnosed mild diabetes mellitus.

Monitor for impotence and libido changes. Monitor for changes in sexual function; a diminished sex drive may be of benefit for hypersexual patients; explore other causes including illness or current conflict with partner.

Monitor for galactorrhea and gynecomastia; changes in body function may be intolerable and require change in drug.

Monitor for weight gain and loss. Monitor for an increase in appetite; monitor caloric intake in relation to loss or gain; molindone may cause weight loss and may be of benefit in obese patients.

Hypothalmic crisis (rare)
Monitor for hyperpyrexia, diaphoresis, drooling, tachycardia, dyspnea, seizures, and unstable blood pressure. If noted, drug should be discontinued and symptoms treated.

Pigmentation of skin and eyes
Assess skin surfaces most often exposed to sunlight (face, hands, arms). Monitor for golden brown coloration progressing to slate grey to metallic blue or purple. Monitor for sunburn. Pigment may also be deposited on eye structures; assess conjunctiva, sclera, lens, and cornea. (There is no visual impairment; pigment is reabsorbed after drug is discontinued.)

Reduction of seizure threshold
Monitor seizure patients carefully. Patients with a preexisting seizure disorder may need increased antiepileptic medication. Patients with no history of seizure activity may have grand mal seizures with increased doses or rapidly administered doses (rare). Treat with antiepileptic medications. If no effect, decrease dose of antipsychotic.

Extrapyramidal effects
Accurate observation and monitoring of patient response to antipsychotic therapy can be significant in recognizing extrapyramidal effects and the prompt initiation of treatment. There is a high incidence of extrapyramidal effects, including drug-induced parkinsonism, dystonic reactions, akathisia, and *dyskinesias* in patients taking these medications. These effects can occur early in therapy (usually during the first few days) and are usually reversible. Their occurrence, however, can be painful and frightening to patients. Tardive dyskinesia is the most severe of the dyskinesias. Unlike the other extrapyramidal effects, it usually occurs after years of treatment with antipsychotic medications, but it can also occur early in treatment. It usually presents after a maintenance dose is discontinued or decreased. There is no cure for this syndrome; however, it can be masked by reinstitution of the antipsychotic drug dosage or by changing to another antipsychotic medication.

Careful assessment and monitoring is required so that extrapyramidal effects are not mistaken for apathy, emotional blunting, psychotic agitation, withdrawal, or a deterioration in the patient's condition. Misdiagnosis can result in an increase in the antipsychotic dose to control the symptoms, resulting in a worsening of effects. When noted, symptoms should be readily discussed with the prescriber, and the patient should be reassured that they are usually reversible. Management of these effects is very important because they may affect the patient's willingness to continue drug therapy.

Extrapyramidal effects may not be constant in strength or appearance and can be missed or misinterpreted. Because they are usually more pronounced in stressful situations, they are affected by the patient's affective state and level of anxiety. It is thus not unusual for symptoms to occur only in the presence of others and to disappear when the patient is alone. These symptoms should not be mistaken for manipulation or avoidance behavior. Restlessness can occur in group therapy, for example, and not be observed when patients are involved in a card game or another activity they enjoy.

Drug-induced parkinsonism
During the first 8 weeks of therapy, monitor for *masklike facies*. Do not mistake masklike facies for the flat affect of schizophrenia. Patient may employ

GENERAL NURSING IMPLICATIONS—cont'd

Nursing of patients requiring antipsychotics—cont'd

Drug-induced parkinsonism—cont'd

other means than facial gestures to indicate a wider range of affect.

Monitor for *resting tremor.* Tremor appears faster and more irregularly than seen with true parkinsonism. Tremor is present during movement and at rest at speeds of about 5 cycles per second. Tremor usually begins in one or both upper extremities and when severe, involves tongue, jaw and lower extremities. Patient may complain of difficulty performing tasks or hobbies requiring fine motor control.

Monitor for *alterations in posture,* such as a rigid posture with slow voluntary movements, or a stooped posture.

Monitor for a *festinating, shuffling somewhat propulsive gait.*

Monitor for *muscle rigidity.* It affects both axial and limb musculature. Do not mistake it for tension or anxiety. Test patient by holding patient's elbow in palm of hand with thumb positioned over flexor tendons. Flex and extend the arm with the other hand and ask patient to relax the arm allowing you to move it. Leadpipe rigidity (smooth resistance to movement) or cogwheel rigidity (ratchet-like phenomena) are evidence of drug-induced rigidity rather than rigidity caused by tension or anxiety.

Monitor for *akinesia:* fatigue, lack of interest in activities, slowness, lack of usual ambition or drive, vague bodily discomfort, apathy, and decreased gestures. Do not mistake for depression or negativism. Patient may complain of feeling like a "robot" or a "zombie." When questioned, patient will state he or she feels "slowed down" or weak; assess muscle strength bilaterally for weakness. Patient is less interested in conversation and lacks spontaneity.

Monitor for a *loss of associated movements:* decreased or absent armswing, and ambulation with forearms perpendicular to trunk. Patient describes self as looking like a puppy begging or like a kangaroo.

Monitor for *hypersalivation and drooling:* patient compains of feeling like a

baby, and carries tissue to wipe mouth or uses sleeve or hand.

Akathisia

During later weeks or months of treatment, in particular, monitor for *motor restlessness:* an inability to sit or stand still without shifting weight, rocking, tapping feet, squirming, or fidgeting. Patient unable to watch television, knit, play quiet games, or read or look at magazines. Patient also unable to resist compulsion to stand and walk around or pace, and to lie down or sleep.

Monitor for *patient complaints of:* "never felt like this before," "feel restlessness inside," "more comfortable standing and walking than sitting," and "muscle quivering."

Monitor for *agitation:* increased desperation, and feelings of terror, fright, anger, or rage. This is especially important because these signs indicate severe akathisia and are associated with suicidal, violent, or homicidal behavior. Do not mistake behavior for anxiety or psychomotor agitation because increased doses of antipsychotics can worsen symptoms. Treat by lowering dose or changing drug; diazepam therapy may be indicated with effect in approximately 3 days.

Dystonic reactions

Especially during the first few days of therapy, monitor for the sudden onset of *severe muscle contractions* (which can be incoordinated, jerking, or spastic) involving the tongue, face, extraocular muscles, torso, and arms or legs. Monitor also for the sudden onset of *protrusion of tongue, torticollis, opisthotonos,* or an *oculogyric crisis.*

Monitor for *patient complaints of* a twisting jaw, an inability to speak or difficulty in talking and swallowing, and of complaints such as "eyes roll back in my head against my will." Also monitor for respiratory distress; there may be a spontaneous remission in 1 to 2 weeks.

Episodes can last for minutes or several hours. Diphenhydramine (25 to 100 mg) or benztropine should be on hand for relief of severe symptoms. Monitor for the effect of PO—60 minutes; IM—

15 minutes; or IV—1 minute. Reassurance is important and the patient should know that this reaction is a common side effect and how soon to expect relief of the frightening symptoms. A prn order for diphenhydramine or benztropine should be obtained in the event of acute dystonic reactions.

Dyskinesias

Especially during the first few days of therapy monitor for the sudden onset of coordinated, involuntary, rhythmic movements of limbs and trunk, especially in male patients.

Tardive dyskinesia

Tardive dyskinesia is the most severe syndrome associated with the use of antipsychotics. There is no known effective treatment for tardive dyskinesia, although it can be reversible if symptoms are detected early. Thus patients, especially elderly females receiving high doses of medication, require careful and frequent monitoring.

Monitor for *rhythmic involuntary movements of the face, mouth, tongue, jaw* (buccolinguomasticatory triad; most commonly described symptom), including: excessive blinking; grimacing; frowning; puffing of the cheeks; fine, vermiform movements of the tongue; tongue protrusion; sucking, lip smacking, chewing movements; pursing movements of the tongue; and puckering of the mouth.

Monitor for *involuntary movements of extremities,* including jerky choreiform movements or twitching involving the upper extremities or the facial muscles. All muscles of the body can be affected (not spastic as movements with dystonias). Monitor also for slow, irregular twisting or writhing or snakelike athetoid movements of arms and legs, especially the upper extremities and hands and fingers. Fingers may alternately flex and extend ("piano playing restlessness").

Monitor for *jerky movements of the head and neck,* including: tense, tonic contractions of the neck and back; axial hyperkinesis or to and fro clonic movements of the spine; and hemibalis-

Continued.

GENERAL NURSING IMPLICATIONS—cont'd

Nursing of patients requiring antipsychotics—cont'd

Tardive dyskinesia—cont'd

tic movements or jerky and twitching movements of one side of the body or swaying from side to side. They are cyclic (lasting 5 to 8 seconds), repetitive, easily modified by attention, emotion, posture, activity, and involve decreased or reduced voluntary activity of affected muscle; there is no decrease with sleep.

Patients on long-term antipsychotics should be screened for tardive dyskinesia at least every 3 months. It is recommended that such tools as the Abnormal Involuntary Movement Scale (Aims Test) be used to facilitate screening and to document patient status. If symptoms are identified, the antipsychotic should be discontinued if clinically possible. The family and the patient should understand the risks involved with continued use of the antipsychotic, if indicated for control of behavior. In some areas, written consent may be required.

When patients who are receiving antipsychotics are admitted to acute hospital settings for treatment of other conditions, they should likewise be assessed for the development of tardive dyskinesia. If medications are to be stopped (e.g., NPO for tests, preoperatively), it should be noted on the care plan to review the patient's neurological status carefully.

PATIENT EDUCATION

The patient and the family, as indicated, should be fully informed about the nature of the patient's condition and treatment plan, and should be involved in health care planning whenever possible. The patient and the family should have a clear understanding of the anticipated course of the therapy and medication regimen, including the exact name of the medication, its general action, purpose, dosage, storage, administration, and adverse side effects. They should know how to monitor therapeutic response, identify and manage common adverse side effects, and to identify signs that indicate the health care provider should be contacted. Patient education should also emphasize the promotion of mental health, prevention of recurrent psychotic episodes, and the risks and benefits of antipsychotic therapy.

Course of therapy

The patient and the family should have a clear idea of the course of therapy. For example, they should know that a low dose of medication will be started and gradually increased until the drug takes effect, with constant monitoring of adverse side effects. They should know that it can take several days, weeks, or months before a clinical response is noted. This is often hard for both the patient and the family, and much support and reassurance are needed. Any questions that the patient or family may have regarding therapy or progress should be answered honestly.

The patient and the family should have a realistic view of what to expect in relation to antipsychotic therapy, recognizing that antipsychotics will not solve all of the patient's problems but will enable the patient to work on problems. The patient and the family should understand that the antipsychotic medication will not improve judgment, poor socialization skills, interpersonal abilities, or change the patient's personality. They can expect, however, that the drug will assist the patient to better focus thoughts and concentrate on a wider range of topics, as well as control hallucinations or other initial symptoms.

Misconceptions should be clarified. Patients and family members should be aware that antipsychotics do not cause drug addiction nor do high doses of medication indicate a more severe mental condition, because dose selection depends on age, weight, metabolism, and other individual factors. The patient and the family should recognize that the patient's participation in other rehabilitative activities along with medication therapy and the maintenance of regular appointments with health care providers are important in treatment. Both patients and families should be taught and encouraged to ask questions about therapy as active consumers of mental health services.

Adverse side effects

Although the therapeutic effects of antipsychotic therapy should be emphasized, the patient and the family should be aware of possible adverse side effects. This is important because these effects can be attributed to emotional distress or relapse.

Patients and families should know that side effects usually diminish over the first few weeks of therapy. The patient should be encouraged to remain on antipsychotic medication despite mild adverse effects. This is difficult because the effect of the medication is usually not seen until later. The management of adverse side effects such as dose reduction, use of alternative drugs, use of antiparkinsonism medication, taking medication before going to bed, and other actions should be explored with the patient and the family if adverse side effects are intolerable. It is often helpful to weigh the discontinuation of the medication because of tolerable adverse effects against the risk of psychotic decompensation.

Patients should understand that if adverse side effects occur, symptoms will be treated quickly. It is important to acknowledge how troublesome, annoying, and uncomfortable they are, and patients should be encouraged to discuss their feelings about them. Because the inability to manage or tolerate adverse side effects is often a major reason for patients to stop taking antipsychotic medication, special attention should be given during patient education to the management of common mild side effects.

Points for managing common and mild adverse side effects

For the anticholinergic effect of *dry mouth,* encourage the patient to do the following: rinse mouth with water frequently through the day; chew sugarless gum or suck on sugarless hard candy or ice chips (sugarless gum and candy is preferred to regular gum or candy because there is less chance of monilial infections of the mouth); and brush teeth at least twice a day with a soft toothbrush.

GENERAL NURSING IMPLICATIONS—cont'd

Nursing of patients requiring antipsychotics—cont'd

Points for managing common and mild adverse side effects—cont'd

For the anticholinergic effect of *blurred vision,* encourage the patient to do the following: avoid reading while vision is blurred; use handrails when going up and down stairs; avoid standing on ladders; be especially careful crossing streets; avoid driving or operating dangerous equipment; and avoid having glasses adjusted until response to medication is determined.

For the anticholinergic effect of *constipation,* encourage the patient to do the following: eat a balanced diet including bran, and fresh fruits and vegetables (diet teaching may be indicated); exercise moderately and participate in other planned activities (exercise planning may be indicated); increase intake of fluids, including water and favorite beverages, avoiding excessive use of alcohol, coffee, or tea; and report severe constipation and discuss use of mild laxatives with health care provider before using them (constipation may be indicative of bowel obstruction).

For the anticholinergic effect of *urinary hesitancy or retention,* encourage the patient to do the following: drink at least 8 to 10 glasses of water or other beverage per day, avoiding excessive use of alcohol, coffee, or tea; notify the health care provider if smaller amounts than usual of urine are passed; and report difficulty urinating, dribbling, burning, need to urinate but cannot, or a firm uncomfortable feeling in the lower abdomen (if retention is acute, catheterization or treatment with bethanechol may be indicated; if a severe problem, antipsychotic medication may require change).

For the anticholinergic effect of *nasal congestion,* encourage the patient to do the following: report nasal discomfort or stuffiness; discuss temporary relief using a nasal decongestant, if not contraindicated; tolerate minor discomfort from nasal congestion until body adapts because there is rebound congestion associated with using nasal decongestants.

For the anticholinergic effect of *orthostatic hypotension,* encourage patient to do the following: change positions slowly; stand from a sitting position slowly after long periods (e.g., group therapy, watching a movie or television program, card or other game); hold onto a chair when getting up from a sitting position; sit back down if faintness is felt; get out of bed slowly in the morning and sit at the edge of the bed for 1 full minute before standing; use handrails when going up and down stairs; report dizziness or lightheadedness to health care provider (discuss use of elastic stocking, which may be helpful in preventing venous pooling); sit down or lie down at the first sign of dizziness; and avoid hot showers or baths.

For the anticholinergic effect of *sedation,* encourage the patient to do the following: get up readily in the morning and get moving in an effort to fight sedation; try to go to bed and get up at the same time every day; set a schedule for the day and keep to it; schedule a rest period if needed with a set time to get up and resume activity schedule; and avoid driving, operating dangerous machinery, or doing jobs that require alertness.

For the anticholinergic effect of *pigmentation of skin and eyes,* encourage the patient to do the following: avoid prolonged exposure to sunlight if medication makes him or her sensitive; wear protective clothing and sunglasses; and use a sunscreen containing paraaminobenzoic acid to prevent sunburn.

For *metabolic and endocrine effects,* encourage the patient to do the following: discuss changes in body function; explore causes of decreased libido, amenorrhea, inhibition of ejaculation, or other noted effect; for galactorrhea, use absorbent breast pads to protect clothing and change frequently to prevent skin irritation; monitor self for increased appetite; weigh self daily and report weight loss or gain of more than 2 kg; select a well-balanced diet (nutrition teaching may be indicated); eat snack foods low in calories; and talk to the health care provider about planning a diet and exercise program.

Points for managing extrapyramidal symptoms

For the extrapyramidal effect of the *buccolinguomasticatory triad,* encourage the patient to do the following: use a lip lubricant to prevent or treat chapping caused by tongue protrusion or licking of lips; if dentures are worn, continue to wear them because not only does wearing dentures toughen gums but patients have found this decreases some oral movements; report pain or irritation caused by dentures to the health care provider (a local anesthetic may be helpful); report difficulty keeping dentures in place (the use of various denture preparations can be explored; it should be assured that the patient is in no danger of aspirating dentures); change to soft foods when dysphagia is a problem (so that nutrition can be maintained, assistance with food selection may be indicated); consciously inhibit movements; wear well-fitting shoes and report irritation, callouses, or blisters if increased movement in lower extremities; speak slowly if dysarthria is a problem; plan rest periods during the day, especially if sleep is affected or increased motor activity is a problem, to replenish energy stores (an increase in calories may be indicated); and discuss feelings about symptoms with the health care provider (support, empathy, and patience are important in helping patients manage symptoms).

Tardive dyskinesia

Patients on maintenance or long-term antipsychotic therapy should be told the risks of tardive dyskinesia, and taught to recognize the early symptoms of this side effect and the importance of early detection.

Patients and family members should recognize that the failure to continue maintenance therapy can result in an increased risk of relapse.

Patients and family members should be taught to recognize symptoms of relapse and report them to the health

Continued.

GENERAL NURSING IMPLICATIONS—cont'd

Nursing of patients requiring antipsychotics—cont'd

Tardive dyskinesia—cont'd

care provider immediately if they note loss of appetite, trouble sleeping, restlessness, preoccupation with one or two thoughts, social withdrawal, paranoia, hallucinations, or recurrence of behaviors *noted* before treatment.

Approaches to patient education

It is often helpful for patients to receive information in writing as an inpatient so that information can be reviewed with the nurse during hospital treatment. This can encourage the patient to discuss therapy with the nurse and reinforce teaching measures before discharge.

To assist patients with self-medication on an outpatient basis after discharge, many approaches can be used. One approach is to use medication groups. These group meetings can help patients understand the purpose of their medication and its role in promoting and maintaining their mental health. Peer support and pressure can help patients to gain insight into their own feelings about taking medication. The group setting enables patients to learn from and be assured by other members' experiences. Discussions validate for the patient that others with the same symptoms also find them uncomfortable, difficult, unpleasant, or painful. Patients can also identify and discuss feelings such as loss of control or self-esteem related to the need for maintenance or long-term antipsychotic therapy. The nurse can serve as an effective resource in these groups.

With individualized instruction and careful preparation, the patient and or the family, as indicated, should be able to do the following. State the exact name of the medication; explain the purpose of the medication; describe the dosage schedule; demonstrate the method of administration (e.g., oral, rectal); demonstrate appropriate storage of medication; describe how long the medication shoud be taken; describe how to obtain more medication appropriately *as needed;* describe common side effects; manage adverse side effects; describe effects that indicate the health care provider should be notified; and discuss taking any other medication with the health care provider before it is taken, recognizing that antipsychotics can interact with numerous prescription and nonprescription medications.

Patient education should begin as soon as possible because the success of antipsychotic therapy depends on the patient's willingness and ability to take the medicaton correctly. Patient education is complex and must be individualized to the needs of patients, their families, and their readiness for learning. The nurse's unique approach is influenced by developed interpersonal skills, empathy and humanistic beliefs, understanding, the selected model of nursing practice, as well as by the patient's behavior pattern. The role of patient education in self-medication cannot be overemphasized in helping patients to resume their social function in the community.

GENERAL INSTRUCTIONS FOR DISCHARGE/OUTPATIENTS

This medication is used to treat your psychosis. This drug is sometimes called a "tranquilizer." It helps you to organize your thoughts and can also help you to feel more relaxed or less frustrated. If you do not understand why you are taking this medication, check with your health care provider.

Follow the instructions on the prescription exactly. If you have any questions about how this medication should be taken, check with your health care provider.

Take this medication with food or a glassful of water to prevent stomach upset.

It may take 2 weeks to 1 month or more for you to see the effect of this medication. Be sure to take the medication as prescribed and try not to miss any doses.

If you miss a dose of medication and you are taking divided doses, add the missed dose to the next dose. If you take only one dose per day, skip the missed dose.

You may feel like stopping or changing your medication schedule. Do not stop taking this medication without checking with your health care provider. Suddenly stopping your medication can cause harmful effects.

If your medication is in
Capsule form: Swallow capsules whole. Do not chew them. Do not open them.

Liquid form: Be sure you know how to measure the dose correctly with the dropper. If you have any questions, check with your health care provider. Be sure to shake suspension medications well.

Store liquid medications in a cool, dark place and avoid getting the medication on skin or clothes, because it is irritating. Liquid medication can be taken mixed in juices, milk, or water.

Tablet form: Swallow tablets whole. Do not chew.

Suppository form: Be sure you know how to insert the suppository. Check with your health care provider if you have any questions, and be sure to obtain written instructions. Store your suppositories in a cool, dry place.

Any medication can cause an unwanted effect or side effects. You may notice some side effects even before you notice the beneficial effects of your medication. Be patient and continue taking your medication. Side effects usually go away as your body adjusts to the medication.

Drowsiness, uncontrollable muscle movements, headache, dryness of the mouth, tremors, skin reactions to excessive sunlight, and stomach upset are some of the side effects that can occur. If these persist or become extreme, notify your health care provider. Your health care provider can also help you with the management of mild side effects.

Until you learn how this medication affects you (usually at least 2 weeks) do not drive, operate any dangerous machinery, or put yourself in situations where decreased mental alertness may cause danger.

If you are pregnant, thinking about becoming pregnant, or nursing an infant, do not take this medication without first discussing this with your health care provider.

Carry a card indicating you are taking this medication, in case of an emergency.

Be sure to tell other health care providers, including your dentist, that you are taking this medication.

Do *not* take high blood pressure medications (especially guanethidine), sleeping pills, pain relievers, laxatives, diet pills, or cough, cold, or allergy medication while taking this medication, because of possible harmful effects. Your health care provider should be notified before any other medications are taken.

Notify your health care provider if you notice a sore throat, fever, sores in your mouth, unusual tiredness or unusual movements of your face, tongue, hands, or stiffness of arms or legs, difficulty urinating, constipation, changes in eyesight, rapid heart rate, yellow color to the eyes or skin, or unusual weakness.

It is recommended that you avoid drinking alcoholic beverages while taking this medication. If you plan to drink alcoholic beverages while taking this drug, drink smaller amounts than usual and observe your response. This medication can decrease your tolerance to alcohol, so you may feel intoxicated by smaller amounts than usual.

This medication has been prescribed especially for you. Do not trade or give this medication to any relatives or friends.

Keep this medication and all other medications out of the reach of children.

In addition to the general instructions, if you are taking *chlorpromazine,* follow these specific instructions.

This medication can cause your urine to turn pink, red, or red-brown. This is not an unusual effect, so do not become alarmed. Your urine color will return to normal when you no longer take this medication.

Exercise only moderately in hot weather and do not get overheated. This medication may effect your body's ability to regulate body temperature.

If you have had a reaction to a phenothiazine, notify your health care provider before taking this medication.

Do not take this medication at the same time as antacids or antidiarrhea medication: they can prevent this medication from being absorbed by your stomach. Take them at least 1 hour apart.

NURSING DRUG DIGEST

Medication (trade name*)	Indication	Usual dosage and administration	Dosage forms, preparation, and storage	Contraindications, cautions, and comments	Monitoring
★ **Acetophenazine** Tindal	Psychoses and severe neuroses	*Adults:* 40-120 mg/24 hr PO in 2-4 divided doses Maximum: 500 mg/24 hr *Children:* 0.8-1.6 mg/kg/24 hr PO t.i.d. Maximum: 80 mg/24 hr—outpatient Maximum: 120 mg/24 hr—inpatient Administer last dose 1 hr before retiring for those patients who have difficulty sleeping	Tablet: 20 mg	*Contraindicated* in comatose patients Commonly causes extrapyramidal reactions Commonly causes atropine-like effects (e.g, dry mouth, decreased GI secretions, urinary retention) Bedside rails and supervision of ambulation for patient who exhibits excessive drowsiness	Monitor for excessive drowsiness Monitor for urinary retention or constipation
★ **Butaperazine** Repoise	Psychoses (rarely used)	*Adults:* Initial, 10-50 mg/24 hr PO in 3 divided doses Increase by 5-10 mg every few days until desired response Maximum: 100 mg/24 hr Maintenance: usually ¼-½ initial dose *Children:* 12 years and older, same as adult dose *Elderly:* Usually require a smaller dose	Tablets: 5, 10, 25 mg	Frequently causes atropine-like effects (e.g., dry mouth, decreased GI secretions, urinary retention) Frequently causes extrapyramidal reactions	Monitor for urinary retention or constipation Monitor for extrapyramidal reactions
★ **Carphenazine** Proketazine	Psychoses (rarely used)	*Adults:* Initial, 50-150 mg/24 hr PO in 2-3 divided doses Increase by 25-50 mg at weekly intervals Maximum: 400 mg/24 hr *Elderly* patients, usually require one-fourth to one-half regular adult dose Concentrate may be mixed with fruit juices	Tablets: 12.5, 25, 50 mg Concentrate: 50 mg/1 ml	*Contraindicated* in comatose patients *Contraindicated* in pregnant patients May take several months for full effect to occur Frequently causes extrapyramidal reactions	Observe for drowsiness and extrapyramidal reactions, especially with higher doses

Drug	Uses	Dosage	Available forms	Cautions/Effects	Nursing implications
Chlorproma-zine Chlorprom Chlor-pro-manyl♣ Chlor-pz Cromedazine Elmarine Hibanil♣ Largactil♣ Megaphen Omazine Ormazine Promachel Promapar Promosol♣ Psychezine Sonazine Thorazine Tranzine	Psychoses	*Adults:* 30-1000 mg/24 hr PO or IM in 3-6 divided doses; or q.h.s. once stabilized. Start with low doses and increase gradually. *Children:* 2 mg/kg/24 hr PO, PR, or IM in 3-4 divided doses. Contact with concentrate can cause contact dermatitis. Monitor blood pressure and watch for extravasation during IV administration. Keep patient in a recumbent position for 1 hr after all parenteral doses to avoid orthostatic hypotension. Give IM injection deeply into upper, outer quadrant of buttock and inject slowly. Rotate injection sites. Dilute concentrate in juice or water. Can mask taste of concentrate with orange juice. Precipitate may form on dilution but this does not affect activity and is okay to administer to patient PO	Tablets: 10, 25, 50, 100, 200 mg. Suppositories: 25, 100 mg. Capsules: 30, 75, 150, 200, 300 mg. Concentrates, oral: 30 mg/1 ml, 100 mg/1 ml. Syrup: 2 mg/1 ml. Injectable: 25 mg/1 ml. Protect liquid preparation from light. *Discard dark yellow solutions.* Keep suppositories refrigerated. Precipitate will form if chlorpromazine mixed with solutions not having a pH of 4-5	*Contraindicated* in comatose patients. *Contraindicated* in blood dyscrasias. *Contraindicated* in liver failure. Does *not* cause respiratory depression. *Frequent* drowsiness, dizziness, parkinsonism, hypotension, and anticholinergic effects; may cause seizures in epileptic patients. May cause jaundice. *Frequently* increases appetite leading to weight gain. May color urine pink or red-brown. May cause *phototoxicity.* Use with extreme caution in epileptic patients	Observe for signs of overdepression. Observe for jaundice with prolonged therapy. Observe for elevated temperature, malaise. Monitor for sore throat, especially in older women during fourth to tenth week of therapy, because this may be a sign of agranulocytosis. Check intake and output for urinary retention and constipation. Monitor blood pressure and pulse until both blood pressure and pulse are stabilized. Monitor caloric intake and weight for possible weight gain. Monitor for convulsions at doses greater than 1000 mg/24 hr, particularly in epileptic patients
	Nausea and vomiting	*Adults:* 100-300 mg/24 hr PO, IM, PR in 3-4 divided doses as needed. *Children:* 25 mg/24 hr PR. Maximum: 6 months-5 years, 40 mg/day; 5-12 years, 75 mg/day			
	Intractible hiccoughs	*Adults:* 100-300 mg/24 hr PO in 3-4 divided doses as needed			

Continued.

NOTE: For additional details regarding the individual agents listed in this table see the text and other tables in this chapter.
*Indicates a multiple active ingredient product. For a complete listing of all active ingredients see the *Drug Reference Guide to Brand Names and Active Ingredients.*
♣ Indicates that drug is generally available only in Canada.
★ Indicates that drug is generally available only in the United States.

NURSING DRUG DIGEST—cont'd

Medication (trade name)	Indication	Usual dosage and administration	Dosage forms, preparation, and storage	Contraindications, cautions, and comments	Monitoring
Chlorprothixene Taractan Tarasan Truxal	Psychoses and neuroses	*Adults:* 45-200 mg/24 hr PO, IM in 3-4 divided doses Maximum: 600 mg/24 hr *Children:* 6-12 years, 30-100 mg/24 hr PO in 3-4 divided doses; 12 years and older, same as adult dose *Elderly:* Usually need lower dose; start with 30-100 mg/24 hr PO, IM in 3-4 divided doses For IM administration inject deeply into large muscle mass Can administer concentrate in orange juice Do *not* administer IV	Tablets: 10, 15, 25, 50, 100 mg Injectable: 12.5 mg/1 ml Concentrate: 20 mg/1 ml Protect solution from light *Discard* darkly discolored solutions	*Contraindicated* in comatose patients *Contraindicated* in circulatory collapse Because of postural hypotension, patient should be supine during IM administration Bedside rails and supervision of ambulation may be required *Frequent* dizziness, drowsiness, atropine-like effects (e.g., dry mouth, decreased GI secretions, urinary retention), lethargy, orthostatic hypotension, and tachycardia Onset of action after IM injection is 10-30 minutes	With prolonged use, hematologic studies are advised to check for blood dyscrasias Monitor intake and output for urinary retention or constipation
Droperidol Droleptan Inapsine Innovar*	Preoperative, adjunct to anesthetic NOTE: *Not* used for antipsychotic effect	*Adults:* 2.5-10 mg IM, IV 30-60 min before induction of anesthesia *Children:* 2-12 years, 0.1-0.15 mg/kg IM, IV 30-60 min before induction of anesthetic *Elderly:* Decrease initial dose Inject IV slowly	Injectable 2.5 mg/1 ml Protect from light Store at room temperature	Rapid onset of action after IM or IV administration (3-10 minutes) Little effect on cardiovascular system *Frequent* incidence of dyskinetic reactions (especially in children) Use with *caution* in patients with liver dysfunction, kidney dysfunction, or parkinsonism	Closely monitor pulse and blood pressure during postoperative phase until stabilized Observe for extrapyramidal reactions
Fluphenazine Dapotom Modecate Moditen Permitil	Psychoses	*Adults: Initial,* 2.5-10 mg/24 hr PO, IM, SC in 3-4 divided doses *Maintenance:* 1-5 mg/24 hr PO, often as single dose Maximum: 20 mg/24 hr	Tablets: 0.25, 1, 2.5, 5, 10 mg Elixir: 0.5 mg/1 ml Injectable: 2.5mg/ml (hydrochloride salt); 25 mg/Ml (decanoate and enanthate salts)	*Contraindicated* in comatose patients *Contraindicated* in blood dyscrasias *Contraindicated* in subcortical brain damage	Monitor for fluctuations in blood pressure Monitor renal function in long-term patients

Drug	Use	Dosage	Preparation	Effects	Nursing Implications
Prolixin, Trancin		*Children:* 0.25-3 mg/24 hr PO in divided doses Maximum: 10 mg/24 hr *Elderly:* Usually require smaller doses, starting at 1-2.5 mg/24 hr PO CAUTION: Note which salt form of fluphenazine is being administered IM The hydrochloride (HCl) form should *not* exceed 10 mg/24 hr IM The decanoate and enanthate form can be given as a 50-100 mg IM maximum single dose at 2-4 week intervals Use dry needle and syringe because moisture will cause solution to become cloudy (to precipitate) Do *not* administer IV Concentrate may be administered with fruit juice	Concentrate: 5 mg/1 ml *Discard* darkly discolored solutions Protect dosage forms from light Store at room temperature; do *not* freeze	*Contraindicated* in severe cardiac disease Onset of action is slow (24-72 hr), but duration is prolonged (up to 3 weeks) Common extrapyramidal reactions and atropine-like effects (e.g., dry mouth, decreased GI secretions, and urinary retention) Less sedation and hypotension than with other phenothiazines	Monitor intake and output for urinary retention or constipation Observe for extrapyramidal effects
Haloperidol Haldol Serenace	Psychoses	*Adults: Initial,* 1-20 mg/24 hr PO, IM in 2-3 divided doses Maintenance: 2-8 mg/24 hr Maximum: 75 mg/24 hr *Children:* 3-12 years, 0.05-0.15 mg/kg/24 hr in 2-3 divided doses; 12 years and older, same as adult dose *Elderly:* Usually require lower doses, starting with 1-4 mg/24 hr PO, IM in 2-3 divided doses Concentrate is colorless, odorless, and tasteless, may be mixed with food or beverage Do *not* administer IV Deltoid muscle recommended for IM administration; use of other sites may result in erratic absorption	Tablets: 0.5, 1, 2, 5, 10, 20 mg Injectable: 5 mg/1 ml Concentrate: 2 mg/1 ml Protect from light *Discard* darkly discolored solutions Do *not* dilute injectable form with normal saline	*Contraindicated* in parkinsonism *Contraindicated* in comatose patients Causes less sedation and hypotension than phenothiazines Peak effect 30-45 min after IM injection; rapidly absorbed from GI tract, reaching peak in 2-3 hr Margin between therapeutic effect and extrapyramidal reactions is very narrow and these reactions occur *frequently* (especially in children) Better than chlorpromazine for rapid tranquilization because of less hypotensive effect	Monitor blood pressure and respirations after first dose and until both dose and patient are stabilized Observe elderly patients for lethargy and decreased thirst Observe for extrapyramidal effects

Continued.

NURSING DRUG DIGEST—cont'd

Medication (trade name)	Indication	Usual dosage and administration	Dosage forms, preparation, and storage	Contraindications, cautions, and comments	Monitoring
Loxapine Daxolin Daxolin C Loxitane Loxapac	Psychoses	*Adults:* 20-100 mg/24 hr IM, PO in 2-4 divided doses Maximum: 250 mg/24 hr Do *not* administer IV Use enclosed calibrated dropper to measure dose of concentrate To mask unpleasant taste, add desired dose of concentrate to 60 ml of orange juice just before administration	Capsules: 5, 10, 25, 50 mg Concentrate: 25 mg/1 ml Injectable: 50 mg/1 ml Store at room temperature Do not freeze	*Contraindicated* in severe depression *Contraindicated* in serious liver impairment *Contraindicated* in circulatory collapse *Contraindicated* in comatose patients *Contraindicated* in blood dyscrasias Common parkinsonism and other extrapyramidal reactions Sedation usually noted 20-30 minutes following administration and persists for up to 12 hours May cause oculogyric crisis Use with caution in epilepsy Use with caution in narrow-angle glaucoma Use with caution in cardiovascular disease	Observe for tardive dyskinesia with prolonged high-dose therapy Monitor for syncope, particularly in the elderly
Mesoridazine Lidanar Serentil	Psychoses	*Adults:* 75-400 mg/24 hr PO, in 3 divided doses, or 25-200 mg/24 hr IM *Children:* 12 years and older, same as adult dose *Elderly:* Usually require one-fourth to one-half usual adult dose Do *not* administer IV	Tablets: 10, 25, 50, 100 mg Injectable: 25 mg/1 ml Concentrate: 25 mg/1 ml Protect from light *Discard* darkly discolored solutions	*Contraindicated* in severe hypertension or heart disease *Contraindicated* in comatose patients *Frequent* drowsiness, hypotension, and anticholinergic effects Maintain patient in supine position for 30 to 60 minutes after IM dose to avoid orthostatic hypotension	Observe for hypotension, especially in elderly or alcoholic patients Monitor intake and output for urinary retention or constipation Observe for vision changes

Drug	Uses	Dosage	Formulations/Administration	Contraindications/Precautions	Nursing Implications
Methotrimeprazine Levoprome Nozinan Veractil	Psychoses, particularly those accompanied by manic symptoms (See also Chapter 17, "Analgesics and Narcotic Antagonists")	*Adults:* Minor psychoses, 6-25 mg/24 hrs PO in 3 divided doses, administered with meals; severe psychoses, 50-100 mg/24 hrs PO in 3 divided doses, administered with meals *or* 75-100 mg/24 hrs IM into large muscle in 3-4 divided doses. Maximum: 1000 mg/24 hr *Children:* 250 µg/kg/24 hrs PO in 3 divided doses, administered with meals; or 62.5-125 µg/kg/24 hrs IM into large muscle in single or divided dose. If IM is used, switch to PO dosage as soon as feasible. Maximum: For children less than 12 years, 40 mg/24 hr	Tablets: 2, 5, 25, 50 mg Liquid: 25 mg/5 ml Drops (oral): 40 mg/1 ml Injectable: 25 mg/1 ml *Protect* liquid formulations from light *Discard* darkly discolored solutions	*Contraindicated* in blood dyscrasias *Contraindicated* in liver failure *Contraindicated* in hypersensitivity Also used as an analgesic and an adjunct to anesthesia May cause varying degrees of CNS depression	May cause weight gain May inhibit ejaculation; *warn* sexually active male patients that the drug may inhibit ejaculation Have patient inform you of any changes in vision Monitor for excessive sedation Observe for hypotension Monitor intake and output for urinary retention and constipation
★ **Molindone** Lidone Moban	Psychoses	*Adults:* Initial, 50-75 mg/24 hr in 3-4 divided doses *Maintenance:* 10-225 mg/24 hr PO in 3-4 divided doses Maximum: 300 mg/24 hr *Elderly:* Usually require lower doses than younger adult May need to decrease dose in renal failure	Capsules: 5, 10, 25 mg Tablets: 5, 10, 25, 50, 100 mg Concentrate: 20 mg/ml	*Contraindicated* in comatose patients *Contraindicated* in hypersensitivity *Contraindicated* in severe CNS depression *Frequent* drowsiness, parkinsonism, and akathisia *Warn* patients about possible drowsiness and avoidance of activities requiring mental alertness *Commonly* causes atropine-like effects (e.g., dry mouth, decreased GI secretions, and urinary retention)	Monitor intake and output for urinary retention and constipation Observe for parkinsonism

Continued.

NURSING DRUG DIGEST—cont'd

Medication (trade name)	Indication	Usual dosage and administration	Dosage forms, preparation, and storage	Contraindications, cautions, and comments	Monitoring
Perphenazine Etrafon Forte* Etrafon* Etrafon-A* Fentazin Phenazine Triavil* Trilafon	Psychoses	*Adults:* 6-64 mg/24 hr PO in 2-4 divided doses, or 1-10 mg IM repeated in 6 hr if necessary *Children:* 12 years and older, give lower range of adult dosage Dilute each 5 ml of oral concentrate with 60 ml of diluent such as carbonated beverage, orange juice, or water Do *not* mix with apple juice, coffee, cola, grape juice, or tea Care in handling because solution can cause contact dermatitis Do *not* administer IV for psychiatric conditions	Tablets: 2, 4, 8, 16 mg Suppositories: 2, 4, 8 mg Concentrate: 16 mg/5 ml Syrup: 2 mg/5 ml Injectable: 5 mg/1 ml Store solution protected from light in an amber bottle Store between 2° and 8° C Shake concentrate well before use	*Contraindicated* in comatose states *Contraindicated* in blood dyscrasias *Contraindicated* in severe liver damage *Common* extrapryamidal reactions with large doses	Observe for orthostatic hypotension in elderly, or alcoholic patients, especially if these patients have cardiovascular disease
	Nausea and vomiting	*Adults:* 8-30 mg/24 hr in 2-4 divided doses PO, IM; or 1-3 mg/24 hr IV *Children:* 1-5 mg/24 hr PO, IM in 1-2 doses IV solution should be diluted with NS to a concentration of 0.5 mg/1 ml and should be administered at a rate *no* greater than 1 mg/min (maximum: 5 mg IV) Do *not* administer IV to children			
Pimozide Orap	Chronic schizophrenia *not* accompanied by manic symptoms	*Adults: Initial*, 2-4 mg/24 hr PO q.h.s. Increase by 2-4 mg weekly until desired response Maximum: 30 mg/24 hr *Children:* Clinical experience is limited, and thus use is *not* recommended	Tablets: 2, 4, 10 mg	*Contraindicated* in patients with CNS depression, parkinsonism, liver dysfunction, blood dyscrasias, hypersensitivity to pimozide or related compounds, or renal insufficiency	NOTE: Because clinical experience in North America with this drug is limited, the nurse should be particularly diligent in monitoring for *any* untoward or adverse effect of this drug, and these should be reported immediately

Drug	Use	Dosage	Preparations/Notes	Nursing Considerations
			Commonly causes extrapyramidal reactions, including akathisia, dystonia (especially torticollis), and parkinsonism / Use with *caution* in patients with cardiovascular disorders because pimozide may cause hypotension, tachycardia, and a prolongation of the Q-T interval of the ECG / Use with *caution* in patients with epileptic disorders because pimozide may decrease the convulsive threshold	Observe for extrapyramidal reactions / If patient is on a cardiac monitor, observe for any early ECG changes
Piperacetazine Actazine Quide	Psychoses	*Adults:* Initial, 20-40 mg/24 hr PO in 2-4 divided doses / Maintenance: increase gradually from initial dose over 3-5 days to 100-160 mg/24 hr / *Children:* 12 years and older, same as adult dose / *Elderly:* usually require one-fourth to one-half the adult dose	Tablets: 10, 25, 50 mg / Protect from light	*Contraindicated* in pregnant patients / *Contraindicated* in comatose states / *Contraindicated* in blood dyscrasias / *Contraindicated* in liver disease / *Frequent* incidence of extrapyramidal reactions and drowsiness / More effective in acute versus chronic schizophrenia
Prochlorperazine Combid Spansule* Combid* Compazine Eskatrol* Stemetil Tementil	Psychoses *(rarely used for this indication)*	*Adults:* 15-150 mg/24 hr PO, IM, PR in 3-4 divided doses / *Elderly:* Usually require a smaller dose / To mask taste, add desired dosage of concentrate to 60 ml of beverage or semisolid food just before administration / Dilute IV with NS or D$_5$W to a concentration of 1 mg/1 ml and administer at a rate of 1 ml/min / IM injection should be made deeply in upper outer quadrant of buttock	Tablets: 5, 10, 25 mg / Injectable: 5 mg/1 ml / Syrup: 1 mg/1 ml / Suppositories: 2.5, 5, 10, 25 mg / Capsules: 10, 15, 30, 75 mg / Concentrate: 10 mg/1 ml / Store all forms of drug in tight closing amber bottles / Suppositories should be kept below 37° C / *Discard* darkly discolored solutions	Observe for extrapyramidal reactions, especially in elderly or alcoholic patients

Nursing considerations column for Piperacetazine: Observe patients with history of convulsive disorders, because this drug may lower their seizure threshold

Remarks column for Prochlorperazine: *Contraindicated* in comatose patients / *Contraindicated* in pregnant patients / *Contraindicated* in blood dyscrasias / *Contraindicated* in severe liver damage / Has greater antiemetic and extrapyramidal effects than most phenothiazines

Continued.

NURSING DRUG DIGEST—cont'd

Medication (trade name)	Indication	Usual dosage and administration	Dosage forms, preparation, and storage	Contraindications, cautions, and comments	Monitoring
Prochlorperazine—cont'd	Nausea and vomiting	*Adults:* 15-40 mg/24 hr PO, IM, IV, PR in 2-4 divided doses. *Children:* Dose is based on body weight and administered in 2-3 divided doses: 9-14 kg receives 2.5-7.5 mg/24 hr PO, PR; 14-18 kg receives 5-10 mg/24 hr PO, PR; 18-39 kg receives 7.5-15 mg/24 hr PO, PR; IM dose is 0.13 mg/kg as a single dose. *Tablets* should be given ½ hr before meals. *Suppositories* should be inserted 1 hr before meals			
Promazine Atarzine Intrazine Norzine Promabec Promagen Promanyl Promazettes Promwill Protactyl Sparine Verophen	Psychoses	*Adults:* 40-1000 mg/24 hr PO, IM, IV in 4-6 divided doses. Maximum: 1000 mg/24 hr. *Children:* 12 years and older, 40-150 mg/24 hr PO in 4-6 divided doses. Taste of concentrate can be masked with flavored drinks, fruit juices, or milk. IV injection should not exceed 25 mg/1 ml concentration and should be given slowly into lumen of the vein. Inject IM deeply into dorsogluteal muscle of buttock. Carefully aspirate before injecting to prevent intraarterial injection and resultant arterial spasm. Rotate injection sites	Tablets: 10, 25, 50, 100, 200 mg. Injectable: 25, 50 mg/1 ml. Syrup: 2 mg/1 ml. Concentrate: 30, 100 mg/1 ml	*Contraindicated* in comatose patients. *Contraindicated* in blood dyscrasias. *Contraindicated* in severe liver damage. Drowsiness and atropine-like effects (e.g., dry mouth, decreased GI secretions, and urinary retention) are common. Hypotensive effects are prominent with large doses. May cause seizures in epileptic patients; use with caution	Monitor IV site for possible cellulitis or thrombophlebitis. Observe for orthostatic hypotension, especially in elderly or alcoholic patients. Monitor intake and output for urinary retention or constipation. Monitor patients receiving large daily doses for convulsions

Thiopropazate Dartal	Psychoses	*Adults: Initial,* 15-30 mg/24 hr PO in 3 divided doses Maintenance: may increase dose by 10 mg at 3-day intervals to maximum 100 mg/24 hr	Tablets: 5 mg	*Contraindicated* in comatose states *Contraindicated* in blood dyscrasias *Contraindicated* in severe liver damage *Commonly* causes extrapyramidal reactions Metabolized to perphenazine	Observe for extrapyramidal reactions with large doses Observe for orthostatic hypotension
Thioridazine Mellaril Mellaril-S Novoridazine Thioril	Psychoses	*Adults:* 30-800 mg/24 hr PO in 2-4 divided doses, or q.h.s. once patient stabilizes Doses greater than 800 mg/24 hr have been associated with pigmentary retinopathy *Children:* 2 years and older, 0.5-3 mg/kg/24 hr PO in 2-4 divided doses *Elderly:* Usually require 75 mg/24 hr PO in 3 divided doses *Dilute* each dose of oral concentrate with water or juice just before administration	Tablets: 10, 15, 25, 50, 100, 150, 200 mg Concentrate: 30, 100 mg/1 ml Suspension: 5, 20 mg/1 ml Protect from light and store in amber colored containers *Discard* darkly discolored solutions	*Contraindicated* in severe liver damage *Contraindicated* in severe hypertension or heart disease *Contraindicated* in comatose states *Contraindicated* in blood dyscrasias Low incidence of extrapyramidal reactions No antiemetic effect Does not affect temperature regulation Drowsiness, hypotension, and anticholinergic effects are common May cause weight gain May inhibit ejaculation; *warn* sexually active male patients that the drug may inhibit ejaculation May cause pigmentary retinopathy NOTE: Severity of side effects appears to be directly related to duration of therapy with thioridazine	Observe for pigmentary retinopathy with long-term use, particularly with doses greater than 800 mg/24 hr Observe patients closely for any signs of diminished visual acuity Observe for orthostatic hypotension Monitor intake and output for urinary retention or constipation Monitor for potential ECG and cardiac disturbances, particularly in hypokalemic patients
Thiothixene Navane Orbinamon	Psychoses	*Adults: Initial,* 6-15 mg/24 hr PO, IM in 2-4 divided doses Maintenance: May gradually increase to maximum of 30 mg/24 hr IM or 60 mg/24 hr PO *Children:* 12 years and older, same as adult dose IM injections should be administered into the gluteus maximus or midlateral thigh Do *not* administer IV	Capsules: 1, 2, 5, 10, 20 mg Concentrate: 5 mg/1 ml Injectable: 2 mg/1 ml solution IM form is also in glass vials; when reconstituted with 2.2 ml of sterile water for injection, each ml contains 5 mg/1 ml; reconstituted solution is stable for 48 hr at room temperature	*Contraindicated* in circulatory collapse *Contraindicated* in comatose patients *Contraindicated* in severe CNS depression *Contraindicated* in blood dyscrasias Parkinsonism, dyskinesias, and insomnia are common	Observe for pigmentary retinopathy and blood dyscrasias with long-term use Observe for precipitation of seizures in patients with past convulsive history

Continued.

NURSING DRUG DIGEST—cont'd

Medication (trade name)	Indication	Usual dosage and administration	Dosage forms, preparation, and storage	Contraindications, cautions, & comments	Monitoring
Trifluoperazine Chem-flurazine Clinazine Fluazine Jatroneural Novoflurazine Pentazine Solazine Stelazine Terfluzine Triflurin Tripazine	Psychoses	*Adults:* Initial, 2-15 mg/24 hr PO in 2-4 divided doses Maintenance: 15-30 mg/24 hr in 3-4 divided doses, or q.h.s. once patient stabilizes Maximum: 10 mg/24 hr IM NOTE: 1 mg IM is equivalent to 3 mg PO *Children:* 6-12 years initial, 1-2 mg/24 hr PO in 1-2 doses Maintenance: Gradually increase to desired effect Maximum: 15 mg/24 hr *Dilute* concentrate with 60 ml of beverage or semisolid food just before administration Do *not* administer IV	Tablets: 1, 2, 5, 10 mg Injectable: 2 mg/1 ml Concentrate: 10 mg/1 ml Suppository: 4 mg Protect liquid forms from light *Discard* darkly discolored solutions Skin contact with the concentrated liquid oral dosage form may cause dermatitis	*Contraindicated* in cardiovascular disease *Contraindicated* in comatose patients *Contraindicated* in blood dyscrasias *Contraindicated* in severe liver damage Takes 2-3 weeks for maximal effect *Frequent* incidence of extrapyramidal reactions and parkinsonism	Observe for extrapyramidal reactions, particularly with large doses
★ **Triflupromazine** Psyquil Siquil Vesprin	Psychoses	*Adults:* 20-150 mg/24 hr PO, IM in 2-3 divided doses *Children:* 20-150 mg/24 hr PO in 3 divided doses or 0.25 mg/kg/24 hr IM in divided doses *Elderly:* Usually require a smaller dose, 15-30 mg/24 hr in 3 divided doses	Tablets: 10, 25, 50 mg Injectable: 3, 10, 20 mg/1 ml Suppositories: 35, 70 mg Concentrate: 10 mg/1 ml Store in amber colored containers to protect from light Store solutions at room temperature	*Contraindicated* in comatose patients *Contraindicated* in blood dyscrasias *Contraindicated* in liver failure *Contraindicated* in subcortical brain damage *Commonly* causes extrapyramidal reactions, sedation, and atropine-like effects	Observe for extrapyramidal reactions, particularly with elderly patients receiving large doses Monitor temperature for hyperthermic reactions, which can occur up to 16 hours after drug administration
	Nausea and vomiting	*Adults:* 20-35 mg/24 hr PO; or 15-60 mg/24 hr IM *Children:* 3 years and older, 0.2 mg/kg/24 hr PO, IM Maximum: 10 mg/24 hr	*Discard* darkly discolored solutions Skin contact with the concentrated liquid oral dosage form may cause contact dermatitis		Monitor intake and output for urinary retention and constipation

BIBLIOGRAPHY

Cohen, M., & Amdur, M. Medication group for psychiatric patients. *American Journal of Nursing,* 1981, *81,* 343-345.

DeVane, C.L., & Ahsanuddin, K.M. Use of psychoactive drugs in children. *Drug Intelligence and Clinical Pharmacy,* 1983, *17,* 562-564.

Drugs for psychiatric disorders. *Medical Letter,* 1983, *25,* 45-52.

Harris, E. Antipsychotic medications. *American Journal of Nursing,* 1981, *81,* 1316-1323.

Harris, E. Extrapyramidal side effects of antipsychotic medications. *American Journal of Nursing,* 1981, *81,* 1324-1328.

Harvey, S. Role of the medicine nurse on the psychiatric team. *Psychiatric Nursing,* 1982, *20,* 16-17.

Itil, T.M., & Soldatos, C. Epileptogenic side effects of psychotropic drugs. *Journal of the American Medical Association,* 1980, *244,* 1460-1463.

Klawans, H., Goetz, C., & Perlik, S. Tardive dyskinesia: review and update. *American Journal of Psychiatry,* 1980, *137,* 900-908.

Kline, N.S. Advances in pharmacological treatment of schizophrenia. *Pharmacy Times,* 1978, *78,* 395-397.

McAfee, H.A. Tardive dyskinesia. *American Journal of Nursing,* 1978, *788,* 395-397.

Priest, R.G. Major tranquillisers. *The Pharmaceutical Journal,* 1981, *226,* 117-119.

Rosal-Greif, V.L.F. Drug-induced dyskinesias. *American Journal of Nursing,* 1982, *82*(1), 66-69.

Skorga, P. How to spot . . . and care for . . . the patient with Lown-Ganong-Levine Syndrome. *Nursing 81,* 1981, *11,* 37-42.

Drugs Used to Treat Affective Disorders

William G. Dewhurst

Medications discussed in this chapter

Tricyclic antidepressants
  Amitriptyline
  Clomipramine
  Desipramine
  Doxepin
  Imipramine
  Nortriptyline
  Protriptyline
  Trimipramine
Lithium carbonate
  Lithium carbonate
Monoamine oxidase inhibitors
  Isocarboxazid
  Phenelzine
  Tranylcypromine

Vitamins
  Pyridoxine
Hormones
  Liothyronine
Miscellaneous antidepressants
  Amoxapine
  Maprotiline
  Nomifensine
  Trazodone

The affective disorders are pathologic disturbances of mood along a continuum from depression to elation. They differ from normal fluctuations of mood in that the disturbances are prolonged, profound, and seriously affect one's life whether at work or leisure. Affective disorders are divided into two broad classes: the depressive illnesses and the hypomanic or manic illnesses. The depressive illnesses, in particular, have been subdivided in various ways: (1) according to supposed etiology (e.g., reactive or exogenous as opposed to endogenous, implying that one group is caused by something in the environment and that the second group is caused by some factor in the biology of the individual); (2) according to severity (e.g., mild as opposed to severe, equating with neurotic and psychotic); or (3) according to the times of life at which they occur (e.g., adolescent depression). For the purposes of this chapter, the depressive disorders can be best regarded as presenting a common syndrome with causes that should be regarded as multifactorial. In other words, depressive disorders are neither reactive nor endogenous, but depend on the biologic, psychologic, and sociologic variables of the individual patient and how these variables interact.

DEPRESSIVE SYNDROME

The depressive syndrome is defined in the box below. The primary change in the depressive disorder is a lowering (depression) of mood. This is best discovered by direct and careful questioning of the patient rather than by relying solely on such signs as psychomotor retardation or appearance.

Secondary to depressed mood, changes occur in thinking (in both rate and judgment), and the IQ may also be diminished as judged by performance tests, although these are reversible on recovery. Low self-esteem and feelings of hopelessness and helplessness may characterize the individual's perception and affect judgment. Certain somatic functions may also be changed (e.g., gastrointestinal [GI] motility may be slowed).

Finally, there is a third category of symptoms, main-

Depressive syndrome		
Primary change	Depression of mood	↓
Secondary changes	Thinking rate	↓
	Judgment	↓
	IQ	" ↓ "
	Somatic	" ↓ "
Associated but independent phenomena	Sleep	↓ ↑
	Appetite	↓ ↑
	Sexual activity	↓ ↑
	Motor activity	↓ ↑

ly hypothalamic or extrapyramidal, in which sleep, appetite, sexual activity, and motor activity are disturbed. Increases or decreases may occur. In mania or hypomania (which is a mild form of mania) the converse occurs.

The essential criterion for diagnosis is *lowering of mood.* The etiology of the depressive symptoms naturally varies according to the individual patient and it is true that some patients' illness may be mainly attributable to the autosomal or perhaps sex-linked dominant gene or genes; others show less genetic predisposition and may be precipitated more by psychologic factors. In Freudian terms, the loss of a love object may be important (e.g., in bereavement). Other depressions seem to have a primarily social determination. Whatever different weights one can attribute to the genetic, physical, and psychosocial precipitants in any depressive syndrome (and it is a matter not of "either-or" but of "how much of each" such factors contribute), experimental facts seem to demonstrate clearly that in all cases there is a final common pathway that has a biochemical basis.

THEORY

There now seems to be overwhelming evidence that implicates a number of comparatively simple amines. This evidence indicates that a deficiency may be responsible for depression and a surplus may well be responsible for mania. There is, however, considerable controversy over which amines are important because for a long time, the most popular views were that either serotonin or norepinephrine were deficient. My own view, which was propounded some 15 years ago, is that the trace amines, phenylethylamine and tryptamine, are important, with recent work increasingly supporting their relevance. Such arguments need not deter the reader from adopting a generally accepted working hypothesis that alterations in various groups of amines occur in affective disorders.

Figure 19-1 depicts a metabolic map showing the formation of two of the amines considered relevant to our topic. In the middle of this map one can recognize an essential amino-acid, L-tryptophan (essential because it has to be ingested and cannot be synthesized by the human body), which is decarboxylated to trypt-

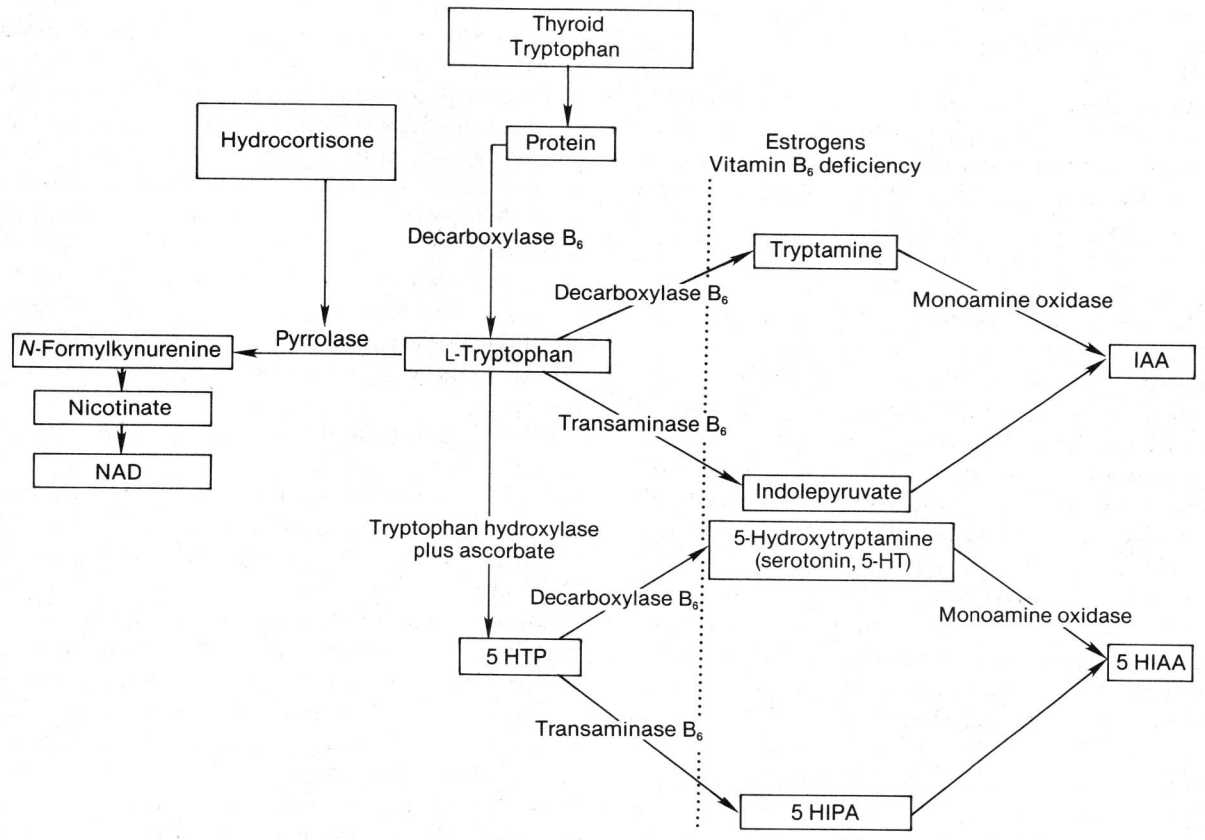

FIGURE 19-1. **Metabolic map that depicts the formation of tryptamine and serotonin.**

amine, one of the trace amines noted previously, and also the hydroxylation of tryptophan to 5-hydroxy-tryptophan (5-HTP), which in turn is decarboxylated to serotonin, which others believe to be important. With this simple scheme in mind, and also taking into account that a deficiency of amines, in general, may underlie depressive illnesses, perhaps this can help in understanding the etiology and treatment of such conditions.

On the right of the metabolic map (Figure 19-1) one can see, at the top, estrogens, and a dotted line descending to the base. In a large study done in Britain under the aegis of the College of Family Practice, questionnaires were distributed to 40,000 subjects taking oral contraceptives, which showed that approximately 25% of the recipients had depressive or *dysphoric* reactions.

In light of the belief that an amine deficiency is responsible, one may see that estrogens, in fact, cause a relative deficiency of Vitamin B₆ (pyridoxine), which is the essential cofactor for the decarboxylase enzyme. Consequently, as the same decarboxylase forms tryptamine, serotonin, and dopamine (and hence noradrenaline) from various amino acids, it is apparent that a deficiency of pyridoxine will cause a diminution in amine content. Furthermore, whether women take the pill, they are still subject to the vicissitudes of fluctuating endogenous estrogen. Production peaks in many cases some 10 days before menses, at which time some women complain of premenstrual syndrome. During this time, mood is depressed, weight goes up mainly because of water retention (both are estrogen-related effects) and epidemiologic studies show that the suicide rate is highest.

If the theory works, one can immediately prescribe a specific treatment for this type of depressive syndrome—pyridoxine. Double-blind controlled trials in premenstrual tension have shown that pyridoxine in a dose of 25 mg or 50 mg a day either given throughout the cycle, or only at the period of highest risk, is more effective than a placebo. For those women on the pill who get depressed, it has been shown by a group from St. Mary's Hospital in London that if evidence of pyridoxine deficiency exists, those women showing such a deficiency within an associated depressive syndrome get better when given pyridoxine. Here then is one situation where a knowledge of the etiology of the syndrome can be linked directly to a specific treatment.

The middle part of the chart indicates the effect of the thyroid hormone or hormones. In general, thyroxin and its congeners are catabolic substances liberating amino acids from proteins and amines from

amino acids. Measuring the amines in the urine of a patient with thyrotoxicosis is almost comparable to measuring the amines in the urine of a patient on *monoamine oxidase inhibitors (MAOI)*, for in both cases the urine is loaded with amines. This also occurs in the peripheral circulation and the essential, integral characteristic of a patient with thyrotoxicosis is the anxiety state almost entirely the result of large amounts of circulating norepinephrine in the peripheral bloodstream. However, because of the phenomenon of the blood-brain barrier, this only reflects a *peripheral* metabolism, and within the confines of the brain a variety of situations can occur.

In the early stages, liberation of amine from stores may lead to excessive amounts of cerebral amines and perhaps a state of *mania*. In the later stages, the inevitable depletion of amine stores will occur and, therefore, depression will result. So the amine idea can explain the various psychiatric pictures that may occur in thyroid disease. Also, as in the case of estrogen-induced changes, it can lead to fresh insights in treatment.

If the thyroid hormone can aid in liberating amines, it should follow that the thyroid hormone might be helpful in treating depression. To confirm this, Prange, et al. (1969) have shown that the thyroid hormone, given as a supplement to the tricyclics, may help in an otherwise tricyclic treatment-resistant patient. Curiously, this phenomenon seems to be sex-influenced, because only women appear to respond. Their work indicates that in women, liothyronine in a dose of 25 μg daily for 2 to 3 weeks maximum will speed up the beneficial effects. The contraindications of such a treatment are cardiovascular disease and thyroid disease. Further, although efficacy is most established in women, Prange, et al. would also have no hesitation in using it in male patients resistant to tricyclic therapy.

On the left of the diagram one may see the effects of cortisone. Although cortisone does not, as in the previous two instances, lead directly to a therapeutic benefit, it does *indirectly* in that recognizing the effects of cortisone may lead to one of the principal aims of all treatment, *primum non nocere* (first do no harm). Acute administration can produce *euphoria*—almost certainly the result of the liberation of amines. In the chronic state (classically exemplified by Cushing's syndrome), the most common psychiatric complication is depressive illness. The way in which cortisone acts (and estrogens may act similarly) almost certainly is by the induction (increase) of an enzyme called tryptophan pyrrolase, which routes more tryptophan down the kynurenine pathway, thus depleting the source of amine production and also incurring a relative pyridoxine deficiency. Some interesting things about cortisone levels are that: (1) they show a diurnal variation, (2) they are higher in women, and (3) they increase in old age. Thus this might, in part, provide a biochemical basis for the following: (1) mood shows a diurnal variation, (2) depression is more common in women and (3) depression is more common in old age. Women are also subject, as we have seen, to the estrogenic mechanism.

Notice the central position of L-tryptophan, the *essential* amino acid, because clearly as a source of amines it might be considered a potential treatment.

One can turn now to Figure 19-2 for a further interpretation of these facts. Here one can see a highly stylized representation of a synapse between a presynaptic neuron and a postsynaptic neuron somewhere in the hypothalamus or the reticular system in the upper brainstem. This diagram is designed to show the normal cycle of amine formation and destruction. Again, the phenomena represented do not depend on any particular theory other than the general idea that an amine deficiency may be responsible for depressive illness. On the left one can see the formation of the amine from the essential amino acid tryptophan.

Tryptophan, which is present in the cell cytoplasm, is decarboxylated to the amine *(1)* (as noted in Figure 19-2) and is almost immediately bound *(2a)* in a storage vesicle by combination with ATP. This binding with ATP in storage vesicles seems to be necessary for at least two reasons. First, without such a combination, free amine would be susceptible to degradation by monoamine oxidase. Second, in emergency situations the rate of formation of amines is too slow to provide all that is required for sudden emergencies that may require a massive and instantaneous release of amines; hence a reserve of preformed amines is necessary.

This process of binding with ATP is blocked by reserpine *(2a)* representing again the etiology and treatment situation. Because this binding is blocked by reserpine, reserpine *in the short term* can be used successfully in combination with tricyclics in treating tricyclic-resistant depression, but by an entirely different mechanism to that by which liothyronine acts. In the long term, however, reserpine can lead to amine depletion and a most severe form of depression.

Following the metabolic cycle still further, after being stored in the vesicle, the amine is normally released by a nerve impulse and after its egress into the synaptic cleft *(3)*, it acts on the postsynaptic receptor, which is stereospecific, and thus activates the postsynaptic neuron. Thereafter, the amine is normally

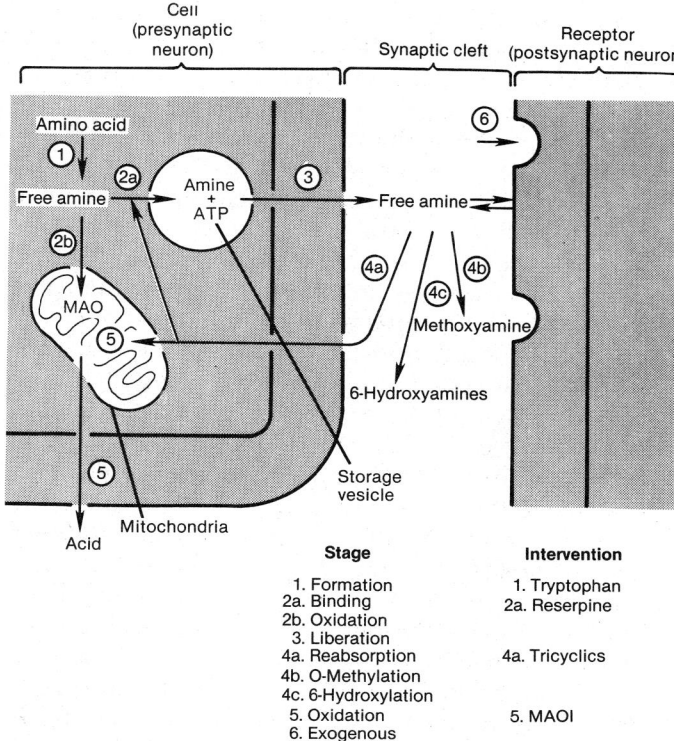

Stage	Intervention
1. Formation	1. Tryptophan
2a. Binding	2a. Reserpine
2b. Oxidation	
3. Liberation	
4a. Reabsorption	4a. Tricyclics
4b. O-Methylation	
4c. 6-Hydroxylation	
5. Oxidation	5. MAOI
6. Exogenous	

FIGURE 19-2. **Normal cycle of amine formation and destruction listing proposed sites of antidepressant drug action.**

reabsorbed into the presynaptic neuron and then is either restored in the vesicle *(4a → 2a)* or destroyed by monoamine oxidase, *(5)*, which is found in the mitochondria. The end product of that activity is the production of an aldehyde acid or glycol, which is then excreted in the urine.

With this scheme in mind, one can see how this helps in understanding and treating a depressed patient. Following the continuing theme that an amine deficiency is responsible, the first step, logically and chronologically, is to give more of the amine precursor. If one believes in the tryptamine or phenylethylamine deficiency theory of depression, then the precursor is tryptophan or phenylalanine. Tryptophan, with or without MAOIs or nicotinamide, has been shown to be an efficacious euphoriant.

There is some evidence that phenylalanine may also be helpful. This underlines one of the tenets of the trace amine theory of the depressive illnesses, which emphasizes substances such as tryptamine and phenylethylamine, as opposed to norepinephrine, serotonin, and dopamine.

If one accepts that giving a precursor makes a patient better, then one must really have difficulty in understanding why tryptophan, the precursor of tryptamine, or phenylalanine, the precursor of phenylethylamine, works, whereas giving 5-hydroxytryptophan, the precursor of serotonin, does not and why giving dopa, the precursor of both dopamine and norepinephrine, does not work either. This, in my view, is one of the many pieces of evidence indicating that it is *not* the macroneurotransmitters such as serotonin, norepinephrine, or dopamine, but the microtransmitters or trace amines, such as tryptamine and phenylethylamine, that are important.

Turning next to the second stage in the cycle, if one believes that amines are deficient in depression, then the most logical thing to do is to give the appropriate amine. The problem is that if one believes that norepinephrine or serotonin are deficient, neither of these gets past the blood-brain barrier. Tryptamine, although it certainly gets past the blood-brain barrier, has a half-life of about 10 minutes biologically and therefore would have to be given by continuous intravenous drip. Furthermore, giving these amines, which are highly active, by such a route would be highly inadvisable because one of the features commonly observed, when one uses these amines in laboratory animals, is sudden cardiovascular death caused by induced dysrhythmias. However, one variation of this mode of attack can be used if one takes the natural molecule and modifies it so it can be absorbed by mouth.

If one puts a methyl group on β-phenylethylamine one produces a substance called α-methylphenylethylamine, perhaps better known as amphetamine. This substance is indeed a euphoriant. The snag with amphetamines as a practical mode of treatment lies in the phenomenon of both addiction and tachyphylaxis (i.e., diminishing effects with repeated doses), although it may be used as a test substance, as I shall discuss shortly. Electroconvulsive therapy (ECT) probably works by mimicking the nerve impulse illustrated by step 3, and perhaps mobilizes amines from reserve areas that are not ordinarily accessible to other modes of treatment.

If one is unable to increase the amounts of amine supposedly deficient in depressive illnesses, what else can one do? We can do the best we can with what we've got and make a little go a long way; this is the manner in which the last two treatments I shall mention in this chapter work. First, if we can inhibit the reuptake of amines into the presynaptic neuron, then amines will remain at receptor sites for a longer time than is customary. This is exactly what the tricyclic antidepressants do. The tricyclic antidepressants are, as the name suggests, big molecules. They are highly

fat soluble—so fat soluble that once they are taken into a cell membrane the reverse is difficult. They thus act as an inert obstacle to the reuptake of amine transmitters. So the tricyclic antidepressants potentiate the biologic life of liberated amines at the synaptic cleft.

Monoamine oxidase inhibitors, the last type of antidepressant discussed in this chapter, inhibit monoamine oxidase and, therefore, potentiate the amines by inhibiting their conversion to aldehydes and acids.

The amine idea can lead to further insights into treatment, as well as into the mechanisms underlying these.

PRACTICE

Management of the depressed patient

The first step in the management of the depressed patient is making sure that the patient is really depressed; the simplest and quickest way is to question the patient closely on this specific topic. Do not be misled by the mask of myxedema, parkinsonism, or anything else. The essential in depressive illness is to have a depressed mood. Accurate diagnosis is the key as it is in all of the rest of therapeutics.

Having assured oneself that the diagnosis is indeed correct, I suggest one proceed as indicated in Figure 19-3. This is a three-stage process, with stages 2 and 3 each being divided into three steps.

Stage 1 is to remove the cause. This is a primary precept in therapeutics, but is not too satisfactory in the depressive syndromes. We may know the cause and can do nothing about it, as in the case of bereavement reactions. Or, we may know the cause, as in a reserpine-induced depression (see box for a list of drugs implicated in causing depression), but removal of the cause (reserpine) may not alleviate the depression because many depressions, no matter how triggered, may still run an autonomous course even when the cause is removed. Or, in many cases, we either have no idea of the cause or we know the cause, but it is so compounded by other factors that we can do nothing about removing it. If indeed the patient is on oral contraceptives it would be wise to consider alternative forms of contraception if practical, or to stop reserpine or, more likely, other hypotensive agents if possible, but this has to be done with circumspection in relation to the physical repercussions; and although I put it first in my list of three, I have to confess that in most cases one can do little about it.

The next stage in treatment is to decide whether one should deal with the patient inside or outside of an appropriate hospital. One cannot easily categorize this as either social, psychologic, or even physical,

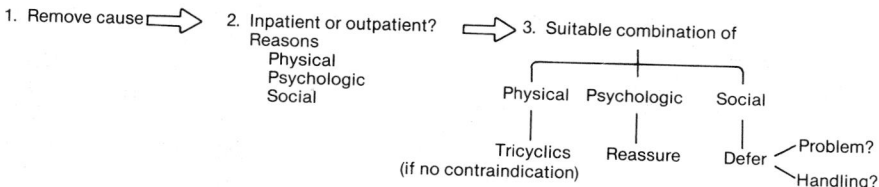

FIGURE 19-3. **A three-stage scheme for the treatment of depression.**

Drugs that can aggravate or cause depression

Alcohol
Amantadine
Antipsychotics
Cimetidine
Corticosteroids
Fenfluramine
Guanethidine
Indomethacin
Levodopa
Methyldopa
Narcotic analgesics
Propranolol
Reserpine
Sedative-hypnotics

---

because all three components play a part in the treatment and one's decision regarding hospitalization. Physical considerations would include serious ailments of which the patient may complain, psychologic components including suicidal risk, and social components, including marital status and the work situation, when it might be helpful to remove the patient from an intolerable social environment.

The third stage in treatment, whether one hospitalizes the patient or not, is to consider a suitable combination of physical, psychologic, and social measures. In the diagram these are put on the same level because the choice between the three modalities is not an either/or one, but *how much of each* is appropriate in a particular case. It is my view that these principles apply to any illness that one may treat.

Social aspects

Now, taking in reverse order these various factors, one can consider the *social* aspects of the treatment of depression. When a patient complains that a work situation or marital situation is bad, my advice is to empathize with the patient. The patient needs to feel genuine concern and to gain an understanding of what is happening. Action should be temporarily deferred. My reasons for suggesting this are twofold. First, many of the life situations described by the depressed patient as being poor may simply reflect the effect of the depression on the patient's judgment. That an individual considers himself or herself a poor worker or a bad parent may well be the depression speaking; if one waits sufficiently until the depression gets better, the problem may resolve itself. Even if the problem is real and has substance, judged independently, the depressed patient in a depressed state may in no way be able to handle counseling. The patient will all too readily concede that he or she is at fault and may do himself or herself a grave injustice. One must elevate the mood before conducting suitable planning and vocational counseling.

Psychologic aspects

Concerning the psychologic aspects of treatment, my advice is very simply one word, "reassurance." I would advise against any tampering with guilt complexes, because these patients have enough trouble. If one attempts deep psychotherapy inappropriately, the incidence of suicides is likely to exceed the average. However, these patients *do* need reassurance from some independent authority figure that they are going to get better and are correspondingly grateful for it.

Physical aspects

As to the physical aspects of treatment, particularly on an outpatient basis, tricyclic antidepressants should be considered. Before tricyclics are administered, however, please recite a small litany of contraindications. They comprise those associated with the anticholinergic effects of tricyclic antidepressants, such as glaucoma or prostatic hypertrophy, which may precipitate a catastrophic event such as acute glaucoma or urinary retention that might threaten life. Another contraindication is pregnancy, particularly in the first trimester, because no one has ever proven, at least to my satisfaction, that tricyclic antidepressants

Sudden unexpected death in patients with cardiac disease
On amitriptyline 13/119 On imipramine 4/87 Nonamitriptyline 3/119 Nonimipramine 2/87

Drug selection	Imipramine	Amitriptyline
Amines affected	NE	5-HT
MHPG	↓ + ↑ −	↓ − ↑ +
Amphetamine +	+	−
Appetite Activity Anxiety Alertness	↓ ↑ ↑ ↑	↑ ↓ ↓ ↓

are completely absolved from the crime of teratogenesis. The final call for caution is for the patient suffering from cardiac disease. The box above is taken from the first warnings by Moir et al. (1972) that amitriptyline is much more likely to cause unexpected cardiac death than imipramine. Later work indicates that possibly the least cardiotoxic tricyclic antidepressant is doxepin.

Drug selection

Assuming, however, that one chooses a tricyclic, which one does one choose? The box above right gives some guidance on the matter. It indicates that, at a theoretical level, substances such as amitriptyline affect serotonin (5-hydroxytryptamine [5-HT]) most, whereas substances such as imipramine affect norepinephrine (NE) most. It further indicates that a low excretion of 3-methoxy, 4-hydroxyphenylglycol (MHPG) and a positive response to short-term oral administration of amphetamine (and vice versa) indicate imipramine might be better than amitriptyline. Aside from such experimental data are four main clinical pointers that might guide drug selection. I call these the four "As": appetite, activity, anxiety, and alertness. In general, the patient with agitated depression and a poor appetite responds best to amitriptyline; the reverse is true for imipramine. Currently I replace amitriptyline with doxepin if in any doubt about the patient's cardiac status; others prefer maprotiline.

Dosage

Having chosen the most appropriate tricyclic or tetracyclic antidepressant, the next consideration must be dosage. It has been shown fairly conclusively in most studies that the minimal dosage for treatment with most tricyclics, such as imipramine, amitriptyline, or doxepin, in adults is a total of 150 to 200 mg a day. Others (e.g., protriptyline) may be used in smaller amounts (see the Nursing Drug Digest). However, because of the side effects previously noted, one would normally give the largest dose of imipramine in the morning (e.g., 75 mg), a medium dose in the middle of the day (e.g., 50 mg), and a smaller dose at 5:00 PM (e.g., 25 mg) to avoid disturbing sleep. In the case of

amitriptyline or doxepin the reverse is true. For amitriptyline, one would normally use something like 25 mg three times a day and 100 mg at bedtime. Many advocate giving *all* of the dose at night in the case of the soporific antidepressants such as amitriptyline and doxepin, using arguments that a one-dose-at-night regimen ensures maximal patient compliance, and the patient sleeps away the side effects. Would that this were true; the side effects, whether one takes the dose during the day in divided doses or in a single large dose at night, persist the next day, and include dry mouth and difficulty in accommodation. Furthermore, the maximum impact of these side effects may indeed occur at night, which can be disadvantageous if a patient has to get up to use the bathroom, feels dizzy, and falls down and breaks a leg. This consideration must be weighed, particularly with the elderly. I prefer to temporize and spread some of the dosage out throughout the day.

How long does one continue on such a regimen? Usually, a minimum of 3 weeks is a necessary trial period before one can judge if the patient is going to respond. Unfortunately, side effects occur immediately, whereas a beneficial response in mood may be delayed, so the nurse must educate patients on this point right from the beginning. Ideally, in the majority of cases the patient will start improving at or before 3 weeks. Then the question arises: does one lower the dose? The answer is *no*. There is no maintenance dose with tricyclic antidepressants. One has to continue at the 150 mg or 200 mg level as long as one is treating the patient. To reduce the dose simply ensures that the patient gets the side effects without any beneficial effects.

Another question is: how long does one continue therapy? The answer must come from what one knows of the natural history of depressive illness. In general it may be assumed that the shortest depressive episode will last at least 3 months. Therefore, tricyclic antidepressants should be continued at therapeutic dosage levels for a minimal 3-month period. Thereafter one may cut the dosage in half and wait 3 or 4 weeks to see if the symptoms return. If they *do,* one resumes the normal therapeutic dosage level and waits another month; by trial and error one can cut the dosage in half without any return of symptoms in the ensuing 3 or 4 weeks. At that stage, one may safely terminate the treatment.

What of those patients who fail to respond? One needs to consider the following and review: (1) diagnosis, (2) compliance, (3) absorption, (4) liver catabolism, (5) therapeutic window, and (6) other factors.

If a patient fails to respond, first review the diagnosis—is one treating a masked myxedema, parkinsonism, or another condition? The next problem is patient compliance (i.e., whether the patient is really following the recommended therapy). In general it has been shown that the more often a patient is required to take a prescribed drug during the day or night, the less frequently the patient complies. Hence, the advocacy for the one shot treatment of depression. One may examine this by discussing it with the patient and in most cases one is able to form an accurate assessment. Lack of compliance may be the result of forgetfulness or of a lack of understanding about how to take the drug. Patient education about the type of drug, dosage, and how to take the drug should be provided individually, because understanding improves compliance.

Another problem is absorption. Because many of the antidepressants are encased in enteric coatings, they may pass straight through the intestine.

Yet another problem is liver metabolism. Those who have ingested a variety of drugs previously may have increased liver oxidases to catabolize antidepressants. Barbiturates are particularly notorious in this regard (see Chapter 5, "Drug Metabolism and Elimination").

A more subtle condition is posed by the therapeutic window, a phrase indicating that one can perhaps give too much of a drug, as well as too little. There may indeed be a curvilinear response to certain tricyclic antidepressants, especially amitriptyline and its demethylated metabolite, nortriptyline. Scandinavian work suggests that one should aim for a blood level between 50 ng/ml and 150 ng/ml plasma, and that both below this level and above this level one does not get a satisfactory response. This has not yet been shown to hold true for other antidepressants.

However, consideration of the last four reasons for failure to respond (compliance, absorption, catabolism, and dosage) indicates that in such nonresponders, without measuring blood levels, one is somewhat at a loss in assessing the situation. Whether to blame the patient, the drug not being absorbed, the liver for metabolizing it too quickly, or oneself for giving too little or too much, can only be decided by knowing the blood levels.

If the patient does not respond despite achieving appropriate blood levels, where does one go next? Perhaps most of us would consider ECT if the depression is severe, but there are other pharmacologic treatments that I have hinted at throughout this chapter. Tricyclic antidepressants may be combined with liothyronine or with reserpine in the short term. Tricyclic antidepressants may not be needed at all in the pyridoxine-deficient depressions, or tricyclic antidepressants may be combined (with great caution) with MAOIs, although this is a combination I believe should only be undertaken initially under hospital conditions.

Finally, what of the patient who has recurrent depressions? In general one has two resources: chronic administration of tricyclic antidepressants, or chronic administration of lithium. In choosing one or the other, one must now be guided more by the etiology of the depression. In patients who either in the family history or in their own history show evidence of episodes of mood elevation (i.e., who have a bipolar disorder), lithium is the drug of choice. On the other hand, patients who neither in their family history nor in their own history show any mood elevation (i.e., unipolar disorders), may be treated with tricyclic antidepressants.

Before starting lithium, a full work-up of the main visceral systems in the body is necessary, specifically the heart, the thyroid, and the kidney. It is now known that long-term lithium administration may be associated with goiters and perhaps hypothyroidism. In the opinion of most experts such manifestations do not preclude stopping the lithium, but suggest that thyroxine or an equivalent be administered in a suitable dosage. Concerning the kidney, the condition called nephrogenic diabetes insipidus may occur, in which patients have considerable polyuria supposedly the result of the inhibition of the antidiuretic hormone. However, evidence has accrued that in a very small proportion of patients interstitial fibrosis may occur, although later work has suggested other etiologies. One is then back to the eternal problem of therapeutic treatment, weighing hazards against benefits. Again, lithium treatment in cardiac failure faces the risk that when there is any salt depletion (which may occur when the patient is on diuretics), lithium will fill the void created by sodium deficiency and lithium toxicity may very easily ensue. If suicidal risk is serious, then lithium is not the drug of choice, because an overdose of lithium may be irreversibly fatal, whereas the treatment of tricyclic-antidepressant overdosage is, on the whole, reasonably satisfactory.

Treatment of tricyclic overdose is really a matter of keeping vital organs functioning for 24 to 48 hours, and usually the patient recovers. For *severe* tricyclic poisoning in adults (manifested by life-threatening anticholinergic effects; i.e., severe hypotension, uncontrollable seizures, or coma with respiratory depression) physostigmine administered intravenously at a rate of 1 mg/min and repeated every 10 to 15 minutes to a maximum of 4 mg or desired response may be used with caution (note: physostigmine can cause bronchospasm, bradycardia, and hypotension). The pediatric dosage is one half the adult dosage, to a maximum of 2 mg. Because the half-life of the tricyclic antidepressants is several days, the patient who overdoses must be closely monitored and the lowest effective dose readministered every 30 to 60 minutes if the life-threatening symptoms recur.

SUMMARY

This chapter has examined the various types and uses of antidepressant medications. The depressive syndrome has been related to the modification or alteration of the level of various amines within the central nervous system. Management or treatment of the depressed patient deals with physical, psychologic, and social variables, as well as with pharmacologic intervention.

With an understanding of the various individual agents, including their actions and side effects, the nurse will be better able to provide optimal care to patients requiring these medications. Patient education can be enhanced, adverse drug effects anticipated, monitored for, and minimized, and clinically significant drug interactions avoided by using the information presented in this chapter.

ADVERSE/SIDE EFFECTS OF THE ANTIDEPRESSANTS*

AUTONOMIC NERVOUS SYSTEM

Blurred vision (change in accommodation is very slight; however, it is noticeable in patients whose accommodation is already impaired by age-related changes)
Confusional reactions
Constipation
Dizziness
Dry mouth
Increased perspiration
Mydriasis
Orthostatic hypotension
Tachycardia
Urinary retention or frequency

BEHAVIOR

Manic episodes

CARDIOVASCULAR SYSTEM

(See Autonomic Nervous System)
Abnormalities in the ECG
First-degree heart block (occurring more often in patients with cardiac disease)
Tachycardia and other dysrhythmias
Ventricular tachydysrhythmias secondary to prolongation of ventricular repolarization and a lengthened Q-T interval

CENTRAL NERVOUS SYSTEM

Confusional episodes, including hallucinations
Drowsiness (particularly with amitriptyline and doxepin)
Epileptiform seizures
Excessive anxiety (often with imipramine-like drugs)
Excessive sweating
Impotence
Increased activity (not unusual with imipramine and related congeners)
Peripheral neuropathy

CUTANEOUS SYSTEM

Rashes (as with most medications) may occur

HEMATOLOGIC SYSTEM

Toxic effects on the bone marrow are fortunately rare, but may on occasion include agranulocytosis and thrombocytopenia

HEPATIC SYSTEM

Cholestatic jaundice (with imipramine)

METABOLIC AND ENDOCRINE SYSTEMS

Craving for carbohydrates
Galactorrhea
Epigastric distress
Unpleasant taste
Weight gain (more common with the sedative-type tricyclics than with the alerting tricyclics)

NEUROMUSCULAR (EXTRAPYRAMIDAL) SYSTEM

Tremor may be prominent, particularly with the nonsedative group of tricyclics

OCULAR SYSTEM

Glaucoma may be exacerbated and an ophthalmologic consultation should be obtained *before* administering the drugs dealt with here

SEXUAL BEHAVIOR

Impotence or decreased libido may be reported

*See Chapter 11, "Drug Toxicity," for an overview of drug toxicity.

CLINICALLY SIGNIFICANT DRUG INTERACTIONS*

Primary drug	Interacting drug	Possible effect(s)	Probable mechanism(s)
Lithium carbonate	Acetazolamide	Impaired therapeutic response to lithium	Impaired reabsorption of lithium in proximal tubules
Lithium carbonate	Indomethacin	Increased lithium effects (toxicity)	Decreased lithium renal excretion
Lithium carbonate	Sodium-depleting agents (e.g., diuretics, especially the thiazides)	Lithium toxicity	Sodium chloride excretion influences lithium retention
Lithium carbonate	Sodium bicarbonate	Impaired therapeutic response to lithium	Increased renal excretion of lithium
Lithium carbonate	Urea	Impaired therapeutic response to lithium	Increased renal excretion of lithium
MAOIs	Amphetamines	Death, hyperpyrexia, hypertension, headache, cardiac dysrhythmias	Potentiation of effects caused by inhibition of amphetamine metabolism
MAOIs	Cold preparations containing metaraminol, phenylpropanolamine, or phenylephrine	Hypertensive reaction	Potentiation of amines causing hypertension
MAOIs	Ephedrine	Hypertensive reaction	Potentiation of amines causing hypertension
MAOIs	Insulin	Excessive hypoglycemia	Unknown
MAOIs	Meperidine	Hyperpyrexic reaction	Potentiation
MAOIs	Methylphenidate	Severe hypertensive reaction	Hypertensive effect of amines enhanced
MAOIs	Tetracyclic antidepressants	Death, hyperpyrexia, tremors, chronic convulsions, delirium	Potentiation of adverse effects of various drugs and amines
Tricyclic antidepressants	Guanethidine (bethanidine, debrisoquine)	Reversal of hypotensive effects	Inhibition of uptake into neuron terminals
Tricyclic antidepressants	MAOIs	Excitation may cause death	Probably via CNS and cardiotoxic mechanisms
Tricyclic antidepressants	Sympathomimetics	Increase in pressor responses with IV infusion of sympathomimetics	Mutual potentiation
Tricyclic antidepressants	Thyroid and TSH	Cardiovascular irritability increased (combined therapy may produce better response—see text)	Neuron sensitivity increased to amines
Tricyclic antidepressants	Tranylcypromine	Hyperplexia, convulsions, sweating, delirium	Probably via CNS and cardiotoxic mechanisms

*See Chapter 10, "Drug Interactions," for an overview of drug interactions.

Nursing of patients requiring antidepressants

ASSESSMENT

Assessment of the patient is extremely important in relation to establishing an accurate diagnosis and in selecting a drug therapy plan. Baseline data is especially helpful in evaluating a patient's response to therapy. A careful drug history should be completed during the initial assessment to identify possible sensitivity to specific medications, contraindications, and cautions as well as to identify the possibility of serious drug interactions (see Clinically Significant Drug Interactions).

SENSITIVITY

Any drug has the potential to cause a hypersensitivity reaction in susceptible individuals. Allergic reactions, including skin rash, petechiae, edema, and drug fever, have been reported with the use of some antidepressants (e.g., imipramine). See the Nursing Drug Digest for further information on specific drugs discussed in this chapter.

CONTRAINDICATIONS

The use of antidepressants is contraindicated in patients with the following conditions.

A history of hypersensitivity to a specific antidepressant. (See the Nursing Drug Digest for specific contraindications to the use of the individual antidepressant medications)

MAOIs are contraindicated in liver disease, pheochromocytoma, glaucoma, impaired renal function, hyperthyroidism, epilepsy, arteriosclerosis, paranoid schizophrenia, hypertension, and cardiovascular disease.

CAUTIONS

Many of the antidepressants can cause drowsiness, and safety precautions should be implemented as indicated. Patients should be warned of this effect and cautioned against operating dangerous or hazardous machinery that requires alertness, until they become familiar with the effect the medication has on them. Because many depressed patients are either suicidal or have the potential for suicide, suicide precautions should be implemented. See the Nursing Drug Digest for cautions related to individual antidepressants.

DRUG INTERACTIONS

Antidepressants have the potential to interact with numerous drugs in a variety of mechanisms causing serious side effects. (See Clinically Significant Drug Interactions.)

ADMINISTRATION

Antidepressants can be administered orally or intramuscularly, depending on individual patient requirements, clinical setting, the severity of the patient's condition, and self-medication abilities.

Starting and stopping antidepressants

During initial treatment, administer medications carefully and assess the individual patient's medication taking attitude and behavior (e.g., is the patient cheeking the medication, possibly for a future suicide attempt?).

Nurses must also know that mild withdrawal reactions have been observed on abrupt termination of imipramine after 2 months of treatment with 300 mg daily. The reactions observed consisted of nausea, vomiting, and malaise. Because a gradual reduction in dosage is usually carried out in preference to an abrupt withdrawal, these reactions should not present a problem. The patient, however, should be warned about the abrupt discontinuation of medication to prevent withdrawal reactions.

During early therapy, drowsiness, orthostatic hypotension, and dizziness are common. Warn the patient, and supervise ambulation. Bedside rails and other precautions may be advised. Monitor recumbent and standing blood pressure. Withhold the medication if the systolic pressure drops more than 20 to 30 mm Hg below normal. Notify the prescriber. Advise the patient not to operate hazardous machinery. If drowsiness persists, the medication can be administered at bedtime because this has worked with some individuals in reducing daytime drowsiness. The prescriber may need to be consulted because the medication may need to be changed to a less sedative antidepressant (e.g., imipramine). Seizure precautions should be observed during initial treatment be-

cause these medications can lower the seizure threshold. Advise the physician if a seizure occurs because an adjustment of anticonvulsant therapy in patients with seizure disorders and perhaps discontinuation of the antidepressant may be warranted. Advise patient of the potential danger of ingesting CNS depressants (e.g., sleeping pills or alcohol) because the sedative property of the antidepressants may be greatly potentiated by these CNS depressants.

Before administering *lithium*, be sure that baseline studies of renal, thyroid, cardiac, and electrolyte status have been completed. Because of its narrow therapeutic index, lithium is considered a potentially dangerous drug.

Suicide precautions associated with the administration of antidepressant medications

(NOTE: See selected psychiatric nursing texts for a more detailed discussion of the nursing care of the suicidal patient.)

Tablets or capsules may not be swallowed and may be hoarded by the suicidal patient until a lethal amount has been accumulated. It has been reported that ingestion of 20 tablets may be lethal (e.g., 1000 mg of imipramine can cause severe tricyclic intoxication, and ingestion of 2000 mg can result in death). To prevent this, mouth checks are often required. This involves directing the patient to open the mouth and, using a tongue depressor, looking thoroughly for tablets hidden in the cheeks or under the tongue. This should be done as an expression of concern and a desire to protect the patient from self-destructive impulses.

Observe the patient's behavior after the medication is given. If the patient goes to the same area following the administration of medication or tries to be alone at that time, it may be that the patient is adding to a cache of drugs. The nurse may confront the patient with these observations with an expression of concern and with a desire to protect the patient from his self-destructive impulses. A search of the patient's room and possessions for a drug cache may be indicated. The patient

Nursing of patients requiring antidepressants—cont'd

Suicide precautions associated with the administration of antidepressant medications—cont'd

should be informed of the procedure and the reason for it, and should be encouraged to observe while the search takes place. Searching the patient's room and possessions has legal implications that vary in relation to areas of practice. Generally, the patient's permission should be obtained, if possible. If this is not possible, there should be clear evidence of a threat to the patient's life. Family members may be involved, if indicated, and may be able to give permission or help with the search. In a psychiatric hospital, it must be recognized that the patient, usually able to move about at will, has innumerable places to hide medications and may be ingenious in doing so. Close observation of the suicidal patient is the best way to prevent self-destructive activity.

Some suicidal patients may refuse oral medications. This may be a more passive means of self-destructive behavior in which the patient invites death by doing nothing to support life. Very withdrawn suicidal patients may accept parenteral medication without resistance, although without giving explicit permission. Others may actively resist injections, in which case the legal implications concerning the patient's right to refuse medications and treatment must be considered by the nurse.

Because of suicide potential, patients should receive no more than 1 week's supply of antidepressants on an outpatient basis until they have been carefully assessed and are responding well to treatment.

MONITORING PATIENT RESPONSE
Therapeutic response

Nurses caring for patients who are placed on antidepressant therapy must be aware that the therapeutic response to the medication may not occur for up to 3 weeks after the first dose is taken. The patient requires much supportive nursing care and much encouragement while waiting for the medication to reach a therapeutically effective level, particularly if side effects are pres-

ent. It is common for patients to become discouraged and to state they are going to stop taking the medication because it is not helping.

Carefully observe the patient for changes in mood. The therapeutic response may result in improved affect, greater interest in surroundings, personal appearance, better sleep, improved appetite, and less psychomotor retardation. When the patient begins to respond to drug therapy, however, the risk of suicide may be the greatest. Therefore, supervise drug ingestion and take environmental precautions, if necessary.

Monitor patients receiving *tetracylic compounds and miscellaneous antidepressants* carefully, because the clinical efficacy and toxicity of these drugs are not yet fully established. Monitor for the onset of therapeutic effects earlier (i.e., after 1 week) than for side effects; however, anticholinergic effects are usually fewer and less severe than with the older antidepressants. Lower dosages are recommended for the elderly.

Lithium

A therapeutic effect does not occur until 1 to 3 weeks after the initial dose of lithium. If the patient is unmanageable during this lag period, antipsychotic therapy may be indicated. If the manic patient shows no clinical response to lithium after 3 weeks with adequate blood levels, the patient is then considered to be refractory to lithium. If the patient is hypomanic and there is no special urgency to control behavior, lithium alone will likely be the drug of choice. In either case, the patient requires intensive supportive and protective nursing care until the therapeutic effect of the drug(s) occurs.

Once the patient's symptoms are in control, including a return to a normal mood state, the patient may often be continued on lithium maintenance at a lower dose. If the dosage is not reduced when symptoms remit, signs of toxicity may develop.

Adverse side effects

Adverse side effects vary widely depending on the chemical family or structure of the particular antidepressant. (See Adverse Side Effects of the Antidepressants for an outline of adverse side effects.) Major adverse side effects can occur during antidepressant drug therapy, and the nurse should have an understanding of the occurrence, severity, and symptoms of these effects and be alert to prevention. Other effects can be minimized with specific nursing assistance, which can do much to promote therapeutic response and compliance.

Monoamine oxidase inhibitors

Careful monitoring of patients receiving MAOIs is essential because of the potential occurrence of *hypertensive crisis* related to their concurrent use with tyramine-containing foods (e.g., aged cheese, Chianti wine) or medications containing sympathomimetics (e.g., epinephrine, isoproterenol). Careful self-medication instruction is essential.

Nursing measures associated with a hypertensive crisis
Death may occur anywhere from 2 to 20 hours after a hypertensive crisis, usually occurring in the following four phases: (1) an increase in blood pressure (BP), sweating, and chills, followed by (2) a severe increase in BP and chest pain, followed by (3) an occipital headache and palpitations, followed by (4) death.

Nursing measures are directed at monitoring vital signs, especially changes in BP. Aspirin is *not* used to cool the patient. Tepid sponge baths and environmental interventions are indicated (e.g., using ice or a fan). The distress subsides in 24 hours. It is important to be supportive to the patient during this time and to explain care and the action of the drug, and to reinforce that the crisis will be over in 24 hours.

Nursing measures to prevent a hypertensive crisis
Patient teaching regarding careful attention to diet and avoidance of pressor drugs and related substances is essential. Patients receiving these medications should have a thorough understanding of the medication and dietary requirements.   *Continued.*

GENERAL NURSING IMPLICATIONS—cont'd

Nursing of patients requiring antidepressants—cont'd

Monoamine oxidase inhibitors—cont'd

Patients should know that the special diet needs to be maintained for 2 to 3 weeks after the MAOI has been discontinued.

Overdose

An overdose of an MAOI can be fatal. Following the ingestion of an overdose, a patient may be symptom-free for 2 to 6 hours. One should not be misled by the absence of symptoms during this period. After the symptom-free period, the patient progressively develops symptoms of overdosage—agitation and restlessness, which may progress to coma, hyperreflexia, and death. The patient who has taken more than three tablets should be observed medically for 24 to 48 hours.

Tricyclic antidepressants

Overdoses of tricyclic antidepressants can be fatal. Early symptoms typically include agitation, confusion, visual hallucinations, and various dysrhythmias. In addition, severe hypotension, dilated pupils, and stupor or coma may occur. Treatment is symptomatic and supportive. Emesis or gastric lavage is performed and respiratory and cardiac support initiated as necessary. Close monitoring of cardiac functioning should continue for at least 1 week. Anticonvulsants may be required to control seizures. Physostigmine (1 to 3 mg IV over 2 minutes) may be needed to reverse the symptoms of a tricyclic antidepressant overdose. Additional doses of 1 to 2 mg IV may be administered every 30 minutes for up to 2 hours, as necessary. Note that physostigmine itself has the potential of inducing seizures and cholinergic crisis (e.g., excessive sweating, nausea, and vomiting) and its administration must be closely monitored.

Psychostimulants

Monitor patients receiving *psychostimulants* for abuse and possible toxic psychosis associated with their use.

Lithium

Monitor patients taking lithium for side effects that can occur as early as 2 hours after the first dose, occurring as isolated symptoms; however, most occur at therapeutic serum levels and subside in the first weeks of treatment (see the Nursing Drug Digest). Side effects are usually innocuous, though they may mask signs of toxicity. The nurse should be aware of the distinction between side effects and intoxication.

Side effects

Side effects are experienced by *most* patients taking lithium. They are never severe and rarely necessitate the cessation of therapy. Those occurring during the first 2 weeks are the most bothersome, but they generally disappear and rarely recur. They may recur, however, if the tissue concentration increases for any reason, such as in the abuse of the drug by the patient, unexpected sodium depletion caused by excessive sweating or vomiting, diuretic therapy, or recurrent infections. Occasionally a side effect may persist, but patient acceptance of the drug is excellent and most do not complain. It is important for the nurse to inform and reassure the patient and the family about the following and assist them in minimizing side effects.

Early side effects include nausea, vomiting, loose stools, and abdominal pain. Patients receiving antidepressants may have nausea masked as an action of these drugs. It is helpful to have the patient take the tablet or capsule with meals and before bedtime. This also assists with compliance. Fine tremor of the hands, fatigue, and muscle weakness are other bothersome effects. The patient can be encouraged to perform gross rather than fine motor activities. Sleepiness, lightheadedness, and feelings of being dazed or restrained are important to monitor. Safety precautions may be indicated, as well as the regulation of activity to the patient's degree of alertness. Extra rest periods can be planned. Polyuria, usually accompanied by thirst, can also be bothersome. Ensure that the patient drinks at least 8 glasses of water or other fluids a day.

Later side effects include edema, weight gain, polydipsia, and polyuria; persistent hand tremors may require dose reduction, especially in the elderly.

Important points for nurses to know regarding side effects include the following.

1. All side effects appear to be fully reversible with discontinuation of the drug.

GENERAL NURSING IMPLICATIONS—cont'd

Nursing of patients requiring antidepressants—cont'd

Side effects—cont'd

2. The occurrence of side effects is not necessarily related to dosage. However, the intensity of the side effects is dose related.
3. Side effects are similar to the early signs of lithium intoxication. The criteria for differentiation include the following.
   a. Side effects, unlike toxic symptoms, are not disabling.
   b. Side effects do not progressively worsen.
   c. Serum levels are not in the toxic range.

Lithium intoxication

Lithium intoxication is a dose-related phenomenon that occurs when more lithium is ingested than can be excreted. It *never* occurs instantaneously, even when massive doses are ingested. Even after a suicidal dose, several hours elapse before signs of toxicity appear. In the usual clinical situations, signs of impending intoxication are visible 4 to 5 days before the clinical picture of intoxication becomes fully developed. At this point it can often be interrupted by discontinuing the drug or reducing the dosage. The nurse should distinguish between early and late symptoms of intoxication.

EARLY SIGNS. The earliest signs of intoxication are essentially *magnified* side effects, including nausea, vomiting, diarrhea, lethargy, confusion, unsteady gait, and slurred speech. The patient's fine hand tremor becomes gross and irregular and is markedly intensified by action. (The patient should also be taught how to monitor for signs of toxicity).

LATER SIGNS. The CNS is the principal target of lithium intoxication, and signs of CNS irritability become even more apparent as intoxification advances. Symptoms include striking muscular irritability with twitching, fasciculation, and clonic contractions of various muscle groups. The EEG is abnormal and there may be convulsive seizures. Confusion progresses to delirium, stupor, and finally coma.

CRITICAL POINT. Some patients who are toxic may have serum electrolyte levels within normal limits. On the other hand, some patients do not become toxic even though their lithium levels may lie within the toxic range (greater than 1.5 mEq/L). Consequently, adequate clinical observation of the lithium patient by nursing staff members and the family during outpatient care cannot be overemphasized.

Nursing measures for lithium intoxication

Provide supportive and protective nursing care. Monitor vital signs and cardiac and pulmonary status, because death is usually caused by cardiac or pulmonary complications. Seizure precautions should be initiated. Prevention of infections is indicated. Recovery takes place gradually over 4 to 5 days in uncomplicated cases. The patient and the family require support to understand the extent of the reactions.

PATIENT EDUCATION

The patient and the family, as indicated, should be involved as early as possible in the patient's individual drug therapy regimen. Thorough teaching and follow-up regarding the storage, administration, and possible side effects, including their influence on activities of daily living and measures to decrease or minimize them, are essential. These should be included on written discharge instructions that have been gone over in detail with the patient and the family. In working with the patient, it is important for the nurse to recognize that many side effects (see Adverse Side Effects of the Antidepressants) can be minimized or avoided by gradual dosage increase to the therapeutic level for the individual patient. Dosing should be discussed with the prescriber, as necessary, in this regard.

Side effects that do occur may be alleviated by nursing measures, thereby increasing patient compliance with the medication regimen and promoting a therapeutic response to the prescribed drug. Careful observations for side effects enable the patient, nurse, and physician to work cooperatively in the care of the patient. Severe side effects (e.g., paralytic ileus or serious dysrhythmia) can be averted by frequent evaluation of the patient's progress and by educating the patient with regard to reporting signs and symptoms accurately.

GENERAL INSTRUCTIONS FOR DISCHARGE/OUTPATIENTS

This medication is an *antidepressant*. It is used to treat depression and should help you. If you do not understand why you are receiving this medication, talk to your nurse or health care provider.

Follow the instructions of the prescription exactly. If you have any questions about how this medication should be used, ask your nurse, pharmacist, or physician.

This medication may cause you to have blurred vision, drowsiness, uncontrollable muscle movements, headache, dryness of the mouth, tremors, skin reactions to excessive sunlight, and gastrointestinal disturbances. If these persist or become extreme, notify your nurse, pharmacist, or physician.

Until you learn how this medication affects you, do not drive, operate any dangerous machinery, or put yourself in situations where decreased mental alertness may cause harm.

Do not take alcohol, high blood pressure medications (especially guanethidine), barbiturates, or narcotics without consulting with your nurse, pharmacist, or physician, because of possible significant additive CNS depressant effects or a serious fall in blood pressure.

Along with the desired effects, this medicine may cause some unwanted effects. Although these side effects do not occur very often, when they do occur they may require medical attention. Check with your nurse, pharmacist, or physician if any of the following occur: sore throat, fever, and malaise; headache; difficulty with urination; mental confusion; excessive anxiety; increased activity; excessive sweating; a change in sexual activity; yellowing of the skin or eyes; or skin rash.

The following three side effects occur more commonly and usually do not require medical attention. However, if they become bothersome to the point where they interfere with daily activities, check with your nurse, pharmacist, or physician. Your nurse can assist you with minimizing some side effects that might occur, as well as help you with your activities of daily living in relation to your drug therapy.

1. Dry mouth, which can usually be relieved by sucking on a sugarless hard candy.
2. Constipation, which can be prevented with a balanced diet including bran, fresh fruits, vegetables, and prunes. An adequate intake of 8 or more glasses of water each day is also helpful. If persistent, report to your nurse, pharmacist, or physician.
3. Weight gain, usually caused by increased appetite. Monitor your weight and eat a well-balanced diet. Avoid sweets. If you need help with diet planning, contact your nurse.

This medication has been prescribed especially for you. Do not trade or give this medication to any relatives or friends.

Notify your nurse, pharmacist, or physician before you start or stop taking any other medications while taking this medication.

Keep this and all other medications out of children's reach.

LITHIUM THERAPY

This medication is used to treat mood swings and should help you.

If you do *not* understand why you are receiving this medication, check with your nurse, pharmacist, or physician.

Because you are on maintenance therapy, you will be required to see your health care provider for periodic physical examinations and laboratory tests to ensure optimal drug therapy.

If you accidentally miss a dose of your medication, never try to make it up. Taking the missed dose can lead to a brief toxic reaction.

GENERAL INSTRUCTIONS FOR DISCHARGE/OUTPATIENTS—cont'd

LITHIUM THERAPY—cont'd

For accurate monitoring of your response to your medication you will require serum lithium or blood lithium tests. Omit the last dose of the drug before these tests. If you have any questions regarding this, ask your health care provider.

Maintain a constant diet in relation to salt intake. This is *very* important for stabilizing your response to your medication. Your nurse can discuss your diet with you if you have any questions.

If you are a woman of childbearing age, effective birth control is recommended, because using this medication can cause risk to your unborn baby even as early as the first few months of pregnancy. Discuss questions you have about birth control with your nurse. If you are considering having children you and your partner should discuss this with your nurse or physician in relation to risks that may be involved if you continue to take lithium. Risks associated with discontinuing this medication at this time can also be explored.

Because lithium appears in breast milk, it is recommended that you do not breast feed. Discuss this with your nurse or health care provider.

Your family should be able to recognize signs of recurrence of mania, including euphoria, decreased sleep, increased talkativeness, increased motor activity, grandiosity, upsurge of sexual interest, distractibility, spending sprees, or racing thoughts. These are signs of relapse that should be reported to your health care provider immediately. Because you may not be aware of these symptoms, be sure family members know how to contact your health care provider. They should also recognize and report such symptoms of depression as your loss of interest in pleasurable activities, lethargy, loss of appetite, crying, and feelings of hopelessness.

You and your family should be able to recognize and report the following symptoms of toxicity: abdominal pain, nausea, dizziness, muscle weakness, excessive thirst, fatigue, and excessive urination. Immediate medical assistance is required if blurred vision, mental confusion, and muscle twitching occur.

For your safety, carry a card that states you are on lithium therapy. If you have fever, weight loss (or begin a weight-loss diet), profuse sweating, decreased fluid or salt intake, loss of appetite, or vomiting and diarrhea, notify your health care provider because these conditions can lead to toxicity.

If you drink alcoholic beverages, limit your alcohol consumption to one drink per day.

Follow the instructions on the prescription exactly. If you have any questions about how this medication should be used, ask your nurse, pharmacist, or physician.

Until you learn how this medication affects you, do not drive, operate any dangerous machinery, or put yourself in situations where decreased mental alertness may cause harm.

This medication has been prescribed especially for you. Do not trade or give this medication to any relatives or friends.

Notify your nurse, pharmacist, or physician before you start or stop taking any other medications while taking this medication.

Keep this and all other medications out of children's reach.

NURSING DRUG DIGEST

Medication (trade name*)	Indication	Usual dosage and administration	Dosage forms, preparation, and storage	Contraindications, cautions, and comments	Monitoring
Amitriptyline Amiline Amitid Amitril Deprex Elatrol Elavil Endep Etrafon Forte* Etrafon* Laroxyl Lovate Maroline Novotriptyn Relazine Saroton SK-Amitriptyline Triavil*	Depression including that accompanied by anxiety	*Adults: Initial.* 75-150 mg/24 hr PO; or 20-30 mg IM q.i.d. A small number of hospitalized patients may require up to 300 mg/24 hr Maintenance: 50-100 mg/24 hr *Children: Not* recommended for children under 12 years *Elderly:* 10 mg PO t.i.d.	Tablets: 10, 25, 50, 75, 100, 150 mg Injectable: 10 mg/ml (for IM use *only*)	*Contraindicated* in patients on antihypertensive medication Use with caution with history of seizures Use with caution in narrow-angle glaucoma Use with caution in cardiovascular disease Use with caution during pregnancy and lactation May impair mental or physical ability to operate machinery such as a car May enhance response to alcohol and CNS depressants May color urine blue-green (rarely)	Closely supervise hyperthyroid patients or those receiving thyroid medication Ensure patient does not have easy access to large quantities of drug Ensure dosage is ingested Observe for mood changes and suicidal tendencies Observe for urinary retention
Amoxapine Asendin	Depression, including that accompanied by anxiety or agitation	*Adults:* 50-100 mg PO t.i.d. May be given q.h.s. *Children: Not* established *Elderly:* The elderly usually respond to lower doses and can be started on 25 mg PO t.i.d.; this can be gradually increased to a *maximum* 100 mg PO t.i.d.; once stabilized, the entire dose can be administered q.h.s.	Tablets: 25, 50, 100, 150 mg	*Contraindicated* in patients receiving MAOIs within the past 14 days *Contraindicated* in hyperpyretic crises Use with caution in angle-closure glaucoma Use with caution in seizure disorder patients Amoxapine has a half-life of approximately 8 hr; It is rapidly absorbed after oral administration, and peak blood levels occur after 90 min	Monitor cardiac patients for development of dysrhythmias

Drug	Indications	Dosage	Supplied	Contraindications and Precautions	Remarks
✦ **Clomipramine** Anafranil	Depression Agitated depression Depression with anxiety	*Adults*: Initial, 75-150 mg/24 hr PO in 3 divided doses Hospitalized patients may require up to 300 mg/24 hr PO *Children and elderly*: 20-30 mg/24 hr PO Increase by 10 mg daily if necessary	Tablets: 10, 25 mg Protect from light and moisture	*Contraindicated* in liver damage *Contraindicated* in history of blood dyscrasias *Contraindicated* in glaucoma *Contraindicated* within 14 days of MAOI treatment *Contraindicated* in women of childbearing potential, particularly during first trimester Caution in convulsive disorders Caution in patients susceptible to hypotensive episodes Caution in urinary pathologic conditions, particularly prostatic hypertrophy Possible initial sedative effect Caution in thyroid conditions	Sedative and anticholinergic side effects are the most common Major depressive symptoms often show improvement within 1 week, and over 80% of responsive patients show improvement within 2 weeks Cardiac toxicity *reportedly is minimal* Observe for constipation in elderly and hospitalized patients Supervise carefully possibly suicidal patients

Continued.

NOTE: For additional details regarding the individual agents listed in this table *see* the text and other tables in this chapter.
*Indicates a multiple active ingredient product. For a complete listing of all active ingredients see the *Drug Reference Guide to Brand Names and Active Ingredients.*
✦ Indicates that the drug is generally available only in Canada.
★ Indicates that the drug is generally available only in the United States.

NURSING DRUG DIGEST—cont'd

Medication (trade name)	Indication	Usual dosage and administration	Dosage forms, preparation, and storage	Contraindications, cautions, and comments	Monitoring
Desipramine Norpramin Pertofrane	Depression	Adults: Initial, 75-100 mg/24 hr PO Increase to 150 mg/24 hr Maintenance: (after 2-3 weeks) 50-100 mg/24 hr PO Children: Not recommended for use in children Elderly: Start with lower dose (i.e., 25 mg/24 hr PO)	Tablets: 10, 25, 50, 75, 100, 150 mg Capsules: 25, 50 mg Store below 30° C	Contraindicated within 14 days of MAOI treatment Contraindicated during recovery from myocardial infarction Caution in conjunction with dibenzepines Caution in cardiovascular disease Caution in urinary retention Caution in glaucoma Caution in thyroid disease Caution in history of seizure disorders Leukocyte and differential counts needed in patients who develop fever and sore throat Caution in women of childbearing potential, during pregnancy, or during lactation Caution because drowsiness may occur Caution in use with alcohol May cause temperature elevation May cause bad taste in mouth Discontinue as soon as possible before elective surgery	Watch for hypomania in manic-depressive patients Observe for urinary retention

Drug	Uses	Dosage	Dosage Forms	Precautions/Contraindications	Nursing Considerations
Doxepin Adapin Aponal Curatin Sinequan	Depression with anxiety Alcoholic patients with anxiety or depression	*Adults: Initial,* 75 mg/24 hr PO Maintenance: 100-150 mg/24 hr; may be given q.h.s. *Children: Not* recommended in children younger than 12 years *Elderly:* Start with lower dosage and increase cautiously Dilute concentrate with 4 oz of milk, water, or fruit juice before administration	Capsules: 10, 25, 50, 75, 100, 150 mg Oral concentrate: 10 mg/ml	*Contraindicated* in glaucoma *Contraindicated* in tendency to urinary retention *Contraindicated* in blood dyscrasias *Contraindicated* in severe liver disease *Contraindicated* within 2 weeks of use of MAOI Caution in use during pregnancy Caution, causes drowsiness initially Caution in cardiovascular disorders Caution in convulsive disorders If sore throat or fever occur, perform leukocyte and differential counts and liver function studies (agranulocytosis)	Closely supervise patients with suicidal risk Observe for urinary retention
Imipramine Antipress Apo-imipramine Impril Janimine Melipramin Novopramine Praminil Presamine Ropramine SK-Pramine Tofranil	Endogenous depression	*Adults: Initial,* 75-150 mg/24 hr; severely ill, hospitalized patients may need up to 300 mg/24 hr Maintenance: Up to 150 mg/24 hr PO in divided doses *Children and Elderly:* 30-40 mg/24 hr; gradual increase by 10 mg/24 hr, if necessary	Tablets: 10, 25, 50, 75, 150 mg Injectable: 25 mg/2 ml (for IM use *only*) Store protected from light Check ampule for formation of crystals; if formed can be dissolved by immersing ampule in hot water for 1-2 min	*Contraindicated* within 2 weeks of MAOI medication *Contraindicated* in first trimester of pregnancy Caution in heart disease Caution in glaucoma Caution in agitation or hyperaction Caution in epilepsy Tinnitus may occur but usually ceases when dose is decreased	Supervise suicidal patients closely Ensure no access to large quantities of drug Observe for seizures and report; seizure precautions may be indicated

Continued.

NURSING DRUG DIGEST—cont'd

Medication (trade name)	Indication	Usual dosage and administration	Dosage forms, preparation, and storage	Contraindications, cautions, and comments	Monitoring
Isocarboxazid Marplan	Depression and chronic debilitating disorders with associated depression	*Adults:* Initial, 30 mg/24 hr PO Maintenance: 10-20 mg/24 hr PO	Tablet: 10 mg	*Contraindicated* in impaired liver or kidney function or hepatic disease *Contraindicated* in cardiac decompensation, congestive heart failure, cerebrovascular disorders, and pheochromocytoma *Contraindicated* in conjunction with other MAOIs, antidepressants, antihypertensives, narcotics, amphetamines, methyldopa, levodopa, dopamine, tryptophan, epinephrine, and norepinephrine Caution, avoid foods with high tryptophan concentration (broad beans) and tyramine (cheese, beer, wine, pickled herring, chicken livers, yeast extract) Caution, discontinue 7 days before change in antidepressant medication Caution, discontinue 1-2 weeks before anesthesia for surgery Caution, avoid self-medication with cough and cold preparations	Observe for frequent headache indicating possibility of hypertensive episodes Observe for suicidal tendencies

Drug	Use	Dosage	Contraindications/Cautions	Nursing Observations
Liothyronine Cynomel Cytomel Cytomine Tertroxin Thyroid strong	See text for use in depression See also Chapter 61, "Thyroid and Antithyroid Medications"	See text Tablets: 5, 25 µg	*Contraindicated* in uncorrected adrenal insufficiency Caution in use in cardiovascular disorders Caution because myxedematous patients are sensitive to thyroid; start at low-level dose	Observe for headaches, irritability, nervousness, sweating, or tachycardia, indicating too high a dosage
Lithium carbonate Camcolit Carbolith Eskalith CR Hypnorex Lithane Lithizine Lithobid Lithonate Lithonate-S Lithotabs Priadel PF1-Lithium	Manic depression	*Adults:* Initial, First day 600–900 mg/24 hr PO in divided doses Second day 1200–1800 mg/24 hr Adjust to obtain serum lithium concentrations between 1–1.5 mEq/L and kept below 2 mEq/L Maintenance: To obtain serum lithium concentrations between 0.6 and 1.2 mEq/L	Tablets: 300 mg Capsules: 150, 300 mg Liquid: 8 mEq/5 ml (8 mEq of lithium is equivalent to 300 mg tablet or capsule of lithium carbonate)	*Contraindicated* in cardiovascular disease *Contraindicated* in renal disease *Contraindicated* if evidence of severe debilitation or dehydration, sodium depletion, or brain damage *Contraindicated* in conditions requiring low sodium intake *Contraindicated* in concomitant use of diuretics *Contraindicated* during pregnancy or in women of childbearing potential Caution, maintain regular check on serum levels (not above 1.5 mEq/L), to avoid toxicity Lithium suppresses thyroid function and may cause hypothyroidism Low-salt or crash diets increase lithium serum levels and may result in toxicity Present in breast milk; should be avoided while breastfeeding	Observe for symptoms of toxicity (fatigue, muscular weakness, drowsiness, coarse tremors, diarrhea, vomiting, and ataxia) Ensure adequate salt and fluid intake Observe for signs of renal toxicity (e.g., excessive thirst, polyuria, or edema) Monitor creatinine and BUN for changes in renal function

Continued.

NURSING DRUG DIGEST—cont'd

Medication (trade name)	Indication	Usual dosage and administration	Dosage forms, preparation, and storage	Contraindications, cautions, and comments	Monitoring
Maprotiline Ludiomil	Endogenous depression	*Adults: Initial,* moderate depression, 25-75 mg/24 hr; increase to maximum 225 mg/24 hr Severe depression with hospitalization, 100 mg/24 hr; increased up to 300 mg/24 hr Maintenance: 75-150 mg q.h.s. *Children: Not* recommended for children *Elderly:* 50-75 mg/24 hr PO	Tablets: 25, 50, 75 mg Store in childproof containers	*Contraindicated* within 14 days of MAOI use *Contraindicated* in severe hepatic damage *Contraindicated* in severe renal damage *Contraindicated* in history of severe blood dyscrasias *Contraindicated* during acute recovery phase from myocardial infarction *Contraindicated* in narrow-angle glaucoma *Contraindicated* in convulsive disorders *Contraindicated* during pregnancy or lactation and for women of childbearing potential Caution in known cardiovascular disease Caution in hyperthyroid conditions or with thyroid medication Caution in history of urinary retention Caution in use with anticholinergic or sympathomimetic drugs Caution in use with alcohol or CNS depressants Caution against driving a vehicle Caution, discontinue as early as possible before elective surgery	Supervise carefully suicidal patients during all phases of treatment Observe for skin rashes Observe for seizures and report; seizure precautions may be indicated

Nomifensine Alival Merital	Depression	*Adults:* 25-100 mg PO b.i.d. *Elderly:* 25 mg PO b.i.d. Reduce dosage in renal impairment	Tablet: 25 mg Capsule: 25, 50 mg	*Not* chemically related to the tricyclic antidepressants Appears to have lower anticholinergic and cardiac side effects than most antidepressants Nomifensine has a mild CNS alerting effect, but appears to have minimal epileptogenic activity Well absorbed after oral administration, reaching a peak plasma concentration within 1 hr, with a half-life of approximately 2 hr Use with caution in renal or hepatic dysfunction	Because clinical experience with this drug is limited, the nurse must be extremely careful to monitor for any untoward reactions
Nortriptyline Acetexa Allegron Altilev Avantyl Aventyl Noritren Pamelor Vividyl	Depression	*Adults:* 30-100 mg/24 hr PO in 3-4 divided doses *Children:* 1-2 mg/kg PO *Elderly:* 30-50 mg/24 hr PO in 3-4 divided doses	Capsules: 10, 25 mg Oral solution: 10 mg/5 ml	*Contraindicated* within 14 days of MAOI dosage *Contraindicated* in conjunction with other dibenzepines *Contraindicated* during acute recovery after myocardial infarction Caution in cardiovascular disease Caution in glaucoma Caution in urinary retention Caution in history of seizures Caution in hyperthyroidism or with thyroid medication Caution in operation of hazardous machinery (e.g., car) Caution in pregnancy or lactation and in women of childbearing potential Caution in use with anticholinergic or sympathomimetic drugs Caution, discontinue several days before elective surgery	Supervise suicidal patients carefully Ensure no access to a quantity of drug Observe for urinary retention

Continued.

NURSING DRUG DIGEST—cont'd

Medication (trade name)	Indication	Usual dosage and administration	Dosage forms, preparation, and storage	Contraindications, cautions, and comments	Monitoring
Phenelzine Monotan Nardelzine Nardil Stinerval	Atypical, reactive, neurotic depression	Adults: 45 mg/24 hr PO in 3 divided doses; may be increased after 2 weeks to maximum 90 mg/24 hr Maintenance: 15 mg/24 hr Children: Not recommended for patients younger than 16 years	Tablet: 15 mg	Contraindicated in pheochromocytoma, congestive heart failure, history of liver disease, or abnormal liver function tests Contraindicated in conjunction with sympathomimetic drugs (e.g., self-administered cold cures), methyldopa, levodopa, dopamine, tryptamine, epinephrine, and norepinephrine Contraindicated in conjunction with foods with high concentrations of tryptamine or tyramine (e.g., broad beans, aged cheeses, beer, wine, pickled herring, chicken livers, yeast extract, excessive caffeine, and excessive chocolate) Contraindicated in conjunction with CNS depressants, alcohol, and narcotics (e.g., meperidine) Contraindicated in conjunction with other MAOIs and dibenzepine derivatives (allow 10 days to elapse between discontinuation and introduction of other antidepressant) Contraindicated in electroconvulsive surgery with anesthesia; discontinue 10 days in advance	Supervise suicidal patients carefully Monitor for possibility of hypertensive reaction: frequent or severe headaches and high blood pressure Monitor foods chosen to avoid prohibited items

Drug	Use	Dosage	Dosage Forms	Contraindications and Cautions	Nursing Implications
				Contraindicated in conjunction with cocaine or vasoconstrictors *Contraindicated* in elderly or debilitated patients, hypertension, cardiovascular disease, cerebrovascular disease, or history of frequent or severe headache Caution in pregnancy, lactation, and in women of childbearing potential Caution in epilepsy Caution in use in conjunction with barbiturates (reduce latter's dose) Caution in use in conjunction with rauwolfia compounds Caution in diabetes	Supervise suicidal patients and ensure no access to large amounts of the drug Monitor vital signs t.i.d. during initiation of therapy
Protriptyline Concordin Maximed Triptil Vivactil	Depression	*Adults:* Initial, patient ambulatory 15–40 mg/24 hr PO in 3–4 divided doses; patient hospitalized 30–60 mg/24 hr (last dose by midafternoon to avoid insomnia) *Children:* Not recommended for use in children *Elderly:* Start with lower dosage (i.e., 5 mg t.i.d.); if total daily geriatric dose exceeds 20 mg/24 hr, be sure to monitor carefully cardiovascular system	Tablets: 5, 10 mg	*Contraindicated* if MAOI used less than 14 days previously *Contraindicated* during acute recovery phase after myocardial infarction *Contraindicated* in congestive heart failure *Contraindicated* in glaucoma or history of urinary retention *Contraindicated* in pregnancy Caution in history of seizures; seizure precautions, may be indicated Caution in history of cardiovascular disease Caution in hyperthyroidism or with thyroid medication	

Continued.

NURSING DRUG DIGEST—cont'd

Medication (trade name)	Indication	Usual dosage and administration	Dosage forms, preparation, and storage	Contraindications, cautions, and comments	Monitoring
Protriptyline—cont'd				Caution when operating machinery or driving a car Caution because use may enhance response to alcohol, barbiturates, and other CNS depressants Caution, discontinue several days before elective surgery	
Pyridoxine Hexa-Betalin Hexa-Vibex	Depression associated with oral contraception See also Chapter 66, "Vitamins, Minerals, and Trace Elements"	*Adults:* 5-10 mg/24 hr PO	Tablet: 5 mg Injectable: 100 mg/ml	Caution in conjunction with levodopa May suppress lactation	
Tranylcypromine Parnate	Moderate to severe depression	*Adults:* Initial, 20 mg/24 hr PO in 2 divided doses; increase after 2-3 weeks to 30 mg/24 hr	Tablet: 10 mg	*Contraindicated* in cardiovascular disease and elevated blood pressure *Contraindicated* in foods containing tyramine or dopa (e.g., aged cheese, Marmite Bovril [yeast extracts], chicken livers, pickled herring, chocolate, sour cream, canned figs, raisins, soy sauce, caffeine in excess, red wine, sherry, beer, pods of broad or fava beans), because concurrent use may cause hypertensive crisis *Contraindicated* in conjunction with all sympathomimetic amines such as those found in proprietary cough and cold preparations	Supervise suicidal patients throughout all phases of treatment Monitor diet to avoid prohibited items Observe for start of hypertensive crisis and frequent or severe headaches

Continued.

Drug	Uses	Dosage	Availability	Contraindications and cautions	Nursing considerations
Trazodone Desyrel	Depression, including that accompanied by anxiety or agitation	*Adults:* 50-100 mg PO t.i.d. Maximum: 600 mg/24 hr *Children: Not* established Administration with meals may *decrease* absorption; administration shortly after meals can increase absorption by as much as 20%	Tablets: 50, 100 mg Protect from light	*Contraindicated* in conjunction with methyldopa and compounds *Contraindicated* in pheochromocytoma *Contraindicated* in conjunction with other MAOIs and antidepressant drugs *Contraindicated* in history of liver disease or abnormal liver function tests *Contraindicated* in history of frequent or recurring headaches Caution by allowing medication-free interval of at least 1 week before administering another antidepressant and then using half the normal dosage Caution with its use in conjunction with CNS depressants (e.g., morphine, meperidine, barbiturates, alcohol, hypotensive agents, and antiparkinsonism drugs) Caution in suspected myocardial ischemia Caution in epilepsy Caution in pregnancy, especially first trimester Caution, discontinue 7 days before elective surgery Caution in impaired renal function	Drowsiness, dry mouth, and dizziness are the most common side effects CNS depression of other drugs may be enhanced Monitor cardiac patients for bradycardia

NURSING DRUG DIGEST—cont'd

Medication (trade name)	Indication	Usual dosage and administration	Dosage forms, preparation, and storage	Contraindications, cautions, and comments	Monitoring
Trazodone—cont'd				Cardiac toxicity appears to be minimal, with no evidence of heart block or rhythm disturbance other than slowing of the normal sinus rhythm	
		Dose does *not* have to be reduced in most cases of renal impairment, because most of the dose is metabolized, and only small amounts are excreted in unchanged form in the urine			
Trimipramine Stangyl Surmontil	Mild to moderate depression	*Adults: Initial,* 75 mg/24 hr; increase up to 150 mg/24 hr, adding to late afternoon or bedtime doses; some patients may need up to 300 mg/24 hr	Tablets: 12.5, 25, 50, 100 mg Capsules: 25, 50, 75, 100 mg	*Contraindicated* within 2 weeks of MAOI treatment	Monitor blood pressure and cardiac rhythm in elderly patients
		Maintenance: Lowest level required for symptomatic relief q.h.s.		*Contraindicated* in acute recovery phase following myocardial infarction	Close supervision of suicidal patients throughout course of treatment
		Elderly: Initial, 12.5-25 mg and then test after 45 min for orthostatic hypotension; then 50 mg/24 hr and slowly increase by 25 mg/week up to 100 mg/24 hr PO		*Contraindicated* in drug-induced CNS depression	
				Contraindicated in conjunction with dibenzepines	
				Extreme caution in cardiovascular disease	
				Caution in urinary retention	
				Caution in glaucoma	
				Caution in thyroid disease or with thyroid medication	
				Caution in seizure disorders	
				Caution in use during pregnancy, lactation, or in women of childbearing potential	
				Caution in use of hazardous machinery (e.g., driving a car)	
				Caution in use in conjunction with anticholinergic or sympathomimetic drugs	
				Caution in use with alcohol	
				Caution, discontinue as soon as possible before elective surgery	

BIBLIOGRAPHY

DeGennaro, M.D., Hymen, R., Crannell, A.M., & Mansky, P.A. Antidepressant drug therapy. *American Journal of Nursing,* 1981, *81*(7), 1304-1310.

Donlon, P.T. Cardiac effects of antidepressants. *Geriatrics,* 1982, *37,* 53-60.

Dugas, J.E., & Weber, S.S. Amoxapine. *Drug Intelligence and Clinical Pharmacy,* 1982, *16,* 199-204.

Feighner, J.P. The new generation of antidepressants. *Journal of Clinical Psychiatry,* 1983, *44*(11), 49-55.

Fields, E.D. Nomifensine maleate. *Drug Intelligence and Clinical Pharmacy,* 1982, *16,* 547-552.

Harris, E. Lithium. *American Journal of Nursing,* 1981, *81*(7), 1310-1315.

Rawls, W.N. Trazodone. *Drug Intelligence and Clinical Pharmacy,* 1982, *16,* 7-13.

Rosenberg, J.M., & Kirschenbaum, H.L. Lithium. *RN,* 1981, *44,* 44-46.

Smith, D.L. Drug-induced xerostomia. *American Pharmacy,* 1983, *NS23*(5), 35.

Trazodone (Desyrel), a new non-tricyclic antidepressant. *The Medical Letter,* 1982, *24,* 47-48.

Antiparkinsonian Medications and Stimulants

Donald R. McLean

Medications discussed in this chapter

Antiparkinsonism medications
- Amantadine
- Benztropine
- Biperiden
- Bromocriptine
- Cycrimine
- Diphenhydramine
- Ethopropazine
- Levodopa
- Levodopa-benserazide
- Levodopa-carbidopa
- Orphenadrine
- Procyclidine
- Trihexyphenidyl

CNS stimulants
- Amphetamine
- Benzphetamine
- Caffeine

CNS stimulants—cont'd
- Chlorphentermine
- Deanol acetamidobenzoate
- Dextroamphetamine
- Diethylpropion
- Fenfluramine
- Methamphetamine
- Methylphenidate
- Pemoline
- Phendimetrazine
- Phenmetrazine
- Phentermine

Miscellaneous
- Doxapram
- Mazindol
- Nikethamide

Parkinson's syndrome refers to a group of diseases that share a common clinical expression reflecting a dysfunction of the extrapyramidal part of the central nervous system (CNS). The major signs and symptoms of Parkinson's syndrome are: (1) *akinesia* (bradykinesia), a slowness in initiating or performing movements; (2) *tremor*, a rhythmic shaking that may involve the hands ("pill rolling tremor"), arms, head, or legs, and that characteristically occurs at rest and is transiently interrupted by action; (3) *rigidity*, a stiffness of muscles with increased resistance to passive movement (the rigidity may have a cogwheel character evident when the limb is passively moved); (4) generally flexed posture, involving the neck, trunk, arms, and legs; and (5) fixed facial expression ("masked facies").

Therapy in Parkinson's syndrome is directed at controlling the symptoms, especially the akinesia, tremor, and rigidity. Unfortunately, drug therapy does not effect the underlying disease responsible for the symptoms and, consequently, the symptoms gradually worsen despite treatment and eventually become relatively unresponsive to therapy.

PARKINSON'S SYNDROME

Parkinson's disease (paralysis agitans)

By far the largest number of parkinsonian patients suffer from Parkinson's disease (paralysis agitans), a disease estimated to occur in 1% of people over 50 years of age. The etiology of the disease is unknown, but the presence of intracytoplasmic inclusion bodies (Lewy bodies) in degenerating cells of the substantia nigra indicates a viral etiology—perhaps one of the so-called slow viruses.

Postencephalitic parkinsonism

Two pandemics occurred concurrently around 1918-1920—influenza and von Economo's disease (encephalitis lethargica). Postencephalitic parkinsonism complicated the latter. Parkinsonian symptoms sometimes followed the acute illness, but could be delayed up to 10 years. The etiologic agent was presumably viral, but this has not been proved. The clinical features indicated widespread brain involvement. Hemiplegia, bulbar or oculomotor palsies, dystonia, or oculogyric crises accompanied the more classical extrapyramidal symptoms of akinesia, rigidity, and tremor. Intracellular inclusion bodies were not seen in the brain biopsies of these patients.

Arteriosclerotic parkinsonism

Arteriosclerotic parkinsonism is misnamed, and is often listed in textbooks as a cause of parkinsonism. Long-standing hypertension produces vascular changes in medium sized end arteries supplying the internal capsule, basal ganglia, thalamus, brainstem, and cerebellum, resulting in tiny infarcts expressed clinically as a small stroke. A series of such small strokes results in a neurologically devastated patient bearing a superficial resemblance to one having advanced parkinsonism. However, the neurologic signs are primarily those of bilateral corticobulbar and corticospinal dysfunctions together with progressive *dementia*. These patients exhibit uncontrolled laughing or crying (pseudobulbar affect), pseudobulbar palsy, bilateral spasticity (*not* rigidity) and weakness. Pronounced hyperreflexia and bilateral Babinski's responses are invariably present—changes not found in parkinsonism. Finally, the symptoms in this condition (more accurately called pseudobulbar palsy or a lacunar state) do *not* respond to antiparkinsonian drugs.

Drug-induced parkinsonism

Phenothiazines, butyrophenones, and high doses of reserpine will produce an extrapyramidal syndrome mimicking Parkinson's disease (see Chapter 18, "Drugs Used to Treat Psychotic Disorders").

In young patients a single dose of a neuroleptic may produce *dystonic* posturing, oculogyric crisis, retrocollis, or forced protrusion of the tongue. In adults, more prolonged administration may cause parkinsonism or tardive dyskinesia. Tardive dyskinesia is a hyperkinetic movement disorder characterized by chewing, lip smacking, grimacing, tongue rolling, choreiform movements of the arms, legs, and trunk, and an uncontrolled restlessness (akathisia). Tardive dyskinesia is refractory to therapy and may persist permanently following the withdrawal of the offending medication. The parkinsonism is typically responsive to either antiparkinsonian medication or to withdrawing the offending medication. Evidence for permanent drug-induced parkinsonism has not yet been clearly demonstrated.

Secondary parkinsonism

Poisoning with carbon monoxide, methanol, or manganese may result in a nonprogressive neurologic disability with clinical features resembling parkinson's disease, called secondary parkinsonism. Antiparkinsonian medication in these situations has a variable response.

Other degenerative diseases with parkinsonian features

A group of rare degenerative diseases have parkinsonian features as part of their clinical presentation. These include striatonigral degeneration, progressive supranuclear palsy (Steele-Richardson-Olszewski's syndrome), olivopontocerebellar degeneration, and Shy-Drager's syndrome. The response to therapy with antiparkinsonian medication is variable, but should be tried if the parkinsonian symptoms are prominent.

Pharmacologic basis of antiparkinsonian therapy

Axons from the substantia nigra project to the corpus striatum. When cells in the substantia nigra degenerate along with their axons, dopamine is reduced in the corpus striatum. This dopaminergic system has a tonic inhibitory influence on the corpus striatum, which in part is antagonized by a cholinergic system (i.e., a system in which acetylcholine is the neurotransmitter). The lesion in Parkinson's disease can be thought of as an imbalance, a decrease in dopaminergic influence, or a relative increase in cholinergic influence. Pharmacologic therapy corrects this imbalance by increasing dopamine with levodopa or decreasing cholinergic activity with anticholinergic drugs.

Early in the course of Parkinson's disease, when the imbalance is slight, these manipulations of neuronal transmissions are effective in controlling symptoms. As the disease worsens, larger doses of medication are required and side effects emerge from overmedication. Therapy becomes a compromise between side effects and therapeutic benefit.

Special problems with levodopa

Because dopamine does not cross the blood-brain barrier, it cannot be used to treat parkinsonism. However, brain dopamine levels can be raised by administering a precursor of dopamine that does cross the barrier: levo-dihydroxyphenylalanine (i.e., levodopa). This drug has been used successfully to treat parkinsonism.

Levodopa is metabolized by decarboxylation outside of the brain and high doses are required to obtain effective brain levels. For this reason, levodopa is now combined with a peripheral decarboxylase inhibitor (e.g., benserazide, carbidopa) that allows higher brain concentrations of dopamine at much reduced levodopa doses (approximately 75% reduced). Nausea and vomiting have been replaced by adventitious movements and dystonia as the major limiting side effects of levodopa because of the introduction of peripheral decarboxylase inhibitors. These adventitious movements seem to bother the clinician more than the patients, who much prefer the involuntary movements to rigidity. Faced with adventitious movements and dystonia, one can either lower the dose, or administer smaller doses more frequently. The balance between satisfactory control and toxicity is sometimes precarious.

Some intoxicated patients develop a hyperkinetic movement disorder characterized by a marked restlessness and continuous movements of the limbs, trunk, or face very similar to those observed in tardive dyskinesia. This side effect requires an adjustment in dose or scheduling.

Several disturbing alterations in therapeutic effectiveness complicate treatment with levodopa alone or with peripheral decarboxylase inhibitors. The on and off effect represents a more or less sudden return of parkinsonian symptoms as the medication wears off. Sudden brief akinetic crises may occur because of a sudden emergence of parkinsonian symptoms or a more protracted akinesia with associated hypotonia (akinesia paradoxica), and may persist for up to a half an hour. These side effects are more difficult to correct, but are commonly dealt with by adjusting the dose of levodopa or adding another drug (e.g., benztropine or trihexyphenidyl) to produce a smoother symptomatic response.

Levodopa sometimes causes a paranoid psychosis resembling paranoid schizophrenia. These patients have highly structured auditory or visual hallucinations, paranoid delusions, and social withdrawal. This side effect tends to occur in the elderly, demented parkinsonian patient.

Patients with akinesia and rigidity as their major symptoms receive the most benefit from levodopa because the tremor is poorly ameliorated and may worsen with therapy.

Levodopa may become ineffective with long-term administration. Side effects also usually become more of a problem. Doses previously well tolerated gradually start producing adventitious movements. The precise pathophysiologic explanation for these phenomena is unknown. Some patients experiencing these problems will benefit from a 2- to 3-week drug holiday when levodopa is replaced by another drug (e.g., benztropine, trihexyphenidyl, or amantadine). Following the drug holiday, symptoms are usually more easily controlled and the side effects are less of a problem. Unfortunately, this benefit is generally short lived.

Surgery in Parkinson's disease

Stereotactic ablation of the ventrolateral nucleus of the thalamus and portions of the globus pallidus is effective in controlling the tremor in the limbs contralateral to the lesion. Bilateral lesions can be made to control a bilateral tremor. The operation has minimal if any effect on rigidity and akinesia. Patients who are primarily bothered by the tremor are chosen for surgery if medical therapy proves ineffective. Hemiplegia from an improperly placed lesion and inadvertent hemorrhage are uncommon surgical complications.

CENTRAL NERVOUS SYSTEM STIMULANTS

Adjunctive therapy in obesity

Apart from being a national preoccupation, obesity does represent a major public health problem. It is well established that obesity increases the risk of developing diabetes mellitus, coronary and cerebrovascular disease, hypertension, osteoarthritis, thrombophlebitis, and stasis ulcers. Reducing excess body weight is a desirable therapeutic goal. However, treatment is extremely frustrating for both the patient and the clinician. Grossly obese patients usually have hypercellular and hypertrophic fat cells, limb and trunk fat accumulation, a history of an obese childhood, and refractoriness to therapy. Although the weight can be reduced, these patients almost universally reaccumulate fat. In contrast, adult-onset obesity is generally associated with hypertrophic, but not hypercellular, fat cells, trunkal obesity (middle age spread), no history of childhood obesity, and a better response to therapy.

CNS stimulants are used in weight reduction programs to capitalize on their appetite suppressing side effects. Most authorities do *not* recommend these medications in weight reduction programs because their anorexic effect is exhausted long before the weight reduction goal has been achieved. The risk of addiction with these drugs is high.

Role of CNS stimulants in the sedated patient

CNS stimulants are sometimes used to counter the soporific side effects of anticonvulsant medication (see Chapter 21, "Drugs Used to Treat Epilepsy"). Indeed, stimulants are useful in this context. However, stimulants should *not* be used to hasten a patient's recovery from anesthetic or drug overdose. Proper management dictates ventilatory and circulatory support until recovery occurs. Stimulants may complicate recovery by inducing cardiac dysrhythmia, hypertension, or violent behavior. The stimulant may wear off before the sedative, resulting in respiratory arrest or hypotensive crises, which may go unnoticed if monitoring was withdrawn during the time of stimulant effectiveness.

CNS stimulants in the hyperactive (hyperkinetic) child

The hyperkinetic child poses both a diagnostic and therapeutic problem. The main clinical features of the hyperkinetic child are hyperactive behavior, impulsivity, easy distractibility, and a limited attention span. This results in an incessant shifting of attention and wandering activity, which becomes a problem when the child is obliged to function in a school. This behavior makes it very difficult for the child to learn and the increased activity is distracting and disrupting to other students. Accordingly, hyperkinesis is also referred to as attention deficit disorder.

There are several conditions associated with hyperkinetic behavior. These include mental retardation, brain damage or brain dysfunction syndromes, seizures, developmental hyperactivity, environmental causes, childhood autism, and progressive neurologic or metabolic disorders. It is important to arrive at a definite diagnosis because the therapeutic implications vary with each cause.

Apart from medication, the management of the hyperkinetic child requires appropriate family counseling and modified educational and environmental management. The drugs most commonly used for the hyperkinetic syndrome are methylphenidate and dextroamphetamine. Although learning improves at a lower dose than does behavior, a higher dose is usually used. Dextroamphetamine is alleged to be twice as potent as methylphenidate, but methylphenidate is generally considered superior because its side effects are fewer.

Long-term use of CNS stimulants may cause a delay in linear growth. This is more of a problem with dextroamphetamine, but may occur with methylphenidate when the dose exceeds 20 mg/day.

Stimulants are not universally successful in treating the hyperkinetic syndrome. Some children may not respond, and their behavior may in fact worsen. The response to therapy must be carefully assessed and the drug dosage chosen after careful observation by the clinician, patients, their families, and teachers. Anorexia and insomnia are rarely a problem because the drug is given in a single dose before morning school. Rarely is a repeat dose at noon required. Children under 6 years of age are generally not treated with medication. Hallucinations, a syndrome resembling Gilles de la Tourette's syndrome, depression, and apathy are less common side effects that may occur with methylphenidate.

Major tranquilizers are sometimes used in the treatment of the hyperkinetic syndrome, but opinions vary about their value. Thiordazine seems more favorable than chlorpromazine. Use is usually reserved for cases in which the diagnosis includes childhood schizophrenia or autism.

CNS stimulants in the treatment of narcolepsy

Narcolepsy is a relatively common disease; more common than epilepsy by some estimates. The two types of narcolepsy, simple and compound, are both characterized by excessive daytime drowsiness and sleep attacks. In compound narcolepsy, cataplexy (i.e., sudden, generalized weakness in response to an emotional stimulus), sleep paralysis (i.e., awakening from sleep unable to move but still able to breathe), and hypnagogic hallucinations (i.e., vivid, often unpleasant dreams on falling asleep) occur along with the daytime drowsiness and sleep attacks that characterize simple narcolepsy.

Narcolepsy must be differentiated from other causes of daytime sleepiness, principally those conditions characterized by sleep apnea, which, by interrupting normal sleep, causes daytime drowsiness.

Research indicates that narcoleptic patients have a restless sleep, interrupted by movements and periods of wakefulness. Night sleep is abnormally fragmented and is often reduced in total duration.

In both simple and compound narcolepsy, it is important for the patient to maintain a regular and adequate night sleep, because disruption of the usual sleep schedule worsens symptoms.

Simple narcolepsy is treated with a CNS stimulant (e.g., methylphenidate, or dextroamphetamine). The dose and schedule must be individualized. Insomnia may complicate therapy if the last dose is given near bedtime. Anorexia with significant weight loss or drug addiction may require interruption of the medication.

Compound narcolepsy is treated with tricyclic antidepressants that control the cataplexy and the sleep paralysis. Stimulant drugs are still needed in individualized doses to control daytime drowsiness and sleep attacks.

Overnight somnographs that monitor cerebral electrical activity, eye movements, and muscle tone have demonstrated abnormalities in night sleep indicating a less efficient sleep pattern in narcolepsy. Therapy with certain experimental drugs such as gamma-hydroxybutyrate, which allows more efficient sleep, has produced an improvement of the symptoms of both compound and simple narcolepsy. This approach to therapy shows considerable promise and may eventually replace more conventional treatments.

SUMMARY

This chapter has examined the various types and uses of antiparkinsonian medications and stimulants. Parkinson's syndrome and related conditions, including drug-induced parkinsonism, have been described and discussed. The pharmacologic basis of antiparkinsonian therapy, including a discussion of the dopaminergic system and individual pharmacologic agents has been presented. The therapeutic use of CNS stimulants in the treatment of a variety of disorders including obesity, hyperactivity, and narcolepsy has also been presented.

With an understanding of the various individual agents, including their actions and side effects, the nurse will be better able to provide optimal care for patients requiring these medications. Patient education can be enhanced, adverse drug effects anticipated, monitored for, and minimized, and clinically significant drug interactions avoided by using the information presented in this chapter.

ADVERSE/SIDE EFFECTS OF ANTIPARKINSONIAN DRUGS*

CARDIOVASCULAR AND RESPIRATORY SYSTEMS

Bizarre breathing patterns
Cough
Feeling of pressure in the chest
Flushing
Hoarseness
Orthostatic hypotension
Phlebitis
Tachycardia

CENTRAL NERVOUS SYSTEM

Agitation
Anxiety
Angle-closure glaucoma
Blurred vision
Delusions
Depression with suicidal tendencies
Disturbed behavior
Dry mouth
Euphoria
Hallucinations
Headache
Hypomania in bipolar depressed
   patients (levodopa)
Increased hand tremor
Mental confusion
Nervousness (many mental side
   effects can be obviated by
   introducing the drug slowly)

Nightmares
Numbness of fingers
Paranoia
Psychotic episodes
Stimulation

GASTROINTESTINAL SYSTEM

Abdominal distress and pain
Anorexia
Bitter taste
Burning sensation of tongue
Constipation
Dilatation of the colon
Duodenal ulcer
Dysphagia
Eructation
Flatulence
Gastrointestinal (GI) bleeding
Hiccup
Nausea
Paralytic ileus
Sialorrhea
Vomiting

HEMATOLOGIC SYSTEM

Agranulocytosis
Hemolytic anemia
Leukopenia

METABOLIC AND ENDOCRINE SYSTEM

Increased libido with antisocial
   behavior

MUSCULOSKELETAL SYSTEM

Bruxism
Low back pain
Muscle spasm and twitching of
   mouth, eyes, or tongue
Oculogyric crisis

RENAL AND URINARY SYSTEMS

Hematuria
Incontinence
Retention
Urinary hesitancy

ABNORMALITIES IN LABORATORY TESTS

Elevation of BUN, SGOT, SGPT, LDH,
   bilirubin, alkaline phosphatase, or
   PBI
Elevation of uric acid with
   colorimetric method
Occasional reduction in WBC,
   hemoglobin, and hematocrit
   Positive Coombs' test

*See Chapter 11, "Drug Toxicity," for an overview of drug toxicity.

ADVERSE/SIDE EFFECTS OF CNS STIMULANTS*

CARDIOVASCULAR SYSTEM

Angina
Changes in blood pressure
Palpitation

CENTRAL NERVOUS SYSTEM

Addiction
Dizziness
Dysphoria
Dyskinesia

Euphoria
Headache
Insomnia
Overstimulation
Psychotic episodes
Restlessness
Tremor

CUTANEOUS SYSTEM

Urticaria

GASTROINTESTINAL SYSTEM

Anorexia
Diarrhea
Dryness of mouth
Nausea
Unpleasant taste
Weight loss

*See Chapter 11, "Drug Toxicity," for an overview of drug toxicity.

CLINICALLY SIGNIFICANT DRUG INTERACTIONS*

Primary drug	Interacting drug	Possible effect(s)	Probable mechanism(s)
Amphetamines	MAO Is	Increased amphetamine effect (headache, hypertensive crisis)	Decreased metabolism
Amphetamines	Sodium bicarbonate	Prolonged amphetamine effect	Reduced urine excretion in alkaline urine
Levodopa	MAO Is	Hypertensive crisis even after prolonged periods of withdrawal of either drug	Decreased dopamine degradation; increased storage and release of dopamine and norepinephrine
Levodopa	Methyldopa	Decreased therapeutic effect	May replace levodopa with a "false" neurotransmitter
Levodopa	Phenothiazines	Decreased therapeutic effectiveness of levodopa	Interferes with dopamine synthesis
Levodopa	Pyridoxine	Inhibits the effect of levodopa; must not be used concurrently	Stimulates metabolism (decarboxylation of levodopa)
Methylphenidate	Guanethidine	Increased hypotensive effect	CNS stimulation

*See Chapter 10, "Drug Interactions," for an overview of drug interactions.

GENERAL NURSING IMPLICATIONS

Nursing of patients requiring antiparkinsonian medications

ASSESSMENT

Assessment of the patient is essential in relation to obtaining baseline data for monitoring the therapeutic drug response and side effects, in addition to formulating an individualized care plan. The presence or absence of the classic signs of parkinsonism and their extent should be noted, including slowness of movement, immobile facial expressions, *festinating gait*, intermittent tremor at rest, speech difficulties (e.g., *palilalia, echolalia*), drooling, excessive perspiration, seborrhea, orthostatic hypotension, constipation caused by hypomotility of the GI tract, other autonomic involvement, and mental depression. Loss of libido and impotence may also be observed.

Assessment should include a detailed drug history to identify the possibility of sensitivity to the selected antiparkinsonian medication, as well as cautions, contraindications, and to identify possible serious drug interactions (see Clinically Significant Drug Interactions).

SENSITIVITY

Any drug has the potential to cause a hypersensitivity reaction in susceptible individuals. The possibility of sensitivity should be carefully explored with the patient, although allergic reactions to antiparkinsonian medications are rare. When antiparkinsonian medications are administered for the first time, patients should be monitored for skin rash, itchiness, fever, and wheeziness.

CONTRAINDICATIONS

The use of antiparkinsonian medications is contraindicated in hypersensitivity and narrow-angle glaucoma.

See the Nursing Drug Digest for specific contraindications associated with individual agents.

CAUTIONS

Because a wide range of chemically diverse drugs are used in the direct and adjunctive management of parkinsonism and the related disorders, see the Nursing Drug Digest for cautions related to each specific medication.

In general, however, pregnant women should be treated only when necessary, particularly during the first trimester of pregnancy. The use of these agents must be weighed against the risk to the mother and the embryo.

DRUG INTERACTIONS

As a wide range of chemically diverse drugs are used in the direct and adjunctive treatment of parkinsonism and related disorders, see Clinically Significant Drug Interactions for clinically significant drug interactions involving antiparkinsonian medications.

Be aware that parkinsonian symptoms may be exacerbated or caused by phenothiazines (e.g., chlorpromazine) or other medications such as butyrophenones and high doses of reserpine.

ADMINISTRATION AND MONITORING PATIENT RESPONSE
During initial therapy

Monitor for nausea and vomiting

Dosage is gradually increased until the patient achieves a therapeutic response or severe side effects develop. Some patients receiving levodopa with a peripheral decarboxylase inhibitor develop anorexia or nausea and vomiting as the dosage is increased. Support is often required because relief of parkinsonian symptoms may not be observed during this time. The nausea and vomiting can be relieved by taking the medication with meals or with milk. It is often helpful for the patient to know that the nausea and vomiting will subside and that an improvement in symptoms can be expected after a few days.

Monitor for othostatic hypotension

Pulse and lying, sitting, and standing blood pressures should be taken every 4 hours during initial therapy. The patient should understand that dizziness on arising is not unusual and will subside. Encourage the patient to get up from a recumbent position slowly and to dangle the legs over the edge of the bed for a few minutes before standing. The patient should be encouraged to stand up and ambulate slowly and to avoid sudden changes in position. Elastic stockings may be beneficial.

Continued therapy

Monitor therapeutic response

Although drug therapy does not halt the progression of the condition, patient mobility should be improved, and akinesia, tremor, rigidity, stooped posture, altered gait, and other symptoms should be relieved to some degree.

Monitor adverse side effects (see Adverse/Side Effects of Antiparkinsonian Drugs) and plan to minimize the following

Dry mouth, constipation, difficult urination (urinary frequency, incontinence, and retention) are common problems associated with anticholinergic drug regimens. Plan for promoting bowel and urinary function with the patient before discharge. Dryness of the mouth can be relieved with sugarless gum or hard candies, ice chips, or increased fluid intake unless contraindicated.

Dyskinesia related to the duration of treatment involving the face, tongue, and mouth, will result in involuntary grimaces or will involve the whole body. The patient should be prepared for this side effect and be able to recognize spasmodic or twitching contractions of the eyelids as early signs of dyskinesia related to prolonged therapy or toxicity.

Behavioral changes can also occur. Hallucinations can occur with higher doses of these medications. Confusion, particularly in the elderly, demented patient may worsen at night, requiring the use of bedside rails, a night light, or other precautions. Nightmares and paranoid delusions can occur in patients receiving bromocriptine alone or in combination with levodopa.

It is important to note that increased or exaggerated side effects can occur if amantadine is used in combination with levodopa or the anticholinergics.

PATIENT EDUCATION

Involve the patient and the family, as indicated, as early as possible in the drug therapy plan and regimen. They should have a knowledge of the medication regimen and a clear under-

GENERAL NURSING IMPLICATIONS—cont'd

Nursing of patients requiring antiparkinsonian medications—cont'd

PATIENT EDUCATION—cont'd

standing of the purpose of the medication, its predictable side effects (see Adverse/Side Effects of Antiparkinsonian Drugs), and what can be done to minimize the side effects. The patient and the family should understand that the medication can help to control the symptoms of this progressive disease and will need support in recognizing the chronic nature of this condition and the continued need for medication.

Patients and their families require continued monitoring and support in relation to adapting to changes in meeting activities of daily living. Support and assistance in promoting self-care in dressing, eating, and socialization is extremely important, in addition to establishing normal gait and balance.

Modification of drug regimens, self-care behaviors, and assistance with compliance are indicated over time as patients show signs of dementia during the course of therapy.

Treatment modifications are often indicated when the benefits are outweighed by the adverse effects. Modifications should be explored so that the patient's ability to minimize adverse effects is enhanced. It may be necessary to explore with the prescriber the possibility of decreasing the dose of the offending agent, changing to another antiparkinsonian medication, or treating the adverse effect with another medication (e.g., treating vomiting with an antiemetic).

Follow-up is especially important after 2 to 3 years of the onset of Parkinson's syndrome, because therapeutic responsiveness tends to decrease after 3 years and the usual progression of the condition tends to accelerate.

Nursing of patients requiring CNS stimulants

ASSESSMENT

Assessment of the patient is essential in relation to obtaining baseline data for monitoring the therapeutic drug response and side effects, in addition to formulating an individualized care plan. Assessment depends on which condition is being treated. In the treatment of narcolepsy, assessment should include a sleep history, identifying the sleep-wakefulness pattern, as well as the frequency and duration of narcoleptic attacks. In the treatment of hyperkinetic disorders in children, the general affect of the child, as well as the level of activity over 24 hours, should be noted. These baseline measures will be indicators with which future comparisons can be made to assess the therapeutic response.

In addition, because the CNS stimulants can cause adverse side effects, including the elevation of blood pressure, insomnia, and weight loss, a baseline assessment should also be made of these related physical parameters to monitor the extent of the adverse side effects caused by using these agents.

Assessment should include a detailed drug history to identify the possibility of sensitivity, cautions, contraindications, and drug interactions before initiating stimulant therapy.

SENSITIVITY

Any drug has the potential to cause a hypersensitivity reaction in susceptible individuals. The possibility of sensitivity should be carefully explored with the patient, although allergic reactions are typically rare.

Allergic rections can include urticaria. Hypersensitivity reactions signified by an unusual response to the CNS stimulant such as extreme CNS excitation or psychotic episodes, although rare, are more likely to occur in the very young, the very elderly, or debilitated patients.

CONTRAINDICATIONS

The use of stimulants is contraindicated in hypersensitivity to specific agents, a history of drug abuse, a hyperexcited CNS state, agitated prepsychotic states, severe cardiovascular disease, severe hypertension, during or within 14 days following the administration of MAOIs, and hyperthyroidism.

See the Nursing Drug Digest for contraindications to specific agents.

CAUTIONS

Pregnant women should be treated only when necessary, particularly during the first trimester of pregnancy. The use of these agents must be weighed against the risk to the mother and the embryo.

Mild to moderate hypertensive patients should receive CNS stimulants cautiously because they have the potential to increase blood pressure.

Because of the possibility of CNS overstimulation, patients should be cautioned regarding the use of dangerous or hazardous machinery requiring alertness until they are aware of the effects the drug may have on them.

For specific cautions and comments associated with specific CNS stimulants, see the Nursing Drug Digest.

DRUG INTERACTIONS

The concurrent use of MOAIs can result in severe hypertension and possible hypertensive crisis. See Contraindications.

See Clinically Significant Drug Interactions, for interactions associated with using CNS stimulants.

Stimulants can influence insulin requirements, and patients with diabetes mellitus should be monitored carefully.

ADMINISTRATION

Stimulants are administered orally and are readily absorbed from the GI tract.

Continued.

GENERAL NURSING IMPLICATIONS—cont'd

Nursing of patients requiring CNS stimulants—cont'd

ADMINISTRATION—cont'd

Onset of action is usually within 1 hour, with the duration of effect lasting from 2 to 10 hours. Because gastric irritation may occur, these medications are commonly administered with food.

Dose and frequency of dose depend on the specific drug's indication for use, as well as on individual patient factors and response.

MONITORING PATIENT RESPONSE
Therapeutic response

Monitoring the therapeutic response depends on the drug's indication for use and is performed in relation to patient parameters identified during assessment.

Adverse side effects

Predominant adverse side effects of the CNS stimulants are related to the cardiovascular system and the CNS. Patients receiving these medications should be monitored for signs of cardiovascular adverse effects including tachycardia, palpitations, and elevated blood pressure. CNS adverse effects include overstimulation, restlessness, insomnia, tremor, headache, dizziness, and euphoria. Anorexia and weight loss may also occur and should be monitored. See Adverse/Side Effects of CNS stimulants and the Nursing Drug Digest for adverse side effects associated with specific CNS stimulants.

PATIENT EDUCATION

The patient and the family, as indicated, should be involved in the drug therapy plan and regimen. They should have a knowledge of the patient's condition and treatment plan, including the name of the medication, its administration, potential adverse side effects, and what can be done to minimize these effects. Continued monitoring and support, as well as assistance with adapting to changes in daily living associated with the condition, are indicated. Modification of drug regimens, self-care behaviors, and assistance with compliance are often needed over time. Treatment modifications are often indicated when the benefits are outweighed by the adverse effects.

Patients and their families should understand the potential for the abuse of these drugs and should be instructed to monitor for signs of dependence, including increased frequency of dosage and refills of medication prescriptions.

GENERAL INSTRUCTIONS FOR DISCHARGE/OUTPATIENTS

ANTIPARKINSONIAN DRUGS

Follow the instructions on the prescription exactly, especially the time when the medication is taken.

Report any urinary problems, blurred vision, dizziness on standing, insomnia, loss of appetite, weight loss, confusion, uncontrollable movements, or extreme restlessness to your health care provider.

Notify your nurse or physician before you start or stop taking any other medication.

Keep this and all other medication out of children's reach.

CNS STIMULANTS

Follow the instructions on the prescription exactly, especially the time when the medication is taken.

Report any problems with insomnia, excessive stimulation, or mental changes to your health care provider.

Notify your nurse or physician before you start or stop taking any medication.

Do not give any of this medication to your friends or members of your family.

Keep this and all other medication out of children's reach.

NURSING DRUG DIGEST

Medication (trade name*)	Indication	Usual dosage and administration	Dosage forms, preparation, and storage	Contraindications, cautions, and comments	Monitoring
Amantadine Symmetrel Virofral	Adjunct in Parkinson's disease to control rigidity, akinesia, and tremor To control extrapyramidal side effects from phenothiazines and butyrophenones when anticholinergic drugs are contraindicated	*Adults:* 100-200 mg/day as single or divided dose PO Maximum: 200 mg/day Last daily dose should *not* be given too late, because this may produce insomnia May need to decrease dose in renal failure	Capsule: 100 mg Syrup: 50 mg/5 ml	Abrupt discontinuation may precipitate parkinsonian crisis Use cautiously in patients with a history of congestive heart failure, orthostatic hypotension, peripheral edema, liver disease, epilepsy, recurrent eczematoid rash, or in patients with psychosis or severe psychoneurosis Amantadine may accumulate when renal function is impaired Excreted in human breast milk Activities requiring mental alertness should be resumed gradually	Monitor, particularly in the elderly, for orthostatic hypotension, dizziness, blurred vision, impaired coordination
Amphetamine Benzedrine Obetrol-10* Obetrol-20*	Hyperkinetic children Narcolepsy To reverse soporific side effects of anticonvulsant drugs Rarely parkinsonism To suppress hunger in the treatment of obesity *Use of amphetamines as a stimulant following sedative overdose is strongly discouraged*	*Adults:* 5-60 mg/day PO as single or divided dose *Children:* 2.5-40 mg/day PO as single dose Always administer last dose at least 6 hr before bedtime to minimize insomnia For weight reduction, patient should be on a reducing program; drug should be taken 30-60 min before meals	Tablets: 5, 10 mg Capsules (extended-release): 10, 15 mg Injectable: 20 mg/1 ml	*Contraindicated* in patients receiving MAOIs *Contraindicated* in active cardiovascular diseases (e.g., dysrhythmias, angina, hypertension) Insomnia may result if last dose is late in the day Anorexia and weight loss require a reduction in dosage Use cautiously in hypertensive or hyperthyroid patients Avoid caffeine drinks	Observe for psychologic dependence Fatigue may result as drug wears off; patient requires more rest Observe for overstimulation of CNS (e.g., dizziness, insomnia, hyperactivity, restlessness) Monitor vital signs for CNS and cardiovascular toxicity

Continued.

NOTE: For additional details regarding the individual agents listed in this table see the text and other tables in this chapter.
*Indicates a multiple active ingredient product. For a complete listing of all active ingredients see the *Drug Reference Guide to Brand Names and Active Ingredients.*
♣ Indicates that the drug is generally available only in Canada.
★ Indicates that the drug is generally available only in the United States.

NURSING DRUG DIGEST—cont'd

Medication (trade name)	Indication	Usual dosage and administration	Dosage forms, preparation, and storage	Contraindications, cautions, and comments	Monitoring
★ **Benzphetamine** Didrex	To suppress hunger in the treatment of obesity	*Adults:* 25-100 mg q.d. PO Administer in midmorning or midafternoon for optimum therapeutic effect and to minimize insomnia *Children:* Use is *not* recommended	Tablets: 25, 50 mg	*Contraindicated* in patients receiving MAOIs, patients with hypertension, angina pectoris, and other severe cardiac disease Avoid caffeine drinks; cola, coffee, and tea	Monitor for symptoms of overstimulation
Benztropine Bensylate Cogentin	Parkinson's disease to control rigidity, tremor, and akinesia To control the extrapyramidal side effects of phenothiazine, rauwolfia, and butyrophenone drugs	*Adults:* individualized Initially 0.5-1 mg q.h.s. increased up to 6 mg/day PO in divided doses In drug-induced parkinsonism, 1-4 mg q.d. or b.i.d. PO Acute dystonic reactions, 2 mg IM or IV	Tablets: 0.5, 1, 2 mg Injectable: 1 mg/ml	*Contraindicated* in children under 3 years of age *Contraindicated* in narrow-angle glaucoma Use cautiously in patients with cardiac disease or urinary or pyloric obstruction May cause drowsiness In large doses may induce an apparent weakness in previously rigid muscles; effects are cumulative and may not be evident until 2-3 days after medication is started	
Biperiden Akineton	Parkinson's disease adjunct to control akinesia, rigidity, and, to a lesser extent, tremor To control the extrapyramidal side effects of phenothiazine, rauwolfia, and butyrophenone drugs	*Adults:* 2-8 mg/day PO in divided dose 2 mg IM or IV or up to q.i.d. May produce transient hypotension when used IV Administer with food or milk to decrease GI irritation	Tablet: 2 mg Injectable: 5 mg/1 ml Store between 15° and 30° C	Use cautiously in patients with glaucoma, cardiac disease, or urinary or pyloric obstruction As spasticity is decreased tremor may increase May cause drowsiness May need to aid ambulation	Observe for hypotension, tremor, and drowsiness

Drug	Uses	Dosage	Preparations	Remarks	Nursing Implications
Bromocriptine Parlodel	Adjunct in Parkinson's disease to produce a smoother response by reducing the on/off effect	*Adults:* Initially, 1.25-2.5 mg PO b.i.d.; increase at 2-4 week intervals by 2.5 mg/day until optimum response Maximum: 100 mg/day Administer with food or milk to decrease GI irritation	Tablets: 2.5 mg Capsule: 5 mg	*Contraindicated* in hypersensitivity to ergot alkaloids High incidence of minor side effects (e.g., dizziness, constipation, headaches, nausea, vomiting) May induce reversible *livedo reticularis* The major side effects limiting use are mental changes, confusion, hallucination and paranoid delusions Safe use during pregnancy has *not* been established	Monitor for orthostatic hypertension
Caffeine Amostat Caffedrine Makoz Nodoz Quick-Pep Tirend Verb T.D. Vivarin	Mainly used in combination with other drugs to treat headache In combination with other drugs to combat their sedative effect To combat drowsiness	*Adults:* 60-1200 mg/day PO in divided dose; or 250-1000 mg IM (parenteral use is *not* recommended)	Tablets: 60, 100, 200 mg Capsules: 100, 200 mg Capsules (extended-release): 100, 200, 250 mg Injectable caffeine sodium benzoate: 250 mg/ml Powder caffeine citrate: 65 mg Plus in combination with numerous other medications	*Contraindicated* in patients with duodenal ulcers Has cardiac, cerebral and respiratory stimulant properties May cause diuresis Note that many beverages contain caffeine (e.g., tea and coffee 40-180 mg/180 ml; cola 20-60 mg/180 ml)	Observe for dose-related side effects, including cardiac dysrhythmias, gastritis, insomnia, irritability, and tremors
Chlorphentermine Chlorophen Lucofen Pre-Sate	To suppress hunger in treatment of obesity	*Adults:* 65 mg PO with or after morning meal *Children:* Use is *not* recommended	Tablet: 65 mg	*Contraindicated* in hyperthyroidism, hypertension, angina pectoris, and other severe cardiac disease *Contraindicated* in patients receiving MAOIs *Contraindicated* in patients with narrow-angle glaucoma The anorexigenic effect is temporary and the drug should be viewed as an adjunct in obesity therapy Habituation or addiction is a problem Should not be used during pregnancy Avoid caffeine drinks	Monitor for symptoms of overstimulation Monitor blood sugar and urine (S & A) because this drug may alter daily insulin requirements

Continued.

NURSING DRUG DIGEST—cont'd

Medication (trade name)	Indication	Usual dosage and administration	Dosage forms, preparation, and storage	Contraindications, cautions, and comments	Monitoring
★ **Cycrimine** Pagitane	Parkinson's disease to control rigidity, tremor, and akinesia	*Adults:* Individualized, starting at 1.25-2.5 mg PO t.i.d. Maximum: 20 mg/day Administration with food or milk may decrease GI distress	Tablets: 1.25, 2.5 mg	Vertigo, disorientation or weakness may require lowering the dose Should *not* be used in glaucoma patients	
❦ **Deanol acetamidobenzoate** Cervoxan Deaner Deaner-100	Adjunct in the treatment of the minimally brain-damaged hyperactive child	*Children:* 300 mg each morning PO for 3 weeks, then reduce to maintenance dose, which varies from 100-300 mg as a single morning dose	Tablets: 25, 100, 250 mg	*Contraindicated* in patients who suffer from generalized tonic-clonic seizures Prolonged use may produce a temporary suppression of normal weight or height patterns Overstimulation is most common side effect	Monitor patient for growth suppression
Dextroamphetamine Biphetamine* Dexampex Dexamyl* Dexedrine Eskatrol* Ferndex Obetrol* Obotan Synatan	Hyperkinetic children Narcolepsy To reverse soporific side effects of anticonvulsant drugs Rarely parkinsonism To suppress hunger in the treatment of obesity *Use of amphetamines as a stimulant following sedative overdose or anesthesia is strongly discouraged*	*Adults:* 5-60 mg/day PO in single or divided dose *Children:* over 3 years of age 2.5-40 mg/day PO in single or divided doses When used for treatment of obesity, administer last dose at least 6 hr before bedtime to minimize insomnia	Tablets: 5, 10 mg Capsules (extended-release): 5, 10, 15 mg Elixir: 5 mg/5 ml (10% alcohol) Injectable: 20 mg/ml Also available in combination with amobarbital with or without aspirin and acetaminophen	*Contraindicated* in patients receiving MAOIs *Contraindicated* in severe hypertension, hyperthyroidism, glaucoma, and advanced arteriosclerosis Insomnia may result if last dose is late in the day Anorexia and weight loss require a reduction in dosage Use cautiously in hypertensive or hyperthyroid patients Higher CNS activity and fewer cardiovascular side effects than amphetamine Avoid caffeine drinks	Monitor for psychologic dependence Monitor for symptoms of CNS and cardiovascular toxicity Monitor diabetic patients' blood sugar and urine S & A because can alter insulin requirements

Drug	Use	Dosage	Preparations	Nursing Implications
Diethylpropion D.I.P., Darfon, Dietic, Nobesine, Regenon, Regibon, Tenuate, Tenuate Dospan, Tepanil, Tepanil Ten-Tab	To suppress hunger in treatment of obesity. Can be used to stop eating at night because will rarely cause insomnia	*Adults:* 25 mg t.i.d. PO before meals, or 75 mg extended-release tablet at midmorning. *Children:* Use is *not* recommended	Tablet: 25 mg. Tablet (extended-release): 75 mg. Capsule (extended-release): 75 mg	*Contraindicated* in patients with glaucoma, hyperthyroidism, hypertension, angina pectoris, or other severe cardiac disease. *Contraindicated* in patients receiving MAOIs or who have narrow-angle glaucoma. Should not be used during pregnancy. Avoid caffeine drinks
Diphenhydramine Allerdryl, Benadryl, Insomnal	Parkinson's disease adjunct in control of rigidity, tremor, and akinesia. Parkinson's disease in the frail, elderly patient who cannot tolerate more potent medication. See also Chapter 29, "Antihistamines, Antitussives, Decongestants, and Expectorants"	*Adults:* individualized. Start at 25 mg t.i.d. PO, IM, IV, increase as necessary up to 200 mg/day in 4 divided doses. Avoid subcutaneous or perivascular injection. Administer with food or milk to decrease GI irritation	Capsules: 25, 50 mg. Oral solution: 10 mg/ml. Elixir: 12.5 mg/5 ml (with 14% alcohol). Injectable: 10, 50 mg/ml	Drowsiness may make driving hazardous. Monitor for drowsiness; can be relieved with caffeine drinks, coffee, or tea
Doxapram Dopram, Doxapril, Stimulexin	To hasten arousal and to treat respiratory depression associated with sedative overdose or anesthesia (*use of doxapram in this manner is discouraged*). Other supportive measures are much more important and necessary in the overly sedated patient, and analeptic drugs should *not* be used	*Adults:* IV 0.5-1 mg/kg body weight; may be repeated twice at intervals of 5 min. Maximum: 3 gm/24 hr. Can also be administered as an IV drip in D_5W or NS at a rate of 5 mg/min	Injectable: 20 mg/ml. Compatible with D_5W, $D_{10}W$, and NS; *not* compatible with alkaline solutions (e.g., sodium bicarbonate)	*Contraindicated* in patients with bronchial asthma, severe cardiac disease, or epilepsy. Overdosage may cause respiratory alkalosis. Doxapram has a narrow margin of safety. May induce tachycardia, hypertension, or generalized tonic-clonic seizures. Have resuscitation equipment on hand. Use seizure precautions. Monitor vital signs for at least 1 hour after patient becomes alert. Monitor arterial blood gas levels for carbon dioxide retention and acidosis

Continued.

NURSING DRUG DIGEST—cont'd

Medication (trade name)	Indication	Usual dosage and administration	Dosage forms, preparation, and storage	Contraindications, cautions, and comments	Monitoring
Ethopropazine Lysivane Parsidol Parsitan	Parkinson's disease to control tremor and rigidity	*Adults:* individualized Start at 10 mg q.i.d. PO Increase slowly every 2-3 days up to 600 mg/day in divided doses	Tablets: 10, 50, 100 mg	*Contraindicated* in glaucoma and prostatic hypertrophy Overall incidence of side effects is high Drowsiness, dizziness and lassitude most commonly limit the dosage used Use cautiously in patients with cardiac disease, or urinary or pyloric obstruction	Observe for drowsiness and dizziness Monitor for urinary retention, especially in older men with a history of prostatic hypertrophy
Fenfluramine Ganal Ponderal Ponderax Pondimin	To suppress hunger in the treatment of obesity	*Adults:* 20 mg t.i.d. PO before meals, which may be increased to 40 mg t.i.d.	Tablet: 20 mg Store between 15° and 30° C	*Contraindicated* in severe hypertension, alcoholism, glaucoma, severe cardiac disease, or patients receiving MAOIs Causes less stimulation and more CNS depression than most other amphetamines Use cautiously in patients with hypertension, depression, or diabetes Not recommended for children The drug should be discontinued when tolerance to anorexigenic effects occurs	Monitor diabetic patients carefully, including blood sugar and urine S & A, because may alter insulin requirements

Drug	Uses	Dosage	Supply	Contraindications/Precautions	Nursing Implications
Levodopa Bendopa Dopaidan Dopar L-Dopa Lardopa Larodopa Lavopa Sinemet*	Parkinson's disease to control rigidity, akinesia, and, to a lesser extent, tremor (this drug has been largely replaced by drugs that combine levodopa with a peripheral decarboxylase inhibitor; e.g., levodopa-carbidopa)	*Adults:* Must be individualized Initially 500 mg-1 gm/day PO in 2-4 doses with meals, gradually increasing in increments of 125-250 mg every 3-4 days to optimal effect, up to 8 gm/day unless intolerable side effects occur Administration with food or milk may decrease GI irritation	Tablets: 100, 125, 200, 500 mg Capsules: 100, 250, 500 mg Protect from heat, light, and moisture If preparations darken, potency is lost and medication should be discarded appropriately	*Contraindicated* in uncompensated cardiovascular, endocrine, hematologic, hepatic, pulmonary, or renal disease, narrow-angle glaucoma, and in patients with a history of melanoma or with suspicious undiagnosed skin lesions MAOIs should be stopped 2 weeks *before* commencing drug Not recommended for drug-induced extrapyramidal symptoms Levodopa *must be* stopped 12 hours before starting levodopa-carbidopa Most common side effects are dose-related choreiform and dystonic movements, oscillation in performance (on/off) effect, psychiatric, and cardiovascular symptoms Nausea and vomiting are prominent side effects May color urine red-brown May color perspiration slightly dark Pyridoxine (Vitamin B_6) can reverse the therapeutic effects of levodopa (dietary assessment may be indicated in relation to use of fortified cereals or multivitamin preparations)	Monitor for orthostatic hypotension Observe for development of depression and suicidal tendencies Monitor for nausea and vomiting, or color changes in urine or perspiration

Continued.

NURSING DRUG DIGEST—cont'd

Medication (trade name)	Indication	Usual dosage and administration	Dosage forms, preparation, and storage	Contraindications, cautions, and comments	Monitoring
Levodopa-benserazide Prolopa	Parkinson's disease to control rigidity, akinesia, and, to a lesser extent, tremor	*Adults:* Initially 100 mg levodopa with 25 mg benserazide PO/24 hr gradually increasing every 3 days until optimal dosage is reached that does not produce dyskinesia When changing patient from levodopa, this drug is stopped 12 hr before starting levodopa-benserazide at a dosage that will provide 15% of the previous levodopa daily dosage Capsules should be swallowed whole and *not* opened or dissolved in liquid Administration with meals may decrease GI distress	Capsules: levodopa 50 mg with benserazide 12.5 mg, levodopa 100 mg with benserazide 25 mg, levodopa 200 mg with benserazide 50 mg	*Contraindicated* in uncompensated cardiovascular, endocrine, hematologic, hepatic, pulmonary, or renal disease; narrow-angle glaucoma, and in patients with a history of melanoma or with suspicious undiagnosed skin lesions Discontinue levodopacarbidopa the night before general anesthesia and reinstitute when patient can take the drug orally MAOIs should be stopped 2 weeks before commencing drug Not recommended for drug-induced extrapyramidal symptoms Levodopa *must be* stopped 12 hours before starting levodopacarbidopa May cause urine to darken slightly on standing Most common side effects are dose related choreiform and dystonic movements, oscillation in performance (on/off) effect, psychiatric, and cardiovascular symptoms	Monitor dietary protein because a high-protein diet may reduce drug effectiveness Observe for signs of drug overdose, which usually develop 3 to 5 years after initiating therapy despite using the same dosage

Levodopa-carbidopa
Sinemet

Parkinson's disease to control rigidity, akinesia, and, to a lesser extent, tremor

Adults: Initially 100 mg levodopa with 25 mg carbidopa PO t.i.d. gradually increasing every 3 days until optimal dosage is reached that does not produce dyskinesia

Usually 750 mg levodopa/75 mg carbidopa q.d. should not be exceeded

When patient is changed from levodopa to levodopa-carbidopa, levodopa is stopped 12 hr *before* starting levodopa-carbidopa (at a dosage of 25% of the previous levodopa daily dosage) to prevent CNS toxicity from levodopa overdose; usually accomplished by administering last levodopa dose at bedtime and starting the combination the following morning

Tablets: 100 mg levodopa with 10 mg carbidopa, 250 mg levodopa with 25 mg carbidopa, 100 mg levodopa with 25 mg carbidopa

Contraindicated in uncompensated cardiovascular, endocrine, hematologic, hepatic, pulmonary, or renal disease, narrow-angle glaucoma, and in patients with a history of melanoma or with suspicious undiagnosed skin lesions

MAOIs should be stopped 2 weeks *before* commencing drug

Not recommended for drug-induced extrapyramidal symptoms

Levodopa *must be* stopped 12 hr before starting levodopa-carbidopa

May cause urine to darken slightly on standing

Discontinue levodopa-carbidopa the night before general anesthesia and reinstitute when patient can take the drug orally

May color perspiration slightly dark

Pyridoxine (Vitamin B₆) does *not* affect this combination product; use of this preparation decreases by 75% the dose of levodopa when used alone

Most common side effects are dose-related choreiform and dystonic movements, oscillation in performance (on/off) effect, psychiatric, and cardiovascular symptoms

Observe for signs of potential overdosage (e.g., involuntary movement), which usually start 3 to 5 years after the initiation of therapy despite using the same dosage

Monitor for orthostatic hypotension

Continued.

NURSING DRUG DIGEST—cont'd

Medication (trade name)	Indication	Usual dosage and administration	Dosage forms, preparation, and storage	Contraindications, cautions, and comments	Monitoring
Mazindol Mazanor Sanorex	To suppress hunger in the treatment of obesity	*Adults:* 1 mg t.i.d. PO before meals or 2 mg 1 hr before lunch in a single dose Administration with food or milk may decrease GI distress *Children:* Use is *not* recommended	Tablets: 1, 2 mg Store below 25° C	*Contraindicated* in patients with severe hypertension, glaucoma, severe cardiac disease, or in patients receiving MAOIs Anorexigenic drugs should be viewed as adjuncts in the treatment of obesity; for most obese patients alteration in eating habits is the most effective therapy Pressor agents should be administered with caution in patients receiving mazindol Safety has not been established in pregnancy	Monitor vital signs Monitor blood glucose and urine S & A because this drug can alter insulin requirements in the diabetic patient
★ **Methamphetamine** Desoxedrine Desoxyn Desyphad Methampex Methedrine Neodrine Norodin Obedrin-LA Semoxydrine Syndrox	Narcolepsy To counteract the sedative effects of anticonvulsants Obesity Parkinsonism Hyperkinetic children	*Adults:* For narcolepsy, 15-60 mg/day PO in single or divided doses For obesity, 2.5-5 mg t.i.d. ½ hr before meals *Children:* 2.5-40 mg/day PO in single or divided doses	Tablets: 2.5, 5, 7.5, 8 mg; (extended-release): 5, 10, 15 mg Injectable: 20 mg/1 ml Elixir: 3.3 mg/5 ml, 5 mg/5 ml Extended-release in various dosages and combinations	*Contraindicated* in patients with hyperthyroidism, nephritis, hypertension, angina pectoris, diabetes, or other severe blood disease *Contraindicated* in patients receiving MAOIs or who have narrow-angle glaucoma The possibility of drug dependence or addiction must be borne in mind when using methamphetamine Should not be used during pregnancy Avoid caffeine drinks	Observe for psychologic dependence Monitor for CNS and cardiovascular toxicity Monitor blood glucose and urine S & A because this drug can alter insulin requirements in the diabetic patient

Drug	Uses	Dosage	Dosage Forms	Remarks	Nursing Implications
Methylphenidate Centedrin Methidate Ritalin	Narcolepsy Hyperkinetic children *Should not be used to reverse the effects of drug overdosage or general anesthetic*	*Adults:* Initially 20-60 mg/day PO in divided doses *Children:* Over 6 years of age, start with 10 mg/day and gradually increase as needed up to 60 mg/day PO in 2 divided doses Administer last dose before 6 PM to avoid interference with sleep	Tablets: 5, 10, 20 mg; extended-release: 20 mg Injectable: 20 mg (lyophilized) Store below 30° C Protect from light	*Contraindicated* in glaucoma and serious heart disease Safe use during pregnancy has not been established Methylphenidate should *not* be viewed as a replacement for important support measures in sedative overdosed patients Has less CNS stimulant activity than the amphetamines May lower seizure threshold May induce psychologic dependence May cause insomnia if last dose given late in the day Avoid caffeine drinks	Monitor for psychologic dependence Observe patient for weight loss Monitor diabetic patients carefully because drug may alter daily insulin requirements; monitor blood sugar and urine S & A
Nikethamide Anacardone Coramine Corvotone Nikethyl Nikorin	Stimulate cardiorespiratory function in patients overdosed with CNS sedatives *(this use is strongly discouraged)*	Analeptic use of nikethamide is strongly *discouraged* (see text)	Injectable: 250 mg/ml Solution (oral): 1.25 gm/5 ml Store in tight, light-resistant container	Nikethamide has a narrow margin of safety, and marked side effects, including convulsions, may occur Patients receiving nikethamide must receive appropriate supportive measures Seizures can be treated with IV diazepam, 5-20 mg Be prepared to ventilate	Monitor vital signs
Orphenadrine Brocasipal Disipal Marflex Mephenamine Myotrol Norflex Norgesic* Norgesic Forte*	Parkinson's disease to control rigidity and akinesia See also Chapter 16, "Muscle Relaxants"	Parkinsonism, individualized, start at 50 mg t.i.d. PO, increase as necessary up to 400 mg/day in divided doses	Tablets: 25, 50 mg Injectable: 60 mg/2 ml Suspension: 8.3 mg/5 ml Tablet (extended-release): 100 mg	Should *not* be used concurrently with propoxyphene because it may result in tremor, confusion, and anxiety Use cautiously in patients with cardiac disease, glaucoma, or urinary or pyloric obstruction As rigidity decreases, tremor may increase	Monitor urinary patterns; causes urinary retention and hesitancy; monitor intake and output

Continued.

NURSING DRUG DIGEST—cont'd

Medication (trade name)	Indication	Usual dosage and administration	Dosage forms, preparation, and storage	Contraindications, cautions, and comments	Monitoring
★ **Pemoline** Cylert Deltamine Kethamed Pioxol Stimul Volital	To treat carefully selected hyperactive children older than 6 years of age	*Children:* Older than 6 years of age, individualized—37.5 mg each morning PO, increase weekly by 18.75 mg to achieve a maintenance dose between 56.25 and 75 mg q.d. Administer in morning to decrease insomnia Maximum: 112.5 mg/24 hr	Tablets: 18.75, 37.5, 75 mg; chewable: 37.5 mg	May produce mental changes with prolonged use May induce anorexia, weight loss, or insomnia Patients may crave pemoline when drug is stopped abruptly May accumulate in renal failure and dose may need to be decreased	Observe and record weight and height measurements because drug may retard growth Monitor carefully for therapeutic effects that may not be evident for 14-21 days
★ **Phendimetrazine** Adphen Anorex Aptrol Bacarate Bontril PDM Bontril Slow Release Dietrol Ex-Obese Limit Melfiat Obepar Obeval Phendimead Plegine Ropledge StatoDex Trimstat Trimtabs	To suppress hunger in the treatment of obesity	*Adults:* 35 mg PO b.i.d. or t.i.d., 1 hr before meals; *or* 105 mg (slow-release capsule) PO 30 min before morning meal *Children:* Use is *not* recommended	Tablet: 35 mg Capsule: 35 mg; slow-release: 105 mg	*Contraindicated* in hyperthyroidism, hypertension, and severe cardiovascular disease *Contraindicated* in patients with glaucoma and patients receiving MAOIs Habituation or addiction may occur with phendimetrazine Avoid caffeine drinks	Monitor for symptoms of overstimulation Monitor diabetic patients carefully because insulin requirements may be altered; monitor blood sugar and urine S & A
★ **Phenmetrazine** Preludin	To suppress hunger in the treatment of obesity	*Adults:* 12.5-25 mg PO b.i.d. or t.i.d., 1 hr before meals; *or* extended-release tablet 75 mg midmorning *Children:* Use is *not* recommended	Tablet: 25 mg; extended-release: 75 mg	*Contraindicated* in hypertension, hyperthyroidism, severe cardiac disease, narrow, angle glaucoma, and in combination with MAOIs Should not be used during pregnancy May cause habituation Avoid caffeine drinks	Monitor for overstimulation

Drug	Action/Indications	Dosage	Dosage Forms / Precautions	Nursing Implications
Phentermine Adipex Adipex-P Duromin Fastin Ionamin Mirapront Obesamead Parmine Phentermyl Phentrol Phermine Pronidin Rolaphant Teramine	To suppress hunger in the treatment of obesity	*Adults*: 8 mg PO t.i.d. ½ hr before meals; *or* 15-30 mg extended-release capsule PO before breakfast *Children*: Use is not recommended	Tablet: 8 mg Capsules (extended-release): 15, 30 mg (resin complex) *Contraindicated* in hyperthyroidism, hypertension, and severe cardiovascular disease *Contraindicated* in patients with glaucoma and patients receiving MAOIs Habituation or dependence may occur with phentermine	Monitor for habituation or dependence
Procyclidine Kemadrin Procyclid	Parkinson's disease to control rigidity, tremor, akinesia To control extrapyramidal side effects of phenothiazine and butyrophenone drugs	*Adults*: individualized Initially 2.5 mg t.i.d. PO after meals, increased to 5 mg t.i.d.; occasionally 5 mg is added q.h.s. Administration with food or milk may decrease GI irritation	Tablets: 2, 5 mg Elixir: 2.5 mg/5 ml (10% alcohol) *Contraindicated* in narrow-angle glaucoma Use cautiously in patients with glaucoma, tachycardia, or urinary or pyloric obstruction	Monitor for anticholinergic effects
Trihexyphenidyl Antitrem Aparkane Apo-Trihex Artane Hexyphen Novohexidyl Pipanol T.H.P. Tremin Trihexane Trihexidyl Trixyl	Parkinson's disease to control rigidity, tremor, akinesia To control extrapyramidal side effects of phenothiazine and butyrophenone drugs	*Adults*: individualized Start with 1 mg/day PO and increase by 2 mg/day every 3-5 days up to 6-10 mg/day depending on response and adverse effects Drug usually given t.i.d. in divided doses at mealtime Causes nausea if given *before* meals	Tablets: 2, 5 mg Capsule (extended-release): 5 mg (1.25 mg released immediately and remainder over 6-8 hr) Elixir: 2 mg/5 ml (5% alcohol) Used cautiously in patients with glaucoma or obstructive disease of bowel or bladder May induce incipient glaucoma Elderly patients must be monitored more closely Drug has a bitter taste followed by tingling and numbness in the tongue	Observe for CNS stimulation (e.g., agitation, delirium, insomnia, restlessness)

BIBLIOGRAPHY

Gresh, C. Helpful tips you can give your patient with Parkinson's disease. *Nursing 80,* 1980, *10*(1), 26-33.

Hahn, K. Management of Parkinson's disease. *Nurse Practitioner,* 1982, January, 13-25.

Jewell, J.A. Tardive dyskinesia, the involuntary movement disorder that no one really understands. *The Canadian Nurse,* 1983, *79,* 20-24.

Rosal-Greif, V.L.F. Drug-induced dyskinesias. *American Journal of Nursing,* 1982, *82*(1), 66-69.

Weber, S.S., Dufresne, R.L., Becker, R.E., & Mastrati, P. Diazepam in tardive dyskinesia. *Drug Intelligence and Clinical Pharmacy,* 1983, *17,* 523-527.

Weiner, M. Update on antiparkinsonian agents. *Geriatrics,* 1982, *37*(9), 81-91.

CHAPTER 21

Drugs Used to Treat Epilepsy

Donald R. McLean

Medications discussed in this chapter

Barbiturates
  Amobarbital
  Mephobarbital
  Metharbital
  Pentobarbital
  Phenobarbital
  Primidone
  Thiopental
Benzodiazepines
  Clonazepam
  Diazepam
Oxazolidinediones
  Paramethadione
  Trimethadione
Hydantoins
  Ethotoin

Hydantoins—cont'd
  Phenytoin
  Mephenytoin
Succinimides
  Ethosuximide
  Methsuximide
  Phensuximide
Miscellaneous
  Acetazolamide
  Carbamazepine
  Corticotropin
  Magnesium sulfate
  Paraldehyde
  Phenacemide
  Valproic acid

Numerous classifications of epilepsy exist, depending on varying guidelines and criteria. Several synonyms are used to identify the same seizure type. *Grand mal, generalized tonic-clonic,* and *centrencephalic* are all terms used to describe essentially the same clinical seizure. Hoping to correct this nomenclature problem, the International League Against Epilepsy met in Marseilles in 1964 and developed a classification system based on clinical and electroencephlographic (EEG) characteristics. The following is an abbreviated updated version of that classification.

CLASSIFICATION

A. Partial seizures beginning locally
  1. Simple partial seizures. Consciousness is *not* impaired
    a. With motor symptoms: jerking movement of the face, arm, or leg; commonly starts in one part of the body and spreads to incorporate other parts (originate frontal lobe)
    b. With special sensory or somatosensory symptoms: usually manifests as a spreading numbness or pins and needles sensation; rarely involves unformed visual phenomena (originate parietal or occipital lobe)
    c. With autonomic symptoms: changes in skin color, sweating, or blood pressure
    d. With psychic symptoms: deja vu, dreamy state, fear, anger, structured hallucinations (originate temporal lobe)
  2. Complex partial seizures. Consciousness *is* impaired. Commonly originate in the temporal lobe. Commonly called temporal lobe or psychomotor epilepsy.
    a. With impaired consciousness only
    b. With cognitive symptomatology, such as disrupted thinking
    c. With affective symptomatology: change in mood, commonly fear, magnanimity, and rarely anger or depression
    d. With psychosensory symptomatology: rising epigastric sensation, hallucination of taste, smell, hearing, or vision
    e. With psychomotor symptomatology: inappropriate activity such as fumbling with clothing, walking about, dressing, or undressing; referred to as automatisms
    f. Compound forms
  3. Partial seizures secondarily generalized. Originate focally in the cortex and spread to the diencephalon and the remainder of the cortex
B. Generalized seizures, bilateral symmetrical seizures without local onset (originate in the diencephalon)
  1. Absence seizures
    a. Simple absence seizures: very brief (2 to 15 seconds) lapse in contact with the environment

b. Complex absence seizures: other phenomena associated with impaired consciousness

2. Bilateral massive epileptic myoclonus seizures: brief whole body jerk, usually a flexion movement of the trunk

3. Infantile spasms: whole body jerk, somewhat more prolonged, generally involving flexion movement of the trunk

4. Clonic seizures: generalized repetitive jerking and loss of consciousness

5. Tonic seizures: generalized stiffening and loss of consciousness

6. Tonic-clonic seizures (grand mal seizures): generalized stiffening followed by generalized jerking of the limbs and the trunk with loss of consciousness

7. Atonic seizures: loss of muscle tone

8. Akinetic seizures: loss of movement without atonia

C. Unilateral or predominantly unilateral seizures (almost exclusively in very young children or newborns; originate in the cortex)

D. Unclassified seizures

SYNOPSIS OF ANTICONVULSANT CHOICE RELATED TO SEIZURE TYPE

Certain seizures are responsive to one medication and not to others. The appropriate drugs for use in the various seizures are as follows.

1. Drugs used for partial seizures or seizures beginning locally and for generalized seizures (bilateral symmetrical seizures without local onset) *except* those associated with either absence or infantile spasm: carbamazepine, phenobarbital, phenytoin, and primidone.

2. Drugs used for absence seizures: ethosuximide, trimethadione, and valproic acid.

3. Drugs used for infantile spasm: clonazepam, corticotropin, and diazepam.

PHARMACOKINETICS

The ability easily and accurately to measure anticonvulsant blood levels has greatly contributed to more effective seizure control. Anticonvulsant drugs are started at a dose expected to result in a therapeutic blood level and the dose is then modified depending on seizure control, side effects, and measured blood level. Therapeutic blood levels should not be viewed as inviolable figures, but rather as starting points to arrive at a rational drug dosage. In particular, the upper limit may often be exceeded in an uncontrolled patient who does not have significant side effects.

Several important considerations determine the dosage schedule of an anticonvulsant. The frequency of drug administration is dictated by its rate of metabolism and by the peak plasma levels achieved following its administration. The drug should be administered at an interval less than or equal to the half-life of the anticonvulsant to avoid wide fluctuations in serum concentration. Some drugs with very long half-lives can theoretically be administered every 2 days, providing that the peak level immediately following administration (before distribution within the body) does not induce intolerable side effects. It should be self-evident that one usually strives for the least number of daily administrations to improve patient compliance.

With the advent of anticonvulsant blood level monitoring, a better understanding of drug interactions has evolved. Multiple drug therapy (polypharmacy) was popular in the past, and was based on the belief that the anticonvulsant effect of drugs administered concurrently would be synergistic and would allow for seizure control with smaller doses of each individual drug. It was believed that adverse side effects could thus be avoided or reduced with the smaller dose. By monitoring anticonvulsant levels, it became clear that seizure control occurred when one of the anticonvulsants achieved therapeutic blood concentrations. Anticonvulsant drugs do not act synergistically and side effects are additive, proportional to the number of drugs used. For these reasons, polypharmacy of anticonvulsants is now discouraged.

Monotherapy, guided by serum levels to ascertain the proper dose and limited only by side effects, represents the appropriate way to treat epileptic patients. There are still occasions when a second drug must be added to a therapeutic program. Usually the dose employed when using polypharmacy must be lower, not because the drugs act synergistically, but because the cumulative side effects preclude a higher dose. Drugs such as carbamazepine, valproic acid, primidone, and clonazepam are started at a low dose, and slowly increased to a maintenance level, allowing tolerance to dose-related side effects. Phenytoin, ethosuximide, and phenobarbital can be inaugurated at their respective maintenance doses. In fact, with phenytoin it is common to commence therapy with a loading dose. A steady state is achieved with any particular dose after the drug has been administered for five times its half-life (see Chapter 6, "Pharmacokinetic Considerations in Drug Response").

With prolonged use, most anticonvulsant drugs enhance their own metabolism by inducing the activity of additional metabolic enzymes in the liver. This has the effect of shortening the drugs' half-lives and unless the dosage regimen is readjusted this may result in the reappearance of seizures. In the past, this phenomenon was interpreted as the development of "tolerance" to the medication, which allowed the epilepsy to break through. The common response at that time was to add a second drug. A more rational approach, based on recognizing the phenomena of enzyme induction (see Chapter 5, "Drug Metabolism and Elimination"), is to increase the dose of the medication, because the blood level will invariably be below the therapeutic concentration.

Similar problems result from drug interactions. A second drug may reduce the therapeutic effectiveness of an anticonvulsant by inducing enzymes that hasten the metabolism and lower the serum concentration of the anticonvulsant. This type of drug interaction is quite common and requires that epileptic patients be monitored closely, both clinically and with serum anticonvulsant levels, whenever a medication is added to or withdrawn from their therapeutic regimen. The appropriate response is usually obvious if serum levels are available. Some drugs enhance anticonvulsant effects (therapeutic and toxic) by displacing protein-bound anticonvulsants or by interfering with metabolism, resulting in toxic levels of the anticonvulsants.

ANTICONVULSANT DRUGS AND PREGNANCY

Many studies have demonstrated a twofold to threefold increase in congenital malformations in the offsprings of mothers receiving anticonvulsant medication. In one prospective study the rate was 23% of 31 pregnancies. Phenytoin, primidone, and phenobarbital are the major offenders and produce similar malformations (e.g., cleft palate, cleft lip, congenital heart defects). Trimethadione is especially dangerous because it consistently produces congenital heart disease in a large number of exposed fetuses.

Whereas a large number of pregnancies with patients receiving carbamazepine have not been recorded to date, no congenital abnormalities have been reported. Neural tube defects may be increased in fetuses exposed to valproic acid. This condition can be diagnosed by measuring amniotic fluid levels of alpha-fetoprotein.

A reasonable policy in patients with very infrequent or minor seizures is to stop anticonvulsant medications before fertilization and for the first trimester of pregnancy. This may prove impossible because seizure propensity is increased during pregnancy. If frequent or severe seizures preclude stopping medication, the patient should be switched to carbamazepine or valproic acid before fertilization and for as long as possible into the pregnancy. If valproic acid is used, amniotic fluid alpha-fetoprotein levels should be measured at 16 weeks gestation.

WHEN CAN ANTICONVULSANT MEDICATION BE STOPPED?

Many patients with seizures, particularly those starting in childhood, will outgrow their disorder. Once this happens, anticonvulsant medication is no longer required. How does one recognize such patients?

Certain kinds of epilepsy are known to remit; benign rolandic epilepsy (partial seizure with motor symptoms) and absence seizures are the best examples. As a general rule, most epilepsy of childhood onset and some epilepsy of adult onset have the potential to remit. Unfortunately, there is no conclusive way, short of stopping medication, to tell whether the epilepsy has remitted. Although the EEG is used as a guide, the presence or absence of seizure activity in the EEG is not a reliable predictor of remittance. Medication is stopped when patients reach the age when their particular epilepsy is expected to remit and their EEG has become nonepileptic. In those epilepsies where remission does not follow a specific pattern, anticonvulsant medication is generally stopped after 4 years of seizure freedom if the patient approves, and if the EEG is nonepileptic. Patients with childhood-onset seizures can be offered a favorable prognosis for remission, but adult-onset seizure patients should be offered a less optimistic outlook. Once the decision is made to stop treatment, the anticonvulsant dose is gradually reduced, usually over a period of 1 month, and finally stopped.

THERAPY OF STATUS EPILEPTICUS

Epileptic patients may suffer a series of recurrent, closely spaced seizures without regaining consciousness. This is called *status epilepticus* and represents a life-threatening situation requiring emergency treatment. One must maintain an airway, support the blood pressure, and stop the seizures.

Diazepam is effective in stopping such seizures (5 to 20 mg IV push at a rate of 5 mg/min). However, intravenous diazepam is rapidly distributed into extravascular compartments and effective blood levels rarely last longer than 30 minutes, at which time the seizures can recur. Consequently, coincident with the IV administration of diazepam, a loading dose of IV phenytoin, 15 mg/kg given at a rate *not* exceeding 50 mg/minute, is administered. This drug dissipates slowly because it has a long half-life (i.e., 7 to 42 hours), and will prevent the recurrence of seizures when the diazepam wears off. Phenytoin should not be administered intramuscularly because absorption is erratic.

Occasionally the diazepam and phenytoin regimen will not be effective. In these cases, a barbiturate such as pentobarbital, amobarbital, or phenobarbital can be used intravenously in a dosage sufficient to control the seizures without producing serious hypotension or respiratory arrest. When barbiturates are used, respiratory depression is a threat and ventilatory support equipment must be immediately available.

ALCOHOL WITHDRAWAL SEIZURES

After prolonged alcohol consumption, some alcoholic patients have generalized tonic-clonic or partial seizures when they reduce or discontinue their alcohol intake. The convulsion generally occurs within 24 hours after reducing the alcohol intake and commonly is the event prompting medical attention. The seizures will rarely be multiple. These patients pose a special problem. They are not truly epileptic because their seizures are essentially drug-related and self-induced.

The convulsions can be avoided if the patient starts anticonvulsant medication in anticipation of a reduction in alcohol consumption. However, an alcoholic patient on a binge rarely has such foresight. Alcoholic patients can be placed on anticonvulsants, but they generally stop taking medication during a binge, so this maneuver is usually unsuccessful. Voluntary admissions to drug withdrawal programs yield the patients most amenable to therapy because they can be started on a drug such as phenytoin and achieve therapeutic blood levels quickly enough to prevent withdrawal seizures. The anticonvulsant can be stopped after 1 week, by which time the seizure risk is minimal.

INFANTILE SPASMS WITH HYPSARRHYTHMIA

Infantile spasms with hypsarrhythmia are sometimes associated with treatable metabolic conditions such as hypoglycemia, pyridoxine deficiency, lead encephalopathy, and phenylketonuria. More commonly, the cause is unknown. Corticotropin gel given daily for 20 days and repeated later if necessary will reduce the number of seizures and normalize the dramatically abnormal (hypsarrhythmia) EEG in these cases. Diazepam is frequently used to control the spasm-type body flexion seizures that characteristically occur. The seizures are difficult to control, although by 3 or 4 years of age, the spasm seizures may be replaced by generalized tonic-clonic seizures. Of these children, 90% are moderately to severely retarded.

ANTICONVULSANT PROPHYLAXIS IN HEAD TRAUMA

Most studies indicate that prophylactic anticonvulsant therapy does not significantly alter the occurrence rate of posttraumatic epilepsy in patients with closed head injuries. Treated or untreated, seizures occurred in approximately 7% of patients. Therefore, most patients with head injuries are not given anticonvulsant medication until they have a convulsion.

PROBLEMS IN BEING EPILEPTIC

The burden placed on the epileptic patient by society is commonly greater than that of the disease. The misunderstanding, prejudice, and rejection by family members and society faced by an epileptic leads to frustration, resentment, and anger. A significant aspect of epilepsy treatment must be directed at these psychologic and social problems. The patient's family and working colleagues must be educated concerning the nature of epilepsy. This can usually be achieved by a visit from a member of a community epilepsy society, a nurse, or a physician. An ongoing community education program should be an integral part of any epilepsy management clinic.

SUMMARY

This chapter has examined the various types and uses of anticonvulsant medications. A classification scheme for epilepsy based on clinical and electroencephalographic characteristics has been presented and the selection of the appropriate drug related to the identified seizure type has been discussed. The importance and clinical application of pharmacokinetic parameters, including blood levels of the anticonvulsant medications, has been presented and the use of this information in monitoring and modifying anticonvulsant drug regimens has been discussed. Various clinical concerns, including drug interactions, teratogenesis, and discontinuation of anticonvulsant drug therapy have also been discussed.

With an understanding of the various individual agents, including their actions and side effects, the nurse will be better able to provide optimal care for patients requiring these medications. Patient education can be enhanced, adverse drug effects can be anticipated, monitored for, and minimized, and clinically significant drug interactions can be avoided by using the information presented in this chapter.

ADVERSE/SIDE EFFECTS OF THE ANTICONVULSANTS*

CARDIOVASCULAR SYSTEM

Aggravation of coronary artery disease
Aggravation of hypertension
Atrial and ventricular conduction
  depression
Cardiac dysrhythmia
Cardiovascular collapse with IV
  phenytoin
Congestive heart failure
Hypotension
Periarteritis nodosa
Recurrence of thrombophlebitis
Stokes-Adams syndrome in patients
  with A-V block
Syncope
Ventricular fibrillation

CENTRAL NERVOUS SYSTEM

Aggression
Anxiety
Ataxia
Behavioral deterioration
Choreiform movements with high
  dose IV phenytoin
Circumoral tingling
Depression
Diplopia
Dizziness
Epigastric pain
Exacerbation of preexisting pain
Hallucinations
Headache
Hemeralopia
Insomnia
Lethargy
Mental confusion
Motor twitching
Myasthenia gravis–like syndrome
Nystagmus
Paradoxic excitation
Paresthesia

Peripheral neuritis
Personality changes
Photophobia
Psychosis
Rage
Sleep disturbance
Sleepiness
Slurred speech
Talkativeness
Tinnitus
Transient nervousness
Vertigo

CUTANEOUS SYSTEM

Alopecia
Bleeding gums
Bullous, exfoliative, or purpuric
  dermatitis
Coarsened facial features
Conjunctivitis
Epistaxis
Erythema multiforme
Facial edema
Gingival hypertrophy
Hirsutism
Lupus erythematosus
Morbilliform or scarlatiniform rash
Photosensitivity
Pruritus
Retinal and petechial hemorrhages
Stevens-Johnson syndrome
Urticaria

ENDOCRINE SYSTEM

Teratogenicity

GASTROINTESTINAL SYSTEM

Anorexia
Constipation
Dry mouth

Glossitis
Hiccups
Indigestion
Nausea
Stomatitis
Toxic hepatitis
Vomiting
Weight loss

GENITOURINARY SYSTEM

Albuminuria
Change in libido
Elevated BUN
Glycosuria
Hematuria
Impotence
Nephrosis
Urinary frequency
Urinary retention

HEMATOLOGIC AND LYMPHATIC SYSTEMS

Agranulocytosis and pancytopenia
Eosinophilia
Granulocytopenia
Hepatosplenomegaly
Hypoplastic anemia
Leukocytosis
Leukopenia
Lymphadenopathy
Macrocytic anemia
Macrocytosis
Thrombocytopenia

MUSCULOSKELETAL SYSTEM

Leg cramps
Polyarthropathy

*See Chapter 11, "Drug Toxicity," for an overview of drug toxicity.

CLINICALLY SIGNIFICANT DRUG INTERACTIONS*

Primary drug	Interacting drug	Possible effect(s)	Probable mechanism(s)
Barbiturates	Alcohol	Increased CNS depression	Potentiation of CNS depressant effect
Barbiturates	Anesthetics (general)	Increased CNS depressant effect, delayed recovery postanesthetic; cardiovascular collapse	Additive effect
Barbiturates	Anticoagulants (oral)	Decreased anticoagulant effect	Enzyme induction; may persist up to 6 weeks after barbiturate withdrawal; may inhibit anticoagulant absorption
Barbiturates	Antidepressants	Potentiates sedative effect of barbiturates; may inhibit tricyclic effects	Enzyme induction
Barbiturates	Corticosteroids	Decreased steroid effect	Enzyme induction
Barbiturates	Griseofulvin	Decreased antifungal activity	Enzyme induction
Barbiturates	Oral contraceptives	Decreased contraceptive effect	Enzyme induction
Barbiturates	Quinidine	Decreased quinidine effect	Enzyme induction
Carbamazepine	Anticoagulants	Decreased anticoagulant effect	Enzyme induction
Carbamazepine	Troleandomycin	Increased carbamazepine effects and toxicity	Inhibition of carbamazepine metabolism by troleandomycin
Carbamazepine	Erythromycin	Increased carbamazepine effects and toxicity	Inhibition of carbamazepine by erythromycin
Carbamazepine	Isoniazid	Increased carbamazepine effects and toxicity	Inhibition of carbamazepine by isoniazid
Carbamazepine	Propoxyphene	Carbamazepine intoxication	Propoxyphene strongly inhibits carbamazepine metabolism
Hydantoins	Chloramphenicol	Increased hydantoin blood levels	Chloramphenicol inhibits hydoxylation of hydantoin
Hydantoins	Cimetidine	Increased hydantoin blood levels	Cimetidine inhibits hydoxylation of hydantoin
Hydantoins	Corticosteroids	Decreased effectiveness of corticosteroids	Enhanced corticosteroid metabolism
Hydantoins	Diazoxide	Decreased hydantoin blood levels	Enhances hydantoin metabolism
Hydantoins	Disulfiram	Increased hydantoin blood levels	Disulfiram inhibits hepatic hydantoin metabolism
Hydantoins	Folic acid	Decreased hydantoin levels and recurrences of seizures; long-term build up of CNS folic acid; decreased hydantoin efficacy	Folic acid enhances hydoxylation of hydantoin
Hydantoins	Isoniazid	Increased hydantoin blood levels	Enzyme inhibition especially in slow acetylators
Hydantoins	Phenylbutazone	Enhanced hydantoin effect	Inhibition of α-hydoxylation and displacement of protein-binding sites (monitor patients closely)
Hydantoins	Quinidine	Decreased quinidine antidysrhythmic effects; increased quinidine effect when hydantoin withdrawn	Decreases quinidine half-life by about 50%, probably by enzyme induction
Hydantoins	Sulfonamides	Potentiates hydantoin	Inhibits metabolism; displaces hydantoin from protein-binding site
Hydantoins	Theophyllines	Decreased blood level of both drugs	Enzyme induction
Hydantoins	Valproic acid	Potentiates effect of hydantoins	Displacement from protein-binding sites
Valproic acid	Barbiturates	Barbiturate intoxication sometimes leading to coma	Inhibits metabolism of barbiturates

*See Chapter 10, "Drug Interactions," for an overview of drug interactions.

GENERAL NURSING IMPLICATIONS

Nursing of patients requiring anticonvulsant drug therapy

ASSESSMENT

Assessment of the patient is extremely important in establishing an accurate diagnosis and in selecting drug therapy because various types of seizures require specific drug therapy. The most important data used in obtaining an accurate seizure diagnosis are descriptions of the attack from the patient, family members, or other witnesses and professionals who have observed the seizure. Diagnostic evaluation confirms the diagnosis and determines treatable causes and precipitating factors. Therapy is usually started with the single drug the neurologist believes will have the best seizure control and the least toxicity. Accurate baseline data are especially helpful in evaluating the patient's response.

A drug history should include information identifying possible drug sensitivity and or serious drug interactions (e.g., valproic acid and phenobarbital; phenobarbital or phenytoin and sodium warfarin) (see Clinically Significant Drug Interactions). This is essential before administering the first dose of an anticonvulsant. If the patient is unable to provide this information, family members or others may be able to provide it.

Although patients with seizure disorders are usually managed on an outpatient basis, hospitalization is usually required for diagnostic evaluation or if seizure activity cannot be controlled. When the patient is hospitalized, seizure precautions are indicated until the seizures are controlled: padded siderails should be in place, and suction equipment and oxygen should be immediately available. Forcing a padded tongue blade or other instrument between the teeth during a seizure is *not* recommended. Showers are recommended for seizure patients, but if a tub bath is preferred by the patient, bathing must be supervised because drowning may result if a seizure occurs while the patient is in the bathtub. If seizures are poorly controlled, rectal, or preferably axillary, temperatures should be taken.

SENSITIVITY

Allergic reactions to anticonvulsants are rare; however, any drug has the potential to cause a hypersensitivity reaction in a susceptible individual. Allergic reactions may be manifest by various dermatologic conditions such as skin rash and purpura, which the nurse should monitor for. See the Nursing Drug Digest for specific medications.

CONTRAINDICATIONS

Anticonvulsants are contraindicated in the presence of hypersensitivity. See the Nursing Drug Digest for contraindications associated with specific individual agents.

CAUTIONS

Anticonvulsants when taken during early pregnancy can cause teratogenic effects. Women of childbearing age who are receiving anticonvulsant medications should be informed about the problems of drug therapy during pregnancy. The patient may need to explore birth control methods with the nurse and may need to discuss feelings about her condition and pregnancy. The nurse can be especially supportive and helpful to the patient in identifying her feelings and helping her to make decisions related to childbearing. Family counseling and other community referral services (planned parenthood) can also be explored. If the patient desires pregnancy, the risks must be understood clearly by the patient in consultation with her physician.

See the Nursing Drug Digest for cautions and comments related to specific individual agents.

DRUG INTERACTIONS

Anticonvulsants have the potential to interact with numerous drugs in a variety of mechanisms, including synergistic pharmacologic effect, displacement from protein-binding sites, and induction of hepatic microsomal enzymes.

See Clinically Significant Drug Interactions for specific interactions involving anticonvulsants.

ADMINISTRATION

Anticonvulsants can be administered orally, intramuscularly, or intravenously by the appropriate dosage form. The selection of the route of administration depends on the severity of the patient's condition, as well as on individual patient factors.

During initial drug therapy, administer medications carefully and monitor the individual patient's response. Observe for signs of hypersensitivity, such as skin rash, fever, ataxia, or wheezy breathing. Observe for any change in level of consciousness or behavior changes, especially after introducing new anticonvulsant drugs (e.g., valproic acid). Monitor for common side effects, including drowsiness and gastrointestinal (GI) disturbances. Warn patients about drowsiness; smoking should not be done without supervision. GI disturbances can be minimized by encouraging patients to take the medication with meals or with one to two full glasses of water.

When anticonvulsant drugs are used intravenously, pulse, blood pressure, and respiration must be monitored closely. The rate of injection instructions must be rigorously followed.

When barbiturates are given by continuous IV infusion, the patient must be observed constantly to obviate the danger of respiratory arrest from an inadvertent overdose. Emergency respiratory support equipment must be immediately available.

MONITORING PATIENT RESPONSE
Therapeutic response

A therapeutic response to anticonvulsants may not occur for up to 4 to 5 times the half-life of the drug. Do not evaluate medication until a steady state is achieved. The patient will need support during this time because seizures may recur and side effects may be observed. Drug adjustment to control recurring seizures may take many months, resulting in patient frustration. *Continued.*

GENERAL NURSING IMPLICATIONS—cont'd

Nursing of patients requiring anticonvulsant drug therapy—cont'd

Therapeutic response—cont'd

It is common for patients who have been seizure-free for a period of time on anticonvulsant therapy to think that they are cured and have no further need for their medication. The patient needs to understand that discontinuing the medication without discussion and evaluation with the health care provider can lead to seizure activity caused by an inadequate concentration of the anticonvulsant drug in the blood. The patient should be aware of and know how to minimize other seizure triggers, including hyperventilation, trauma, fever, illness, lack of sleep, photosensitivity, emotional stress, hormonal changes such as those occuring with menses, fluid and electrolyte imbalances, as well as alcohol and drug use.

Children often grow out of the need for anticonvulsant therapy, depending on the specific etiology of their seizures and adults after 5 years of seizure-free therapy are usually weaned off of medication. The patient and the family should understand what to monitor and will require much support during this time.

Adverse side effects

Adverse side effects vary widely depending on the chemical family or structure of the particular anticonvulsant. (See Adverse/Side Effects of the Anticonvulsants for a summary of the adverse side effects of these medications). Major adverse side effects encountered in patients on anticonvulsant therapy include blood dyscrasias. The nurse should have an understanding of the occurrence, severity, and symptoms of these effects because they frequently have an insidious onset and require immediate attention. Other common adverse side effects, although less severe and dangerous, require recognition and appropriate treatment to enhance the course of therapy. One such commonly encountered effect is drowsiness, which is seen with virtually all of the anticonvulsants.

Monitor for dose-related toxicity, usually affecting the CNS, including diplopia, ataxia, drowsiness, and mental dulling (see the Nursing Drug Digest for specific toxic effects of anticonvulsant drugs).

Nurses must be diligent to differentiate between the side effects of the anticonvulsants and the symptoms associated with the seizure disorder being treated (e.g., ataxia can be caused by an overdose of phenytoin, or it can be a symptom of a grand mal seizure). As noted in the body of this chapter, serum levels can often aid the nurse in differentiating between the progression of the condition and an adverse side effect of the anticonvulsant medication. For this reason, nurses must familiarize themselves with the therapeutic and toxic blood levels of the anticonvulsant medications and use them in monitoring patient response. See the Nursing Drug Digest for specific information on the adverse side effects, as well as the therapeutic blood levels, of specific anticonvulsant agents.

PATIENT EDUCATION

The patient and the family should be involved as early as possible in care. They should have a clear understanding of the drug regimen, storage, administration, possible side effects, signs of toxicity, what to do if a dose is missed, and when to notify the health care provider. They should also know how to minimize side effects and what to do in case a seizure occurs. Activities of daily living often need to be adjusted, and nursing assistance is often needed here. The patient and the family should recognize the importance of taking medications consistently. Because a danger of recurrent seizures exists if the medication is not taken as prescribed, dosing according to an individual's lifestyle can be helpful in maintaining compliance.

Psychosocial aspects of care should not be underemphasized, because the nurse can contribute much to this aspect of care.

Discharge planning is important in increasing the patient's and family's self-care abilities. Fear and anxiety regarding recurrent seizures and complications are not unusual at discharge and they need much support.

In addition to monitoring and minimizing side effects, patients and families must recognize when to seek assistance from the health care provider or to go to the hospital, what to do for a missed dose, and what to do if a seizure occurs. The patient will require assistance in planning adjustments in lifestyle, which may include employment change, driving restrictions, changes in sport or recreation participation, bathing, and alcohol use.

Patients should be encouraged to wear Medic-Alert bracelets or medallions and should carry identification with the following information: name and phone number, name of primary clinician, name of hospital for emergency treatment, medication schedule, names and telephone numbers of persons to be notified in case of an emergency, and a list of allergies.

Before discharge patients should understand their complete medication regimen and should be able to monitor therapy and record seizures and other observations. This is especially important for patients receiving long-term anticonvulsant drug therapy.

GENERAL INSTRUCTIONS FOR DISCHARGE/OUTPATIENTS

ANTICONVULSANTS

This medication is an anticonvulsant used to control seizures. If you do not understand why you require this medication, check with your health care provider.

This medication regimen has been specially developed to meet your individual needs. Follow the instructions on the prescription exactly. If you have any questions, please contact your health care provider.

Drowsiness and gastrointestinal disturbances can occur with this medication. Do not operate dangerous machinery or participate in activities that require alertness. Gastrointestinal disturbances can be relieved by taking your medication with meals or with 1 to 2 glasses of water.

Report any imbalance, sleepiness, altered vision, double vision, difficulty concentrating, weight gain, skin rash, loss of appetite, nausea, weight loss, hiccups, fever, sore throat, or easy bruising to your health care provider.

Notify your nurse or physician before starting or stopping any other medication, because whenever a medication is added or withdrawn the effects of your anticonvulsant medication can be altered.

Many anticonvulsant medications can cause birth defects if taken during early pregnancy. Birth control should be practiced. Talk to your nurse or physician about the risks involved if you plan to become pregnant.

Tolerance to alcohol is reduced by anticonvulsant medication. Be cautious with alcohol consumption. It is best to abstain from alcohol, because it can aggravate your condition. Over-the-counter elixirs containing alcohol (e.g., cough syrup, cold preparations) should be avoided.

Keep this medication and all other medications in a safe place out of children's reach.

This medication is prescribed especially for you. Do not share it with friends or family.

NURSING DRUG DIGEST

Medication (trade name*)	Indication	Usual dosage and administration	Dosage forms, preparation, and storage	Contraindications, cautions, and comments	Monitoring
Acetazolamide Acetazolam Diamox Hydrazol Dedemin Rozolamide	Adjunctive therapy in absence seizures	*Adults and children:* 8-30 mg/kg/24 hr PO in 3-4 divided doses Maximum: 1000 mg/24 hr Administer IV push at a rate of 250-500 mg/min Parenterally, the direct IV route is preferred IM administration is painful	Tablets: 125, 250 mg Capsules (sustained-release): 500 mg Injectable: 500 mg to be diluted with 5 ml sterile water for injection Refrigerate reconstituted solution and discard after 24 hr	*Contraindicated* in patients hypersensitive to the sulfonamides *Contraindicated* in angle-closure glaucoma Therapeutic blood level is 2.2 µg/ml May cause drowsiness Chronic use usually results in tolerance Drug also has diuretic properties	Monitor patients' fluid status because of drug's diuretic properties • Observe for hypokalemia • Observe for hyperglycemia, especially in diabetic and prediabetic patients • Observe for signs of acidosis during long-term therapy
Amobarbital Amytal Isobec Novamobarb	Status epilepticus See also Chapter 15, "Sedative-hypnotics"	*Adults and children:* Anticonvulsant dose in status epilepticus individualized depending on patient's response The rate of injection should *not* exceed 100 mg/min in adults or 60 mg/m² of body surface area per min in children Superficial IM or SC injection may be painful and may produce sterile abscess or sloughing of tissue Ensure that IM injections are deep No more than 5 ml of reconstituted amobarbital should be injected at any one adult site Amobarbital should be administered IV at a rate *not* exceeding 100 mg/min	Elixir: 22 or 44 mg/5 ml Tablets: 15, 30, 50, 100 mg Capsules: 65, 200 mg Injectable: 125, 250, 500, 1000 mg Reconstitute with sterile water for injection Gently rotate vial; do not shake vial	Equipment for respiratory support must be immediately available Prolonged use may induce physical and psychologic dependence	Respiration, pulse, and blood pressure must be closely monitored during IV administration and for several hours afterwards

Carbamazepine Mazepine Tegretol	Partial seizures, including complex partial seizures Generalized tonic-clonic seizures To replace hydantoins or barbiturates in epileptic women contemplating pregnancy	Adults: 200 mg PO b.i.d. to q.i.d. Maximum: 1600 mg/day Children: 6-12 years of age, 100 mg PO b.i.d. to q.i.d. Maximum: 1000 mg/day	Tablet: 200 mg; chewable: 100 mg Protect from moisture	Contraindicated in patients with a hepatic disease or serious blood disorder Therapeutic blood level is 6-12 µg/ml Should not be administered immediately before, in conjunction with, or immediately after an MAOI Should not be administered to patients with atrioventricular block Should not be given to patients with a known hypersensitivity to tricyclic antidepressant drugs May cause urinary retention May cause drowsiness Abrupt withdrawal may precipitate seizures May cause fatal blood dyscrasias; thus complete pretreatment blood counts, including platelet, should be obtained	Monitor hematologic values Observe for fever, sore throat, or bruising (i.e., signs of bone marrow depression) Monitor renal and hepatic function tests Observe for changes in mental status (especially in psychotic and elderly patients) and report ataxia, diplopia, blurred vision, drowsiness, dizziness, nausea and vomiting, and lens opacities Monitor for signs of toxicity: diplopia, dizziness, bone marrow depression, cardiovascular collapse, Stevens-Johnson syndrome, ataxia, nausea, and vomiting

Continued.

NOTE: For additional details regarding the individual agents listed in this table, see the text and other tables in this chapter.
*Indicates a multiple active ingredient product. For a complete listing of all active ingredients see the *Drug Reference Guide to Brand Names and Active Ingredients.*
★ Indicates that the drug is generally available only in the United States.

NURSING DRUG DIGEST—cont'd

Medication (trade name)	Indication	Usual dosage and administration	Dosage forms, preparation, and storage	Contraindications, cautions, and comments	Monitoring
Clonazepam Clonopin Iktorivil Rivotril	Absence seizures Myoclonic epilepsy See also Chapter 15, "Sedative-hypnotics"	*Adults:* Initially 1.5 mg/day PO in 3 divided doses Increase by 0.5-1 mg every third day until seizures controlled or adverse effects preclude further increase; usual maintenance dose is 8-10 mg/day Maximum: 20 mg/day *Children:* Up to age 10 years, initially 0.01-0.03 mg/kg/day PO in 2-3 divided doses increasing by 0.25-0.50 mg/day every third day	Tablets: 0.5, 1, 2 mg	*Contraindicated* in severe hepatic disease *Contraindicated* in sensitivity to the benzodiazepines Therapeutic blood level is .013-.072 µg/ml Drowsiness and ataxia are prominent side effects Tends to lose effectiveness after 2-4 months' use May precipitate grand mal seizures or status epilepticus if abruptly withdrawn May be excreted in human breast milk Concomitant use of clonazepam and valproic acid may produce petit mal seizures Should *not* be used in patients with acute narrow-angle glaucoma	Monitor for oversedation Monitor for drowsiness, ataxia, as well as blurred vision, diplopia, dizziness, nausea, and vomiting Monitor for signs of toxicity: ataxia, CNS depression, sedation, confusion, tremors, piloerection, motor activity, thick speech, hypersalivation, hypotonia, and hyperactivity
Corticotropin Actest Acthar ACTH Cortrophin Cortrophin-Zinc Depo-Acth Duracton H.P. Acthar	Infantile spasms with hypsarrythmia See also Chapter 65, "Corticosteroids and Adrenal Steroid Inhibitors"	*Children:* 25 units/day IM for 20 days	Injectable: 25, 40 IU/ml Repository Gel, sterile, injectable: 40, 80 IU/ml Reconstitute immediately before use with NS or sterile water for injection Refrigerate reconstituted solution Discard unused portion after 24 hr	*Contraindicated* in severe CHF, severe hypertension; and systemic fungal infections Except for hypersensitivity reactions, short-term administration is unlikely to produce harmful effects For long-term effects see Chapter 65	Monitor for fluid and electrolyte disturbances (i.e., hypocalcemia, hypokalemia, hypernatremia, and fluid retention)

Drug	Uses	Dosage and administration	Pharmaceutical preparations	Contraindications and precautions	Nursing implications
Diazepam Neo-Calme Novodipam Valium Vivol E-Pam Meval	Status epilepticus See also Chapter 15, "Sedative-hypnotics"	*Adults:* 5-20 mg IV May repeat in *10-15 min* Maximum: 50 mg *Children:* 30 days-5 years of age, 0.2-0.5 mg IV slowly q2-5 min; 5 years and older, 1 mg IV slowly q2-5 min Maximum: 10 mg Should be injected into large vein Should be administered IV *no faster than 5 mg/min*	Injectable: 5 mg/ml (combined with 40% propylene glycol, 10% alcohol, 5% sodium benzoate and 1.5% benzyl alcohol) Do *not* mix with other IV medications unless compatibility is assured	*Contraindicated* in sensitivity to the benzodiazepines and narrow-angle glaucoma May cause drowsiness Rare reports of apnea and cardiac arrest in elderly or severely ill patients Use cautiously in combination with other respiratory depressants Excreted in human breast milk in sufficient quantity to cause sedation in the neonate After IV use ambulation should be delayed 1-2 hrs until patient is alert Ventilatory support should be available when diazepam is used to treat status epilepticus Seizure precautions should be observed	Monitor pulse, blood pressure, and respiratory status before, during, and following IV administration
Ethosuximide Capitus Petinimid Suxinutin Thilopemal Zarontin	Absence seizures (petit mal)	*Adults:* 15-30 mg/kg/day PO in divided doses b.i.d. Maximum: 1.5 gm/day *Children:* 20 mg/kg/day PO in divided doses Administration with food or milk may decrease GI distress	Capsule: 250 mg Elixir: 250 mg/5 ml Syrup: 250 mg/5 ml Store below 30° C Protect from light	*Contraindicated* in hypersensitivity to the succinimides Therapeutic blood level is 40-100 µg/ml Administer with caution in patients with known hepatic or renal disease Should *not* be used during pregnancy or given to nursing mothers unless the expected benefits warrant the possible risk Abrupt withdrawal may precipitate seizures May cause systemic lupus erythematosus Seizure precautions should be observed	Monitor hepatic and renal function Observe for personality changes, especially for signs of depression Monitor for other side effects, including headache, nausea, euphoria, vomiting, dizziness, anorexia, erythema multiforme, pancytopenia, and hiccups Monitor for signs of toxicity: skin reactions, nausea, dizziness, parkinson-like syndrome, behavior changes, vomiting, drowsiness, leukopenia, and hiccups

Continued.

NURSING DRUG DIGEST—cont'd

Medication (trade name)	Indication	Usual dosage and administration	Dosage forms, preparation, and storage	Contraindications, cautions, and comments	Monitoring
★ **Ethotoin** Peganone	Generalized tonic-clonic seizures Partial seizures Myoclonic seizures	*Adults:* Start with 1-3 gm/day PO in 4-6 divided doses *Children:* 500-1000 mg/day PO in divided doses Administration with food or milk may decrease GI distress	Tablets: 250, 500 mg	*Contraindicated* in hepatic dysfunction and hematologic abnormalities Ataxia and gingival hypertrophy less common than with phenytoin May produce lymphoma-like syndrome; drug should be stopped Should *not* be used during pregnancy or given to nursing mothers unless the expected benefits warrant the possible risk May cause drowsiness	Monitor for ataxia, gingival hypertrophy, lymphoma-like syndrome, and drowsiness
Magnesium sulfate Adlerika Epsom Salt Mag-5	To prevent and control severe preeclampsia and eclampsia To treat seizures associated with various medical conditions (usually other antiepileptic drugs are preferred) See also Chapter 41, "Laxatives and Antidiarrheals"	For severe preeclampsia and eclampsia, dose is individualized Initial, 4 gm IV and 4-5 gm IM into each buttock q.4h. depending on the response For controlling seizures associated with epilepsy or glomerulonephritis, 1 gm IV; to counteract muscle-stimulating effect of barium poisoning, 1-2 gm IV *Children:* In hypertensive encephalopathy associated with acute nephritis in children; 20-40 mg/kg IM q.4-6h. (20% solution)	Crystals: 100 mg/ml (10%), 250 mg/ml (25%), 500 mg/ml (50%) Unused portion should be discarded	*Contraindicated* in patients with heart block or myocardial damage Knee jerk disappears with intoxication; this reflex should be present, the respiratory rate should be more than 16/min and urine output should be more than 100 ml in the preceding 4 hr *before* administering additional magnesium sulfate parenterally	Monitor patients for flushing, sweating, hypotension, depressed reflexes, paralysis, hypothermia, and cardiac or CNS depression because these precede fatal respiratory paralysis Monitor patellar reflex (i.e., knee jerk) *before* each dose

Drug	Uses	Dosage	Preparations	Nursing considerations
		In severe cases 100-200 mg/kg IV over 1 hr (½ given over first 15-20 min) (1%-3% solution)		The drug should *not* be administered for 2 hours before delivery to prevent respiratory depression in the newborn
		IV rate of administration should not exceed 150 mg/min		Calcium gluconate should be available for IV injection to reverse serious toxicity
		Decrease dose in renal failure		The drug should be used cautiously in patients with renal failure
				Magnesium sulfate should be used cautiously with sedative drugs, anesthetic agents, neuromuscular blocking agents, and digitalis
Mephenytoin Mesantoin Phenantoin	Generalized tonic-clonic seizures and partial seizures *refractory* to other medications	*Adults:* 200-600 mg/day PO	Tablet: 100 mg	Monitor WBC monthly; more frequently if WBC is below 2500
	Should *not* be used if other less toxic drugs are effective	*Children:* 5-12 years 100-400 mg/day PO		Monitor for drowsiness, and exfoliative dermatitis
				Contraindicated in hypersensitivity to the hydantoins
				Because of relatively high incidence of fatalities linked with mephenytoin from exfoliative dermatitis, aplastic anemia, pancytopenia and hepatitis, the drug is *contraindicated* unless patient is refractory to other medications
				Therapeutic blood level is 5-20 µg/ml
				Stop medication if WBC falls below 1600/mm^3
				Should *not* be used in pregnancy nor given to nursing mothers
				May cause systemic lupus erythematosus

Continued.

NURSING DRUG DIGEST—cont'd

Medication (trade name)	Indication	Usual dosage and administration	Dosage forms, preparation, and storage	Contraindications, cautions, and comments	Monitoring
Mephobarbital Mebaral Mebroin* Menta-Bal Mephoral Phemitone Prominal	Generalized tonic-clonic seizures Partial seizures, except complex partial seizures See also Chapter 15, "Sedative-hypnotics"	*Adults:* 400-600 mg/day PO *Children:* Under 5 years of age, 16-32 mg PO t.i.d. to q.i.d.; over 5 years of age, 32-64 mg PO t.i.d to q.i.d. Administer at bedtime for nocturnal seizures *Elderly:* Start with lower doses May need to decrease dose in renal impairment	Tablets: 32, 50, 100, 200 mg Protect from light	*Contraindicated* in hypersensitivity to the barbiturates and porphyria Should *not* be used during pregnancy or giving en to nursing mothers unless expected benefits warrant the possible risk Approximately 75% of an absorbed dose is metabolized to phenobarbital Use with caution in presence of hepatic dysfunction	Monitor prothrombin times for patients receiving concurrent anticoagulant therapy Observe same precautions as for phenobarbital
★ **Metharbital** Gemonil	Generalized tonic-clonic seizures Partial seizures, except complex partial seizures	*Adults:* 100 mg q.d. to t.i.d, increasing if necessary up to 800 mg/day in divided doses *Children:* 50-100 mg q.d. to t.i.d.	Tablets: 100 mg	*Contraindicated* in hypersensitivity to the barbiturates and porphyria Should *not* be used during pregnancy or giving en to nursing mothers unless expected benefits warrant the possible risk	Monitor prothrombin times for patients receiving concurrent anticoagulant therapy
Methsuximide Celontin Petinutin	Absence seizures (petit mal)	*Adults:* 300 mg/day PO Maximum: 1.2 gm/day *Children:* 150-300 mg/day PO	Capsules: 150, 300 mg Store between 15° and 30 ° C Protect from light and excessive heat Discard capsules that are not full or that appear melted	*Contraindicated* in hypersensitivity to the succinimides Therapeutic blood level is 40-100 μg/ml May color urine pink or brown Abrupt withdrawal may precipitate seizures Administer with caution in patients with known hepatic or renal disease	Observe skin for rashes, urticaria, and Stevens-Johnson syndrome

Drug	Uses	Dosage	Preparations	Contraindications/Precautions	Nursing considerations
Paraldehyde Paral	Anticonvulsant in status epilepticus (largely replaced by other drugs) Acute agitation or alcohol, barbiturate, or narcotic withdrawal (use in this regard has been largely replaced by chlordiazepoxide and diazepam) See also Chapter 15, "Sedative-hypnotics"	*Adults:* 5-10 ml IM or 0.2-0.4 ml/kg IV *Children:* 0.1-0.15 ml/kg IV or IM To control convulsions in the newborn, 0.1 mg/kg IM Status epilepticus in childhood may be managed by rectal paraldehyde 1 ml per year of age up to 5 ml; this dose may be repeated in 1 hr if needed; additional administration may be given by gastric tube in a dose of 2-5 ml every 2-4 hr; however, *rectal* administration is not recommended because dosage is difficult to control *Adults:* 5-10 ml PO or 5 ml IM q.4-6h.; the oral route is preferred; the dose should be reduced as agitation lessens IM administration is extremely painful and may produce nerve damage at injection site, sterile skin abscesses, sloughing of skin, fat necrosis, and muscular irritation Great care should be taken in choosing the correct injection site and needle length The drug should *not* be administered subcutaneously Oral paraldehyde should be diluted with milk or iced fruit juice to disguise the odor and taste and to minimize gastric irritation Rectal paraldehyde should be diluted with 200 ml of 0.9% sodium chloride or with 2 proportionate volumes of olive oil or cottonseed oil to reduce rectal irritation	Capsule: 1 gm (approx 1 ml) Liquid: 30 ml Injectable: 2, 5, 10 ml Should be stored in well-filled, tight, light-resistant glass container with capacity no larger than 30 ml at temperature not exceeding 25° C Unused contents of a container should be discarded after 24 hr Dilute *before* IV administration with several proportionate volumes of NS	Should *not* be used during pregnancy or given to nursing mothers unless the expected benefits warrant the possible risk *Contraindicated* in patients with gastroenteritis or severe hepatic impairment Preparations having a brownish color or odor of acetic acid (vinegar) should *not* be used IV administration may cause pulmonary edema, pulmonary hemorrhage, right heart failure, and collapse Decomposed paraldehyde may cause erosion of the stomach or rectum Paraldehyde should be used with great caution in patients with asthma, bronchopulmonary disease, or impaired hepatic function Paraldehyde should *not* be used in obstetrics because neonates may be born with marked respiratory depression Prolonged use may produce physical or psychologic dependence	Monitor injection sites for sterile abscess and irritation Monitor anal area for irritation if administered PR Monitor respiratory function; bronchial secretions may be increased; position patient on side to prevent aspiration; suction equipment should be readily accessible

Continued.

NURSING DRUG DIGEST—cont'd

Medication (trade name)	Indication	Usual dosage and administration	Dosage forms, preparation, and storage	Contraindications, cautions, and comments	Monitoring
★ **Parametha-dione** Alondra Dilar Paradione	Absence seizures (petit mal) NOTE: Should *not* be used if other less toxic drugs are effective	*Adults*: 300-600 mg PO t.i.d. to q.i.d. *Children*: 100-300 mg PO t.i.d. Dilute oral solution with water, milk, or juice before administration	Capsules: 150, 300 mg Solution: 300 mg/ml (65% alcohol)	Therapeutic blood level is 600-800 μg/ml (as dimethadione, the active metabolite May cause drowsiness May cause nephrosis and various hematologic abnormalities May cause sensitivity to bright light Should *not* be used during pregnancy or given to nursing mothers unless expected benefits warrant the possible risk Less toxic than trimethadione, but also less effective	Monitor for drowsiness and sensitivity to bright light
Pentobarbital Butylone Carbrital* Dorsital Hypnotal Ibatal Nebralin Nembutal Nembutal Sodium Nova-Rectal Pentanca Pentogen WANS*	Status epilepticus See also Chapter 15, "Sedative-hypnotics"	The IV dose is individualized to control seizures without producing respiratory depression unless the patient is intubated with respiratory assistance No more than 250 mg or 5 ml solution of pentobarbital should be injected IM at any one site in adults May need to decrease dose in renal impairment	Capsules: 30, 50, 100 mg Elixir: 20 mg/5 ml Injectable: 50, 125, 300 mg/ml Suppositories, rectal: 15, 30, 60, 100, 120, 200 mg Tablets: 30 mg	*Contraindicated* in hypersensitivity to the barbiturates *Contraindicated* in porphyria Respiratory support equipment must be immediately available when pentobarbital is used intravenously Rapid IV administration may cause respiratory depression, apnea, laryngospasm, bronchial spasm, or hypotension	Monitor respiratory function Patient must be observed for 20-30 min after IM injection to assure that narcosis has not been excessive Monitor blood pressure
★ **Phenacemide** Epiclase Phenurone	Phenacemide is extremely toxic and should *not* be used until all other appropriate medication has been proved ineffective	*Adults and children*: 1.5 gm daily in three divided doses Increase 500 mg weekly to maintenance dose of 2-3 gm daily in divided doses	Tablet: 500 mg	Toxic drug (may produce fatal hepatic necrosis, severe bone marrow depression, nephrosis or severe psychosis) Liver function tests, blood counts, and urinalysis must be performed regularly during treatment	Monitor renal and hepatic function Observe for signs of serious adverse effects (e.g., sore throat, persistent fever, easy bruising, epistaxis, seizures, and skin rashes) and report

Drug	Uses	Dosage	Supply	Remarks	Nursing Implications
	Generalized tonic-clonic seizures Partial seizures Effective in some patients with absence seizures			Should *not* be used during pregnancy or giving to nursing mothers unless the expected benefits warrant the possible risk Often causes personality changes ranging from mild depression to severe psychosis and suicidal tendencies Complete blood counts should be obtained before initiating therapy	Observe for personality changes (e.g., depression, psychosis) and report
Phenobarbital Barbenyl Barbita Barbivis Gardenal Hypnolone Liquital Luminal Mediphen Nova-Pheno Pheno-Squar Phenonyl Solfoton Solu-Barb Stental SK-Phenobarbital Talpheno	Generalized tonic-clonic seizures Partial seizures Less effective in complex partial seizures; less effective for myoclonic seizures Absence seizures See also Chapter 15, "Sedative-hypnotics"	*Adults:* 50-100 b.i.d. to t.i.d. *Children:* 15-50 mg b.i.d. to t.i.d. Not to exceed 60 mg/min when injected IV Status epilepticus 120-240 mg IV	Tablets: 8.5, 15, 30, 50, 60, 100 mg Capsules: 16, 65 mg Drops: 16 mg/ml Injectable: 120 mg/ml Elixir: 4 mg/ml Dissolve powder in sterile water for injection; 1 ml for IM and SC; 3 ml for IV Discard injectable solution if it contains a precipitate	*Contraindicated* in hypersensitivity to the barbiturates, porphyria, and severe hepatic impairment Therapeutic blood level is 10-40 µg/ml May cause excitability in children and the elderly Should *not* be used during pregnancy or giving to nursing mothers unless expected benefits warrant the possible risk Overdose may cause respiratory arrest or significant hypotension Equipment for respiratory support must be immediately available when used IV to control status epilepticus May cause sedation, rash, psychic changes, and physical dependence *Toxicity:* Sedation, psychic changes, nystagmus, and ataxia	Observe for signs of overdose (e.g., cyanosis, clammy skin, hypotension) Monitor prothrombin times for patients receiving concurrent anticoagulant therapy Monitor phenobarbital levels closely if valproic acid is added to drug regimen because phenobarbital levels can rise significantly

Continued.

NURSING DRUG DIGEST—cont'd

Medication (trade name)	Indication	Usual dosage and administration	Dosage forms, preparation, and storage	Contraindications, cautions, and comments	Monitoring
Phensuximide Lifene Milontin	Absence seizures (petit mal)	*Adults:* 500-1000 mg b.i.d. to t.i.d. *Children:* 250-1000 mg b.i.d. to t.i.d.	Capsules: 250, 500 mg Suspension: 300 mg/5 ml	*Contraindicated* in hypersensitivity to succinimides Therapeutic blood level is 40-80 µg/ml Abrupt withdrawal may precipitate seizures Administer with caution in patients with known hepatic or renal disease Should *not* be used during pregnancy or given to nursing mothers unless the expected benefits warrant the possible risk May cause muscle weakness May cause alopecia May color urine red-brown to pink Less toxic than other succinimides but also less effective	
Phenytoin Dantoin Dilantin Epanutin Eptoin Mebroin* Novophenytoin	Generalized tonic-clonic seizures Partial seizures Myoclonic seizures Status epilepticus See also Chapter 32, "Antidysrhythmics"	*Adults:* 300-400 mg/day PO *Children:* 4-8 mg/kg/day PO in 2-3 divided doses *Adults:* 150-250 mg IV slowly, followed by 100-150 mg after 30 min if necessary *Children:* 250 mg/m² IV slowly Do *not* exceed 50 mg/min IV Do *not* administer IM because absorption is too erratic	Tablet: 50 mg Capsules: 30, 100 mg Injectable: 50 mg/ml with propylene glycol (40%) and alcohol (10%) in water for injections Suspension: 30, 125 mg/ml Can be mixed with 60-100 ml NS Do *not* mix with D₅W—will form precipitate	*Contraindicated* in hypersensitivity to the hydantoins *Contraindicated* in sinus bradycardia, Adams-Stokes syndrome, and sinoatrial block Therapeutic blood level is 10-20 µg/ml	Monitor pulse when administering IV Monitor for hyperplasia and skin disorders, including exfoliative dermatitis Monitor blood sugar Monitor for megaloblastic anemia

IM and SC injections are painful and may cause tissue necrosis

Avoid continuous infusion; alkalinity of solution causes venous irritation

Administer with food or milk to decrease GI upset

When administering oral suspension, shake bottle vigorously before pouring to ensure uniform distribution of drug

Not compatible with acidic solutions

Discard cloudy solutions

Should *not* be used during pregnancy because of high incidence of teratogenicity, especially cleft lip and cleft palate

Should *not* be given to nursing mothers unless benefits warrant potential risk

Ataxia is major side effect; other side effects include drowsiness, nystagmus, tremor, nausea, fever, and leukopenia

May color the urine reddish brown or pink

May cause various skin disorders, including hirsutism, facial coarsening, exfoliative dermatitis, lupus erythematosus, and Stevens-Johnson syndrome

May cause hyperplasia of the gums; encourage meticulous oral hygiene including brushing, flossing, and gum massage

May cause hyperglycemia

Teach patient about side effects to expect, including gum hyperplasia and coloring of urine

Patients should receive dietary supplements of folic acid and pyridoxine to prevent drug-induced deficiency

Avoid abrupt discontinuation

Continued.

NURSING DRUG DIGEST—cont'd

Medication (trade name)	Indication	Usual dosage and administration	Dosage forms, preparation, and storage	Contraindications, cautions, and comments	Monitoring
Primidone Mylepsine Mysoline Ro-Primidone Sertan	Partial seizures, especially complex partial seizures Generalized tonic-clonic seizures	Adults: 250-500 mg PO t.i.d. to q.i.d. Maximum: 2 gm/day Children: Less than 8 years of age, 10-25 mg/kg/day in 3-4 divided doses PO Maximum: 1 gm/day	Tablets: 50, 250 mg Suspension: 250 mg/5 ml	Contraindicated in porphyria and hypersensitivity to phenobarbital Therapeutic blood level is 5-15 µg/ml May cause alopecia, impotence, or drowsiness Some patients develop profound ataxia from a single dose Not a true barbiturate but has similar chemical structure and mode of action Should not be used during pregnancy or given to nursing mothers unless expected benefits warrant possible risk Partially metabolized to phenobarbital; phenobarbital levels should therefore be drawn, along with primidone levels Toxicity: ataxia, sedation, psychic changes, nystagmus, and GI disturbances Observe same precautions as for phenobarbital	Monitor for alopecia, ataxia, impotence, drowsiness, GI disturbances, and psychic changes Monitor for rash, and physical dependence

| **Thiopental** Pentothal | Status epilepticus See also Chapters 14, "General Anesthetics," and 15, "Sedative-hypnotics" | For status epilepticus dose is individualized; assisted respiration is commonly required 2.5% solution is administered by continuous IV administration | Injectable: 0.5, 1, 5 gm Discard solutions that are discolored or contain a precipitate Rectal suspension: 400 mg/gm with anhydrous sodium carbonate in mineral oil Reconstitute injectable with sufficient D_5W, NS, or sterile water for injection to yield a concentration between 2% and 5% for IV use Discard unused reconstituted portions after 24 hr | *Contraindicated* in patients hypersensitive to barbiturates, with status asthmaticus or porphyria Emergency respiratory support equipment must be immediately available Use with great caution in hypotension or shock, hepatic or renal disease, myxedema, Addison's disease, severe anemia, severe cardiovascular disease, increased intracranial pressure, asthma, and myasthenia gravis Rectal suspension should not be used in inflammatory ulcerative or neoplastic lesions of the lower bowel Laryngospasm may occur during induction Avoid intraarterial injection because thiopental may cause severe arterial spasms Must not be administered via varicose veins | Children given thiopental PR must be constantly attended and monitored Monitor respiratory function |

Continued.

NURSING DRUG DIGEST—cont'd

Medication (trade name)	Indication	Usual dosage and administration	Dosage forms, preparation, and storage	Contraindications, cautions, and comments	Monitoring
★ **Trimethadione** Tridione Trimedone	Absence seizures (petit mal) refractory to treatment with other drugs	*Adults:* 300-600 mg PO t.i.d. to q.i.d. *Children:* 100-300 mg PO t.i.d.	Tablet (chewable): 150 mg Capsule: 300 mg Solution: 40 mg/ml	*Contraindicated* during pregnancy because of teratogenicity Therapeutic blood level is 600-800 µg/ml (as dimethadione, the active metabolite of trimethadione) Should *not* be given to nursing mothers unless expected benefits warrant the possible risk Teratogenesis in the neonate includes congenital heart defects, V-shaped eyebrows, low-set ears, and phalangeal hypoplasia	Monitor CBC Observe for grand mal seizures
Valproic acid Depakene Epilim Ergenyl Urekene	Absence seizures Myoclonic epilepsy Generalized tonic-clonic seizures	*Adults:* 15-30 mg/kg/day PO in divided doses Maximum: 60 mg/kg/day *Children:* 15 mg/kg/day PO	Capsule: 250 mg Syrup: 250 mg/5 ml (as sodium salt)	*Contraindicated* during first trimester of pregnancy because 1% of exposed fetuses may develop spina bifida	Patients must be monitored closely when valproic acid is added to regime of other drugs

Capsules should be swallowed whole; chewing may cause irritation of mouth and throat
Administration with food or milk may decrease GI side effects

Contraindicated in hepatotoxicity
Therapeutic blood level is 50-100 µg/ml
Will rarely cause coma when used with other anticonvulsants, especially phenobarbital
Serum phenobarbital levels must be monitored closely when used with valproic acid
Excreted in breast milk and should *not* be given to nursing mothers
Concomitant use of valproic acid and clonazepam may produce petit mal status
May cause tremors, asterixis, nausea, vomiting, weight gain, diarrhea, transient hair loss, hepatic toxicity, thrombocytopenia, and inhibition of platelet aggregation
May affect platelet function; report any abnormal bleeding
Toxicity: drowsiness, nausea, vomiting, and diarrhea

Monitor hepatic function because fatal hepatic failure has been reported usually within first 6 mo of therapy
Monitor for bruising and unusual bleeding

BIBLIOGRAPHY

Andermann, E. Teratogenic effects of anticonvulsant medication. In P. Robb (Ed.). *Epilepsy updated: causes and treatment.* Miami: Symposia Specialists, 1980.

Caveness, W.F., et al. Natural history of posttraumatic epilepsy. In J.A. Wada & K.F. Penry (Eds.). *Advances in epileptology Xth Epilepsy International Symposium.* New York: Raven Press, 1978.

Delgado-Escueta, A.V., Treiman, D.M., & Walsh, G.O. The treatable epilepsies (part I). *The New England Journal of Medicine,* 1983, *308*(25), 1508-1514.

Delgado-Escueta, A.V., Treiman, D.M., & Walsh, G.O. The treatable epilepsies (part II). *The New England Journal of Medicine,* 1983, *308*(26), 1576-1584.

Hawken, M., & Ozuna, J. Practical aspects of anticonvulsant therapy. *American Journal of Nursing,* 1979, *79*(6), 1062-1068.

MacDougall, V. Teaching children and families about seizures. *The Canadian Nurse,* 1982, *78*(4), 30-36.

Norman, S., & Browne, T. Seizure disorders. *American Journal of Nursing,* 1981, *81*(5), 984-994.

Trekas, J. Managing epilepsy, don't forget the patient. *Nursing 82,* 1982, *12*, 63-65.

SECTION IV

PERIPHERAL NERVOUS SYSTEM MEDICATIONS

Medications discussed in this section

CHAPTER 23

Acetylcholine
Anisotropine methylbromide
Atropine
Belladonna
Bethanechol
Carbachol
Clidinium
Cyclopentolate
Glycopyrrolate
Hexocyclium methylsulfate
Homatropine methylbromide
Hyoscyamine
Isopropamide
Mepenzolate
Methantheline
Methscopolamine
Oxyphencyclimine
Oxyphenonium
Pilocarpine
Propantheline
Scopolamine
Tridihexethyl
Tropicamide

CHAPTER 24

Albuterol
Bretylium
Dobutamine
Dopamine
Debrisoquine
Ephedrine
Epinephrine
Ethylnorepinephrine
Fenoterol
Guanethidine
Hydroxyamphetamine
Isoproterenol
Mephentermine
Metaproterenol
Metaraminol
Methoxamine
Metoprolol
Naphazoline
Norepinephrine
Nylidrin
Oxymetazoline
Phenylephrine
Phenylpropanolamine
Phenoxybenzamine
Phentolamine
Prazosin
Propranolol
Propylhexedrine
Pseudoephedrine
Reserpine
Terbutaline
Tetrahydrozoline
Timolol
Xylometazoline

CHAPTER 25

Ambenonium
Atropine
Demecarium
Echothiophate
Edrophonium
Isoflurophate
Neostigmine
Physostigmine
Pralidoxime
Pyridostigmine

CHAPTER 26

Atracurium
Gallamine
Hexaflorenium
Lobeline
Mecamylamine
Metocurine
Nicotine
Pancuronium
Succinylcholine
Trimethaphan
Tubocurarine

Review of the Anatomy, Physiology, and Assessment of the Peripheral Nervous System

David F. Biggs

The nervous structures of the body can be divided into the central and the peripheral nervous systems. The central nervous system (CNS) is made up of the brain and spinal cord (see Chapter 13). The peripheral nervous system (PNS) is made up of all the nerves that lie outside the CNS. Thus the PNS consists of the 12 paired cranial nerves, which emerge from the brain, and the 31 pairs of spinal nerves, which exit from the spinal cord. This division is summarized in the box on p. 434.

The nerves of the PNS that carry impulses *toward* the CNS are called *afferent* nerves. In general, all afferent nerves subserve sensory structures, and the terms *afferent* and *sensory* are often used synonymously. Nerves of the PNS that carry impulses *away* from the CNS are called *efferent* nerves. All cranial and spinal nerves contain both afferent and efferent nerve fibers. These data are summarized in the box on p. 434.

AFFERENT NERVES

The afferent nerves of the PNS can be subdivided into three major groups: the somatic, the visceral, and the proprioceptive subdivisions.

Somatic subdivision

The *somatic* subdivision includes neurons that are associated primarily with the anatomic framework of the body. Impulses that originate in the sensory structures near or at the surface of the body are carried along pathways referred to as *general* somatic afferent nerves. The latter subserve three types of sensations detected by separate groups of receptors. The three types of sensation are: pain; temperature, including both hot and cold; and touch, which is usually subdivided into light touch (reflecting surface changes) and deep touch (reflecting pressure). The latter implies the activation of receptors that lie much below the surface. Sensory function is assessed by asking the patient to close the eyes and applying stimuli to areas on the forehead, cheek, hand, lower arm, abdomen, foot, and lower leg. It is not necessary to evaluate the entire skin surface if stimuli are applied strategically so that the dermatomes and the major peripheral nerves are tested symmetrically. In screening the nerve may be assumed to be intact if sensation is felt at the most peripheral extent. Variation in sensitivity of skin areas including the palm of the hand as compared to the dorsal aspect of the hand is normal.

Light touch is tested by brushing the skin lightly with a wisp of cotton or with a small soft brush, avoiding the hair of the skin to prevent undue stimulation. With the eyes closed, the patient is instructed to identify when touch is felt. Tactile localization can be assessed by having the patient point to the spot touched.

Superficial pain and pressure are usually tested together with the use of the sharp and dull points of a safety pin or hypodermic needle. The patient is instructed to describe the sensation as "sharp," "dull," or "can't tell" when the skin is touched. Deep pressure is tested over the eyeball, achilles tendon, calf, and forearm.

Vibratory sensation is also tested. A tuning fork vibrating between 200 and 400 cycles per second is used. The patient, with eyes closed, is instructed to identify when vibrations are felt and when they dissappear as the fork is applied to the clavicles, elbows, ankles, finger joints, and toes. Assessment of the most distal joint is completed moving to more proximal joints as needed.

Temperature is tested with tubes of hot and cold water that are touched to or rolled over skin dermatome areas. The patient is instructed to identify "hot," "cold," or "can't tell." Temperature is not usually tested if pressure, pain, and vibration are normal.

Other somatic sensory neurons include those involved in hearing and vision subserving receptors for

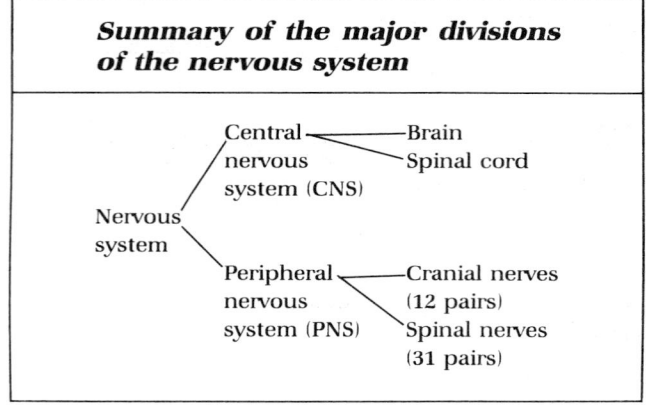

Summary of the major divisions of the nervous system

- Nervous system
  - Central nervous system (CNS)
    - Brain
    - Spinal cord
  - Peripheral nervous system (PNS)
    - Cranial nerves (12 pairs)
    - Spinal nerves (31 pairs)

Summary of the major divisions of the peripheral nervous system (PNS)

- Peripheral nervous system
  - Afferent nerves (impulses *to* CNS)
  - Efferent nerves (impulses *from* CNS)

sound and light, respectively. These nerves are referred to as the *special* somatic afferent system. (See Chapter 13 for assessment of hearing and vision.)

Visceral subdivision

The visceral subdivision includes all afferent nerves that carry impulses arising in or around the viscera. The *general* visceral afferent system contains nerves that subserve receptors found in and on mucous membranes and in the walls of most organs. These receptors detect physical or chemical changes within an organ and also the degree of distention of the wall of an organ.

In addition, two specialized receptor systems are served by nerves commonly referred to as the *special* visceral afferent system. These are the receptor systems for taste and smell, and they respond to chemical stimuli. (See Chapter 13 for assessment of taste and smell.)

Proprioceptive subdivision

The proprioceptive subdivision contains afferent nerves that are concerned with the position and movement of the body. The *general* proprioceptive afferent system contains nerves that subserve receptors of the pressure or tension type, which are associated with the muscles, tendons, and capsules of diarthroidal joints.

Perception of position, orientation, and motion of limbs and body parts is obtained from kinesthetic sensations and is tested by moving the finger or toe with the patient's eyes closed from a neutral position to another position. The patient is asked to identify how the position was changed.

Because of the integration of the peripheral nervous system with the cerebellum and the posterior columns of the spinal cord, cerebellar tests are utilized to test

the proprioceptive system in relation to posture, balance, and coordination. Tactile discrimination requires cortical integration and is assessed by stereognosis, two-point discrimination, and extinction tests. Deep tendon reflexes are assessed to identify integrity of sensory pathways from the tendons and muscles. Damage to a peripheral nerve results in loss of movement and sensation in the innervated area distal to the lesion.

The organs associated with the detection of equilibrium and acceleration are subserved by the *special* proprioceptive afferent system. Neither the general nor special proprioceptive system is under conscious control, but these systems make possible all forms of normal movement.

The subdivisions of the afferent division of the PNS are summarized in Table 22-1.

EFFERENT NERVES

The efferent nerves of the PNS, those nerves that carry impulses *away* from the brain or spinal cord, can be classified similarly. The term *motor* is often applied to this system since impulses passing through these nerves cause contraction or relaxation. The efferent system can be divided into the *somatic* and *visceral* efferent systems.

Somatic subdivision

The somatic efferent system is generally distributed throughout the body and hence the term *general* is frequently applied to it. However, since no "special" efferent system exists, the term is superfluous. The somatic efferent system innervates the motor endplates of all skeletal muscles. The fibers of this system originate in the ventral columns of gray matter in the spinal cord or in the nuclei of the cranial nerves III, IV, VI, and XII (see Table 22-2).

TABLE 22-1

The major subdivisions of the afferent division of the peripheral nervous system (PNS)

Major division	Subdivision	Nerve type	Function
Afferent (sensory) nerves	Somatic	General	Pain
			Temperature
			Touch
		Special	Hearing
			Vision
	Visceral	General	Chemical content
			Distention
		Special	Taste
			Smell
	Proprioceptive	General	Mechanoreceptors in skeletal muscle, tendons, joint capsules
		Special	Equilibrium
			Acceleration

TABLE 22-2

List of the cranial nerves

Cranial nerve no.	Name
I	Olfactory
II	Optic
III	Oculomotor
IV	Trochlear
V	Trigeminal
VI	Abducens
VII	Facial
VIII	Acoustic
IX	Glossopharyngeal
X	Vagus
XI	Accessory
XII	Hypoglossal

Visceral subdivision

The visceral efferent system can be divided into the general and special divisions. The *general* efferent division regulates the functions of the viscera (the organs) of the body and controls all smooth, involuntary muscle, cardiac muscle, and the glands. The term *autonomic* is often applied to this system. This term means "characterized by autonomy" and implies that this system regulates visceral function without the need for conscious control. The visceral efferent system is concerned with the maintenance of homeostasis and regulates heart rate, blood pressure, temperature, glandular secretion, peristalsis, sphincter tension, and pupil size and accommodation.

The *special* visceral efferent system has only a small distribution. It innervates the facial muscles, muscles involved in mastication, and the muscles of the pharynx and larynx. The muscles innervated are typical skeletal muscles but are embryonically related to visceral systems such as the digestive and respiratory tracts. They are therefore classified as visceral. Efferent impulses for this system originate in the brainstem and pass through the V, VII, IX, X, and XI cranial nerves. (Assessment of the cranial nerves is discussed in Chapter 13.)

The various subdivisions of the efferent nervous division of the PNS are summarized in Table 22-3.

GANGLIA

Ganglionic stimulants and blockers, as their name implies, act on ganglia. A ganglion (pl. ganglia) consists of a collection of nerve cell bodies found outside the CNS. A ganglion appears as a node, series of nodules, or a swelling on a nerve. Ganglia can be classified into two groups: sensory ganglia and motor ganglia. Sensory ganglia can be subdivided into cranial and spinal groups. The motor ganglia comprise those found in the autonomic, or general visceral efferent, system.

Sensory ganglia

Cranial sensory ganglia. These are the sensory ganglia associated with afferent fibers in the various cranial nerves. Each ganglion contains the cell bodies of unipolar (monopolar) afferent (sensory) neurons. Ganglia in this subdivision can contain neurons from more than one cranial nerve, although this is not the general rule. Table 22-4 sets out the names of the gan-

TABLE 22-3

The major subdivisions of the efferent division of the peripheral nervous system (PNS)

Major division	*Subdivision*	*Nerve type*	*Location (end-organ)*
Efferent (motor) nerves	Somatic	General	Motor endplates of skeletal muscle
	Visceral	General (autonomic)	Smooth muscle, heart, and exocrine glands
		Special	Muscles for facial expression, mastication, pharynx, larynx

TABLE 22-4

Afferent (sensory) ganglia associated with the various cranial nerves

Cranial nerve	*Associated sensory ganglia*
I Olfactory	None. Bipolar neuron serves as both receptor and afferent neuron and synapses directly in the olfactory bulb.
II Optic	None. Bipolar cells contact rods and cones in the retina. These bipolar cells synapse with ganglion cells in the retina, and the axons of these neurons form the optic nerve and enter the CNS in the optic chiasma.
III Oculomotor	None. Course of afferent neurons is uncertain.
IV Trochlear	None. Cell bodies are found in the mesencephalic nucleus of the trigeminal nerve.
V Trigeminal	Trigeminal (gasserian, semilunar) ganglion (paired)
VI Abducens	None. Cell bodies are found in the mesencephalic nucleus of the trigeminal nerve.
VII Facial	None. Cell bodies are found in the mesencephalic nucleus of the trigeminal nerve.
VIII Acoustic	Spiral (Corti's) ganglion (paired)
IX Glossopharyngeal	Petrosal ganglion (paired). Consists of two parts: superior, the upper; and the inferior, the lower; of two ganglia formed as the IX nerve traverses the jugular foramen. "Petrosal" sometimes only refers to the inferior ganglion.
X Vagus	Nodose (inferior vagal) ganglion (paired) and jugular (superior vagal) ganglion (paired). Both are found adjacent to the jugular foramen.
XI Accessory	None known
XII Hypoglossal	None. Location of the cell bodies is uncertain.

glia associated with afferent neurons in each cranial nerve. It is important to note that these ganglia are bilaterally symmetrical and that none of them contain synapses.

Spinal sensory ganglia. These are the paired ganglia found on the *dorsal* sides of the spinal cord (Figure 22-1). All spinal afferent nerves have cell bodies in the dorsal root ganglia.

Using the previous classification of the afferent nerves, the pathways of the various divisions can be set out as follows.

General somatic afferent nerves. The pathways for the afferent neurons for pain and temperature are shown in Figure 22-2. The pathway for light (crude) touch is shown in Figure 22-3.

General visceral afferent nerves. The pathways for

these neurons are shown in Figure 22-4. It is important to note here that afferent nerve fibers can pass through other ganglia, such as the prevertebral ganglia or the ganglia of the sympathetic chain. However, they do not synapse in these ganglia, and the cell bodies of these afferent neurons are always found in the dorsal root ganglia.

General proprioceptive afferent nerves. The pathways for these afferent nerves are shown in Figure 22-5. Note again that *all* afferent neurons have their cell bodies in the dorsal root ganglia.

Motor ganglia

These are all associated with the general visceral efferent system, or the autonomic nervous system (ANS) as it will now be called (see Table 22-3). It is

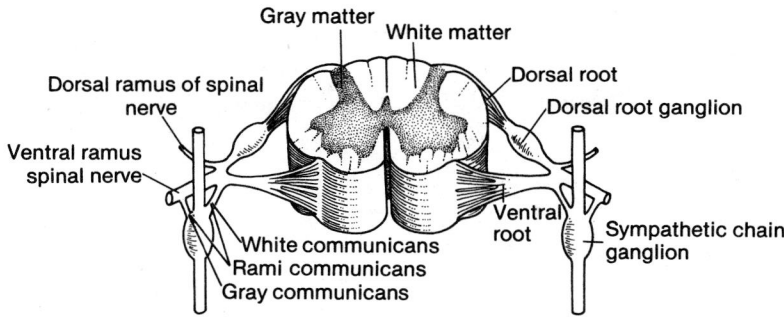

FIGURE 22-1. **A transverse section of the spinal cord showing the dorsal ganglia, dorsal and ventral roots, and the spinal nerves.**

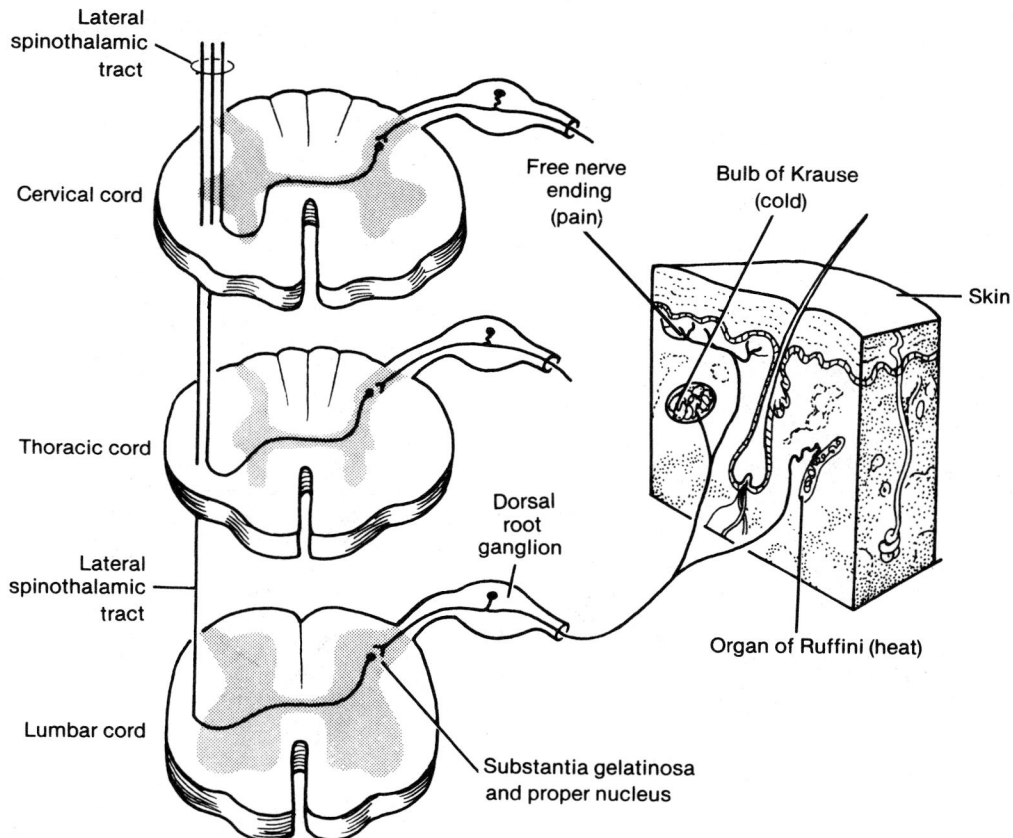

FIGURE 22-2. **The conscious pathway for pain and temperature, including the types of receptors.**

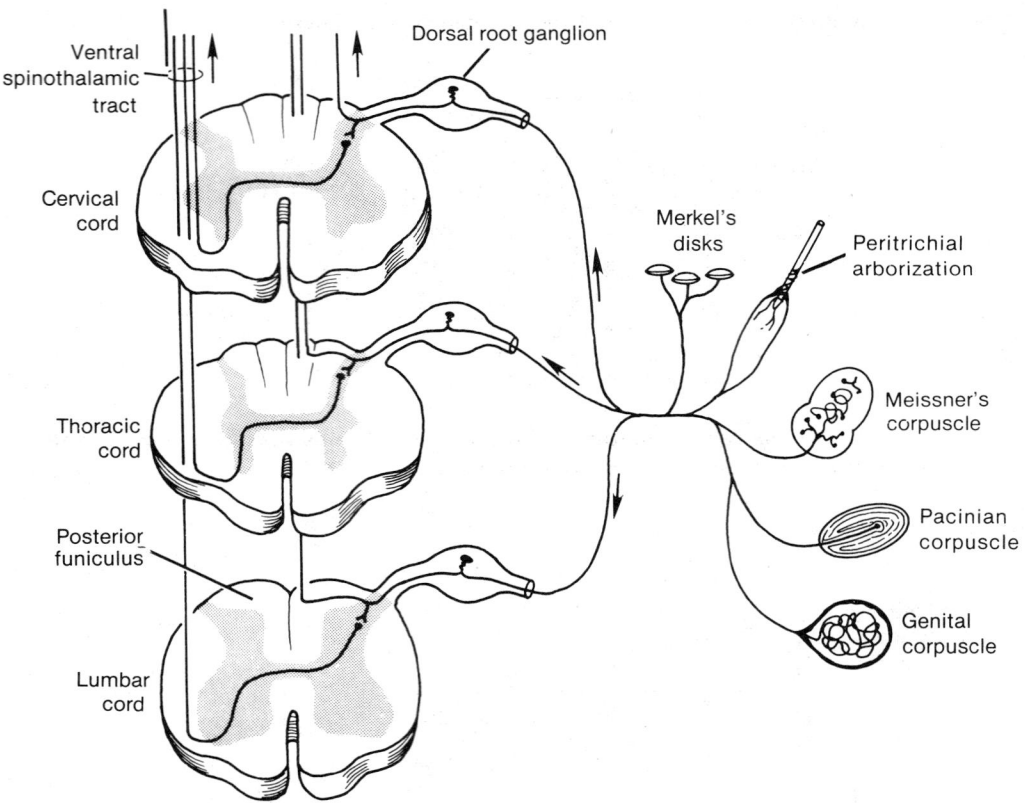

FIGURE 22-3. **The pathway for light touch.**

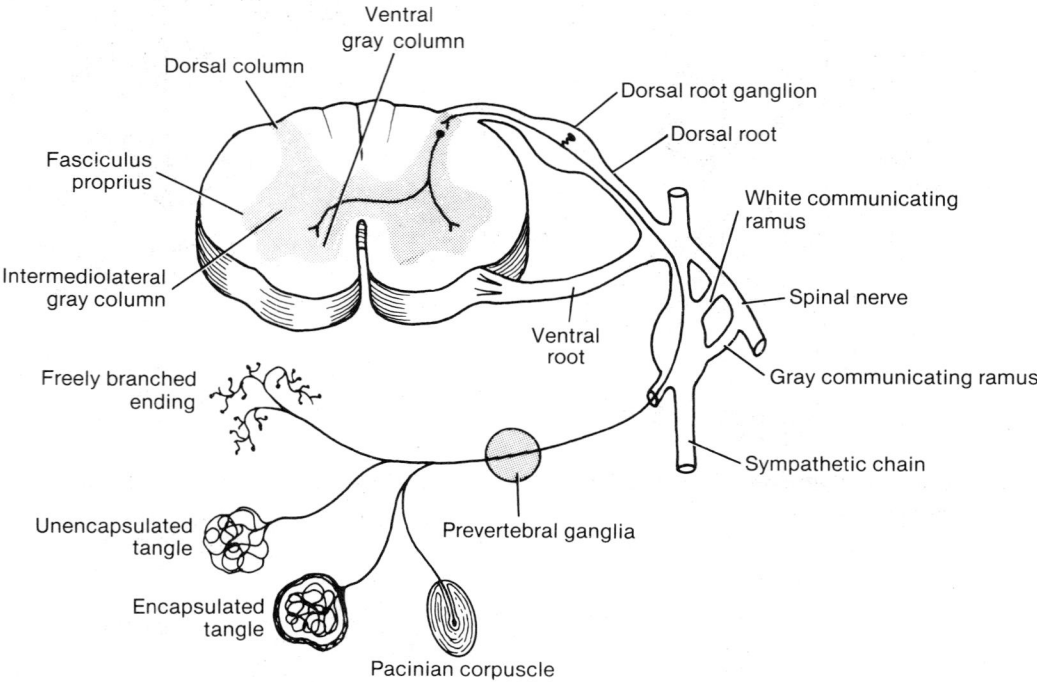

FIGURE 22-4. **The visceral afferent pathway for impulses entering the CNS through the spinal nerves.**

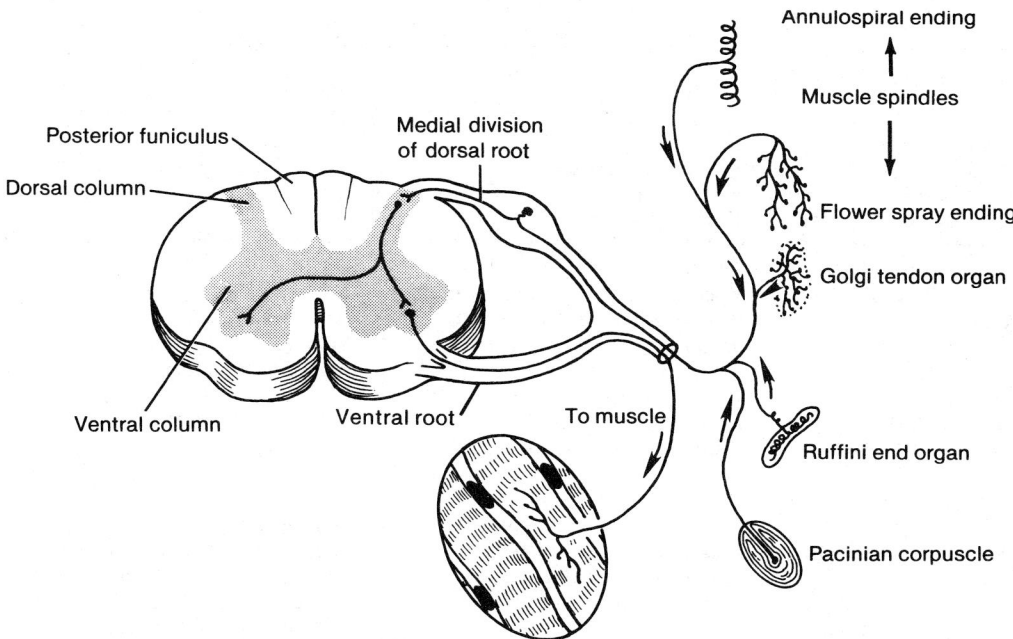

FIGURE 22-5. **General proprioceptive afferent pathways for impulses entering the CNS through the spinal nerves.**

important to have a good understanding of this system because medications that are ganglionic stimulants and blockers exert many of their effects on the ANS.

AUTONOMIC NERVOUS SYSTEM

The ANS regulates the functions of the viscera of the body. In general, the viscera receive two opposing sets of nerve fibers: one stimulates or increases the activity of that organ; the other inhibits or reduces its activity. One unique feature of the ANS is the fact that both the stimulatory and inhibitory mechanisms have a two-neuron chain between their site of origin in the CNS and their peripheral site of action. This means that there is a *synapse* between two neurons; this synapse is found outside the CNS in a motor ganglion. It is customary to refer to the nerve fiber or neuron closer to the CNS as the *preganglionic* fiber. The cell bodies of the preganglionic nerve fibers are small and multipolar and are found in the intermediolateral columns of the spinal cord or in the nuclei of the brainstem. The second nerve fiber, whose cell body lies within a motor ganglion and that innervates the organ, is referred to as the *postganglionic* fiber. The termination of these postganglionic nerve fibers is characteristic and not all smooth muscle fibers or gland cells receive innervation. This "skipping" pattern is called a *synapses en passant.* Postganglionic nerve fibers rely on humoral transmission to produce their effects. The

major chemical transmitters are norepinephrine and acetylcholine.

The ANS is divided into two divisions depending on the site of origin of the preganglionic nerve fibers. The preganglionic fibers arising from the thoracic and lumbar spinal cord are called the *thoracolumbar* or *sympathetic* division. The preganglionic fibers arising in the cranial nerve nuclei or the sacral section of the spinal cord are called the *craniosacral* or *parasympathetic* division.

Sympathetic division

The ganglia of this division are located opposite each spinal segment and are adjacent to the lateral face of each vertebra. These ganglia are connected by longitudinal fibers and form a continuous chain on each side of the spinal cord. These ganglia are called chain or paravertebral ganglia and form the thoracic and lumbar sympathetic trunk. No sympathetic fibers emerge from the cervical section of the spinal cord. Instead, the thoracic sympathetic trunk continues rostrally (toward the head) and forms the cervical sympathetic trunk. Three ganglia on each side are associated with this trunk: the inferior, the middle, and the superior cervical ganglia. The caudal end (tail) of the chain continues as far as the coccyx, but no fibers join it from the sacral section of the spinal cord. The organs affected and the outflows involved are summarized in Tables 22-5 and 22-6.

TABLE 22-5

Innervation of the viscera*

Organ	Sympathetic division		Action	ACh/NE/E
	Preganglionic	Postganglionic		
Arrector pili	All levels	All ganglia of trunk and chain	Erects hair	NE
Bladder	T-11 to L-2	Hypogastric ganglion and plexus	Relaxes	NE
Cavernous tissue	L-2	Hypogastric ganglion and plexus	Deturgescence	NE
Ciliary muscle	C-8 to T-2	Superior cervical ganglion	Relaxes	NE
Colon	T-6 to T-10	Superior and inferior mesenteric ganglia and plexuses	Inhibits peristalsis	NE
Coronary vessels	T-1 to T-5	Cervical and thoracic ganglia	Dilates	ACh
Heart muscle	T-1 to T-5	Cervical and thoracic ganglia	Accelerates rate	NE
Iris of eye	C-8 to T-3	Superior cervical ganglion	Dilates pupil	NE
Kidney	T-10 to T-11	Renal ganglion and plexus	Constricts pelvis and vessels	NE
Lacrimal gland	T-1 to T-3	Superior cervical ganglion	Vasoconstricts to reduce secretion	NE
Liver	T-5 to T-6	Celiac ganglion and plexus	Glycogenolysis	NE
Lung	T-2 to T-5	Thoracic ganglia	Relaxation of bronchial muscle	NE
Mammary gland	T-2 to T-6	Thoracic ganglia	Constricts ducts	NE
Nasal and oral glands	T-1 to T-3	Superior cervical ganglion	Vasoconstricts to reduce secretion	NE
Pancreas	T-5 to T-6	Celiac ganglion and plexus	Vasoconstricts to reduce secretions	NE
Parotid gland	T-1 to T-3	Superior cervical ganglion	Vasoconstricts to reduce secretions	NE
Small intestine	T-6 to T-10	Celiac and superior mesenteric ganglia and plexus	Inhibits peristalsis, vasoconstriction, reduces secretions	NE
Sphincters				
Anal	L-2	Hypogastric ganglia and plexus	Constricts	
Pyloric	T-6 to T-10	Celiac ganglion and plexus	Constricts	
Urethral	L-2	Hypogastric ganglia and plexus	Constricts	
Stomach	T-6 to T-10	Celiac ganglion and plexus	Inhibits peristalsis, vasoconstriction, reduces secretions	NE
Sublingual and submandibular glands	T-1 to T-3	Superior cervical ganglion	Vasoconstricts to reduce secretions	
Sweat glands	All levels	All trunk and chain ganglia	Stimulates secretion	

*The table shows the origin of the preganglionic fibers, the site of the ganglionic synapse, the action produced, and the transmitter involved (*ACh*, acetylcholine;

Parasympathetic division		Action	ACh/NE/E
Preganglionic	Postganglionic		
Not present	Not present	None	—
S-2 to S-4	Intrinsic ganglia	Contracts	ACh
S-2 to S-4	Vesical plexus	Turgescence	ACh
EW nucleus	Episcleral ganglion	Contracts	ACh
Dorsal motor nucleus of X	Myenteric and submucosal plexuses	Excites peristalsis	ACh
Dorsal motor nucleus of X	Cardiac plexus and ganglia	Constricts	ACh
Dorsal motor nucleus of X, Right X, SA node Left X, AV node	Cardiac plexus and ganglia	Decelerates rate	ACh
EW nucleus	Ciliary ganglion	Constricts pupil	ACh
Not present	Not present	None	—
Lacrimal or superior salivatory nucleus	Pterygopalatine ganglion	Stimulates secretion	ACh
Dorsal motor nucleus of X	Unknown	Contracts gall bladder	ACh
Dorsal motor nucleus of X	Pulmonary plexus	Constricts bronchi	ACh
Not present	Not present	None	—
Lacrimal or superior salivatory nucleus	Pterygopalatine ganglion	Stimulates secretion	ACh
Dorsal motor nucleus of X	Intrinsic ganglia	Increases secretion	ACh
Inferior salivatory nucleus	Otic ganglion	Stimulates secretion	ACh
Dorsal motor nucleus of X	Myenteric and submucosal plexi	Stimulates peristalsis and secretions	ACh
S-2 to S-4	Intrinsic ganglia	Relaxes	ACh
Dorsal motor nucleus of X	Myenteric ganglia	Relaxes	ACh
S-2 to S-4	Intrinsic ganglia and plexus	Relaxes	ACh
Dorsal motor nucleus of X	Myenteric and submucosal plexi	Stimulates peristalsis and secretions	ACh
Inferior salivatory nucleus	Pterygopalatine and submandibular ganglia	Stimulates secretion	ACh
Not present	Not present	None	—

NE, norepinephrine; E, epinephrine).

TABLE 22-6

The origin, destination, and action of the sympathetic outflow*

Spinal nerve roots carrying outflow	Destination	Action
T-1	Iris	Produces dilation
T-1 to T-5	Head and neck	Produces vasoconstriction and sweating
T-2 to T-9	Upper limbs	Produces vasoconstriction and sweating
T-2 to T-6	Heart	Increases rate and force of contraction
T-5 to T-9	Lungs	Produces bronchodilation
T-5 to T-9	Adrenal medulla	Produces secretion
T-6 to L-2	Abdominal viscera	Inhibits motility; inhibits secretions; constricts sphincters
T-4 to L-2	Lower limbs	Produces vasoconstriction and sweating
L-1 to L-2	Genitourinary	Contracts seminal vesicles or uterus; relaxes bladder

*The levels of the outflow can vary from individual to individual. Striated muscle in limbs receives both sympathetic adrenergic and cholinergic postganglionic fibers.

Preganglionic neuron. The cell bodies are located in the intermediolateral column of the thoracic and upper lumbar sections of the spinal cord (T-1 to T-12, L-1 to L-3). The axons leave this column ventrally and emerge as myelinated fibers along with the somatic efferent fibers, where together they form the ventral root. These nerves travel in the ventral root to just beyond the point where the dorsal and ventral roots merge to form the spinal nerve trunk. Here the sympathetic fibers leave the spinal nerve trunk as white rami communicantes. The latter enter the sympathetic trunk in the region of the nearest chain or paravertebral ganglion. A fiber entering the sympathetic trunk can:

1. Synapse with cell bodies in the chain ganglion at the level of entry
2. Pass up or down in the sympathetic trunk and synapse with cell bodies in a chain ganglion above or below the point of entry
3. Pass rostrally in the cervical sympathetic trunk and synapse with cell bodies in one of the cervical ganglia
4. Pass transversely through the sympathetic trunk forming nerves that run ventrocaudally and synapse with cell bodies in ganglia that lie in front of the spinal cord (These ganglia are called prevertebral ganglia, and the preganglionic fibers form the splanchnic nerves. Note that prevertebral ganglia are *not* paired.)
5. Pass through the sympathetic trunk, through a prevertebral (collateral) ganglion, and synapse in the adrenal medulla
6. Pass through the sympathetic trunk, through a prevertebral ganglion, and synapse with cell bodies in the wall of the organ innervated

TABLE 22-7

Names of the prevertebral ganglia

Name	Single/Paired
Celiac ganglion	Single
Superior mesenteric ganglion	Single
Inferior mesenteric ganglion	Single
Adrenal medulla	Paired

It should be noted that preganglionic nerve fibers can pass through many ganglia but will synapse only once.

The names of the prevertebral ganglia are summarized in Table 22-7. Again, it must be noted that these are not paired ganglia except in the case of the adrenal medulla. The various possible courses of the preganglionic fibers are summarized in Figure 22-6.

Postganglionic neuron. These are small multipolar cells, and their cell bodies are located in any of the ganglia mentioned. Axons arising from the chain ganglia reenter the spinal nerve trunk through gray rami communicantes. These rami leave the sympathetic trunk at all levels, including the cervical sympathetic trunk, and follow the course of the spinal nerves, eventually terminating in the walls of the peripheral blood vessels, the sweat glands, and the piloerector muscles. In the upper thorax some fibers pass from the chain ganglia to supply the bronchi and lungs. Fibers from the cervical ganglia pass caudally to the heart and rostrally, following the carotid artery and its branches, to the blood vessels in the head, sweat glands in the face and scalp, piloerector mus-

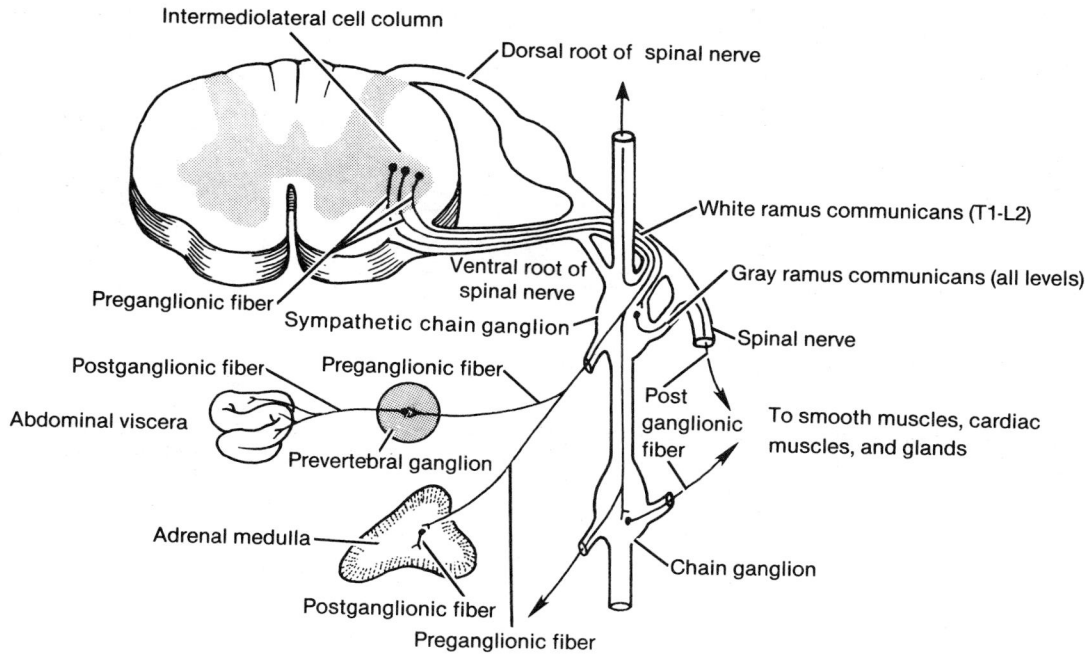

FIGURE 22-6. **A section of the spinal cord showing two sympathetic chain ganglia, a paravertebral ganglion, and connecting nerves illustrating the distribution of the preganglionic and postganglionic nerve fibers.**

cles, salivary glands, and dilator muscles of the pupils. Axons from the prevertebral ganglia follow the mesenteric blood vessels and send fibers to the walls of these vessels and the muscular coats of the viscera.

Ganglionic synapses in the sympathetic division. It has been recognized for some years that humoral transmission in ganglia is a complex process that cannot be completely described by assuming a single transmitter/receptor system. In the sympathetic division the primary pathway involves acetylcholine (ACh) as transmitter. The acetylcholine is released from the preganglionic nerve ending and acts on receptor sites located on the dendritic processes of the postganglionic neuron. The receptors are referred to as *nicotinic* since they can be stimulated by the drug nicotine, cannot be stimulated by methacholine, and can be blocked by the nondepolarizing blocking agent hexamethonium. The activation of this primary pathway gives rise to an excitatory postsynaptic potential (EPSP). An action potential is generated in the axon of the postganglionic neuron when the initial EPSP attains a certain critical amplitude. In general, an EPSP that exceeds a certain critical value excites more than one postganglionic neuron because of the multipolar nature of pre- and postganglionic neurons.

Secondary pathways are also found in sympathetic ganglia. These include both excitatory and inhibitory pathways. An inhibitory postsynaptic potential (IPSP)

and a late excitatory postsynaptic potential (late EPSP) can be observed (Figure 22-7). These potentials are of longer duration and smaller amplitude than the EPSP. The IPSP is unaffected by hexamethonium but is sensitive to block by atropine. There is evidence that catecholamines such as epinephrine or dopamine cause or are involved in the IPSP. Characteristically, the IPSP consists of a hyperpolarization and a similar hyperpolarization can be induced by exogenous norepinephrine or dopamine. Both hyperpolarization and the IPSP can be abolished by α-adrenergic antagonists. Since both atropine and α-adrenergic antagonists block the production of IPSP's, it has been suggested that the atropine-sensitive sites could be found on a catecholamine-releasing interneuron, which in turn generates the IPSP.

The EPSP can be produced by agents that mimic the muscarinic actions of acetylcholine. The *late* EPSP is not blocked by hexamethonium but is blocked by atropine. This pathway may serve to facilitate the transmission of impulses through the primary pathway. The various pathways of transmission through sympathetic ganglia are summarized in Figure 22-8. It must be stressed that the secondary pathways probably serve only to modulate synaptic events. Agents that block the primary pathway can completely inhibit ganglionic transmission. Atropine and α-adrenergic antagonists cannot do this.

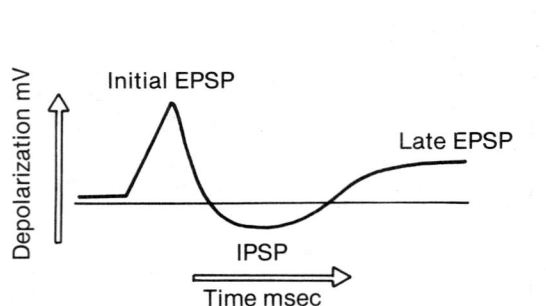

FIGURE 22-7. **Postganglionic synaptic potentials seen in mammalian sympathetic ganglia.**

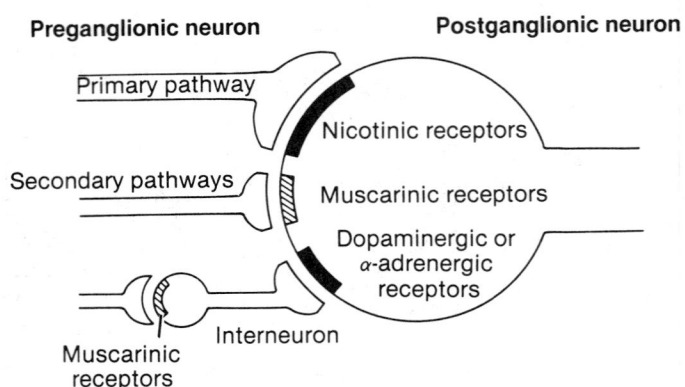

FIGURE 22-8. **The transmission pathways through a mammalian sympathetic ganglion.**

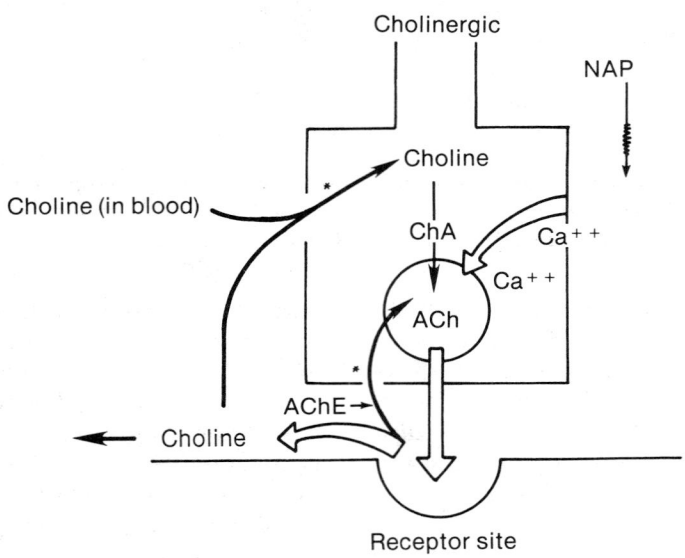

FIGURE 22-9. **The processes involved in the synthesis and release and disposal of acetylcholine at cholinergic nerve terminals and receptor sites.** ACh, **Acetylcholine;** ChA, **choline acetyltransferase;** AChE, **acetylcholinesterase;** NAP, **nerve action potential;** *, **site of active transport.**

The process of acetylcholine synthesis and release in sympathetic ganglia is similar to that seen at other sites at which acetylcholine functions as a transmitter. The processes are summarized in Figure 22-9.

Postganglionic synapses in the sympathetic division. The transmitter released at the sites where these axons synapse with their effector organs is norepinephrine. The processes involved in the synthesis and release of this transmitter are summarized in Figure 22-10. Norepinephrine is released from synapses en passant. These appear as varicosities of the postganglionic nerve fiber, which project onto the smooth muscle fibers and cells of the effector organs. The norepinephrine then acts on receptors on the cells of the end organ. These receptors are classified as either α or β. Subclasses of both α- and β-receptors exist, but, in general, α-receptors are excitatory and β-receptors inhibitory.

The adrenal medulla differs from the scheme outlined above. In the adrenal medulla the postganglionic fibers are the secretory cells of the medulla itself. The preganglionic fibers reaching this organ through the splanchnic nerves and the celiac ganglion synapse with the secretory cells. The release of acetylcholine

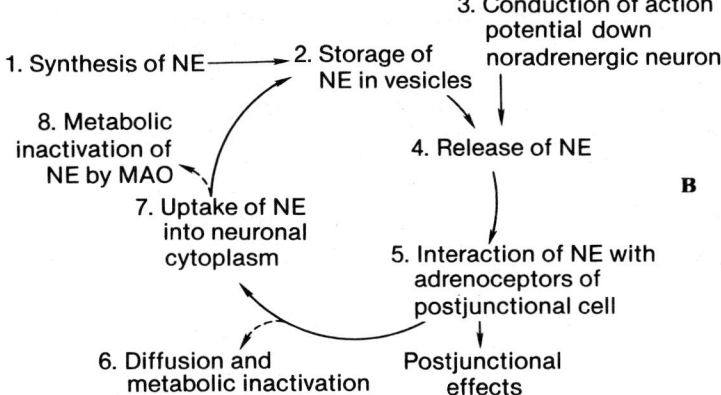

FIGURE 22-10. *A,* **Steps in the enzymatic synthesis of dopamine, norepinephrine, and epinephrine. The enzymes are shown in parentheses, essential factors in italics.** *B,* **Adrenergic transmission.** NE, **Norepinephrine.**

from the presynaptic neuron affects nicotinic receptors on the secretory cells resulting in the release of epinephrine. The synthesis and release processes for epinephrine are similar to those for norepinephrine.

Not all postganglionic neurons release catecholamines such as norepinephrine or epinephrine. Cholinergic postganglionic sympathetic nerves also exist in the body. These are not widely distributed and are found only in three areas:

1. Most of the postganglionic fibers innervating the sweat glands
2. Vasodilator fibers ending in the blood vessels of skeletal muscle
3. Vasodilator fibers leading to the coronary vessels

The transmitter released at these synapses is acetylcholine, and it acts on muscarinic receptors located on the effector organs. The effect of acetylcholine are blocked by atropine at these sites.

Parasympathetic division

This system differs from the sympathetic division in that there are large gaps or interruptions in the system in the CNS. Thus there are considerable gaps between the nuclei involved in the system in the brainstem, and there is a very large distance between the nucleus of the vagus and the outflow from the second segment of the sacral spinal cord. Because of this discontinuity, it is easier to describe the cranial and sacral outflows separately. The organs affected and the outflows involved are summarized in Tables 22-5 and 22-8.

Cranial outflow

Preganglionic neurons. The small cell bodies of the preganglionic neurons are located in a series of nuclei. The nuclei include the Edinger-Westphal (EW) nucleus associated with cranial nerve III; the oculomotor nucleus, the superior salivatory nucleus, and possibly the lacrimal nucleus associated with cranial nerve VII; the inferior salivatory nucleus associated with cranial nerve IX; and the dorsal motor nucleus of the vagus (X). The latter is a particularly large group of cells. The preganglionic fibers enter a series of ganglia where they synapse with postganglionic neurons. Table 22-8 summarizes the nuclei of origin of the preganglionic fibers, their associated cranial nerves, the names of the ganglia associated with the various nerves, and the organs innervated. Note that the ganglia in this outflow are paired with the exception of the vagus.

Postganglionic neurons. The cell bodies of these neurons lie in the ganglia named in Table 22-8 The course of these fibers is variable. From the ciliary ganglion short ciliary nerves emerge, reach the eye, penetrate the sclera, and innervate the ciliary and sphincter pupillae muscles. From the pterygopalatine ganglion fibers follow several paths innervating the lacrimal glands and the glands in the mucous membranes of the nose and the palate (Figure 22-11). From the submandibular ganglion short fibers emerge and innervate the submandibular and sublingual glands. From the otic ganglion the postganglionic fibers follow

TABLE 22-8

The origin, destination, and action of the parasympathetic outflow

Origin	*Cranial nerve (ganglion)*	*Destination*	*Action*
Edinger-Westphal nucleus	III (Ciliary)	Ciliary muscle	Accommodation for near vision
		Iris	Constricts pupil
Superior salivatory nucleus	VII (pterygopalatine; chorda tympani)	Lacrimal glands	Produces tears
		Nasal mucosa	Produces secretion
		Submandibular and sublingual salivary glands	Produces secretion
Inferior salivatory nucleus	IX (otic)	Parotid salivary gland	Produces secretion
Dorsal motor nucleus of vagus	X	Heart	Slows rate and conduction
		Bronchi	Produces constriction
		Alimentary canal down to proximal colon	Stimulates peristalsis and secretions
Spinal cord sacral segments S-2 to S-4	Splanchnic nerves	Distal colon and rectum	Produces contraction
		Bladder	Produces contraction
		Genitalia	Produces contraction

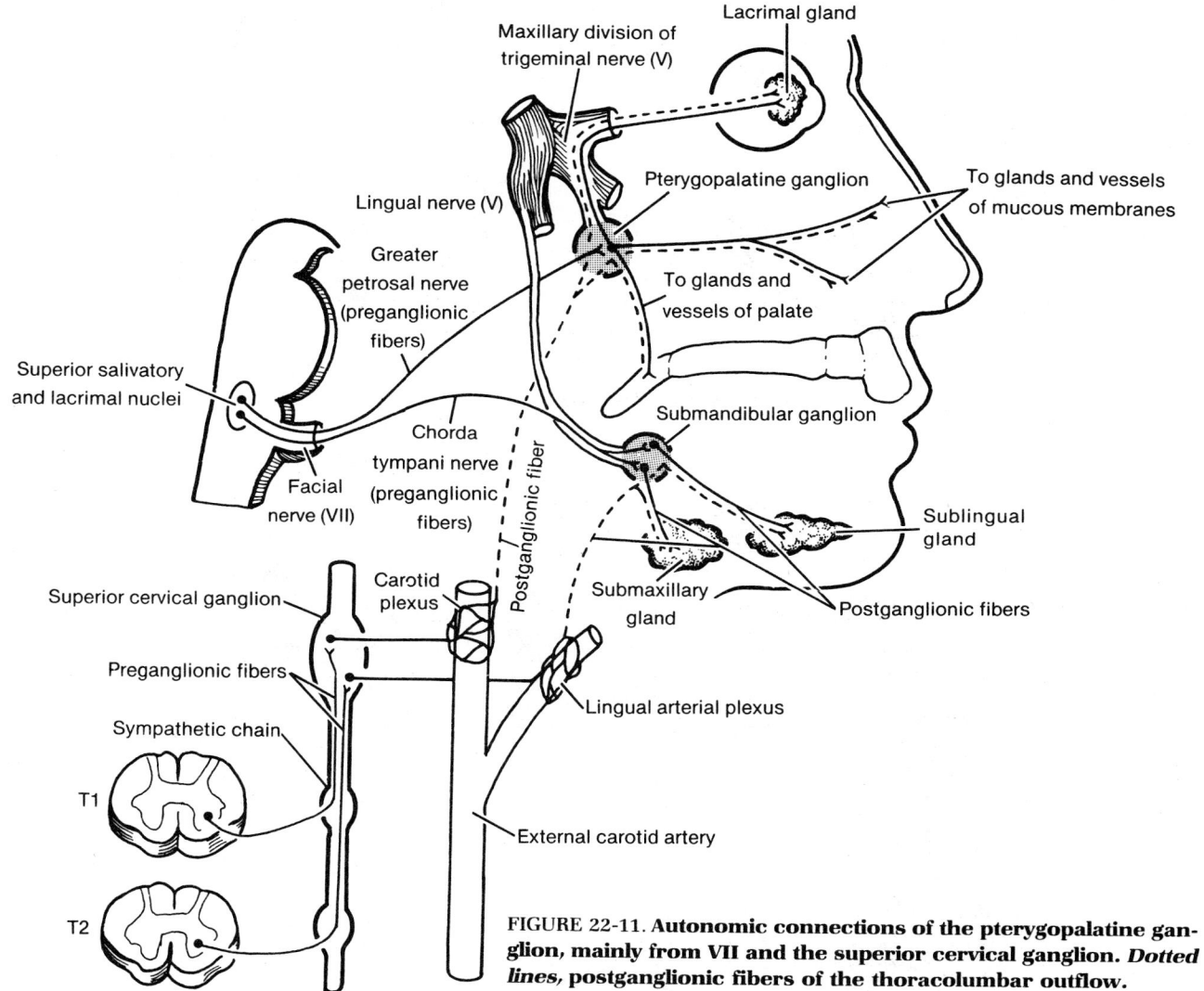

FIGURE 22-11. **Autonomic connections of the pterygopalatine ganglion, mainly from VII and the superior cervical ganglion.** *Dotted lines,* **postganglionic fibers of the thoracolumbar outflow.**

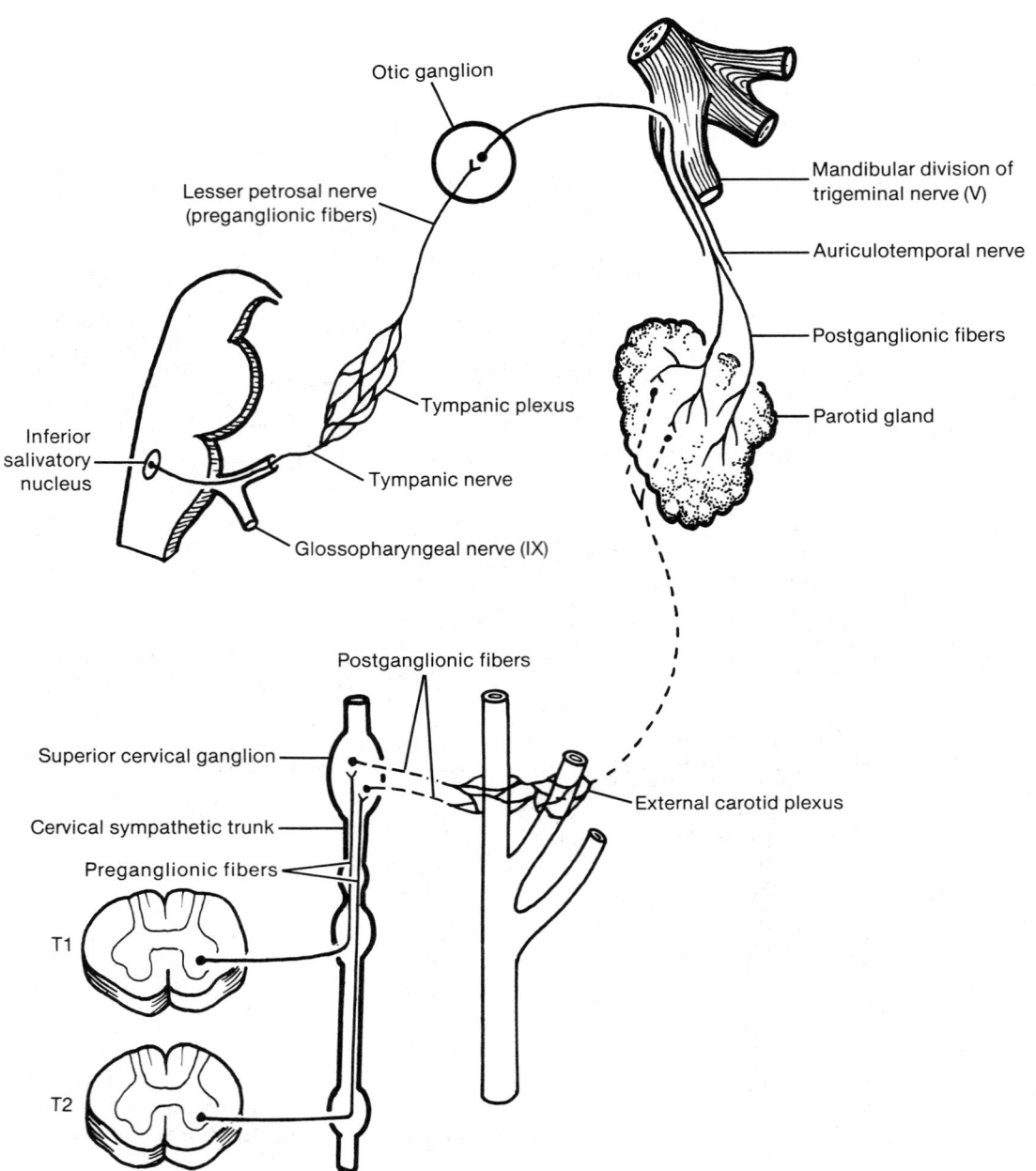

FIGURE 22-12. **Cranial autonomic nerves, with special emphasis on the connections of the otic ganglion, chiefly through IX and the superior cervical ganglion.** *Dotted lines,* **postganglionic fibers of the thoracolumbar outflow.**

the course of cranial nerve V and innervate the parotid glands (Figure 22-12).

In contrast to these distinct and discrete ganglia, terminal ganglia also exist at other sites. These form more diffuse collections of ganglia, or plexuses, from which short postganglionic fibers emerge. Examples are the episcleral ganglia, which are involved in reflex constriction of the pupil for near vision and accommodation; the cardiac and pulmonary plexuses in which the postganglionic fibers arise from ganglia on the heart and bronchi; and Auerbach's (myenteric) and Meissner's (submucosal) plexuses, which lie between the smooth muscle coats of the viscera and in the submucosal coat, respectively. Terminal ganglia, unlike the other ganglia named, are not paired. Also, in ganglia such as the ciliary ganglion, a preganglionic neuron will synapse with only a few postganglionic neurons. In terminal ganglia a much greater degree of amplification exists; for example, in Auerbach's plexus it has been estimated that amplification factors of approximately 8000:1 can exist.

Sacral outflow

Preganglionic neuron. The cell bodies of this outflow lie in the intermediolateral cell columns of the spinal cord, specifically at S-2, S-3, and S-4. The fibers leave the spinal cord ventrally with the ventral roots of S-2, S-3, and S-4 as white rami communicantes and form the pelvic nerves. These nerves pass ventrally across the lower abdomen and end in terminal ganglia in or on the pelvic viscera and the lower part of the colon.

Postganglionic neuron. The cell bodies lie in the terminal ganglia associated with the connective tissue covering the pelvic viscera and colon. The axons are short and innervate the smooth muscle and glands of the effector organs.

Ganglionic synapses in the parasympathetic division.

As in the sympathetic division, the nervous pathways involved in the transmission at the ganglionic synapses can be divided into primary and secondary pathways. The primary pathway is essentially the same as that found in the sympathetic division. Acetylcholine released from preganglionic fibers acts on receptors on the postganglionic processes of the cell to produce an EPSP. When an EPSP reaches a critical level, an action potential is generated in the postganglionic neuron. The acetylcholine receptors are "nicotinic" in character and the effects of acetylcholine on these receptors can be blocked by hexamethonium. (See Chapter 26, "Ganglionic Stimulants and Blockers and Neuromuscular Blockers.")

The secondary pathways are less well defined compared to sympathetic ganglia. Receptor sites for serotonin and catecholamines have been described, but their function is not well understood. As in sympathetic ganglia, they probably serve to modulate the primary pathway. A schematic diagram of the synapse in a parasympathetic ganglion is shown in Figure 22-13.

The process of acetylcholine synthesis and release is similar to that seen in sympathetic ganglia (Figure 22-9).

Postganglionic synapses in the parasympathetic division.

The transmitter released at these sites is acetylcholine and it acts on "muscarinic" receptors located on the effector organs. The effects of acetylcholine at these sites can be blocked by atropine and atropine-like drugs. (See Chapter 23, "Parasympathomimetics and Parasympatholytics"). The synthesis and release of acetylcholine are similar to that described previously.

Types of control exerted by the ANS

Three major types of control can be identified:

1. *On-off:* Here only sympathetic fibers reach the effector organ. An example is the blood vessels of the skin and viscera. The diameter of these vessels is dependent on hemodynamic pressure and the constrictor action of the sympathetic nerves.

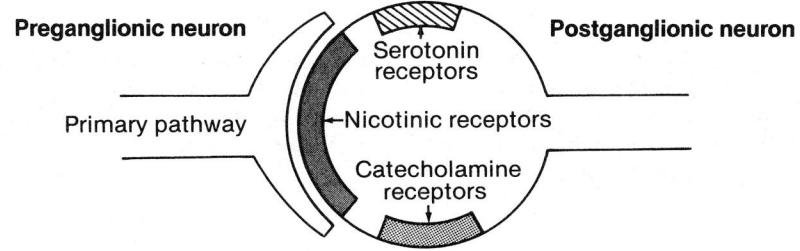

FIGURE 22-13. **Transmission pathways in a mammalian parasympathetic ganglion.**

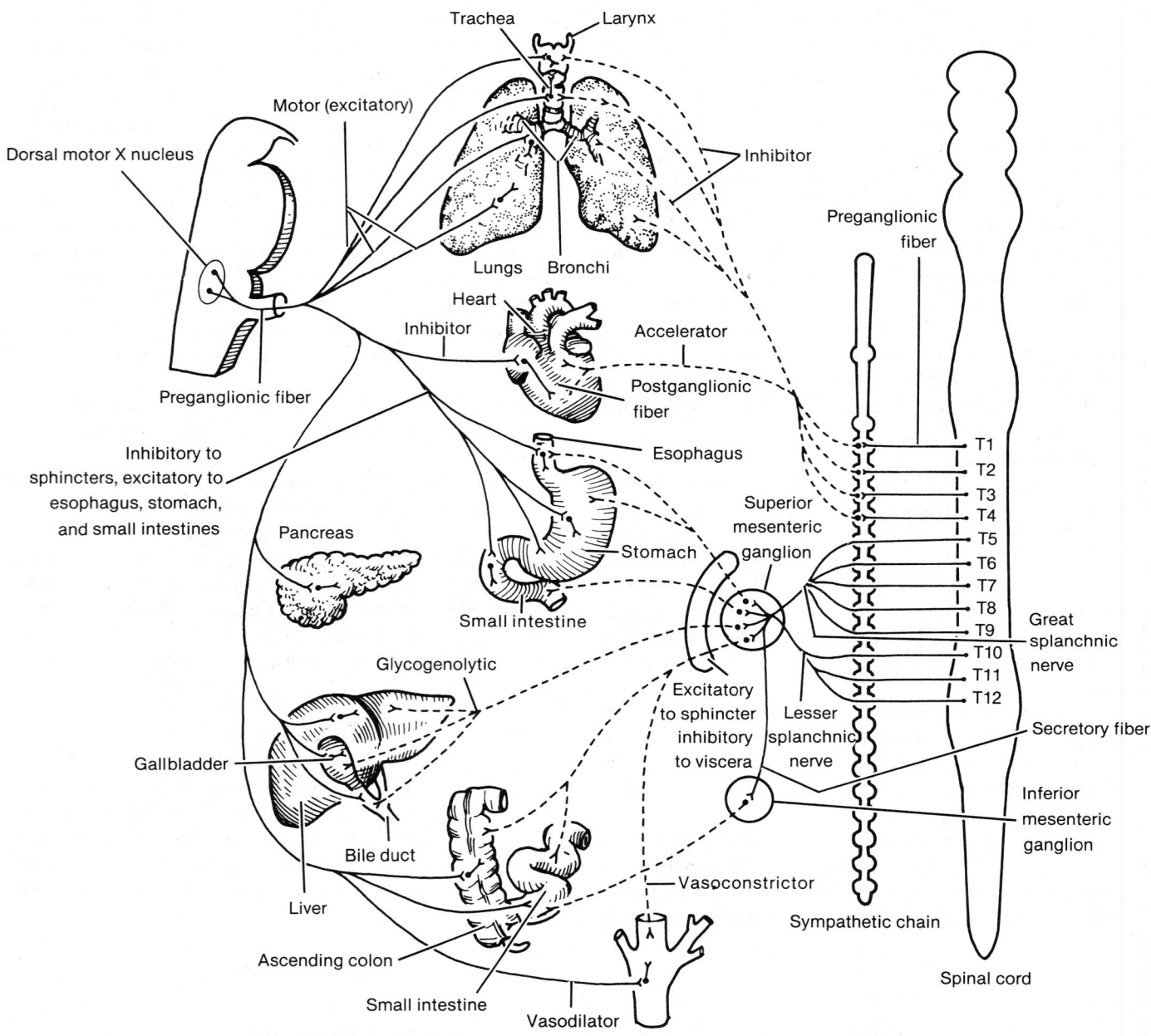

FIGURE 22-14. **The autonomic nerve supply to the thoracic and abdominal viscera.** *Dotted lines,* postganglionic fibers of the thoracolumbar outflow. The postganglionic fibers of the craniosacral outflow are represented by *short solid lines,* usually on or in the walls of the structures innervated. Some functional values have been assigned to some of the fibers shown.

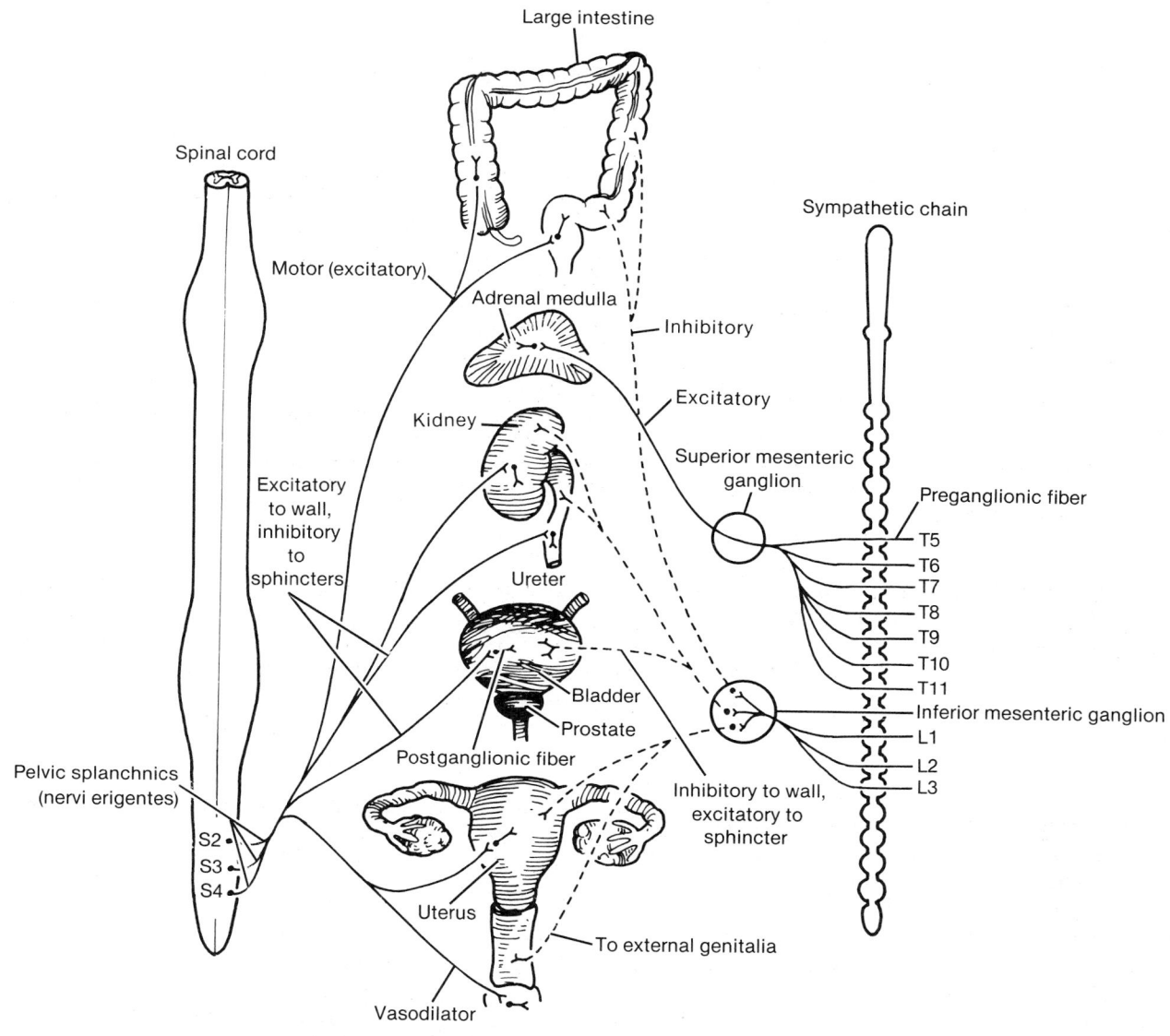

FIGURE 22-15. **The autonomic nerve supply to the viscera of the lower abdomen and pelvis.** *Dotted lines,* postganglionic fibers of the thoracolumbar outflow. The postganglionic fibers of the craniosacral outflow are indicated by *short lines* usually in or on the walls of the structures innervated. Some functional values have been assigned to some of the fibers shown.

2. *Reciprocal:* Organs receive two sets of fibers, one sympathetic, the other parasympathetic. An example is the iris of the eye. The dilator muscle receives sympathetic fibers, the constrictor muscles parasympathetic fibers.

3. *Antagonistic:* In these situations the same smooth muscle groups receive fibers from both divisions. One division is excitatory, the other inhibitory. Examples are the heart, in which the sympathetic is excitatory and the parasympathetic inhibitory; and the lungs, in which the

sympathetic is inhibitory and the parasympathetic excitatory. Other examples are shown diagrammatically in Figures 22-14 and 22-15.

As a result of these various interactions, each effector organ will display the net result of the two systems opposing one another. Thus either sympathetic or parasympathetic effects can dominate in a given organ. The dominance of one system over another will result in a state of partial activity in a particular organ; this is termed *tone*. Tone is manifested as baseline secretion of the gland or partial contraction of the

TABLE 22-9

The predominance of sympathetic (adrenergic) or parasympathetic (cholinergic) tone at various effector sites*

Effector site	Predominant tone	Effect of ganglionic blockade
Arterioles	Sympathetic (NE)	Vasodilation; increased peripheral blood flow; hypotension
Ciliary muscle	Parasympathetic (ACh)	Cycloplegia
Gastrointestinal tract	Parasympathetic (ACh)	Reduced tone and motility; constipation
Heart	Parasympathetic (ACh)	Tachycardia
Iris	Parasympathetic (ACh)	Mydriasis
Salivary glands	Parasympathetic (ACh)	Xerostomia
Sweat glands	Sympathetic (ACh)	Anhydrosis
Urinary tract	Parasympathetic (ACh)	Urinary retention
Veins	Sympathetic (NE)	Dilation; pooling of blood; decreased venous return; decreased cardiac output

*The predominance was determined by blocking motor ganglia with a ganglionic blocking drug. The postganglionic transmitter involved is shown as NE, norepinephrine; ACh, acetylcholine.

organ. Table 22-9 summarizes the various states of tone of some organ systems. The data were obtained by blocking transmission through both sympathetic and parasympathetic ganglia, thus inducing a state of zero tone.

the following chapters. In addition, this should provide a sound basis for better understanding of the peripheral nervous system side effects and toxicity associated with medications discussed in other sections of this text.

SUMMARY

Many drugs affect the peripheral nervous system directly and indirectly. Those drugs directly affecting this system are discussed in the following chapters in this section. The brief overview presented in this chapter describing the anatomy, physiology, and assessment of the peripheral nervous system should assist the nurse in better understanding the mechanisms of action and the effects of the medications discussed in

BIBLIOGRAPHY

Foster, R.W., & Cox, B. (Eds.). *Basic pharmacology.* London: Butterworths, 1980.

Goodman, A.G., Goodman, L.S., & Gilman, A. (Eds.). *The pharmacological basis of therapeutics* (6th ed.). New York: Macmillan, 1980.

House, E.L., Pansky, B., & Siegal, A. *A systematic approach to neuroscience* (3rd ed.). New York: McGraw-Hill, 1979.

Mountcastle, V.B. *Medical physiology* (vol. 1 and 2) (14th ed.). St. Louis: The C.V. Mosby Co., 1980.

Parasympathomimetics and Parasympatholytics

Abram J.D. Friesen

Medications discussed in this chapter

Muscarinic agonists	*Muscarinic blockers—*
Acetylcholine	*cont'd*
Bethanechol	Homatropine methylbro-
Carbachol	mide*
Pilocarpine	Hyoscyamine
Muscarinic blockers	Isopropamide*
Anisotropine methyl-	Mepenzolate*
bromide*	Methantheline*
Atropine	Methscopolamine*
Belladonna	Oxyphencyclimine
Clidinium*	Oxyphenonium*
Cyclopentolate	Propantheline*
Glycopyrrolate*	Scopolamine
Hexocyclium methylsul-	Tridihexethyl*
fate*	Tropicamide

AUTONOMIC NERVOUS SYSTEM

The autonomic nervous system (ANS) consists of two divisions—the parasympathetic and the sympathetic nervous systems—which exert involuntary homeostatic control over a number of functions including heart activity, maintenance of blood pressure, digestion, respiration, and vision. Many organs receive innervation from both divisions of the ANS, and the effects produced by each are usually opposite (e.g., stimulation of sympathetic nerves increases heart rate whereas stimulation of the parasympathetic nerves decreases heart rate). Notable exceptions to the dual innervation phenomenon are blood vessels, most of which receive only sympathetic nerves, and the *ciliary muscle* of the eye, which receives only parasympathetic nerves. See Chapter 22, "Review of the Anatomy, Physiology, and Assessment of the Peripheral Nervous System."

Cholinergic and adrenergic nerves

The *efferent*, or motor, nerves of the ANS are classified according to the neurotransmitter substance re-

*Quaternary ammonium derivatives.

leased. *Cholinergic nerves* are those that release acetylcholine (ACh) and include all preganglionic nerves and all postganglionic parasympathetic nerves. All *somatic* motor nerves, which innervate skeletal muscle, are also cholinergic (Figure 23-1). *Adrenergic nerves* are those that release norepinephrine (NE) as their neurotransmitter substance and include most postganglionic sympathetic nerves. A small percentage of the postganglionic sympathetic nerves, however, are cholinergic and innervate structures such as the sweat glands. The adrenal medulla represents a special case. It consists of chromaffin cells, which receive cholinergic innervation and release epinephrine (adrenalin) and smaller amounts of NE directly into the bloodstream. While the adrenal medulla actually represents an *endocrine* organ, it is considered to be part of the sympathetic nervous system (Figure 23-1).

Cholinergic and adrenergic receptors

When the neurotransmitters ACh and NE are released upon excitation or stimulation of appropriate nerves, they diffuse across a synaptic cleft and interact with specific receptor molecules located on *postsynaptic* organs or neurons. This interaction in turn triggers a sequence of events leading to an observable response. *Cholinergic receptors* are those that are activated by ACh. They are classified as *muscarinic* and *nicotinic* receptors because historically one type was found to be selectively stimulated by muscarine and the other by nicotine. Muscarinic receptors are located mainly in organs innervated by postganglionic parasympathetic nerves and are selectively blocked by atropine. Some important exceptions are the presence of muscarinic receptors in the smooth muscle of blood vessels, most of which do not receive cholinergic innervation, and their presence in those sweat glands receiving input from cholinergic sympathetic fibers. Nicotinic receptors are really of two distinct types: (1) those located in all autonomic ganglia and in the ad-

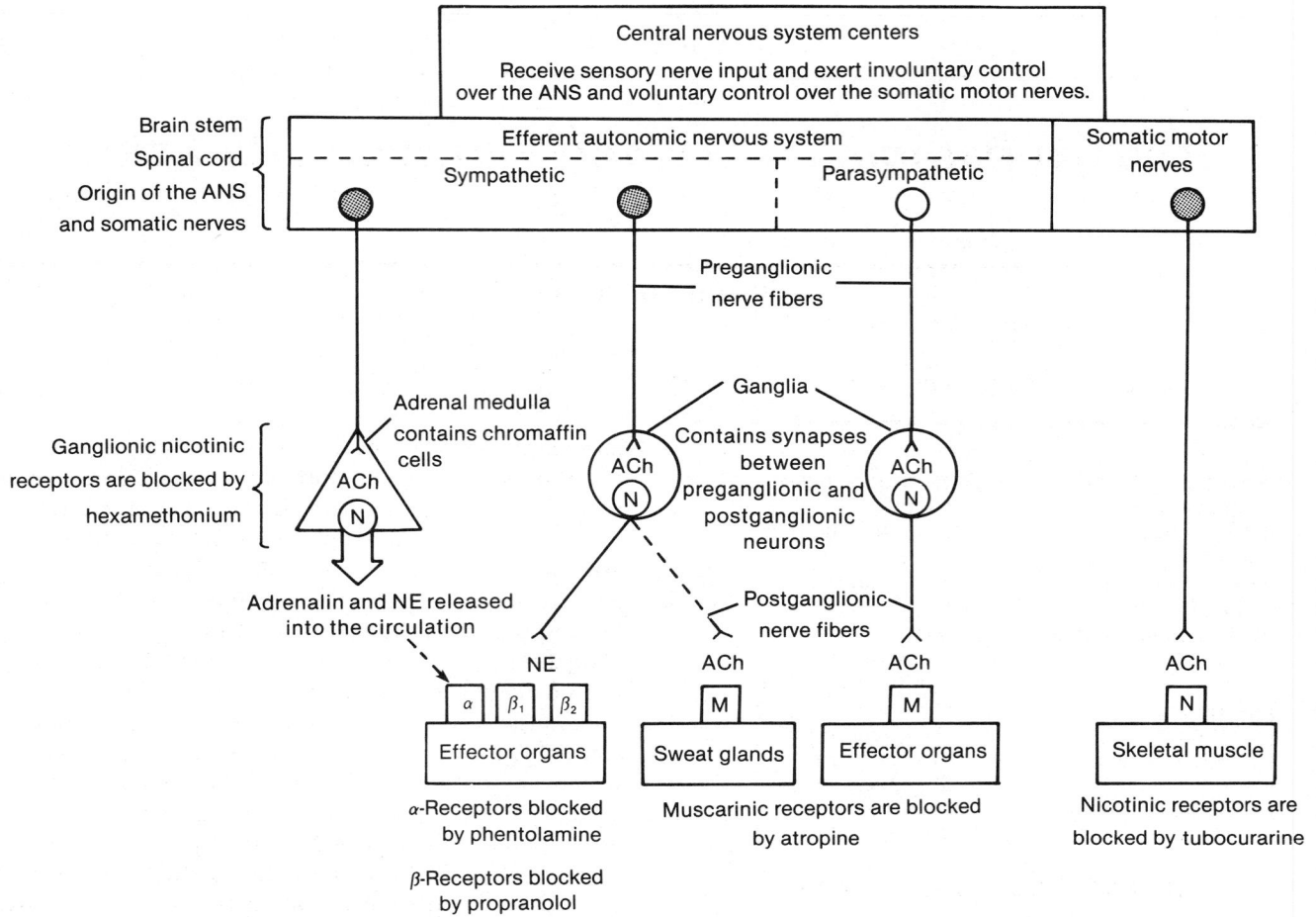

FIGURE 23-1. **Schematic representation of the autonomic nervous system and related structures.** *NE,* **Norepinephrine;** *ACh,* **acetylcholine;** *N,* **nicotinic receptors;** *M,* **muscarinic receptors;** *ANS,* **autonomic nervous system.**

renal medulla, which are selectively blocked by hexamethonium; and (2) those located in skeletal muscle, which are selectively blocked by tubocurarine.

Adrenergic receptors are those that are activated by NE and epinephrine. The α-adrenergic receptors are selectively activated by phenylephrine and blocked by phentolamine. In contrast, β-adrenergic receptors are selectively activated by isoproterenol and blocked by propranolol. More recently, β-receptors have been further subdivided into β_1 and β_2 receptors on the basis of their responses to different agonists and blocking drugs. For example, β_1 receptors are involved in mediating increases in heart activity; β_2 receptor activation leads to a relaxation of bronchial smooth muscle. The adrenergic receptors are primarily located in organs innervated by postganglionic sympathetic nerves (see Chapter 22, "Review of the Anatomy, Physiology, and Assessment of the Peripheral Nervous System").

Typical responses of various organs to adrenergic or cholinergic nerve stimulation are presented in Table 23-1 together with the type of receptor involved. On the basis of the information given one can predict most of the important effects of drugs affecting the ANS provided their mechanism of action is known. For example, an α-adrenergic *agonist* would be expected to raise the blood pressure and to dilate the pupil. It is also important to know which type of nerve exerts dominant control or tonic effects on a particular organ. This latter information is particularly useful in predicting the effects of drugs that selectively block or suppress nerve activity. For example, atropine, a muscarinic receptor blocking agent, would be expected to dilate the pupil, increase the heart rate, decrease *exocrine gland* secretions, and reduce gut and bladder tone or motility.

Since ACh and NE are also neurotransmitters in the

TABLE 23-1

Responses of some effector organs to autonomic nerve stimulation

| Effector organ | Adrenergic nerves | | Cholinergic nerves (muscarinic receptors) |
	Receptor type	Responses	Responses
BLOOD VESSELS			
Most vascular beds	α	Constriction*	Innervation is poor, but dilation occurs with administered muscarinic agonists
Skeletal muscle beds	β_2	Dilation*	
EYE			
Ciliary muscle	—	Not significant	Contraction (near vision)*
Pupil	α	Dilation (mydriasis)	Contraction (miosis)*
FAT CELLS	β_1	Lipolysis	None
GASTROINTESTINAL TRACT			
Exocrine glands	—	Not significant	Increased secretion*
Motility and tone	α, β_1	Decreased	Increased*
Salivary glands	—	Not significant	Increased secretion*
Sphincter tone	α	Increased	Decreased*
HEART (Direct effects)†			
Conduction of impulses	β_1	Increased	Decreased*
Force of contraction	β_1	Increased*	Decreased
Rate of beating	β_1	Increased†	Decreased*†
LIVER			
Glucose release	β_2	Increased (glycogenolysis and gluconeogenesis increased)*	Decreased (glycogen synthesis increased)
LUNGS			
Bronchial muscles	β_2	Dilated	Constricted*
Bronchial secretions	—	None	Increased*
PANCREAS			
Exocrine secretions	α	Decreased	Increased*
Insulin secretion	α	Decreased*	Not significant
	β_2	Increased	
SEX ORGANS			
Male organs	α	Ejaculation*	Erection of penis*
Nonpregnant uterus	β_2	Relaxation*	Not significant
Pregnant uterus	α	Contraction*	Not significant
SWEAT GLANDS			
Most glands	—	None	Increased secretion*
Palms and soles of feet	α	Increased secretions*	None
URINARY BLADDER			
Detrusor muscle	β	Relaxation	Contraction*
Trigone and sphincter	α	Contraction	Relaxation*

*Denotes dominant effect or tone under most circumstances.
†Effects may be modified by subsequent initiation of cardiovascular reflexes (e.g., the rise in blood pressure caused by adrenergic stimulation may cause a reflex slowing of heart rate).

central nervous system (CNS), some drugs affecting the ANS may also cause CNS effects if they are sufficiently lipid soluble to diffuse across the *blood-brain barrier* or if they are transported by selective carriers across this barrier. *Quaternary ammonium* compounds, such as propantheline, bethanechol, carbachol, or other lipid-insoluble drugs, such as epinephrine, isoproterenol, and guanethidine, do not readily penetrate into the brain and therefore generally do not produce significant CNS effects. In contrast, more lipid-soluble agents, such as atropine, scopolamine, ephedrine, and reserpine do produce CNS effects in addition to their effects on the ANS.

In this chapter the drugs affecting the parasympathetic division of the ANS—the parasympathomimetics and the parasympatholytics—are presented. The reader is referred to Chapter 24, "Sympathomimetics and Sympatholytics," for a discussion of the medications affecting the sympathetic division.

DRUGS AFFECTING THE PARASYMPATHETIC NERVOUS SYSTEM

Parasympathomimetics are agents that *mimic* or produce effects similar to that seen after activation of the parasympathetic nervous system. Parasympatholytics are drugs that *inhibit* the responses normally seen when parasympathetic nerves are stimulated.

Parasympathomimetics

Parasympathomimetics can be subdivided into drugs that activate muscarinic receptors and drugs that inhibit cholinesterase enzymes

Agents that activate muscarinic receptors. Drugs such as bethanechol, carbachol, and pilocarpine selectively interact with muscarinic receptors located on organs innervated by postganglionic parasympathetic nerve fibers and produce effects similar to those seen after parasympathetic nerve stimulation (e.g., bradycardia, exocrine gland secretions, constriction of bronchioles, and increased gastrointestinal motility). These agents are referred to as *muscarinic agonists* in this chapter. Less precise terms, such as cholinergic drugs, are also used to describe this group of agents.

Agents that inhibit cholinesterase enzymes. Cholinesterases are a group of enzymes that are involved in the rapid hydrolysis and inactivation of acetylcholine (ACh). Physostigmine, neostigmine, and related drugs inhibit these enzymes, thus allowing the nerve-released ACh to accumulate in the synaptic cleft. In this manner ongoing parasympathetic activity is enhanced. Although these cholinesterase inhibitors

produce important effects on other cholinergic synapses, their predominant or overt effects are parasympathomimetic. It should be obvious from the foregoing information that anticholinesterase agents can markedly potentiate the effects of ACh and prolong its action. The concurrent use of bethanechol, carbachol, aceclidine, or pilocarpine with anticholinesterases, however, will only cause additive muscarinic effects because these latter drugs are resistant to enzymatic attack by cholinesterases. A more detailed discussion of anticholinesterase agents is presented in Chapter 25, "Anticholinesterases and Cholinesterase Reactivators."

Parasympatholytics

Currently there is only one group of drugs available for therapeutic purposes that produces selective parasympatholytic effects—the atropine-like agents. They selectively interact with muscarinic receptors, but this interaction does not excite or activate the receptor. The presence of these drugs on the receptors prevents endogenously released ACh from combining with muscarinic receptors, thereby inhibiting ongoing parasympathetic nerve activity. This results in such effects as *mydriasis*, decreased GI motility, inhibition of exocrine gland secretions, and increased heart rate. These agents are referred to as muscarinic blockers in this chapter. Less precise terms, such as anticholinergics, are also used to describe this group of drugs.

SIGNS AND SYMPTOMS OF POISONING BY PARASYMPATHOLYTICS (i.e., ATROPINE-LIKE DRUGS AND BELLADONNA ALKALOIDS)

Dry mouth, thirst, and difficulty in swallowing

Rapid heart rate, palpitations; blood pressure may be elevated initially and then fall

Dilated pupils, *photophobia*, and blurring of near vision

Difficulty in urinating

Hot, flushed skin; a rash may appear over the face, neck, and upper trunk (more likely to occur in children and may resemble the rash associated with measles)

Elevated body temperature especially in children because of blockage of heat loss via perspiration and a poorly developed temperature regulatory system

CNS excitement (e.g., restlessness, agitation, and hallucinations; less likely with quaternary ammonium derivatives)

Behavior and mental symptoms resembling organic psychoses (less likely with quaternary ammonium derivatives)

Muscle incoordination with disturbed gait and speech; quaternary ammonium derivatives in high doses may cause skeletal muscle paralysis Death resulting from respiratory depression caused by a CNS or PNS depressant effect or cardiovascular collapse

SUMMARY

This chapter has examined the various types and uses of the parasympathomimetic and parasympatholytic medications. A brief review of the autonomic nervous system including a differentiation between the cholinergic and adrenergic aspects has been presented as a basis for understanding the mechanisms of action and effects of the parasympathomimetics (muscarinic agonists) and parasympatholytics (muscarinic blockers).

With an understanding of the various individual agents, including their actions and side effects, the nurse will be better able to provide optimal care to patients requiring these medications. Patient education can be enhanced; adverse drug effects can be anticipated, monitored for, and minimized; and clinically significant drug interactions can be avoided by utilizing the information presented in this chapter.

ADVERSE/SIDE EFFECTS OF MUSCARINIC AGONISTS AND MUSCARINIC BLOCKERS*

Muscarinic agonists†
CARDIOVASCULAR SYSTEM

Bradycardia (contraindicated in patients with sinus bradycardia)
Dysrhythmias, atrial flutter, or fibrillation, and various degrees of heart block (contraindicated in patients with hyperthyroidism or heart block)
Hypotension (contraindicated in patients with coronary artery disease)
Reflex tachycardia

CENTRAL NERVOUS SYSTEM

Headache
Malaise

GASTROINTESTINAL SYSTEM

Abdominal cramps/diarrhea/ involuntary defecation (contraindicated if there is an abdominal obstruction or if the strength of the walls of the GI tract is in question)
Epigastric distress, increased gastric secretions (contraindicated in peptic ulcers)
Nausea
Salivation

OCULAR SYSTEM‡

Conjunctival vascular congestion
Local hypersensitivity reactions
Myopia
Ocular pain
Visual acuity decreased in dim light

RESPIRATORY SYSTEM

Bronchospasms (contraindicated in asthma)
Bronchosecretions, increased (contraindicated in asthma)

UROGENITAL SYSTEM

Urinary urgency/involuntary urination (contraindicated when there is an obstruction in the urinary tract or if the strength of the walls of the bladder is in question)

OTHER EFFECTS

Lacrimation
Perspiration
Rhinorrhea

Muscarinic blockers§
CARDIOVASCULAR SYSTEM

Flushing
Mild bradycardia in low doses (with atropine, scopolamine, and related preparations, but absent in quaternary ammonium derivatives)
Tachycardia in larger doses (use with caution in patients with coronary artery disease or heart failure)

CENTRAL NERVOUS SYSTEM

Excitement, agitation, irritability, mental confusion (with atropine and related compounds, but absent in quaternary ammonium derivatives)
Sedation, amnesia, euphoria, and dreamless sleep (with scopolamine only)

GASTROINTESTINAL SYSTEM

Bloated feeling and constipation (contraindicated in patients with paralytic ileus, pyloroduodenal stenosis, megacolon, and severe ulcerative colitis)
Dry mouth (very common, can be relieved by sucking on a sugarless hard candy)
Nausea/vomiting

---

*See Chapter 11, "Drug Toxicity," for an overview of drug toxicity.
†The effects listed are more likely to occur when excessive systemic doses are used. The contraindications listed are for systemically used agents only. Agents applied topically to the eye are less likely to cause serious effects, but should be used with caution in patients who are more likely to suffer an adverse reaction. Atropine is an effective antidote for overdosages of muscarinic agonists.
‡Effects may occur on topical application to the eye.
§Physostigmine is an effective antidote for overdosages. Infants and young children are more susceptible to the toxic effects of muscarinic blockers mainly because of their immature temperature regulation systems.   *Continued.*

ADVERSE/SIDE EFFECTS OF MUSCARINIC AGONISTS AND MUSCARINIC BLOCKERS—cont'd

NEUROMUSCULAR SYSTEM

Neuromuscular transmission decreased (with quaternary ammonium derivatives at higher dosage; these agents are therefore contraindicated in myasthenia gravis because these patients are very sensitive to neuromuscular blocking drugs)

OCULAR SYSTEM

Blurring of near vision (especially after topical use)
Conjunctivitis, edema, hyperemia, and hypersensitivity reactions (with topical application to eye)

Increased intraocular pressure in susceptible persons (contraindicated especially in narrow-angle glaucoma)
Photophobia (especially after topical use; instruct patient to wear sunglasses)

RESPIRATORY SYSTEM

Bronchial secretions decreased (may cause mucus plugs; use with caution in patients with asthma or chronic obstructive lung disease)

UROGENITAL SYSTEM

Impotence (may occur with larger doses of the quaternary ammonium derivatives)
Urinary retention (contraindicated in patients with prostatism; patients should be instructed to void just prior to administration of each dose)

OTHER EFFECTS

Perspiration decreased (high environmental temperature can cause heat prostration especially in infants and young children because of their immature temperature regulation systems)

CLINICALLY SIGNIFICANT DRUG INTERACTIONS*

Primary drug	*Interacting drug*	*Possible effect(s)*	*Probable mechanism(s)*
Muscarinic agonists (e.g., bethanechol, pilocarpine)	Adrenergic agonists	Decreased muscarinic effects†	Functional antagonists in many organ systems
Muscarinic agonists	Anticholinesterases	Increased muscarinic effects†	Additive/inhibition of the metabolism of choline esters
Muscarinic blockers (e.g., atropine, scopolamine)	Adrenergic agonists	Increased adrenergic muscarinic blocking effects (e.g., tachycardia, hypertension, and mydriasis)	Additive effects on the same organ systems
Muscarinic blockers	Antihistamines (H₁-blockers) Antidepressants, tricyclic Meperidine Phenothiazines	Increased muscarinic blocking effects (e.g., tachycardia, dry mouth, urinary retention, mydriasis, and constipation)	Additive effects with agents that possess some muscarinic blocking activities

*See Chapter 10, "Drug Interactions" for an overview of drug interactions.
†Bradycardia, hypotension, increased tone and motility of GI and urinary tracts, miosis, increased exocrine gland secretions, and bronchoconstriction are examples of muscarinic effects.

GENERAL NURSING IMPLICATIONS

Nursing of patients requiring muscarinic agonists (systemic and ophthalmic agents)

ASSESSMENT

A complete nursing assessment is essential to establish a baseline from which to monitor therapeutic response, side effects, and adverse reactions. Assessment should include a careful drug history to identify sensitivity, contraindications, cautions, and potential drug interactions (see Clinically Significant Drug Interactions) before the first dose is taken.

Assessment of the patient's condition and need for this class of medication should be completed and documented. This is important because there are several indications for this class of drug. For example, if bethanechol is required for postoperative urinary retention, the patient should be carefully assessed for dysuria and bladder distention, and intake and output monitored.

SENSITIVITY

Generally, allergic reactions to muscarinic agonists are rare; however, any drug has the potential to cause a hypersensitivity reaction in a susceptible individual.

Cholinergic overstimulation manifested by circulatory collapse, hypotension, abdominal cramps, shock, and cardiac arrest may occur with hypersensitivity or overdose particularly when administered systemically.

When applied topically, hypersensitivity results in sensitization of the eyelids or conjunctiva.

Allergic reactions are rare but require discontinuation of the drug when they do occur. When possible, another drug may be selected by the prescriber (e.g., carbachol is used by patients allergic to pilocarpine).

CONTRAINDICATIONS

Muscarinic agonists are contraindicated in patients with known hypersensitivity. In addition, when used systemically, it is important to recognize that these medications are contraindicated in patients with hyperthyroidism, heart block, history of dysrhythmia, coronary artery disease, abdominal obstruction, peptic ulcers, asthma, or urinary tract obstruction. Systemically, muscarinic agonists are contraindicated in parkinsonism and patients with hypotension. They should not be used if the integrity of the bladder or gastrointestinal wall is in question or there is obstruction.

See Nursing Drug Digest for specific contraindications associated with individual agents.

CAUTIONS

Special caution must be taken when these medications are used systemically in patients receiving ganglionic blocking compounds as this can cause severe abdominal symptoms and critical hypotension.

Ophthalmic solutions (e.g., carbachol) should be used with caution if the epithelial barrier of the conjunctiva or cornea has been denuded, abraded, or decreased because of the use of topical anesthetics or tonometry.

See Nursing Drug Digest for cautions related to each specific agent.

DRUG INTERACTIONS

Muscarinic agonists, especially those given systemically, have the potential to interact with other medications including anticholinesterases (e.g., neostigmine, pyridostigmine) and adrenergic agonists (e.g., epinephrine). See Clinically Significant Drug Interactions for specific drug interactions and mechanisms.

ADMINISTRATION

Muscarinic agonists are available in various preparations including oral, subcutaneous, and ophthalmic preparations.

These agents must *never* be administered IM or IV because of the likelihood of eliciting violent muscarinic effects such as cardiovascular collapse and severe bronchospasms.

Dosage and route of administration must be individualized (see Nursing Drug Digest) depending on type and severity of condition being treated. Oral preparations (e.g., bethanechol) should be given when the stomach is empty to prevent nausea and vomiting, which can occur if the drug is taken after eating.

Ophthalmic preparations are supplied in various percentage solutions for selected therapeutic use. For example, carbachol is available in a 0.75%, 1.5%, or 3% ophthalmic solution and pilocarpine, the drug most widely used for the treatment of open-angle glaucoma, is available in 0.5%, 1%, 2%, 3%, and 4% solutions. When administering these medications, special attention should be given to solution strengths. Because these preparations are associated with slight hyperemia, aching eyes, and headache during the first few days of therapy, it is recommended that the cornea be gently massaged through the eyelids after administration of the drops as ordered to increase ocular penetration and decrease these effects. After administration it is also recommended that all excessive solution be wiped away to prevent systemic absorption by the lacrimal system.

MONITORING PATIENT RESPONSE
Therapeutic response

Because these agents can be used for the treatment of a variety of different conditions monitoring for therapeutic effect must be individualized to the patient and indication for drug therapy. For example, ophthalmic preparations of this class of drugs when applied topically to the eye contract the *sphincter muscle* of the iris causing *miosis*. This effect should be monitored in relation to drug action and expected effect. For example, carbachol's action lasts 4 to 8 hours, and the drug is given 2 to 3 times a day whereas with pilocarpine miosis and accommodation spasms begin within 15 minutes of drug use and last 30 to 60 minutes with the pupil remaining constricted for 20 hours while fixation of the lens disappears within 3 hours. While some of these effects are observable, others are not as readily observable in the treatment of glaucoma. Tonometry and follow-up are required to monitor the effect of these medica-

Continued.

GENERAL NURSING IMPLICATIONS—cont'd

Nursing of patients requiring muscarinic agonists (systemic and ophthalmic agents)—cont'd

Therapeutic response—cont'd

tions on vasodilation and control of intraocular fluid pressure. Symptoms (e.g., decreased visual field, eye pain) should be monitored in relation to the monitoring of therapeutic effect.

See Nursing Drug Digest for monitoring as related to specific agents.

Adverse side effects

Systemic effects

Because the pharmacologic effects of the muscarinic agonists are related to receptors in several organ systems and thus not organ specific, the nurse must be alert to monitor for effects that may in some cases be the desired principal effect but in the patient being cared for is an unwanted or adverse effect. For example, if bethanechol is administered as adjunctive therapy in the treatment of gastroesophageal reflux with pylorus, then increased urination would be considered an adverse effect, whereas in a patient with postoperative urinary retention, this would be a desired effect. The monitoring of side effects is essential (see Adverse/Side Effects of the Muscarinic Agonists). Planning for the minimization of these effects with the patient and family promotes compliance and avoids undue problems associated with side effects.

Monitor for signs of toxicity, hold the medication, and advise the prescriber if the following are noted: hypotension, bradycardia, increased salivation and perspiration, bronchospasms, GI tract distress/diarrhea, and urinary urgency.

Atropine should be readily available to treat signs and symptoms of overdosage; it is an effective antidote for overdose of muscarinic agonists. The adult dose is 0.5 to 1 mg of atropine IM or IV.

Ophthalmic effects

Observe and report any systemic effects, such as bronchospasm, gastrointestinal tract distress/diarrhea, urinary urgency, or increased salivation or sweating.

Monitor for local ophthalmic effects including conjunctival vascular congestion, signs of local hypersensitivity reactions, myopia, ocular pain, and decreased visual acuity in dim light.

PATIENT EDUCATION

The patient and family as indicated should be involved as early as possible in the prescribed drug regimen. They should have a clear understanding of the purpose of the medication, possible side effects to expect, what to do to minimize side effects (especially those that may occur when the medication is taken systemically), adverse reactions to report, and proper administration, especially if the patient is to administer his or her own medication in the hospital or at home.

For ophthalmic medications, instruct the patient on proper method for instillation, including corneal massage through the eyelids and the use of finger pressure on the lacrimal apparatus

to ensure desired response and to minimize systemic absorption resulting in systemic side effects (see Chapter 2 "Preparation, Administration, and Monitoring of Medications").

The patient should be able to demonstrate correct administration of eyedrops before discharge. Patients also require a sound knowledge about their condition and therapy. This is essential especially for patients such as those requiring muscarinic agonists for the treatment of glaucoma. These patients need to be aware that glaucoma is a chronic condition and that they will need to continue their medication as well as require supervision and follow-up so that their individual therapy program can be modified or changed as needed to maintain and promote optimal visual ability. Safety should also be emphasized with these patients because the pupil does not dilate in response to diminished light or darkness. This makes it difficult for the patient to see at night or in darkened areas. The nurse should explore aspects of environmental safety with these patients so that they are aware that stairways should be well lighted and free of clutter, for example, and other environmental changes can be made as needed. Patients should also be cautioned about driving or walking at night because of problems associated with loss of accommodation (see Instructions for Discharge/Outpatients).

Nursing of patients requiring muscarinic blockers

ASSESSMENT

A complete nursing assessment is essential to establish a baseline from which to monitor therapeutic response, side effects, and adverse reactions. Assessment should include a careful drug history to identify sensitivity, cautions, contraindications, and potential drug interactions (see Clinically Significant Drug Interactions) before the first dose is taken.

Because these medications are used for the treatment of a variety of conditions (e.g., relaxation of the gastrointestinal, biliary, and genitourinary tracts; prophylaxis of syncope from Stokes-Adams syndrome; *mydriatic* effects; suppression of salivary, gastric, and respiratory tract secretions; and as antidotes for muscarinic agonists [i.e., atropine] and anticholinesterases, assessment must be made for the

individual condition being treated. Documentation of this assessment is essential in monitoring patient response.

SENSITIVITY

Generally, allergic reactions to muscarinic blockers are rare; however, any drug has the potential to cause a hypersensitivity reaction in susceptible individuals. See Nursing Drug Digest for specific agents.

GENERAL NURSING IMPLICATIONS—cont'd

Nursing of patients requiring muscarinic blockers—cont'd

CONTRAINDICATIONS

These drugs are contraindicated in individuals with known hypersensitivity.

These medications are contraindicated in patients with a history of *paralytic ileus*, pyloroduodenal stenosis, megacolon, ulcerative colitis, narrow-angle glaucoma, and *prostatism*. See Nursing Drug Digest for each specific agent.

CAUTIONS

Special caution is required when administering muscarinic blockers to patients with a history of coronary artery disease, heart failure, asthma, or chronic obstructive lung disease. See Nursing Drug Digest for each specific agent.

DRUG INTERACTIONS

Muscarinic blockers have the potential to interact with antihistamines, phenothiazines, and adrenergic agonists. See Clinically Significant Drug Interactions for specific details concerning drug interactions with these agents.

ADMINISTRATION

Various muscarinic blockers can be given by oral, rectal, subcutaneous, intramuscular, intravenous, and ophthalmic routes. See Nursing Drug Digest for each individual drug.

Use the proper method of instilling these medications ophthalmically including the use of finger pressure on the lacrimal apparatus to ensure desired response and to minimize systemic side effects (see Chapter 2, "Preparation, Administration, and Monitoring of Medications").

MONITORING PATIENT RESPONSE
Therapeutic response

Because these medications can be given for a variety of conditions, monitoring of response is essential in relation to specific indication so that therapy can be adjusted or modified in order to optimize therapy according to the individual patient's needs.

Adverse side effects

Adverse side effects of the muscarinic blockers include blurred vision, brady-cardia, flushing, mydriasis, urinary retention, and xerostomia. In addition, overdoses may cause delirium, fever, tachycardia, coma, respiratory failure, and death. Treatment of overdose is with physostigmine. The dose for adults is 0.5 to 2 mg by slow IV at a rate not to exceed 1 mg per minute; or the dose can be given IM. If necessary 1 to 4 mg may be repeated at the occurrence (recurrence) of serious life-threatening signs such as convulsions, dysrhythmias, or coma. Conventional supportive measures must also be initiated.

Systemic agents

When muscarinic blockers are administered, the monitoring of side effects is essential (see Adverse/Side Effects of Muscarinic Blockers). Planning for the minimization of these effects with the patient and family promotes compliance and avoids undue problems associated with troublesome adverse effects especially when long-term therapy is indicated.

Monitor for signs of toxicity. Hold the medication and advise the prescriber if the following are noted: skin flushing, skin rash, elevated body temperature, tachycardia, or CNS excitement. Infants and young children are more sensitive to the toxic effects of these medications than adults because they have a poorly developed temperature regulatory system.

Monitor for signs of an acute attack of glaucoma, such as severe, throbbing pain in the eyes, sudden loss of vision, or the phenomenon of seeing colored halos around lights, accompanied by nausea and vomiting. Because those patients with narrow-angle glaucoma are particularly susceptible to this adverse effect, these drugs are contraindicated in such patients.

Monitor for signs of urinary retention. If noted, advise prescriber. Instruct patient to void prior to the administration of each dose.

High environmental temperatures should be avoided as they may cause heat prostration because these drugs inhibit heat loss by suppressing perspiration. This is especially important to monitor with infants and young children because of their immature temperature regulation systems, as well as in the elderly.

Ophthalmic agents (see also systemic agents)

Monitor for any systemic effect including skin flushing or rash, elevated body temperature, tachycardia, and signs of CNS excitement. Infants and young children are more sensitive to the toxic effects of these drugs than adults mainly because they have immature temperature regulation systems.

Monitor for signs of an acute attack of glaucoma, such as severe throbbing pain in the eyes, sudden loss of vision, or the phenomenon of seeing colored halos around lights, accompanied by nausea and vomiting. Patients with a family history of glaucoma, those over 40 years of age, diabetics, and those who have sustained a recent eye injury should have their intraocular pressure checked *before* these drugs are administered topically to the eye.

Monitor for suspected allergic reaction in the eyes from the medication: conjunctivitis, local vascular congestion, and edema.

Monitor for blurring of near vision and photophobia. Sunglasses may relieve photophobia.

PATIENT EDUCATION

The patient and family as indicated should be involved as early as possible in the prescribed drug regimen. They should have a clear understanding of the purpose of the medication, possible side effects, adverse reactions to report, and proper administration of the medication especially if the patient is to be administering his or her own medication in the hospital or at home (see General Instructions for Discharge/ Outpatients).

GENERAL INSTRUCTIONS FOR DISCHARGE/OUTPATIENTS

MUSCARINIC AGONISTS
Ophthalmic medication

This medication is used for the treatment of various eye conditions including glaucoma. If you do not understand why you require this medication, check with your health care provider.

Follow instructions for instillation and frequency of administration exactly.

Systemic side effects can be minimized by exerting pressure on the lacrimal sac for about 1 minute during and following instillation.

Regular checks of your intraocular pressure and vision, as scheduled by your health care provider, are very important to control your glaucoma and prevent loss of vision or blindness.

Ocular pain that may occur shortly after instillation can be relieved by local application of cold compresses (ice cubes).

Distant vision may be impaired for several hours after instillation. Driving a car during this period may be hazardous.

Vision in dim light or at night may be somewhat impaired. Avoid driving a car at night if this effect is noted.

Notify your health care provider if persistent redness or irritation occurs in your eyes. This may be a sign that an allergic reaction has developed and will require a change in your medication.

Keep this and all medications out of the reach of children.

MUSCARINIC BLOCKERS
Ophthalmic medication

This medication is used for the treatment of the eyes. If you do not understand why you require this medication, check with your health care provider.

Follow instructions for instillation and frequency of administration exactly.

Systemic side effects can be minimized by exerting pressure on the lacrimal sac for about 1 minute during and after instillation.

Notify your health care provider immediately if you experience a throbbing pain in the eyes, a sudden loss of vision, or if you are seeing colored halos around lights.

Notify your health care provider immediately if you develop a skin rash, your skin becomes hot and flushed (red), your body temperature increases, your heart is beating fast, or if you experience signs of excessive mental excitement or agitation.

Your ability to read or see near objects may be impaired by this medication.

Wear sunglasses if photophobia becomes troublesome.

Notify your health care provider if your eyes become red, swollen, or are excessively irritated by this medication.

Keep this and all medication out of the reach of children.

Oral medication

This medication is used for the treatment of various conditions, including stomach and urinary tract conditions. If you do not understand why you require this medication, check with your health care provider.

Follow instructions carefully and do not exceed the recommended dosage.

Notify your health care provider immediately if you experience a throbbing pain in the eyes, a sudden loss of vision, or if you are seeing colored halos around lights.

Notify your health care provider immediately if you develop a skin rash, your skin becomes hot and flushed (red), your body temperature increases, your heart is beating fast, or if you experience signs of excessive mental excitement or agitations.

Urinate just prior to taking each dose to avoid urinary retention and possible bladder infection.

This medication may cause impotence in some men. If you note any change in sexual function, discuss this with your health care provider. Reducing the dosage or changing the drug to one that is not a quaternary ammonium derivative will usually solve this problem.

This medication will tend to cause dry mouth and difficulty in swallowing. Sucking on a hard sugarless candy, chewing sugarless gum, or increasing water intake will relieve this condition.

Keep this and all medications out of the reach of children.

NURSING DRUG DIGEST

Medication (trade name*)	Indication	Usual dosage and administration	Dosage forms, preparation, and storage	Contraindications, cautions, and comments	Monitoring
Acetylcholine Acecoline Miochol	Miotic in eye surgery	*Adults:* 0.5-2 ml of 1% solution instilled in the anterior chamber of the eye Follow special instructions for preparation of solution and its administration listed in the package insert	Vial: 20 mg with 2 ml sterile water for injection as diluent Fresh solution must be prepared just before use with aseptic technique Immediately before use, remove dust cap from vial and completely immerse vial in 70% alcohol or other sterilizing solution for at least 30 min	*Contraindicated* in acute iritis Systemic effects are unlikely on topical use; however, its effects can be markedly potentiated by anticholinesterases Acetylcholine is rapidly destroyed by cholinesterases; its effects are rapid in onset and last only minutes, but can be prolonged and intensified by anticholinesterases In cataract surgery use *only after delivery of lens*	Observe eye for signs of infection or continued irritation (slight hyperemia may occur at onset of therapy)
Anisotropine methylbromide Valpin Valpin 50 Valpin 50-PB*	Adjunctive in peptic ulcer therapy	*Adults:* 10-50 mg PO before meals and q.h.s.	Tablets: 10, 50 mg	See Atropine *Contraindicated* in patients with myasthenia gravis	

Continued.

NOTE: For additional details regarding the individual agents listed in this table, see the text and other tables in this chapter.
*Indicates a multiple active ingredient product. For a complete listing of all active ingredients see the *Drug Reference Guide to Brand Names and Active Ingredients.*
★Indicates that the drug is generally available only in the United States.

NURSING DRUG DIGEST—cont'd

Medication (trade name)	Indication	Usual dosage and administration	Dosage forms, preparation, and storage	Contraindications, cautions, and comments	Monitoring
Atropine Alisod* Atrobarb* Atropisol Barbidonna* Butabell HMB* Comhist* Diaction* Di-Atro* Masp* Mybephen* Isopte Atropine Kinesed* Loflo* Lomotil* Lonox* Pylora* Ru-Tuss Setamine* Trac Tabs* Urised*	Adjunctive therapy of peptic ulcers Hypermotility/spasms of GI, biliary, and urogenital tracts	*Adults:* 0.4-0.6 mg PO 30 min before meals and q.h.s.; increase dosage *gradually* to obtain desired response; 0.4 to 0.6 mg IM or IV if rapid effects desired *Children:* 0.1-0.4 mg PO 30 min before meals and q.h.s.; increase dosage *gradually* to obtain desired response	Tablets: 0.3, 0.4, 0.6 mg Injectable: 0.05, 0.1, 0.3, 0.4, 0.5, 1, 1.2 mg/ml Ophthalmic solution: 0.125%-4% Ophthalmic ointment: 0.5%-1%	*Contraindicated* in patients with narrow-angle glaucoma, paralytic ileus, severe ulcerative colitis, megacolon, prostatism, pyloroduodenal stenosis, or adhesions between the lens and iris *Use with caution* in patients over 40 years of age because of increased incidence of glaucoma, and in patients with prostatic hypertrophy, coronary artery disease, cardiac failure, asthma or chronic lung disease High environmental temperatures may cause heat prostration, especially in children under 6 years	Monitor for antimuscarinic effects (e.g., dry mouth, blurred vision, urinary retention) Observe for signs of atropine poisoning (see pp. 456-457) Physostigmine is an effective antidote: 1-4 mg by slow IV injection (*less than* 1 mg/min) for adults and 0.5-1 mg for children Children are more susceptible to toxic effects of overdoses When used topically in eye, minimize absorption by compressing the lacrimal sac for 1 min during and following instillation; effects on the eye may last for several days With low doses (0.4-0.6 mg) the most usual side effect is dry mouth; may be relieved by chewing gum or sucking on ice chips or hard sugarless candy Instruct patient to void before each dose to minimize urinary retention Blurred vision and photophobia can be expected on topical use in eye
	Preanesthetic medication to inhibit bronchial secretions and to block cardiac vagal reflexes	*Adults:* 0.4-0.6 mg IM 30-60 min before anesthetic *Children:* 0.1-0.4 mg IM depending on age (0.01 mg/kg) 30-60 min before anesthetic			
	Mydriatic/cycloplegic	*Adults:* 1-2 drops of 1% ophthalmic solution into eye(s) up to t.i.d. if required *Children:* 1-2 drops of 0.5% ophthalmic solution into eye(s) up to t.i.d. if required			
	Iritis	*Adults:* 1-2 drops of 1% ophthalmic solution or small amount of ophthalmic ointment applied b.i.d. to t.i.d. *Children:* Same as adults			
	Antidote to cholinesterase inhibitors	*Adults:* Initially 2-4 mg IV, followed by 2 mg q.5-10 min until muscarinic symptoms disappear or atropine toxicity *Children:* One fourth of adult dose			
	Syncope from Stokes-Adams syndrome Type I AV conduction deficits	*Adults:* 0.4-1 mg IV, repeat if necessary to a maximum of 2 mg *Children:* 0.01-0.03 mg/kg IV May need to decrease dose in renal impairment			

Drug	Uses	Dosage	How Supplied	Nursing Implications	
	Severe bradycardia associated with hyperactive carotid sinus reflex	Administer IV dose slowly			Instruct patients to wear sunglasses Instruct patient to use caution while operating motor vehicle
Belladonna Belap Belladenal* Belladenal-S* Bellergal* Bellergal-S* Bellermine-D.D.* Chardonna-2* O & B Suppository*	Adjunctive peptic ulcer therapy Hypermotility/spasms of the GI, biliary, and urogenital tracts NOTE: Use is generally not recommended	*Adults:* 10.8-21.6 mg PO 30 min before meals and q.h.s. NOTE: *Do not confuse with belladonna tincture, the dosage of which is 0.2-0.3 mg t.i.d. to q.i.d.*	Tablets: 10.8, 15 mg	See Atropine Do *not* confuse with belladonna tincture Belladonna is a botanical preparation that contains several antimuscarinic alkaloids including atropine and scopolamine	See Atropine
Bethanechol Duvoid Mictrol Myotonachol Urecholine Urolax Vesicholine	*Atony* of urinary bladder or GI tract Postoperative and postpartum nonobstructive urinary retention See also Chapter 37, "Drugs Used to Treat Urinary Tract Disorders"	*Adults:* 20-200 mg/24 hr PO in 2-4 divided doses on an empty stomach; or 2.5-5 mg SC q.4-8h Start with lower doses, then increase gradually to obtain the desired response Individualization of dosage is required to minimize the number and severity of side effects Should *never* be given IM or IV because of the possibility of eliciting violent muscarinic effects, including cardiovascular collapse	Tablets: 5, 10, 25, 50 mg Injectable: 5 mg/ml Parenteral solutions are rendered harmful if frozen	*Contraindicated* in patients with bradycardia, hyperthyroidism coronary artery disease, obstruction of GI or urinary tracts or if strength of walls of these structures is in question, peptic ulcers, peritonitis, epilepsy, parkinsonism, asthma, and pregnancy Atropine should be readily available as an antidote: the adult dose is 0.5-1 mg IM or IV; epinephrine may be of additional benefit, 0.1-1 mg SC Bronchospasms, marked hypotension, and bradycardia are the most feared adverse effects Additive hypotensive effects can be expected with other agents capable of lowering blood pressure	Monitor heart rate, respiratory status, and blood pressure

Continued.

NURSING DRUG DIGEST—cont'd

Medication (trade name)	Indication	Usual dosage and administration	Dosage forms, preparation, and storage	Contraindications, cautions, and comments	Monitoring
Bethanechol—cont'd				May cause nausea and vomiting Additive muscarinic effects can be expected with anticholinesterase agents	
Carbachol Carbacel Carcholin Doryl Isopto Carbachol Lentin Miostat Mistura C P. V. Carbachol	Miotic in eye surgery Glaucoma	*Adults:* Instill 0.5 ml of 0.01% solution in anterior chamber *Adults:* 1-2 drops of 0.75%-3% solution in eyes b.i.d. or t.i.d.	Ophthalmic solutions: 0.75%, 1.5%, 2.25%, 3%	See Bethanechol Varying degrees of myopia may develop In cataract surgery, use carbachol *only after* delivery of lens Because of miosis, visual acuity in dim light will be reduced Individualize dosage to minimize adverse effects Lower doses should be used if the epithelial barrier of the conjunctiva or cornea has been reduced by topical anesthetics, tonometry, or trauma Not the first drug of choice; is generally considered an alternative agent in those resistant or intolerant to pilocarpine	
★ Clidinium Chlordinium Sealets* Clipoxide* Librax* Lidinium* Quarzan	Adjunctive peptic ulcer therapy Hypermotility/spasms of the GI, biliary, and urogenital tracts	*Adults:* 2.5-5 mg PO before meals and q.h.s. Maximum: 20 mg/day *Elderly:* 2.5 mg PO t.i.d.	Capsules: 2.5, 5 mg	See Atropine *Contraindicated* in patients with myasthenia gravis	

Cyclopentolate Ak-Pentolate Cyclogyl Cyclomydril* Mydplegic Mydrilate Novo-Cyclo Optopento- late	Mydriatic and cy- cloplegic	*Adults:* 1-2 drops of 0.5% for those with blue irises; 1-2 drops of 1% or 2% for those with brown irises *Children:* One half of adult dose	Ophthalmic solution: 0.5, 1, 2%	*Contraindicated* in glau- coma Maximum effects occur in 30 to 60 min and may last for 24 hr May increase intraocular pressure Use has been associated with behavioral distur- bances in young chil- dren, particularly un- der 6 years of age
Glycopyrrolate Nodapten Robinul Robinul Forte Robinul-PM Forte* Robinul-PM* Tarodyl	Adjunctive peptic ulcer therapy Hypermotility/ spasms of the GI, biliary, and urogenital tracts Preanesthetic medication to reduce respira- tory secretions	*Adults:* 3-6 mg/24 hr PO in 3 divided doses; or 0.1 mg SC, IM, or IV q.4h. *Children:* Use is *not* recom- mended Burning sensation may occur at injection site *Adults:* 0.004-0.005 mg/kg IM 30-60 before anesthetic *Children:* Same as adults	Tablets: 1, 2 mg Injectable: 0.2 mg/ml The parenteral solution is *incompatible* with sodium bicarbonate, diazepam, pentobarbital, phenothia- zines, dimenhydrinate, chloramphenicol, and so- dium chloride	See Atropine *Contraindicated* in pa- tients with myasthenia gravis
★ **Hexocyclium methylsul- fate** Tral Filmtab Tral Gradu- met	Adjunctive peptic ulcer therapy Hypermotility/ spasms of the GI, biliary, and urogenital tracts	*Adults:* 25 mg PO before meals and q.h.s.; or timed-release tablets, 50-75 mg PO before lunch and q.h.s.	Tablet: 25 mg; timed-release: 50, 75 mg	See Atropine *Contraindicated* in pa- tients with myasthenia gravis *Contraindicated* in chil- dren
Homatropine hydrobro- mide Homapin Homatrisol Homatrocel Isopto Hom- atropine Malcotran Matropinal* Mesopin Novatrin Novatropine Probilagol Ru-Spas No. 2	Mydriatic and cy- cloplegic	*Adults:* 1-2 drops of 1-5% solu- tion in eyes up to q.i.d. if re- quired *Children:* Same as adults	Ophthalmic solution: 1%, 2%, 5% Protect from light	See Atropine

Continued.

NURSING DRUG DIGEST—cont'd

	Indication	Usual dosage and administration	Dosage forms, preparation, and storage	Contraindications, cautions, and comments	Monitoring
Hyoscyamine Anaspaz Anaspaz PB* Barbidonna* Comhist* Cystospaz Digestamic* Dolonil* Donnagel* Donnagel-PG* Donnatal* Donnatal Extentabs* Donnazyme* Donphen* Hasp* Hybephen* Kinesed* Levamine Levsin Sedralex* Setamine* Sidonna* Spalix* Spasmolin* Spasmorel* Trac Tabs* Urised*	Adjunctive peptic ulcer therapy Hypermotility/ spasms of the GI, biliary, and urogenital tracts	*Adults:* 0.125-0.5 mg PO before meals and q.h.s.; or 0.375 mg of timed-release capsules q.12h.; or 0.25-0.5 mg SC, IM, or IV as required q.4-6h. *Children:* 2-10 years, one half of adult dose; infants and up to 2 years, one fourth of adult dose	Tablet: 0.125, 0.15, 0.25 mg Capsule timed-release: 0.375 mg Injectable: 0.25, 0.5 mg/ml Elixir: 0.125 mg/5 ml Drops: 0.125 mg/ml	See Atropine Causes fewer CNS stimulating effects than atropine	
Isopropamide Combid* Combid Spansule* Darbid Decan-Aid TR* Decon-Tuss TR* Ornade* Priamide Tyrimide	Adjunctive peptic ulcer therapy Hypermotility/ spasms of the GI, biliary, and urogenital tracts	*Adults:* 5-10 mg PO b.i.d. *Children: Not* recommended for children under 12 years	Tablet: 5 mg	See Atropine *Contraindicated* in patients with myasthenia gravis Unless contraindicated, increase fluid intake to prevent constipation	

Drug	Use	Dosage	Supplied	Considerations
★ **Mepenzolate** Cantil	Adjunctive peptic ulcer therapy Hypermotility/ spasms of the GI, biliary, and urogenital tracts	*Adults*: 25-50 mg PO before meals and q.h.s.	Tablet: 25 mg Liquid: 25 mg/5 ml	See Atropine *Contraindicated* in patients with myasthenia gravis Monitor for dizziness and postural hypotension Monitor bowel function and increase fluid if necessary unless contraindicated
★ **Methantheline** Banthine	Adjunctive peptic ulcer therapy Hypermotility/ spasms of the GI, biliary, and urogenital tract	*Adults*: 200-400 mg/24 hr PO in 4 divided doses *Children*: newborns, 25 mg/24 hr PO in 2 divided doses; 1-12 months, 50-100 mg/24 hr PO in 4 divided doses; over 1 year, 50-200 mg/24 hr PO in 4 divided doses Do *not* chew tablets, because they are bitter	Tablet: 50 mg	*See* Atropine *Contraindicated* in patients with myasthenia gravis
★ **Methscopolamine** Dallergy* Extendryl* Histaspan-D* Histeral* MSC Triaminic* Pamine Sinovan Timed* Skopyl	Adjunctive peptic ulcer therapy Hypermotility/ spasms of the GI, biliary, and urogenital tracts	*Adults*: 2.5 mg PO 30 min before meals and q.h.s.	Tablet: 2.5 mg	*See* Atropine *Contraindicated* in patients with myasthenia gravis
Oxyphencyclimine Daricon Enarax* Gastrix Naridan Setrel Vio-Thene Vistrax* W-T Anticholinergic Zamanil	Adjunctive peptic ulcer therapy Hypermotility/ spasms of the GI, biliary, and urogenital tracts	*Adults*: 10-20 mg/24 hr PO in 2 divided doses *Children: Not* recommended for children under 12 years	Tablet: 10 mg	See Atropine
★ **Oxyphenonium** Antrenyl	Adjunctive peptic ulcer therapy Hypermotility/ spasms of the GI, biliary and urogenital tracts	*Adults*: 20-40 mg/24 hr PO in 4 divided doses *Children: Not* recommended for children	Tablet: 5 mg	See Atropine *Contraindicated* in patients with myasthenia gravis

Continued.

NURSING DRUG DIGEST—cont'd

Medication (trade name)	Indication	Usual dosage and administration	Dosage forms, preparation, and storage	Contraindications, cautions, and comments	Monitoring
Pilocarpine Adsorbocarpine Almocarpine E-Carpine* E-Pilo* Isopto Carpine Miocarpine Mi-Pilo Mistura P Ocusert Ocusert Pilo Optopilo Pilocar Pilocel Pilomiotin Pilovisc P. V. Carpine P1E1* P2E1* P3E1* P4E1* P5E1*	Glaucoma	*Adults:* 1-2 drops in eyes up to 6 times daily; dosage must be individualized, start with solution of lower concentrations	Ophthalmic solutions: 0.25%, 0.5%, 1%, 1.5%, 2%, 3%, 4%, 5%, 6%, 8%, 10% Ocusert Pilo-20 Ocusert Pilo-40 Protect solutions from light Store Ocusert systems between 2° and 8° C	See Bethanechol Discontinue use if local hypersensitivity reactions occur; these are rare Varying degrees of myopia may develop Because of miosis, visual acuity in dim light will be reduced Instruct patient to check for presence of Ocusert q.h.s. and q.a.m.	Monitor for blurred vision or headaches
		Ocuserts are placed in the cul-de-sac of eye; it is recommended that they be replaced once a week, and that this be done q.h.s. because the initial release rates of the drug tend to be higher and cause myopia			
Propantheline Banlin Giquel Norpanth Novopropanthil Pro-Banthine	Adjunctive peptic ulcer therapy Hypermotility/ spasms of GI, biliary, and urogenital tracts	*Adults:* 7.5-15 mg PO with meals and 15-30 mg q.h.s.; or 30 mg PO long-acting tablets b.i.d. or q.8-12h. IM or IV: 30 mg q.6h. initially and then a maintenance dose of 15 mg q.6h.	Tablets: 7.5, 15 mg; prolonged-acting, 30 mg Injectable: 30 mg/vial Reconstitute with 1 ml sterile water for injection for IM use, and 10 ml sodium chloride for injection for IV use	See Atropine *Contraindicated* in patients with myasthenia gravis	

Generic/Trade Names	Uses	Preparations	Administration/Dosage	Remarks
Pro-Banthine w/Phenobarbital* / Propanthel / Robantaline / Ropanth		Reconstituted solution is stable for 7 days when stored between 2° and 8° C	*Children:* Use is *not* recommended	Monitor level of consciousness; side rails and other precautions may be indicated
Scopolamine / Comhist L.A.* / Comhist* / Donnagel* / Donnagel-PG* / Isopto Hyoscine / Kinesed* / Kwells / Plexonal* / Ru-Tuss* / Sidonna* / Transderm-scop / Transderm-V	Preanesthetic medication Prevention of motion sickness Treatment of motion sickness Mydriatric and cycloplegic	Tablets: 0.4, 0.6 mg Injectable: 0.3 to 1 mg/1 ml Ophthalmic solution: 0.2%, 0.25% Ophthalmic ointment: 0.2% Transdermal patch: 1.5 mg	*Adults:* 0.2-0.6 mg PO, SC, or IM 30-60 min before anesthetic *Children:* 0.006 mg/kg IM, IV, or SC 30 min before anesthetic *Adults:* 0.1 mg PO 30-60 min before traveling. Transdermal patch applied behind ear releases 0.5 mg over a period of 3 days *Children:* Use is *not* recommended *Adults:* 0.2-0.6 mg IM, IV, SC; or 0.4-0.8 mg PO t.i.d. to q.i.d. *Adults:* 1-2 drops in eyes as required. Adjust dosage to specific requirements	See Atropine Sedation is a major side effect Is an effective prophylactic agent against motion sickness Use with caution in patients with glaucoma Transdermal form may cause unilateral dilation of pupil
★ **Tridihexethyl** / Claviton / Milpath* / Pathibamate* / Pathilon	Adjunctive peptic ulcer therapy Hypermotility/spasms of GI, biliary, and urogenital tracts	Tablet: 25 mg Capsule (sustained-release): 75 mg Injectable: 10 mg/1 ml	Adult: 75-200 mg/24 hr PO in 3-4 divided doses; or 75 mg of sustained-release capsules q.12h. 10-20 mg SC, IM, or IV q.6h. Substitute oral therapy as soon as feasible	See Atropine *Contraindicated* in patients with myasthenia gravis
Tropicamide / Mydriacyl	Mydriatic and cycloplegic	Ophthalmic solution: 0.5%, 1%	*Adults:* 1-2 drops 0.5%-1% in eyes; repeat in 20-30 min if required	See Atropine Tropicamide has a much shorter duration of action than atropine when used topically in the eye

BIBLIOGRAPHY

Avery, G.S. (Ed.). *Drug treatment: principles and practice of clinical pharmacology and therapeutics* (2nd ed.). New York: Adis, 1980.

Black, C.D. Transdermal drug delivery systems. *U.S. Pharmacist, 1982, 7,* 49.

Compendium of pharmaceuticals and specialties (19th ed.). Ottawa: Canadian Pharmaceutical Association, 1984.

Cooper, J.R., Bloom, F.E., & Roth, R.H. *The biochemical basis of neuropharmacology* (3rd ed.). New York: Oxford University Press, 1978.

Day, M.A. *Autonomic pharmacology: experimental and clinical aspects.* New York: Churchill Livingston, 1979.

Gever, L.N. Cholinergics. *Nursing 84,* 1984, *14*(5), 41.

Gilman, A.G., Goodman, L.S., & Gilman, A. (Eds.). *Goodman and Gilman's the pharmacological basis of therapeutics* (6th ed.). New York: Macmillan, 1980.

Quail, C. & Waddleton, C. Treating the glaucomas. *Nurses' Drug Alert,* 1980, September, 93-96.

Sympathomimetics and Sympatholytics

Abram J.D. Friesen

Medications discussed in this chapter

Sympathomimetics
  α-Adrenergic agonist
    Metaraminol
    Methoxamine
    Naphazoline
    Oxymetazoline
    Phenylephrine
    Phenylpropanolamine
    Propylhexedrine
    Pseudoephedrine
    Tetrahydrozoline
    Xylometazoline
  β-Adrenergic agonists
    Albuterol
    Dobutamine
    Ethylnorepinephrine
    Fenoterol
    Isoproterenol
    Metaproterenol
    Nylidrin
    Terbutaline
  α- and β-Adrenergic agonists
    Dopamine

Sympathomimetics—cont'd
  Ephedrine
  Epinephrine
  Hydroxyamphetamine
  Mephentermine
  Norepinephrine
Sympatholytics
  α-Adrenergic blockers
    Phenoxybenzamine
    Phentolamine
    Prazosin
  β-Adrenergic blockers
    Metoprolol
    Propranolol
    Timolol
  Adrenergic neuron blockers
    Bretylium
    Debrisoquine
    Guanethidine
    Reserpine

TABLE 24-1

Common therapeutic uses of sympathomimetics and sympatholytics

Sympathomimetics	*Sympatholytics*
Bronchospasms or asthma	Angina pectoris
Albuterol	Metoprolol
Ephedrine	Propranolol
Epinephrine	Timolol
Ethylnorepinephrine	Cardiac dysrhythmias
Fenoterol	Bretylium
Isoproterenol	Propranolol
Metaproterenol	Hypertension
Methoxyphenamine	Bethanidine
Terbutaline	Debrisoquine
Heart block or cardiac decompensation	Guanethidine
Dobutamine	Metoprolol
Isoproterenol	Prazosin
Hypotensive states not caused by hypovolemia	Propranolol
Dopamine	Reserpine
Ephedrine	Timolol
Levarternol	Pheochromocytoma
Mephentermine	Phenoxybenzamine
Metaraminol	Phentolamine
Methoxamine	Propranolol
Phenylephrine	Prophylaxis of migraine
Nasal congestion	Ergotamine
Ephedrine	Propranolol
Naphazoline	Wide-angle glaucoma
Oxymetazoline	Timolol
Phenylephrine	
Phenylpropanolamine	
Propylhexedrine	
Pseudoephedrine	
Tetrahydrozoline	
Tuaminoheptane	
Xylometazoline	
Wide-angle glaucoma or as mydriatic	
Epinephrine	
Hydroxyamphetamine	
Phenylephrine	

Sympathomimetics are drugs that mimic or produce effects similar to those seen after activation of the sympathetic division of the autonomic nervous system (ANS) (e.g., increased heart rate, constricted blood vessels, and increased blood pressure). In contrast, the *sympatholytics* are agents that inhibit or suppress ongoing sympathetic activity and decrease smooth muscle tone in peripheral vessels thereby increasing peripheral circulation and decreasing blood pressure. Thus these drugs have many therapeutic uses (Table 24-1).

A better understanding of the pharmacology and therapeutic potential of these agents can be achieved by first reviewing the anatomy and physiology of the ANS (see Chapter 22). In addition, in Chapter 23 a review of the parasympathetic and sympathetic nervous systems is presented as well as a discussion of drugs that mimic the parasympathetic nervous system (i.e., parasympathomimetics and parasympatholytics). The reader is advised to review these sections before proceeding to the more detailed information presented in this chapter.

DRUGS AFFECTING THE SYMPATHETIC NERVOUS SYSTEM

Sympathomimetics

Sympathomimetics can be subdivided into drugs that activate α- and β-adrenergic receptors and drugs that release norepinephrine (NE) from adrenergic neurons.

Agents that activate α- and β-adrenergic receptors. Certain sympathomimetics interact with postsynaptic adrenergic receptors and produce responses similar to those seen after sympathetic nerve stimulation. For example, phenylephrine selectively activates α-adrenergic receptors, and isoproterenol interacts primarily with β-adrenergic receptors. In addition, there are sympathomimetics (e.g., NE, epinephrine, and ephedrine) that are capable of exciting both types of receptors. These drugs are referred to as *adrenergic agonists.*

Agents that release NE from adrenergic neurons. Tyramine, an agent present in certain foods and beverages, is a classic example of a sympathomimetic that produces its effects by releasing NE from adrenergic nerves. Such agents are referred to as *indirect-acting sympathomimetics.* Amphetamines also release NE from peripheral adrenergic nerves. However, because they produce powerful CNS stimulatory effects, they are primarily used therapeutically for these effects (see Chapter 20, "Antiparkinsonian Medications and Stimulants."). Although few therapeutically useful agents act primarily by this mechanism, certain drugs (e.g., ephedrine, metaraminol, phenylpropanolamine, and pseudoephedrine) possess some ability to induce the release of NE, but also directly excite α- and β-adrenergic receptors.

Sympatholytics

Sympatholytics can be subdivided into drugs that selectively block α- or β-adrenergic receptors and drugs that cause NE depletion or directly inhibit its release.

Agents that selectively block α- or β-adrenergic receptors. Some sympatholytics are capable of selectively interacting with α- or β-adrenergic receptors. This interaction, however, does not activate the receptor to initiate a response. The physical presence of these drugs on the receptor prevents the NE released by the nerve endings from combining with the receptor; therefore the α- or β-adrenergic effects of NE are blocked. Phentolamine is an example of a selective α-adrenergic blocker; propranolol is a β-adrenergic blocker.

Many of the ergot alkaloids produce some degree of α-adrenergic blockade, but they also produce many other effects unrelated to α-blockade. Most notable of these other actions are vasoconstriction, which makes some of them useful in the treatment of migraine headaches (e.g., ergotamine) and contraction of the uterus (e.g., ergonovine is of value in treating uterine hemorrhage). Ergot alkaloids are discussed in more detail in Chapter 71, "Unclassified Miscellaneous Agents."

Agents that cause NE depletion or directly inhibit its release. Reserpine is an example of a sympatholytic that interferes with the storage of NE in adrenergic nerves, thereby causing NE depletion. Therefore less NE is released when sympathetic nerves are activated, which leads to a reduction in sympathetic effects (tone) on organ systems. Guanethidine interferes with NE storage in a manner similar to reserpine but, in addition, directly inhibits NE release. This latter effect becomes evident even before significant NE depletion has occurred. Bretylium, on the other hand, causes no NE depletion but acts solely by directly inhibiting NE release from adrenergic neurons. These drugs are referred to as *adrenergic neuron blocking agents* (Figure 24-1).

IMPORTANT ASPECTS OF THE DISPOSITION AND METABOLISM OF NOREPINEPHRINE

Disposition and metabolism of NE occur primarily by a "reuptake" mechanism and by enzymatic inactivation.

Reuptake

When NE is released from adrenergic nerves, the major mechanism responsible for terminating its effects is reuptake into the adrenergic nerve terminal and its subsequent entry into the storage vesicles (Figure 24-1). This process serves a dual purpose: it rapidly reduces NE concentration in the vicinity of adrenergic receptors, and it rapidly replenishes the store of NE in nerve terminals. This specialized NE transport system, however, is not specific, and other drugs, even if they differ significantly in chemical structure, can be transported into the adrenergic nerve. Important examples are guanethidine and bretylium, which gain access to their site of action via the NE reuptake sys-

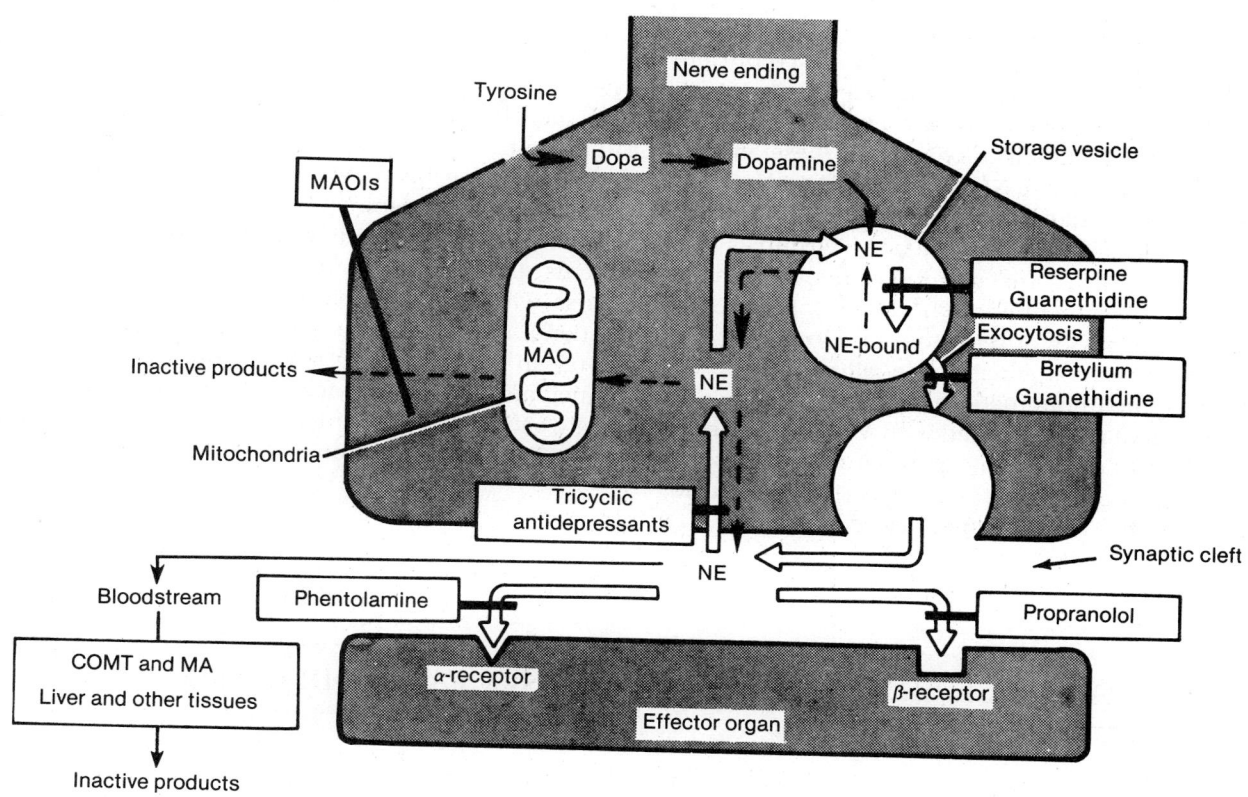

FIGURE 24-1. **Schematic representation of the events that occur at an adrenergic synapse. Tyrosine is actively transported into the nerve ending and is converted by a sequence of enzymatic steps to norepinephrine (NE). NE is stored in the bound form in vesicles. When an action potential reaches the nerve ending, excytosis occurs. This process involves the fusion of vesicles to the presynaptic membrane and the discharge of NE into the synaptic cleft. The released transmitter then activates α or β receptors in the postsynaptic effector organ. Active reuptake of NE into the nerve ending is the major mechanism for terminating the action of NE. Any excess NE that cannot be stored in vesicles is inactivated by MAO located in mitochondria of the adrenergic nerve terminal. A less important mechanism involves the diffusion of NE from the synaptic cleft into the bloodstream, where it is subsequently inactivated by COMT/MAO located in the liver and other tissues. Examples of drugs that can block or inhibit various processes are indicated in boxes.**

tem. The tricyclic antidepressants are capable of inhibiting this process and therefore can interfere with the action of guanethidine and bretylium. It should also be noted that tricyclic antidepressants can potentiate the action of most sympathomimetic amines; although this effect may be partly the result of inhibition of the NE reuptake mechanism, the main reason for this adverse drug interaction is unknown.

Enzymatic inactivation

In contrast to endogenously released NE, enzymatic inactivation by *catechol-O-methyltransferase* (COMT) and by monoamine oxidase (MAO) assumes a more important role than the reuptake process in terminating the action of injected NE. COMT is present in high concentration in the liver. Smaller amounts are found in other tissues. Compounds that have the 3,4-catechol group on the benzene ring, (e.g., the catecholamines, NE, epinephrine, isoproterenol, and dopamine) are good substrates for this enzyme. However, since catecholamines are also subject to inactivation by MAO, COMT inhibitors do not significantly potentiate the effects of these catecholamines.

Many tissues contain some *monoamine oxidase* (MAO), but the liver and adrenergic nerve endings contain the highest concentrations of this enzyme. Phenethylamines lacking α-methyl groups are good substrates for this enzyme: these include the catecholamines mentioned as well as drugs such as tyramine and phenylephrine. MAO inhibitors (MAOIs) represent a potential hazard in terms of adverse drug interactions with the sympathomimetic amines. They not only inhibit the metabolism of some of these amines, but also they allow more NE to be stored in adrenergic nerves thereby enhancing the action of those agents capable of releasing NE from the nerve terminals (e.g., tyramine, ephedrine, metaraminol, phenylpropanolamine, and pseudoephedrine). MAOIs may also increase the sensitivity of receptors to adrenergic agonists. Therefore, as a general rule, all adrenergic agonists or sympathomimetic amines are contraindicated in patients being treated with MAOIs. MAOIs are used therapeutically in the treatment of depression and are discussed in greater detail in Chapter 19, "Drugs Used to Treat Affective Disorders."

SUMMARY

This chapter has examined the various types and uses of sympathomimetic and sympatholytic medications. The agents have been differentiated according to receptor (i.e., α, β, specificity, and the mechanisms of action have been related to the disposition and metabolism of norepinephrine.

With an understanding of the various individual agents, including their actions and side effects, the nurse will be better able to provide optimal care to patients requiring these medications. Patient education can be enhanced; adverse drug effects can be anticipated, monitored for, and minimized; and clinically significant drug interactions can be avoided by utilizing the information presented in this chapter.

ADVERSE/SIDE EFFECTS OF THE SYMPATHOMIMETICS*

α-Adrenergic agonists
ALLERGIC REACTIONS

Ocular hypersensitivity (may occasionally occur on topical application to eye)

CARDIOVASCULAR SYSTEM

Bradycardia (use with caution in patients with bradycardia or partial heart block)

Hypertension (use with caution in patients with a history of stroke, hypertension, or hyperthyroidism; phentolamine, 5 to 10 mg IV, can be used as an antidote)

Vasoconstriction (Use a large vein for IV infusions and check periodically for free flow. Infiltrate 5 to 10 mg of phentolamine into ischemic area at the first sign of extravasation to prevent necrosis of tissue. Repeated SC or IM injections in the same area should be avoided to prevent necrosis. Use with caution in patients with peripheral arteriosclerosis.)

CENTRAL NERVOUS SYSTEM

Cerebral hemorrhage (may develop in susceptible patients if excessive hypertension develops)

METABOLIC AND ENDOCRINE SYSTEMS

Hyperglycemia (may develop in patients with maturity-onset diabetes)

OCULAR SYSTEM

Hypersensitivity (may develop with repeated topical usage)

Increased intraocular pressure (will develop in patients with narrow-angle glaucoma [prior to iridectomy] and could precipitate an acute attack of glaucoma; these agents are therefore contraindicated in such patients)

Pigmentary deposits in conjunctiva (may develop with prolonged topical use of epinephrine)

Reactive conjunctival hyperemia (may develop with topical use)

Transitory stinging or pain (can be expected with topical use)

RESPIRATORY SYSTEM

Rebound nasal congestion or rhinitis (May occur with prolonged excessive topical use. Avoid the use of topical nasal decongestants for more than 3 to 4 consecutive days. Allow several drug-free days before resumption of medication. Systemic absorption from overdose has caused deep sleep or coma [children].)

UROGENITAL SYSTEM

Contraction of pregnant uterus (avoid during pregnancy)

Spasms of vesical sphincter (may result in painful urination or urinary retention in males with prostatism)

*See Chapter 11, "Drug Toxicity," for an overview of drug toxicity.

ADVERSE/SIDE EFFECTS OF THE SYMPATHOMIMETICS—cont'd

β-Adrenergic agonists
BEHAVIOR*

Anxiety
Confusion
Excitability
Hallucinations
Insomnia

CARDIOVASCULAR SYSTEM†

Angina pain
Dysrhythmias
Flushing of face
Palpitations
Tachycardia

CENTRAL NERVOUS SYSTEM

Anxiety
Dizziness
Excitability
Hallucinations
Headache
Nausea/vomiting
Tremor

METABOLIC AND ENDOCRINE SYSTEMS

Hyperglycemia (may develop in diabetics)

RESPIRATORY SYSTEM

Paradoxical airway resistance (may occasionally occur on repeated excessive inhalation therapy; discontinue aerosol use immediately and use alternate form of therapy)

α-, β-Adrenergic agonists
These agents will tend to produce adverse side effects similar to the *combined* effects of α-agonists and β-agonists discussed previously

*More likely to occur in the elderly, especially with ephedrine
†Use with caution in patients with coronary artery disease, dysrhythmias, and hyperthyroidism.

ADVERSE/SIDE EFFECTS OF THE SYMPATHOLYTICS*

α-Adrenergic blockers
CARDIOVASCULAR SYSTEM

Acute hypotension†
Cutaneous flushing
Dysrhythmias†
Orthostatic hypotension (common)
Palpitations
Tachycardia†

CENTRAL NERVOUS SYSTEM

Dizziness
Feeling of tiredness/weakness
Sedation

GASTROINTESTINAL SYSTEM

Abdominal discomfort (common, especially with phentolamine)
Diarrhea
Exacerbation of peptic ulcers (especially with phentolamine)
Nausea and vomiting

RESPIRATORY SYSTEM

Nasal congestion/stuffiness (common)

UROGENITAL SYSTEM

Inhibition of ejaculation (especially with phenoxybenzamine)

β-Adrenergic blockers
BEHAVIOR‡

Emotional lability
Hallucinations
Lassitude
Mental depression
Short-term memory loss

CARDIOVASCULAR SYSTEM§

Bradycardia
Exacerbation of heart block
Exacerbation of heart failure
Orthostatic hypotension (uncommon)

CENTRAL NERVOUS SYSTEM‡

Emotional lability
Hallucinations
Lassitude
Mental depression
Short-term memory loss
Visual disturbances

GASTROINTESTINAL SYSTEM

Abdominal cramps
Diarrhea/constipation (uncommon)
Epigastric distress

METABOLIC AND ENDOCRINE SYSTEMS

Hypoglycemia (use with caution in diabetics and those subject to hypoglycemic episodes)

RESPIRATORY SYSTEM

Bronchospasm (in susceptible patients; contraindicated in patients with asthma, bronchitis, or emphysema)

Continued.

*See Chapter 11, "Drug Toxicity," for an overview of drug toxicity.
†May occur especially after parenteral injection and may lead to anginal attacks, myocardial infarction, cerebrovascular spasm, or cerebrovascular occlusion. Contraindicated in patients with a history of myocardial infarction or coronary artery disease.
‡Effects are uncommon.
§Contraindicated in patients with sinus bradycardia or greater than first-degree heart block, heart failure, or myocarddial infarction.

ADVERSE/SIDE EFFECTS OF THE SYMPATHOLYTICS—cont'd

Guanethidine-like drugs
CARDIOVASCULAR SYSTEM

Bradycardia (common)

Edema (common, can be controlled with a diuretic)

Exacerbation of congestive heart failure (contraindicated in patients with frank congestive failure)

Increased sensitivity to direct-acting sympathomimetics (may cause excessive hypertension/dysrhythmias; use sympathomimetics with caution; for similar reasons, guanethidine-like drugs are contraindicated in pheochromocytoma)

Postural and exertional hypotension (common; worse on arising from sleep and accentuated by hot weather or alcohol; may be associated with cerebral/myocardial ischemia in susceptible patients)

GASTROINTESTINAL SYSTEM

Diarrhea (common; can usually be controlled with small doses of atropine-like drugs)

Exacerbation of peptic ulcers

Nausea/vomiting

RESPIRATORY SYSTEM

Exacerbation of asthma (best avoided in such patients)

UROGENITAL SYSTEM

Decreased libido/inhibition of ejaculation (may lead to impotence; reduce the dosage or try an alternate class of drugs if this becomes a problem)

Decreased renal function (may further compromise renal function in patients with preexisting renal disease)

Edema (common; can be controlled with a diuretic)

Reserpine
BEHAVIOR

Depression (about 6% of patients may develop this effect; discontinue medication because patient may become suicidal; contraindicated in patients with a history of mental depression)

Impaired mental acuity (caused by sedation, which is worse during the first few days of treatment)

CARDIOVASCULAR SYSTEM

Angina-like symptoms

Bradycardia (common)

Edema (common; can be controlled with a diuretic)

CENTRAL NERVOUS SYSTEM

Extrapyramidal symptoms (rare, except in high doses)

Nightmares

Paradoxical anxiety

Sedation (common, especially during the first few days of treatment)

GASTROINTESTINAL SYSTEM

Abdominal cramps and diarrhea (fairly common; not recommended for patients with ulcerative colitis or related conditions)

Bleeding (ulcerogenic effects)

Nausea/vomiting

Peptic ulcerations (discontinue when symptoms appear; not recommended for patients with a history of peptic ulcers)

Salivation (low doses of atropine will prevent this if it becomes troublesome)

HEMATOLOGIC SYSTEM

Purpura with thrombocytopenia (occasionally occurs; discontinue medication)

METABOLIC AND ENDOCRINE SYSTEMS

Gynecomastia

Inhibits ovarian cycle (may lead to infertility while on drug)

Pseudolactation

RESPIRATORY SYSTEM

Asthma (in susceptible patients)

Nasal congestion (common)

UROGENITAL SYSTEM

Edema (can be controlled with a diuretic)

Decreased libido/impotence (reduce the dosage or switch to another class of drugs if this becomes a problem)

Inhibition of ovarian cycle (may lead to infertility while on this drug)

CLINICALLY SIGNIFICANT DRUG INTERACTIONS*

Primary drug	Interacting drug	Possible effect(s)	Probable mechanism(s)
α-Adrenergic agonists (e.g., phenylephrine, pseudoephedrine)	Guanethidine-like drugs (e.g., bethanidine, debrisoquine)	Excessive hypertension	Increased adrenergic receptor sensitivity
α-Adrenergic agonists	MAOIs (e.g., tranylcypromine, phenelzine)	Excessive hypertension Increased adrenergic effects	Decreased metabolism Increased adrenergic receptor sensitivity Increased norepinephrine content of adrenergic neuron
β-Adrenergic agonists (e.g., albuterol, isoproterenol)	β-Adrenergic blockers (e.g., propranolol, timolol)	Decreased β-adrenergic effects Decreased bronchodilation in asthmatic patients	Competitive antagonism at receptor level
α- and β-Adrenergic agonists (e.g., ephedrine, epinephrine)	β-Adrenergic blockers (e.g., propranolol, timolol)	Increased hypertension, reflex bradycardia	Block only β-adrenergic effects leaving α-adrenergic (pressor) effects predominating
α- and β-Adrenergic agonists	Guanethidine-like drugs (e.g., bethanidine, debrisoquine)	Excessive hypertension, cardiac dysrhythmias	Increased adrenergic receptor sensitivity Decreased norepinephrine uptake into adrenergic neurons
α- and β-Adrenergic agonists	MAOIs (e.g., tranylcypromine, phenelzine)	Excessive hypertension, cardiac dysrhythmias	Decreased metabolism Increased adrenergic receptor sensitivity Increased norepinephrine content of adrenergic neurons
α- and β-Adrenergic agonists	Tricyclic antidepressants (e.g., imipramine, amitriptyline)	Excessive hypertension	Not established
β-Adrenergic blockers (e.g., propranolol, timolol)	α- and β-Adrenergic agonists (e.g., epinephrine, ephedrine)	Increased hypertension, reflex bradycardia	Only β-adrenergic effects blocked, leaving α-effects (pressor) predominating
β-Adrenergic blockers	Antidiabetic drugs (e.g., insulin, tolbutamide)	Increased hypoglycemia Masks tachycardia and tremor associated with hypoglycemia	Decreased glycogenolysis Blocks β-adrenergic effects of the hypoglycemia-induced released catecholamines
β-Adrenergic blockers	β-Adrenergic agonists (e.g., isoproterenol, albuterol)	Decreased β-adrenergic effects Decreased bronchodilation in asthmatic patients	Block β-adrenergic receptors
β-Adrenergic blockers	Clonidine	May aggravate any rebound hypertension on withdrawal of clonidine therapy	Block only β-effects of catecholamines released on withdrawal of clonidine leaving α-adrenergic (pressor) effects predominating

*See Chapter 10, "Drug Interactions," for an overview of drug interactions.

Continued.

CLINICALLY SIGNIFICANT DRUG INTERACTIONS—cont'd

Primary drug	Interacting drug	Possible effect	Probable mechanism
Guanethidine-like drugs	Amphetamines, ephedrine, doxepin, haloperidol, phenothiazines, tricyclic antidepressants	Decreased antihypertensive effect of guanethidine-like drugs	Block uptake of guanethidine-like drugs into site of action (the adrenergic nerve terminal)
Reserpine	Anesthetics, spinal and general	Increased hypotensive effects	Additive effects
Reserpine	Levodopa	Decreased antiparkinsonism effect	Reserpine tends to deplete levels of dopamine in the brain

GENERAL NURSING IMPLICATIONS

Sympathomimetics

Nursing of patients requiring adrenergic agonists

ASSESSMENT

A complete nursing assessment is essential to establish a baseline from which to monitor therapeutic response, side effects, and adverse reactions. Assessment should include a careful drug history to identify sensitivity, contraindications, and potential drug interactions (see Clinically Significant Drug Interactions) before the first dose is taken.

Because adrenergic agonists are used in the treatment of a variety of different conditions assessment must be completed in relation to the indication for which the medication is being used in the individual patient. For example, when these medications are used in the treatment of asthma, respiratory assessment is indicated.

SENSITIVITY

Any drug has the potential to cause a hypersensitivity reaction in a susceptible individual. Hypersensitivity to the sympathomimetics has been noted; thus this should be carefully evaluated in the nursing and drug histories. This is especially important since hypersensitivity to any of the sympathomimetic amines constitutes a contraindication to the use of all drugs in this class.

CONTRAINDICATIONS

The use of adrenergic agonists is contraindicated in patients with known hypersensitivity to the sympathomimetics. The use of adrenergic agonists is generally contraindicated in cardiac tachydysrhythmias not caused by atrial-ventricular nodal block and in patients receiving monoamine oxidase inhibitors (MAOI's).

It is important to recognize that these medications are contraindicated in patients with a history of narrow-angle glaucoma and could precipitate an acute attack of glaucoma.

See Nursing Drug Digest for specific contraindications of each drug.

CAUTIONS

These agents should be used with caution in the elderly and in individuals with heart disease, hypertension, or hyperthyroidism. Caution should also be exercised when administering these drugs during pregnancy.

Special caution is required when administering β-adrenergic agonists to patients with a history of coronary artery disease, dysrhythmias, and hyperthyroidism.

The adrenergic agonists phenylephrine, phenylpropanolamine, and ephedrine are used as nasal decongestants because of their vasoconstrictor effects. Cold remedies containing these drugs should be given cautiously to hypertensive and cardiac patients. Caution should also be exercised in dealing with patients receiving tricyclic antidepressants or monoamine oxidase inhibitors because of the danger of a hypertensive crisis.

See Nursing Drug Digest for cautions related to specific agents and routes of administration.

DRUG INTERACTIONS

Adrenergic agonists have the potential to interact with numerous drugs in a variety of mechanisms. In addition, interactions are often specific depending upon whether the drug is an α-adrenergic agonist, β-adrenergic agonist, or α- and β-adrenergic agonist.

See Clinically Significant Drug Interactions.

ADMINISTRATION

Adrenergic agonists are available in a variety of dosage forms for administration by various routes depending upon

GENERAL NURSING IMPLICATIONS—cont'd

Nursing of patients requiring adrenergic agonists—cont'd

ADMINISTRATION—cont'd

the indication for use and individual patient factors. For example, the same drug can be applied topically (e.g., ephedrine) for the treatment of nasal congestion or systemically for the treatment of specific cardiac conditions.

See Nursing Drug Digest for specific information in relation to dosage forms and routes of administration associated with the individual adrenergic agonists.

Systemic agents

When administering these agents IM or SC, rotate the injection sites carefully when repeated injections are indicated to prevent tissue necrosis. Record sites carefully and examine sites for signs of irritation.

These agents are to be administered carefully when given intravenously. Use a large vein, such as the antecubital for IV infusions. Infiltrate 5 to 10 mg of phentolamine into the ischemic area at the first sign of extravasation. Infusions of levarterenol, dopamine, and dobutamine require constant monitoring. Infusion of heparin at the same time (100 to 200 units heparin/hour for an adult) has been reported to decrease the incidence of venous thrombosis. Monitor blood pressure, cardiac rhythm, ECG, and other vital signs when these agents are used parenterally. With some of these medications (e.g., dopamine, dobutamine) blood pressure should be monitored continuously. Phentolamine should be kept on hand during infusion as an effective antidote for excessive hypertension.

Store all solutions in a cool place protected from light and discard brownish solutions or those containing a precipitate (see Nursing Drug Digest).

Ophthalmic medications

The proper method of instillation of ophthalmic preparations should be utilized (see Chapter 2, "Preparation, Administration, and Monitoring of Medications") including the exertion of finger pressure on the lacrimal apparatus for about 1 minute after instilla-

tion. This minimizes systemic absorption.

Transitory stinging or pain can be expected following instillation of ophthalmic preparations. Monitor for signs of persistent eye irritation since this may indicate the patient has developed a local allergic reaction to the medication.

Monitor for systemic effects.

Inhalation agents

The proper method of administering inhalation products should be used (see Chapter 28, "Bronchodilators and Respiratory Gases").

Avoid excessive repeated inhalations in patients with lung conditions since this may lead to a paradoxical increase in airway resistance.

Nasal agents

The proper technique for administering these medications should be used (see Chapter 2).

Patients should also be made aware of the dangers of overusing nasal medications. Encourage them to use these nasal preparations only during the acute stages of their condition. These medications should not be used more than 3 to 5 consecutive days since this may cause drug-induced rhinitis or "rebound" effects. Allow several drug-free days prior to resumption of medication use.

MONITORING PATIENT RESPONSE
Therapeutic response

Because these medications are used for a variety of indications (see Table 24-1), monitoring must be tailored to the condition for which the adrenergic agonist was prescribed. See Nursing Drug Digest for specific information regarding the monitoring of the individual agents.

Adverse side effects

The monitoring of side effects is essential (see Adverse/Side Effects). Planning for the minimization of these effects with the patient and family promotes compliance and avoids undue prob-

lems associated with potentially troublesome side effects.

Adverse effects vary depending on whether the drug is an α-adrenergic agonist, a β-adrenergic agonist, or an α-, β-adrenergic agonist.

See Adverse/Side Effects of the Sympathomimetics for general adverse/side effects and Nursing Drug Digest for effects associated with specific drugs. In addition it is important to:

Monitor blood pressure, cardiac rhythm, ECG, and other vital signs when these agents are used parenterally. A β-adrenergic blocker, such as propranolol, is an effective antidote for treating symptoms of overdosages of β-adrenergic agonists.

Monitor for signs of toxicity or overdose. Hold the medication and advise the prescriber if aggravation of diabetes, cardiac status, or glaucoma is noted.

Monitor blood glucose levels in all diabetic patients since these drugs can cause hyperglycemia.

Observe any signs of excessive cardiac stimulation such as dizziness, tachycardia, angina pain, or cardiac dysrhythmias.

Monitor for signs of acute attacks of glaucoma such as severe throbbing eye pain, sudden loss of vision, or the phenomenon of seeing colored halos around lights.

PATIENT EDUCATION

The patient and family as indicated should be involved as early as possible in the prescribed drug regimen. They should have a clear understanding of the purpose of the medication, possible side effects and what to do to minimize them, which adverse reactions to report, and proper administration especially if the patient is to be administering his or her own medication in the hospital or at home.

See General Instructions for Discharge/Outpatients.

Continued.

GENERAL NURSING IMPLICATIONS—cont'd

Nursing of patients requiring α- and β-adrenergic agonists

These agents tend to produce adverse effects similar to the *combined* effects of α-agonists and β-agonists discussed previously. Therefore the precautions and monitoring procedures listed under α-agonists and β-agonists should be applied to this group of drugs since they possess both types of pharmacologic activity.

Sympatholytics

Nursing of patients requiring adrenergic blockers

ASSESSMENT

A complete nursing assessment is essential to establish a baseline from which to monitor therapeutic response, side effects, and adverse reactions. Assessment should include a careful drug history to identify sensitivity, contraindications, cautions, and potential drug interactions (see Clinically Significant Drug Interactions) before the first dose is administered.

Because adrenergic blockers are used in the treatment of a variety of different conditions (see Table 24-1), assessment must be completed in relation to the indication for which the medication is being used in the individual patient. For example, when these medications are used in the treatment of hypertension, blood pressure and related assessments are indicated.

SENSITIVITY

Any drug has the potential to cause a hypersensitivity reaction in a susceptible individual.

See Nursing Drug Digest for information related to specific agents.

CONTRAINDICATIONS

Adrenergic blockers are contraindicated in known hypersensitivity.

See Nursing Drug Digest for specific contraindications of each drug.

CAUTIONS

These drugs should be used with caution in the elderly and in pregnant patients.

See Nursing Drug Digest for cautions related to the use of specific agents.

DRUG INTERACTIONS

Adrenergic blockers have the potential to interact with numerous drugs in a variety of mechanisms and occur primarily with β-adrenergic blockers. See Clinically Significant Drug Interactions.

ADMINISTRATION

Adrenergic blockers are available in a variety of dosage forms for administration by various routes depending upon the indication for use and individual patient factors. For example, propranolol is administered orally in the treatment of hypertension and intravenously in the treatment of emergent cardiac dysrhythmias.

See Nursing Drug Digest for specific information in relation to dosage forms and routes of administration associated with the individual adrenergic blockers.

MONITORING PATIENT RESPONSE

Therapeutic response

Because adrenergic blockers are used for a variety of indications (see Table 24-1), monitoring must be tailored to the indication for which the agent was prescribed.

See Nursing Drug Digest for specific information regarding the monitoring of the individual adrenergic blockers.

Adverse side effects

The monitoring of side effects is essential. (See Adverse/Side Effects of the Sympatholytics for an overview of adverse effects of adrenergic blockers). Planning for the minimization of troublesome effects with the patient and family as indicated promotes compliance and avoids undue problems associated with potentially troublesome side effects.

Adverse side effects vary depending upon whether the drug is an α-adrenergic blocker, a β-adrenergic blocker, or an adrenergic neuron blocker.

α-Adrenergic blockers

Monitor blood pressure, ECG, and other vital signs, especially when these agents are used parenterally. Norepinephrine or an α-adrenergic agonist can be used to combat excessive hypotension. A β-adrenergic blocker, such as propranolol, can be used to reduce excessive tachycardia if this occurs in *normotensive* patients.

Assist patients out of bed until a maintenance dose has been established and they are able to deal with the orthostatic hypotension.

Monitor and report any signs of exacerbation of peptic ulcers, especially with phentolamine.

β-Adrenergic blockers

Observe and report any signs of heart failure, asthma, or severe bradycardia.

Monitor blood glucose levels in all diabetics and in those patients who suffer from hypoglycemic episodes. These drugs may mask symptoms of hypoglycemia.

Avoid abrupt withdrawal of these agents once the patient has been on this medication for more than several days, since this may precipitate severe anginal attacks or even a myocardial infarction.

Guanethidine-like drugs

Assist patients out of bed until the maintenance dose has been established and they are able to deal with orthostatic hypotension.

Observe and report any signs of peptic ulcers, severe diarrhea, asthma, heart failure, or bradycardia.

GENERAL NURSING IMPLICATIONS—cont'd

Nursing of patients requiring adrenergic blockers—cont'd

Guanethidine-like drugs—cont'd

Use drugs possessing α-adrenergic activity with caution since they may cause excessive hypertension in patients on guanethidine-like drugs.

Reserpine

Observe and report any signs of depression or personality change as some patients may develop suicidal tendencies when receiving this medication.

Observe and report any signs of peptic ulcers, severe diarrhea, or asthma.

Assist patients out of bed until the maintenance dose has been estab-

lished and until they have been educated to deal with orthostatic hypotension.

Observe and report any signs of purpura with thrombocytopenia.

Sedation, especially during the first few days of treatment, and nasal congestion are common side effects and can be expected in a high percentage of patients.

See Adverse/Side Effects for general effects listed according to these categories and Nursing Drug Digest for adverse side effects associated with specific drugs.

PATIENT EDUCATION

The patient and family as indicated should be involved as early as possible in the prescribed drug regimen. They should have a clear understanding of the purpose of the medication, possible side effects to expect, what to do to minimize side effects, adverse reactions to report, and proper administration especially if the patient is to be administering his or her own medication in the hospital or at home.

See General Instructions for Discharge/Outpatients.

GENERAL INSTRUCTIONS FOR DISCHARGE/OUTPATIENTS

SYMPATHOMIMETICS
α-Adrenergic agonists

Follow instructions for use exactly and do not exceed the recommended dose or frequency of administration.

Notify your health care provider immediately if you experience throbbing eye pain, sudden loss of vision, or if you are seeing colored halos around lights.

When applied to the eyes, this drug may cause initial pain or a stinging sensation.

If you are a diabetic, this medication may necessitate changes in your dose of insulin or oral hypoglycemic agent; therefore check your urine/blood glucose levels more frequently until these adjustments can be made.

Avoid using nasal preparations for more than 3 to 5 consecutive days as this may paradoxically make nasal congestion worse. Allow several drug-free days before resumption of this medication.

Store all solutions in a cool place protected from light, and discard brownish solutions or those containing a precipitate.

Keep this medication and all medications out of the reach of children.

β-adrenergic agonists

Notify your health care provider if your heart is beating at an unusually fast rate or if you experience chest pains or dizziness after taking this medication.

If you are a diabetic, this medication may necessitate changes in your dose of insulin or oral hypoglycemic agent; therefore check your urine/blood glucose levels more frequently until these adjustments can be made.

Follow instructions for inhalation therapy exactly and do not exceed the number of inhalations since this may overstimulate your heart and also lead to a temporary loss of effectiveness of the medication for controlling your bronchial condition.

Store solutions in a cool place protected from light and discard brownish solutions or those containing a precipitate.

Keep this medication and all medications out of the reach of children.

α- and β-Adrenergic agonists

Since these agents possess both types of adrenergic activity, instructions to patients will be similar to those listed previously for α-adrenergic agonists and β-adrenergic agonists. The specific information or instructions transmitted will depend on the intended use of the drug, the type of preparation used, and the route of administration.

SYMPATHOLYTICS
α-Adrenergic blockers

To avoid dizzy spells or fainting, sit up in bed slowly before arising and sit on the edge for a few minutes before standing up. Also avoid making sudden changes in posture during the remainder of the day. Excessive exercise, exposure to heat, or drinking alcohol may also cause dizzy spells.

Report any unusual increase in your heart rate to your health care provider.

Report any persistent abdominal discomfort to your health care provider (especially with phentolamine)

This medication may cause nasal congestion. Consult your physician for treatment if this becomes troublesome.

Continued.

GENERAL INSTRUCTIONS FOR DISCHARGE/OUTPATIENTS—cont'd

α-Adrenergic blockers—cont'd

These drugs (especially phenoxybenzamine) may inhibit ejaculation in some men. If this becomes a problem for you, report it to your health care provider. A reduction in dosage may resolve this problem.

Keep this and all medication out of the reach of children.

β-adrenergic blockers

Do not discontinue this medication abruptly as this may lead to potentially serious heart problems.

Report any unusual slowness of your heart beat (less than 50 beats per minute) or shortness of breath to your health care provider.

Patients with diabetes and those who suffer from hypoglycemic episodes should check urine/blood glucose levels more frequently until adjustments are made in their diet or diabetic drug doses.

Keep this and all medications out of the reach of children.

Guanethidine-like drugs

To avoid dizzy spells or fainting, sit up in bed slowly before arising and sit on the edge for several minutes before standing up. Also avoid making sudden changes in posture during the remainder of the day. Excessive exercise, exposure to heat, or drinking alcohol may also cause dizzy spells. Sleeping with head of bed elevated and wearing elastic stockings may be helpful.

Report any persistent abdominal discomfort, diarrhea, fluid retention (edema), or unusual shortness of breath to your health care provider.
Avoid taking cold or allergy remedies (containing sympathomimetics) unless directed by your physician since these may cause excessive hypertension.

This medication may cause impotence in some men. If this becomes a problem, discuss it with your health care provider. Reducing the dosage or changing to another class of drugs usually resolves this problem.

Keep this and all other medications out of the reach of children.

Reserpine

This medication may cause sedation, especially during the first few days of treatment. Avoid driving a car or operating complicated machinery until your system has adjusted to this effect.

Report any nightmares, changes in sleep patterns, or persistent changes in mood or personality, especially depression, to your health care provider.

To avoid dizzy spells or fainting, sit up in bed slowly before arising and sit on the edge for several minutes before standing up. Also avoid making sudden changes in posture during the remainder of the day. Excessive exercise, exposure to heat, or drinking alcohol may also cause dizzy spells.

Report any signs of persistent abdominal discomfort, diarrhea, edema, or unusual shortness of breath to your health care provider.

This medication may cause nasal congestion. If this becomes a problem consult your physician for appropriate measures to treat this condition. Do not self-medicate.

This medication may cause impotence in some men. If this becomes a problem, discuss it with your health care provider. Reducing the dosage or changing to another class of drugs usually resolves this problem.

Report any unusual slowness of your heart beat (less than 50 beats per minute) to your health care provider.

Keep this medication and all medication out of the reach of children.

NURSING DRUG DIGEST

Medication (trade name*)	Indication	Usual dosage and administration	Dosage forms, preparation, and storage	Contraindications, cautions, and comments	Monitoring
Albuterol Proventil Ventolin	Bronchospasms or asthma See also Chapter 28, "Bronchodilators and Respiratory Gases"	*Adults:* 6-16 mg/24 hr PO in 3 or 4 divided doses or 1-2 inhalations up to a maximum of 8/day *Children:* 6-12 years, 6-8 mg/24 hr PO in 3 or 4 divided doses *Elderly:* start with half the recommended adult dosage, then increase to optimal dosage over a period of days May need to decrease dose in renal impairment	Tablet: 2, 4 mg Respirator solution: 0.6% Metered-dose aerosol: 100 μg/inhalation Store in light-resistant container	Similar to isoproterenol Tends to cause fewer cardiac adverse effects than isoproterenol May cause headache, dizziness, nausea, and palpitations	Monitor heart rate and blood pressure
Bretylium Bretylate ♦ Bretylin ♦ Bretylol Darenthin ♦	Life-threatening ventricular dysrhythmias See also Chapter 32, "Antidysrhythmics"	*Adults:* Initially 5-10 mg/kg IM increase to 10 mg/kg at 15-min intervals until a maximum of 30 mg/kg has been given Maintenance: 5-10 mg/kg q.8h. IM IV infusion *not* recommended because of the occurrence of vomiting and severe hypotension; onset is no faster than IM *Elderly* patients and those with impaired renal function usually require smaller doses Use is usually restricted to life-threatening ventricular dysrhythmias that have *not* responded to conventional therapy Switch patient to oral antidysrhythmic as soon as possible	Injectable: 50 mg/ml Must be diluted to a *minimum* of 50 ml with D_5W or NS *before* IV administration	*Contraindicated* in aortic stenosis and pulmonary hypertension Rotate IM injection site to prevent necrosis; do not inject near large nerves because damage may result Keep patient in supine position until tolerance to orthostatic hypotension develops Transient hypertension and worsening of dysrhythmias may occur during the first hour Antidysrhythmic effects are delayed in onset and may become evident only 20 min to 6 hr after initiation of therapy Dosage should be reduced or discontinued after 3 to 5 days and an alternate antidysrhythmic drug substituted if required	Monitor for orthostatic hypotension, particularly in elderly patients Monitor ECG

Continued.

NOTE: For additional details regarding the individual agents listed in this table, see the text and other tables in this chapter.
*Indicates a multiple active ingredient product. For a complete listing of all active ingredients see the *Drug Reference Guide to Brand Names and Active Ingredients.*
♦ Indicates that the drug is generally available only in Canada.
★ Indicates that the drug is generally available only in the United States.

NURSING DRUG DIGEST—cont'd

Medication (trade name)	Indication	Usual dosage and administration	Dosage forms, preparation, and storage	Contraindications, cautions, and comments	Monitoring
❦ **Debrisoquine** Declinax	Hypertension See also Chapter 33, "Antihypertensives"	*Adults: initially* 5-10 mg/day PO Allow 1-2 weeks before increasing dosage to achieve desired response Maintenance: 10-30 mg/day PO; if more than 10 mg is required, give in 2 or more divided doses before meals Maximum: 140 mg/day *Children: not* recommended because of lack of clinical experience	Tablets: 10, 20 mg	See Guanethidine *Contraindicated* in severe cerebral, coronary, or renal impairment *Contraindicated* in pheochromocytoma Most *common* side effect is orthostatic hypotension Avoid concurrent use of MAOIs	Monitor blood pressure, especially standing blood pressure in the elderly
Dobutamine Dobutrex	Cardiac decompensation	*Adults:* 2-10 µg/kg/min by IV infusion, usually for several hr Maximum duration of treatment is 72 hr	Injectable: 12.5 mg/ml; 250 mg powder in 20 ml vial Reconstitute with 10-20 ml D₅W May be diluted with D₅W or NS Should be used within 24 hr if refrigerated and 6 hr if kept at room temperature Store solutions in cool place protected from light Destroyed by alkaline solutions such as 5% sodium bicarbonate	*Contraindicated* in patients with cardiac dysrhythmias and in idiopathic hypertrophic subaortic stenosis Usually increases both heart rate and blood pressure Use with caution in patients with coronary artery disease, hyperthyroidism, or hypertension Rapid onset of action (1 to 2 min) with peak in 10 min	Individualize the dosage by careful monitoring for adverse effects Monitor pulmonary artery wedge pressure (PAWP) Monitor blood pressure and ECG
Dopamine Intropin Revimine	Hypotensive states *not* caused by hypovolemia	*Adults: initially,* 2-5 µg/kg/min by IV infusion; gradually increase as required up to 20-50 µg/kg/min Dilute with 250 or 500 ml of sterile NS, lactated Ringer's solution, or D₅W just *before* use and *infuse into large vein* of the antecubital fossa to prevent extravasation; check periodically for free flow Extravasation may cause sloughing and necrosis	Injectable: 200 mg/5 ml Must be diluted before administration with 250 or 500 ml of sterile IV solution Store in cool place protected from light Is destroyed by alkalis such as sodium bicarbonate, and by oxidizing agents (e.g., oxygen, nitrites, and ferric salts) Diluted solutions are stable for only 24 hr	*Contraindicated* in pheochromocytoma and ventricular fibrillation Correct hypovolemia *before* administration Less likely than epinephrine to raise diastolic blood pressure Dopamine may also produce a beneficial increase in renal blood flow and hence improve renal function	Monitor PAWP and urine output Monitor IV site for extravasation Also check extremities for changes in temperature, pulse, and color, because significant changes in these parameters may indicate decreased circulation to the extremities

Drug/Trade names	Uses	Dosage	Preparations	Nursing implications	Assessment
		Infiltrate 5-10 mg of phentolamine into ischemic area at first sign of extravasation		Improvement in renal blood flow is thought to result from an interaction with dopamine receptors	Monitor urine flow, cardiac output, and blood pressure during infusion
Ephedrine Amesec*, Asthmagyl*, Benadryl with Ephedrine*, Bronkaid*, Bronkotabs*, Efedron Nasal Jelly, Ephedsol, I-Sedrin Plain, Marax*, Mudrane GG*, Nasdro No. 3, Nyquil Nighttime Colds Medicine*, NyQuil*, Phedral*, Primatene M*, Primatene P*, PBZ Expectorant w/ Ephedrine*, Quibron Plus*, Quiet-Nite*, T.E.P.*, Tedral SA*, Tedral*, Theophedrizine*, Theophedri-Theotabs*, Va-Tro-Nol, Vatronol Nose Drops*	Bronchospasms or asthma Hypotensive states not caused by hypovolemia Enuresis Nasal congestion See also Chapter 29, "Antihistamines, Antitussives, Decongestants, and Expectorants"	*Adult:* 150-300 mg/24 hr PO in 4-5 divided doses *Children:* 6-12 years, 25-50 mg/24 hr PO in 3-4 divided doses; 2-6 years, 1.2-2 mg/kg/24 hr PO in 3-4 divided doses *Adults:* 25-50 mg IM, IV, or SC Maximum: 150 mg/24 hr IV doses should be lower and given slowly *Children:* 25-100 mg/m²/24 hr IM or SC in 4-6 divided doses *Children:* 25-50 mg q.h.s. PO *Adults:* 2-3 drops of 0.5%-3% solution or a small amount of nasal jelly into each nostril b.i.d. to t.i.d. *Children:* Over 6 years of age, same as adults	Tablet: 25 mg Syrup: 11, 20 mg/5 ml Capsule: 25, 50 mg Injectable: 25, 50 mg/ml Nasal solution: 0.5%, 1%, 3% Nasal jelly: 0.6%	*Contraindicated* in narrow-angle glaucoma, severe hypertension, and patients anesthetized with cyclopropane or halothane More CNS stimulation than epinephrine *Elderly* are particularly sensitive to CNS stimulation Urinary retention may develop in men with prostatic hypertrophy May cause painful urination *Caution* older male patients to report difficulty voiding Tolerance to the drug may develop on continuous use; temporary cessation (3 to 4 days) of therapy will restore original response Do not use as topical nasal decongestant for more than 3 to 5 consecutive days Excessive topical nasal use may cause drug-induced rhinitis; allow several days before resumption of medication	Monitor heart and respiratory rate
Epinephrine Adrenalin, Adrenatrate, Asmatane Mist, Asmolin, AsthmaHaler, AsthmaNefrin	Anaphylactic shock Acute bronchospasms Serum sickness Hypersensitivity to insect stings or bites	*Adults:* 0.2-1 mg SC or IM, or 0.1-0.25 mg IV *Children:* 0.01 mg/kg SC to a maximum dose of 0.5 mg Use tuberculin syringe to ensure accuracy of small IV doses	Injectable: 0.1, 1 mg/ml Injectable: 1:400, 1:200 suspension for IM and SC only *Shake well* before using Injectable: 1:1000, 1:10,000 NOTE: 1:1000 solution contains 1 mg/ml	*Contraindicated* in patients with narrow-angle glaucoma and in those receiving cyclopropane or halogenated hydrocarbon anesthetics, guanethidine-like drugs, or tricyclic antidepressants	Individualize the dosage by careful monitoring for adverse effects (e.g., during parenteral use monitor blood pressure and ECG frequently q.2-5 min until stable)

Continued.

NURSING DRUG DIGEST—cont'd

Medication (trade name)	Indication	Usual dosage and administration	Dosage forms, preparation, and storage	Contraindications, cautions, and comments	Monitoring
Epinephrine —cont'd Breatheasy Bronitin Mist Bronkaid Mist Dysne-Inhal E-Carpine* E-Pilo* Epifrin Epitrate Lyophrin Medihaler- Epi Micronefrin Mistura-E Murocoll Mytrate Primatene Mist Simplene Sus-Phrine Vaponefrin	Cardiac arrest	*Adults:* 0.1-0.5 mg intracardiac, 0.5 mg IV q.5 min during resuscitation	Inhalation solution: 1-3, 5% Inhalation aerosols: 0.2, 0.25, 0.3 mg/spray or inhalation Ophthalmic solutions: 0.1%, 0.25%, 0.5%, 1%, 2% Nasal solution: 0.1% Store solutions in a cool place protected from light Drug is *destroyed by alkalis* (e.g., sodium bicarbonate and sodium lactate) and by oxidizing agents (e.g., oxygen, nitrites, and ferric salts) Dilute with D₅W or NS Discard brownish solutions or those containing a precipitate	Use with caution in patients with peripheral/ coronary artery disease, hyperthyroidism, cardiac dysrhythmias, a history of strokes, and during pregnancy Use with caution in patients on digitalis because dysrhythmias may be produced Excessive hypertension/ peripheral vasoconstriction may develop in patients on ergot alkaloids, vasopressin (ADH) or oxytocin This drug may cause hyperglycemia in diabetic patients Phentolamine in a dose of 5- 10 mg IV can be used as an antidote for excessive hypertension An increase in the dosage of insulin or oral hypoglycemic agent may be required Transitory stinging or pain can be expected when applied topically to the eye Paradoxical airway resistance may develop on repeated excessive inhalations; if this occurs, substitute an alternate form of therapy	Monitor extremities for changes in temperature, pulse and color, because significant changes in these parameters may indicate decreased circulation to the extremities
	Bronchospasms or asthma	*Adults:* 1 or 2 inhalations; no more than 8 such doses/24 hr *Children:* Use lower-strength inhalation preparations			
	Wide-angle glaucoma	*Adults:* 1 or 2 drops ophthalmic solution in eyes q.d. to b.i.d.			
	Conjunctivitis	*Adults:* 1 or 2 drops of 0.1% ophthalmic solution in eye(s) as needed			
	Nasal congestion	*Adults:* 1-2 drops of 0.1% nasal solution in each nostril q.4-6h. *Children:* Over 6 years of age, same as adults			
★ **Ethylnorepinephrine** Bronkephrine	Acute bronchospasms	*Adults:* 1-2 mg IM or SC *Children:* 0.2-1 mg IM or SC according to weight/age	Injectable: 2 mg/ml	*Contraindicated* in patients with cardiac dysrhythmias	Monitor heart rate and blood pressure

Drug	Use	Dosage	Availability	Side effects and contraindications	Nursing considerations
Fenoterol Berotac Berotac Inhaler Partusisten	Bronchospasms or asthma	*Adults:* 5-15 mg/24 hr PO in 2-3 divided doses; do not exceed 15 mg/24 hr 1-2 puffs inhaled *not* more often than q4h. up to a maximum of 4 such doses/day *Children:* safety and efficacy not established	Metered dose aerosol: 0.2 mg/inhalation Respirator solution: 1 mg/ml Tablet: 25 mg	Use with caution in patients with coronary artery disease, hyperthyroidism, or hypertension	Monitor heart rate and blood pressure
Guanethidine Esimil Ismelin Ismelin-Esidrix* Visutensil	Hypertension See also Chapter 33, "Antihypertensives"	*Adults, ambulatory: initially,* 10 mg PO/24 hr for 5-7 days; adjust dosage upward at weekly intervals until desired response is obtained Maintenance: 25-50 mg PO/24 hr Patients with impaired renal function usually require lower doses *Adults, hospitalized: initially,* 25-50 mg PO/24 hr; increase daily by 25 mg until the desired response is obtained Maintenance: 1/7 of loading dose PO/24 hr	Tablets: 10, 25 mg	*Contraindicated* in patients with frank congestive heart failure, pheochromocytoma, or patients receiving MAOIs Antihypertensive effects are slow in onset and may last for weeks after cessation of therapy *Use with caution* in patients with peptic ulcers or asthma. Potentiation of the pressor effects of sympathomimetic drugs may interfere with its antihypertensive action (see Clinically Significant Drug Interactions) If possible, discontinue drug 2 to 3 weeks before elective surgery to prevent vascular collapse or cardiac arrest during anesthesia	Monitor lying, sitting, and standing blood pressure, and if possible after light exercise Monitor weight regularly Observe for edema (may require use of diuretic to control edema)

Contraindicated in patients with cardiac dysrhythmias
Use with caution in patients with coronary artery disease, hyperthyroidism, or hypertension

Additive hypotensive effects can be expected with other hypotensive drugs
Patient should avoid strenuous exercise and standing for long periods
Retrograde ejaculation may occur

Continued.

NURSING DRUG DIGEST—cont'd

Medication (trade name)	Indication	Usual dosage and administration	Dosage forms, preparation, and storage	Contraindications, cautions, and comments	Monitoring
★ **Hydroxy-ampheta-mine** Paredrine	To produce mydriasis	*Adults:* 1-2 drops in conjunctival sac	Ophthalmic solution: 1%	*Contraindicated* in narrow-angle glaucoma	Individualize the dosage by careful monitoring for adverse effects (e.g., during parenteral use)
Isoproterenol Aerolone* Aludrin Duo-Medihaler* Duohaler* Iprenol Isonorin Isuprel Isuprel-Neo Mistometer* Luf-Iso Medihaler-Iso Neo-Epinine Norisodrine Prenomiser Forte Proternol Saventrine Vapo-Iso Vapo-N-Ise	Shock-hypoperfusion syndrome	*Adults:* 0.5 to 5 µg/min IV to obtain desired response; lower dosage if heart rate exceeds 110 beats/min *Children:* Approximately half of adult dose	Injectable: 1:5000 solution Tablets: 10, 15, 30 mg for sublingual or rectal use Nebulizer solutions: 0.25%, 0.5%, 1% Inhalation aerosol: 45-125 µg/metered spray *Store* solutions in a cool place protected from light. The drug is *destroyed* by alkalis (e.g., sodium bicarbonate and sodium lactate) and by oxidizing agents (e.g., oxygen, nitrites, and ferric salts) *Discard* brownish solutions or those containing a precipitate	*Contraindicated* in patients with cardiac dysrhythmias and in those receiving cyclopropane or halogenated hydrocarbon anesthetics *Use with caution* in patients with coronary artery disease, hyperthyroidism, or hypertension; those on digitalis may experience dysrhythmias Propranolol is an effective antidote for overdoses; the usual dose is 1-3 mg given by slow IV injection; if necessary, repeat this dosage after 5 min May increase heart rate; therefore *decrease* rate of infusion if heart rate exceeds 110 beats/min May cause hyperglycemia in diabetic patients CNS excitatory effects of the drug are more prominent in the *elderly* Absorption from rectal or sublingual preparations may be irregular An increase in the dosage of insulin or oral hypoglycemic drug may be required	Monitor blood pressure and ECG frequently Monitor diabetics carefully Monitor for respiratory distress resulting from refractory reaction; drug may need to be withdrawn temporarily
	Partial heart block Cardiac arrest	*Adults:* Initially, 20-60 µg IV, subsequently 10-200 µg Alternatively give 200 µg IM *initially* and 20-1000 µg IM subsequently; lower dosage if heart rate exceeds 110 beats/min *Children:* Approximately half of adult dosage			
	Mild heart block Adams-Stokes syndrome	*Adults:* Initially 5 mg PR; or 10 mg sublingually; subsequently, 5-15 mg PR *or* 5-50 mg sublingually q.4-6h. as required *Children:* Approximately half of adult dose			

Drug	Uses	Dosage	Preparations	Remarks	Nursing considerations
	Cardiac arrest	*Adults:* 20 µg intracardiac *Children:* Approximately half of adult dose		Paradoxical airway resistance may develop on repeated excessive inhalation Substitute an alternate form of therapy if this occurs Sublingual tablets should be allowed to disintegrate under the tongue; saliva should not be swallowed during this process because the drug is rapidly metabolized in the small intestine and liver	Monitor blood pressure
	Acute bronchospasms	*Adults:* 10-20 µg IV *Children:* Approximately half of adult dose			
	Bronchospasms or asthma	*Adults:* 30-45 mg/24 hr sublingually in 3 divided doses; alternatively, 1-2 inhalations; no more than 8 such doses/24 hr One aerosol treatment is usually sufficient to control asthma attack *Children:* Approximately half of adult dose			
Mephentermine Biocidin Wyamine	Acute hypotension *not* caused by hypovolemia See also Chapter 28, "Bronchodilators and Respiratory Gases"	*Adults:* 30-45 mg IV or IM *initially;* then 30 mg q.1-2h. as required NOTE: Correct hypovolemia before administration	Injectable: 15, 30 mg/ml May be diluted in D₅W	*Contraindicated* in hypotension caused by chlorpromazine and in patients receiving MAOIs Reserpine and guanethidine cause depletion of norepinephrine, thereby reducing the effects of drugs such as mephentermine Acts mainly by releasing norepinephrine from adrenergic nerves; therefore reserpine and guanethidine-like drugs may render this drug ineffective	
Metaproterenol Alupent Dosalupent Metaprel	Bronchospasms or asthma See also Chapter 28, "Bronchodilators and Respiratory Gases"	*Adults:* 60-80 mg/24 hr PO in 3-4 divided doses; alternatively, 1-2 inhalations q.4h. up to maximum of 12 inhalations/day *Children:* Over 9 years or 60 lb, 60-80 mg/24 hr PO in 3-4 divided doses; 6-9 years or less than 60 lb, 30-40 mg/24 hr PO in 3-4 divided doses Aerosol not recommended for children Drug is not recommended for children under 6 years	Tablets: 10, 20 mg Syrup: 10 mg/5 ml Metered-dose aerosol: 0.65 mg/inhalation Respirator solutions: 0.6%, 5% Inhalation solution: 5% Discard solutions that have turned brown or contain a precipitate	Similar to isoproterenol Tends to produce fewer cardiac adverse effects than isoproterenol Encourage increased fluid intake to liquefy secretions	Monitor blood pressure and pulse before and after first treatment to evaluate cardiac response Auscultate lung fields to evaluate effectiveness of medication after treatment

Continued.

NURSING DRUG DIGEST—cont'd

Medication (trade name)	Indication	Usual dosage and administration	Dosage forms, preparation, and storage	Contraindications, cautions, and comments	Monitoring
Metaraminol Aramine Pressonex Pressoral	Acute hypotensive states not caused by hypovolemia	*Adults:* 0.5-5 mg IV *initially,* followed by IV infusion with dilute solution, containing 15-100 mg in 500 ml of D_5W or NS at a rate to maintain blood pressure; or 2-10 mg IM or SC Advisable to use larger veins to avoid possibility of extravasation (see Norepinephrine)	Injectable: 10 mg/ml	Similar to phenylephrine *Contraindicated* in circulatory disorders and in patients receiving cyclopropane or halothane anesthesia Differs from phenylephrine in that it may cause significant CNS excitement	Monitor blood pressure, ECG, and urinary output Monitor color and temperature of extremities
Methoxamine Vasoxyl	Paroxysmal supraventricular tachycardia Prevent hypotension caused by spinal anesthetics Acute hypotensive states not caused by hypovolemia	*Adults:* 5-10 mg IV injected slowly *Adults:* 10-15 mg IM, allow 15 min before repeating dose *Adults:* 3-5 mg IV injected slowly, followed by 10-15 mg IM; allow at least 15 min before repeating IM dose Infiltrate 5-10 mg of phentolamine into ischemic area at first signs of extravasation	Injectable: 10, 20 mg/ml	*Contraindicated* in severe heart disease *Not recommended* for prolonging the effects of *local* anesthetics Can cause tissue necrosis/gangrene because of excessive vasoconstriction when injected with local anesthetics in fingers or toes May cause projectile vomiting, bradycardia, or urinary urgency Use with caution in patients with a history of strokes, hypertension, hyperthyroidism, bradycardia, partial heart block, or peripheral arteriosclerosis	Monitor color and temperature of extremities Monitor blood pressure
Metoprolol Betaloc Lopressor Seloken	Hypertension Angina pectoris	*Adults:* Initially, 100 mg/24 hr PO in 2 divided doses; increase at weekly intervals if required Maintenance: 100-450 mg/24 hr PO in 2 divided doses When *discontinuation* of therapy is planned, discontinue gradually over 2 weeks	Tablets: 50, 100 mg; slow-release: 200 mg	*Contraindicated* in heart failure, sinus bradycardia, and cardiogenic shock Possesses a *negative* inotropic effect Abrupt cessation of therapy has resulted in angina, myocardial infarction, and ventricular dysrhythmia	Monitor heart rate and respiratory status

Drug	Indication	Dosage	Preparation	Remarks	Monitoring
Naphazoline Albalon Albalon Liquifilm Albalon-A* Antistine-Privine* Clear Eyes Degest-2 Naphcon Naphcon Forte Optozoline Privine Rhino-Mex Rhino-Mex-N Vaso Clear Vasocon Vasocon A* Vasocon Regular Zincfrin-A* 20/20 Eye Drops 4-Way Nasal Spray* 4-Way*	Nasal congestion As an ocular vasoconstrictor	*Adults:* 2 drops or sprays in nostrils q.4-6h. *Children:* Over 6 years of age, same as adults *Adults:* 1-2 drops of ophthalmic solution in conjunctival sac q.3-4h. as required *Children:* Use *not* recommended	Nasal drops: 0.05% Nasal spray: 0.05% Ophthalmic solution: 0.1%	*Contraindicated* in narrow-angle glaucoma *Overdose* (particularly in children) may result in hypothermia, CNS depression, respiratory depression, and cardiovascular collapse May cause rebound nasal congestion Similar to phenylephrine topical preparations	Monitor blood pressure and heart rate Monitor for overuse (abuse) particularly of nasal products in young patients
Norepineph-rine Levophed	Acute hypotensive states *not* caused by hypovolemia	*Adults:* 8-12 µg/min by IV infusion *initially* and then 2-4 µg/min to desired response *Dilute before usage* Infuse into large vein such as the antecubital to minimize chance of extravasation; check periodically for free flow; infiltrate 5-10 mg of phentolamine into ischemic area at first signs of extravasation NOTE: Correct hypovolemia *before* administration	Injectable: 1 mg/ml *Store* in cool place protected from light Destroyed by alkalis (e.g., sodium bicarbonate) and by oxidizing agents (e.g., oxygen, nitrites, and ferric salts) Dilute 4 mg in 1000 ml of D_5W	*Contraindicated* in blood volume deficits and during cyclopropane or halothane anesthesia Use with caution in patients receiving tricyclic antidepressants or MAOIs Tends to cause a greater elevation of diastolic pressure and more reflex bradycardia than epinephrine; also causes less cardiac stimulation than epinephrine Produces more peripheral vasoconstriction than epinephrine	Monitor blood pressure every 2 min initially, then every 5 min after it has stabilized Monitor IV site for extravasation and free flow

Continued.

NURSING DRUG DIGEST—cont'd

Medication (trade name)	Indication	Usual dosage and administration	Dosage forms, preparation, and storage	Contraindications, cautions, and comments	Monitoring
Nylidrin Arlidin Circlidrin Dilatyl Perdilatal Pervadil Rolidrin	Peripheral vascular diseases	*Adults:* 12-48 mg/24 hr PO in 3-4 divided doses	Tablets: 6, 12 mg	*Contraindicated* in acute myocardial infarction, paroxysmal tachycardia, and thyrotoxicosis. Use with caution in congestive heart failure and tachycardia. Beneficial effect may take several weeks	Monitor for palpitations (chief side effect) Monitor extremities for relief of pain, increased temperature, improved color, and healing of tissue
Oxymetazoline Afrin Afrin Pediatric Drixine Duration Duration Mentholated Vapor Spray Hazol Nafrine Neo-Synephrine 12-Hour Ocuclear St. Joseph Decongestant for Children St. Joseph Nasal Spray/Drops	Nasal congestion As an ocular vasoconstrictor	*Adults:* 2-3 drops or sprays of the 0.05% solution in each nostril b.i.d. *Children:* 2-5 years of age 2-3 drops or sprays of the 0.025% solution in each nostril b.i.d., over 6 years of age, same as adult *Adults:* 1-2 drops of ophthalmic solution in conjunctival sac t.i.d. to q.i.d. *Children:* Over 6 years of age, same as adults	Nasal drops: 0.025%, 0.05% Nasal spray: 0.025%, 0.05% Ophthalmic solution: 0.025%	Similar to phenylephrine nasal preparations May cause rebound nasal congestion Use with caution in patients with hypertension or diabetes mellitus	Monitor for rebound nasal congestion
★ **Phenoxybenzamine** Dibenzyline	Hypertension resulting from inoperable pheochromocytoma	*Adults:* Initially, 10 mg/24 hr PO Increase by 10 mg/24 hr at 4-day intervals Maintenance: 20-60 mg/24 hr PO	Capsule: 10 mg	*Contraindicated* in patients with a history of myocardial infarction or angina *Warning:* can cause severe orthostatic hypotension and tachycardia or a hypotensive state	Monitor blood pressure in lying, sitting and standing positions daily until stable

Drug	Uses	Dosage	Preparations	Nursing Considerations
Phentolamine Regitine Rogitine	Control hypertensive episodes caused by pheochromocytoma or drugs possessing α-adrenergic activity	*Adults:* 200-300 mg/24 hr PO in 4-6 divided doses *Children:* 100-150 mg/24 hr PO in 4-6 divided doses Reduce dosage in patients with renal impairment	Tablet: 50 mg Injectable: 5 mg/1 ml To reconstitute, add 1 ml of sterile water for injection to the 5 mg in vial Use solution *immediately after* reconstitution	Monitor heart rate and blood pressure until maintenance dosage is established Teach patient how to manage hypotension This agent has a slow onset of action and its effects may last for several days after cessation of therapy Individualize dosage for each patient Norepinephrine (2-4 µg/min IV) or an α-adrenergic agonist is recommended as an antidote; do not use epinephrine because it will excessively stimulate the heart (β-adrenergic effects are more prominent)
	Test for pheochromocytoma	*Adults:* 5 mg IV *Children:* 1 mg IV A fall in blood pressure by more than 35 mm Hg systolic or 25 mm Hg diastolic confirms the diagnosis		*Contraindicated* in patients with a history of myocardial infarction or angina *Warning:* can cause severe hypotensive states, especially after parenteral administration; orthostatic hypotension is common; teach patient how to manage hypotension Norepinephrine, (2-4 µg/min IV) or an α-adrenergic agonist is recommended as an antidote; do not use epinephrine because it produces more prominent cardiac stimulation Determination of urinary catecholamine levels is now the preferred method for diagnosing pheochromocytoma Monitor blood pressure, particularly after IM or IV administration

Continued.

NURSING DRUG DIGEST—cont'd

Medication (trade name)	Indication	Usual dosage and administration	Dosage forms, preparation, and storage	Contraindications, cautions, and comments	Monitoring
Phenylephrine Alamine* Allerest Nasal Citra* Citra Forte* Clistin-D* Codimal PH* Colrex* Comhist* Conar* Congespirin* Contac Nasal Mist Coricidin Nasal Spray Degest Dimetane Expectorant* Dimetapp Elixir* Dristan* Isuprel-Neo Mistometer* Naldecon* Neo-Synephrine Novahistex* Novahistine LP* NTZ P-V Tussin Syrup* Prefrin Pyracort-D Romex* Romilar* Ru-Tuss* Sinarest Nasal Spray* Sinex Super Anahist Nasal Spray Vacon	Acute hypotension not caused by hypovolemia	*Adults:* Usual mode is SC or IM, up to 2 mg *initially*, then 2-5 mg *not more often than* q.1h. *In emergency:* 0.1-0.5 mg IV *not more often than* q.10-15 min	Injection: 2, 10 mg/ml Nasal solution: 0.125% to 1% Nasal spray: 0.25% and 0.5% Nasal jelly: 0.5% Ophthalmic solutions: 0.12%, 2.5%, 10% *Store* solutions in cool place protected from light *Discard* brownish solutions or those containing a precipitate	*Contraindicated* in patients with narrow-angle glaucoma, severe hypertension, ventricular tachycardia, and in those receiving MAOIs, tricyclic antidepressants, or guanethidine-like drugs Phentolamine in a dose of 5-10 mg IV can be used as an antidote for excessive hypertension	Individualize the dosage, especially during parenteral use by monitoring blood pressure, urine output, and ECG frequently Monitor diabetics carefully, especially urine sugar and acetone and blood sugars Monitor for fullness in head or tingling of extremities
	Paroxysmal supraventricular tachycardia	*Adults: initially,* 0.1-0.5 mg IV; increase dosage if required, but do not exceed 1 mg		Use with caution in patients with a history of stroke, hypertension, hyperthyroidism, bradycardia, partial heart block, or peripheral arteriosclerosis	
	Prolong spinal anesthesia	*Adults:* add 2-5 mg to anesthetic solution		Use in pregnancy should be avoided	
	Nasal congestion	*Adults:* 1-2 drops or sprays of 0.25%-1% solution in each nostril q.3-4h. *Children:* Under 6 years of age, 1-2 drops of 0.125%-0.2% nasal solution in each nostril q.2-4h.; over 6 years of age, 1-2 drops of 0.25% in each nostril q.3-4h.		Excessive peripheral vasoconstriction/hypertension may develop in patients on ergot alkaloids, vasopressin (ADH), or oxytocin	
	Wide-angle glaucoma	*Adults:* 1 drop of 10% solution to upper cornea as required, not more often than q.30-60 min		An increase in the dosage of insulin or oral hypoglycemic drug may be required in diabetics	
	To produce mydriasis	*Adults:* 1 drop of 2.5%-10% ophthalmic solution in each eye		May cause hyperglycemia in diabetics	
	As an ocular vasoconstrictor See also Chapter 29, "Antihistamines, Antitussives, Decongestants, and Expectorants"	*Adults:* 1-2 drops of 0.12% ophthalmic solution in conjunctival sac q.3-4h. as required		Excessive topical nasal use may cause drug-induced rhinitis; allow several days before resumption of medication Avoid the use of topical nasal preparations for more than 3-5 consecutive days	

Drug	Use	Dosage	Preparations	Nursing implications
Vicks Sinex Decongestant Nasal Spray* 4-Way Cold*				Transitory stinging or pain can be expected when applied topically to the eye Teach correct administration to patient/family and to use only as directed
★ **Phenylpropanolamine** A.R.M. Allergy Relief Medicine* Allerest* Ayds Weight Suppressant Bayer Decongestant* Breacol* Comtrex* Congesprin* Contac* Coricidin "D"* Daycare* Dexatrim Dietac Dimetane Expectorant* Formula 44-D* Head & Chest Cold Medicine* Propadrine Sinarest* Sine-Aid* Sine-Off* Sinutab* Triaminic*	Nasal decongestant Adjunct in weight reduction (together with caloric restriction) See also Chapter 29, "Antihistamines, Antitussives, Decongestants, and Expectorants"	*Adult:* 25 mg q.4h. PO; or timed-release capsule 75 mg PO q.12h. *Children:* 6-12 years, 12.5 mg PO q.4h.; 2-6 years, 6.25 mg PO q.4h. *Adults:* 25 mg PO t.i.d.; or 75-150 mg PO (timed-release) once daily	Tablets: 25, 50, 100 mg Capsules: 25, 37.5, 50 mg Timed-release capsules: 75, 150 mg Elixir: 20 mg/5 ml Syrup: 12.5 mg/5 ml	Monitor blood pressure Similar to phenylephrine nasal preparation More vasoconstrictive action and less CNS stimulation than with ephedrine Older men may have difficulty voiding

Continued.

NURSING DRUG DIGEST—cont'd

Medication (trade name)	Indication	Usual dosage and administration	Dosage forms, preparation, and storage	Contraindications, cautions, and comments	Monitoring
Prazosin Hypovase Minipress Minizide*	Hypertension See also Chapter 33, "Antihypertensives"	*Adults:* Initially 1 mg PO q.h.s.; gradually increase to 3 mg/24 hr in 3 divided doses over a few days Maintenance dose should be arrived at gradually and should not exceed 20 mg/24 hr PO in 3 divided doses	Capsules: 1, 2, 5 mg	Dosage must be increased gradually to avoid syncopal reactions and excessive tachycardia; these reactions occur especially during the first few days of therapy and then tolerance to them usually develops Additive or potentiated hypotensive effects can be expected if the patient is already receiving other antihypertensive drugs Because of the tendency of this agent to cause tachycardia, prazosin is best avoided in patients with angina pectoris Most effective if used with a diuretic *Caution* not to withdraw medication suddenly Dizziness or drowsiness may decrease alertness	Monitor for dizziness, drowsiness, and headache
Propranolol Avlocardyl Detensol Inderal Inderal-LA Inderide* Noropranol Panolol	Cardiac dysrhythmias Angina pectoris	*Adults:* 40-120 mg/24 hr PO in 4 divided doses, before meals, and q.h.s. *In emergencies:* 1-3 mg IV at the rate of 1 mg/min; second dose after 2 min if necessary; subsequent doses at 4-hr intervals if necessary *Adults: Initially,* 40 to 80 mg/24 hr PO in 4 divided doses, before meals, and q.h.s.; increase dosage if needed at 3 to 7-day intervals Maintenance: 160-320 mg/24 hr PO in 2-4 divided doses	Tablets: 10, 20, 40, 60, 80 mg Capsules (controlled-release): 80, 120, 160 mg (for once-daily dosing) Injectable: 1 mg/ml	*Contraindicated* in patients with bradycardia, heart failure, myocardial infarction, asthma, bronchitis, or emphysema Individualize dosage to obtain optimal therapeutic effects with minimal side effects Use with caution in patients on anesthetics, phenothiazines, antidiabetic drugs, or clonidine	Monitor heart rate, blood pressure, and respiration Monitor ECG and central venous pressure during IV administration Monitor blood glucose in diabetic patients and in patients subject to hypoglycemic episodes

Hypertension	Adult: Initially, 80 mg/24 hr PO in 2 divided doses; increase dosage at weekly intervals if needed Maintenance: 160-480 mg/24 hr PO in 2-4 divided doses	Use with caution in patients subject to hypoglycemic episodes Do not discontinue abruptly; this may cause severe angina attacks or even induce myocardial infarction in susceptible patients
Pheochromocytoma with an α-adrenergic blocker	Adults: 30-60 mg/24 hr PO in 3-4 divided doses, before meals, and q.h.s.	Diabetics may require decreased dosage of insulin or oral hypoglycemic drugs; signs of hypoglycemia may be masked Additive hypotensive effects can be expected with other hypotensive agents Onset of maximal antihypertensive effects may take several weeks
Hypertrophic subaortic stenosis	Adults: 80-160 mg/24 hr PO in 4 divided doses, before meals, and q.h.s.	If drug-induced, excessive sinus bradycardia develops, it can be treated with 0.25 to 1.0 mg of atropine PO or IV
Prophylaxis of migraine headache See also Chapters 32, "Antidysrhythmics" and 33, "Antihypertensives"	Adults: Initially, 80 mg/24 hr PO in 2 divided doses; gradually increase at weekly intervals if required Maintenance: 80-160 mg/24 hr PO in 2 divided doses Maximum: 240 mg/24 hr	Should not be used without an α-adrenergic blocker in pheochromocytoma; otherwise excessive hypertension may occur Used to control some of the cardiovascular and other symptoms of hyperthyroidism, such as tremor, anxiety, and stare May mask some of the signs and symptoms of hyperthyroidism and make diagnosis more difficult

Continued.

NURSING DRUG DIGEST—cont'd

Medication (trade name)	Indication	Usual dosage and administration	Dosage forms, preparation, and storage	Contraindications, cautions, and comments	Monitoring
Propylhexedrine Benzedrex Dristan Inhaler Eventin	Nasal congestion	*Adults:* Insert tube into nostril, close other nostril, and inhale twice; use only as needed	Plastic inhaler tube: 250 mg Once opened, the active ingredient is lost by evaporation in 2-3 months	*Contraindicated* in narrow-angle glaucoma May cause rebound congestion	Observe for drug abuse (propylhexedrine is removed from inhaler and injected IV by addicts)
Pseudoephedrine Actifed* Afrinol Repetabs Benylin Decongestant* Chlor-Trimeton Decongestant* CoTylenol Cold Formula* Drixoral* Fedahist* First Sign Multi-Symptom* Novahistine Sinus* Nucofed* Robitussin-PE* Sinufed Sudafed Sudafed S.A.	Nasal or eustachian tube congestion See also Chapter 29, "Antihistamines, Antitussives, Decongestants, and Expectorants"	*Adults:* 60 mg tablet q.4h. PO; or 60 to 120 mg timed-release capsule q.8-12h. Maximum: 240 mg/24 hr *Children:* 6-12 years, 30 mg q.4h. PO; or 60 mg timed-release capsule q.8-12h.; 2-5 years, 15 mg PO q.6h. Maximum: 60 mg/24 hr	Tablets: 30, 60 mg; repeat-action: 120 mg Timed-release capsules: 60, 120 mg Syrup: 30 mg/5 ml	Similar to phenylephrine nasal preparations Use with caution in hypertensive patients	Monitor blood pressure

Drug	Uses	Dosage	Precautions	Nursing Implications
Reserpine Butiserp-azide* Demi-Regro-ton* Ebserserp Geneserp Hiserpia Lemiserp Neo-Serp R-HCTZ-H* Rau-Sed Rauloydin Raurine Regroton* Relaserp-S Renese-R* Resercen Resercrine Reserfia Reserjen Reserpanca Reserpoid Roxinoid Salutensin* Sandril Ser-Ap-Es* Serfin Seroalan Serpanray Serpasil Serpasil-Apresoline* Serpate SK-Reserpine Triserp Vio-Serpine Vioserp Zepine	Hypertension Hypertensive crises See also Chapter 18, "Drugs Used to Treat Psychotic Disorders," and Chapter 33, "Antihypertensives"	*Adults:* Initially, 0.5 mg/24 hr PO for 1-2 weeks Maintenance: 0.1-0.25 mg/24 hr PO *Adults:* 0.5-1 mg IM followed by 2 to 4 mg IM q.3h as required Tablets: 0.1-1 mg Capsule: 0.5 mg Elixir: 0.2 mg/4 ml Injectable: 2.5 mg/1 ml	*Contraindicated* in patients with a history of depression Discontinue drug if patient becomes depressed; this may progress to a suicidal tendency Use with caution in patients with peptic ulcers, ulcerative colitis, or asthma Use with caution in patients receiving other antihypertensive agents Additive hypotensive effects can be expected when used with other agents capable of lowering blood pressure Now seldom used for psychiatric disorders because of the availability of more effective agents (see also Chapter 18, "Drugs Used to Treat Psychotic Disorders") The onset of maximum antihypertensive action may take several weeks After cessation of therapy, reserpine's effects may last for several weeks; therefore discontinue therapy, if possible, 2 weeks before elective surgery to avoid possible cardiovascular collapse or cardiac arrest during anesthesia	Monitor blood pressure lying, sitting and standing at regular intervals Monitor weight twice weekly for fluid retention and edema Monitor for signs of drug-induced depression

Continued.

NURSING DRUG DIGEST—cont'd

Medication (trade name)	Indication	Usual dosage and administration	Dosage forms, preparation, and storage	Contraindications, cautions, and comments	Monitoring
Terbutaline Brethine Bricanyl Filair	Acute bronchospasms	*Adults:* 0.25 mg SC into lateral deltoid area; repeat same dose if necessary in 15-30 min; if no response, consider other agents Maximum: 2.5 mg/24 hr	Tablets: 2.5, 5 mg Injectable: 1 mg/1ml Discard discolored solutions Store in light-resistant containers	Tends to produce fewer adverse cardiac effects than isoproterenol Prolonged use may cause tolerance May cause nervousness and tremor Use with caution in patients with diabetes, hypertension, or seizure disorders	
	Bronchospasms or asthma See also Chapter 28, "Bronchodilators and Respiratory Gases"	*Adults:* 7.5-15 mg/24 hr PO in 3 divided doses *Children:* Use is *not* recommended			
★ **Tetrahydrozoline** Murine Plus Murine 2 Ocusol Drops Soothe Eye Drops Tyzine Visine Eye Drops	Nasal congestion	*Adults:* 2-4 drops or sprays of 0.1% into each nostril not more often than q.3h. *Children:* 6-12 years, 2 drops or sprays of 0.1%; 2-6 years, 2 drops of 0.05%; do not repeat doses more often than q.3h.	Nasal solution: 0.05, 0.1% Nasal spray: 0.1% Ophthalmic solution: 0.05%	Similar to phenylephrine topical preparations *Contraindicated* in narrow-angle glaucoma May cause rebound nasal congestion	
	As an ocular vasoconstrictor	*Adults:* 1-2 drops ophthalmic solution in each eye b.i.d. to t.i.d.			
Timolol Betim Blocadren Tamserin Timolide* Timoptic Timoptol	Wide-angle glaucoma	*Adults:* 1 drop of 0.25%-0.5% ophthalmic solution in each eye b.i.d.	Ophthalmic solution: 0.25%, 0.5% Tablets: 5, 10 mg	*Contraindicated* in COPD, cardiogenic shock, sinus bradycardia, and heart failure When used topically, it may occasionally produce ocular irritation Local hypersensitivity reactions are rare Can be used concurrently with miotics, epinephrine, or carbonic anhydrase inhibitors to treat wide-angle glaucoma	Monitor for development of congestive heart failure and dyspnea Continued, regular intraocular measurements by an ophthalmologist should be completed to monitor response
	Prophylaxis maintenance *after* myocardial infarction	*Adults:* 10 mg PO b.i.d.			
	Angina pectoris	*Adults:* Initially 10-15 mg/24 hr PO in 2-3 divided doses; increase dose if required at 3-day intervals Maximum: 45 mg/day			

	Hypertension	*Adults:* Initially, 10-20 mg/24 hr PO in 2 divided doses; increase dose if required at 2-week intervals Maximum: 60 mg/day		May cause congestive heart failure, dyspnea, hypotension, headache, vomiting, and diarrhea
Xylometazoline Dristamead Long Dristan Long Lasting Nasal Mist Dristan Long Lasting Vapor Nasal Mist Duramist PM Hydra-Spray Neo-Synephrine II Otrivin Sine-Off Once-A-Day Sinex-L.A. Sinus Spray Sinutab Long-lasting Decongestant Sinus Spray Sinutab Nasal Spray Sustaine Vicks Sinex Long-Acting Decongestant Nasal Spray 4-Way Long Acting Nasal Spray	Nasal congestion See also Chapter 29, "Antihistamines, Antitussives, Decongestants, and Expectorants"	*Adults:* 2-3 drops or sprays of 0.1% in each nostril q.8-12h. *Children:* 1-3 drops or sprays of 0.05% in each nostril q.8-12h.	Nasal solution: 0.05%, 0.1% Nasal spray: 0.05%, 0.1%	Similar to phenylephrine nasal preparations Decongestant effect lasts 6-12 hr

BIBLIOGRAPHY

Avery, G.S. (Ed.). *Drug treatment: principles and practice of clinical pharmacology and therapeutics* (2nd ed.). New York: Adis, 1980.

Barrows, J.J. Shock demands drugs. *Nursing 82,* 1982, *12,* 34-41.

Compendium of pharmaceuticals and specialties (19th ed.). Ottawa: Canadian Pharmaceutical Association, 1984.

Cooper, J.R., Bloom, F.E., & Roth, R.H. *The biochemical basis of neuropharmacology* (3rd ed.). New York: Oxford University Press, 1978.

Day, M.A. *Autonomic pharmacology: experimental and clinical aspects.* New York: Churchill Livingston, 1979.

Rivera-Calimlim, L. A short review of adrenergic drug therapy. *Nurses' Drug Alert,* 1981, *5,* 25-27.

Smith-Collins, A. Dobutamine a new inotropic agent. *Nursing 80,* 1980, *10,* 62.

Anticholinesterases and Cholinesterase Reactivators

David F. Biggs

Medications discussed in this chapter

Reversible anticholinester-ases
Ambenonium
Demecarium
Distigmine
Edrophonium
Galantamine
Neostigmine
Physostigmine
Pyridostigmine

Irreversible anticholinester-ases
Echothiophate
Isoflurophate
Antagonist of irreversible anticholinesterases
Atropine
Cholinesterase reactivator
Pralidoxime

This chapter describes the effects and uses of drugs that inhibit cholinesterases. *Cholinesterases*, which were discovered by Hunt and Taveaux in 1906, is the term applied to a family of enzymes that catalyze the hydrolysis of choline esters, particularly acetylcholine (ACh). From their biochemical properties and physiologic functions, cholinesterases (ChEs) can be classified into two major groups: true, or acetylcholinesterase (AChE), and pseudocholinesterase, butyryl-cholinesterase, or cholinesterase (ChE).

ACETYLCHOLINESTERASE

AChE is one of the most efficient enzymes known; its tetrameric basic unit has a molecular weight of about 320,000. The active center of the enzyme consists of a negatively charged (anionic) site that attracts the quaternary nitrogen of acetylcholine and an esteratic site that attracts and attacks the acyl carbon of the substrate. Anticholinesterases can inhibit the enzyme through interaction at either or both sites.

AChE is found in high concentrations in the gray matter of the brain, in autonomic ganglia, at the *motor endplates*, and in erythrocytes. It is most effective at hydrolyzing acetylcholine, and much less effective

against other choline esters. Its major physiologic function is inactivation of the neurotransmitter acetylcholine.

CHOLINESTERASE

ChE is located in the intestinal mucosa, the liver, the white matter of the brain, and in the plasma. It is capable of hydrolyzing many aliphatic choline esters and several aromatic esters. Its function in the body is not entirely known, but it is believed to play a role in the homeostasis of plasma choline levels. Several variants of ChE are known to occur in humans. Many people who possess these "atypical" ChEs may be especially sensitive to skeletal muscle relaxants such as succinylcholine and suxethonium because of the inability of these patients' ChE to hydrolyze these drugs. Sensitivity can be moderately or markedly increased; the major clinical feature observed is prolonged apnea after administration of the muscle relaxant succinylcholine. The incidence of this phenomenon is highly variable and ranges from 1 in 200 to 1 in 200,000 individuals depending on the ChE variant involved. (See Chapter 9, "Genetic Factors Affecting Drug Response").

ANTICHOLINESTERASES

Anticholinesterases (antiChE), as the term implies, inhibit the hydrolysis of choline esters by ChEs. The first anticholinesterase discovered, physostigmine, was isolated in the mid-nineteenth century from the calabar bean, the dried seed of *Physostigmina venenosum*. Interestingly, physostigmine was known and used in the treatment of glaucoma before cholinesterases were described. Physostigmine is sometimes referred to as "eserine," the name given to it by the second group to isolate this alkaloid. In the 1930's, synthetic anticholinesterases such as neostigmine and edrophonium were prepared, and the former was used in the treatment of myasthenia gravis. *Organo-phosphate* anticholinesterases were developed initially in Germany as insecticides and then during World War II as chemical warfare agents (i.e., "nerve gases"). Extensive research after the war resulted in more than 30 selectively toxic, commercially available insecticides. In the mid-1950's aromatic carbamates (e.g., carbaryl) were introduced, also as insecticides. Today the majority of anticholinesterase agents are used as insecticides; the clinical use of these agents is limited to a few specific indications.

Anticholinesterases can be conveniently divided into two major groups: (1) reversible anticholinesterases and (2) irreversible anticholinesterases. This division reflects more the duration of inhibition observed than the actual mechanism involved in inactivating the enzyme. Anticholinesterases classified as *reversible* include ambenonium, benzpyrinium, demecarium, distigmine, edrophonium, galantamine, neostigmine, physostigmine, and pyridostigmine. Of these only edrophonium and ambenonium interact noncovalently with the enzyme. The other drugs carbamylate the enzyme's esteratic site. The carbamylated enzyme is much more stable than the normal acetylated form, and inhibition, dependent on the rate of hydrolysis of the carbamyl-enzyme, results. Clinically, agents that carbamylate the enzyme induce inhibition for 3 to 4 hours.

Irreversible anticholinesterases include echothiophate and isoflurophate. Also most of the organophosphate insecticides (e.g., malathion, parathion) and so-called nerve gases (e.g., sarin, soman, tabun) fall into this category. These agents phosphorylate the esteratic site. Unlike carbamylated enzyme, the rate of hydrolysis of phosphorylated enzyme back to its normal form is often extremely slow—so slow, in fact, that reactivation does not occur to a significant degree, and the return of cholinesterase activity depends entirely on the biosynthesis of new enzyme. The stability of the phosphorylated enzyme is also increased by "aging," a process resulting from the loss of an alkyl group from the phosphorylator.

Summary of effects of anticholinesterases

All anticholinesterases have similar systemic effects: they prevent breakdown of the neurotransmitter acetylcholine, which then accumulates causing an enhancement and prolongation of its physiologic effects. If poisoning caused by overdose occurs, it is characterized by signs of overactivity of the parasympathetic division of the autonomic nervous system (ANS) (see Chapter 23, "Parasympathomimetics and Parasympatholytics") including miosis, salivation and lacri-

mation, bronchospasm and wheezing, cramping and diarrhea, and involuntary urination. These signs and symptoms may be accompanied by muscular weakness and convulsions depending on the degree of poisoning and the anticholinesterase involved.

The physicochemical properties of the anticholinesterase drugs determine to a large degree their clinical use. Quaternary ammonium salts, such as the reversible anticholinesterases neostigmine and pyridostigmine, are 100% ionized in plasma and do *not* cross the blood-brain barrier to an appreciable extent, rendering them suitable for use peripherally. By contrast, physostigmine, a tertiary amine, even though it is more than 90% ionized at plasma pH, readily crosses the blood-brain barrier. In general, organophosphate anticholinesterases readily penetrate the skin and mucous membranes and are rapidly and completely absorbed on inhalation.

Clinical indications

Myasthenia gravis. Anticholinesterases are used to increase acetylcholine levels at the skeletal neuromuscular junction. The quaternary drugs neostigmine and pyridostigmine are most commonly used to avoid central nervous system (CNS) side effects. The result of therapy is an increase in muscle power and decreased fatigability. Drugs commonly used are neostigmine, pyridostigmine, ambenonium, and, outside North America, galantamine. Edrophonium, a short-acting drug, is used in the diagnosis of myasthenia gravis.

Reversal of neuromuscular blockade. Edrophonium, neostigmine, and pyridostigmine are effective in reversing neuromuscular paralysis resulting from the use of *nondepolarizing* muscle relaxants such as tubocurarine and pancuronium. They are not effective against depolarizing relaxants such as succinylcholine and decamethonium.

Gastrointestinal disorders. Anticholinesterases are used occasionally to treat paralytic ileus and for expelling flatus before x-ray examination of the gallbladder, kidneys, or ureters.

Genitourinary disorders. These drugs are used to treat postoperative urinary retention and to modulate bladder function in paraplegics and quadraplegics.

Glaucoma. Physostigmine, echothiophate, demecarium, and isoflurophate are used in the treatment of simple glaucoma and glaucoma following cataract extraction. The drugs are always applied topically to the eye for treatment of glaucoma.

Reversal of anticholinergic and tricyclic antidepressant poisoning. Physostigmine and occasionally other anticholinesterases are used systemically to reverse poisoning from anticholinergic drugs (e.g., atropine, hyoscine) and tricyclic antidepressants (e.g., amitriptyline, imipramine).

Other uses. Anticholinesterases, in particular physostigmine, have been used topically to reverse the effects of anticholinergic agents in the eye; and systemically to treat some forms of ataxia, mania, tardive dyskinesia, Gilles de la Tourette's syndrome, constipation in megacolon, atrial tachycardia and fibrillation, and to improve memory in Alzheimer's disease. Edrophonium is used to treat supraventricular tachycardias (e.g., atrial tachycardia and fibrillation).

Antagonism of anticholinesterase poisoning

Organophosphate anticholinesterases (e.g., parathion) were one of the new classes of insecticides that emerged after World War II. Unlike chlorinated hydrocarbons such as DDT, organophosphates do not persist in the environment. However, they do cause acute poisoning in animals and humans when used improperly. The *carbamates* (e.g., carbaryl), another class of insecticides with anticholinesterase activity, also poses no environmental problems but can cause acute poisoning if misused. The *sulfonates*, a less common class of insecticides, have properties similar to the organophosphates.

Poisoning most frequently results from the use of these classes of compounds in agriculture. Victims have usually been exposed by dermal absorption or by inhalation during spraying of fields, crops, and buildings. Poisoning has also occurred by these routes in industrial and scientific workers. Occasionally, people ingest large quantities of these insecticides in attempts to commit suicide. The toxicity of these agents results from their ability to inhibit cholinesterases and, in particular, acetylcholinesterase. The actions of acetylcholine have been described previously. Inhibition of cholinesterases results in the accumulation of acetylcholine and enhancement, augmentation, and prolongation of its effects.

Rapid appraisal of the severity of poisoning can be achieved by observing if the patient is: (1) able to walk, (2) unable to walk but conscious, or (3) unconscious. This is a rough guide of mild, moderate, or severe poisoning. In mild poisoning signs and symptoms reflect hyperactivity of the parasympathetic division of the autonomic nervous system. The sympathetic division may be involved in moderate and severe poisoning.

Signs and symptoms of parasympathetic hyperactivity include bronchospasm (mild dyspnea with some wheezing), increased lacrimation, increased salivation, increased sweating, vomiting, bradycardia, invol-

untary defecation, involuntary urination, abdominal cramps, and miosis. In addition, muscle weakness, *fasciculations*, and twitching may be seen. Organophosphates, sulfonates, and many carbamates cross the blood-brain barrier. Here their actions cause excessive dreaming, nightmares, emotional lability, tension, anxiety, restlessness, dizziness, impairment of memory, and speech defects. At moderate and severe levels of poisoning, convulsions and coma may occur. Death results from respiratory failure caused by respiratory muscle weakness and paralysis, central depression of respiration, and airway obstruction.

To understand the therapy of acute anticholinesterase poisoning, one must first examine the mechanism of the inhibitory effects of these agents. Acetylcholine is hydrolyzed to acetate and choline by ChEs. The important enzyme is *acetylcholinesterase* (AChE); it is the inhibition of this enzyme—not ChE—that results in toxicity. Inhibition of AChE by organophosphates, sulfonates, and carbamates occurs by a similar mechanism. Inhibition is regarded as irreversible for organophosphates and sulfonates because the covalent bond formed between the phosphates or sulfonate is very stable and difficult to hydrolyze. In addition, with some organophosphates, aging may increase the stability of the bonding and further decrease the reversibility of the blockade. Inhibition by carbamates gives a covalent bond that is hydrolyzable but at a much slower rate than acetylcholine. The inhibitory product of AChE and a carbamate is generally not a significant therapeutic problem since hydrolysis of the product takes place over 4 to 8 hours, making the poisoning self-limiting. Emergency treatment usually consists of the use of atropine and the maintenance of respiration.

CHOLINESTERASE REACTIVATORS

The stable, nonhydrolyzable product of AChE and organophosphates or sulfonates is a different therapeutic problem. Inhibited enzyme is hydrolyzed back to AChE at a slow and comparatively insignificant rate. Reactivators can be used to achieve measurable conversion of inhibited enzyme to AChE. Cholinesterase reactivators include diacetyl monoxime, pralidoxime, obidoxime, and trimedoxime. These compounds contain an oxime group that attacks the phosphorus (or sulfur) atom and combines with it to form an oxime-phosphonate. This is then released by the enzyme regenerating the AChE. The oxime-phosphonate then decomposes to give a nitrile and phosphate, avoiding the possibility of an undesirable reverse reaction.

If the AChE-inhibitor complex has undergone aging

(further chemical change), the phosphorylated enzyme may be resistant to the actions of reactivators.

The emergency treatment of organophosphate or sulfonate poisoning involves administration of atropine, maintenance of respiration, and administration of a cholinesterase reactivator (e.g., pralidoxime). In addition, it is important to prevent or reduce further absorption of the toxic material.

PROCEDURE FOR TREATMENT OF ACUTE POISONING BY ORGANOPHOSPHATE, SULFONATE, AND CARBAMATE ANTICHOLINESTERASES AND INSECTICIDES

Order of priority

1. Establish airway, and administer artificial respiration.
   a. Air or oxygen must be supplied continuously.
   b. Be prepared to maintain artificial respiration for many hours.
2. Give atropine.
   a. Give atropine sulfate, 2 mg IM, and repeat every 3 to 8 minutes until signs of atropinization (dilated pupils, fast pulse) appear. Repeat 2 mg of atropine sulfate to maintain dilated pupils and pulse rate greater than 80 beats per minute.
   b. As much as 12 mg of atropine has been given safely in the first 2 hours, and 50 mg in the first 24 hours.
   c. Interruption of atropine therapy may be rapidly followed by fatal pulmonary edema or respiratory failure.
3. Give cholinesterase reactivator (e.g., pralidoxime).
   a. Do *not* use for carbamate poisoning.
   b. Use *only* with atropine.
   c. Give pralidoxime, 1 gm in aqueous solution (20 to 25 ml), IV *slowly*, not to exceed a rate of 500 mg per minute. Repeat after 30 minutes if respiration does not improve. This dose may be repeated twice within each period of 24 hours.
4. If victim's eyes are contaminated, they should be washed with running water or saline.
5. Remove all contaminated clothing and wash affected skin with soap and water.
   a. Wear gloves to avoid contamination.
   b. Using a cloth soaked in water, rub soap over the contaminated area firmly enough to remove any residues of the insecticide, as well as dirt and oil, but not so hard as to abrade the skin or produce reddening because this will increase percutaneous absorption. Rinse off soap with more water.
6. Lavage or emesis (for oral exposure)
   a. Remove ingested material by gastric lavage with water or by induction of emesis using syrup of ipecac, depending upon circumstances of poisoning and patient condition (e.g., conscious or unconscious).
   b. Induce emesis by giving 15 ml of syrup of ipecac orally followed by half a glass of water and repeat in 20 minutes if not effective initially.
7. General measures
   a. Pulmonary secretions are removed by postural drainage or by catheter suction.
   b. Avoid morphine, aminophylline, barbiturates, phenothiazines, and other respiratory depressants.
   c. Treat convulsions with diazepam, 2-10 mg IV at 1 mg per minute, or with trimethadione, 1 gm IV slowly up to maximum of 5 gm.

SUMMARY

This chapter has examined the various types and uses of the anticholinesterases and the cholinesterase reactivators. A brief review of the cholinesterases has been presented as a basis for understanding the mechanisms of action and effects of the anticholinesterases and the cholinesterase reactivators.

With an understanding of the various individual agents, including their actions and side effects, the nurse will be better able to provide optimal care to patients requiring these medications. Patient education can be enhanced; adverse drug effects can be anticipated, monitored for, and minimized; and clinically significant drug interactions can be avoided by utilizing the information presented in this chapter.

ADVERSE/SIDE EFFECTS OF THE ANTICHOLINESTERASES AND CHOLINESTERASE REACTIVATORS*

Reversible anticholinesterases†

CARDIOVASCULAR SYSTEM

Bradycardia
Hypotension
Paradoxical tachycardia

CENTRAL NERVOUS SYSTEM

Agitation
Coma
Convulsions
Fear
Hallucinations
Increased/excessive dreaming
Nystagmus
Restlessness

CUTANEOUS SYSTEM

Flushing
Increased perspiration

OCULAR SYSTEM (topical use)

Cataract formation (after long-term
    use)
Conjunctival congestion
Iris cyst formation
Lacrimation
Miosis (common)
Retinal detachment

GASTROINTESTINAL SYSTEM

Abdominal cramps (common)
Belching
Diarrhea (common)
Increased salivation (sialorrhea)
    (common)
Involuntary defecation
Nausea and vomiting (common)

GENITOURINARY SYSTEM

Involuntary urination
Urinary frequency

MUSCULOSKELETAL SYSTEM

Cholinergic crisis
Fasciculations
Increased fatigability

Muscle cramps
Muscle weakness
Twitching

RESPIRATORY SYSTEM

Bronchoconstriction
Dyspnea
Increased secretions
Rhinorrhea
Wheezing

Irreversible anticholinesterases

Used in medicine
    Echothiophate and isoflurophate;
        see Adverse/Side Effects of
        Reversible Agents and the
        Nursing Drug Digest
Not used in medicine
    Carbamates, organophosphates,
        and sulphonates used as
        insecticides

Antagonists of irreversible anticholinesterases and cholinesterase reactivators

Atropine
CARDIOVASCULAR SYSTEM

Circulatory depression
Tachycardia

CENTRAL NERVOUS SYSTEM

Coma
Confusion
Delirium
Excitement
Hallucinations
Hyperpyrexia
Pyrexia
Respiratory depression

CUTANEOUS SYSTEM

Dryness
Flushing

GASTROINTESTINAL SYSTEM

Constipation
Difficulty in swallowing
Dry mouth
Thirst

GENITOURINARY SYSTEM

Difficulty in urinating

OCULAR SYSTEM

Increased intraocular pressure
Loss of accommodation
Mydriasis

Pralidoxime and related compounds
CARDIOVASCULAR SYSTEM

Tachycardia

CENTRAL NERVOUS SYSTEM

Dizziness
Drowsiness
Headache
Visual disturbance

GASTROINTESTINAL SYSTEM

Nausea
Vomiting

MUSCULOSKELETAL SYSTEM

Hyperventilation
Muscular paralysis
Muscle weakness
NOTE: When pralidoxime and related
compounds are given together with
atropine, the signs of atropinization
can appear at lower doses of atropine
than when the drug is given alone.
Large doses of pralidoxime
intravenously have been reported to
cause transient neuromuscular
blockade.

*See Chapter 11, "Drug Toxicity," for an overview of drug toxicity.
†In myasthenia gravis, the primary symptom of overdosage is muscular weakness or increased fatigability.

CLINICALLY SIGNIFICANT DRUG INTERACTIONS*

Primary drug	Interacting drug	Possible effect(s)	Probable mechanism(s)
Anticholinesterases	Aminoglycoside antibiotics (e.g., streptomycin, gentamicin) Local anesthetics (e.g., lidocaine) Antidysrhythmic drugs, (e.g., procainamide, quinidine) Polymyxin antibiotics	Decreased therapeutic effect of anticholinesterase†	Neuromuscular blocking action antagonizes effects
Anticholinesterases	Depolarizing neuromuscular blockers, (e.g., succinylcholine)	Prolongation of neuromuscular blockade	Synergism with depolarizing neuromuscular blockers
	Nondepolarizing neuromuscular blockers, (e.g., tubocurarine, pancuronium)	Reduced effect of neuromuscular blockers Respiratory depression with apnea	Antagonism of neuromuscular blockers

*See Chapter 10, "Drug Interactions," for an overview of drug interactions.
†These interactions are *not* clinically significant in *normal* persons, but in patients suffering from myasthenia gravis who are poorly controlled or whose control is "brittle," these interactions are significant and potentially life threatening.

GENERAL NURSING IMPLICATIONS

Nursing of patients requiring reversible anticholinesterase medication

ASSESSMENT

Assessment of the patient is extremely important in relation to the specific condition that is being treated with this medication, because these medications can be used in the treatment of various conditions including myasthenia gravis, paralytic ileus, urinary retention, and for various x-ray procedures. They can be used in the treatment of simple glaucoma and glaucoma after cataract extraction. Drugs in this class can also be used to reverse poisoning from anticholinergic drugs (e.g., atropine, scopolamine) or antidepressants (e.g., amitriptyline, imipramine) as well as other medications.

In addition to general assessment and nursing history data, the initial data base should include specific data related to the patient's condition and a detailed drug history to identify sensitivity, contraindications, cautions, potential drug interactions, and drug-taking patterns before drug therapy is initiated.

SENSITIVITY

Any drug has the potential to cause a hypersensitivity reaction in susceptible individuals.

Because some of the anticholinesterases are formulated as iodide salts (see Nursing Drug Digest), careful assessment and monitoring of patients for iodide sensitivity (e.g., sensitivity to shellfish) should be performed. Such sensitivity constitutes a contraindication to use of these agents. Ambenonium may be of value in patients who cannot tolerate neostigmine or pyridostigmine.

CONTRAINDICATIONS

The use of reversible anticholinesterases is contraindicated in known hypersensitivity.

Routine administration of atropine with ambenonium to counter muscarinic side effects is contraindicated as symptoms of overdosage may be suppressed until the more serious nicotinic complications of muscle fasciculations and paralysis appear.

All anticholinesterases are contraindicated when mechanical intestinal or urinary obstruction exists.

CAUTIONS

These drugs should be used cautiously in patients with bradycardia, bronchial asthma, cardiac disease, epilepsy, hypotension, Parkinson's disease, or peptic ulceration.

If physostigmine is used to counteract atropine, homatropine, or cocaine mydriasis it can induce pain and irritation due to spasm.

Patients with recent bowel resections may be particularly at risk if neostigmine and related compounds are given to reverse the effects of a skeletal muscle relaxant even if atropine has been given.

Anticholinesterases should not be used in conjunction with *depolarizing* muscle relaxants (e.g., succinylcholine).

GENERAL NURSING IMPLICATIONS—cont'd

Nursing of patients requiring reversible anticholinesterase medication—cont'd

CAUTIONS—cont'd

These drugs should not be used *during* cyclopropane or halothane anesthesia. They may be used when anesthesia is withdrawn.

Anticholinesterases should not be given by injection to patients with diabetes or gangrene.

Acute cholinergic crisis may develop with the use of these agents.

DRUG INTERACTIONS

Anticholinesterases have the potential to interact with several drugs. See Clinically Significant Drug Interactions.

ADMINISTRATION

Anticholinesterases are available in either oral or parenteral (intramuscular or intravenous) forms.

See Nursing Drug Digest for specific administration of the various drugs in this class.

MONITORING PATIENT RESPONSE
Therapeutic response

The onset of anticholinesterase effect is largely dependent on the dosage form and route of administration as well as on individual patient factors. (See Nursing Drug Digest for specific drugs.) When monitoring therapeutic response, observations related to the patient's need for the medication should be observed for and documented. For example, if the drug is given for myasthenia gravis, the patient should be observed for increased muscle power and decreased fatigability. When given for treatment of Alzheimer's disease, improvement in memory should be monitored.

Adverse side effects

Adverse side effects occurring with anticholinesterases are outlined in Adverse/Side Effects. The nurse should have an understanding of the occurrence of these effects and plan to minimize troublesome common effects as well as monitor for more severe effects requiring the administration of counteractants.

Miotics such as physostigmine may induce retinal detachment in patients predisposed to this condition.

Patients receiving edrophonium should be monitored for cardiac abnormalities, respiratory muscle failure, and excessive bronchial secretions.

Toxic alopecia has been reported following the administration of pyridostigmine.

Toxic effects of physostigmine are usually more severe than those of quaternary anticholinesterases because of its ability to enter the brain.

Atropine sulfate can be given to counteract the undesirable parasympathomimetic actions of anticholinesterases in patients with myasthenia gravis.

PATIENT EDUCATION

The patient and family as indicated should have a clear understanding of the medication regimen as well as the exact name of the medication, its general action, dosage, storage, administration, and therapeutic effect. The patient should be made aware of common side effects and should be assisted with the minimization of these effects. The patient should be able to monitor therapeutic response as well as be able to identify signs that indicate the prescriber should be contacted (see General Instructions for Discharge/Outpatients).

Nursing of patients requiring irreversible anticholinesterase medication

ASSESSMENT

Assessment of the patient is important in relation to the specific condition that is being treated because these medications can be used in the treatment of various conditions. In addition to general assessment and nursing history data, the initial data base should include a detailed drug history to identify possible sensitivity, contraindications, cautions, drug interactions, and drug-taking patterns before drug therapy is initiated.

SENSITIVITY

Any drug has the potential to cause a hypersensitivity reaction in susceptible individuals.

CONTRAINDICATIONS

The use of irreversible anticholinesterases is contraindicated in patients with known hypersensitivity.

CAUTIONS

These drugs should be used cautiously in such conditions as asthma, bradycardia, parkinsonism, and peptic ulcer. See Nursing Drug Digest for cautions associated with the use of specific agents.

DRUG INTERACTIONS

Irreversible anticholinesterases have the potential to interact with other medications. See Clinically Significant Drug Interactions.

ADMINISTRATION

Irreversible anticholinesterases are available in dosage forms for specific indications including ophthalmic solutions. For example, irreversible anticholinesterases are sometimes used to treat certain forms of strabismus (esotropia).

See Nursing Drug Digest for information regarding the administration of specific medications in this class as well as other information. Medically used organophosphates such as echothiophate are often given with a systemic carbonic anhydrase inhibitor.

Continued.

GENERAL NURSING IMPLICATIONS—cont'd

Nursing of patients requiring irreversible anticholinesterase medication—cont'd

MONITORING PATIENT RESPONSE

Therapeutic response

The onset of action is largely dependent on the dosage form and route of administration as well as on individual patient factors. (See Nursing Drug Digest for specific drugs). When monitoring therapeutic response, observations related to the patient's need for the medication should be observed and documented.

Adverse side effects

Adverse side effects occurring with this class of drugs are outlined in Adverse/Side Effects. It is important to recognize that:

Miotics of these types may induce retinal detachment in patients predisposed to this condition.

Pain, headache, and dimming of vision have been reported during the first days of treatment with isoflurophate.

Acute iritis or precipitation of acute glaucoma occasionally follow the ophthalmic use of these agents.

The effects of irreversible anticholinesterases can be antagonized by giving neostigmine or physostigmine beforehand.

PATIENT EDUCATION

The patient and family as indicated should have a clear understanding of the medication regimen as well as the exact name of the medication, its general action, dosage, storage, administration, and therapeutic effect. The patient should be made aware of common side effects and should be assisted with the minimization of these effects. The patient should be able to monitor therapeutic response as well as be able to identify signs that indicate the prescriber should be contacted (see General Instructions for Discharge/Outpatients).

GENERAL INSTRUCTIONS FOR DISCHARGE/OUTPATIENTS

ANTICHOLINESTERASES

Oral

This drug is generally used to treat myasthenia gravis. If you do not understand why you require this medication, check with your health care provider.

Take medication only as directed to reduce the possibility of side effects.

Take this medication with food or milk to reduce the possibility of side effects.

Keep a record of your signs and symptoms to help your doctor adjust the dose as required.

Report any side effects that occur to your health care provider.

Do not omit any dose. If you forget to take a dose, take it as soon as possible, then go back to your usual schedule

unless it is nearly time for your next dose. In this case, just take the next dose as usual. *Do not* double the next dose.

Keep this medication and all medications out of the reach of children.

Ophthalmic

This drug is generally used to treat glaucoma. If you do not understand why you require this medication, check with your health care provider.

Do not apply this medication more often than directed or use more of it than directed. This will reduce the amount of drug absorbed into the body and reduce the chance of side effects.

If you miss a dose: If you were to apply the medicine every other day and remember it on the same day, apply the dose and continue your schedule. If

you have missed the dose and the day, apply the dose, miss a day, and then continue your schedule. If it was to be applied daily, apply it as soon as possible and continue your schedule. If you forget a day, continue your schedule. Do not apply the missed dose.

You may experience a stinging sensation, tearing, and a dull ache when you apply the medication. This should disappear in a few minutes and is not harmful. If it persists, contact your health care provider.

These agents constrict the pupil and may affect your ability to see clearly at night. If affected, do not drive at night.

Keep this medication and all other medications out of the reach of children.

NURSING DRUG DIGEST

Medication (trade name)	Indication	Usual dosage and administration	Dosage forms, preparation, and storage	Contraindications, cautions, and comments	Monitoring
Ambenonium Mysuran Mytelase	Myasthenia gravis	*Adults:* 5-25 mg PO t.i.d. or q.i.d. Increase dosage gradually as indicated Maximum: 200 mg/day	Tablet: 10 mg Store in airtight containers	*Contraindicated* in mechanical obstruction of intestinal or urinary tracts Longer duration of action than neostigmine Sometimes useful in patients with myasthenia gravis who cannot tolerate neostigmine Atropine can be used to counteract excessive parasympathomimetic effects *Routine* administration of atropine is *contraindicated*	Patients receiving drug should be observed carefully for the development of unwanted side effects
★ **Demecarium bromide** Tosmilen Humorsol Tonilen Tosmilen Visumiotic	Glaucoma	*Adults:* 1-2 drops of a 0.125%-0.5% solution instilled twice weekly (preferably at bedtime) to 1-2 drops/day Gently remove (wipe) any excess solution after administration to minimize or prevent any possible systemic absorption; to avoid systemic absorption patient should press finger to lacrimal sac during and for 1-2 min after instillation	Sterile ophthalmic solution: 0.125, 0.25% Store in airtight containers; protect from light	Stronger concentrations may be required in patients with dark irises than in those with blue or light-colored irises Miotic action begins in 20 min and may last for more than 1 week Used topically as an antiglaucoma agent and cyclostimulant in strabismus Tolerance can develop with prolonged use May be given with phenylephrine to reduce the incidence of iris cyst formation	Patients receiving drug should be observed carefully for the development of unwanted side effects Observe patient for signs of systemic absorption, (e.g, diarrhea, weakness) Observe eyes for irritation and development of cataracts (chronic administration)

Continued.

NOTE: For additional details regarding the individual agents listed in this table, see the text and other tables in this chapter.
* Indicates that the drug is generally available only in Canada.
★ Indicates that the drug is generally available only in the United States.

NURSING DRUG DIGEST—cont'd

Medication (trade name)	Indication	Usual dosage and administration	Dosage forms, preparation, and storage	Contraindications, cautions, and comments	Monitoring
Echothiophate Ecofilina Echodide Phospholine iodide	Glaucoma Accommodative esotropia	1 drop of a 0.03%-0.25% solution to affected eye(s) q.d. to b.i.d. 1 drop of a 0.03%-0.125% solution to affected eye(s) q.d.	Sterile powder and diluent for ophthalmic solution: 0.03%, 0.06%, 0.125%, and 0.25% Solution must be freshly prepared with diluent supplied by manufacturer Store at 2°-8° C in airtight containers Protect from light Reconstituted solution is stable 12 months if refrigerated, but recommend use within 1 month	*Contraindicated* in uveal inflammation Systemic cholinesterase inhibition occurs with prolonged use Carbonic anhydrase inhibitor (e.g., acetazolamide) may be added for antiglaucoma effect Has been used occasionally to treat myasthenia gravis Should be used with caution in patients with a history of retinal detachment Generally miosis occurs within 10-45 min and can persist for up to 30 days	Observe patient for signs of systemic absorption (e.g., diarrhea, weakness) Observe eyes for irritation and the development of cataracts (chronic administration) Monitor for cardiac, respiratory, or gastrointestinal problems
Edrophonium Tensilon	Diagnosis of myasthenia gravis Reversal of nondepolarizing muscle relaxants	*Adults:* 2-10 mg IV; 10 mg IM In the diagnosis of myasthenia gravis, inject 2 mg; if no adverse reactions occur within 30 seconds inject remainder of dose; if IV injection is difficult, 10 mg can be injected IM *Adults:* 5-10 mg IV repeated q.5-10 min up to 40 mg maximum	Injectable: 10 mg/ml	*Contraindicated* in mechanical obstruction of intestinal or urinary tracts Drug has a short duration of action, usually less than 10 min Atropine injection should always be available when the drug is being used Can be used to distinguish cholinergic crisis from undertreatment in myasthenia gravis Edrophonium ameliorates symptoms and improves function at once in undertreated patients	Patients should be observed for the reappearance of signs and symptoms present before treatment Observe patient carefully for signs of excessive salivation and bronchial secretions

★ | Drug | Use | Dosage | Preparation/Storage | Cautions | Nursing Considerations |
|---|---|---|---|---|---|
| **Isoflurophate** DFP Diflupyl Floropryl | Glaucoma | *Adults:* Apply ¼ inch of ointment to eye q.8-72 h. as indicated | Sterile ophthalmic ointment: 0.25% Protect from moisture | *Use cautiously if patient has a history of bronchial asthma or is receiving cardiac glycosides, (e.g., digoxin)* | Observe patient for signs of systemic absorption (e.g., diarrhea, weakness) |
| | Accommodative esotropia | *Adults:* Apply ¼ inch of ointment to eye q.1-7 days at bedtime *Children:* Same as adults | | *Should be used carefully in patients with a history of retinal detachment* *For other cautions see Echothiophate* | Observe for eye irritation and development of cataracts (with chronic use) |
| **Neostigmine** Intrastigmina Juvastigmina Prostigmin Prostigmina Prostigmine | Myasthenia gravis | *Adults:* 1 to 25 mg q.d. in divided doses SC, IM; or 75 to 300 mg PO in divided doses Doses of neostigmine should be divided throughout the day; more of total daily dose can be given at times of greatest fatigue *Children:* 0.01-0.04 mg/kg IM or SC q.2-4h.; or 2 mg/kg/day PO in 6-8 divided doses | Injectable (methylsulfate): 0.25, 0.5, or 1 mg/ml Tablets (bromide): 15 mg Store in airtight containers; protect from light | *Contraindicated* in asthma or mechanical obstruction of the intestinal or urinary tracts Atropine or other anticholinergics can be given up to t.i.d. to reduce muscarinic side effects Ephedrine (30 mg t.i.d.) may increase the effectiveness of neostigmine in myasthenia gravis *Cautious use of the drug is essential in patients with bradycardia, bronchial asthma, cardiac disease, epilepsy, parkinsonism, or peptic ulcer* Use of drug in conjunction with depolarizing muscle relaxants, (e.g., succinylcholine) should be avoided Note which salt of the drug is being ordered and the actual amount of drug in each | Patients receiving drug should be observed carefully for the development of unwanted side effects Monitor patients for signs of cholinergic crisis (weakness, fatigue, difficulty in swallowing) Monitor for cardiac, respiratory, and gastrointestinal problems |
| | Reversal of nondepolarizing muscle relaxants | *Adults:* 0.5-2 mg injected slowly IV; atropine 0.6-1.2 mg is usually given at the same time *Children:* 0.04 mg/kg IV; atropine 0.02 mg/kg is usually given at the same time | | | |
| | Prevention of postoperative atony | *Adults:* 0.25 mg SC or IM after surgery; may repeat q.4-6h. as indicated | | | |

Continued.

NURSING DRUG DIGEST—cont'd

Medication (trade name)	Indication	Usual dosage and administration	Dosage forms, preparation, and storage	Contraindications, cautions, and comments	Monitoring
Physostigmine Antilirium Eserine Fisostin Geneserine Isopto-eserine	Miotic/glaucoma	*Adults:* Instillation of 0.25%-0.5% solution b.i.d. or t.i.d.; 0.25% ointment applied b.i.d. or t.i.d.	Sterile ophthalmic solution in water or oil: 0.25%, 0.5% Eye ointment 0.25%, 0.5% Injectable: 1 mg/ml *Do not use colored solutions*	Physostigmine base is used for oily eye drops Physostigmine readily enters the CNS Drug must be used cautiously and conservatively in treatment of anticholinergic and antidepressant poisoning Drug has been used for the treatment of many central nervous system disorders (see text for examples)	Ophthalmic use: Observe eyes for irritation and development of cataracts Patients receiving drug should be observed carefully for the development of unwanted side effects Observe patient for signs of systemic absorption, (e.g., diarrhea, weakness)
	Reversal of anticholinergic or antidepressant poisoning	*Adults:* 2 mg IM or slow IV; repeat dose if life-threatening signs recur IV should not be administered at a rate greater than 1 mg/min *Children:* 0.5 mg slow IV over 1 min; repeat q.5-10 min if indicated Maximum: 2 mg total dose			
Pyridostigmine bromide Mestinon Regonol	Myasthenia gravis	*Adults:* 0.3-1.5 gm PO daily in divided doses; extended-release tablet is swallowed whole; or 2 mg SC, IM, or IV q. 2-4h. Dose should be divided throughout day; more of daily dose can be given at times of greatest fatigue	Tablets: 60 mg; extended-release tablets, 180 mg Syrup: 60 mg/5 ml Store in airtight containers and protect from light Injectable: 5 mg/ml	*Contraindicated* in obstruction of the intestinal or urinary tracts Pyridostigmine has a slower onset and longer duration of action than neostigmine Anticholinergics are usually needed less frequently than with neostigmine Can be combined with neostigmine	Patients receiving drug should be observed carefully for the development of unwanted side effects Patients should be observed for signs of cholinergic crisis and muscarinic side effects
	Reversal of nondepolarizing muscle relaxants	*Adults:* 10-20 mg IV (with 0.6-1.2 mg atropine)			

DRUGS USED TO TREAT ANTICHOLINESTERASE POISONING

Drug	Use	Dosage	Preparations	Remarks
Atropine	Anticholinesterase poisoning See also Chapter 23, "Parasympathomimetics and Parasympatholytics"	*Adults:* 2-4 mg IM or IV initially; then 2 mg every 3-8 min until signs of atropinization appear (pulse rate > 80, dilated pupils), or muscarinic symptoms disappear; repeat as necessary. Up to 12 mg has been given in first 2 hr and 50 mg in the first day. Dose is adjusted in accordance with the needs of the patient. *Children:* 1 mg IM or IV initially, followed by 0.5-1 mg q.3-8 min as indicated	Injectable: 0.5 mg/ml	See Chapter 23. In anticholinesterase poisoning atropine is the drug of first choice and can be life-saving; see text for details of the treatment of anticholinesterase poisoning
Pralidoxime Protopam	Adjunct to treatment of irreversible anticholinesterase poisoning in conjunction with atropine (2 to 4 mg)	*Adults:* 1 to 2 gm given by slow IV injection over at least 5 min as a 5% solution. Dose may be repeated twice after periods of 1 hr; or 1-3 gm PO q.5h. Rapid injection may cause neuromuscular block, blurred vision, nausea, and tachycardia. Do *not* administer at a rate greater than 500 mg/min. Decrease dosage in renal impairment. *Children:* 20-40 mg/kg by slow IV as a 5% solution over at least 5 min	Injectable: 50 mg/ml Tablets: 0.5 gm	Pralidoxime is not effective against all irreversible anticholinesterases; ineffective against carbamate insecticides; unlikely to be effective if given more than 36 hr after exposure. Carry out decontamination procedures. Ensure patient is atropinized. Patients should not be permitted to smoke. May cause drowsiness, dizziness, disturbances of vision, nausea, tachycardia, headache, and transient muscular block. Monitor vital signs frequently. Observe patient for at least 24 hr

BIBLIOGRAPHY

Das, P.K. On genetically determined human serum cholin-esterases. *Enzyme,* 1976, *21,* 253.

Namba, T., Cholinesterase inhibition by organophosphorous compounds and its clinical effects. *Bulletin of the World Health Organization,* 1971, *44,* 289.

Quail, C., & Waddleton, C. Treating the glaucomas. *Nurses' Drug Alert,* September, 1980, 93.

Reynolds, J.E.F. (Ed.). *Martindale, the extra pharmacopoeia,* (28th ed.). London: The Pharmaceutical Press, 1982.

Spencer, E.Y. *Guide to the chemicals used in crop protection,* Publication 1093, (7th ed.), Ottawa, Ministry of Supply and Services Canada, 1982.

Taylor, P. Anticholinesterase agents. In A.G. Goodman, L.S. Goodman, and A. Gilman, (Eds.), *The pharmacological basis of therapeutics,* (6th Ed.). New York: Macmillan, 1980.

1984 USPDI, Drug Information for the health care provider, Rockville: The United States Pharmacopoeia Convention Inc., 1983.

CHAPTER 26

Ganglionic Stimulants and Blockers and Neuromuscular Blocking Agents

David F. Biggs

Medications discussed in this chapter

Ganglionic stimulants	Nondepolarizing neuro-
Lobeline	muscular blocker
Nicotine	Atracurium
Ganglionic blockers	Gallamine
Mecamylamine	Hexafluorenium
Trimethaphan	Metocurine
Depolarizing neuromuscu-	Pancuronium
lar blocker	Tubocurarine
Succinylcholine	

This chapter discusses two groups of drugs, ganglionic stimulants and blockers and neuromuscular blocking agents, that are used for certain specific clinical purposes. Both groups of drugs have a long history, and many compounds with these types of activities are known. The drugs currently used clinically represent those that have proved themselves over many years to be acceptable in terms of safety and efficacy.

GANGLIONIC STIMULANTS AND BLOCKERS

Before one can understand how these drugs produce their effects in the body, one must understand the functional anatomy and physiology of the peripheral nervous system. The reader is referred to Chapter 22 for this information.

Ganglionic transmission is dependent upon the integrity of the nervous system pathways for the synthesis, storage, and release of acetylcholine (ACh). Thus any drug affecting these processes will affect ganglionic transmission in both the parasympathetic and sympathetic divisions of the autonomic nervous system (ANS). Also, because acetylcholine is the neurotransmitter between the postganglionic neuron and the effector organ in the parasympathetic division, transmission will be affected here too.

Ganglionic stimulants

Ganglionic stimulants described in this chapter all cause initial stimulation of autonomic ganglia followed by blockade. Agents that induce only ganglionic stimulation are known (e.g., dimethylphenylpiperazinium, tetramethylammonium) but have no clinical uses. Note that even acetylcholine in excess can block ganglionic transmission. Some ganglionic stimulants enter the central nervous system (CNS) and induce effects, and all ganglionic stimulants can affect the sensory receptors of the peripheral nervous system (PNS). Many of these agents also affect neuromuscular transmission.

Nicotine. In humans and animals nicotine causes tremor; with larger doses this progresses to convulsions. Small amounts of nicotine, such as that contained in a cigarette, cause an alerting pattern to appear in the electroencephalogram (EEG), decreased muscle tone, and reduced deep tendon reflexes. Nicotine has been reported to reduce aggression and irritability and to improve attention and facilitate memory. The drug can induce nausea and vomiting by an effect on the chemoreceptor trigger zone and by enhancing the vagal reflexes involved in vomiting. It has also been reported to increase blood concentrations of growth hormone, cortisol, antidiuretic hormone, and norepinephrine and epinephrine.

Nicotine stimulates most peripheral sensory receptors, including pain, temperature, and touch, pressoreceptors and chemoreceptors, and mechanoreceptors involved in proprioception. Many of these effects have little pharmacologic significance, but the stimulant effect of nicotine on chemoreceptors causes an increase in the rate and depth of respiration.

Nicotine stimulates and then blocks all autonomic ganglia, the physiologic effect representing the result of the removal of nervous tone from the effector organs.

Nicotine induces rapidly developing neuromuscular paralysis, usually preceded by stimulant effects (e.g., twitching, *fasciculations*). The varied effects of nicotine on nervous and organ systems account for the unpredictability and complexity of the changes seen after nicotine administration.

Nicotine and smoking. Smoking tobacco results in the absorption of significant quantities of nicotine. The nicotine is present in smoke in suspension together with tar and other materials. When inhaled in this form, the drug is rapidly absorbed at a rate equivalent to intravenous administration. Absorption via the buccal cavity is not as rapid, and absorption from the stomach is minimal because of the low gastric pH and the pKa of nicotine (i.e., 8.5). Peak concentrations of nicotine after smoking an "average" cigarette are 25 to 50 ng/ml plasma; the drug has a plasma half-life of 30 to 60 minutes. Nicotine is mostly metabolized to inert products in the body; only small amounts of the drug are excreted unchanged in the urine. Nicotine crosses the placenta and is excreted in pharmacologically significant amounts in breast milk.

Tolerance develops to many of the effects of nicotine (e.g., nausea and vomiting) but its effects on the cardiovascular system and on hormone concentrations persist. Smokers metabolize nicotine more rapidly than nonsmokers, the result of nicotine inducing hepatic microsomal enzymes. This may affect the metabolism and the half-life of other drugs. These effects are more pronounced in young and middle-aged smokers than in older ones.

Stopping the administration of nicotine (stopping smoking tobacco) results in a highly variable withdrawal syndrome. Major signs and symptoms include tremor, restlessness, and irritability, together with an often overwhelming desire to smoke a cigarette. These effects can be prevented by the administration of nicotine. The only clinical use for nicotine is in the treatment of the nicotine withdrawal syndrome. Solutions of nicotine are still used occasionally as insecticides.

Lobeline. This drug has many of the pharmacologic effects of nicotine but has less effect on the central nervous system (CNS). Lobeline can substitute for nicotine during withdrawal but must be given in adequate dosage. It stimulates peripheral sensory receptors and has particularly pronounced effects on chemoreceptors. Like nicotine, this drug stimulates then blocks autonomic ganglia and blocks neuromuscular transmission, but is less potent.

Lobeline was formerly used as a respiratory stimulant. Controlled trials of the drug as a smoking substitute have shown the drug to be effective if given in adequate dosage, but generally results have been disappointing. Lobeline (in the form of the herb, *Lobelia*) has been smoked as a folk remedy for asthma and bronchitis.

Ganglionic blockers

Ganglionic blockers are usually classified as antihypertensives, and they were the first synthetic drugs to be used for hypertension. They were soon replaced by more effective agents that produced fewer side effects (see Chapter 33, "Antihypertensives"). Drugs in this category include azamethonium, dicolinium, hexamethonium, mecamylamine, pempidine, pentamethonium, pentolinium, tetraethylammonium, trimethaphan, and trimethidinium. Of these, only trimethaphan, mecamylamine, and pentolinium are used to any extent. Their major use is in the production of controlled hypotension in patients undergoing surgical procedures.

All of these drugs block transmission by competing with acetylcholine for receptors on the postganglionic neuron. They block all autonomic ganglia, affecting both the sympathetic and parasympathetic divisions. The fall in blood pressure that results is largely postural in origin and results from the failure of the efferent pathways for normal homeostasis. Ganglionic blockers are occasionally used to treat hypertension, hypertensive encephalopathy, and eclampsia.

NEUROMUSCULAR BLOCKING AGENTS

Curare, a South American arrow poison, has been known for many years. It was introduced into medicine in the 1930's in a purified form as tubocurarine to induce muscle relaxation during surgery. Many compounds with neuromuscular blocking properties have been prepared synthetically and from natural sources. Of these, six to eight are used clinically. Agents currently in use can be divided into two groups: depolarizing agents and nondepolarizing agents.

Depolarizing agents

These agents block neuromuscular transmission and induce muscle relaxation by producing a prolonged partial depolarization of the *motor endplate* by an action on acetylcholine nicotinic receptors. The endplate is then unresponsive to normal amounts of the neurotransmitter acetylcholine. The effect of these agents is not reversed by anticholinesterases (e.g., neostigmine, edrophonium), and use of these agents in combination with a depolarizing agent can result in greater muscle paralysis or prolonged recovery times. Agents included in this group are succinylcholine, suxethonium, and decamethonium.

Nondepolarizing agents

These agents compete with the neurotransmitter acetylcholine for its receptors at the motor endplate, thus preventing endplate depolarization by the transmitter. Neuromuscular blockade of this type is reversed by anticholinesterases. Agents included in this group are gallamine, metocurine, pancuronium, tubocurarine, alcuronium, and fazadinium.

Both groups show some selectivity for the skeletal muscle groups paralyzed, at least during the early stages of block; the intercostal muscles and the diaphragm are usually affected last.

Dual block can occur after repeated doses of depolarizing agents or after an infusion. It is sometimes referred to as *desensitization block.* Clinically, it is characterized by prolonged apnea or continued paralysis after the drug is withdrawn. This block can often be reversed, paradoxically, by anticholinesterases.

Mixed block can occur when depolarizing and nondepolarizing agents are given at the same time. The cause of this phenomenon is not known.

When nondepolarizing agents are given in the presence of metabolic acidosis, neostigmine-resistant paralysis can occur.

Neuromuscular blocking agents are used as an adjunct to anesthesia to induce muscle relaxation, during electroconvulsive therapy, during the treatment of muscle spasms in tetanus and similar conditions, and for endotracheal intubation.

None of the neuromuscular blocking drugs affect consciousness or mentation, and none affect pain threshold or have any analgesic action.

SUMMARY

This chapter has examined ganglionic stimulants and blockers and neuromuscular blocking agents. Ganglionic stimulants are used clinically as an aid to stop smoking. Ganglionic blockers have been largely superseded by more pharmacologically specific agents but are still used to induce controlled hypotension during some surgical procedures. Depolarizing and nondepolarizing neuromuscular blockers are important adjuncts to anesthesia and are also used in electroconvulsive therapy, minor manipulative procedures, and in some forms of muscle spasm.

It is important that nurses understand the mechanisms of action of these agents and the rationale behind their uses. Knowledge of the actions, uses, and side effects of these drugs will aid nurses in providing better patient care. Careful observation and monitoring of patients will enable potential adverse reactions to be avoided or minimized and clinically significant drug interactions anticipated and prevented.

ADVERSE/SIDE EFFECTS OF THE GANGLIONIC STIMULANTS AND BLOCKERS*

Ganglionic stimulants

CARDIOVASCULAR SYSTEM

Blood pressure changes
Heart rate changes

CENTRAL NERVOUS SYSTEM

Drowsiness
Irritability
Nausea and vomiting

CUTANEOUS SYSTEM

Sweating increased

GASTROINTESTINAL SYSTEM

Constipation
Diarrhea
Salivation

GENITOURINARY SYSTEM

Urinary frequency
Urinary urgency
Urinary retention

MUSCULOSKELETAL SYSTEM

Muscle weakness
Tremor

OCULAR SYSTEM

Blurring of vision

RESPIRATORY SYSTEM

Bronchial relaxation
Bronchospasm
Bronchial secretions increased/
  decreased
Respiratory rate and depth increased

---

*See Chapter 11, "Drug Toxicity," for an overview of drug toxicity.

Continued.

ADVERSE/SIDE EFFECTS OF THE GANGLIONIC STIMULANTS AND BLOCKERS—cont'd

Ganglionic blockers
CARDIOVASCULAR SYSTEM

Anginal attacks
Heart rate changes
Homeostatic reflexes absent
Postural hypotension

CENTRAL NERVOUS SYSTEM

Drowsiness
Mental confusion
Nausea

CUTANEOUS SYSTEM

Sweating decreased

GASTROINTESTINAL SYSTEM

Constipation
Diarrhea
Paralytic ileus

GENITOURINARY SYSTEM

Impotence
Leaky sphincters
Urinary retention

MUSCULOSKELETAL SYSTEM

Muscle weakness
Tremors

OCULAR SYSTEM

Blurring of vision
Paralysis of accommodation
Pupillary reflexes absent

RESPIRATORY SYSTEM

Bronchodilation
Dry mouth

ADVERSE/SIDE EFFECTS OF THE NEUROMUSCULAR BLOCKERS*

Depolarizing neuromuscular blockers
CARDIOVASCULAR SYSTEM

Bradycardia
Dysrhythmias
Hypotension

CENTRAL NERVOUS SYSTEM

Hyperpyrexia

MUSCULOSKELETAL SYSTEM

Fasciculations
Myoglobinemia
Postoperative muscle pain
Twitching

OCULAR SYSTEM

Transient rise in intraocular pressure

RESPIRATORY SYSTEM

Apnea prolonged
Bronchospasm

OTHER EFFECTS

Hyperkalemia

Nondepolarizing neuromuscular blockers
CARDIOVASCULAR SYSTEM

Dysrhythmias
Hypotension

CENTRAL NERVOUS SYSTEM

Hyperpyrexia

RESPIRATORY SYSTEM

Apnea
Bronchospasm

OTHER EFFECTS

Hypersensitivity

*See Chapter 11, "Drug Toxicity," for an overview of drug toxicity.

CLINICALLY SIGNIFICANT DRUG INTERACTIONS*

Primary drug	Interacting drug	Possible effect(s)	Probable mechanism(s)
GANGLIONIC STIMULANTS			
Nicotine (smoking)	Theophylline	Decreased serum concentrations of theophylline	Increased metabolism resulting from enzyme induction†
Nicotine (smoking)	Pentazocine	Decreased analgesic effect	Increased metabolism resulting from enzyme induction†
Nicotine (smoking)	Imipramine	Decreased serum concentrations of imipramine	Increased metabolism resulting from enzyme induction†
GANGLIONIC BLOCKERS			
Ganglionic blockers	Pressor agents (e.g., epinephrine)	Increased pressor response and tachycardia	Loss of homeostatic control
Ganglionic blockers	Depolarizing neuromuscular blockers	Decreased neuromuscular block	Pharmacologic antagonism of depolarizing drugs
Ganglionic blockers	Nondepolarizing neuromuscular blockers	Increased neuromuscular block	Pharmacologic potentiation of nondepolarizing drugs
Trimethaphan	Spinal anesthetics (e.g., lidocaine)	Enhanced hypotension	Loss of homeostatic control
Trimethaphan	Antihypertensive drugs	Enhanced hypotension	Loss of homeostatic control
NEUROMUSCULAR BLOCKERS			
Depolarizing neuromuscular blockers	Anticholinesterases, including insecticides and antimalarials	Increased neuromuscular block; prolonged apnea	Pharmacologic potentiation; decreased metabolism (succinylcholine)
Neuromuscular blockers	Aminoglycoside antibiotics, (e.g., streptomycin) Clindamycin Lincomycin Polymyxin antibiotics	Increased neuromuscular block; apnea when given postoperatively	Pharmacologic potentiation of both depolarizing and nondepolarizing agents
Neuromuscular blockers	General anesthetics (e.g., enflurane, ether, isoflurane, methoxyflurane, cyclopropane, halothane)	Increased risk of hyperpyrexia Increased neuromuscular block; dose of blocker must be reduced	Not established Pharmacologic potentiation
Neuromuscular blockers	Quinidine, quinine	Increased neuromuscular block; prolonged apnea	Pharmacologic potentiation

*See Chapter 10, "Drug Interactions," for an overview of drug interactions.
†The enzyme induction is most pronounced in heavy and moderate smokers.

GENERAL NURSING IMPLICATIONS

Nursing of patients requiring ganglionic stimulants

Ganglionic stimulants include a variety of chemical structures that, except for the treatment or maintenance of nicotine addiction, have no essential therapeutic uses. They are, however, used widely as experimental drugs in basic pharmacology laboratory research.

ASSESSMENT

Assessment of the patient is important in relation to the monitoring of response. A drug history should include the identification of possible sensitivity, contraindications, cautions, and potential drug interactions before the drug is administered.

Ganglionic stimulants (e.g., nicotine, lobeline) are used for the temporary aid in helping smokers to stop smoking cigarettes as they decrease nicotine withdrawal. The efficacy of lobeline in this regard had been refuted by controlled studies and was not recommended. However, it has now been found to be effective when given in adequate dosages (see Nursing Drug Digest). When required for the cessation of smoking, baseline data should include a smoking history identifying the number of pack years and lifestyle patterns associated with smoking (e.g., smoking after dinner, when anxious, etc.). This information is helpful in planning with the patient an individualized stop smoking program.

SENSITIVITY

Generally, allergic reactions to ganglionic stimulants are rare; however, any drug has the potential to cause a hypersensitivity reaction in susceptible individuals.

CONTRAINDICATIONS

These medications are contraindicated in patients with known hypersensitivity.

The use of nicotine is contraindicated in pregnancy because of known adverse effects on the fetus. Women of childbearing age should be warned about the risks involved with smoking or the use of this medication during pregnancy. These medications are contraindicated in women who are breast feeding since nicotine is excreted in breast milk and can cause CNS excitation in the infant. See Nursing Drug Digest for contraindications to specific agents in this class.

CAUTIONS

Ganglionic stimulants are contraindicated in patients with gastritis, peptic ulceration, or inflammation of the mouth since these drugs can cause exacerbation of related symptoms.

Nicotine should be used with caution in patients with angina, coronary artery disease, or peripheral vascular disease.

See Nursing Drug Digest for cautions related to the use of specific ganglionic stimulants.

DRUG INTERACTIONS

Ganglionic stimulants have the potential to interact with other drugs.

See Clinically Significant Drug Interactions.

ADMINISTRATION

Ganglionic stimulants are administered orally for buccal absorption. Nicotine is available in chewing gum form since its pharmacokinetic mechanism favors buccal rather than gastrointestinal absorption. It is more rapidly absorbed buccally and avoids rapid hepatic inactivation by this route.

Nicotine is available in 2 mg and 4 mg strengths. One piece of the medicated gum is chewed for 30 minutes when the patient desires a smoke, and this can be repeated as needed to 10 a day. Dosage is decreased on a day-to-day basis after the first phase of cigarette withdrawal is completed. Dosage is individualized.

The effect of gum preparations is affected by the amount of chewing and frequency with which pieces of gum are chewed.

See Nursing Drug Digest for further information regarding the administration of specific ganglionic stimulants.

MONITORING PATIENT RESPONSE
Therapeutic response

Because ganglionic stimulants (e.g., lobeline, nicotine) are usually given in quit smoking programs, monitor for change in smoking habits as related to the smoking history and frequency of use of this medication. Nicotine is not a substitute for smoking and should not be required for use over a long period. The patient should be able to decrease the use of this medication 1 to 2 weeks after the smoking habit has been successfully broken. The gum should be carried in the pocket for 3 months after cigarette smoking has ceased, however, as an available aid for the craving of a cigarette that can occur.

Adverse side effects

During initial therapy, administer medication carefully and monitor patient response. Observe for signs of aphthous ulcers, throat irritation, excessive salivation, and hiccups, which can occur especially with nicotine in 4-mg dosages. Weight gain has been observed in patients receiving ganglionic stimulants such as nicotine for the cessation of smoking, and patients should be monitored for weight gain at regular intervals. Diet modification as well as an exercise program may be indicated.

Monitor for CNS stimulation, nausea, vomiting, and diarrhea.

Monitor for dose-related overdose or toxicity.

Monitor for signs of acute poisoning (nicotine): abdominal pain, diarrhea, dizziness, headache, mental confusion, hypotension, and vomiting. Death can result from respiratory paralysis.

Treatment of overdose is evacuation of stomach contents followed by the use of activated charcoal if necessary. Comatose patients require the establishment and maintenance of an airway and supportive measures including gastric lavage.

GENERAL NURSING IMPLICATIONS—cont'd

Nursing of patients requiring ganglionic stimulants—cont'd

PATIENT EDUCATION

The patient and family as indicated should have a clear understanding of the medication regimen as well as the exact name of the medication, its action, dosage, storage, administration, and side effects as well as how these effects can be minimized. Patients on smoking cessation programs require much support and encouragement. Assisting patients with smoking cessation is extremely important. Patients should be aware of signs that indicate the health provider should be notified.

Patients should be advised to give up smoking. Appropriate support and referral services should be made available to the patient as he or she desires.

Excessive smoking should be actively discouraged.

Heavy or moderate smokers should be observed to ensure that drugs such as theophylline or pentazocine are having their desired therapeutic effect. Dosage adjustments may be necessary.

Nursing of patients requiring ganglionic blockers

ASSESSMENT

These drugs are used mostly in basic pharmacology laboratory research. The only two in clinical use in North America are mecamylamine and trimethaphan. Although they can be employed as adjunctive therapy in the treatment of various conditions, their main use is related to their hypotensive effect in the treatment of hypertensive cardiovascular disease. Because of the wide range of indication, assessment data when these drugs are given should include baseline assessment of the specific patient factors associated with the administration of these medications. These data are important in monitoring patient response to drug therapy.

Initial assessment should include a drug history to identify possible sensitivity, contraindications, cautions, potential drug interactions, and drug-taking patterns.

SENSITIVITY

Generally, allergic reactions to ganglionic blockers are rare; however, any drug has the potential to cause a hypersensitivity reaction in susceptible individuals.

Because some of the ganglionic blockers are formulated as iodide salts (see Nursing Drug Digest), assessment of patients for a history of iodide sensitivity (e.g., sensitivity to shellfish) should be completed. Such sensitivity constitutes a contraindication to the use of these agents. Patients without a known history of iodide sensitivity should be monitored carefully.

CONTRAINDICATIONS

The use ganglionic blockers is contraindicated in: patients with known hypersensitivity, patients with inadequate blood volume associated with any cause, coronary disease, severe renal or hepatic dysfunction, later months of pregnancy and childbirth, severe anemia, glaucoma

See Nursing Drug Digest for specific contraindications to each drug.

CAUTIONS

Postural hypotension is the major caution associated with the use of these agents.

See Nursing Drug Digest for cautions related to each agent.

DRUG INTERACTIONS

Ganglionic blockers have the potential to interact with other drugs. See Clinically Significant Drug Interactions.

ADMINISTRATION

The two clinically utilized ganglionic blockers, mecamylamine and trimethaphan are administered orally and intravenously, respectively. It is important to note that trimethaphan, available in 10-ml ampules for intravenous administration, should *not* be mixed with other medications. In solution it is not compatible with thiopental, thiamylal, gallamine triethiodide, strongly alkaline solutions, iodides, or bromides. In addition, simultaneous administration of other drugs in the same infusion fluids should not be done. See Nursing Drug Digest for administration information on these medications.

MONITORING PATIENT RESPONSE
Therapeutic response

Individual patient response varies and the rate of intravenous administration must be adjusted to the patient's requirements. Since these drugs can be used for various therapeutic reasons including neurosurgery where hypotensive effect is indicated (e.g., brain tumor, thoracic vascular surgery) and hypertensive crisis, monitor for hypotensive effects and rapid onset and short duration of action.

Adverse side effects

These drugs are rarely used, however, when used, monitor for the following adverse side effects, including anhidrosis, anorexia, constipation, cycloplegia, hypotension, mydriasis, nausea, reduced tone of gastrointestinal tract, subjective chilliness, syncope occurring without warning, tachycardia, urinary retention, and xerostomia

It is important to monitor for signs of *overdose*, including hypotension, respiratory depression, and tachycardia. Overdose is generally treated with vasopressor agents. (See Adverse/Side Effects and Nursing Drug Digest for adverse/side effects of each agent.)

Caution the patient to get up in stages to minimize the possibility of postural hypotension.

Do not administer pressor agents to these patients without considering the possibility of an exaggerated therapeutic response.

Continued.

GENERAL NURSING IMPLICATIONS—cont'd

Nursing of patients requiring ganglionic blockers—cont'd

Adverse side effects—cont'd

Do not place the patient in abnormally hot environments, such as a hot bath, since vasodilation can result.

Caution the patient regarding the possible ocular effects of these agents.

Monitor for the development of tolerance to the hypotensive actions of these agents.

PATIENT EDUCATION

The patient and family as indicated should have a clear understanding of the medication use, its action, administration, and adverse effects in relation to individual need and drug therapy plan. Safety precautions related to syncope and untreated hypertension or other medical indications for treatment should be discussed. (See Chapter 33, "Antihypertensives," for further discussion of patient education as related to hypertension.)

Nursing of patients requiring neuromuscular blockers

ASSESSMENT

Neuromuscular blockers are indicated for adjunctive use with anesthetics and electroconvulsive therapy (ECT). In addition to baseline assessment related to these conditions, a detailed drug history identifying possible sensitivity, contraindications, cautions, potential drug interactions, and drug-taking patterns should be obtained before the administration of these medications.

SENSITIVITY

Generally, allergic reactions to neuromuscular blockers are rare; however, any drug has the potential to cause a hypersensitivity reaction in susceptible individuals. It is important to note that some individuals are extremely hypersensitive to succinylcholine because of a genetic alteration of their plasma cholinesterase (see Chapter 9, "Genetic Factors Affecting Drug Response").

CONTRAINDICATIONS

The use of neuromuscular blockers is contraindicated in patients with glaucoma, myasthenia gravis, pulmonary disorders, renal dysfunction, and respiratory insufficiency

See Nursing Drug Digest for specific contraindications to individual agents.

CAUTIONS

Because of the potential for respiratory blockade, these drugs should be administered in a controlled clinical setting where respiratory and cardiac support is readily available.

Potassium depletion as a result of thiazide diuretics can increase sensitivity to neuromuscular blocking agents, and it is important to ensure adequate serum potassium levels or discontinue diuretic therapy with thiazide diuretics at least 4 days before elective surgery and use of this class of medication.

Use these drugs with caution in the elderly or debilitated patient.

See Nursing Drug Digest for specific cautions related to the use of individual neuromuscular blockers.

ADMINISTRATION

Because the neuromuscular blocking agents are poorly absorbed from the gastrointestinal tract, they are usually given by intravenous route, although tubocurarine may be given intramuscularly. Dosage is highly individualized. See Nursing Drug Digest for specific information on administration of each neuromuscular blocker.

MONITORING PATIENT RESPONSE
Therapeutic response

Because neuromuscular blockers are given for a variety of indications, monitoring should be completed in relation to the specific indication for the drug therapy.

Ulnar nerve stimulation can be used to assess the degree of neuromuscular blockade.

Adverse side effects

See Adverse/Side Effects of the Neuromuscular Blockers for a summary of effects associated with the neuromuscular blockers. Also see Nursing Drug Digest for side effects associated with specific agents.

It is important to monitor for signs of overdose or toxicity. Monitor for prolonged apnea, cardiovascular collapse (caused by respiratory paralysis and histamine release), progressive fall in blood pressure, and symptoms of shock. Neostigmine (0.5 mg for adults) is helpful in treating overdose when respiratory depression is not great.

PATIENT EDUCATION

The patient and family should be involved in care as indicated. They should have a clear understanding of the drug regimen whenever possible. Special attention should be given to patient teaching related to the patient's individual condition and the need for neuromuscular blockers.

GENERAL INSTRUCTIONS FOR DISCHARGE/OUTPATIENTS

GANGLIONIC STIMULANTS FOR CESSATION OF SMOKING

This medication is used to help you with your stop smoking program. The use of this medication will help you with your craving for a cigarette.

This medication is to be chewed. It is intended to substitute for smoking a cigarette. When you feel the need to smoke, chew a piece of this medicated gum. If you do not understand why you are taking this medication, check with your health care provider.

Follow the instructions on the prescription exactly. If you have any questions about how this medication should be taken, check with your health care provider.

This medication is to be chewed. Do not swallow the gum. It is ineffective when swallowed. For the best results, chew it as directed.

Chew the gum for 10 to 30 minutes. After 30 minutes it will be exhausted and can be discarded.

Do *not* use more than 10 pieces of gum a day. If you find that you need more, notify your health care provider. Support groups are also helpful to people who need help with stopping smoking. Your health care provider can discuss these groups with you and refer you to community resources.

Any medication can cause unwanted effects or side effects. You may notice that chewing the medicated gum may make you salivate more than usual. This effect will go away after awhile and is not harmful. In some people, chewing this gum can make their mouth sore. If this happens, try to use the gum less frequently. If the soreness persists, notify your health care provider.

Until you learn how this medication affects you, do not drive, operate any dangerous machinery, or put yourself in situations where a change in your alertness may cause danger.

If you are pregnant, thinking about becoming pregnant, or are nursing an infant, do not take this medication without first discussing this with your health care provider. The use of nicotine, including smoking cigarettes, has been associated with harmful effects on unborn children. Nicotine is also passed into breast milk and can have harmful effects on infants who are breast feeding.

This medication has been prescribed especially for you. Do not trade or give this medication to any relatives or friends.

Children who have accidently taken this medicated gum and swallowed it have had harmful reactions. Keep this medication and all other medications out of the reach of children.

GANGLIONIC BLOCKERS

This medication is used to treat your high blood pressure. If you do not understand why you are taking this medication, check with your health care provider.

Follow the instructions on the prescription exactly. If you have any questions about how this medication should be taken, check with your health care provider.

Any medication can cause unwanted effects or side effects such as dizziness.

Do not get out of bed or stand up quickly or you may faint. Get up gradually and change positions from sitting to standing slowly to prevent this side effect. If you find dizziness a problem, even with these measures, notify your health care provider.

Avoid excessively hot environments (e.g., hot baths) because this can cause your veins to dilate and increase the effect of the medication. Shower with warm water and be alert to environmental temperature.

You may become constipated from this medication. Eating a balanced diet including roughage and bran and a moderate exercise program can be helpful in preventing this. It is also helpful to drink at least 8 glasses of water a day unless you are directed not to by your health care provider. If constipation occurs, use a mild laxative. If you do not have a bowel movement for 2 to 3 days or if constipation persists and is bothersome, contact your health care provider.

Your mouth may become dry with this medication; if this happens, suck hard, sugar-free candy.

Your vision may become blurred on this medication and dizziness may also occur. Until you know how this medication affects you, do not drive, operate dangerous machinery, or put yourself in situations where blurred vision, dizziness, or a change in mental alertness may cause danger.

This medication has been prescribed especially for you. Do not trade or give this medication to any relatives or friends.

Keep this and all other medication out of the reach of children.

GENERAL INSTRUCTIONS FOR NEUROMUSCULAR BLOCKERS—INPATIENTS

Neuromuscular blockers are used for various reasons. If you have any questions about why you require this medication, check with your nurse or physician.

Any medication can cause unwanted effects or side effects. If these should occur or become bothersome, notify your nurse or physician. If you are taking a depolarizing neuromuscular blocker, you may notice pain in your muscles when you come back from your operation. This is common after use of these drugs. It is nothing to be alarmed about and will go away in 1 to 2 days. There are no significant side effects associated with nondepolarizing muscle relaxants.

NURSING DRUG DIGEST

Medication (trade name)	Indication	Usual dosage and administration	Dosage forms, preparation, and storage	Contraindications, cautions, and comments	Monitoring
GANGLIONIC STIMULANTS					
Lobeline Habit-X Lobatox Lobidan Nikoban Unilobin	Smoking substitute	*Adults:* 0.5-2 mg PO t.i.d. to q.i.d. Maximum: 20 mg/day	Tablets: 0.5 mg	Formerly used as a respiratory stimulant	Observe patient for signs of overdosage (e.g., tremor)
Nicotine Nicorette	Smoking substitute	*Adults:* Chew 2-4 mg for 15-30 min; repeat as necessary Reduce dose and terminate over a 1-week period Maximum: 40 mg/day Do *not* swallow gum	Chewing gum: 2, 4 mg	Patients can become addicted to gum May cause GI distress	Observe patients for signs of overdosage (e.g., tremor, palpitations, nausea and vomiting)
GANGLIONIC BLOCKERS					
★ **Mecamylamine** Inversine Mevasine	Hypertension	*Adults:* 2.5 mg PO b.i.d., increasing by 2.5 mg q. 2 days until control is obtained Administration with food or milk may decrease GI distress	Tablets: 2.5, 10 mg	*Contraindicated* in myocardial infarction, coronary insufficiency, glaucoma, and uremia Use with caution in patients with renal insufficiency Well absorbed PO *Must not be given with* ambenonium May cause postural hypotension, caution patient not to stand up quickly and to avoid hot baths	Observe patient for signs of angina, tremors, convulsions, and mental aberrations Monitor patient's bowel activity (paralytic ileus) Monitor for urinary retention
Trimethaphan Arfonad	Controlled hypotension during surgery	*Adults:* Initially, 3-4 mg/min by IV infusion (0.1% solution) according to response	Injectable: 50 mg/ml Store between 2° and 8° C	May release histamine Short duration of action; used with postural tilting during surgery	Monitor patient for excessive fall in blood pressure

Drug	Use	Dosage	Preparation/Administration	Nursing Considerations
	Hypertensive crises	Maintenance: 0.2-6 mg/min IV *Children:* 0.1 mg/min IV adjusted according to response *Adults:* Initially, 0.5-1 mg/min by IV infusion (0.1% solution) according to response Maintenance: 1-15 mg/min IV *Children:* 0.1 mg/min IV adjusted according to response *Decrease* dose (and use with caution) in renal impairment	Dilute 500 mg ampule immediately *before* administration with 500 ml D₅W to yield a 1 mg/ml solution Prepared solution is stable for 24 hr at room temperature Discard any unused solution	Use with caution in patients receiving other antihypertensive drugs and neuromuscular blocking agents Large doses may cause respiratory paralysis Monitor circulatory status Monitor rate and depth of respiration

NEUROMUSCULAR BLOCKING AGENTS

Drug	Use	Dosage	Preparation/Administration	Nursing Considerations
Atracurium Tracrium	Adjunct to general anesthetic	*Adults: After* induction of anesthetic, 0.4-0.5 mg/kg IV; if necessary 0.08-0.1 mg/kg IV may be administered at 15-30 min intervals as indicated *Children:* Same as adults May need to decrease dose in cardiovascular disease Do *not* administer IM	Injectable: 10 mg/ml Discard solutions that are discolored or contain a precipitate Incompatible with alkaline solutions (e.g., barbiturates)	May release histamine All patients receiving muscle relaxants should have their vital signs monitored frequently during the postoperative period
Gallamine triethiodide Flaxedil Miowas Relaxan	Adjunct to surgical anesthetic Adjunct to electroconvulsive therapy	*Adults:* Initially 1-1.5 mg/kg IV; if necessary, 0.5-1 mg/kg IV may be administered at 45-90 min intervals *Children:* Same as adults Maximum: 100 mg *Adults:* 40-60 mg IV *Decrease* dose (and use with caution) in renal impairment	Injectable: 20 mg/ml Protect from light Discard discolored (yellow) solutions Do *not* mix with anesthetics because a precipitate may form	*Contraindicated* in myasthenia gravis, hypersensitivity to either gallamine or iodide, and severe renal impairment May induce tachycardias and dysrhythmias Not to be used in patients with renal failure Onset of effect: 1-2 min Duration: 20-30 min Reversed by anticholinesterases May cause anaphylactic reactions All patients receiving muscle relaxants should have their vital signs monitored frequently during the postoperative period

NOTE: For additional details regarding the individual agents listed in this table see the text and other tables in this chapter.

★ Indicates that the drug is generally available only in the United States.

Continued.

NURSING DRUG DIGEST—cont'd

Medication (trade name)	Indication	Usual dosage and administration	Dosage forms, preparation, and storage	Contraindications, cautions, and comments	Monitoring
★ **Hexafluorenium bromide** Mylaxen	Adjunct to succinylcholine neuromuscular blockade	*Adults:* After induction of anesthetic, 0.4 mg/kg IV (followed in 3 min by 0.2 mg/kg succinylcholine)	Injectable: 20 mg/ml	*Contraindicated* in hypersensitivity to either hexafluorenium or bromides Use with caution in patients with significant cardiovascular, hepatic, pulmonary, or renal disorders Used to increase and prolong effect of succinylcholine Possesses anticholinesterase activity Onset of effect: 1 to 2 min Duration: 20 to 30 min	All patients receiving muscle relaxants should have their vital signs monitored frequently during the postoperative period
Metocurine iodide Metubine	Adjunct to anesthetic Adjunct to electroconvulsive therapy	*Adults:* 0.2-0.4 mg/kg IV over 30-60 sec *Adults:* 1.75-5.5 mg IV over 30-60 sec Do not administer IM Decrease dose in renal impairment	Injectable: 2 mg/ml Incompatible with alkaline solutions, barbiturates, meperidine, and morphine	*Contraindicated* in hypersensitivity to either metocurine or iodides Incompatible with alkaline solutions Onset of effect: 1-2 min Duration: 25-90 min Reversed by anticholinesterases Less histamine-releasing effect than tubocurarine	All patients receiving muscle relaxants should have their vital signs monitored frequently during the postoperative period
Pancuronium bromide Pavulon	Adjunct to anesthetic	*Adults:* 0.04-0.1 mg/kg IV *Children:* Same as adults NOTE: A test dose of 0.02 mg/kg IV is recommended for administration to neonates in order to determine response to drug	Injectable: 1, 2 mg/ml	*Contraindicated* in hypersensitivity to either pancuronium or bromides Approximately 5 times as potent as tubocurarine Minimal histamine-releasing activity Onset of effect: 2-3 min Duration: 40-45 min Reversed by anticholinesterases	All patients receiving muscle relaxants should have their vital signs monitored frequently during the postoperative period

Drug	Use	Dosage	Supplied/Storage	Side Effects/Contraindications	Nursing Considerations
Succinylcholine Anectine Celocurin Celocurin-Chlorid Celocurin-Klorid Curacit Curalest Lysthenon Midarine Myoplegnine Myotenlis Pantolax Paranoval Quelicin Scoline Succinolin Succinyl Succinyl-Asta Sucostrin Suxamethonium Sux-Cert	Adjunct to anesthetic	*Adults:* *After* induction of anesthetic, 25-75 mg IV, repeat as indicated; or 2.5-4.3 mg/min by IV infusion of 0.1% solution *Children:* 1-5 years of age, *after* induction of anesthetic, 2 mg/kg IV; 6-12 years of age, *after* induction of anesthetic, 1 mg/kg IV	Injectable: 20, 50, 100 mg/ml Store between 2° and 8°C Powder for injection: 500, 1000 mg/vial Dilute to 0.1% with D5W or NS Prepared solution is stable for 24 hr	*Contraindicated* in hypersensitivity, narrow-angle glaucoma, myopathy, history of malignant hyperthermia, and atypical pseudocholinesterase Induces fasciculations and twitching Causes postoperative muscle pain Prolonged apnea in patients with atypical pseudocholinesterase May cause cardiac dysrhythmias May be associated with malignant hyperpyrexia (rarely); have dantrolene (IV) available for treatment Hypersensitivity reactions have occurred as has bronchospasm Myoglobinuria may occur after use of this drug May cause a transient rise in intraocular pressure Onset of effect: 0.5-1 min Duration 2 to 5 min *Not* reversed by anticholinesterases	All patients receiving muscle relaxants should have their vital signs monitored frequently during the postoperative period
Tubocurarine Curarin Curarine Intocostrin-T Intocostrine-T Jexin Tubarine Tubarine Miscible Tubocuran	Adjunct to anesthetic Adjunct to electroconvulsive therapy	*Adults:* 0.1-0.3 mg/kg IV *Adults:* 0.1-0.2 mg/kg IV	Injectable: 3 mg/ml Discard discolored solutions Incompatible with barbiturate solutions	*Contraindicated* in myasthenia gravis May cause histamine release Onset of effect: 3-5 min Duration: 20-40 min Use with caution in pulmonary disorders, renal impairment, and hepatic impairment Neostigmine (0.5 mg IV) can be used to treat tubocurarine overdose	Patients receiving muscle relaxants should have their vital signs monitored frequently during the postoperative period

BIBLIOGRAPHY

Compendium of pharmaceuticals and specialties 1984 (19th ed.). Ottawa: Canadian Pharmaceutical Association, 1984.

Nicotine gum. *The Medical Letter,* 1984, *26*(661), 47-48.

Reynolds, J.E.F. (Ed.). *Martindale, the extra pharmacopoeia,* (28th Ed.). London: The Pharmaceutical Press, 1982.

Taylor, P. Ganglionic blocking and stimulating agents. In A.G. Goodman, L.S. Goodman, & A. Gilman, (Eds.). *The pharmacological basis of therapeutics* (6th Ed.). New York: Macmillan, 1980.

Taylor, P. Neuromuscular blocking agents. In A.G. Goodman, L.S. Goodman & A. Gilman (Eds.), *The pharmacological basis of therapeutics* (6th Ed.). New York: Macmillan, 1980.

1984 USPDI, Drug information for the health care provider. Rockville: The United States Pharmacopoeia Convention Inc., 1983.

RESPIRATORY AND RELATED MEDICATIONS

Medications discussed in this section

Review of the Anatomy, Physiology, and Assessment of the Respiratory System

Richard L. Jones

The primary function of the lungs is to add oxygen to and remove carbon dioxide from the blood. These two seemingly simple processes are affected by many factors such as (1) the resistance of the airways to gas movement into and out of the lungs; (2) the stiffness of the lungs, which in some instances requires excessive work during inspiration and in others extra work during expiration; (3) the matching of pulmonary blood flow and ventilation; (4) the thickness of the barrier between alveolar air and capillary blood; and (5) the sensitivity of the chemoreceptors to maintain homeostatic partial pressure of oxygen and carbon dioxide. These factors affecting the primary function of the lung will be the subject of this chapter.

ANATOMY

The right and left lungs are encased in the airtight thorax composed of 12 thoracic vertebrae, 12 pairs of ribs, the sternum, the diaphragm, and intercostal muscles (Figure 27-1), with the trachea and its branches supplying atmospheric air for oxygen and carbon dioxide exchange. The right lung has three lobes (superior, middle, and inferior), whereas the left lung has only two lobes (superior and inferior). In spite of the structural difference there is a nearly equal distribution of ventilation and perfusion with each lung receiving approximately 50% of the totals. Assessment of respiratory efficiency depends on direct and indirect observation of the chest and underlying structures.

During normal breathing the thoracic cage is expanded symmetrically by contraction of the diaphragm, which causes the diaphragm to move from its resting dome shape (Figure 27-1) to a flatter configuration. The diaphragmatic excursion is assessed by way of percussion at the scapular line during inspiration and expiration; excursion is usually 3 to 5 cm bilaterally. This expansion of the thorax causes

pressure in the pleural space to become more negative (relative to atmospheric pressure), which causes the lungs to inflate to fill the void created by the larger chest cavity. The external intercostals and accessory muscles can also expand the thorax, but these are used only when large volumes of air must be moved rapidly, as during exercise, or by patients with lung disease who have lost the effectiveness of their diaphragm.

When respiratory muscles are relaxed, the lungs have approximately one-half their maximum volume. The lungs are able to maintain this volume because their tendency to collapse is balanced by the tendency for the chest wall to expand. Inspiration causes additional stretch on the lungs. When inspiration is complete and the inspiratory muscles are relaxed, expiration proceeds as the lungs recoil back to their resting volume. Thus muscular effort is not required for expiration during normal breathing, but during exercise and in patients with certain lung diseases expiration must be assisted by the abdominal muscles and the internal intercostal muscles of the chest wall. The abdominal muscles assist expiration by forcing the abdominal contents against the diaphragm, pushing it up into the thoracic cavity.

The lung is an extremely well designed organ. The surface area available for diffusion is more than 40 times that of the skin, and oxygenation and carbon dioxide removal can be maintained at resting levels even during heavy exercise.

Inhaled air travels through airways that divide approximately 16 times before there is any chance for it to participate in gas exchange with the pulmonary capillary blood. The smallest non–gas-exchanging airways are called terminal bronchioles, of which the average adult has in excess of 65,000. Each terminal bronchiole gives rise to a respiratory unit that consists of respiratory bronchioles, alveolar ducts, and alveolar sacs with their numerous alveoli (Figure 27-2). The

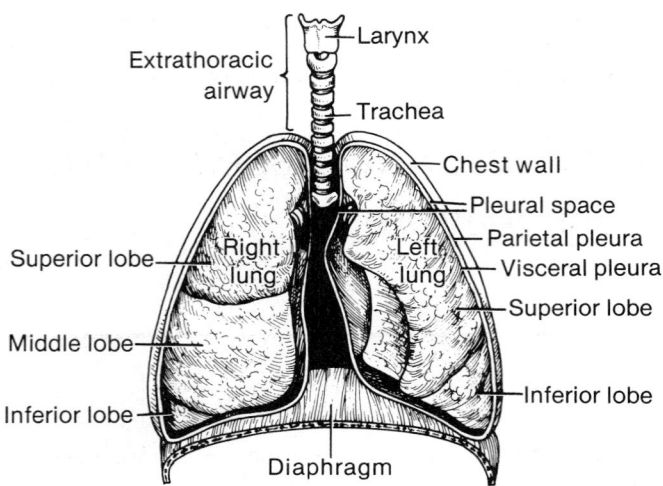

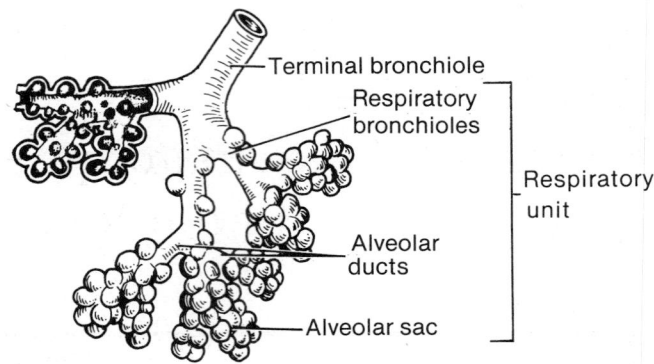

FIGURE 27-2. **A terminal bronchiole with a portion of its respiratory unit extending from it.**

FIGURE 27-1. **Relationship of lungs with chest wall. The various lobes of each lung are identified. The pleural space is really only a fluid layer separating the parietal pleura of the chest wall from the visceral pleura of the lung. The extrathoracic airway consists of that portion of the trachea outside the chest wall as well as the larynx.**

respiratory bronchioles are tubular airways with alveoli protruding at intervals from their walls. There are about three divisions of respiratory bronchioles with progressively greater alveolarization of the walls with each division. The alveolar ducts extend distal to the respiratory bronchioles and the walls are completely covered with alveoli. After approximately three divisions each alveolar duct terminates in an alveolar sac. The average adult lung contains at least 300 million alveoli for gas exchange.

LUNG VOLUMES

Perhaps the best way to acquaint oneself with the various lung volumes is to inflate and deflate your own lungs. Fill your lungs as much as possible; the volume is defined as total lung capacity (TLC). Now exhale as much as possible; really squeeze the last little bit of air out. No matter how hard you tried to empty your lungs there will be some volume remaining, and this is called the residual volume (RV). The volume of air exhaled from TLC to RV is defined as vital capacity (VC). If you exhale from TLC to RV as fast as possible, then we would define the volume exhaled as the forced vital capacity (FVC).

Since you are now breathing normally, stop at the end of a normal expiration. The volume in your lungs at this point is called functional residual capacity (FRC), and it is determined by a balance of the elastic

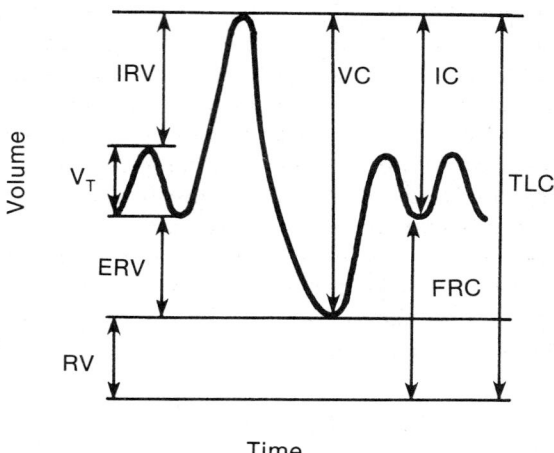

FIGURE 27-3. **A spirogram illustrating the various lung volumes and capacities.**

forces where the tendency for chest wall expansion is matched by the tendency for lung collapse. The "functional" component of FRC was derived from the fact that even at the end of a normal expiration there is sufficient volume in the lung to maintain oxygen flow into and carbon dioxide flow out of the blood. The volume of a normal breath is called the tidal volume (V_T). If you inhale from FRC to TLC, you have taken an inspiratory capacity (IC) breath. The amount you can inhale over and above a normal tidal volume is called inspiratory reserve volume (IRV); the amount you can exhale from FRC is called expiratory reserve volume (ERV).

Figure 27-3 shows a spirogram, which is a recording of air movement into and out of the lungs. Note that there are four volumes and four capacities, and that a lung capacity incorporates two or more of the four volumes, e.g., ERV + RV = FRC.

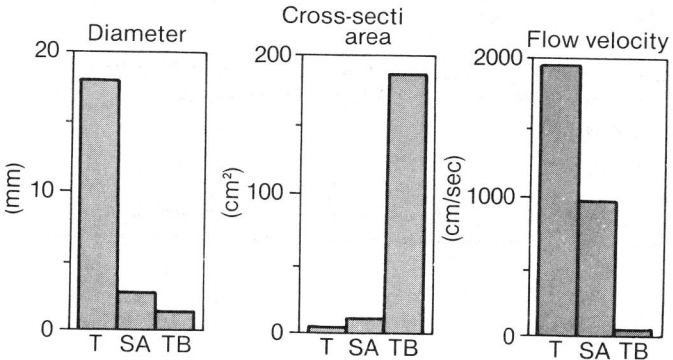

FIGURE 27-4. **Data for the trachea (T), small airways (SA) 2mm in diameter, and terminal bronchioles (TB) 0.6 mm in diameter. When the individual area of the approximately 65,000 terminal bronchioles are summed, the result is a large total cross-sectional area compared with the individually larger trachea. During a forced expiration the velocity of flow through airways of various sizes is inversely proportional to cross-sectional area.**

AIRWAY OBSTRUCTION

Intrathoracic obstruction

The most common lung diseases are those that affect the airways within the thorax. These diseases normally begin their development in bronchioles less than 2 mm in diameter but at this stage there is little discomfort.

The reason patients are, for the most part, unaware of disease affecting their small airways is that the small airways have a large cross-sectional area compared to the larger airways such as the trachea. At first this seems ironic since we know the trachea has a large diameter, and large tubes offer less flow resistance than small ones. However, when we consider that there are hundreds of airways 2 mm in diameter and that the flow of air is divided among these numerous small airways, then the velocity of air flow through the small airways is low. It takes little pressure to move air slowly so that an increase in the resistance of small peripheral airways adds only a slight, and largely unnoticed, increase in the overall effort required to move air into or out of the lung. Figure 27-4 shows data for the trachea, small airways 2 mm in diameter, and terminal bronchioles 0.6 mm in diameter. It is clear that the larger the airway the smaller is its cross-sectional area and the greater the velocity of flow.

An increase in resistance of large airways is detected by the patient, since the work of breathing is increased because of the greater pressures required to move air through airways having relatively low cross-sectional area. Note the effort needed when breathing through a soda straw.

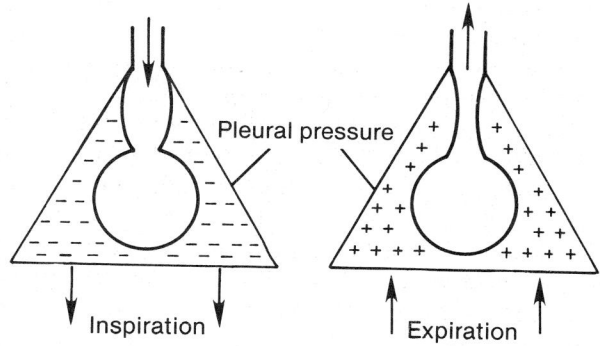

FIGURE 27-5. **The effects of pleural pressure on airway size. Airway resistance is lower during inspiration than during expiration.**

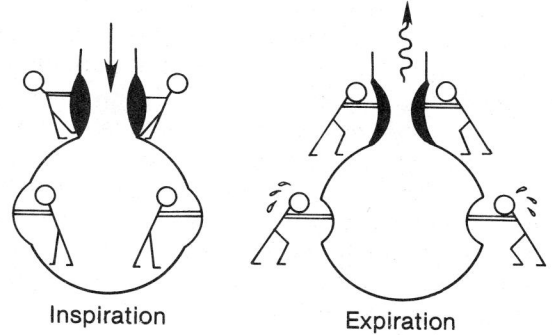

FIGURE 27-6. **The relative work required during expiration and inspiration in patients with severe airway obstruction. Because of the high resistance, positive pressure may be exerted on the lung's exterior in order to exhale at a reasonable rate. This positive pleural pressure compresses the already narrowed airway, resulting in excessive work with each expiration. During inspiration the negative pleural pressure tends to dilate airways, making the work of inspiration less than that during expiration.**

In patients with intrathoracic airway obstruction it is more difficult to exhale than to inhale. Figure 27-5 shows that during inspiration the more negative intrapleural pressure widens airways and lowers airway resistance, and thus the work of inspiration. On the other hand, during expiration pleural pressure becomes less negative and may even swing to positive (relative to atmospheric pressure), causing a force that narrows the airways, increases airway resistance, and therefore the work required to exhale. Figure 27-6 shows diagrammatically the relative work required to inhale and exhale in a patient with clinically significant airway obstruction. Rhonchi can be heard on auscultation as the air passes through the narrowed airways.

In people with normal lungs, work is required to inhale because we have to expand the elastic lungs. However, we accomplish a normal tidal expiration simply by relaxing the muscles of inspiration (mainly the diaphragm), and the energy stored in the elastic lung (like a stretched spring) is sufficient to permit expiration back to FRC without additional muscular work.

However, because of the high airway resistance, patients with obstructive lung diseases have to perform extra work to exhale. On palpation, expansion is diminished and there is decreased tactile-fremitus. There is not enough elastic energy stored in the lung after a normal inspiration to force air out in a short enough time to allow for adequate ventilation. This added expiratory work can be so high in some patients (e.g. those in *status asthmaticus*) that they tire to the point where ventilation actually decreases. The amount of expiratory work required in patients with emphysema can also be high, since the lungs of these patients have little elastic recoil. There is permanent hyperinflation of the lung beyond the terminal bronchioles with destruction of alveolar walls. The loss of elastic recoil makes it relatively easy for patients with emphysema to inhale but the aid to expiration from elastic recoil is diminished and this, along with the usually high airway resistance, causes excessive expiratory work after each tidal inspiration.

Patients normally seek medical help after they notice an increase in their work of breathing (usually during exertion), and in most cases the obstructive defect is so far advanced at this point that complete reversal is probably not possible except in patients with asthma.

Extrathoracic obstruction

In contrast to obstructive disorders affecting airways within the chest cavity where inspiration is relatively easy, patients with narrowing in the extrathoracic segment of the airway (Figure 27-1) have difficulty both inhaling and exhaling. Extrathoracic airway obstruction can result from things such as a traumatic neck injury and a healed tracheostomy.

The increased airway resistance to both inspiration and expiration occurs because the narrowed portion acts as a fixed resistance, which is unaffected by the pressure within the pleural space. Intrathoracic airways are narrower during expiration than inspiration because of the less negative pleural pressure.

Intrathoracic versus extrathoracic obstruction

The typical changes in lung function seen in patients with intrathoracic and extrathoracic airway ob-

TABLE 27-1

Comparison of pulmonary function between intrathoracic and extrathoracic airway obstruction

Function	Intrathoracic	Extrathoracic
TLC	+	N
VC	−	N
FRC	+	N
RV	+ +	N
FEV_1	−	−
FIF	N	−

N, normal; +, above normal; −, below normal.

struction are illustrated in Table 27-1. The increased work required to exhale in patients with intrathoracic obstruction causes the patient to breathe at a higher FRC because a large lung offers greater elastic assistance during expiration. In addition, elevated FRC decreases airway resistance, as illustrated in Figure 27-7, where the elastic properties of the lung are shown as a set of springs attached at one end to the visceral pleura (outer surface of the lung) and the other end to an airway. Expansion of the lung also causes the airway to expand and this decreases airway resistance. Therefore an increased FRC aids breathing in patients with intrathoracic airway obstruction by offering an increased elastic force during expiration and by decreasing airway resistance.

Intrathoracic airway obstruction causes increased RV because narrowed airways tend to collapse at higher volumes than in a normal lung. If some airways are closed during normal breathing there will be no ventilation to gas exchange areas served by those airways, and this causes a shunt (see below). An increased FRC tends to keep airways open and this permits better blood oxygenation.

When performing a FVC, the forced expiratory volume in the first second (FEV_1) gives a good indication of airway function. Patients with a significant amount of intrathoracic or extrathoracic airway obstruction have decreased FEV_1. Forced inspiratory flow rate (FIF) is relatively normal in patients with intrathoracic airway obstruction but is decreased in extrathoracic airway obstruction.

Pulmonary fibrosis

There are many insults and factors that can cause pulmonary fibrosis. As fibrotic tissue builds up, the lung becomes stiffer and less compliant than normal. Because of the lung's stiffness, patients with pulmo-

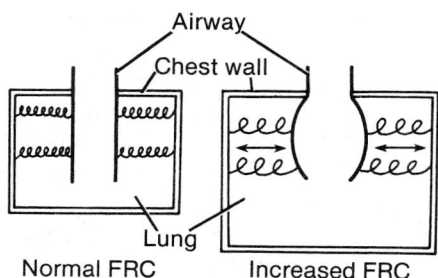

FIGURE 27-7. **How the lung's elastic tissue supports airways. Airway diameter varies directly with lung volume.**

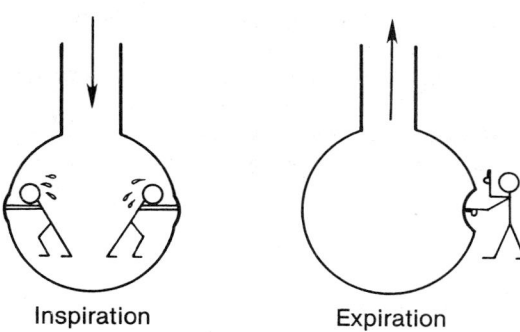

FIGURE 27-8. **The relative work during expiration and inspiration in patients with pulmonary fibrosis. It is difficult to inhale because of the increased elastic recoil, but once the breath has been taken, expiration is effortless because of the large amount of elastic energy stored in the lung.**

nary fibrosis have to do more than a normal amount of work to inhale (Figure 27-8). However, as in the normal lung, there is an excess of energy stored in the lungs' elastic tissue at the end of a tidal inspiration to allow passive expiration back to FRC. These patients may demonstrate dyspnea on exertion and tachypnea and diminished thoracic expansion with assessment. Cyanosis may be observed, and on palpation the trachea may be deviated to the most effective side. Percussion is resonant to dull, and the breath sounds reduced or absent, bronchovesicular or bronchial. Increased vocal fremitus may be noted along with increased whisper pectoriloquy. Inspiratory and expiratory rales may be noted.

Since FRC is determined by the balance of elastic forces between lung collapse and chest wall expansion, a stiff lung causes a lower than normal FRC. Also TLC and VC are decreased, but RV may be normal. The stiff lung aids expiration, and the FEV_1 of these patients approaches their FVC.

BLOOD GASES

Defects in the mechanical function of the lung do not always interfere with the exchange of oxygen and carbon dioxide between alveolar air and blood, but this is a common consequence. There are three basic causes of gas exchange problems: (1) a generalized decrease in alveolar ventilation ($\dot{V}_A$); (2) localized defects in the matching of ventilation with pulmonary perfusion; and (3) defects in the gas exchange surface.

Figure 27-9 shows a sketch of the terminal portion of a respiratory unit. A cross section taken through the alveolar sac reveals a pulmonary capillary embedded between two alveolar walls composed of alveolar epithelium. The capillary itself is enclosed in endothelium. The epithelium and endothelium are in contact on one side, and the contact surface is called the *basement membrane.* On the other side the endothelium and epithelium are separated by an interstitial

space, which probably serves as a channel for fluid removal. The thin side containing the basement membrane is thought to be the major site for gas exchange with little or no gas exchange occurring through the thicker interstitial space.

Before normal values for blood gases are discussed, it is important to understand how altitude affects barometric pressure and the partial pressures of gases. Figure 27-10 shows that barometric pressure decreases with increasing altitude. Partial pressures of gases have a similar relationship to altitude, since a partial pressure of a gas is nothing more than the percentage of barometric pressure occupied by that gas. For instance, a gas mixture containing 21% oxygen would have a partial pressure of oxygen (Po_2) at sea level ($P_B = 760$ mm Hg) of $0.21 \times 760 = 160$ mm Hg. In other words, 160 mm Hg is 21% of 760 mm Hg. As altitude increases, the Po_2 in alveolar air (Pao_2) and in arterial blood (Pao_2) decreases. Therefore any single set of normal values would exist for only a given altitude. You must know the altitude of your hospital in order to interpret the normality of a Pao_2. For instance, in Vancouver a normal Pao_2 would be near 90 mm Hg, but in Denver a Pao_2 of about 65 mm Hg would be normal.

Figure 27-11 shows a normal set of values for Po_2 and carbon dioxide partial pressure (Pco_2). The atmosphere has a Po_2 of 160 mm Hg, but as that air is inhaled into the airways it is warmed to 37°C, and relative humidity increases to 100%. The addition of water vapor, which is a gas, decreases the contributions of all other gases to barometric pressure. For this reason the Po_2 decreases to 150 mm Hg. About 70% of an inhaled breath reaches the alveoli, which already contain some gas (FRC) at a lower Po_2 than 150 mm Hg, and, in addition, carbon dioxide is present in the

FIGURE 27-9. **The ultrastructure of an alveolar wall. The alveolar epithelium is separated from capillary endothelium on one side by the basement membrane and on the other side by an interstitial space. The arrow shows that gas exchange occurs between alveolar air and capillary blood primarily across the thinnest side.**

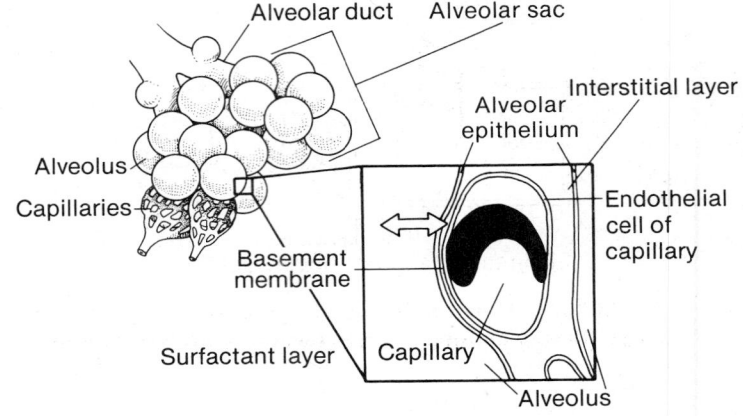

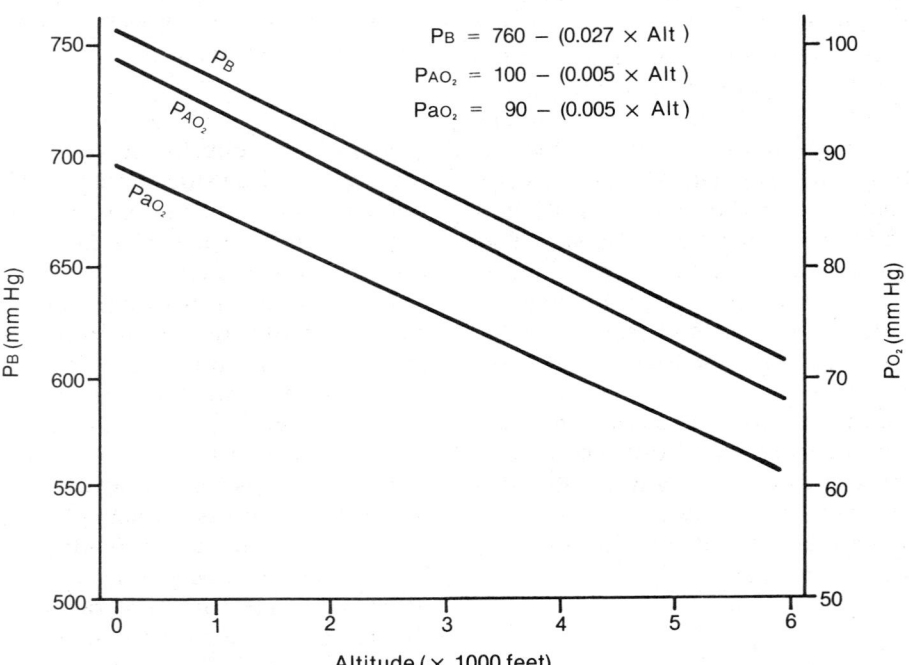

$$P_B = 760 - (0.027 \times Alt)$$
$$P_{AO_2} = 100 - (0.005 \times Alt)$$
$$Pa_{O_2} = 90 - (0.005 \times Alt)$$

FIGURE 27-10. **The relationships of barometric pressure (P_B), alveolar P_{O_2} (P_{AO_2}), and arterial P_{O_2} (Pa_{O_2}) to altitude. The linear regression equations permit calculation of P_B, P_{AO_2} and Pa_{O_2} for altitudes between sea level and 6000 ft.**

alveolar air, which decreases the P_{O_2}. Alveolar air has a P_{O_2} near 100 mm Hg and P_{CO_2} of 40 mm Hg. The systemic arteries carry blood that has just left the lung. If there were perfect gas exchange, the P_{O_2} in arterial blood and alveoli would be the same. But pulmonary gas exchange is not perfect, and thus arterial P_{O_2} is lower than alveolar P_{O_2}, although alveolar and arterial P_{CO_2} are the same (40 mm Hg). The metabolizing tissues use oxygen and produce carbon dioxide. Therefore venous blood returning to the lungs has an average P_{O_2} of 40 mm Hg and P_{CO_2} of 46 mm Hg.

If a patient underventilates, there will be less fresh air bathing the alveolar gas exchange area. Since the carbon dioxide partial pressure in arterial blood (Pa_{CO_2}) is inversely proportional to $\dot{V}_A$, patients who underventilate will have higher than normal Pa_{CO_2}. Figure 27-12 shows that doubling the $\dot{V}_A$ halves the Pa_{CO_2}, whereas halving the $\dot{V}_A$ doubles the Pa_{CO_2}. Therefore the measurement of Pa_{CO_2} provides information about the adequacy of $\dot{V}_A$. In most patients Pa_{CO_2} is nearly the same as alveolar P_{CO_2} (P_{ACO_2}), but this is not the case for P_{AO_2} and Pa_{O_2}.

Also shown in Figure 27-12 is the effect of $\dot{V}_A$ on P_{AO_2} and Pa_{O_2} in young normal individuals living at sea

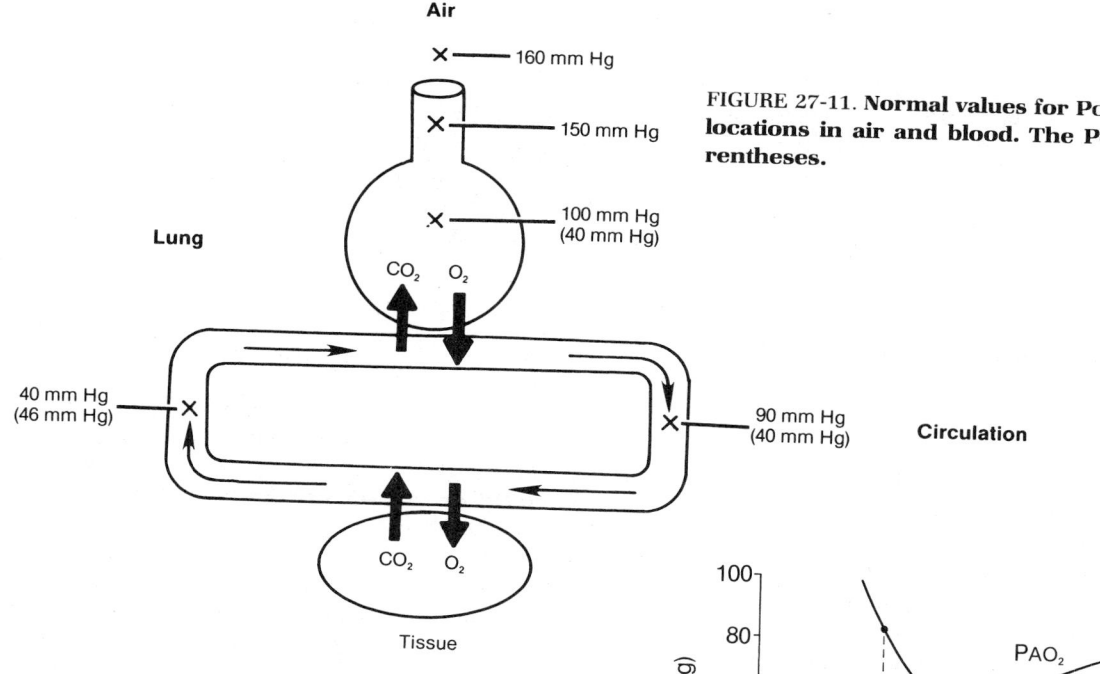

FIGURE 27-11. Normal values for P_{O_2} and P_{CO_2} at various locations in air and blood. The P_{CO_2} values are in parentheses.

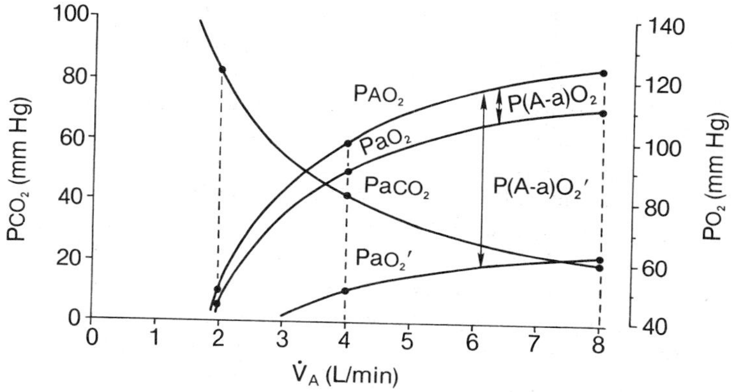

FIGURE 27-12. The changes in Pa_{CO_2}, PA_{O_2} and Pa_{O_2} with changes in $\dot{V}_A$. In this example a $\dot{V}_A$ of 4 L/min would yield a Pa_{CO_2} of 42 mm Hg and a Pa_{O_2} of 90 mm Hg. If $\dot{V}_A$ falls to 2 L/min, Pa_{CO_2} increases to 84 mm Hg and Pa_{O_2} falls to 43 mm Hg, but if $\dot{V}_A$ increases to 8 L/min, Pa_{CO_2} will decrease to 21 mm Hg and Pa_{O_2} will rise to 112 mm Hg. These data were obtained assuming a CO_2 production of 232 ml/min (at body temperature) and a ratio of Pa_{O_2}/PA_{O_2} of 0.9. At a $\dot{V}_A$ of 4 L/min, the $P(A-a)O_2$ would be 10 mm Hg. If there is a Pa_{O_2}'/PA_{O_2} ratio of 0.5 because of lung disease, then the Pa_{O_2}' would be lower at a given $\dot{V}_A$; at a $\dot{V}_A$ of 4 L/min, the $P(A-a)O_2$ would be 50 mm Hg.

level. The difference between PA_{O_2} and Pa_{O_2}, or the alveolar-arterial difference for oxygen—$P(A-a)O_2$—at any given $\dot{V}_A$ would be greater in older individuals.

Even in the most healthy lungs there is imperfect matching of ventilation and perfusion, and this is largely responsible for the $P(A-a)O_2$. Although both ventilation and perfusion increase from the top to the bottom of the lung, in the lower one third of the lung perfusion exceeds ventilation, and there is incomplete oxygenation of the venous blood returning to the lung. When this is mixed with well-oxygenated blood from the upper regions, the end result is a reduction in Pa_{O_2} and an increased $P(A-a)O_2$.

The decrease in lung elastic recoil with age causes some airways to collapse during normal breathing with a resultant increase in $P(A-a)O_2$. The amount of airway closure in the elderly increases when they lie down, since in the supine position abdominal contents push against the diaphragm and lower the FRC. Younger people also have a drop in FRC in the supine position, but this drop normally is not sufficient to place their lung at a volume where airway closure occurs. The rate at which $P(A-a)O_2$ increases with age is shown in Figure 27-13.

The most common cause for higher than expected $P(A-a)O_2$ is underventilation in relation to the amount of blood flowing ($\dot{Q}$) through some lung regions. This defect, known as low $\dot{V}/\dot{Q}$ ratio, is common in persons with airway obstruction. If a lung region is perfused but not ventilated (zero $\dot{V}/\dot{Q}$ ratio), then a widened $P(A-a)O_2$ will also result. This condition is known as a

shunt, since there is no chance for oxygenating that portion of the blood flowing through the unventilated regions.

Another potential cause for abnormally large $P(A-a)O_2$ is a widened membrane separating alveolar gas from pulmonary capillary blood. In various interstitial lung diseases leading to pulmonary fibrosis the membrane (both thin and thick sides, Figure 27-9) is thickened, and this decreases the rate at which oxygen

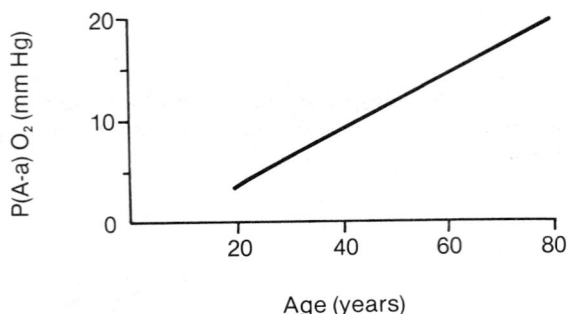

FIGURE 27-13. **The approximate increase in P(A-a)O₂ with increasing age.**

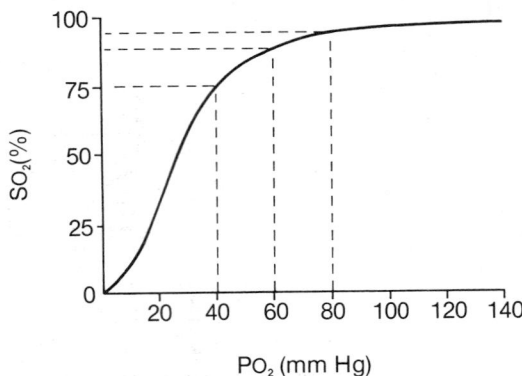

FIGURE 27-14. **The oxygen dissociation curve. At PO_2 levels above 60 mm Hg there is little change in the saturation of hemoglobin with oxygen (SO_2). If PO_2 falls below 60 mm Hg, there is a more dramatic drop in SO_2. At PO_2 values of 40, 60, and 80 mm Hg, SO_2 is 75%, 91%, and 95%, respectively.**

flows into the blood. The effect of increased diffusion distance is exaggerated during exercise, since venous blood returning to the lungs has a lower PO_2, and the time available for gas exchange is decreased. The lowered oxygen-diffusion rate can be insufficient to completely oxygenate the blood. The result is a drop in PaO_2 during exercise compared with rest. In normal individuals PaO_2 is maintained at the resting level during exercise.

Although PaO_2 gives information about the efficiency of lung gas exchange, it is not necessarily an indicator of the amount of oxygen in arterial blood. It is important to remember that about 99% of blood's oxygen content is carried on hemoglobin and that a PaO_2 of 100 mm Hg causes nearly complete saturation of the oxygen-binding sites on hemoglobin. If PaO_2 increases from 100 to 200 mm Hg, the amount of oxygen in arterial blood will increase by only 6%. However, doubling the PaO_2 from 40 to 80 mm Hg will result in a 29% increase in arterial oxygen content. This discrepancy between PaO_2 and oxygen content is caused by the shape of the oxygen dissociation curve (Figure 27-14). A drop in PO_2 below about 60 mm Hg causes an accelerated loss of oxygen from hemoglobin, whereas an increase in PO_2 above 60 mm Hg adds little oxygen to the hemoglobin. (Remember that hemoglobin carries nearly all the oxygen, so that the percent saturation gives an indication of the relative amounts of oxygen in blood at different PO_2 values.) A patient with a PaO_2 of 60 mm Hg still has 91% of the available oxygen-binding sites on hemoglobin filled, and this (providing there is not a severe anemia) provides plenty of oxygen to meet resting tissue demands.

CHEMOSENSITIVITY

In normal individuals there is little variation in PaO_2 and PaCO_2 during the waking hours or during sleep.

However, in some patients with chronic bronchitis there are marked reductions in PaO_2 and increases in PaCO_2 at various times during sleep. These blood gas abnormalities during sleep are caused by periodic decreases in alveolar ventilation and by the poor matching of ventilation and blood flow in the lung.

The ability to maintain consistent arterial blood gases hinges on the proper function of chemosensitive tissues that can detect alterations in PaO_2 and PaCO_2 and adjust ventilation in an attempt to correct the abnormality. It appears that many patients with airway obstruction have altered chemosensitivity.

Adjacent to the carotid arteries are specialized cell masses called the carotid bodies. The carotid bodies receive a high blood flow so that their venous PO_2 is only slightly below the arterial level. The carotid bodies sense decreases in PaO_2 and by some poorly understood mechanism excite nerves that cause stimulation of the respiratory control center in the brainstem. This stimulation causes ventilation to increase in an attempt to raise PaO_2 and therefore PaO_2 (see Figure 27-12).

The carotid bodies also cause increased ventilation when they are exposed to increased PaCO_2. However, the primary detectors of alterations in PaCO_2 are the central chemoreceptors that are located on the ventral surface of the medulla near the respiratory center. The central chemoreceptors are surrounded by cerebral spinal fluid (CSF) and are separated from the blood by the so-called blood-brain barrier. Therefore carbon dioxide must diffuse from the blood, through the blood-brain barrier, and into the CSF before the receptor is stimulated. Carbon dioxide diffuses readily across membranes so that it easily enters the CSF from blood. When carbon dioxide arrives in the CSF, it reacts with water to produce hydrogen ions, which are the actual stimulators of the central chemoreceptor. As in the case of the carotid body, the central chemoreceptors have nervous connections to the respiratory control center that controls ventilation.

If $Paco_2$ increases, ventilation increases and this causes $Paco_2$ to decrease. The opposite is also true; if we hyperventilate, $Paco_2$ falls, and there is less chemoreceptor stimulation so that ventilation decreases causing $Paco_2$ to increase. Remember, $Paco_2$ is inversely proportional to ventilation so that a change in ventilation causes opposite changes in $Paco_2$ (see Figure 27-12).

Some patients have altered sensitivity to carbon dioxide and fail to show the normal response of increasing ventilation when their $Paco_2$ rises. Other patients have such poor lung function that they are unable to increase ventilation in response to chemoreceptor stimulation. These patients often have wide fluctuations in Pao_2 and $Paco_2$ during acute respiratory tract infections.

Changes in ventilation have predictable effects on $Paco_2$, even in patients with severe lung disease. However, increasing ventilation alone will rarely increase Pao_2 to a normal value in a lung containing regions where ventilation and perfusion are poorly matched (Figure 27-12). The inability to increase Pao_2 to normal by increasing ventilation stems from the fact that Pao_2 is determined by the mixture of blood oxygen contents emerging from the various lung regions. If one region continues to be poorly ventilated even though overall ventilation is increased, then the lower oxygen content of blood emerging from that region tends to lower the oxygen content (and Pao_2) of the mixture. Regions that are overventilated produce blood with an increased Po_2 but the oxygen content is not proportionately increased because of the shape of the oxygen dissociation curve (Figure 27-14), which is nearly flat at high Po_2 levels. Therefore Pao_2 will be decreased if only a portion of the lung fails to normally oxygenate its blood.

SUMMARY

Normal individuals rarely notice their breathing because the amount of work done is small. However, patients with lung disease are often preoccupied with the extra work they do during the approximately 17,000 breaths taken each day. Disorders leading to increased work of breathing include narrowed airways and stiff lungs.

When airways within the thorax are narrowed, more work is done during expiration than during inspiration. However, if the site of increased airway resistance is in the extrathoracic airway, there is increased work required during both inspiration and expiration. When the lungs are stiff the extra work occurs only during inspiration when the lungs have to be stretched.

Most lung diseases cause decreased Pao_2, but it is important to recall that a lower than normal Pao_2 does not necessarily produce the same magnitude of decrease in the amount of oxygen carried in the blood. Hemoglobin is still 91% saturated with oxygen at a Po_2 of 60 mm Hg.

Blood gases are maintained at consistent levels by chemoreceptors. The carotid bodies detect alterations in Pao_2 and $Paco_2$, but the primary sensors for altered $Paco_2$ are the central chemoreceptors. The result of chemoreceptor stimulation is increased ventilation, which is more effective in decreasing $Paco_2$ than it is in raising Pao_2 in a diseased lung.

BIBLIOGRAPHY

Bates, D.V. Chronic bronchitis and emphysema: The search for their natural history. In P.T. Macklen & S. Permutt (Eds.). *The lung in the transition between health and disease.* New York: Marcel Dekker, 1979.

Craig, D.B., Wahba, W.M., Don, H.F., Courter, J.G., & Becklake, M.R.: Closing volume and its relationship to gas exchange in seated and supine positions. *Journal of Applied Physiology,* 1971, *31,* 717-721.

Douglas, N.J., Leggett, R.J., Calverley, P.M., & others. Transient hypoxaemia during sleep in chronic bronchitis and emphysema. *Lancet,* 1979, *1,* 1-4.

Hughes, J.M., Hoppin, F.G., & Mead, J. Effect of lung inflation on bronchial length and diameter in excised lungs. *Journal of Applied Physiology,* 1972, *32,* 25-35.

Knudson, R.J. & Burrows, B. Early detection of obstructive lung diseases. *Medical Clinics of North America,* 1973, *57,* 681-690.

Macklem, P.T. Obstruction in small airways: A challenge to medicine. *American Journal of Medicine,* 1972, *52,* 721-724.

Malasanos, L., Barkauskas, V., Moss, M., & Stoltenberg-Allen, K. *Health Assessment* (3rd ed.). St. Louis: The C.V. Mosby Co., 1985.

Mellemgaard, K. Alveolar-arterial oxygen difference: Size and components in normal man. *Acta Physiologica Scandinavica,* 1966, *67,* 10-20.

Murray, J.F. *The normal lung: the basis for diagnosis and treatment of pulmonary disease.* Philadelphia: W.B. Saunders, 1976.

CHAPTER 28

Bronchodilators and Respiratory Gases

Margaret A. Peterson
David F. Biggs

Medications discussed in this chapter

Adrenergics (sympathomimetics)
  Albuterol
  Ephedrine
  Epinephrine
  Ethylnorepinephrine
  Fenoterol
  Isoetharine
  Isoproterenol
  Metaproterenol
  Terbutaline
Anticholinergic (parasympatholytic)
  Ipratropium

Phosphodiesterase inhibitors
  Aminophylline
  Dyphylline
  Oxtriphylline
  Theophylline
Inhibitor of mediator release
  Cromolyn sodium
Respiratory gas
  Oxygen

Bronchodilators and respiratory gases, particularly oxygen, are commonly used in the treatment of various respiratory conditions. Often bronchodilators and oxygen or other respiratory gases are used together to promote respiratory function in hospitals or in the home setting. A sound knowledge of the use of these medications is required for planning individualized patient care and for helping patients and their families participate in their own care both in the hospital and in the home.

BRONCHODILATORS

Bronchodilators are drugs used to reverse respiratory obstruction caused by the narrowing of airways from muscle contraction, thickening of airway walls, or the formation of mucous plugs associated with such conditions as asthma, chronic bronchitis, emphysema, or chronic obstructive lung disease.

Before individual bronchodilating agents are discussed, some anatomy and physiology of the airways will be reviewed so that the mechanisms involved in bronchoconstriction can be understood. Both the use-

fulness and the limitations of the many bronchodilators that are available may then be more fully appreciated.

The trachea is the largest of the airways and divides to form the major bronchi. The major bronchi repeatedly subdivide, becoming progressively shorter and of smaller diameter with each division. The bronchi of smallest diameter are referred to as bronchioles; two types are important: terminal bronchioles and respiratory bronchioles (see Chapter 27 "Review of the Anatomy, Physiology, and Assessment of the Respiratory System").

Terminal bronchioles lie between the airways, which are concerned chiefly with the exchange of oxygen and carbon dioxide. The terminal bronchioles branch into the respiratory bronchioles. The respiratory bronchioles open directly into an alveolus or form several alveolar ducts, which in turn open into alveoli. The alveoli are the major sites of gas exchange within the lungs.

All of the airways from the trachea to the alveolar ducts contain smooth muscle. The muscle is arranged in a geodesic pattern, and therefore muscle contraction produces both shortening and narrowing of the airways. Muscle hypertrophy accompanies many chronic lung conditions and causes the lumen of the airways to narrow.

The lungs are innervated by both the parasympathetic and the sympathetic nervous systems. The innervation pattern is complex, and some anatomic crossing between the two systems occurs. However, in general the parasympathetic system is thought to cause constriction of airway smooth muscle, whereas the sympathetic system is thought to cause dilation of airway smooth muscle.

The predominant neural influence is parasympathetic and is derived chiefly from the vagus nerve. Vagal mediated effects are important to maintain normal tone in the airways.

Changes in the tone of the airways can be used to

divide the airways into two relatively distinct groups: conducting airways and peripheral airways. Although most pulmonary function tests are more sensitive to changes occurring in the first group, responses within each group can be used to measure airway function and are therefore useful in determining the following.

1. Type of lung disease
2. Severity of lung disease
3. Effectiveness of drug therapy

The first group, the large, or conducting, airways, technically extends from the trachea to the terminal bronchioles. Clinically, however, this group is more commonly defined as airways with a diameter greater than 2 mm. Changes in the tone of the large airways primarily affect the ability of air to flow through the lungs. These changes are referred to as changes in flow resistance or its reciprocal, airway conductance.

The second group, the small, or peripheral, airways, extends from the large airways to the alveoli. Changes in tone occurring in the small airways chiefly affect the ease with which the lungs expand and deflate. These changes are referred to as changes in lung compliance or its reciprocal, elastance.

Many drugs interact with specific receptors to produce either constriction or dilation of the airways by changing the tone of airway smooth muscle. For example, acetylcholine interacts with specific receptors to produce constriction of airway smooth muscle. In contrast, the catecholamines interact with β_2-receptors to produce relaxation of airway smooth muscle. Some evidence also exists to suggest that β_1-receptors may mediate airway smooth muscle relaxation, especially in the large airways.

Histamine interacts with histamine H_1-receptors to produce constriction and with histamine H_2-receptors to produce relaxation of airway smooth muscle. In humans H_1-receptors predominate in airway smooth muscle. Many of the prostaglandins and the structurally related leukotrienes also have been shown to affect the tone of airway smooth muscle. The prostaglandin $PGF_{2\alpha}$ and the leukotrienes, slow-reacting substances of anaphylaxis, are the most important of the constrictors, whereas the prostaglandins PGE_1 and PGE_2 are the most important of the relaxants of these groups of compounds. In addition, the tone of airway smooth muscle can be affected indirectly by actions that cause the release of substances that can alter tone or by stimulation of reflexes that affect the airways.

Both chemical and immunologic stimuli cause release of active substances within the lungs. Although some of these agents can cause relaxation of airway smooth muscle, most, such as histamine or slow-

---

Some agents producing release of histamine

Acetylcholine
Antigen (reaction with IgE)
Morphine
Nicotine
Pancuronium
Plasma expanders—dextran, hetastarch
Polymyxin B
Promethazine
Succinylcholine
Thiopental

---

reacting substances of anaphylaxis (SRS-A or leukotrienes C_4 and D_4), produce bronchoconstriction. A variety of agents that produce histamine release are listed in the box above. Also, many drugs, including some that produce airway constriction, stimulate the release of catecholamines from the adrenal medulla. The effects of the catecholamines facilitate relaxation of airway smooth muscle and therefore can modulate the degree of airway constriction.

Several reflexes are involved in the regulation of airway smooth muscle tone, and most of these produce bronchoconstriction. Reflex constriction resulting from stimulation of irritant receptors, carotid chemoreceptors, or carotid baroreceptors is particularly important because it may be involved in the airway *hyperreactivity* commonly associated with obstructive lung disease.

The vagus nerve provides both the afferent and efferent pathways for reflex constriction resulting from stimulation of the irritant or "cough" receptors. These receptors are located in the large airways and are most numerous in the trachea and major bronchi.

Carotid chemoreceptors and baroreceptors are located in the carotid bodies and carotid sinus areas. Stimulation of these receptors activates afferent fibers forming part of the glossopharyngeal nerves. Species differences have complicated the identification of the efferent pathways of these reflexes; both vagal and nonvagal pathways have been implicated. In addition to producing bronchoconstriction, some of these reflexes may produce changes in the frequency and depth of breathing. Alterations in the pattern of breathing may in turn affect smooth muscle tone.

Reflexes with efferent pathways mediated by the vagus nerve have more pronounced effects in the large airways than in the small airways because of the pat-

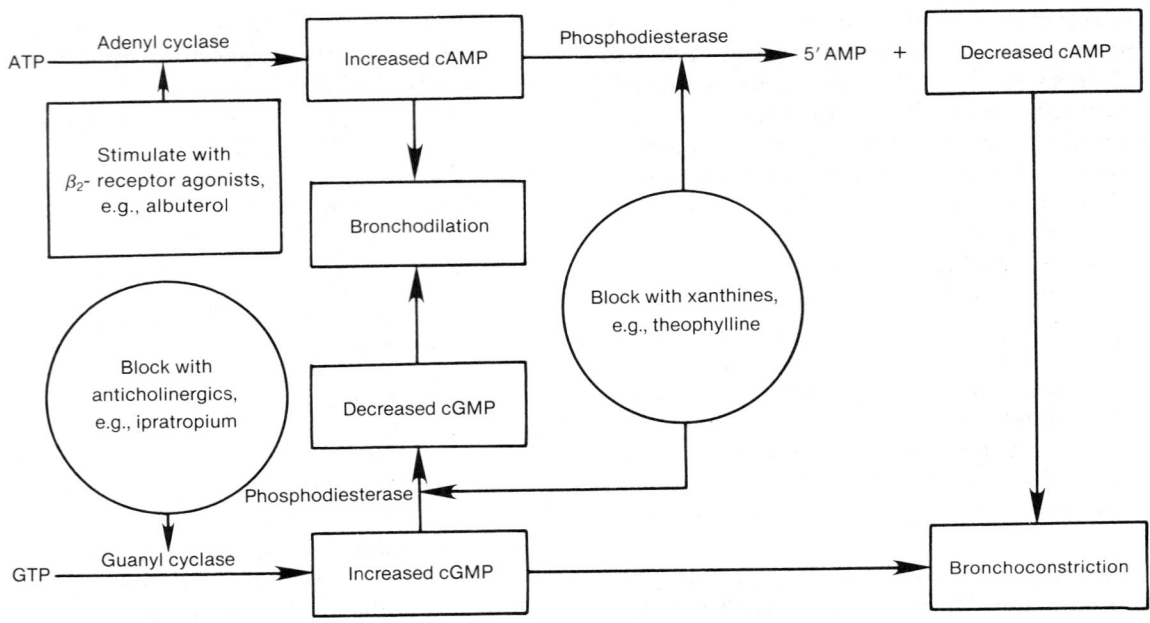

FIGURE 28-1. **Actions of bronchodilators.**

tern of innervation. Reflex constriction of this type is particularly susceptible to blockade by cholinergic antagonists.

At the cellular level changes in the tone of airway smooth muscle produced by either neural or humoral stimuli are caused by changes in the balance between cyclic adenosine-3',5'-monophosphate (cAMP) and cyclic guanosine monophosphate (cGMP). Cyclic AMP produces smooth muscle relaxation, whereas cGMP causes smooth muscle contraction (Figure 28-1).

The actions of cilia, goblet cells, and bronchial glands also affect the caliber of the airways. The cilia are found in the airway mucosa to the level of the terminal bronchioles, although they may be absent from large portions of the airways of some asthmatic patients. Normally the cilia beat in a rhythmic fashion to propel secretions and inhaled particles toward the mouth. The cilia are independent of nervous control but have been shown to be inhibited by a variety of factors (box) and drugs, especially those with atropine-like activity. In general, ciliary activity is stimulated by cholinergic agonists; ions of sodium, calcium, and potassium; and some bronchodilating agents, which will be discussed.

Most airway secretions arise from goblet cells and bronchial glands. The goblet cells are most numerous in the larger bronchi and disappear at the level of the bronchioles. These cells secrete a relatively viscous mucus. Although independent of nervous control,

Some factors inhibiting cilia	
Cold	High concentrations of
Dehydration	oxygen
Drugs (e.g., atropine,	Infection
codeine)	Low humidity
Dust	Mediators of allergic
High concentrations of	reactions
carbon dioxide	Smoke

both the number and the activity of goblet cells are increased in the presence of airway irritation. Unlike cilia, goblet cells are affected by drugs only insofar as the drugs cause or reduce airway irritation.

The bronchial glands extend from the trachea to the bronchioles and are embedded deeper in the airway wall than are goblet cells. Secretions from the glands are composed of both mucous and serous components and reach the lumen by means of a secretory duct. Bronchial gland activity is influenced by the parasympathetic nervous system and is also affected by cholinergic drugs. In general, cholinergic agonists stimulate secretions, whereas cholinergic antagonists inhibit secretions.

Normally airway secretions and ciliary activity are

balanced to provide a demulcent coating over the airways, which is constantly flowing toward the mouth helping to remove foreign particles and cellular debris. Inflammation, increased viscosity of secretions, and a reduction in the number or activity of cilia can all interrupt the normal balance and contribute to obstruction of the airways by causing reduction in mucociliary clearance, development of mucosal edema, and/or formation of mucous plugs.

The secretions form a sol-layer, which envelops the cilia, and also a more superficial and more viscous gel-layer. The effects of drugs on these layers and on mucociliary clearance will be considered in the discussion of expectorants and mucolytic agents (Chapter 29, "Antihistamines, Antitussives, Decongestants, and Expectorants").

The lungs receive a rich blood supply. The large airways are supplied primarily by the bronchial arteries, whereas the small airways are supplied chiefly by the pulmonary arteries. The pulmonary veins receive blood from both groups of airways. Changes in pressure or permeability of the pulmonary vasculature directly influence the development of edema and congestion within the airways. The vasculature supplying the lungs, in contrast to that supplying skeletal muscle, constricts in response to *hypoxia*. This response is important to the maintenance of an effective ventilation-perfusion ratio and must be considered when treating bronchospasm with β-receptor stimulants.

The drugs in this chapter can be classified into the following groups, which will be considered separately: adrenergic drugs (sympathomimetics), anticholinergics (parasympatholytics), phosphodiesterase (PDE) inhibitors, corticosteroids, and other agents that inhibit mediator release. Finally, respiratory gases will be discussed.

The major action of bronchodilators is to relax airway smooth muscle. However, many of these drugs have additional effects on blood vessels and the airway mucosa that must be considered. Although not true bronchodilators, drugs that inhibit mediator release are also used to treat conditions characterized by obstruction of the airways.

PDE inhibitors and β-receptor agonists act by raising the levels of cAMP. Stimulation of β-receptors activates adenyl cyclase, the enzyme that converts ATP to cAMP. Phosphodiesterase is the enzyme responsible for breakdown of cAMP within the cell. Thus both increases in adenyl cyclase activity and decreases in PDE activity cause accumulation of cAMP and produce muscle relaxation (Figure 28-1). Most of the β-receptors in airway smooth muscle are of the β$_2$ subtype.

Nonselective adrenergic (sympathomimetic) bronchodilators

The first two adrenergic drugs used as bronchodilators were ephedrine and epinephrine. Each drug stimulates α- and β-receptors and produces central nervous system stimulation. Ephedrine is less potent but has a longer duration of action and unlike epinephrine is effective orally. However, much of the peripheral activity of ephedrine is due to the release of noradrenaline. Thus tachyphylaxis develops readily with frequently repeated doses because of a depletion of stored noradrenaline. In addition, ephedrine produces a more marked central nervous system stimulation than epinephrine and may produce anxiety, nervousness, or insomnia. Ephedrine has often been prescribed in combination with a sedative (e.g., phenobarbital), or suboptimal dosages of ephedrine have been combined with another bronchodilator such as theophylline to reduce the central nervous system effects. Because of the greater safety and efficacy of the many newer agents, the use of ephedrine is *not* recommended.

Epinephrine, a catecholamine, is rapidly inactivated in the gastrointestinal tract and is therefore not effective after oral administration. When used intravenously the cardiovascular effects of epinephrine limit its use as a bronchodilator, but it has been used extensively as a bronchodilator when administered subcutaneously or by inhalation. For many years epinephrine given subcutaneously has been the treatment of choice for severe bronchospasm associated with status asthmaticus or anaphylaxis. More recently agents with a greater selectivity for β$_2$-receptors (e.g., albuterol) have been increasing in favor for the treatment of status asthmaticus. Epinephrine is also available as the active medication in several nonprescription bronchodilator products.

Trade names of products containing these and other drugs used to treat obstruction of the airways are listed in Nursing Drug Digest.

Most of the adrenergic bronchodilators available possess some degree of β-receptor selectivity with little or no stimulation of α-receptors at therapeutic dosages. Older drugs of this type such as isoproterenol stimulate both β-receptor subtypes (i.e., β$_1$—primarily heart and β$_2$—primarily lung). Newer agents such as albuterol are more selective and preferentially stimulate the β$_2$-receptors, which mediate relaxation of airway smooth muscle.

β-Receptor selective bronchodilators

Inhalation of isoproterenol produces rapid and marked bronchodilation, but stimulation of cardiac β-receptors (i.e., β₁-receptors) also occurs and may produce dysrhythmias, dizziness, or hypotension. The development of dysrhythmias is a major side effect that limits therapy with isoproterenol. The cardiac effects together with β₂-mediated vessel dilation may be sufficient to reverse hypoxic vasoconstriction in the lungs. Such a reversal produces an increase in the perfusion of poorly ventilated lung regions and could explain the initial worsening of the ventilation-perfusion ratio experienced by some patients despite bronchodilation.

Some patients have been observed to experience paradoxic responses of increased bronchospasm or refractoriness to further bronchodilation after an initial dose of isoproterenol. The mechanisms of these responses are not fully understood but may be aggravated by metabolism of isoproterenol to the 3-methoxy derivative, which possesses some β-blocking activity. However, similar reactions have been reported after administration of other β-receptor agonists that are not metabolized in a similar way.

The major advantage of the newer agents is that little or no cardiac stimulation occurs at therapeutic dosages. However, β₂-receptor selectivity is lost with high dosages, and cardiac effects are a particular risk if such agents are administered parenterally.

In addition to cardiac effects all β-receptor agonists may cause central nervous system stimulation, resulting in symptoms such as tremor, nervousness, headache, anxiety, or nausea. Most of the side effects produced by these agents decrease with continued use or may be minimized by a reduction in dosage. However, hyperthyroidism, diabetes, hypertension, or other cardiac disease presents either relative or absolute contraindications and must be considered carefully before therapy is initiated with β-receptor agonists.

Another problem common to all of the β-receptor agonists is the development of tolerance. Although more marked with agents such as ephedrine and isoproterenol, tolerance to the newer agents has also been reported. As tolerance develops, patients require larger or more frequent doses of these agents to achieve the same degree of bronchodilation. If this situation arises, the patient must be advised to seek assistance from the health care provider because overuse of these agents increases the risk of toxicity. Alternatively the lack of response to these drugs may indicate that the condition is deteriorating and other therapy is required.

α-Receptor antagonists

Investigational studies with moxisylyte (thymoxamine) and indoramin have suggested that α-receptor antagonists may produce bronchodilation and enhance β-receptor–mediated bronchodilation by eliminating possible α-receptor–mediated bronchoconstriction. However, the bronchodilation reported may not have involved actions on α-receptors, and the use of α-receptor antagonists as bronchodilators requires further evaluation.

In contrast to possible bronchoconstriction, stimulation of α-receptors produces decongestion of the bronchial mucosa and may in fact reduce obstruction of the airways. However, drugs that produce marked stimulation of α-receptors cause mydriasis and should therefore be avoided in patients with narrow-angle glaucoma.

Adrenergic drugs also affect the release of mediators from mast cells. In general, the release of spasmogens induced by the interaction of antigen and IgE is increased by α-receptor stimulation and decreased by β-receptor stimulation.

Phosphodiesterase inhibitors

Theophylline and its various salts and dyphylline are the most common phosphodiesterase inhibitors used as bronchodilators (Table 28-1). Unlike the adrenergic bronchodilators, the use of phosphodiesterase inhibitors is not accompanied by tolerance. Theophylline is only poorly soluble in water and is therefore usually administered in a micronized solid dosage form or as an alcoholic elixir. Aminophylline, the ethylenediamine salt of theophylline, is administered intravenously to treat episodes of acute bronchospasm. These agents relax bronchial smooth muscle, stimulate the respiratory center, and are particularly useful in patients with a tolerance to adrenergic bronchodilators.

Optimal bronchodilation occurs when levels of theophylline range between 10 and 20 μg/ml of serum. As gastric irritation and anxiety appear with serum levels near 20 μg/ml, some practitioners prefer to limit the therapeutic levels of theophylline to between 10 and 15 μg/ml. Cardiac effects of theophylline, including dysrhythmias and hypotension, generally occur when serum concentrations reach 30 μg/ml, and convulsions are likely to occur with serum levels exceeding 40 μg/ml, (Figure 28-2).

Other effects that may occur at therapeutic dosage levels include a short-lived diuretic effect, headache, increases in cardiac output, release of catecholamines from the adrenal medulla, and relaxation of other smooth muscles. The diuretic effect results from a combination of the cardiovascular effects, which increase glomerular filtration rate, and a direct effect on the renal tubules to decrease reabsorption. In some patients excessive potassium may be excreted, leading

TABLE 28-1

Theophylline content of various theophylline salts

Theophylline salt	Theophylline content (% anhydrous theophylline)
Calcium salicylate	48
Cholinate (oxtriphylline)	65
Dyphylline (dihydroxypropyl-theophylline)	0 (not a simple salt, but a true chemical derivative of theophylline)
Ethylenediamine (aminophylline)	78 to 86 (depends on relative amounts of anhydrous and hydrous aminophylline)
Monoethanolamine	75
Sodium acetate	65
Sodium glycinate (aminoacetate)	50

to hypokalemia. Although most blood vessels are dilated by theophylline, cerebral vasoconstriction may occur and produce headache.

Approximately 90% of an oral dose of theophylline is metabolized by demethylation or oxidation by liver microsomal enzymes. The rate of metabolism shows large variations among individuals, but the average serum half-life in adults is approximately 8 hours. Factors affecting the rates of theophylline metabolism have been extensively studied because of the slight difference between the therapeutic and toxic serum levels. In general, young children metabolize theophylline more quickly than adults but are more sensitive to the toxic effects of theophylline. Similarly, patients who consistently eat diets high in protein have increased clearance rates and may require higher doses of theophylline. Chronic smoking induces the enzymes responsible for theophylline metabolism and results in a shorter half-life and reduced serum levels. Thus any change in smoking habits may require an adjustment in maintenance dosages of theophylline.

In contrast the half-life of theophylline is prolonged in elderly patients or patients with impaired hepatic function. Similarly, cardiac disease may reduce theophylline clearance, and average dosages may then produce toxic serum levels.

Serum levels of theophylline should be monitored and used to adjust dosages in any patients in whom adequate bronchodilation is not obtained or in whom bronchodilation is accompanied with signs of theophylline toxicity. Serum levels of theophylline may be estimated from the levels of theophylline found in saliva. Salivary levels are usually about 50% lower than serum levels, but the exact relationship should be determined for each individual patient before such levels are used.

Theophylline is well absorbed after oral adminis-

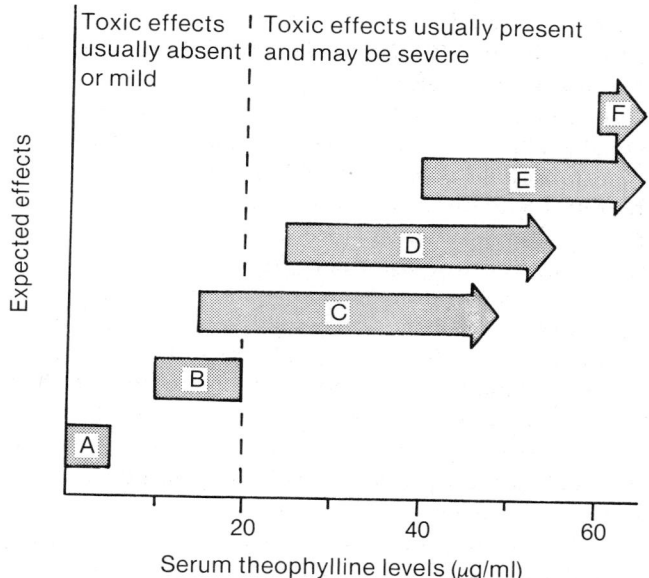

FIGURE 28-2. **Correlation between serum theophylline levels and pharmacologic effects.** *A*, **Effects rarely present (therapeutic or toxic).** *B*, **Optimal bronchodilation with minimal side effects expected.** *C*, **Gastric side effects expected to be prominent.** *D*, **Effects on CNS expected to be prominent.** *E*, **Cardiac effects expected to be prominent.** *F*, **Convulsions expected.**

tration, but the bioavailability from different products may differ widely (i.e., 50% to 100%) in the same individual. Because of its solubility in alcohol, many oral preparations have been formulated as alcoholic elixirs with an alcohol concentration as high as 20%. The alcoholic concentration of such products must be considered before selecting products for diabetics, children, alcoholics, or those patients receiving other medications known to interact with alcohol.

Theophylline is available in products for rectal administration. However, absorption from these products is difficult to predict, and therefore they are not recommended. Aqueous solutions of theophylline produced for inhalation are too weak to be recommended, and the alcoholic solutions of this type are *not* recommended because of their irritant properties when inhaled.

As mentioned earlier theophylline has been marketed in products containing ephedrine or ephedrine plus a sedative (e.g., theophylline, ephedrine, and phenobarbital compound). The rationale for these products was to provide adequate bronchodilation and minimize side effects resulting from central nervous system stimulation. However, many safer products are available, and such combination products are *not* recommended.

However, theophylline or one of its derivatives is often prescribed in combination with a selective β-adrenergic bronchodilator. Since both these agents increase cAMP by different mechanisms, it is hoped that simultaneous use of these agents will produce a synergistic effect and increased bronchodilation. However, if optimal dosages of either drug are used, it is doubtful whether further bronchodilation will be produced after addition of the second agent. Furthermore, administration of two drugs increases the risk of side effects. In practice many patients tolerate such combinations well, and they may be useful in patients susceptible to developing tolerance to adrenergic bronchodilators. In patients unable to tolerate full therapeutic dosages combinations containing suboptimal dosages of the individual agents may provide adequate bronchodilation without producing intolerable side effects.

Caffeine and theobromine have been used as bronchodilators. However, they are less potent than theophylline and are not used extensively. They are still included in some combination preparations that are available.

Anticholinergics (parasympatholytics)

Atropine and other anticholinergic drugs relax airway smooth muscle by inhibiting vagal nerve activity and by reducing cellular levels of cGMP. However, cholinergic blockade can produce effects such as dry mouth, mydriasis, cycloplegia, and urinary retention, which limits the use of anticholinergics as bronchodilators. Even when administered by inhalation, atropine has been reported to reduce sputum production and depress ciliary activity. More recently drugs such as ipratropium bromide and oxitropium bromide have renewed interest in the use of parasympatholytics as bronchodilators. Administered by inhalation, these drugs are well tolerated by patients and have minimal effects on sputum production or ciliary activity.

Corticosteroids

Although not true bronchodilators, the corticosteroids are of major importance in the management of a variety of lung conditions. Products for inhalation or for oral administration are available and are used for both short- and long-term therapy. In addition, steroids often are administered parenterally to help control acute exacerbations and status asthmaticus.

The major benefits of steroid therapy in respiratory diseases are derived from three types of actions.
1. Antiinflammatory effects
2. Inhibition of the formation, storage, and release of histamine
3. Enhancement of β-receptor stimulation, particularly in patients who have become tolerant and unresponsive to β-receptor stimulants

The sensitizing of the β-receptors is usually referred to as the "permissive effect" of the steroids. Improvement of ciliary clearance and production of euphoria or a sense of well-being are some additional actions of steroids that may contribute to their effectiveness. The effects of steroid therapy may require 8 to 12 hours to develop. Even after intravenous administration peak effects may not be experienced for approximately 5 hours.

Therapy with steroids is limited by the risk of the many serious side effects, including sodium retention and Cushing's syndrome, which are reviewed in Chapter 65, "Corticosteroids and Adrenal Steroid Inhibitors." The use of new steroid inhalation products minimizes systemic absorption and therefore adverse reactions. For this reason inhalation products should be tried whenever possible before resorting to systemic therapy with oral steroids.

Drugs affecting mediator release

Cromolyn sodium prevents release of mediators from mast cells induced by both immunologic and nonimmunologic stimuli. However, the drug has no bronchodilating or antiinflammatory effects and is only useful if given prophylactically. Absorption from the gastrointestinal tract is poor, and therefore oral therapy is not used in the treatment of respiratory disease although the drug is marketed in oral capsule form (Nalcrom) for the treatment of gastrointestinal disorders. For respiratory therapy cromolyn sodium is marketed as a powder (e.g., Aarane, Inostral, Intal, Lomudal, Lomusol, and Nasmil), which is inhaled from a Spinhaler device, but can be dissolved in saline solution and used with a nebulizer. A newer inhaler form (i.e., Fivent) is being marketed. The drug is also available as a powder for insufflation into the nostrils (Rynacrom), a solution for nasal instillation (Rynacrom 2% Nasal Solution), and as eyedrops (Opticrom).

A disadvantage to therapy with cromolyn sodium is that some patients may require therapy for 6 to 8 weeks before benefit is obtained. However, cromolyn sodium is the least toxic of drugs used for the treatment of respiratory diseases. Cough and a slight degree of bronchoconstriction related to irritation by the powder form are the most common side effects and generally can be avoided by using cromolyn sodium after inhalation of a bronchodilator. Some patients complain of a dry mouth, which is usually relieved with a glass of water. More serious side effects are rare, but dermatitis, gastroenteritis, myositis, and true allergic reactions have been reported.

The prostaglandins PGE$_1$ and PGE$_2$ may modulate mediator release but have been investigated chiefly because of their ability to produce bronchodilation. However, to date formulations of these agents have produced local irritation and bronchospasm and are therefore not used routinely.

When bronchodilator therapy is indicated, the objective of therapy is to restore and maintain the patient's pulmonary function as close as possible to normal. Selection of the appropriate therapy depends chiefly on the situation (emergency or maintenance therapy) and the patient (i.e., age, concurrent medications or diseases, and ability to use metered-dose aerosol). However, selection is affected by the type of disease or condition. Asthma, for example, is characterized by a large reversible component and generally would be expected to respond well to a bronchodilator. In contrast, emphysema and chronic bronchitis are characterized by large irreversible components and are therefore more likely to require steroids.

Initially, intermittent therapy (when symptoms develop) with a selective β$_2$-receptor stimulant (e.g., albuterol) administered by metered-dose aerosol may be sufficient for a patient with infrequent episodes of wheezing, shortness of breath, or bronchospasm. However, many patients have more frequent attacks or have abnormal lung function between attacks. These patients should be instructed to use the metered aerosol on a regular basis. If symptoms persist, systemic therapy with a selective β$_2$-receptor stimulant is indicated. If control remains inadequate or if tolerance develops, an oral phosphodiesterase inhibitor (e.g., theophylline) might be helpful. Patients noticing a decreased response to sympathomimetics should be advised to consult with their health care provider because mucous plugging and bronchial edema, rather than tolerance, may be developing.

Therapy with both a sympathomimetic and a phosphodiesterase inhibitor may be tried in an effort to produce maximal bronchodilation by raising cAMP levels by two separate mechanisms. Although the combined therapy may be well tolerated, the potential for toxicity is high, and patients should be carefully monitored.

Any patient receiving bronchodilators, especially atopic patients, may benefit from cromolyn sodium. If no benefit is noticed after 6 to 8 weeks, cromolyn sodium should be discontinued.

Patients with markedly impaired pulmonary function despite optimal use of bronchodilators and cromolyn sodium require the addition of a steroid to their drug regimen. Initially an inhalation product should be tried if at all possible to minimize systemic absorption. Administration of the steroid after inhalation of a bronchodilator aids the deposition of the steroid into the smaller airways. If systemic therapy becomes necessary, alternate-day dosing should be tried before daily steroids are prescribed. All patients maintained on steroids should be advised that their steroid requirements will rise during acute exacerbations of respiratory disease or other stressful periods.

Emergency therapy depends to some extent on the patient's usual maintenance therapy. If normally maintained with sympathomimetics, the patient may be relatively unresponsive to further adrenergic therapy, and the risks of cardiotoxicity are increased. In these patients intravenous aminophylline is recommended. Similarly administration of aminophylline to a patient usually maintained with a theophylline compound must be monitored carefully to avoid toxic serum concentrations of theophylline. Parenteral administration of epinephrine or preferably a selective β$_2$-receptor stimulant (e.g., terbutaline) may be safer in these patients.

Steroids are indicated for emergency treatment. After parenteral administration some effect may be noted after 1 hour, but peak effects are delayed approximately 5 to 8 hours. Therefore patients able to take drugs by mouth may be given oral steroids that produce peak effects between 8 and 12 hours after administration.

RESPIRATORY GASES

Oxygen, carbon dioxide, nitrogen, carbon monoxide, helium, and xenon can all be considered respiratory gases. The most important, however, are the first two, oxygen and carbon dioxide, and these will be discussed in detail. Although helium has special uses in diving, the others are used only for diagnostic purposes and will not be considered.

Oxygen (O_2) transport from the lungs to the tissues depends largely on the partial pressure of oxygen in the alveoli (PAO_2). The partial pressure of oxygen (PO_2) in dry air at sea level (air pressure = 1 atmosphere = 760 mm Hg) is equal to the concentration of oxygen in the air (21%) times the pressure, or approximately 160 mm Hg. In the alveoli the PAO_2 is reduced to about 100 mm Hg by the contributions of water vapor and carbon dioxide to the total pressure. The value of PAO_2 is slightly decreased when in a supine position because of changes both in dead space and in regional ventilation. Similarly the PAO_2 decreases with age because of associated increases in ventilation-perfusion inequalities. The normal venous admixture, pathologic shunts, hypoventilation, pathologic ventilation-perfusion inequalities, and diffusion defects are all factors that cause additional decreases in the PAO_2. In contrast, hyperventilation, increasing the concentration of oxygen in inspired air, and use of hyperbaric oxygen are all factors that produce increases in PAO_2.

Although oxygen rapidly diffuses from the alveoli into the pulmonary circulation, the partial pressure of oxygen in the arteries (PaO_2) leaving the lungs is lower than the partial pressure of oxygen in the alveoli because of a combination of normal venous admixture and incomplete equilibration of oxygen between the alveoli and capillaries. Most of the oxygen that diffuses into the capillaries reacts with hemoglobin to form oxyhemoglobin and is transported to the tissues in that form. The relationship between PO_2 and the saturation of hemoglobin for a young adult, assuming a temperature of 37° C, blood pH of 7.4, and a normal hemoglobin level of 15 gm/dl, is shown in Figure 28-3. Because of the sigmoid nature of the curve, only slight changes in the degree of saturation are noted after small decreases from a normal PaO_2. However, at lower values of PO_2 the curve is steep, and even small reductions in pressure markedly impair the ability of hemoglobin to bind oxygen. Thus normal venous blood with a PO_2 of 40 mm Hg readily releases oxygen to the tissues.

The affinity of oxygen for hemoglobin is affected by a variety of other factors that displace the hemoglobin saturation curve to the right or left. A shift to the right is produced by increases in temperature or decreases in pH. The pH-dependent shift is known as the Bohr effect. Carbon dioxide and molecules such as 2,3-diphosphoglycerate, a byproduct of anaerobic glycolysis, also bind to the reduced form of hemoglobin,

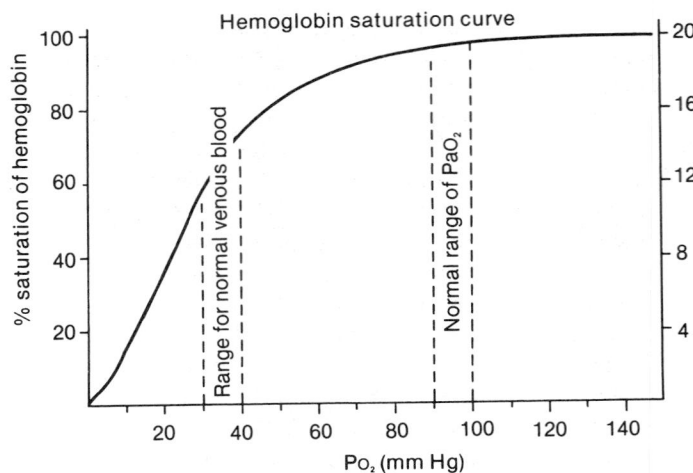

FIGURE 28-3. **Hemoglobin saturation curve.**

decrease its ability to bind oxygen, and shift the curve to the right. In contrast, decreases in temperature, increases in pH, decreases in carbon dioxide, and other factors that increase the affinity of oxygen for hemoglobin impair subsequent dissociation in the tissues and shift the curve to the left.

A small amount of oxygen that diffuses into the pulmonary circulation dissolves in the plasma instead of combining with hemoglobin. The total amount of dissolved oxygen is directly proportional to the PaO_2. For each mm Hg PaO_2, 0.003 ml of oxygen dissolves in each 100 ml of blood, producing a total of about 0.3 ml at a normal PaO_2. If 100% oxygen is substituted for inspired air, the PaO_2 increases, and approximately 2 ml of oxygen dissolve in each 100 ml of blood. Similarly, if air is inspired at a pressure of 3 atmospheres, each 100 ml of blood contains about 1 ml of oxygen. Thus PaO_2 can be increased effectively by either increasing the concentration of inspired oxygen or by increasing inspiration pressure. If both techniques are used simultaneously, enough oxygen can be dissolved in the blood to meet the tissue demands of a normal, healthy, resting adult. Although the response to oxygen is affected by the cause of the oxygen deficiency, the administration of oxygen for therapeutic purposes is an important aspect of respiratory therapy. However, since oxygen tensions are closely related to those of carbon dioxide (CO_2), this gas will be considered before the therapeutic uses of oxygen are reviewed.

Carbon dioxide

Ventilation serves the dual purpose of delivering oxygen to and eliminating carbon dioxide from the body. Generally, the carbon dioxide tension ($PaCO_2$) is near 40 mm Hg when ventilation is sufficient to maintain Pa_{O_2} within normal limits. Most of the carbon dioxide produced by the body rapidly diffuses into red blood cells where it either combines with hemoglobin or is converted to carbonic acid, which dissociates to free hydrogen and bicarbonate ions. A small amount of carbon dioxide is bound to plasma proteins, and, like oxygen, some remains dissolved in the plasma. The amount of dissolved carbon dioxide (mmol CO_2/L) can be calculated as 0.03 Pa_{CO_2}. This value is particularly useful because it is equivalent to the effective concentration of carbonic acid, the major acid of the arterial buffer system. The bicarbonate ion provides the chief arterial base, and arterial blood pH can be shown to be directly affected by the level of carbon dioxide using the following formulas:

$$pH = pK + \log \frac{base}{acid}$$

$$pH = pK + \log \frac{[HCO_3^-]}{[H_2CO_3]}$$

$$pH = pK + \log \frac{[HCO_3^-]}{0.03 \, Pa_{CO_2}}$$

In the alveoli dissolved carbon dioxide, carbon dioxide bound to plasma proteins, and bicarbonate ions are all made available as free carbon dioxide, which is excreted during ventilation. Since this is a rapid process, ventilation not only affects Pa_{O_2} but also provides a direct and sensitive control of pH and Pa_{CO_2}.

The regulatory role of the lungs is strengthened by the activities of the respiratory center in the central nervous system and by peripheral chemoreceptors sensitive to changes in Pa_{CO_2}. Stimulation of the respiratory center by increases in carbon dioxide with the ensuing acidosis and stimulation of the chemoreceptors results in increased ventilation. Although a potent respiratory stimulant, carbon dioxide is more generally used as a diagnostic agent to evaluate the degree of control exercised by the respiratory center.

The levels of bicarbonate ion are chiefly controlled by the kidney. Although the renal system is slower than the respiratory system to adapt to changes in Pa_{CO_2}, arterial pH may be maintained within normal limits by the increased renal retention of bicarbonate in the presence of higher values of Pa_{CO_2}. Thus ventilation, Pa_{O_2}, Pa_{CO_2}, or pH must be manipulated carefully with a view to their complex interactions.

Impaired ventilation is characterized by reduced Pa_{O_2} values (*hypoxemia*) with or without raised Pa_{CO_2} levels (*hypercapnia*). Individuals may compensate for mild to moderate hypoxemia with increased rates of ventilation and/or the development of polycythemia. More severe hypoxia, or hypoxia of sudden onset, is characterized by a variety of other symptoms (see box,

---

Symptoms of hypoxia

Shortness of breath, tachypnea, progressive dyspnea, and respiratory depression

Pulmonary hypertension leading to cor pulmonale, tachycardia, dysrhythmias, hypotension, myocardial insufficiency, cardiac failure, circulatory collapse, and shock

Headache, impaired judgment and intellectual functioning, depression or other neuroses, lethargy, restlessness, loss of coordination, irritability, tremor, convulsions, and coma

Sodium and fluid retention, renal insufficiency, edema, pulmonary edema, and cerebral edema

Lactic acidosis, cyanosis, nausea and vomiting, clubbing, polycythemia, and increased tendency for venous thrombosis

---

Symptoms of hypercapnia

Vasodilation of peripheral blood vessels followed by reflex vasoconstriction

Initial vasoconstriction of pulmonary vessels

Cardiac dysrhythmias and hypertension

Headache, anxiety, confusion, tremors, convulsions, and coma

Weakness, fatigue, visual disturbances, nausea and vomiting, and cyanosis*

*Blood gas analyses should be performed to confirm cases of suspected hypercapnia because cyanosis is an unreliable index. Factors such as anemia or dark skin pigmentation can mask cyanosis, whereas polycythemia can enhance cyanosis.

---

above, top). In general, the milder symptoms are associated with chronic hypoxia, whereas the more serious symptoms accompany acute, severe hypoxia. The degree of hypoxia required to produce symptoms varies among individuals, but most persons will experience symptoms of hypoxia when the Pa_{O_2} falls below 50 mm Hg.

Similarly, mild hypercapnia may produce no other sign than an increased ventilation rate. However, carbon dioxide retention can result in toxic Pa_{CO_2} levels and then respiration is depressed. Other symptoms of carbon dioxide toxicity are listed in the box above, bottom.

Most cases of hypoxia respond well to the administration of oxygen. However, the degree and rate of response to oxygen therapy depends chiefly on the cause of the hypoxemia and also on the method of oxygen administration. In addition, overzealous administration of oxygen may remove a patient's ventilatory drive, resulting in depressed respiration and carbon dioxide retention. For these reasons blood gas analyses should be used to assess and monitor all patients given oxygen. However, in some situations such as after carbon monoxide poisoning tissue oxygenation primarily depends on the concentration of dissolved oxygen, and therefore the overall Pao_2 becomes a less reliable guide.

Oxygen administration

Oxygen is used to treat the effects of hypoxia that can occur with such conditions as anemia, shock, pulmonary edema, pneumonia, and other conditions in which insufficient oxygen is carried by the blood to the tissue. Oxygen can also be used as a vehicle for the administration of general anesthetics or medications such as bronchodilators and steroids.

Oxygen is supplied either from wall outlets such as those found in hospital settings or from portable oxygen tanks or cylinders. It is administered in liters per minute or by percentage, depending on the oxygen delivery system and device.

To relieve hypoxia, oxygen must be administered continuously at concentrations of 70% to 100% at rates required to increase oxygen content of inspired air to 50%. To attain or maintain adequate blood levels, oxygen therapy must not be interrupted for care, transport, eating, or ambulation. Withdrawal of the oxygen source for any reason can cause reflex hypoxemia in some patients, resulting in a Pao_2 less than the pretherapy level.

Oxygen can be administered by various delivery systems such as hyperbaric chambers and devices such as catheter, tent, mask, nasal cannula, Plexiglas hood, or T-piece. Although an effective means of increasing Pao_2, the use of hyperbaric oxygen is accompanied by a greater risk of oxygen toxicity. In addition, specific indications for hyperbaric oxygen are limited, and the facilities are expensive and generally not available.

The choice of device depends on individual patient factors as well as on the degree of hypercapnia and the risk of removing the patient's hypoxic respiratory drive.

Although more commonly used in the past, the oxygen tent is now generally restricted to infants and young children with respiratory conditions, fever, or postoperative nasopharyngeal irritation. Oxygen tents are also used in home settings by adult patients, especially during sleep. The major disadvantage to the use of tents is that high oxygen flow rates of 10 L or more a minute are required to maintain the desired concentration of inspired oxygen. This amount of oxygen can be expensive when chronic use is indicated. Because the maintenance of oxygen concentration depends on an undisturbed canopy, nursing care and monitoring are also difficult, and the patient's level of activity is restricted.

Oxygen masks are commonly used for the administration of oxygen therapy. Masks vary in the degree to which the patient's pattern of breathing affects the concentration of inspired oxygen and in the degree of rebreathing that is possible. Several types of simple masks are available, including some with ports that allow oxygen mixture with room air and some with valves that prevent mixing of room air as well as rebreathing exhaled air. Masks with reservoirs (e.g., Venturi mask) increase the amount of rebreathing. These masks must be used with caution to avoid carbon dioxide narcosis in patients likely to develop carbon dioxide retention. The administration of oxygen by simple mask is safer in these patients because the concentration of inspired oxygen can be more carefully controlled.

The major disadvantage of using masks is the inconvenience to patients. Because the mask interferes with activities of daily living, patients often remove them, temporarily making it difficult to control the actual amount of oxygen delivered. A mask is also irritating to the area around the nose and mouth where it comes into contact with the skin. The area should be checked carefully for irritation and excessive moisture. A mask, although supplied with elastic headbands that can be adjusted to the patient's head, often slips down and off the face.

The nasal cannulas are generally preferred by adult patients because they do not interfere with activities such as eating and conversation. Patients usually experience less of a feeling of suffocation with cannulas than with masks, and they are more comfortable. They also allow the patient more activity. For this reason nasal cannulas are being used more in the care of infants and young children. Cannulas allow more interactive play, socialization, and greater physical mobility. This freedom is especially important for the child who requires chronic therapy. Nasal cannulas for infants, which are made from nasogastric tubes and carefully secured to the face, enhance feeding and interaction with parents and caretakers.

When oxygen is administered by nasal cannulas, flow rates are adjusted to the patient's age and condition. Young infants can receive such low flow rates as 0.125 to 0.25 L per minute. When oxygen is administered to adults by nasal cannulas, flow rates of 2 to 3 L per minute are well tolerated and provide an inspired oxygen concentration near 30%. Higher flow rates may be indicated (6 L per minute or more) for hypoxic patients who do not have carbon dioxide retention. However, higher flow rates can increase nasal irritation and drying. In addition, when flow rates greater than 7 L per minute are used, the concentration of inspired oxygen is more difficult to predict. Patients with chronic obstructive lung disease can usually tolerate flow rates of 2 to 3 L per minute.

The actual concentration of inspired oxygen depends on the patient's tidal volume, the proper positioning of the cannula prongs, and patent nasal passages. The large tidal volumes commonly found in dyspneic patients lower the inspired oxygen concentration because of increased dilution with room air. Similarly, incorrect placement of the cannula prongs or obstructed nasal passages can reduce the concentration of inspired oxygen by decreasing the amount of oxygen obtained by the patient. Oral breathing has been thought to affect oxygen concentration as well, and the use of cannulas has been contraindicated in oral breathing patients. However, apparently a decrease in the concentration of oxygen delivered by this method has not been seen because oxygen from the nasal airways is drawn into the mouth.

Oxygen in all circumstances requires cautious use because it promotes combustion. Smoking in the area of oxygen administration is strictly prohibited. Signs indicating oxygen in use should be clearly posted, and other environmental precautions (e.g., control of static electricity) should be taken. Oxygen clings to bedclothes, patient gowns, and curtains for 3 to 6 hours after use. Flammable products (e.g., oil-based lip balm, body lotion, and rubbing alcohol) should not be used in patient care, and the use of electric equipment (e.g., electric beds, heating pads, or electric razors) should be avoided.

Oxygen tanks should be carefully secured to prevent them from being knocked over, causing personal injury or damage to seals or valves, which might result in leakage of gas. Because oxygen is stored under pressure, a damaged valve can be catapulted, resulting in serious injury. Oxygen wall outlets should likewise be carefully checked for leakage. In addition, because oxygen concentrations and flow rates must be accurate and because oxygen is often required for emergency therapy, wall outlets and tanks as well as delivery devices require routine monitoring for proper function.

In addition to the hazards associated with combustion, oxygen administration is associated with two major types of adverse reactions: those that are secondary to the delivery of the oxygen and those that result from the toxic effects of oxygen.

Adverse effects of oxygen delivery. Because oxygen is a dry gas, it must be administered with humidification to prevent drying and irritation of the mucous membranes of the respiratory tract. Various humidifiers (e.g., cold bubble–diffusion and Cascade humidifiers) and nebulizers (e.g., large-volume, ultrasonic, and sidestream nebulizers and mininebulizers) are used to add the desired amount of water vapor to the inspired gas not only to prevent its drying effects, but also to liquefy thick or tenacious secretions so that they can be more easily removed. Sidestream nebulizers and mininebulizers are also commonly used with oxygen in the administration of various medications, including bronchodilators and steroids.

Each humidifier and nebulizer has a reservoir that is filled with sterile distilled water to the fill line. It is important that the reservoir not be overfilled because water can collect in the tubing and decrease oxygen flow to the patient. Commercially prepackaged sterile distilled water bottles are also available. The water level in the reservoir must be frequently checked and not allowed to run low or dry. This step is especially important when heated treatments are administered because burning of the respiratory mucosa and excessive drying and irritation can result. When water is low, it should be discarded and the reservoir refilled with fresh sterile distilled water. When commercial prepackaged preparations are used, the empty unit is discarded and replaced with a new one.

Sterile equipment, water, and tubing must be used and changed daily or more frequently as indicated using aseptic technique. Equipment should not be shared among patients. Unless equipment is cared for appropriately and changed often, the water and moist tubing can become reservoirs for bacteria (e.g., *Pseudomonas aeruginosa*) and other pathogens capable of causing infection when distributed through the airways. When patients are receiving low flow rates of oxygen, reservoirs should be emptied and refilled or replaced at least once a day to prevent bacterial growth.

In addition to respiratory infections, the use of humidifiers and large-volume nebulizers can cause excessive humidification, which can lead to overhydration in some patients because large quantities of water are delivered to the lungs and insensible losses are decreased. Infants and patients with fluid balance problems or cardiac and renal dysfunction are particularly at risk.

Overhydration of the respiratory system can create a barrier to effective oxygen diffusion and can complicate therapy in the presence of edema or conditions characterized by copious airway secretions. Patients receiving warm-mist therapy from Cascade humidifiers or Ultrasonic nebulizers should be monitored carefully for weight gain over several days of therapy, pulmonary edema, and fluid and electrolyte imbalance. Cardiac work load can be increased by overhydration, which is serious in patients whose cardiac reserve is limited. Therapy with these nebulizers can cause bronchospasm and dyspnea in susceptible patients, and irritation and burning of the mucous membranes if the reservoir is not filled appropriately. Bronchospasm can also be caused paradoxically by administration of medications (e.g., bronchodilators) with sidestream nebulizers and mininebulizers as a result of an adverse side effect of the medication or aerosolization of the sterile distilled water or isotonic saline solution used for inhalation. Inhaled medications can cause other adverse effects. (See Adverse Side Effects of the Bronchodilators and Nursing Drug Digest.)

Additional risks are encountered when ventilation involves intubation of the patient. Trauma to the mucosa, particularly of the larynx and trachea, may occur during intubation. *Atelectasis* has occurred following misplacement or occlusion (crimping or blockage with mucus, blood, or other secretions) of endotracheal and tracheostomy tubes. Because these patients cannot verbalize distress, careful monitoring is essential. Intubated patients are more susceptible than others to the development of oxygen toxicity because all of their inspired air is received from the ventilator system and high oxygen levels are easily achieved. This risk can be minimized by keeping the concentration of inspired oxygen below 40% to 50% when patients are ventilated through endotracheal or tracheostomy tubes for periods of 2 days or longer. Because of the bypass of the upper airway, these patients are especially prone to the drying and irritating effects of oxygen, and humidification is important.

Another adverse side effect associated with the use of oxygen is physical and psychologic dependence. Weaning is often required for patients who have been receiving mechanical ventilation or other oxygen therapy for a prolonged period. Weaning is indicated when therapy is no longer required and should be planned individually. The patient and family should be involved in the physician's decision along with the nurse and the respiratory therapist. Because it can be stressful and frightening, weaning should not be started at night, and the patient should as much as possible be free from infection or other major problems. Much support and reassurance are required as well as careful and constant monitoring.

Special risks are associated with oxygen therapy when positive pressure is used (Table 28-2). These risks are similar for all three of the major systems that use positive pressure.

1. Intermittent positive pressure breathing (IPPB). Positive pressure is applied during inspiration, but the lungs are allowed to deflate passively.
2. Positive end-expiratory pressure (PEEP). A small positive pressure is maintained at the end of expiration.
3. Continuous positive airway pressure (CPAP). A small constant positive pressure is applied.

To avoid these types of adverse reactions, patients should be closely monitored, caution should be ex-

TABLE 28-2

Adverse effects of positive pressure ventilation

Effect	Mechanism(s)
Increased anatomic dead space	Increased radial pressure within airways
Increased functional dead space	Diversion of blood away from ventilated areas because of increased pressure resulting in capillary collapse
	Reduced blood flow to lung (see ventilation-perfusion inequalities)
Increased ventilation-perfusion inequalities in some lung regions—particular risk with PEEP	Reduced blood flow to lung due to reduced venous return and subsequent reduction in cardiac output
Cardiac dysrhythmias	Low serum potassium levels resulting from metabolic effects of rapidly reduced P_{CO_2}
Overdistention of lungs and emphysema	Excessive tidal volumes and rupture of alveoli

ercised when initiating therapy, and apparatus should be subjected to regular maintenance and cleaning routines.

Adverse effects of oxygen. The major adverse side effects related to the use of oxygen are drying and irritation of mucous membranes, respiratory depression, especially in patients with chronic obstructive pulmonary disease, and oxygen toxicity.

Drying and irritation of mucous membranes can cause decreased ciliary action and increased thickening of secretions, resulting in difficult removal and formation of mucous plugs. Humidification helps to prevent these adverse effects, which occur especially when oxygen is delivered under pressure.

Respiratory depression, or oxygen-induced apnea, can occur when high concentrations of oxygen are administered to patients in whom hypoxia provides the major stimulus for breathing, such as those patients with impaired respiratory control of ventilation. In these patients the stimulus for respiration is no longer the central receptor sites in the medulla and pons, but rather the peripheral chemoreceptors located in the arch of the aorta and carotid arteries. These receptors are sensitive to oxygen lack. The administration of oxygen may dampen this secondary stimulus, resulting in hypoventilation and respiratory failure. Thus correction of hypoxia in these patients results in hypoventilation and hypercapnia. Hyperventilation may be produced by the increase in $PaCO_2$, but if the respiratory center responsiveness is impaired, carbon dioxide retention may increase and produce severe carbon dioxide toxicity and narcosis.

Oxygen toxicity, progressive failure of the ventilation of the lungs, occurs when pure oxygen is administered for a prolonged period at high flow rates. Oxygen toxicity does not occur when oxygen is administered at low flow rates.

Maintenance of high concentrations of inspired oxygen may lead to atelectasis, particularly in patients with significant ventilation-perfusion inequalities or excessive mucus production. In these patients alveolar nitrogen concentrations are washed out by the excessive oxygen. The oxygen is quickly absorbed, producing negative pressures and atelectasis. Even if excessive oxygen concentrations are not reached, mucous plugging of the airways may result in oxygen being absorbed more quickly than it can be delivered to the alveoli.

As mentioned earlier, oxygen can dry and irritate the nasal mucosa. Such irritation can occur throughout the airways. With higher oxygen concentrations cellular damage occurs and can result in pulmonary edema. Failure of ventilation causes a decrease in oxygen tension in the blood. Early recognition of the signs of oxygen toxicity is essential because this condition is time and dose related, taking 24 to 48 hours to become evident. In the acute stage structural damage to the pulmonary tissue occurs, resulting in interstitial edema, thickened alveolar capillary membranes, intraalveolar hemorrhage, and the development of edema and atelectasis. Oxygen transport is impaired, and damage increases with hyaline membrane formation in the alveoli. In the end stage atelectasis is progressive, and consolidation and fibrosis of the lung occurs. Breath sounds are diminished, and rales may be audible.

Oxygen toxicity is not restricted to the lungs. Other adverse side effects associated with the therapeutic use of high concentrations of oxygen include retrolental fibroplasia, especially in premature infants receiving oxygen, and tearing, edema, and visual impairment in older children and adults as a result of its effects on the cornea and lens (Table 28-3).

TABLE 28-3

Adverse effects of oxygen

Effect(s)	Monitoring
Decreased respiration, apnea, and coma	Watch for in all hypoxic patients receiving oxygen, especially those with hypercapnic respiratory failure
Atelectasis	Patient may complain of substernal pain, cough, or increased dyspnea—headache occurring in inner ear or sinus area may indicate atelectasis
Irritation of airway mucosa, swelling, and inflammation	Initial sore throat and cough and nasal congestion may lead to decreased mucociliary clearance and increase risk of atelectasis
Circulatory changes—constriction of most vessels and dilation of conjunctival and pulmonary vessels	Look for conjunctivitis and development of mild hypertension
Tissue and blood vessel damage, pulmonary edema, decreased compliance, and increased shunting	Perform respiratory assessment
Central nervous system irritation, damage, and seizures	Hyperbaric oxygen administration is most likely form to be associated with central nervous system effects

The risk of oxygen toxicity increases with prolonged use of high oxygen concentrations but can be reduced by careful monitoring with the aid of blood gas determinations.

SUMMARY

Bronchodilators are used to treat conditions that cause narrowing of the airways. Sympathomimetics, phosphodiesterase inhibitors, parasympatholytics, cromolyn sodium, and steroids are used individually or in combination to treat and prevent bronchial constriction and maintain respiratory function.

Although numerous gases can be used for various therapeutic or diagnostic reasons, oxygen is used most often. Although oxygen is generally used to relieve hypoxia, hyperbaric oxygen can be used for cardiac surgery, treatment of anaerobic infections (e.g., gas gangrene), bends, or carbon monoxide poisoning.

The use of these medications requires attention to patient assessment, monitoring, and individualized teaching to ensure appropriate and effective drug therapy and to prevent and minimize adverse side effects. Because conditions affecting the respiratory system can cause psychologic as well as physical concerns to patients and their families, the nurse's role in providing support, teaching, and understanding cannot be overemphasized.

ADVERSE/SIDE EFFECTS OF THE BRONCHODILATORS*

Sympathomimetics
CARDIOVASCULAR SYSTEM

Dysrhythmias
Palpitations
Tachycardia†

CENTRAL NERVOUS SYSTEM

Agitation
Anxiety†
Dizziness
Euphoria
Headache
Insomnia
Psychosis
Restlessness†
Sweating
Tremor† (also caused by direct actions on β-receptors in muscle)

GASTROINTESTINAL SYSTEM

Nausea
Vomiting

METABOLISM

Aggravation of diabetes mellitus or hyperthyroidism

RESPIRATORY SYSTEM

Dry mouth and throat
Paradoxic bronchospasm

MISCELLANEOUS SYSTEMS

Aggravation of narrow-angle glaucoma
Pallor
Urinary retention

Parasympatholytics
CARDIOVASCULAR SYSTEM

Bradycardia followed by
Dysrhythmia
Palpitations
Tachycardia

GASTROINTESTINAL SYSTEM

Constipation
Nausea
Vomiting

OCULAR SYSTEM

Blurred vision
Increased intraocular pressure
Loss of accommodation
Mydriasis
Photophobia

RESPIRATORY SYSTEM

Dry mouth†
Drying of bronchial secretions

MISCELLANEOUS SYSTEMS

Difficulty in swallowing
Thirst

Phosphodiesterase inhibitors
CARDIOVASCULAR SYSTEM

Dysrhythmias
Palpitation
Peripheral vascular constriction and vasomotor collapse
Tachycardia†

CENTRAL NERVOUS SYSTEM

Convulsions
Excitement
Headache
Insomnia
Irritability
Nervousness†
Restlessness†
Tremor

GASTROINTESTINAL SYSTEM

Anorexia
Diarrhea
Epigastric pain
Gastric bleeding and reactivation of ulcer disease
Gastric irritation†
Nausea†
Vomiting

INTEGUMENTARY SYSTEM

Dermatitis
Generalized pruritus
Urticaria

MISCELLANEOUS SYSTEMS

Increased diuresis

Cromolyn sodium

See Nursing Drug Digest

Steroids

See Chapter 65, "Corticosteroids and Adrenal Steroid Inhibitors."

---

*See Chapter 11, "Drug Toxicity," for an overview of drug toxicity.
†Most common effects.

CLINICALLY SIGNIFICANT DRUG INTERACTIONS*

Primary drug	Interacting drugs	Possible effect(s)	Probable mechanism(s)
Epinephrine	Tricyclic antidepressants	Increased pressor effect of epinephrine with possibility of severe hypertension and cardiac dysrhythmias	Not established
Epinephrine	β-blockers	Bronchospasm, bradycardia, and hypotension	Blockage of β-receptors mediating dilation and possible stimulation of α-receptors mediating constriction
Epinephrine	Halogenated anesthetics	Cardiac dysrhythmias	Anesthetic sensitizes myocardium to effects of epinephrine
Ephedrine	Monoamine oxidase (MAO) inhibitors	Severe hypertension	MAO inhibitors increase amounts of norepinephrine in nerve storage sites that are released by ephedrine
Theophylline	Sympathomimetics	Increased bronchodilation Increased side effects	Cause increases in cAMP concentrations by separate mechanisms Additive actions
Theophylline	β-blockers	Antagonized bronchodilation	Blockage of β-receptors mediating bronchodilation
Theophylline	Cimetidine	Increased theophylline toxicity	Inhibition of microsomal enzymes
Theophylline	Nondepolarizing muscle relaxants	Decreased effect of the nondepolarizing muscle relaxants	Not established

*See Chapter 10, "Drug Interactions," for an overview of drug interactions.

GENERAL NURSING IMPLICATIONS

Nursing of patients requiring bronchodilators or oxygen

ASSESSMENT

A complete nursing assessment is essential in establishing a baseline from which to plan individualized drug therapy regimens and to monitor patient response. Assessment should include a detailed drug history to identify sensitivity, contraindications, cautions, potential drug interactions, and drug-taking patterns before drug therapy is initiated. Because bronchodilators are commonly abused or misused, use of over-the-counter preparations and self-care practices should be carefully explored when assessing, planning, and monitoring therapeutic regimens.

Assessment should include detailed baseline data related to fluid and electrolyte balance, acid-base balance, and nutritional status. Anorexia and weight loss should be noted. Laboratory data should include blood counts, arterial blood gases, chest x-ray examination, electrocardiogram, spirometry or full pulmonary function tests, and sputum cultures as indicated. These results should be obtained initially and at regular intervals during therapy. Laboratory values, including hematocrit and hemoglobin, can be falsely elevated because of hemoconcentration if dehydration or fluid volume deficit is presenting. Polycythemia is not uncommon in patients with chronic respiratory conditions.

Physical assessment of the patient should be completed carefully. Respiratory distress or failure requires systematic assessment completed quickly and calmly so that emergency measures can be implemented immediately. Baseline data including the rate, rhythm, and pattern of respiration should be recorded as well as the heart rate, blood pressure, and temperature so that changes in respiratory status or response to therapy can be readily identified.

The shape and symmetry of the thorax should be noted. This observation is especially important if an obstructed airway or chronic obstructive pulmonary disease (COPD) is suspected and oxygen therapy is to be administered. In the presence of COPD the anteroposterior diameter may be increased with the chest appearing rounded and the ribs horizontal. Slight kyphosis of the thoracic spine, a prominent sternal angle, and a widened costal angle as well as other deviations may be seen.

Breathing may be labored with the use of accessory muscles, and supraclavicular, substernal, or intercostal retractions may be present. Shortness of breath, complaints of dyspnea, orthopnea, audible respirations, or nasal flaring should be noted. The presence or

Continued.

GENERAL NURSING IMPLICATIONS—cont'd

Nursing of patients requiring bronchodilators or oxygen—cont'd

ASSESSMENT—cont'd

absence of chest pain and its relationship to breathing or exercise should be recorded. Cyanosis may be present and is a late sign of hypercapnia or hypoxia. Clubbing of the fingers and toes may be present, particularly in COPD patients.

Palpation should be completed over all chest areas. Thoracic expansion and vocal fremitus may be decreased. Resonance to hyperresonance may be noted with percussion, and diaphragmatic excursion may be small.

The chest should be auscultated carefully for absent or decreased breath sounds, and adventitious sounds including rales, rhonchi, stridor, and pleural friction rub should be identified and their exact location and occurrence in relation to inspiration and expiration noted. The presence of a productive or nonproductive cough or pain associated with coughing should be assessed. The amount, color, and character of sputum should be recorded.

Special attention should be given to the assessment of mental status and activity tolerance, since changes in mentation including apathy, irritability, fatigue, and weakness can be excellent indicators of respiratory status. These baseline measurements are essential in monitoring therapy.

Other information should include a family history, an occupational history, and a smoking history identifying number of pack years (i.e., number of packs smoked per day times years of smoking). Past surgery of the respiratory tract as well as the presence of allergies that produce respiratory symptoms should be identified and recorded. Because bronchodilators are contraindicated in certain conditions and because diuretics, antibiotics, and heart medications can interact with some bronchodilators, the health history should also include the identification of such conditions as heart disease, hypertension, and renal or hepatic dysfunction. Pregnancy should also be identified.

Because some drugs can cause pulmonary reactions that closely resemble respiratory conditions, a careful drug history is especially important. Bronchospasm may result from the drug itself (e.g., β-blockers), a stabilizing agent, or drug impurities. Asthma is the most common drug-induced respiratory condition and can be caused by medications such as aspirin, penicillin, or isoproterenol. Gases can also produce respiratory conditions such as congestive atelectasis, which can occur from prolonged oxygen use.

Anxiety is common in the patient suffering from respiratory distress because difficult breathing is frightening to both the patient and family. In addition to pharmacologic measures, a calm, supportive, and understanding approach is essential. Dyspneic patients should not be left alone, and measures to conserve energy and maximize oxygenation should be readily implemented. The patient in respiratory distress may be encouraged to perform learned breathing exercises or coached to breathe more effectively as well as assisted to positions that promote maximal chest expansion. Patients generally know their most effective breathing positions and assume these positions when in distress. However, assistance is required to conserve energy. Assistance with pillows to support the patient's arms and to position the overbed table is usually required. These measures are helpful adjuncts to pharmacologic therapy.

Patients in respiratory distress should not be oversedated. If in doubt about the use of a sedative to relieve anxiety or to promote rest and conserve energy requirements, consult with the prescriber. The presence of the nurse and the utilization of adjunct measures to promote comfort and enhance breathing can be effective. The presence of family may also be helpful. However, in some instances family presence may not relieve anxiety and may cause tension. In such cases the family should be asked to leave until the patient is feeling better. They should, however, also receive support and assistance

from the nursing staff as needed. This help is especially important because the family is often instrumental in planning and managing therapeutic measures in the home setting.

In the presence of hypoxia with apnea or dyspnea at rest the patient may require manual or mechanical ventilation. Emergency respiratory equipment and suction apparatus should be readily available. Because patients cannot verbalize needs or distress when mechanically ventilated, careful monitoring and anticipation of needs are essential. Nurses should talk with patients during care, explain procedures, and work out communication plans as the patient is able.

BRONCHODILATORS
Sensitivity

All drugs have the potential to induce hypersensitivity reactions in susceptible individuals. Whenever a bronchodilator is administered for the first time, the patient should be carefully questioned regarding reactions to the specific or related medications and should be monitored carefully for early signs of allergic reaction including increased difficulty in breathing, rash, or any other unusual effect. Cromolyn sodium has produced true allergic reactions in sensitive patients, and patients should be questioned carefully about previous use of this medication. Because cromolyn sodium capsules contain 20 mg of cromolyn sodium mixed with lactose, the capsule form should not be used by patients with a history of allergic reaction to lactose, milk, or milk products. In these patients use of cromolyn solution may be an appropriate substitute.

All patients should be closely monitored for hypersensitivity when receiving bronchodilators as well as oxygen for the first time.

Contraindications

Bronchodilators are contraindicated in patients with a history of hypersensitivity to the specific or related medication. Other contraindications are as follows.

GENERAL NURSING IMPLICATIONS—cont'd

Nursing of patients requiring bronchodilators or oxygen—cont'd

Contraindications—cont'd

Sympathomimetics are contraindicated in patients with the following.
Hypersensitivity to sympathomimetic amines
Predisposition to narrow-angle glaucoma, which can be aggravated by these agents
Shock
History of cardiac disease, diabetes, hypertension, or hyperthyroidism
General anesthesia with halogenated hydrocarbons or cyclopropane
History of receiving MAO inhibitors within past 3 weeks—or concomitant administration of MAO inhibitors (in addition, sympathomimetic therapy is contraindicated because hypertensive crises may be precipitated)

Phosphodiesterase inhibitors are contraindicated in patients with the following.
Hypersensitivity to xanthine agents, including theophylline and its salts (e.g., aminophylline), caffeine, and theobromine
Coronary artery disease aggravated by myocardial stimulation because these agents can stimulate the heart
Peptic ulcer disease because these agents can induce or aggravate ulcer disease, gastric bleeding, and gastritis

Cromolyn sodium is contraindicated in patients with the following.
Known hypersensitivity to cromolyn sodium
Acute asthma during an attack

Cautions

Bronchodilators should be used with caution in patients during/with the following.
Pregnancy or women with childbearing potential
Cardiovascular disorders
Diabetes mellitus
Prostate hypertrophy
Glaucoma

Following are additional cautions.

Sympathomimetics
Tachyphylaxis, or acute tolerance, can occur readily with the β-receptor agonists, especially ephedrine, isoproterenol, and newer agents. Patients require larger and more frequent doses to achieve the same degree of bronchodilation (i.e., tachyphylaxis). Overuse increases risk of toxicity, and lack of response may indicate deterioration of condition and the need for other therapy.

Elderly patients are more likely to develop adverse reactions because of reduced metabolism and clearance of these agents.

Phosphodiesterase inhibitors
Patients with cardiac insufficiency or decreased hepatic function are more likely to develop adverse reactions because the resulting reductions in metabolism and clearance can result in drug accumulation and high serum levels.

Cromolyn sodium
Caution must be exercised if cromolyn sodium is discontinued in patients in whom its use allowed reduction in maintenance doses of steroids. Steroid doses should be restored to previous levels before withdrawal of cromolyn sodium to avoid risk of acute relapse.

Drug interactions
Bronchodilators can interact with numerous other drugs, foods, and alcohol. In addition, smoking can also affect drug action.

Sympathomimetics
Ephedrine can antagonize the antihypertensive effect of bethanidine or guanethidine, resulting in the need for increased dosage or use of additional antihypertensive agents.

Severe hypertension may occur with concurrent use of ephedrine with furazolidone and MAO inhibitors, which potentiate pressor effects.

Use of OTC metered-dose inhalers unless specifically prescribed can increase the side effects of sympathomimetics such as palpitations and tachycardia, since many contain epinephrine.

Phosphodiesterase inhibitors
An increased diet of protein can increase the clearance rate of theophylline, requiring higher dosage to maintain desired effects. Chronic smoking can cause decreased enzyme response for metabolism of theophylline, leading to a shorter half-life of the drug and decreased serum levels. A change in smoking habits can necessitate an adjustment in maintenance dose.

Erythromycin, some tetracyclines, and cimetidine can prolong the half-life of these preparations.

Cardiac disease such as congestive heart failure can decrease theophylline clearance, leading to toxic levels with average doses.

Liver and hepatic dysfunction can slow metabolism. Dosage adjustment may be indicated. Dosage should be adjusted for the elderly with diminished hepatic or renal function related to aging. (See Clinically Significant Drug Interactions for important clinical drug interactions.)

Administration

The different bronchodilators are available in a variety of dosage forms, including oral (capsule, tablet, granule, or elixir), inhalation (metered-dose inhaler or solution for inhalation), parenteral, and rectal (enema or suppository).

The inhalation forms, except for cromolyn preparations, are generally used to provide prompt, immediate relief of bronchospasm. The oral dosage forms and cromolyn inhalation are used primarily for prophylaxis. Parenteral forms are typically used to treat acute respiratory distress and are usually administered in the hospital setting.

When administration schedules with patients are planned, it is important that pharmacodynamic parameters and the potential for drug interactions be carefully considered. Patients with chronic pulmonary conditions who are admitted to hospitals should not be expected to change their home medication schedules to fit the hospital rou-
Continued.

GENERAL NURSING IMPLICATIONS—cont'd

Nursing of patients requiring bronchodilators or oxygen—cont'd

Administration—cont'd

tine. If the patient's home schedule is not optimal, adjustments should be made with the knowledge of the patient so that reasons for change are understood. Patients should be allowed to keep their own medications and take them as indicated until their hospital supply of medication is received from the pharmacy so that undue anxiety, missed doses, or the hiding of medications by patients is prevented. Following is additional information about administration of specific bronchodilators.

Sympathomimetics

Sympathomimetics are available in various dosage forms: oral preparations, metered-dose inhalers, solution for inhalation, and parenteral forms for subcutaneous or intramuscular injection.

If two sympathomimetics must be given, they should be dosed alternately instead of concurrently to prevent additive effects that can result in the increased risk of toxic reactions, especially reactions involving the cardiovascular system.

It is not uncommon for patients to require both a sympathomimetic and a phosphodiesterase inhibitor. Administration times should be spaced to allow more constant bronchodilation and fewer side effects.

Patients receiving both a sympathomimetic and a steroid preparation by aerosol should be advised to use the sympathomimetic before the steroid to increase deposition of the steroid within the small airways.

Epinephrine should be administered subcutaneously or intramuscularly for bronchodilator effect. Inadvertent intravenous administration can cause pulmonary edema or cerebral hemorrhage because of the sharp increase in blood pressure that can occur.

Phosphodiesterase inhibitors

Phosphodiesterase inhibitors are available in oral short-acting (effective 4 hours) or sustained release (effective 8 to 12 hours) dosage forms. Granule preparations (e.g., TheoDur Sprinkles) are available for patients who have difficulty swallowing tablets. Intravenous forms are also available. Rectal forms (enema and suppository) are not recommended because absorption may be erratic and local irritation is common.

Oral phosphodiesterase inhibitors are irritating to the gastric mucosa and should be taken with meals, milk and crackers, or an antacid. Elixirs can be mixed with a little water and taken with a full glass of water to decrease gastric irritation.

Some oral preparations are better tolerated than others, and sometimes an alternate brand or other oral dosage form may be helpful if gastric irritation or vomiting is a problem associated with the administration of this medication.

Phosphodiesterase inhibitors should be administered evenly spaced throughout a 24-hour period. These medications are most effective when serum levels remain constant within the therapeutic range (e.g., theophylline serum levels of 10 to 20 μg/ml).

This medication should be administered early during an asthmatic attack to prevent a mild attack from becoming severe.

Cromolyn sodium

Cromolyn sodium is available in powder form in single-dose Spincap capsules for use with a Spinhaler. Solution for inhalation is also available.

Ensure that the patient understands the correct use of the Spinhaler so that the entire contents of the single dose capsule is used (Figure 28-4).

A common complaint associated with use of the Spinhaler treatment is irritation of the throat. This problem can be prevented or relieved if the patient drinks a glass of water after the treatment.

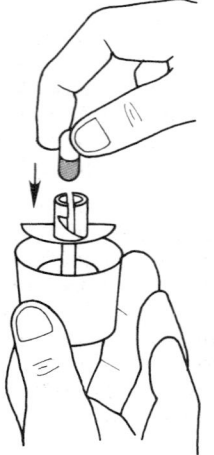
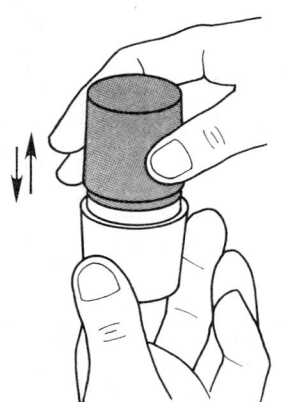

FIGURE 28-4. **Use of Spinhaler for administration of cromolyn sodium.**

GENERAL NURSING IMPLICATIONS—cont'd

Nursing of patients requiring bronchodilators or oxygen—cont'd

Cromolyn sodium—cont'd
In addition, transient bronchospasm and coughing occasionally occur after inhalation of the powdered form. Inhalation of a bronchodilator aerosol before the Spinhaler treatment can prevent or minimize this problem. If necessary, the solution form may be used, which is easier for some patients to take and is less likely to cause dyspnea and coughing.

Ipratropium bromide
Dry mouth is the usual complaint associated with this medication, and it can be minimized by advising the patient to drink water after use.

Sidestream nebulizers and mininebulizers can be used to deliver aerosolized medication (Figure 28-5, C and D). A mask or mouthpiece should be selected in relation to patient need.

Patients should be positioned in a sitting or high Fowler's position to encourage full lung expansion and aerosol dispersion through the lungs. Pressurized oxygen is used to administer the treatment, although mixtures of oxygen and room air can be used if indicated. The medication is drawn up into a sterile syringe. A diluent such as sterile normal saline solution or distilled water is also drawn up, depending on the medication to be administered. The sterile saline solution or distilled water is also available in premeasured containers that can be poured into the reservoir of the nebulizer.

The patient is positioned after the procedure is explained and the medication and saline solution or water are placed into the reservoir and held in an upright position to prevent leakage.

The oxygen flow rate is usually set at 4 to 6 L per minute. The patient is told to take slow deep even breaths and to hold each breath 2 to 3 seconds for full benefit of the medication. The treatment usually takes from 15 to 20 minutes, and the nurse should remain with the patient during treatment to monitor response as well as self-medication ability. The patient should be encouraged and assisted with coughing and expectoration. Breath sounds and sputum character and amount should be assessed after the treatment. If the patient becomes tired during the treatment, a rest period should be allowed. Chest physiotherapy is best completed after the treatment. In addition, baseline vital signs, including blood pressure, should be completed before therapy when drugs that can affect heart rate or blood pressure (e.g., sympatho-

Continued.

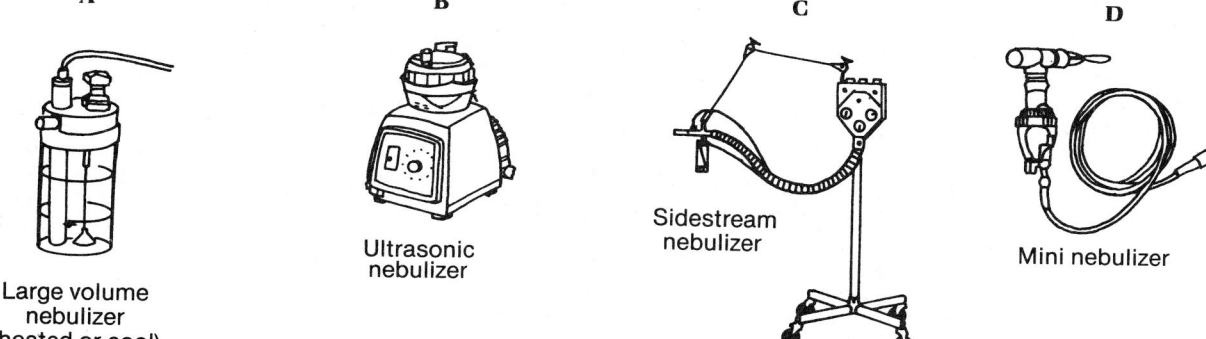

A Large volume nebulizer (heated or cool)

B Ultrasonic nebulizer

C Sidestream nebulizer

D Mini nebulizer

FIGURE 28-5. **Administration of bronchodilators by nebulizer. A and B, Large-volume nebulizers are generally used for humidification of oxygen and not for administration of bronchodilators. C, Sidestream nebulizers are used to deliver medication with IPPB treatment or with respirator. The ordered dose of medication is diluted 1:3 with normal saline or other diluent and is placed in the reservoir. The treatment usually lasts for 15 to 20 minutes. For the IPPB, although individualized to each patient, the inspiratory flow rate is adjusted between 6 and 30 L/min at a cycling pressure of 10 to 15 cm H_2O. The sensitivity is adjusted individually. D, Mininebulizers are often used to administer bronchodilators. The inhalant solution form of the bronchodilator is poured into the nebulizer reservoir with a duluent such as sterile water for inhalation. A mask or mouth piece can be used for the treatment. The patient should slowly inhale. The breath is held 3 seconds. This is repeated until the medication is used. For young children, the mist is held 1 to 2 inches from the mouth if the mask is refused until the treatment is completed. The ordered flow rate of oxygen used for aerosolization is usually 4 to 6 L/minute over a period of 15 to 20 minutes.**

GENERAL NURSING IMPLICATIONS—cont'd

Nursing of patients requiring bronchodilators or oxygen—cont'd

Ipratropium bromide—cont'd
mimetics) are administered. Vital signs should be reevaluated when therapy is completed.

Monitoring patient response

Therapeutic response
The goal of bronchodilator therapy is to restore and maintain pulmonary function as close as possible to normal by dilating narrowed airways. Monitoring patient response is essential in planning appropriate and effective therapy. Bronchodilation occurs rapidly after the administration of these drugs. Immediate response can be observed in the patient's breathing, including increased flow rates and vital capacity, as small muscles of the respiratory tract relax and bronchospasm is relieved. The patient will appear less distressed and anxious. Inhalation and exhalation will be less labored. The respiratory rate should decrease to the normal range, and adventitious sounds indicating bronchoconstriction diminish. Coloring should improve as well as socialization and ability to perform self-care.

Sympathomimetics
Dyspnea should be relieved, and the bronchodilator should not be required more often than every 4 hours. When response is monitored, it is important to note that oral short-acting preparations should be effective for at least 4 hours. Oral sustained-release preparations should be effective for 8 to 12 hours. Subcutaneous or intramuscular routes are used for severe bronchospasm, and effectiveness should be noted immediately or within 15 minutes.

Phosphodiesterase inhibitors
Ideally, all patients receiving phosphodiesterase inhibitors should have serum theophylline levels determined routinely. However, this evaluation is not usually practical, and the patient's general condition, clinical response, and the time required to achieve steady-state kinetics must all be considered when deciding how often serum levels should be determined. Serum theophylline levels should be used whenever one adjusts dosages in patients showing signs of theophylline toxicity or lack of therapeutic response. Dosage is highly individualized; however, therapeutic response is usually attained with serum concentrations of 5 to 20 µg/ml.
Generally

4 to 5 µg/ml	Bronchodilation begins
10 to 20 µg/ml	Optimal bronchodilation
>20 µg/ml	Adverse reactions increasingly common

Cromolyn sodium
Therapeutic effects with daily use may take 6 to 8 weeks to occur. Because cromolyn sodium is given prophylactically to prevent asthmatic attack, patient management of condition and prevention of attacks are important indicators of therapeutic response. Cromolyn sodium will not relieve symptoms once an attack has started.

Teenagers and younger children with allergic asthma as well as adults with exercise-induced asthma usually respond better than other patients to this medication.

Adverse side effects
Except for allergic effects, most adverse effects are dose related. Adverse side effects decrease with continued use or may be minimized by decreasing the medication dosage. (See Adverse/Side Effects of the Bronchodilators.) Following are additional adverse side effects.

Sympathomimetics
Tachycardia occurs as an adverse effect of β$_1$-stimulants, and vasoconstriction occurs with the use of α-adrenergics. Selective β$_2$-stimulants have fewer adverse side effects than β$_1$-stimulants when given in recommended doses.

Monitor for symptoms of central nervous system stimulation, including dizziness, confusion, anxiety, restlessness, and hallucinations, especially when nonselective agents are used.

If overuse is suspected, observe for tremor and tachycardia, palpitations, headache, restlessness, and insomnia. Question the patient about sleepless-ness, nausea, vomiting, headache, or any increase in use of medication or lack of relief after use, since patients may take medication more often than every 4 hours if ineffective.

Shakiness and hand tremor may develop when taking oral sympathomimetics but usually diminish with continued use of the drug.

Phosphodiesterase inhibitors
Adverse effects should be reported to the prescriber. However, medication should not be stopped unless symptoms are severe, indicating dosage should be changed or a different drug prescribed.

Question the patient about loss of appetite, headache, insomnia, tinnitus, irritability, flushing, nausea, vomiting, and increased diuresis or thirst.

Monitor for nausea and vomiting, gastrointestinal pain, and restlessness. Restlessness may be first sign of toxicity. Because infants and young children cannot report adverse side effects, they require careful monitoring. Theophylline preparations have a low therapeutic index. Since children require higher dosages than adults to offset their higher clearance rates, they should be observed carefully for signs of toxicity: rapid pulse rate, rapid breathing, signs of central nervous system excitation, or dehydration.

Hyperreflexia and fasciculations preceding convulsions are most likely observed in infants with toxic serum levels.

Toxicity usually occurs at serum concentrations *greater* than 20 µg/ml. Central nervous system or cardiovascular reactions are more indicative of overdose because gastrointestinal reactions may be caused by local irritation.

In cases of overdose report to prescriber. Discontinue drug immediately and avoid administration of sympathomimetics. Emergency equipment including oxygen, diazepam, and intravenous fluids should be readily available to treat overdose.

GENERAL NURSING IMPLICATIONS—cont'd

Nursing of patients requiring bronchodilators or oxygen—cont'd

Cromolyn sodium

Inhalation of dried powder form in capsule for use with Turboinhaler or Spinhaler may cause bronchospasm from local irritation or irritation of the throat and cough. These effects can be minimized by having the patient drink a glass of water after the treatment or by administering a sympathomimetic aerosol before treatment.

Parasympatholytics

Atropine-like effects including dry mouth, mydriasis, cycloplegia, and urinary retention can occur with the use of parasympatholytics. When inhaled, these drugs can cause decreased ciliary action and decreased sputum production.

OXYGEN

Contraindications

Oxygen delivered at flow rates greater than 2 to 3 L per minute is contraindicated and can be fatal to patients with carbon dioxide retention, in which hypoxia provides the major stimulus for breathing.

To prevent carbon dioxide narcosis, administer only low concentrations (25% to 35%) of oxygen at flow rates of 2 to 3 L per minute.

Cautions

Oxygen, even when administered at flow rates of 2 to 3 L per minute, should be administered cautiously to patients with carbon dioxide retention because these patients are especially prone to oxygen toxicity.

Prolonged use of oxygen at high concentrations can cause serious eye defects, including irreversible damage to infants' eyes (retrolental fibroplasia) and tearing and corneal damage in older children and adults.

Inhalation of high concentrations of oxygen under pressure may cause irritation to respiratory mucosa, decreased vital capacity, and neurologic symptoms.

Although oxygen itself is not flammable or explosive, it supports combustion. Fire and explosion are potential hazards whenever oxygen is in use. Safety precautions should be implemented before therapy is started. Signs should be posted clearly warning that oxygen is in use. Smoking, open flames, and use of electric equipment and flammable substances such as rubbing alcohol or lanolin lotions for patient care should be avoided. Lemon glycerine swabs and lotions can be used if necessary.

All-cotton thermal blankets should be used. Silk, wool, and synthetics, because they generate static electricity, should *not* be allowed. These precautions are especially important when concentrations of 100% oxygen are used. All valves should be turned off when oxygen is not being administered, and fire extinguishers should be readily available. Patients as well as family and visitors should be advised regarding safety precautions when oxygen is in use.

Administration

Oxygen is administered at concentrations that reverse hypoxia without causing undesired and harmful adverse side effects. Oxygen should be administered *only* after arterial blood gases have been assessed. Arterial blood gases should be frequently monitored during oxygen therapy, and patient response must be observed carefully and documented. The monitoring of oxygen effect on Pao_2 is especially important.

Oxygen is supplied from wall outlets or portable tanks and cylinders. It is administered in liters per minute or by percentage, depending on the oxygen delivery system or device (e.g., cannula, mask, or ventilator). Oxygen must be administered humidified.

Monitoring patient response

Therapeutic response

Half-hourly or more frequent monitoring is required when patients are receiving oxygen for treatment of acute hypoxia until their condition is stable. Monitoring can then be less frequent, depending on the individual patient's condition. The date, type of therapy, delivery device, and patient response should be recorded. Patients should be carefully monitored for relief of symptoms of hypoxia.

When humidified oxygen is used, loosened productive coughing and increased sputum production should be observed with improvement in breath sounds. Some patients may require assistance with clearing respiratory passages. Nasal and oral hygiene is important in maintaining respiratory function and patient comfort. Suctioning may be necessary for patients with copious amounts of mucus but should be used only if the patient is unable to adequately cough and expectorate or clear air passages.

Adverse side effects

Patients should be monitored for general adverse side effects related to oxygen therapy including drying and irritation of mucous membranes and thickening of secretions especially when oxygen is delivered under pressure or at higher flow rates. When large-volume humidifiers (e.g., Cascade humidifier) or nebulizers (e.g., Ultrasonic nebulizer) are used to increase airway hydration, patients should be monitored for overhydration and pulmonary edema. Monitoring is especially important when treatments are heated or if the patient has a condition in which fluid balance is an existing or potential problem (e.g., congestive heart failure or renal dysfunction). Because the temperature control of heated treatments can malfunction and cause irritation or burning of the respiratory mucosa as a result of breathing hot, dry air, especially if the correct water level is not maintained in the reservoir, it is particularly important to monitor the patient for complaints of warmth or discomfort and to check tubing for warmth as well as maintain adequate water volume in reservoirs. As a precaution a thermometer can be placed in the tubing to better monitor temperature.

Other effects are related to the oxygen delivery device used. For example, nasal cannulas can cause local irritation to the nares, and oxygen masks can cause irritation where they make contact around the nose and mouth. Skin areas should be assessed for irritation and equipment selected carefully in relation to the individual patient's needs.

Continued.

GENERAL NURSING IMPLICATIONS—cont'd

Nursing of patients requiring bronchodilators or oxygen—cont'd

Adverse side effects—cont'd

When oxygen is used to deliver medications with sidestream nebulizers or mininebulizers, adverse effects such as bronchospasm can occur as a result of the aerosolization of water, isotonic saline solution, or medication.

More serious adverse side effects can occur. Patients should be carefully monitored for respiratory depression, especially the patient with COPD and oxygen toxicity.

Respiratory depression

Carefully monitor patients for the following.

Decreased rate or depth of respiration

Change in level of consciousness

Increased hypercapnia

If noted, notify the physician at once. These signs indicate that the oxygen flow rate should be lowered. Manual ventilation may be required, and equipment should be readily available.

Oxygen toxicity

Carefully monitor patients, especially during the first 24 to 48 hours of oxygen therapy, for the following.

Complaints of a tickling feeling near carina tracheae where the trachea bifurcates

Occasional coughing that becomes progressively more frequent and severe because of tracheal irritation

Complaints of a burning feeling in the lungs

Uncontrollable coughing

Increased substernal irritation with dyspnea at rest

Reduced vital capacity

Decreased Pao_2

Decreased breath sounds

Decreased lung compliance resulting in increased inspiration airway pressure needed to deliver tidal volume

Other symptoms may be noted including anorexia, nausea and vomiting, fatigue, headache, orthostatic fainting, sore throat, and paresthesia.

Monitoring of arterial blood gases is especially important in preventing oxygen toxicity as well as its early recognition because patients receiving high concentrations of oxygen over a prolonged period are usually critically ill, intubated, and unable to communicate discomfort. It is also difficult to differentiate many signs of oxygen toxicity from many primary respiratory conditions (e.g., adult respiratory distress syndrome, ARDS). If oxygen toxicity is suspected, notify the physician at once. Provide emotional support to the patient as well as monitor fluid and electrolytes, vital capacity, inspiratory force, tidal volume, and arterial blood gases. A chest x-ray examination is indicated to identify effects of toxicity. The patient should be protected from infection because risk is increased because of damage to the respiratory system. Continue to monitor for signs of hypoxia.

To prevent oxygen toxicity, maintain the lowest possible oxygen flow rate to maintain a Pao_2 range of 60 to 90 mm Hg unless otherwise indicated. (Higher oxygen flow rates are indicated in the treatment of carbon monoxide intoxication.)

PATIENT EDUCATION

The patient and family should know the importance of following the therapeutic plan developed with the health care provider. Patient education should be individualized to the needs of the patient and family and should include information about normal respiratory function. Self-care measures to promote respiratory function should be included such as the avoidance of smoke, irritants, cold, or allergens; maintenance of adequate nutrition and hydration; identification of exercise and activity tolerance levels and how activities can be completed within these levels; utilization of chest physiotherapy techniques (e.g., postural drainage, deep breathing, and coughing) and breathing exercises (e.g., diaphragmatic breathing, pursed lip breathing, and dyspneic positions); and the prevention of respiratory infections (care of sputum, care of inhalers or other respiratory equipment, avoidance of others with respiratory infections, and dressing appropriately for weather).

The patient and family should understand the importance of regular follow-up clinic visits or health care appointments and the need for pulmonary function and laboratory tests as indicated.

Respiratory tract infections are common in patients with chronic pulmonary conditions and can lead to serious complications. Patients should be taught to recognize early signs of respiratory tract infections so that appropriate treatment can be implemented readily. This is important because bacterial infections respond best when antibiotic therapy is started early. Patients should be able to monitor sputum for changes in amount, color, or viscosity. The patient should recognize that an increase or decrease in the usual amount or thickness of sputum, a yellow or green tinge to the sputum, or an elevated temperature and heart rate can indicate the presence of infection.

The patient should be taught to take the predetermined antibiotic medication (e.g., ampicillin or tetracycline) for the entire prescribed time (usually for 7 to 10 days). Patients using tetracycline should be reminded not to take this medication with milk or antacids because absorption is impaired. The patient should be able to recognize when antibiotic therapy is ineffective and when to consult with the health care provider so that sputum cultures can be obtained and alternate therapy selected (e.g., chloramphenicol, cephalosporin, or sulfonamide).

In addition to these general areas of patient therapy education, the patient and family should understand how to handle emergency respiratory situations (e.g., acute asthma attacks or reversible bronchospasm).

Bronchodilators

The patient and family should have a clear understanding of the medication regimen as well as the exact name of the medication, its action, dosage, storage, administration, adverse side effects, and how these effects can be managed or minimized. The patient and family should know how to mon-

GENERAL NURSING IMPLICATIONS—cont'd

Nursing of patients requiring bronchodilators or oxygen—cont'd

Bronchodilators—cont'd

itor therapeutic effects as well as be able to identify signs that indicate that the health care provider should be contacted.

With careful individualized teaching, the patient and family as indicated should be able to do the following.

Monitor respiratory status, including respiratory and pulse rates, and recognize signs of hypercapnia or hypoxemia.

Describe the medication schedule, including foods, beverages, or other medications that should be avoided when taking the medication.

Demonstrate the correct administration of the medication (e.g., swallow sustained-release products whole without crushing or chewing; and do not swallow sublingual tablets or Spinhaler capsules) and not exceed or change the dosage or frequency of administration of the medication without first consulting with the health care provider.

Discuss the use of other medications with the health care provider before they are taken, recognizing that some drugs can cause harmful effects if taken with bronchodilators (e.g., propranolol or other β-blockers).

Report adverse effects or decrease in effectiveness of the medication.

Demonstrate the correct care and cleaning of metered aerosols, Spinhalers, or other equipment used in administering bronchodilator medication.

Use of Spinhaler for administration of cromolyn sodium

With mouthpiece downward, place the colored end of the cromolyn capsule into the propeller cup of the inhaler (Figure 28-4, A).

Screw on the top and push the gray sleeve of the inhaler down to pierce the capsule. Pull the sleeve up to the original position (Figure 28-4, B).

Have patient exhale to empty the lungs and place the mouthpiece into the mouth. Close the teeth and lips around the mouthpiece and inhale as rapidly as possible. Inhalation causes the propeller to rotate, and the powder is aerosolized.

Have patient hold breath for a few seconds and exhale.

Remind patient not to breathe into the inhaler because moisture can interfere with aerosolization of powder.

Repeat until all the powder is inhaled and the capsule is empty.

Take apart and wash all parts in warm water at least once a week. Reassemble after thoroughly dry.

Spinhaler should be replaced after 6 months of use.

Use of metered-dose inhaler

Sympathomimetic bronchodilators, steroids, and cromolyn sodium can be administered by metered-dose inhaler. Explain the administration procedure carefully to the patient and ensure that the patient is capable of self-adminis-

tration. The patient should also be taught to monitor the amount of medication remaining by placing the canister in water (Figure 28-6). Instruction should begin when first prescribed. Reteaching may be necessary for patients who have been using metered-dose inhalers. Follow-up should include assessment of how well the patient uses the metered-dose inhaler, how effective treatments are, and adverse side effects experienced.

Put the inhaler together, and shake to mix the medication with the propellant.

Remove the cap from the mouthpiece and have the patient hold the canister with the index finger on the top and the thumb on the bottom (Figure 28-7, A).

Continued.

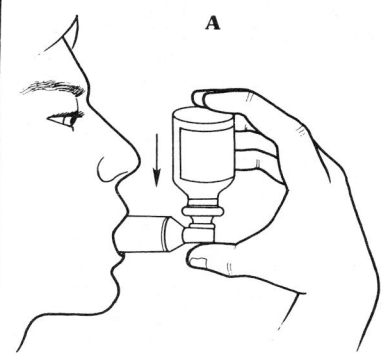

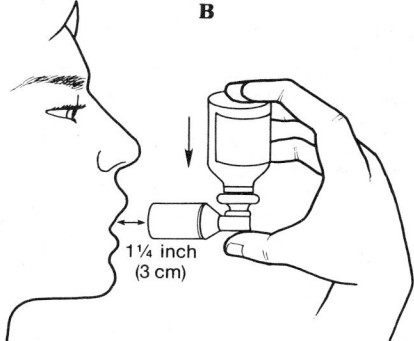

FIGURE 28-7. **Use of metered-dose inhaler.**

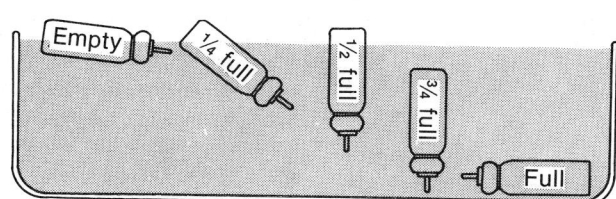

FIGURE 28-6. **Estimating remaining medication in inhalers. Metered-dose inhalers contain approximately 200 puffs. Patients can estimate remaining medication in canisters by floating the canister in a pan of water.**

GENERAL NURSING IMPLICATIONS—cont'd

Nursing of patients requiring bronchodilators or oxygen—cont'd

Use of metered-dose inhaler—cont'd

The patient should place the inhaler in the mouth keeping the tongue away from the opening of the inhaler. If the patient initially has difficulty, the mouthpiece may be gently gripped with the teeth until the patient is comfortable with the technique.

The patient should exhale gently through the mouth.

Depress the medication canister with the index finger while inhaling deeply. It is important that each dose is completely inhaled because the inhaler delivers exact doses of the medication. The patient should remove the inhaler from the mouth and hold a breath for 10 seconds or for as long as the patient comfortably can and then exhale through pursed lips.

If preferred (Figure 28-7, *B*), advise patient to position the tip of the pressurized inhaler 1 to 1¼ inches in front of the widely opened mouth. This position prevents medication from being deposited at the back of the throat. The patient should breathe normally, and following a relaxed expiration, inhale slowly and as deeply as possible. About halfway through the inspiration the canister should be depressed, and the patient should continue to inhale to maximum. The airways are widely dilated at this time, which ensures increased distribution of the medication. The patient should hold the breath for 5 to 10 seconds and exhale normally. If two puffs are required, repeat the procedure approximately 30 seconds after the first puff.

For *sympathomimetic* preparations the following information should be taught.

Sympathomimetic preparations are used for immediate relief during acute episodes of breathlessness. Patients should be able to use the metered-dose inhaler readily because they may be panicky when breathless.

If two puffs are prescribed, encourage the patient to wait 1 to 5 minutes between inhalations so that the airway can dilate and the medication can be inhaled more deeply into the lungs.

For *steroid* preparations the following information should be taught.

Encourage the patient to wait at least 1 minute between puffs of steroid preparations to allow first dose to take effect and enhance the effect of subsequent inhalations.

Encourage patients to take bronchodilator before corticosteroid, if prescribed, so that passages are dilated, allowing corticosteroid to be inhaled more deeply into the lungs.

If beclamethasone is taken, remind the patient to rinse the mouth to prevent fungal infections in the mouth and throat, which can result from this medication because it suppresses normal flora.

In addition, patients should clean inhaler daily. First remove the metal medication canister by pulling up firmly, and then rinse the plastic container under warm running water. The container should be dried well.

Reteaching and follow-up are indicated. In addition, the nurse should ascertain the following.

    How well the patient is able to use
      the inhaler.
    How often the inhaler is used.
    How effective the inhaler is.
    What adverse side effects are caused
      by the use of the inhaler.

Advise patients not to use over-the-counter inhalants, especially those that contain epinephrine, without first checking with their health care provider. Patients may overdose themselves by using these inhalers too frequently in an attempt to maintain relief, because, although effective readily, their effects last only a short while. Overuse can cause rebound bronchospasm.

Patients should be warned specifically against the overuse of aerosol bronchodilators to minimize the development of toxic reactions (e.g., epinephrine in many bronchodilators can increase such adverse effects as palpitation and tachycardia) and tachyphylaxis, thus avoiding delay in seeking alternative therapy when required.

Store container in a cool place and do not place the container in hot water or near radiators, stoves, or other sources of heat. Do not puncture, burn, or incinerate container even when empty because it is under pressure and could explode.

Patients requiring steroid therapy should be carefully advised that steroid requirements may be increased by coughs, colds, and flu or other stress. If wheezing or bronchospasm occurs or worsens, the steroid dosage should be increased according to a predetermined regimen and the advice of the health care provider should be sought.

Patients should be taught to avoid antihistamines, which can dry airway secretions and make expectoration of secretions difficult, cough suppressants, which can prevent expectoration of mucus, and sedatives, which can decrease respirations and cause hypoventilation. If allergy is a problem or if cough is persistent and interrupts sleep, the health care provider should be contacted so that adjustments in the drug regimen can be made or appropriate medications selected to treat these problems.

Patients who require bronchodilators for acute asthmatic attacks or reversible bronchospasm and their family members should be able to administer epinephrine subcutaneously for a severe attack. The medication and equipment should be readily available in the home for emergency use. Emergency telephone numbers should be posted clearly on the telephone.

Oxygen

The patient and family should have a clear understanding of the benefits of oxygen therapy to decrease any fear or anxiety related to the need for its use. They should clearly understand the safe procedure for its administration and storage. The patient and family should be able to monitor therapeutic effects as well as be able to recognize signs that indicate that the health care provider should be notified.

Assistance with securing oxygen equipment for home use may be necessary

GENERAL NURSING IMPLICATIONS—cont'd

Nursing of patients requiring bronchodilators or oxygen—cont'd

Oxygen—cont'd

as well as financial aid in some instances. Referrals should be completed before discharge, and follow-up is indicated to ensure action.

Instructions should be given carefully in the hospital with an opportunity for patients and family members to ask questions as they arise and to demonstrate care of equipment needed and oxygen administration. Written instructions should be provided and should include telephone numbers of health care provider and equipment suppliers for patients to contact when needed. A visiting nurse should be involved early in care planning to assist in the assessment of the home if home therapy is indicated.

With individualized teaching the patient and family should be able to do the following.

Monitor respiratory status, including respiratory rate and pulse rate, and recognize signs of hypercapnia or hypoxia.

Maintain a patent airway using positioning, suctioning, productive coughing, oral and nasal care, and chest physiotherapy (i.e., postural drainage) if indicated.

Describe the equipment used for oxygen administration.

Demonstrate correct administration of oxygen and not exceed specified flow rate or percentage without consulting the health care provider.

Detect malfunction of equipment using oxygen meter.

Describe precautions to be used when oxygen is being used, and demonstrate the promotion of a safe environment (e.g., no smoking when oxygen is being used).

When oxygen therapy is indicated for home use, identify hazards in the home and make environment safe for oxygen therapy.

Secure oxygen tank to prevent falling, which would result in damage or injury.

Store oxygen tanks in well-ventilated area away from open flame.

Ground electric appliances and keep at least 5 feet (2 m) from oxygen source.

Post signs indicating oxygen is in use to remind visitors.

Allow no smoking in area of oxygen administration.

Observe kitchen safety when portable oxygen in ambulatory use.

Care for oxygen tubing and devices to prevent bacterial infection and maintain correct function.

GENERAL INSTRUCTIONS FOR DISCHARGE/OUTPATIENTS

BRONCHODILATORS

This medication is a bronchodilator. It is used to open the air passages in your lungs and will help to make you breathe easier.

If you have an allergy to, or are taking any cough or cold remedies or heart or weight-reducing medications, notify your health care provider before taking this medication.

Take this medication as directed. Do not change the amount of medication you take without checking with your health care provider.

Do *not* use this medication more often than recommended by your health care provider.

Call your health care provider immediately if your breathing problem becomes worse or if this medication does not relieve your breathing problem.

Do *not* take any additional medications, either prescription or nonprescription, while taking this medication without first checking with your health care provider. This medication can interact with other drugs and cause unwanted or harmful effects.

Call your health care provider if you notice a change in the amount, color, or thickness of your sputum. These changes are early signs of an infection in your lungs, and it should be treated with an appropriate medication to prevent more problems with your breathing.

Few people experience adverse side effects from this medication. However, notify your health care provider if you have chest pain, headache, sweating, fast heart beats, or dizziness.

This medication has been prescribed especially for you. Do not give this medication to anyone else.

If you are pregnant, thinking about becoming pregnant, or nursing an infant, discuss this with your health care provider *before* taking this medication. This discussion is important because some medications can be harmful to unborn children or can be passed into breast milk and affect breast-fed infants.

Keep this and all other medications out of the reach of children.

Following is additional information about your medication.

Sympathomimetics

Too frequent use of sympathomimetics can cause your heart to beat fast or cause pounding heart beats. The medication can also lose its effectiveness if overused. Use this medication only as discussed with your health care provider.

Continued.

GENERAL INSTRUCTIONS FOR DISCHARGE/OUTPATIENTS—cont'd

Sympathomimetics—cont'd

Shakiness and hand tremors can develop when taking this medication by mouth. These effects usually decrease with continued use of the drug. If shakiness and tremors persist or become bothersome and interfere with your activities, notify your health care provider so that an adjustment in dosage can be made or another drug selected.

It is helpful when taking this medication by mouth to eat food or drink a glass of water along with it to prevent nausea or stomach upset.

If you are taking this medication by inhaler, be sure to obtain written instructions from your health care provider and be sure you know the proper use of the inhaler. If you have any questions, ask your nurse before leaving.

If your medication is *isoproterenol*, remember the following.

Do not be concerned if your saliva turns pink or red in color after inhalation of this medication. This color is not harmful and occurs occasionally, so do not be alarmed.

Rinse your mouth after inhalation.

If you are taking this medication by sublingual tablet, place the tablet under your tongue or in the pouch of your cheek. Do *not* swallow until the tablet is completely dissolved. Rinse your mouth and brush your teeth after the tablet has dissolved because when used over a period of time damage to your teeth may result from contact with the dissolved medication.

It is not unusual to have flushing of the face or notice a faster heart beat just after taking this medication.

Notify your health care provider if you notice the appearance of swollen glands or a skin rash.

Phosphodiesterase inhibitors

Take tablets or liquid forms of this medication with food or a full glass of water to prevent stomach upset.

If this drug is being taken by rectal suppository, obtain written instructions from your nurse and be sure you know how to insert the suppository correctly. If you have any questions, ask your nurse before leaving.

Call your health care provider if you notice your bowel movements are black or if you notice a skin rash.

Never take this medication at the same time as other medications containing *aminophylline, oxtriphylline,* or *theophylline* unless specifically told to do so by your health care provider. When taken together, unwanted or harmful effects can occur.

Take this medication as directed equally spaced throughout the day so that you can obtain the best effect of the medication. Remember to take this medication even if you are feeling well.

Report adverse side effects to your health care provider, but do not stop taking this medication unless symptoms are severe.

CORTICOSTEROIDS AND CROMOLYN SODIUM

If you are taking this medication by inhaler, be sure to obtain written instructions from your nurse and be sure you know the proper use of the inhaler. If you have any questions, ask your nurse before leaving.

This medication must be taken regularly as directed to work effectively. It will not relieve acute attacks but will help to prevent them from occurring.

For corticosteroids remember the following.

Rinse your mouth and gargle after use of the inhaler. Do not swallow the water.

Notify your health care provider if you notice white patches in your mouth or on your throat or if you develop a sore mouth or throat.

For cromolyn sodium remember to drink a glass of water to prevent or relieve throat irritation that can occur after the use of this medication.

NURSING DRUG DIGEST

Medication (trade name*)	Indication	Usual dosage and administration	Dosage forms, preparation, and storage	Contraindications, cautions, and comments	Monitoring
Albuterol Proventil Ventolin	Reversible obstruction of the airways See also Chapter 24, "Sympathomimetics and Sympatholytics"	Aerosol *Adults:* 1 or 2 inhalations q.4-6h. *Children:* Less than 12 years, dosage not established; 12 years and older, same as adult dose Maximum daily dose is 8 inhalations/day Tablet *Adults:* 2-4 mg PO t.i.d. to q.i.d. *Children:* 6-12 years, 2 mg PO t.i.d. to q.i.d.; 12 years and older, same as adult dose *Elderly:* 2 mg PO t.i.d. to q.i.d. to initiate therapy NOTE: Recommended initial dosage for cardiac patients same as the recommended elderly dose Respirator solution The respirator solution should be used only under supervision and should be administered with IPPB (recommended diluents: normal saline solution or sterile distilled water) *Adults:* 0.25-0.50 ml of solution diluted with minimum of 5 ml of diluent *Children: Not recommended* for those under 12 years; 12 years and older, single dose of 0.25 ml of solution diluted as for adult With respirator solution the optimum duration of therapy is 10-15 min The treatment should not be repeated within 3 hr	Aerosol, metered: 90, 100 μg/inhalation Respirator solution: 0.6% Tablet: 2, 4 mg Store all products away from light and heat (storage between 15° and 30°C is usually best) Aerosol and solution formulations are for oral inhalation *only*; aerosol should be well shaken immediately before use	When 2 aerosol inhalations are used, patients should be advised to wait 1-5 min between inhalations Overuse may indicate serious worsening of patient's condition and need for medical reassessment May cause dizziness, nervousness, headache, and tremor	Patients using high doses should be monitored for cardiac effects: dysrhythmia, palpitations, tachycardia Observe for muscle tremors, which may require reduction in dosage Patients with coronary artery disease should have pulse taken before and during initial therapy to determine response to drug Arterial blood gas levels should be monitored during therapy

Continued.

NOTE: For additional details regarding the individual agents listed in this table, see the text and other tables in this chapter.
*Indicates a multiple active ingredient product. For a complete listing of all active ingredients see the *Drug Reference Guide to Brand Names and Active Ingredients.*
♦ Indicates that the drug is generally available only in Canada.
★ Indicates that the drug is generally available only in the United States.

NURSING DRUG DIGEST—cont'd

Medication (trade name)	Indication	Usual dosage and administration	Dosage forms, preparation, and storage	Contraindications, cautions, and comments	Monitoring
Aminophylline Amosac* Aminoaur Dura-Tabs Aminophyl Amoarines Amphylline Chomphyl Corophyllin Corphyllin Ethophylline Lixaminol Mini-Lix Phylarox Phyllocontin Quinite* Rectalad-Aminophylline Relasma* Roamphed* Somophyllin Theolamine	Reversible obstruction of the airways	Oral See Theophylline for PO dosage NOTE: Anhydrous aminophylline contains 86% theophylline; hydrous aminophylline contains 79% theophylline Patients should be advised to swallow enteric-coated and extended-release tablets whole without crushing or chewing Parenteral Adults: Loading dose of 6 mg/kg body weight IV at a rate of 25 mg/min, followed by 700 μg/kg body weight/hr for 12 hr, then 500 μg/kg body weight/hr in otherwise healthy, nonsmoking patients Adult smokers: Loading dose 6 mg/kg IV, followed by 1 mg/kg body weight/hr for 12 hr, then 800 μg/kg body weight/hr	Elixir: 33.3 mg/5 ml, 83.3 mg/5 ml (anhydrous) Enema: 60 mg/ml (anhydrous), 100 mg/ml (hydrous) Injectable: 25 mg/ml (hydrous) Oral solution: 105 mg/5 ml (anhydrous) Suppository: 125, 250, and 500 mg (hydrous) Tablet: 100, 200 mg (anhydrous) Tablet, enteric-coated: 100, 200 mg (hydrous) Tablet, extended-release: 225, 300 mg (hydrous) Store in tightly closed containers between 15° and 30° C; protect from freezing	*Contraindicated* in hypersensitivity to ethylenediamine See Theophylline Increased sensitivity in children and patients sensitive to phosphodiesterase inhibitors If patient has mild throat irritation, suggest a lozenge	See Theophylline

Elderly: Loading dose 6 mg/kg IV, followed by 600 μg/kg body weight/hr for 12 hr, then 300 μg/kg body weight/hr IV

Patients with congestive heart failure or liver failure: Loading dose 6 mg/kg IV followed by 500 μg/kg body weight/hr for 12 hr, then 100 to 200 μg/kg body weight/hr

Patients with cor pulmonale: See elderly dosage

Children: 6 months old to 16 years, loading dose of 6 mg/kg body weight IV, followed by one of the following: 6-month-old to 9-year-old, 1.2 mg/kg body weight/hr for 12 hr, then 1 mg/kg body weight/hr; 9- to 16-yr old, 1 mg/kg body weight/hr for 12 hr, then 800 μg/kg body weight/hr

IM administration is painful and is *not* recommended

NOTE: For IV administration, concentration should *not* exceed 25 mg/ml and should *not* be administered at a rate greater than 25 mg/min

Continued.

NURSING DRUG DIGEST—cont'd

Medication (trade name)	Indication	Usual dosage and administration	Dosage forms, preparation, and storage	Contraindications, cautions, and comments	Monitoring
Cromolyn sodium Aarane Intal Lomudal Lasmil Nalcrom Nasalcrom Opticrom Rynacrom	Prophylactic management of bronchoconstriction associated with allergic asthma	Aerosol *Adults:* 1 to 2 inhalations q.i.d. up to 8 inhalations daily at regular evenly spaced intervals *Children:* See adult dosage Spinhaler *Adults:* 20 mg q.i.d. up to 160 mg daily at regular evenly spaced intervals *Children:* See adult dosage Respirator solution *Adults:* As for Spinhaler *Children:* As for Spinhaler Nasal solution *Adults:* 1 spray in each nostril t.i.d. to q.i.d. *Children:* Over 6 years of age, same as adults NOTE: Medication should be taken daily regardless of attacks May need to *decrease* dosage in renal impairment Do *not* administer parenterally	Aerosol, metered-dose inhaler: 1 mg/inhalation Spincap: 20 mg for use with Spinhaler Respiratory solution: 10 mg/ml (for use with power-operated nebulizer with face mask) Nasal solution spray: 40 mg/ml (for use with Nasalmatic metered-spray device)	This medication is *not* indicated for the relief of severe, acute asthma Cough or bronchospasm produced by irritant effects of inhaled powder (Spinhaler) can be minimized or prevented by prior use of aerosol bronchodilator Withdrawal of cromolyn therapy should be done gradually over a period of 1 week; if steroid dosage was reduced while using cromolyn, the original steroid dosage should be restored before withdrawal of cromolyn May take up to 4 weeks for effect of treatment to be seen Not recommended in pregnancy Peak plasma level obtained in 15 min Oral preparations are not well absorbed Because initial treatment effects are not seen readily, patient needs support and reassurance to continue daily use of drug	
Dyphylline Aerophylline Airet Asminyl Dillin Dilor Dyflex Iphyllin	Reversible obstruction of the airways	Oral *Adults:* 5-15 mg/kg PO q.i.d. *Children:* 5 mg/kg body weight PO t.i.d. Maximum: 600 mg/day Doses may be taken with meals or antacids to decrease gastric irritation	Elixir: 100 mg/15 ml Injectable: 250 mg/1 ml Excessive cold may cause injectable formulation to precipitate; may be redissolved by autoclaving 10 min at 120° C Suppository: 400, 500 mg	*Contraindicated* in hypersensitivity to xanthines. Parenteral administration is *contraindicated* in myocardial infarction and severe angina pectoris	See Theophylline Monitor for early signs of overdose: nausea, vomiting, headache, palpitations, CNS stimulation Monitor *dyphylline* serum levels

	Uses	Dosage and administration	Preparations available	Side effects and nursing considerations
Lufyllin Neophyl Neothylline Neothylline cc Neutraphylline Oxystat Protophylline		Parenteral *Adults:* 200-500 mg IM slowly up to t.i.d. *Children:* 4-6 mg/kg/day IM in divided doses q.8h. as indicated Rectal *Adults:* 400-500 mg PR t.i.d. NOTE: IV administration generally *not* recommended	Syrup: 20 mg/1 ml Tablets: 200, 250, 400 mg Store all products in airtight containers, between 15° and 30° C Protect from light and freezing Recommended diluent for syrup is simple syrup	May cause urinary retention; monitor intake/output Monitor blood pressure repeatedly during first 5 min of IV administration and every 3-5 min until stable Monitor patient for insomnia, especially with continued therapy; a change in dosage or time may be indicated Monitor for maximum bronchodilator effect 1 hour after administration; effect lasts up to 3 hr
Ephedrine Asthmagyl* Benadryl with Ephedrine* Bronitin* Bronkaid* Bronkotabs* Bronicolixir* Chemfedral* Co-xan Syrup* Efedron nasal jelly Histadyl EC* Mudrane GG Elixir* Mudrane GG* Nasdro No 3 NyQuil Nighttime Colds Medicine* NyQuil* Quelidrine* Quibron Plus* Roamphed* Rynatuss* Tedral SA* Tedral* Thalfed* Theotabs* Vicks Vatronal Nose Drops*	Reversible obstruction of the airways See also Chapter 29, "Antihistamines, Antitussives, Decongestants, and Expectorants"	Oral *Adults:* 25-50 mg PO q.3-4h. or 15-60 mg extended-release formulation q.8-12h. *Children:* 25 mg/m² body surface q.4-6h.; or 15-30 mg extended-release form q.8-12h. Parenteral *Adults:* 25-50 mg IM or SC (or 5-25 mg slow IV) q.3-4h. Patients must be monitored closely during IV administration *Children:* 500 µg/kg body weight or 16.7 mg/m² body surface q.4-6h. SC or IV Tolerance is a common problem; after 2-4 weeks of therapy, dosage may have to be increased or sensitivity may be recovered by discontinuing therapy for 2-3 days The last daily dose should be taken a few hours before bedtime to prevent insomnia *Elderly:* No specific dosage is recommended, but elderly patients may require less than average adult dose of all sympathomimetics	Capsule: 25, 50 mg Capsule, extended-release: 15, 30, 60 mg Injectable: 25, 50 mg/ml Syrup: 10, 20 mg/5 ml Tablet: 25 mg Store away from light, in tightly closed containers, between 15° and 30° C; protect from freezing	*Contraindicated* in patients receiving MAOIs currently or within 3 weeks of starting ephedrine therapy because of risk of hypertensive crisis and death Acidification of the urine significantly increases excretion May antagonize antihypertensive effects of bethanidine or guanethidine Ephedrine is secreted in breast milk in concentrations that can affect infants Confusion, hallucinations, CNS depression, or respiratory depression may indicate overdose Drug is commonly abused Use with caution in patients with coronary disease

Continued.

NURSING DRUG DIGEST—cont'd

Medication (trade name)	Indication	Usual dosage and administration	Dosage forms, preparation, and storage	Contraindications, cautions, and comments	Monitoring
Epinephrine Adrenalin Adrenalin in Oil Adrenaline Chloride Adrenatrate Asmatane Mist Asmolin Asthma Haler AsthmaNefrin Breatheasy Bronitin Mist Bronkaid Mist Bronkaid Mistometer Dysne-Inhal Lyophrin Medihaler-Epi Micronefrin Misture-E Murocoll Mytrate Primatene Mist Simplene Suprarenin Sus-Phrine Vaponefrin	Reversible obstruction of the airways See also Chapter 24, "Sympathomimetics and Sympatholytics"	Aerosol *Adults:* 1 or 2 inhalations, may be repeated after 4 hr *Children:* 6 years and older, see adult dosage Metered aerosols should be well shaken immediately before use Aerosols and respirator solutions are for oral inhalation use only When more than one inhalation is to be used, patients should be advised to wait 1-5 min between inhalations If no relief or a worsening of patient's condition is noted 20 min after inhalations, discontinue medication and consult prescriber Respirator solution *Adults:* 1-2 inhalations of 0.5%-2.25% solution from hand nebulizer; may be repeated after 4-5 min, then up to 4 or 6 times daily; or with respirator, 5 ml of 0.1% solution over 15 min q.3-4h. *Children:* 4 years and older, see adult dosage Respirator solutions may be diluted according to manufacturer's directions	Aerosol, metered: 160, 200, 250 µg/inhalation Injection, solution: 100 µg/ml, 1 mg/ml Injection, suspension: 5 mg/ml Respirator solution: 0.5%, 1%, 2%, 2.25% Store all products away from light; protect from freezing Injectable suspensions should be stored between 2° and 8° C; all other products should be stored between 15° and 30° C Do *not* use solutions if pink or brown discoloration has developed or if precipitate has formed Protect from light	*Contraindicated* in patients receiving MAOIs, general anesthesia with cyclopropane or halogenated hydrocarbons, narrow-angle glaucoma, severe hypertension, shock, or tachycardia Treatment should start with first symptoms Patients may become unresponsive, especially if acidotic Tolerance can occur with prolonged use Dosage should be checked extremely carefully especially with premade minijets because only a portion of vial may be required Note different strengths—1:100, 1:1000, 1:10,000—and routes Use cautiously in patients with a history of coronary artery disease, cerebrovascular accident, or diabetes Toxicity treated with α- and β-adrenergic	Monitor patients for dysrhythmias, hypertension and tachycardia; severe cardiac and other adverse reactions have followed inadvertent intraarterial injection Monitor serum glucose levels of diabetics because drug may inhibit peripheral glucose uptake and promote glycogenolysis. Least number of inhalations for relief should be used Obtain initial blood pressure and heart rate; monitor status during therapy Monitor respiratory response, mentation Monitor for bronchodilator effect 3-5 min following SC injection of 1:1000 solution with maximum effects occurring in 20 min; or 1 min after oral use; suspensions provide rapid and sustained response for 8-10 hr

	Dosage		Remarks
	Injectable: solution *Adults:* 200-500 µg SC or IM repeated every 20 min to 4 hr; single dose may be increased to maximum of 1 mg *Children:* 10 µg/kg body weight or 300 µg/m² body surface SC repeated after 15 min and then q. 4h. Injectable suspension *Adults:* 500 µg SC, then 500 µg-1.5 mg q.6h. It is recommended that tuberculin syringes with 26-gauge needles be used with injectable suspensions to ensure accuracy; suspensions must be well shaken before use and should be injected promptly after withdrawing into syringe to avoid settling *Children:* 5 µg/kg body weight SC q.6h. Maximum single dose: 150 µg *Elderly:* No specific dosage is recommended, but elderly patients may require less than the average adult dose of all sympathomimetic drugs		blockers for pressor and cardiac or bronchodilator effects, respectively Dryness of mouth and gastric irritation related to swallowing residual drug after oral inhalation can be decreased by rinsing the mouth immediately after inhalation treatment If used concurrently, isoproterenol should *not* be used within 4 hr of epinephrine
★ **Ethylnorepinephrine** Bronkephrine	Reversible obstruction of the airways See also Chapter 24, "Sympathomimetics and Sympatholytics"	*Adults:* 1-2 mg SC or IM *Children:* 200 µg-1 mg SC or IM *Elderly:* No specific dosage is recommended, but elderly patients may require less than the average dose of all sympathomimetics	Injectable: 2 mg/ml Protect from light and freezing; store between 15° and 30° C Do *not* use solutions if brown discoloration has developed or a precipitate has formed	See Isoproterenol Less hyperglycemic, pressor, and analeptic effects than most sympathomimetics; therefore, may be useful in children, diabetics, and patients with heart disease See Isoproterenol

Continued.

NURSING DRUG DIGEST—cont'd

Medication (trade name)	Indication	Usual dosage and administration	Dosage forms, preparation, and storage	Contraindications, cautions, and comments	Monitoring
Fenoterol Berotec Pertusisten	Reversible obstruction of the airways	Aerosol *Adults:* 1 or 2 inhalations t.i.d. to 2 inhalations q.4h. with a maximum of 8 inhalations daily Tablet *Adults:* 2.5 mg PO b.i.d. to maximum of 5 mg q.6h. Respirator solution (for use in motorized nebulizers and IPPB) *Adults:* 0.5-1 ml of solution in 5 ml diluent q.6h. Maximum of 2.5 ml solution in 5 ml of diluent Total volume should be administered over 15 min *Children:* Use is *not* recommended *Elderly:* No specific dosages recommended, but elderly patients may require less than the average adult doses of all sympathomimetics	Aerosol, metered-dose inhaler: 200 µg/inhalation Respirator solution: 0.1% Tablet: 2.5 mg Protect from light; store between 15° and 30° C Recommended diluent for respirator solution is saline	See Albuterol *Contraindicated* in tachycardia	See Albuterol
Ipratropium Atrovent	Reversible obstruction of the airways	Aerosol *Adults:* 1 or 2 inhalations t.i.d. to q.i.d. q.4h. Some patients may require doses of 4 inhalations when therapy is initiated Maximum: 8 inhalations/day *Children:* Less than 6 years old, 1 inhalation t.i.d.; 6 to 12 years old, 1 or 2 inhalations t.i.d.	Aerosol, metered: 20 µg/inhalation Store between 15° and 30° C	Dry mouth may be relieved with glass of water	Patients on high doses should be monitored for mydriasis and urinary retention Monitor fluid intake and output
Isoetharine Bronkometer Bronkosol	Reversible obstruction of the airways See also Chapter 24, "Sympathomimetics and	Aerosol *Adults:* 1 or 2 inhalations q.4h. Respirator solution *Adults:* 4 inhalations (diluted or undiluted)	Aerosol, metered: 0.34 mg/inhalation Respirator solution: 0.125% and 0.25%, used undiluted; 0.5% and 1%, diluted up to 1:3	See Isoproterenol Tolerance may develop with prolonged or excessive use	See Isoproterenol

Drug / Uses	Dosage / Administration	Preparations / Storage	Side effects / Precautions	Nursing considerations
Sympatholytics" (cont'd)	*Children:* Not established *Elderly:* No specific dosage is recommended, but elderly patients may require less than the average adult doses of all sympathomimetics	Store all products in airtight containers; protect from light and freezing; store between 15° and 30° C Recommended diluents include sterile water, 0.45% and 0.9% sterile saline solution Do *not* use if brown discoloration has developed or precipitate has formed		
Isoproterenol Aerolone* Aludrin Duo-Medihaler* Iprenol Isuprel Isuprel-Neo-Mistometer* Luf-Iso Medihaler-Iso Neo-Epinine Norisodrine Prenomiser Forte Proternol Saventrine Vapo-Iso Vapo-N-Iso Reversible obstruction of the airways See also Chapter 24, "Sympathomimetics and Sympatholytics"	Aerosol *Adults:* 1-2 inhalations q4-6h. to a maximum of q.3h. *Children:* Dosage as for adult because smaller ventilations limit drug deposition Inhalation powder (sulfate only) *Adults:* 2-4 inhalations repeated after 5 min then after 10 min if necessary; no more than 3 treatments recommended *Children:* Dosage as for adult because smaller ventilations limit drug deposition Patients should be advised to wait 1-5 min between inhalations Respirator solution *Adults:* 5-15 inhalations of 0.25% solution or 3-7 inhalations of 1% solution from nebulizer q3-4h.; if administered with IPPB or compressed air or oxygen, 2 ml of 0.125% or 2.5 ml of 0.1% solution over 15-20 min up to 5 times daily *Children:* 6-12 inhalations of 0.25% nebulized solution up to 3 times every 15 min with a maximum of 8 times daily; if administered with IPPB or compressed air or oxygen, 2 ml of 0.0625% or 2.5 ml of 0.05% solution over 10-15 min with a maximum of 5 times daily	Aerosol, metered: 80, 120, 125 μg/inhalation Injectable: 20, 200 μg/ml Powdered inhalation (sulfate): 45, 75, 110 μg/inhalation Nebulizer solution: 0.125%, 0.25%, 0.5%, 1% Tablets sublingual: 10, 15 mg Store in tightly closed containers away from light, between 15° and 30° C	*Contraindicated* in tachycardia Administration by inhalation or sublingual tablet may cause saliva to turn pink-red/brown Excessive or prolonged use has been associated with severe, paradoxical bronchospasm Patients should be advised not to chew or swallow sublingual tablets which should be dissolved under the tongue Tremor may require dosage reduction Absorption from sublingual tablet often unreliable and unpredictable If condition worsens or no relief is obtained after 3-5 treatments within 6-12 hr, consult prescriber Patients should be advised to avoid deep, forced inhalations when using powdered aerosol (sulfate) to prevent excessive irritation of the airways Warn patient sputum can appear pink in color after inhalation treatment and not to be alarmed	Monitor cardiac and respiratory status Patients receiving more than 3 aerosol treatments daily should be closely monitored Monitor for exaggerated systemic drug effects after oral inhalation Watch for hypotension, tachycardia, dysrhythmias, headache, nausea, insomnia Monitor for bronchodilation effect: *inhalation and sublingual 1-2 hr* Oral assessment is indicated at routine intervals when sublingual tablets are used chronically because damage to teeth has been reported related to acidity of medication; rinsing between doses is helpful Monitor for parotid swelling with prolonged use

Continued.

NURSING DRUG DIGEST—cont'd

Medication (trade name)	Indication	Usual dosage and administration	Dosage forms, preparation, and storage	Contraindications, cautions, and comments	Monitoring
Isoproterenol —cont'd		Sublingual *Adults:* 10-15 SL mg t.i.d. to q.i.d. Maximum: 60 mg/24 hr *Children:* 5-10 mg SL t.i.d. Maximum: 30 mg 24 hr Advise patient not to chew or suck sublingual tablets and to avoid swallowing saliva until medication is dissolved Warn patient that facial flushing, chest pain, and palpitation can occur and not to be alarmed *Elderly:* No specific geriatric dosage is specified, but elderly patients may require less than the average adult dose of all sympathomimetic drugs		Emergency respiratory equipment should be readily available	
Metaproterenol Alupent Dosalupent Metaprel	Reversible obstruction of the airways See also Chapter 24, "Sympathomimetics and Sympatholytics"	Aerosol *Adults:* 1-3 inhalations, which can be repeated after 3 hr to maximum of 12 inhalations/day *Children:* Less than 12 years, *not recommended;* 12 years and older, see adult dose Oral *Adults:* 20 mg PO t.i.d. to q.i.d. *Children:* 6 to 9 years, 10 mg PO t.i.d. to q.i.d.; over 9 years, see adult dose	Aerosol, metered-dose inhaler: 650, 750 µg/inhalation Injectable: 500 µg/ml Respiratory solution: 5% Syrup: 2 mg/ml Tablets: 10, 20 mg Store all products in airtight containers, between 15° and 30° C Protect from light Discard solutions that have turned brown or contain a precipitate	See Albuterol *Contraindicated* in tachycardia Drug may have shorter duration of action after long-term use Peak effect in 1 hr with effects persisting to 4 hr after oral dose and 1-5 hr following inhalation	See Albuterol Monitor for bronchodilation within 15 min of oral administration and within 1 min of inhalation

Drug	Uses	Dosage	Preparations	
		Respirator solution *Adults:* 5-10 inhalations from hand nebulizer; *or* 0.3 ml (5% solution) diluted in 2.5 ml NS by IPPB q.4-6h. as indicated *Elderly:* No specific dosage is recommended, but elderly patients may require less than average adult dose of any sympathomimetic drug		See Theophylline
Oxtriphylline Brondecon* Choledyl Choledyl Expectorant* Choledyl SA Chophylline	Reversible obstruction of the airways	See Theophylline NOTE: Oxtryphylline contains 64% theophylline *Adults:* 200 mg PO q.i.d.; or 400-600 mg (sustained-action tablets) q.12h. *Children:* 2-12 years, 3.7 mg/kg PO q.i.d.	Elixir: 100 mg/5 ml Syrup: 50 mg/5 ml Tablets: 100, 200 mg Tablets, sustained-action: 400, 600 mg Store in tightly closed containers, between 15° and 30° C; protect liquids from freezing and light	See Theophylline
Terbutaline Brethine Bricanyl Filair	Reversible obstruction of the airways See also Chapter 24, "Sympathomimetics and Sympatholytics"	Aerosol *Adults:* 1 or 2 inhalations q.4h. to a maximum of 12 inhalations/24 hr Oral *Adults:* 2.5-5 mg PO b.i.d. to t.i.d. Maximum: 15 mg/24 hr Parenteral *Adults:* 250-500 µg SC up to q.i.d.; injections may be repeated at intervals of 15-30 min to a maximum of 500 µg/4 hr Recommended parenteral administration is into lateral deltoid area SC *Children: Use is not recommended*	Aerosol, metered-dose inhaler: 250 µg/inhalation Injectable: 1 mg/ml Syrup (sugar-free): 1.5 mg/5 ml Tablets: 2.5, 5 mg Store all products between 15° and 30° C Protect from light Recommended diluent for solution is saline Do *not* use discolored solutions	See Albuterol *Contraindicated* in tachycardia See Albuterol

Continued.

NURSING DRUG DIGEST—cont'd

Medication (trade name)	Indication	Usual dosage and administration	Dosage forms, preparation, and storage	Contraindications, cautions, and comments	Monitoring
Theophylline Accurbron* Acet-Am Acet-AM Expectorant* Aerolate Liquid Aerolate Sr & Jr & III Aqualin Suprettes Asbron G Inlay* Asma-Lief* Asmalix Asminyl* Asthmophylline Bronitin* Bronkaid* Bronkodyl Bronkodyl S-R Bronkolixir* Bronkotabs* Chemfedral* Co-Xan* Dixurin Procaine* Dorsaphyllin Elixicon Elixophyllin Elixophyllin SR Entair* Labid 250mg Lanophyllin Marax* Mudrane GG Elixir* Phedral* Physpan Primatene M* Primatene P*	Reversible obstruction of the airways	NOTE: Dosage must be individualized based upon serum concentrations and therapeutic response Dosage should generally be calculated on the basis of lean body weight NOTE: All doses quoted are for *anhydrous theophylline;* see Table 28-1 for conversions **Chronic therapy** *Adults:* Initially the lesser of 400 mg/day PO or 15 mg/kg body weight/day PO, then up to a maximum of the lesser of 900 mg/day or 13 mg/kg body weight/day in 3 or 4 evenly spaced doses of regular formulation Suspension: should be well shaken before administration Chewable tablets should be well chewed before swallowing Extended release capsules and tablets must be swallowed without chewing or crushing Tablets: should be taken with at least 240 ml of water Administer after meals to decrease GI irritation *Children:* Same initial dosage as for adults, then up to the following maximum: less than 9 years old, 16-24 mg/kg body weight/day PO; 9 to 12 years old, 12-20 mg/kg body weight/day PO; 12 to 16 years old, 12-18 mg/kg body weight/day PO; 16 years and older; see adult dosage	Capsule: 100, 200, 250 mg Capsule, extended release: 60, 65, 125, 130, 250, 260, 300 mg Elixir: 27, 37.5, 50 mg/5 ml Solution: 27, 53 mg/5 ml Suspension: 100 mg/5 ml Syrup: 27 mg/5 ml Tablets: 100, 125, 200, 225, 250, 300 mg Tablet, chewable: 100 mg Tablets, extended-release: 100, 200, 250, 300, 500 mg All products should be stored in tightly closed containers, between 15 and 30° C; tablets should be protected from moisture	*Contraindicated* in severe peptic ulcer *Contraindicated* in hypersensitivity to xanthines Advise patients that dizziness is often experienced when therapy is started The recommended maximum dosages may be exceeded *if* theophylline serum levels are monitored and remain below 15 to 20 μg/ml (does *not* apply to dyphylline) When dosages are increased, dose should be raised gradually, (i.e. 25% every 2-4 days) Advise patient of expected diuresis after IV administration Breast feeding while receiving theophylline is *not* recommended because the drug is secreted into breast milk in concentrations high enough to affect infant Use with caution in children Toxicity is uncommon when serum levels remain below 20 μg/ml	Monitor theophylline serum levels Monitor for diuretic effect after IV administration Monitor children for CNS excitation Serious cardiac toxicity may develop without prior less serious side effects; patients should be monitored for dysrhythmias and tachycardia Monitor pulmonary function tests

Quadrinal*
Quibron Plus*
Quibron*
Salyrgan-Theophylline*
Slo-Phyllin
Slo-Phyllin GG*
Slo-Phyllin 80
Somophyllin-T
Sustaire
Synophylate
Synophylate-GG*
T.E.P.*
Tedral SA*
Tedral*
Thalfed*
Theo-Dur
Theo-Dur Sprinkle
Theo-Guaia*
Theo-Organidin*
Theobid & Theobid Jr. Durcap
Theocap
Theoclear
Theoclear L.A.
Theocyne
Theolair
Theolixir
Theophedrizine*
Theophyl Chewable
Theophyl-SR
Theophyl-225
Theospan SR
Theospan
Theospan 80
Theotabs*
Theovent Long-Acting
Veraquad*
Verquad*

Adults: 4 mg/kg every 8 to 12 hour up to the lesser of 13 mg/kg body weight or 900 mg/day of extended release formulation
Children: Same total daily dosage as for regular formulation except dosed q.6-12h.
May administer with food or antacids to decrease gastric irritation

Acute attack
Parenteral
See aminophylline for IV dosage
Oral
Adults: Loading dose of 6 mg/kg body weight PO, followed by 3 mg/kg body weight PO q.6h. for 12 hr, then 3 mg/kg body weight PO q.8h. for otherwise healthy, non-smoking patients
Adult smokers: Same loading dose as above, then 3 mg/kg body weight PO q.4h. for 12 hr followed by 3 mg/kg body weight PO q.6h.
Adults with congestive heart failure or liver disease: Same loading dose as above, then 2 mg/kg body weight PO q.8h. for 2 doses, then 1 to 2 mg/kg body weight PO q.12h.
Elderly and cor pulmonale patients: Same loading dose as above, then 2 mg/kg body weight PO q.6h. for 2 doses, followed by 2 mg/kg body weight PO q.8h.
Children: 6 months-16 years, 6 mg/kg body weight PO loading dose, then the following: 6 months-9 years, 4 mg/kg body weight PO q.4h. for 3 doses, then 4 mg/kg PO q.6h.; 9-16 years, 3 mg/kg body weight q.4h. for 3 doses, then 3 mg/kg body weight q.6h.
NOTE: May need to decrease dose in renal impairment

BIBLIOGRAPHY

Breslin, A.B.X. Chronic asthma: which treatment? *Drugs,* 1979, *18,* 103-112.

Casterline, C.L., Evans, R., III, & Ward G.W. Jr. The effect of atropine and albuterol aerosols on the human bronchial response to histamine. *Journal of Allergy and Clinical Immunology,* 1976, *58,* 607-613.

D'Agostino, J.S. Set your mind at ease on oxygen toxicity. *Nursing 83,* 1983, *13*(7), 55-56.

Dunlap, C.I. Help your COPD patient take a better breath—with inhalers. *Nursing 83,* 1983, *13*(5), 42-43.

Ellmyer, P., & Thomas, N.J. A guide to your patient's safe home use of oxygen. *Nursing 82,* 1982, *12*(1), 56-57.

Fantozzi, R., Moroni, F., Masini, E., Blandini, P., & Mannaioni, P.F. Modulation of the spontaneous histamine release by adrenergic and cholinergic drugs. *Agents and Actions,* 1978, *8,* 347-348.

Kirilloff, L.H., & Tibbals, S.C. Drugs for asthma—a complete guide. *American Journal of Nursing,* 1983, *83*(1), 55-61.

Lorenz, W., & Doenicke, A. Histamine release in clinical conditions. *Mount Sinai Journal of Medicine,* 1978, *45,* 357-386.

Meier-Sydow, J., & Gonsior, E. The physiologic regulation of bronchial tone. *Triangle,* 1978, *17,* 97-101.

Nadel, J.A. Autonomic control of airway smooth muscle and airway secretions. *American Review of Respiratory Disease,* 1977, *115*(6, Pt. 2), 117-126.

Paintal, A.S. Effect of drugs on chemoreceptors, pulmonary and cardiovascular receptors. *Pharmacology and Therapeutics; Part B: General and Systematic Pharmacology,* 1977, *3,* 41-63.

Persson, C.G.A., Ekman, M., & Erjefalt, I. Terbutaline preventing permeability effects of histamine in the lung. *Acta Pharmacologia et Toxicologica,* 1978, *42,* 395-397.

Pierson, D.J., Hudson, L.D., Stark, K., & Hedgecock, M. Cardiopulmonary effects of terbutaline and a bronchodilator combination in chronic obstructive pulmonary disease. *Chest,* 1980, *77,* 176-182.

Piper, P.J. Anaphylaxis and the release of active substances in the lungs. *Pharmacology and Therapeutics; Part B: General and Systematic Pharmacology,* 1977, *3,* 75-98.

Richardson, J.B. Nerve supply to the lungs. *American Review of Respiratory Disease,* 1979, *119,* 785-802.

Rifas, E.M. Teaching patients to manage acute asthma—the future is now. *Nursing 83,* 1983, *13*(7), 11-15.

Simonsson, B.G., & Svedmyr, N. Bronchoconstrictor drugs. *Pharmacology and Therapeutics; Part B: General and Systemic Pharmacology,* 1978, *3,* 239-303.

Svedmyr, N., & Simonsson, B.G. Drugs in the treatment of asthma. *Pharmacology and Therapeutics; Part B: General and Systematic Pharmacology,* 1978, *3,* 397-440.

Voyles, J.B. Bronchopulmonary dysplasia. *American Journal of Nursing,* 1981, *81*(3), 510-513.

Webb-Johnson, D.C., & Andrews, J.L. Bronchodilator therapy. *New England Journal of Medicine,* 1977, *297*(Pt. 1), 476-482.

Webber-Jones, J.E., & Bryant, M.K. Over-the-counter bronchodilators. *Nursing 80,* 1980, *10*(1), 34.

Wilson, A.F., & McPhillips, J.J. Pharmacological control of asthma. *Annual Review of Pharmacology and Toxicology,* 1978, *18,* 541-561.

Zorychta, E., & Richardson, J.B. Control of smooth muscle in human airways. *Bulletin European de Physiopathologie Respiratoire,* 1980, *16,* 581-586.

Antihistamines, Antitussives, Decongestants, and Expectorants

Margaret A. Peterson
David F. Biggs

*Medications discussed in this chapter**

Antihistamines	Antitussives—cont'd
Ethanolamines	Nonnarcotic
Bromodiphen-	Benzonatate
hydramine	Chlophedianol
Carbinoxamine	Dextromethorphan
Chlorphenoxamine	Levopropoxyphene
Diphenhydramine	Noscapine
Diphenylpyraline	Decongestants
Ethylenediamines	Ephedrine
Antazoline	Naphazoline
Pyrilamine	Oxymetazoline
Tripelennamine	Phenylephrine
Alkylamines	Phenylpropanolamine
Brompheniramine	Propylhexedrine
Chlorpheniramine	Pseudoephedrine
Dexchlorpheniramine	Tetrahydrozoline
Pheniramine	Xylometazoline
Triprolidine	Expectorants
Miscellaneous antihista-	Acetylcysteine
mine	Ammonium chloride
Terfenadine	Guaifenesin
Antitussives	Iodides (potassium io-
Narcotic	dide)
Codeine	Ipecac
Hydrocodone	Terpin hydrate
Hydromorphone	

The drugs discussed in this chapter comprise the major ingredients of many combination medication products marketed for the treatment of "coughs and colds" and are used extensively in the treatment of *allergic rhinitis* or hay fever.

---

*NOTE: Only agents that are primarily used to treat allergic rhinitis or that are commonly included in cough and cold products are included. Most piperazine and phenothiazine antihistamines are usually used for other purposes (see Chapter 18, "Drugs Used to Treat Psychotic Disorders").

Numerous products containing various combinations of these and other drugs are available. However, it is recommended that individual agents or products containing no more than two agents be selected whenever possible. This approach provides two advantages. First, the use of unnecessary drugs is limited while relief from specific symptoms is provided, and second, it is easier to adjust dosages to meet the needs of individual patients. In keeping with this recommendation only individual agents are discussed.

Many viruses are known to cause cold symptoms. The "common cold" is usually caused by one of the many different types of rhinoviruses. A typical common cold begins with a tickling or feeling of dryness in the throat. Sneezing may occur, and the eyes may be inflamed. This phase lasts from 1 to 3 days. The symptoms may subside then or progress further. If the latter occurs, a coryza, or running nose, develops, often quite abruptly. Coryza is accompanied by malaise, aches and pains in the joints, headache, and a mild fever. Mucous secretion from the nose may be copious. The secretion is clear and watery. This represents the second phase. The third phase is a period of consolidation—the mucous membranes swell and become hyperemic; mucous secretions mix with cellular cell debris, and the mucus becomes thick, viscous, and often colored yellow or green. A secondary infection, usually bacterial, may occur. The nasal passages are often blocked, and it is not possible to clear them by blowing the nose. Coughing becomes prominent, often with the expectoration of thick yellow or green sputum signifying bacterial infection. The final or fourth phase is the phase of recovery. The symptoms slowly disappear, excessive secretion of thick mucus and coughing usually being the last symptoms to go. The average cold lasts from 7 to 14 days, but recovery may be prolonged if secondary infection develops.

Although the symptoms are the same for all colds, the severity of the symptoms varies greatly and provides a basis for the classification of colds. Following are the usual five classifications.

CLASSIFICATION OF COLDS

Designation	Symptoms
Abortive cold	Respiratory symptoms appear and subside within 24 hours. No definite increase in nasal secretions.
Doubtful mild cold	Symptoms persist for several days. Not severe enough to permit definite diagnosis.
Mild cold	Definite upper respiratory symptoms. Significant increase in nasal secretions. Duration: 2 to 4 days.
Moderate cold	Local symptoms of increased severity. Definite constitutional symptoms such as headache and malaise. Possibly fever. Duration: Up to 1 week.
Severe cold	Marked upper respiratory symptoms. Fever and loss of appetite. Bed rest indicated. Constitutional symptoms. Cough.

Some antiviral drugs have been developed, but the use of these agents generally is restricted to more serious conditions. Thus treatment of the common cold remains symptomatic. The agents most commonly used to treat colds include *antihistamines, antitussives, decongestants,* and *expectorants.* The routine use of products that include an analgesic/antipyretic should be discouraged. Fever associated with the common cold is mild. High fever may indicate the presence of a more serious disorder or the development of a secondary infection. The use of products containing an analgesic/antipyretic may mask the fever and delay recognition and proper treatment of such conditions.

ANTIHISTAMINES

The antihistamines discussed in this chapter are competitive antagonists of histamine H_1-receptor sites. The major action of these agents is to prevent the effects of histamine by binding to the receptors and thus preventing the binding of histamine. They do not prevent the release of histamine or reverse any actions of histamine. They are, therefore, of greatest benefit when treating conditions in which histamine is the major mediator and in which they are administered before contact with the allergen producing the release of histamine. They are effective in the treatment of allergic rhinitis, moderately effective during the early stages of a cold, less effective against allergic dermatitis, and practically ineffective in the treatment of asthma. In fact, the antihistamines can aggravate symptoms of airway obstruction and must be used with care in asthmatic patients.

In addition to their primary action, the antihistamines possess varying degrees of anticholinergic, antiserotonergic, and cocainelike activities. These secondary actions provide the basis for the use of antihistamines in the treatment of motion sickness, carcinoid syndrome, Parkinsonism, and a variety of other conditions. Antihistamines such as chlorpheniramine, which possesses cocainelike activity, may prolong the effects of sympathetic nerve stimulation and increase response to noradrenaline. As a result these agents may appear to enhance responses to other sympathomimetics.

The anticholinergic activity of antihistamines produces a drying effect on nasal mucosa, which may be beneficial during the early stages of a cold. When more pronounced, such activity may produce marked drying and thickening of airway secretions, thus inducing or aggravating symptoms of airway obstruction. For this reason it is recommended that these agents be used with caution by asthmatic patients, although the overall effect of antihistamines in this group remains unclear.

Adverse reactions to the antihistamines are listed in Adverse/Side Effects of Antihistamines, Antitussives, Decongestants, and Expectorants. The most usual side effects experienced with therapeutic concentrations of these agents include sedation, dryness of the mucous membranes (particularly of the nose, mouth, and throat), and gastric irritation. Toxic levels produce symptoms similar to atropine poisoning (dilated pupils, fever, and flushed face) as well as excitement, ataxia, loss of coordination, hallucinations, and muscular tremors with or without intermittent tonic-clonic seizures. Children are particularly prone to central nervous system stimulation associated with antihistamine toxicity, and some adolescents have purposely abused antihistamines to achieve this "high."

Some side effects are most likely to occur after treatment with an agent from a particular chemical grouping. For example, ethanolamines often have pronounced sedative and anticholinergic side effects but minimal gastric irritation. Ethylenediamines commonly produce gastric irritation, but have fewer CNS side effects than the other groups, whereas alkylamines more commonly cause CNS stimulation in children. However, variability within groups occurs, and, in addition, individuals differ greatly in their responses to the same agent. For these reasons selection of an appropriate antihistamine for a particular patient often may require trial and error. Several antihistamines, some from the same class, may have to be tried before a suitable agent is obtained. Initially an agent may be selected on the likelihood of its producing or not producing a particular side effect. For example, diphenhydramine may be chosen for administration at bedtime because of its sedative properties. Alternatively, it may be chosen in an effort to avoid gastric irritation. Next, the patient's response must be determined so that the dosage can be adjusted to provide maximum benefit with minimum side effects. If the drug is not well tolerated, a second agent should be selected and tested in the same manner.

The antihistamines are metabolized chiefly in the liver. As a result infants and young children are more sensitive to the effects of these agents than adults. Because of diminished hepatic function associated with normal aging, the elderly also may experience increased sensitivity to these agents.

The antihistamines are excreted in breast milk and therefore should be used with caution in nursing mothers. A clear link between human teratogenicity and antihistamine usage has not been established. Although some of these agents have been prescribed as antiemetics during pregnancy, the potential risks must now be considered. Antihistamines of the piperazine group have been shown to produce teratogenic effects in animals and are therefore contraindicated during pregnancy.

Caution also is required when antihistamines are used by patients with hyperthyroidism, hypertension, or other cardiovascular disease because these agents may produce dysrhythmias, hypertension, or tachycardia. In addition, the anticholinergic actions of these agents may exacerbate symptoms of narrow-angle glaucoma, bladder neck distention, and prostatic hypertrophy.

ANTITUSSIVES

Coughing is an effective method for removing cellular debris, excessive secretions, or foreign materials from the airways. In patients such as chronic smokers with impaired mucociliary clearance it becomes the most important method of clearing the airways. Cough that serves to clear the airways is called *productive cough*. Alternatively, cough may occur but not remove secretions or materials from the airways. This type of cough is called *nonproductive cough* and often is associated with colds that are not complicated by secondary bacterial infection.

Both types of cough are symptoms of underlying conditions that may or may not be of a serious nature (see box above). The cause of the cough should be investigated and identified before it is suppressed. Also, the desirability of suppressing the cough, particularly a productive cough, should be considered

Common causes of cough	
Allergy	Persistent cough may indicate asthma, nasal polyps, or allergic alveolitis
Anatomy and physiology	Anatomic abnormalities, trauma, or carcinoma
Environment	Dryness, cold, and irritants such as smoke or fumes
Infection	Viral, bacterial, or parasitic infections of upper or lower respiratory tract
Medication	Drugs with prominent anticholinergic activity produce dry mouth and throat (see Chapter 23, "Parasympathomimetics and Parasympatholytics")
	Cromolyn sodium see (Chapter 28, "Bronchodilators and Respiratory Gases")

carefully before any antitussive is used. Indications for the use of antitussives are listed in the box on p. 588 and various antitussive agents are listed in the Nursing Drug Digest.

Antitussives may suppress cough through central or peripheral actions and are classified as either narcotic or nonnarcotic cough suppressants. All of the narcotic and some of the nonnarcotic agents act centrally to depress activity of the cough center in the medulla. Other agents act by suppressing peripheral nerve activity or nerve receptors in the respiratory tract. Antitussives with peripheral actions in theory can affect either afferent or efferent pathways of the cough reflex. In practice only agents that reduce activity in the afferent pathways are used as cough suppressants.

The narcotic antitussives usually are more effective than the nonnarcotic agents. However, the efficacy of dextromethorphan, a nonnarcotic antitussive, is equal to that of codeine, which is the most widely used cough suppressant.

The selection of an antitussive chiefly depends on its efficacy and the adverse side effects experienced by the patient. Although addiction is possible with any narcotic agent, the risk is not great when these agents are used for short periods of time. Dextromethorphan may be a better choice for long-term use.

Some indications for the use of antitussives

1. Cough leading to nausea, emesis, or urinary incontinence
2. Cough resulting in fractures or tearing of ligaments, muscles, or veins
3. Cough inducing bronchospasm, asthmatic attacks, or ventilation-perfusion abnormalities leading to severe hypoxia
4. Cough resulting in fainting, reduced cardiac output, atrioventricular block, or other cardiac dysrhythmias
5. Cough interrupting or preventing sleep, thus resulting in fatigue or irritability (The benefit/risk ratio should be carefully considered before suppressing a productive cough for this reason.)
6. Cough that is dry and nonproductive
7. Cough that is nonproductive and secondary to lung cancer

DECONGESTANTS

The decongestants discussed in this chapter are all sympathomimetics (see Chapter 24, "Sympathomimetics and Sympatholytics"), which act by stimulating α-adrenergic receptors of blood vessels in the nose, producing constriction and relieving nasal congestion. Stimulation may be produced by direct effects on the receptors or indirectly by the release of noradrenaline. Cocaine also is an effective decongestant. However, since it is not used *therapeutically* for this purpose, it is not discussed.

Decongestants are available for either oral or topical administration. The oral products are available as tablets, capsules, or elixirs. The topical preparations have been formulated in jelly, liquid drops, and spray products for nasal instillation. All of the products reduce congestion through vasoconstrictor effects on the nasal mucosa. Unfortunately, the vasoconstrictor effects of these agents are followed by vasodilation, which may cause *rebound congestion,* particularly after prolonged use. For this reason decongestants should be used for only short periods of time. Individuals should not use decongestant therapy for longer than 5 to 7 days unless directed by their health care provider.

Topical preparations produce a more intense vasoconstriction within the nasal mucosa than do oral decongestants. The local vasoconstriction further serves to limit systemic absorption. In addition, the topical preparations can be used for agents that are poorly absorbed from the gastrointestinal tract. However, rebound congestion is more probable and generally is more severe after topical administration of decongestants. In cases of pronounced congestion topical preparations may not penetrate to all parts of the nasal mucosa, and systemic administration may be required.

Adverse reactions to the decongestants generally are the result of stimulation of α-adrenergic receptors outside the nasal mucosa following systemic absorption. These effects may include hypertension, tachycardia, hyperglycemia, mydriasis, and central nervous system stimulation. Therefore patients with heart disease, diabetes, hypertension, hyperthyroidism, or a predisposition to narrow-angle glaucoma should avoid using decongestants whenever possible. If these agents must be used by patients with any of these conditions, topical preparations should be recommended and the patient should be carefully monitored.

Some products combine an antihistamine with a decongestant to reduce central nervous system stimulation. Although the sedative properties of the antihistamine should theoretically antagonize any central nervous system stimulation produced by the decongestant, this interaction has not been demonstrated to be clinically significant, especially with the concentrations of drugs usually found in combination products. In addition, the antihistamine may produce central nervous system stimulation rather than sedation in some patients. Drugs that interact with the decongestants to produce effects of clinical importance are listed in Clinically Significant Drug Interactions.

EXPECTORANTS

Expectorants are drugs that aid the elimination of mucus and other secretions from the airways. These agents may act by increasing the watery secretions of the sol-layer. The secretions are increased either by direct effects on the bronchial glands and mucosa or reflexly by irritation of the gastric mucosa. Alternatively, expectorants may affect the more viscous sol-layer by causing proteolytic liquefaction of the secretions. Thus expectorants are used to decrease the viscosity of airway secretions and make them easier to expel from the airways. However, although numerous agents have been marketed for this purpose, their efficacy is questionable and therefore the use of expectorants is controversial.

Optimal mucociliary clearance requires adequate airway hydration whether or not expectorants are used. Fever and "mouth breathing" associated with colds and nasal congestion are factors that promote dehydration. The hyperventilation that accompanies an asthmatic attack also produces generalized dehydration and thus results in a drying and thickening of airway secretions.

Hydration

In a patient experiencing a severe asthmatic attack, adequate hydration may necessitate the use of intravenous fluid replacement. However, in most instances hydration can be achieved and maintained by increasing the patient's oral fluid intake.

In addition to systemic hydration inhalation of humidified air also may aid expectoration. Large-volume nebulizers are effective and are used routinely in some chronic conditions. However, most persons suffering from colds can obtain relief from a hot, steamy shower or from a portable vaporizer. Steam-mist and cool-mist vaporizers are available and both provide similar humidification. The cool-mist systems may have a safety advantage, particularly when used with small children, who might upset the vaporizer. Often adequate hydration eliminates any need for additional expectorants. In the event that additional agents are used, care should be taken to maintain adequate hydration to derive maximal benefit from the selected expectorant.

Iodides

Inorganic iodides (i.e., supersaturated potassium iodide—SSKI) remain some of the most effective expectorants available. Organic iodides may be less effective but better tolerated. The iodides produce effects by all three of the mechanisms discussed: direct and indirect stimulation of secretions and some proteolytic liquefaction. Their use is limited chiefly by adverse side effects, which are listed in Adverse/Side Effects of Antihistamines, Antitussives, Decongestants, and Expectorants.

Ammonium salts

The ammonium salts produce their effects reflexly through an irritant mechanism on the gastric mucosa. Ammonium chloride is the most extensively used salt for this purpose. However, the efficacy of this and the other ammonium salts is questionable, and at best only a mild expectorant effect is produced. Because of potentially serious adverse side effects, the use of ammonium salts is generally no longer recommended. Dosages contained in most of the available multiingredient products are in the subtherapeutic range and are thus of doubtful efficacy.

Guaifenesin

Guaifenesin is one of the most popular expectorants and is often included in combination preparations marketed for the treatment of coughs and colds. However, as with the ammonium salts the clinical efficacy of guaifenesin has not been proven. Large doses may promote muscle relaxation and reduce platelet adhesiveness, but the clinical significance of these actions is questionable.

Adverse side effects and dosages of these and other expectorants are listed in Adverse/Side Effects of Antihistamines, Antitussives, Decongestants, and Expectorants and the Nursing Drug Digest. Those agents that act chiefly as mucolytic or proteolytic expectorants are used in patients with chronic obstruction of the airways. Both adverse side effects and unnecessary expense do not warrant the use of these agents for the relief of symptoms of the common cold.

SUMMARY

The medications discussed in this chapter provide only *symptomatic* relief. They do not effect cures or shorten the duration of colds and allergies. Most of the agents reviewed in this chapter are available for self-medication without a prescription. However, if symptoms persist longer than 10 to 14 days, a clinician should be consulted.

Whenever possible, therapy should consist of a single drug (e.g., antitussive for cough or antihistamine for *rhinorrhea*), and multiingredient products should be avoided.

ADVERSE/SIDE EFFECTS OF THE ANTIHISTAMINES, ANTITUSSIVES, DECONGESTANTS, AND EXPECTORANTS*

Antihistamines
CARDIOVASCULAR SYSTEM

Decreased or increased blood
  pressure
Dysrhythmias
Palpitations
Tachycardia

CENTRAL NERVOUS SYSTEM

Blurred vision
Confusion
Diplopia
Hallucinations
Headache
Insomnia
Irritability
Muscle weakness
Paresthesia
Sedation† (decreased ability to
  concentrate, drowsiness, and loss
  of coordination)

GASTROINTESTINAL SYSTEM

Anorexia (except for cyproheptadine,
  an agent not discussed in this
  chapter—see Chapter 55,
  "Antiseptics and Local
  Anesthetics")
Constipation or diarrhea
Epigastric pain
Generalized gastric irritation†
Nausea and vomiting

GENITOURINARY SYSTEM

Difficult urination
Urinary frequency or retention

RESPIRATORY SYSTEM

Cough
Dry mouth
Drying of bronchial, nasal, tracheal
  secretions
Wheezing

MISCELLANEOUS SYSTEMS

Agranulocytosis
Excessive sweating
Hypersensitivity
Leukopenia
Photosensitivity

Antitussives
Benzonatate
CENTRAL NERVOUS SYSTEM

Convulsions
Dizziness†
Drowsiness†
Headache

CUTANEOUS SYSTEM

Pruritus
Rash
Urticaria

GASTROINTESTINAL SYSTEM

Constipation†
Nausea and vomiting

MISCELLANEOUS SYSTEMS

Nasal congestion
Hypersensitivity
Numbness of mouth, throat, and
  tongue

Chlophedianol
CENTRAL NERVOUS SYSTEM

Confusion
Excitation
Hallucinations
Insomnia
Nightmares

GENITOURINARY SYSTEM

Difficult urination
Urinary retention

RESPIRATORY SYSTEM

Drying of airway secretions

MISCELLANEOUS SYSTEMS

Dry mouth
Hypersensitivity
Rash

Dextromethorphan
CENTRAL NERVOUS SYSTEM

Confusion
Dizziness†
Drowsiness†
Excitation

GASTROINTESTINAL SYSTEM

Generalized upset

RESPIRATORY SYSTEM

Respiratory depression with very high
  dosages

Levopropoxyphene
CENTRAL NERVOUS SYSTEM

Agitation
Dizziness
Drowsiness†
Headache
Nervousness†
Visual disturbances

GASTROINTESTINAL SYSTEM

Diarrhea
Epigastric pain
Nausea and vomiting

GENITOURINARY SYSTEM

Urinary frequency and urgency

MISCELLANEOUS SYSTEMS

Skin rash

Narcotic antitussives
CARDIOVASCULAR SYSTEM

Bradycardia
Hypotension
Palpitations

CENTRAL NERVOUS SYSTEM

Confusion
Dizziness
Drowsiness†
Insomnia
Irritability
Hypothermia
Miosis
Restlessness
Sweating
Visual disturbances

GASTROINTESTINAL SYSTEM

Constipation†
Dry mouth
Nausea†
Vomiting

*See Chapter 11, "Drug Toxicity" for an overview of drug toxicity.
†Most common effects.

ADVERSE/SIDE EFFECTS OF ANTIHISTAMINES, ANTITUSSIVES, DECONGESTANTS, AND EXPECTORANTS—cont'd

GENITOURINARY SYSTEM

Biliary spasm
Difficult urination

SKIN

Facial flushing
Pruritus
Rash
Urticaria

MISCELLANEOUS SYSTEMS

Respiratory depression
Dependence

Noscapine
CENTRAL NERVOUS SYSTEM

Dizziness
Drowsiness†
Headache

GASTROINTESTINAL SYSTEM

Nausea

MISCELLANEOUS SYSTEMS

Allergic rhinitis
Conjunctivitis
Skin rash

Decongestants
CARDIOVASCULAR SYSTEM

Hypertension
Increased cardiac output
Tachycardia

CENTRAL NERVOUS SYSTEM

Agitation
Anxiety
Headache†
Insomnia
Restlessness†

GASTROINTESTINAL SYSTEM

Discomfort
Nausea

MISCELLANEOUS SYSTEMS

Hyperglycemia
Mydriasis
Rebound congestion

Expectorants
Acetylcysteine
GASTROINTESTINAL SYSTEM

Nausea†
Vomiting

RESPIRATORY SYSTEM

Bronchospasm†
Dyspnea
Hemoptysis
Rhinorrhea
Wheezing

MISCELLANEOUS SYSTEMS

Chills
Fever
Stomatitis

Ammonium chloride
CENTRAL NERVOUS SYSTEM

Confusion
Drowsiness
Mild diaphoresis
Headache

GASTROINTESTINAL SYSTEM

Gastric irritation†
Nausea†

GENITOURINARY SYSTEM

Increased diuresis
Hypokalemia

MISCELLANEOUS SYSTEMS

Hyperventilation
Metabolic acidosis
Thirst

Guaifenesin
CENTRAL NERVOUS SYSTEM

Drowsiness

GASTROINTESTINAL SYSTEM

Gastric discomfort
Nausea
Vomiting

Iodides
CUTANEOUS SYSTEM

Pruritus
Rash
Urticaria

GASTROINTESTINAL SYSTEM

Gastric irritation†
Nausea†
Vomiting

MISCELLANEOUS SYSTEMS

Bitter, metallic aftertaste
Excessive salivation
Hypothyroidism and goiter
Nasal congestion
Parotitis

Ipecac
CARDIOVASCULAR SYSTEM

Bradycardia
Dysrhythmia
Vasomotor collapse

GASTROINTESTINAL SYSTEM

Bloody diarrhea
Gastric irritation†
Mucosal erosion
Vomiting

MISCELLANEOUS SYSTEMS

Albuminuria

Terpin hydrate
GASTROINTESTINAL SYSTEM

Epigastric pain
Gastric irritation†

CLINICALLY SIGNIFICANT DRUG INTERACTIONS*

Primary drug	Interaction drug	Possible effect(s)	Probable mechanism(s)
Ammonium chloride	Spironolactone	Acidosis	Acidifying effect of ammonium chloride combined with spironolactone-induced decrease in hydrogen ion secretion by kidney
Codeine and other narcotic antitussives	Alcohol and other CNS depressants	CNS depression, respiratory depression	Additive pharmacologic effect
Codeine and other narcotic antitussives	MAOIs	Increased CNS depression	Not yet established
Decongestants	MAOIs	Hypertensive crisis, headache, hyperpyrexia	Increased storage of noradrenaline leading to increased release by indirectly acting sympathomimetics (e.g., ephedrine, phenylpropanolamine); increased metabolism of phenylephrine

*See Chapter 10, "Drug Interactions," for an overview of drug interactions.

GENERAL NURSING IMPLICATIONS

Nursing of patients requiring antihistamines, antitussives, decongestants, or expectorants

ASSESSMENT

A complete nursing assessment is essential in establishing a baseline from which to plan individualized drug therapy regimens and to monitor patient response. Assessment should include a detailed drug history to identify possible sensitivity, contraindications, cautions, potential drug interactions, and self-medication abilities before drug therapy is initiated. This assessment is important because many allergy and cough and cold products contain multiple ingredients, including habit-forming or narcotic ingredients. Because antihistamines and decongestants can be abused or misused, use of over-the-counter preparations and self-care practices should be carefully explored when assisting patients with self-medication.

In addition to the patient's general condition assessment should include a history of the symptoms and their severity as well as duration. The presence of conditions such as asthma, hypertension, heart disease, diabetes mellitus, or thyroid disease should be identified as well as current medications being taken to treat such conditions.

Self-care measures that were tried and their results should also be ascertained as well as medications used for the treatment of the cold or allergy.

Assessment should include inspection of the external nose for color of skin, presence of swelling, pain, or irritation. The nares should be inspected for shape and symmetry. The presence of nasal discharge from one or both nares should be noted along with its character and amount. The base of the nose and columella can be reddened and irritated from nasal discharge and frequent wiping. The skin can appear inflamed and scaly.

The nose should be palpated for loss of support, presence of underlying tissues, and patency of nostrils. The patient may have dry, cracked lips from oral breathing resulting from nasal congestion and blocked nasal passages. Sneezing can also be present. The nasal mucosa should be inspected for color and character. The mucosa normally appears deep pink and is firm in consistency. The mucosa can appear pale when congested by a cold, and the inferior turbinates of allergic patients can appear bluish gray or pale pink,

often with a boggy consistency. Nasal polyps are also common and should be noted along with perforations.

Many patients with common cold symptoms complain of the ears feeling plugged. This feeling of plugged ears can occur as a result of the eustachian tubes becoming blocked by edema of the oropharynx. Blockage of the sinus passages can cause sinus pain or headache. The frontal and maxillary sinuses should be palpated, gently percussed for tenderness, and transluminated to identify mucous consolidation.

Postnasal discharge can irritate bronchial passages, causing persistent hacking cough, hoarseness, and a scratchy throat. As the cold progresses, coughing can become productive. The presence of cough should be identified and the amount and character of sputum noted. The posterior oropharynx should be assessed for the presence of inflammation or exudate as well as for white, yellow, or red patches. The condition of the tonsils should also be noted.

In addition to these common symptoms of cold and allergy, fever, malaise,

GENERAL NURSING IMPLICATIONS—cont'd

Nursing of patients requiring antihistamines, antitussives, decongestants, or expectorants—cont'd

ASSESSMENT—cont'd

anorexia, fatigue, and dehydration may be present. The patient's general health state should be carefully assessed. Dark discoloration under the eyes is not uncommon in allergic patients, and patients suffering from allergic rhinitis often complain of sneezing and inflamed or burning eyes. Children often have vomiting and diarrhea associated with cold symptoms. When allergy is the presenting problem, identification of the allergen is also indicated whenever possible.

SENSITIVITY

Many nonprescription cough and cold preparations contain additional ingredients (e.g., aspirin) to which the patient may be hypersensitive. A detailed history of drug and food allergies as well as familiarity with *all* the ingredients in the cough and cold preparations is required by the nurse to provide optimal care.

Antihistamines

Hypersensitivity reactions are extremely rare with antihistamines. However, use of these agents should be avoided in individuals who display such reactions (usually if the antihistamine is administered parenterally).

Antitussives

Patients may experience hypersensitivity reactions to antitussives, especially those containing codeine.

Decongestants

Some patients display a hypersensitivity to the sympathomimetic (pressor) amines (e.g., phenylephrine and pseudoephedrine), and use of this class of agents should be avoided in these individuals.

Expectorants

Rarely, iodides produce serious hypersensitivity reactions in highly sensitive individuals. Such individuals typically report a sensitivity to shellfish, which contains iodides. Use of iodide expectorants is usually contraindicated in these individuals, although reactions at recommended dosages, even in sensitive individuals, rarely appear.

CONTRAINDICATIONS
Antihistamines

Any antihistamine is *contraindicated* in patients with known hypersensitivity to that particular agent.

Antihistamines are contraindicated in patients receiving MAOIs because anticholinergic effects are prolonged and intensified.

Patients with a history of severe asthma should not use antihistamines because they can, because of their drying effects, aggravate symptoms of airway obstruction.

In addition, infants or children less than 2 years of age should not be given antihistamines *unless* dosage is individualized by the prescriber. Although some products do have specific dosage recommendations for patients in these age groups, they are generally *not* recommended. Antihistamines are metabolized in the liver; therefore infants and young children are more sensitive to the effects of these agents than are adults. The elderly may also experience increased sensitivity to these agents.

Although no clear link between antihistamines and human teratogenesis has been shown, the risks and benefits must be assessed by the prescriber before administering antihistamines to pregnant patients or women with childbearing potential. (Piperazine group of antihistamines has been associated with teratogenic effects in animals and is contraindicated in pregnancy or in women of childbearing age.)

Antihistamines can be excreted in breast milk in concentrations high enough to affect infants and are thus contraindicated in nursing mothers.

See Nursing Drug Digest for contraindications to individual agents.

Antitussives

Antitussives are *contraindicated* in conditions that require coughing to maintain clear respiratory passages (i.e., productive coughs). The cause of the coughing should be established before antitussives are utilized.

Antitussives are contraindicated in patients with known hypersensitivity to their ingredients.

Decongestants

Decongestants are relatively *contraindicated* in patients with diabetes, hypertension, hyperthyroidism, and ischemic heart disease because symptoms may be aggravated or induced. If a decongestant is necessary, use with extreme caution and monitor patient carefully.

Expectorants

Ammonium chloride is *contraindicated* in patients with renal, hepatic, or pulmonary insufficiency.

Iodide preparations are contraindicated in patients with known sensitivity to iodide.

CAUTIONS
Antihistamines

Because of anticholinergic effects, antihistamines should be used cautiously in patients with history of or predisposition to asthma, cardiovascular disease, hypertension, hyperthyroidism, narrow-angle glaucoma, or prostatic hypertrophy.

Children are especially prone to central nervous system stimulation and toxicity with antihistamines.

Antihistamines have been abused, particularly by adolescents, to achieve a "high."

Most antihistamines are metabolized in the liver and excreted by the kidney in 24 hours. Tolerance to antihistamines after prolonged use can develop because they induce their own enzymatic metabolism. Switching to an antihistamine of a different chemical group is often effective.

Antitussives

Narcotic antitussives have the potential for addiction with chronic use.

Decongestants

Decongestants should be used cautiously because misuse or abuse can

Continued.

GENERAL NURSING IMPLICATIONS—cont'd

Nursing of patients requiring antihistamines, antitussives, decongestants, or expectorants—cont'd

Decongestants—cont'd

cause rebound congestion. Patients should be advised that prolonged use or overuse of decongestants, particularly topical agents, can lead to rebound congestion.

Topical decongestants are generally recommended because oral decongestants are systemically absorbed in higher concentrations, resulting in a higher incidence of systemic adverse side effects, which require careful monitoring.

Expectorants

Expectorants should be used cautiously in patients who have difficulty coughing up mucus or clearing respiratory passages.

DRUG INTERACTIONS

The possibility of clinically significant drug interactions should be carefully evaluated because many over-the-counter products contain multiple ingredients that can interact with medications patients may be taking for the treatment of other conditions.

Antihistamines

Antihistamines can potentiate central nervous system depressant effects of alcoholic beverages, antidepressants, narcotic analgesics, sedative-hypnotics, antipsychotics, and other CNS depressants, resulting in excessive drowsiness with possible impairment of motor coordination and judgment.

Antihistamines can intensify atropine-like effects (e.g., dry mouth and constipation) of MAOIs (e.g., isocarboxazid, pargyline, phenelzine, and tranylcypromine) and antidepressants (e.g., amitriptyline, doxepin, and imipramine) as well as other drugs with anticholinergic effects. This effect can be especially a problem for patients with narrow-angle glaucoma, cardiovascular disease, prostatic hypertropy, and hyperthyroidism.

Diphenhydramine can interfere with absorption of aminosalicylic acid (PAS) and cause lowered blood plasma levels.

If needed, space dosage schedule so that they are not given together. Diphenhydramine can also depress labyrinthine function and can mask signs of ototoxicity caused by aminoglycosides, loop diuretics, high dosages of aspirin, or other ototoxic drugs.

Antitussives

Antitussives containing codeine or other narcotics can increase central nervous system depressant effects of alcohol, antihistamines, barbiturates, or other depressant drugs.

Decongestants

Decongestants, can react with MAOIs causing hypertensive crisis, occipital headache, stiff neck, nausea and vomiting, dysrhythmias, and palpitations.

Expectorants

Potassium iodide and lithium can interact to produce synergistic hypothyroid activity and resultant hypothyroidism in the patient.

See Clinically Significant Drug Interactions.

ADMINISTRATION
Antihistamines

Antihistamines are available in tablets, capsules, elixirs, syrups, and sprays as well as in the form of nasal drops and eyedrops. Nasal drop and eyedrop preparations should not be confused.

Oral liquid forms can be given well diluted in juice or water. Tablets and capsules can be taken with milk or food to prevent gastrointestinal upset. Elixirs can be administered with simple syrup for convenience or palatability. Patients should be advised to swallow extended-release tablets and capsules whole without crushing or chewing them. Tablets should not be allowed to dissolve in the mouth, and capsules should not be taken apart.

Nasal sprays are not recommended for use in children because of the risk of overdosage; nasal drops are preferred.

Recommendation for dosage in the elderly is usually not specified, but elderly patients may require less than the usual adult dosages.

Most agents are available in numerous combination products.

Discard unused solutions and diluted elixirs 14 days after opening. Store dosage forms, except for elixirs, between 15° and 30° C in tightly closed containers, and protect from light.

Antitussives

Narcotic and nonnarcotic antitussives are available in tablet, capsule, or liquid forms (i.e., syrup, solution, and suspension) as an ingredient in liquid cough preparations.

Syrup forms should be administered undiluted and to maximize their soothing effect on the throat should not be immediately followed with water or fluid.

Nonnarcotic antitussive capsules should be swallowed whole and not chewed. Temporary anesthesia of the oral mucosa can occur if the drug is released in the mouth.

Some products (e.g., dextromethorphan) are available in lozenge form combined with benzocaine for control of spasmodic coughing and should be sucked slowly.

Drug effects should be enhanced with adjunct measures including adequate hydration, cessation of smoking, and sucking on sugarless hard candy to help control nonproductive coughing. Increased fluid intake decreases tenacity of secretions. Throat irritation from constant coughing can be soothed with throat lozenges or sugarless hard candy.

Do not administer to children under 2 years of age.

Do not administer to patients with productive cough.

Do not administer to vomiting patients because aspiration can result.

GENERAL NURSING IMPLICATIONS—cont'd

Nursing of patients requiring antihistamines, antitussives, decongestants, or expectorants—cont'd

Antitussives—cont'd

Shake suspensions *well* before pouring medication to ensure accurate dosage. Store antitussives safely between 15° and 30° C in tightly closed containers, and protect from light.

Decongestants

Decongestants are available in tablet, extended-release capsule, syrup, solution, and elixir oral forms. They are also available for topical administration in nasal drops, jellies, sprays, and inhalation forms.

Specific dosages for the elderly are not established, but elderly patients generally require less than the average adult dose of all sympathomimetic preparations.

Administration of oral preparations

Tablets and capsules should be swallowed whole with a full glass of water or juice and *not* chewed or crushed. Capsules should not be taken apart. This caution is especially important for time-release tablets or capsules. To minimize the insomnia associated with oral decongestants, the last dose should be administered 3 to 4 hours before bedtime.

Administration of topical preparations

See General Instructions for Discharge/Outpatients for the administration of nasal drops, sprays, and jellies.

Do *not* confuse nasal preparations with otic or ophthalmic preparations.

Nasal sprays and jellies are well tolerated by older children and adults, but are *not* recommended for children under 6 years of age because of their smaller nasal passages and the risk of overdosage. Nasal drops should be used for younger children when necessary.

To prevent infection by fungi and bacteria, rinse droppers and spray tips in hot water after use. Avoid contact with the nares when administering nasal

drops and use only for individual patients as specified. Advise patients that containers of nasal drops or sprays should be used by *only* one person.

Store safely between 15° and 30° C in tightly closed containers, and protect from light.

Discard unused solutions 14 days after opening.

Recap inhaler preparations immediately after use to prevent evaporation.

Expectorants

Expectorants are available for oral administration in tablet, capsule, syrup, or elixir forms. They are also available in solution for direct instillation through tracheostomy, bronchoscope, intratracheal catheter, or nebulizer.

Oral preparations should be taken with a full glass of water or juice. Providing humidification, increasing fluid intake to 8 to 10 glasses per day, and advising patients to stop or decrease smoking are helpful measures to enhance the effect of the medication.

Tablets and capsules should be swallowed whole and *not* chewed, crushed, or allowed to dissolve in the mouth. Capsules should not be taken apart.

Solutions should be stored in airtight containers. Opened or diluted solutions should be stored in the refrigerator and used within 96 hours. Discoloration of acetylcystine solution will occur if it comes into contact with rubber, iron, or copper, but this will *not* impair the effectiveness of the medication. Potassium iodide solution, however, should be discarded if discolored brown. Crystallization of potassium iodide solutions can also occur. Warming and gently shaking will dissolve the crystals.

Oral preparations should not be refrigerated. Store safely between 15° and 30° C and protect from light.

NOTE: *Never* administer potassium iodide *tablets* for expectorant effect. Potassium iodide *tablets* are used for thy-

roid blocking in a radiation emergency *only*. (See Chapter 61, "Thyroid and Antithyroid Medications.")

MONITORING PATIENT RESPONSE

Therapeutic response

Antihistamines

Monitor for symptomatic relief of allergic or vasomotor *rhinitis.*

Antihistamines are included in many "cough and cold" products, but their effectiveness in treating the common cold is largely unsubstantiated.

Monitor for drying effect on nasal mucosa (i.e., anticholinergic action).

Antihistamines provide symptomatic relief of allergy by inhibiting the effect of histamine at the receptor site. They are helpful in managing seasonal allergic rhinitis. The slight drying effect on mucous membranes may help to alleviate associated symptoms of runny nose and watery eyes.

It is important in determining patient response to adjust the dosage to provide maximal benefit with minimal side effects. If the first product tried is not well tolerated, another agent may be effective.

Antitussives

Antitussives provide symptomatic relief of cough.

Monitor for decreased cough frequency and severity.

Therapeutic response can be noted 10 to 30 minutes after oral administration with effect lasting 3 to 6 hours.

Decongestants

Decongestants provide symptomatic relief of nasal congestion or acute rhinitis. NOTE: Some agents have additional uses not covered in this chapter. (See Chapter 24, "Sympathomimetics and Sympatholytics.")

Monitor for reduced congestion through vasoconstriction effects on nasal mucosa, especially topical application.

Continued.

GENERAL NURSING IMPLICATIONS—cont'd

Nursing of patients requiring antihistamines, antitussives, decongestants, or expectorants—cont'd

Decongestants—cont'd

Alpha-adrenergic sympathomimetic amines provide rapid and dramatic relief of nasal congestion by facilitating drainage of sinus cavities. They are available in both topical and oral forms. The topical form constricts dilated blood vessels in the nasal mucosa, resulting in decrease or elimination of congestion and airway obstruction. The oral preparations produce a less intense pharmacologic response but a longer duration of action than do the topical preparations.

Expectorants

Monitor for facilitation of removal of viscous mucus from the respiratory tract, increased flow of secretions, and decreased viscosity of thickened secretions (especially effective with humidification of air and increased fluids to promote drug effect).

The use of expectorants is controversial. Adequate patient hydration is a significant factor.

Adverse side effects

Antihistamines

Sedation is the most common adverse side effect, especially with ethanolamines, and may pose a problem for the mobile patient, particularly the elderly, because mind and reflexes may be dulled to a point where accidents can occur. Safety measures should be implemented in the hospital setting (e.g., bedside rails and assistance with ambulation) as indicated, and patients in home settings should be advised not to drive or participate in activities that require alertness until they know how the specific medication affects them.

Gastric irritation is another common adverse side effect associated with antihistamines. Monitor for anorexia, diarrhea, constipation, nausea, and vomiting.

Monitor for adverse side effects associated with anticholinergic effects of antihistamines, including excessive drying of nose, mouth, and throat and thickening of secretions, which can ag-gravate airway obstruction. Urinary frequency or retention are also associated with anticholingergic effects as well as blurred vision.

Antihistamines also can cause central nervous system effects, including dizziness, fatigue, incoordination, lassitude, or tinnitus. Monitor for these effects.

Patients should be advised to avoid alcoholic beverages while receiving antihistamines because depressant effects on the central nervous system are ad ditive. Dosage reductions should be considered if concomitant therapy with other central nervous system depressants is necessary.

The elderly are most likely to experience dizziness, hypotension, and weakness as well as sedation and should be monitored carefully and assisted with precautionary measures as indicated.

Toxicity

Monitor for atropine-like poisoning signs: ataxia, dilated pupils, fever, flushed face, excitement, hallucinations, loss of coordination, and muscle tremors with or without tonic-clonic seizures.

Children, especially with overdosage, are likely to develop paradoxic excitation of the central nervous system and should be observed for nervousness, sleeplessness, and tremor. They should also be monitored for tachycardia.

Sedative and anticholingergic side effects of ethanolamines are often pronounced; gastric irritation usually is minimal, and some agents are used as antiemetics. Gastric side effects are common with ethylenediamines, but their central nervous system effects are usually *not* as pronounced as the other groups of antihistamines. The alkylamines are some of the most potent antihistamines; usually they cause less sedation than other groups, but central nervous system stimulation is more common.

See Adverse/Side Effects of the Antihistamines, Antitussives, Decongestants, and Expectorants and the Nursing Drug Digest.

Antitussives

Narcotic antitussives can cause nausea, vomiting, constipation, lightheadedness, and somnolence.

Monitor for overdose: hypotension, tachycardia, central nervous system depression, and respiratory depression. Naloxone can reverse central nervous system and respiratory depression.

Narcotic antitussives have abuse potential. Monitor for dependence.

Nonnarcotic antitussives (e.g., dextromethorphan) possess few adverse side effects (i.e., slight drowsiness, nausea, and dizziness).

Patients may become drowsy and should be advised to avoid driving and other activities that require mental alertness or precise motor coordination until their individual response is known. In the hospital patients may need assistance with ambulation, bedside rails or other safety precautions. Supervision with smoking is indicated. These agents are not likely to induce dependence because they have no analgesic action and do not produce euphoria.

Large doses may cause central nervous system and respiratory stimulation. Monitor patients for signs of nervousness, irritability, or sleeplessness.

Decongestants

Topical preparations

Few systemic adverse side effects occur with topical preparations because the amount absorbed is usually minimal. However, rebound congestion is more prevalent, especially after prolonged use. Advise patients not to use more frequently than recommended or longer than 5 to 7 days. Monitor for continued congestion and abuse or misuse.

Overdose of tetrahydrozoline and naphazoline can cause CNS depression, particularly in children.

Oral preparations

Oral preparations can cause pronounced adverse side effects in other

GENERAL NURSING IMPLICATIONS—cont'd

Nursing of patients requiring antihistamines, antitussives, decongestants, or expectorants—cont'd

Oral preparations—cont'd

organ systems because they are systemically absorbed. Monitor patients for nervousness, dizziness, insomnia, transient hypertension, palpitations, central nervous system stimulation, and increased blood glucose levels.

Although oral preparations are less likely to cause rebound congestion, monitor for abuse or misuse of medication and this adverse side effect.

Expectorants

Monitor for adverse side effects as specified in Adverse/Side Effects of the Antihistamines, Antitussives, Decongestants, and Expectorants and the Nursing Drug Digest, because effects vary with each individual agent (e.g., iodism can occur with potassium iodide therapy, and gastrointestinal upset and inhibition of platelet aggregation can occur with high doses of guaifenesin).

PATIENT EDUCATION

Patient teaching is extremely important in enhancing self-care abilities in the prevention and management of common colds and allergies. Patient education should include information about the causes and prevention of common colds and allergies as well as their treatment, including the use of self-care measures and prescription and nonprescription medications.

The patient and family should understand that the use of antihistamines, antitussives, decongestants, and expectorants in the management of common cold and allergy is directed at relieving annoying symptoms of runny nose, watery eyes, cough, congestion, and postnasal drip. Headache, malaise, and fever associated with common colds may require the use of an analgesic/antipyretic such as aspirin or acetaminophen. Patients and family members should be able to recognize the common symptoms of cold and allergy and how they differ from more severe respiratory conditions. They should be aware of the hazards associated with the unnecessary use or abuse of nonprescription medications

used in the treatment of these conditions and should be encouraged to utilize their health care providers to enhance optimal self-care.

Patients requiring medications for the treatment of common cold or allergy symptoms should have a clear understanding of the exact use of the medication, its exact name, action, dosage, storage, administration, and adverse side effects. Patients and family should know how to monitor drug effectiveness and be able to identify signs that indicate that the health care provider should be contacted.

Patients should recognize that it is best *not* to self-medicate for the treatment of common cold symptoms if they have asthma, chronic rhinitis, diabetes, heart disease, hypertension, pneumonia, pharyngitis, sinusitis, or thyroid disease. The health care provider should be consulted because complications can occur with the use of over-the-counter medications in these patients.

Patients who self-medicate should be advised to avoid multiingredient products so that only presenting symptoms are treated and unnecessary adverse side effects are avoided. They should be encouraged to read and follow the manufacturer's recommendations and not increase the dosage or take the medication more frequently than recommended. If they have any questions about self-medication, they should readily discuss them with their health care providers.

Prevention of common colds

The patient and family should recognize that cold viruses are spread through person-to-person contact by droplets sprayed into the air when a person coughs, sneezes, and talks or by direct hand contact. The incubation period is 1 to 4 days with rapid onset and progression of symptoms.

The mouth should be covered when coughing, and tissues should be flushed down the toilet. Dishes used by a family member who has a cold should be washed separately, and glasses or utensils should not be used

by other family members unless washed in a dishwasher with hot water. Handwashing after sneezing or coughing is important in the prevention of the spread of cold viruses.

Because susceptibility to catching a cold is increased when one is overtired or physically exhausted, emotionally upset, or malnourished, in addition to avoiding crowded areas, patients should be encouraged to maintain adequate nutrition and rest and to avoid undue stress.

Self-care measures for treating the common cold

Stay home to prevent spread of cold virus.

Get plenty of sleep.

Drink 8 to 10 glasses of water, juice, soup, and other beverages, especially if fever is present. Warm beverages such as tea with lemon and honey are especially soothing to the throat, and hot soup is helpful in liquefying secretions.

Avoid chilling and fatigue, especially if you must care for children or do other work.

Eat lightly but maintain adequate nutrition.

Because decreased humidity can aggravate cold symptoms by drying air passages and secretions, increase room humidity with a cool-mist or hot-mist vaporizer. Medications such as camphor can be used with hot-mist vaporizers to soothe respiratory passages. Safety precautions are essential to prevent burns. A warm, steamy shower is just as effective.

To soothe irritated and inflamed mucous membranes or a scratchy throat, gargle with a glassful of warm water in which ½ teaspoon (2.5 ml) of salt has been dissolved or suck on hard sugarless candy, cough drops, or throat lozenges.

Stop or decrease smoking because it can further irritate respiratory passages.

Continued.

GENERAL NURSING IMPLICATIONS—cont'd

Nursing of patients requiring antihistamines, antitussives, decongestants, or expectorants—cont'd

Self-care measures for treating the common cold—cont'd

Apply petroleum jelly if nares are irritated by nasal discharge, and use soft tissues.

Muscle aches and mild fever (less than 38.5° C) can be treated with aspirin or acetaminophen unless contraindicated. If unsure, check with your health care provider.

Self-medication

Antihistamines

Patients should understand that allergy-like symptom responses to a cold virus are caused by an excessive amount of histamine released in the body. Antihistamines relieve symptoms by blocking the action of histamine on nasal passages and tear ducts. Anticholinergic drugs can also dry up mucous membranes.

Antitussives

Patients should know that antitussives are used to treat dry, harsh cough caused by irritation of postnasal drip or congestion. A productive cough should not be suppressed because it clears passages. A dry hacking cough is nonproductive and can irritate passages; an antitussive can be used for relief.

Some antitussives contain codeine and have abuse potential and thus may need prescription in some states and provinces.

Decongestants

Patients should understand that a decongestant can break up nasal congestion, unplug ears, and help dry up a runny nose. Patients should understand how to take the decongestant (e.g., nasal spray, nasal drops, inhaler, capsule, or tablet) and when selecting a decongestant recognize that topical preparations have fewer adverse side effects than oral preparations. They should also recognize, however, that topical preparations are more habit-forming. It is important that patients know that because decongestants can be habit-forming and that overuse can cause rebound congestion, they should not be used regularly. These medications should not be used more often than recommended on the package and no longer than 3 to 5 days. If symptoms persist or are bothersome, patients should contact their health care provider.

Expectorants

Expectorants are thought to facilitate removal of irritants from the air passages and promote thinning or liquefaction of mucus and phlegm so that it can be more easily coughed up. Patients should recognize the importance of maintaining adequate hydration to promote the effect of this medication.

Follow-up care

The patient should understand that the health care provider should be notified in the following instances.

The patient's temperature is greater than 100° F because this is indicative of respiratory infection requiring treatment with a specific antibiotic. Although flu can produce elevated temperature and overwhelming fatigue and weakness, high fever is not usually associated with viral cold infections.

Chills or sweating recur.

Coughing increases or becomes more severe.

Chest pain increases or becomes more severe.

Breathing becomes more difficult or shortness of breath occurs.

Earache or toothache develops, or skin over the sinuses is tender.

White, yellow, or red patches appear on the throat or tonsils.

Sputum or phlegm becomes thicker or yellow, green, or gray, or a change in the amount of sputum is noted, because these signs can indicate a secondary bacterial infection that will require treatment with an antibiotic.

If pneumonia is suspected, it must be treated by a physician; pneumonia is most likely to occur just as the cold seems to be going away.

GENERAL INSTRUCTIONS FOR DISCHARGE/OUTPATIENTS

COUGHS AND COLDS

If selecting your own product, be sure to select products that only contain agents indicated for particular symptoms. In general, products containing two or more active ingredients should be avoided unless specifically indicated. Do not use a "shotgun" approach.

Be sure to use the proper technique for instilling nasal drops, jellies, and sprays. Gently blow your nose *before* instillation to aid penetration of the drug, but avoid blowing the nose, if possible, for several minutes after nasal administration.

Nasal drops: Tilt head backward (this may be easier if lying with head over edge of bed). The dropper should be inserted slightly into the nostril and the correct number of drops released. Keep head tilted back for approximately 3 minutes to allow medication to penetrate properly.

Nasal jellies: A small amount of jelly should be placed on the finger and instilled into nostril. The jelly should then be sniffed deeply into the nostril. Procedure is repeated for second nostril.

Nasal sprays: Spray container should be held to nostril opening. While holding the other nostril closed, squeeze container firmly and sniff the released medication into the nostril. The procedure should be repeated for the correct number of sprays and then repeated for the other nostril.

Rinse droppers or the tips of spray containers in hot water and dry with a clean tissue after each use.

Containers of nasal drops or sprays should not be used by more than one person.

No product should be used more frequently than directed. Products should not be used longer than 10 days without consulting the health care provider.

If sustained-action capsules are used, they should be swallowed whole.

These medications may cause side effects such as drowsiness; do not drive a car or operate hazardous machinery until you know what effect the medication has on you.

Keep this and all medications out of children's reach.

ANTIHISTAMINES

This drug is an *antihistamine.* It is used to relieve symptoms such as watery eyes or runny nose that occur with common cold or allergic conditions such as hayfever.

Take tablets, capsules, or liquid forms of this medication with food to prevent stomach upset. Take only as recommended.

Do *not* take a larger or smaller dose of this medication than recommended. Do *not* take this medication more often than recommended.

Some people experience side effects such as dry mouth, difficult urination, constipation, skin rash, dizziness, inability to concentrate, muscle weakness, incoordination, restlessness, or headache while taking this medication. If these occur and are bothersome, stop taking this medication, and notify your health care provider.

Antihistamines can cause you to feel drowsy. Avoid driving or performing jobs that require you to be alert until you know how this drug affects you.

Do not take alcoholic beverages (beer, wine, or liquor) with this medication because the antihistamine may make you more drowsy and less alert than usual, since it increases the effects of alcohol. Do not drive or operate dangerous machinery or do jobs that require alertness.

Do not take this medication if you are taking sleeping pills, tranquilizers, or pain killers without first checking with your health care provider.

If you have diabetes, high blood pressure, glaucoma, peptic ulcer disease, angina, hyperthyroidism, heart disease, or trouble passing your water or bladder obstruction, do *not* take this medication without talking with your health care provider.

If you are pregnant, thinking about becoming pregnant, or nursing an infant, do *not* take this medication without first talking with your health care provider. This medication can have effects on your baby.

You may not require *all* of this medication. Contact your health care provider immediately if you have any questions. Do not give this medication to anyone else. When no longer needed, do *not* save this medication; flush it down the toilet.

Keep this medication and all other medication out of the reach of children.

DECONGESTANTS

This drug is a *decongestant.* It is used to relieve symptoms such as stuffy nose that can occur with colds or allergies such as hayfever.

Read the label on your medication carefully. If you have any questions, ask your health care provider. Do *not* use this medication more often than recommended and do *not* use more than the recommended amount.

Notify your health care provider if this medication does not relieve your stuffy nose in 3 to 5 days when used as directed.

Be sure you know how to use nasal sprays or nasal drops. If you are not sure how to take the medication, check with your health care provider before leaving. Your nurse can give you a direction sheet for the use of nasal drops or nasal sprays as well as show you how to take this medication correctly.

Do *not* use *adult* strength for children under 6 years of age.

Do *not* use this medication for children under 1 year of age.

Store this medication in a dry, dark place. Refrigeration is not necessary.

Keep this and all other medication out of the reach of children.

Take the tablet, capsule, or liquid form of this medication with food to prevent upset stomach, which can occur in some people.

If you are a diabetic or have high blood pressure, glaucoma, angina, hyperthyroidism, heart disease, or trouble passing your water (urinating), do *not* take this medication without talking with your health care provider.

Continued.

GENERAL INSTRUCTIONS FOR DISCHARGE/OUTPATIENTS—cont'd

DECONGESTANTS—cont'd

Call your health care provider immediately if you notice any restlessness, insomnia, headache, weakness, or confusion while taking this medication.

Do *not* take any other medication when taking this medication because they may interact, causing unwanted or harmful effects.

If you are pregnant or thinking about becoming pregnant, do not take this medication without discussing this with your health care provider. Some decongestants are not safe to take during pregnancy.

Do not take this medication if you are breast-feeding an infant because some of the medication can be passed into breast milk, affecting your infant. Discuss this with your health care provider.

ANTITUSSIVES

This drug is an *antitussive* and it is used to relieve coughs.

Do not take this medication if you have ever had an allergic reaction to cough medicine.

Swallow tablets whole with a glass of water. Do *not* dissolve tablets in your mouth or chew them.

Do not take syrup with water. Do not follow the medication immediately with water because this can decrease its soothing effect on your throat.

This drug may cause drowsiness in some people. Do *not* drive, operate dangerous equipment, or do jobs that require alertness until you know how this medication affects you.

Notify your health care provider if your cough lasts longer than 1 week or if you develop fever, skin rash, or a headache.

Do *not* use this medication longer than 1 week. Check with your health care provider.

If you are pregnant, considering pregnancy, or breastfeeding an infant, do *not* take this medication without discussing this with your health care provider.

This medication should not be given to children less than 1 year of age. If you have any questions, check with your health care provider.

Store this medication in a dry, dark place. Refrigeration is not necessary.

Keep this and all other medication out of the reach of children.

In addition to the general instructions, if your cough medicine contains *codeine* remember the following.

This drug could become habit forming. Do *not* take this medication more often or longer than prescribed.

Do *not* take *any* other medications, especially sleeping pills, tranquilizers, pain relievers, or cold and hay fever medications, without checking with your health care provider. These medication can cause harmful effects when taken together.

This medication can cause constipation in some people. Be sure to drink at least 8 to 10 glasses of water a day; eat a well-balanced diet including breads, salads, cereals, and bran; and exercise moderately. These measures will help to prevent constipation.

NURSING DRUG DIGEST

Medication (trade name*)	Indication	Usual dosage and administration	Dosage forms, preparation, and storage	Contraindications, cautions, and comments	Monitoring
ANTIHISTAMINES NOTE: Only those agents chiefly used to treat allergic and vasomotor rhinitis and those commonly included in "cough and cold" preparations are included in this table	Symptomatic relief of allergic or vasomotor rhinitis Included in many "cough and cold" products, but effectiveness in treating the common cold is largely unsubstantiated	Specific recommendations for geriatric dosages are not always specified, but elderly patients may require *less* than the usual adult dosages May be administered with food to minimize gastric irritation	Only dosage forms used in the treatment of coughs, colds, and rhinitis are listed in this table; most agents are also available in numerous combination products	*Contraindicated* in nursing mothers and neonates *Contraindicated* in patients receiving MAOIs because anticholinergic effects are prolonged and intensified Also *contraindicated* in patients with known hypersensitivity to particular agent in question Because of anticholinergic side effects, should be used cautiously in patients with history of or predisposition to asthma, cardiovascular disease, hypertension, hyperthyroidism, narrow-angle glaucoma, or prostatic hypertrophy These agents generally are *not* recommended for infants or children less than 2 years old unless dosage is individualized by prescriber, although some products do have specific dosage recommendations for patients in these age groups	Children, especially with overdosage, are likely to develop paradoxic excitation of the central nervous system and should be observed for nervousness, sleeplessness, and tremor and monitored for tachycardia. See also individual agents

NOTE: For additional details regarding the individual agents listed in this table, see the text and other tables in this chapter.
*Indicates a multiple active ingredient product. For a complete listing of all active ingredients see the *Drug Reference Guide to Brand Names and Active Ingredients*.
♦ Indicates that the drug is generally available only in Canada.
★ Indicates that the drug is generally available only in the United States.

NURSING DRUG DIGEST—cont'd

Medication (trade name)	Indication	Usual dosage and administration	Dosage forms, preparation, and storage	Contraindications, cautions, and comments	Monitoring
ANTIHISTA-MINES—cont'd				Risks and benefits must be assessed by prescriber before administering to pregnant patients or women of childbearing age; these medications may be secreted in breast milk in concentrations high enough to affect infants See also individual agents Sedation is a common side effect; patients should be advised not to drive or engage in other acivities requiring mental alertness or precise motor coordination until individual response is determined Patients should be advised to avoid alcoholic beverages while receiving antihistamines because depressant effects on central nervous system are additive; dosage reductions should be considered if concomitant therapy with other central nervous system depressants is necessary Elderly patients are most likely to experience dizziness, sedation, hypotension, and weakness	

Drug	Use	Dosage	Dosage Forms/Storage	Comments
Antazoline Albalon-A* Antastan Antistine Antistine-Privine* Histostab Vasocon A* Zincfrin-A*	Symptomatic relief of allergic or vasomotor rhinitis	*Adults:* 100-200 mg PO t.i.d. to q.i.d.; may be increased to a *maximum* of 1200 mg/day. Administration with food or milk may decrease GI distress	Tablet: 100 mg Store between 15° and 30° C in tightly closed containers and protect from light Discard unused solutions 14 days after opening	The nasal spray (nebulizer) is *not* recommended for use in children because of the risk of overdosage. Oral dosage is *not* commonly used. Patients should be advised to discontinue nasal instillation after 3 to 5 days to avoid rebound nasal congestion See Antihistamines See Naphazoline	Topical use of antihistamines commonly leads to allergic reactions; after ocular use observe for increased redness or inflammation (if allergic reaction develops, discontinue medication and consult prescriber) See Antihistamines See Naphazoline
Bromodiphenhydramine Ambenyl Expectorant* Ambodryl Deserol	Symptomatic relief of allergic or vasomotor rhinitis	*Adults:* 25 mg PO t.i.d. to q.i.d.; may be increased to a maximum of 150 mg/day *Children:* 6-12 years of age 6.25-25 mg PO t.i.d. to q.i.d. up to a maximum of 2.5 mg/kg body weight/24 hr	Capsule: 25 mg Elixir: 12.5 mg/5 ml Store between 15° and 30° C in tightly closed containers	Sedation can be marked with this agent, particularly with elixir, which contains 12% to 15% alcohol May produce fewer anticholinergic side effects than other ethanolamines See Antihistamines	Monitor for sedative effects
Brompheniramine Brocon C.R.* Brocon Chewable* Bromphen Dimetane Dimetane Expectorant* Dimetapp Elixir* Dimetapp Extentabs* Dynehist S.A.* Histatapp Elixirs* Histatapp T.D.* Ilvin Poly-Histine-DX*	Symptomatic relief of allergic or vasomotor rhinitis	*Adults:* 4-8 mg PO t.i.d. to q.i.d. up to a *maximum* of 24 mg/day *Children:* 2-6 years old, 1-2 mg PO t.i.d. to q.i.d.; 6-12 years old, 2-4 mg PO t.i.d. to q.i.d. Extended-release *Adults:* 8-12 mg PO q.8-12h. *Children:* Less than 6 years old, *not* recommended; 6 years and older, 8-12 mg q.12h.	Elixir: 2 mg/5 ml Recommended diluent for elixir is simple syrup Tablet: 4 mg Tablets, extended-release: 8, 12 mg Injectable: 10 mg/ml Store between 15° and 30° C in tightly closed containers and protect from light	Patients should be advised to swallow extended-release tablets whole without crushing or chewing See Antihistamines	See Antihistamines

Continued.

NURSING DRUG DIGEST—cont'd

Medication (trade name)	Indication	Usual dosage and administration	Dosage forms, preparation, and storage	Contraindications, cautions, and comments	Monitoring
Brompheniramine—cont'd Puretane Puretane DC Expectorant* Puretane Expectorant* Symptom 3 Veltane					
★ **Carbinoxamine** Allergefon Clistin Clistin-D* Rondec* Rondec-DM*	Symptomatic relief of allergic or vasomotor rhinitis	*Adults:* 4-8 mg PO t.i.d. to q.i.d. *Children:* 1-3 years old, 2 mg PO t.i.d. to q.i.d.; 3-6 years old, 2-4 mg PO t.i.d. to q.i.d.; 6 years and older, 4 mg PO t.i.d. to q.i.d. Extended-release *Adults:* 8 or 12 mg q.8-12h. *Children: Not* recommended *Not* recommended in newborn or premature infants because limited ability to metabolize and clear drug is likely to result in accumulation and toxicity	Elixir: 4 mg/5 ml; contains 6.5% to 8% alcohol Tablet: 4 mg Tablet, extended-release: 8, 12 mg Store between 15° and 30° C in tightly closed containers and protect from light	Patients should be advised to swallow extended-release tablet whole without crushing or chewing See Antihistamines	See Antihistamines
Chlorpheniramine A.R.M. Allergy Relief Medicine* Alka-Seltzer Plus* Allerbid Allerest Regular & Children's* Allergesic* Allorphen 12 Aspirin Free Dristan* Atlachlor AL-R	Symptomatic relief of allergic or vasomotor rhinitis	*Adults:* 4 mg PO t.i.d. to q.i.d., may be increased to a *maximum* of 24 mg/day *Children:* 6-12 years old, 2-4 mg t.i.d. to q.i.d. Extended-release *Adults:* 8 or 12 mg b.i.d. to t.i.d. *Children:* Less than 12 years old, *not* recommended; 12 years and older, 8 mg b.i.d.	Capsules, extended-release: 8, 12 mg Elixir: 10 mg/ml Recommended diluent for elixir is simple syrup Patients should be advised to discard any unused, diluted elixir after 2 weeks Syrup: 2 mg/5 ml Tablet: 4 mg Tablet, chewable: 2 mg Tablet, extended-release: 8, 12 mg Injectable: 10, 20, 100 mg/ml Store all products except elixirs between 15° and 30° C in tightly closed containers	One of most potent antihistamines, but may be less sedating than most Patients should be advised to swallow extended-release capsule or tablet whole without crushing or chewing See Antihistamines	See Antihistamines

Elixirs should be stored between 15° and 25° C; protect all products from light

Bayer Decongestant*
Breacol*
Cheracol Plus*
Chlorfen
Chlor-Trimeton
Chlor-Tripolon
Citra*
Co Tylenol*
Colrex*
Comhist*
Comtrex*
Conex*
Contac*
Coricidin*
Coryban-B*
Covanamine*
Covangesic*
C3 Cold Cough*
Duadacin*
Duradyne-Forte*
Efricon*
Extendac*
Extendryl*
Fedahish*
Fedahist*
H-Stadur
Headway*
Histalon
Histaspan
Historal*
Hot Lemon
Hycomine Compound
Ibioton
Midran Decongestant*
Naldecon*
Nilcol*
Nolamine*
Norel Plus
Noscosed
Novafed A*
Novahistine*
Novopheniram
Ornade*

Continued.

NURSING DRUG DIGEST—cont'd

Medication (trade name)	Indication	Usual dosage and administration	Dosage forms, preparation, and storage	Contraindications, cautions, and comments	Monitoring
Chlorpheniramine—cont'd Piriton Polaronil Romex* Romilar* Ru-Tuss* Sinarest* Sine-Off* Sinurex* Spantac* Sudafed Plus* Supercetin* Teldrin Telodron Triaminic Syrup* Triaminicin* Tymcaps* Valihist*					
Clemastine Tavegil Tavist Tavist-1	Symptomatic relief of allergic or vasomotor rhinitis	*Adults:* 1 mg PO b.i.d., may be increased to a *maximum of* 6 mg/day *Children: Not* established *Not* recommended in newborn or premature infants because limited ability to metabolize and clear drug is likely to result in accumulation and toxicity Tablet should be taken with water before meals	Liquid, pediatric: 0.25 mg/5 ml Tablet: 1.34, 2.68 mg fumarate salt (equivalent to 1, 2 mg) Store between 15° and 30° C in tightly closed containers	May be less sedating than most agents See Antihistamines	See Antihistamines
Dexchlorpheniramine Polaramine Expectorant* Polaramine	Symptomatic relief of allergic or vasomotor rhinitis	*Adults:* 2 mg PO t.i.d. to q.i.d. *Children:* 0.5-1 mg t.i.d. to q.i.d. Extended-release *Adults:* 4 or 6 mg PO b.i.d. to t.i.d. *Children: Not* recommended *Not* recommended in newborn or premature infants because limited ability to metabolize and clear drug is likely to result in accumulation and toxicity	Syrup: 2 mg/5 ml Tablet: 2 mg Tablet, extended-release: 4, 6 mg Store between 15° and 30° C in tightly closed containers and protect from light	See Antihistamines	See Antihistamines

Drug	Use	Dosage	Preparations	Remarks
Diphenhydramine Allerdryl Ambenyl Expectorant* Benadryl Benadryl with Ephedrine* Bendylate Benylin Benylin Decongestant* Benylin Pediatrics Benylin Cough Syrup Diahist Eldadryl Fenylhist Nautamine Standryl SK-Diphenhydramine	Symptomatic relief of allergic or vasomotor rhinitis See also Chapter 15, "Sedative-Hypnotics"	*Adults:* 25-50 mg PO t.i.d. to q.i.d., may be increased to *maximum* of 400 mg/day *Children:* 1 to 5 years old, 12.5-25 mg PO t.i.d. to q.i.d.; 6 to 12 years old, 25-50 mg PO t.i.d. *Not* recommended in newborn or premature infants because limited ability to metabolize and clear drug is likely to result in accumulation and toxicity	Capsule: 25, 50 mg Elixir: 12.5, 50 mg/5 ml Elixir formulation contains 14% alcohol Syrup: 12.5 mg/5 ml Tablet: 50 mg Injectable: 10, 50 mg/ml Store between 15° and 30° C in tightly closed containers and protect from light	An isomer, phenyltoloxamine, also has antihistaminic activity but is only available in combination products See Antihistamines Patients should be advised to swallow extended release tablet whole without crushing or chewing See Antihistamines
★ **Diphenylpyraline** Diafen Hispril Hista-Nil Novahistex*	Symptomatic relief of allergic or vasomotor rhinitis	*Adults:* 2 mg PO q.4-6h. *Children:* 2-6 years old, 1-2 mg PO q.8h. up to a *maximum* of 4 mg/day; 6 years and older, 2 mg PO q.6h. up to a maximum of 6 mg/day Extended-release *Adults:* 5 mg PO q.12h. *Children:* Less than 6 years old, *not* recommended; 6-12 years old, 5 mg/day *Not* recommended in newborn or premature infants because limited ability to metabolize and clear drug is likely to result in accumulation and toxicity	Capsule, extended-release: 5 mg Tablet: 2 mg Tablet, extended-release: 5 mg Store between 15° and 30° C in tightly closed containers and protect from light	Extended-release formulations are the only products used frequently; patients should be advised to swallow whole without crushing or chewing See Antihistamines

Continued.

NURSING DRUG DIGEST—cont'd

Medication (trade name)	Indication	Usual dosage and administration	Dosage forms, preparation, and storage	Contraindications, cautions, and comments	Monitoring
★ **Pheniramine** Citra* Citra Forte Dristan Nasal Spray* Extendac* Fiogesic* Inhisten Poly-Histine-D* Ru-Vert* S-T Forte Syrup* Timed Cold* Triaminic Expectorant with Codeine* Triaminic Expectorant* Triaminic* Triaminicol Triaminicol Decongestant Cough Syrup* Triaminicol Trimeton Tussagesic Tussaminic Suspension* Tussagesic* Tussaminic* Ursinus* Vasominic TD* Verstat*	Symptomatic relief of allergic or vasomotor rhinitis	*Adults:* 25-50 mg (aminosalicylate) PO t.i.d., may be increased to a maximum of 40 mg PO t.i.d. *Children:* 1-5 years old, 7.5-15 mg (maleate) PO up to t.i.d.; 6 years and older, 5-22.5 mg (maleate) PO up to t.i.d. Extended-release *Adults:* 75 mg (maleate) PO q.d. to b.i.d.; or 150 mg PO q.h.s. Extended-release tablets *not* recommended for patients with Crohn's disease because of increased risk of intestinal obstruction and stricture Patients should be advised to swallow extended-release tablet whole without crushing or chewing *Children: Not* recommended	Elixir: 15 mg/5 ml (maleate) Tablet: 50 mg (aminosalicylate) Tablet, extended-release: 75 mg (maleate)	See Antihistamines	See Antihistamines
★ **Pyrilamine** Allerest* Alleroc Anthisan Bronitin* Citra Forte*	Symptomatic relief of allergic or vasomotor rhinitis	*Adults:* 25-50 mg PO t.i.d. to q.i.d., may be increased up to a maximum of 1 gm/day *Children:* 6 years and older, 12.5-25 mg PO t.i.d. to q.i.d	Elixir: 12.5 mg/5 ml Tablet: 25 mg Store between 15° and 30° C in tightly closed containers and protect from light	Pyrilamine has been reported to inhibit actions of guanethidine, therefore caution is advised during concomitant therapy	See Antihistamines

See Antihistamines

Codimal DM*
Codimal PM*
Compoz*
Copsamine
Dorantamin
Duadacin*
Enrumay
Fiogesic*
Histalet
  Forte*
Histan
Kriptin
Miles Nervine
Minihist
Napril Pla-
  teau
Neo-Antergan
P-V Tussin
  Syrup*
Pamprin*
Paraminyl
Primatene-H*
Pyma
Pymafed
Pyra-Maleate
Pyramal
Quiet World*
Rynatan
Sleep-Eze
  Tablets
Stamine
Sunril*
Thylogen
Triaminic Ex-
  pectorant*
Triaminic*
Triaminicol*
Tussagesic
  Suspen-
  sion*
Tussagesic
Tussaminic*
Zem-Histine
4-Way Nasal
  Spray*

Continued.

NURSING DRUG DIGEST—cont'd

Medication (trade name)	Indication	Usual dosage and administration	Dosage forms, preparation, and storage	Contraindications, cautions, and comments	Monitoring
Terfenadine Seldane	Symptomatic relief of allergic or vasomotor rhinitis	*Adults:* 60 mg PO b.i.d.	Tablet: 60 mg	*Contraindicated* in hypersensitivity Adverse side effects are generally minimal	See Antihistamines
Tripelennamine Benzoxal Poly-Histine-D* Poly-Histine-D Elixir* Pyribenzamine Pyrizil PBZ PBZ w/ Ephedrine* PBZ Expectorant w/ Ephedrine* PBZ Lontabs PBZ-SR Rholinist* Ro-Mist* Tri-Tomine*	Symptomatic relief of allergic or vasomotor rhinitis	*Adults:* 25-50 mg PO q.4-6h., may be increased to a *maximum* of 600 mg/day *Children:* 1.25 mg/kg body weight PO q.6h. up to a *maximum* of 300 mg/day Extended-release *Adults:* 100 mg q.8-12h. *Children:* Less than 5 years old, *not* recommended; 5 years and older, 50 mg q.8-12h. *Not* recommended in newborn or premature infants because limited ability to metabolize and clear drug is likely to result in accumulation and toxicity Patients should be advised to swallow extended-release tablets whole without crushing or chewing NOTE: All doses quoted refer to HCl salt form (see Dosage forms, preparation, and storage)	Elixir: 37.5 mg/5 ml (citrate) (equivalent to 25 mg/5 ml [HCl]) Tablet: 25, 50 mg (HCl) Tablet: Tablet: 25.50 mg extended release: 50, 100 mg (HCl) Store between 15° and 30° C in tightly closed containers and protect from light	See Antihistamines	See Antihistamines
Triprolidine Acridil Acti-Pron* Actidil Actidilon Actifed Expectorant* Actifed* Actifed-C* Pro-Actidil	Symptomatic relief of allergic or vasomotor rhinitis	*Adults:* 2.5-5 mg PO t.i.d. to q.i.d., up to a *maximum* of 15 mg/day *Children:* Less than 2 years old, 0.3-1 mg PO up to t.i.d.; 2-6 years old, 1 mg PO up to t.i.d.; 6-12 years old, 1.25 mg up to t.i.d. Extended-release *Adults:* 10 mg 5 to 6 hours before bedtime, may be increased to 10 mg b.i.d.	Elixir: 2 mg/5 ml Syrup: 1.25 mg/5 ml Tablet: 2.5 mg Tablet, extended release: 10 mg Store between 15° and 30° C in tightly closed containers and protect from light Recommended diluent for elixir is simple syrup; discard any unused diluted elixir after 14 days	See Antihistamines	See Antihistamines

		Children: Use *not* recommended *Not* recommended in newborn or premature infants because limited ability to metabolize and clear drug is likely to result in accumulation and toxicity Patients should be advised to swallow extended-release tablet whole without crushing or chewing			
ANTITUSSIVES					
Benzonatate Tessalon Ventussin	Symptomatic relief of cough (has been reported to relieve intractable hiccup)	*Adults:* 100 mg PO q.4-6h. daily; *maximum* 600 mg/day	Capsule: 50, 100 mg Store between 15° and 30° C in airtight containers and protect from light	*Contraindicated* in patients with known hypersensitivity to benzonatate Patients should be warned about possible drowsiness, dizziness, or headache; until individual response is determined, patients should be advised not to drive or engage in other activities requiring mental alertness or precise motor coordination Risks and benefits must be assessed by prescriber before use during first trimester of pregnancy Local anesthetic actions may produce numbness or tingling sensation of the mouth, tongue, and pharynx; nasal congestion may occur	Convulsions have been reported, therefore patients should be observed for signs of muscle tremor
Chlophedianol Detigon Ulo Ulone	Symptomatic relief of cough	*Adults:* 25 mg PO t.i.d. to q.i.d. *Children:* 2-6 years old, 12.5 mg PO t.i.d. to q.i.d.; 6-12 years old, 12.5-25 mg PO t.i.d. to q.i.d.	Syrup: 25 mg/5 ml Store between 15° and 30° C	Mouth and throat dryness and irritation generally can be relieved with candy or gum This agent may enhance effects of other CNS depressants *and* stimulants	Observe patients for nervousness and other signs of central nervous system stimulation

Continued.

NURSING DRUG DIGEST—cont'd

Medication (trade name)	Indication	Usual dosage and administration	Dosage forms, preparation, and storage	Contraindications, cautions, and comments	Monitoring
Codeine Actifed-C* Acutuss Expectorant with Codeine* Alamine Expectorant* Alamine-C* Ambenyl Expectorant* Broncho-Tussin* Cerose* Cetro-Cirose* Cheracol* Coastaldyne* Codalan* Codasa*	Symptomatic relief of cough that does not respond to non-narcotic antitussives	*Adults:* 10-20 mg PO q4-6h. *Children:* 2-6 years old, 2.5-5 mg PO q4-6h.; 6-12 years old, 5-10 mg PO q4-6h.	Solution: 10 mg/ml Syrup: 25 mg/5 ml Tablet: 15 mg Store in airtight containers and protect from light	*Contraindicated* in patients with known hypersensitivity to codeine or preexisting respiratory depression; the respiratory center of young children is particularly sensitive to depressant effects of codeine Also used as analgesic in higher doses *Not* recommended for use during pregnancy because it crosses placental barrier Prolonged use or high dosages may lead to dependency	Monitor respiratory signs in patients receiving codeine concomitantly with MAOIs, phenothiazines, tricyclic antidepressants, or other central nervous system depressants because respiratory depression may be markedly enhanced. Monitor cardiovascular signs in patients receiving codeine concomitantly with MAOIs either hypotension and coma or hypertensive crisis may develop

Codimal DM*
Codophen*
Conex with Codeine*
Copavin*
Coryphen-Codeine*
Cotussis*
C 3*
C 4*
Dimetapp with Codeine*
Lo-Tussin*
Noratuss*
Novahistine DM*
Novahistine Expectorant*
Nucofed*
Paveral*
Pediacof*
Pruni-codeine*
Tussar SF*
Tussar-2*
Tussi-Organidin*

Drying effect on airway secretions and depressant effect on cough reflex may aggravate asthma or emphysema

Patients should be advised not to drive or engage in other activities requiring mental alertness or precise motor coordination because sedation may be marked

Advise patients that constipation is likely to be experienced

Monitor for constipation

Continued.

NURSING DRUG DIGEST—cont'd

Medication (trade name)	Indication	Usual dosage and administration	Dosage forms, preparation, and storage	Contraindications, cautions, and comments	Monitoring
Dextromethorphan Ambenyl-D Decongestant Cough Formula* Balminil DM Bayer Cough Syrup for Children* Benylin DM Breacol* Cerose DM* Cheracol D* Cheracol Plus* Children's Hold 4-Hour Cough Suppressant* Chloraseptic DM Cough Control Lozenges* Colrex Antitussive* Comtrex* Contac Jr. Children's Cold Medicine* Coryban-D Antitussive* CoTylenol Liquid Cold Formula* C3 Cold Cough Capsules*	Symptomatic relief of cough	*Adults:* 10-30 mg PO t.i.d. to q.i.d.; *maximum* 120 mg/day *Children:* 2-6 years old, 3.5 mg PO up to q.i.d.; 6-12 years old, 6.75 mg PO up to q.i.d. Controlled-release liquid *Adults:* 60 mg PO b.i.d. *Children:* 2-5 years old, 15 mg PO b.i.d.; 6-12 years old, 30 mg PO b.i.d.	Syrup: 10 mg/5 ml, 15 mg/5 ml, 25 mg/5 ml Store in tightly closed containers and protect from light Lozenges: 7.5, 10 mg Liquid, controlled-release: 30 mg/5 ml	The higher dosages prolong rather than increase antitussive action Respiratory depression unlikely unless high dosages are used This agent has no analgesic activity and only slight sedative properties	

Delsym
Dristan Antitussive*
DM Syrup
Formula 44 Cough Discs
Formula 44*
Formula 44-D*
Halls*
Histalet DM Syrup*
Hold Liquid Cough Suppressant*
Hold 4-Hour Cough Suppressant
Hold*
Methorate
Naldetuss*
Novahistine DMX*
Nyquil Nighttime Colds Medicine*
Ornacol*
Orthoxicol*
Quiet-Nite*
Robitussin-DM Cough Calmers
Robitussin-DM*
Romex*
Romilar
Romilar Capsules*
Romilar Children's
Sedatuss
Silence is Golden

Continued.

NURSING DRUG DIGEST—cont'd

Medication (trade name)	Indication	Usual dosage and administration	Dosage forms, preparation, and storage	Contraindications, cautions, and comments	Monitoring
Dextromethorphan—cont'd					
Spec-T Sore Throat/Cough Suppressant*					
St. Joseph Cough Syrup for Children					
Sucrets Cough Control Formula					
Sudafed Cough*					
Triaminic-DM Cough Formula*					
Triaminicol*					
Trind DM*					
Tussagesic*					
Tussaminic*					
Tussorphan					
Vicks Cough Silencer					
Vicks Cough Syrup*					
Vicks Formula 44 Cough Mixture*					
Vicks Nyquil Nighttime Cold Medicine*					
2/G-DM*					
Diphenhydramine	See Antihistamines, p. 607				

Drug	Use	Dosage	Preparations	Remarks	
Hydrocodone Citra Forte* Citra Forte Syrup* Codone Corutel DH Dicodid Entuss Expectorant* Hycodan Hycomine Compound* Hycomine* Hycotuss* Mercodinone Norcet* P-V Tussin Syrup* P-V Tussin* Pseudo-Mist Expectorant* Robidone S-T Forte Syrup* Tussene Expectorant* Tussend* Tussionex* Vicodin	Symptomatic relief of cough that does not respond to nonnarcotic antitussives	*Adults:* 5 mg PO q.4-6h.	Syrup: 5 mg/5 ml Tablet: 5 mg Store in tightly closed containers and protect from light	*Contraindicated* in patients with known hypersensitivity to hydrocodone or preexisting respiratory depression This agent has *no* real advantages over codeine in treatment of cough, but has higher dependency risk See Codeine	See Codeine
Hydromorphone Dilaudid Hymorphan	Symptomatic relief of cough that does not respond to nonnarcotic antitussives	*Adults:* 1 mg PO q.3-4h. *Children:* Not established	Tablets: 1, 2, 3, 4 mg Store in tightly closed containers and protect from light	See Codeine	See Codeine
★ **Levopropoxyphene** Novrad Regretos	Symptomatic relief of cough	*Adults:* 50-100 mg PO q.4h. *Children:* 1 mg/kg PO q.4h.	Capsule: 50, 100 mg Suspension: 50 mg/5 ml Store in tightly closed containers between 15° and 30° C and protect from light	Patients should be advised not to drive or engage in other activities requiring mental alertness or precise motor coordination until individual response is determined. Does *not* induce physical dependence This agent has no analgesic activity	

Continued.

NURSING DRUG DIGEST—cont'd

Medication (trade name)	Indication	Usual dosage and administration	Dosage forms, preparation, and storage	Contraindications, cautions, and comments	Monitoring
Noscapine Actoe Expectorant* / Conar Expectorant* / Conar* / Coscopin / Coscotabs / Nectadon / Noscatuss / Tusscapine	Symptomatic relief of cough	*Adults:* 15-30 mg PO q.i.d. *Children:* 2-6 years old, 7.5-15 mg PO t.i.d.; 6-12 years old, 15 mg PO t.i.d. to q.i.d.	Suspension: 15 mg/5 ml; Syrup: 15 mg/5 ml; Tablet, chewable: 15 mg; Store in tightly closed containers	Patients may become drowsy and should be advised to avoid driving and other activities that require mental alertness or precise motor coordination until their individual response is known. *Not* likely to induce dependence because this agent has no analgesic action and does not produce euphoria; patients should be advised to chew tablets well before swallowing. Large dosages may cause central nervous system and respiratory stimulation	Observe patients for signs of nervousness, irritability, or sleeplessness
DECONGESTANTS Relief of nasal congestion or rhinitis (NOTE: some agents have additional uses *not* covered in this chapter)		*Elderly:* Specific geriatric dosages *not* established, but elderly patients may require less than average adult dosage of all sympathomimetic drugs	Only dosage forms used to treat allergic rhinitis or colds are listed. See individual agents. Discard unused nasal solutions 14 days after opening	*Contraindicated* in patients with diabetes, severe hypertension, hyperthyroidism, and ischemic heart disease because symptoms are aggravated or induced. *Contraindicated* in patients receiving MAOIs within 3 weeks of decongestant therapy because hypertensive crisis may be provoked. Patients should be advised that prolonged use or overuse, particularly with topical agents, can lead to rebound congestion	See individual agents. Observe for rebound nasal congestion, particularly with *topical* use

Drug	Use	Dosage	Available forms	Remarks
				Advise patients of proper techniques for using nasal sprays, drops, or jellies (see General Instructions for Discharge/Outpatients) Use with caution in cardiovascular disease Patients should be advised that containers of nasal sprays or drops should be used by one person only Observe for tolerance or dependence
Ephedrine Ephedron Ephedsol Vatronol Nose Drops	Relief of nasal congestion or rhinitis See also Chapter 28, "Bronchodilators and Respiratory Gases"	Adults: 15-30 mg PO t.i.d. to q.i.d. Children: 0.5 mg/kg body weight PO t.i.d. to q.i.d. Extended-release Adults: 15-60 mg q.8-12h. Children: 15 mg q.8-12h. Topical Adults: 2-4 drops or sprays of 1% or 3% solution into each nostril b.i.d. to q.i.d. Children: 2-4 drops of 0.25% or 0.5% solution into each nostril b.i.d. to q.i.d.	Capsule: 25, 50 mg Capsule, extended release: 15, 30, 60 mg Elixir: 15 mg/5 ml Recommended diluent for elixir is simple syrup Discard any unused diluted elixir after 14 days Solution, nasal drops: 0.25%, 0.5%, 1%, 3% Solution, nasal spray: 1%, 3% Syrup: 10 mg/5 ml Tablet: 25 mg Nasal jelly: 0.6% Store between 15° and 30° C in tightly closed containers and protect from light	Contraindicated in patients receiving MAOIs because of risk of hypertensive crisis Tolerance and dependence have been reported after prolonged use Paranoid psychosis has been reported in cases of abuse See Decongestants
Naphazoline Optozoline Privine Rhino-Mex Rhino-Mex-N 4-Way Nasal Spray* 4-Way*	Relief of nasal congestion or rhinitis See also Chapter 24 "Sympathomimetics and Sympatholytics"	Topical Adults: 1-3 drops or sprays into each nostril up to q.i.d. Children: Over 6 years of age, same as adults Sprays not recommended for children because of risk of overdosage	Nasal drops: 0.05%, 1% Nasal spray: 0.05% Store in tightly closed containers and protect from light	CNS depression more common than excitation after systemic absorption See Decongestants

Continued.

NURSING DRUG DIGEST—cont'd

Medication (trade name)	Indication	Usual dosage and administration	Dosage forms, preparation, and storage	Contraindications, cautions, and comments	Monitoring
Oxymetazoline Afrin Dristan Long Lasting Drixine Duration Hazol Nafrine Neo-Synephrine 12-Hour St. Joseph Decongestant for Children St. Joseph Nasal Spray/ Drops	Relief of nasal congestion or rhinitis See also Chapter 24, "Sympathomimetics and Sympatholytics"	Topical *Adults:* 1-3 drops or sprays of 0.05% solution into each nostril q.12h. *Children:* Less than 6 years old, 1 or 2 drops of 0.025% solution into each nostril q.12h.; 6 years and older, see adult dosage	Nasal drops: 0.025%, 0.05% Nasal spray: 0.05%	Rebound congestion less likely than with agents instilled t.i.d. to q.i.d. See Decongestants	See Decongestants
Phenylephrine Allerest Nasal Al-Tuss* Anatuss* Anodynos Forte* Aspirin Free Dristan* Biomydrin Cerose DM* Cerose* Chlor-Trimeton Expectorant with Codeine* Chlor-Trimeton Expectorant* Citra* Citra Forte* Colrex Antitussive*	Relief of nasal congestion or rhinitis See also Chapter 24, "Sympathomimetics and Sympatholytics"	*Adults:* 10 mg PO q.4h. *Children:* 2-6 years old, 2.5 mg PO q.4h.; 6-12 years old, 5 mg PO q.4h. Topical, nasal drops *Adults:* 1-3 drops of 0.25% or 0.5% solution into each nostril q.4h. *Children:* 2-6 years old, 1-3 drops of 0.125% solution q.4h.; 6-12 years old, 1-3 drops of 0.25% solution q.4h. Topical, nasal jelly *Adults:* 1 instillation (see General Instructions for Discharge/Outpatients) into each nostril q.4h. *Children: Not* recommended Topical, nasal spray *Adults:* 1 or 2 sprays into each nostril q.4h.	Elixir: 1 mg/ml Nasal drops: 0.125%, 0.25%, 0.5%, 1% Nasal jelly: 0.5% Nasal spray: 0.25%, 0.5% Store in tightly closed containers and protect from light	This agent may induce or aggravate irritation of the nasal mucosa; if irritation is experienced, drug should be discontinued See Decongestants	See Decongestants

Children: *Not* recommended

NOTE: Nasal jellies and sprays are *not* recommended for children because of risk of overdosage

Colrex*
Comhist L.A.*
Comhist*
Conar*
Congespirin*
Contac Nasal Mist
Coricidin Nasal Spray
Coryban-D Antitussive*
Covanamine*
Covangesic*
Degest
Demazin*
Dimetane Expectorant*
Dimetapp
Dimetapp Elixir*
Dimetapp Extentabs*
Dristan*
Duohaler*
Duradyne-Forte*
Efricel
Epicel
Fendol*
Histaspan-D*
Hydra
Isuprel-Neo Mistometer*
Mistura D
Mydfrin
Naldecon*
Naso-X
Naso Mist
Neo-Synephrine
Neozin
Novahistex*
Pediacof*
Pediaqull*
Phenatapp Extend*
Puretapp Elixir*
Pyracert-D

Continued.

NURSING DRUG DIGEST—cont'd

Medication (trade name)	Indication	Usual dosage and administration	Dosage forms, preparation, and storage	Contraindications, cautions, and comments	Monitoring
Phenylephrine—cont'd Romex* Romilar* Rynatuss* Sinaphen-Nasal Sinarest Nasal Spray* Sinex Super Anahist Nasal Spray Triminicin Nasal Spray* Tussar DM* Vacon Vicks Sinex Decongestant Nasal Spray* Zincfrin 4-Way Cold* 4-Way Nasal Spray*					See Decongestants
★ **Phenylpropanolamine** A.R.M. Allergy Relief Medicine* Alka-Seltzer Plus* Allerest* Allergesic* Anatuss* Bayer Decongestant* Breacol*	Relief of nasal congestion or rhinitis	*Adults:* 25 mg PO q.4h.; or 50 mg PO q.8h. *Children:* 2-6 years old, 6.25 mg PO q.4h. or 12.5 mg PO q.8h.; 6-12 years old, 12.5 mg PO q.4h. or 25 mg PO q.8h. Extended-release *Adults:* 75 mg q.12h. *Children: Not* recommended To minimize insomnia, last dose should be administered 3-4 hours before bedtime	Capsule: 25, 50 mg Capsule, extended-release: 50, 75 mg Elixir: 20 mg/5 ml Syrup: 12.5 mg/5 ml Tablet: 25, 50 mg Store between 15° and 30° C in tightly closed containers and protect from light	Similar to ephedrine but slightly less likely to produce stimulation of central nervous system See Decongestants	

Patients should be advised to swallow extended-release capsule whole without crushing or chewing

Brocon Chewable*
Cheracol Plus*
Codimal Expectorant*
Coldecon
Comtrex*
Conex*
Congesprin*
Contac*
Control Capsules
Coricidin Antitussive*
Coryban-D*
Covanamine*
Covangesic*
C3 Cold Cough Capsules*
Diadax
Dimetane Expectorant*
Halls*
Head & Chest Cold Medicine*
Headway*
Naldecon*
Novahistine*
Ornacel*
Ornex*
Prolamine
Propadrine
Puretapp Elixir*
Rhindecon
Robitussin-CF*
Romilar 111*
Ru-Tuss*

Continued.

NURSING DRUG DIGEST—cont'd

Medication (trade name)	Indication	Usual dosage and administration	Dosage forms, preparation, and storage	Contraindications, cautions, and comments	Monitoring
Phenylpropanolamine —cont'd Sinarest* Sine-Aid* Sine-Off* Sinubid* Sinustat* Sinutab* Soltice* St. Joseph Cold for Children* Super Anahist* Super Odrinex* Timed Cold* Triaminic* Triaminicin* Triaminicin* Trind* Tuss-Ornade* Tussagesic* Tussaminic* Vicks Formula 44D Decongestant Cough Mixture* 4-Way*					See Decongestants
Propylhexedrine Benzedrex Dristan Inhaler Eventin	Relief of nasal congestion or rhinitis	*Adults:* 1 or 2 inhalations with each nostril q2-3h. (NOTE: Each inhalation provides approximately 0.25 mg) *Children: Not recommended*	Inhaler: 250 mg Store in cool place in tightly closed containers; recap immediately after use to minimize evaporation	Tolerance and dependence have been reported after prolonged use; because of high abuse potential, (when removed from inhaler and injected IV), other agents and formulations are recommended	See Decongestants

★ **Pseudo-ephedrine**
Actifed*
Afrinol
Ambenyl-D Decongestant Cough Formula*
Benylin Decongestant*
Besan
Conafed
Chlor-Trimeton Decongestant*
Codimal*
CoTylenol*
D-Feda
Disophrel*
Drixoral*
Eltor
Emprazil*
Fedahist*
Fedrazil*
First Sign
Histalet Syrup*
Historal*
Kodet SE
Naldegesic*
Nasalspan*
Novafed
Novahistine Sinus*
Polaramine
Pseudofrin Expectorant*
Pseudofrin
Robitussin-PE*
Rondec*
Sinufed
Sudadrine
Sudafed
Sudo-60
Sudodrin
Sudrin
Symptom 2
Tussend*

For relief of nasal congestion or rhinitis

Adults: 60 mg PO t.i.d. to q.i.d. up to a maximum of 240 mg q.d.
Children: 2-6 years old, 15 mg PO q.6h.; 6-12 years old, 30 mg PO q.6h.
Extended-release
Adults: 120 mg q.8-12h.
Children: Less than 6 years old, *not* recommended; 6-12 years old, 60 mg q.8-12h.
To minimize insomnia, last dose should be administered 3 to 4 hours before bedtime
Patients should be advised to swallow extended-release capsule whole without crushing or chewing

Capsule, extended-release: 60, 120 mg
Elixir: 30 mg/5 ml
Syrup: 30 mg/5 ml
Tablet: 30, 60 mg
Tablet, extended-release: 120 mg
Store between 15° and 30° C in tightly closed containers and protect from light

See Decongestants

See Decongestants

Continued.

NURSING DRUG DIGEST—cont'd

Medication (trade name)	Indication	Usual dosage and administration	Dosage forms, preparation, and storage	Contraindications, cautions, and comments	Monitoring
★ **Tetrahydrozoline** Tyzine	Relief of nasal congestion or rhinitis See also Chapter 24, "Sympathomimetics and Sympatholytics"	*Adults:* 2-4 drops or sprays of a 0.1% solution instilled into each nostril q.3-4h. *Children:* 2-6 years old, 2-3 drops of a 0.05% solution instilled into each nostril q.3-4h.; over 6 years old, see adult dose	Nasal drops: 0.05%, 0.1% Nasal spray: 0.1% Store in tightly closed containers	See Decongestants	See Decongestants
Xylometazoline Dristamead Long Dristan Long-Lasting Nasal Mist Dristan Long-Lasting Vapor Nasal Mist Duramist PM Hydra-Spray Neo-Synephrine 11 Otrivin Sine-Off Once-A-Day Sinex-L.A. Sinus Spray Sinutab Long-lasting Decongestant Sinus Spray Sinutab Nasal	Relief of nasal congestion or rhinitis	*Adults:* 2 or 3 drops or sprays of 0.1% solution into each nostril q.8-12h. *Children:* 2-12 years old, 2 or 3 drops of 0.05% solution into each nostril q.12h.	Nasal drops: 0.05%, 0.1% Nasal spray: 0.1% Store between 15° and 30° C in tightly closed containers and protect from light	Similar to oxymetazoline See Decongestants	See Decongestants

Spray
Sustaine
Vicks Sinex Long-Acting Decongestant Nasal Spray
4-Way Long-Acting Nasal Spray

EXPECTORANTS

Acetylcysteine
Airbron
Mucomyst
MAC

To promote productive cough and prevent accumulation of tenacious airway secretions (also given PO in experimental treatment of hepatotoxicity associated with acetaminophen overdosage)

Direct instillation: 1 to 2 ml of 10% or 20% solution instilled through tracheostomy, bronchoscope, or intratracheal catheter, may repeat hourly
Nebulization: 1 to 10 ml of 10% or 20% solution q.4-6h. with face mask, mouthpiece, or tracheostomy tube; 50 to 300 ml (enough to maintain heavy mist) of 10% or 20% solution in oxygen tent, head tent, or croup tent

Solution: 10%, 20%
Store in airtight containers; opened or diluted solution should be stored in refrigerator in tightly closed containers and used within 96 hours (NOTE: a light purple color may develop but will not impair effectiveness of solution)
Discoloration will occur if solution comes in contact with rubber, iron, or copper

Always have a bronchodilator ready for use because severe bronchospasm and dyspnea may develop
Following use, rinse face and equipment with water to remove sticky coating left by drug
Encourage fluid intake and maintenance of adequate hydration
Advise patient that foul odor is to be expected
If coughing is inadequate, mechanical aspiration should be considered to facilitate expectoration
Hand-operated nebulizers should *not* be used because droplet size produced in this manner is too large

Continued.

NURSING DRUG DIGEST—cont'd

Medication (trade name)	Indication	Usual dosage and administration	Dosage forms, preparation, and storage	Contraindications, cautions, and comments	Monitoring
Ammonium chloride Amchlor Ammoneric Baby Cough Syrup Chlor-Trimeton Expectorant* Colrex Expectorant* Coricidin Antitussive* DeWitt's Baby Cough Syrup* Dextrotussin Syrup* Endotussin-NN* Histadyl EC* Noratuss* Pinex Wild Cherry Pre-Mens Forte* PBZ Expectorant with Ephedrine* Rhinex DM Syrup* Romilar CF* Triaminicol Decongestant Cough Syrup*	Use as expectorant *no* longer recommended	*Formerly* used as expectorant	Tablet: 500 mg More commonly included in combination preparations Store in tightly closed containers Enteric-coated tablet *not* used as expectorant because gastric irritation decreases, and therefore expectorant activity is decreased	Encourage fluid intake and maintenance of adequate hydration	Monitor respiratory signs because dyspnea and hyperventilation may signify development of acidosis (see Chapter 67, "Fluids and Electrolytes")

Guaifenesin Actifed Expectorant* Actifed-C* Adatuss D.C. Expectorant* Ambenyl-D Decongestant Cough Formula* Anatuss* Anti-Tuss Balminil Expectorant Biotussin Bronchicide Broncho-Grippex Brondecon* Bronitin* Cheracol D* Cheracol* Chlor-Trimeton Expectorant* Choledyl Expectorant* Colrex Expectorant* Conar Expectorant* Conex* Coricidin Antitussive* Corutol Expectorant Coryban-D Antitussive* Demo-Cineol Demo-Cineol Expectorant Syrup Dimacol Dimetane Expectorant*	To promote productive cough and prevent accumulation of tenacious airway secretions (efficacy *not* clearly demonstrated)	*Adults:* 100-400 mg PO q.4-6h. up to a *maximum* of 2400 mg/day *Children:* 2-6 years old, 50 mg PO q.4h.; 6-12 years old, 50-100 mg PO q.4-6h.	Capsule: 100, 200 mg Syrup: 100 mg/5 ml Tablet: 100, 200 mg Store in tightly closed containers	Relaxant effect on skeletal muscle may be observed with high dosage Encourage fluid intake and maintenance of adequate hydration May decrease platelet aggregation, caution suggested when administered to patients receiving anticoagulants

Continued.

NURSING DRUG DIGEST—cont'd

Medication (trade name)	Indication	Usual dosage and administration	Dosage forms, preparation, and storage	Contraindications, cautions, and comments	Monitoring
Guaifenesin—cont'd					
Donaril Anti-cough*					
Dorcol Pedi-atric*					
Entuss Ex-pectorant*					
Fedahist Ex-pectorant*					
Formula 44-D*					
G.L. Tussin					
Gaiapect					
Glycotuss					
Glytuss					
Gualanesin					
GG-Con					
Histalet X*					
Hycotuss*					
Hytuss					
Hytuss 2X					
Motussin					
Mudrane GG*					
Naldecon-CX*					
Nortussin					
Novahistine DMX*					
Novahistine Expecto-rant*					
Pertussin Cough Syrup for Children*					
Polaramine Expecto-rant*					
Pseudo-Bid*					

Pseudo-Mist
Expecto-
rant*
Queltuss*
Quibron Plus*
Quibron*
Resyl
Rhinex DM
Syrup*
Robitussin
Robitussin-
CP*
Robitussin-
DM*
Robitussin-
PE*
Romex*
Sedatuss Ex-
pectorant
Slo-Phyllin
GG*
Soltice*
Sorbutuss*
Sudafed
Cough*
Triaminic Ex-
pectorant*
Tussanca
Tussar-SF*
Tussar-2*
Tussciden
Expecto-
rant
Tussend Ex-
pectorant*
Vicks Cough
Syrup*
Vicks Formula
44D Decon-
gestant
Cough Mix-
ture*
2/G
2/G-DM*

Continued.

NURSING DRUG DIGEST—cont'd

Medication (trade name)	Indication	Usual dosage and administration	Dosage forms, preparation, and storage	Contraindications, cautions, and comments	Monitoring
Iodides (potassium iodide) Iodo-Niacin* Isuprel Compound Elixir* KI KIE* Mudrane* Mudrane-2* Pediacof* Pima Syrup Quadrinal Rum-K SSKI	To promote productive cough and prevent accumulation of tenacious airway secretions when less toxic agents are ineffective	*Adults:* 250-500 mg PO q,4-6h. *Children: Not* established Liquid formulation should be well diluted with water or juice before administration and should be taken with food to minimize irritation NOTE: Use of enteric-coated tablets has been associated with small bowel lesions, and use is *not* recommended	Solution: 167 mg/5 ml Syrup: 325 mg/5 ml Tablets: enteric-coated: 300, 650 mg Store between 15° and 30° C in tightly closed container and protect from light; do *not* refrigerate Solutions with brown discoloration should be discarded Crystallization of solution may occur; warming and shaking will redissolve crystals	*Contraindicated* in patients with hypersensitivity to iodine and in patients with hyperthyroidism or goiter because of increased risk of thyrotoxicosis or myxedema *Contraindicated* in hyperkalemia Encourage fluid intake and maintenance of adequate hydration May aggravate acne, particularly in adolescents *Not* recommended for use during pregnancy; may be secreted into breast milk in concentrations high enough to affect infant To reduce risk of iodism, therapy should be short-term and recommended dosages should not be exceeded	Monitor patients for signs of iodism including rash, fever, acne, parotitis, and metallic aftertaste; if symptoms develop, discontinue use and consult prescriber Monitor for GI distress

Drug	Use	Dosage	Remarks	Nursing Implications
Ipecac Cerose DM* Cerose* Cetro Cirose* Dr. Drake's* Quelidrine* Sorbutuss*	Use as expectorant *no longer* recommended (see Chapter 40, "Emetics and Antiemetics")	*Formerly* used as expectorant	Syrup contains not less than 123 mg and not more than 157 mg of total ether soluble alkaloids of ipecac. NOTE: Fluidextract, approximately 14 times stronger than syrup, is still available in some areas. Store in tightly closed containers and protect from light	*Risk* of acute toxicity and death if fluidextract used in place of syrup. Large dosages may cause persistent vomiting, bloody diarrhea, dehydration, and vasomotor collapse. See Chapter 40, "Emetics and Antiemetics"
Terpin hydrate Broncho-Tussin* Cotussis* Creo-Terpin* Mycinettes Sugar Free* Noratuss* Prunicodeine* Terpo-Diomin* Toclonol with Codeine* Toclonol Expectorant* Tricodene C-V* Tussagesic Suspension* Tussagesic* Tussaminic*	To promote productive cough and prevent accumulation of tenacious airway secretions; efficacy *not* clearly demonstrated	*Adults:* 50-150 mg PO q4h.	Elixir: 85 mg/5 ml (NOTE: 39% to 44% alcohol content). Slight warming and shaking should redissolve any formed crystals. Store between 15° and 30° C in tightly closed containers. Generally found in combination products (e.g., terpin hydrate and codeine)	Encourage fluid intake and maintenance of adequate hydration. High alcoholic content may cause drowsiness; patients should be advised not to drive or engage in other activities requiring mental alertness or precise motor coordination until individual response is known

BIBLIOGRAPHY

Chasnoff, I.J., Diggs, G., & Schnoll, S.H. Fetal alcohol effects and maternal cough syrup abuse. *Amercian Journal of Diseases of Children*, 1981, *135*, 968.

Connell, J.T., Williams, B.O., Allen, S., Cato, A, & Perkins, J.G. A double-blind controlled evaluation of Actifed and its individual constituents in allergic rhinitis. *Journal of International Medical Research*, 1982, *10*, 341-347.

Crutcher, J.E., and Kantner, T.R. The effectiveness of antihistamines in the common cold. *Journal of Clinical Pharmacology*, 1981, *21*, 9-15.

Diwan, J., Dhand, R., Jindal, S.K., Malik, S. K., & Sharma, P.L. A comparative randomized double-blind clinical trial of isoaminile citrate and chlophedianol hydrochloride as antitussive agents. *International Journal of Clinical Pharmacology, Therapy, and Toxicology*, 1982, *20*, 373-375.

Eigen, H. The clinical evaluation of chronic cough. *Pediatric Clinics of North America*, 1982, *29*, 67-78.

Empey, D.W., Laitinen, L.A., Young, G.A., Bye, C.E., & Hughes, D.T. Comparison of the antitussive effects of codeine phosphate 20 mg, dextromethorphan 30 mg and noscapine 30 mg using citric acid-induced cough in normal subjects. *European Journal of Clinical Pharmacology*, 1979, *16*, 393-397.

Empey, D.W., & Medder, K.T. Nasal decongestants. *Drugs*, 1981, *21*, 438-443.

Empey, D.W., Young, G.A., Letley, E., John, G.C., Smith, P., McDonnell, K.A., Bagg, L.R., & Hughes, D.T. Dose-response study of the nasal decongestant and cardiovascular effects of pseudoephedrine. *British Journal of Clinical Pharmacology*, 1980, *9*, 351-358.

Escobar, J.I., & Karno, M. Chronic hallucinosis from nasal drops. *Journal of the American Medical Association*, 1982, *247*, 1859-1860.

Gwaltey, J.M., Jr. Epidemiology of the common cold. *Annals of the New York Academy of Sciences*, 1980, *353*, 54-60.

Hamilton, L.H. Nasal decongestant effect of propylhexedrine. (Pt. 1), *Annals of Otology, Rhinology and Laryngology*, 1982, *1*, 106-111.

Hamilton, M., Bush, M., Bye, C., & Peck, A.W. A comparison of triprolidine and cyclizine on histamine (H1) antagonism, subjective effects and performance tests in man. *British Journal of Clinical Pharmacology*, 1982, *13*, 441-444.

Howard J.C., Jr., Katner, T.R., Lilienfield, L.S., Princiotlo, J.V., Krum, R.E., Crutcher, J.E., Belman, M.A., & Danzig, M.R. Effectiveness of antihistamines in the symptomatic management of the common cold. *Journal of the American Medical Association*, 1979, *242*, 2414-2417.

Irwin, R.S., & Pratter, M.R. Treatment of cough. *Chest*, 1982, *82*, 662-663. (Editorial)

Kuhn, J.J., Hendley, J.O., Adams, K.F., Clark, J.W., & Gwaltney, J.M., Jr. Antitussive effect of guaifenesin in young adults with natural colds. Objective and subjective assessment. *Chest*, 1982, *82*, 713-718.

Leighton, K.M. Paranoid psychosis after abuse of Actifed. *British Medical Journal*, 1982, *284*, 789-790.

Lewiston, N.J., Johnson, S., & Sloan, E. Effect of antihistamine on pulmonary function of children with asthma. *Journal of Pediatrics*, 1982, *101*, 458-460.

Middleton, R.S. Double blind trial in general practice comparing the efficacy of "Benylin Day and Night" and paracetamol in the treatment of the common cold. *British Journal of Clinical Practice*, 1981, *35*, 297-300.

Mullan, P.A. Cough/cold preparations. *American Pharmacy*, 1981, *21*, 42-45.

Petruson, B. Treatment with xylometazoline (Otrivin) nosedrops over a six-week period. *Rhinology*, 1981, *19*, 167-172.

Reed, S.E. The common cold. *Practitioner*, 1979, *223*, 753-757.

Reed, S.E. The aetiology and epidemiology of common colds, and the possibilities of prevention. *Clinical Otolaryngology*, 1981, *6*, 379-387.

Reinhardt, D., & Borchard, U. H1-receptor antagonists: comparative pharmacology and clinical use. *Klinische Wochenschrift*, 1982, *60*, 983-990.

Richardson, P.S. The principles of drug action on cough and on sputum characteristics. *European Journal of Respiratory Diseases*, 1980, *61*(110), 67-79. (Suppl.)

Secher, C., Kirkegaard, J., Borum, P., Maansson, A., Osterhammel, P., & Mygind, N. Significance of H1 and H2 receptors in the human nose: rationale for topical use of combined antihistamine preparations. *Journal of Allergy and Clinical Immunology*, 1982, *70*, 211-218.

Simons, F.E., Frith, E.M., & Simons, K.J. The pharmacokinetics and antihistaminic effects of brompheniramine. *Journal of Allergy and Clinical Immunology*, 1982, *70*, 458-464.

Svedmyr, N. General aspects on evaluation of drug effects on cough and expectoration. *European Journal of Respiratory Diseases*, 1980, *61*(110), 81-92. (Suppl.)

Toohill, R.J., Lehman, R.H., Grossman, T.W., & Belson, T.P. Rhinitis medicamentosa. *Laryngoscope*, 1981, *91*, 1614-1621.

Van de Donk, H.J., Van den Heuel, H.G., Zuidema, J., & Merkus, F.W. The effects of nasal drops and their additives on human nasal mucociliary clearance. *Rhinology*, 1982, *20*, 127-137.

Virtanen, H. The effect of an oral combined preparation (antihistamine and decongestant) on Eustachian tube function in the common cold. *Journal of Oto-Rhino-Larnygology and Its Related Specialties*, 1982, *44*, 268-276.

Zanjanian, M.H. Expectorants and antitussive agents: are they helpful? *Annals of Allergy*, 1980, *44*, 290-295.

CARDIOVASCULAR MEDICATIONS

Medications discussed in this section

Review of the Anatomy, Physiology, and Assessment of the Cardiovascular System

Loren W. Kline

The cardiovascular system is composed of the heart and blood vessels. The functions of the cardiovascular system are to deliver nutrients, oxygen, and hormones to the tissues and to remove the waste products of metabolism.

ANATOMY OF THE HEART

The movement of the blood throughout the body requires the rhythmical pumping action of the heart. The heart is a hollow organ that lies in the thoracic cavity within the mediastinum. The base of the heart lies in the top of the thoracic cavity behind the upper portion of the body of the sternum; the lower portion, the apex, is directed downward and to the left midclavicular line. Figure 30-1 shows the four chambers of the heart, the heart valves, and other related structures. The heart is divided into right and left halves. Each half is composed of a receiving chamber, or atrium, and a ventricle. The right atrium receives unoxygenated blood from the venae cavae and the left atrium receives oxygenated blood from the lungs via the pulmonary vein. Below the atria are the ventricles. The right ventricle pumps the unoxygenated blood, received from the right atria, through the pulmonary artery to the lungs and the pulmonary circulation. The left ventricle pumps oxygenated blood, received from the left atria, to the body by way of the aorta and the systemic circulation.

The direction of blood flow is controlled by valves. The valves are located between the atria and ventricles and at the base of the aorta and pulmonary artery. The bicuspid or mitral valve separates the left atrium and ventricle. The tricuspid valve separates the right atrium and ventricle. The bicuspid valve is composed of two triangular flaps of connective tissue; the tricuspid valve of three flaps. These valves open when the atria contract and force blood into the ventricles. These valves close during ventricular contraction and thereby prevent backflow of blood into the atria. The valve flaps are anchored to the ventricle heart wall by chordae tendinae and papillary muscles that prevent the atrioventricular valves from being inverted during ventricular contraction.

The valves at the base of the pulmonary and aortic arteries are called semilunar valves (Figure 30-2). These valves open during ventricular contraction to allow the blood to flow to the lungs or to the body. The semilunar valves close after ventricular contraction to prevent backflow into the ventricles.

The cardiac cycle begins with the return of blood from the systemic circulation to the right atrium, where it is pumped into the right ventricle. The blood leaving the right ventricle travels via the pulmonary artery to the lungs. The blood passes through the capillaries of the lungs to remove carbon dioxide in exchange for oxygen. The oxygenated blood is pumped to the left atrium, where it is pumped to the left ventricle and through the aorta and is pumped throughout the body via the systemic circulation. Oxygenated blood travels to all regions of the body and exchanges oxygen for carbon dioxide. This blood returns to the right heart and the circuit is complete (Figures 30-3 and 30-4).

Before the peripheral parts of the circulatory system are discussed, the mechanisms involved in coordinating the actions of the heart are considered.

The heart is composed of cardiac muscle, nodal tissue, and connective tissue. Cardiac muscle has a striated appearance similar to that of skeletal muscle (Figure 30-5). The fibers branch and interconnect with each other, forming a latticework or syncytium. In the heart are two separate muscle syncytia. One makes up the atria, and the other constitutes the ventricles. These two muscle masses are separated by a disk of connective tissue that surrounds the valves between the atria and the ventricles.

The individual muscle fibers are separated from the

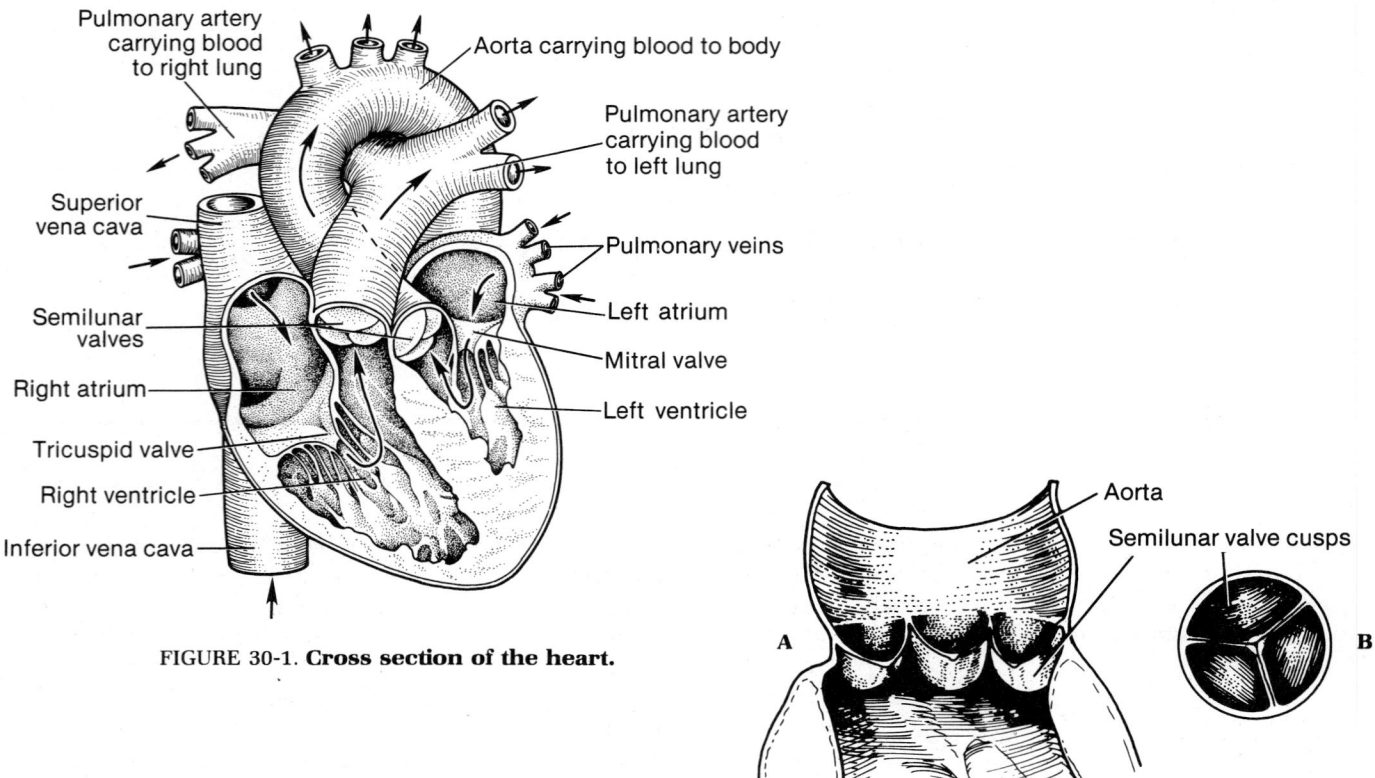

FIGURE 30-1. **Cross section of the heart.**

FIGURE 30-2. *A,* **Aortic valve cross section.** *B,* **Aortic valve closed, viewed from above.**

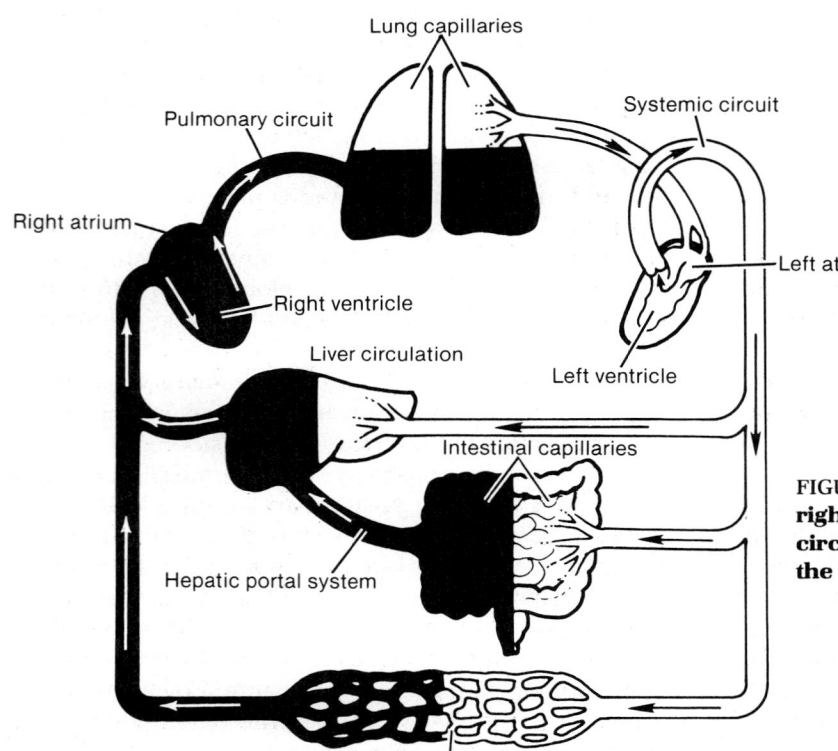

FIGURE 30-3. **Schematic diagram of the circulation. The right side of the heart pumps blood into the pulmonary circulation. The left side of the heart pumps blood into the systemic circulation.**

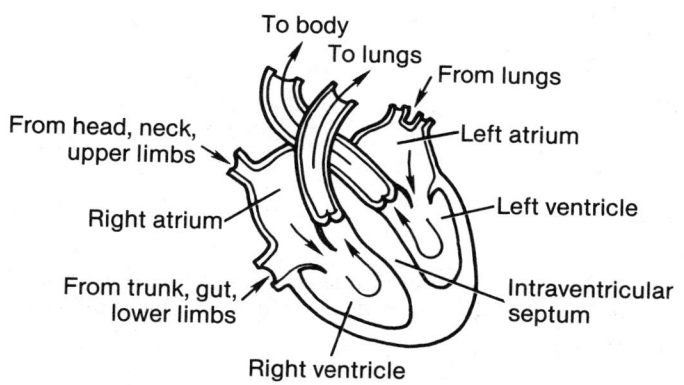

FIGURE 30-4. **Blood flow through the heart.**

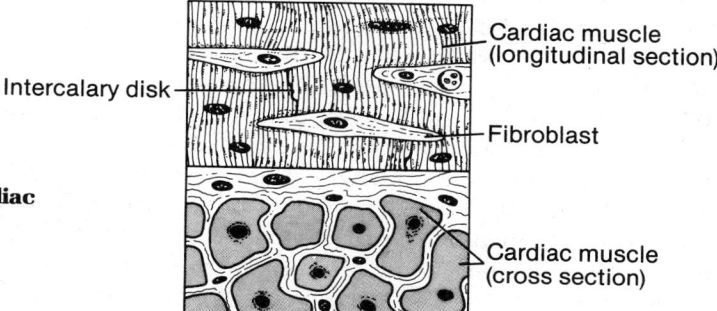

FIGURE 30-5. **Longitudinal and cross sections of cardiac muscle.**

neighboring cells by intercalated disks. These areas are tight junctions of low electrical resistance between the cells that facilitate the spread of action potentials (APs) through the muscle.

PHYSIOLOGY OF THE HEART
Mechanical properties of cardiac muscle

Cardiac muscle follows several general principles of muscle function, such as the All-or-None Law and the length-tension relationship. The All-or-None Law states that an adequate stimulus initiates a maximal contractile response, the strength depending on the conditions present at the time of stimulation. The length-tension relationship as applied to the heart has been called the law of the heart or Starling's law. Starling's law states that the more the cardiac fibers are stretched, within limits, the more forcefully they will contract. Thus, as more blood enters the ventricle, the muscle is stretched and the force to pump the blood out increases.

Like skeletal muscle, cardiac muscle undergoes a series of electrical events before contraction. An AP sweeps over the muscle depolarizing it and initiating the events that lead to a mechanical change in muscle length. Cardiac muscle repolarizes more slowly than skeletal muscle. This gives rise to a period when no stimulus will cause a second response. This period is called the absolute refractory period. This is followed by a relative refractory period, a period when a stronger than normal stimulus may initiate a response. The absolute refractory period is so long that it lasts into the relaxation phase of cardiac muscle activity. This ensures the muscle will be partially relaxed and allows for filling the ventricles before the next contraction. This long refractory period prevents tetany from normally occurring and assures that the normal cardiac cycle is maintained.

Electrical properties of cardiac muscle

The heart has the characteristic property of rhythmic self-excitation known as autorhythmicity. This property is the result of specialized cardiac muscle known as nodal tissue. Whereas all fibers of the heart can conduct APs, the nodal tissue has a faster conduction velocity than the general cardiac muscle fibers. Not only does nodal tissue have a faster rate of conduction, but it also spontaneously depolarizes cyclically.

The nodal tissue is present in the form of bundles

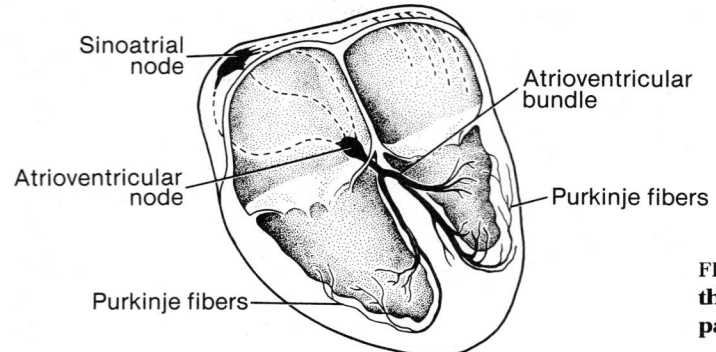

FIGURE 30-6. **The conducting system, Purkinje system, of the heart. The dotted lines represent the internodal pathway.**

and fibers within the heart and includes (Figure 30-6) the sinoatrial (SA) node and the atrioventricular (AV) node. The SA node initiates the rhythmic impulses and is termed the pacemaker. The cause of this rhythmicity is the permeability of the SA node fibers to sodium. At rest the membrane is permeable to sodium. Sodium ions continually leak into the fibers, causing the resting potential to rise toward a positive value. When the membrane reaches the threshold value, an AP is generated. As the AP ends, the membrane becomes highly permeable to potassium ions. As the positive potassium ions leak out of the fibers, the inside membrane potential becomes more negative. This condition lasts for a fraction of a second and then disappears as the membrane returns to its normal state of permeability. The leakiness to sodium ions is reestablished and the cycle continues. The other node, the atrioventricular node (AV node), may also generate APs; however, the frequency of the SA node–generated APs is usually greater than the AV-node rate, thus the SA node initiates the sequence of events giving rise to the heart beat.

The APs generated by the SA node travel through the atrial muscle wall and are carried to the left atrium at the rate of 1 m/sec. These specialized pathways called internodal pathways serve to conduct the APs directly from the SA node to the AV node. These pathways are composed of a mixture of ordinary myocardial cells and Purkinje fibers that are similar to those in the ventricle.

The conduction velocity is slow near the AV node, and there is a conduction delay at the AV node. The delay is necessary to coordinate the pumping action of the heart. The distance from the SA to the AV nodes is shorter than from the SA node to the most distant part of the left atrium. It is necessary to slow the passage of the APs through the nodal tissue until both atria have completed their contraction, which allows for emptying the atria and filling the ventricles.

The AP is transmitted in the ventricles through the Purkinje fibers, which originate in the AV node, form the AV bundle, divide into left and right bundle branches, curve around the ventricular apex, and spread to the base of the ventricles. Only about 0.06 seconds elapses between the arrival of the AP at the AV node and excitation of the ventricular muscle. Whereas only adjacent cardiac muscle is directly stimulated by the Purkinje fibers, the AP spreads throughout the muscle mass.

The function of the Purkinje system is to transmit the cardiac APs rapidly throughout the atria and then throughout the ventricles. Rapid conduction allows all portions of each cardiac syncytium to contract in unison so that each will exert a coordinated pumping effort. Without the Purkinje system conduction would be slow and some parts of the syncytium would contract before others, giving rise to an uncoordinated contraction generating little force.

ELECTROCARDIOGRAM

The electric potential changes in the heart may be recorded from the body surface by way of an electrocardiogram (ECG). The ECG is a useful diagnostic aid. The characteristics of the ECG (Figure 30-7) are the following.

1. P wave represents atrial depolarization. The P wave is about 0.25 mV in strength and lasts for about 0.1 seconds.
2. QRS complex is the result of ventricular depolarization. The QRS complex is about 1 mV in strength and has a duration of about 0.08 seconds.
3. T wave is the result of ventricular repolarization.

The time intervals between the different waves provide valuable information about the conduction of the depolarization through the cardiac muscle. The two important intervals routinely used are the P-R and Q-T intervals.

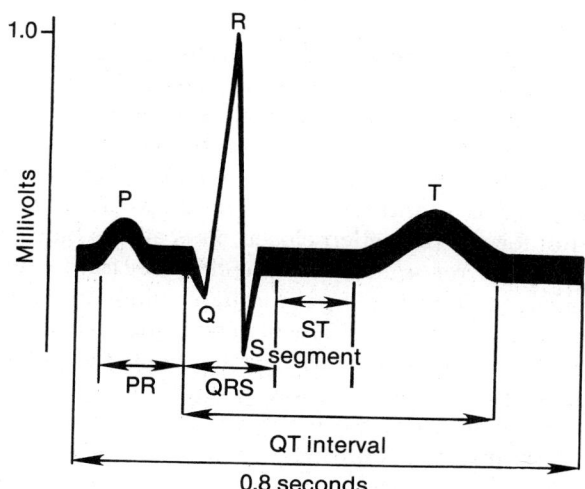

FIGURE 30-7. **Normal electrocardiogram.**

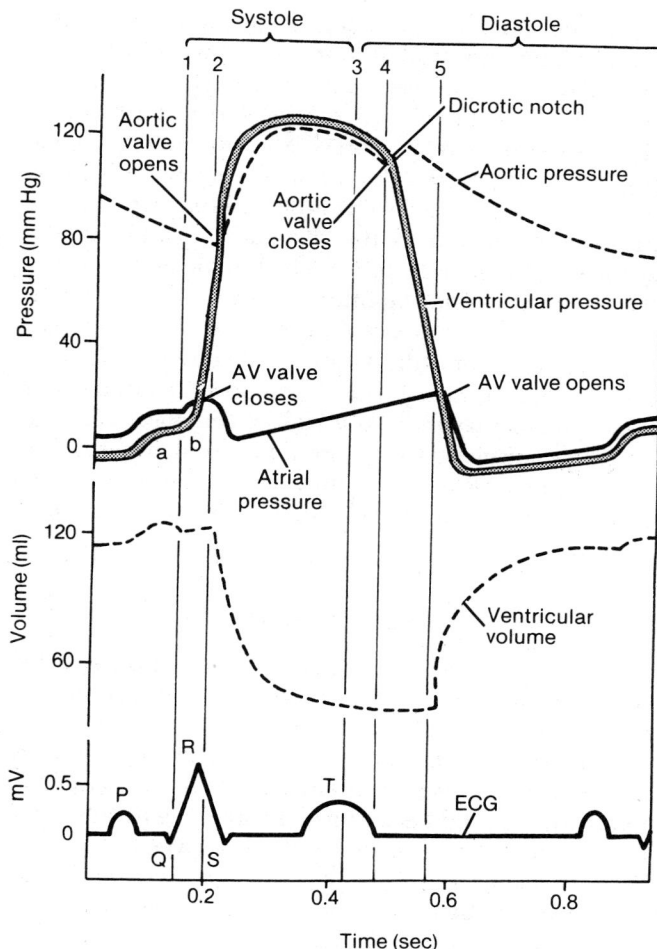

FIGURE 30-8. **Wigger's chart illustrating pressure and volume changes, valve action, and electric events during a single cardiac cycle.**

The P-R interval is measured from the beginning of the P wave to the beginning of the R wave. It represents the time taken from the start of the excitation at the SA node to the beginning of ventricular depolarization (i.e., depolarization of the atrium, conduction through the AV node and the Purkinje system to the ventricular muscle). This is normally 0.16 to 0.20 seconds. An increase in this interval indicates a slowing of the conduction system, usually in the AV node.

The Q-T interval represents the total time for the ventricular muscle to depolarize and repolarize. This interval is longer for men and children than for women, and is usually reduced as the heart rate increases. Speeding of the heart is accomplished more by shortening the period of electric activity.

CARDIAC CYCLE

A cardiac cycle is defined as one complete series of events during heart activity. Figure 30-8 illustrates the major events of the cycle, including pressure changes, the ECG, and the phonogram. The beginning of the cardiac cycle is usually considered as the initiation of an AP by the SA node. The depolarization spreads over the atria, giving rise to the P wave. The mechanical events quickly follow. The atria begin to contract, raising the pressure exerted on the blood within the atria. The pressure rises until the pressure exerted opens the AV valves, and the blood enters the ventricles. Meanwhile the AP has passed through the AV node and the AV bundles. The AP spreads rapidly over the ventricles causing the QRS complex of the ECG and stimulates the ventricular muscle to contract. The rising ventricular pressure closes the AV valves, thereby generating the first heart sound (S₁). The ven-

tricles continue to contract against a constant volume of blood. This phase is called the isovolumetric systolic period. This period lasts until the pressure generated by the contracting ventricles opens the semilunar valves. The blood is then forced out of the ventricles under pressure and the blood volume in the ventricles decreases. The muscles relax (T wave) and the pressure behind the blood falls. The semilunar valves close, giving rise to the second heart sound (S₂). The muscle continues to relax. This phase of relaxation is called the isovolumetric relaxation period. Pressure in the aorta, and to a lesser extent in the pulmonary artery, remains high while the ventricular pressure rapidly decreases. The ventricles never completely eject all the blood within them (end diastolic volume). The pressure in the ventricle drops below the atrial pressure. The AV valves open and blood again flows into the ventricles. Each cycle takes, at rest, only 0.8 seconds.

The period of the cardiac cycle when the ventricles are contracting is called systole. Systolic blood pressure is the pressure generated by ventricular contraction. The normal value is considered to be 120 mm Hg. The period of relaxation is called diastole. Diastolic pressure is the arterial blood pressure when the heart is relaxed. The normal value is 80 mm Hg. The diastolic pressure is related to the distensible nature of the aorta and the major arteries. The blood ejected by the left ventricle cannot be immediately passed throughout the system because of peripheral resistance (i.e., the resistance of a fluid to pass through a tube). As the blood is pumped into it, the aorta distends. The heavy muscle layers in the wall of the aorta contract and force the blood throughout the circulatory system.

The pulse pressure is the difference between the systolic pressure and diastolic pressure. It is normally 40 mm Hg.

HEART SOUNDS

Heart sounds are generated as the heart pumps the blood. Because of the alternating cycle of contraction and relaxation the movement of the blood occurs in spurts. The abrupt increase in ventricular pressure closes the AV valves. This causes vibrations or turbulence that can be heard through the chest walls with auscultation. This closure of the AV valves causes the first heart sound (S_1). The second sound (S_2) occurs as the ventricles begin to relax and the aortic and pulmonary semilunar valves close.

Anatomically, the valves are in close proximity. However, they can be best heard with a stethoscope over different areas of the chest wall. The pulmonic valve is best auscultated in the second left intercostal space at the sternal border. The aortic valve is heard at the second right intercostal space at the sternal border. When auscultating the tricuspid valve, one hears the sound best along the lower left sternal border at the fourth left intercostal space. The closure of the mitral valve is best heard at the apex in the fifth intercostal space at the midclavicular line or at the apical impulse—point of maximum impulse (PMI). Other heart sounds can also be auscultated. The third heart sound (S_3) can be heard at the apex with the bell of the stethoscope during early diastole as the ventricles are filled passively with blood. The fourth heart sound (S_4) can be heard during late diastole because rapid ventricular filling occurs just before S_1. S_4 is also heard best at the base with the bell of the stethoscope. Extra sounds (e.g., the opening snap of the mitral valve and the ejection click) are caused by diseased valves and are abnormal, as are sounds produced by pericardial friction rub.

Heart murmurs may arise if the valves become deformed. The murmurs result from the development of turbulence in the rapidly flowing blood. Prolonged sounds during systole and diastole are produced resulting in systolic or diastolic murmurs. Two conditions of the valves cause heart murmurs. Valvular insufficiency is a condition where the cusps of the valves do not form a seal when closed. This allows blood to leak back or regurgitate into the chamber from which it had been pumped. The regurgitated blood interferes with the incoming stream of blood and causes detectable turbulence. Murmurs are often best heard around the area of the involved valve.

Insufficiency of a valve may be the result of deformity, rigidity, retraction, fusion of the cusps or chordae tendinae, the presence of a particular orifice, or valvular growths or scar tissue. Some of these problems may be congenital; others may be caused by disease. Rheumatic endocarditis is the most common disease leading to abnormalities of the heart valves. Other causes of valvular disease include syphilis, bacterial endocarditis, calcification of the valves, and trauma. Stenosis or valvular growths that may narrow the opening, interfering with the blood flow through it, constitute the second cause of heart murmurs. One result of a stenosis is that the heart must work harder to overcome the increased resistance to blood flow through the restricted opening. Stenosis of the valves is caused by fusion of the leaflets, rigidity of the cusps because of fibrosis or shortening, and adherences of the chordae tendinae. Often the causes of a murmur are present simultaneously.

Functional murmurs of a nonpathologic origin often occur in children and young people. These murmurs are often detected at times of increased blood-flow rate (e.g., after heavy exercise).

BLOOD PRESSURE

Many factors may affect arterial blood pressure. These include factors that affect blood pressure on a moment-to-moment basis, including the generalized factors of age, sex, stress, body build, diet, exercise, and emotional status.

Age exerts a definite influence on blood pressure. From birth to puberty the blood pressure rises rapidly at first and then undergoes a steady gradual rise. At puberty a sudden rise occurs. A steady, though not great, rise in blood pressure occurs from adolescence to old age. Women have an additional abrupt rise in blood pressure at menopause. The systolic pressure in women is usually 4 to 5 mm Hg lower than in men until the rise at menopause. The values for women are then slightly higher than for men (Table 30-1).

TABLE 30-1

Mean blood pressure and standard deviations in apparently healthy persons

Age group (yr)	Men		Women	
	Systolic	**Diastolic**	**Systolic**	**Diastolic**
20-24	123 ± 13.7	76 ± 9.9	116 ± 11.8	72 ± 9.7
25-29	125 ± 12.6	78 ± 9.0	117 ± 11.4	74 ± 9.1
30-34	126 ± 13.6	79 ± 9.7	120 ± 14.0	75 ± 10.8
35-39	127 ± 14.2	80 ± 10.4	124 ± 13.9	78 ± 10.0
40-44	129 ± 15.1	81 ± 9.5	127 ± 17.1	80 ± 10.6
45-49	130 ± 16.9	82 ± 10.8	131 ± 19.5	82 ± 11.6
50-54	135 ± 19.2	83 ± 11.3	137 ± 21.3	84 ± 12.4
55-59	138 ± 18.8	84 ± 11.4	139 ± 21.4	84 ± 11.8
60-64	142 ± 21.1	85 ± 12.4	144 ± 22.3	85 ± 13.0
65-69	143 ± 26.0	83 ± 9.9	154 ± 29.0	85 ± 13.8
70-74	145 ± 26.3	82 ± 15.3	159 ± 25.8	85 ± 15.3
75-79	146 ± 21.6	81 ± 12.9	158 ± 26.3	84 ± 13.1
80-84	145 ± 25.6	82 ± 9.9	157 ± 28.0	83 ± 13.1
85-89	145 ± 24.2	79 ± 14.9	154 ± 27.9	82 ± 17.3
90-94	145 ± 23.4	78 ± 12.1	150 ± 23.6	79 ± 12.1
95-106	146 ± 27.5	78 ± 12.7	149 ± 23.5	81 ± 12.5

Obese persons have a pronounced increase of systolic pressure in comparison with persons of normal weight of the same age. The incidence of abnormally high blood pressure (hypertension) is greater in overweight persons.

Emotional status, such as fear, anxiety, and shock markedly affect blood pressure, especially the systolic pressure. The effects are the result of increased cardiac action and changes in vasomotor tone.

Of all physiologic conditions, strenuous exercise has the most dramatic effect on the arterial blood pressure. During the muscular effort the systolic pressure may rise 60 to 80 mm Hg. The diastolic pressure usually undergoes a slight increase of 10 mm Hg and in light exercise there is no change. Diastolic pressure is affected by peripheral resistance. During exercise there is greater blood flow through the skeletal muscle. This is matched by a marked decrease in the amount of blood flowing through the gut and other visceral organs; consequently, there is little change in peripheral resistance.

Five other factors may affect the arterial blood pressure. These tend to be short term, and include (1) cardiac output (CO), (2) viscosity of the blood, (3) elasticity of the arterial walls, (4) volume of blood in the arterial system, and (5) caliber of the arterial lumen.

If the CO is increased suddenly, the arterial blood pressure increases. More blood is pumped into the arterial system than can exit, and the arterial walls are stretched. The pressure will rise until the flow becomes balanced again by increasing the outflow to the capillary and venous systems.

The caliber of the arterial system and the viscosity of the blood affect peripheral resistance. Under normal conditions, the viscosity of the blood does not vary appreciably. The caliber of the arteries, especially the arterioles, can vary and are under both neural and chemical control (this is discussed in the section on vasomotor control).

The quantity of blood in the arterial system affects the blood pressure in cases where the volume suddenly increases in the case of increased CO or when too much fluid is added during a transfusion. In cases of hemorrhage, if the volume of fluid loss is great, the pressure will fall.

The elasticity of the vessels contributes to the origin and maintenance of the diastolic pressure, as well as to sustaining the mean pressure at a higher level than would be possible in a rigid system (these properties are referred to in the section on diastolic pressure).

REFLEX CONTROL OF HEART RATE

Whereas the heart does not require nervous input to initiate contraction, the heart receives both sympathetic and parasympathetic innervation to aid in the fine control of the heart rate (Figure 30-9). The sensory receptors responsible for this fine control are called baroreceptors and are located in the walls of the heart, in the aortic arch, in the carotid sinus, in the superior

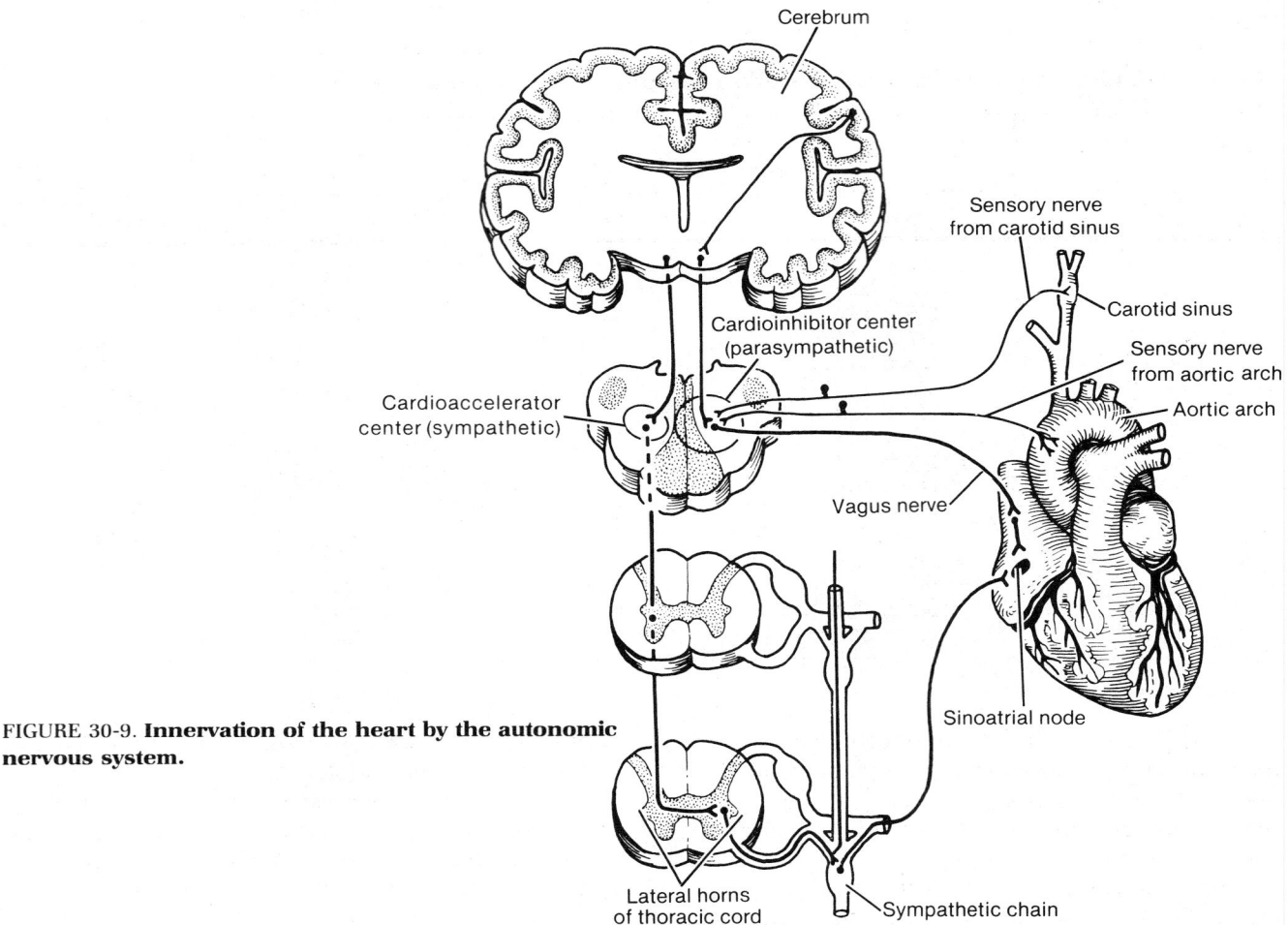

FIGURE 30-9. **Innervation of the heart by the autonomic nervous system.**

and inferior venae cavae as they enter the right atrium, and in the left atrium at the entrance of the pulmonary veins. These receptors respond to the distention or stretching of the structures in which they are located.

The sensory fibers pass in the glossopharyngeal (IX) and vagus (X) nerves to the cardioinhibitory center (CIC) of the medulla. When the structures are stretched, APs travel to the medulla and excite the CIC. The CIC is reciprocally innervated with the cardioaccelerator center (CAC). When the CIC is activated, the CAC is inhibited. In addition, vagal activity to the heart is increased. The right vagus sends more fibers to the SA node than does the left vagus, whereas the converse is true for the AV node. Thus vagal stimulation decreases the heart rate, decreases the force of contraction, decreases the conduction rate through the AV node, and decreases the blood flow through the coronary blood vessels. The blood pressure falls. When the pressure falls below normal within the carotid sinus, activity within the receptors decreases. This de-

creased activity inhibits the action of the CIC, and the CAC becomes active. The outflow from the CAC is carried by sympathetic fibers. These innervate both nodes and all parts of the myocardium. Sympathetic stimulation of the heart has the opposite effects of parasympathetic stimulation (i.e., increased heart rate, increased force of contraction, and increased blood flow to the coronary blood vessels). The heart rate may double or even triple under sympathetic stimulation.

Chemoreceptors, sensory receptors sensitive to carbon dioxide or lactic acid, are located in the carotid body. An increase in either carbon dioxide or lactic acid in the blood will stimulate these receptors. Activation of these receptors inhibits the cardioinhibitory center and the heart rate will increase.

Other chemicals may affect the heart rate. Epinephrine, a hormone secreted by the adrenal medulla and at the endings of postganglionic sympathetic fibers, acts on the cardiac muscle and the nerve fibers that innervate them. Epinephrine will increase the

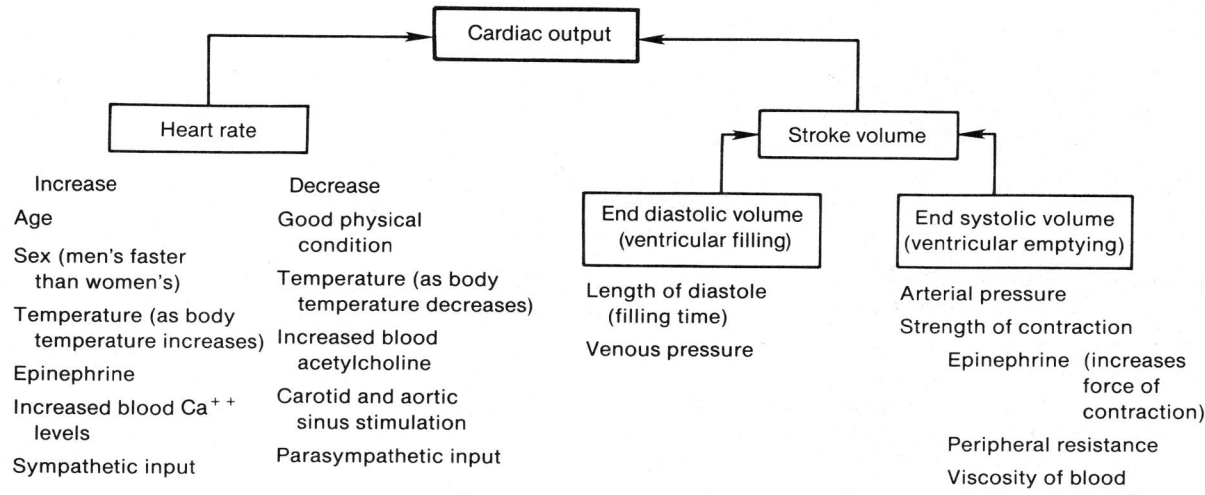

FIGURE 30-10. **Factors regulating cardiac output.**

TABLE 30-2

Mean heart rate and range in apparently healthy children

Age group	Mean heart rate (beats/min)	Range
0-30 hours	123	95-155
1-7 days	138	100-188
8-30 days	162	115-194
1-3 months	156	95-200
3-6 months	144	115-195
6-12 months	137	105-188
1-3 years	121	100-178
3-5 years	102	70-140
5-8 years	101	75-150
8-12 years	87	65-120
12-15 years	83	50-120

heart rate and the force of contraction. Plasma levels of calcium ions (Ca^{++}) also affect the heart. Decreased Ca^{++} levels lead to a weakness of the heart muscles. The duration of systole decreases, and the heart dilates excessively during diastole. Excess Ca^{++} promotes overcontraction of the heart. The muscle contracts too forcefully during systole and does not relax enough during diastole to allow for adequate filling of either the atria or ventricles. Age also affects heart rate (Table 30-2).

CARDIAC OUTPUT

Cardiac output (CO) is the amount of blood pumped by the heart in 1 minute. The volume of blood pumped in each ventricular contraction is called the stroke volume. The CO is then the product of the stroke volume and the heart rate. The stroke volume at rest is 70 ml and the heart rate 72 beats per minute. Hence, the CO = 70 ml × 72/min = 5 L/min. As the heart rate increases, the cardiac cycle shortens. This is accomplished by shortening both the systoles and the diastoles; however, the diastoles shorten more. This reduces the ventricular filling time as the heart rate increases. Increasing the heart rate beyond a certain point does not result in an increased CO. The diastoles are so shortened that the ventricles do not have time to adequately fill with blood. This point is seldom reached in normal activity, but does occur with severe ventricular tachycardia. To increase the heart rate to these limits requires sympathetic input to the heart. This input stimulates not only the increased heart rate but also the force of contraction that, coupled with increased venous return, prevents the stroke volume from decreasing much until the diastolic period is greatly shortened (i.e., until the heart rate is about 160 beats per minute) (Figure 30-10).

Venous return is the amount of blood returning from the peripheral vessels to the heart. At rest this is about 5 L per minute, which is also the resting CO. If a large volume of blood were suddenly to attempt to return to the heart, the excess amount, over 25 L per minute, would pool in the veins rather than be pumped into the arteries.

The factor that often controls venous return is the vascular resistance. If a large proportion of the peripheral vessels become widely opened without compensating vasoconstriction elsewhere, the vascular resistance decreases, and large amounts of extra blood

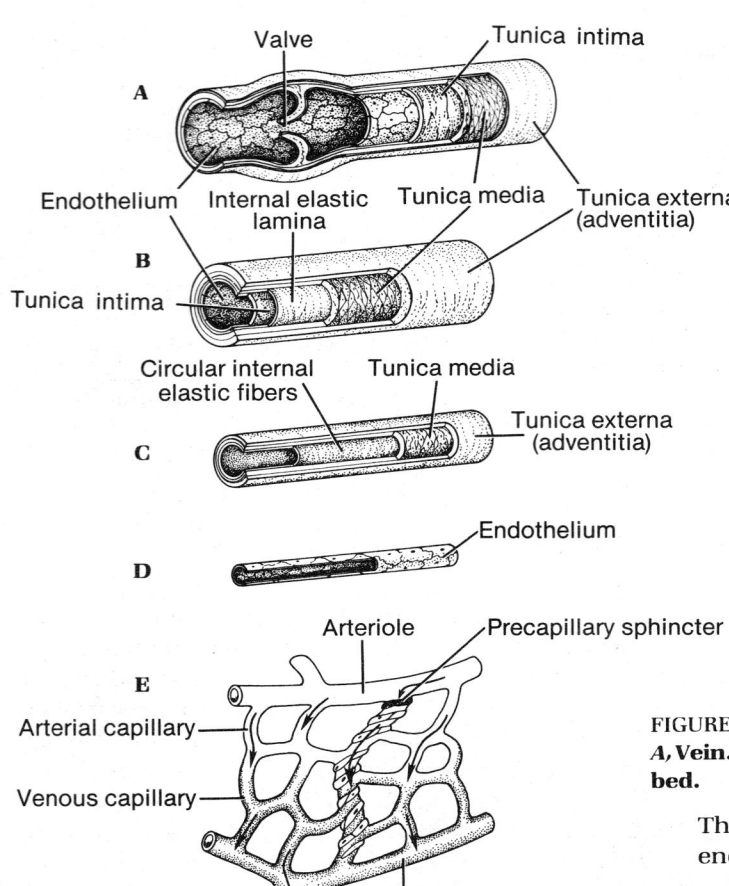

FIGURE 30-11. **Comparison of the structure of blood vessels.** *A,* **Vein.** *B,* **Elastic artery.** *C,* **Arteriole.** *D,* **Capillary.** *E,* **Capillary bed.**

will flow from the arteries to the veins. This decreases the rate of venous return and decreases the CO.

VASOMOTOR CONTROL OF THE BLOOD VESSELS

Most arterial blood vessels of the body receive nervous input. These nerves are part of the autonomic nervous system (ANS) (see also Section IV of this text) and influence the caliber of the vessels by their action. This input regulates the state of contraction of the muscular layers of the vessels (Figure 30-11). This direct nervous control of the luminal diameter of the vessels is one of the most important factors that determine the arterial blood pressure and the rate of flow in different parts of the systemic circulation. These nerve fibers are referred to as vasomotor nerves and are divided into two groups: vasoconstrictors, which are primarily of sympathetic origin, and vasodilators, which are primarily of parasympathetic origin. Stimulation of the vasoconstrictors produces constriction or narrowing of the caliber of the vessels.

These fibers are used to exert a continued tonic influence and maintain vessel tone.

The vasodilators produce dilation, or enlarging, of the caliber of the vessels. These fibers do not exert a tonic effect, and are activated by reflex action. Their effects are primarily local, and activation of any one set of fibers produces little or no effect on the vascular system in general.

Sympathetic vasodilator fibers probably exist along with those nerves that contain vasoconstrictors. These vasodilator fibers originate in the cerebral cortex, pass through the medulla, and enter the spinal cord. Vessels of the skeletal muscle are innervated by these fibers and although they travel with sympathetic vasoconstrictors that are adrenergic, these fibers are cholinergic. Stimulation of this system by exercise or emotional stimuli such as anxiety, stress, or fear produces vasodilation in skeletal muscle. Because exercise or emotional stimuli also produce vasoconstriction in other parts of the body, the blood pressure does not usually change, but may rise somewhat.

Dilation may also be affected by an inhibition of vasoconstrictor impulses. When the vascular area so affected is small, the effects are local, and more blood is distributed through the area. An increase in the circulating levels of lactic acid or carbon dioxide will reflexly cause vasodilation in skeletal muscle.

The inhibition of tonic constrictor impulses may affect large portions of the vascular tree. When such inhibitions occur, a marked fall in general blood pressure may be observed. Fainting is one example of such a reaction. A powerful emotional stimulus can stimulate a severe nervous outflow from the brain that inhibits the vasoconstrictor tone. Large numbers of blood vessels undergo dilation, the blood pressure drops dramatically, the brain is not adequately oxygenated, and fainting results.

The control of the volume of blood flow through the capillary bed is controlled by precapillary sphincters at the distal end of the arteriole. These sphincters are sensitive to nervous input, epinephrine, and local chemical conditions within the tissues in which they are located. A rise in local lactic acid tends to stimulate the opening of the sphincters to allow more blood flow to the area.

SUMMARY

Many drugs affect the cardiovascular system directly and indirectly. Those drugs that directly affect this system are discussed in the following chapters in this section. The brief overview presented in this chapter describing the anatomy, physiology, and assessment of the cardiovascular system should help the nurse better understand the mechanism of action and the effect of these agents, as well as the cardiovascular toxicity associated with drugs discussed in other sections of this text.

BIBLIOGRAPHY

Adolph, E.F. The heart's pacemaker. *Scientific American,* 1967, *216,* 32-37.

Berne, R.M., & Levy, M.N. *Cardiovascular physiology* (4th ed.). St. Louis: The C.V. Mosby Co., 1981.

Braunwald, E. Regulation of the circulation. *New England Journal of Medicine,* 1974, *290,* 1420-1425.

Folkow, B., & Neil, E. *Circulation.* London: Oxford University Press, 1971.

Mellander, S., & Johansson, B. Control of resistance exchange and capacitance functions in the peripheral circulation. *Pharmacological Reviews,* 1968, *20,* 117-196.

Mountcastle, V.B. *Medical physiology* (vols. 1 & 2) (14th ed.). St. Louis: The C.V. Mosby Co., 1980.

Wood, J.E. The venous system. *Scientific Systems,* 1968, *218,* 88-96.

Zweifach, B.W. The microcirculation of the blood. *Scientific American,* 1959, *200,* 54-60.

Cardiac Glycosides

D. George Wyse

Medications discussed in this chapter

Cardiac glycosides
Digitoxin
Digoxin
Ouabain

A large number of cardiac glycosides are found in different parts of a variety of plants, although other sources in nature are also known (e.g., toad skins). Only a limited number, however, are used in clinical therapeutics today. The most well known of the cardiac glycosides are the digitalis glycosides. In fact, the terms *digitalis* and *digitalis glycosides* are often used interchangeably with the term *cardiac glycosides.* The first detailed description of the clinical usefulness of these drugs is usually credited to William Withering, who 200 years ago described the use of the foxglove *(Digitalis purpura)* leaf for the treatment of *dropsy* or generalized edema (see also the discussion in Chapter 1, "Pharmacologic Aspects of Nursing: A Historical Overview").

At the present time, single, pure glycosides are used, but it was not long ago that crude preparations made from leaves were still in wide use. The few glycosides presently used are obtained from the leaf of *Digitalis lanata* (digoxin and digitoxin) and the seed of *Strophanthus gratus* (ouabain). Other glycosides are only of historical interest and are seldom used in North America. It is of practical toxicologic importance that some common garden flowers such as foxglove *(Digitalis purpura)* and lily of the valley *(Convallaria majalis)* contain these glycosides.

CHEMISTRY

Chemically, each of the cardiac glycosides consists of two parts, the aglycone, or genin, and one to four molecules of a sugar such as glucose. The aglycone is the part of the molecule that confers pharmacologic activity, and its structural base is a steroid ring system. Many of the older and now seldom-used glycosides are precursors of the more commonly used glycosides (i.e., they contain one or two additional sugar molecules). Lanatoside-C is a precursor of digoxin. Semisynthetic compounds have been made but have not gained wide clinical use. Acetylstrophanthidin is such a compound that finds limited use as a research tool because of its rapid onset and short duration of action.

MECHANISM OF ACTION AND PHARMACOLOGIC EFFECTS

The mechanism of action and pharmacologic effects are identical for all cardiac glycosides. The most important effects of these drugs are to increase the force of the contraction of myocardial muscle (i.e., a *positive inotropic effect*) and to slow conduction through the atrioventricular (AV) node. The mechanism(s) that explains these pharmacologic effects is incompletely understood, despite many years of intensive investigation. Among the various pharmacologic agents that have a positive inotropic effect, the cardiac glycosides are unique in that they increase the force of the contraction and, at least in heart failure, there is often a less than proportional increase in myocardial oxygen consumption. The mechanism for the inotropic action is probably a direct result of more calcium being made available at the intracellular sites where it is used in the process of *excitation–contraction coupling.* Whether the calcium comes from outside or inside the cell, or both, and exactly how its movement occurs are not known with any certainty.

The cardiac glycosides inhibit an enzyme in myocardial cell walls called sodium, potassium ion–activated adenosine triphosphatase (Na^+, K^+ − ATPase). Whether this enzyme is the receptor for cardiac glycosides and its inhibition explains all of the actions of these drugs remain unanswered at the present time. Na^+, K^+ − ATPase is intimately involved in the movement of sodium and potassium across myocardial cell membranes, and the movement of these ions is to a large degree the explanation of resting and action potentials (APs) of cardiac cells (see Chapter 30, "Review of the Anatomy, Physiology, and Assessment of the Cardiovascular System"). Alteration in the movement of these ions alters cardiac APs, and this effect explains some of the electrophysiologic actions of the cardiac glycosides, particularly their toxic effects. There is also a striking, although incomplete, parallel between the inotropic effect of cardiac glycosides and the inhibition of this enzyme. How the inhibition of Na^+, K^+ − ATPase would bring about changes in the availability of calcium for excitation–contraction coupling is unknown.

As a result of their enhancement of *contractility*, the cardiac glycosides increase the cardiac output of the failing heart at any given *filling pressure* (Figure 31-1). This action is the basis for the beneficial effect of these drugs in congestive heart failure. Cardiac glycosides also increase the contractility of the normal heart, but the cardiac output is unchanged, and this is usually attributed to increased impedance to left ventricular emptying as a result of a direct and sympathetically mediated (i.e., indirect) increase in arteriolar tone. The actions of cardiac glycosides on the heart rate are complex. Results from animal studies have demonstrated a slowing effect on heart rate that is partly mediated through the vagus nerve, but this effect is not prominent in normal humans. In congestive heart failure, however, there is usually a reflex tachycardia, and when the heart failure improves following the administration of these drugs, the heart rate will slow. A slow heart rate as a sign of digitalis excess has probably been overemphasized in the past. It must be recalled, however, that the pulse rate is determined by ventricular contraction and that occasionally excessive impairment of AV node conduction by the cardiac glycosides can result in heart block and a slow pulse rate.

The effects of cardiac glycosides on the conduction system of the heart are complex and a composite of both a direct action (i.e., Na^+, K^+ − ATPase inhibition) and an indirect action caused by increased vagal tone. The single most clinically important electrophysiologic effect is the slowing of AV node conduction velocity caused by a summation of both direct and vagal actions. Other parts of the conduction system are affected differently by these drugs. Vagal effects may predominate in those areas of the conduction system with dense vagal innervation, and direct effects may predominate in areas with sparse vagal innervation. Direct and vagal effects may compete, rather than summate as they do at the AV node. Therefore the observed effects on refractory periods, automaticity, and conduction velocity in various parts of the heart will also differ under different conditions of inherent vagal tone.

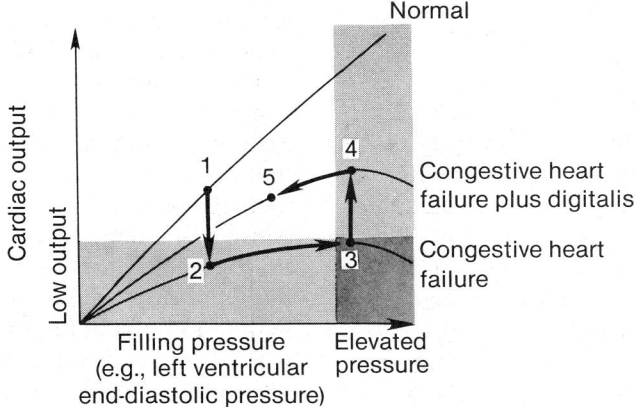

FIGURE 31-1. **A schema to illustrate the benefit of digitalis in congestive heart failure. 1, Normal cardiac output and filling pressure. 2, Low cardiac output at normal filling pressure in the failing heart. 3, Compensatory mechanisms (e.g., salt and water retention) raise filling pressure until it is elevated (e.g., dyspnea occurs) but cardiac output remains low. 4, Digitalis increases contractility, and cardiac output becomes normal, although filling pressure remains elevated. 5, Compensatory mechanisms (e.g., diuresis) lower filling pressure to the normal range with a normal cardiac output.**

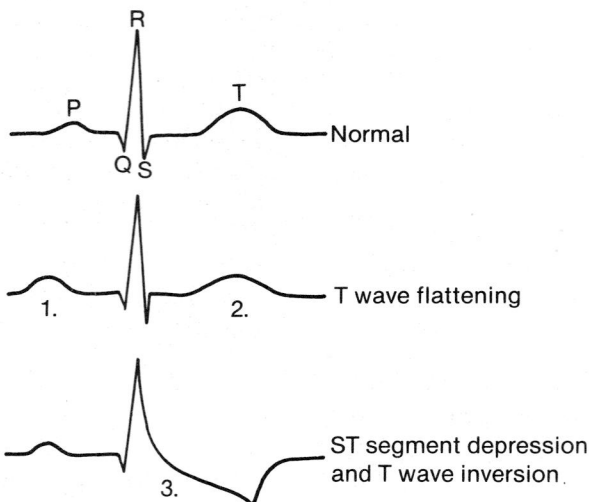

FIGURE 31-2. **Effects of digitalis on ECG.** 1, **Increased PR interval.** 2, **Decreased T-wave amplitude.** 3, **ST segment shortened, depressed.**

Rapid intravenous administration of the glycosides can raise the blood pressure because of an action via a central mechanism, but this is not seen if the drugs are given slowly (i.e., over 15 minutes). These drugs are not themselves diuretics but can cause a diuresis to occur in patients with congestive heart failure because they improve renal blood flow secondary to their positive inotropic effect. The cardiac glycosides can produce several nonspecific changes in the ECG, which include T wave flattening or inversion, ST segment depression, and shortened QT and longer PR intervals (Figure 31-2).

PHARMACOKINETICS

The major differences between the three agents discussed in this chapter are the result of differences in pharmacokinetics (see Chapter 6, "Pharmacokinetic Considerations in Drug Response") and metabolism (Table 31-1). Digitoxin is used almost solely as an oral agent, whereas ouabain is used only intravenously, primarily because its absorption by the oral route is unreliable. Digoxin, by far the most commonly used cardiac glycoside, can be given either orally or parenterally. The preferred parenteral route is intravenous.

Digitoxin is the glycoside most completely absorbed (i.e., nearly 100%) after oral administration. Of an oral dose of digoxin, 60% to 85% is absorbed. Digitoxin is highly bound to plasma proteins, whereas the other two agents are not. This accounts for the higher therapeutic plasma levels of digitoxin (i.e., 15 to 30 ng/ml) compared with those of digoxin (i.e., 1.0 to 2.0 ng/ml).

The onset of action and peak effect of these drugs are quite different; ouabain has the shortest onset and earliest peak effect, and digitoxin is at the opposite end of the spectrum. Ouabain, as previously mentioned, is used only intravenously, and after a single *digitalizing dose* (i.e., 0.015 mg/kg), an effect is observed within 5 to 10 minutes and the patient is fully *digitalized* in 45 minutes. Intravenously administered digoxin begins to have an effect within 15 to 30 minutes and has its peak action at approximately 3 hours. Comparative times of onset and peak effects for digitoxin are approximately twice those for digoxin, but digitoxin is seldom used intravenously.

Digoxin and ouabain (in particular) are primarily eliminated unchanged in the urine; therefore the maintenance dose largely depends on the patient's renal function. Digitoxin, on the other hand, is first metabolized in the liver, and then the primarily inactive metabolites are excreted in the urine. Therefore the maintenance dose of digitoxin is much less dependent on the patient's renal function. Approximately 15% of the total amount of digoxin in the body will be metabolized in the liver and excreted in the bile, although some is reabsorbed via enterohepatic circulation (see Chapter 5, "Drug Metabolism and Elimination"). The liver has a tremendous functional reserve capacity to metabolize digoxin and it is unusual to have to take account of liver function in arriving at a digoxin maintenance dose.

There is a remarkable difference in the half-lives of these agents. The plasma half-life of a digitalization dose of each of these agents follows: ouabain, 21 hours; digoxin, 36 hours; and digitoxin, 5 to 7 days. All of

TABLE 31-1

Summary of the pharmacokinetics of cardiac glycosides

Drug	Gastro-intestinal absorption	Onset	Peak effect	Plasma protein binding (%)	Therapeutic plasma level	Average half-life	Route of elimination
Digitoxin	90%-100%	Oral 3-6 hr IV 20-120 min	Oral 6-12 hr IV 4-8 hr	90	15-30 ng/ml	5-7 days	Metabolized in liver and metabolites excreted in urine
Digoxin	60%-85%	Oral 1.5-6 hr IV 15-30 min	Oral 4-6 hr IV ½-3 hr	25	1.0-2.0 ng/ml	36 hr	Mostly unchanged in urine; some liver metabolism
Ouabain	Unreliable	IV 5-10 min	IV ½-2 hr	25	—	21 hr	Unchanged in urine

these agents are eliminated from the body at a rate best approximated by first-order kinetics (i.e., a fixed percentage of the total body level is excreted per unit of time).

The cardiac glycosides are often administered by a regimen that will quickly establish a total body drug level within the therapeutic range (i.e., a digitalization dose), and then a daily dosage scheme is selected to keep the drug at that level (i.e., a maintenance dose). The digitalization dose is given over a time period dictated by the clinical circumstances; this may be minutes (ouabain) to hours or days (digoxin or digitoxin). For these glycosides, whose elimination is described by first-order kinetics, it can be recognized that a steady-state body level of drug will be achieved in approximately 4 to 5 half-lives, if a daily maintenance dose scheme is followed without initial rapid digitalization.

Thus, digitalization can be accomplished by giving the daily maintenance dose and requires approximately 1 week with digoxin or 1 month with digitoxin. Once the total body level has achieved a steady state, approximately 10% of that amount of digitoxin and 30% to 40% of that amount of digoxin will be excreted per 24 hours; these percentages will thus determine the maintenance dose. It must be emphasized that these percentages vary markedly in individual patients and are dependent on renal (digoxin) and hepatic (digoxin and digitoxin) function.

A single daily dose usually results in better *patient compliance* and is satisfactory for most patients. However, twice daily administration results in a slightly higher average drug level at the steady state, in addition to lower peak and higher trough drug levels between doses; for certain patients, this may be a more appropriate regimen.

USES

Clinical indications for using the cardiac glycosides are relatively few, but extremely common, which accounts for their wide use. The most common clinical indication is congestive heart failure (CHF) from a variety of causes. Congestive heart failure caused by coronary artery disease or hypertensive cardiovascular disease responds best. High-output heart failure states, such as thyrotoxicosis, are not helped by cardiac glycosides but should be treated by correcting the underlying condition. Congestive heart failure secondary to certain types of heart disease, because of their hemodynamic nature, may not respond dramatically to cardiac glycosides. Examples include mitral stenosis with sinus rhythm and regurgitant valvular lesions (i.e., mitral and aortic).

These drugs are often useful in the CHF of dilated cardiomyopathies, but obstructive cardiomyopathy (i.e., idiopathic hypertrophic subaortic stenosis [IHSS]) is a relative contraindication to using the cardiac glycosides. This is because the obstruction is of a dynamic nature and an increase in force of contraction and reduction in heart size will *increase* outflow obstruction. Notwithstanding the general discussion above, some patients with congestive cardiac failure who would be expected to improve with administration of digitalis glycosides do not respond. It has been noted that patients with more chronic and severe heart failure, greater left ventricular dilatation, and greater reduction in systolic function are more likely to respond to digitalis glycosides. The presence of a third heart sound may be useful in predicting which patients will respond to digitalis glycosides. Isolated right-sided heart failure (cor pulmonale) is not usually improved by the cardiac glycosides for reasons that are unknown.

Responses to the glycosides may be blunted in elderly patients. The exact reason for this is uncertain but may reflect a diminished ability of the senescent myocardium to respond.

The other clinical indication for using cardiac glycosides is in treating certain supraventricular tachycardias; in particular, atrial fibrillation, atrial flutter, and paroxysmal atrial tachycardia. In approximately one half of the cases of these dysrhythmias, when an adequate dose of a cardiac glycoside is administered, the rhythm will be converted back to a normal sinus rhythm. In the remaining half, the ventricular rate will be controlled by the drugs' actions at the AV node, but the abnormal rhythm will remain. In chronic atrial fibrillation and flutter, the cardiac glycosides are often used simply to control the ventricular rate. The dosage of digoxin required to control atrial fibrillation is sometimes higher than that required to obtain a positive inotropic effect. Cardiac glycosides are particularly efficacious when CHF causes, or is the result of, one of these dysrhythmias.

The choice of agent will depend on the clinical circumstances. Digoxin is by far the most commonly used agent. Ouabain is generally reserved for those instances when a rapid effect is needed. Digitoxin is much less commonly used, probably partly because of its long half-life, which may be more troublesome if the patient develops toxicity, but offers at least some theoretic advantage in the patient with chronic renal failure because it is primarily metabolized by the liver.

ADVERSE EFFECTS AND TOXICITY

A recent multicenter survey of in-hospital medical deaths where drug toxicity was implicated as a factor showed that in one half of these instances digoxin was the suspected offending agent. Digoxin is reputed to be the fourth most commonly prescribed drug in the United States, and this frequency of use and the narrow therapeutic index of cardiac glycosides results in the common occurrence of digitalis toxicity. Therefore the dangers of intoxication from cardiac glycosides cannot be overstated. Anorexia, nausea, and vomiting are prominent features of intoxication by the cardiac glycosides. Nausea and vomiting are mediated through the chemoreceptor trigger zone in the medulla oblongata. Diarrhea may occur along with other gastrointestinal symptoms, and abdominal discomfort or pain may also be present. The other prominent feature of cardiac glycoside excess is cardiac dysrhythmia. Toxic concentrations of these drugs can cause virtually every dysrhythmia known, but the most common ones are ventricular extrasystoles, often bi-

geminy or multiform, atrial tachycardia with block, and junctional tachycardia.

Fatigue, malaise, drowsiness, and headache are also commonly seen. Visual disturbances such as *chromatopsia* for yellow or green are often written about, but simple blurred vision is the most common visual side effect. Mild mental confusion or disorientation may be seen, particularly in the elderly, but in extreme cases aphasia, hallucinations, and frank dementia have been noted. Rarely, skin rashes (e.g., urticaria), eosinophilia, and *gynecomastia* have been reported.

DRUG INTERACTIONS

An important reciprocal relationship exists between the serum potassium level and cardiac glycoside intoxication. Low serum potassium levels will potentiate the toxic effects of these agents. The importance of this interaction is that many cardiac patients who are taking cardiac glycosides are also taking diuretics that can, and often do, lower the serum potassium level secondary to renal loss of K^+. Administering potassium to maintain the serum level in the high normal range is one of the first steps in treating digitalis glycoside intoxication.

A potential exists for an interaction between cardiac glycosides and Ca^{++} but this is rarely of any practical importance. An increase in Ca^{++} will enhance glycoside effects and may contribute to toxicity, but a change in the amount of *ionized* calcium in the serum rarely occurs, although *total* calcium may often be abnormally low or high. Hypocalcemia may nullify the effects of digitalis; the drug may be ineffective until a normal serum calcium level is restored. Hypomagnesemia is associated with an increased sensitivity to digitalis. The mechanism involved may be the result of enhanced myocardial uptake of digitalis in the presence of hypomagnesemia.

Another important interaction is that between digoxin and quinidine. These two drugs are commonly administered concurrently to the same patient. It has been noted in patients taking digoxin on a regular basis whose plasma digoxin is at a steady state that the institution of quinidine therapy often results in a twofold to threefold increase in the plasma digoxin level. In some cases this change has resulted in clinical digitalis toxicity. The mechanism of this effect is unclear and may be caused by an altered elimination of the glycoside or an alteration of the volume of distribution of digoxin. There is conflicting evidence about whether quinidine similarly interacts with digitoxin, with one study reporting no interaction and a second noting an effect of quinidine similar to that seen with digoxin. It is presently unclear whether other antidysrhythmics similar to quinidine (e.g., procainamide and disopyramide) have the same effect, although thus far it appears to be seen only with quinidine. It is generally recommended that the dose of digitalis be halved when quinidine therapy is initiated. Now that Ca^{++} entry blockers are becoming so widely used for a variety of cardiac conditions, it is important to point out that verapamil can also raise the serum digoxin level. Thus far this interaction has not been shown to have the same degree of clinical relevance as the digoxin-quinidine interaction.

In passing it is worthwhile to comment on measuring plasma or serum digoxin levels and their relationship to glycoside intoxication. A spectrum of plasma digoxin levels exists that results in an increasing likelihood of clinical toxicity as the level increases above 2 ng/ml. Cardiac glycoside toxicity, however, is a clinical diagnosis based on the presence of symptoms and the dysrhythmias referred to earlier. No absolute plasma level makes this diagnosis. An elevated level is corroborative data. Patients can have frank digitalis intoxication with plasma digoxin levels substantially less than 2 ng/ml (particularly when the serum K^+ level is low), and many patients will be free of any toxicity with plasma levels in the 2.5 to 3.0 ng/ml range. Recall that blood for the determination of a serum digoxin level should be collected 6 to 8 hours after the last oral dose of the drug to allow adequate time for absorption and distribution (see Chapter 4, "Drug Availability and Distribution").

SUMMARY

The terms *glycoside* and *cardiac glycoside* are often used to mean digitalis glycoside; however, the cardiac glycosides currently used include digoxin, digitoxin, and ouabain. Of the three, digoxin and digitoxin (i.e., the digitalis glycosides) are the most widely used. The cardiac glycosides increase the force of the contraction of the heart (i.e., a positive inotropic effect) and slow conduction through the AV node. The primary clinical use of the cardiac glycosides is in treating CHF. They are also used in treating certain supraventricular tachycardias. Because the cardiac glycosides are used in treating relatively serious conditions, and because they have a relatively narrow *therapeutic index*, dosage and monitoring their effects in the patient must be done with care and caution. Familiarity with both the therapeutic and toxic effects of these drugs should enable the nurse to provide optimal care to patients requiring these agents.

ADVERSE/SIDE EFFECTS OF THE CARDIAC GLYCOSIDES*

ALLERGIC REACTIONS

Urticarial skin rash—rare

AUTONOMIC NERVOUS SYSTEM

Decreased sympathetic "tone" usual but perhaps increased in some situations and body systems (see gastrointestinal system)
Increased vagal "tone"

BEHAVIOR

Confusion
Delirium
Disorientation

CARDIOVASCULAR SYSTEM

Atrioventricular block
Extrasystoles—all types
Nonspecific ST and T changes in ECG

Virtually every type of cardiac dysrhythmia has been reported (ventricular bigeminy and atrial tachycardia with atrioventricular block are particularly common)

CENTRAL NERVOUS SYSTEM

Aphasia
Convulsions—rare
Drowsiness
Fatigue
Hallucinations
Headache
Malaise
Neuralgic pain (cranial nerve V)

GASTROINTESTINAL SYSTEM

Anorexia
Abdominal pain (possible mesenteric ischemia because of increased sympathetic vasoconstriction)
Diarrhea

Nausea (caused by a central effect on chemoreceptor trigger zone)
Vomiting (caused by a central effect on chemoreceptor trigger zone)

HEMATOLOGIC SYSTEM

Eosinophilia—rare
Possible increased coagulability

METABOLIC AND ENDOCRINE SYSTEMS

Gynecomastia—rare

OCULAR SYSTEM

Amblyopia
Blurred Vision
Disturbed color vision
Dyplopia
Halos around dark objects
Scotomas

*See Chapter 11, "Drug Toxicity," for an overview of drug toxicity.

CLINICALLY SIGNIFICANT DRUG INTERACTIONS*

Primary drug	Interacting drug	Possible effect(s)	Probable mechanism(s)
Cardiac glycoside	Amphotericin B	Increased glycoside toxicity	Hypokalemia
Cardiac glycoside	Calcium preparations (parenteral)	Increased glycoside toxicity	Increased ionized calcium levels increase effect of glycoside on the myocardium
Cardiac glycoside (oral)	Cholestyramine	Decreased glycoside effect	Decreased oral absorption
Cardiac glycoside	Diuretics (except spironolactone and triamterene)	Increased glycoside toxicity	Hypokalemia
Cardiac glycoside	Propylthiouracil	Increased glycoside effect	Not established
Cardiac glycoside	Quinidine	Increased glycoside toxicity	Decreased volume of distribution and decreased clearance
Cardiac glycoside	Thyroid hormones	Decreased glycoside effect	Not established
Cardiac glycoside	Verapamil	Increased glycoside effect	Reduced clearance and additive effect

*See Chapter 10, "Drug Interactions," for an overview of drug interactions.

GENERAL NURSING IMPLICATIONS

Nursing of patients requiring cardiac glycosides

ASSESSMENT

A complete nursing assessment is essential in establishing a baseline from which to individualize drug therapy and to monitor therapeutic response, adverse side effects, and signs of digitalis toxicity. Assessment should include a careful drug history to identify sensitivity, contraindications, and potential drug interactions before the first dose is taken. Assessment may also reveal prior use or preconceived misconceptions regarding the digitalis glycosides.

SENSITIVITY

When cardiac glycosides are administered to patients who have not received them before, monitoring for hypersensitivity is extremely important. Hypersensitivity may not be observed for 5 to 7 days after the onset of therapy. It is especially important to monitor elderly patients, because allergic reactions, although rare, occur more often among this age group.

CONTRAINDICATIONS

It is important to recognize that cardiac glycosides are contraindicated in patients with the following conditions: atrioventricular block, digitalis toxicity, hypersensitivity to cardiac glycosides, obstructive cardiomyopathy (IHSS), and ventricular fibrillation.

CAUTIONS

Caution is required when these medications are used with patients who have a history of the following: acute myocarditis, Adams-Stokes syndrome, cardiac amyloidosis, carotid sinus syndrome, cyanotic heart or pulmonary disease, angina, acute myocardial infarction, hypoxia, ischemic heart disease, myxedema, ventricular tachycardia, or impaired renal or hepatic function.

Caution is also advised when cardiac glycosides are used in pregnant women or nursing mothers; neonates, because of their immature renal and hepatic function and potential increased sensitivity; premature infants, because they are particularly sensitive to the effects of these medications; and the elderly. In addition, caution is required when cardiac glycosides are used concurrently with quinidine.

DRUG INTERACTIONS

Caution is required with cardiac glycosides because a potential exists for numerous drug interactions (see Clinically Significant Drug Interactions).

ADMINISTRATION

Initially digitoxin and digoxin are administered at higher doses (digitalization or loading doses) to achieve desired effects. Maintenance doses are then employed to replace daily losses and should be administered at the same time each day. Elderly patients usually require lower individualized doses because of hepatic, renal, and lean body mass changes. Digitoxin and digoxin can be given orally or parenterally. Ouabain is for emergency use only. Do not give to patients who have received digitalis during the previous 3 weeks. Intravenous administration results in an onset of action within 3 to 10 minutes with a maximal effect of 30 to 60 minutes.

GENERAL NURSING IMPLICATIONS—cont'd

Nursing of patients requiring cardiac glycosides—cont'd

Oral

Any medication given by the oral route can cause nausea. This can be minimized by the patient taking the medication near mealtime. Be sure *not* to confuse this with the nausea associated with cardiac glycoside overdosage.

Intramuscular

NOTE: This route of administration is *not* recommended.

It is important to recognize that *digitoxin* should *not* be administered subcutaneously because it is irritating to the subcutaneous tissues. It should be injected deeply into healthy muscle tissue and the site vigorously massaged to enhance absorption. Sites require careful rotation. *Digoxin* should likewise be administered deep intramuscularly. When cardiac glycosides are administered by the intramuscular route, it is important to recognize that this route should be avoided in severe CHF because absorption may be delayed or erratic and the effect prolonged as a result of diminished blood circulation to the site of injection and the fat solubility of the digitalis glycosides.

Intravenous

Monitoring is essential during intravenous administration of cardiac glycosides. These medications must be administered *slowly* by this route over 15 minutes. Hypertension can occur if intravenous administration is too rapid.

MONITORING

Initial therapy: The ECG is used and emergency equipment should be available.

Maintenance therapy: Apical rates should be obtained for 1 full minute before the administration of a cardiac glycoside and the medication held and the prescriber advised if a change in rate, quality, or rhythm other than expected are noted (e.g., excessive slowing of heart to less than 60 beats per minute, tachycardia, or missed beats).

Monitor weight (at the same time each day), intake and output, and cardiac status as indicated (e.g., monitor for signs of fluid retention, ankle edema, distention of neck veins, and rales for CHF).

Monitor laboratory results for hypokalemia and hypercalcemia, and monitor the patient for signs of these imbalances, including weakness, flaccid paralysis (hypokalemia); and confusion, anorexia, abdominal pain, muscle pain, and weakness (hypercalcemia).

Therapeutic response

Inotropic effects include slowing and strengthening of heart rate, relief of symptoms of CHF, or correction of a specific dysrhythmia. Although not diuretics per se, these medications have a diuretic effect secondary to a positive inotropic effect and the resulting improved renal perfusion.

Side effects and adverse reactions

Monitoring side effects is essential (see Adverse/Side Effects of the Cardiac Glycosides), as is planning to minimize these effects with the patient and the family. Involving the patient and the family promotes compliance and does much to avoid undue and serious problems associated with the side effects that can occur with using cardiac glycosides. Because side effects are closely related to signs of toxicity, the patient must be monitored carefully and should have an understanding of which signs indicate that consultation with the health care provider is necessary, especially on discharge.

Toxicity

Toxicity caused by cardiac glycosides can be the result of: the patient taking more digitalis than prescribed; CHF resulting in diminished renal and hepatic perfusion and thus reduced excretion; renal or hepatic failure; and concurrent use of quinidine, which can decrease the renal excretion of these medications increasing their concentration within days to toxic levels in some patients. The most common cause of toxicity is, however, decreased levels of serum potassium resulting in increased sensitivity of the myocardium to digitalis even though the blood levels of the drug remain unchanged. Monitor patients carefully, especially those prone to potassium losses (e.g., patients with vomiting, diarrhea, nasogastric suction, large amounts of wound drainage, or those patients receiving potassium-wasting diuretics concurrently [e.g., furosemide, thiazides, ethacrynic acid]). Monitoring is essential because the signs of toxicity develop gradually. Hold the medication and advise the prescriber if the following are noted: gastrointestinal disturbances including anorexia, epigastric discomfort, nausea, and vomiting; pain in lower third of the face and the lumbar areas; visual disturbances (blurring or clouding of vision, changes in color vision, yellow vision [xanthopsia], the phenomena of seeing yellow or green halos around objects, or white vision); loss of energy, malaise, headache, fatigue, drowsiness, mental disorders, and other CNS effects; changes in heart rate, rhythm or irritability, including excessive slowing, extrasystoles, bigeminal pulse, ectopic beats, ventricular tachycardia, or sinus dysrhythmia; or convulsions (extreme situations).

It is important to recognize that the signs of toxicity may vary in relation to age. *Neonates* will show a slowing of sinus rate, and a prolongation of the P-R interval. The *elderly* experience CNS symptoms early and may have confusion, disorientation, hallucinations, or psychosis. Anorexia is a more common complaint than is nausea or vomiting. In addition, dysrhythmias may occur before gastrointestinal, visual, or mental symptoms.

Not only is age an important consideration in monitoring, but special care should also be used when monitoring *obese* patients because digitalis glycosides are highly fat soluble and in these patients may be cleared slowly.

Patients with signs of toxicity should receive ECG monitoring as indicated, and digitalis should be held. The patient should be kept quiet. Potassium

Continued.

GENERAL NURSING IMPLICATIONS—cont'd

Nursing of patients requiring cardiac glycosides—cont'd

Toxicity—cont'd

should be readily available for infusion, and antidysrhythmic drugs should be on hand.

PATIENT EDUCATION

The patient and the family, as indicated, should be involved as early as possible in the prescribed drug regimen. They should have a clear understanding of the purpose of the cardiac glycoside, possible adverse side effects and how to report these, what to do to minimize adverse side effects, signs of toxicity, and how the medication modifies activities of daily living. If the patient is to continue cardiac glycoside use on a long-term basis, he or she should understand the potency of these medications and their proper storage and administration. These medications should be taken only as directed, because taking more than the prescribed dosage can lead to toxicity. The patient also needs to understand how changes in health state (e.g., nausea, vomiting, and diarrhea) can cause changes in body chemistry (e.g., hypokalemia) and influence medication requirements.

The patient should be taught how to recognize signs of CHF, including moist cough, difficulty in breathing, shortness of breath, swollen feet or ankles, and poor sleep (e.g., inability to find a comfortable position at night). The patient should understand that these signs indicate he or she may need to have the medication adjusted and that he or she should notify the health care provider.

Patients receiving cardiac glycosides are often receiving additional medications for CHF and associated cardiovascular disorders. Not only will the patient and the family require careful instruction about the medications, but they will also require assistance with adapting to changes in activities of daily living, including stress management, exercise, diet (e.g., low sodium), and activity adjustments. Follow-up after discharge is important, and referral to respective lay groups is often beneficial in helping the patient and the family accept the condition as well as the therapeutic regimen.

Patients should be encouraged either to avoid or to moderate alcohol consumption.

GENERAL INSTRUCTIONS FOR DISCHARGE/OUTPATIENTS

CARDIAC GLYCOSIDES

This medication is a cardiac glycoside generally used to help your heart beat stronger and more slowly. If you do not understand why you require this medication, check with your nurse or physician.

Try to take this medication at the same time each day. Do *not* change the dose or timing without consulting with your nurse or physician.

Do *not* begin taking any other medications while you are on this medication, especially diuretics (water pills), potassium supplements, or quinidine, without consulting with your nurse or physician. This includes drugs you can get without a prescription, even antacids.

Report promptly any unusual sensations, palpitations, loss of appetite, headaches, changes in your vision, or any extended gastrointestinal flulike symptoms to your nurse or physician.

This medication has been prescribed especially for you; do *not* trade or give this medication to any relatives or friends.

This is a very potent medication. Keep this medication, as well as all other medications, out of the reach of children.

Remember, even though this medication will make you feel better, you must continue to take it *as directed*. Do *not* discontinue this medication or change the dose without consulting with your nurse or physician.

NURSING DRUG DIGEST

Medication (trade name*)	Indication	Usual dosage and administration	Dosage forms, preparation, and storage	Contraindications, cautions, and comments	Monitoring
Digitoxin Cardidigin Crystodigin Digisidin Digitaline Na-tivelle Purodigin Unidigin	Congestive heart failure Supraventricular tachycardias	*Adults:* Digitalizing 1.0-1.6 mg PO or IV; maintenance 0.05 to 0.20 mg/day PO or IV. NOTE: Administer 50% of digitalization dose, followed by 2 additional doses of 25% at 4-6 hr intervals as indicated. *Children:* Digitalizing, new-borns, 0.022 mg/kg; 1 month-1 year, 0.045 mg/kg; 1-2 years, 0.04 mg/kg; over 2 years, 0.03 mg/kg PO or IV; maintenance, 10% of digital-izing dose. NOTE: Administer 50% of digitalization dose, followed by 2 additional doses of 25% at 4-6 hr intervals as indicated. *Elderly:* Start with lower doses. Do *not* administer by IM route because absorption is er-ratic. Reduce dose in severe liver disease. NOTE: Neonates and the elder-ly commonly require lower doses, whereas infants (1 month to 2 years) often re-quire a 50% higher than normal adult dose *based on body weight*	Tablets: 0.05, 0.1, 0.15, 0.2 mg Injectable: 0.2 mg/ml Protect solution from light	*Contraindicated* in digi-talis toxicity, beriberi, heart disease, and ventricular fibrillation Less caution in renal failure than digoxin Toxicity potentiated by hypokalemia Administration of paren-teral calcium salts may cause serious toxicity Therapeutic serum levels are generally 14-26 ng/ml	Take apical pulse be-fore administration; monitor serum po-tassium and serum calcium Observe for signs of toxicity (e.g., anorex-ia, nausea, blurred vision, dysrhythmias) Monitor ECG, especial-ly in neonates Monitor for therapeutic serum levels

NOTE: For additional details regarding the individual agents listed in this table see the text and other tables in this chapter.
★Indicates that the drug is generally available only in the United States.

Continued.

NURSING DRUG DIGEST—cont'd

Medication (trade name)	Indication	Usual dosage and administration	Dosage forms, preparation, and storage	Contraindications, cautions, and comments	Monitoring
Digoxin Lanoxicaps Lanoxin Natigoxine Novodigoxin SK-Digoxin Winoxin	Congestive heart failure Supraventricular tachycardias	*Adults:* Digitalizing 0.5-1 mg (8-15 μg/kg) IV; or 1-1.5 mg PO over 24 hr; maintenance 0.125 to 0.5 mg/day NOTE: Administer 50% of digitalizing dose, followed by 2 additional doses of 25% each at 4-6 hr intervals as indicated *Children:* Digitalizing, newborns, 25-40 μg/kg IV (or 40-60 μg/kg PO); 1 month-2 years, 35-50 μg/kg IV (or 60-80 μg/kg PO); 2-10 years, 25-40 μg/kg IV (or 40-60 μg/kg PO); over 10 years, same as adult dose; maintenance 20%-30% of digitalizing dose per 24 hr NOTE: Administer 50% of digitalizing dose, followed by 2 additional doses of 25% each at 4-6 hr intervals as indicated Neonates require lower doses, whereas infants (1 month to 2 years) usually require higher digitalizing doses; after 2 years of age the required dose usually decreases *Elderly:* Because of reduced renal function, start with lower doses	Capsules: 0.05, 0.1, 0.2 mg Tablets: 0.125, 0.25, 0.375, 0.5 mg Elixir: 0.05 mg/ml Parenteral: 0.05, 0.1, 0.25 mg/ml For IV use dilute in small amount (5-10 ml) of D₅W or NS and inject slowly over 10 to 15 min Protect solution from light	*Contraindicated* in digitalis toxicity and ventricular fibrillation Toxicity potentiated by hypokalemia A potential cause of accidental poisoning in children In children the first signs of toxicity are *not* anorexia, nausea, and blurred vision, as are seen in adults, but usually a cardiac dysrhythmia Administration of parenteral calcium salts may cause serious toxicity Therapeutic serum levels are generally 0.8-1.6 ng/ml	Monitor serum potassium and serum calcium Take apical pulse before administration Observe for signs of toxicity (e.g., anorexia, nausea, blurred vision, dysrhythmias) Monitor serum levels

	Intravenous: 80% of oral dose (*except* for PO Lanoxicaps, which because of greater bioavailability are dosed the same as the IV injection) NOTE: IM injection is poorly absorbed and is *not* recommended Reduced dose in renal failure and perhaps also in severe liver disease NOTE: Monitoring of ECG and serum concentration may be necessary to avoid or monitor for toxicity NOTE: Dosage based on lean body weight		
★ **Ouabain**	Rapid effect given IV (use *only* for digitalization, *not* for maintenance)	*Adults:* 0.25–0.5 mg slow IV, followed by 0.1 mg q.h. as indicated Maximum: 1 mg/24 hr *Children:* 0.005–0.01 mg/kg; administer by slow IV infusion NOTE: ECG monitoring is essential during administration to newborn infants NOTE: Usually *not* recommended for children Reduce dose in renal impairment IM administration is painful and is *not* recommended	Injectable: 0.25 mg/ml Protect solution from light	*Contraindicated* in digitalis toxicity and ventricular fibrillation Toxicity potentiated by hypokalemia and hypomagnesemia Use with caution in hypertensive patients because a transient rise in blood pressure may occur When administered IV, ouabain is the most rapidly acting cardiac glycoside available Use with extreme caution in patients who have received a digitalis preparation within the previous 3 weeks	Take apical pulse before administration Monitor patient closely during administration Observe for signs of toxicity (e.g., nausea, anorexia, blurred vision, dysrhythmias) Monitor serum magnesium and serum potassium levels Monitor ECG, particularly in neonates

BIBLIOGRAPHY

Adverse interactions of drugs. *The Medical Letter,* 1975, *17,* 17.

Adverse interactions of drugs. *The Medical Letter,* 1977, *19,* 5.

Adverse interactions of drugs. *The Medical Letter,* 1979, *21,* 5.

Brown, D.D., Spector, R., & Juhl, R.P. Drug interactions with digoxin. *Drugs,* 1980, *20,* 198-206.

Dickstein, E.S. Digitalis toxicity mistaken for jaundice. *Geriatrics,* 1982, *37*(4), 33-138.

Doering, W. Quinidine-digoxin interaction: pharmacokinetics, underlying mechanism, and clinical implications. *New England Journal of Medicine,* 1979, *301,* 400-404.

Doering, W., Fichtl, B., Herrmann, M., & Besenfelder, E. Quinidine-digoxin interaction: evidence for involvement of an extrarenal mechanism. *European Journal of Clinical Pharmacology,* 1982, *21,* 281-285.

Doherty, J.E. How and when to use the digitalis serum levels. *Journal of the American Medical Association,* 1978, *239,* 2594-2596.

Drugs used in the care of the cardiac patient. *Nursing Clinics of North America,* 1978, *13*(3), 473-497.

Fenster, P.E., Powell, J.R., Graves, P.E., Conrad, K.A., Hager, W.D., Goldman, S., & Marcus, F.I. Digitoxin-quinidine interaction: pharmacokinetic evaluation. *Annals of Internal Medicine,* 1980, *93,* 698-701.

Goldberg, P.B. How do digitalis tolerance and toxicity change with age? *Geriatric Nursing,* 1980, *1,* 142-144.

Gómez-Arnau, J., Maseda, J., Burgos, R., Cordón, J., Domínguez, R., Criado, A., & Avello, F. Cardiac arrest due to digitalis intoxication with normal serum digoxin levels: effects of hypokalemia. *Drug Intelligence and Clinical Pharmacy,* 1982, *16,* 160-161.

Gordon, F.S. Geriatric medications, tailoring cardiovascular therapy to the patient. *RN,* 1978, *41*(3), 56-61.

Hammond, C. Is digitalis the solution or cause of this problem? *RN,* 1981, *44*(10), 51-53.

Heinz, N., & Rietbrock, N. Relationship between dose and plasma level of digoxin and patient characteristics. *European Journal of Clinical Pharmacology,* 1979, *15,* 109-114.

Kim, D.H., Akera, T., & Brody, T.M. Tissue binding sites involved in quinidine-cardiac glycoside interactions. *Journal of Pharmacology and Experimental Therapeutics,* 1981, *218,* 357-362.

Klein, H.O., Lang, R., Weiss, E., DiSegni, E., Libhaber, C., Guerrero, J., & Kaplinsky, E. The influence of verapamil on serum digoxin concentration. *Circulation,* 1982, *65,* 998-1003.

Leahey, E.B., Jr., Reiffel, J.A., Heissenbuttel, R.H., Drusin, R.E., Lovejoy, W.P., & Bigger, J.T., Jr. Enhanced cardiac effect of digoxin during quinidine treatment. *Archives of Internal Medicine,* 1979, *139,* 519-521.

Lee, D.C.S., Johnson. R.A., Bingham, J.B., Leaky, M., Dinsmore, R.E., Goroll, A.H., Newell, J.B., Strauss, H.W., & Haber, E. Heart failure in outpatients: a randomized trial of digoxin versus placebo. *New England Journal of Medicine,* 1982, *306,* 699-705.

MacCannell, K.L., & Wyse, D.G. Pharmacologic management: cardiovascular drugs. In N.K. Wenger, J.W. Hurst, & M.C. McIntyre (Eds.). *Cardiology for nurses.* New York: McGraw-Hill Book Co., 1980.

Ochs, H.R., Pabst, J., Greenblatt, D.J., & Dengler, H.J. Noninteraction of digitoxin and quinidine. *New England Journal of Medicine,* 1980, *303,* 672-674.

Owens, J.F., McCann, C., & Huteimyer, C.M. Cardiac rehabilitation: a patient education program. *Nursing Research,* 1978, *27*(3), 148-150.

Waldorff, S., & Buch, J. Serum digoxin and empiric methods in identification of digitoxicity. *Clinical Pharmacology and Therapeutics,* 1978, *23,* 19-24.

CHAPTER 32

Antidysrhythmics

D. George Wyse

Medications discussed in this chapter

Antidysrhythmic/anti-cholinergic
  Disopyramide
  Quinidine
  Procainamide
Antidysrhythmic/local anesthetic/anticonvulsant
  Lidocaine
  Phenytoin

Antidysrhythmic/antiadrenergic
  Bretylium
Antidysrhythmic/calcium antagonist
  Verapamil

Antidysrhythmic drugs include all of those medications used to maintain a regular cardiac rhythm with a normal rate. Several agents used for this purpose are not discussed in this chapter because they are fully covered in other sections. These include drugs such as cardiac glycosides (Chapter 31, "Cardiac Glycosides"), beta-adrenergic blocking agents and phenylephrine (Chapter 24, "Sympathomimetics and Sympatholytics"), atropine (Chapter 23, "Parasympathomimetics and Parasympatholytics"), and edrophonium (Chapter 25, "Anticholinesterases and Cholinesterase Reactivators"). No completely satisfactory pharmacologic classification scheme for the antidysrhythmics exists, and that presented above has its own weaknesses.

The pharmacology of this group of drugs is among the most complex to be found for any drugs. There are several reasons for this complexity: (1) the basic electrophysiologic properties of the heart (i.e., excitability, automaticity, conduction velocity, refractoriness) have a complex interrelationship and classification is based on the effects on these properties; (2) drug effects are not seen in all parts of the heart or may be different in different parts; (3) drug effects on normal tissue are not the same as those on diseased tissue; and (4) many drugs have both direct and indirect effects.

Each agent may be discussed in terms of the four basic electrophysiologic properties of the heart: *excitability, automaticity, conduction velocity,* and *refractoriness.* It is important to recognize, however, that measurable variables used to assess these properties and the effects of drugs on them have a complex interrelationship. Excitability is assessed by measurements such as *threshold,* rate of *phase 4 depolarization,* and *resting membrane potential;* automaticity is assessed by the same measurements; conduction velocity is related to the rate of depolarization (i.e., *phase O, [dV/dt]),* which in turn depends on the resting membrane potential and the closeness of two heart beats to one another (i.e., heart rate [RR interval]; and refractoriness is determined by the duration of the *action potential* (AP) *(phases 2* and *3),* which also can depend on the resting membrane potential. At an even more basic level, all of these measurements are in turn determined by complex and incompletely understood movements of ions such as Na^+, K^+, Ca^{++}, and Cl^- across cell membranes.

The heart is not a monolithic organ, and these processes and the effects of drugs on them may differ in *sinoatrial (SA) node,* atrial muscle, *atrioventricular (AV) node,* specialized conduction tissue *(His-Purkinje* [HP] *system),* and ventricular muscle. These processes are altered in disease states that lead to dysrhythmias, and thus the effects of drugs in healthy, normally functioning cardiac tissue are probably different from those in diseased tissue. As corollaries to this point, the actual mechanism(s) of cardiac dysrhythmias is known in only a very few instances and relatively few studies have been done with human tissue, which may react differently than that of experimental animals. Finally, many of these agents have both direct and indirect actions.

The indirect actions of the antidysrhythmics are usually mediated via the autonomic nervous system and may be caused by drug effects on that system itself or on the central nervous system (CNS) or various

TABLE 32-1

Summary of effects of selected antidysrhythmic drugs on electrophysiologic properties of cardiac tissue

Type of cardiac tissue	Quinidine Procainamide Disopyramide	Lidocaine Mexiletine Phenytoin Tocainide	Verapamil	Amiodarone Bretylium
SA NODE				
Automaticity	0	0	?↓	↑*,↓
AV NODE				
Conduction	↑,0,↓	↑,0,↓	↓↓↓	↑,0,↓
PURKINJE FIBERS				
AP duration	↑	↓	0	↑
Effective refractory period	↑	↓	0	↑
Membrane responsiveness	↓↓↓	↓↓	0	0
Automaticity	↓	↓	?↓	↑*,0

0, no effect; ↑, increase; ↓, decrease; ?, uncertain; more than one arrow in one direction indicates prominent effect and in different directions indicates variability; *, this effect caused by catecholamine release.

TABLE 32-2

Summary of effects of selected antidysrhythmic drugs on the ECG

	P-R	QRS	QTc*	Ventricular rate in atrial fibrillation
Quinidine	0,↑	↑↑	↑↑	↑
Procainamide	0,↑	↑↑	↑↑	↑
Disopyramide	0,↑	0,↑	↑	↑
Lidocaine	0	0	0,↓	↑,0,↓
Phenytoin	0,↓	0	0,↓	↑,0,↓
Verapamil	0,↑	0	0	↓↓↓
Bretylium	0,↑	0	0,↓	↑,↓

0, no effect; ↑, increase; ↓, decrease; more than one arrow in one direction indicates prominent effect and in different directions indicates variability; QTc* is QT corrected for heart rate by dividing by √R-R.

homeostatic reflex arcs. The direct and indirect effects may be competing or additive, and in the intact heart the predominant effect in any one instance will depend on the pattern of innervation and the amount of tone present.

Keeping these considerations in mind, an overview is presented here that focuses on what are thought to be the major pharmacologic properties of these agents (Tables 32-1 and 32-2). The reader will be helped by a brief review of the basic electrophysiology of the heart at this time (see Chapter 30, "Review of the Anatomy, Physiology, and Assessment of the Cardiovascular System").

MECHANISM OF ACTION AND PHARMACOLOGIC EFFECTS

Quinidine, procainamide, disopyramide. The group of drugs composed of quinidine, procainamide, and disopyramide is one of the most commonly used for pharmacologic control of the heart rhythm. Although they differ in relation to pharmacokinetic properties and the relative frequency and type of some side effects, they may be considered identical in terms of their mechanism of action and pharmacologic effects. They have effects on all portions of the conduction system (i.e., SA node, atria, AV node, HP system, and ventricles). A prominent portion of their actions (and side effects) are indirect and caused by an atropine-like (antivagal) effect and reflex sympathetic activation secondary to hypotension.

In general, the direct actions of these drugs may be thought of as depressant (i.e., decreased phase 4 depolarization, increased threshold, slowed dV/dt, and prolongation of the AP). Thus automaticity and excitability are decreased, conduction velocity is slowed, and refractoriness is increased. In the intact heart, however, competing indirect effects can predominate in areas where there is dense autonomic innervation, particularly the SA and AV nodes. For this reason the heart rate will often increase slightly and conduction through the AV node is facilitated rather than slowed. All three agents are myocardial depressants and cause peripheral vasodilatation.

Lidocaine, phenytoin, mexiletine,* tocainide,* encainide,* flecainide,* lorcainide,* aprindine.* The second major group of antidysrhythmic agents all have prominent local anesthetic or anticonvulsant properties. This group of drugs is pharmacologically far less homogeneous than the others. In fact, certain of these drugs, particularly aprindine, encainide, flecainide, and lorcainide may be more appropriately grouped with quinidine, procainamide, and disopyramide.

The prototype drugs in this group are lidocaine and phenytoin. Although these two drugs have striking differences in their pharmacokinetics and side effects, these two drugs have virtually identical pharmacologic cardiac properties. In the usual therapeutic concentrations, the effects are confined to the HP system and the ventricular muscle and there are no important indirect effects. Like the quinidine group, these agents depress phase 4 depolarization and dV/dt. Thus, when present, automaticity of the HP system and the ventricular muscle (automaticity is not normally present in these tissues) is decreased and conduction velocity is slowed. Unlike the quinidine group, lidocaine and phenytoin shorten—or at least do not prolong—the AP duration and the threshold remains unchanged. These two drugs then do *not* alter excitability, but do

shorten the refractoriness of the HP system and the ventricular muscle. It has always been difficult to reconcile such effects with the known efficacy of lidocaine in suppressing ventricular dysrhythmias in acute myocardial infarction. Recent evidence suggests that lidocaine has a potent depressant effect on ischemic ventricular muscle cells, and this action would certainly be more in keeping with its known ability to suppress ventricular dysrhythmias in this setting. Such observations emphasize the point that normal and abnormal myocardial tissue do not necessarily respond in the same fashion when exposed to drugs.

Several newer drugs are also assigned to this group, and some are quite similar pharmacologically to lidocaine and phenytoin, with only minor differences. Others are quite different from lidocoaine and phenytoin, their effects are also largely confined to the HP system and the ventricular muscle, although aprindine has been reported to have some benefit in supraventricular dysrhythmias and thus may have more widespread effects. There are no apparent or important indirect effects thus far identified for the newer agents in this group.

Tocainide and mexiletine may be considered pharmacologically identical to lidocaine. Aprindine, encainide, and lorcainide are slightly different in an unusual fashion. These last three agents *shorten* the AP duration, as do the other agents in this group, but unlike the others, they *increase* refractoriness, but this effect may be more pronounced in the ventricular muscle than in the HP system (except for lorcainide, which has marked effects on the HP system). Flecainide, on the other hand, prolongs the AP duration and may be more appropriately grouped with quinidine. All agents in this group are myocardial depressants and peripheral vasodilators, but these are less prominent effects than those in the quinidine group.

Bretylium, amiodarone.* Bretylium and amiodarone are interesting agents whose actions are incompletely understood. They are both antiadrenergics, and this action has been most widely studied with bretylium, which was initially introduced as an antihypertensive agent. The antidysrhythmic action of these drugs may be the result of a combination of both the antiadrenergic mechanism and an ill-defined direct effect. Bretylium and amiodarone have effects on all electrically active parts of the heart. The antiadrenergic effects of bretylium are biphasic and consist of an initial inhibition of release of neuronal norepinephrine combined with a blockade of neuronal reuptake (can potentiate catecholamine effects). Potentiation of catecholamine effects may partly explain increased automaticity (i.e., increased rate of phase 4

---

*These drugs are experimental agents and *not* yet approved for general use in the United States or Canada.

depolarization) seen early after administration (hypotension and reflex sympathetic activation via baroreceptors may also play a role). In time, however, tissue norepinephrine levels fall, similar effect to guanethidine and reserpine, and in this second phase the antiadrenergic action becomes evident and probably adds to the direct depressant action. Except for the early phase, these drugs are depressants and decrease the slope of phase 4, decrease dV/dt, and lengthen the AP. The correlates of changes in these measurements are decreased automaticity and conduction velocity and increased refractoriness. There is thus a superficial resemblance to the quinidine group, but the mechanism of action is different and there are no anticholinergic effects; therefore, except for an early transient phase, heart rate and conduction through the AV node are slowed rather than increased, as they are with the quinidine group.

Verapamil, diltiazem. These agents represent an interesting and entirely new class of drugs that are used for a wide variety of conditions including certain dysrhythmias. The full extent of their usefulness remains unknown at present and they are discussed in other chapters (see Chapter 34, "Vasodilators, Antilipemics, Anticoagulants, and Platelet Aggregation Inhibitors"), but because the oldest agent, verapamil, is primarily an antidysrhythmic, they are also discussed here. Many additional drugs with the same mechanism are being actively developed by various drug companies. These drugs inhibit a slow inward current caused by Ca^{++} ion movement. This current is important in the plateau phase (i.e., phase 2) of the cardiac AP and in some areas of the heart in the slow diastolic depolarization (i.e., phase 4). Even though phase 2 is not prominent in the SA and AV nodes, these agents have prominent effects on refractoriness at these sites, and this striking action at the AV node is the basis for their major indication as antidysrhythmics. The observed electrophysiologic effects are decreased automaticity and slowed conduction. Although the entire heart is affected, effects at the SA and AV nodes are much more prominent.

These drugs have come to be referred to as Ca^{++} *entry blockers* or *slow current blockers* but they do not block all effects of Ca^{++} at all sites; therefore another popular term, Ca^{++} *blockers*, is incorrect. The slow Ca^{++} current is also important in vascular and other smooth muscle, and in cardiac muscle its inhibition affects both contraction and relaxation. These drugs also therefore are vasodilators (smooth muscle relaxants), and they alter cardiac mechanical function. These actions form the basis of their use in several other conditions. It is interesting that the various

agents appear to have a predilection for certain of their actions. Verapamil has a prominent effect at the AV and SA node and is a less potent vasodilator. Diltiazem has a more balanced effect. The basis for these differences is presently unknown.

These drugs have no well-recognized indirect actions. As the above discussion would suggest, they are myocardial depressants, but this effect is probably less than that of the quinidine groups.

PHARMACOKINETICS

Quinidine, procainamide, disopyramide. The differences between drugs *within* the various groups lies in their absorption, distribution, metabolism, and excretion. These factors will often determine the clinical circumstances in which one particular drug will be chosen over another. The quinidine group of drugs is easily and relatively completely absorbed from the gastrointestinal tract. The maximal effect by this route is usually seen at approximately 1 hour for procainamide and slightly later for the other two agents. By the intravenous route the effects of these agents are not instantaneous but take several minutes. This may reflect time required for accumulation in cardiac tissue. Quinidine is more highly bound to plasma proteins than procainamide. Quinidine binding decreases in patients on dialysis, and this may be caused by displacement by heparin. Protein binding of disopyramide is complicated by its being concentration dependent, and at higher concentrations the proportion of free drug is greater. It is also complicated by the fact that there are two separate sites, and one of these is α_1-acid glycoprotein, which is also important in lidocaine pharmacokinetics (see below).

Active metabolites (see Chapter 5, "Drug Metabolism and Elimination") of both quinidine (3-hydroxyquinidine, 2-oxo-quinidinone) and procainamide (N-acetylprocainamide) are known and, at least for quinidine, the amount of these agents formed is highly variable from patient to patient. Individual variation in amount and rate of formation of metabolites may partly explain the variability between patients in their therapeutic responses to these agents. Metabolism of disopyramide has not been fully determined, but the major metabolite is a mono-N-dealkylated compound. The active metabolites of quinidine and disopyramide may have slightly different rates of excretion than the parent compounds. It is definitely known that N-acetylprocainamide is excreted more slowly than procainamide.

All three drugs and their metabolites are largely excreted via the kidneys, and in the presence of impaired renal function the dosage interval must be altered. Drug accumulation in patients with renal impairment seems to be less of a problem with procainamide. Clearance of disopyramide is unaltered in patients with uncomplicated myocardial infarction but is slowed in patients with heart failure, and this may partly explain why this drug has such a marked myocardial depressant effect in patients with heart failure. Quinidine and disopyramide have similar half-lives (approximately 4 to 5 hours), and thus the oral dosage frequency is usually 6 to 8 hours. Procainamide has a considerably shorter half-life (approximately 2 to 3 hours) and must be administered orally every 3 to 4 hours. Such a short half-life means patients must awaken for a dose in the middle of the night if it is crucial to maintain a therapeutic drug level. Significant accumulation of the active metabolite N-acetylprocainamide, which has a longer half-life, may explain why some patients on long-term treatment with procainamide have a therapeutic response with a dosage frequency of 6 hours, although the blood levels of N-acetylprocainamide achieved would not seem sufficient to have a significant antidysrhythmic effect. N-Acetylprocainamide is being actively investigated as an antidysrhythmic drug in its own right.

A constant infusion of disopyramide and procainamide is the best technique to maintain adequate blood levels of these agents when the intravenous route is used. Quinidine has a reputation of being difficult to use via the parenteral routes (e.g., sudden cardiovascular collapse), and intravenous use is *not* recommended except in emergency situations. Patients receiving oral quinidine who need a temporary suspension of oral medication for elective surgery should be given intravenous procainamide or disopyramide.

Measurement of plasma drug levels of any of the three drugs may be helpful in selected patients who have difficult problems, such as a patient who does not respond to seemingly adequate oral doses but did respond to intravenous administration, or a patient with impaired renal function. It is important to know the technique of analysis used, however, because older techniques measure both the parent compound and the metabolites. The usually accepted therapeutic levels are based on older techniques. Therapeutic plasma levels are procainamide 4.0 to 8.0 µg/ml, disopyramide 2.0 to 4.0 µg/ml, and quinidine 2.0 to 6.0 µg/ml.

Lidocaine, phenytoin, mexiletine, tocainide, encainide, flecainide, lorcainide, aprindine. Lidocaine and phenytoin have remarkably different pharmacokinetic profiles and illustrate some important pharmacologic principles. Lidocaine is administered parenterally because it is highly subject to the "first-pass effect"; when given orally, the major portion (approximately 70%) of the absorbed drug is metabolized to an inactive form the first time it passes through the liver via the portal circulation, and thus therapeutic blood levels cannot be achieved by the oral route. The preferred route for this drug is the intravenous route, but therapeutic levels can also be achieved via the intramuscular route.

Following intravenous administration of a single bolus dose, lidocaine demonstrates a prominent redistribution phase in the plasma level curve, and even when an infusion is begun at the same time, the level may be less than therapeutic at 30 to 120 minutes. This phenomenon has led to a multitude of different schedules for administering this agent, the simplest of which is the second bolus technique. In this technique, a second bolus ½ to 1 times the size of the first is given 30 minutes after the first bolus, and a constant infusion is begun with the first bolus.

The elimination phase of the plasma level curve indicates a half-life of approximately 90 minutes for lidocaine. A variable amount (40% to 80%) of lidocaine is bound to plasma protein. Lidocaine is primarily bound to α_1-acid glycoprotein, and this protein is released following myocardial infarction. Variation in levels of this protein may explain variability in the amount of protein-bound lidocaine and also partly explain why total lidocaine levels rise during steady-state in patients with myocardial infarction. Metabolism of lidocaine, as mentioned previously, is primarily by the liver and is critically dependent on hepatic blood flow. The consequences of this are that in low-flow states such as shock and congestive heart failure the dose used must be *reduced*. The dose must also be reduced in patients with extensive parenchymal liver disease (e.g., hepatitis and cirrhosis). Renal failure does not substantially alter lidocaine pharmacokinetics. One of the major lidocaine metabolites, monoethylglycinexylidide, has antidysrhythmic properties and anticonvulsant properties, and at least one other metabolite has anticonvulsant properties. The role of these metabolites in relation to the clinical usefulness and toxicity of lidocaine remains unknown at present. The therapeutic plasma level of lidocaine is usually stated to be 1.4 to 6.0 µg/ml.

The metabolism of phenytoin presents a special problem. The kinetics of phenytoin blood levels versus time are nonlinear (i.e., dose-dependent) and cannot be described by linear compartment models (see Chapter 5, "Drug Metabolism and Elimination"). The pharmacokinetics of this drug are also highly variable among patients. The excretion rate of phenytoin actually increases as the blood level rises. It is metabolized in the liver by microsomal enzymes, conjugated, and excreted in the urine. It is highly bound (i.e., more than 90%) to plasma protein. There are several practical consequences of these properties of phenytoin. First, the oral dose may be given as a single amount or divided over a 24-hour period, whichever is most convenient. Second, steady-state plasma levels take longer to achieve and are unpredictable. Thus, for this drug, monitoring plasma levels is important. Third, metabolism by microsomal enzymes and a high degree of binding to plasma protein are properties that make this drug highly subject to a wide variety of interactions with other drugs. The therapeutic level of this agent is generally considered to be 10 to 20 μg/ml (see also Chapter 21, "Drugs Used to Treat Epilepsy").

Only scattered and incomplete pharmacokinetic data exist on the other newer agents in the lidocaine–phenytoin group. Tocainide is structurally similar to lidocaine, but the slight difference makes it much less subject to the first-pass effect, and thus its major difference from lidocaine is that it can be administered via the oral route. It is reasonably well absorbed after an oral dose, and peak levels are seen after 60 to 90 minutes. Approximately one half of the tocainide in the blood is protein bound, and because less of the drug is metabolized in the liver, renal function may be a factor in its use; 35% is excreted unchanged in the urine. Therapeutic plasma levels of tocainide are in the 5.0 to 10.0 μg/ml range. The elimination half-life of tocainide is 13 to 14 hours. Tocainide has no active metabolites. Mexiletine is well absorbed orally, and approximately 70% is bound to plasma protein. The elimination half-life of mexiletine is 5 to 7 hours in healthy volunteers. Metabolism is largely by the liver; less than 10% of an administered dose is excreted unchanged in the urine. The therapeutic level is 1.0 to 2.0 μg/ml.

Aprindine is also well absorbed orally but is more highly protein bound (85% to 95%). A high proportion (95%) of this drug is hydroxylated in the liver by microsomal enzymes, and most (65%) is excreted in the urine, although a substantial portion (35%) appears in the feces. This metabolism pattern again makes aprindine subject to interaction with other agents affecting microsomal enzymes. The elimination half-life is variable, but usually within the 15 to 30 hour range for most patients. This means aprindine can be given with a less frequent dosing interval (e.g., every 12 hours). A small amount of an active metabolite appears in the blood of patients receiving chronic treatment with aprindine. The therapeutic plasma level is 1.0 to 3.0 μg/ml.

Little pharmacokinetic information is currently available on lorcainide, flecainide, or encainide. Encainide apparently has a half-life of approximately 3 hours, and that of lorcainide is approximately 30 hours. Encainide has active metabolites.

Bretylium, amiodarone. Amiodarone is slowly and incompletely absorbed orally and there is a good deal of variability in absorption among patients. The drug apparently builds up in highly perfused and adipose tissues with chronic use, and serum concentrations rise slowly. Tissue buildup may explain the persistent effect observed for 30 to 45 days after it is discontinued. The elimination half-life, although not accurately known, is long (i.e., 15 to 60 days). Pathways of metabolism are currently unknown. Therapeutic blood levels are in the range of 1 to 3.5 μg/ml.

Bretylium is not effectively absorbed by the oral route and must be given parenterally. It is excreted by the kidneys largely unchanged, and there are no known active metabolites. The elimination half-life of bretylium is 5 to 10 hours.

Verapamil, diltiazem. Verapamil is rapidly and completely absorbed after oral administration. Approximately 90% is bound to plasma protein. The drug is almost completely metabolized in the liver, and little is excreted unchanged in the urine (i.e., less than 4%). Thus verapamil is subject to a prominent first-pass effect, and the intravenous dose is much lower (i.e., ⅛ to ⅒) than the corresponding oral dose. Metabolites accumulate, but they are only weakly active. The major active metabolite is norverapamil. The peak therapeutic effect after oral administration occurs somewhat after the peak plasma level, and the explanation for this observation is presently unclear. Therapeutic blood levels for verapamil are believed to be in the range of 100 to 300 ng/ml. The elimination half-life of verapamil is 4 to 6 hours, but with chronic use, it increases and may become as long as 8 hours. Little information is available on the agent, diltiazem.

USES

The antidysrhythmic drugs are used to treat a wide variety of cardiac dysrhythmias (see box p. 667 and Table 32-3). The objectives of therapy with antidysrhythmic drugs are decreased morbidity and mortality because of irregularities of the heartbeat. The mere documentation that a dysrhythmia exists does not in itself constitute an indication for treatment. Other factors such as the presence or absence of cardiac disease or symptoms must also be considered.

In some cases the need for treatment is well defined, as are the specific objectives of treatment. In

> ## A classification of cardiac dysrhythmias
>
> ### Ectopic beats
>
> Atrial premature beats (APB)
> Junctional premature beats (JPB)
> Ventricular premature beats (VPB)
>
> ### Tachycardias
> *Atrial*
>
> Paroxysmal atrial tachycardia (PAT)
> Atrial flutter
> Atrial fibrillation
> Multifocal atrial tachycardia (MAT)
>
> *Junctional*
>
> Accelerated junctional rhythm
> Junctional tachycardia
>
> *Ventricular*
>
> Accelerated idioventricular rhythm
> Ventricular tachycardia
> Ventricular fibrillation
>
> ### Bradycardias and heart block
> *Sinus*
>
> Sinus bradycardia
> Sinoatrial (SA) block
> Sinus arrest
>
> *Atrioventricular (AV) block*
>
> First degree
> Second degree
> Advanced AV block
> Third degree

other situations the need or specific objectives of treatment are not known with any certainty. It is important to keep this in mind when discussing the use of these agents. These drugs have a high incidence of side effects, and one must constantly strive to keep a balance among the need for treatment, therapeutic efficacy, and adverse affects.

Supraventricular dysrhythmias are only rarely life-threatening. The initial goal is usually to control the ventricular rate. The traditional agents used for this purpose, digitalis (see Chapter 31, "Cardiac Glycosides") and beta-adrenergic blocking agents (see Chapter 24, "Sympathomimetics and Sympatholytics"), are

discussed in other chapters. The newer calcium current antagonists, of which verapamil is the prototype, are a significant development for this indication. Given intravenously, this agent can almost always, except in some forms of ventricular preexcitation, rapidly control the heart rate, and in a significant proportion of those forms with organized rhythms (e.g., atrial tachycardia and flutter) will convert the rhythm to sinus. Atrial fibrillation is not as readily converted to sinus rhythm by verapamil, but the ventricular rate is easily controlled. Verapamil works more rapidly than the digitalis glycosides and has less of a myocardial depressant effect than do beta-adrenergic blocking agents.

Once the ventricular rate is controlled, further success at reversion to sinus rhythm may often be achieved by adding another agent, such as one from the quinidine group. The quinidine group will help to suppress extrasystoles, which are often the trigger for supraventricular tachycardias, or alter the conduction properties of the heart in a fashion that makes it less likely that a tachycardia will be sustained. The quinidine drugs are generally not given alone for supraventricular tachycardias because they often improve conduction through the AV node and thus, during the tachycardia, the ventricular rate may be faster than it was when the patient was not taking drugs.

Some patients with *Wolff-Parkinson-White* (W-P-W) *syndrome* will have difficulty in controlling supraventricular dysrhythmias because of the conduction properties of their accessory pathways to the ventricles. Aprindine and amiodarone are particularly useful in patients with these problems. Generally, however, the lidocaine group of drugs is not used for supraventricular tachycardias because either these drugs have no effect or they have side effects that are too troublesome. One other exception to this rule of thumb is that phenytoin is reputed to be particularly efficacious in junctional tachycardia because of digitalis excess. Occasionally, when lidocaine is given to patients with supraventricular tachycardia, there may be an alarming increase in the ventricular rate, but this is a much less common occurrence than is the case with the quinidine group.

Ventricular dysrhythmias are often more worrisome, particularly with acute myocardial ischemia such as myocardial infarction and some types of angina. In an emergency, intravenous lidocaine is usually the drug of choice for this problem. If long-term oral therapy is needed, the most commonly used of the presently available agents are quinidine and disopyramide. Procainamide is also fairly widely used, but because it must be given much more frequently (i.e., every 3 to 4 hours) and because long-term use has

TABLE 32-3

Use of selected antidysrhythmic agents in treating some common dysrhythmias

Dysrhythmia	Quinidine	Procain-amide	Disopyr-amide	Lido-caine	Phenytoin	Verapamil	Bretylium
SUPRAVENTRICULAR							
Conversion of atrial fibrillation	+ +	+ +	+	0	0	0	0
Conversion of atrial flutter	+	+	?	0	0	+	0
Conversion of par-oxysmal atrial tachycardia	+ + +	+ + +	+ + +	0	+	+ + + +	0
Prophylaxis of above rhythms	+ + + +	+ + + +	+ + + +	0	0	?	0
Atrial premature beats	+ + +	+ + +	+ + +	0	+	0	0
VENTRICULAR							
Ventricular prema-ture beats	+ + +	+ + +	+ + +	+ + + +	+ +	?	+
Ventricular tachy-cardia	+ +	+ + + +	+ + +	+ + + +	+ +	0	+ + +
DIGITALIS-INDUCED							
Atrial tachycardia with block	+	+	+	+ + +	+ + +	−	−
Junctional tachy-cardia	+	+	+	+ + +	+ + +	−	−
Ventricular dys-rhythmias	+	+	+	+ + +	+ + +	−	−

+, beneficial (more than one indicates prominent effect); 0, no effect; ?, unknown; −, probably *contraindicated*

some troublesome side effects, the other two agents are often selected first. Bretylium is only used for short periods, usually in patients with an acute myocardial infarction, or who have life-threatening dysrhythmias resistant to the more standard agents. The newer agents in the lidocaine group are also usually reserved for those patients in whom conventional drugs have failed. The calcium current antagonists have some effect in ventricular dysrhythmias, but, at present, must be considered secondary agents for this purpose. The Ca^{++} entry blockers, as indicated previously, have a much wider use for other conditions in addition to dysrhythmias. These include angina pectoris—both vasospastic and regular types, systemic hypertension, pulmonary hypertension, hypertrophic obstructive cardiomyopathy, and heart failure; probably several other uses will become apparent with time.

ADVERSE EFFECTS AND TOXICITY

Quinidine, procainamide, disopyramide. As can be seen on reviewing Adverse/Side Effects of the Antidysrhythmics, antidysrhythmic drugs cause a wide variety of adverse side effects and some of these are potentially serious. Therefore, use of these drugs should never be undertaken without carefully considering the possible adverse side effects.

Side effects from using the quinidine group of drugs are quite common and are very similar with all three agents, although some exceptions will be noted. Gastrointestinal side effects are extremely common, and these occur most often with quinidine itself. Atropine-like effects (e.g., dry mouth, blurred vision, urinary retention) are also extremely common, particularly at higher doses, and disopyramide seems to cause these effects more often than the other agents in this group.

Other side effects, which are less common but potentially more dangerous, include drug-induced dysrhythmias, (particularly when the QT interval becomes markedly prolonged), thrombocytopenia, hemolytic anemia, and dementia.

Quinidine is related to quinine and therefore is chemically classified as a cinchona alkaloid. In sensitive patients, it can cause a toxic syndrome called cinchonism, which in its mild form consists of tinnitus, headache, nausea, and disturbed vision. In many patients receiving long-term treatment with procainamide, a syndrome similar to *lupus erythematosus* can occur, including arthralgia, arthritis, rash, myalgia, fever, pleuritic chest pain, and pericarditis. Fortunately, nephritis is not a feature of this syndrome, and it generally resolves when the drug is discontinued.

A high percentage of patients receiving chronic procainamide will have serologic evidence of lupus (i.e., a positive antinuclear antibody [ANA]), but only a few develop the symptoms. The lupuslike syndrome is more likely to occur in patients who are slow acetylators who may have had similar reactions to other drugs.

All drugs in the quinidine group will cause myocardial depression and vasodilatation. Because of *idiosyncratic* responses to quinidine, a test dose of this drug is recommended before beginning chronic treatment. Disopyramide has been implicated in sudden cardiovascular collapse when given to patients in congestive heart failure; congestive heart failure is probably a relative contraindication for this agent.

Others. The side effects of the lidocaine group of drugs are more likely to be manifest as neurologic symptoms such as tremor, confusion, restlessness, paresthesias, sedation, and seizures. Those taken orally also commonly cause gastrointestinal upset. Phenytoin is a folate antagonist and can cause a macrocytic anemia. In addition, it causes a peculiar hyperplasia of the gums. The incidence of side effects is extremely high in patients taking tocainide and aprindine, but, in spite of this, these agents are often well tolerated for long periods. Cholestatic jaundice and *agranulocytosis* have been reported with aprindine, and like several other antidysrhythmics it has been reported to cause psychoses in rare instances. Tocainide can rarely cause alveolitis. The major side effect of bretylium is hypotension. Amiodarone causes a peculiar slate-blue discoloration of the skin and microdeposits in the cornea that disappear when the drug is discontinued. Amiodarone can also interfere with thyroid function. It is important to emphasize that virtually all antidysrhythmics can cause dysrhythmias or make them worse. The incidence of side effects

with verapamil is fairly low. Most are related to hypotension and bradycardia. Verapamil's most common gastrointestinal side effects are nausea and constipation. Intravenous calcium can be given in emergencies to try to counteract the adverse effects of verapamil.

DRUG INTERACTIONS

Many of the antidysrhythmic agents have not been in use for a sufficient period of time to have developed an extensive list of other agents with which they interact. Phenytoin, because it is metabolized by microsomal enzymes (a property shared by many other agents), interacts with a large group of drugs (see Clinically Significant Drug Interactions). For cardiac patients, the most important of these is the interaction between phenytoin and the oral anticoagulants. Quinidine also interacts with oral anticoagulants; the quinidine-digoxin and quinidine-digitoxin interactions are discussed in Chapter 31, "Cardiac Glycosides." Amiodarone will also prolong bleeding time in patients taking warfarin. The combination of verapamil or diltiazem and a beta-adrenergic blocking agent is at least relatively contraindicated because it can cause complete heart block and profound bradycardia. These particular combinations have been used, however, in patients with angina pectoris and no apparent preexisting conduction problems, and the risk seems low. As noted previously, verapamil also increases plasma levels of digoxin. Bretylium can potentiate the effects of catecholamines, and caution should be exercised when these drugs are being used concurrently. Propranolol can cause an increase in plasma levels of lidocaine, and caution should be used when these two drugs are combined.

SUMMARY

The antidysrhythmics are used to maintain a regular cardiac rhythm and rate. These agents elicit their pharmacologic effect by affecting the excitability, automaticity, conduction velocity, and refractoriness of the cardiac tissue.

A wide variety of agents is found that possess antidysrhythmic activity. For purposes of convenience and comparison the agents discussed in this chapter were categorized into four major groups: (1) antidysrhythmic and anticholinergic; (2) antidysrhythmic, local anesthetic and anticonvulsant; (3) antidysrhythmic and antiadrenergic; and (4) antidysrhythmic and calcium antagonist. Although drugs within the various groups differ in relation to their pharmacokinetic properties (i.e., absorption, distribution, metabolism, and elimination) and the relative frequency and type of some side effects, they are usually closely related or identical in relation to their mechanism of action and pharmacologic effect. The pharmacokinetic and toxicologic differences of the various drugs within the antidysrhythmic groups are often used to determine which particular drug will be chosen over another in a given clinical circumstance with a particular patient.

Familiarity with both the therapeutic and toxic effects of the antidysrhythmics should enable the nurse to provide optimal care to patients who require these medications.

ADVERSE/SIDE EFFECTS OF THE ANTIDYSRHYTHMICS*

ALLERGIC REACTIONS

Angioedema
Asthma
Itching
Lupus erythematosus
Lymphadenopathy
"Serum sickness" (fever, chills,
    malaise, myalgia)
Stevens-Johnson syndrome
Urticaria (hives) and numerous other
    skin rashes, including purpura

AUTONOMIC NERVOUS SYSTEM

Anticholinergic effects (dry mouth,
    eyes, nose; urinary hesitancy and
    retention)

BEHAVIOR

Anxiety
Confusion
Dementia and memory impairment
Giddiness
Mental depression and other mood
    alterations
Personality changes
Psychosis (including hallucinations)

CARDIOVASCULAR SYSTEM

Bradycardia
Cardiac arrest
Congestive heart failure

Flushing
Heart block
Hypotension
Nonspecific ST-T changes
QT prolongation
QRS widening
Sudden death
Tachycardia
Ventricular dysrhythmias

CENTRAL NERVOUS SYSTEM

Ataxia
Altered hearing
Coma (lidocaine)
Convulsions
Drowsiness
Dysarthria
Headache
Nervousness
Paresthesia
Restlessness
Tinnitus
Tremor
Vertigo
Weakness

GASTROINTESTINAL SYSTEM

Abdominal discomfort and dyspepsia
Anorexia
Bitter taste
Diarrhea
Nausea
Vomiting

HEMATOLOGIC SYSTEM

Agranulocytosis
Anemia (megaloblastic and aplastic)
Eosinophilia
Hypoprothrombinemia
Leukopenia

HEPATIC SYSTEM

Cholestatic jaundice

**METABOLIC AND ENDOCRINE
SYSTEMS**

Gingival hyperplasia
Hyperthyroidism
Hypothyroidism
Impaired ADH release
Impaired glucose tolerance
Osteomalacia
Skin discoloration

NEUROMUSCULAR SYSTEM

Peripheral neuropathy

OCULAR SYSTEM

Blurred vision
Corneal microdeposits
Diplopia
Nystagmus

*See Chapter 11, "Drug Toxicity," for an overview of drug toxicity.

CLINICALLY SIGNIFICANT DRUG INTERACTIONS*

Primary drug	Interacting drug	Possible effect(s)	Probable mechanism(s)
Bretylium	Digitalis glycosides (toxicity)	Aggravation of digitalis toxicity	Initial release of norepinephrine caused by bretylium
Lidocaine	Cimetidine	Increased lidocaine effect	Decreased lidocaine clearance
Lidocaine	Propranolol	Increased lidocaine effect	Decreased lidocaine clearance
Phenytoin	Anticoagulants (oral)	Increased phenytoin effect	Inhibition of microsomal enzymes and displacement from binding sites
Phenytoin	Chloramphenicol	Increased phenytoin effect	Inhibition of microsomal enzymes
Phenytoin	Corticosteroids	Decreased effect of corticosteroids	Induction of microsomal enzymes
Phenytoin	Disulfiram	Increased phenytoin effect	Inhibition of metabolism
Phenytoin	Isoniazid	Increased phenytoin effect	Inhibition of microsomal enzymes
Procainamide	Parasympathomimetics	Decreased parasympathomimetic effect on skeletal muscle	Neuromuscular blocking properties of procainamide antagonize parasympathomimetic effect on skeletal muscle
Quinidine	Anticoagulants (oral)	Increased anticoagulant effect	Decreased prothrombin levels
Quinidine	Barbiturates	Decreased quinidine effect	Induction of microsomal enzymes
Quinidine	Digoxin	Increased digoxin serum levels and effect	Displacement of digoxin from tissue stores and decreased clearance
Quinidine	Phenytoin	Decreased quinidine plasma levels and effect	Induction of microsomal enzymes
Quinidine	Tubocurarine	Increased curariform effect (unresponsiveness and apnea)	Additive
Quinidine	Urine alkalinizers (e.g., sodium bicarbonate, acetazolamide)	Increased quinidine effect and potential toxicity	Increased tubular reabsorption of quinidine
Verapamil	Beta-adrenergic blocking agents	Heart block	Additive effect at AV node
Verapamil	Digoxin	Increased digoxin serum levels and effect	Decreased volume of distribution and decreased clearance of digoxin

*See Chapter 10, "Drug Interactions," for an overview of drug interactions.

GENERAL NURSING IMPLICATIONS

Nursing of patients requiring antidysrhythmics

ASSESSMENT

A complete nursing assessment is essential to establish a baseline from which to individualize drug therapy and to monitor the therapeutic response, adverse side effects, and signs of toxicity. Assessment should include a careful drug history to identify sensitivity, contraindications, and potential drug interactions before the first dose of an antidysrhythmic is administered. The nurse's role in assessment cannot be overemphasized, because the recognition and successful treatment of life-threatening cardiac dysrhythmias and the selection of appropriate antidysrhythmic agents are based on correct and precise identification of the dysrhythmia, as well as on its cause or precipitating factors.

In assessment of patients the nurse should be aware of correctable conditions that can bring about dysrhythmias: hypoxia, hypercapnia, hypothermia, electrolyte imbalances, and the use of antidysrhythmic agents themselves. The nurse must also be alert to assess cardiac diagnoses that may predispose a patient to dysrhythmias, such as cardiomyopathies, coronary atherosclerotic heart disease, preexcitation syndromes, and antidysrhythmic agents.

SENSITIVITY

In administration of antidysrhythmic agents to patients who have not received them before, monitoring for hypersensitivity is extremely important. For some of these drugs (e.g., quini-

Continued.

GENERAL NURSING IMPLICATIONS—cont'd

Nursing of patients requiring antidysrhythmics—cont'd

SENSITIVITY—cont'd

dine), a test dose is recommended before proceeding with therapy. Antidysrhythmic agents have specific signs of hypersensitivity, and these must be carefully monitored. For example, thrombocytopenia and platelet lysis may indicate hypersensitivity to quinidine (see the Nursing Drug Digest).

CONTRAINDICATIONS

Antidysrhythmics are contraindicated in patients with a known sensitivity to a specific antidysrhythmic agent. In addition, certain conditions also indicate contraindications to using specific drugs in this class (see the Nursing Drug Digest).

CAUTIONS

These agents should be used with caution in heart block, severe hypotension, hepatic or renal impairment, and in elderly patients. See the Nursing Drug Digest for additional cautions associated with individual agents.

DRUG INTERACTIONS

Various drug interactions have been reported involving the antidysrhythmics (see Clinically Significant Drug Interactions). For example, cimetidine and propranolol are known to decrease the clearance of lidocaine, requiring lower doses to maintain therapeutic blood levels without toxicity; and quinidine, when given with digitalis, can produce digitalis toxicity if the dosage is not reduced.

ADMINISTRATION
Initial therapy

The ECG is used to monitor carefully individual patient responses and emergency equipment should be readily available. Most of these medications can be given orally or parenterally, however, some are given by only one route. Be alert to the recommended route of administration.

In addition, many, if not most, antidysrhythmics (e.g., bretylium, phenytoin, procainamide) can produce severe hypotension when administered intravenously and thus careful monitoring of both rhythm and blood pressure is indicated.

Phenytoin, when administered intravenously, requires flushing of the vein with normal saline after administration to prevent irritation of the vein. This must be done carefully or a precipitate will form. In addition, phenytoin should *not* be given intramuscularly, because it is erratically absorbed and can cause tissue necrosis and sterile abscesses. (See the Nursing Drug Digest for specific information regarding the administration of individual antidysrhythmic agents.)

Maintenance therapy

The efficacy of many antidysrhythmics depends on maintenance of plasma levels within a narrow therapeutic range, and this requires careful attention and close adherence to dosage and administration frequency as specified by the prescriber. The medication should be taken as scheduled in the hospital, as well as on discharge.

Gastrointestinal adverse side effects can often be alleviated by administering oral medication forms with food, milk, or juice (see the Nursing Drug Digest).

A change in clinical status of the patient or the patient's concurrent medication may necessitate a change in the dosage or administration frequency of antidysrhythmic drugs.

MONITORING
Therapeutic response

Monitoring patient compliance and response is essential. Monitor for normal rate, sinus rhythm, and termination of the original dysrhythmia. ECG monitoring is indicated during initial therapy and at regular intervals with continued long-term use of these medications. The specific response varies with each group of antidysrhythmic agents (see the Nursing Drug Digest).

Adverse side effects

Monitoring side effects is essential (see Adverse/Side Effects of the Antidysrhythmics), as is planning to minimize these effects with the patient and the family, especially if the patient is to continue the antidysrhythmic therapy at home.

When antidysrhythmic agents are administered, continuous ECG monitoring is essential for all patients, except for those taking the drugs orally on a long-term or prophylactic basis. These patients should be monitored periodically. Pulse, blood pressure, apical rate, and signs of cardiac decompensation should be monitored because antidysrhythmics may cause hypotension and cardiac depression. Some dysrhythmias are characterized by a pulse deficit, so that the peripheral pulse is less per minute than the apical heartbeat.

Patients receiving long-term procainamide therapy (3 to 6 months) will have an elevated antinuclear antibody titer, and some may develop a systemic lupus erythematosus syndrome, particularly if therapy extends over 6 months. These patients must be warned to monitor for systemic infection and abnormal bleeding episodes. Patients should have routine ECGs and be instructed to report immediately any symptoms of dizziness or syncope.

Toxicity

Toxicity associated with the use of the antidysrhythmics can be caused by the patient taking more medication than prescribed, diminished renal or hepatic function (see the Nursing Drug Digest), and concurrent use with certain other medications (see Clinically Significant Drug Interactions). Close monitoring of patients receiving antidysrhythmic agents for signs of toxicity is essential because patient response can be idiosyncratic (as with quinidine) and

GENERAL NURSING IMPLICATIONS—cont'd

Nursing of patients requiring antidysrhythmics—cont'd

Toxicity—cont'd

result in sudden death. If signs of toxicity are noted, the medication should be stopped and the prescriber notified. Patients should also be able to monitor themselves for signs of toxicity related to their individual drug regimen.

PATIENT EDUCATION

The patient and the family, as indicated, should be involved as early as possible in the prescribed drug regimen. They should have a clear understanding of the purpose of the specific antidysrhythmic agent required, possible adverse side effects, signs of toxicity, and how the medication modifies activities of daily living. If the patient is to continue on the antidysrhythmic agent on a long-term basis, he or she should understand that it must be taken specifically as directed, and that continued monitoring by both the pa-

tient and the health care provider is required. The patient needs to know how best to take the medication, how to maintain compliance with the drug regimen, and what to do if a dose is missed inadvertently. The patient must understand that antidysrhythmics interact with numerous medications and that he or she should not begin or discontinue any other medications without first consulting with the health care provider.

Involving the patient and the family in care planning will do much to promote compliance and to avoid serious problems that can occur through the misuse of the medication. Research has also demonstrated that helping patients minimize side effects can enhance compliance (e.g., taking quinidine-like antidysrhythmics with meals

prevents the more common gastrointestinal side effects, which have been reported to be the cause of many patients' discontinuing the use of their medication).

Patients should have a sound understanding of the monitoring of their condition and the effects of medication. They should know what signs indicate they should notify their health care provider. Patients receiving antidysrhythmic agents often receive additional medications and usually require assistance with adapting to changes in activities of daily living and lifestyle, including stress management, exercise, diet, and activity adjustments. Follow-up after discharge is important, and referral to respective lay groups is often beneficial in helping the patient and the family accept the condition, as well as the therapeutic regimen required.

GENERAL INSTRUCTIONS FOR DISCHARGE/OUTPATIENTS

This drug is an antidysrhythmic used to control an irregular heartbeat. Follow the instructions on the prescription exactly. If you do not understand why you require this medication or if you have any questions, check with your health care provider.

Do not stop taking this medication before consulting with your health care provider. It is important that you do not miss any doses.

Do not drink alcohol while taking this medication.

This medication can interact with other medicines to cause severe reactions; do *not* start any new medicine, prescription or nonprescription, without first checking with your health care provider.

This medication can cause certain side effects. Report any unusual effects of this medicine to your health care provider.

This medication has been prescribed especially for you. Do *not* trade or give this medication to any relatives or friends.

Keep this and all medications out of children's reach.

NOTE: This list of instructions can be modified for each specific antidysrhythmic as needed; see Adverse/Side Effects of the Antidysrhythmics, Clinically Significant Drug Interactions, and the Nursing Drug Digest.

NURSING DRUG DIGEST

Medication (trade name)	Indication	Usual dosage and administration	Dosage forms, preparation, and storage	Contraindications, cautions, and comments	Monitoring
Bretylium tosylate Bretylate Bretylin Bretylol Darenthin	Ventricular tachycardia and fibrillation resistant to standard drugs	*Adults:* Used only 3-5 days IV, loading: 5-10 mg/kg over 10-20 min; repeat in 1-2 hr if necessary Maintenance: 5-10 mg/kg IV over 10-20 min q.6h.; or 1-2 mg/min constant IV infusion IV dose should be diluted before administration, except when treating life-threatening ventricular fibrillation IM, loading: 5-10 mg/kg; repeat in 1-2 hr if necessary Maintenance: 5-10 mg/kg q.6h. IM Do *not* dilute before IM injection Do not administer more than 5 ml per site Rotate IM injection sites Patients should be switched to an oral antidysrhythmic as soon as possible Bretylium is excreted primarily unchanged by the kidneys; therefore, dosage must be decreased in renal insufficiency *Elderly:* Start with lower doses	Injectable: 50 mg/ml Prepare solution for IV infusion by diluting one ampule (500 mg) to a *minimum* 50 ml with either dextrose solution for injection or sodium chloride solution for injection	*Contraindicated* in digitalis-induced dysrhythmias and recent myocardial infarction Postural hypotension can be marked; slowly and cautiously change patient from supine to upright posture Patients should generally be kept in a supine position during therapy until tolerance develops to the hypotensive effects Rapid IV administration of undiluted drug may cause nausea and vomiting Use with caution in aortic stenosis, sinus bradycardia, and pulmonary hypertension Initial onset of action may not occur for ½-6 hr after the initiation of therapy	Observe for orthostatic hypotension Monitor heart rate Monitor ECG continuously during loading dose

Drug	Uses	Dosage	Preparations	Remarks	Nursing implications
Disopyramide Rythmodan (base—oral) (phosphate—injectable) Norpace (phosphate) Norpace CR (phosphate)	Ventricular and supraventricular dysrhythmias	*Adults:* IV, loading dose: 2 mg/kg over 10-15 min; if necessary, an additional 1-2 mg/kg by slow IV over the next 45 min. Maintenance: 0.003 to 0.007 mg/kg/min for up to 24 hr 100-200 mg PO q.6h. (base); or 150-300 mg PO q.6h. (phosphate salt) *Children:* Less than 1 year of age, 10-30 mg/kg/24 hr PO in divided doses q.6h.; 1-4 years of age, 10-20 mg/kg/24 hr PO in divided doses q.6h.; 4-12 years of age, 10-15 mg/kg/24 hr PO in divided doses q.6h.; 12-18 years of age, 6-15 mg/kg/24 hr PO in divided doses q.6h. NOTE: Children's dosages are presented in terms of disopyramide base *Reduce dosage in both renal and hepatic impairment* NOTE: Be sure to check whether the base or phosphate	Injectable: 10 mg/ml (base) Capsule: 100, 150 mg (base and phosphate) Capsules (controlled-release): 100, 150 mg A pediatric suspension can be prepared by adding cherry syrup to the base to obtain a concentration of 1-10 mg/ml; this suspension is stable for 1 month if refrigerated	*Contraindicated* in heart block *Contraindicated* in cardiogenic shock and congestive heart failure Use caution in shock states Manage constipation with fluids and bulk laxatives Anticholinergic side effects are common Therapeutic plasma levels of disopyramide (base) are generally 3-6 µg/ml May cause congestive heart failure or hypotension	Observe for anticholinergic side effects (e.g., blurred vision, constipation, dry mouth, urinary retention) Check apical pulse before administration Monitor blood pressure at least t.i.d. for hypotensive effects Monitor plasma levels of drug Monitor ECG: if greater than 25% widening of QRS complex or Q-T interval occurs, discontinue medication and notify prescriber Monitor IV infusion rates

NOTE: For additional details regarding the individual agents listed in this table see the text and other tables in this chapter.

Continued.

NURSING DRUG DIGEST—cont'd

Medication (trade name)	Indication	Usual dosage and administration	Dosage forms, preparation, and storage	Contraindications, cautions, and comments	Monitoring
Lidocaine LidoPen Auto-Injector Xylocaine Xylocard	Ventricular dysrhythmias See also Chapter 55, "Antiseptics and Local Anesthetics"	*Adults:* IV, loading: 1-1.5 mg/kg over 2-5 min; after 10 min repeat 1-1.5 mg/kg over 2-5 min if indicated Particularly important to give second bolus over 2-5 min to avoid seizures Maximum: 300 mg/hr Maintenance: 0.015 to 0.05 mg/kg/min IM, 300 mg (4.3 mg/kg); may repeat in 60 to 90 min (use IM *only* when IV is not available or not possible) May cause pain at injection site Deltoid muscle is the preferred site for IM injection, to obtain optimal absorption; use 10% solution NOTE: The LidoPen Auto-Injector is self-administered by the patient into the vastus lateralis muscle May need to decrease dosage in hepatic failure May need to decrease dose in renal impairment Drug is ineffective if orally administered *Elderly:* May require *lower* loading and maintenance doses, particularly in presence of congestive heart failure Patients should be switched to an oral antidysrhythmic as soon as possible	Use *only* lidocaine hydrochloride injectable without preservatives that is clearly labeled for IV use Injectable: 0.2%, 0.4%, 0.8%, 1%, 2%, 4%, 10%, 20% Injectable: 100 mg/ml IM Prepare solutions for IV infusions by adding 1 or 2 gm of lidocaine to 1 L of D₅W to obtain a solution containing 1 or 2 mg/ml Stable for 24 hr Do *not* add lidocaine to blood transfusion assemblies Discard unused solutions	*Contraindicated* in heart block, Adams-Stokes syndrome, and Wolff-Parkinson-White syndrome *Contraindicated* in patients hypersensitive to amide-type local anesthetics May cause neonatal depression if administered during labor May cause hypertension and bradycardia Use with caution in congestive heart failure, shock, and reduced cardiac output Therapeutic serum levels are generally 1.5-5 μg/ml	Monitor blood pressure Observe for respiratory depression Monitor via ECG for signs of excessive cardiac depression (e.g., prolongation of P-R interval and QRS complex); if observed, stop drug and notify prescriber Monitor IV infusion rates

Drug	Uses	Dosage	Preparations	Contraindications/Cautions	Nursing Implications
Phenytoin Dantoin Dilantin Diphenylan Ditan Epanutin Eptoin Novophenytoin	Ventricular and supraventricular dysrhythmias, particularly if caused by digitalis excess NOTE: Although commonly used, this indication is not FDA or HPB approved See also Chapter 21, "Drugs Used to Treat Epilepsy"	*Adults:* 100 to 300 mg by slow IV; *no faster than 50 mg/min;* may repeat in 30 min 100 to 600 mg/24 hr PO may be given as single or divided dose *Children:* 250 mg/m²/24 hr IV; or 4-8 mg/kg/24 hr PO *Elderly:* Start with lower doses NOTE: The parenteral solution is highly alkaline and should be administered into a large vein if possible; administration of PO dose with food or milk may decrease GI irritation; flush IV line with normal saline before and after administration Do not administer IM	Injectable: 50 mg/ml Dilute with normal saline Do *not* mix with D₅W Tablet: 50 mg Capsule: 30, 100 mg Suspension: 30 mg/5 ml, 125 mg/5 ml	*Contraindicated* in heart block, sinus bradycardia, and Adams-Stokes syndrome Rapid administration can cause heart block *Teratogenic:* may cause cleft lip or palate if administered during first trimester of pregnancy Therapeutic serum levels are generally 10-20 µg/ml	Monitor *vital signs* for bradycardia and respiratory depression Observe for gingival hyperplasia Monitor serum levels
Procainamide Novocamid Procan SR Pronestyl Pronestyl SR Sub-Quin	Ventricular and supraventricular dysrhythmias	*Adults:* IV, loading: 10-12 mg/kg as boluses of 100 mg every 5 min at a rate *not* exceeding 50 mg/min; or 500 mg IV administered at a constant rate over 30 min followed by 2-6 mg/min IV Maintenance: 2-6 mg/min IV infusion; or 500-1000 mg IM q.3-8h. (this route may be preferable for patients who are NPO or who are vomiting); or 250-500 mg (i.e., 6 mg/kg) PO q.3h. Administration with food or milk may decrease GI irritation Oral administration must be on a 24 hr basis (i.e., have to awaken patient at night) 500-1000 mg PO q.6h. (sustained-release tablet) Reduce dosage in renal impairment Monitor and adjust dosage if necessary via plasma levels of procainamide (therapeutic: 3-10 µg/ml)	Injectable: 100, 500 mg/ml Capsule: 250, 375, 500 mg Tablets (sustained-release): 250, 500, 750 mg Store parenteral solutions at room temperature and protect from light Yellow discoloration occurs, but this does not prevent use Discard if darker than light amber or any other color Dilute with D₅W *before* IV administration	*Contraindicated* in myasthenia gravis *Contraindicated* in heart block *Contraindicated* in patients hypersensitive to procaine and related drugs *Prolonged* administration often causes a positive antinuclear antibody (ANA) test with or without symptoms of a lupus erythematosus-like syndrome Hemodialysis may be used in cases of overdosage to significantly increase the rate of procainamide elimination Rapid onset of action May cause hypotension Maintain patient in a supine position during IV administration	Frequent monitoring of blood pressure necessary during IV administration Monitor ECG during infusion for signs of toxicity (e.g., excessive widening greater than 25% of QRS complex, prolongation of P-R interval) Patient should be attended and blood pressure monitored at all times during infusion Observe for symptoms of lupus erythematosus-like syndrome (e.g., arthritis, fever, myalgia) Monitor serum levels

Continued.

NURSING DRUG DIGEST—cont'd

Medication (trade name)	Indication	Usual dosage and administration	Dosage forms, preparation, and storage	Contraindications, cautions, and comments	Monitoring
Quinidine sulfate (contains 83% anhydrous quinidine alkaloid) Cin-Quin Novoquinidin Quinicardine Quinidex Extentabs Quinora SK-Quinidine **Quinidine bisulfate** (contains 66% anhydrous quinidine alkaloid) Biquin Durules **Quinidine gluconate** (contains 62% anhydrous quinidine alkaloid) Duraquin	Ventricular and supraventricular dysrhythmias	*Adults:* IV, gluconate 300-800 mg slowly over 45-60 min NOTE: It is recommended that the *diluted gluconate* solution be administered slowly at a rate of 1 ml/min IM, initially 600 mg gluconate followed by 400 mg IM q2-6h. as indicated Maximum: 4 gm/24 hr Maintenance: Sulfate 200-400 mg PO q.6-8h. (NOTE: The extended-release tablets can be dosed q.8-12h.) Administration with food or milk may decrease GI distress NOTE: Differences in the amount of quinidine alkaloid in the various salt preparations necessitates differences in dosage Test dose of 200 mg PO or IM is recommended because of idiosyncratic response (e.g., allergic reaction)	Injectable: 190 mg/ml (sulfate), 80 mg/ml (gluconate) Tablet (sulfate): 200 mg Tablet (bisulfate): 250 mg Tablet (gluconate): 325 mg Tablet (polygalacturonate): 275 mg *Discard* discolored (brownish) solutions Parenteral solution of the gluconate salt can be diluted to 16 mg/ml using D₅W as the diluent (e.g., dilute 10 ml to 50 ml with D₅W)	*Contraindicated* in heart block, myasthenia gravis, and digitalis intoxication with AV conduction defects *Contraindicated* in patients hypersensitive to quinidine Effects are potentiated by potassium (hyperkalemia) and reduced by hypokalemia (NOTE: this is exactly opposite of the effects that potassium has on the action of the digitalis cardiac glycosides—see Chapter 31) Therapeutic serum levels are generally 3-6 µg/ml Use with caution in atrial flutter Quinidine syncope may occur, particularly with long-term therapy	Watch for diarrhea, an early sign of toxicity Monitor for quinidine cardiotoxicity (50% widening of QRS complex and frequent ectopic beats); if observed, discontinue medication and continue ECG monitoring Monitor blood pressure Monitor ECG, particularly during IV administration and with PO doses greater than 2 gm/24 hr Monitor serum levels Observe for signs of cinchonism (e.g., dizziness, nausea, headache, fever, tinnitus)

Drug	Uses	Dosage	Preparation	Nursing Implications	Monitoring
Quinaglute Dura-Tabs Quinate **Quinidine polygalacturonate** (contains 60% anhydrous quinidine alkaloid) Cardioquin					
Verapamil Calan Cordilox Iproveratril Isoptin Vasolan	Supraventricular dysrhythmias See also Chapter 34, "Vasodilators, Antilipemics, Anticoagulants, and Platelet Aggregation Inhibitors"	*Adults:* 0.075-0.15 mg/kg IV over 2 min with continuous ECG and blood pressure monitoring; may repeat in 30 min *Children:* 1 month-1 year of age, 0.1-0.2 mg/kg IV over 2 min (may repeat if indicated after 30 min); 1-15 years of age, 0.1-0.3 mg/kg IV over 2 min (may repeat if indicated after 30 min) Maximum single dose: 10 mg *Elderly:* Administer lower adult dose over a minimum of 3 min Reduce dosage in hepatic failure	Injectable: 2.5 mg/ml Compatible with D₅W, Ringer's, and NS Store between 15° and 30° C Protect from light Discard any solutions that contain a precipitate	*Contraindicated* in acute myocardial infarction, heart block, cardiogenic shock, and severe hypotensive states *Contraindicated* in patients taking beta-blocker (e.g., propranolol) because of danger of complete heart block Bradycardia and hypotension are the most commonly observed side effects IV calcium may be given to treat toxicity Therapeutic serum levels are generally 0.08-0.3 µg/ml	Monitor blood pressure and discontinue verapamil if severe hypotension is observed Monitor heart rate for bradycardia Monitor serum levels Monitor ECG during IV administration

BIBLIOGRAPHY

Adverse reactions of drugs. *The Medical Letter,* 1975, *17,* 17-24.

Adverse reactions of drugs. *The Medical Letter,* 1977, *19,* 5-12.

Adverse reactions of drugs. *The Medical Letter,* 1979, *21,* 5-12.

Antman, E.M., Stone, P.H., Muller, J.E., & Braunwald, E. Calcium channel blocking agents in the treatment of cardiovascular disorders. Part I: Basic and clinical electrophysiologic effects. *Annals of Internal Medicine,* 1980, *93,* 875-885.

Befeler, B., & Lazzara, R. Clinical pharmacology of the antiarrhythmic agent disopyramide phosphate (Norpace). *Heart and Lung,* 1980, *9,* 475-482.

Brown, J.E., & Shand, D.G. Therapeutic drug monitoring of antiarrhythmic drugs. *Clinical Pharmacokinetics,* 1982, *7,* 125-148.

Bryson, S.M.,, Cairns, C.J., & Whiting, B. Disopyramide pharmacokinetics during recovery from myocardial infarction. *British Journal of Clinical Pharmacology* 1982, *13,* 417-421.

Budassi, S.A. Management of cardiopulmonary arrest. *Nursing Clinics of North America,* 1981, *16*(1), 37-53.

Canada, A., Lesko, L., Haffajee, C., Johnson, B., & Asdourian, G. Amiodarone for tachyarrhythmias: pharmacology, kinetics, and efficacy. *Drug Intelligence and Clinical Pharmacy,* 1983, *17,* 100-104.

Carrasco, H.A., Fuenmayor, A., Barboza, J.S., & Gonzalez, G. Effect of verapamil on normal sinoatrial node function and on sick sinus syndrome. *American Heart Journal,* 1978, *96,* 760-771.

Cocco, G., & Strozzi, C. Initial clinical experience of lorcainide (R013-1042), a new antiarrhythmic agent. *European Journal of Clinical Pharmacology,* 1978, *14,* 105-109.

Danilo, P. Jr. Aprindine. *American Heart Journal,* 1979, *97,* 119-124.

Danilo, P. Jr. Tocainide. *American Heart Journal,* 1979, *97,* 259-262.

Danilo, P. Jr. Mexiletine. *American Heart Journal,* 1979, *97,* 399-403.

Dhurandhar, R.W., Pickron, J., & Goldman, A.M. Bretylium tosylate in the management of recurrent ventricular fibrillation complicating acute myocardial infarction. *Heart and Lung,* 1980, *9,* 265-270.

Drayer, D.E., Hughes, M., Lorenzo, B., & Reidenberg, M.M. Prevalence of high (3S)-3-hydroxyquinidine/quinidine ratios in serum, and clearance of quinidine in cardiac patients with age. *Clinical Pharmacology and Therapeutics,* 1980, *27,* 72-75.

Ellrodt, G., & Singh, B. Adverse effects of disopyramide (Norpace): toxic interactions with other antiarrhythmic agents. *Heart and Lung,* 1980, *9,* 469-474.

Federman, J., & Vlietstra, R.E. Antiarrhythmic drug therapy. *Mayo Clinic Proceedings,* 1979, *54,* 531-542.

Feigl, D., & Ravid, M. Electrocardiographic observations on the termination of supraventricular tachycardia by verapamil. *Journal of Electrocardiology,* 1979, *12,* 129-136.

Flecainide-Quinidine Research Group. Flecainide versus quinidine for treatment of chronic ventricular arrhythmias. *Circulation,* 1983, *67,* 1117-1123.

Freedman, S.B., Richmond, D.R., Ashley, J.J., & Kelly, D.T. Verapamil kinetics in normal subjects and patients with coronary artery spasm. *Clinical Pharmacology and Therapeutics* 1981, *30,* 644-652.

Graboys, T.B. Clinical pharmacology of antiarrhythmic agents. *Heart and Lung,* 1979, *8,* 706-710.

Graffner, C., Conradson, T.B., Hofuendahl, S., & Ryden, L. Tocainide kinetics after intravenous and oral administration in healthy subjects and in patients with acute myocardial infarction. *Clinical Pharmacology and Therapeutics,* 1980, *27,* 64-71.

Hamer, A., Peter, T., Mandel, W.J., Scheinman, M.M., & Weiss, D. The potentiation of warfarin anticoagulation by amiodarone. *Circulation,* 1982, *65,* 1025-1029.

Harper, R.W., Olsson, S.B., & Varnauskas, E. Effect of mexiletine on monophasic action potentials recorded from right ventricle in man. *Cardiovascular Research,* 1979, *13,* 303-310.

Harper, R.W., & Olsson, S.B. Effect of mexiletine on conduction of premature ventricular beats in man: a study using monophasic action potential recordings from the right ventricle. *Cardiovascular Research,* 1979, *13,* 311-319.

Heger, J.J., Prystowsky, E.N., & Zipes, D.P. New drugs for treatment of ventricular arrhythmias. *Heart and Lung,* 1981, *10,* 475-483.

Henry, P.D. Comparative pharmacology of calcium antagonists: nifedipine, verapamil and diltiazem. *American Journal of Cardiology,* 1980, *46,* 1047-1058.

Jahnchen, E., Bechtold, H., Kasper, W., Kersting, F., Just, H., Hezkants, J., & Meinertz, T. Lorcainide. I. Saturable presystemic elimination. *Clinical Pharmacology and Therapeutics,* 1979, *26,* 187-195.

Johnston, A., Henry, J.A., Warrington, S.J., & Hamer, N.A.J. Pharmacokinetics of oral disopyramide phosphate in patients with renal impairment. *British Journal of Clinical Pharmacology,* 1980, *10,* 245-248.

Kaltenbach, M., Hopf, R., Kober, G., Bussmann, W.D., Keller, M., & Petersen, Y. Treatment of hypertrophic obstructive cardiomyopathy with verapamil. *British Heart Journal,* 1979, *42,* 35-42.

Kambara, H., Fujimoto, K., Wakabayashi, A., & Kawai, C. Primary pulmonary hypertension beneficial therapy with diltiazem. *American Heart Journal,* 1981, *101,* 230-231.

Kasper, W., Meinertz, T., Kersting, F. Lollgen, H., Lang, K., and Just, H. Electrophysiological actions of lorcainide in patients with cardiac disease. *Journal of Cardiovascular Pharmacology,* 1979, *1,* 343-352.

Kates, R.E., Keefe, D.L.D., Schwartz, J., Harapat, S., Kirsten, E.B., & Harrison, D.C. Verapamil disposition kinetics in chronic atrial fibrillation. *Clinical Pharmacology and Therapeutics,* 1981, *30,* 44-51.

Keefe, K.L., Yee, Y.G., & Kates, R.E. Verapamil protein binding in patients and in normal subjects. *Clinical Pharmacology and Therapeutics,* 1981, *29,* 21-26.

Kessler, K.M., & Perez, G.O. Decreased quinidine plasma protein binding during hemodialysis. *Clinical Pharmacology and Therapeutics*, 1981, *30*, 121-126.

Kesteloot, H., & Stroobandt, R. Clinical experience of encainide (MJ 9067): a new anti-arrhythmic drug. *European Journal of Clinical Pharmacology*, 1979, *16*, 323-326.

Klotz, U., Müller-Seydlitz, P.M., & Heimburg, P. Lorcainide infusion in the treatment of ventricular premature beats. *European Journal of Clinical Pharmacology*, 1979, *16*, 1-6.

Klotz, U., Müller-Seydlitz, P., & Heimburg, P. Pharmacokinetics of lorcainide in man: a new antiarrhythmic agent. *Clinical Pharmacokinetics*, 1978, *3*, 407-418.

Landmark, K., Bredesen, J.E., Thaulow, E., Simonsen, S., & Amlie, J.P. Pharmacokinetics of disopyramide in patients with imminent to moderate cardiac failure. *European Journal of Clinical Pharmacology*, 1981, *19*, 187-192.

Landmark, K., Storstein, L., & Larsen, A. Disopyramide plasma levels in cardiac patients on maintenance therapy. *Acta Medica Scandinavica*, 1979, *206*, 385-389.

Leak, D., & Eydt, J.N. Control of refractory cardiac arrhythmias with amiodarone. *Archives of Internal Medicine*, 1979, *139*, 425-428.

Leon, M.B., Rosing, D.R., Bonow, R.O., Lipson, L.C., & Epstein, S.E. Clinical efficacy of verapamil alone and combined with propranolol in treating patients with chronic stable angina pectoris. *American Journal of Cardiology*, 1981, *48*, 131-139.

Lertora, J.J.L., Atkinson, A.J., Jr., Kushner, W., Nevin, M.J., Lee, W.K., Jones, C., & Schmid, F.R. Long-term antiarrhythmic therapy with N-acetyl-procainamide. *Clinical Pharmacology and Therapeutics*, 1979, *25*, 273-282.

Lima, J.J., Boudoulas, H., & Blanford, M. Concentration-dependence of disopyramide binding to plasma protein and its influence on kinetics and dynamics. *Journal of Pharmacology and Experimental Therapeutics*, 1981, *219*, 741-747.

Lima, J.J., Conti, D.R., Goldfarb, A.L., Golden, L.H., & Jusko, W.J. Pharmacokinetic approach to intravenous procainamide therapy. *European Journal of Clinical Pharmacology*, 1978, *13*, 303-308.

Llett, K.F., Madsen, B.W., & Woods, J.D. Disopyramide kinetics in acute myocardial infarction. *Clinical Pharmacology and Therapeutics*, 1979, *26*, 1-7.

Ludden, T.M., & Crawford, M.H. N-Acetylprocainamide kinetics after single and repeated oral doses. *Clinical Pharmacology & Therapeutics*, 1982, *31*, 343-349.

MacCannell, K.L., & Wyse, D.G. Pharmacologic management: cardiovascular drugs. In N.K. Wenger, J.W. Hurst, & M.C. McIntyre (Eds.). *Cardiology for nurses*. New York: McGraw-Hill Book Co., 1980.

Man, R.Y.K., & Dresel, P.E. A specific effect of lidocaine and tocainide on ventricular conduction of mid-range extrasystoles. *Journal of Cardiovascular Pharmacology*, 1979, *1*, 329-342.

McMahon, M., & Sheaffer, S. Verapamil. *Drug Intelligence and Clinical Pharmacy*, 1982, *16*, 443-447.

Meinertz, T., Kasper, W., Kersting, F., Just, H., Bechtold, H., & Jahnchen, E. Lorcainide II plasma concentration effect relationship. *Clinical Pharmacology and Therapeutics*, 1979, *26*, 196-204.

Ochs, H.R., Greenblatt, D.J., & Woo, E. Clinical pharmacokinetics of quinidine. *Clinical Pharmacokinetics*, 1980, *5*, 150-168.

Phillips, R.E., & Feeney, M.K. *The cardiac rhythms: a systematic approach to interpretation* (2nd ed.). Philadelphia: W.B. Saunders Co., 1980.

Pottage, A., Campbell, R.W.F., Achuff, S.C., Murray, A., Julian, D.G., & Prescott, L.F. The absorption of oral mexiletine in coronary care patients. *European Journal of Clinical Pharmacology*, 1978, *13*, 393-399.

Ryan, W.F., & Karliner, J.S. Effects of tocainide on left ventricular performance at rest and during acute alterations in heart rate and systemic arterial pressure. *British Heart Journal*, 1979, *41*, 175-181.

Scheinman, S.J., Poll, D.S., & Wolfson, S. Acute cardiac failure and hepatic ischemia induced by disopyramide phosphate. *Yale Journal of Biology and Medicine*, 1980, *53*, 361-366.

Selzer, A. Quinidine in perspective: the rise and fall of quinidine. *Heart and Lung*, 1982, *11*(1), 20-23.

Shand, D.G., Hammell, S.C., Aanonsen, L., & Pritchett, E.L.C. Reduced verapamil clearance during long-term oral administration. *Clinical Pharmacology and Therapeutics*, 1981, *30*, 701-703.

Slack, J.D., Rizk, Assad E., & Wright, K.E. Successful long-term suppression of previously refractory paroxysmal ventricular tachycardia with bretylium tosylate. *Heart and Lung*, 1979, *8*, 721-727.

Sonnhag, C., & Karlsson, E. Comparative antiarrhythmic efficacy of intraveous *N*-acetylprocainamide and procainamide. *European Journal of Clinical Pharmacology*, 1979, *15*, 311-317.

Stanford, J.L., Felner, J.M., & Arensberg, D. Antiarrhythmic drug therapy. *American Journal of Nursing*, 1980, *80*(7), 1288-1295.

Stavenow, L., Hanson, A., & Johansson, B.W. Mexiletine in treatment of ventricular arrhythmias. *Acta Medica Scandinavica*, 1979, *205*, 411-415.

Stone, P.H., Antman, E.M., Muller, J.E., & Braunwald, E. Calcium channel blocking agents in the treatment of cardiovascular disorders. Part II: Hemodynamic effects and clinical applications. *Annals of Internal Medicine*, 1980, *93*, 886-904.

Story, J.R., Abdulla, A.M., & Frank, M.J. Cardiogenic shock and disopyramide phosphate. *Journal of the American Medical Association*, 1979, *242*, 654-655.

Swedberg, K., Pehrson, J., & Ryden, L. Electrocardiographic and hemodynamic effects of tocainide (W-36095) in man. *European Journal of Clinical Pharmacology*, 1978, *14*, 15-19.

Velebit, V., Podrid, P., Lown, B., Cohen, B.H., & Graboys, T.B. Aggravation and provocation of ventricular arrhythmias by antiarrhythmic drugs. *Circulation*, 1982, *65*, 886-894.

Waleffe, A., Bruninx, P., & Kulbertus, H.E. Effects of amiodarone studied by programmed electrical stimulation of the heart in patients with paroxysmal re-entrant supraventricular tachycardia. *Journal of Electrocardiology*, 1978, *11*, 253-260.

Whiting, B., Holford, N.H.G., & Sheiner, L.B. Quantitative analysis of the disopyramide concentration-effect relationship. *British Journal of Clinical Pharmacology,* 1980, *9,* 67-75.

Winkle, R.A., Glantz, S.A., & Harrison, D.C. Pharmacologic therapy of ventricular arrhythmias. *American Journal of Cardiology,* 1975, *36,* 629-650.

Woodcock, B.G., Rietbrock, I., Vohringer, H.F., & Rietbrock, N. Verapamil disposition in liver disease and intensive-care patients: kinetics, clearance, and apparent blood flow relationships. *Clinical Pharmacology and Therapeutics,* 1981, *29,* 27-34.

Yamaguchi, I., Obayashi, K., & Mandel, W.J. Electrophysiological effects of verapamil. *Cardiovascular Research,* 1978, *12,* 597-608.

Zipes, D.P., & Troup, P.J. New antiarrhythmic agents. *American Journal of Cardiology,* 1978, *41,* 1005-1024.

Antihypertensives

D. George Wyse

Medications discussed in this chapter

Alpha-adrenergic blocking
agents
  Phenoxybenzamine
  Phentolamine
  Prazosin
Alpha- and beta-adrenergic
blocking agent
  Labetalol
Antiadrenergic/adrenergic
neuron blocking agents
  Debrisoquine
  Guanethidine
  Reserpine
Beta-adrenergic blocking
agents
  Atenolol
  Metoprolol
  Nadolol
  Oxprenolol

Beta-adrenergic blocking
agents—cont'd
  Pindolol
  Propranolol
  Timolol
Central-acting alpha-adren-
ergic agonists
  Clonidine
  Methyldopa
Ganglionic blocking agent
  Trimethaphan
Inhibitor of angiotensin
converting enzyme
  Captopril
Vasodilators
  Diazoxide
  Hydralazine
  Minoxidil
  Nitroprusside

A simple classification scheme for hypertension

Primary, essential, or idiopathic hypertension
  (90%)
Secondary hypertension (10%)
  Renal hypertension
    Renal parenchymal disease (e.g.,
      glomerulonephritis)
    Renovascular disease (e.g., renal artery
      stenosis)
  Endocrine hypertension
    Adrenal cortical disease (e.g., Cushing's
      syndrome, primary aldosteronism)
    Adrenal medullary disease (e.g.,
      pheochromocytoma)
    Other (e.g., acromegaly)
  Neurogenic hypertension (e.g., increased
    intracranial pressure)
  Miscellaneous
    Coarctation of the aorta
    Toxemia of pregnancy
    Carcinoid syndrome
    Drug- or food-induced

A wide variety of medications are used to lower elevated blood pressure, including some discussed in other chapters. Many of these agents have additional cardiovascular and noncardiovascular indications. This chapter will discuss all of the major agents used in treating hypertension, except for the diuretics, which are discussed in Chapter 36, "Diuretics and Antidiuretics." The calcium antagonist drugs (e.g., diltiazem, nifedipine, verapamil) are newer agents but most certainly will play a role in treating hypertension, and are discussed as antidysrhythmics in Chapter 32. Some drugs formerly used to treat hypertension such as the monoamine oxidase inhibitors (MAOIs) and the rauwolfia alkaloids, *cannot* be recommended for this purpose at the present time and are not discussed here. The one exception is reserpine, which continues to be used fairly widely.

Drugs are a prominent aspect of the treatment of an elevated blood pressure. Treatment of hypertension is important for two reasons. First, it is an extremely common condition, affecting about 15% of adult North Americans. Second, the presence of hypertension increases the risk that a person will subsequently have a myocardial infarction, stroke, or experience other target organ damage. Lowering even mildly elevated blood pressure to the normal range reduces this risk.

There are a variety of etiologies for hypertension, but in over 90% of patients the exact mechanism is incompletely understood. These patients are referred to as having *primary* or *essential hypertension* (see box above). To understand the pharmacology of these

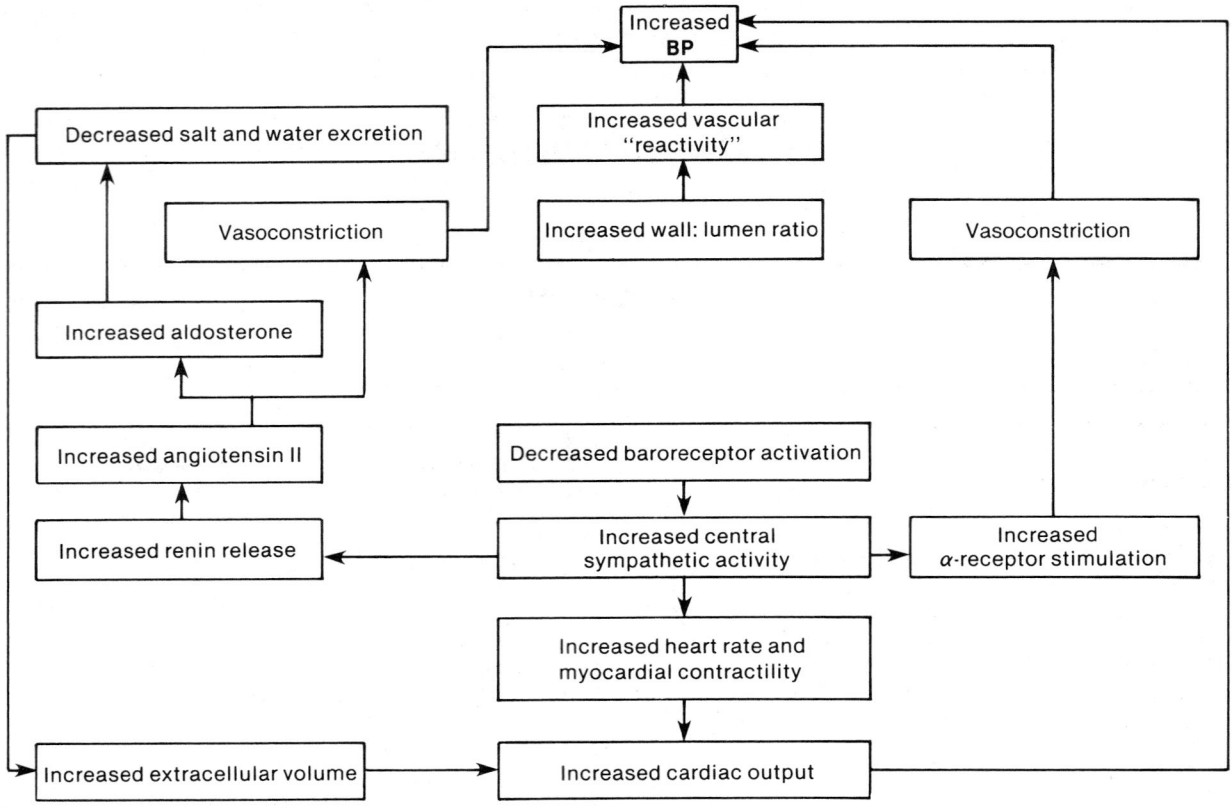

FIGURE 33-1. **Simplified schema to illustrate some of the factors involved in control of blood pressure.**

agents, it is advisable to review the physiology of the control of blood pressure, particularly the role of the autonomic nervous system and the renin-angiotensin system (Figure 33-1). As will be seen, the mechanism of action of most of these agents involves inhibition at various points in these systems.

MECHANISM OF ACTION AND PHARMACOLOGIC EFFECTS

Guanethidine, bethanidine, debrisoquine, reserpine. The antiadrenergic agents guanethidine, bethanidine, debrisoquine, and reserpine interfere with the functioning of the sympathetic (adrenergic) component of the autonomic nervous system but *not* through a direct blockade of receptors on the effector organ (e.g., arterioles and heart). It is unclear how much of the effect is caused by an antiadrenergic effect in the vasomotor centers of the CNS and how much is caused by an effect on peripheral postganglionic sympathetic neurons. Guanethidine and bethanidine have identical pharmacologic effects. Their action depends on their being taken up into the nerve ending, where they displace norepinephrine. Over a period of

time, tissue norepinephrine levels fall. Adrenergic neuron function is inhibited before the tissue levels decrease, however, and the reason for this is uncertain.

Because the active uptake mechanism into the neuron, which is an important factor in terminating the action of *catecholamines* at many sites, is used by guanethidine, it can potentiate the effects of exogenous catecholamines, as well as the endogenous catecholamines released from the adrenal medulla. Guanethidine does not deplete catecholamine levels in the adrenal medulla and this, plus the potentiation phenomenon, *contraindicates* using this drug to treat pheochromocytoma.

Guanethidine penetrates the CNS poorly; thus most of its actions are probably on the peripheral adrenergic neurons. Guanethidine's cardiovascular effects are the result of a reduction in both alpha-mediated and beta-mediated adrenergic responses. There is vasodilation of both *resistance* and *capacitance* vascular beds. The cardiac output may initially rise, but with chronic administration it returns to normal and the heart rate may be slowed. Most of the reflexes that maintain blood pressure with changes in posture are blunted; thus postural hypotension can be a problem. Plasma renin activity is decreased by guanethidine. Debriso-quine is similar to guanethidine and bethanidine but in addition inhibits the enzyme monoamine oxidase in sympathetic neurons and platelets. This additional action probably does not play any role in the drug's antihypertensive action.

Reserpine (and other similar drugs, such as alse-roxylon rescinnamine and rauwolfia serpentina) also depletes catecholamines from postganglionic sympathetic nerve endings, but, unlike guanethidine, it also depletes the adrenal medulla and CNS neurons. The mechanism of displacement and release is not via the physiologic mechanism (i.e., no exocytosis and dopamine-β-hydroxylase release), but, like guaneth-idine, the active catecholamine uptake mechanism into neurons is blocked by reserpine. The effect on the adrenal medulla is much slower to develop. In general, the effects of reserpine are slow to occur and recovery following discontinuation of the medication is prolonged. Tissues are also depleted of 5-hydroxy-tryptamine by reserpine. Clinical manifestations of re-serpine's central effects include sedation and tran-quilization. As with guanethidine, the blood pressure is lowered because of vasodilation, and the heart rate and cardiac output fall. These effects are caused by a loss of sympathetic tone. The homeostatic reflexes that maintain the blood pressure are inhibited, but usually not to the same degree as is seen with guanethidine, and postural hypotension is less of a problem. It must be recognized, however, that only low doses of reser-pine are usually used, and if the dose used is sufficient to cause an equivalent lowering of blood pressure, *postural hypotension* can also be a problem.

Trimethaphan. Several ganglionic blocking agents exist (see Chapter 26, "Ganglionic Stimulants and Blockers and Neuromuscular Blocking Agents"), but only trimethaphan is used to treat hypertension. Tri-methaphan's effects are the result of a blockade of the peripheral autonomic ganglia and are thus the combined effects of inhibition of the sympathetic and para-sympathetic nervous systems. The exact effect in any one patient depends on the existing balance of tone in these two systems. Usually, both arteriolar and ve-nous dilatation occur because of an inhibition of the sympathetic system, and the consequences of this are a fall in blood pressure. Unless there is a preexisting tachycardia, the heart rate usually increases slightly. If heart failure is present, the cardiac output can increase, but more often the cardiac output decreases.

Because the entire autonomic nervous system is affected, there are widespread effects throughout the body. Generally, body secretions (e.g., gastric, pan-creatic, intestinal, perspiration) are decreased, motility of the gastrointestinal (GI) tract is reduced, and visual

accommodation, male sexual function, and emptying of the urinary bladder are impaired.

Phentolamine, phenoxybenzamine, prazosin. The alpha-adrenergic blocking agents phentolamine and phenoxybenzamine are of limited use in treating hypertension, whereas the newer drug prazosin is of more widespread use. Phentolamine is a competitive equilibrium antagonist of catecholamines at the alpha-adrenergic receptor and thus produces a surmount-able blockade of the vasoconstrictor effect of these amines. The effects of 5-hydroxytryptamine are also inhibited by this agent. Phentolamine is a relatively weak blocking agent and the effects are transient. Blockade of alpha-adrenergic receptors results in di-lation of both arteries and veins, and this results in a fall in blood pressure.

Phentolamine may also have some direct vasodi-lating properties in addition to that caused by the alpha-adrenergic blockade. It has a stimulating effect on the heart, probably somehow mediated through endogenous catecholamines, which results in an in-creased heart rate and cardiac output. Body secretions (e.g., gastric, pancreatic, intestinal) are increased, as is GI motility.

Phenoxybenzamine produces a noncompetitive, nonequilibrium blockade of alpha-adrenergic recep-tors, which is a blockade difficult to overcome; how-ever, there may be some reversibility of the effect in the early stages of the blockade. The blockade is slow to develop and slow to wane. Phenoxybenzamine is not a particularly specific antagonist, and responses to 5-hydroxytryptamine, histamine, and acetylcholine are also inhibited. Administration of this agent causes a fall in blood pressure and an increase in cardiac output. There is usually a compensatory tachycardia. It also has a number of noncardiovascular effects, but these are unpredictable.

Prazosin is a much newer agent, and when it was first introduced it was thought to have direct vaso-dilatory effects, but it now seems clear its effects are solely the result of an alpha-adrenergic blockade. It lowers blood pressure through a blockade of the alpha-adrenergic receptors in both the arteries and the veins. Cardiac output is increased. The heart rate does not change; the reasons for this are unclear, al-though it has been suggested that it is because the presynaptic alpha-receptors, which inhibit catechol-amine release, are not blocked by prazosin.

All of the alpha-adrenergic blocking agents can cause postural hypotension.

Beta-adrenergic blocking agents. The beta-adrenergic blocking agents are one of the main classes of drugs used in treating hypertension. Propranolol is the prototype agent, but a multitude of newer agents are being introduced into the North American market. It is presumed the blood pressure–lowering effect is the same for all of these agents. The exact mechanism for the blood pressure–lowering effect of these agents is uncertain. It has been variously ascribed to: (1) lowering the cardiac output, (2) inhibition of sympathetically-mediated renin release, and (3) an unspecified central effect resulting in an inhibition of the *vasomotor centers*. It is most likely that the blood pressure falls because of a combination of such effects. The blockade induced by these agents is an equilibrium, competitive effect, and can be overcome by administering an agonist drug such as isoproterenol. As mentioned previously, the cardiac output falls and there is also a decrease in the heart rate. Beta-adrenergic receptors elsewhere in the body are also blocked and this can result in bronchial constriction (bronchospasm) or vasoconstriction in the skeletal muscle beds. The cardiovascular effects are naturally more marked when there is an increased sympathetic tone. Postural hypotension does not appear to be a major problem with these agents.

In connection with the pharmacologic properties of the beta-adrenergic blocking agents, two additional features must be noted: intrinsic sympathomimetic activity (also called partial agonist activity) and cardioselectivity. The two subcategories of beta-adrenergic receptors are those that mediate the cardiac effects, called beta$_1$, and the others, called beta$_2$. Some agents have a *relative* selectivity for beta$_1$ receptors and thus at low doses have fewer effects outside of the cardiovascular system (e.g., less likely to produce bronchospasm). It must be emphasized that such selectivity is only *relative* and that at higher doses it disappears.

Of the agents currently available in North America, only metoprolol and atenolol have relative cardioselectivity; all others are nonselective blockers of beta-adrenergic receptors. Acebutolol, which is currently available in Europe, also has cardioselective properties, but in addition it has intrinsic sympathomimetic activity. Several of the beta blockers have been found to have intrinsic sympathomimetic activity (i.e., they are beta *agonists*, as well as beta *antagonists*). With such agents there may be a blunting of some of the effects of beta-adrenergic antagonists, such as bradycardia, bronchoconstriction, and lethargy, apparently without significant diminution of antihypertensive effects. They may also have less depressant effect on the heart. Of the agents currently on the market in North America, pindolol and oxprenolol (only in Canada) have significant intrinsic sympathomimetic activity. It has already been mentioned that acebutolol has *both*

cardioselectivity and intrinsic sympathomimetic activity but is currently available only in Europe. Alprenolol also has intrinsic sympathomimetic activity but is not available in North America. Alprenolol does not have cardioselectivity. Timolol may be considered to be identical to propranolol in beta blocking properties. Nadolol, although similar to propranolol on a pharmacologic basis, differs for pharmacokinetic reasons. In the past much has been written about another property of some beta-adrenergic blocking agents, their membrane-stabilizing or quinidine-like property. It is thought by some to play a role in the drugs' antidysrhythmic effect. However, the membrane-stabilizing effect is observed only at higher concentrations, and the present consensus is that it is not usually a clinically important property. The following agents mentioned above have membrane-stabilizing effects: acebutolol, alprenolol, oxprenolol, pindolol, and propranolol. Sotalol, which is not generally available, is a nonselective beta-blocker without intrinsic sympathomimetic or membrane-stabilizing effects but with some electrophysiologic effects similar to those of amiodarone and bretylium (see Chapter 32).

Labetalol. Labetalol is a newer agent that blocks both alpha-adrenergic and beta-adrenergic receptors. Relatively little is known about this agent at present, but it can be predicted that its effects will be similar to those of a combination of a beta-adrenergic blocker such as propranolol, and an alpha-adrenergic blocker such as prazosin.

Clonidine, methyldopa. The pharmacology of clonidine is complex. It is both an alpha-adrenergic agonist and antagonist and has some direct vasodilatory effects. The major action of clonidine seems to be within the CNS, and it has been postulated that it is the result of a stimulation of the alpha-adrenergic receptors that have an inhibitory effect on vasomotor centers. There is also a bradycardic effect that is probably also the result of an effect in the CNS. Other CNS effects of clonidine include sedation, inhibition of salivation, and a theoretically very interesting effect of preventing narcotic withdrawal symptoms. With acute administration the cardiac output usually falls, but with chronic administration it remains unchanged. Postural hypotension can occur, but is not a major problem with clonidine. Plasma renin levels are reduced by clonidine.

The mechanism of action of methyldopa has undergone an interesting evolution. It was first thought to deplete tissue catecholamines because of an inhibition of the enzyme dopa decarboxylase, an enzyme necessary for the biosynthesis of these amines. Later it was felt to act as a false transmitter because methyldopa can be incorporated into the catecholamine biosynthetic pathway, resulting in formation of methylnorepinephrine, which was postulated to have little agonist activity. Both of these hypotheses have subsequently been shown not to explain the blood pressure–lowering effect of this agent.

It now seems clear that the action of methyldopa is in the CNS and is the result of the formation of methylnorepinephrine, which probably acts on alpha-adrenergic receptors with an inhibitory effect on the vasomotor centers. However, some peripheral component of this drug's effect has not been completely ruled out. Methyldopa causes a fall in the blood pressure and the heart rate. The cardiac output may initially fall, but subsequently returns to normal, although the drug's effect on this measurement is by no means clear. Postural hypotension is not a major problem. Methyldopa has a number of other CNS effects, including sedation, sleep disturbances, and an increased prolactin release leading to lactation.

Diazoxide, hydralazine, minoxidil, nitroprusside. Diazoxide is chemically related to the thiazide diuretics and has some actions that are qualitatively similar to them. Intravenous administration results in a marked arteriolar dilation and a rapid fall in blood pressure. This change is usually accompanied by an increase in the cardiac output and some increase in the heart rate. There is little effect on large veins and *homeostatic reflexes* are not interfered with. Therefore, postural hypotension is not a major problem. The other pharmacologic properties of diazoxide are of some interest. Unlike other thiazides, it causes salt and water retention, and for this reason it is often necessary to administer a potent diuretic concurrently with diazoxide. Similar to the other thiazides, it can cause hyperglycemia and hyperuricemia. It has been used therapeutically for its hyperglycemic effect.

Hydralazine is the only one of a family of related vasodilator agents that is widely used in North America, although minoxidil, a newer agent, is a distant chemical relative. The major antihypertensive action of these agents is a direct relaxation of the vascular smooth muscle. Arterioles are affected more than veins. The cardiac output usually increases and there is almost always a tachycardia; these factors can limit the blood pressure–lowering effect. Thus, a beta-adrenergic blocking agent is usually given with these agents. Plasma renin is increased and salt and water retention commonly occur. A diuretic is thus often needed, particularly with minoxidil.

Nitroprusside's effects are very similar to the nitrites (see Chapter 34, "Vasodilators, Antilipemics, Anticoagulants, and Platelet Aggregation Inhibitors"), but is

discussed in this chapter because one of its major uses is in treating hypertensive emergencies. It is an agent whose use has waxed and waned over many years and currently is being widely used in several emergency situations when an agent with a rapid onset but short duration of action is needed to control blood pressure or loading (i.e., *preload* and *afterload*) conditions of the left ventricle. It is a powerful vasodilator that acts directly on the smooth muscle. It dilates both the arterial and the venous sides of the circulation. The cardiac output is increased and the effect on the heart rate is variable. When tachycardia is present, the heart rate may fall, but more often there is a slight increase or no change.

Captopril. Several agents at various stages of development and intended for treating hypertension have as one of their major actions the ability to inhibit the angiotensin converting enzyme. The angiotensin converting enzyme is responsible for catalyzing the conversion of angiotensin I to angiotensin II, the latter peptide being the more potent vasoconstrictor. Angiotensin II is thought to play a role in controlling blood pressure (see Figure 33-1). Captopril is the prototype agent in this group. Although it is a potent inhibitor of the angiotensin converting enzyme, this does not appear to be the only mechanism by which the blood pressure is lowered. Although it would seem reasonable that this agent is most efficacious in those forms of hypertension, such as *renovascular hypertension*, where angiotensin is thought to play a direct role in the elevation of blood pressure, captopril also lowers the blood pressure in essential hypertension and this effect is seemingly independent of renin status.

Another group of agents that interfere with the actions of angiotensin are the peptide analogs, which act at the angiotensin receptor as competitive, equilibrium antagonists. Saralasin is the prototype agent of this group. It is unlikely that these agents will have a wide therapeutic use, because they must be given intravenously.

PHARMACOKINETICS

Guanethidine, bethanidine, debrisoquine, reserpine. The absorption of guanethidine after oral administration is relatively constant in any one patient, but varies from 3% to 30% among patients. It is partly metabolized by microsomal enzymes in the liver, and the parent compound and its less active metabolites are rapidly cleared by the kidneys. Small amounts of guanethidine, however, remain in the body for extended periods of up to 2 weeks. Debrisoquine is almost identical to guanethidine in its metabolism.

Bethanidine has a shorter duration of action than gua-nethidine but is otherwise very similar. Reserpine is well absorbed from both the GI tract and sites of parenteral administration. The effects of reserpine develop only slowly (over 2 to 3 weeks) and also wane slowly after the drug has been discontinued.

Trimethaphan. Trimethaphan is erratically absorbed from the GI tract and thus is only given intravenously. It is a quaternary ammonium salt and does not penetrate the blood-brain barrier. Its effects are immediate and wane rapidly over a few minutes when it is discontinued. Trimethaphan is excreted essentially unchanged by the kidney.

Phentolamine, phenoxybenzamine, prazosin. Very little is known about the pharmacokinetics of phentolamine. An effective amount of this drug can be absorbed via the oral route, but it is used almost exclusively in the intravenous form. The oral dose is 5 to 10 times the intravenous dose, suggesting either poor absorption or a substantial first-pass effect. Only one tenth of an intravenous dose can be recovered in the urine in an active form.

Phenoxybenzamine is absorbed orally, although somewhat erratically (20% to 30%), but is now seldom administered by that route. The only parenteral route used for phenoxybenzamine is intravenous, because of the substantial irritant properties by other routes. The metabolic fate and excretion are poorly understood. Over 80% is excreted within 24 hours, but small amounts remain in tissues for 1 week or more. Delayed excretion may be related to sequestration in body fat. The prolonged action of this drug (several hours to days) is partly the result of slow metabolism and excretion, which in turn are the result of the formation of a stable covalent bond with the alpha-adrenergic receptor.

Data on the pharmacokinetics of prazosin are also incomplete at present. Enough prazosin is adequately absorbed from the GI tract (approximately 50%) for it to be useful via the oral route. Once absorbed, it is highly bound to plasma protein (97%). The drug is nearly completely metabolized by demethylation and conjugation and is then excreted in the bile and feces with only negligible amounts of unchanged drug appearing in the urine. The plasma elimination half-life of prazosin is 2 to 3 hours, but no clear relationship exists between plasma levels and the hypotensive effect. A hypotensive effect can still be observed for 2 or 3 half-lives after the drug has been discontinued. In patients with congestive heart failure the pharmacokinetics of orally administered prazosin are altered, and higher plasma levels and a longer half-life are seen.

Beta-adrenergic blocking agents. Aside from their differences in pharmacologic properties (e.g., cardioselectivity, intrinsic sympathomimetic activity) there are important differences in pharmacokinetics among the beta-adrenergic blocking agents. Only those agents available in North America are mentioned in this section. Except for nadolol, 90% or more of an orally administered dose of all of the other beta-adrenergic blocking agents is rapidly absorbed. Only 37% of an orally administered dose of nadolol is absorbed, and the absorption is much slower. Several of the beta-adrenergic blocking agents are metabolized in the liver by a high affinity, but saturable mechanism, and thus are subject to the first-pass effect. Approximately 70% of absorbed propranolol is removed on the first pass through the liver; the corresponding figure for metoprolol and timolol is 50% and for atenolol is 60%.

Binding to plasma proteins is also variable among these agents. More than 90% of propranolol is bound to plasma proteins and corresponding figures, where known, for the other agents are alprenolol 85%, metoprolol 12%, nadolol 30%, and timolol 80%.

Because of the variability in degree of liver metabolism, there are different amounts (i.e., percent of oral dose) of unchanged drug excreted in the urine, from a low of 1% to 3% for propranolol, alprenolol, and metoprolol, to a high of 20% and 40% for timolol and pindolol, respectively. Of an administered dose of nadolol, 70% appears in the feces and only 20% in the urine. Approximately 65% of an administered dose of timolol appears in the urine, but more than 90% of the other four agents (alprenolol, metoprolol, pindolol, propranolol) is excreted in the urine.

Metoprolol, nadolol, and pindolol have no known active metabolites, whereas 4-hydroxypropranolol, a metabolite of propranolol, has activity similar to the parent compound, and alprenolol has clinically significant active metabolites. Except for nadolol and atenolol, the elimination half-life of all of the other beta-adrenergic blocking agents discussed here is the same and is approximately 3 to 4 hours. The elimination half-life of nadolol and atenolol is approximately 25 hours.

There is an unclear relationship between plasma level and beta-adrenergic blockade with these drugs. The degree of blockade appears to correlate with the plasma level achieved, but when the drugs are discontinued, the blockade persists after the level of drug in the plasma has fallen well below a level that initially had no effect. This phenomenon is unexplained at present.

One of the consequences of the properties of these

agents is that those (e.g., alprenolol, metoprolol, propranolol, timolol) metabolized to a high degree in the liver can be expected to accumulate in patients with liver failure. Although it is unclear what happens with most of these agents in renal failure, it is assumed that a cumulative effect would be expected in those agents (e.g., nadolol, pindolol, timolol) where greater amounts of the unchanged drug are excreted in the urine. Although only a small amount (1%) of an orally administered dose of propranolol is excreted in the urine, a cumulative effect of this agent is seen in renal failure, most likely because of an accumulation of the active metabolite, 4-hydroxypropranolol.

Because of the differences in their half-lives, dosage frequency varies among agents. Nadolol and atenolol are given as a single daily dose. In spite of their short half-lives, the other agents can be efficacious when given as two or three divided doses per day.

Labetalol. Because of its newness, no substantial information is available on the pharmacokinetics of the combined alpha-adrenergic and beta-adrenergic blocking agent labetalol.

Clonidine, methyldopa. Clonidine appears to be well-absorbed from the intestine and peak plasma levels are reached in about 3 hours. There is accumulation in some tissues, and it is not clear if the plasma levels have significance in relation to the pharmacologic effects. An enterohepatic circulation has been described in rats but it is unknown whether this exists in humans, and interspecies variability is common with this drug. The exact details of metabolism and excretion of clonidine are incompletely understood at present, partly because such small amounts are given. Approximately 65% of an orally administered dose of clonidine is excreted in the urine and the estimated fecal excretion is 30%. There are four known metabolites, and 40% to 50% of the drug excreted in the urine is unchanged clonidine. The plasma elimination half-life of this drug is 7 to 8 hours and increases to 20 to 40 hours in renal failure.

Approximately 50% of an orally administered dose of methyldopa is absorbed and it is excreted mostly (90%) in the urine, largely unchanged except for conjugation. The elimination curve seems to have two components, and the first accounts for about 90% of the administered dose. In patients with normal renal function, this first elimination half-life is approximately 100 minutes. With impaired renal function, the half-life is considerably prolonged and significant accumulation can occur. There is considerable variation in the metabolism and excretion of methyldopa between patients and even from day to day in the same patient. It should be noted that methyldopa and its metabolites significantly cross react in several tests for urinary catecholamines used to diagnose pheochromocytoma, and this can cause a false positive test.

Diazoxide, hydralazine, minoxidil, nitroprusside. In the treatment of hypertension, diazoxide is only given intravenously, but it is used orally for its hyperglycemic effect, and thus appreciable oral absorption can occur. The drug is not appreciably metabolized and is excreted by glomerular filtration in an unchanged form. More than 90% of an administered dose is bound to plasma protein, and this has been used in the past to justify the need for rapid intravenous administration. As mentioned previously, however, it has been clearly demonstrated that the hypotensive effect after slow infusion is equal to that of a bolus injection. The elimination half-life of diazoxide is approximately 28 hours.

Hydralazine is rapidly and completely absorbed via the oral route, and peak levels are reached in 1 to 2 hours. Approximately 85% of hydralazine is bound to plasma proteins. Hydralazine is almost completely metabolized before excretion and the major mechanism is acetylation in the liver. This has clinical significance because so-called slow acetylator patients (see Chapter 9, "Genetic Factors Affecting Drug Response") can accumulate remarkably high levels of the drug and are thus more subject to side effects. Most of the metabolized drug is rapidly excreted in the urine. Accumulation of drug is known to occur in renal failure, and because little unchanged drug is excreted in the urine, it is assumed the metabolism is altered by uremia. The elimination half-life is 1.7 to 3 hours, but as with many antihypertensive drugs the relationship between the plasma level and the antihypertensive effect is unclear, and a hypotensive effect is still present after much of the drug is excreted. This may be partly the result of an accumulation of hydralazine in the arterial walls.

More than 90% of orally administered minoxidil is absorbed, and maximum plasma concentrations are reached within the first hour. Minoxidil does not bind significantly to plasma proteins. It is largely metabolized in the liver and excreted in the urine (more than 90%), with a half-life of elimination of approximately 4 hours. Dosage should normally be reduced in renal impairment. Although plasma levels fall rapidly, the hypotensive effect lasts for at least 12 hours and the total duration of the effect is close to 72 hours. At least one metabolite (minoxidil-o-glucuronide) has some antihypertensive effect, although it is less active than the parent compound.

Sodium nitroprusside is only given intravenously and it has an immediate effect, probably because of the nitroso (−N:0) group. Because the effect is transient, caused by sodium nitroprusside's rapid conversion to thiocyanate that is inactive as a vasodilator, a constant infusion must be given. When the drug is discontinued, the hypotensive effect rapidly wanes in 1 to 10 minutes. Thiocyanate is then predominantly excreted in the urine, although a small amount is subsequently metabolized to cyanide. Cases of cyanide poisoning have been known to occur, particularly with the prolonged use of high doses. With prolonged use thiocyanate can also accumulate and cause hypothyroidism. After the first 48 hours, thiocyanate levels should be monitored, and are generally felt to be safe if they are less than 10 mg/dl.

Captopril. Approximately 75% of an oral dose of captopril is absorbed on an empty stomach. The presence of food in the GI tract can reduce absorption by as much as 40%. Between 40% and 50% of unchanged drug is eliminated in the urine, and dosage must be adjusted in renal impairment. Effects begin within 1 to 2 hours and last about 6 hours, although with high doses the effects can last for 12 hours. The half-life of elimination from the blood has been estimated to be less than 3 hours.

USES

The use of the antihypertensive medications is quite obviously to lower the blood pressure when it is elevated. The reason for treating high blood pressure is that it is an important risk factor for stroke and myocardial infarction and lowering the blood pressure, even when it is only mildly elevated, lessens that risk. It is important to note that mild hypertension can often be controlled by nondrug treatments such as salt restriction, weight reduction, and exercise. If these measures are not successful, drugs are then used.

Selection of which drug to use is based on the degree of elevation of blood pressure, the suspected etiologic or pathophysiologic factors involved, and the urgency to lower the pressure. There are also the personal preferences of the prescriber in selecting the exact drug to be used; these are based on experience and familiarity with the various drugs. A stepped-care approach is often used (Figure 33-2). Combinations of drugs are used, and the patient can end up on two or three different medications to control the blood pressure.

Often the initial medication in a stepped-care approach is a diuretic (see Chapter 36, "Diuretics and Antidiuretics"), and if this is not successful, other agents are added. Some prescribers would initially use a beta-adrenergic blocking agent rather than a diuretic. For mild to moderate hypertension the initial drug added to a diuretic is chosen from reserpine, prazosin, the beta-adrenergic blocking agents, clonidine, methyldopa, or hydralazine. Reserpine is probably used less now because of its troublesome side effects (e.g., nasal stuffiness, depression, peptic ulcer disease) and also because there is now a selection of more useful drugs. Other rauwolfia alkaloids are only of historical use and probably should *not* be used at

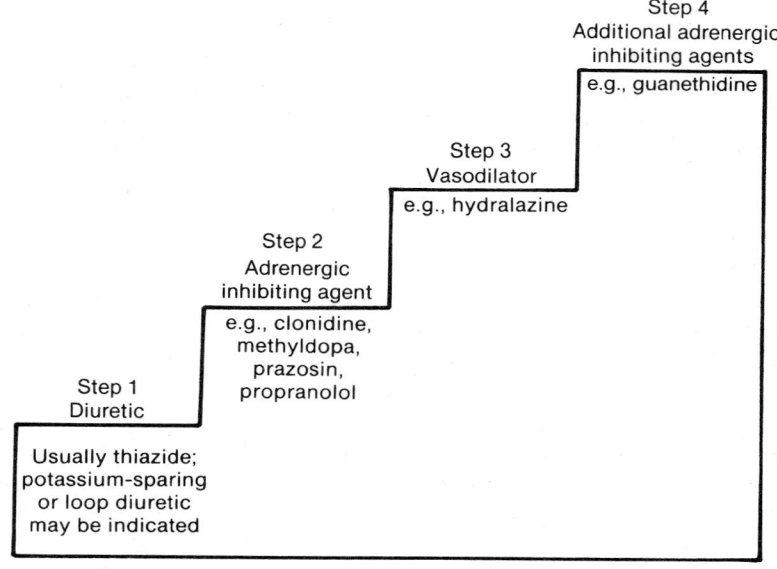

FIGURE 33-2. **Stepped-care approach for the treatment of hypertension.**

present. Sometimes two drugs will be added, and in this case, a beta-adrenergic blocking agent is usually combined with one of the others. A beta-adrenergic blocking agent usually will have to be added if hydralazine is used, because this vasodilator produces a reflex tachycardia and an increase in cardiac output that limits its hypotensive effect.

In severe hypertension increased amounts or combinations of up to four medications can be used. The dosages used are usually limited by the side effects. The general principle is that as little drug as necessary to control the blood pressure is used. Therefore, a low starting dose is used and is gradually increased as required. In severe hypertension when the other drugs fail, guanethidine or bethanidine can be added, or minoxidil can be used in place of hydralazine. Using minoxidil almost always requires concurrently using a potent loop diuretic and a beta-adrenergic blocking agent because of fluid retention and tachycardia. The full place of labetalol and captopril in the treatment of hypertension remains to be determined although they are primarily used as adjunctive therapy, particularly when patients have not responded satisfactorily to the other agents. A diuretic is almost always required with captopril.

The remainder of the drugs discussed in this chapter have very specific and limited use in treating hypertension (Table 33-1). Trimethaphan, diazoxide, and nitroprusside are used only in treating hypertensive emergencies. All three are given intravenously. Trimethaphan and nitroprusside must be given as constant infusions because of their very short durations of action. This can be an advantage if the blood pressure becomes too low, for within a few minutes of discontinuing the infusion, the drug effects will wane and the pressure will begin to rise. Once diluted for use, nitroprusside is chemically unstable and a fresh solution must be prepared every 4 hours. Exposure to light accelerates the chemical decomposition of nitroprusside and precautions must be taken to protect it from light. This is usually done by wrapping the bottle and tubing with aluminum foil. The dosage of nitroprusside or trimethaphan is highly variable between patients and *tachyphylaxis* (i.e., development of resistance to the drug's effect) can develop with both. Onset of tachyphylaxis can be particularly rapid with trimethaphan.

Diazoxide has an immediate effect when given intravenously as a single bolus, and this effect can last for 3 to 24 hours and the dose may then be repeated. Although much of the literature on diazoxide states that the drug must be given rapidly over 15 to 30 seconds, it has now been clearly shown that a slow in-

fusion will produce the same resultant blood pressure and that the rapid bolus technique should generally be abandoned because it often produces a transient precipitous fall in blood pressure. Diazoxide also causes marked salt and water retention (opposite to the effect of other thiazides), and this can limit the hypotensive effect when second and subsequent doses are needed. The usual technique used to overcome this problem is concurrently to administer a potent loop diuretic, such as furosemide, with the second and each subsequent dose of diazoxide.

Phentolamine and phenoxybenzamine are really only used to control blood pressure temporarily in patients with pheochromocytoma until the tumor can be removed surgically. This is particularly necessary during any invasive tests the patient might undergo and during the surgery itself. A beta-adrenergic blocking agent may also be necessary to control those effects of excessive catecholamines. Intravenous administration of phentolamine has also been described as a test for pheochromocytoma, but there are better diagnostic tests for this condition (e.g., urinary metanephrine level).

Many of the drugs discussed in this chapter have a number of other cardiac and noncardiac uses and

TABLE 33-1

Schema for management of selected hypertensive emergencies

Syndrome	*Drugs*
Malignant hypertension (untreated)	Nitroprusside or diazoxide (occasionally trimethaphan)
Hypertensive encephalopathy	Nitroprusside or diazoxide (occasionally trimethaphan)
Hypertension with:	
Pulmonary edema	Nitroprusside
Intracranial hemorrhage	Nitroprusside
Aortic dissection	Nitroprusside ± propranolol (occasionally trimethaphan)
Ischemic chest pain	Nitroprusside + propranolol
Eclampsia	Diazoxide or nitroprusside
Pheochromocytoma	Phentolamine or phenoxybenzamine ± propranolol
Withdrawal of antihypertensive*	Propranolol + phentolamine or phenoxybenzamine or nitroprusside

*In less acute situations, the withdrawn drug can be administered.

some of these are listed in the Nursing Drug Digest. Reserpine was once used as an antipsychotic (see Chapter 18, "Drugs Used to Treat Psychotic Disorders"), but has now been replaced by other agents. Drugs used for hypertensive emergencies, such as nitroprusside and trimethaphan, are used in the acute management of dissection of the aorta, whether or not there is hypertension. Prazosin, hydralazine, and captopril have been used in congestive heart failure or for low cardiac output states of several etiologies to reduce the loading conditions on the left ventricle and to improve the forward cardiac output. Nitroprusside and phentolamine have also been used in acute situations for this purpose. The beta-adrenergic blocking agents have a wide variety of cardiac and noncardiac uses. They are one of the mainstays in the treatment of angina pectoris (see Chapter 34, "Vasodilators, Antilipemics, Anticoagulants, and Platelet Aggregation Inhibitors"). They are also used in *idiopathic hypertrophic subaortic stenosis (IHSS)*, some supraventricular tachycardias, and in symptomatic *mitral valve prolapse*. The newest use for beta-blockers is based on several large clinical trials, which have shown a reduction in mortality and reinfarction when these agents are given in the first year following myocardial infarction. Many patients who have had a myocardial infarction are taking these drugs for this reason. Noncardiac uses of the beta-adrenergic blocking agents include prophylaxis of migraine headaches and the treatment of some forms of tremor. Several of these drugs, including phentolamine, diazoxide, and hydralazine, have been used to treat primary pulmonary hypertension. The hyperglycemic effect of diazoxide has been used to treat some forms of hypoglycemia.

ADVERSE EFFECTS AND TOXICITY

Certain side effects are common to almost all antihypertensive agents, although they may be more prominent with one drug rather than with another. These side effects include excessive lowering of blood pressure, usually manifested as symptomatic postural or exertional hypotension, salt and water retention, and an excessive hypertensive rebound when the drug is discontinued.

Guanethidine, bethanidine, debrisoquine, reserpine. The adrenergic neuron blocking agents bethanidine, guanethidine, and reserpine cause the same general types of side effects. One of the most common problems is postural or exertional hypotension, and symptoms include dizziness, fatigue and *syncope*. Unopposed parasympathetic activity can result in bradycardia, increased GI secretions, and diar-

rhea. Ejaculation may be interfered with. There can be a tendency to retain salt and fluid resulting in edema. Nasal congestion caused by vasodilation occurs with all three but is particularly a problem with reserpine. Reserpine is also more likely to cause mental depression and its use is contraindicated in depressed patients with suicidal tendencies. In addition, reserpine can aggravate peptic ulcer disease and ulcerative colitis. Reserpine has also recently been implicated by retrospective epidemiologic studies as a factor associated with breast cancer. This finding has been disputed and is presently a very controversial issue. These agents have been known to cause a multitude of problems, which include nausea, vomiting, anorexia, flushing, cardiac dysrhythmias, several CNS symptoms (e.g., nightmares, tremors), skin rashes (e.g., *thrombocytopenic purpura*), and asthma. It is partly because of the wide variety and number of side effects that these agents are now used less commonly.

Trimethaphan. The ganglionic blocking agent trimethaphan is generally only used for a short period of a few hours to a few days, and adverse effects are directly related to the hypotensive effect. These include excessive hypotension, tachycardia, and headache. Tachyphylaxis to this agent, which can limit its usefulness, can develop quite rapidly.

Phentolamine, phenoxybenzamine, prazosin. The alpha-adrenergic blocking agents phentolamine and phenoxybenzamine have a rather limited use and the major side effects are directly related to the hypotensive effects. These include postural or exercise-induced hypotension and tachycardia. Such effects are manifested as symptoms of dizziness, headache, and fatigue. Excessive lowering of the blood pressure and tachycardia can be dangerous in patients with *coronary artery disease* and can lead to an exacerbation of angina or even the precipitation of a myocardial infarction. Sedation can also occur when phentolamine and phenoxybenzamine are used. Phentolamine has been associated with GI symptoms such as abdominal pain, nausea, vomiting, and diarrhea. Prazosin has been reported to cause syncopal episodes, often early when the drug is first begun, and most of these are believed to be caused by hypotension. Prazosin is used on a more extended basis than the other two drugs, and problems of alpha-blockade, in addition to those noted earlier, include impairment of ejaculation. Prazosin has also been noted to cause some skin rashes, urinary frequency, visual disturbances, tinnitus, and CNS symptoms such as depression and nervousness.

Beta-adrenergic blocking agents. The major side effects of the beta-adrenergic blocking agents are directly related to their pharmacologic action. Depression of myocardial function is an important side effect, and although oral administration does not lead to sudden decompensation, heart failure can develop insidiously. Compensatory mechanisms are also interfered with in situations of stress, such as the administration of a general anesthetic. Another major problem is the development of increased airway resistance, which can lead to decompensation in patients with chronic obstructive pulmonary disease, and acute asthmatic attacks in certain susceptible patients. Bradycardia can also be a problem. Although less of a problem with beta-adrenergic blockers than with some of the other agents, hypotension can occur. These last two effects can lead to lightheadedness, dizziness, and occasionally syncope. Patients frequently complain of fatigue and lassitude. Sexual function can be interfered with (i.e., impotence) and a few cases of *Peyronie's disease* have been noted with propranolol. Some patients develop partial or even classical *Raynaud's phenomenon* and the symptoms of *intermittent claudication* can be aggravated. As with most drugs taken orally, some patients will experience GI side effects (e.g., abdominal distress, nausea, vomiting, diarrhea, constipation) and an assortment of skin rashes have been noted. The CNS side effects include mental dullness, insomnia, drowsiness, dizziness, vertigo, and anxiety. Despite this long list of adverse effects, the beta-blockers are well tolerated by many patients.

The newer agents, particularly those with cardioselectivity (e.g., alprenolol, atenolol, metoprolol) or intrinsic sympathomimetic activity (e.g., pindolol, oxprenolol) are touted as having fewer of these side effects, but their use is too limited at present to be sure of this. Certainly individual patients who have difficulties tolerating one of these agents may do very well with an alternative drug, and therefore the availability of a selection of agents is a distinct advantage.

Two particular adverse effects noted with propranolol, and that may also apply to the others, should be specifically mentioned. First, in insulin-dependent diabetic patients, many of the symptoms of hypoglycemia are blunted by beta-blockade and the compensatory catecholamine mechanisms for hypoglycemia (i.e., glycogenolysis, lypolysis, gluconeogenesis) are inhibited. Therefore, these agents are *contraindicated* in such patients. Second, the sudden withdrawal of propranolol can result in a precipitous rebound of symptoms, particularly in patients with some forms of angina. The rebound occurs from the second to the eighth day and is probably caused by transient supersensitivity to catecholamines. Pindolol has been reported to have less of this type of rebound. When

possible, therefore, these agents should always be discontinued *gradually*, or perhaps patients should be continued on a small dose (e.g., 10 mg propranolol per day) for 2 to 3 weeks before stopping the drug.

Practolol is a cardioselective beta-adrenergic blocking agent that was at one time available in Europe but was withdrawn because it caused a high incidence of a peculiar immune-type reaction called oculomucocutaneous syndrome, and a few of these patients developed a devastating sclerosing peritonitis. There remains some concern that this problem could also be induced by other beta-adrenergic blockers (oxprenolol, propranolol), albeit with a low incidence.

Labetalol. The combined alpha-adrenergic and beta-adrenergic blocking agent labetalol is too new for its adverse effects to be well cataloged. It is to be fully expected there will be a mixture of the adverse effects noted earlier in the discussion of those agents with similar pharmacologic effects.

Clonidine, methyldopa. The central-acting alpha-adrenergic agonists clonidine and methyldopa have some side effects in common (and in common with many other antihypertensives) and some side effects that are unique to each individual agent. Among the frequent adverse effects these two agents share are sedation and dry mouth, both probably caused by CNS effects. These two effects are often transient and occur only at the initiation of treatment or when the dose is increased. Other CNS effects of these two drugs include headache, mood alteration (e.g., euphoria and depression with clonidine; depression with methyldopa), sleep disturbances, and decreased mental acuity. Both drugs should be used with caution in depressed patients. Methyldopa also can cause abnormal choreoathetotic movements, Bell's palsy, and parkinsonism.

As is the case with many antihypertensive agents, there may be problems with postural or exertional hypotension. Low blood pressure is probably at least partly the basis for symptoms such as lethargy and fatigue. Bradycardia is a side effect of methyldopa, and fluid retention can occur with both agents. Clonidine has caused Raynaud's phenomenon. Both agents can cause the usual GI side effects of abdominal discomfort, nausea, vomiting, diarrhea, and constipation.

Abrupt withdrawal of clonidine (and to a lesser degree, of methyldopa) has been associated with a precipitous rise in blood pressure and hypertensive crisis. In this situation, the blood pressure can be controlled by alpha-adrenergic and beta-adrenergic antagonists. Therefore this drug should never be suddenly discontinued.

Methyldopa has a number of side effects with an

apparent immunologic basis. They include hepatitis, arthralgia, myalgia, *myocarditis*, drug fever, hemolytic anemia, and combination syndromes resembling *lupus erythematosus.* As with other agents with similar properties, serologic tests, notably *Coombs' test* and antinuclear antibody test, may be positive even in the absence of symptoms. Methyldopa may also cause a cholestatic jaundice and a number of hematologic abnormalities in addition to hemolytic anemia (e.g., *thrombocytopenia, leukopenia,* and *granulocytopenia).* Skin rashes of various types occur with both agents. Methyldopa can cause a number of endocrine problems, such as gynecomastia, lactation, impotence, and decreased libido. Some of these effects may be related to dopamine being an inhibitor of prolactin release (perhaps methyldopamine is a partial antagonist). Clonidine has also been noted to cause impotence. It must be stated that the experience with clonidine is considerably briefer than with methyldopa and the full range of side effects may not yet be appreciated.

Diazoxide, hydralazine, minoxidil, nitroprusside.
The side effects of diazoxide are related to its hypotensive action, to its thiazide-like effects of hyperglycemia and hyperuricemia, and to salt and water retention. Hypotension can be profound, although usually transient, when the drug is given as a rapid bolus, and can lead to serious problems, such as stroke and myocardial infarction. As mentioned previously, the drug does *not* have to be given very rapidly to have a therapeutic effect. Hyperglycemia commonly occurs and can be particularly troublesome with repeated injections, especially in patients with diabetes. Hyperuricemia and salt and water retention are also common, particularly with the repeated use of diazoxide and salt and water retention can be averted by the concurrent administration of a potent loop diuretic (e.g., furosemide). Less severe vasodilator phenomena such as flushing, headaches, and postural hypotension commonly occur. Cardiac dysrhythmias, usually tachycardias, occur and are probably secondary to hypotension in most cases. If diazoxide is inadvertently injected subcutaneously, it can cause cellulitis. Nausea, vomiting, and abdominal discomfort are relatively common, even though diazoxide is given intravenously. The prolonged oral use of diazoxide for its hyperglycemic effect has resulted in hypertrichosis.

Hydralazine also has a wide variety of adverse effects. Many of these are reflex-induced and secondary to the vasodilator effects. Such effects include palpitation, headache, sweatiness, and dizziness. These may be controlled by the concomitant use of a beta-adrenergic blocking agent. Anorexia, nausea, vomiting, and diarrhea are fairly common with hydralazine. There are a number of CNS effects, including depression, disorientation, and anxiety. Peripheral nervous system effects of numbness, tingling, and tremors are probably caused by a pyridoxine deficiency and can be corrected by administering the vitamin. Cardiovascular effects, in addition to those previously mentioned, include flushing, nasal congestion, and fluid retention. A number of immunologic or hypersensitivity reactions occur with hydralazine, such as drug fever, rashes, *eosinophilia,* and, rarely, hepatitis. Slow acetylator patients can develop a number of syndromes that partially or completely mimic lupus erythematosus. Such syndromes are rare or unheard of with doses of less than 200 mg/day. The typical serologic changes (e.g., positive antinuclear antibody test) are present in these patients, but, as with methyldopa, asymptomatic patients often have a positive serology. Anemia, leukopenia, and thrombocytopenia, with or without purpura, have occurred in patients on hydralazine.

Minoxidil is a relatively new drug and a complete listing of its side effects is yet to be developed. It is, however, a potent vasodilator and thus has many of the same side effects as hydralazine. Using this agent always requires concomitantly using a beta-adrenergic blocking agent to control reflex effects (e.g., tachycardia, sweatiness) caused by vasodilation and a potent diuretic to combat salt and water retention. As with most hypotensive agents, an excessive lowering of the blood pressure can occur with minoxidil, and the most serious consequence of this is the occurrence or exacerbation of symptoms caused by myocardial or cerebral ischemia. Hypertrichosis is a common side effect with chronic use and can be very distressing for female patients.

Nitroprusside's adverse effects are directly related to the excessive lowering of the blood pressure or the accumulation of toxic metabolites such as thiocyanate, resulting in hypothyroidism, or cyanide, resulting in tissue hypoxia and anoxia. The effects of the metabolites were previously discussed in the pharmacokinetics section, and the excess hypotensive effects are similar to those mentioned earlier for other agents in this group.

Captopril. Captopril is a new agent and little is known about its side effects. Incidence of adverse effects with this agent is generally stated to be low. The most common side effects are urticarial rash, fever, and loss of taste. Some other more disturbing side effects may now be appearing, but whether they are clearly caused by the drug is uncertain. Neutropenia and agranulocytosis have been reported in patients on this drug. Proteinuria (enough to be called a nephrotic syndrome) and renal failure have also occurred in patients taking captopril, but in hypertension it is uncertain whether this is solely the result of the drug.

DRUG INTERACTIONS

Interactions of the antihypertensive agents with other drugs are listed in Clinically Significant Drug Interactions. As would be expected with such a diverse group of drugs, these are fairly numerous. It should be emphasized that many of the agents discussed in this chapter are fairly new drugs and the listing must be regarded as incomplete.

The mechanism of action of the antiadrenergic agents revolves around the uptake and release of endogenous catecholamines, and thus other agents that also rely on these processes for their actions will interact with the antiadrenergics. Such drugs include amphetamines, tricyclic antidepressants, phenothiazines, and sympathomimetic amines.

Prazosin has been reported to interact with a number of other drugs in isolated instances, but because the drug is new and no clear pattern has emerged, it is presently unclear if any of these are clinically important. The list includes cardiac glycosides, oral hypoglycemics, antidysrhythmics (e.g., procainamide, quinidine), phenobarbital and benzodiazepine sedatives, some nonsteroidal antiinflammatory agents, and drugs used to treat gout (e.g., allopurinol, colchicine, probenecid).

The beta-adrenergic blocking agents interact with insulin and the oral hypoglycemic agents because of the blockade of catecholamine-mediated responses to hypoglycemia. This was referred to in the discussion of the adverse effects of these agents. The interaction between calcium antagonists such as verapamil and the beta-adrenergic blocking agents (heart block) is referred to in Chapter 32.

The central-acting alpha-adrenergic agonists interact with a variety of agents. Tricyclic antidepressants and tolazoline decrease the effects of clonidine by an unknown mechanism. Clonidine interacts with oral hypoglycemics in a similar way to beta-adrenergic blocking agents (i.e., blunting of the catecholamine response to hypoglycemia). Clonidine can inhibit the effects of levodopa, but the mechanism of this effect is unknown. Another interesting interaction of clonidine for which the mechanism is unknown is the blockade of the effects of narcotic withdrawal. Methyldopa increases haloperidol and lithium toxicity by unknown mechanisms.

Diazoxide will decrease the anticonvulsant effect of phenytoin, but the mechanism for this interaction is unknown.

Many drugs used primarily for other purposes can also lower the blood pressure by various mechanisms, and such agents interact with all of the antihypertensives by having an additive effect that can lead to excessive hypotension. Such interacting agents include the general anesthetics, phenothiazines, and thiothixenes.

SUMMARY

Pharmacologic treatment of primary or essential hypertension includes the individual and stepped-care approaches using diuretics, CNS agents, alpha-adrenergic and beta-adrenergic blockers, and vasodilators. Newer investigational drugs are also being used to achieve lower blood pressure. Individualized drug therapy regimens and the involvement of patients in planning their care are essential.

The nurse's role is expanding, especially at the nurse practitioner levels where there is specialized preparation in the management of the patient with hypertension. All nurses, however, should be involved in screening and identifying high-risk individuals who are unaware that they may be developing or have hypertension. Nurses will become increasingly involved in counseling and supporting patients so they can responsibly follow their treatment plans, which are usually lifelong and require the incorporation of lifestyle changes to prevent target organ damage leading to stroke, heart disease, and renal failure. Teaching patients about their condition will increase success in its control. Monitoring patient response is a major role for the nurse in managing hypertensive care.

ADVERSE/SIDE EFFECTS OF THE ANTIHYPERTENSIVES*

ALLERGIC REACTIONS

Angioedema
Asthma
Fever
Hemolytic anemia
Lupus erythematosus
Oculomucocutaneous syndrome
Pruritus
Sclerosing peritonitis
Serologic abnormalities (positive
   antinuclear antibody test, Coombs'
   test, rheumatoid factor)
Urticaria (hives) and other skin rashes

AUTONOMIC NERVOUS SYSTEM

Antiadrenergic (bradycardia,
   bronchospasm, decreased cardiac
   output, impaired ejaculation,
   postural hypotension)
Anticholinergic (constipation, dry
   mouth and eyes, impotence,
   urinary retention)

BEHAVIOR

Apprehension
Depression
Lassitude
Sedation
Weakness

CARDIOVASCULAR SYSTEM

Bradycardia
Congestive heart failure
Decreased cardiac output
Fluid retention, edema
Flushing
Heart block
Hypertensive crisis in combination
   with other drugs or some foods
Hypotension

Increased angina
Intermittent claudication
Nasal congestion
Raynaud's phenomenon
Rebound hypertension on withdrawal
Stroke
Tachycardia

CENTRAL NERVOUS SYSTEM

Dizziness
Hallucinations
Headache
Nightmares
Paresthesias
Sleep disturbances
Tremor
Vertigo

GASTROINTESTINAL SYSTEM

Abdominal cramps
Anorexia
Bitter taste
"Bloating"
Constipation
Diarrhea
Dyspepsia
Eructation
Hemorrhage
Increased acid secretion
Nausea and vomiting
Peptic ulcer

HEMATOLOGIC SYSTEM

Anemia
Granulocytopenia
Pancytopenia
Purpura
Thrombocytopenia

**METABOLIC AND ENDOCRINE
SYSTEMS**

Possibly carcinogenic (e.g., breast
   cancer and reserpine)
Coarsening of facial features
Cyanide intoxication
Decreased libido
Hirsutism
Hyperglycemia
Hypertrichosis
Hyperuricemia
Hypothyroidism
Increased insulin release
Increased prolactin release—
   galactorrhea
Loss of taste
Masking of hypoglycemia
Peyronie's disease
Potentiation of insulin
Weight gain

NEUROMUSCULAR SYSTEM

Muscle cramps
Parkinsonism
Polyneuritis
Weakness

OCULAR SYSTEM

Blurred vision
Conjunctivitis
Dry eyes
Impaired accommodation
Lacrimation
Miosis
Mydriasis

MISCELLANEOUS

Chilliness
Piloerection
Sweating

*See Chapter 11, "Drug Toxicity," for an overview of drug toxicity.

CLINICALLY SIGNIFICANT DRUG INTERACTIONS*

Primary drug	Interacting drug	Possible effect(s)	Probable mechanism(s)
All antihypertensives	Anesthetics, general	Hypotension	Additive effects
All antihypertensives	Phenothiazines	Hypotension	Additive effects
Debrisoquin, gua-nethidine	Antidepressants (tricyclic)	Decreased antihy-pertensive effect	Blockage of debrisoquine and guanethidine uptake
Debrisoquin, gua-nethidine, reser-pine	Sympathomimetic amines	Hypertensive crisis	Blockade of amine uptake
Clonidine	Antidepressants (tricyclic)	Decreased antihy-pertensive effect	Not established
Clonidine	Levodopa	Decreased levodo-pa effect	Stimulation of adrenergic receptors
Clonidine	Hypoglycemics (oral)	Hypertension, hy-poglycemia	Increased circulating catecholamine (e.g., epinephrine) levels
Diazoxide	Hydralazine	Hypotension	Additive effects
Guanethidine	Alcohol	Hypotension	Vasodilation
Guanethidine	Amphetamines	Decreased antihy-pertensive effect	Antagonism of guanethidine's adrenergic blockade
Guanethidine	Levarterenol	Increased pressor effects	Antagonism of guanethidine's adrenergic blockade
Guanethidine	Phenothiazines	Decreased antihy-pertensive effect	Blockade of guanethidine up-take
Minoxidil	Guanethidine	Severe orthostatic hypotension	Additive and potentiated ef-fects
Propranolol	Hypoglycemics (oral)	Hypertension, hy-perglycemia	Increased circulating cate-cholamine (e.g., epineph-rine) levels

*See Chapter 10, ''Drug Interactions,'' for an overview of drug interactions.

GENERAL NURSING IMPLICATIONS

Nursing of patients requiring antihypertensives

ASSESSMENT

A complete nursing assessment is essential in establishing a baseline from which to identify risk factors, as well as to individualize drug therapy and to monitor therapeutic response, adverse side effects, and signs of hypertensive crisis. This is important in both inpatient and outpatient settings. Assessment should include a careful drug history to determine sensitivity, contraindications, and cautions before drug therapy is initiated. In addition, potential drug interactions should be identified, including medications currently taken by the patient that can cause hypertension (e.g., oral contraceptives, amphetamines, cocaine) or that may diminish the effectiveness of some antihypertensives, including prescription drugs (e.g., tricyclic antidepressants) and over-the-counter drugs (e.g., sympathomimetic amines such as ephedrine), require identification.

SENSITIVITY

When antihypertensives are taken by patients who have not received them before, monitoring for hypersensitivity reactions is extremely important. Skin rash, fever, laryngeal edema (although uncommon), or asthma-like symptoms should be reported immediately to the prescriber. Outpatients should monitor and report these signs to the health care provider immediately.

CONTRAINDICATIONS

Antihypertensives, because of their actions and effects on various body systems, are contraindicated in the presence of various conditions. See the Nursing Drug Digest for contraindications to each specific agent.

CAUTIONS

Caution should be used when antihypertensives, including diuretics (see

Continued.

GENERAL NURSING IMPLICATIONS—cont'd

Nursing of patients requiring antihypertensives—cont'd

CAUTIONS—cont'd

Chapter 36, "Diuretics and Antidiuretics"), are administered to elderly patients. Elderly patients are more sensitive to fluid volume depletion and sympathetic inhibition than are younger patients because of reduced cardiovascular function, and are more prone to hypotensive effects. Potassium regulation may also be a problem with elderly patients and requires careful monitoring. Dosage should be smaller and spaced at longer intervals. The blood pressure should be lowered slowly so that weakness, faintness, or syncope are avoided, because many elderly patients have poor baroreceptor control.

Caution should also be used when antihypertensives are administered to children and to pregnant women because data on their effects in such patients are limited.

Caution should be used when patients receiving antihypertensive therapy require surgery or dental procedures. It is important that the anesthesiologist is aware that the patient is receiving antihypertensive therapy.

It is important for nurses to recognize that the sedative-hypnotics (see Chapter 15) do not directly lower the blood pressure and should *not* be used as primary therapy in treating hypertension.

DRUG INTERACTIONS

Antihypertensives can interact with numerous medications, including prescription and nonprescription drugs (see Clinically Significant Drug Interactions). Newer antihypertensives have limited drug interaction information available and their use with other medications should be monitored closely.

ADMINISTRATION
Initial therapy

Patients with moderate and severe hypertension, as well as certain patients with mild hypertension (e.g., those patients with the presence of target organ damage or elevated cholesterol levels), are usually placed on an individualized drug regimen or a stepped-care program (see Figure 33-2). When administering medications according to this regimen or when teaching the patient to do so, one must be alert to possible reasons for a lack of responsiveness to therapy before proceeding to the next step or altering the drug plan. Ineffective drug therapy is often a result of poor adherence to therapy, insufficient dose of current drug(s), excessive sodium intake, weight gain, or the concomitant use of competing drugs (e.g., oral contraceptives, sympathomimetic decongestants).

Maintenance

When the blood pressure is reduced to the goal level, doses of medications are stabilized at maintenance levels. To simplify drug therapy regimens and to increase compliance, combination preparations (e.g., Aldactazide, the hydrochlorothiazide and spironolactone combination, Ser-Ap-Es, the reserpine, hydralazine, hydrochlorothiazide combination) are sometimes used.

Cautiously stepping down drugs may be attempted with individual patients in uncomplicated mild hypertension; however, long-term therapy is usually indicated.

Follow-up and reassessment at regular intervals are important for reinforcement in relation to blood pressure control and adherence to therapy. The patient's blood pressure is the indicator of the therapeutic response and should be recorded at regular intervals during visits. The nurse should explore the difficulties of long-term therapy with the patient, including lifestyle changes, difficulty remembering medications, and consequences of poor control. Providing simple written instructions of the medication plan, common side effects, and therapeutic goals can do much to help patients manage their drug regimens. Progress should be emphasized during visits, and a willingness to discuss the possibility of drug change to avoid side effects does much to communicate genuine concern as does individualized treatment.

Other techniques found by nurses working with patients with hypertension that can be used to increase self-maintenance of drug regimens are clear reminders of appointments, setting appointments up at each visit, a short waiting time, telephone reminders for missed appointments, and increasing the frequency of visits (especially if the patient is having difficulty following a prescribed regimen). The use of other resources, including family members, in the patient's care has also been shown to be helpful.

Specific information regarding the administration of these agents can be found in the Nursing Drug Digest.

MONITORING PATIENT RESPONSE
Therapeutic response

Monitoring the patient's therapeutic response is especially important in adjusting antihypertensive therapy regimens to attain optimal blood pressure control with minimal side effects. Response determines the titration of various antihypertensives and determines individualized patient antihypertension drug regimen planning. All findings should be recorded carefully to document patient response and to facilitate planning. In addition to blood pressure changes, psychologic changes that occur as the blood pressure is lowered are important and should be related to patient symptoms.

Adverse side effects

Monitoring side effects is essential (see Adverse/Side Effects of the Antihypertensives), as is planning to minimize these effects with the patient and the family as indicated. Involving the patient and the family promotes decision making in relation to the drug regimen and promotes compliance, thus avoiding the potential of undue serious problems associated with the patient discontinuing medication because of an inability to live with side effects.

Common side effects include symptomatic postural and exertional hypotension. The blood pressure should be measured, especially with guanethi-

GENERAL NURSING IMPLICATIONS—cont'd

Nursing of patients requiring antihypertensives—cont'd

Adverse side effects—cont'd

dine therapy, in both lying and standing positions to monitor this effect. The patient should be prepared to manage this effect at home.

Impotence has been found to be the major side effect next to dry mouth and drowsiness with methyldopa and clonidine therapy. This side effect is often difficult for many male patients to discuss and requires special nursing consideration. Nurses working with patients receiving these medications recommend that this side effect not be suggested to patients to avoid psychosomatic complaint, but that the patient be carefully questioned regarding any new problems or concerns after the initiation of methyldopa, clonidine, or guanethidine therapy. It is also important to identify other possible causes of the condition (e.g., marital discord) with the patient before changes in medication are sought.

All antihypertensives can cause excessive hypertensive rebound when discontinued abruptly and require gradual discontinuation. See the Nursing Drug Digest for specific implications for monitoring side effects of each antihypertensive agent.

It is also important when monitoring side effects to differentiate between those that can be minimized and those that indicate the medication should be discontinued.

Toxicity

Patients requiring antihypertensive therapy should be monitored for the excessive lowering of blood pressure, or symptomatic postural or exertional hypotension manifested by dizziness, fatigue, and syncope. Toxic side effects are identified in the Nursing Drug Digest for each specific agent. Patients should be monitored for these effects in relation to their individual drug regimens and findings should be communicated to the prescriber so the drug plan can be adjusted as required.

PATIENT EDUCATION

Most patients requiring antihypertensive drug therapy are outpatients and are responsible for their own medication regimens related to controlling their hypertension. Patient teaching is essential to promote their ability to make choices about drug regimens, follow planned drug therapy, modify activities of daily living as needed, and to reduce risk factors in controlling their condition. Nurses play an important part in this aspect of care and it cannot be overemphasized. The family should be involved, as indicated, because their understanding of the patient's care and condition is essential in coping with changes that can occur in relation to the patient's hypertensive condition. Their assistance and support can be invaluable in dietary planning (e.g., low cholesterol, low sodium). In addition, because of the hereditary aspects of hypertension, family members should be taught to recognize the need for screening and monitoring their own blood pressures.

Patients should know the exact names of their medications, how they work, the dosage and frequency of administration, side effects, when to seek assistance from the health care provider, and how side effects can be minimized. For example, patients receiving beta-adrenergic blockers should be advised of the possible bradycardia, anorexia, nausea, lightheadedness, fatigue, and insomnia that can occur with this medication. The nurse should help the patient plan what to do if any of these occur, including stopping the medication. If either or all of these occur, they will require assistance in managing the effects.

It is also important that the patient recognize which side effects are transient or need to be minimized and those that are not side effects at all. Many patients require support in waiting out transient side effects.

In addition, the patient should know what precautions to take while on medications, especially when beginning new medications, and to report side effects such as drowsiness and nasal stuffiness that can be eliminated by a change in medication. The patient should also know the following: the prevalence and etiology of their condition; the seriousness of high blood pressure and the risks of uncontrolled hypertension; the lack of symptoms and thus the inability to estimate their blood pressure by how they feel; the importance of following an individualized regimen and of maintaining a drug treatment record. Patients should also know how to monitor their own blood pressure at home or know where to get their blood pressure monitored in the community. They should understand the importance of looking at trends rather than relying on one reading, and know dangerous blood pressure levels. The need for follow-up and the probability of lifelong treatment even after the blood pressure stabilizes should be carefully discussed as should the reasons for changing or discontinuing certain medications.

Not only does nurse monitoring of patient medication schedules and simplifying regimens represent a major aspect of promoting patient management, but counseling can be another important nursing function. The development and use of hypertensive assessment and treatment tools to ensure comprehensive care and the continuity of care can also do much to ensure success. In addition, patients and their families often require assistance in setting realistic health care goals and support in adapting their lifestyles to minimize risk factors. Behavioral approaches to lower blood pressure should be taught and reinforced, such as the following: weight loss if the patient is overweight; reducing alcohol intake if it averages more than one to two drinks a day; reducing salt intake and foods that cause sodium retention, such as black licorice; limiting caffeine intake; exercising regularly; regular use of relaxation exercises or biofeedback; and reducing stress. Reducing dietary cholesterol is indicated if lipids are elevated. Family involvement is essential. Referral to lay counseling groups is often beneficial in helping patients and their families accept the condition and the therapeutic regimen.

GENERAL INSTRUCTIONS FOR DISCHARGE/OUTPATIENTS

ANTIHYPERTENSIVES

This drug is an antihypertensive, and it is used to lower your high blood pressure.

Follow the instructions on the prescription exactly. Even if you feel well and do not notice any signs of need for this medication, take it exactly as directed. Do *not* miss any doses and do *not* take more medicine than directed.

If this medication is irritating to your stomach, take it with or immediately following meals or with a glassful of milk, unless you are told it should be taken on an empty stomach.

To help you remember to take your medicine, take it at the same time each day. It is often helpful to take it in relation to an everyday routine (e.g., with a certain meal, after brushing your teeth).

If a dose is missed, take it as soon as possible and then go back to your regular dosing schedule. If you remember the missed dose close to the time of the next dose, do *not* take the missed dose and do *not* double the next one. Go back to your regular dosing schedule. Call your health care provider if you have any questions.

Do *not* discontinue this medication or change your dosage regimen without consulting your health care provider. Your health care provider may want you to reduce the amount of medication you are taking gradually before stopping it completely because some conditions can worsen if the medication is stopped suddenly.

It is important that you take this medication, even if you feel healthy, exactly as instructed. Remember this medication will not cure your high blood pressure, but it will help to control it. You may have to take this medication for the rest of your life to prevent the problems that can occur with your hypertension. It is important not to miss any doses, and when your supply of this medication runs low, order a refill from your pharmacist or check with your health care provider. You may want to carry an extra dose in your wallet or purse.

Be careful when drinking alcohol because the combination may make you very sleepy. You should modify your alcohol intake to one to two drinks per day if you use alcohol.

Do *not* change posture suddenly while taking this medication because this can cause lightheadedness. Get up slowly from a sitting or lying position, particularly when arising in the morning.

Drowsiness, uncontrolled muscle movements, dryness of mouth and eyes, skin rashes, GI upset, and mood changes are some side effects that can occur when this medication is taken. Although not all of these side effects occur very often, when they do occur or become bothersome or extreme, notify your health care provider.

This medicine may cause you to become dizzy, lightheaded, or less alert than usual. Until you learn how this medication affects you, usually about 1 week, do not drive, drink excessive alcohol, operate machinery requiring alertness, or do jobs that require alertness. If this problem continues or becomes extreme, notify your health care provider. In addition, use caution when going up and down stairs.

It is important that you keep appointments with your health care providers so they can check your progress at regular times and adjust your medication dosage if necessary so your medication will work best for you.

You should carry a medication card stating that you are taking this medication.

If you are going to have surgery, dental procedures, or emergency treatment, tell the physician or dentist in charge that you are taking this medication.

This medication has *not* been tested extensively in pregnancy. If you are pregnant or intend to become pregnant, discuss this with your health care provider.

If you are breast feeding or plan to breast feed your infant, discuss this with your health care provider, because there may be a chance that this medication can pass into your breast milk and affect your infant.

Your health care provider may have planned a special diet with you to follow. Your medicine will be more effective if you follow this diet. Do not make any changes unless you consult your health care provider.

Do *not* begin to take any other medications while you are taking this medication without consulting with your health care provider.

Remember, this medication has been prescribed especially for you and your need to reduce your high blood pressure. Do *not* trade or give this medication to any relatives or friends.

Keep this and all medications out of children's reach.

NURSING DRUG DIGEST

Medication (trade name*)	Indication	Usual dosage and administration	Dosage forms, preparation, and storage	Contraindications, cautions, and comments	Monitoring
Atenolol Tenormin	Mild to moderate hypertension	*Adults:* 50-100 mg PO daily as a single dose Decrease dose in severe renal impairment	Tablets: 50, 100 mg Protect from heat and moisture	*Contraindicated* in cardiogenic shock, heart block, right ventricular failure, and sinus bradycardia May cause bradycardia, dizziness, and GI distress Adverse effects are generally mild and transient	Monitor blood pressure and heart rate
Captopril Capoten	Hypertension not responsive to conventional medication (particularly renovascular but also essential hypertension)	*Adults:* 75-450 mg/day PO in 3 divided doses, administered 1 hr before meals (to increase absorption) Reduce dosage in renal impairment	Tablets: 25, 50, 100 mg Store at room temperature protected from moisture	May increase serum potassium Captopril is excreted primarily by the kidneys May cause proteinuria, alteration in taste perception, or skin rash	Monitor blood pressure Monitor for neutropenia (fever, sore throat, reduced neutrophil count) Monitor renal function for increased serum creatinine or increased blood urea nitrogen, especially in patients with preexisting renal disease
Clonidine Catapres Combipres* Dixarit	Moderate to severe hypertension	*Adults:* Initially, 0.1 mg PO b.i.d. Maintenance: 0.2-0.8 mg/day in divided doses Maximum: 2.4 mg/day Dosage should be low initially and increased gradually *Dangerous* to discontinue abruptly because may result in hypertensive crisis	Tablets: 0.1, 0.2, 0.3 mg	Less drug is usually required in patients with renal failure; caution should be used in depressed patients; can aggravate or precipitate Raynaud's phenomenon Postural hypotension can be a problem	Monitor for signs of fluid retention (e.g., weight gain, edema), drowsiness, dry mouth, fatigue, and dizziness Monitor blood pressure

Continued.

NOTE: For additional details regarding the individual agents listed in this table see the text and other tables in this chapter.
*Indicates a multiple active ingredient product. For a complete listing of all active ingredients see the *Drug Reference Guide to Brand Names and Active Ingredients.*
✦ Indicates that the drug is generally available only in Canada.
★ Indicates that the drug is generally available only in the United States.

NURSING DRUG DIGEST—cont'd

Medication (trade name)	Indication	Usual dosage and administration	Dosage forms, preparation, and storage	Contraindications, cautions, and comments	Monitoring
Debrisoquine Declinax	Moderate to severe hypertension	*Adults:* 5-30 mg/day PO (if total daily dose exceeds 10 mg, then generally administered in 2-3 divided doses) Maximum: 140 mg/day Start with low doses and increase *gradually* by 5-10 mg/week May need to decrease dose in renal impairment	Tablets: 10 mg	*Contraindicated* in hypersensitivity, patients receiving MAOIs, pheochromocytoma, and severe circulatory impairment May cause orthostatic hypotension, GI distress, and mild CNS excitation Pharmacologic effect of debrisoquine can be potentiated by fever, hot weather, or strenuous physical exertion Tolerance to the pharmacologic effect may develop in some patients over time Discontinue 24 hours before elective surgery to avoid possibility of cardiovascular collapse	Observe for orthostatic hypotension If discontinued before elective surgery, blood pressure must be carefully monitored
Diazoxide Hyperstat Proglycem	Hypertensive crises	*Adults:* 1-3 mg/kg by rapid IV (maximum 150 mg/dose); repeat at 5-15 min intervals as indicated *Children:* 2.5-10 mg/kg/dose IV Once stabilized, patient should be switched to other antihypertensives Contrary to package insert, does *not* have to be given over 30 sec or less	Injectable: 300 mg/20 ml Protect from light, heat and freezing Store between 2° and 30° C	*Contraindicated* in patients sensitive to thiazides and in compensatory hypertension (e.g., that associated with aortic coarctation) Salt retention occurs, and second and subsequent doses should be administered with a loop diuretic (e.g., furosemide)	Hyperglycemia can occur with repeated use, and blood sugar should be monitored (daily in diabetic patients) Monitor weight daily for fluid retention and weight gain Monitor for signs of congestive heart failure

Drug	Uses	Dosage	Remarks	Nursing considerations
		Administer undiluted. Patients should be in a recumbent position during administration and for 30 min following; extravascular injection is irritating to the tissues and may cause pain and inflammation; inject *only* into a peripheral vein and monitor blood pressure closely during administration	Postural hypotension can be a problem. Frequent administration may cause edema and congestive heart failure. Diazoxide crosses the placenta. May interrupt labor—if this occurs labor can be reestablished with oxytocic agents (e.g., pitocin). May cause significant hyperglycemia in diabetic patients	Observe for postural hypotension, depression, diarrhea, weakness, and nasal stuffiness. Monitor blood pressure
Guanethidine * Ismelin Ismelin-Esidrix* Visutensil	Moderate to severe hypertension	*Adults:* 10-60 mg/day PO. Head of bed should be elevated to have antihypertensive effect if patient is confined to bed. Tablets: 10, 25 mg	*Contraindicated* in pheochromocytoma and congestive heart failure (*not* secondary to hypertension). Onset of action may take 1-3 weeks. Avoid concurrent use of MAOIs; MAOIs should be discontinued at least 1 week before starting guanethidine. Caution patients to be cautious with alcohol intake until they determine tolerance to combining the two agents	Monitor blood pressure. Observe for orthostatic hypotension

Continued.

NURSING DRUG DIGEST—cont'd

Medication (trade name)	Indication	Usual dosage and administration	Dosage forms, preparation, and storage	Contraindications, cautions, and comments	Monitoring
Hydralazine Apresazide* Apresoline Apresoline-Esidrix* Dralserp* Dralzine Lopress Mydrap-ES Myser Plus* Nor-press R-MCTZ-M* Ser-Ap-Es* Serpasil-Apresoline* Unipres	Moderate hypertension Hypertensive emergencies Some forms of congestive heart failure or low cardiac output	*Adults:* 10-50 mg IM or IV over 10-20 min; repeat as necessary q.3-6h. 40-200/mg day PO in 4 divided doses	Injectable: 20 mg/ml Tablets: 10, 25, 50, 100 mg	*Contraindicated* in hypersensitivity, coronary artery disease, and mitral valvular rheumatic heart disease Use with caution in patients who have previously had drug-induced lupus erythematosus Doses greater than 200 mg/day should not be used Effects greater in slow-acetylator patients Tachycardia and salt retention almost always occur, and a diuretic and beta-adrenergic blocking agent may enhance the effect	Monitor for signs of lupus erythematosus (e.g., fever, joint pain), tachycardia, fluid retention, palpitations, headache, and nausea Monitor blood pressure
Labetalol Trandate	Moderate to severe hypertension (usually used with a thiazide diuretic)	*Adults:* 100-400 mg PO b.i.d. Maximum: 1200 mg/day Administration with food or milk may decrease GI distress	Tablets: 100, 200 mg	*Contraindicated* in severe congestive heart failure, sinus bradycardia, heart block (greater than first degree), and cardiogenic shock	Monitor blood pressure Observe for postural hypotension

| **Methyldopa***\
Aldoclor\
Aldomet\
Aldoril*\
Dopamet\
Medimet-250\
Novomedopa\
Presinol\
Seebrine*\
Supres* | Mild to moderate hypertension | *Adults:* 250-1000 mg IV q.4-8h.; initial dose of up to 3 gm may be necessary; *or* 500 mg-2 gm/day PO in 2-4 divided doses\
Children: 10-65 mg/kg/day PO in 2-4 divided doses, but *not more than 3 gm/day; or* 20-40 mg/kg/24 hr IV divided into 4 doses | Injectable: 50 mg/ml\
Tablets: 125, 250, 500 mg\
Oral suspension: 250 mg/5 ml | *Contraindicated* in active hepatitis or history of drug-induced lupus erythematosus\
Use with caution in depressed patients because can cause worsening of depression\
Advise patient that drug may color urine blue (or dark) on rare occasions, but that this effect is *not* harmful\
Can cause lupus erythematosus and Coombs' positive hemolytic anemia\
Less required in patients with renal failure\
Dosage should be low initially and increased gradually\
Postural hypotension can be a problem\
Can cause false-positive urine test for pheochromocytoma\
If administered with alcohol may cause excessive hypotension\
Advise patient that drowsiness may occur and caution should be used in operating equipment or machinery requiring alertness | Monitor blood studies for hemolytic anemia, granulocytopenia, and thrombocytopenia\
Observe for fever, myalgias, and flulike symptoms when drug is initiated or dose increased; if observed, hold medication and notify prescriber\
Monitor blood pressure\
Observe for postural hypotension, drowsiness |

Continued.

NURSING DRUG DIGEST—cont'd

Medication (trade name)	Indication	Usual dosage and administration	Dosage forms, preparation, and storage	Contraindications, cautions, and comments	Monitoring
Metoprolol Betaloc Lopresor Lopressor Seloken	Mild to moderate hypertension See also Chapter 24, "Sympathomimetics and Sympatholytics"	*Adults:* Initially, 100 mg/24 hr PO Maintenance: 100-450 mg/24 hr PO in single or divided doses Dosage should be low initially and be increased gradually. High doses can precipitate bronchospasm in susceptible patients; abrupt discontinuance may exacerbate angina and MI and cause hypertensive crisis Reduce dosage in renal impairment	Tablets: 50, 100 mg	*Contraindicated* in marked sinus bradycardia or atrioventricular block, congestive heart failure, with concurrent verapamil use, and in insulin-dependent diabetic patients Can aggravate or precipitate Raynaud's phenomenon	Monitor apical pulse; if less than 50 beats/min, hold medication and notify prescriber Monitor for symptoms of congestive heart failure (e.g., edema, dyspnea) Monitor blood pressure
Minoxidil Loniten	Severe hypertension resistant to conventional agents	*Adults:* 5-40 mg/day PO as single or 2 divided doses Maximum recommended daily dose is 100 mg *Children:* 0.2 mg/kg/day PO initially in two divided doses Maximum recommended daily dose is 1 mg/kg	Tablets: 2.5, 10 mg	*Contraindicated* in hypersensitivity, pheochromocytoma and pulmonary hypertension Tachycardia and salt retention always occur and a potent diuretic and beta-adrenergic blocking agent are often given concurrently Reversible hirsutism occurs in many patients Periodic effusion may occur and should be monitored by echocardiography	Observe for fluid retention Monitor for signs and symptoms of pericardial effusion Monitor heart rate for tachycardia and blood pressure for orthostatic hypotension Monitor blood pressure
Nadolol Corgard Corzide*	Mild to moderate hypertension See also Chapter 24, "Sympathomimetics and Sympatholytics"	*Adults:* 80-240 mg PO; occasionally up to 320 mg PO q.d. as a single dose Dosage should be low initially and be increased gradually Dangerous to discontinue abruptly because may result in hypertensive crises, angina, or MI Decrease dosage in renal impairment	Tablets: 40, 80, 120, 160 mg	*Contraindicated* in asthma or severe chronic obstructive pulmonary disease, marked sinus bradycardia, atrioventricular block, congestive heart failure with concurrent verapamil use, and in insulin-dependent diabetic patients	Monitor respiratory function, particularly in patients with chronic bronchitis and emphysema Monitor for sinus bradycardia Monitor blood pressure

Drug	Uses	Dosage	Preparations	Comments	Nurse's Implications
				May cause CHF, AV block, or bronchospasm; Can aggravate or precipitate Raynaud's phenomenon	
Nitroprusside Nipride Nitropress	Hypertensive crises	*Adults:* 0.25-10 µg/kg/min as a continuous IV infusion; *Children:* same as adults; Dosage is highly variable; Do *not* inject undiluted solution; *Elderly:* use lower doses initially; Freshly prepared, diluted solution should be administered with the aid of an infusion pump or a microdrip regulator	Injectable: 10 mg/ml; Store in dark; avoid freezing; To prepare IV solution: add 2 ampules (100 mg) to 1 L of D_5W; Dilute *only* with D_5W, and do not use same line for any other medication; Use *only* freshly prepared solution and *discard* every 4 hr or if highly discolored; Protect solution from light with opaque material such as aluminum foil	*Contraindicated* in compensatory hypertension; Cyanide poisoning can occur with prolonged use of a high dose; Patient should be closely supervised in ICU if possible	Observe for thiocyanate toxicity (e.g., blurred vision, delirium, tinnitus); Thiocyanate levels should be monitored if used longer than 48 hr; Monitor infusion site carefully because tissue irritation can occur with extravasation; Monitor blood pressure every 15-30 min (ideally with an arterial line)
Oxprenolol Slow-Trasicor Trasicor	Mild to moderate hypertension; See also Chapter 24, "Sympathomimetics and Sympatholytics"	*Adults:* 60-480 mg/day PO given in 3 divided doses; an equivalent dose of the extended-release tablet (Slow-Trasicor) can be administered q.a.m. Extended-release tablets must be swallowed whole to be effective	Tablets: 20, 40, 80 mg; Extended-release tablets: 80, 160 mg	*Contraindicated* in bronchospasm, AV block, CHF, and cardiogenic shock	Monitor for sinus bradycardia and symptoms of CHF; Monitor blood pressure
Phenoxybenzamine Dibenzyline	Pheochromocytoma (to control hypertension)	*Adults:* 20-60 mg/day PO in 2 divided doses	Capsule: 10 mg	Profound hypotension and tachycardia can occur and are managed with IV fluids and beta-adrenergic blocking agents; Postural hypotension can be a problem; Full therapeutic response may take several weeks to develop	Monitor vital signs and respiratory status; Monitor blood pressure; Observe for hypotension

Continued.

NURSING DRUG DIGEST—cont'd

Medication (trade name)	Indication	Usual dosage and administration	Dosage forms, preparation, and storage	Contraindications, cautions, and comments	Monitoring
Phentolamine Regitine Rogitine	Pheochromocytoma (to control hypertension preoperatively and during surgery)	*Adults:* 5 mg IV *or* IM, repeat as necessary to control blood pressure; *or* 50 mg PO q.4-6h. *Children:* 1 mg IV *or* IM, repeat as necessary to control blood pressure; *or* 25 mg PO q. 4-6h.	Injectable: 5 mg/ml Tablet: 50 mg For phentolamine test dissolve 5 mg in 1 ml of sterile water for injection Use solution after reconstitution; discard any unused solution	*Contraindicated* in angina, coronary artery disease, and history of MI Postural hypotension can be a problem Do *not* use epinephrine as an antidote because this may result in a further fall in blood pressure Tachycardia is common and can be controlled with beta-adrenergic blocking agents	Monitor blood pressure and heart rate
Pindolol Visken	Mild to moderate hypertension See also Chapter 24, "Sympathomimetics and Sympatholytics"	*Adults:* 10-60 mg/day PO given in two or three divided doses with meals Dosage should be low initially and increased gradually Dangerous to discontinue abruptly because may result in angina or MI May need to decrease dose in hepatic impairment	Tablets: 5, 10, 15 mg	*Contraindicated* in marked sinus bradycardia or AV block, CHF, with concurrent verapamil use, and in insulin-dependent diabetic patients Asthma and severe chronic obstructive pulmonary disease are also *contraindications* to use, but pindolol is less of a problem than some beta-adrenergic blockers Can aggravate or precipitate Raynaud's phenomenon	Observe for sinus bradycardia and symptoms of CHF Monitor for aggravation of CHF, diabetes, hyperthyroidism, and asthma
Prazosin Hypovase Minipress Minizide*	Mild to moderate hypertension	*Adults:* 0.5-1 mg PO b.i.d. or t.i.d. gradually increasing to a total daily dose of 20 mg; occasionally up to 40 mg Dosage should be low initially and be increased only gradually Give first dose at bedtime immediately before retiring	Capsules: 0.5, 1, 2, 5 mg	Several interactions with other drugs have been reported as isolated cases thus far Postural hypotension or syncope can occur, usually when the drug is being started or when dosage is increased	Monitor for hypotension (e.g., dizziness, palpitations, lightheadedness, syncope, headache, drowsiness, weakness, nausea) Monitor pulse and blood pressure frequently

Drug	Uses	Dosage	Dosage Forms	Cautions/Side Effects	Nursing Implications
Propranolol Avlocardyl Inderal Inderal-LA* Inderide* Novopranol Panolol	Mild to moderate hypertension See also Chapter 24, "Sympathomimetics and Sympatholytics"	*Adults:* 40-240 mg/day PO in 2 divided doses Maximum: 640 mg/day Patients on maintenance doses of 160 or 320 mg/day can be dosed *once daily* with the controlled-release capsule Dosage should be low initially and increased gradually *Dangerous* to discontinue abruptly in patients with a history of angina or if on a large dose; may cause hypertensive crisis, MI, or angina	Tablets: 10, 20, 40, 60, 80, 120 mg Capsules: 80, 120 160 mg controlled-release (Inderal-LA)	*Contraindicated* in asthma and severe chronic obstructive pulmonary disease, marked sinus bradycardia or AV block, CHF, with concurrent verapamil use, and in insulin-dependent diabetic patients Can aggravate or precipitate Raynaud's phenomenon If administered during pregnancy, may cause bradycardia and hypoglycemia in the neonate May cause CHF and bronchospasm Anorexia, nausea, and vomiting are common side effects	Monitor for bradycardia, CHF, bronchospasm, anorexia, nausea, and vomiting
Reserpine Alkarau Butiserpazide* Chloreserpine* Diupres* Diutensen-R* Ebserpine Eskaserp Geneserp Hydropres* Hydroserpine* Lemiserp Metatensin* Naquival* Rauloydin Salutensin* Sandril Serpasil Serpate Triserp Unipres* Zepine	Mild to moderate hypertension	*Adults:* 0.5-1.0 mg IM followed by 2 and 4 mg at 3-hr intervals as needed up to a total of 8 mg; if this regimen fails, use other agents; *or* 0.5 mg/day PO for 1 week, then 0.1-0.25 mg/day, occasionally up to 1.0 mg/day usually in 2 or 3 divided doses Administration as single dose can often reduce flushing and nasal congestion Administer with food or milk to decrease GI irritation *Elderly:* Use lower dosage NOTE: Parenteral form is used *only* to treat hypertensive emergencies (crises)	Injectable: 2.5 mg/ml Tablets: 0.1, 0.25 mg	*Contraindicated* in mental depression, particularly if patient is suicidal, and in active peptic ulcer disease Chronic use of this drug has been associated with breast cancer but causality is not established Parenteral IM form is often erratically absorbed Administration with alcohol may cause excessive hypotension	Observe for early signs of depression (e.g., nightmares, personality changes) Monitor for nasal stuffiness and lethargy

Continued.

NURSING DRUG DIGEST—cont'd

Medication (trade name)	Indication	Usual dosage and administration	Dosage forms, preparation, and storage	Contraindications, cautions, and comments	Monitoring
Timolol Betim Blocadren Temserin Timcacor Timolide*	Mild to moderate hypertension See also Chapter 24, "Sympathomimetics and Sympatholytics"	*Adults:* 10-60 mg/day PO given in 2 divided doses Dosage should be low initially and increased gradually Dangerous to discontinue abruptly because may cause hypertensive crises, angina, or MI	Tablets: 5, 10, 20 mg	*Contraindicated* in asthma and severe chronic obstructive pulmonary disease, marked sinus bradycardia, AV block, CHF, with concurrent verapamil use, and in insulin-dependent diabetic patients Can aggravate or precipitate Raynaud's phenomenon	Monitor respiratory status because dyspnea and bronchospasm are common adverse effects Observe for bradycardia and CHF Monitor blood pressure
Trimethaphan Arfonad	Hypertensive crisis Acute dissection of aorta	*Adults:* 0.3-10 mg/min IV infusion Do *not* coadminister with any other drugs because trimethaphan solution is incompatible with a wide variety of drugs and solutions Position patient to avoid cerebral anoxia NOTE: Individual dosage and response are highly variable	Injectable: 50 mg/ml Dilute *before* administration to 0.1% concentration with D₅W	*Contraindicated* in some forms of asthma, severe anemia, severe renal or hepatic disease, advanced arteriosclerosis, and coronary disease Tachyphylaxis can develop over several hours Action of drug may be enhanced by placing patient in a reversed Trendelenburg position	Monitor blood pressure and vital signs frequently Observe for respiratory depression Observe for signs of peripheral vascular collapse

BIBLIOGRAPHY

AYM Update. Timolol. *About Your Medicines Newsletter,* 1982, *2,* 7-8.

Baughman, R.A., Arnold, S., Benet, L.Z., Lin, E.T., Chatterjee, K., & Williams, R.L. Altered prazosin pharmacokinetics in congestive heart failure. *European Journal of Clinical Pharmacology,* 1980, *17,* 425-428.

Chau, N.P., Flouvat, B.L., LeRoux, E., & Safar, M.E. Prazosin kinetics in essential hypertension. *Clinical Pharmacology and Therapeutics,* 1980, *28,* 6-11.

Cohen, M.L., Wiley, K.S., & Slater, I.H. *In vitro* relaxation of arteries and veins by prazosin: alpha-adrenergic blockade with no direct vasodilation. *Blood Vessels,* 1979, *16,* 144-154.

Davis, J.C., Reiffel, J.A., & Bigger, J.T., Jr. Sinus node dysfunction caused by methyldopa and digoxin. *Journal of the American Medical Association,* 1981, *245,* 1241-1243.

Dreyfuss, J., Griffith, D.L., Singhvi, S.M., Shaw, J.M., Ross, J.J., Jr., Vukovich, R.A., & Willard, D.A. Pharmacokinetics of nadolol, a beta-receptor antagonist: administration of therapeutic single- and multiple-dose regimens to hypertensive patients. *Journal of Clinical Pharmacology,* 1979, *19,* 712-720.

Ferguson, R.K., & Vlasses, P.H. Clinical pharmacology and therapeutic applications of the new oral angiotensin converting enzyme inhibitor, captopril. *American Heart Journal,* 1981, *101,* 650-656.

Foster, S., & Kousch, D.C. Promoting patient adherence. *American Journal of Nursing,* 1978, *78,* 829-832.

Frishman, W.H. *Clinical pharmacology of the beta-adrenoceptor blocking drugs.* New York: Appleton-Century-Crofts, 1980.

Gangnon, R.M., Morissette, M., Presant, S., Savard, D., & Lemire, J. Hemodynamic and coronary effects of intravenous labetalol in coronary artery disease. *American Journal of Cardiology,* 1982, *49,* 1267-1269.

Geyskes, G.G., Boer, P., & Mees, E.J.D. Clonidine withdrawal: mechanism and frequency of rebound hypertension. *British Journal of Clinical Pharmacology,* 1979, *7,* 55-62.

Hobbs, D.C., Twomey, T.M., & Palmer, R.F. Pharmacokinetics of prazosin in man. *Journal of Clinical Pharmacology,* 1978, *18,* 402-406.

Hutchins, L.N. Drug treatment of high blood pressure. *Nursing Clinics of North America,* 1981, *16,* 365-377.

Koch-Weser, J. Metoprolol. *New England Journal of Medicine,* 1979, *301,* 698-703.

Koch-Weser, J., & Pettinger, N. (Eds.). Symposium on prazosin. *Journal of Cardiovascular Pharmacology,* 1979, *1.*

Kornerup, H.J., Pedersen, E.B., Christensen, N.J., Pedersen, A., & Pedersen, G. Labetalol in the treatment of severe essential hypertension: relationship between arterial blood pressure, plasma catecholamines, plasma renin activity, plasma aldosterone and body weight. *Acta Medica Scandinavica,* 1979, *205* (Suppl. 625), 59-64.

Kripalani, K.J., McKinistry, D.N., Singhvi, S.M., Willard, D.A., Vukovich, R.A., & Migdalof, B.H. Disposition of captopril in normal subjects. *Clinical Pharmacology and Therapeutics,* 1980, *27,* 636-641.

Laragh, J.H. (Ed.). Hypertension symposium. *American Journal of Medicine,* 1976, *60,* 733.

Laragh, J.H. (Ed.). Hypertension symposium. *American Journal of Medicine,* 1976, *61,* 721.

Lijnen, P., Fagard, R., Staessen, J., Verschueren, L.J., & Amery, A. Dose reponse in captopril therapy of hypertension. *Clinical Pharmacology and Therapeutics,* 1980, *28,* 310-315.

Loustau, A., & Blair, B.J. A key to compliance. *Nursing 81,* 1981, *11,* 36-39.

Lowther, N.B., & Carter, V.D. How to increase compliance in hypertensives. *American Journal of Nursing,* 1981, *81,* 963.

MacCannell, K.L., & Wyse, D.G. Pharmacologic management: cardiovascular drugs. In N.K. Wenger, J.W. Hurst, & M.C. McIntyre (Eds.). *Cardiology for nurses.* New York: McGraw-Hill Book Co., 1980.

Marcinek, M.B. Hypertension—what it does to the body. *American Journal of Nursing,* 1980, *80,* 928-932.

Maruyama, A., Ogihara, T., Naka, T., Mikami, H., Hata, T., Nakamaru, M., Iwanaga, K., & Kumahara, Y. Long-term effects of captopril in hypertension. *Clinical Pharmacology and Therapeutics,* 1980, *28,* 316-323.

McKenney, J.M. Methods of modifying compliance behavior in hypertensive patients. *Drug Intelligence and Clinical Pharmacy,* 1981, *15,* 8-14.

Moser, M. Hypertension—how therapy works. *American Journal of Nursing,* 1980, *80,* 937-941.

Packer, M., Meller, J., Medina, N., Yushak, M., & Gorlin, R. Hemodynamic characterization of tolerance to long-term hydralazine therapy in severe chronic heart failure. *New England Journal of Medicine,* 1982, *306,* 57-62.

Pettinger, W. (Ed.) Symposium on minoxidil. *Cardiovascular Pharmacology,* 2: (Suppl. 2), 1980.

Rangno, R.E., Langlois, S., & Lutterodt, A. Metoprolol withdrawal phenomena: mechanism and prevention. *Clinical Pharmacology and Therapeutics,* 1982, *31,* 8-15.

Rangno, R.E., Nattel, S., & Lutterodt, A. Prevention of propranolol withdrawal mechanism by prolonged small dose propranolol schedule. *American Journal of Cardiology,* 1982, *49,* 829-833.

Roberts, R.H. (Ed.) *Theories and use of β-blockade in hypertension and angina.* Chicago: Year Book Medical Publishers, 1979.

Schoof, C.S. Hypertension—common questions patients ask. *American Journal of Nursing,* 1980, *80,* 926-927.

Sklar, J., Johnston, D., Overlie, P., Gerber, J.G., Brammell, H.L., Gal, J., & Nies, A.S. The effects of a cardioselective (metoprolol) and a nonselective (propranolol) beta-adrenergic blocker on the response to dynamic exercise in normal man. *Circulation,* 1982, *65,* 894-899.

Taylor, S.H., Silke, B., & Lee, P.S. Intravenous beta-blockade in coronary heart disease. Is cardioselectivity or intrinisic sympathomimetic activity hemodynamically useful? *New England Journal of Medicine*, 1982, *306*, 631-635.

U.S. Department of Health and Human Services. *The 1980 report of the joint national committee on detection, evaluation, and treatment of high blood pressure* (NIH Publication No. 81-1088). Washington, D.C.: U.S. Government Printing Office, 1980.

U.S. Department of Health, Education, and Welfare. *Guidelines for educating nurses in high blood pressure control* (reprint) (NIH Publication No. 80-1241). Washington, D.C.: U.S. Government Printing Office, 1980.

Vidt, D.G., Bravo, E. L., & Fouad, F.M. Captopril. *New England Journal of Medicine*, 1982, *306*, 214-219.

Ward, G.W., Bandy, P., & Fink, J.W. Treating and counseling the hypertensive patient. *American Journal of Nursing*, 1978, *78*, 824-828.

Wilber, J.A. (Ed.). Symposium on clonidine. *Journal of Cardiovascular Pharmacology*, 1980, *2* (Suppl. 1),

Vasodilators, Antilipemics, Anticoagulants, and Platelet Aggregation Inhibitors

D. George Wyse

Medications discussed in this chapter

Vasodilators
  Nitrite/nitrate vasodila-
    tors
    Amyl nitrite
    Erythrityl tetranitrate
    Isosorbide dinitrate
    Nitroglycerin
    Pentaerythritol tetrani-
      trate
    Erythrityl tetranitrate
  Miscellaneous vasodila-
    tors
    Cyclandelate
    Dipyridamole
    Isoxsuprine
    Niacin
    Nicotinyl alcohol
    Nylidrin
    Prenylamine
    Tolazoline
  Calcium channel blocker
    vasodilators
    Diltiazem
    Nifedipine
    Verapamil
Antilipemics
  Hormone and vitamin
    antilipemics
    Dextrothyroxine
    Niacin
  Ion-exchange resin antili-
    pemics

Antilipemics—cont'd
    Cholestipol
    Cholestyramine
  Metabolic antagonist an-
    tilipemics
    Clofibrate
    Probucol
Anticoagulants
  Heparin-like anticoagu-
    lants
    Heparin
  Vitamin K–antagonist an-
    ticoagulants
    Acenocoumarol
    Dicumarol
    Phenindione
    Phenprocoumon
    Warfarin
Platelet aggregation inhibi-
tors
  Prostaglandin synthesis
    and platelet aggrega-
    tion inhibitors
    Aspirin
    Sulfinpyrazone
  Other platelet aggrega-
    tion inhibitors
    Clofibrate
    Dipyridamole

In this chapter a diverse group of drugs used in a variety of cardiovascular conditions is discussed. The reader will note that several of these agents fall into more than one group. Dipyridamole is both a vaso-dilator and a platelet aggregation inhibitor, niacin is both an antilipemic and a vasodilator, and clofibrate is both an antilipemic and a platelet aggregation in-hibitor. This is an opportune moment therefore to point out again that most drugs are neither organ specific nor system specific in their effects or toxicity. Sometimes a relative selectivity can be obtained at low-er doses, but there is great individual variability. This principle must not be forgotten by those who admin-ister drugs to patients.

VASODILATORS

As implied by their name, vasodilators are agents that cause dilation of blood vessels, and as will be seen, this effect can be accomplished through a number of different mechanisms. It will be obvious that the agents discussed in Chapter 33 as "antihypertensives" could be classified as "vasodilators" under such a broad definition. However, because these particular vasodilators find their major use in the treatment of hypertension and because they form such a large group of drugs, they are placed in a separate chapter. The calcium channel blockers (e.g., verapamil, nifed-ipine, and diltiazem) are also vasodilators, but are dis-cussed with the antidysrhythmics in Chapter 32. There remains the nitrite/nitrate group and a miscel-laneous group of vasodilators that are discussed in this chapter. Additional information concerning the calcium channel blockers is considered together with the miscellaneous group of vasodilators.

Chemistry

The nitrite/nitrate group of vasodilators is probably among the oldest group of drugs used for their va-sodilator effect. The pharmacologic property of vaso-dilation is thought to be the result of the nitrite ion, and it is generally accepted that only those nitrates that can be converted to nitrite in vivo are useful va-sodilators. This reaction depends on sulfhydryl groups that may form an intimate part of the "nitrite" receptor, and the depletion of sulfhydryl groups may be partly responsible for the tolerance that can develop to these agents. There are no particular distinguishing chemical features of the miscellaneous group of vasodilators.

Mechanism of action and pharmacologic effects

The basic pharmacologic action of the nitrites is the relaxation of smooth muscle, the consequence of which is vasodilation. The effect, however, is not specific for vascular smooth muscle, and smooth muscle elsewhere, such as the biliary tree and ureters, is also relaxed. The effect on the vasculature is not homogeneous. In general, venodilation is more prominent than arterial dilation and, on the arterial side, large arteries are dilated more than small arteries and arterioles. In addition, certain vascular beds appear to be more susceptible to the effects of the nitrites/nitrates. The cutaneous vessels in the "blush zone" (i.e., meningeal, splanchnic, pulmonary, and coronary beds) appear to be among those affected most by the nitrites/nitrates.

The preponderance of effects on the veins is one of the reasons that hypotension with these agents is usually postural, and the predilection for the meningeal bed is the explanation for the side effect of headache. Blood pressure, even in the supine position, can fall because of the effects of these agents. There are no direct effects on the heart, but vasodilation and a fall in the filling pressure of the heart (i.e., *preload*) can cause a reflex tachycardia.

The effects on cardiac output will depend on the "loading" conditions of the heart and reflexes activated by a fall in pressures. Most commonly, the cardiac output increases because of a reduction of *afterload* and reflex sympathetic stimulation. Reduction of preload may also contribute to an increase in cardiac output if it is increased beyond the optimum (i.e., marked elevated left ventricular end-diastolic pressure) (see Figure 31-1).

However, an excessive lowering of preload, if it is greater than the offsetting reduction of afterload, can lead to a fall in cardiac output. In the absence of other measures or changes, the effect of nitrites/nitrates on cardiac output is transient.

In congestive heart failure (CHF), when there is a tachycardia, administration of the nitrite/nitrates can *lower* the heart rate if the drug improves forward cardiac output and lessens CHF. Nitrite/nitrates are devoid of action in organs without smooth muscle. An abnormal spasm in any hollow viscus containing smooth muscle within its walls (e.g., biliary tree, ureters, esophagus) can be relieved by the nitrites/nitrates.

Miscellaneous vasodilators

The miscellaneous vasodilators act through several different mechanisms. Cyclandelate, dipyridamole, niacin, and prenylamine are nonspecific vasodilators (i.e., they relax vascular smooth muscle via mechanisms not involving any interference with autonomic nervous system functions or activation or blockade of receptors for known *neurohumors*).

Dipyridamole inhibits the enzyme phosphodiesterase and thus interferes with the breakdown of adenosine and adenine nucleotides, which are smooth muscle relaxants. The effects of this agent seem to be more prominent in the small arteries and arterioles, and there is a fall in blood pressure coupled with an increase in the heart rate and the cardiac output.

Cyclandelate and niacin are weak vasodilators similar to dipyridamole in effects, although their pharmacologic mechanism is unclear. Niacin has a particularly prominent effect in the cutaneous vessels of the blush area. In fact, little evidence exists that niacin causes vasodilation outside of the cutaneous vascular bed. How prenylamine works is not established but is thought by some to be a calcium channel blocker.

Isoxsuprine and nylidrin, on the other hand, are drugs that seem to be beta-adrenergic agonists and thus cause vasodilation, primarily in the skeletal muscle vascular beds, and cardiac stimulation through the activation of beta-adrenergic receptors. Cardiac stimulation results in both an increase in the rate and the force of the contraction of the heart. The effects of these agents, however, are somewhat resistant to blockade by propranolol.

Tolazoline is an alpha-adrenergic blocking agent that is similar to phentolamine but is a weaker agent in this regard. Like phentolamine, it has some nonspecific vasodilator properties. Tolazoline causes both vasodilation and cardiac stimulation (rate and force increases), and the net effect on blood pressure depends on which effect predominates.

The calcium channel blockers (e.g., diltiazem, nifedipine, verapamil) dilate both coronary arteries and peripheral arterioles. Diltiazem causes less peripheral vasodilation than does nifedipine. All of the calcium channel blockers diminish cardiac contractility. In this regard verapamil has the greatest activity.

Pharmacokinetics

The nitrites/nitrates can be absorbed by a variety of routes. Amyl nitrite, which is a volatile liquid, is rapidly absorbed through the mucosa of the nasopharynx and the lungs. All of the organic nitrates are readily absorbed via the sublingual or buccal mucosa, as well as directly through the skin. Nitroglycerin is the only agent currently given via the transdermal route. A number of different pharmaceutical formulations have been devised to use the transdermal route. The oldest is a 2% ointment that is applied to the skin. More recently several products have been marketed that contain nitroglycerin in a bandagelike patch to be applied to the skin. These patches come in several different strengths and are generally more convenient than the ointment. The organic nitrates are readily absorbed from the GI tract, but there is a substantial first-pass effect, and much larger amounts must be administered via this route to have an effect.

Although it is thought that conversion to nitrite is necessary for nitrates to be active, there is no substantial delay in the onset of the effects of nitrates given intravenously. Nitroglycerin can in fact be given intravenously, and intravenous infusion has recently become a popular route of administration in certain conditions where a rapid and controlled effect is needed. It is difficult to detect the parent compounds in the blood, and little in the way of active metabolites can be detected. These observations suggest that a rapid conversion takes place at the site of action (i.e., the receptor) and that the active compounds are then rapidly denitrated and become inactive. The inactive metabolites are usually mononitrates or dinitrates that are excreted in the urine.

The duration of action of any agent primarily depends on the route of administration. Intravenous nitroglycerin has an immediate effect that wanes over a few minutes when it is discontinued. Given by the sublingual route, the effects last ½ to 1½ hours. Larger doses administered via the oral route or as a topical application to the skin can act as a reservoir for continued absorption, and effects may be typically seen for 4 or 5 hours. A newer transdermal delivery system for nitroglycerin provides effective concentrations for 24 hours. It should be noted that the transdermal route results in stable blood levels, but effects wane anyway, and in this instance tolerance can be a problem.

Tolerance to the use of these agents is almost invariable, and cross-tolerance also occurs. Therapeutically, however, this seems to be of little consequence (except for transdermal) and perhaps even of some benefit, because in many patients the headache caused by meningeal vasodilation tends to wane with time. A withdrawal rebound effect may occur, however, and this is an important factor for workers continuously exposed to organic nitrates in their work.

Except for the calcium channel blockers, there is little noteworthy about the pharmacokinetics of the miscellaneous vasodilators. All of these agents are effective by the oral route and have a reasonably long duration of action.

The calcium channel blockers are all well absorbed following oral administration (i.e., greater than 90%). However, because of the first-pass effect a significant amount of both diltiazem and verapamil (i.e., 60% to 75%) is rapidly metabolized during the first pass through the liver. Thus, the bioavailability (see Chapter 4, "Drug Availability and Distribution") of these two agents is only 20% to 30%. The bioavailability of nifedipine is significantly higher at approximately 65%. All of these agents are highly protein bound (i.e., 80% to 90%) and all are extensively metabolized in the liver. Less than 5% of the administered dose of the calcium channel blockers is excreted unchanged in the urine. The half-life of elimination for these agents ranges from 4 to 10 hours. When administered intravenously, verapamil has an onset of action of less than 3 minutes.

Uses

The nitrates are mostly used in treating angina pectoris and in alterating loading conditions of the left ventricle (in selected cases of left ventricular failure or low cardiac output). Intravenous nitroglycerin is being used increasingly in acute myocardial infarction and unstable angina to obtain rapid and controlled relief of pain. It is also used in these two conditions and following myocardial infarction to lower elevated blood pressure. Nitrates are given to terminate an attack of angina (the major use for sublingual nitroglycerin), or they can be given prophylactically to reduce the frequency of attacks. Angina can be averted by taking sublingual nitroglycerin or isosorbide dinitrate just before physical exertion, which usually provokes chest pain (this can be viewed as a short-term prophylaxis). Alternatively, topical nitroglycerin or oral isosorbide dinitrate or pentaerythritol tetranitrate can be given on a regular basis around the clock as a long-term prophylaxis.

The exact mechanism by which nitrates relieve the pain of myocardial ischemia is unclear. It is not simply the result of vasodilation because agents such as dipyridamole cause a much greater decrease in coronary vascular resistance and yet are not particularly effective against angina. There may in fact be several contributing mechanisms, including (1) a reduction of preload, thereby decreasing wall tension (a major determinant of myocardial oxygen need), (2) sustained and selective dilation of large coronary arteries, or (3) a promotion of the flow through the collateral vessels.

The nitrates are particularly useful in angina pectoris, which has a vasospastic component. The effect of lowering the preload through venodilation and blood pooling is also useful in some forms of CHF or low cardiac output. Nitrites/nitrates also cause a slight reduction in afterload, but usually another dilator is used concurrently to achieve a greater reduction of afterload. The objective is to achieve a left ventricular filling pressure (left ventricular end-diastolic pressure) that will optimize the cardiac output and minimize the pulmonary congestion.

Nitrates are sporadically used for other conditions when vasodilation or relaxation of other types of smooth muscle is required. For example, topical nitrates have been used to treat *Raynaud's phenomenon.*

One of the side effects of excessive nitrate use is a reduction of hemoglobin to *methemoglobin,* and in cyanide poisoning this can be a useful effect because cyanide is preferentially bound to methemoglobin, leaving regular hemoglobin free for oxygen transport.

The miscellaneous vasodilators are promoted for a wide variety of conditions of reduced blood flow such as *intermittent claudication,* reduced cerebrovascular flow in elderly patients, angina, and Raynaud's phenomenon. There would seem to be little rationale for such use in the presence of fixed obstructive lesions caused by atherosclerosis. If the etiologic factor is vasospasm, the rationale would be more secure. Few studies have carefully differentiated between these conditions on an etiologic basis, and therapeutic benefits have not been clearly demonstrated. Dipyridamole has some use as a platelet aggregation inhibitor. This is discussed later in the chapter. Tolazoline finds a limited and specialized use as a pulmonary vasodilator in treating persistent fetal circulation in the newborn.

The calcium channel blockers are being used and examined for treating a variety of conditions. All of the calcium channel blockers (e.g., diltiazem, nifedipine, verapamil) have been approved for treating angina, particularly vasospastic angina. Verapamil has been approved for paroxysmal supraventricular tachycardias (PSVT) (see Chapter 32, "Antidysrhythmics"). All of these agents are under study and have produced encouraging results in treating hypertension. Because this is a relatively new class of medications, only future study and use will determine the extent of use and success that the calcium channel blockers have in treating any of the various conditions.

Adverse effects and toxicity

The adverse effects of the nitrites/nitrates are almost entirely related to their major therapeutic effect on the cardiovascular system (i.e., vasodilation). One of the most common of these is headache, which can be severe. Commonly patients will develop tolerance to the headache, but some patients will be unable to take nitrites/nitrates because of this problem. It can be managed by reducing the dosage or starting with a very low dose and gradually increasing the dosage or by administering standard analgesic agents.

Postural hypotension can be a problem, particularly in elderly patients and in those patients concurrently taking beta-adrenergic blocking agents, which can blunt the compensatory reflexes. Excessive lowering of the blood pressure, particularly if coupled with a tachycardia, can be an unfavorable change in the balance between myocardial oxygen supply and demand and thus the nitrites/nitrates can sometimes cause a seemingly paradoxic worsening of the angina.

It is a common belief that these agents increase intraocular pressure, and it is frequently stated that glaucoma is a contraindication to their use, but there is little evidence to support such a notion. As with most drugs, the organic nitrates can cause skin rashes, but this is not common. Isosorbide dinitrate can cause a peculiar drug rash that occurs only on those parts of the body exposed to sunlight. Exfoliative dermatitis may also rarely occur with the use of isosorbide dinitrate. In excessive amounts the nitrites/nitrates can cause the formation of significant amounts of methemoglobin.

The miscellaneous vasodilators cause a variety of adverse effects. As with all oral agents, they can cause several types of GI distress (e.g., nausea, vomiting, diarrhea). They can also cause side to effects related to vasodilation such as flushing, headache, tachycardia, and postural hypotension.

Niacin is particularly likely to cause a flushing of the blush area and pruritus in the upper half of the body. Niacin, when used in large doses, has also been reported to decrease glucose tolerance, activate peptic ulcers, cause toxic amblyopia, and result in liver dysfunction. Skin rashes (e.g., increased pigmentation, pruritus, keratosis) have also been reported.

The adverse effects and toxicity observed with the calcium channel blockers have, for the most part, been associated with their pharmacologic effect. Signs and symptoms of peripheral vasodilation, which have been reported, include dizziness, headache, hypotension, flushing, and tachycardia. Bradycardia and heart block can also occur. Life-threatening reactions have been observed (e.g., asystole) in patients (less than 1%) receiving IV verapamil. Most of these patients had been receiving concomitant beta-adrenergic blockers (e.g., propranolol) also by the IV route. Using IV verapamil is contraindicated in these circumstances. Whenever verapamil is to be administered intravenously, monitoring and resuscitation equipment, including DC-cardioversion, should be immediately available.

Drug interactions

All agents in this group can interact with one another and with the antihypertensive agents to cause excessive falls in the blood pressure through additive effects. Dipyridamole can interact with the anticoagulants to promote bleeding because of its platelet aggregation inhibiting properties.

ANTILIPEMICS

The antilipemics are used to treat various types of elevation in blood lipids. The major lipids of concern are cholesterol and triglycerides. The metabolism of these fats is complex (Figure 34-1). A brief review of the classification scheme for the hyperlipidemias (Table 34-1) will assist in understanding the use and mechanism of action of the antilipemics. One of the importances of lipid metabolism is that some of these disorders are a predisposing factor in the development of accelerated and premature atherosclerosis.

Mechanism of action and pharmacologic effects

Niacin (nicotinic acid) appears to act by decreasing the synthesis of *very low density lipoproteins (VLDLs)* in the liver, and thus triglyceride levels fall. The fall in VLDL in turn causes a fall in *low density lipoproteins (LDLs)* and cholesterol. Niacin also inhibits lipolysis in fatty tissue. The effect of niacin therefore is to cause a fall in both triglycerides and cholesterol.

Dextrothyroxine apparently acts through the stimulation of liver metabolism and the breakdown of cholesterol with the excretion of the bile salt breakdown products in the bile and feces. Dextrothyroxine does not affect cholesterol synthesis. Thus dextrothyroxine causes a fall primarily in the level of cholesterol in the blood.

Cholestyramine and colestipol have virtually identical mechanisms of action and effects. They are both ion-exchange resins that are not absorbed when taken orally and thus remain within the GI tract. There they bind the bile salts that are breakdown products of

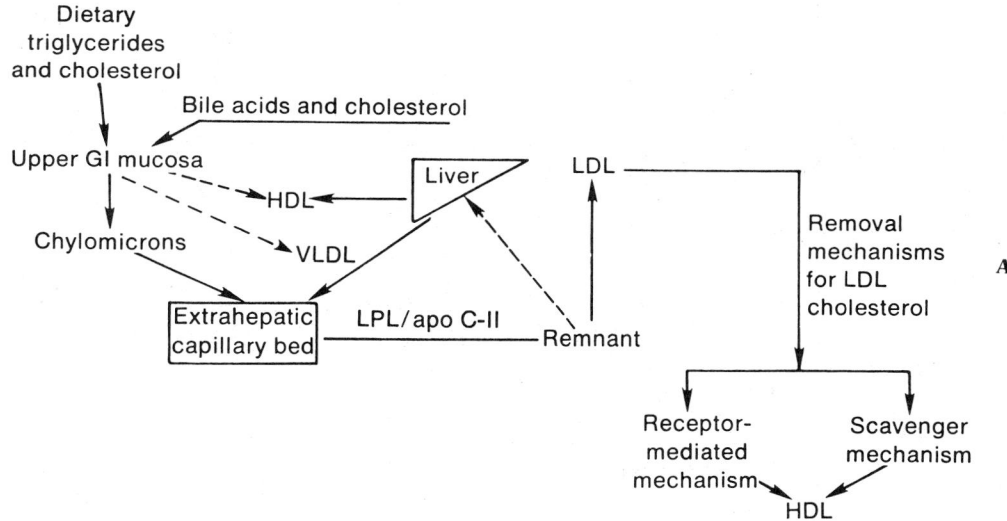

FIGURE 34-1. **A. Formation and degradation of plasma lipoproteins. After the ingestion of triglycerides and cholesterol from the diet, bile acids, biliary cholesterol, and pancreatic lipase enter the upper intestinal lumen. Chylomicrons and to a lesser extent VLDL and HDL are also produced by upper intestinal mucosal cells. VLDL and HDL are synthesized and secreted into the bloodstream by the liver as their quantitatively major source. Triglycerides of chylomicrons and VLDL are removed in extrahepatic capillary beds, mainly of adipose tissues and muscle, after hydrolysis by LPL, activated by its apo C-II cofactor. The triglyceride-depleted remnants thereby formed are then further metabolized to LDL by lipolytic and remodeling processes that may involve both LPL and hepatic triglyceride lipase. Extrahepatic tissues remove and catabolize LDL as a source of cholesterol both by a specific, receptor-mediated, endocytotic, high-affinity uptake process and by a nonspecific, low-affinity, scavenger mechanism. It is speculated that HDL and LCAT subsequently remove cellular cholesterol from extrahepatic tissues and return sterol to the liver for excretion. (A from Kaye, D., & Rose, L. Fundamentals of internal medicine. St. Louis: The C. V. Mosby Co., 1983.)**

Continued.

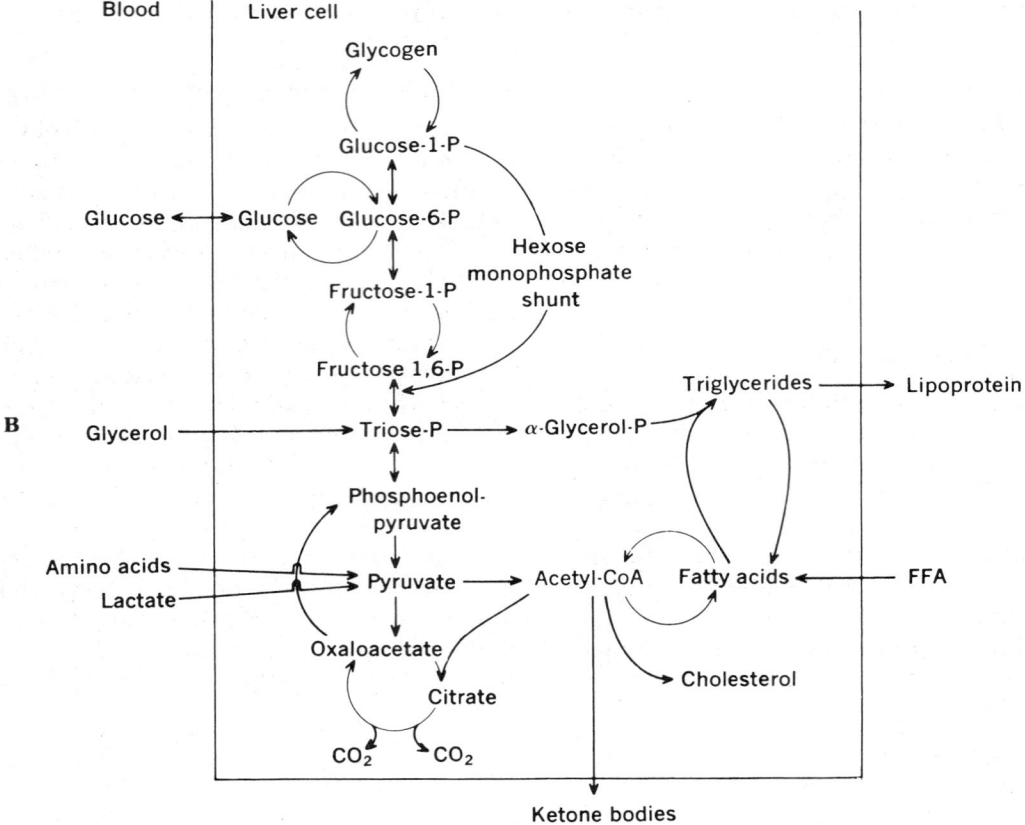

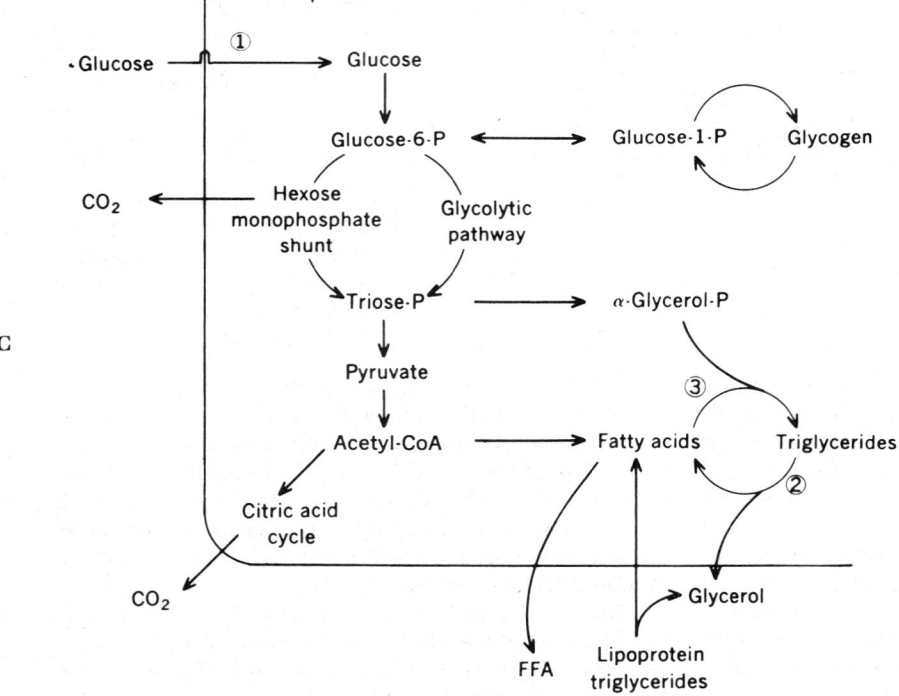

FIGURE 34-1, cont'd. *B,* Schematic representation of carbohydrate and lipid metabolism in liver. *C,* Schematic representation of carbohydrate and lipid metabolism in adipose tissue. Important rate-limiting reactions controlling fatty acid production are, 1, transport of glucose into adipose cell, 2, cleavage of triglyceride into fatty acids and glycerol, and 3, fatty acid esterification. (*B* and *C* from Mountcastle, V. *Medical physiology.* St. Louis: The C. V. Mosby Co., 1980.)

TABLE 34-1

Summary of types of primary lipoproteinemias

Type	Name	Incidence	Lipids elevated	Lipoproteins elevated	Premature coronary artery disease association	Appearance of plasma after exposure to cold*	General treatment
I	Fat induced (exogenous) hyperlipidemia	Rare	Triglycerides	Chylomicrons	No	Creamy supernatant and clear infranatant	Low fat diet; Treatment of underlying condition (e.g., diabetes, hypothyroidism); Substitution of unsaturated fats in diet
IIa	Familial (sporadic) hypercholesterolemia	Common	Cholesterol	LDL	Yes	Clear	Drug therapy (see text); Substitution of unsaturated fats in diet
IIb	Combined hyperlipoproteinemia	Common	Cholesterol Triglycerides	LDL VLDL	Yes	Turbid	Drug therapy (see text); Weight reduction; Reduced carbohydrates
III	Broad beta disease	Uncommon	Cholesterol Triglycerides	"Abnormal" IDL	Yes	Slightly creamy supernatant and turbid infranatant	Drug therapy (see text); Weight reduction; Reduced carbohydrates
IV	Endogenous (carbohydrate induced) hypertriglyceridemia	Common	Triglycerides	VLDL	No/Yes	Turbid	Drug therapy (see text); Weight reduction; Reduced carbohydrates
V	Mixed hyperlipidemia (types I & IV)	Uncommon	Triglycerides	Chylomicrons VLDL	No/Yes	Creamy supernatant and turbid infranatant	Drug therapy (see text)

IDL, Intermediate density lipoproteins; LDL, Low density lipoproteins; VLDL, Very low density lipoproteins; Chylomicrons, *Exogenous* triglyceride concentration.
*Stand upright in refrigerator overnight (i.e., 12 hours at 4° C).

cholesterol. This prevents bile salt reabsorption and thus interrupts the enterohepatic circulation and leads to the excretion of greater amounts of bile salts. This in turn leads to further catabolism of cholesterol to form bile salts. There may also be an increase in cholesterol synthesis, but this does not usually overcome the effect of increased catabolism. These two agents will therefore primarily lower the level of cholesterol in the blood.

Clofibrate acts by inhibiting the production or release of VLDL by the liver. This effect is manifested by a decrease in plasma triglyceride levels. Clofibrate is much less effective in reducing LDL and cholesterol levels, although it does have some effect on these substances. Its action is not the result of clofibrate itself but of a metabolite called clofibric acid.

Probucol is a newer agent that appears to be structurally and mechanistically different from all of the other agents. Its major effect is to lower total cholesterol by lowering all subfractions (VLDL, LDL, and HDL). At present it is unclear exactly how the drug accomplishes this effect. It would seem to act by inhibiting lipoprotein formation or the intestinal mucosal transport of cholesterol. Lowering HDL cholesterol levels may not be a desireable effect because high levels of HDL cholesterol have a *negative* correlation with coronary heart disease. Gemfibrozil lowers VLDL and LDL cholesterol and triglycerides and may in fact raise HDL cholesterol. The latter effect, if confirmed by further studies, would be unique. The mechanism of action of gemfibrozil is unknown at present.

Pharmacokinetics

Niacin is readily absorbed after oral administration, even though very large amounts are given, and reaches a peak level in ½ to 1 hour. A fall in triglyceride level is not seen for 4 to 6 hours, although the elimination of niacin is rapid, with a half-life of about 45 minutes. There seems to be an avid uptake of niacin into the liver and this, plus the fact that some time is required to use the VLDL already synthesized, explains the delayed effect and the prolonged action. About one third of an orally administered dose of niacin is excreted unchanged in the urine.

Oral absorption of dextrothyroxine is incomplete and variable, particularly when given with food, and therefore the drug should be taken before meals. Over 99% of what is absorbed is protein bound, primarily to specific thyroid-binding proteins.

Thyroxine has a half-life of 6 or 7 days in healthy humans. Therefore the effects of this drug begin slowly and dissipate slowly. The drug is metabolized to thyroacetic acid and thyronine, which are conjugated to glucuronide or sulfate and excreted in the urine.

The ion-exchange resins, cholestyramine and colestipol, have no pharmacokinetics to speak of because these agents are insoluble and are not absorbed from the GI tract.

Little is known about the pharmacokinetics of probucol. Absorption appears to be limited (i.e., less than 7%) and variable. The onset of effect is slow, and a steady state is not reached for 3 or 4 months. It appears that probucol may be sequestered somewhere in the body (most likely in adipose tissue) because it disappears only very slowly from the plasma when the drug is discontinued, and over 1 month is required for halving the plasma level.

Clofibrate is hydrolyzed to clofibric acid either in the gut lumen during absorption or on its first passage through the liver and, as mentioned previously, clofibric acid is the active form of the drug. Absorption is slow but complete, and peak plasma levels of clofibric acid are seen 2 to 6 hours after an oral dose. Most of the clofibric acid appears to remain in the vascular space because the apparent volume of distribution is only 0.13 L/kg. Approximately 90% of the plasma clofibric acid level achieved with the usual dose is protein bound. The binding sites appear to be saturable, however, because a lower percentage is protein bound as the total plasma level rises. There is a marked variability among patients in the elimination of clofibric acid, with half-lives that vary from 6 to 25 hours. Renal elimination is the major route of excretion, but only 10% is unchanged. The dose of clofibrate must be reduced if there is impaired renal function. Gemfibrozil is apparently well absorbed and reaches its peak blood levels in 1 to 2 hours. Most of the drug is excreted unchanged in the urine (approximately 70%).

Uses

The various *hyperlipidemias* are either primary or secondary and regardless of type they can cause problems in their own right, such as abdominal pain, neuropathies, and *xanthomas* (Table 34-1). However, one of the major reasons for treating these conditions is that some are felt to be factors that predispose patients to premature atherosclerosis. Of the five major types of hyperlipidemia, *only* type I can be clearly stated *not* to be a factor contributing to premature atherosclerosis. Type IV and type V probably are relatively weak contributing factors, and the connection is most clear for types II and III.

In spite of this clear relationship between some forms of hyperlipidemia and atherosclerosis, there is considerable controversy about whether a reduction of an elevated lipid level changes the prognosis with respect to developing atherosclerosis. A moderate view would be that some benefit is to be expected from lowering lipid levels in those patients who are clearly in a very high risk group, such as those with the familial form of type II.

Diet is an integral part in treating all hyperlipidemias, and drugs are used to augment dietary changes. The correct approach to diet therapy involves both restricting total calorie intake and adjusting diet composition, paying particular attention to carbohydrate, cholesterol, and fat content.

The mechanism of action of the various drugs will be a major determinant in their use in the various types of hyperlipidemia. Drugs that act by different mechanisms can be combined to have an additive effect. Niacin can be used in almost all instances (except type I) because it decreases the levels of both VLDL and LDL. Dextrothyroxine is used only for type II, and because of numerous side effects its use is limited to young and otherwise healthy patients. The ion-exchange resins (e.g., cholestyramine and colestipol) are used for type II hypercholesterolemia. Clofibrate primarily affects VLDL and triglycerides and therefore is used in types IIb, III, and IV. Gemfibrozil has uses similar to clofibrate although it is primarily indicated as adjunctive treatment for type IV hyperlipidemia. Probucol is used only for type II at present, but this is still a relatively new agent and the full extent of its effects and usefulness remains unknown.

Adverse effects and toxicity

The adverse effects of niacin are discussed with the vasodilators earlier in this chapter and appear to be largely the result of vasodilation. There are, however, some less common, but more worrisome, side effects from niacin, including decreased glucose tolerance, activation of peptic ulcer, abnormalities of liver function, and toxic amblyopia.

The adverse effects of dextrothyroxine are a major factor in limiting its usefulness. These effects are basically the effects of excess thyroid hormone (see Chapter 61, "Thyroid and Antithyroid Medications"). Problems seemingly similar to those of hyperthyroidism include insomnia, nervousness, palpitations, weight loss, tremors, flushing, and heat intolerance. There can be a considerable increase in the frequency of angina in patients with coronary artery disease who take dextrothyroxine. In addition, a number of patients may have supraventricular tachydysrhythmias, such as atrial fibrillation.

The adverse effects of the ion-exchange resins (e.g., cholestyramine and colestipol) are largely confined to the GI tract. Nausea, vomiting, and abdominal discomfort are fairly common. Constipation is also common and in elderly patients this can progress to obstipation

and fecal impaction. Diarrhea is less common, and with higher doses steatorrhea can occur.

The usual GI complaints of nausea, vomiting, abdominal discomfort, and diarrhea also occur with clofibrate use. Less commonly clofibrate causes a multiplicity of side effects in several other systems. Myositis, gallstones, liver dysfunction, and ventricular ectopy are among the more common side effects.

Probucol is such a new agent that the full range of its side effects remains to be defined. Diarrhea seems to be the most common side effect of probucol, occuring in about 10% of patients. Flatulence, abdominal pain, nausea, and vomiting have also been reported. Less common adverse effects include angioneurotic edema, fetid sweat, and hyperhidrosis; these effects occur in less than 0.5% of patients treated.

Drug interactions

There are some important drug interactions in this group of agents (see Clinically Significant Drug Interactions). Dextrothyroxine is a physiologic antagonist of insulin and thus can diminish the hypoglycemic effects of insulin and the oral hypoglycemic agents. This drug can also increase the anticoagulant effect of the vitamin K antagonists by an unknown mechanism.

The ion-exchange resins can bind a number of drugs and thus decrease their absorption and desired effects. Drugs that can be significantly affected in this fashion include digoxin, thyroid hormone, and the oral anticoagulants.

Clofibrate also interacts with the oral anticoagulants, but *increases* their effects by displacement from protein binding sites. By a similar mechanism, clofibrate can cause augmentation of the hypoglycemic effects of the oral hypoglycemic agents. The effect of clofibrate is blunted by the oral contraceptives via an unknown mechanism. Gemfibrozil can also increase the effects of oral anticoagulants. Although they probably have different mechanisms of action, clofibrate and probucol should not be used together because this combination *causes* hypertriglyceridemia.

ANTICOAGULANTS

The cascading systems involved in the coagulation of the blood are reviewed in Figure 34-2. Heparin is a naturally occurring substance found within mast cells and thus can be isolated from those organs that contain an abundance of such cells (e.g., liver and lung). There has been much discussion over the years about the physiologic function of heparin, but there is no convincing evidence of what it might be. The initial discovery of the oral anticoagulants is an interesting

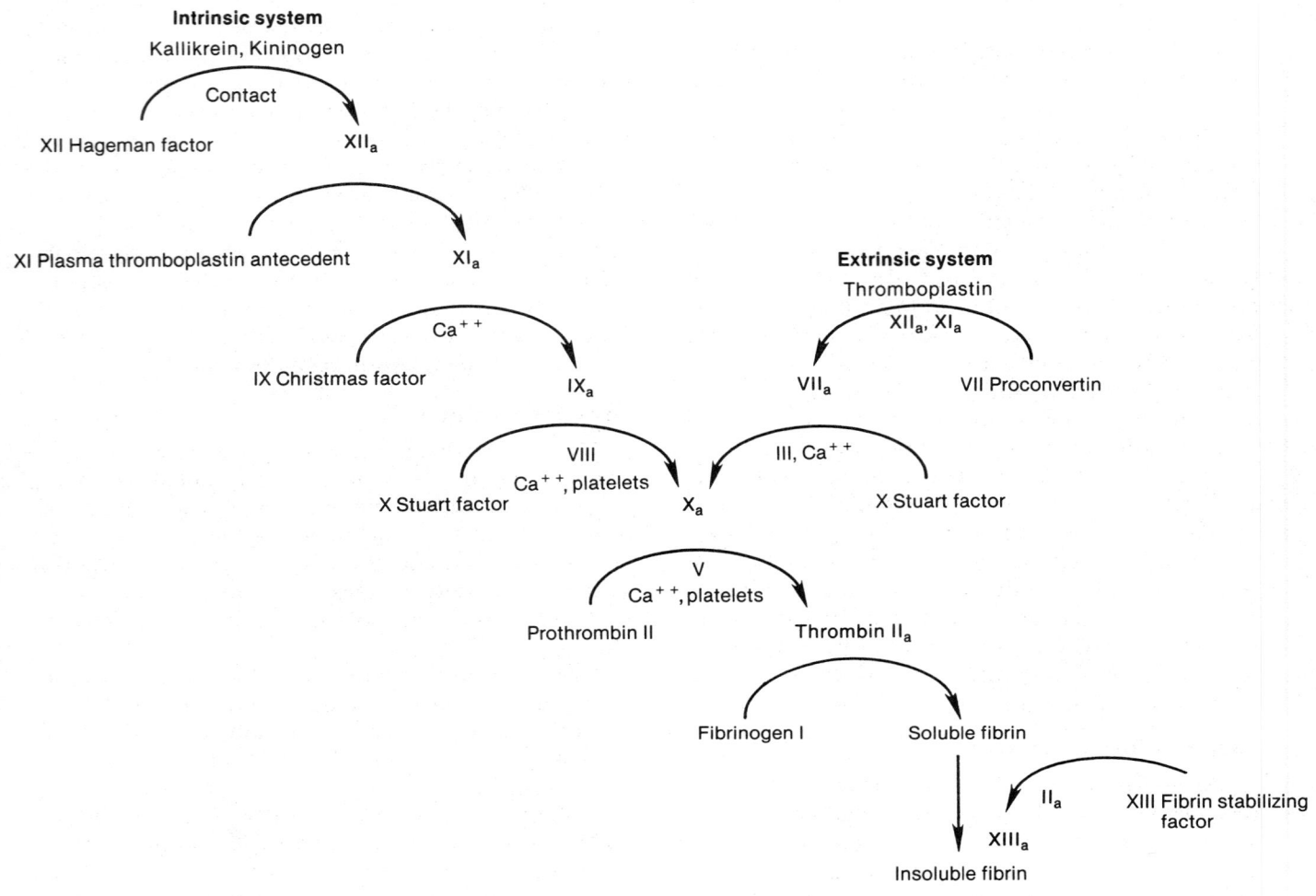

Blood Clotting Factors

Factor I	Fibrinogen.
Factor II	Prothrombin.
Factor III	Tissue thromboplastin.
Factor IV	Calcium.
Factor V	Proaccelerin; labile factor; accelerator globulin.
Factor VI	No longer recognized as a clotting factor.
Factor VII	Proconvertin; stable factor: serum prothrombin conversion accelerator (SPCA).
Factor VIII	Antihemophilic factor (AHF): antihemophilic globulin (AHG).
Factor IX	Plasma thromboplastin component (PTC): Christmas factor.
Factor X	Stuart-Prower factor.
Factor XI	Plasma thromboplastin antecedent (PTA).
Factor XII	Hageman factor.
Factor XIII	Fibrin-stabilizing factor.

FIGURE 34-2. **Simplified schema of intrinsic and extrinsic systems of blood coagulation. Subscript "a" refers to activated form.**

anecdote. In the early part of this century "sweet clover disease" of cattle was a severe bleeding disorder that occurred in cattle who ate spoiled sweet clover hay. In 1934 the disease was proved to be caused by the oral anticoagulant dicumarol, which was formed during spoilage of sweet clover hay. Thrombolysis (as opposed to anticoagulation) is a treatment that actually dissolves (lyses) clot rather than preventing its formation. Several enzymes can be used for this purpose; those currently in use are urokinase and streptokinase. These agents are infused in certain life-threatening circumstances such as pulmonary embolus and, experimentally at least, in acute myocardial infarction. Agents for thrombolysis are not discussed in this chapter (see Chapter 71).

Chemistry

Heparin is a mucopolysaccharide composed of many subunits of sulfated D-glucosamine and D-glucuronic acid. Heparin's molecular weight is somewhere between 6000 and 20,000, and it is the strongest organic acid occurring within the body. The anticoagulant effect of heparin is related to the sulfuric acid content and the conformation of the molecule; when these are altered, activity is lost.

The oral anticoagulants, although numerous, have only two simple structural forms. They are derivatives of either 4-hydroxycoumarin or indan-1,3-dione. Although these are structurally simple compounds, it has proved to be a difficult task to elucidate the portion of these molecules that is essential for anticoagulant activity.

Mechanism of action and pharmacologic effects

The anticoagulant effect of heparin requires a plasma alpha-globulin referred to as the heparin cofactor, which appears to be identical to antithrombin III. The drug does not block the synthesis of prothrombin or other clotting factors. The anionic groups of heparin appear to attach to each of the activated factors IX, X, XI, and XII, and thrombin, and facilitate their interaction with antithrombin III, which inhibits the normal physiologic function of these factors. A much smaller amount of heparin is needed to inactivate the first four factors mentioned and this is probably the primary anticoagulant effect of heparin. The net result is that coagulation is inhibited because of an inhibition of the conversion of prothrombin to thrombin. Heparin also inhibits platelet aggregation to a limited degree.

Lipoprotein lipase is activated by heparin and thus the drug can accelerate the clearing of chylomicrons from the plasma, but there appears to be little therapeutic usefulness in this effect. Because of its mechanism of action, heparin will inhibit coagulation both in vitro and in vivo. The oral anticoagulants will only inhibit coagulation in vivo; this is because their mechanism of action is to inhibit the synthesis of those coagulation factors that require vitamin K. The site of action is the liver, and the factors whose formation is inhibited are II, VII, IX, and X. The inhibition is competitive and can be overcome by administering high doses of vitamin K. Thus, vitamin K_1 (phytonadione) is used as an antidote for an overdose of the oral anticoagulants.

Pharmacokinetics

Heparin is not effective when given by the oral or sublingual routes; it must be given parenterally. There is marked variability in patient sensitivity to heparin, and each patient's dose must be adjusted individually. The variability is related to body weight, gender, duration from onset of symptoms to treatment, and smoking history, but the reasons for this are unclear. The subcutaneous, intramuscular, and intravenous routes have all been used, but for the full anticoagulation effect, the intravenous route is best. When administered intramuscularly, heparin can cause local irritation, mild pain, or hematoma at the injection site. In addition, tissue sloughing has been related to intramuscular administration of heparin, and thus this route is *not* recommended.

Heparin is distributed between both white blood cells and plasma, and after administration of a single dose, the plasma level falls exponentially at a rate dependent on the dose. The usual therapeutic doses have a half-life of 1 to 3 hours. Heparin is partly metabolized by the liver, and the much less active metabolite (i.e., uroheparin) is excreted in the urine. A portion of unchanged heparin is also excreted in the urine, and this portion increases with the dose, suggesting that the metabolism is saturable. Heparin does not cross the placenta and is the preferred form of anticoagulation in pregnancy for this reason, although caution should be used, especially during the last trimester.

The pharmacokinetics of each of the oral anticoagulants is similar with only slight differences in the onset and duration of action. In all cases there is a lag of at least 1 day between administration of the drug or change in the dosage and the observed effect on coagulation. The reason for the delay is that time is required for the depletion of clotting factors that have already been synthesized.

There is some variability in the degree of absorption

of each of the agents. Dicumarol is poorly and erratically absorbed, whereas the others are reasonably well absorbed, with warfarin being the most completely absorbed. There is, however, considerable interindividual variation in the absorption of each of these agents, and this is part of the reason therapeutic dosages vary so much among patients.

Phenindione is generally considered to be a shorter acting agent and has a half-life in plasma of approximately 6 hours. A therapeutic effect with this agent is seen in 20 to 30 hours, full anticoagulation in 2 to 3 days, and a return to normal in a similar period of time after the drug has been discontinued. Acenocoumarol, dicumarol, and warfarin have durations of action intermediate to those of phenindione and phenprocoumon. Maximal plasma concentrations of these agents are reached in 2 to 8 hours, and their plasma half-lives vary between 10 to 60 hours depending on the dose. The lag between the administration of the drug and an observation of an effect for these agents can be 24 to 72 hours. When these drugs are discontinued, 6 to 10 days may be required for clotting factors to return to normal levels. Phenprocoumon is similar to the other agents except that up to 14 days may be required for the anticoagulant effect to wane completely.

The oral anticoagulants are almost completely, but loosely, bound to plasma proteins. All of these drugs are hydroxylated to inactive forms by enzymes in the endoplasmic reticulum of the liver (i.e., microsomal enzymes), and these metabolites are eliminated in the urine. These drugs readily cross the placenta and thus have direct effects on the fetus.

Uses

Anticoagulants are used in treating and preventing thromboembolism of both the arterial and venous systems. The most common venous thromboembolic conditions treated with these agents are deep venous thrombophlebitis and pulmonary embolus. On the arterial side, several forms of atherosclerotic heart disease, particularly that of the carotid and femoral systems, are treated with anticoagulants.

Patients with valvular heart disease and left ventricular aneurysm who are at a high risk for systemic emboli are given anticoagulants. Prosthetic devices of various kinds, particularly mechanical artificial heart valves, require permanent anticoagulation therapy.

Heparin is used in acute situations because its effects are *immediate*. It is also preferred for pregnant women because it does not cross the placenta, and in those clinical situations when anticoagulation may need to be discontinued temporarily. In this situation, a return to normal coagulation can be hastened by

giving the heparin antagonist protamine sulfate. Protamine sulfate is also used as an antidote in cases of heparin overdose.

The degree of anticoagulation achieved with heparin must be closely followed through the partial thromboplastin time (PTT), which should be kept 2 to 2½ times the control value. Heparin is often given in low doses subcutaneously as a prophylaxis against venous thromboembolic disease, and under these circumstances the PTT is usually normal or slightly prolonged. Occasionally, however, patients, particularly elderly patients, can become fully anticoagulated with subcutaneous heparin.

The oral agents are used for more prolonged periods of anticoagulation and often are begun following an initial period of anticoagulation with heparin. For the vitamin K antagonist (i.e., oral) anticoagulants, the prothrombin time (PT) is used to follow therapy and should be kept approximately twice the control value.

Adverse effects and toxicity

The adverse side effects of the anticoagulants may be stated in a few words: bleeding, bleeding, bleeding, and more bleeding. The problem most often arises with excessive anticoagulation, but it also can occur when the coagulation tests are well within the normal therapeutic range.

If bleeding occurs while coagulation tests are therapeutic, a careful search must be made for underlying pathologic conditions. In patients with artificial heart valves, the risk of a major bleeding complication has been estimated to be 2% to 7% *per year*. This risk must be weighed against the benefits to be achieved from therapy.

Advanced age, difficulty in controlling hypertension, active peptic ulcer disease, and bleeding disorders are considered to be relative contraindications to using anticoagulants.

Patients receiving oral anticoagulants must be completely reliable in carefully following instructions about their medication, and a patient who is incapable of such compliance cannot be given this type of medication.

Other side effects of the anticoagulants are much less of a problem. Heparin has been known to cause various types of allergic reactions. Thrombocytopenia and alopecia have occurred with short-term use, and osteoporosis has been reported with the long-term use of heparin. Discontinuation of heparin therapy has been associated with aldosterone suppression and transient hyperlipidemia.

There are few side effects, other than bleeding, with the oral anticoagulants. Allergic-type responses (particularly skin rashes), alopecia, and GI upset occur. A rare complication is a hemorrhagic infarction of the skin.

Drug interactions

The anticoagulants can interact with each other, and the antagonism between protamine sulfate and heparin and between vitamin K and the oral anticoagulants has already been mentioned. However, drug interactions between the oral anticoagulants and other agents (see Clinically Significant Drug Interactions) are some of the major pharmacologic points about these drugs. Almost every conceivable kind of medication will interact with the oral anticoagulants. The reader is referred to Clinically Significant Drug Interactions. A safe assumption is that *any* drug will interact with this group of agents, and one must be prepared for changes in PT whenever a new medication is begun, a dosage change is made, or a concurrent medication is discontinued.

The extensiveness of these interactions is based to a large degree on two aspects of the pharmacology of the oral anticoagulants. First, these drugs are highly but loosely bound to plasma proteins and can be easily displaced by many drugs. Second, they are metabolized by microsomal enzymes that are influenced by a large number of other agents. In addition, factors that alter vitamin K availability such as diet and antibiotics (some vitamin K is synthesized by gut bacteria) can influence the effects of these anticoagulants. Patients who take these drugs must be made acutely aware of these problems.

PLATELET AGGREGATION INHIBITORS

Platelet aggregation is thought to play a role in the pathogenesis of certain forms of thromboembolic disease, particularly in the arterial circulation. All of the agents to be discussed in this section also have other properties and thus are also discussed elsewhere: aspirin with nonsteroidal antiinflammatory agents (Chapter 58); sulfinpyrazone with uricosuric agents (Chapter 59); dipyridamole with vasodilators (earlier in this chapter); and clofibrate with antilipemics (earlier in this chapter). Because drug therapy for this objective remains ill defined at present and because these drugs are discussed elsewhere, only a few highlights are covered in this section.

Mechanism of action and pharmacologic effects

Platelets aggregate under a number of conditions to form platelet thrombi and initiate coagulation. In clinical medicine probably the most important situation where this occurs is when there is a break in the continuity of the endothelial layer of arteries. Plate-

let aggregation is probably the first step in true thrombus formation, but in some instances, for reasons incompletely understood, it does not progress beyond the formation of the initial aggregate.

In vitro, platelets can be induced to aggregate by a number of agents including adenosine diphosphate, catecholamines, and the antibiotic ristocetin (which is no longer in clinical use in North America). All platelet aggregation inhibitors inhibit the formation of the initial platelet aggregates. One of the final steps in the cascade leading to activated platelets is thought to be a reduction in levels of cyclic adenosine monophosphate (Figure 34-3). Therefore, high levels of cyclic adenosine monophosphate (cAMP) in the platelets inhibit platelet aggregation.

Dipyridamole raises cAMP levels by inhibiting the enzyme phosphodiesterase that normally inactivates cAMP. This may be the mechanism of action of dipyridamole, but other agents that also inhibit phosphodiesterase (e.g., theophylline) are not platelet aggregation inhibitors. There is some evidence that dipyridamole potentiates the effects of prostacyclin, which is a naturally occurring prostaglandin formed in the endothelial cells of the blood vessels and is an antiaggregant. Aspirin and sulfinpyrazone also raise the level of cAMP in platelets.

Two prostaglandins have competing effects on adenylate cyclase. Prostacyclin is located in the endothelial cells of the blood vessels, and it stimulates adenylate cyclase and the formation of cAMP and thus is an antiaggregant. Thromboxane A_2 is located in the platelets themselves, inhibits adenylate cyclase and the formation of cAMP, and thus is an aggregant. Low doses of aspirin and sulfinpyrazone selectively inhibit the formation of thromboxane A_2 and thus are antiaggregants. Higher doses of aspirin probably also inhibit prostacyclin formation, but there is some controversy over whether prostacyclin is even formed in diseased blood vessels. If it is not formed, then the dose of aspirin is less important.

A lack of formation of prostacyclin would also compromise the action of dipyridamole if it acts by potentiating prostacyclin. The inhibition of prostaglandin formation by aspirin is noncompetitive, whereas that by sulfinpyrazone is competitive; this will influence the way in which the two drugs are used. The mechanism of action of clofibrate as a platelet aggregation inhibitor is unknown at present.

Pharmacokinetics

Clofibrate has already been discussed in the section on antilipemics in this chapter. Because its mechanism of action is not currently known, the relevance of its pharmacokinetics is unclear. The pharmacoki-

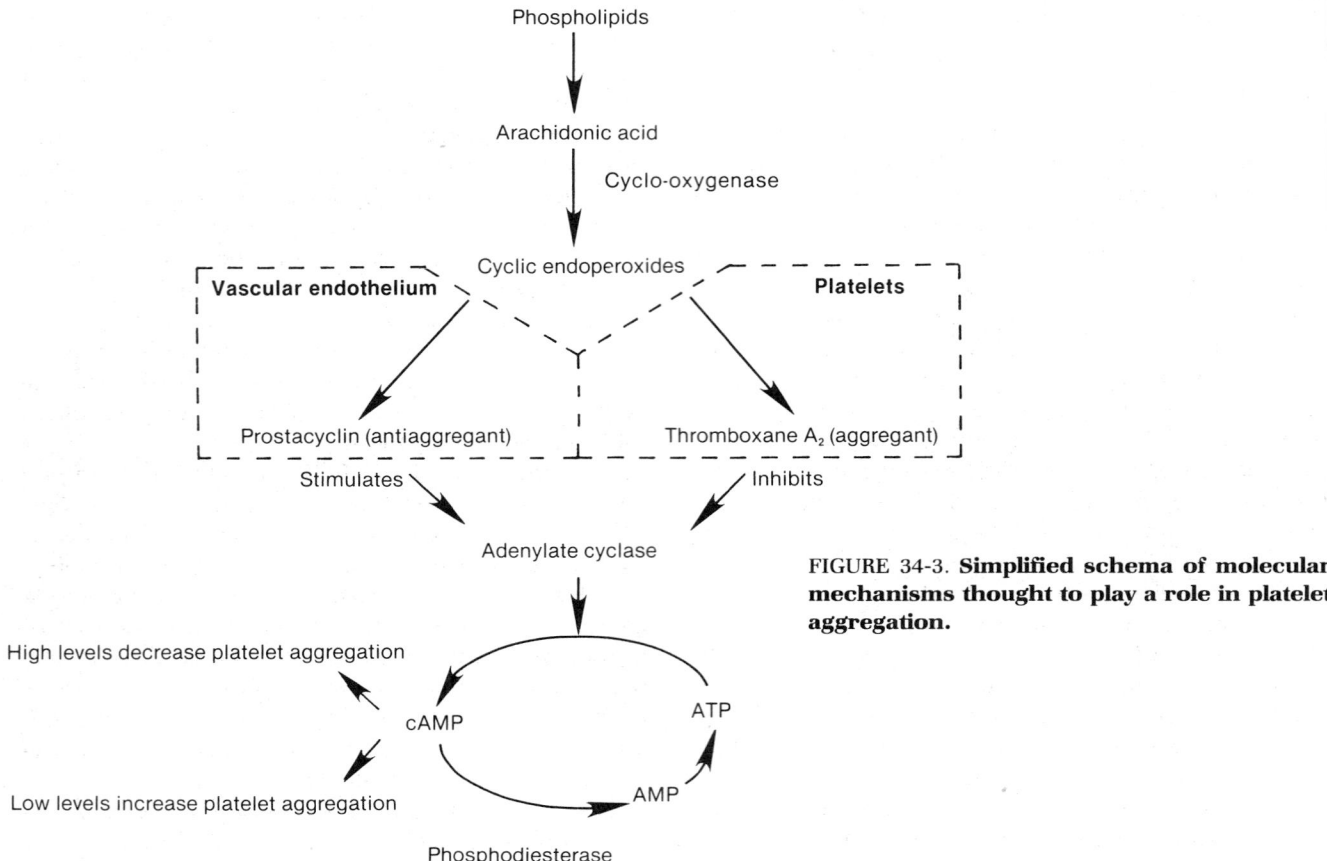

FIGURE 34-3. **Simplified schema of molecular mechanisms thought to play a role in platelet aggregation.**

netics of clofibrate may be important, however, because much larger concentrations must be used in vitro for platelet aggregation inhibition than are achieved in vivo.

Little is known about the pharmacokinetics of dipyridamole. It is adequately absorbed via the oral route. Dipyridamole undergoes extensive enterohepatic recirculation and is conjugated to the glucoronide form (i.e., metabolized) in the liver. It does *not* cross the blood-brain barrier. It is usually given more frequently (i.e., 4, rather than 3 times per day) for platelet aggregation inhibition than it is for vasodilation, but there is no clear reason for such a difference.

All salicylates, including aspirin, are absorbed from the stomach and upper small intestine. The peak level is usually reached in about 2 hours. The pH of various body fluids can alter the absorption and the excretion rates of aspirin because it is a weak acid. Tablet formulation may also be important in absorption. From 50% to 90% of aspirin is bound to plasma protein. Aspirin is widely distributed throughout the body, including the brain, and it crosses the placenta. Only a small portion of aspirin is metabolized (everywhere, but chiefly in the liver), and the majority is excreted

unchanged in the urine. The plasma half-life for aspirin is approximately 20 minutes. However, because platelet half-life is approximately 10 hours and platelet aggregation inhibition is noncompetitive, the drug does not need to be given more than 2 or 3 times per day (see also the discussion on aspirin in Chapter 17, "Analgesics and Narcotic Antagonists," and Chapter 58, "Nonsteroidal Antiinflammatory Drugs").

Sulfinpyrazone is well absorbed via the oral route and is approximately 99% bound to plasma protein. The elimination half-life is approximately 3 hours, and 90% is excreted unchanged in the urine. It is excreted by active secretion in the proximal tubule. Unlike aspirin, the platelet antiaggregant effects of sulfinpyrazone are competitive, and the agent must be given 4 times per day to maintain an effective plasma level.

Uses

The evidence that the inhibition of platelet aggregation has clinical usefulness is incomplete and fragmentary. The major reasons for its proposed use are for patients with coronary disease, particularly if there has been a recent myocardial infarction, for transient ischemic attacks caused by cerebrovascular disease, and for thromboembolism caused by intravascular or intracardiac prosthetic devices (usually combined with a regular anticoagulant). The evidence of usefulness of these agents can be briefly summarized.

In patients with angina pectoris, but without an antecedent myocardial infarction, one study has demonstrated that clofibrate will reduce the incidence of the first myocardial infarction independent of its lipid lowering effect. In a controversial study, sulfinpyrazone started shortly after a recent myocardial infarction was believed to reduce the incidence of sudden death over the next 7 months. This last study has been harshly criticized, but reanalysis of the data by an independent panel has supported the conclusions of the investigators. A second trial with sulfinpyrazone after myocardial infarction has shown the drug to reduce the incidence of reinfarction but not sudden death. Several other studies have produced evidence of no clear effect in this condition with various aggregation inhibitors, and the proponents on either side continue to criticize the design of each other's studies. In patients with prosthetic heart valves who continue to have problems with thromboembolism despite adequate anticoagulation, *adding* aspirin or dipyridamole seems to reduce the incidence of these complications. It must be emphasized that these agents *cannot* replace anticoagulation in patients with prosthetic heart valves. Aspirin, but not sulfinpyrazone, has been claimed to reduce the incidence of transient ischemic attacks (small strokes), but, curiously, the effect appears to be restricted to male patients.

Adverse effects and toxicity

Adverse effects and toxicity are reviewed in Adverse/Side Effects of Vasodilators, Antilipemics, Anticoagulants, and Platelet Aggregation Inhibitors and are discussed elsewhere with each of the agents discussed in this section. There are the usual problems of a variety of GI and allergic reactions, particularly skin rash-

es. All of these agents can potentiate the bleeding problems that occur with anticoagulants. Sulfinpyrazone is a uricosuric agent and can precipitate urolithiasis and renal colic in susceptible patients if adequate measures are not taken to prevent this problem. Rarely, sulfinpyrazone has been associated with transient profound renal failure. Aspirin (i.e., salicylate) toxicity is a common form of poisoning.

Drug interactions

The interaction of all of these agents with the anticoagulants to enhance bleeding tendencies has been previously mentioned. This is particularly important for aspirin, which is additive by two different mechanisms. Other interactions are listed in Clinically Significant Drug Interactions, and those for clofibrate and dipyridamole are discussed earlier in this chapter. The interaction between alcohol and aspirin is important one with which all patients should be familiar. Aspirin is a uricosuric agent in its own right at lower doses and can interfere with the uricosuric effect of other agents such as probenecid. Aspirin can also interfere with the excretion of other drugs, such as methotrexate, which are secreted via the same mechanism.

SUMMARY

The nurse's role in relation to administering and monitoring vasodilators, antilipemics, anticoagulants, and platelet aggregation inhibitors is complex, and because these medications are often used in treating life-threatening conditions, the nurse needs to have a sound knowledge of the pharmacology of these drugs. In addition, because conditions requiring the use of these medications are often chronic and require changes in the patient's lifestyle, the nurse's role in patient education, support in modifying risk factors, and assistance in adjusting to life changes cannot be overemphasized.

ADVERSE/SIDE EFFECTS OF VASODILATORS, ANTILIPEMICS, ANTICOAGULANTS, AND PLATELET AGGREGATION INHIBITORS*

Vasodilators

ALLERGIC REACTIONS	BEHAVIOR	CARDIOVASCULAR SYSTEM
Dermatitis	Anxiety	Angina
Photosensitivity	Depression	Dysrhythmias (e.g., supraventricular
Variety of skin rashes (e.g., pigmentation, urticaria)	Nervousness	tachycardias)
		Flushing

*See Chapter 11, "Drug Toxicity," for an overview of drug toxicity.

Continued.

ADVERSE/SIDE EFFECTS OF VASODILATORS, ANTILIPEMICS, ANTICOAGULANTS, AND PLATELET AGGREGATION INHIBITORS—cont'd

Vasodilators—cont'd

CARDIOVASCULAR SYSTEM—cont'd

Tachycardia
Widened QRS and QT intervals

CENTRAL NERVOUS SYSTEM

Dizziness
Drowsiness
Headache
Syncope
Weakness

GASTROINTESTINAL SYSTEM

Abdominal discomfort
Activation of peptic ulcer disease
Belching
Diarrhea
Nausea
Vomiting

HEMATOLOGIC SYSTEM

Methemoglobin formation

HEPATIC SYSTEM

Abnormal liver function tests
Jaundice

METABOLIC AND ENDOCRINE SYSTEMS

Decreased glucose tolerance
Hyperuricemia

NEUROMUSCULAR SYSTEM

Piloerection

OCULAR SYSTEM

Toxic amblyopia

Antilipemics

ALLERGIC REACTIONS

Pruritus
Variety of skin rashes (e.g., pigmentation, urticaria)

BEHAVIOR

Mood changes
Nervousness

CARDIOVASCULAR SYSTEM

Dysrhythmias (e.g., supraventricular tachycardias)
Flushing
Hypertension
Hypotension
Increased angina

CENTRAL NERVOUS SYSTEM

Dizziness
Fatigue
Headache
Insomnia
Syncope
Tinnitus

GASTROINTESTINAL SYSTEM

Abdominal discomfort
Activation of peptic ulcer disease
Constipation
Diarrhea
Fecal impaction
Flatulence
Nausea
Steatorrhea
Vomiting

HEMATOLOGIC SYSTEM

Hypothrombinemia

HEPATIC SYSTEM

Abnormal hepatic function tests
Jaundice

METABOLIC AND ENDOCRINE SYSTEMS

Alopecia
Decreased glucose tolerance
Decreased libido
Gynecomastia
Hyperthyroidism
Hyperuricemia
Impotence
Menstrual irregularities
Osteoporosis
Sweatiness

NEUROMUSCULAR SYSTEM

Arthralgia
Myalgia
Paresthesia

OCULAR SYSTEM

Toxic amblyopia

Anticoagulants

ALLERGIC REACTIONS

Asthma
Chills
Fever
Hemorrhagic infarction and necrosis of skin
Lacrimation
Local skin reaction

ADVERSE/SIDE EFFECTS OF VASODILATORS, ANTILIPEMICS, ANTICOAGULANTS, AND PLATELET AGGREGATION INHIBITORS—cont'd

Anticoagulants—cont'd
ALLERGIC REACTIONS—cont'd

Pruritus
Rhinitis
Variety of skin rashes (e.g., urticaria, petechiae, purpura)

CARDIOVASCULAR SYSTEM

Hemorrhage

CENTRAL NERVOUS SYSTEM

Hemorrhage

GASTROINTESTINAL SYSTEM

Diarrhea
Hemorrhage
Steatorrhea
Vomiting

HEMATOLOGIC SYSTEM

Agranulocytosis
Eosinophilia
Hemorrhage
Leukopenia
Thrombocytopenia

HEPATIC SYSTEM

Hepatitis
Jaundice

METABOLIC AND ENDOCRINE SYSTEMS

Aldosterone suppression
Alopecia
Osteoporosis

NEUROMUSCULAR SYSTEM

Hemorrhage

OCULAR SYSTEM

Conjunctivitis
Hemorrhage
Paralysis of accommodation

RENAL SYSTEM

Albuminuria
Hemorrhage

Platelet aggregation inhibitors
ALLERGIC REACTIONS

Pruritus
Variety of skin rashes (e.g., urticaria, petechiae, erythema multiforme)

CARDIOVASCULAR SYSTEM

Dysrhythmias (e.g., supraventricular tachycardias)
Flushing
Increased angina

CENTRAL NERVOUS SYSTEM

Confusion
Dizziness
Drowsiness
Headache
High-tone deafness
Syncope
Tinnitus

GASTROINTESTINAL SYSTEM

Abdominal discomfort
Activation of peptic ulcer disease
Diarrhea
Gastritis
Hemorrhage
Nausea
Vomiting

HEMATOLOGIC SYSTEM

Agranulocytosis
Anemia
Eosinophilia
Hypoprothrombinemia
Leukopenia
Thrombocytopenia

HEPATIC SYSTEM

Abnormal liver function tests

METABOLIC AND ENDOCRINE SYSTEMS

Acidosis (metabolic)
Alkalosis (respiratory)
Alopecia
Decreased libido
Hyperuricemia
Impaired glucose tolerance
Impotence

NEUROMUSCULAR SYSTEM

Arthralgia
Myalgia

RENAL SYSTEM

Dysuria
Precipitation of urolithiasis and renal colic
Proteinuria

RESPIRATORY SYSTEM

Hyperventilation

CLINICALLY SIGNIFICANT DRUG INTERACTIONS*

Primary drug	Interacting drug	Possible effect(s)	Probable mechanism(s)
VASODILATORS			
All vasodilators	Alcohol	Hypotension	Additive
All vasodilators	All antihypertensives	Hypotension	Additive
Dipyridamole	All anticoagulants and platelet aggregation inhibitors	Increased anticoagulant effect	Additive (platelet effect)
ANTILIPEMICS			
Cholestyramine and colestipol	Digoxin	Decreased digoxin effect	Decreased absorption
Cholestyramine and colestipol	Thyroid hormone	Decreased thyroid effect	Decreased absorption
Cholestyramine and colestipol	Vitamins A, D, E, and K	Vitamin deficiency	Decreased absorption
Cholestyramine and colestipol	Vitamin K antagonist anticoagulants	Decreased anticoagulant effect	Decreased absorption
Clofibrate	Other platelet aggregation inhibitors	Increased platelet dysfunction	Additive
Clofibrate	Vitamin K antagonist anticoagulants	Increased anticoagulant effect	Displacement from binding sites, additive pharmacologic effects
Colestipol	Chlorothiazide	Decreased diuretic effect	Decreased absorption
Dextrothyroxine	Oral hypoglycemics and insulin	Decreased hypoglycemic effect	Physiologic antagonist
Dextrothyroxine	Vitamin K antagonist anticoagulants	Increased anticoagulant effect	Not established
ANTICOAGULANTS			
Vitamin K antagonists	Acetaminophen (chronic use)	Increased anticoagulant effect	Not established
Vitamin K antagonists	Alcohol	Decreased anticoagulant effect with chronic alcohol use	Increased metabolism
Vitamin K antagonists	Allopurinol	Increased anticoagulant effect	Inhibition of microsomal enzymes
Vitamin K antagonists	Amiodarone	Increased anticoagulant effect	Not established
Vitamin K antagonists	Anabolic and androgenic steroids	Increased anticoagulant effect	Not established
Vitamin K antagonists	Aspirin	Increased anticoagulant effect	Displacement from protein binding sites and inhibition of platelet aggregation by aspirin
Vitamin K antagonists	Barbiturates	Decreased anticoagulant effect	Induction of microsomal enzymes
Vitamin K antagonists	Carbamazepine	Decreased anticoagulant effect	Induction of microsomal enzymes
Vitamin K antagonists	Chloral hydrate	Increased anticoagulant effect	Displacement from binding sites
Vitamin K antagonists	Chloramphenicol	Increased anticoagulant effect	Inhibition of microsomal enzymes
Vitamin K antagonists	Cholestyramine	Decreased anticoagulant effect	Decreased absorption
Vitamin K antagonists	Cimetidine	Increased anticoagulant effect	Inhibition of microsomal enzymes

*See Chapter 10, "Drug Interactions," for an overview of drug interactions.

CLINICALLY SIGNIFICANT DRUG INTERACTIONS—cont'd

Primary drug	Interacting drug	Possible effect(s)	Probable mechanism(s)
ANTICOAGULANTS—cont'd			
Vitamin K antagonists and heparin	Clofibrate	Increased anticoagulant effect	Displacement from binding sites and additive (platelet effect)
Vitamin K antagonists	Dextrothyroxine	Increased anticoagulant effect	Not established
Vitamin K antagonists	Dipyridamole	Increased anticoagulant effect	Additive (platelet effect)
Vitamin K antagonists	Disulfiram	Increased anticoagulant effect	Not established
Vitamin K antagonists	Glutethimide	Decreased anticoagulant effect	Induction of microsomal enzymes
Vitamin K antagonists	Griseofulvin	Decreased anticoagulant effect	Induction of microsomal enzymes
Vitamin K antagonists	Hypoglycemics (oral)	Increased hypoglycemic effect	Inhibition of microsomal enzymes
Vitamin K antagonists	Indomethacin	Increased anticoagulant effect	Additive (platelet effect)
Vitamin K antagonists	Metronidazole	Increased anticoagulant effect	Inhibition of microsomal enzymes
Vitamin K antagonists	Oral contraceptives	Decreased anticoagulant effect	Increased activity of clotting factors
Vitamin K antagonists	Oxyphenbutazone	Increased anticoagulant effect	Displacement from binding sites
Vitamin K antagonists	Phenylbutazone	Increased anticoagulant effect	Displacement from binding sites and inhibition of microsomal enzymes
Vitamin K antagonists	Phenytoin	Increased phenytoin toxicity	Inhibition of microsomal enzymes
Vitamin K antagonists	Rifampin	Decreased anticoagulant effect	Induction of microsomal enzymes
Vitamin K antagonists	Salicylates	Increased anticoagulant effect	Additive because of hypoprothrombinemic and platelet effect
Vitamin K antagonists	Sulfonamides	Increased anticoagulant effect	Inhibition of microsomal enzymes
Vitamin K antagonists	Thyroid hormones	Increased anticoagulant effect	Increased clotting factor catabolism
Vitamin K antagonists	Triclofos sodium	Increased anticoagulant effect	Displacement from binding sites
Vitamin K antagonists	Vitamin K	Decreased anticoagulant effect	Antagonism of anticoagulant effect
Heparin	Aspirin	Increased anticoagulant effect	Additive
Heparin	Ethacrynic acid	Increased anticoagulant effect	Not established
PLATELET AGGREGATION INHIBITORS			
All platelet aggregation inhibitors	Anticoagulants	Increased anticoagulant effect	Additive
Aspirin	Alcohol	Increased GI bleeding	Additive
Aspirin	Antacids	Decreased salicylate levels	Increased renal clearance
Aspirin	Anticoagulants	Increased anticoagulant effect	Additive hypoprothrombinemic effect
Aspirin	Hypoglycemics (oral) and insulin	Increased hypoglycemia	Displacement from binding sites Additive
Aspirin	Methotrexate	Increased methotrexate toxicity	Decreased renal clearance
Aspirin (chronic moderate doses)	Probenecid	Decreased uricosuric effect Salicylate toxicity	Not established Decreased excretion

GENERAL NURSING IMPLICATIONS

Nursing of patients requiring vasodilators

ASSESSMENT

A complete nursing assessment is essential in establishing a baseline from which to monitor drug therapy. Assessment should include a careful drug history to determine sensitivity, contraindications, and potential drug interactions before drug therapy is initiated. The nurse should also be alert to identifying risk factors.

If the vasodilator is required for angina, the patient's pain must also be carefully assessed before initiating the drug therapy to ensure that the angina is not a myocardial infarction or an infarct extension. Assessment should be carried out as quickly as possible so that the pain can be controlled. Assessment of the patient's chest pain should include the following: the location of the pain; a description of discomfort (many patients may identify discomfort such as squeezing, tearing, and deny pain); the emotional stressors associated with the onset of the pain; the activity the patient was engaged in when the pain started; and whether the pain is relieved by rest.

It should also be ascertained whether a medication was taken to relieve the pain or discomfort. If so, the medication, the dosage, and how it was taken should be identified. It should also be noted if the medication was effective. In addition to pain assessment, baseline data related to cardiac function must also be obtained, including heart rate, respiratory rate, blood pressure, chest sounds, heart sounds, and rhythm. The nurse may also be involved in acute cases in obtaining more specific baseline data related to hemodynamic status, including an electrocardiogram and intraarterial and venous pressures.

If the vasodilator is used in relation to CHF management, specific assessment in relation to CHF should be performed (e.g., presence or absence of peripheral edema, pulmonary edema, orthopnea, or cyanosis).

Patients requiring a vasodilator for a vasospasm, including Raynaud's phenomenon, should be assessed carefully so the therapeutic response can be monitored in relation to cyanotic discoloration, coldness, or peripheral sweating, especially in the hands. Data related to the precipitation of the arterial spasm should also be recorded in the baseline assessment (e.g., cold, emotional stress).

SENSITIVITY

When vasodilators are taken by patients who have not received them before, monitoring for hypersensitivity reactions is extremely important. Observe for skin rash. Patients should be encouraged to report any unusual signs such as these to the health care provider immediately.

CONTRAINDICATIONS

Vasodilators, because of their actions and effects on various body systems are contraindicated in the presence of some conditions. These are specified for each agent in the Nursing Drug Digest. These agents are contraindicated in the presence of hypotension.

CAUTIONS

Caution should be used when vasodilators are administered to elderly patients taking beta-adrenergic blockers and ambulatory patients. Caution should also be used when vasodilators are used in patients who have compromised respiratory function, such as severely hypoxic patients (e.g., hypoxic pulmonary vasoconstriction [HPV]). The nurse should be aware that the following conditions can trigger HPV: myocardial infarct, pulmonary fibrosis, emphysema, mitral valve disease, right ventricular failure, pulmonary vein thrombosis, or high altitude location.

DRUG INTERACTIONS

Vasodilators can interact not only with each other, but also with numerous other medications including prescription and nonprescription drugs (see Clinically Significant Drug Interactions). The nurse should be especially alert not to administer medications that can potentiate the hypotensive effects of these drugs (e.g., antihypertensives) without checking with the prescriber.

ADMINISTRATION
Initial therapy

Patients requiring vasodilators are placed on individualized regimens. When administering these medications or when teaching the patient to self-medicate, one must be alert to correct administration. Some vasodilators (e.g., nitroglycerin) are taken as needed and others (e.g., isosorbide dinitrate) are taken in scheduled doses throughout the day. The patient must be clear on the route of administration because many of these drugs can be taken by various routes (e.g., sublingually, orally, topically). Patients who are receiving more than one vasodilator need a clear understanding of how and when to take their medications.

Allow the inpatient to keep the medication (e.g., nitroglycerin) at the bedside. Instruct the patient to report the following to the nurse: how much of the drug the patient requires to relieve angina, how frequently the drug is taken, whether the pain is relieved, the length of time before relief is obtained, and whether any side effects are experienced.

Observe the patient for tolerance, which may begin several days after treatment is started, and is typically manifested as a lack of response to the usual dose. NOTE: A lack of response may also indicate that the medication has lost its potency and that a new supply should be ordered, or that the patient is suffering from another condition (e.g., acute myocardial infarction).

Administration of nitroglycerin

Nitroglycerin can be administered sublingually, intravenously, and topically.

Sublingual
Nitroglycerin tablets are absorbed rapidly via the sublingual route. Inpatients are provided with tablets to keep at their bedside after they are taught how to use the sublingual tablets. Patients should sit down if they have angina pain and place a tablet under the tongue. A burning sensation should be felt if the medication is active. Monitoring of pain frequency, use of drug, side effects (especially headache, flushing, and hypotension), and response is

GENERAL NURSING IMPLICATIONS—cont'd

Nursing of patients requiring vasodilators—cont'd

Sublingual—cont'd

important. The sublingual route allows rapid absorption into the bloodstream. The patient should be encouraged *not* to swallow saliva for about 1 minute to ensure absorption.

Intravenous

Intravenous administration of nitroglycerin is useful in caring for the patient with unstable angina. It is usually administered in intravenous dextrose and water solutions and infused according to patient response at doses of approximately 5 μg/minute initially (see the Nursing Drug Digest). Headaches, tachycardia, chills, nausea, vomiting, hypotension, and lightheadedness can occur. Vital signs should be monitored closely and should be taken before initiating the therapy. When preparing intravenous infusion solutions, do not use plastic bags or polyethylene tubing, because this can result in considerable loss of drug potency via adsorption to the surface of the plastic. Use glass intravenous solution bottles and the special tubing supplied with the medication. Use of an intravenous infusion pump is recommended.

Topical

Nitroglycerin ointment is applied topically to the chest, forearm, abdomen, or thigh. Research indicates that the chest is the most effective site. It has been found that the forehead can increase the chance of headache and that the ankle is the least effective site. The ointment should be applied as ordered to a clean, dry area free from as much body hair as possible. The ointment is measured out using the enclosed ruler for accuracy and then spread with a tongue blade thinly over a 10 to 15 cm area. The nurse should be careful not to use the fingers because the medication can be absorbed. The ointment should not be rubbed in, because this can increase the rate of absorption and reduce the sustained effectiveness. It has been found that absorption is best when the skin is moist. Therefore, it is recommended that the site be carefully covered with plastic wrap and secured with tape. This also prevents the ointment from being rubbed off on clothing or bed linen. Application sites should be rotated and thoroughly cleansed of ointment residues. Side effects should be monitored, as should the patient response. The blood pressure should be taken 1 hour after administration of the medication. A drop in blood pressure of 20 mm Hg should be reported to the prescriber immediately. If a drop in blood pressure is greater than this, the ointment should be removed immediately. A 10 mm Hg fall in pressure or increase of the heart rate by 10 beats per minute is within the therapeutic range. The ointment should be stored in a tightly closed tube at room temperature.

A newer delivery device for the topical administration of nitroglycerin is the transdermal therapeutic system (e.g., Transderm-Nitro). These systems typically contain a *total* amount of 25 mg or 50 mg of nitroglycerin, which is released at a constant rate of either 5 mg/ 24 hours or 10 mg/24 hours, respectively. Any area of skin on the body, except the extremities below the elbow or knee, can be used. The preferred site, however, is either the chest or back because these areas are usually free of hair, skin folds, and excessive movement.

The transdermal therapeutic system is removed from its package and applied to the selected area of dry skin. The exposed, adhesive side of the system is then firmly pressed against the selected area and held in place for 10 to 15 seconds. To ensure optimum adhesion, circle the outside edge of the system with one or two fingers after it is in place.

Once the system is in place, contact with water (e.g., bathing, swimming) will *not* affect the operation of the system or its correct delivery of medication. If, however, the system should become detached or fall off, it should be discarded and a new system applied to a different skin site.

The system should be removed and a new one applied to a different skin site *every* 24 hours.

Maintenance

Follow-up and reassessment at regular intervals are important in relation to helping patients self-medicate with vasodilators. Patients who have been taking vasodilators for a period of time who are then hospitalized maintain the responsibility, as they are able, for self-medication. They should be encouraged to report anginal episodes and the use of their medication to the nurse. The medication should be stored carefully, and the nurse should be sure that the supply is adequate.

MONITORING PATIENT RESPONSE

Therapeutic response

Angina. To monitor accurately the patient's therapeutic response, the nurse may be required to remain with the patient for 10 minutes after a vasodilator is taken during the initial therapy involving such drugs as nitroglycerin.

Note the alleviation of pain as reported by the patient, including how soon relief occurred after the drug was taken and whether the relief was partial or complete. The blood pressure should be monitored 1 to 2 minutes after the administration of the drug and then every 3 minutes to assess the systolic pressure, which should gradually decline.

CHF. If the vasodilator is given for CHF or diminished cardiac output, monitor for improved pulmonary congestion and cardiac output.

Vasospasm. Monitor for relief of acrocyanosis, including mottling and increasing warmth of the extremities.

Monitoring the therapeutic response is especially important in adjusting initial vasodilator therapy regimens to attain optimum pain control with minimum side effects. Response determines the titration of various vasodilators and determines the individualized patient drug therapy plan. All assessment data should be recorded carefully to document patient response and to facilitate treatment decisions.

Adverse side effects

Monitoring side effects (see Adverse/ Side Effects of Vasodilators, Antilipemics, Anticoagulants, and Platelet Aggregation Inhibitors) and planning to min-

Continued.

GENERAL NURSING IMPLICATIONS—cont'd

Nursing of patients requiring vasodilators—cont'd

Adverse side effects—cont'd

imize these effects with the patient and the family are indicated. The most common side effects of the vasodilators are headache and hypotension. The patient should be reminded to report any dizziness or faintness, especially with nitroglycerin. The duration and severity of the headache (caused by the dilation of the cerebral vessels) should be recorded and nursing measures should be used to minimize this effect, including exploring the use of a common analgesic. The patient should be supported and should be made aware that tolerance to the effects of nitroglycerin and a decrease in headaches usually occur. The headache can also be managed by reducing the dose or by starting at low doses of medication and increasing the dosage gradually. Patients should be encouraged to change position slowly to prevent problems related to the hypotensive effect.

Toxicity

Patients requiring vasodilator therapy should be monitored for excessive lowering of the blood pressure manifested by postural hypotension, dizziness, fatigue, tachycardia, and syncope. Toxic effects for each specific agent can be found in the Nursing Drug Digest. If toxicity is identified, the prescriber should be advised so the drug plan can be adjusted as required.

Tolerance

Tolerance is invariable, and cross-tolerance occurs; however, this is of little significance therapeutically. Nitroglycerin is not habit forming, and tolerance to the vasodilating or antianginal effects develops rarely, except with the transdermal route. The therapeutic effect of vasodilators does not decrease over time.

PATIENT EDUCATION

Most patients requiring vasodilators will be responsible for self-medication related to controlling their conditions. Patient teaching is essential in promoting self-medication. Drug therapy, however, is only part of the treatment of many conditions related to coronary artery disease and other vascular conditions. Modification of lifestyle and activities of daily living is often necessary. Nurses play an important part in helping patients identify and reduce risk factors in controlling their conditions, including weight and smoking control, limiting alcohol consumption, and reducing or avoiding activities that trigger the problem (e.g., smoke-filled rooms; sudden physical stress; temperature change, especially cold). Family members should be involved in education because their understanding of the patient's care and control of the condition is essential.

Patient teaching should be individualized. The patient should have a clear understanding of the medication regimen, as well as the exact name(s) of medication(s), action, dosage, storage, administration, dosing frequency, and side effects. The patient should know how to minimize side effects and know which effects should be readily reported to the health care provider. The patient should also know the etiology and prevalence of the condition, the seriousness of not modifying identified risk factors, the importance of following the drug regimen as planned with the health care provider, and the need for follow-up and the probability of lifelong therapy. The nurse should be alert to explore difficulties of long-term therapy with patients, including changes related to lifestyle. Patients need support in controlling symptoms so they can live as normally as possible.

Counseling may also be indicated because some patients (e.g., patients with coronary artery disease), often fearful of recurrent pain episodes and of the possibility of sudden death, needlessly curtail normal activities. The patient and the family may need help in understanding that although restraint may be necessary in some activities, most activities can be resumed or modified.

Advise patients receiving nitrates *not* to drink alcohol because alcohol syncope may occur.

Providing simple written instructions concerning the medication plan and common side effects can do much to reinforce home care.

Nursing of patients requiring antilipemics

ASSESSMENT

A complete nursing assessment is essential in establishing a baseline from which to identify risk factors as well as to individualize drug therapy and to monitor therapeutic response, adverse side effects, sensitivity, contraindications, and potential drug interactions before drug therapy is initiated. Assessment of blood cholesterol and triglyceride levels is also indicated before therapy is initiated to monitor response appropriately.

SENSITIVITY, CONTRAINDICATIONS, AND CAUTIONS

See the Nursing Drug Digest for specific information regarding each agent

DRUG INTERACTIONS

Antilipemics can interact with numerous medications, including prescription and nonprescription drugs (see Clinically Significant Drug Interactions).

MONITORING PATIENT RESPONSE

Therapeutic response

Monitoring the patient's therapeutic response is especially important in adjusting antilipemic therapy regimens to obtain optimum blood triglyceride and cholesterol levels.

Adverse side effects

Monitoring side effects is essential (see Adverse/Side Effects of Vasodilators, Antilipemics, Anticoagulants, and

GENERAL NURSING IMPLICATIONS—cont'd

Nursing of patients requiring antilipemics—cont'd

Adverse side effects—cont'd

Platelet Aggregation Inhibitors) as is planning to minimize such effects (e.g., abdominal pain, neuropathies, and xanthomas).

See the Nursing Drug Digest for monitoring side effects of specific antilipemics.

PATIENT EDUCATION

Patients requiring antilipemics require careful education about their drug therapy regimen. The drug therapy augments dietary changes to control blood triglyceride and cholesterol levels. Patients may require support and guidance in drug regimens and dietary modifications. Patients should have a clear understanding of the etiology of their condition, the control of risk factors, and the need for follow-up care. The names of medication(s), actions, side effects, what to do to minimize side effects, administration, and storage should be discussed as indicated.

Nursing of patients requiring anticoagulants

ASSESSMENT

A complete nursing assessment is essential in establishing a baseline from which to individualize drug therapy and to monitor response. Baseline clotting profiles should be completed to rule out any hemostatic abnormality. This is important for both inpatients and outpatients. The assessment should also include a careful drug history to determine sensitivity, contraindications, and potential drug interactions before drug therapy is initiated.

SENSITIVITY

When anticoagulants are taken by patients who have not received them before, monitoring for hypersensitivity is extremely important. Heparin has been known to produce various types of allergic reactions (e.g., chills, fever, burning of feet, lacrimation, skin eruptions, osteoporosis, and even anaphylactic shock). The oral anticoagulants can also produce allergic reactions, especially skin rashes, alopecia, and GI upset.

CONTRAINDICATIONS

Anticoagulants are *contraindicated* in certain conditions, including known sensitivity, patients with uncontrolled hypertension, active peptic ulcer disease, in women over 60 years of age, and in patients with bleeding disorders (e.g., hemophilia). These medications are also contraindicated in brain, spinal, or eye surgery. Low-dose heparin therapy is contraindicated in patients having major orthopedic surgery, brain surgery, and abdominal prostatectomy.

CAUTIONS

Caution should be used when anticoagulants are administered to elderly patients, pregnant and lactating women, to patients during and following major surgery, and to patients who have continuous nasal gastric suction of the stomach or small intestine. Caution should also be used in the immediate postpartum period and with patients who have conditions associated with increased bleeding tendency (e.g., thrombocytopenia). To avoid possible cerebral hemorrhage, it is generally recommended that heparin therapy be delayed for at least 3 days following cerebral embolism, and then administered only when the computerized tomographic brain scan indicates *no* evidence of intracranial bleeding.

Caution is indicated with the concurrent use of platelet inhibitors (e.g., aspirin, dipyridamole) because anticoagulant effects can be potentiated.

DRUG INTERACTIONS

Anticoagulants can interact with each other and with a wide variety of other drugs (see Clinically Significant Drug Interactions). The clotting times should be monitored carefully whenever a new drug is started, when a patient is receiving an anticoagulant, or when a dosage of a concurrent drug is changed or discontinued.

As mentioned previously, platelet inhibitors can interact with anticoagulants and can generally potentiate anticoagulant effects.

ADMINISTRATION
Initial therapy

Patients requiring anticoagulant therapy are often started on heparin and as needed are gradually switched over to oral anticoagulants if long-term therapy is indicated, as is required in relation to clotting conditions. The patient may be receiving both heparin and an oral anticoagulant at the same time until the oral anticoagulant therapeutic blood levels are established.

Low-dose heparin therapy is administered prophylactically usually in doses of 5000 units every 8 to 12 hours for 7 consecutive days or until the patient is ambulatory. In the surgical patient, the initial dose is given 2 hours preoperatively and then continued. Low-dose heparin is administered subcutaneously in the lower abdomen fat pads between the iliac crests (see Chapter 2, "Preparation, Administration, and Monitoring of Medications"). The lateral upper thigh can also be selected in relation to rotating sites.

Maintenance

When anticoagulant effects are established at the goal level, doses of medication are stabilized. Follow-up in anticoagulant clinics for outpatients is important at regular intervals to adjust the therapy and to monitor response. The patient's PTT (for heparin) or PT (for the oral anticoagulants) is the indicator of therapeutic response and should be measured regularly. The nurse should be alert to explore difficulties of long-term therapy, including modifications in activities of daily liv-

Continued.

GENERAL NURSING IMPLICATIONS—cont'd

Nursing of patients requiring anticoagulants—cont'd

Maintenance—cont'd

ing, remembering to take medications according to individualized plan, and the consequences of poor control.

Specific information regarding the administration of these agents can be found in the Nursing Drug Digest.

Administration of heparin

Heparin can be administered intramuscularly, intravenously, or subcutaneously. The intramuscular route is *not* recommended, however, because irritation, mild pain, and hematoma can occur at the injection site, and the literature suggests that this route shortens drug action because of irregular absorption from the muscle. In addition, bleeding in the muscle mass following injection has resulted in tissue sloughing, so this route should be *avoided* when administering heparin. If this route is ordered by the prescriber, the nurse should discuss these aspects with the prescriber before administering the heparin. Intramuscular injections of any kind should be completed with caution in patients receiving heparin or any other anticoagulant and are *not* recommended.

Intravenous

Heparin is often administered continuously via intravenous infusion. This route has less of a tendency to cause bleeding than the subcutaneous route. Heparin can also be administered by bolus IV push. This method is common with higher concentrations of heparin doses. When heparin is administered intravenously, the IV site requires careful monitoring, especially with the higher concentrations, because heparin tends to be irritating. The drug concentration should be carefully checked to ensure accuracy, and it is recommended that heparin doses be counterchecked by another registered nurse for safety. Continuous IV heparin should be administered by way of an infusion pump to ensure maximal safety.

Heparin should always be administered on time, and doses should not be missed. Monitoring IV sites is essential to maintain patency and drug regimen schedules. Piggybacking other IV medications into the continuous heparin infusion line should be avoided because of the number of drugs that can interact with the heparin, as well as because of the increased irritation that can occur to the vein wall.

Subcutaneous

Low-dose heparin (e.g., administering doses of 5000 units every 8 to 12 hours for prophylaxis of deep vein thrombophlebitis [DVT]) is usually administered subcutaneously. Landmarking injection sites should be done carefully. A dry needle should be used when the injection is made, and it is recommended that the skin roll be gently picked up and *not* pinched. The site is prepared as for other subcutaneous injections (see Chapter 2, "Preparation, Administration, and Monitoring of Medications"); however, the literature suggests that ice be used at the site to reduce hematoma before and after the injection is given. The application of ice (wrapped in a piece of plastic or in a rubber glove) also tends to reduce the pain of the injection. The ice is held against the site for 1 to 2 minutes after the injection. As with other subcutaneous injections, fat pads of the lower abdomen between the iliac crests 5 cm away from the umbilicus or lateral thigh areas are recommended. The site should be free of hematoma, scars, or irritation. Special attention should be given to the rotation of sites, especially if therapy is prolonged. When heparin is administered subcutaneously, it is important that the needle tip not be moved after insertion. Some references suggest that the plunger be carefully aspirated, whereas others recommend that the plunger not be pulled back before the injection of the heparin. A 25-gauge, 1-inch or ⅝-inch needle is used depending on the patient's size. After the heparin is injected, the needle should be carefully withdrawn at the same angle that it was inserted. The skin roll is released and an alcohol swab or sterile gauze is gently pressed to the site for a few minutes to minimize blood oozing. The area should *not* be rubbed, and the patient should be reminded not to rub it.

MONITORING PATIENT RESPONSE
Therapeutic response

Monitoring therapeutic response is especially important in relation to anticoagulant therapy. Monitoring PT for oral anticoagulants and monitoring PTT for heparin are essential in assessing the therapeutic effect and in preventing adverse effects. Heparin PTT should generally be 2 to 2½ times the control value; oral anticoagulants should usually be maintained at a PT of 2 times the control value.

If the patient is receiving intermittent heparin therapy, blood should be drawn for PTT ½ hour before the next dose is scheduled to avoid falsely high readings; blood can be drawn any time after 8 hours of continuous IV heparin therapy using the opposite arm to avoid falsely high readings. A pressure dressing should be applied to the site after the blood is withdrawn. Frequent PTT monitoring is generally not required during low-dose heparin therapy, although incision sites of postoperative patients receiving this therapy prophylactically should be monitored for hematoma formation. They should also be monitored for postoperative complications, including embolism.

Adverse side effects

Monitoring adverse side effects is essential, as is planning to minimize these effects together with the patient and the family, as indicated. Patients receiving anticoagulant therapy should be monitored for early signs of bleeding (e.g., bleeding gums, bruises on the arms and legs, epistaxis, tarry stools, hematuria, hemoptysis, and hematemesis). Any signs indicating bleeding should be readily reported to the prescriber and usually indicate that the drug therapy regimen requires adjustment.

Bleeding can be minimized by encouraging patients to prevent undue injury to themselves by modifying activities (e.g., contact sports) and self-care activities (e.g., using an electric razor for shaving, wearing slippers or shoes at all times when up, using a soft bristle tooth brush).

GENERAL NURSING IMPLICATIONS—cont'd

Nursing of patients requiring anticoagulants—cont'd

Adverse side effects—cont'd

Nurses should be alert to recognize that patients receiving subcutaneous heparin may be more likely to bleed than patients receiving continuous IV heparin therapy. Injection sites should be carefully monitored for hematoma.

Toxicity

Patients requiring anticoagulants should be monitored, and taught to monitor themselves, for excessive anticoagulation resulting in excessive bleeding or hemorrhage. This can occur even when clotting times are within the normal therapeutic range. The patient should know what to do if excessive bleeding should occur including notifying the health care provider immediately and applying firm pressure, if appropriate, to the site. The drug should be discontinued and the excessive bleeding reported to the prescriber immediately. Protamine sulfate should be readily available when patients are receiving heparin, and vitamin K$_1$ (phytonadione) should be readily available for emergency intravenous use for oral anticoagulants (see the Nursing Drug Digest).

PATIENT EDUCATION

Patients receiving anticoagulant therapy in the hospital should be involved as much as possible in their individual drug regimen planning and in monitoring their therapeutic response. Patients requiring long-term anticoagulant therapy as outpatients require careful assessment in relation to their self-medication abilities. Some elderly, psychotic, or alcoholic patients may not be able to be relied on to safely follow their drug therapy regimen without assistance. Most patients, however, are responsible and should be helped to control their conditions and drug regimens. These patients require individualized teaching in relation to their drug regimen and in relation to adaptations in lifestyle that may be indicated. It has been found that careful patient education in these areas has done much to decrease hospital admissions for bleeding and clotting complications.

Patient education should include the following: the prevalence and etiology of the condition, including the importance of clot formation control to prevent serious effects; the generic names of the drugs, how they work, dosage and frequency of administration, side effects, and how side effects can be minimized; the importance of following the drug regimen as planned with the health care provider to maintain control of clot formation; the need for follow-up clinic visits, clotting studies, and check-ups in relation to the control of the condition; the probability, in some instances, of the need for long-term anticoagulant therapy; storage of medications and the importance of checking expiration dates; the modifications of lifestyle indicated; and the signs that indicate the primary health care provider should be notified immediately.

Some of these areas will be discussed in more detail.

Drug schedules

Patients receiving long-term anticoagulant therapy often have confusing drug schedules (e.g., patients on long-term warfarin therapy may be on one of three dosing plans, including a multiple dosage plan, a 5 mg plan, or a 2 mg and 5 mg plan). These patients often need assistance in using calendars and other drug record plans to follow these schedules. Helping the patient to associate medication taking with rituals (e.g., reading the evening newspaper) is often helpful. Patients on these schedules should be warned about mixing various strengths of tablets in the same container and should be encouraged to identify tablets by looking at the number on each tablet to ensure accurate and safe dosage.

Missed dose

Patients sometimes miss a dose and should know what to do if this occurs. Patients receiving long-term coumadin therapy should only take a missed dose if they remember before midnight. If they do not remember until the following morning, the dose should be missed and reported to the clinic. The patient should be warned *not* to make up a missed dose in the same waking day (i.e., they should *not* take an extra dose).

Storage

Storage of anticoagulants should be discussed because potency can be affected by extreme heat. Thus, oral anticoagulants should *not* be stored in the glove compartment of a car when patients are traveling. They also require careful storage out of the reach of children.

Drug interactions

Drug interactions are a major concern because anticoagulants interact with both prescription and nonprescription medications. The patient should be warned about taking other medications without first checking with the clinic or prescriber. In addition, the patient should be warned about using aspirin, which can potentiate anticoagulant effects and cause GI bleeding. Acetaminophen (Tylenol) should be recommended to control mild pain if not contraindicated. Patients should be made aware that aspirin can be found in many nonprescription products.

In addition, patients should be warned to report that they are taking anticoagulant therapy before accepting treatment for other conditions from other health care providers, including nurses, physicians, pharmacists, and dentists. Patients should be encouraged to carry an identification card or to wear a Medic-Alert bracelet stating that they are taking this medication to alert medical or paramedical personnel should an accident or excessive bleeding occur or if emergency surgery is required.

Modifications in lifestyle

Self-care activities require modification to minimize the side effects of anticoagulants and to prevent undue patient injury. The patient should be encouraged to use an electric shaver, to use the softest tooth brush available, to wear shoes or slippers whenever up, to wear gloves while gardening, and to be alert to avoid injury. If an injury occurs, such as a small cut or a bump, the patient should know how to apply firm

Continued.

GENERAL NURSING IMPLICATIONS—cont'd

Nursing of patients requiring anticoagulants—cont'd

Modifications in lifestyle—cont'd

pressure for 5 minutes with a clean gauze or cloth to control and stop the bleeding or to apply an ice pack to the bump to decrease hematoma or bruising. The benefits of vitamin K are questionable because it requires time to act when taken orally; however, patients are sometimes given a supply to control bleeding if necessary. For more serious injury or if bleeding does not stop, the patient should readily seek emergency treatment.

Patients should also be given information about adapting dietary regimens to their anticoagulant therapy. Patients should eat well-balanced diets with normal sized portions of most foods. Patients should not take vitamin preparations containing vitamin K because this can affect the action of the anticoagulant. Patients should consult with their primary health care provider before making dietary changes such as increasing bran in the diet or going on a reducing diet high in fish, dark leafy green vegetables, tomatoes, cauliflower, beef liver, or other vitamin K–rich foods.

Alcohol intake should be limited to 1 or 2 drinks a day (1 drink equals 5 ounces of wine, 1.5 ounces of hard liquor, or 12 ounces of beer). Some clinicians recommend that alcohol be avoided completely.

Patients should be encouraged to limit vigorous physical activity when injury can occur and sports such as horse-back riding or contact sports. Patients should also be cautioned about sitting for long periods, crossing their legs, and wearing constricting clothes.

Patients should know that they should report illness, especially fever, vomiting, or diarrhea to the prescriber or clinic because these conditions can modify anticoagulant absorption. Patients should monitor themselves for early signs of excessive bleeding, including bleeding gums, bruising on the arms and legs, bloody nose, black stools, darkened urine, increased menstrual flow, joint pain, coughing up blood, or vomiting blood. If these are noticed, the prescriber or clinic should be notified immediately and the medication should be stopped.

Nursing of patients requiring platelet aggregation inhibitors

See the Nursing Drug Digest for each specific agent and refer to the section on anticoagulant therapy in this Table for general nursing implications.

GENERAL INSTRUCTIONS FOR DISCHARGE/OUTPATIENTS

VASODILATORS

Take this medication exactly as prescribed.

Do *not* take any other medications without first consulting with your prescriber.

This medication has been prescribed especially for you. Do *not* trade or give this medication to any relatives or friends.

This medication may cause side effects in some people; however, most people experience few if any side effects. Some will disappear after your body gets used to the medication. If side effects are noticed, continue taking your medication. Do not stop taking the medication. If you develop other symptoms or the side effects become severe, notify your primary health care provider.

Until you know how this medication effects you, do *not* drive, operate dangerous machinery that requires alertness, or work in high places.

Keep this and all medication out of the reach of children. It is important that this medication be stored in a tightly closed container and away from heat, in a cool, dry place.

When you are down to your last 2 to 3 days' supply of medication, contact your pharmacist or prescriber to ensure that you do not run out of this medication and that you have a fresh supply.

In addition to the above, if you are taking *nitroglycerin tablets* for chest pain or angina, do not wait until the pain is severe. Sit down immediately. Place one nitroglycerin tablet under your tongue and let it dissolve. Do not chew or swallow the tablet. It is best not to swallow saliva for about 1 minute so the medication can be fully absorbed. You should be able to feel a slight burning

GENERAL INSTRUCTIONS FOR DISCHARGE/OUTPATIENTS—cont'd

VASODILATORS—cont'd

or stinging sensation as the medication dissolves. This indicates that the tablet is still potent. Rest for 15 to 20 minutes to prevent dizziness or fainting, especially if you are elderly.

The nitroglycerin may cause you to feel dizzy or lightheaded. This medication can also cause flushing, rapid heart beat, or headache. The use of alcohol can aggravate these symptoms. If these do occur, they usually do not last long. If they persist or become extreme, notify your nurse or prescriber because you may need to have the dosage changed.

If your pain is not relieved after 3 to 5 minutes, take another nitroglycerin tablet. Do not take more than 3 nitroglycerin tablets for an attack. If the pain persists, notify your nurse or prescriber or go to an emergency room as soon as possible. Keep a record of your attacks, the number of tablets required for relief, and any side effects noted. If the attacks increase or worsen, notify your prescriber.

Store your medication in its original container. Keep it tightly capped and away from heat, light, and moisture, because these can affect the potency of your medication. Remove and discard the cotton plug. Do not store your medication in the bathroom medicine cabinet and do not carry tablets close to your body. Take them with you in a jacket pocket or purse. Do *not* wrap them in tissue or carry them loosely. Carry tablets with you in their original container at all times. Stored carefully, tablets need to be *replaced* only every 3 months.

Take nitroglycerin as directed before any activity that may cause an angina attack, such as physical, sexual, or emotional activities.

Carry an identification card or wear a Medic-Alert bracelet to alert others to your nitroglycerin therapy in case of an emergency.

If you require *nitroglycerin ointment*, administer your ointment exactly as directed on a regular basis regardless of your angina pain. This method of administration should help to prevent the occurrence of angina, help you rest through the night if nocturnal angina is a problem, and also increase your exercise capacity.

Keep a record of your medication use and its effectiveness. Headache, dizziness, and lightheadedness can occur. If these become severe or if fainting occurs, contact your prescriber or clinic nurse immediately.

Your chest, forearm, thighs or abdomen can be used for applying this medication. Try to use a different site with each application. Be sure the skin is clean and dry. Try to use a site with little hair. Measure the desired length of ointment as directed using the special ruler provided and spread it thinly with a tongue depressor over a 4- to 6-inch square area (10 to 15 cm). Do *not* rub the ointment into the skin because this will increase absorption and decrease the sustained effect. Apply plastic wrap over the area and secure it gently with tape. This will keep the ointment from being rubbed off by your clothing and will help it to be absorbed.

Store the tube of nitroglycerin ointment at room temperature. Be sure it is tightly capped and out of the reach of children.

Do not stop taking this medication. If it is to be discontinued it must be done slowly over 4 to 6 weeks according to your prescriber's directions.

ANTILIPEMICS

Follow the instructions on the prescription exactly.

Gastrointestinal upset can be a side effect of many drugs, including this medication. It may help to take this medication along with some food. If the gastrointestinal upset persists, becomes extreme, or if you have nausea, diarrhea, gas, skin rashes, dizziness, or weight gain, notify your clinic nurse or prescriber.

Notify your nurse or prescriber before you start or stop taking any other medications, even over-the-counter medication, while you are taking this medication. Taking other medications with these medications can sometimes cause harmful effects.

Pregnant women or women who are breastfeeding should generally *not* take this medication. Discuss this with your nurse or prescriber before taking this medication. Your nurse can help you explore birth control methods if desired while you are taking this medication to prevent pregnancy.

Store this medication in a dry, dark place. Refrigeration is not required. Keep out of the reach of children.

This medication has been prescribed especially for you. Do not trade or give this medication to any relatives or friends.

In addition to the above, if you are taking *cholestyramine* to reduce the amounts of cholesterol and other naturally occurring fats in the blood, do not take this drug in dry form. Always mix this medication with water, juice, milk, or applesauce. It is best to take this medication before meals. Because this medication can decrease the absorption of certain other medications check with your health care provider about the dosing schedule for other medications you may be taking. Sometimes it is necessary to take vitamin supplements of vitamins A, D, K when you are taking cholestyramine; however, do not take any vitamin preparations unless told to do so by your nurse or prescriber. Your nurse can help you to maintain a balanced diet and help you to select foods in relation to your condition. If you are required to be on a special diet, it is important that you follow it carefully.

ANTICOAGULANTS

Follow the instructions on the prescription exactly. This medication can make you bleed more easily. Use a soft toothbrush, an electric razor, wear shoes or slippers at all times, and avoid contact sports such as football. Take each day's dose at the same time of day. Never take more *or* less medication per day than prescribed.

If you miss a dose, take your medication as soon as you realize that the dose was missed. However, if you do not remember until the next day, do *not* double the doses. Report the missed dose to your clinic nurse or prescriber and

Continued.

GENERAL INSTRUCTIONS FOR DISCHARGE/OUTPATIENTS—cont'd

ANTICOAGULANTS—cont'd

ask for additional information if necessary.

Many drugs can prevent this medication from working the way it is supposed to. Do not stop, start, or change the amount of drugs you are also taking without consulting with your prescriber or clinic nurse.

Aspirin can increase the chance of excessive bleeding while you are taking this medication. Do *not* take aspirin. Do not take any cold medications or non-prescription medications without first talking with your prescriber or clinic nurse, because many of these preparations contain aspirin.

While you are taking this medication you should watch for bleeding of the gums, bruising on the arms and legs, dark urine (pink or brown), black or bloody bowel movements, lower back pain, joint pain or swelling, or heavy bleeding during your menstrual period. If any of these are noted, contact your clinic nurse or prescriber immediately.

While taking this medication you should limit your drinking to 1 to 2 drinks a day (1 drink is 1 glass of wine, 1 beer, or 1 shot of hard liquor).

Eat a balanced diet. Notify your clinic nurse or prescriber before changing your diet. The following foods should be eaten in moderation: dark leafy green vegetables, fish, beef liver, and cauliflower. Do *not* use vitamin preparations that contain vitamin K without consulting with your clinic nurse or prescriber.

If you become ill, have a fever, vomiting, or diarrhea, let your clinic nurse or prescriber know, because these conditions can affect your medication.

Remember to keep clinic appointments or appointments with your prescriber. These are important in relation to monitoring this medication's effects. It is also important that you keep your laboratory appointments so that your blood clotting can be checked accurately.

NURSING DRUG DIGEST

Medication (trade name*)	Indication	Usual dosage and administration	Dosage forms, preparation, and storage	Contraindications, cautions, and comments	Monitoring
VASODILATORS Amyl nitrite	Angina pectoris Cyanide poisoning	*Adults:* Inhale vapors from one ampule, which is crushed in a handkerchief or gauze Have a patient in sitting position during administration Do not administer by parenteral injection	Ampules: 0.18 ml, 0.3 ml (for inhalation)	*Contraindicated in hypersensitivity to nitrites* Repeated use may result in tolerance Vapors are highly flammable and should be kept away from heat or flame (e.g., lighted cigarette) Characteristic pleasant odor Effective within 30 sec, but duration only 4-8 min May increase both intracranial and intraocular pressure and should be used with extreme caution in conditions (e.g., cerebral trauma, glaucoma) that may be adversely affected Dizziness, headache, and flushing of the face are common side effects	Observe for hypotension, tachycardia, and syncope

Continued.

NOTE: For additional details regarding the individual agents listed in this table see the text and other tables in this chapter.
*Indicates a multiple active ingredient product. For a complete listing of all active ingredients see the *Drug Reference Guide to Brand Names and Active Ingredients.*
♦ Indicates that the drug is generally available only in Canada.
★ Indicates that the drug is generally available only in the United States.

NURSING DRUG DIGEST—cont'd

Medication (trade name*)	Indication	Usual dosage and administration	Dosage forms, preparation, and storage	Contraindications, cautions, and comments	Monitoring
Cyclandelate Cyclanfour Cyclospasmol Cydel	Vasospastic impairment of the circulation	*Adults:* 400-1600 mg/day PO in 2 to 4 divided doses Administer 1 hr before or 2 hr after meals to facilitate absorption If severe GI distress occurs, administer with an antacid	Tablets, capsules: 100, 200, 400 mg	*Contraindicated* in hypersensitivity	
Diltiazem Cardizem	Angina pectoris caused by coronary artery spasm and in those patients refractory to treatment with the beta-adrenergic blockers and organic nitrates	*Adults:* 30-60 mg PO q.i.d. Maximum: 360 mg/24 hr	Tablets: 30, 60 mg	*Contraindicated* in hypersensitivity, patients with second- or third-degree AV block, sick sinus syndrome (in the absence of a functioning pacemaker), and severe hypotension May cause hypotension Adverse effects include dizziness, flushing, and headaches	Monitor for bradycardia
Dipyridamole Persantine	Vasospastic impairment of the circulation (see also below)	*Adults:* 50 mg PO t.i.d. Administer 1 hr before or 2 hr after meals to facilitate absorption Administer with a glassful of liquid; if GI distress occurs, administer with a glassful of milk	Tablets: 25, 50, 75 mg	Clinical improvement may not be observed for several months May cause dizziness, headache, or nausea Side effects caused by vasodilation Concurrent use of anticoagulants increases risk of bleeding	Observe for bleeding complications when combined with anticoagulants Observe for hypotension, especially with larger doses
Erythrityl tetrinitrate Cardilate Cardilate-P*	Angina pectoris	*Adults:* 10 mg PO t.i.d. to q.i.d.; or 5-10 mg SL or chewable before emotional or physical stress and at bedtime (for nocturnal angina) as indicated Administer PO dose 1 hr before or 2 hr after meals to facilitate absorption	Tablets: 5, 10, 15 mg Available in oral, sublingual, and chewable forms	*Contraindicated* in hypersensitivity to nitrates	Observe for hypotension

Drug	Uses	Dosage	Dosage forms	Side effects/contraindications	Nursing considerations
Isosorbide dinitrate Carasin Coronex Dilatrate-SR Isoket Isordil Isordil Tembids Isordil Titradose Isotrate Isotrate Timecelles Laserdil Onset Riosordan Sorate Sorbide Sorbitat Sorbitrate Sorbitrate SA Sorquad	Angina pectoris Alteration of loading conditions on left ventricle	*Adults:* Sublingual, 2.5-10 mg q.2-4h; or 10-30 mg PO q.4-6h. Administer with food or milk to decrease GI irritation. Administration with food may also decrease the occurrence of headaches	Tablets, sublingual: 2.5, 5 mg Tablets, chewable: 5, 10 mg Tablets: 5, 10, 20, 30, 40 mg Capsule: 40 mg	*Contraindicated* in the presence of cardiogenic shock *Contraindicated* in hypersensitivity to nitrites. Headache is common. Postural hypotension can be a problem. Prolonged use may result in tolerance. May increase both intracranial and intraocular pressure and should be used with extreme caution in conditions (e.g., cerebral trauma, glaucoma) that may be adversely affected	NOTE: The chewable tablet should be thoroughly chewed and *retained* in the mouth for as long as possible for optimum effect. Monitor blood pressure for hypotension
Isoxsuprine Dilavase Duvadilin Nasodilan Vasodilan Vasoprine	Vasospastic impairment of the circulation. Arrest of premature labor (NOTE: *not* FDA approved use)	*Adults:* 5-10 mg IM b.i.d. to t.i.d.; or 10-20 mg PO t.i.d. to q.i.d. Premature labor, dilute 80 mg in 250 ml D₅W and administer IV at 0.2 mg/min with patient in a left-lateral or semi-Fowler's position; if contractions are not decreased, increase dose every 15 min by 0.1 mg/min until therapeutic response or a maximum dose of 1 mg/min; if contractions stop, decrease dose slowly over 48 hr. Do *not* administer IV to treat cerebrovascular disorders because of increased risk of side effects	Injectable: 5 mg/ml Tablets: 10, 20 mg	*Contraindicated* in immediate postpartum period. Discontinue if severe skin rash develops. Increases blood glucose. Decreases serum potassium	Observe for hypotension and tachycardia with IM use. Monitor contractions (frequency, intensity, duration) when given for premature labor. If administered to manage premature labor; monitor for maternal pulmonary edema and adult respiratory distress syndrome. Monitor maternal blood pressure for hypotension and both mother and fetus for tachycardia. Monitor fluid and electrolyte status, including blood glucose and potassium levels

Continued.

NURSING DRUG DIGEST—cont'd

Medication (trade name)	Indication	Usual dosage and administration	Dosage forms, preparation, and storage	Contraindications, cautions, and comments	Monitoring
Niacin A.C.M.* Cardioguard Nicolar Nico-Metra-zol* Nico-Span Nicobid Nicocap Nicolar Niconacid Nicotinex Nicozol* Novonlacin SK-Niacin Wampocap	Vasospastic impairment of circulation (NOTE: *Not FDA approved use*) See also Antilipemics, p. 749 See also Chapter 66, "Vitamins, Minerals, and Trace Elements"	*Adults:* 0.25-1.0 gm PO t.i.d. or q.i.d. Begin with low dose and increase over several days	Tablets: 50, 100 mg Capsules: 125, 200, 250, 300, 400, 500 mg Oral solution: 50 mg/5 ml Injectable: 10, 50, 100 mg/ml	*Contraindicated* in active peptic ulcer disease, liver dysfunction, and gouty arthritis Flushing of the skin is extremely common	Monitor uric acid levels in patients with gout Observe for hypotension
Nicotinyl alcohol Niacol Radecol Roniacol	Vasospastic impairment of circulation	*Adults:* 150-300 mg PO b.i.d. morning and evening (extended-release tablets); or 50-100 mg t.i.d. (elixir or tablets)	Tablets (extended-release): 150 mg Tablets: 50 mg Elixir: 50 mg/5 ml	*Contraindicated* in active peptic ulcer disease Flushing of the skin is extremely common Use with caution in pregnancy	
Nifedipine Adalat Procardia	Angina pectoris resulting from coronary artery spasm and in patients *not* responsive to beta-adrenergic blockers or organic nitrates	*Adults:* 10-20 mg PO t.i.d. Maximum: 120 mg/24 hr *Elderly:* Start with low dose and gradually increase as tolerated and indicated	Capsule: 10 mg	*Contraindicated* in hypersensitivity; severe hypotension, and pregnancy May cause hypotension Use with caution in patients with heart failure or aortic stenosis Elderly patients may be more susceptible to adverse effects Most common adverse effects include dizziness, headache, nausea, and vomiting Peripheral edema, fluid retention, flushing and heat sensation are also frequently reported	Monitor for hypotension Monitor for fluid retention and edema

Nitroglycerin Angised Cardabid Klavi Cordal Myocon Nitro-Bid Nitro-Dur Nitrobon Nitrodisc Nitroglyn Nitrol Nitrong Nitrospan Nitrostabilin Nitrostat Nitrostat IV Nitrotest Ro-Nitro Susadrin Transderm- Nitro Trates Tridil	Angina pectoris	*Adults:* Sublingual, 0.15–0.6 mg at onset of anginal attack and repeat 5 min apart to a maximum 3 doses per attack (if relief is not obtained, notify prescriber) Maximum: 10 mg/24 hr Sublingual tablets are ineffective if swallowed; proper patient education is necessary Oral (buccal): Dissolve 1 mg in mouth as needed up to q.2h.; *or* (extended-release) 1.3–9 mg PO q.8-12h. as needed Parenteral: 5-150 µg/min IV; start with lowest dose and gradually increase as indicated at 5 min intervals; monitor heart rate and blood pressure continuously during IV infusion Topical, ½-2 inches of 2% ointment; spread evenly over skin (do *not* rub in) Rotate sites of ointment administration to decrease incidence of skin inflammation Wear rubber gloves to prevent absorption while applying ointment Transdermal: Apply 1 unit (containing a 24 hr supply of nitroglycerin) to a clean, hairless, dry area on the upper body at the same time each day Rotate transdermal sites to decrease incidence of skin irritation	Tablets, sublingual: 0.15, 0.3, 0.4, 0.6 mg Transdermal systems: 12.5, 16, 25, 32, 50, 75, 77, 105 mg Tablets, buccal: 1, 2, 3 mg Tablets, extended-release: 1.3, 2.6, 6.5 mg Capsules, extended-release: 2.5, 6.5, 9 mg Topical: 2% ointment in 20, 30, 60 gm tubes Injectable: 10 ml of 1 mg/ml in 9.5% alcohol IV solution must be diluted with sterile NS or D₅W for injection *before* administration Store in dark, dry place with temp 15°-30° C Remaining tablets should be discarded 3 months after opening container; because of loss of potency Do *not* put any packing material (e.g., cotton or tissues) in tablet container because this material may absorb the nitroglycerin and thus reduce the potency of the tablets	*Contraindicated* in severe anemia *Contraindicated* in hypersensitivity to nitrites Headache is common Tingling under tongue and headache indicate medicine is working Postural hypotension can be a problem Do *not* suddenly terminate therapy because withdrawal reactions may occur; should be gradually reduced over 1 month period May increase both intracranial and intraocular pressure and should be used with extreme caution in conditions (e.g., cerebral trauma, glaucoma) that may be adversely affected Tolerance can develop to the effects of nitroglycerin patches (transdermal delivery systems)	Monitor blood pressure for hypotension Observe for development of tolerance with use of transdermal patches
Nylidrin Arlidin Circlidrin Dilatyl Perdilatal Pervadil Rolidrin	Vasospastic impairment of circulation	*Adults:* 6-12 mg PO t.i.d. or q.i.d.	Tablets: 6, 12 mg	*Contraindicated* in thyrotoxicosis, angina pectoris, paroxysmal tachycardia, and acute myocardial infarction Palpitations usually subside as therapy continues	

Continued.

NURSING DRUG DIGEST—cont'd

Medication (trade name)	Indication	Usual dosage and administration	Dosage forms, preparation, and storage	Contraindications, cautions, and comments	Monitoring
Pentaerythritol tetranitrate Angitrate Antora Cartrax* Dilanca Duotrate Plateau El Petn Miltrate* Myocardol Neo-Corvas Pentafin Pentritol Pentryate Peritrate SDM No. 22 SDM No. 23 SDM No. 35 Vasitol Vasodiatoe	Angina pectoris	*Adults:* 10-40 mg PO t.i.d. to q.i.d.; *or* 30-80 mg extended-release formulation PO b.i.d. Administer 1 hr before or 2 hr after meals to facilitate absorption	Tablets: 10, 20, 40 mg Tablets, extended release: 30, 80 mg Capsules, extended-release: 30, 45, 60, 80 mg	*Contraindicated* in hypersensitivity to nitrites May increase both intracranial and intraocular pressure and should be used with extreme caution in conditions (e.g., cerebral trauma, glaucoma) that may be adversely affected Severe persistent headaches may develop in some patients and necessitate discontinuing the medication	Observe for rash; if develops, discontinue medication Observe for hypotension
❦ **Prenylamine** Mostaginan Sedolatan Segontin Synadrin	Vasospastic impairment of the circulation *Long-term management of angina pectoris*	*Adults:* 60 mg PO b.i.d. to q.i.d. Begin with a low dose and increase gradually Administer with food or milk to decrease GI irritation	Tablet: 60 mg	*Contraindicated* in CHF, ventricular conduction disorders, renal and hepatic insufficiency, and hypokalemia Do not administer with MAO inhibitor May cause drowsiness	Monitor renal and hepatic function Monitor pulse and blood pressure Monitor serum potassium
Tolazoline Priscoline Tolzol	Vasospastic impairment of the circulation	*Adults:* 25-50 mg PO q.3-4h.; *or* 10-50 mg IM, IV, SC q.i.d.; *or* 1-2 mg/kg IV over 10 min, then 1-2 mg/kg/hr infusion Begin with a low dose and increase gradually	Tablets: 25, 80 mg Injectable: 25 mg/ml	*Contraindicated* in cerebrovascular accidents *Contraindicated* in active peptic ulcer disease *Contraindicated* in coronary artery disease	Monitor pulse and blood pressure

Flushing of the skin is common
Interaction with alcohol may cause disulfiram-like reaction
Keep patient warm to increase effect of drug

Drug	Uses	Dosage	How Supplied	Remarks	Nursing Implications
Verapamil Calan Cordilox Iproveratril Isoptin Vasolan	Angina pectoris See also Chapter 32, "Antidysrhythmics"	*Adults:* 80-120 mg PO t.i.d. to q.i.d. Maximum: 480 mg/24 hr	Tablets: 80, 120 mg	*Contraindicated* in patients receiving beta-adrenergic blockers (e.g., propranolol) because of the danger of complete heart block. *Contraindicated* in acute myocardial infarction, heart block, severe hypotensive states, and hypersensitivity. Bradycardia, constipation, and hypotension are the most commonly observed side effects. May cause lethargy and edema	Monitor blood pressure and discontinue verapamil if severe hypotension is observed. Monitor heart rate for bradycardia. Observe patient intake and output for signs of constipation. Observe for signs of edema
ANTILIPEMICS **Cholestyramine** Cuemid Questran	Hypercholesterolemia (type IIa) Bile-salt diarrhea	*Adults:* 4-12 gm PO t.i.d. *Must be mixed with juice, milk, or pureed fruit before administration. Interacts with a variety of drugs (see Clinically Significant Drug Interactions); other medication should not be given within 1 hr before or 4 hr after cholestyramine administration. Doses that exceed 24 gm/24 hrs are associated with increased side effects. Do not administer in dry form	Packets: 9 gm. Cans (with measuring scoop): 378 gm. Each level scoop contains 9 gm of cholestyramine resin, equivalent to 4 gm of the anhydrous chloride salt. Powder contains the dye tartrazine that some patients may be allergic to	*Contraindicated* in bile duct obstruction	Observe for signs of vitamin A, D, or K deficiency. Observe for constipation

Continued.

NURSING DRUG DIGEST—cont'd

Medication (trade name)	Indication	Usual dosage & administration	Dosage forms, preparation, and storage	Contraindications, cautions, and comments	Monitoring
Clofibrate Amotril Atromid-S Atromidin Azionyl Claripex Liposid Liprinal Novofibrate Skleromexe	Mixed hypercholesterolemia and hypertriglyceridemia (types IIb, III, and IV)	*Adults:* 1 gm PO b.i.d.	Capsules: 0.5, 1 gm	*Contraindicated* in liver or renal failure *Contraindicated* in pregnancy based on animal studies (e.g., accumulation of drug in rabbit fetus) Interacts with a variety of drugs (see Clinically Significant Drug Interactions) Use extreme caution when anticoagulants are administered concomitantly with clofibrate because a reduction in anticoagulant dose (up to 50%) is required Commonly causes nausea	Observe diabetic patients for hyperglycemia and glycosuria Monitor hepatic function tests (e.g., serum transaminase) Monitor prothrombin time frequently for patients taking anticoagulation medications when clofibrate is started *or* discontinued Monitor serum lipid levels
★ **Colestipol** Colestid	Hypercholesterolemia (type IIa) Bile-salt diarrhea	*Adults:* 5-10 gm PO t.i.d. *Must* be mixed with juice, milk, or pureed fruit before administration Interacts with a variety of drugs (see Clinically Significant Drug Interactions); other medications should not be given within 1 hr before or 4 hr after colestipol administration	Packets: 5 gm Bottle: 500 gm	*Contraindicated* in bile duct obstruction	Observe for signs of vitamin A, D, or K deficiency Observe for constipation
Dextrothyroxine Choloxin	Hypercholesterolemia (type IIa)	*Adults:* 1-8 mg/day as a single dose Administer 1 hr before or 2 hr after meals to facilitate absorption Maximum for patients receiving digitalis glycosides, 4 mg/24 hr	Tablets: 1, 2, 4, 6 mg	*Contraindicated* in hypertension or heart disease *Contraindicated* in iodism *Contraindicated* in severe renal or hepatic disease	Observe for signs of hyperthyroidism (e.g., insomnia, nervousness, weight loss) Observe for angina

Drug and Uses	Dosage and Administration	Supply and Storage	Remarks
	Children: 0.05 to 1 mg/kg/24 hr PO Maximum: 4 mg/24 hr NOTE: Start dosage low and increase slowly at *monthly* intervals		*Contraindicated* in pregnancy and in nursing mothers Can produce syndrome identical to hyperthyroidism and interacts with anticoagulants, digitalis cardiac glycosides, and hypoglycemics May precipitate cardiac dysrhythmias during surgery and is usually discontinued 2 wks before elective surgery in euthyroid patients
Niacin A.C.M.* Cal-M* Magacin* Nicamin Nico-Metra-zol* Nico-Span Nico-400 Nicobid Nicocap Nicolar Niconacid Nicotinex Nicozol* Novoniacir SK-Niacin Wampocap Hypercholesterolemia and mixed hypercholesterolemia (types IIa, IIb, III, IV and V) See also Vasodilators, p. 744 See also Chapter 66, "Vitamins, Minerals, and Trace Elements"	*Adults:* 0.25 to 1.0 gm PO t.i.d. or q.i.d. Administer with food or milk to decrease gastric irritation and flushing Administer, if necessary, with *cold* water to facilitate swallowing Begin with a low dose and increase gradually Maximum: 6 gm/day	Tablets: 25, 50, 100, 200, 250, 300, 500, 625 mg Capsules: 25, 50, 100, 200, 250, 300, 500, 625 mg	*Contraindicated* in active peptic ulcer disease, liver dysfunction, and gouty arthritis Flushing of the skin is common Observe for hypotension Monitor uric acid levels of patients with gout
Probucol Lorelco Hypercholesterolemia and mixed hypercholesterolemia (types IIa and IIb)	*Adults:* 0.5 gm PO b.i.d. with AM and PM meals *Children: Not* recommended	Tablets: 0.25 gm Store in dark, dry place with temperature 15°-30°C (60°-85° F) Dispense in light-resistant containers	*Contraindicated* in hypersensitivity Should *not* be combined with clofibrate Diarrhea occurs in approximately 10% of patients Observe for diarrhea

Continued.

NURSING DRUG DIGEST—cont'd

Medication (trade name)	Indication	Usual dosage and administration	Dosage forms, preparation, and storage	Contraindications, cautions, and comments	Monitoring
ANTICOAGULANTS					
Acenocoumarol Sinthrome Sintrom	Thromboembolic disease and other indications for anticoagulation	*Adults:* Maintenance, 2-10 mg/day given as a single dose to keep PTT 2-2½ times control value. Administer dose at same time each day. When therapy is discontinued, it is usually recommended to gradually taper off the dose over 3-4 weeks	Tablets: 1, 4 mg	*Contraindicated* in active bleeding states, severe hypertension, and pericarditis. *Contraindicated* in recent or planned CNS or eye surgery. Interacts with a wide variety of medications (see Clinically Significant Drug Interactions). Patient understanding and compliance are crucial and must be assured through proper education	Prothrombin time must be monitored especially whenever other drugs are started *or* discontinued. Monitor patient for over anticoagulation (e.g., bleeding gums, tarry stools, bruises) and notify prescriber at first signs
Dicumarol Dicuman Dufalone	Thromboembolic disease and other indications for anticoagulation	*Adults:* Maintenance, 25-200 mg/day as a single dose to keep prothrombin time 1½-2 times control value	Tablets: 25, 50, 100 mg Capsules: 25, 50 mg	Minor overdose may be treated with 2.5-10 mg PO of vitamin K₁ (phytonadione). If minor bleeding persists, vitamin K₁ 5-25 mg may be administered parenterally, preferably IV slowly *not* exceeding a rate of 1 mg/min. In severe cases of bleeding (overdose) it may be necessary to transfuse whole blood or fresh-frozen plasma. See Acenocoumarol	See Acenocoumarol

Heparin Calciparine Depo-Heparin Hepalean Heparinar Hepathrom Lipo-Hepin Liquaemin Minihep Panheprin	Thromboembolic disease and other indications for anticoagulation	*Adults:* IV bolus (5000-10,000 units) and IV infusion (500-2000 units/hr) to keep PTT 2-2½ times control value; or bolus (5000-10,000 units) and intermittent infusion (3000-6000 units) q.4h. to keep PTT 2-2½ times control value SC 5000-20,000 units q.8-12h. keep PTT 2-2½ times control value *Children:* 50 units/kg IV initially, followed by 50 units/kg IV q.4h. to keep PTT 2-2½ times control value Administration of *large* doses should normally be delayed for 4 hr following surgery Administer by deep SC injection to minimize irritation IM administration *not* recommended	Do *not* freeze Injectable: 100, 1000, 5000, 10,000, 15,000, 20,000, 25,000, 30,000, 40,000 units/ml	*Contraindicated* in hypersensitivity *Contraindicated* in active bleeding disorders and severe hypertension Does *not* cross placenta and is thus the anticoagulant of choice during pregnancy Apply pressure dressings after taking blood samples Use of a small test dose (1000 units) is recommended in patients with a history of allergies Protamine sulfate (1 mg/100 units heparin) is an effective antidote for heparin overdose Administer protamine sulfate by slow IV; use a 1% solution and do *not* administer more than 50 mg in any 10 min period May cause thrombocytopenia, usually mild during first few days of therapy When used IV, PTT must always be monitored (especially when *any* other drug is started *or* discontinued) Monitor patient for over anticoagulation (e.g., bleeding gums, bruises, tarry stools) and notify prescriber at first sign Observe for delayed-onset thrombocytopenia

Continued.

NURSING DRUG DIGEST—cont'd

Medication (trade name)	Indication	Usual dosage and administration	Dosage forms, preparation, and storage	Contraindications, cautions, and comments	Monitoring
Phenindione Danilone Hedulin Indon	Thromboembolic disease and other indications for anticoagulation	*Adults:* Maintenance, 50-150 mg/day PO given in divided doses (b.i.d.) to keep prothrombin time 1½-2 times control value	Tablet: 50 mg	See Acenocoumarol	See Acenocoumarol
★ **Phenprocoumon** Liquamar Marcumar	Thromboembolic disease and other indications for anticoagulation	*Adults:* Maintenance, 0.75-6 mg/day given as a single dose to keep prothrombin time 1½-2 times control value	Tablet: 3 mg	See Acenocoumarol	See Acenocoumarol
Warfarin Athrombin-K Coufarin Coumadin Marevan Panwarfin Warcoumin Warfilone Warnerin	Thromboembolic disease and other indications for anticoagulation	*Adults:* Maintenance: 2-10 mg/day given as a single dose to keep prothrombin time 1½-2 times control value	Tablets: 2, 2.5, 5, 7.5, 10 mg	See Acenocoumarol Use during first trimester of pregnancy is associated with teratogenesis of nasal cartilage Use during last trimester of pregnancy must be stopped 1 mo before delivery to prevent fetal hemorrhage	See Acenocoumarol
PLATELET AGGREGATION INHIBITORS					
Aspirin Acetophen Acetyl-Sal Anacin* Arthritis Pain Formula* A.S.A. Asasantine* Ascodeen-30* Ascriptin A/D* Ascriptin* Astrin ASA	Some forms of thromboembolic disease See also Chapter 17, "Analgesics and Narcotic Antagonists," and Chapter 58, "Nonsteroidal Antiinflammatory Drugs"	*Adults:* 0.3 to 1.0 gm/day PO as single or divided dose (t.i.d.) Should be administered with food or milk to decrease GI irritation	Tablets, capsules: 65, 75, 81, 160, 325, 425, 500, 600, 650 mg Suppositories: 65, 130, 195, 325, 650, 1300 mg Packet: 850 mg	*Contraindicated* in active bleeding *Contraindicated* in hypersensitivity to salicylates *Contraindicated* in G-6-PD deficiency Concurrent use of alcohol is dangerous, as is administration to patients taking oral anticoagulants because of increased risk of bleeding	Observe for hypersensitivity reactions Observe for bleeding tendencies

Drug	Uses	Form / Dosage	Contraindications / Interactions	Nursing Considerations
Bayer Aspirin, Bayer Timed Release Aspirin, Bufferin*, Easprin, Ecotrin, Empirin Compound*				May cause GI irritation
Clofibrate Amotril, Atromid-S, Atromidin, Azionyl, Claripex, Liposid, Liprinal, Novofibrate, Skleromexe	Some forms of thromboembolic disease (NOTE: Not FDA approved use) (see also Antilipemics, p. 748)	Capsules: 0.5, 1 gm; *Adults:* 1 gm PO b.i.d.	*Contraindicated* in significant liver or renal impairment; *Contraindicated* in pregnancy; Interacts with a wide variety of drugs (see Clinically Significant Drug Interactions); Concurrent use of anticoagulants increases risk of bleeding	Observe diabetic patients for hyperglycemia and glycosuria; Monitor hepatic function tests (e.g., serum transaminase); Monitor prothrombin time frequently for patients taking anticoagulation medications when clofibrate is started or stopped
Dipyridamole Persantine	Some forms of thromboembolic disease (NOTE: Not FDA approved use) (see also Vasodilators, p. 742)	Tablets: 25, 50, 75 mg; *Adults:* 100 mg PO q.i.d. Administer 1 hr before or 2 hrs after meals to facilitate absorption; Administer with a glassful of milk if GI distress occurs	Side effects caused by vasodilation; Concurrent use of anticoagulants increases risk of bleeding	Observe for hypotension
Sulfinpyrazone Anturan, Anturane, Anturidin, Enturen, Zynol	Some forms of thromboembolic disease (NOTE: Not FDA approved use) See also Chapter 37, "Drugs Used to Treat Urinary Tract Disorders"	Tablets: 100, 200 mg; *Adults:* 200 mg PO t.i.d. or q.i.d. Should be administered with food or milk to decrease GI irritation; Maximum: 1000 mg/day	*Contraindicated* in hypersensitivity to pyrazole derivatives (e.g., phenylbutazone), and active peptic ulcer disease	Monitor blood counts; Observe for skin rash; if occurs, discontinue medication

BIBLIOGRAPHY

Abrams, J. Usefulness of long-acting nitrates in cardiovascular disease. *American Journal of Medicine*, 1978, *64*, 183-186.

Abrams, J. Nitrate tolerance and dependence. *American Heart Journal*, 1980, *99*, 113-123.

Anturan Reinfarction Italian Study. Sulfinpyrazone in postmyocardial infarction. *Lancet*, 1982, *1*, 237-242.

Bourbonnais, F. Nitroglycerin, using a familiar drug in new ways. *The Canadian Nurse*, 1981, *77*, 24-26.

Butler, J.D., & Harrison, B.L. Keeping pace with calcium channel blockers. *Nursing 83*, 1983, *13*, 38-43.

Chamberlain, S.L. Low-dose heparin therapy. *American Journal of Nursing*, 1980, *80*, 1115-1117.

Chatterjee, K., & Parmley, W.W. Vasodilator treatment for acute and chronic heart failure. *British Heart Journal*, 1977, *39*, 706-720.

Cipolle, R.J., Seifert, R.D., Neilan, B.A., Zaske, D.E., & Haus, E. Heparin kinetics: variables related to disposition and dosage. *Clinical Pharmacology and Therapeutics*, 1981, *29*, 387-393.

Danagy, D.T., Burwell, D.T., Aronow, W.S., & Prakash, R. Sustained hemodynamic and antianginal effect of high dose oral isosorbide dinitrate. *Circulation*, 1977, *55*, 381-387.

Dossey, B., & Passons, J.M. Pulmonary embolism—preventing it, treating it. *Nursing 81*, 1981, *11*, 26-33.

Drake, M., & Shin, C. Conversion of ischemic to hemorrhagic infarction by anticoagulant administration: report of two cases with evidence from serial computed tomographic brain scans. *Archives of Neurology*, 1983, *40*, 44-46.

Fuller, E.O. The effect of antianginal drugs on myocardial oxygen consumption. *American Journal of Nursing*, 1980, *80*, 250-254.

Fung, H.L., McNiff, E.F., Ruggirello, D., Darke, A., Thadani, U., & Parker, J.O. Kinetics of isosorbide dinitrate and relationships to pharmacological effects. *British Journal of Clinical Pharmacology*, 1981, *11*, 579-590.

Gronim, S.S. Helping the client with unstable angina. *American Journal of Nursing*, 1978, *78*, 1677-1680.

Hansen, M.S., & Woods, S.L. Nitroglycerin ointment—where and how to apply it. *American Journal of Nursing*, 1980, *80*, 1122-1124.

Heel, R.C., Brogden, R.N., Pakes, G.E., Speight, T.M., & Avery, G.S. Colestipol: a review of its pharmacological properties and therapeutic efficacy in patients with hypercholesterolaemia. *Drugs*, *1980*, *19*, 161-180.

Heparin clots: a dangerous anomaly. *Nurses' Drug Alert*, 1984, *8*, 41-42.

Hill, N.S., Antman, E.M., Green, L.H., & Alpert, J.S. Intravenous nitroglycerin: a review of pharmacology, indications, therapeutic effects and complications. *Chest*, 1981, *79*, 69-76.

Howard, T., Hoy, R.H., Warren, S., Georgiev, M., & Selinger, H. Acute renal dysfunction due to sulfinpyrazone therapy in postmyocardial infarction cardiomegaly: reversible hypersensitive interstitial nephritis. *American Heart Journal*, 1981, *102*, 294-295.

Leonard, R.G., & Talbert, R.L. Calcium-channel blocking agents. *Clinical Pharmacy*, 1982, *1*, 17-33.

Lundin, D.V. You can inject heparin subcutaneously. *RN*, 1978, *41*(12), 51-54.

MacCannell, K.L., & Wyse, D.G. Pharmacologic management: cardiovascular drugs. In N.K. Wenger, J.W. Hurst, & M.C. McIntyre (Eds.). *Cardiology for Nurses*. New York: McGraw-Hill Book Co., 1980.

Mason, D.T. (Ed.). Symposium on vasodilator and inotropic therapy of heart failure. *American Journal of Medicine*, 1978, *65*, 101.

Mehta, J., & Mehta, P. Topical nitroglycerin for ischemic heart disease. *Journal of the American Medical Association*, 1979, *241*, 2649-2651.

Milner, J.A., & Conti, R. Status of antiplatelet drugs in coronary heart disease. *Journal of the American Medical Association*, 1978, *239*, 2166-2167.

Nitroglycerin patches. *The Medical Letter*, 1984, *26*, 59-60.

Patras, A.Z., Palce, J.A., & Lanigan, K. Managing GI bleeding: it takes a two-tract mind. *Nursing '84*, 1984, *14*, 26-33.

Purcell, J.A., & Holder, C.K. Intravenous nitroglycerin. *American Journal of Nursing*, 1982, *82*, 254-259.

Report of the Anturane Reinfarction Trial Policy Committee. The anturane reinfarction trial: reevaluation of outcome. *New England Journal of Medicine*, 1982, *306*, 1005-1008.

Rosenberg, J.M., & Kirschenbaum, J.L. What to watch for with heparin. *RN*, 1981, *44*, 50-52.

The Anturane Reinfarction Trial Research Group: Sulfinpyrazone in the prevention of sudden death after myocardial infarction. *New England Journal of Medicine*, 1980, *302*, 250-256.

Thompson, D.A. Teaching the client about anticoagulants. *American Journal of Nursing*, 1982, *82*, 278-281.

Vanbree, N.S., Hollerbach, A.D., & Brooks, G.P. Clinical evaluation of three techniques for administering low-dose heparin. *Nursing Research*, 1984, *33*(1), 15-19.

Verstraete, M. Antiplatelet agents in coronary disease: are they of prophylactic value? *Drugs*, 1978, *15*, 464-471.

Warren, S.E., & Francis, G.S.: Nitroglycerin and nitrate esters. *American Journal of Medicine*, 1979, *65*, 53-62.

Wessler, S., & Gitel, S.N. Warfarin: from bedside to bench. *New England Journal of Medicine*, 1984, *311*, 645-652.

Worthington de Toledo, L. How vasodilators backfire (and when to expect it). *RN*, 1982, *45*, 41-45.

Yacone, L.A. Is it an MI? *RN*, 1981, *44*, 53-59, 100.

RENAL MEDICATIONS

Medications discussed in this section

Review of the Anatomy, Physiology, and Assessment of the Renal System

John B. Dossetor
Thavisakdi Kovithavongs

The renal system is involved in the regulation of many body functions and in the excretion of waste products and numerous drugs. Renal function can be affected directly and indirectly by many medications such as diuretics and antidiuretics, and numerous drugs are used in treating urinary tract disorders. An understanding of the anatomy, physiology, and assessment of the renal system is essential to understand the mechanism of action of drugs affecting renal function and of the drugs used in treating urinary tract disorders. Because numerous drugs are excreted by the kidneys, it is especially important that the nurse be able to assess normal renal function and to identify signs of dysfunction readily, because renal dysfunction can affect drug selection and dosing. In addition, renal toxicity can be caused by certain drugs, including aminoglycosides. The nurse's role in monitoring patient response and promoting renal function when these drugs are required is essential so that toxicity or dysfunction can be prevented or minimized as much as possible.

This chapter presents a brief overview of the assessment of the renal system, including a discussion of the anatomic structures included in this system. The physiologic functions of the kidney are then reviewed. Following this chapter, diuretics and antidiuretics and drugs used to treat urinary tract disorders are discussed.

ANATOMY AND ASSESSMENT REVIEW

The kidneys are two bean-shaped organs located in the dorsal part of the abdomen in the retroperitoneal space at each side of the vertebral column. The upper pole of each kidney is approximately at the level of the twelfth thoracic vertebra, with the caudal aspect at the level of the third lumbar vertebra. The right kidney is usually in a slightly lower position than the left kidney.

Each kidney in the adult measures approximately 11 cm in length and is 6 cm wide and 2.5 cm thick. Each kidney weighs from 115 to 170 gm depending on body size and sex (approximately 1% of body weight). The kidneys are, however, proportionately 3 times larger in the neonate, compared with the adult.

The function of the kidneys is to produce and eliminate urine through a complex filtration system comprised of approximately 2 million nephrons. Each nephron is composed of glomeruli and renal tubules that regulate water and salt balance. Renal function can be measured by means of various laboratory tests, including creatinine clearance (CrCl), serum creatinine, blood urea nitrogen (BUN), and serum electrolyte determinations, as well as by urinalysis. Aspects of health assessment (e.g., pitting edema) can also be used to determine renal function.

The kidneys and related structures are assessed during examination of the abdomen during the health assessment, although general inspection of the patient can identify renal function, including excesses and deficits in fluid and electrolyte balance. Signs such as moist rales, orthopnea, edema (e.g., periorbital, sacral, dependent), elevated blood pressure, and ascites can alert the nurse to fluid excess, whereas signs such as poor skin turgor, deep furrowed tongue, depressed fontanel in the infant, and dry mucous membranes can alert the nurse to fluid volume deficit.

The right and left adrenal gland and the upper poles of the right and left kidneys are found in the right and left upper quadrants, respectively, or the right and left hypochondriac regions if a nine-region approach is used as opposed to dividing the abdomen into quadrants. The lower poles or caudal aspects of the right and left kidneys can be found in the right and left lower quadrants or right and left lumbar regions. The right and left ureters are found in the right and left lower quadrants with the bladder at the midline. In the nine region approach, the right and left ureters would be found in the right and left inguinal or iliac regions and the bladder in the hypogastric region.

Inspection of the abdomen should be completed carefully because distention of the abdomen can be caused by gas or fluid in the bowel or abdominal cavity. Prolonged distention can cause the abdomen to appear tense, smooth, and shiny. If the distention is caused by fluid, the flanks may bulge when the patient is supine and the lower abdomen may protrude when the patient stands or sits. Inspection should be followed by auscultation with special attention to the renal arteries.

The renal arteries bifurcate from the aorta at approximately the tenth rib. The renal arteries should be auscultated for bruits. Soft medium- to low-pitched murmurs may be heard with the bell of the stethoscope in the area over the upper midline or toward the flank on either side of the abdomen. If heard, these sounds may be indicative of renal arterial stenosis. If the patient has a history of hypertension, the area over the center and posterior flanks should be carefully auscultated for bruit in the arterial tree.

Percussion follows auscultation in examining the abdomen. Beginning at the sternum, tympany is heard to the symphysis pubis where the sound normally changes to dullness. Dullness directly above the symphysis pubis is indicative of a full or distended bladder. Percussion is used to define the outline of the distended bladder, which may extend up to the umbilicus. Flatness is an abnormal sound. A dull sound above the symphysis pubis may indicate fluid in the abdomen. The examiner can percuss for a fluid wave to determine the presence or absence of fluid. One can find free floating intraabdominal fluid or encapsulated fluid within the bowel through percussion of the abdomen with the patient in different positions. Fluid within the abdominal cavity should be mobile and shift in the direction of gravity pull. Excessive fluid within the bowel does not significantly shift in the direction of gravity pull when the patient's position is changed.

Palpation can be used to assess kidney tenderness and is best performed with the patient in the supine position. Light palpation should precede deep palpation.

Palpation of the kidney is performed by pressing directly upward beneath the costal margin at the midclavicular line while the patient is asked to take a deep breath. As the diaphragm is displaced downward, the inferior margin of the kidney is likewise depressed and

may be felt. Because it is anatomically lower than the left kidney, the right kidney is more apt to be palpated with this technique.

Deep palpation of the kidneys can also be performed by having the patient in the supine position with the examiner at the right side. For the left kidney, the examiner reaches across the patient with the left arm and places the hand behind the patient's left flank. The left flank is then elevated with the examiner's fingers so the kidney is displaced anteriorly. The right palmar surface of the examiner's hand is used in deep palpation through the abdominal wall. The examiner remains on the patient's right side and then examines the right kidney, which is similarly elevated with the left hand. The lower pole of the right kidney may be felt with deep palpation as a smooth rounded mass that descends on inspiration. In general, the kidneys are not palpable in the normal adult, although the lower pole of the right kidney, when the abdominal musculature is relaxed, may be felt in the neonate, a thin child or adult, or a thin elderly person who has lost muscle tone and elastic fibers. The left kidney is generally not palpable. Located behind the symphysis pubis, the bladder is not normally palpable in the adult unless it is distended with urine. When distended it may be felt as a smooth, round, tense mass.

The final step in the abdominal assessment of the kidney is an inspection of the back with the patient in a sitting position. The flanks are inspected for symmetry. Fullness of the flanks or asymmetry may be indicative of renal disorders. Direct or indirect fist percussion at the costovertebral margin may also be completed at this time to further assess tenderness.

PHYSIOLOGY REVIEW

The three major physiologic functions of the kidney are (1) the excretion of nitrogenous end products of metabolism, (2) the maintenance of salt concentrations and the volume of body fluids (homeostasis of the body internal environment), and (3) certain hormonal and metabolic functions, including metabolism, production of renin and erythropoietin, and the final step in making 1,25-di-OH-cholecalciferol (see Chapter 62, "Parathyroid Hormone, Calcitonin, and Related Medications").

A fourth aspect, of importance to the subject matter of this text, is the excretion of drugs and their metabolic derivatives. Thus, when kidney function is impaired, it is of great clinical importance to reduce the dose of certain drugs (i.e., those excreted through the kidney) whereas the dose of others (i.e., those not excreted by the kidney) is unaffected (see boxed material).

Partial list of drugs excreted through the kidneys for which either (1) a decrease in dose or (2) an increase in the interval between doses should be considered in the presence of decreased renal function.

Amiloride	Flucytosine
Ampicillin	Furosemide
Carbenicillin	Gentamicin
Cefazolin	Kanamycin
Cephacetrile	Methicillin
Cephalexin	Nafcillin
Cephaloridine	Oxacillin
Cephalothin	Penicillin G
Chlorpropamide	Procainamide
Clindamycin	Streptomycin
Cloxacillin	Sulfadimethoxine
Colchicine	Sulfamethazine
Colistimethate	Sulfamethoxazole
Diazoxide	Sulfamethoxypyridazine
Dicloxacillin	Tetracycline
Digoxin	Tobramycin
Erythromycin	Trimethoprim
Ethambutol	Vancomycin

Modified and reproduced with permission from Pagliaro, L., & Benet, L. Critical compilation of terminal half-lives, percent excreted unchanged, and changes of half-life in renal and hepatic dysfunction for studies in humans with references. *Journal of Pharmacokinetics and Biopharmaceutics*, 1975, *3*, 333-383.

The principal nitrogenous substances requiring excretion in the urine are (1) urea, (2) uric acid, and (3) creatinine. There are, of course, many other substances being excreted as by-products of other metabolic processes, but quantitatively they are much less than these three. On occasion carbohydrate is excreted as glucose or pentose, or, rarely, as galactose. Fat metabolism, when incomplete, may be reflected in the urine as acetoacetate or ketoacid anion (β-OH-butyrate). When this occurs, hydrogen ions (H^+) are also produced and, to avoid progressive acidosis, these also require excretion.

Figure 35-1 gives the ionic composition of the extracellular fluid (ECF) and intracellular fluid (ICF) and from these concentrations the osmolarity can be calculated or measured by osmometry. Disturbances in body electrolytes, the result of a loss of these fluids, cause not only electrolyte depletion states, but also altered acid-base balance with a change in the free

hydrogen ion concentration [H^+] (see Chapter 67, "Fluids and Electrolytes").

The whole question of hydrogen ions in the body is made more complex because the end product of so much of the body's fat and carbohydrate metabolism is carbon dioxide. This forms free hydrogen ions when it comes to react with body water molecules under the catalysis of carbonic anhydrase:

$$CO_2 + HOH \rightarrow CO_2OH^- \text{ (or } HCO_3^-) + H^+$$

All of the hydrogen cations formed in this way come from body water (they do *not* come from energy metabolism) and eventually recombine at the lungs with their appropriate hydroxyl ion, when the hydroxyl ion-bound CO_2 is released again.

Thus, excretion of CO_2 *does not* represent hydrogen ion excretion. How can it, when no hydrogen ions are in fact excreted at the lungs? But during transport of CO_2 from the tissues to lungs many hydrogen ions are temporarily generated (i.e., 14,400 mmole in 24 hours or 10 mmole per minute) and can thus cause profound changes in the acid-base balance when there is any imbalance in the rate at which the 10 mmole per minute of OH^- is generated at the lung alveolar membrane. The reaction is

$$HCO_3^- \text{ (or } CO_2 \times OH^-) \rightarrow OH^- + CO_2 \uparrow$$

The only hydrogen ions the body produces from metabolism are sulfuric acid (from oxidation of protein sulfhydril, -SH, groups) phosphoric acid (from organic phosphate), lactic acid, or β-OH-butyric acid (Figure 35-2). Thus, hydrogen ion metabolism, although complicated by the CO_2 transport effects, should be looked on as part of the cation control of the body. The renal excretion of hydrogen ions, therefore, is just another cation excretion system.

In addition to high concentrations of anions and cations in ECF and ICF, there is a small, but vitally important, concentration of H^+ cation present in such a low concentration of 40 nEq/L (i.e., 40×10^{-6} mEq/L) that it cannot be drawn in a diagram such as Figure 35-1.

The concentration of this cation is generally expressed in pH units; however, it may be better to express the acidity of a solution in terms of its free H^+ concentration in nEq/L. This concentration of free hydrogen ions is in equilibrium with the anions that readily accept or give up H^+ ions. Such anions are also termed buffer anions, or more simply just buffers. In plasma, the important hydrogen ion acceptor anions are HCO_3^-, HPO_4^{--}, and proteinate. It is difficult adequately to represent the free hydrogen ion component of plasma accurately in such a diagram as Figure 35-1, and Figure 35-3 is an attempt to show this.

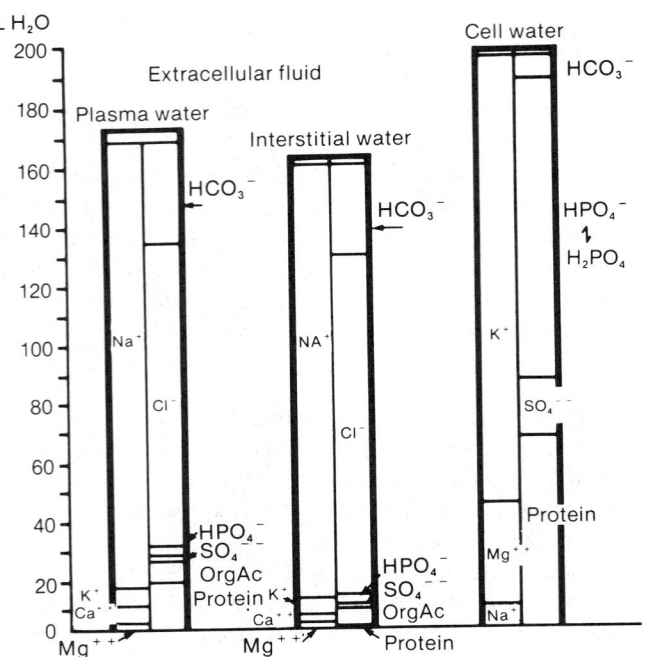

mEq/L H₂O

For plasma water, mEq/L

Na⁺	145	HCO₃⁻	26.5
K⁺	5	Cl⁻	100
Ca⁺⁺	5	Oth	20
Mg⁺⁺	1.5	Prot⁻	10
	156.5		156.5
	Cations		Anions

For cell water, mEq/L

		HCO₃⁻	8
K⁺	160	HPO₄⁻	120
Mg⁺⁺	35	SO₄⁻⁻	20
Na⁺	10	Prot	57
	205		205
	Cations		Anions

FIGURE 35-1. **Ionic composition of the extracellular fluid, which includes the plasma water and the interstitial water, and the intracellular fluid (cell water).**

CO₂ and H⁺

Production and Excretion

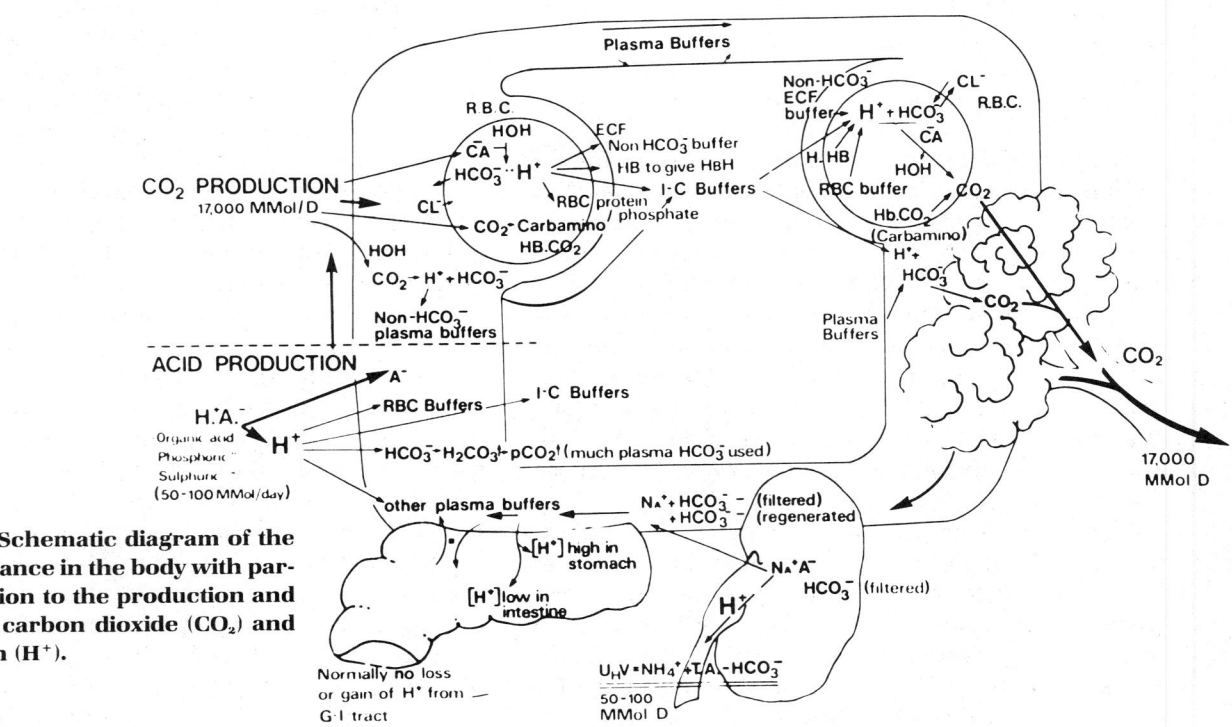

FIGURE 35-2. **Schematic diagram of the acid-base balance in the body with particular attention to the production and excretion of carbon dioxide (CO₂) and hydrogen ion (H⁺).**

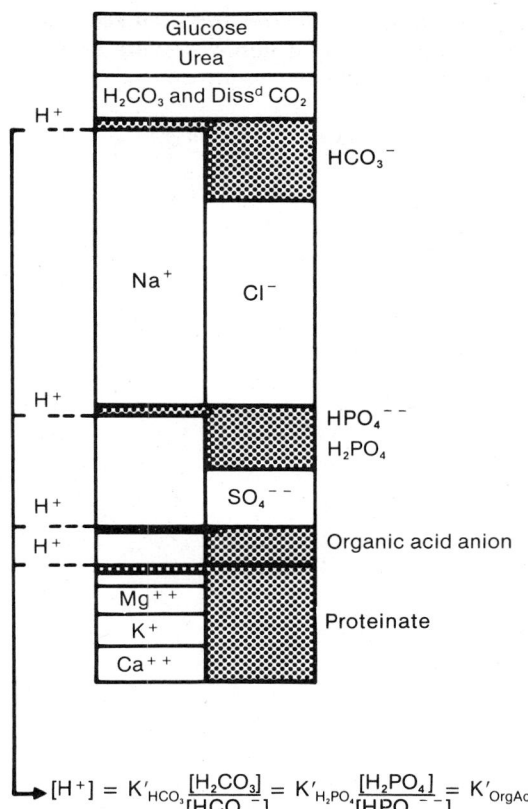

FIGURE 35-3. **Principal electrolytes found in the body fluids represented in terms of cation-anion balance (see also Chapter 67, "Fluids and Electrolytes").**

$$[H^+] = K'_{HCO_3}\frac{[H_2CO_3]}{[HCO_3^-]} = K'_{H_2PO_4}\frac{[H_2PO_4]}{[HPO_4^{--}]} = K'_{OrgAc}\frac{[H_{OrgAc}]}{[OrgAc]} = K'_{Prot}\frac{[HPROT]}{[PROT^-]}$$

Similar reversible cation binding occurs with sodium, too, in bone, and the same principle is employed in cation exchange resins. From a knowledge of the actual concentration and of the acid dissociation constants, or K' values, it is possible to calculate exactly which basic anion is in equilibrium with which portion of the free hydrogen ions. It pays to think of the hydrogen ion as just another cation with certain unique properties that are responsible for keeping its concentration in plasma and cells between the absolute extremes of 20 and 100 nEq/L, with a norm about 40 nEq/L.

An understanding of the renal physiology of salt and water is quite important in the following disease states or abnormal conditions: salt or water deprivation, excessive administration of intravenous infusions or blood transfusions, abuse of diuretic agents (most of which are natriuretics), the effects on body fluids of sustained osmotic diuresis (such as uncontrolled glycosuria in diabetes mellitus), the important homeostatic limitations imposed by chronic renal failure, the nature of electrolyte disturbances in the diuretic phase of acute renal failure, and the effects of excessive endogenous secretion of the antidiuretic hormone.

We may now turn attention to the way by which the kidney maintains homeostasis. We will look first at *renal blood flow*, because it has some unusual features. Why does one quarter of the heart's output of blood go through two structures that together do not weigh more than about 1% of the body weight? Certainly the blood flow to the kidneys is far in excess of that required for renal metabolism. Thus, even when the tubules are reabsorbing maximally from a copious amount of filtrate, under maximal stimuli for salt and water conservation, so little of the oxygen is removed that the renal veins are bright red (arterial) in color. This fact is used by radiologists when attempting to catheterize renal veins for investigative purposes. This unusual blood flow of 500 to 580 ml/min is responsible for the formation of 100 to 120 ml/min of glomerular filtrate of which over 99% is usually absorbed. This filtrate is a low-protein ultrafiltrate of plasma.

Reabsorption of glomerular filtrate in the nephron

The two types of nephron, as seen in Figure 35-4, are an outer set and a deeper set of cortical glomeruli. Most filtration occurs in the outer two thirds of cortical glomeruli where the blood flow is rapid, whereas the innermost one third of glomeruli (so-called juxtamedullary) appear to be adapted for more rapid transit of blood across to the venous side where it passes down

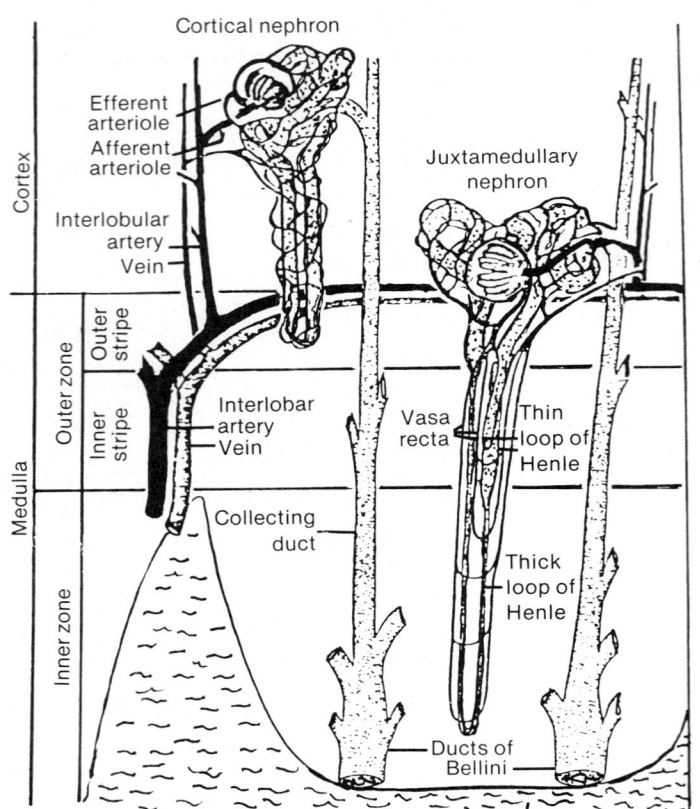

Cortical nephron

Efferent
arteriole
Afferent
arteriole

Interlobular
artery
Vein

Juxtamedullary
nephron

Cortex

Outer stripe

Outer zone

Inner stripe

Medulla

Inner zone

Interlobar
artery
Vein

Collecting
duct

Vasa
recta

Thin
loop of
Henle

Thick
loop of
Henle

Ducts of
Bellini

FIGURE 35-4. **Diagram of the cortex and medulla of the kidney, illustrating two types of nephrons, the cortical nephron and the juxtamedullary nephron.**

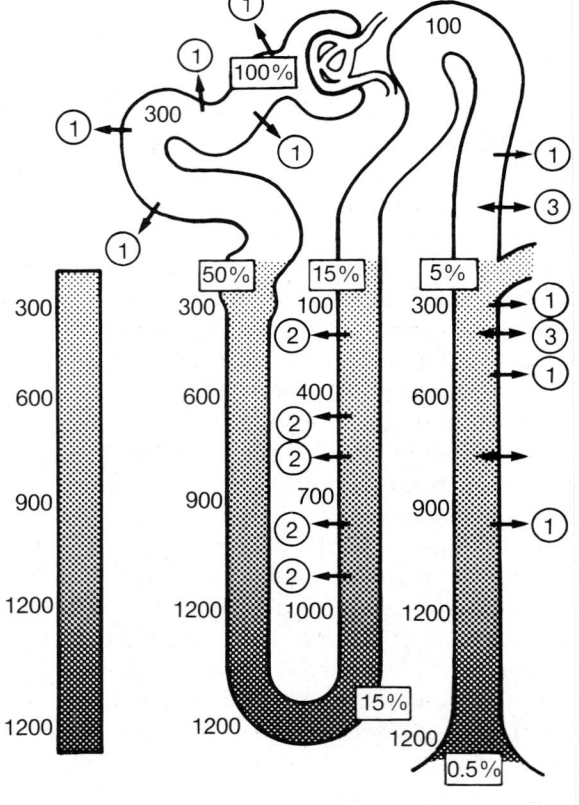

FIGURE 35-5. **The selective movement of anions and cations as the urine flows through the loops of Henle in the medulla of the kidney.**

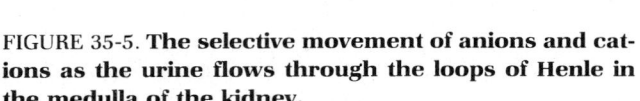

①--Na$^+$ ②--Cl$^-$ ③--Na$^+$ ⟷ K$^+$ or H$^+$

into the medullary capillary loops. Normally medullary blood flow is sluggish compared with the cortex and plays a part in maintaining high osmolarity (i.e., up to 4 times that of plasma in the renal papilla) used in the concentration of urine.

The factors that control the distribution of renal blood flow between the outer two thirds and inner one third of the cortical nephrons are poorly understood, but important. Locally released renin and renal prostaglandins are two factors.

As urine flows through the nephrons, more than 99% (i.e., 100% → 0.5%) of the filtrate is removed (Figure 35-5). Most reabsorption of sodium and water (55% to 65%) takes place in *proximal* tubules. The exact mechanism and its control are not well understood. This mechanism is largely independent of hormones such as aldosterone and antidiuretic hormone (ADH). Some bulk reabsorption occurs into spaces between tubule cells. Peritubular plasma oncotic pressure (increased after the glomerular filtrate has been removed) may also be an important factor because no osmotic gradients can be established or maintained across the cells of the proximal tubules, as shown by several techniques. With the removal of isotonic fluid at this site, the concentration of poorly reabsorbed solutes (e.g., urea, or any glucose that gets past the early glucose reabsorption site) gradually increases and sodium and chloride concentrations decrease, but the sum of all osmotically active particles in the proximal tubules remains approximately 300 mOsm/L. About 80% of the proximally reabsorbed sodium ions are accompanied by chloride ions; the remaining sodium is cation exchanged for a hydrogen ion that combines with filtrate bicarbonate to form intraluminal H_2CO_3. Thus, the Na^+, Cl^-, HCO_3^-, ratios are maintained. Hence the free H^+ ion concentration (i.e., pH) in this region is also unchanged. The active process is an outward pumping of sodium ions. Certain diuretic drugs (actually, natriuretics) act on these sodium pump mechanisms (see Chapter 36, "Diuretics and Antidiuretics"). The H^+ ions are secreted under the catalyst of an enzyme, carbonic anhydrase; blocking this enzyme is one site of diuretic drug action.

Interference with proximal sodium absorption also occurs if there is an increased concentration *in the filtrate* of compounds (e.g., urea, glucose, mannitol, certain radiologic agents) that are poorly reabsorbed. Such agents retain water in the proximal tubule (remember it is permeable to water and is isotonic with plasma) and increase the urine flow. This is called osmotic diuresis and the substances are osmotic diuretics. Urine, in this form of diuresis, has the osmolarity of plasma and the composition of the fluid leaving proximal tubules.

In uncontrolled diabetes the polyuria is an osmotic diuresis and the body can become severely depleted of sodium, chloride, and water. The mechanism of *osmotic diuresis* (i.e., interference with bulk sodium reabsorption in proximal tubules) is quite different from *water diuresis*, caused by an interference with the reabsorption of water, without interference with sodium chloride balance, far down in the last or terminal section of the nephron. In osmotic diuresis so much extra water *and solute* may be delivered to distal sites, where normally the fine tuning of salt and water balance occurs, as to overload or swamp them. The composition of the urine then approaches that in the distal part of the proximal tubule—isosthenuria. This characterizes the urine of chronic renal failure.

The urine in the deeper nephrons now dips down into the medulla via the loops of Henle and passes into a progressively concentrated area (Figure 35-5), losing water and solute passively and becoming concentrated as it passes on downward. After turning the corner at the tip of the loops of Henle, the now concentrated urine becomes progressively diluted again toward, and even below, the osmolarity of plasma. The special mechanisms operating in the thick portion of the ascending limb (medullary and cortical) of the loops of Henle follow. There is an outward active pumping of chloride ions in a region impermeable to water. This makes the surrounding interstitial fluid *more* concentrated and the luminal fluid *less* concentrated.

In Chapter 36 the reader will find that some diuretics (e.g., thiazide diuretics) act selectively at this active chloride transport site.

In the physiologic control of urinary concentration mechanisms of the renal medulla, the loops of Henle are responsible for the *creation* of increased ion concentrations in the peritubular interstitial fluid by a process of solute transport without accompanying water, and the medullary blood vessels are responsible for the *maintenance* of these gradients, which they can only do if they are capillary in nature throughout their length and if medullary blood flow is slow. The major constituents of medullary hyperosmolality are sodium, chloride, and urea. This hyperosmolar medullary tissue, when ADH is present, is responsible for osmotically pulling out the last few milliliters per minute of filtrate in making urine concentrated in the collecting ducts.

There are two interesting facts about the early portion of the distal convoluted tubule, where the thick segment of Henle emerges into the cortex again: (1) the urine is always hypotonic to plasma even under conditions of dehydration (testimony to the efficiency of active solute removal without water in the water-impermeable ascending limb of the loop, which is sometimes referred to as the diluting segment); and (2) the nephron comes into intimate contact with the juxtaglomerular apparatus of *its own* nephron in a specialized area called the macula densa. Various intrinsic feedback regulatory hypotheses have been based on this anatomic fact. The exact mechanism of feedback control awaits elucidation; either osmolality or sodium concentration in the distal tubule effects glomerular filtration by renin release from specialized cells in the afferent glomerular arteriole.

In the distal tubule and active collecting duct regions, sodium extraction can occur even against large sodium gradients from urine to peritubular plasma, but the amount that can be absorbed per unit time is quite small in comparison with the proximal processes. Under normal conditions the distal tubule provides the *fine regulation* of water and salt homeostasis, responding to aldosterone and antidiuretic hormone (ADH). As already mentioned, this fine regulation is impossible, however, if the load being delivered is excessive, such as occurs with marked osmotic diuresis.

In the absence of ADH, urine in the distal convoluted tubule remains dilute, with osmolality well below that of plasma, all the way to the bladder. Salt (i.e., sodium, chloride, potassium, hydrogen ion) control is not affected by the urine remaining dilute in this way. This is known as *water diuresis.*

When ADH is present, as in normal dehydration, the wall of the distal nephron becomes permeable to water and water is removed, so that urine in the most distal region becomes concentrated. As the urine now passes down through the medulla to the tip of the papilla, water is removed by the osmotic pull of the concentrated medullary interstitial fluid, giving urine that may be up to 4 times more concentrated than plasma. Only 3% to 5% of residual fluid is removed at this site.

All of these facts can be pulled together to give an appreciation of the role of the kidney in body water and salt homeostasis through the various neurohumoral and direct humoral pathways that are *extrinsic* to the kidney (e.g., acting through aldosterone and ADH), as well as certain mechanisms that are *intrinsic* to the kidney (e.g., changes in intrarenal blood flow, the macular densa feedback system).

Evidence for the precision of salt and water control is reflected in the following statement: there is no such thing as a normal urinary sodium concentration. The normal kidney is characterized by the wide range of sodium concentrations that can be found in the urine. Sodium deprived, a healthy adult may excrete less than 1 mEq/day of Na^+; salt loaded, the adult may excrete up to 400 mEq/day. The same is true of chloride. For potassium the range is about 10 to 300 mEq/day. This wide range of urinary composition characterizes normality. The urine is the final pathway that reflects the efficacy of the homeostatic regulation.

In the distal tubule much of the sodium ion transported is exchanged for potassium or hydrogen ions, which are excreted (Figure 35-5). Quantitatively this is a more significant K^+ transport process than in the proximal tubules, and is critical to potassium homeostasis and hydrogen balance in the body.

Excretion of acid (hydrogen ions and their anions)

In addition to completing bicarbonate reabsorption, hydrogen ions secreted into the distal tubular fluid combine with ammonia molecules to form *ammonium ions.* This is a form of H^+ ion buffering; it enables much hydrogen excretion to occur without much change in the free hydrogen ion concentration (e.g., urine of pH 5 has a 100 times increase in hydrogen ion concentration $[H^+]$ over that at pH 7 even though it only has 0.1 mEq/L of free H^+). The other mechanism of hydrogen ion excretion is by being buffered by urinary phosphate ($HPO_4^{--} + H^+ \rightarrow H_2PO_4^-$); this is measured as *titratable acidity.* Acid excretion (mEq/day) is measured as: NH_4^+ + Titratable acid $- HCO_3^-$ (all in mEq/day).

The average person, on an average diet, produces 60 to 100 mEq/day of H^+ to be excreted each day, usually about one half as titratable acidity and one half as urinary ammonium. The daily hydrogen ion excretion can vary between $+400$ mEq/day and -150 mEq/day (mainly bicarbonate ions). All of these excreted amounts are small compared with the total hydrogen ions *secreted* to reabsorb bicarbonate in; 180 L of glomerular filtrate in 24 hours, each liter of which may contain 25 mEq/L of bicarbonate, about 4500 mEq/day.

Phosphate reabsorption

Of filtered phosphate, 85% to 95% is reabsorbed, mainly in the proximal tubules. This is partly interfered with by the parathyroid hormone. Depressed urine phosphate reabsorption can be used diagnostically when overactivity of the gland is suspected.

Uric acid

Although uric acid is one of the nitrogenous end products of metabolism, it is largely reabsorbed in the proximal tubule and secreted again further down the nephron. The reason for this apparently unprofitable exercise is not clear. But the secretion process can be affected by drugs. Thus, chlorothiazides may cause hyperuricemia and may even precipitate attacks of clinical gout.

A small proportion of nitrogenous end products are excreted as uric acid (i.e., 500 to 800 mg/day or 5% to 10% of nitrogen excretion). The clearance is only about 10 ml/min, or approximately 10% of the glomerular filtration rate.

Probenecid, phenylbutazone, and salicylic acid, in small doses, increase urate absorption probably because they suppress urate secretion. In higher doses there is an inhibition of urate reabsorption and uricosuria results. Benzothiazides and their derivatives often decrease urate excretion by unknown mechanisms.

Organic acid secretion

The proximal tubule has a transport system that rapidly excretes certain organic acids such as para-amino-hippurate (PAH), penicillins, phenolsulfonphthalein (PSP), or iodopyracet, which after being labeled with iodine can be used to visualize the urinary tract. Probenecid was originally developed to interfere with penicillin secretion in the renal tubules by competitive inhibition on this common secretion system.

Organic base secretion

Such substances as guanidine, methylguanidine, thiamine, histamine, tetraethylammonium, and related bases (e.g., hexamethonium and tolazoline) are all excreted by a common tubular system for which each has a differing affinity. The system is distinct from that for organic acids, and there is no competitive inhibition between the two. Thus different drugs may interact because of effects on the other's secretion.

Diffusion trapping

Excretion of some substances is markedly altered by the difference in free hydrogen ion concentration [H^+] in the urine compared with the blood. Let us suppose that the *undissociated* form of a weak acid is in a simple diffusion equilibrium across the cell wall of the nephron. [HA] in the cell = [HA] in the lumen. If the urine is alkaline, for every molecule of [HA] there will be a greater number of dissociated molecules H^+ and A^- than there is in association with each [HA] in the cell or in plasma. Thus, under stable excretion conditions more of A^- will be excreted if the urine is maintained alkaline than if it is allowed to become acid, even though the concentration of urine [HA] (undissociated) may not have altered. Suppose that an alkaline urine has a ratio of salicylic acid to salicylate ion of 1:3 compared with 1:1 in plasma or the cell.

Then if undissociated salicylic acid approaches diffusion equilibrium across the cell wall, twice as much will be excreted as would occur if the urine had the same free H^+ as the cell.

1. *Urine alkaline to cell*

Cell	Lumen
$1A^- + [1HA]$	$= [1HA] + 3A^-$ (*or* 4 unit quantities)

2. *Urine same H^+ as cell*

Cell	Lumen
$1A^- + [1HA]$	$= [1HA] + 1A^-$ (*or* 2 unit quantities)

Amino acid reabsorption

The three transport systems for reabsorption of filtered amino acids are as follows: (1) for lysine, arginine, ornithine, cystine, and histidine; (2) for glutamic and aspartic; and (3) for the remaining amino acids. Within each group there is transport competition, but each is otherwise separate. Any drug that interferes with any of these might cause aminoaciduria.

Comparison of renal excretion of urea and creatinine

The metabolic production and renal handling of *urea* and *creatinine* are important because, contrary to what many people think, creatinine is a much more accurate indicator than urea of renal disease.

On a normal diet the urine contains about 20 gm/day of urea. This could fall to about 8 gm/day on a low-protein diet and rise to 35 gm/day on a very high-protein diet. The qualitative aspects of urea metabolism, the net effect of the liver in balancing anabolism and catabolism of amino acids in the body amino acid pool is summarized in Figure 35-6.

Creatinine, by contrast, is produced by muscles by a metabolic pathway that is remarkably independent of muscle anabolism or catabolism, and production is relatively constant (Figure 35-6). There is less than 10% variation from day to day in an individual, and dietary protein has little effect. Thus, the kidney is presented with a much more constant daily load of creatinine than of urea.

Renal handling of these filtered loads is much less variable for creatinine than urea. Filtered creatinine, in normal health, is neither absorbed nor added to by secretion. Filtered urea is reabsorbed 30% to 60% depending on flow rates and the medullary urea concentration gradient. Thus, creatinine clearance (CrCl) is an excellent clinical measure of GFR and urea clearance has very little value. It is true that creatinine is

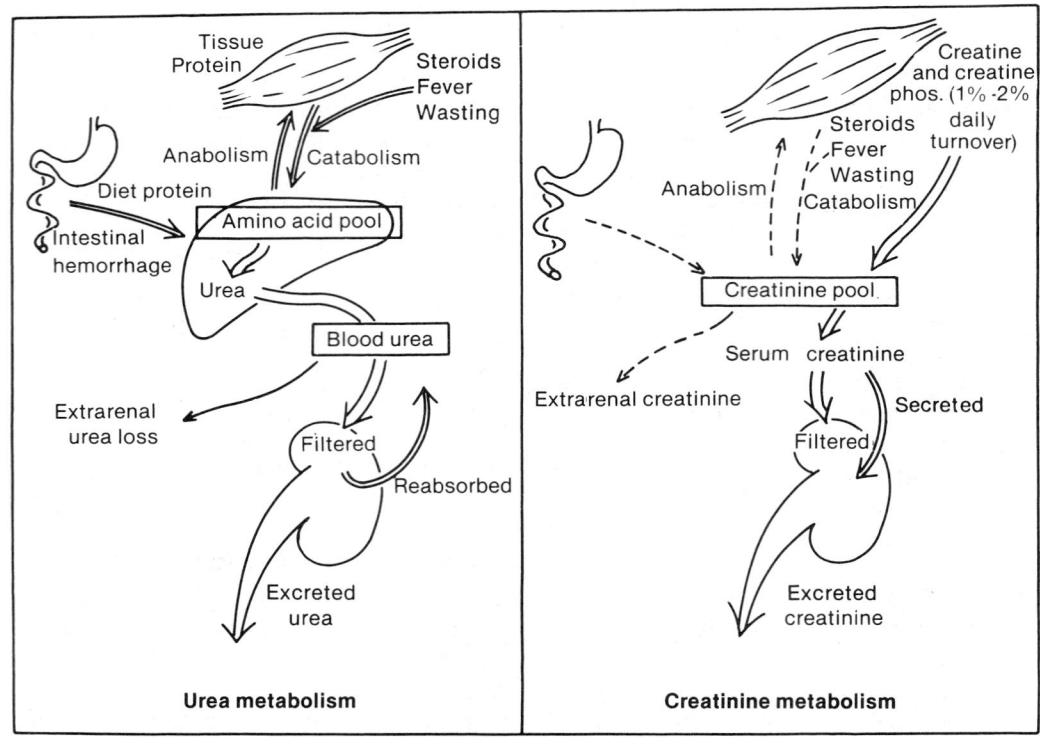

FIGURE 35-6. **Comparison of the production and metabolism of urea and creatinine.**

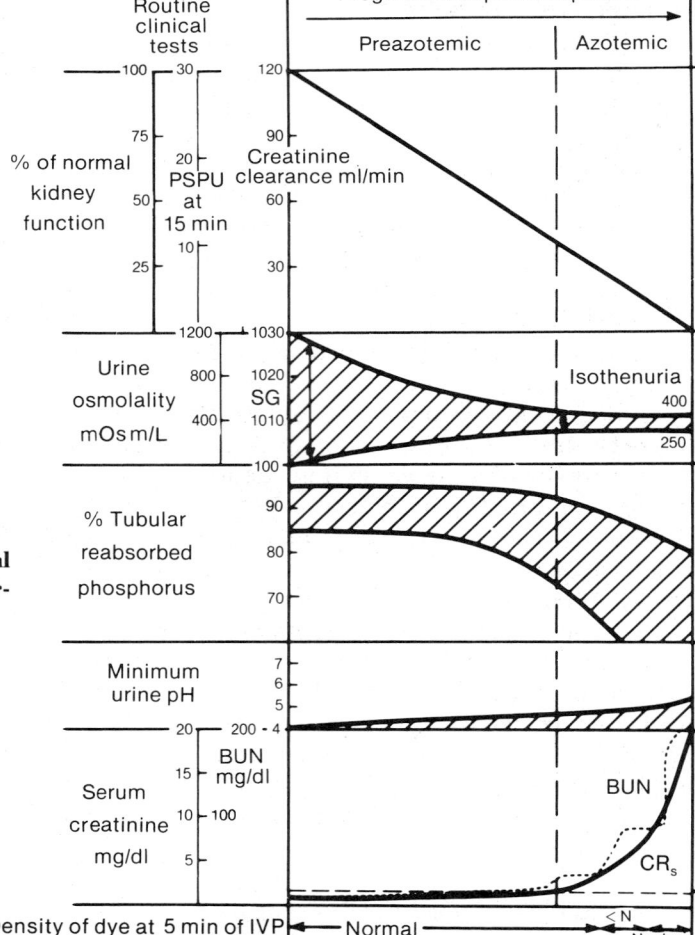

FIGURE 35-7. **Summary of selective changes in renal function parameters as a patient progresses from normal renal function to renal failure.**

secreted by the tubule wall in renal failure as serum creatinine rises so that CrCl becomes less accurate as a measure of GFR once the blood level is *above* 2 to 3 mg/dl. However, this in no way detracts from the value of CrCl as a measure of GFR during early functional deterioration when renal function is decreasing from 100% down to about 33%. Indeed, accurate serial measurements of serum creatinine are also useful as measurements of renal function, but BUN, by itself, is notoriously unreliable, particularly because of the possibility of prerenal azotemia (Figure 35-6).

Figure 35-7 summarizes some changes in various parameters of renal function as a patient goes progressively into renal failure. Frank uremia or creatininemia occurs only after two thirds of the renal function has been destroyed. In assessing the effect of renal dysfunction on drug dosing, the nurse must be aware of which tests show changes in early renal dysfunction (such as the maximum urine specific gravity or osmolality, and creatinine clearance). These detect less drastic changes and yet may indicate that the drug dose needs to be reduced.

SUMMARY

Not only is the renal system involved in the homeostatic balance of fluid and electrolytes and metabolic functions, but it is involved with the excretion of numerous drugs from the body. An understanding of the anatomy, physiology, and assessment of the renal system will enable the nurse to better understand affecting the renal system directly and indirectly. Those drugs that directly affect the renal system and are used for the therapeutic treatment of conditions affecting this system are discussed in the following chapters of this section. The brief overview presented in this chapter should enable the nurse to assess patients requiring these medications and assist them with drug therapy regimens. The nurse's role in monitoring patient response cannot be overemphasized in relation to the promotion of renal function. An understanding of the anatomy, physiology, and assessment of the renal system will also enable the nurse to prevent or minimize toxic effects of other medications, as well as recognize the importance of renal dysfunction or toxicity in drug selection and dosing.

BIBLIOGRAPHY

Gottschalk, C.W., & Lassiter, C.W. Mechanisms of urine formation. In V.B. Mountcastle (Ed.). *Medical physiology.* St. Louis: The C.V. Mosby Co., 1980.

Malasanos, L., Barkauskas, V., Moss, M., & Stoltenberg-Allen, K. *Health assessment.* (3rd ed.). St. Louis: The C.V. Mosby Co., 1985.

Orr, M.L. Drugs and renal disease. *American Journal of Nursing*, 1981, *81*, 969-971.

Pagliaro, L.A., & Benet, L.Z. Critical compilation of terminal half-lives, percent excreted unchanged, and changes of half-life in renal and hepatic dysfunction. *Journal of Pharmacokinetics and Biopharmaceutics*, 1975, *3*, 333-383.

Stark, J.L. BUN/creatinine: your keys to kidney function. *Nursing 80*, 1980, *10*, 33-38.

CHAPTER 36

Diuretics and Antidiuretics

Thavisakdi Kovithavongs
John B. Dossetor

Medications discussed in this chapter

Diuretics
  Benzothiadiazines or
    thiazide diuretics
    Bendroflumethiazide
    Benzthiazide
    Chlorothiazide
    Chlorthalidone
    Cyclothiazide
    Hydrochlorothiazide
    Hydroflumethiazide
    Indapamide
    Methyclothiazide
    Polythiazide
    Quinethazone
    Trichlormethiazide
  Quinazoline diuretic
    Metolazone

Diuretics—cont'd
  Loop diuretics
    Bumetanide
    Ethacrynic Acid
    Ethacrynate
    Furosemide
  Potassium-sparing di-
    uretics
    Amiloride
    Spironolactone
    Triamterene
  Osmotic diuretics
    Mannitol
    Urea
Antidiuretics
    Chlorpropamide
    Desmopressin
    Lypressin
    Vasopressin

Diuretics are drugs that promote urine flow by mechanisms that increase sodium excretion from the kidney. This definition implies that enhanced water excretion accompanies increased sodium excretion and excludes agents that do not have a direct effect on renal tubular sodium reabsorption. In patients with congestive heart failure (CHF), digitalis may improve cardiac function and increase cardiac output, renal blood flow, and sodium and water excretion. But digitalis is not considered a diuretic because it has no direct action on renal tubules in influencing sodium excretion. In another instance, in healthy individuals, water or alcohol consumption in large quantities would be followed by passage of large volumes of urine, but sodium excretion hardly increases. Water and alcohol are also not diuretics, but act by inhibiting antidiuretic hormone (ADH) secretion from the hypothalamus, and in the absence of ADH, water reabsorption in the distal renal tubules and collecting ducts fails to occur, giving rise to *diuresis*.

SODIUM REGULATION

Normally we take in about 5 to 10 gm of salt each day, roughly 170 mEq of sodium and 170 mEq of chloride. With almost 200 L of plasma being filtered by the glomeruli each day, the sodium filtered amounts to approximately 25,000 mEq, but the amount excreted comes to less than 1%. The majority of filtered sodium, some 67%, is reabsorbed along the proximal tubules, and the remaining is reabsorbed by Henle's loops (25%), the distal tubules (5%) and the collecting ducts (3%).

The amount of sodium excreted each day is roughly equal to intake, no matter how drastically it is increased or decreased, so as to ensure that an individual is not volume overloaded to the point of CHF, or dies of severe dehydration. Thus, the kidney is equipped with an efficient system for maintaining sodium balance, obviously influenced by hemodynamic and neurohumoral mechanisms elsewhere in the body that are incompletely understood.

It is well known that two factors influence sodium reabsorption. One is *glomerular filtration:* the more sodium that is filtered at the glomerulus, the more that is reabsorbed by the renal tubules—the so-called glomerulotubular balance. The other factor is aldosterone, a potent mineralocorticoid produced by the adrenal cortex, which is influenced by renal blood flow through a renin angiotensin-aldosterone mechanism that acts on the distal renal tubules to increase sodium reabsorption. It is also known that additional factors are involved, but the nature of these factors has never been completely elucidated. Normally, an expanded extracellular fluid volume would provide a stimulus to diuresis. In sodium-retaining states, notably CHF, liver cirrhosis, and nephrosis, in addition to increased aldosterone levels responsible for sodium retention and edema formation, these additional factors may be in operation to interfere with the control mechanisms so that diuresis fails to occur. In these conditions diuretics can be used to intervene with sodium reabsorption at different sites of the renal tubule to promote diuresis.

TYPES OF DIURETICS

The six groups of diuretics, classified according to their mechanisms of action, are (1) carbonic anhydrase inhibitors, (2) thiazide and nonthiazide sulfonamide diuretics, (3) organomercurials, (4) loop diuretics, (5) potassium-sparing diuretics, and (6) osmotic diuretics. The reader is referred to Chapter 35, "Review of the Anatomy, Physiology, and Assessment of the Renal System," for details regarding the renal tubular handling of sodium reabsorption.

Mechanisms of action, routes of administration, and uses of diuretics

Carbonic anhydrase inhibitors. Normally, carbon dioxide in proximal renal tubular cells is hydrated to carbonic acid in the presence of the enzyme carbonic anhydrase. Carbonic acid then dissociates into hydrogen and bicarbonate ions. Hydrogen is secreted into the luminal tubular fluid in exchange for sodium, which is reabsorbed, combines with filtered bicarbonate, and dissociates into carbon dioxide and water, again by the action of carbonic anhydrase, but now along the brush border of the tubule. Carbon dioxide that is freely diffusible across the cell membrane gets inside the cell and the cycle is repeated. Sodium, once inside the cell, neutralizes bicarbonate ion and enters the blood as the ions of sodium bicarbonate. Thus, most of the filtered bicarbonate is reclaimed in the proximal tubule, and with it a fraction of sodium is also reabsorbed.

In the presence of a carbonic anhydrase inhibitor, this process cannot take place, resulting in a loss of bicarbonate and some sodium in the urine and transient diuresis. In addition, carbonic anhydrase inhibitors cause an increase in potassium secretion in the distal tubule because potassium competes with hydrogen distally for sodium exchange by the same transport system, and when less hydrogen is available for exchange, more potassium is excreted.

The natriuretic and diuretic effects produced by carbonic anhydrase inhibitors are small and transient, because the bulk of sodium reabsorption in association with chloride is unaffected. In addition, as the amount of filtered bicarbonate decreases, sodium excretion, as affected by this group of drugs, also decreases. Thus, carbonic anhydrase inhibitors have been replaced by more potent and efficient compounds and are *no longer used as diuretics.* But their action as inhibitors of carbonic anhydrase elsewhere in the body continues in the presence of systemic acidosis, and they are useful for treating certain types of glaucoma by reducing aqueous humor formation, thus reducing intraocular pressure. The prototype of this group of diuretics is acetazolamide. Other members include dichlorphenamide and methazolamide.

Thiazide diuretics. Thiazide diuretics are also sulfonamides originally synthesized in an attempt to create more potent inhibitors of carbonic anhydrase. Thus all thiazide diuretics have some carbonic anhydrase inhibitory activity. They inhibit proximal tubular bicarbonate reabsorption to some extent, and the appearance of bicarbonate in the urine makes it alkaline. However, the main effect of thiazide diuretic action is on the cortical portion of the thick ascending limb of Henle's loop where they inhibit active chloride transport. In the distal tubules and collecting ducts, thiazides cause an increased secretion of potassium by increasing the delivery of sodium to these sites and therefore increasing sodium-potassium exchange and potassium excretion. Thiazide diuretics may also have some action on the medullary portion of the thick ascending limb of Henle's loop where a further fraction of sodium is normally reabsorbed secondary to active chloride transport, at least for brief periods and with high doses.

Thiazides are the most widely used diuretics. Their indications for use include edematous states and hypertension, alone or in combination with other antihypertensives. They are also effective in preventing recurrent calcium stones in the kidney and in treating *diabetes insipidus.* Thiazides are well absorbed from the GI tract, and the diuretic effect takes place within 1 hour of oral administration. Most are rapidly excreted within 3 to 6 hours.

Organomercurials. The diuretic effect of inorganic mercury was noted as early as the sixteenth century. However, the introduction of organic mercurial compounds as diuretic agents was made only after it was accidentally discovered that merbaphen, an antisyphilitic agent, had a potent diuretic property. Their major site of action appears to be in the thick ascending limb of Henle's loop where they inhibit active chloride transport and therefore interfere with passive sodium reabsorption. Their effect on the distal tubular handling of potassium is complex, and they can either enhance or inhibit distal tubular potassium secretion under different conditions. In general, potassium depletion with organomercurials is not a problem as it is with other potent diuretics.

The organomercurials were once the most potent

diuretic agents available. However, they have now been replaced by the thiazides and loop diuretics because of their poor absorption following oral administration, GI irritation, and the need to be administered parenterally. They are also *nephrotoxic* and are contraindicated in renal insufficiency. Organomercurials are sometimes used in emergency situations or in patients resistant to other forms of diuretics but are not generally recommended. Their action occurs within 1 to 2 hours after an intramuscular injection and lasts for 6 to 9 hours. They are completely excreted by the kidney in 24 hours.

Loop diuretics. The most potent diuretics available today are the loop diuretics furosemide, bumetanide, and ethacrynic acid, which are chemically quite different but appear to act in the same sites of the nephron. Furosemide is a sulfonamide like the thiazides, but in addition to acting on the cortical portion of the thick ascending limb of Henle's loop, it also affects chloride reabsorption along the medullary portion of the thick ascending limb. Thus passive sodium reabsorption is blocked along the entire length of the thick portion of the ascending limb of Henle's loop. In addition, furosemide may also inhibit active sodium transport in the proximal tubule, but this effect is minor compared with its total diuretic action. Ethacrynic acid is an unsaturated ketone derivative of aryloxyacetic acid and is structurally unrelated to any other diuretics, but it has the same potency as furosemide and similar sites of action.

In addition to their inhibitory effect on active chloride reabsorption and, secondarily, sodium reabsorption, these drugs are believed to be capable of altering intrarenal hemodynamics that may contribute to their action. Because of the increased load of sodium to the distal tubules, there is increased potassium and hydrogen ion excretion, and the resultant hypokalemic alkalosis is observable in patients treated with these drugs.

The loop diuretics can be given orally or in emergency situations intravenously. The diuretic effect occurs within 30 minutes after oral administration and lasts 6 to 8 hours. With IV injection the diuretic action occurs within a few minutes and peaks in 1 hour. These diuretics can induce a marked increase in urine volume, containing as much as 30% to 40% sodium chloride of the filtered load. Deafness, usually reversible, can occur when these agents are administered in high doses in the presence of renal insufficiency or with ototoxic drugs, but occurs more often with ethacrynic acid. In patients with chronic renal failure where thiazides are ineffective, furosemide is the drug of choice to induce or maintain urine flow.

Potassium-sparing diuretics. Potassium-sparing diuretics in themselves have little diuretic effect other than by interfering with sodium-potassium and sodium-hydrogen exchange in the collecting ducts. They are effective, however, in sodium-retaining states where aldosterone plays a major role, as in CHF, liver cirrhosis, and the *nephrotic syndrome.* Spironolactone is a specific inhibitor of aldosterone and acts by competing directly for receptor sites intracellularly. It is effective, however, only in the presence of high levels of aldosterone.

In contrast, triamterene and amiloride, two nonsteroidal agents, can effect these cation exchanges by their direct action on tubular cells in the absence of aldosterone. Triamterene and amiloride are used primarily for their potassium-sparing effect, rather than as diuretics. They are usually used in combination with other diuretic agents. They are contraindicated in renal failure with decreasing urine output, and are used only with care in association with potassium supplementation.

Osmotic diuretics. Osmotic diuretics, which are usually not metabolized after administration, are filtered unchanged at the glomerulus and are not reabsorbed by the renal tubules. They act by their osmotic effect, which interferes with solute and water reabsorption in the proximal tubule. They also dissipate the hyperosmolality of the medullary interstitium and therefore interfere with the reabsorption of water (descending limb) and sodium chloride (ascending limb) in Henle's loop. They also increase the renal plasma flow and glomerular filtration. They are not used in edematous states and could be dangerous in CHF. But they are useful in promoting diuresis in drug intoxication to enhance the elimination of drugs, to relieve cerebral edema, and in preventing renal failure in cases of severe trauma and burns.

SIDE EFFECTS AND COMPLICATIONS OF DIURETIC THERAPY

The most common side effect of diuretic therapy is a disturbance in the acid base balance, such as hypochloremic alkalosis, but this is usually mild and does not require treatment. *Hypokalemia* may require potassium supplementation. On the other hand, *hyperkalemia* may result from the use of potassium-sparing agents in the presence of oliguria with or without potassium supplementation. Magnesium depletion occurs with all diuretics except carbonic anhydrase inhibitors, and this along with hypokalemia may aggravate digitalis toxicity.

Depletion of the intravascular volume as manifested

by excessive thirst, a fall in blood pressure, orthostatic hypotension, and a rise in BUN and serum creatinine indicates that the regimen is too aggressive and should be modified. *Hyperuricemia* can occur with all diuretics that reduce extracellular fluid volume by decreasing urate clearance from increased proximal tubular reabsorption of urate. Carbohydrate intolerance can be induced by the thiazides and perhaps furosemide. *Ototoxicity*, generally reversible, has been reported with ethacrynic acid and furosemide. Organomercurials are nephrotoxic and should not be used in patients with renal failure or acute nephritis. The use of furosemide concomitantly with gentamicin or cephaloridine (no longer available in the United States) should be avoided because it can potentiate their nephrotoxicity. Pancreatitis and allergic vasculitis have been reported with the thiazide diuretics, but this must be extremely rare considering how frequently these drugs are used.

RESISTANCE TO DIURETIC THERAPY

The best guide to the effectiveness of diuretic therapy is to follow daily weight changes. Recording intake and output is also helpful in monitoring response, but it is cumbersome and less accurate, especially when patients have difficulty maintaining fluid restriction, when there is extrarenal loss such as diarrhea, or when the patient is at home. Pharmacologic resistance to treatment with diuretics (in removing extra salt and water) is evident when there is no weight loss and no increase in urinary output, when pitting edema persists, and sometimes when the blood pressure is persistently elevated. Resistance to diuretic therapy can occur in certain circumstances; however, resistance or nonresponse to therapy may be the result of the following factors.

Noncompliance to diet or drug therapy. Noncompliance to diet or drug therapy often occurs with outpatients when the patients could be taking in too much salt. It is also possible that because of the inconvenience of frequent visits to the bathroom, the patients may not be taking the medication at all or taking it at a smaller dose (i.e., a lack of compliance rather than resistance).

Renal failure resulting in the inability of the kidneys to respond to the diuretic. Patients with renal failure are more resistant to diuretics because of decreased renal blood flow, glomerular filtration, and tubular reabsorptive mass. There is less sodium reabsorption taking place, and it is harder to block it. Some diuretics may not work at all, such as the thiazides. In a situation such as this, the best drug is furosemide,

which can be increased in dose to several hundred milligrams per day, under close supervision, until a response is obtained.

Malabsorption. Patients—for example, patients with *anasarca* infestation—may not be absorbing the drug adequately from the GI tract.

Alterations in normal hemodynamics. Certain patients may have severe hypoalbuminemia and decreased cardiac output and renal blood flow. For these patients it may be necessary to administer the drug intravenously and to administer albumin infusion at the same time.

Alteration in electrolyte and acid-base balance. The use of the diuretic may have caused a severe electrolyte imbalance such as *hyponatremia, hypochloremia,* alkalosis, or potassium depletion. The action of diuretics depends on the presence of certain electrolytes and a specific acid-base balance. When these are altered, the diuretic effect will be diminished or nonexistent.

Alteration in fluid balance. The edematous state may be caused by surgically correctable disorders such as mitral stenosis or constrictive pericarditis, and surgical intervention may be indicated.

Under such conditions just listed, it is best to keep the patient hospitalized and to investigate the reasons for the refractoriness. Confining patients to bed rest may promote diuresis by mobilizing fluid from the peripheral tissues into the circulation. Monitor for severe anemia, hypercatabolic states, cardiac dysrhythmias, or pulmonary embolism, which may account for the diuretic resistance, and plan to help meet this problem as indicated.

ANTIDIURETICS

Antidiuretics are medications used for treating polyuria secondary to the deficiency of ADH arginine vasopressin (central form of diabetes insipidus), or because of the unresponsiveness of the distal renal tubules and collecting ducts to the effect of ADH (nephrogenic diabetes insipidus). The central form of diabetes insipidus can be partial or complete. In the partial form there is some hormonal activity still present, and drugs that potentiate the hormonal activity or stimulate the release of more hormone are effective. In the complete form this is not possible, and replacement therapy is necessary.

The drug of choice for hormonal replacement is now desmopressin (DDAVP) (1-desamino-8-D-arginine vasopressin), which is a synthetic peptide with a high antidiuretic-to-pressor activity and a prolonged duration of action. The drug can be applied intranasally with a calibrated plastic applicator that comes with the medication. The antidiuretic action occurs within 1 hour and lasts 6 to 20 hours. Side effects are rare except for nausea and headache at higher doses, compared with the parent compounds that are still available (see the Nursing Drug Digest).

Nonhormonal therapy includes drugs that potentiate the effect of ADH (e.g., chlorpropamide), or stimulate the release of residual ADH (e.g., clofibrate and carbamazepine). These drugs are effective only in the partial or incomplete form of central diabetes insipidus. The thiazide diuretics, when used in conjunction with sodium restriction, can reduce extracellular fluid volume and glomerular filtration rate, enhance fluid reabsorption in the proximal tubules, and decrease urine volume in all forms of diabetes insipidus. These nonhormonal preparations can be used in combinations to reduce their individual side effects.

SUMMARY

This chapter has discussed the use and pharmacologic classes of the various diuretics and antidiuretics. Mechanisms of action, adverse side effects, and drug interactions have been presented.

With this information the nurse will be able to provide optimum care to patients who require treatment with either diuretics or antidiuretics.

ADVERSE/SIDE EFFECTS OF DIURETICS*

ALLERGIC REACTIONS

Drug fever
Drug rash
Eczema
Exfoliative dermatitis (mercurials)
Necrotizing vasculitis (thiazides)
Photosensitivity (thiazides)
Urticaria

CARDIOVASCULAR SYSTEM

Potentiation of digitalis toxicity
Ventricular fibrillation (IV mercurials)
Volume depletion, shock (mercurial and loop diuretics)

CENTRAL NERVOUS SYSTEM

Blurred vision
Deafness (ethacrynic acid and furosemide)
Dizziness
Drowsiness
Headache
Lethargy

Paresthesia
Restlessness
Vertigo

GASTROINTESTINAL SYSTEM

Anorexia
Cholestatic jaundice (thiazides)
Constipation
Diarrhea
Epigastric distress
GI bleeding (ethacrynic acid)
Nausea
Pancreatitis (thiazides)
Vomiting

HEMATOLOGIC SYSTEM

Agranulocytosis
Aplastic anemia
Leukopenia
Thrombocytopenia

METABOLIC AND ENDOCRINE SYSTEMS

Glucose intolerance (thiazides)
Gynecomastia (spironolactone)
Hypercalcemia (thiazides)
Hyperkalemia (spironolactone, triamterene)
Hyperuricemia (thiazides)
Hypokalemia (thiazides, mercurials, loop diuretics)
Hyponatremia (thiazides, mercurials, loop diuretics)

NEUROMUSCULAR SYSTEM

Fatigue
Muscle cramps
Muscle weakness

RENAL SYSTEM

Hematuria (ethacrynic acid)
Increasing *azotemia*
Renal stones (carbonic anhydrase inhibitors)
Renal tubular necrosis (mercurials)
Urinary retention (mercurials and loop diuretics)

---

*See Chapter 11, "Drug Toxicity," for an overview of drug toxicity.

CLINICALLY SIGNIFICANT DRUG INTERACTIONS*

Primary drug	Interacting drug	Possible effect(s)	Probable mechanism(s)
Amiloride	Hydrochlorothiazide	Hyperkalemia	Increased sodium excretion and potassium retention
Amiloride	Lithium	Lithium toxicity	Decreased renal clearance of lithium
All diuretics except spironolactone and triamterene	Digitalis	Predisposition to digitalis toxicity	Hypokalemia, hypomagnesemia
Ethacrynic acid	Aminoglycosides	Enhances ototoxicity, impairs renal function	Destruction of cochlea hair cells, damage to nephrons
Ethacrynic acid	Oral anticoagulants	Increased GI bleeding in renal failure and hypoalbuminemia	Ethacrynic acid displaces warfarin from albumin binding sites
Furosemide	Aminoglycosides	Ototoxicity	Damage to cochlea hair cells
Furosemide	Tubocurarine	Enhances neuromuscular blockade	Not established
Loop diuretics	Lithium carbonate	Lithium intoxication	Marked sodium depletion decreases lithium excretion, hence toxicity
Potassium-sparing diuretics (e.g., spironolactone, triamterene)	Potassium chloride	Severe hyperkalemia	Additive effect
Potassium-sparing diuretics (e.g., spironolactone, triamterene)	Salt substitutes (contain large amounts of potassium)	Severe hyperkalemia	Additive effect
Thiazides	Antidiabetics	Worsening of diabetic control	Diabetogenic effect of thiazides
Thiazides	Oral anticoagulants	Thiazides antagonize effect of oral anticoagulants	Increased clotting factors by improving hepatic function
Triamterene	Indomethacin	Kidney failure with severely decreased creatinine clearance	Not established, but believed to be related to suppression of the protective influence of the renal prostaglandins by indomethacin

*See Chapter 10, "Drug Interactions," for an overview of drug interactions.

GENERAL NURSING IMPLICATIONS

Nursing of patients requiring diuretics

ASSESSMENT

A complete nursing assessment is essential in establishing a baseline from which to plan individualized drug therapy regimens and to monitor patient response. Assessment should include a detailed drug history to identify sensitivity, contraindications, cautions, potential drug interactions, and drug-taking patterns before drug therapy is initiated.

Assessment should also include detailed baseline data related to fluid and electrolyte balance and renal function tests before diuretic therapy is started. It is important to note that laboratory values, including hematocrit and hemoglobin, can be falsely low in relation to hemodilution if vascular volume excess is present. Laboratory data should include urinalysis with specific gravity, culture and sensitivity; 24-hour urine for urea and creatinine; serum potassium, sodium, chloride, glucose, uric acid, calcium; diagnostic tests (intravenous pyelogram, KUB film), and BUN. These should be obtained initially and at regular intervals during diuretic therapy.

Physical assessment of the patient should be completed carefully and the presence of local or generalized edema

Continued.

GENERAL NURSING IMPLICATIONS—cont'd

Nursing of patients requiring diuretics—cont'd

ASSESSMENT—cont'd

should be recorded as quantitatively as possible. If peripheral edema is noted, ankle widths and extent of pitting if present should be included. The chest should be auscultated for moist rales and any moist cough or difficulty laying flat should be noted. The abdomen should be inspected, auscultated, percussed, and palpated to determine the presence and extent of fluid. Measurement of abdominal girths is indicated if ascites is noted. Blood pressure, pulse (including strength and regularity), extent of neck vein distention, and central venous pressure when possible should be carefully measured and recorded. Intake and output should be established and special attention should be given to measuring the patient's weight, because this is probably the most significant parameter in determining fluid volume excess. In addition, attention should be given to the assessment of mental status because changes in mentation, including lethargy, apathy, and disorientation can signify fluid, acid-base, and electrolyte imbalance (see Chapter 67, "Fluids and Electrolytes"). These baseline measurements are essential in monitoring therapy.

SENSITIVITY

Diuretics, especially the thiazides, can cause certain sensitivity reactions in sensitive individuals, including rashes, with the initiation of therapy (see the Nursing Drug Digest for each specific agent).

Patients who have not received diuretic therapy before require careful monitoring. It is also important to recognize that because the thiazide and loop diuretics are related to sulfonamides, they should *not* be given to patients who have a history of allergy to sulfa drugs.

CONTRAINDICATIONS

The thiazide and loop diuretics are contraindicated in patients who have a history of sensitivity to these drugs or to sulfonamides, because they are closely related.

Potassium-sparing diuretics are contraindicated in renal insufficiency or renal failure because dangerously elevated potassium levels can result.

(See the Nursing Drug Digest for contraindications to individual agents.)

CAUTIONS

The thiazide and loop diuretics should be used with caution during pregnancy because they can cross the placental barrier. Thiazides should also be used with caution in lactating mothers because these diuretics can be excreted in breast milk, and electrolyte disturbance and thrombocytopenia in the nursing neonate have been reported.

Because the thiazide and loop diuretics can cause hyperuricemia, they should be used with caution in those patients with gout.

Because hyperglycemia is related to the use of the thiazide, loop, and potassium-sparing diuretics, they should be used with caution in patients with diabetes because they may necessitate an adjustment in insulin requirements.

Diuretics should be used with caution in patients with hepatic conditions (e.g., cirrhosis) because hepatic coma may be precipitated by minor alterations in the fluid and electrolyte balance or in serum ammonia. Early signs of hepatic coma should be monitored, including confusion, drowsiness, or the flapping tremor of the outstretched hand.

Diuretics should also be used cautiously with patients who are concurrently taking digitalis glycosides (e.g., digoxin) because the hypokalemia that may result secondary to diuresis with the loop and thiazide diuretics can potentiate the effects of digoxin, creating digitalis toxicity. A potassium supplement or the inclusion of potassium-rich foods (citrus fruits, prunes, bananas) in the daily diet can prevent this.

The patient should also be monitored for and taught to report extreme fatigue, muscle cramps (especially in the calf regions) immediately because these are signs of hypokalemia. Hypokalemia may cause cardiac dysrhythmias. Monitor for and encourage the patient to report the sudden onset of an irregular pulse or heart rate.

DRUG INTERACTIONS

Diuretics can interact with a number of medications, including prescription and nonprescription drugs, resulting in serious effects (e.g., the loop diuretic furosemide can interact with aminoglycosides, causing nephrotoxicity).

Long-term thiazide therapy, when concurrent with lithium therapy, can produce lithium toxicity because it reduces the renal clearance of lithium. Concurrent use of thiazide diuretics with alcohol, narcotics, and barbiturates can aggravate orthostatic hypotensive effects.

Potassium-sparing diuretics may be inhibited by salicylates, including aspirin.

For other important drug interactions, see Clinically Significant Drug Interactions.

ADMINISTRATION

Diuretics are given orally or intravenously (see the Nursing Drug Digest for each specific agent). The administration of diuretics should be scheduled to allow for diuresis during daytime hours so that sleep is not disrupted. Oral diuretics prescribed once per day are best taken in the morning with breakfast because this also decreases GI irritation and upset. Diuretics given in acute situations should be administered intravenously when a rapid response is indicated. When edema is severe, intravenous sites are often hard to locate and cutdowns are often required. Site monitoring is essential to prevent an undue loss of infusion sites. It is also important that injections not be made into edematous tissues because circulation is impaired and the medication will be poorly absorbed.

MONITORING PATIENT RESPONSE
Therapeutic response

Monitoring of therapeutic response, including weight loss, increased urine output, and lowered blood pressure, is especially important in adjusting diuretic therapy regimens to meet the individual patient's requirements. All data should be recorded carefully to document the patient's response and to facilitate treatment decisions. It is

GENERAL NURSING IMPLICATIONS—cont'd

Nursing of patients requiring diuretics—cont'd

Therapeutic response—cont'd

also important to be alert to monitoring drug resistance (no weight loss, oliguria, elevated blood pressure, persistent edema); thus, knowledge of drug peak(s) and duration of action is important in monitoring effects.

The patient should know that the diuretic will cause frequent urination and that this is desired. If nonambulatory, the patient should have a call light and a urinal or bedpan readily available. Urinary incontinence may be a distressing problem for elderly patients who may need assistance in preventing this occurrence. Bed linens should be protected for nonambulatory patients.

The body weight can indicate whether the patient is losing fluid too quickly or if the patient is resistant to the diuretic and should be monitored carefully at the same time under the same conditions (e.g., same clothing, same scale) each day. Intake and output should be measured and recorded accurately. Inpatients should be involved in this aspect of care, especially if they are on fluid restriction, because this will enable their participation in planning fluid intake through the day and will increase their ability for self-monitoring at home if the need for long-term diuretic therapy is indicated.

It is especially important to monitor the blood pressure and the pulse during periods of rapid diuresis. This should be done with the patient in the recumbent and standing positions. Rapid diuresis, especially in the elderly patient, may result in cardiovascular side effects related to a sudden decrease in extracellular fluid volume. Thus, orthostatic hypotension, tachycardia, and circulatory collapse can occur. Thrombus formation is another potential problem associated with rapid diuresis.

Diuretic therapy may be too stringent, leading to fluid volume deficit, as well as to electrolyte imbalance. The patient should be monitored for excessive thirst, weakness, lethargy, oliguria, low grade fever, flushed dry skin, dry mucous membranes, and poor skin turgor. When observed, these indicate that a change in regimen is indicated. It is also important that losses from nasogastric suction, wound drainage, recurrent vomiting, and diarrhea be monitored closely because these can potentiate hypokalemia in patients receiving loop or thiazide diuretic therapy.

Adverse side effects

Monitoring side effects is essential. The most common side effect associated with diuretic therapy is a disturbance in fluid and electrolyte balance. With the loop and thiazide diuretics, the side effects include hypokalemia, hyponatremia, and hyperuricemia. With the potassium-sparing diuretics, hyperkalemia with the presence of oliguria is common. With the loop, thiazide, and potassium-sparing diuretics, side effects include hyperglycemia, magnesium depletion (with the presence of hypokalemia, can aggravate digitalis toxicity), and hypotension (related to the depletion of intravascular fluid volume manifested by thirst, orthostatic hypotension, and elevated BUN and serum creatinine). When such effects are identified, it indicates that the regimen is too aggressive and should be modified.

In addition to disturbances in fluid and electrolyte balance, the effects involving the loop diuretics to be monitored include reversible deafness with increased doses in the presence of renal insufficiency or when used concurrently with ototoxic drugs (e.g., aminoglycosides). It is also important to note that because loop diuretics are more potent than other diuretics, side effects are likely to be more severe and to occur earlier in treatment.

With thiazide diuretics, one should monitor for photosensitivity (warn patients to shade skin or use a sun screen especially if therapy is long term) and ototoxicity (rare).

With potassium-sparing diuretics, one should monitor for gynecomastia, impotence, menstrual irregularities, and decreased libido. The nurse must be especially sensitive to monitoring these side effects because patients may have difficulty discussing problems related to sexuality.

The nurse's role in monitoring for side effects, helping the patient and the family, as indicated, to do so, and helping them to minimize these effects, cannot be overemphasized.

PATIENT EDUCATION

The patient and the family should have a clear understanding of the medication regimen, as well as the exact name of the medication, its action, dosage, storage, administration, and side effects (including what can be done to minimize them). The patient should know how to monitor therapeutic effects and to identify signs that indicate the prescriber should be contacted. The importance of helping patients and their families plan individualized drug therapy regimens and adapt to changes in lifestyle that are often indicated with diuretic therapy (e.g., low-salt diet, weight control, fluid restriction) cannot be overemphasized. With careful preparation, the patient should be able to do the following:

Keep an accurate record of daily weight, obtained under the same conditions each day, and report any increase or loss of 1 to 2 pounds in any one day to the prescriber

Recognize that the medication regimen can be influenced by increased or decreased fluid intake, vomiting, diarrhea, anorexia (if over 24 hours), or high environmental temperatures.

Monitor urinary patterns for changes in frequency, amount, or color of urine, and report any excessive change from usual patterns

Recognize signs of dehydration (e.g., marked thirst, excess dryness of the skin or mouth, decreased urine output, darker colored urine, constipation)

Monitor areas of fluid accumulation for edema or swelling (e.g., ankles, abdomen)

Maintain a low-sodium diet, as indicated, eating a well-balanced diet avoiding foods that are high in sodium

State signs and symptoms of gout

Continued.

GENERAL NURSING IMPLICATIONS—cont'd

Nursing of patients requiring diuretics—cont'd

PATIENT EDUCATION—cont'd

Recognize the signs of low-salt syndrome (anorexia, nausea, vomiting, diarrhea, fatigue, dulled mental function, muscle cramps) and notify the prescriber if these should occur

Know the importance of following the drug regimen as planned with health care providers and the importance of regular follow-up clinic visits during long-term therapy to assess current status and evaluate response, including the need for blood tests (e.g., sodium, potassium, chloride, uric acid, calcium, creatinine, and BUN)

Patients receiving thiazide and loop diuretics often require potassium supplements. They should know the purpose, administration, and storage of these medications, as well as the monitoring of their effects. Potassium supplements are often unpleasant to take and can cause gastric irritation. Potassium supplements are best taken with meals along with a full glass of water or juice. Patients may be able to control potassium balance by including potassium-rich foods in their diets.

Certain diuretics require specific additional information in relation to patient education (e.g., thiazide and potassium-sparing diuretics can lead to hyponatremia when excess water is taken). See the Nursing Drug Digest for specific information regarding diuretics that should be incorporated into teaching plans.

Providing simple written instructions of medication regimens can do much to reinforce care at home.

Nursing of patients requiring antidiuretics

See individual agents as specified in the Nursing Drug Digest.

GENERAL INSTRUCTIONS FOR DISCHARGE/OUTPATIENTS

DIURETICS

Follow the instructions on the prescription exactly and take this medication as directed. This medication can cause stomach upset, so it is best to take it with food, milk, or with a meal. If you take one dose of this medication each day, take the dose with your breakfast. Always take this medication at the same time each day. Taking it with breakfast will help you to remember to take it and will also prevent stomach upset.

This medication will cause you to urinate or pass water more often. You may also pass more water at a time than usual. This is the desired effect of this drug so do not be concerned.

Avoid taking alcohol, barbiturates, or narcotics while you are on this medication because together they may cause your blood pressure to become too low, causing you to faint or fall down.

Avoid eating salty foods such as pretzels, potato chips, salted peanuts, ham, canned soups, and peanut butter. Your nurse can give you a list of foods to avoid, as well as a list of foods you can eat that are low in salt. It is best not to salt your food at the table. If you find that you have difficulty not using salt, you may be able to use a salt substitute. Do *not* use a salt substitute, however, without first checking with your prescriber, because salt substitutes contain potassium and you may get too much potassium if you are taking a potassium-sparing diuretic.

This drug may cause you to lose some potassium from your body. If you are not taking a potassium supplement, eat one or more portions of fruits daily (e.g., oranges, grapefruit, bananas, cantaloupe, prunes) or fruit juices (e.g., orange, grapefruit, pineapple, prune) that are good sources of potassium. Tomatoes, brussel sprouts, beef steak, hamburger, and turkey are also good sources of potassium.

Muscle cramps, weakness, dry mouth, and lightheadedness are side effects of this medication. If these persist or become worse, notify your prescriber.

Weigh yourself every day at the same time. Notify your nurse or prescriber if excessive weight change occurs.

Store your medication in a dry, dark place. Remember, this medication has been prescribed especially for you. Do not trade or give this medication to any relatives or friends. Keep this and all medications out of children's reach.

Notify your prescriber before you start or stop taking any other medications while taking this medication. This medication can interact with some drugs and cause harmful effects. Stopping another medication may necessitate a change in the dose of your diuretic.

If you are taking *triamterene*, it may color your urine blue (rarely). In addition, this medication can also make your skin more sensitive to sunlight. Wear a sunscreen or shade your skin from the sun when outside.

Thiazide and loop diuretics may cause blood glucose levels to increase. Diabetic patients should monitor their blood glucose.

NURSING DRUG DIGEST

Medication (trade name*)	Indication	Usual dosage and administration	Dosage forms, preparation, and storage	Contraindications, cautions, and comments	Monitoring
Amiloride Midamor Moduret* Moduretic*	Conserving potassium in conjunction with other diuretics in hypertension, CHF, or liver cirrhosis	*Adults:* 5-20 mg PO/24 hr in 1-2 doses Administer with food or milk to decrease GI irritation May need to decrease dose in renal impairment because 50% is usually excreted unchanged in the urine	Tablet: 5 mg	*Contraindicated* in acute renal failure, anuria, hyperkalemia or sensitivity to the drug Headache and dizziness are common Use with caution in patients predisposed to acidosis (e.g., uncontrolled diabetes, severe COPD) Use with extreme caution in patients taking potassium supplements ECG changes associated with hyperkalemia include peaked T waves, widening of QRS complex, prolongation of P-R interval, and ST depression	Monitor urine output, serum electrolytes, and ECG for hyperkalemia (other symptoms include fatigue, muscular weakness, bradycardia, and shock)

Continued.

NOTE: For additional details regarding the individual agents listed in this table see the text and other tables in this chapter.
*Indicates a multiple active ingredient product. For a complete listing of all active ingredients see the *Drug Reference Guide to Brand Names and Active Ingredients.*
★Indicates that the drug is generally available only in the United States.

NURSING DRUG DIGEST—cont'd

Medication (trade name)	Indication	Usual dosage and administration	Dosage forms, preparation, and storage	Contraindications, cautions, and comments	Monitoring
Bendroflu-methiazide Aprinox Benuron Bukozide Bristuron Centyl Corzide* Naturetin Neo-Naclex Rauzide* Sodiuretic	Edema associated with CHF, corticosteroid therapy, estrogen therapy, hepatic cirrhosis, or renal dysfunction Hypertension	*Adults:* 2.5-20 mg/24 hr PO Administer with food or milk to decrease GI irritation Administer in the morning to prevent nocturia *Elderly:* Start with lower dosage	Tablets: 2.5, 5, 10 mg	*Contraindicated* in renal failure, hepatic failure, or hypersensitivity to the drug or to sulfonamides Combined use of potassium-sparing agents or potassium supplements may be necessary in individual patients When used in combination with digitalis, may potentiate digitalis toxicity Use during the third trimester of pregnancy may cause thrombocytopenia in the neonate Use with caution during pregnancy and lactation Use with caution in patients predisposed to gout Use with caution in patients receiving lithium therapy May cause various fluid and electrolyte disturbances, including hypokalemia, hypochloremia, hyponatremia, hyperuricemia, and hyperglycemia	Observe for signs of hypokalemia and digitalis toxicity in patients receiving digitalis glycosides Monitor serum electrolytes, blood glucose, and serum uric acid levels Check BP for postural hypotension Check body weight and fluid intake and output at daily intervals Check for signs of fluid and electrolytes imbalance: dry mouth, thirst, weakness, muscle cramps, restlessness, lethargy, drowsiness, hypotension, tachycardia, and GI disturbance

Drug	Uses	Dosage	Availability	Comments	
★ **Benzthiazide** Aquastat Aquatag Benzide Exna-R Exna Hydrex Marazide Naclex Proaque Rola-Benz S-Aqua Urazide Urese	See Bendroflume-thiazide	*Adults:* 50-200 mg/24 hr PO in 2-3 divided doses	Tablet: 50 mg		See Bendroflumethia-zide
★ **Bumetanide** Bumex	Edema associated with CHF and hepatic and renal disease	*Adults:* 0.5-2 mg/24 hr PO, IM, *or slow IV* (over 1-2 min) Maximum: 10 mg/24 hr Administer PO whenever feasible	Tablets: 0.5, 1 mg Injectable: 0.25 mg/ml	*Contraindicated* in anuria, hepatic coma, and hypersensitivity See Furosemide Bumetanide is strongly bound to plasma proteins and may displace other highly protein-bound drugs (e.g., phenylbutazone)	See Furosemide
Chlorothiazide Aldoclor* Chlores-erpine* Chlotride Diupres* Diupres-250* Diuril Ro-Chloro-Serp* Ro-Chloro-zide Saluric Supres* SK-Chloro-thiazide	See Bendroflume-thiazide	*Adults:* 500-1000 mg PO *or IV* q.d. to b.i.d. *Children:* 20-25 mg/kg/24 hr PO in 2 divided doses	Tablets: 250, 500 mg Injectable: 500 mg/vial Dilute with 18 ml of sterile water; D₅W, or NS for injection		See Bendroflumethia-zide

Continued.

NURSING DRUG DIGEST—cont'd

Medication (trade name)	Indication	Usual dosage and administration	Dosage forms, preparation, and storage	Contraindications, cautions, and comments	Monitoring
Chlorpropamide Chloromide Chloronase Diabetoral Diabinese Insulase Mellinese Novopropamide Stabinol	Diabetes insipidus (incomplete) See also Chapter 60, "Insulin and Related Medications"	*Adults:* 250 mg PO initially, 500-750 mg/24 hr as a single dose	Tablets: 100, 250 mg	*Contraindicated* in severe hepatic, renal, or thyroid impairment Potentiates the effect of low levels of arginine-vasopressin (AVP) on collecting tubules; may also increase AVP release from the neurohypophysis Use in combination with thiazides Ineffective in complete central and nephrogenic forms of diabetes insipidus	Observe for signs of hypoglycemia (see Chapter 60)
Chlorthalidone Combipres* Demi-Regroton* Hygroton Hygroton-Reserpine Igroton Novothalidone Regroton* Uridon	See Bendroflumethiazide	*Adults:* 25-100 mg PO initially, then 100-200 mg 3 times a week Long-acting, no need to divide dosage Maximum: 200 mg/24 hr	Tablets: 25, 50, 100 mg	See Bendroflumethiazide	See Bendroflumethiazide
★ **Cyclothiazide** Anhydron Fluidil	See Bendroflumethiazide	*Adults:* 1-2 mg/24 hr PO Maximum: 2 mg PO t.i.d.	Tablet: 2 mg	See Bendroflumethiazide	See Bendroflumethiazide
Desmopressin DDAVP Minirin	Central diabetes insipidus	*Adults:* 10-40 μg/24 hr intranasally in a single or divided dose *Children:* 5-30 μg/24 hr intranasally in a single or divided dose *Elderly:* Start with lower doses Administer *intranasally* only	Nasal solution: 0.1 mg/ml Store under refrigeration at 4° C (do *not* freeze) Protect from light Stable for 3 weeks at room temperature	Drug of choice for the treatment of central (neurogenic) diabetes insipidus; *not* effective in nephrogenic diabetes insipidus Adjust fluid intake to decrease risk of water intoxication	Monitor fluid intake and output Observe for water intoxication Monitor serum electrolytes, particularly for hyponatremia, which can result from excess administration Monitor urine samples for volume and osmolality

Drug	Uses	Dosage	How Supplied/Remarks	Contraindications/Cautions	Nursing Considerations
Ethacrynate Ethacrynic acid Edecrin Hydromedin Reomax Taladren	CHF, acute pulmonary edema, severe edema from nephrotic syndrome, cirrhosis of liver with ascites	*Adults:* 50-200 mg PO/24 hr, daily or every other day. Maximum: 200 mg PO b.i.d. Administration with food or milk may decrease GI distress. Administer in morning to prevent nocturia. 50-100 mg IV over several minutes as an emergency measure. IV administration may cause thrombophlebitis. Do *not* administer SC or IM. *Children:* Over 5 years, 25 mg PO/24 hr; increase by 25 mg daily to desired effect. *Elderly:* Start with lower dosage.	Tablet: 50 mg. Injectable: 50 mg powder. Dilute injectable with at least 50 ml of D₅W or NS. Discard solutions that are cloudy or that contain a precipitate. Discard unused solution after 24 hr. Ethacrynate is the injectable form of ethacrynic acid.	*Contraindicated* in anuria. Transient or permanent deafness may occur in patients with severe renal insufficiency receiving IV doses in excess of the recommended dosages. Use with caution in pregnancy and lactation.	Monitor blood pressure and pulse, body weight, and intake and output. Check for signs of fluid and electrolyte imbalance (e.g., hypokalemia). Monitor serum uric acid levels for symptoms of gout. Observe for watery diarrhea—if observed, discontinue drug and notify prescriber.
Furosemide Furoside Fursemide Lasilix Lasix Laxur Neo-Renal Novosemide Seguril Uritol	CHF, acute pulmonary edema, severe edema from nephrotic syndrome, cirrhosis of liver with ascites. Hypertension	*Adults:* 20-200 mg PO/24 hr. Administer in morning to prevent nocturia. 20-80 mg IM, IV; repeat in 2 hr if necessary. Administer IV *slowly* at a rate of 20 mg/min (10 mg/min or less in the presence of renal impairment). Do *not* add furosemide to the tubing of a running infusion solution or mix with other drugs. *Children:* 1-2 mg/kg q.6-24h. as indicated; or 1 mg/kg IV slowly q.2-24h. as indicated. Maximum: 6 mg/kg/dose. *Elderly:* Start with lower dosage. For *adult* patients with severe renal impairment with GFR *between* 5 and 20 ml/min, who have *not* responded to conventional diuretic doses: 250-1000 mg/24 hr PO or IV (*not* to exceed 4 mg/min) can be administered under *strict* supervision.	Tablets: 20, 40, 500 mg. Injectable 10 mg/ml. Oral solution: 10 mg/ml. Protect from light. *Discard* discolored (yellow) solutions. The 250 mg ampule can be diluted with 250 ml of D₅W or NS.	*Contraindicated* in complete renal shutdown, hypersensitivity, severe hypokalemia, severe hypovolemia, and hepatic cirrhosis. May enhance cephaloridine nephrotoxicity; avoid concomitant use of these two drugs. Transient deafness may occur in patients with severe renal failure or receiving drugs that are ototoxic. Enhances calcium excretion and may be used as an adjunct in the treatment of hypercalcemia.	Monitor BP and pulse, body weight, and intake and output. Check for signs of fluid and electrolyte imbalance. Monitor serum uric acid levels for symptoms of gout. Closely monitor serum glucose levels of diabetic patients because they may be greatly increased. Observe for tinnitus or hearing loss, particularly with high-dose parenteral use.

Continued.

NURSING DRUG DIGEST—cont'd

Medication (trade name)	Indication	Usual dosage and administration	Dosage forms, preparation, and storage	Contraindications, cautions, and comments	Monitoring
Hydrochlorothiazide Aldoril* Diaqua Diuchlor H Dyazide* Esidrix Esimil* Hydrodiuril Hydrozide Manuril Moduretic* Natrimax Oretic Thiuretic Unipres	See Bendroflumethiazide	*Adults:* 25-100 mg PO q.d. to b.i.d. *Children:* 2-2.5mg/kg/24 hr PO in 2 divided doses	Tablets: 25, 50, 100 mg	See Bendroflumethiazide	See Bendroflumethiazide
★ **Hydroflumethiazide** Di-Ademil Duicardin Hydrenox Saluron Salutensin Salutensin-Demi	See Bendroflumethiazide	*Adults:* 25-200 mg/24 hr PO	Tablet: 50 mg	See Bendroflumethiazide	See Bendroflumethiazide
Indapamide Lozide Lozol	See Bendroflumethiazide	Adults: 2.5 mg/24 hr PO as a single morning dose Maximum: 2.5 mg/24 hr	Tablet: 2.5 mg	See Bendroflumethiazide In addition to its renally mediated antihypertensive effect, indapamide apparently also has a direct effect on blood vessels Incidence and severity of fluid and electrolyte side effects increase markedly with doses higher than 2.5 mg/24 hr	See Bendroflumethiazide

Drug	Uses	Dosage	How Supplied	Remarks	Nursing Considerations
★ **Lypressin** Diapid	Diabetes insipidus (nonnephrogenic)	*Adults:* 1-2 sprays in each nostril q.4-6h. Children: Same as adults Dose is highly individualized based on thirst and frequency of urination Administer *intranasally* only	Nasal solution: 0.185 mg/ml NOTE: 0.185 mg lypressin is equivalent to 50 Posterior-pituitary Units	Used as an adjunct to parenteral therapy for diabetes insipidus	
Mannitol Isotol Osmitrol	Cerebral edema, prophylaxis of oliguria in surgical procedures and trauma, glaucoma	*Adults:* 100 gm/24 hr IV Do *not* administer SC or IM Maximum: 6 gm/kg/24 hr *Children:* Start with low dose and increase gradually based on clinical status (generally 1-2 gm/kg IV) Administer as a 5%-25% solution by IV infusion *only*	Injectable: 5%, 10%, 15%, 20%, 25% If crystals have formed, immerse bottle in hot water for 1-2 min, then shake vigorously and allow solution to cool to *body temperature;* discard solution if crystals do not dissolve	*Contraindicated* in anuria, severe dehydration, intracranial bleeding, and CHF Administer fluids as permitted to relieve thirst Mannitol, 1 gm, is equivalent to 5.5 mOsm	Observe for pulmonary edema, hypertension, hypotension, dehydration, and urinary retention Check IV site for infiltration into soft tissue Monitor renal function, serum electrolytes Monitor vital signs at least hourly
Methyclothiazide Aquatensen Diutensen* Diutensen-R* Duretic Enduron Enduronyl Forte* Enduronyl Eutron	See Bendroflumethiazide	*Adults:* 5-10 mg/24 hr PO	Tablets: 2.5, 5 mg	See Bendroflumethiazide	See Bendroflumethiazide
Metolazone Diulo Zaroxolyn	See Bendroflumethiazide	*Adults:* 2.5-20 mg/kg/24 hr PO *Elderly:* Start with lower doses	Tablets: 2.5, 5, 10 mg	See Bendroflumethiazide	See Bendroflumethiazide
Polythiazide Drenusil Lotense Nephril Renese Renese-R*	See Bendroflumethiazide	*Adults:* 1-4 mg/24 hr PO	Tablets: 1, 2, 4 mg	See Bendroflumethiazide	See Bendroflumethiazide
Quinethazone Aquamox Hydromox	See Bendroflumethiazide	*Adults:* 50-100 mg/24 hr PO Maximum: 200 mg/24 hr	Tablet: 50 mg	See Bendroflumethiazide	See Bendroflumethiazide

Continued.

NURSING DRUG DIGEST—cont'd

Medication (trade name)	Indication	Usual dosage and administration	Dosage forms, preparation, and storage	Contraindications, cautions, and comments	Monitoring
Spironolactone Aldactazide* Aldactone	Edema ascites, primary aldosteronism Hypertension	*Adults:* 25-50 mg PO q.i.d. Up to 400 mg/24 hr for hypertension Some patients may be controlled on once daily dosing using the 100 mg tablet *Children:* 3.3 mg/kg/24 hr PO in single or divided doses *Elderly:* Start with lower dosage Administration with food or milk may decrease GI irritation	Tablets: 25, 50, 100 mg	*Contraindicated* in acute renal failure, anuria, hyperkalemia, or sensitivity to the drug Use with extreme caution in patients receiving potassium supplements Use of potassium supplements in patients receiving spironolactone is *not* recommended Gynecomastia may develop particularly after high doses have been administered for prolonged periods	Monitor urine output, serum electrolytes, and ECG for hyperkalemia
Triamterene Dyazide* Dyrenium Dytac Jatropur Novotriamzide*	Conserving potassium in conjunction with other diuretics Edema associated with CHF, cirrhosis, or nephrotic syndrome	*Adults:* 100-200 mg PO/24 hr Maximum: 300 mg/24 hr Administer with food or milk to decrease GI disturbance	Capsules: 50, 100 mg	*Contraindicated* in acute renal failure, anuria, hyperkalemia, or sensitivity to the drug May impart a pale blue fluorescent color to urine (rarely) Use with extreme caution in patients receiving potassium supplements	Monitor urine output, BUN, serum electrolytes, and ECG for hyperkalemia
★ **Trichlormethiazide** Aquex Diurese Iperdiuren Kirkrinal Metahydrin Metatensin* Naqua Naquival* Ropres*	See Bendroflumethiazide	*Adults:* 2-8 mg/24 hr PO	Tablets: 2, 4 mg	See Bendroflumethiazide	See Bendroflumethiazide

Drug	Uses	Dosage	Preparation	Contraindications/Precautions	Nursing considerations
★ **Urea** Ureaphil	Cerebral edema Prophylaxis of oliguria in surgical procedures, trauma and burns; promotes urine flow following prostatic surgery Glaucoma	*Adults:* 0.5-1.5 gm/kg by *slow IV* Maximum: 2 gm/kg/24 hr IV *Children:* Less than 2 years of age, 0.1-1 gm/kg by *slow IV*; greater than 2 years of age, same as adults Used as 30% solution for cerebral edema; 4% solution for oliguria or promotion of urine flow Use only *slow* infusion (3-4 mg/min); do *not* administer through the same set through which blood is being given *Elderly:* Do *not* infuse through veins of lower extremities because of increased risk of phlebitis and thrombosis For IV infusion *only*	Injectable 40 gm powder in 150 ml bottle for reconstitution Reconstitute with 105 ml D₅W to yield 135 ml of 30% (300 mg/ml) solution Use only freshly reconstituted solution up to 48 hr stored refrigerated; discard unused portion	*Contraindicated* in dehydration, renal failure, liver failure, and CHF	Observe for pulmonary edema, hypertension, hypotension, dehydration, and urinary retention; check IV site for infiltration into soft tissue Monitor renal function, serum electrolytes, especially for hypokalemia and hyponatremia Monitor vital signs at least hourly
Vasopressin Insipidin Pitressin Pitressin Tannate in Oil	Diabetes insipidus (nonnephrogenic) Abdominal distention caused by bowel gas	*Adults:* 5-10 units IM or SC b.i.d. to q.i.d. (aqueous); *or* 1.5-5 units/24 hr IM or SC (in oil) q. 1-3 days Repeat dose only after symptoms of polyuria begin to occur to prevent water retention and dilutional hyponatremia *Children:* Start with proportionately smaller adult dose and titrate to clinical response Do *not* administer IV	Injectable: 20 units/ml (aqueous); 5 units/ml (in oil) (for IM use *only*) Warm vial in hands and shake to mix well before administration	*Contraindicated* in advanced arteriosclerosis, angina pectoris, epilepsy, hypertensive cardiorenal disease, coronary thrombosis, and toxemia of pregnancy Preparation in oil must be emulsified by vigorous shaking and warming Use with caution in patients with coronary artery disease and hypertension Restore water balance in dehydrated patients *before* administration	Observe for chest pain, abdominal cramps, drowsiness, confusion, and seizures Check for hypertension Observe for signs of water intoxication

BIBLIOGRAPHY

Burg, M.B. Mechanisms of action of diuretic drugs. In B.M. Brenner and F.C. Rector (Eds.). *The kidney.* Philadelphia: W.B. Saunders Co., 1976.

Burg, M., & Green, N. Effect of ethacrynic acid on the thick ascending limb of Henle's loop. *Kidney International,* 1973, *4,* 301-308.

Burg, M., Stoner, L., Cardinal, J., & Green, N. Furosemide effect on isolated perfused tubules. *American Journal of Physiology,* 1973, *225,* 119-124.

Earley, L.E., & Forland, M. Nephrotic syndrome. In L.E. Earley and C.W. Gottschalk (Eds.). *Strauss and Welt's diseases of the kidney.* Boston: Little, Brown and Co., 1979.

Freis, E.D. Salt in hypertension and the effects of diuretics. *Annual Review of Pharmacology and Toxicology,* 1979, *19,* 13-23.

Jacobsen, J.R., & Kokko, J.P. Diuretics: sites and mechanisms of action. *Annual Review of Pharmacology,* 1976, *16,* 201-214.

Kemp, G., & Kemp, D. Diuretics. *American Journal of Nursing,* 1978, *78*(6), 1006-1010.

Lassiter, W.E. Disorders of sodium metabolism. In L.E. Earley and C.W. Gottschalk (Eds.). *Strauss and Welt's diseases of the kidney.* Boston: Little Brown and Co., 1979.

Lowenthal, D.T., Gould, A., Shirk, J., Mazella, J., Affrime, M.B., Walker, F., & Onesti, G. Effects of amiloride on oral glucose loading, serum potassium, renin, and aldosterone in diet-controlled diabetes. *Clinical Pharmacology and Therapeutics,* 1980, *27,* 671-676.

Madias, N.E., & Zelman, S.J. What are the metabolic complications of diuretic treatment? *Geriatrics,* 1982, *37*(2), 93 96, 99, 103-104.

Nussbaum, P.B. Diabetes insipidus, in H.F. Conn (Ed.). *1980 Current therapy.* Philadelphia: W.B. Saunders Co., 1980.

Orr, M.L. Drugs and renal disease. *American Journal of Nursing,* 1981, *81*(5), 969-971.

Stark, J.L. BUN/creatinine—your keys to kidney function. *Nursing 80,* 1980, *10*(5), 33-38.

Todd, B. Drugs and the elderly—when the patient is on diuretics. *Geriatric Nursing,* 1981, *2*(2), 149-150.

Drugs Used to Treat Urinary Tract Disorders

Lynn M. Paulsen

Medications discussed in this chapter

Urinary acidifiers
  Ammonium biphosphate,
    sodium biphosphate,
    and sodium acid pyro-
    phosphate
  Ammonium chloride
  Ascorbic acid
  Potassium acid phos-
    phate
  Potassium acid phos-
    phate and sodium acid
    phosphate
  Racemethionine
Urinary analgesics
  Ethoxazene
  Phenazopyridine
Urinary antiseptics
  Cinoxacin
  Methenamine
  Methenamine hippurate

Urinary antiseptics—cont'd
  Methenamine mandelate
  Methylene blue
  Nalidixic acid
  Nitrofurantoin
Urinary antiseptic irrigants
  Acetic acid
  Benzalkonium chloride
  Chlorhexidine gluconate
  Neomycin and polymyxin
    B
  Oxychlorosene sodium
  Silver nitrate
Urinary antispasmodics
  Flavoxate
  Oxybutynin
Urinary cholinergics
  Bethanechol
  Neostigmine methylsul-
    fate

Numerous drugs are used specifically for treating urinary tract disorders. These drugs include urinary acidifiers, urinary tract analgesics, urinary tract *antiseptics*, urinary antispasmodics, and urinary cholinergics. These agents are often used in combination with each other for maximum effect.

URINARY ACIDIFIERS

Urinary acidification is used as an adjunct to some urinary antiseptics either to activate them (e.g., methenamine compounds) or to increase their activity (e.g., nitrofurantoin). Acidification of the urine can also be used to increase the renal elimination of some drugs (e.g., in the case of amphetamine overdose).

The urine is normally more acidic (pH 6) than the blood (pH 7.4). This is because of the amount of acid produced from a normal diet containing animal protein and the kidneys' preservation of the acid-base balance of the body by selectively excreting or conserving hydrogen ions. Urinary acidification greater than pH 6 (pH 5.5 or less) is difficult to attain and maintain over prolonged periods of time without a resultant compensation by the kidney or the occurrence of systemic acidosis.

Urinary acidification is produced by the ingestion of organic acids to achieve a urine pH of 5.5 or less. Because the kidney can vary the amount of acid excreted, the urine must be tested regularly with *nitrazine paper*.

Acidification of the urine should be attempted only in patients with normal renal function as determined by serum creatinine and blood urea nitrogen (BUN) assays, because any impairment of renal function puts the patient at a significant risk of getting metabolic acidosis. Acidification of the urine decreases the solubility of uric acid and may precipitate kidney stones.

Ammonium biphosphate, sodium biphosphate, and sodium acid pyrophosphate

Ammonium biphosphate, sodium biphosphate, and sodium acid pyrophosphate acidify the urine by increasing the amount of phosphate buffer that can trap the hydrogen ions in the urine to form titratable acid. Saturation of the sodium pump in this system will limit the ability of this compound to acidify the urine further.

Dosage and administration. The usual adult dose of this combination product ranges from 4 to 12 gm orally per 24 hours in 4 divided doses. The dose for a particular patient will depend on the patient's dietary intake and initial response to the drug. Urine pH should be measured 4 times a day until acidification is achieved, then twice a day thereafter.

Toxicity. This ammonium and sodium phosphate combination is associated with systemic acidosis in high doses (i.e., greater than 6 gm per day), especially in patients with impaired kidney function. Hyperphosphatemia can also occur, especially in renally impaired patients, which is usually manifested by muscle cramps or shortness of breath. Hyperphosphatemia exhibits these toxicities usually by decreasing the serum calcium concentration. Each 500 mg tablet contains 1.7 mEq of sodium so that given a total daily dose of 12 gm, an extra 40.8 mEq or 960 mg of sodium would be ingested. This would present a problem to patients with strict salt restrictions (e.g., CHF). The ammonia content of each 500 mg tablet is approximately 27 mg, with a 12 gm daily dose providing 640 mg of ammonia. Patients with moderate to severe liver disease can progress to hepatic coma with even small doses of ammonia. This combination should *never* be used in patients with kidney or liver dysfunction or in hypocalcemic states (e.g., osteomalacia, hypoparathyroidism). The phosphate content of this product causes significant laxative effects.

Ammonium chloride

Ammonium chloride produces an excess of chloride anion in the glomerular filtrate by the biochemical conversion of ammonium cation to the neutral compound, urea. Accompanying the excess concentration of chloride is an increase in sodium, but a greater increase in hydrogen ion concentration, leading to acidification of the urine. This process is short-lived because the liver soon begins to compensate by synthesizing more ammonium ion for excretion, negating the acidification. Urinary acidification with ammonium chloride is seldom successful for more than 3 to 5 days.

Dosage and administration. The usual adult dose is 2 to 12 gm per day in 2 to 4 divided doses. The dose necessary to acidify the urine in a particular patient will be variable, and the pH of the urine should be measured with nitrazine paper 4 times daily for the duration of therapy.

Toxicity. The usual toxicity of ammonium chloride is severe metabolic acidosis in patients with inadequate renal reserves. The inability of the kidney to excrete the hydrogen ions into the urine causes an increased concentration of hydrogen ions in the blood with a decrease in serum pH. An even more severe toxicity occurs when the liver is unable to convert ammonia to urea so that increased serum levels of ammonia occur and cause the neurologic consequences (e.g., somnolence, confusion) and hepatic coma. This drug is absolutely contraindicated in kidney or liver failure. The nausea produced by ammonium chloride is reduced when the drug is taken with meals.

Ascorbic acid

Ascorbic acid is a water-soluble vitamin structurally similar to the sugars (see Chapter 66, "Vitamins, Minerals, and Trace Elements"). It is excreted unchanged in the urine, where it is capable of acidifying the urine. The amount excreted in the urine depends on the tissue concentrations of ascorbic acid. Patients likely to have low normal tissue concentrations (e.g., nursing home patients and elderly patients) will not excrete enough ascorbic acid adequately to acidify the urine. The variability in patient response makes regular testing of the urine pH essential. Ascorbic acid does have an advantage of not normally causing systemic acidosis; however, urate and oxalate stones are reported regularly.

Dosage and administration. The usual adult dose is 12 gm orally per day in 4 divided doses.

Toxicity. Megadose ascorbic acid therapy proves to be free of toxicity in most patients. Acidification of the urine can lead to urate and oxalate stones, so painful micturition should always be evaluated. Sodium ascorbate is a form of ascorbic acid that provides vitamin activity, but does *not* acidify the urine. Orange juice provides only 60 mg of ascorbic acid per 120 ml dose, which is not usually adequate to acidify the urine.

Racemethionine

Racemethionine is an essential amino acid found in normal diets. With increased supplementation, 80% of racemethionine is converted in the liver to inorganic sulfates and excreted in the urine. Inorganic sulfates buffer the urine by increasing the hydrogen ion excreted as titratable acid similar to the phosphates discussed earlier.

Dosage and administration. The usual adult dose is 12 gm orally per day in 4 divided doses. Like all amino acids, racemethionine has a rather strong odor that may cause patients to become nauseous. Crushing the tablets and mixing them in food may overcome this problem. Because racemethionine undergoes biodegradation in the liver, toxic levels of racemethionine or its metabolites may build up in severe liver disease.

Potassium acid phosphate

Potassium acid phosphate acidifies the urine by providing additional phosphate buffers in the glomerular filtrate to trap hydrogen ions for excretion.

Dosage and administration. The usual adult dose is 4 gm per day in 4 divided doses. Because potassium salts are caustic and may erode the gastric mucosa, this particular product is supplied as a tablet to be dissolved in 180 to 240 ml (6 to 8 oz) of water. The tablets dissolve easier if left to soak for 5 minutes and are then stirred vigorously.

Toxicity. Both the potassium and the phosphate components are associated with systemic toxicity. Each 500 mg tablet of potassium acid phosphate contains 3.67 mEq of potassium, so a maximum adult daily dose would supply an additional 30 mEq of potassium per day. This would present problems in any disease state that was associated with increased potassium levels (e.g., renal failure, Addison's disease, hyperkalemia). The major toxicity of the phosphate is the production of saline catharsis.

Potassium acid phosphate and sodium acid phosphate

Potassium acid phosphate and sodium acid phosphate produce the same effects of the potassium acid phosphate alone, with decreased toxicity.

Dosage and administration. The usual adult dose is 2 to 8 gm per day in 4 divided doses. Because of the decreased amount of potassium in the combination, it is well tolerated in oral tablets.

URINARY TRACT ANALGESICS

Urinary tract analgesics are often used in conjunction with urinary tract antiseptics and antibiotics for symptomatic relief of *dysuria* arising from the irritation of the bladder and of the urethral mucosa. The urinary tract analgesics are azo dyes that are excreted in the urine where they exert topical analgesic effects on the lining of the urinary tract. Because these drugs are dyes, the urine becomes red-orange and the colored urine can stain clothes and bedding.

Phenazopyridine

Phenazopyridine is the most commonly prescribed urinary tract analgesic. It has no antibacterial properties and is *not* used as the sole agent in urinary tract infections. Because the dysuria associated with urinary tract infections dissipates as the antibacterial agent decreases the bacterial count, phenazopyridine is rarely required for more than 3 days.

Dosage and administration. Phenazopyridine is administered orally, with the usual adult dose being 600 mg per day in 3 divided doses. It is often used in combination products containing a sulfonamide (e.g., Azo-Gantanol).

Toxicity. The azo dye phenazopyridine is associated with nausea in approximately 10% of patients. An overdose of phenazopyridine has been reported to cause methemoglobinemia. The dye causes the urine

and sometimes the stools to become red-orange and can stain clothes.

Ethoxazene

Ethoxazene is an azo dye urinary tract analgesic similar to phenazopyridine. It is also used only in conjunction with antibacterial agents because it has no intrinsic antibacterial activity.

Dosage and administration. Ethoxazene is administered orally, with the usual adult dose being 200 mg per day in 2 divided doses.

Toxicity. Gastrointestinal irritation is more prominent with ethoxazene than with phenazopyridine, and for this reason is rarely used. Methemoglobinemia would probably occur if sufficient amounts of drug were taken in an overdose.

URINARY TRACT ANTISEPTICS

Urinary tract antiseptics are drugs synthesized chemically rather than derived from microorganisms as are the antibiotics (see Section X, "Antibacterial, Antifungal, and Antiviral Medications"). These antiseptic drugs reach therapeutic levels only in the urine and are thus limited to use in treating urinary tract infections.

Cinoxacin

Cinoxacin is an organic acid similar to nalidixic acid. It appears to work by interfering with the conversion of intermediate DNA fragments into high-molecular-weight DNA in bacteria. Bacterial resistance to cinoxacin occurs with high frequency in gram-negative bacteria, but the acquired resistance, a result of spontaneous chromosomal mutations, is not transferrable against other classes of antibacterial agents. Serum concentrations attained are only 3% to 4% of the urine concentrations, and prostatic concentrations are even less. Considering the distribution of this drug in the body, cinoxacin is used solely to treat lower urinary tract infections.

Sensitive organisms. Cinoxacin is active against most of the enteric bacteria that commonly cause urinary tract infections (e.g., *E. coli, Proteus, Klebsiella,* and *Enterobacter*) at concentrations easily attained in the urine. *Pseudomonas* and all gram-positive organisms are normally resistant. Inadequate doses of cinoxacin favor an emergence of resistant strains. Cross-resistance with nalidixic acid would be expected.

Dosage and administration. Cinoxacin is administered orally and is rapidly and completely absorbed. The adult dose is 1 gm per day in 2 or 4 divided doses. Because resistance emerges within 48 hours, repeat cultures and sensitivity tests are indicated for patients whose urine is not clear of bacteria in 48 hours or if a relapse occurs.

Excretion. Cinoxacin is 25% to 50% metabolized in the liver and all metabolites and active drug are excreted in the urine within 24 hours. Cinoxacin urine concentrations are decreased and the drug accumulates in patients with impaired renal function, rendering the drug inappropriate in these patients.

Toxicity. Despite the limited clinical experience with cinoxacin, its chemical similarity to nalidixic acid would indicate certain toxicities. Neurotoxicity with cinoxacin has been limited to reports of agitation, dizziness, headache, and visual disturbances in less than 1% of patients treated.

Skin reactions to cinoxacin include allergic skin rashes and urticaria. Because severe photosensitivity reactions have been reported with nalidixic acid, patients receiving cinoxacin should be cautioned to avoid sun exposure and to use sunscreens during the summer months.

In comparative trials, cinoxacin has appeared slightly more effective and produced fewer side effects than nalidixic acid.

Methenamine compounds

Methenamine and its salts, methenamine hippurate and methenamine mandelate, liberate *formaldehyde* when exposed to acid in the urine. Methenamine is combined with mandelic acid and hippuric acid to form methenamine mandelate and methanamine hippurate, respectively. The combination of methenamine with these organic acids was originally thought to promote the acidification of the urine and enhance the liberation of formaldehyde from methenamine, but although this has been refuted clinically, methenamine mandelate remains the most commonly used methenamine salt.

Urinary acidification. The amount of formaldehyde liberated by the decomposition of methenamine depends on the pH of the urine. Adequate levels are achieved only at a urine pH of 5.5 or less. Because the normal pH of urine varies from 4.5 to 8.0, with the average slightly acidic at pH 6, some patients will have adequately acidic urine, whereas many will not. For this reason, urinary pH must be tested with nitrazine paper while patients are receiving methenamine. Because the urinary pH can change depending on food and water intake, the urine pH is measured throughout therapy. Acidification of the urine is achieved by the administration of poorly metabolized acids, especially ascorbic acid, sodium biphosphate, acid-producing foods such as cranberry juice, and the amino acid racemethionine. Upward of 6 to 12 gm per day of these acids may be required to adequately acidify the urine. Unlike the urinary tract antiseptics, the urinary acidifiers do not confine their action to the urine (e.g., ammonium chloride is an excellent urinary acidifier; however, large doses can result in metabolic acidosis, and thus it is rarely used).

Sensitive organisms. Because all microorganisms are susceptible to formaldehyde, methenamine can be used to treat gram-positive and gram-negative bacterial and fungal urinary tract infections. Bacterial resistance to methenamine has not been reported and is unlikely to occur.

Dosage and administration. Methenamine mandelate is administered orally and is well absorbed even from enteric-coated tablets. The adult dose is 4 gm per day in 4 divided doses. Higher doses have been given, but should be reduced when the urine is sterile.

Excretion. Methenamine is totally excreted unchanged in the urine, where it is degraded into ammonia and formaldehyde. It is *not* used in renal failure because inadequate urine concentrations are achieved, and problems (e.g., metabolic acidosis) can result from using urinary acidifiers. Methenamine is *not* used in the presence of liver disease because of the liberation of ammonia in the blood that cannot be converted to urea by the diseased liver. High serum ammonia concentrations are associated with CNS disturbances (e.g., tremor, hyperreflexia, and EEG changes) and severe metabolic acidosis.

Toxicity. Gastrointestinal disturbances, especially nausea and vomiting, are common with methenamine. Dermatologic reactions (e.g., rashes and urticaria) have been reported. Doses of about 6 gm daily are associated with bladder irritation and resultant *hematuria*, *albuminuria*, and dysuria. Patients with high uric acid levels or gout should avoid methenamine because the urinary acidification may precipitate urate crystals in the urine.

Methylene blue

Methylene blue is a bacteriostatic dye that is only *rarely* used as a urinary antiseptic. Methylene blue exerts its weak antiseptic action by oxidation reduction actions. The major value of methylene blue is in treating methemoglobinemia, as occurs in cyanide poisoning. Specific sensitive organisms are not reported, and the sole use of methylene blue in urinary tract infections would be for prophylaxis.

Dosage and administration. Methylene blue is poorly absorbed from the GI tract and is excreted in the reduced form in both the urine and the bile. The adult dose for urinary tract infection prophylaxis ranges from 195 to 390 mg per day in 3 divided doses.

Toxicity. Methylene blue has two opposite effects on hemoglobin. Low concentrations (oral) of methylene blue hasten the conversion of methemoglobin to hemoglobin, except in patients with G-6-PD deficiency. In high concentrations (IV), methylene blue oxidizes the ferrous iron of hemoglobin to ferric ion, producing methemoglobin. The oral administration of methylene blue will cause both the urine and the stools to turn blue-green. The availability of more effective agents precludes all but the extremely rare use of this agent in the prophylaxis of urinary tract infections.

Nalidixic acid

The only approved use of nalidixic acid is for treating urinary tract infections, although inadequate levels are achieved in prostatic fluid to treat prostatitis. Nalidixic acid appears to work by interfering with the conversion of intermediate DNA fragments into high-molecular-weight DNA in bacteria. Bacterial resistance to nalidixic acid occurs with high frequency in gram-negative bacteria, but the acquired resistance, a result of spontaneous chromosomal mutations, is not transferable against other antibacterial agents.

Sensitive organisms. Most gram-negative organisms common in urinary tract infections (e.g., *E. coli, Proteus, Klebsiella,* and *Enterobacter*) are initially sensitive to nalidixic acid. *Pseudomonas* and all gram-positive organisms are usually resistant. Inadequate doses of nalidixic acid favor an emergence of resistant strains. Cross-resistance with cinoxacin and oxolinic acid regularly occurs.

Dosage and administration. Nalidixic acid is administered orally and is completely absorbed. The adult dose is 4 gm per day in 4 divided doses. Because resistance emerges usually within 48 hours, repeat cultures and sensitivity tests are indicated for patients whose urine is not clear of bacteria in 48 hours or if a relapse occurs.

Excretion. Nalidixic acid is partially metabolized in the liver, and all metabolites and the active drug are excreted in the urine within 24 hours. Adequate urine concentrations of nalidixic acid are achieved in patients with renal dysfunction; however, an accumulation of metabolites occurs in the serum, rendering the drug inappropriate for therapy in renal failure.

Toxicity. Neurotoxicity with nalidixic acid, although uncommon, is dramatic when it occurs. Visual disturbances, excitement, depression, confusion, and hallucinations appear most commonly; but headache, syncope, and convulsions have been described. Severe neurotoxicity occurs usually in conjunction with excessive doses; however, most clinicians avoid using the drug in patients with seizure disorders or with preexisting mental instability.

Intracranial hypertension has been reported in in-

fants and young children, so the drug is usually avoided in this age group.

An overdose with nalidixic acid can provoke metabolic disturbances resembling diabetic ketoacidosis without plasma ketones. Standard fluid and electrolyte therapy for metabolic acidosis is used to treat this problem.

Skin reactions to nalidixic acid include allergic skin rashes, urticaria, and severe photosensitivity reactions. Patients receiving nalidixic acid should be warned to avoid sun exposure and to use sunscreens during the summer months.

Nitrofurantoin

The only use of nitrofurantoin is in treating urinary tract infections, including *urethritis, prostatitis, cystitis,* and *pyelonephritis,* because after either oral or intravenous administration therapeutic concentrations are found only in the urine. The precise mechanism of action has not yet been determined for nitrofurantoin, although it is known to interfere with some bacterial enzymes and to inhibit carbohydrate metabolism in human nervous tissues. Despite this, the bacterial sensitivities are well known and, more importantly, acquired resistance has not been a problem with nitrofurantoin.

Sensitive organisms. The organisms sensitive to nitrofurantoin include the common gram-negative urinary tract pathogen, *E. coli;* however, most species of *Proteus, Klebsiella, Enterobacter,* and *Pseudomonas* are resistant. Gram-positive organisms that occasionally cause urinary tract infections, such as *Streptococcus faecalis, Staph. pyogenes,* and *Staph. epidermis,* are sensitive to nitrofurantoin. The activity of nitrofurantoin against sensitive bacteria is increased in acid urine (pH 5.5 or less).

Dosage and administration. Nitrofurantoin is usually administered orally. The macrocrystalline form is absorbed more slowly and may thus produce fewer GI side effects, but like the crystalline form it is completely absorbed. The dose is the same for both the crystalline and the macrocrystalline forms. The adult dose is 200 to 400 mg per day in 4 divided doses with the lower dose used for acute, uncomplicated cystitis and the higher doses reserved for more severe, chronic, or recurrent infections. Long-term suppressive therapy usually consists of a single daily dose of 50 to 100 mg. A single dose of 50 to 100 mg after intercourse is often prescribed for preventing honeymoon cystitis. Nitrofurantoin can also be administered intravenously, although this route is rarely used. Studies suggest that IV nitrofurantoin is indicated only in treating urinary tract infections in acutely ill patients unable to tolerate oral drugs. There is no therapeutic advantage to parenteral nitrofurantoin, and it cannot be used to treat systemic infections.

Excretion. Nitrofurantoin is rapidly excreted in the urine, with about 30% of the administered dose appearing in a therapeutically active form. Concentrations in the renal medulla are approximately equal to concentrations in the urine, allowing the drug to be used in pyelonephritis. Because patients with *uremia* do not excrete the drug into the urine in therapeutic concentrations and neurotoxicity increases, nitrofurantoin is not used in patients with renal failure.

Toxicity. Nausea and vomiting, but not diarrhea, are common reactions to oral and parenteral nitrofurantoin. A controversy exists over whether this is related to a local irritation of the GI tract or to the effects of the rapidly absorbed drug on the CNS. Probably both effects are causing the nausea and vomiting, because although the macrocrystalline form causes slower absorption and a decrease in the nausea and vomiting, it does not eliminate them completely.

Hypersensitivity reactions occur in approximately 5% of treated patients, usually as a skin rash, eosinophilia, or drug fever, which disappear as soon as the drug is discontinued.

One of the most serious side effects of nitrofurantoin is peripheral neuropathy, which occurs primarily in patients with impaired renal function and is a direct effect of nitrofurantoin interference with carbohydrate metabolism in nervous tissue. This effect is usually seen within the first 2 months of chronic therapy and can be reversed if the drug is stopped. Patients should be cautioned to report paresthesias, should they occur.

Therapy with nitrofurantoin has been associated with the following two types of pulmonary reactions.

1. Acute pneumonitis is characterized by the onset of fever, chills, dyspnea, eosinophilia, and pulmonary infiltrates hours to days after the initiation of therapy. This pneumonitis is allergic and subsides within hours of discontinuing the drug.
2. Interstitial pulmonary fibrosis is a more insidious reaction to nitrofurantoin that occurs after prolonged therapy. These changes are only partially reversible when therapy is stopped.

Hematologic side effects of nitrofurantoin exhibit the following two types of disorders.

1. Hemolytic anemia can be precipitated in patients with G-6-PD deficiency and in infants younger than 1 month of age because of the immaturity of the glucose-6-phosphate-dehydrogenase enzyme system.
2. Megaloblastic anemia has been attributed to chronic nitrofurantoin therapy based on its chemical similarity to phenytoin and the development of a folic acid deficiency.

URINARY TRACT ANTISEPTIC IRRIGANTS

Urinary tract infection subsequent to using indwelling catheters remains a major problem in the medical care of hospitalized patients. Patients are then at an increased risk for contracting sepsis. Improvements in catheter systems have helped; however, it is established that bacteria enter the system during the placement of the catheter. The length of catheterization and the manipulation of the catheter (i.e., irrigation) correlate with an increasing opportunity for the introduction of bacteria. Despite the introduction of closed catheter systems, approximately 50% of these patients acquire a urinary tract infection within 2 weeks.

Irrigation of the bladder with antiseptic or antimicrobial agents is a common practice in an attempt to prevent a urinary tract infection in catheterized patients. Despite the widespread use of continuous antiseptic irrigators, the efficacy of the antiseptic agents has not been adequately evaluated in conjunction with the closed catheter systems in current use. Efficacy has been demonstrated in the obsolete, open catheter drainage systems and in intermittent instillations following a single catheterization. In most reports, closed drainage systems alone compare favorably with closed drainage systems with continuous antiseptic irrigation.

Even in the most favorable reports, antiseptic irrigations are successful only in preventing or delaying the occurrence of urinary tract infections, *never* in treating established infections.

Prevention of urinary tract infections among catheterized patients is influenced more by the aseptic technique of the health care providers than by the reassuring presence of an antiseptic in the system. Attention to catheter care procedures appears to yield lower infection rates.

Acetic acid

Acetic acid is employed as a 0.25% solution in water in a continuous irrigation. The control of the urine pH may account for any activity of acetic acid, because only about 30% of gram-positive cocci and gram-negative bacteria are affected by this concentration of acetic acid. Therefore, the urine pH is always measured and should remain less than pH 5. Some patients may develop hematuria with the 0.25% solution, and in these cases the concentration is dropped to 0.125%. Other side effects have not been reported.

Benzalkonium chloride

Benzalkonium chloride (BAC) is a quaternary ammonium compound active against gram-positive and some gram-negative bacteria. As a urinary irrigant, BAC is used as a continuous irrigation of 0.005% solution. BAC is inactivated by most soaps, detergents, and organic material such as bacteria and white blood cells. Some cases of hypersensitivity reactions have been reported, with a blistering of the mucosa. Moderate chemical burns can result from inadequate dilution. Therefore, if a patient being treated with BAC complains of burning sensations, irrigation should be discontinued.

Chlorhexidine gluconate

Chlorhexidine gluconate is used in urinary irrigation solutions in a 0.02% concentration, which must be prepared by the nurse or pharmacist from the commercially available 1% solution (see the Nursing Drug Digest). Concentrations greater than this may irritate the bladder. At this concentration (0.02%), chlorhexidine has minimal activity against gram-negative organisms; epidemic infections by species of *Pseudomonas* have been traced to a contaminated 4% chlorhexidine solution.

Neomycin and polymyxin B

Neomycin and polymyxin B irrigation has been shown to decrease the rates of infection in open urinary drainage systems. The same results have not been shown in closed urinary drainage systems. Several studies suggest an increase in infections resistant to neomycin and polymyxin B after their use in irrigation solutions. The major problem with this irrigation solution lies not so much with its efficacy as an antibacterial, but in the propensity for neomycin to elicit allergic reactions. Hypersensitivity reactions, primarily rashes, occur in 6% to 8% of patients receiving topical neomycin.

Oxychlorosene sodium

Oxychlorosene sodium is a mixture of sodium hypochlorite and alkylbenzene sulfonates. Sodium hypochlorite is one of the oldest of the chlorine disinfectants. It is a proved germicidal agent and deodorizing agent. One of the most useful properties of sodium hypochlorite is its ability to dissolve necrotic tissue. The alkylbenzine sulfonates have detergent properties and allow the sodium hypochlorite better penetration. This irrigation solution is used only intermittently, alternating with saline to remove debris. Antibiotic resistance is not a problem, and toxicity has not been reported.

Silver nitrate

Soluble silver nitrate precipitates with proteins to inactivate most bacteria. It has been used in dilute concentrations as a urinary irrigation solution and is an effective antiseptic; however, routine use is limited by the irritation silver nitrate causes. Intermittent irrigation is recommended despite the increase in breaches of a closed irrigation system. Silver nitrate stains the skin, mucous membranes, and clothing black, so handling can become a problem.

URINARY ANTISPASMODICS

Inflammation or infection of the lower urinary tract (e.g., cystitis, prostatitis, urethritis, urethrocystitis) is often accompanied by dysuria, urgency, nocturia, frequency, and incontinence. These symptoms often include the urgent desire to micturate when the bladder contains as little as 50 ml of urine.

Symptomatic relief of these problems is provided by using systemic anticholinergic agents. This therapy is indicated with the concurrent treatment of the causative disease (e.g., infection) and is not usually continued long term.

In the normal bladder, distention of the bladder walls (400 to 500 ml urine) stimulates the nerves to the cerebral cortex, where the desire to urinate arises. During urination the detrusor muscle of the bladder and the longitudinal muscle of the bladder neck and urethral orifice contract as a result of activity in the parasympathetic nerves. If, instead of a full bladder, irritation of the bladder walls by infection or inflammation stimulates the afferent neurons, inappropriate parasympathetic activation of micturition will occur, causing frequent, small voiding.

All of the anticholinergic drugs (see Chapter 23 "Parasympathomimetics and Parasympatholytics"), such as atropine, cause a relaxation of the urinary bladder, and in high doses they can cause an inability of the bladder to contract. Systemic side effects preclude using atropine for this indication. Although all of the systemic parasympatholytic drugs affect the relaxation of the urinary bladder, two are used primarily for their antispasmodic effects on the genitourinary system: flavoxate and oxybutynin.

Flavoxate

Flavoxate is a popular urinary antispasmodic for the symptomatic treatment of dysuria, urgency, and frequency.

Dosage and administration. The usual adult doses range from 300 to 800 mg per day orally in 3 to 4 divided doses. It is normally well tolerated.

Toxicity. Because the parasympatholytic activity of flavoxate is systemic, the effects are not restricted to the urinary tract (see Chapter 23 "Parasympathomimetics and Parasympatholytics"). Visual disturbances, dizziness, and blurred vision result from the anticholinergic effects on the eyes. Nausea, vomiting, and ileus result from the lysis of a parasympathetic activity. Tachycardia and mental confusion occur predominantly in elderly patients. Overdoses are treated with physostigmine 0.5 to 2 mg IV repeated to a maximum dose of 5 mg. CNS excitement is treated with such sedatives as diazepam.

Oxybutynin

Oxybutynin claims significant increases in antispasmodic activity as compared with atropine, although oxybutyrin has only 20% of the anticholinergic activity of atropine. Whereas these claims are difficult to substantiate because direct measurements are seldom done, oxybutynin remains a popular urinary antispasmodic.

Dosage and administration. The usual adult dose is 10 to 15 mg orally per 24 hours in 2 to 3 divided doses. Do not exceed 20 mg in 24 hours.

URINARY CHOLINERGICS

Urinary retention is a common problem after surgery or parturition, and although the problem often resolves without medical intervention, cholinergic therapy is often employed. The effects of general anesthesia or indwelling Foley catheters or the pressure of the infant on the ureters during delivery causes atony of the detrusor muscles of the bladder and a lack of parasympathomimetic activity.

Because the urinary bladder can be stimulated to empty with the administration of parasympathomimetic or cholinergic drugs, patients who do not resolve their urinary retention shortly after surgery or parturition are given small doses of these drugs. The doses of these drugs normally used produce only the effects of micturition, defecation, and increased peristalsis of the GI tract. Because the activity of these drugs is not limited to the urinary tract, systemic effects of these drugs limit their usefulness and contradict their use in specific groups of patients. Patients with hyperthyroidism tolerate the cholinergic agents poorly because they already have increased parasympathomimetic activity. Patients with peptic ulcers are not good candidates for this type of therapy because the increased GI secretions and the increased gastric emptying time aggravate the ulcer healing. Any obstruction of the GI or urinary tract is a contraindication in cholinergic therapy because increased pressure may rupture the structure or organ involved. Additionally, cholinergic therapy in men with prostatic hypertrophy is not rational because this is a problem with a partial obstruction, not with muscle control of the bladder itself.

The two drugs used in treating postoperative or postpartum urinary retention are bethanechol and neostigmine methylsulfate.

Bethanecol

Bethanecol is the more commonly used cholinergic agent in urinary retention. It is a synthetic derivative of acetylcholine that produces its effects via the stimulation of the parasympathetic nervous system, increasing the time of the detrusor muscle of the urinary bladder, stimulating the motility of the GI tract, and increasing gastric tone.

Dosage and administration. Bethanecol comes in oral tablets usually restricted for use in patients with long-term problems of neurogenic bladder with retention. Acute therapy for postoperative and postpartum patients is more commonly given parenterally. The injectable form of bethanechol is for *subcutaneous use only*. The usual adult dose is 2.5 to 5 mg subcutaneously with repeated doses in 6 to 8 hours only if still needed. The accidental administration of bethanechol intramuscularly or intravenously is a serious problem. Symptoms of overdose include flushing, salivation, sweating, nausea, and asthmatic attacks, especially in patients with known asthma. Atropine is the specific antidote and should be available when the bethanechol injectable is used. Atropine is given subcutaneously except in extreme emergencies, when it is given intravenously. Doses of atropine range from 0.6 to 1.2 mg for adults with proportionately smaller doses for children.

Therapy with oral bethanechol is generally given about 2 hours after meals to avoid GI upset and vomiting. The usual adult dose ranges from 20 to 200 mg in 2 to 4 divided doses each day. The large doses are achieved by starting the patient on lower doses and titrating the dose to the desired effect. Doses above 200 mg per day do not appear to be more efficacious than the 200 mg.

Toxicity. The toxicities of bethanechol are associated primarily with overdose whether by inappropriately high doses or by inadvertent IM or IV injection of the subcutaneous product. The usual symptoms of overdose are flushing, salivation, defecation, nausea, and asthmatic attacks. Fainting and cardiac arrest, brief periods of complete heart block, and orthostatic hypotension have been associated with more serious overdose. Treatment is always initiated with atropine 0.6 to 1.2 mg subcutaneously in an adult. Intravenous atropine in 1 mg increments is employed in severe cases of cardiac dysrhythmias.

Patients receiving any of the ganglionic blocking agents for hypertension should never receive bethanechol because of the possibility of acute drops in blood pressure (see Chapter 26 "Ganglionic and Neuromuscular Stimulants and Blockers"). Patients receiving procainamide or quinidine (see Chapter 32 "Antidysrhythmics") require additional attention because these drugs may antagonize the cholinergic effects of bethanechol.

Neostigmine methylsulfate

Neostigmine methylsulfate is occasionally used for atony of the detrusor muscle of the urinary bladder to relieve postoperative dysuria and to decrease the time interval from surgery to spontaneous urination. Neostigmine blocks the breakdown of acetylcholine by antagonizing the enzyme acetylcholinesterase, thus providing an indirect cholinergic effect (see Chapter 25, "Anticholinesterases and Cholinesterase Reactivators").

Dosage and administration. Neostigmine is administered only as a subcutaneous injection because the drug is destroyed in the GI tract after oral administration. The usual adult dose is 0.5 to 1 mg subcutaneously every 3 hours as needed to a maximum of 5 doses. Inadvertent IM or IV injection of neostigmine is a serious problem and requires immediately notifying the prescriber and treating with atropine.

Toxicity. Like the cholinergic agent bethanechol, neostigmine has certain similar symptoms of overdose: salivation, lacrimation, involuntary urination and defecation, and bradycardia, in some instances. With serious overdoses, paralysis of the respiratory muscles may occur, requiring mechanical ventilation. As with bethanechol, specific treatment of neostigmine overdose is subcutaneous administration of atropine in doses of 0.6 to 1.2 mg for an adult. Serious cases of overdosage will require intravenous atropine (see Chapter 25, "Anticholinesterases and Cholinesterase Reactivators").

SUMMARY

This chapter has examined the use and dosage of various drugs used to treat urinary tract disorders. These drugs include urinary acidifiers, urinary tract analgesics, urinary tract antiseptics, urinary antispasmodics, and urinary cholinergics. Often these agents are used in combination in treating urinary tract disorders to take advantage of their additive or synergistic actions.

With a knowledge of the dosage, adverse effects, and clinically significant drug interactions associated with these various urinary tract agents, the nurse will be better able to provide optimum care to patients who require them, and will be able to anticipate, monitor for, and minimize preventable adverse side effects associated with these drugs.

ADVERSE/SIDE EFFECTS OF THE URINARY TRACT DRUGS*

ALLERGIC REACTIONS

Angioedema (cinoxacin, nalidixic acid, neomycin, nitrofurantoin, methenamine)
Bullae on exposed skin (cinoxacin, nalidixic acid)
Drug fever (nitrofurantoin)
Eosinophilia (cinoxacin, nalidixic acid, neomycin, nitrofurantoin, methenamine)
Erythema (cinoxacin, nalidixic acid)
Photosensitivity (cinoxacin, nalidixic acid)
Pruritus (cinoxacin, nalidixic acid, neomycin, nitrofurantoin, methenamine)

Rash (cinoxacin, nalidixic acid, neomycin, nitrofurantoin, methenamine)
Urticaria (cinoxacin, nalidixic acid, neomycin, nitrofurantoin, methenamine)

CENTRAL NERVOUS SYSTEM

Confusion (anticholinergics, cinoxacin, nalidixic acid)
Convulsions (nalidixic acid)
Drowsiness (nalidixic acid, nitrofurantoin)
Headache (nalidixic acid, nitrofurantoin)
Hallucinations (anticholinergics, cinoxacin, nalidixic acid)

Increased intracranial pressure in children (nalidixic acid)
Peripheral neuropathy (nitrofurantoin)
Toxic psychoses (anticholinergics, cinoxacin, nalidixic acid)
Vertigo (nalidixic acid, nitrofurantoin)

GASTROINTESTINAL SYSTEM

Delayed gastric emptying (antispasmodics)
Laxative action (phosphate-containing acidifiers)
Nausea (ethoxazene, flavoxate, methenamine, nitrofurantoin)
Vomiting (ethoxazene, flavoxate, methenamine, nitrofurantoin)

*See Chapter 11, "Drug Toxicity," for an overview of drug toxicity.

Continued.

ADVERSE/SIDE EFFECTS OF THE URINARY TRACT DRUGS—cont'd

HEMATOLOGIC SYSTEM

Hemolytic anemia in glucose-6-phosphate dehydrogenase deficiency (methylene blue [large doses], nitrofurantoin)

HEPATIC SYSTEM

Cholestatic jaundice (nalidixic acid, nitrofurantoin)

Hepatic coma in patients with preexisting hepatic disease (ammonium chloride)
Hepatic necrosis (nitrofurantoin)

METABOLIC SYSTEM

Acidosis (urinary acidifiers, cinoxacin, naladixic acid)

OCULAR SYSTEM

Difficulty focusing (cinoxacin, nalidixic acid)

Double vision (cinoxacin, nalidixic acid)
Overbrightness of lights (cinoxacin, nalidixic acid)

RESPIRATORY SYSTEM

Interstitial pulmonary fibrosis (nitrofurantoin)
Pneumonitis, acute (nitrofurantoin)

CLINICALLY SIGNIFICANT DRUG INTERACTIONS*

Primary drug	Interacting drug	Possible effect(s)	Probable mechanism(s)
Methenamine compounds	Acetazolamide	Decreased antibacterial effect of methenamine	Alkalinization of the urine
Methenamine compounds	Sulfonamides	Sulfonamide crystals in urine	Decreased solubility of sulfonamides in acid urine
Urinary acidifiers	Salicylates	Increased salicylate levels	Increased tubular reabsorption of salicylate
Urinary acidifiers	Spironolactone	Systemic acidosis	Inhibition of aldosterone impairs ability of kidney to excrete hydrogen ions

*See Chapter 10, "Drug Interactions" for an overview of drug interactions.

GENERAL NURSING IMPLICATIONS

Nursing of patients requiring drugs used to treat urinary tract disorders

ASSESSMENT

A complete nursing assessment is essential in establishing a baseline from which to plan individualized drug therapy regimens and to monitor patient response. Assessment should include a detailed drug history to identify sensitivity, contraindications, cautions, potential drug interactions, and drug-taking patterns before initiating drug therapy.

Assessment should also include detailed baseline data related to urinary dysfunction, including polyuria, hesitancy, frequency, dysuria, nocturia, incontinence, and history of urinary tract dysfunction. Assessment of urinary self-care behaviors that can prevent chronic urinary tract infections (women wiping from front to back, hygiene practices) should also be identified. Assessment of fluid and electrolyte balance and renal function tests should be completed before drug therapy is begun. Laboratory tests should include urinalysis, urine culture and sensitivity, serum creatinine, and BUN.

Special attention should be given to documenting the patient's description of urinary discomfort or difficulty.

SENSITIVITY

Although hypersensitivity to the urinary tract agents is generally rare, any drug has the potential to cause these reactions in susceptible individuals.

See the Nursing Drug Digest for sensitivity associated with the use of each specific agent.

Contraindications, cautions, and toxicity

Various drugs used to treat urinary tract disorders are contraindicated in certain patients and should be used with caution in others. See the Nursing Drug Digest for each specific agent. Toxicity can result from the use of these drugs and is also specified in the Nursing Drug Digest for each individual agent.

Drug interactions

See Clinically Significant Drug Interactions for important drug interactions.

ADMINISTRATION

Drugs used in treating urinary tract disorders can be given by various routes of administration including instillation by way of continuous catheter irrigation. See the Nursing Drug Digest for each specific agent.

MONITORING PATIENT RESPONSE

Monitoring therapeutic response and adverse side effects is especially important in adjusting drug therapy to meet the individual patient's requirements. All data should be recorded carefully to document patient response and to facilitate treatment decisions. The patient should be able to void normal volumes of clear urine at regular times without pain or retention of urine. Monitoring urinary patterns is essential. In addition, for each group of drugs used to treat urinary tract disorders, the following should be monitored.

Urinary acidifiers

Monitor the urine pH at least twice a day (4 times a day is more desirable), and observe patients for signs of systemic acidosis (e.g., hypotension, tachypnea, almond mouth odor, disorientation, Kussmaul breathing), diarrhea (with phosphate acidifiers), and liver dysfunction while on ammonium chloride.

Urinary antiseptics
Cinoxacin, nalidixic acid
Observe for drowsiness, headache, vertigo, increased sensitivity to light, photosensitivity, rashes, convulsions in seizure patients, and bulging fontanels in children. Monitor kidney and liver function tests.

Methenamine
Monitor the urine pH with nitrazine paper, and observe for hematuria.

Nitrofurantoin
Monitor the urine pH with nitrazine paper, and monitor patients for peripheral neuropathy, nystagmus, crystalluria, cough, chest pain, fever, chills, and dyspnea (which may herald the onset of a pulmonary hypersensitivity reaction).

Urinary antiseptic irrigants

Monitor for turbidity or increased urine odor (which may signal infection), irritation of the mucosal areas proximate to the catheter, and hematuria.

Urinary antispasmodics

Monitor for signs of overdose (tachycardia, blurred vision, vomiting, vertigo), mental confusion (especially in elderly patients), and monitor blood pressure and pulse until the patient's physiologic responses are stabilized. Observe for signs of heatstroke in hot weather.

Urinary cholinergics

Observe for bronchoconstriction, and monitor blood pressure and pulse until the patient's physiologic responses are stabilized. Observe for cardiac dysrhythmias, increased salivation, sweating, abdominal cramping, and flushing.

PATIENT EDUCATION

The patient and the family should have a clear understanding of the medication regimen, as well as the exact name of the medication, its action, dosage, storage, administration, and side effects, including what can be done to minimize them. Patients should know how to monitor themselves for the therapeutic effects of the medication and for adverse side effects. The patient should be aware of signs that indicate that the prescriber or nurse should be contacted. Because urinary tract dysfunction can contribute to kidney damage and even renal failure, healthy self-care practices in this area should be promoted. The nurse's role in preventing and managing urinary dysfunction cannot be overemphasized.

Follow-up is often indicated in chronic conditions. Patients who are discharged with medication, or outpatients, often find it helpful if verbal instructions are reinforced with a written plan. In addition to the usual discharge instructions, see General Instructions for Discharge/Outpatients for specific information that should be included and discussed with patients in relation to their individual drug requirements.

GENERAL INSTRUCTIONS FOR DISCHARGE/OUTPATIENTS

URINARY ACIDIFIERS

This drug is used to treat a urinary tract disorder. If you do not understand why you require this medication, check with your health care provider.

For this medication to work, the urine must be acidic (pH 5 or less). Check your urine with nitrazine paper to see if it is acidic. If your urine is not acidic, check with your nurse or physician for further directions.

To decrease gastrointestinal irritation, take this medication with food.

Ammonium biphosphate, sodium biphosphate, sodium acid pyrophosphate, potassium acid phosphate, or sodium acid phosphate may cause diarrhea; if this occurs, notify your nurse or physician.

With potassium acid phosphate, do *not* take tablets whole, but dissolve them first. Dissolve tablets in 6 to 8 ounces (180-240 ml) of water, let set for 2 to 5 minutes, then stir vigorously. This drug may cause diarrhea; if it does, notify your nurse or physician.

Keep this and all medications out of children's reach.

URINARY ANALGESICS

To decrease gastrointestinal irritation, take this medication with food. This medication turns the urine red-orange and may stain clothes.

Keep this and all medications out of children's reach.

URINARY ANTISEPTICS

Make sure that you follow the instructions on the prescriptions exactly. Continue taking this medication for as long as directed to completely clear up your infection. If you do not feel better in 2 to 3 days, or if your symptoms get worse, consult your nurse or physician.

This medication has been prescribed especially for your urinary tract infection. Do not trade or give this medication to any relatives or friends.

Keep this and all medications out of children's reach.

Methenamine compounds can cause nausea or an upset stomach; take after meals.

For methenamine compounds to work, the urine must be acidic (pH 5 or less). Check your urine with nitrazine paper to see if it is acidic. If your urine is not acidic, check with your nurse or physician for further directions. Side effects that should be reported to your nurse or physician include blood in the urine, low back pain, or pain on urination, all of which may result from the drug not working adequately or from drug side effects.

Cinoxacin, nalidixic acid, and oxolinic acid are best taken with a full glass of water on an empty stomach 1 hour before or 2 hours after meals. If nausea or upset stomach occurs, the drug may be taken with food.

Some patients are more likely to suffer sunburn with cinoxacin, nalidixic acid, or oxolinic acid, so use a chemical sunscreen or protective clothing (in summer months) until you see how this drug affects you.

If cinoxacin, nalidixic acid, or oxolinic acid makes you drowsy, do not drive a car or operate machinery that requires alertness.

Nitrofurantoin is best taken with food or milk to avoid stomach upset and to increase the absorption of the drug.

Nitrofurantoin is more active when the urine is acidic, so your urine should be checked with nitrazine paper to make sure the pH is less than 5.5. If your urine is not acidic, check with your nurse or physician for further instructions.

Nitrofurantoin may cause the urine to turn brown, which is a normal effect.

Do not drink alcohol while taking nitrofurantoin, because a few patients experience a severe reaction to alcohol with facial flushing and fainting (disulfiram-like reaction).

If you experience chest pain, trouble breathing, or coughing, notify your nurse or physician.

The liquid form of nitrofurantoin may be mixed with a small amount of water, juice, milk, or infant formula to make the administration of the drug easier. Do not put in an infant bottle.

Keep this and all medications out of children's reach.

URINARY ANTISPASMODICS

To decrease gastrointestinal irritation, take these medications with food. These drugs can cause blurred vision, dry mouth, and palpitations; do not drive a car or operate machinery until you determine how these drugs affect you.

Difficulty in concentrating, mental confusion, or dizziness should be reported to your nurse or physician.

These drugs suppress sweating; therefore, during hot weather care must be taken to avoid heatstroke.

Keep these and all medications out of children's reach.

URINARY CHOLINERGICS

Take on an empty stomach, 1 hour before or 2 hours after meals to avoid nausea and vomiting.

Abdominal cramping, excessive salivation, or flushing should be reported to your nurse or physician.

Keep this and all medications out of children's reach.

NURSING DRUG DIGEST

Medication (trade name*)	Indication	Usual dosage and administration	Dosage forms, preparation, and storage	Contraindications, cautions, and comments	Monitoring
URINARY ACIDIFIERS					
Ammonium chloride	Urinary acidifier See also Chapter 67 "Fluids and Electrolytes"	*Adults:* 2-12 gm/24 hr PO in 2-6 divided doses *Children:* 75 mg/kg/24 hr PO in 4 divided doses Administer with food or milk to decrease GI irritation Normally used for 3 days or less because after that the kidney may compensate	Tablets: 325, 500 mg regular and enteric-coated Syrup: 500 mg/5 ml	*Contraindicated* in renal or hepatic insufficiency Acidosis occurs with high doses May cause nausea and vomiting	Monitor urine pH with nitrazine paper
★ **Ammonium biphosphate, sodium biphosphate, sodium acid pyrophosphate** Phos-phaid	Urinary acidifier	*Adults:* 4-12 gm/24 hr PO q.i.d. Each dose should be followed with a glassful of water	Tablets: 250, 500 mg 250 mg tablet contains ammonium biphosphate 95 mg, sodium biphosphate 100 mg, sodium acid pyrophosphate 55 mg	*Contraindicated* in renal failure Nausea occurs with high doses; large doses may also cause diarrhea	Monitor urine pH with nitrazine paper
Ascorbic acid Cemil Civalin Cevita Flavorcee Vitacee Viterra	Urinary acidifier See also Chapter 66, "Vitamins, Minerals, and Trace Elements"	*Adults:* 12 gm/24 hr PO in 6 divided doses *Children:* 2 gm/24 hr PO in 4 divided doses	Tablets: 25, 50, 100, 250, 500 mg, 1 gm Drops: 35 mg/0.6 ml, 100 mg/ml Syrup: 20 mg/ml; 500 mg/5 ml	Controversy concerning actual efficacy as urinary acidifier Do not confuse with sodium ascorbate Diarrhea is common	Monitor urine pH with nitrazine paper

Continued.

NOTE: For additional details regarding the individual agents listed in this table see the text and other tables in this chapter.

*Indicates a multiple active ingredient product. For a complete listing of all active ingredients see the *Drug Reference Guide to Brand Names and Active Ingredients.*

★ Indicates that the drug is generally available only in the United States.

NURSING DRUG DIGEST—cont'd

Medication (trade name)	Indication	Usual dosage and administration	Dosage forms, preparation, and storage	Contraindications, cautions, and comments	Monitoring
★ **Potassium acid phosphate** K-Phos M.F.* K-Phos Neutral* K-Phos No. 2* K-Phos Original	Urinary acidifier	*Adults:* 4 gm/24 hr dissolved PO in 4 divided doses *Always* dissolve tablets in 180-240 ml water; let soak 2-5 min before stirring vigorously	Tablet: 500 mg	*Contraindicated* in renal failure, severe hepatic disease, hyperkalemia, and Addison's disease Potassium content is 3.67 mEq/500 mg tablet Has a laxative effect Also used in conjunction with low-calcium, low-vitamin D diet to reduce urinary excretion of calcium	
★ **Potassium acid phosphate and sodium acid phosphate** K-Phos MF* K-Phos Neutral* K-Phos No. 2* Uro-Phosphate*	Urinary acidifier	*Adults:* 2-8 gm/24 hr PO in 4 divided doses Maximum: 1 gm PO q.2h.	Tablets: 500 mg, 1 gm	*Contraindicated* in renal failure, severe hepatic disease, hyperkalemia, and Addison's disease Has a laxative effect	
Racemethionine A-D-R Dequasine* Meonine Monile Ninol Pedameth Uracid Uranap	Urinary acidifier for control of diaper rash and urinary odor	*Adults:* 12 gm/24 hr PO in 4 divided doses *Children:* 250 mg/kg/24 hr PO in 3-4 divided doses May be crushed and mixed with food	Tablets: 250, 500 mg	*Contraindicated* in liver disease Odor of tablets is strong and may be objectionable to patient	Monitor protein intake and body weight, particularly in children, because weight gain may be below normal

URINARY TRACT ANALGESICS

Drug	Uses	Dose Ranges	Remarks
★ **Ethoxazene** Serenium	Pain associated with urinary tract infections	Tablet: 100 mg	*Adults:* 300 mg/24 hr PO in 3 divided doses *Children:* Under 8 years, 200 mg/24 hr PO in 2 divided doses Administration with food or milk may decrease GI irritation	*Contraindicated* in severe liver disease, uremia, and chronic pyelonephritis Use with caution in patients with GI disorders May cause nausea and vomiting This drug has no antibacterial action and does *not* treat cystitis—only the pain; turns urine orange-red; may stain clothes Monitor for hypersensitivity Monitor for yellowing of the skin or sclera, which indicates overaccumulation of the drug, necessitating a decrease in dose or discontinuation of the drug
Phenazopyridine Azo Gantrisine Azo-Standard Azomine Azosult* Azotrex* Di-Azo Dolonil* Mallophene Microsul-A* Phenaze Phenazo Pyridium Sedural Suladyne Suldiazol* Thiosulfil-A* Uremide* Uro-Gantanol*	Pain and irritation of the lower urinary tract	Tablets: 100, 200 mg	*Adults:* 600 mg/24 hr PO in 3 divided doses *Children:* 12 mg/kg/24 hr PO in 3 divided doses; 9-12 years, 300 mg/24 hr PO in 3 divided doses Administration with food or milk may decrease GI irritation	*Contraindicated* in hepatitis and renal failure Turns urine orange or red; may stain clothes May cause nausea and vomiting May alter Tes-Tape results for urinary glucose This drug has no antibacterial action and does *not* treat cystitis—only the pain

Continued.

NURSING DRUG DIGEST—cont'd

Medication (trade name)	Indication	Usual dosage and administration	Dosage forms, preparation, and storage	Contraindications, cautions, and comments	Monitoring
URINARY TRACT ANTISEPTICS					
★ **Cinoxacin** Cinobac	Cystitis and urinary tract infections caused by susceptible gram-negative organisms, including *E. coli, Klebsiella pneumonia, Enterobacter* species, *Proteus mirabilus,* and *P. vulgaris*	*Adults:* 1 gm/24 hr PO in 2 or 4 divided doses *Children:* Not recommended for children under 12; over 12 years use adult dose Administer with food or milk to decrease GI irritation Dosage may need to be *decreased* in renal impairment	Capsules: 250, 500 mg	*Contraindicated* in history of convulsive disorder; pregnancy or breast feeding; CNS damage, liver disease, renal failure (serum creatinine > 2.5), infants under 3 mo, or hypersensitivity to nalidixic or oxolinic acid Insomnia, agitation and dizziness are signs of CNS toxicity May cause increased sensitivity of eyes to light May cause nausea	Monitor kidney and liver function Observe for signs of CNS toxicity and report to prescriber
Methenamine Cystex* Formin Methandine Prosed* Trac Tabs* Urised Uritone Uro-Phosphate* Urotropin	Prophylaxis or suppressive treatment of urinary tract infections after eradication of infection by other agents	*Adults:* 4 gm/24 hr PO in 4 divided doses Maximum: 12 gm/24 hr *Children:* 12 years and older, same as adult dose; 6-12 years, 2 gm/24 hr PO in divided doses; under 6 years, 75 mg/kg/24 hr PO in 4 divided doses Administer with food or milk to decrease GI irritation NOTE: Large doses (8 gm daily for 4 weeks) have caused bladder irritation (painful and frequent micturition and hematuria)	Tablet: 500 mg	*Contraindicated* in renal insufficiency, liver disease, and severe dehydration *Not* to be used *alone* in acute infections of the kidney causing systemic symptoms such as fever and chills Urine *must* be acidic (pH = 5.5 or less) for methenamine to work (i.e., to generate formaldehyde) May cause nausea or diarrhea	Monitor fluid intake and output Monitor urine pH with nitrazine paper Observe for skin rash and report

Drug	Use	Dosage	Preparations	Remarks	Nursing Implications
Methenamine hippurate Nip-Rex Niprex Urex	See Methenamine	*Adults:* 2 gm/24 hr PO in 2 divided doses; Maximum: 4 gm/24 hr; *Children:* 12 years and older, same as adult dose; 6-12 years, 1-2 gm/24 hr PO in 2 divided doses	Tablet: 1 gm	Coadministration with sulfonamides may cause precipitation of the sulfonamides in the urine and should be avoided	See Methenamine
Methenamine mandelate Azo-Mandelamine* Mandalay Mandelanine Mandelets Prov-U-Sep Renelatt Sterine Thiacide* Uroqid-Acid* Uroqid-Acid No. 2*	See Methenamine	*Adults:* 4 gm/24 hr PO in 4 divided doses; Maximum: 12 gm/24 hr; *Children:* 6-12 years, 2 gm/24 hr PO in 4 divided doses; under 6 years, 75 mg/kg/24 hr PO in 4 divided doses; Suspensions have vegetable oil base, so administer with caution to elderly and debilitated patients to avoid lipid pneumonia	Tablets: 250, 500 mg, 1 gm; Tablets: (enteric-coated) 250, 500 mg, 1 gm; Granules: 500 mg, 1 gm; Suspension: 250 mg/5 ml; Suspension: (forte) 500 mg/5 ml; *Shake* suspension well before use; Granules *must* be dissolved in 60-120 ml water before administration	See Methenamine	See Methenamine
Methylene blue M-B tabs MG-Blue Prosed* Trac-Tabs* Urised* Urolene Blue	Mild urinary tract antiseptic for cystitis and urethritis (seldom used for these indications and use is not recommended)	*Adults:* 130 to 390 mg/24 hr PO in 2-3 divided doses with a glassful of water; Administration with food or milk may decrease GI irritation	Tablet: 65 mg	*Contraindicated* in renal disease and allergy to methylene blue; Imparts blue-green color to urine and stools; May induce hemolysis in G-6-PD-deficient patients; Long-term treatment (>10 days) may cause anemia; May cause bladder irritation; Large doses may cause fever	Monitor for cyanosis; Monitor fluid intake and output

Continued.

NURSING DRUG DIGEST—cont'd

Medication (trade name)	Indication	Usual dosage and administration	Dosage forms, preparation, and storage	Contraindications, cautions, and comments	Monitoring
Nalidixic acid Cybis NegGram Nogram Wintomylon	Acute and chronic urinary tract infections caused by most gram-negative bacilli, including *E. coli, Proteus, Klebsiella,* and *Enterobacter* species	*Adults:* 4 gm/24 hr PO in 4 divided doses With prolonged therapy, dose may be reduced to 2 gm/24 hr PO in 4 divided doses *Children:* 3 mo-12 years, 55 mg/kg/24 hr in 4 divided doses With prolonged therapy, dose may be reduced to 33 mg/kg/24 hr in 4 divided doses Administer with food or milk to decrease GI irritation	Tablets: 250, 500, 1000 mg Suspension: 250 mg/5 ml (protect from freezing) *Shake* suspension well before use	*Contraindicated* in history of convulsive disorder; first trimester of pregnancy or breast-feeding, CNS damage, liver disease, renal failure, infants under 3 mo, or hypersensitivity May cause drowsiness May cause photosensitivity Brief convulsions have occurred rarely with this drug, especially in elderly patients; reversible with discontinuance of drug Nitrofurantoin may antagonize the effect of nalidixic acid; thus, these two agents should *not* generally be used together Cross-resistance with oxolinic acid may occur	Question patient regarding blurred vision and overbrightness of lights Observe for drowsiness after initial doses Monitor renal and hepatic function Use Tes-Tape or Clinistix to monitor urinary glucose in diabetes because may cause false positive result with Clinitest Monitor blood counts for patients on chronic therapy Monitor for photosensitivity; if observed, drug should be discontinued
Nitrofurantoin Chemiofuran Cyantin Dantafur Fua-Med Furadantin Furalan Furanex Furatine Furatoin Ituran Ivadantin J-Dantin Macrodantin	Cystitis, pyelitis, and pyelonephritis caused by susceptible organisms, including *E. coli, Staphylococcus pyogenes, S. epidermis, Streptococcus faecalis*	*Adults:* 200-400 mg/24 hr PO in 4 divided doses (*Maximum:* 600 mg/24 hr); prophylaxis, 50-100 mg q.h.s. IV, 6.6 mg/kg IV to a maximum 360 mg/24 hr IM may cause severe pain at injection site and is *not* recommended *Children:* Over 3 mo, 5-7 mg/kg/24 hr PO in 4 divided doses; prophylaxis, 1-2 mg/kg PO q.h.s. Administer with food or milk to minimize gastric irritation	Tablets: 50, 100 mg Capsules: 25, 50, 100 mg Suspension: 25 mg/5 ml Injectable: 180 mg/vial Reconstitute with sterile water for injection and dilute to 500 ml with appropriate IV solution (i.e., D_5W, NS, or sterile water for injection [without preservatives]) before administering Store in amber-colored nonmetal containers Protect from light	*Contraindicated* in significant renal dysfunction (CrCl < 40 ml/min), pregnant patients at term, infants less than 3 mo, peripheral neuropathy, pulmonary disease, G-6-PD deficiency May cause nausea, anorexia, vomiting, and diarrhea May impart a brownish color to urine Macrocrystal form asso-	Monitor for pulmonary sensitivity reactions: fever, chills, cough, dyspnea Monitor fluid intake and output Observe for any signs of peripheral neuropathy and report to prescriber Monitor laboratory tests for hemolysis

Drug	Use	Dosage	Remarks		
N-Toin Nephronex Nifuran Nitrex Novofuran Parfuran Sarodant			Suspension can stain teeth, so have patient rinse with water immediately after taking dose Therapy should generally *not* exceed 14 days, to minimize toxicity	Contact with metal (except aluminum) and stainless steel may cause precipitation *Shake* suspension well before use	...ciated with less GI irritation Nitrofurantoin may antagonize the effect of nalidixic acid; thus, these two agents should *not* generally be used together Peripheral neuropathy may occur, and if the drug is not discontinued may become severe and irreversible Drug should be discontinued at first signs of drug-induced hemolysis Chronic therapy may cause interstitial pulmonary fibrosis

URINARY ANTISEPTIC IRRIGANTS

Drug	Use	Dosage	Remarks		
Acetic acid 0.25%	Chronic or short-term prophylaxis of bacteriuria with indwelling catheters (*not* for systemic use)	*Adults:* 1500 ml/24 hr, 1 ml/min through Y-tube Allow to drain every 2 hr	Solution: 0.25% in 1 L irrigation bottle	Some patients may develop hematuria; in this case the concentration of acetic acid is normally reduced to 0.125%	Urine must be less than pH 5 Check with nitrazine paper; if pH is >5, the rate should be increased until pH drops to 5
Benzalkonium chloride 0.005% Benzachloro-50 Cetylcide Solution* Germ-i-Tol Germicin Hyamine 3500 Ionax Sabol Spensomide Theranac Scrub Zephiran chloride	Chronic or short-term prophylaxis of bacteriuria with indwelling catheters (*not* for systemic use) See also Chapter 55, "Antiseptics and Local Anesthetics"	*Adults:* 1500 ml/24 hr; 1 ml/min through Y-tube Lower concentration is used in cases of irritation	Solution: 0.0025% to 0.005% compounded by pharmacist (0.3 ml of 17% benzalkonium chloride to 1 L irrigation fluid for 0.005%); mixed only with sterile water for irrigation		*Contraindicated* in hypersensitivity; do *not* use concentrate on any mucous membrane Benzalkonium chloride is inactivated by soaps Incompatible with silver nitrate solution

Continued.

NURSING DRUG DIGEST—cont'd

Medication (trade name)	Indication	Usual dosage and administration	Dosage forms, preparation, and storage	Contraindications, cautions, and comments	Monitoring
Chlorhexidine gluconate 0.02% Bactigras Hibicare Hibiclens Hibitane Hibitane Tincture*	Chronic or short-term prophylaxis of bacteriuria with indwelling catheters (*not* for systemic use) See also Chapter 55, "Antiseptics and Local Anesthetics"	*Adults:* 1000 ml/24 hr (0.7 ml/min) through Y-tube, or 60 ml following single catheterization	Solution: 0.02% compounded by pharmacist (20 ml of 1% chlorhexidine per 1 L irrigation fluid)	*Contraindicated* in hypersensitivity	
Neomycin and polymyxin B solution for irrigation Neosporin G.U. Irrigant	Short-term (10-day) prophylaxis of bacteriuria with indwelling catheters (*not* for systemic use)	*Adults:* 1000 ml/24 hr via continuous catheter irrigation Maximum: 2000 ml/24 hr *Not* to be injected Rinse of the bladder must be continuous; the inflow should not be interrupted for more than a few minutes	Solution: 1 ml ampule, 20 ml vial containing 40 mg neomycin and 200,000 units of polymyxin B per ml Dilute 1 ml with 1000 ml of NS to prepare irrigation solution	*Contraindicated* in patients hypersensitive to any of the components Use *caution* in administration to avoid any reflux of the irrigation solution up the ureters because the neomycin may cause renal toxicity	
Oxychlorosene sodium Clorpactin WCS-90	Treatment of bacteriuria with indwelling catheter (*not* for systemic use) See also Chapter 55, "Antiseptics and Local Anesthetics"	*Adults:* Intermittent irrigation with 0.1% to 0.2% solution; alternate with saline for irrigation to remove debris	Crystal: 2 gm bottle Solution: 0.1% to 0.2% in water or saline for irrigation; compounded by pharmacist (2 gm per 1 L irrigation fluid for 0.2%) Keep dry crystal under refrigeration until reconstitution	Effective in cases of antibiotic resistance Nontoxic and nonallergenic in concentrations used	

Drug	Use	Dosage	Preparations	Side/Adverse effects	Nursing implications
Silver nitrate 0.25%	Treatment of bacteriuria with indwelling catheter (*not* for systemic use) See also Chapter 55, "Antiseptics and Local Anesthetics"	*Adults:* Intermittent irrigation with 0.25% solution	Solution: 0.25% compounded by pharmacist (2.5 gm silver nitrate per 1 L irrigation fluid)	Stains skin and clothing brown Because solution can be irritating, it is used as intermittent rather than continuous irrigation	
URINARY ANTISPASMODICS					
★ **Flavoxate** Urispas	Symptomatic relief of dysuria, urgency, frequency, and incontinence that result from urinary tract infections	*Adults:* 300-800 mg/24 hr PO in 3 to 4 divided doses *Children:* Over 12 years, use adult doses	Tablet: 100 mg	*Contraindicated* in pyloric obstruction, ileus, GI hemorrhage, and glaucoma Nausea, vomiting, dry mouth, vertigo, headache, tachycardia, and mental confusion in elderly patients	Observe for confusion and blurred vision
Oxybutynin Ditropan	Symptomatic relief of dysuria, urgency, frequency, and incontinence resulting from urinary tract infections	*Adults:* 10-15 mg/24 hr PO in 2 to 3 divided doses; do *not* exceed 20 mg/24 hr *Children:* Over 5 years, 10 mg/24 hr PO in 2 divided doses (*not* to exceed 15 mg/24 hr) *Elderly:* Start with lower dose and increase with caution	Tablet: 5 mg Syrup: 5 mg/5 ml	*Contraindicated* in glaucoma, GI obstruction, myasthenia gravis, intestinal atony of elderly patients, and severe colitis Fever and heat stroke can occur during hot weather Symptoms of hyperthyroidism, coronary heart disease, CHF, dysrhythmias, tachycardia, hypertension, and prostatic hypertrophy may be aggravated Can cause dry mouth, decreased sweating, blurred vision, and dilation of pupils Administer with caution to patients with hiatal hernia because the condition may be exacerbated	Observe for agitation, flushing, or drop in BP Monitor for fever or heat stroke Monitor bowel movements because drug may precipitate or aggravate toxic megacolon

Continued.

NURSING DRUG DIGEST—cont'd

Medication (trade name)	Indication	Usual dosage and administration	Dosage forms, preparation, and storage	Contraindications, cautions, and comments	Monitoring
URINARY CHOLINERGICS					
Bethanechol Duvoid Mictrol Myotonachol Urecholine Urolax Vesicholine	Urinary retention after surgery or parturition and neurogenic atony of the bladder See also Chapter 23, "Parasympathomimetics and Parasympatholytics"	*Adults:* 20-200 mg/24 hr PO in 2-4 divided doses Start with 5 mg q.1h. to effect, then give total dose q.i.d. SC, 2.5-5 mg q.6-8h.; *not* to be given IM or IV Inadvertent IM or IV administration might cause circulatory collapse, shock, and cardiac arrest; this should be treated immediately with 1 mg atropine SC (IV in acute emergencies) To be taken on an empty stomach 1 hr before or 2 hr after meals to avoid nausea and vomiting	Tablets: 5, 10, 25, 50 mg Injectable: 5 mg/ml Do *not* freeze Solution may be autoclaved at 120° C for 20 min without loss of potency	*Contraindicated* in hyperthyroidism, hypersensitivity, peptic ulcer, asthma, danger of rupture of bladder wall, hypotension, epilepsy, parkinsonism, hypertension, pregnancy, or recent GI or bladder surgery Patients receiving quinidine or procainamide will not get adequate cholinergic effects Abdominal discomfort, salivation, sweating, or flushing may occur	Monitor for cardiorespiratory status, pulse, BP, bronchoconstriction, and dysrhythmia (keep atropine available)
Neostigmine methylsulfate Prostigmin	Prevention and treatment of postoperative urinary retention See also Chapter 25, "Anticholinesterases and Cholinesterase Reactivators"	*Adults:* 0.25-0.5 mg SC or IM q.3-4h. for 5 doses IV administration is *not* recommended	Injectable: 1:1000 (1 mg/ml), 1:2000 (0.5 mg/ml), 1:4000 (0.25 mg/ml)	*Contraindicated* in hypersensitivity, and in mechanical intestinal or urinary obstruction Cholinergic crisis may result from overdose, increasing muscle weakness leading to death from paralysis of respiratory muscles; discontinue drug and administer atropine 1 mg SC or IV Use with caution in asthmatic patients Keep atropine on hand for emergencies	Monitor muscle tone

BIBLIOGRAPHY

Bone, R.C., Wolfe, J., & Sobonya, R.E. Desquamative interstitial pneumonia following long term nitrofurantoin therapy. *American Journal of Medicine*, 1976, *60*, 967-968.

Burman, L.G. Apparent absence of transferable resistance to nalidixic acid in pathogenic gram-negative bacteria. *Journal of Antimicrobial Chemotherapy*, 1977, *3*, 509-512.

Dudley, M.N., & Barriere, S.L. Antimicrobial irrigations in the prevention and treatment of catheter-related urinary tract infections. *American Journal of Hospital Pharmacy*, 1981, *38*, 59-65.

Gleckman, R., Alvarez, S., Joubert, D.W., & Matthews, S.J. Drug therapy reviews: methenamine mandelate and methenamine hippurate. *American Journal of Hospital Pharmacy*, 1979, *36*, 1509-1512.

Gould, S. Urinary tract disorders: clinical comparisons of flavonate and phenazopyridine. *Urology*, 1975, *5*, 612-615.

Hamilton-Miller, C.L., & Brumfitt, W.M. Methenamine and its salts as urinary tract antiseptics: variables affecting the antibacterial activity of formaldehyde, mandelic acid and hippuric acid in vitro. *Investigative Urology*, 1977, *14*, 287-298.

Kershaw, N.J., & Leigh, D.A. The antibacterial and pharmacological activity of oxolinic acid (Prodoxol). *Journal of Antimicrobial Chemotherapy*, 1975, *1*, 311-320.

Simonson, W., Stennett, D.J., & Hall, C.A. Nitrofurantoin pneumonitis. *Drug Intelligence and Clinical Pharmacy*, 1977, *2*, 624-628.

Stamey, T.A., & Bragonjie, J. Resistance to nalidixic acid: a misconception due to underdosage. *Journal of the American Medical Association*, 1976, *236*, 1857-1859.

Stamm, W.E. Guidelines for prevention of catheter associated urinary tract infections. *Annals of Internal Medicine*, 1975, *82*, 386-390.

Vainrub, B., & Musher, D.M. Lack of effect of methenamine in suppression of, or prophylaxis against, chronic urinary tract infection. *Antimicrobial Agents and Chemotherapy*, 1977, *12*, 625-631.

Veterans Administration Ad Hoc Interdisciplinary Advisory Committee on Antimicrobial Drug Use. Indwelling urinary catheters. *Journal of the American Medical Association*, 1977, *237*, 1859.

Warren, J.W., Platt, R., & Thomas, R.J. Antibiotic irrigation and catheter associated urinary tract infections. *New England Journal of Medicine*, 1978, *299*, 570-573.

Westwood, G.P.C., & Hooper, W.L. Antagonism of oxolinic acid by nitrofurantoin. *Lancet*, 1975, *1*, 460-462.

GASTROINTESTINAL MEDICATIONS

Medications discussed in this section

Review of the Anatomy, Physiology, and Assessment of the Gastrointestinal System

Walter W. Yakimets

The gastrointestinal tract (Figure 38-1) is a hollow tube extending from the mouth to the anus. Its main functions are to take in fluids and food, to absorb water, and to process the ingested materials so that necessary nutrients can be assimilated and residues stored and eliminated.

The mouth receives fluids and food, and the teeth break the larger food particles into smaller ones to facilitate the digestive process. The esophagus conveys the mouth contents into the stomach where further mixing occurs. The digestive process starts in the mouth and stomach, but is mainly carried out in the small intestine. Digestive juices, mainly enzymes, are secreted by the mouth, stomach, liver, pancreas, and small intestine. Some absorption, mainly water, occurs in the stomach, but most of the absorptive process of nutrients takes place in the small intestine. The colon absorbs some water; however, its main function is the storage of the residues (fecal material) until a suitable time and place are found for evacuation of these residues through the anus.

MOUTH

The mouth, including the lips, teeth, and tongue, is used in speech, facial expression, *mastication*, a minor degree of starch digestion, and in the initiation of the swallowing mechanism (Figure 38-2).

The teeth break food into smaller pieces and together with the activity of the tongue mix them with saliva. Swallowing is facilitated if food is moist or moistened with saliva.

Saliva consists mainly of water, but also contains electrolytes, mucus, and the enzyme amylase. The volume of saliva in the adult is about 1500 ml per day. Submandibular glands, located just below the middle third of the mandible, secrete about 25% of the saliva.

The remainder of saliva is produced by the minor salivary glands, which open directly into the oral cavity. The submandibular ducts drain at the base of the tongue on either side of the frenulum, and the parotid ducts drain through a papilla in the cheek, opposite the second molars. Parotid gland secretions are serous, whereas submandibular gland secretions are both serous and mucous and, therefore, more *viscid*. The flow of saliva is mainly under neural (parasympathetic and sympathetic systems) control, and there is little evidence of *hormonal* influence.

Saliva both facilitates swallowing, especially of dry foods, and initiates splitting of starches into maltose by the enzyme amylase. In addition saliva is necessary for taste. Since taste is chemically mediated, food must be moist for the taste buds (located on the tongue) to determine this sensation.

The chewed, moistened food is propelled by the tongue into the pharynx, where the constriction of the pharyngeal muscles pushes the food into the esophagus. The act of swallowing is mediated by the glossopharyngeal, *vagal*, and the hypoglossal nerves under the coordination of the medullary swallowing center.

The mouth and its related structures are assessed in a systematic manner. The skin, lips, and facial expression are noted as are the patient's ability to smile, frown, clench the teeth, and puff the cheeks. The temporal and masseter muscles are palpated, and the patient is asked to open and close the mouth while the examiner's fingers assess the temporomandibular joint. Oral assessment follows, usually proceeding from front to back with inspection of the teeth, gums, tongue, buccal mucosa, floor of the mouth, hard and soft palates, salivary ducts, tonsils, and uvula. The gag reflex and the patient's ability to swallow are also tested. The presence of caries, mouth odor, areas of plaque, or other deviations are noted.

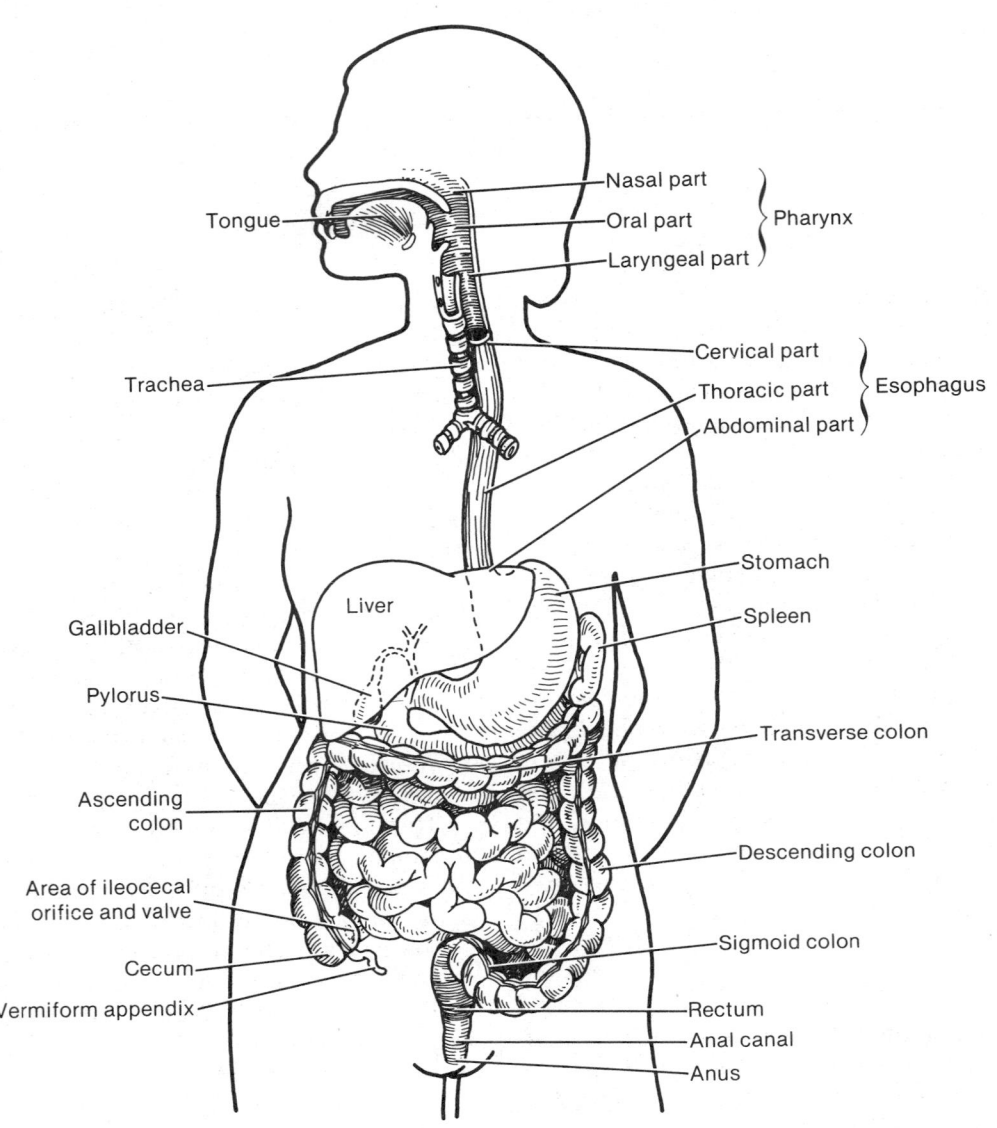

FIGURE 38-1. **The alimentary tract from the mouth to the anus.**

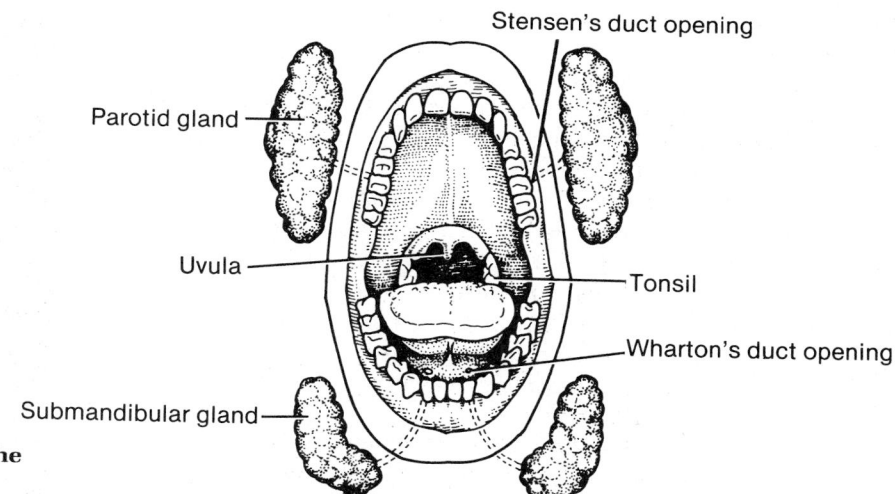

FIGURE 38-2. **The oral cavity and the main salivary glands.**

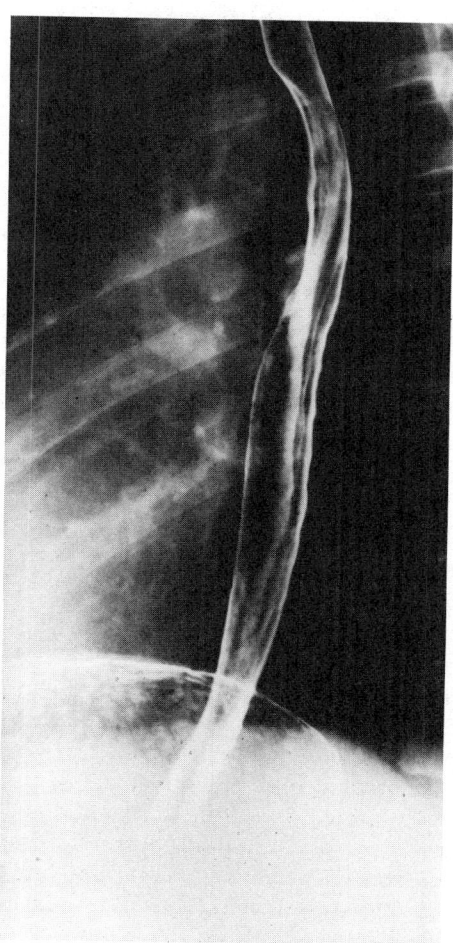

FIGURE 38-3. **Barium swallow showing a normal esophagus. (Courtesy Dr. Ann Conrad.)**

Altered physiology

Salivary secretion may be decreased by calculi obstructing a major salivary duct, especially the submandibular; by surgical removal of the gland(s) for *neoplasms* and infection; by radiation for head and neck tumors; and by preoperative use of medications such as atropine or other anticholinergic drugs given in peptic ulcer therapy. Increased salivary secretion may occur with nausea, reflux esophagitis, and the ingestion of citric fruit juices. Esophageal obstruction causes an unpleasant drooling of saliva.

ESOPHAGUS

The esophagus is a muscular tube lined with squamous epithelium, which extends from the pharyngeal constrictors to the stomach (Figure 38-3). In the adult, the gastroesophageal junction is approximately 40 cm from the upper incisors. The esophagus conveys saliva, foods, and liquids from the mouth and pharynx to the stomach.

Pain from esophagitis, motility disorders, and obstruction may be referred to the high *epigastrium*, retrosternal area, or the base of the neck, depending on the site of the problem.

Esophageal sensation is mediated by the sympathetic and parasympathetic (vagus) nerves. Esophageal motility and swallowing are predominantly under vagal control. Hormonal influence on motility, involving the body of the esophagus, seems to be limited, but *hormones* definitely influence motility in the lower esophageal sphincter (LES).

The pharyngeal constrictor muscles, with which esophageal musculature is continuous, bring foods and liquids to the esophagus. The food is conveyed down the esophagus by peristalsis. Gravity aids but is not necessary for swallowing.

Another important function of the esophagus is the prevention of *reflux* of gastric contents. The reflux preventive mechanisms are not fully understood, but the functional rather than anatomic LES plays the most important role. The LES function occurs in the circular muscle at the lower end of the esophagus. The LES is under vagal and hormonal influence. The hormone gastrin increases LES tone. Foods such as chocolate and alcohol decrease LES tone. *Progesterones* also decrease LES tone and may partly explain the heartburn of pregnancy. Anatomic factors that may aid in preventing esophageal reflux are the right crus of the diaphragm, intraabdominal esophagus, and the mucosal rosette at the esophagogastric junction.

Altered physiology

A disorder of pharyngoesophageal muscular coordination may result in a pharyngeal *diverticulum*. Abnormal esophageal contractions may result in epigastric and retrosternal pain and may be alleviated by smooth muscle relaxants and nitroglycerin. Achalasia, or failure of LES relaxation, causes progressive dysphagia. Reflux of gastric contents into the esophagus causes such symptoms as heartburn and regurgitation and may progress to stricture formation and dysphagia (Figure 38-4). Treatment of reflux *esophagitis* is usually medical, but surgical intervention may be required in difficult cases. Collagen diseases such as scleroderma impair esophageal motility. Tumors and foreign bodies may cause obstruction with marked drooling of saliva. Ingestion of corrosive chemicals may lead to stricture formation and dysphagia or to complete obstruction.

STOMACH

Embryologically the stomach is a foregut derivative (Figure 38-5), and pain from stomach disorders is referred to the epigastrium.

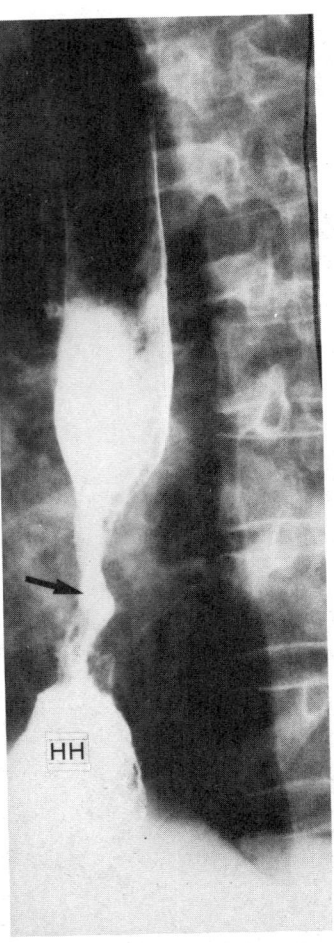

FIGURE 38-4. **Barium swallow showing the lower esophagus. The arrow marks the site of a benign stricture. HH illustrates a sliding hiatus hernia. In a hiatus hernia a portion of the stomach moves into the chest through the esophageal hiatus. (Courtesy Dr. Ann Conrad.)**

The bulk of the stomach is located in the left upper quadrant of the abdomen. It consists of the cardia, fundus, body, antrum, and pyloric canal (Figure 38-6). The cardia, a small area just inferior to the esophagogastric junction, is the site of mucus-producing glands. The fundus and body of the stomach contain glands that secrete hydrochloric acid (HCl), pepsin, *intrinsic factor*, and mucus. The distal one third of the stomach, the antrum, is the site of mucus secretion and also the site of secretion of the hormone *gastrin*. Secretions from the stomach are emptied into the duodenum through a controlling valve, the pyloric sphincter (Figure 38-7).

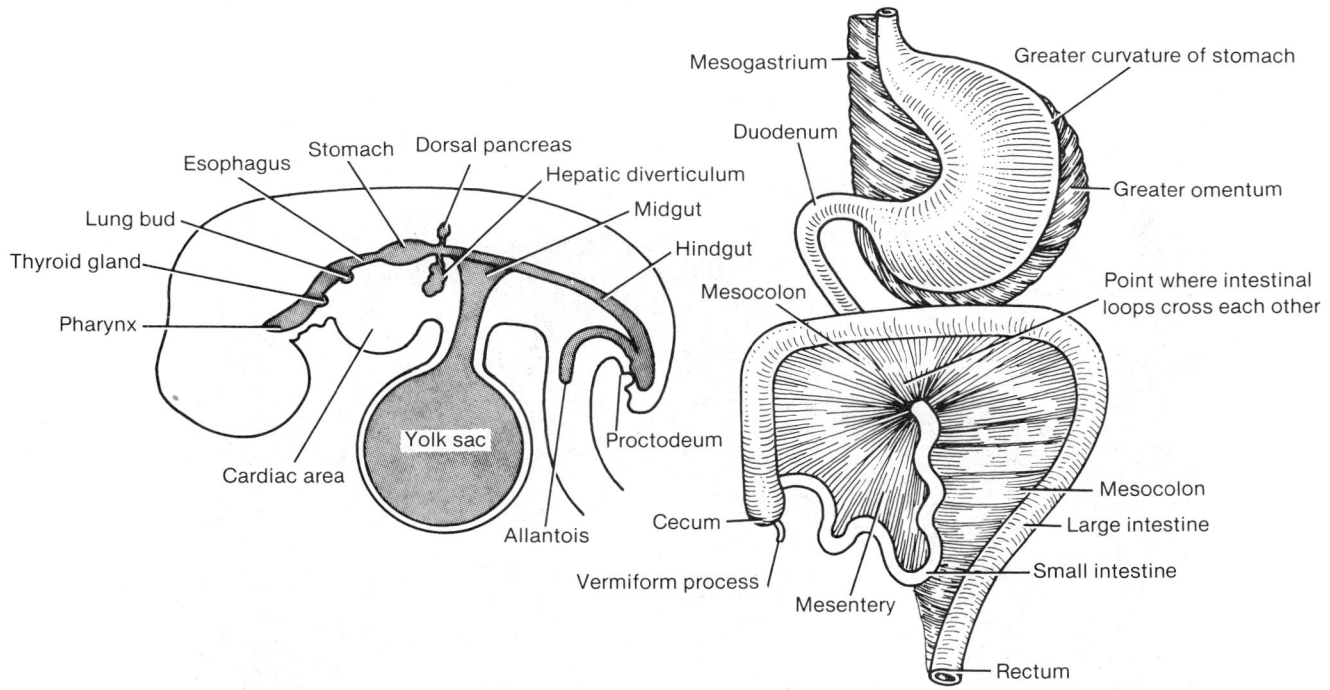

FIGURE 38-5. **Diagram of the foregut, midgut, and hindgut. The stomach, biliary tree, pancreas, and the proximal duodenum just distal to the ampulla of Vater are foregut derivatives. The remainder of the duodenum, the whole of the small intestine, and the colon up to the splenic flexure are midgut derivatives. The splenic flexure and colon extending up to the anus are hindgut derivatives.**

Food and fluids received from the esophagus are temporarily stored in the stomach. Gastric contents are then mixed with pepsin and hydrochloric acid, and protein digestion is initiated. Water, alcohol, some drugs, but little else may be absorbed from the stomach into the circulatory system. Gastric motility under the control of a regional pacemaker moves the contents into the duodenum. The volume of partially digested food entering the duodenum is further controlled by the pyloric sphincter.

Pepsin is secreted in its inactive form, pepsinogen, by the chief cells. Pepsinogen is activated into pepsin by hydrochloric acid. Pepsin, a proteolytic enzyme, breaks down protein into *peptones.*

Hydrochloric acid and intrinsic factor are produced by parietal cells. Hydrochloric acid is necessary for the activation of pepsin and may play a role in reducing the number of viable ingested bacteria. Gastric secretion of HCl and pepsin is under the control of nerves and hormones.

The nervous, vagal, or *cephalic* phase of gastric secretion is initiated by the sight, smell, and taste of food (Figure 38-8). Vagal stimulation also results in the re-

lease of gastrin. The vagal postsynaptic transmitter is acetylcholine, and this phase of gastric secretion may be blocked by anticholinergic drugs such as atropine (see Chapter 23, "Parasympathomimetics and Parasympatholytics").

The hormonal phase of gastric secretion has a major gastric and minor intestinal component. The gastric component of the hormonal phase is caused by gastrin, which is released from the antrum when it is distended or when the antral mucosa is in contact with proteases and peptones. The circulating gastrin induces parietal cells to produce acid and chief cells to produce pepsinogen. Although data are far from complete, histamine may be a potentiating or final transmitter agent, acting on H_2 receptors, in both gastrin- and possibly vagal-induced HCl secretion. The H_2 sites can be blocked by the drug cimetidine and other H_2 blockers with the result that acid secretion is impaired. Gastrin release can be inhibited by an antral acidification, release of secretin from the duodenum and upper jejunum, and enterogastrone (small intestinal gastric inhibitory substances).

The stomach protects itself from acid-pepsin diges-

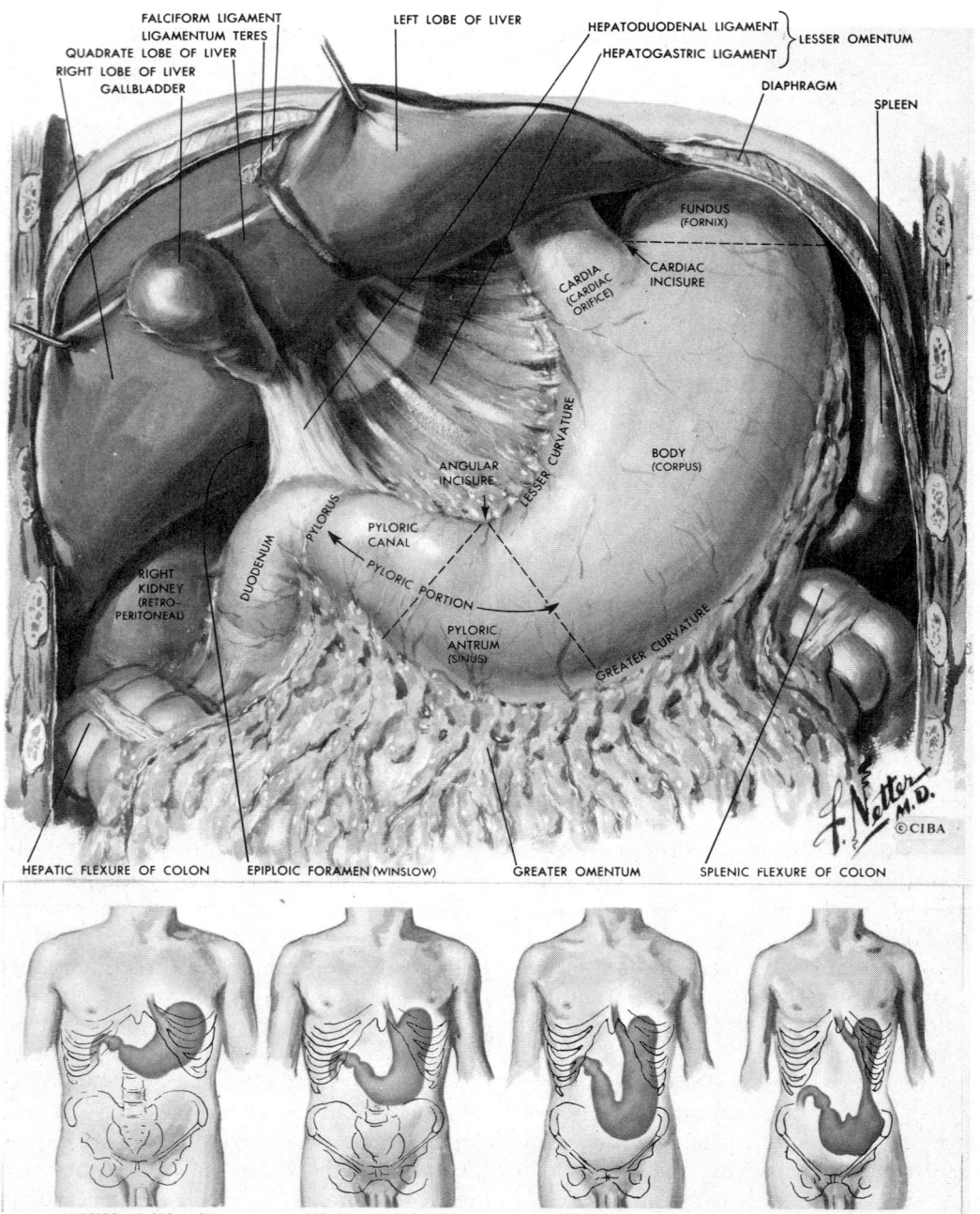

FIGURE 38-6. **External anatomy of the stomach.** (© Copyright 1959, CIBA Pharmaceutical Company, Division of CIBA-GEIGY Corporation. Reprinted with permission from THE CIBA COLLECTION OF MEDICAL ILLUSTRATIONS, illustrated by Frank H. Netter, M.D. All rights reserved.)

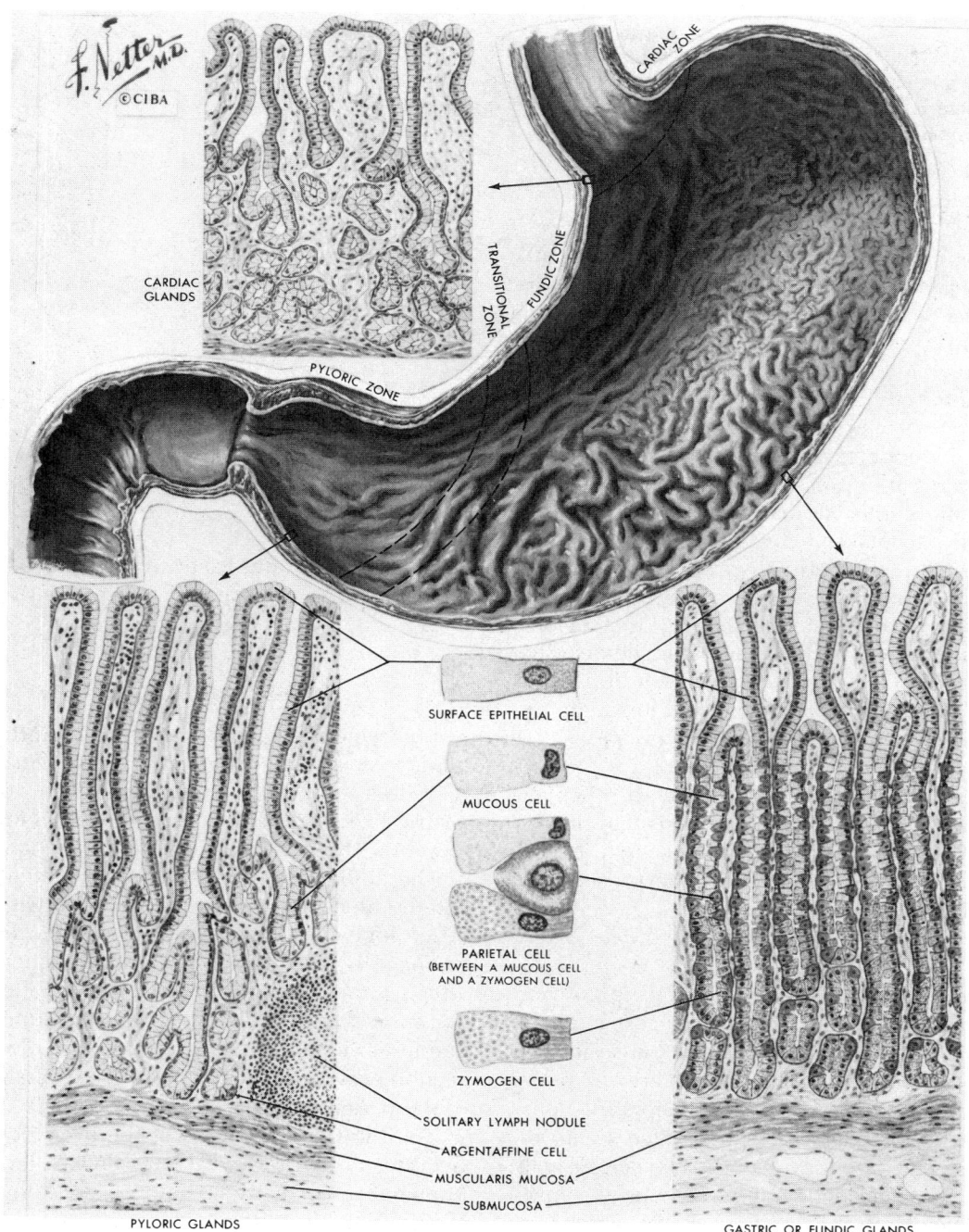

FIGURE 38-7. **Internal anatomy of the stomach.** (© Copyright 1959, CIBA Pharmaceutical Company, Division of CIBA-GEIGY Corporation. Reprinted with permission from THE CIBA COLLECTION OF MEDICAL ILLUSTRATIONS, illustrated by Frank H. Netter, M.D. All rights reserved.)

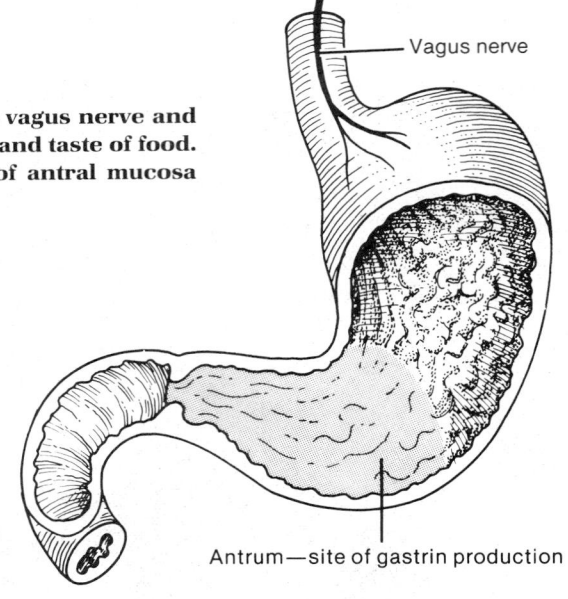

FIGURE 38-8. **Gastric secretion is controlled predominantly by the vagus nerve and the hormone gastrin. Vagus nerves are stimulated by sight, smell, and taste of food. Gastrin release is stimulated by gastric distention and contact of antral mucosa with food, especially proteins.**

tion by secreting a tenacious, somewhat alkaline mucus, which coats the mucosal surface. Drugs such as aspirin, cortisone, and other antiinflammatory agents may alter gastric mucus, which could result in gastritis or cause exacerbation of an ulcer.

Gastric motility is under vagal control and is possibly affected by gastric inhibitory hormones. The stomach accommodates ingested food without a proportionate increase in pressure (receptive relaxation). Slow contractions of the stomach, regulated by a proximally placed pacemaker (which is under vagal control), mix the food and gradually propel it to the duodenum. The volume of gastric contents reaching the duodenum is partially controlled by the pyloric sphincter. Hormones such as secretin, cholecystokinin, and motilin, and hyperosmolar solutions tend to decrease the volume of food going through the sphincter, whereas gastric distention increases the amount.

The stomach is assessed in relation to other abdominal structures, with the patient usually in the supine position. Peristalsis may be observed in thin individuals or infants, especially in the presence of pyloric obstruction or hunger.

Altered physiology

Hypersecretion of hydrochloric acid by the stomach may result in duodenal and prepyloric gastric ulcers in susceptible individuals (Figure 38-9). Causes of gastric hypersecretion resulting in ulcers are unknown but may be related to stress. Gastric ulcers may possibly be initiated by bile reflux. Stress ulcers with resulting gastric bleeding may occur in the seriously ill, including those suffering from severe burns, sepsis, trauma, and head injuries. Erosive gastritis, which may be associated with bleeding, can occur when the protective mucus or some other protective mechanism is altered by antiinflammatory drugs such as aspirin and possibly cortisone. Treatment of ulcers and gastritis includes the use of antacids and cimetidine. If ulcer surgery is necessary, the common procedures include a *truncal vagotomy* and distal gastrectomy or drainage.

Vagotomy denervates gastrin-producing cells, and distal gastrectomy removes the gastric gastrin-producing cells.

LIVER AND BILIARY TREE

Embryologically the biliary tree, including the gallbladder, is a foregut derivative (see Figure 38-5), and disorders, especially those of motility, result in epigastric pain. If inflammation follows, as in acute cholecystitis, the pain is felt in the upper right quadrant.

The adult liver weighs 1200 to 1500 gm and is located under the right hemidiaphragm, with the smaller left lobe extending to the left of the midline. Liver drainage is through the left and right hepatic ducts, which join to form the common hepatic duct. The common bile duct extends from the juncture of the common hepatic and cystic ducts and drains into the second part of the duodenum after traversing the head of the pancreas (Figure 38-10).

The multiple functions of the liver include carbohydrate, protein, and fat metabolism, detoxification (metabolism) of many substances including drugs, and excretion of bile. The adult liver produces 1000 to 1200 ml of bile per day. Bile contains water, electrolytes, bile salts, bile acids, cholesterol, phospholipids, and detoxified products. The gall bladder stores and concentrates bile and expels it in response to the hormone cholecystokinin (i.e., pancreozymin), which is produced by the duodenum and upper jejunum in response to a fatty meal. Bile is necessary for the emul-

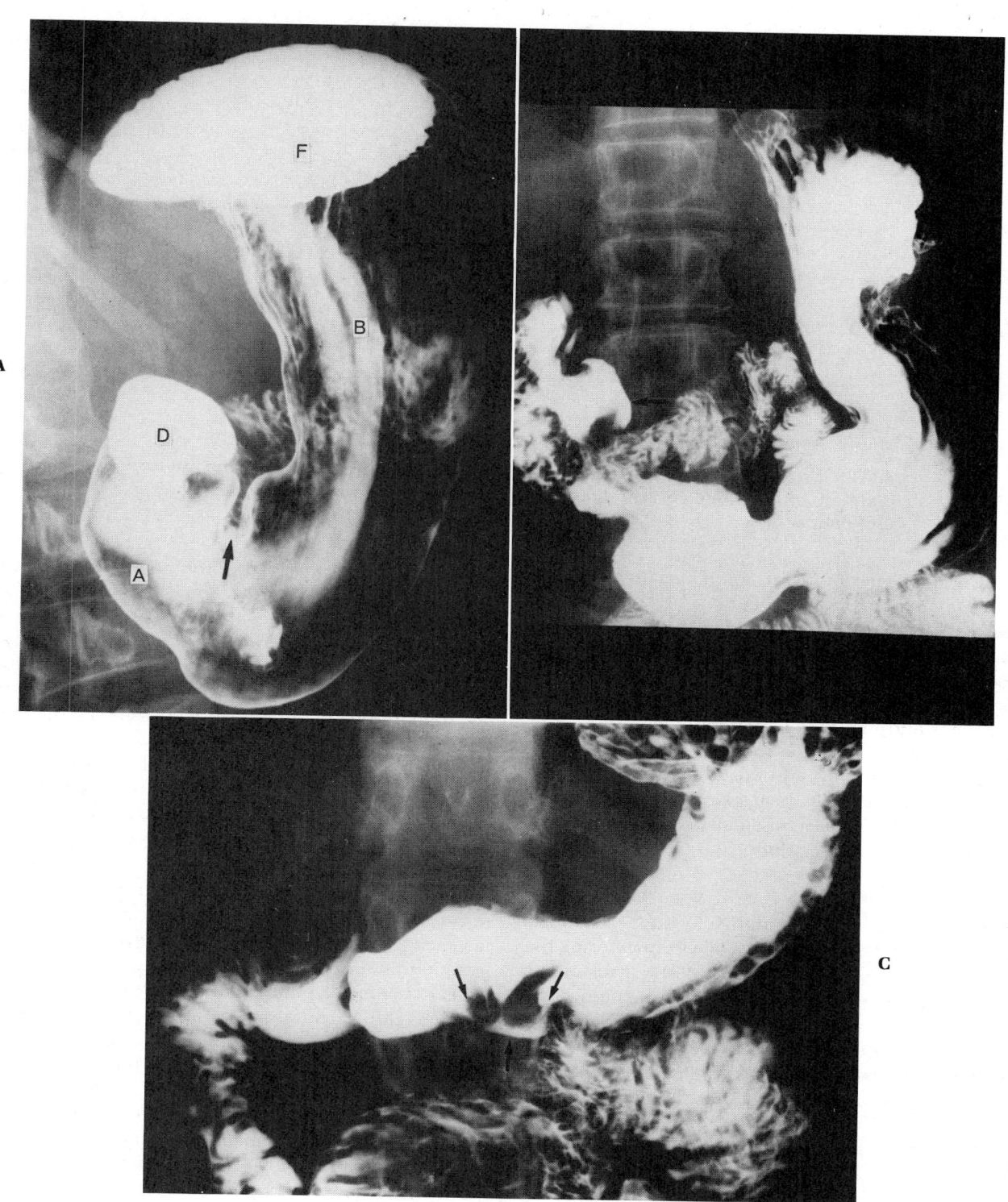

FIGURE 38-9. *A,* Barium meal showing a normal stomach (oblique view). F, Fundus; B, **body, arrow indicates the incisura angulris; D, duodenal bulb; A, antrum. *B,* A huge duodenal ulcer. *C,* A large prepyloric gastric ulcer. (Courtesy Dr. Ann Conrad.)**

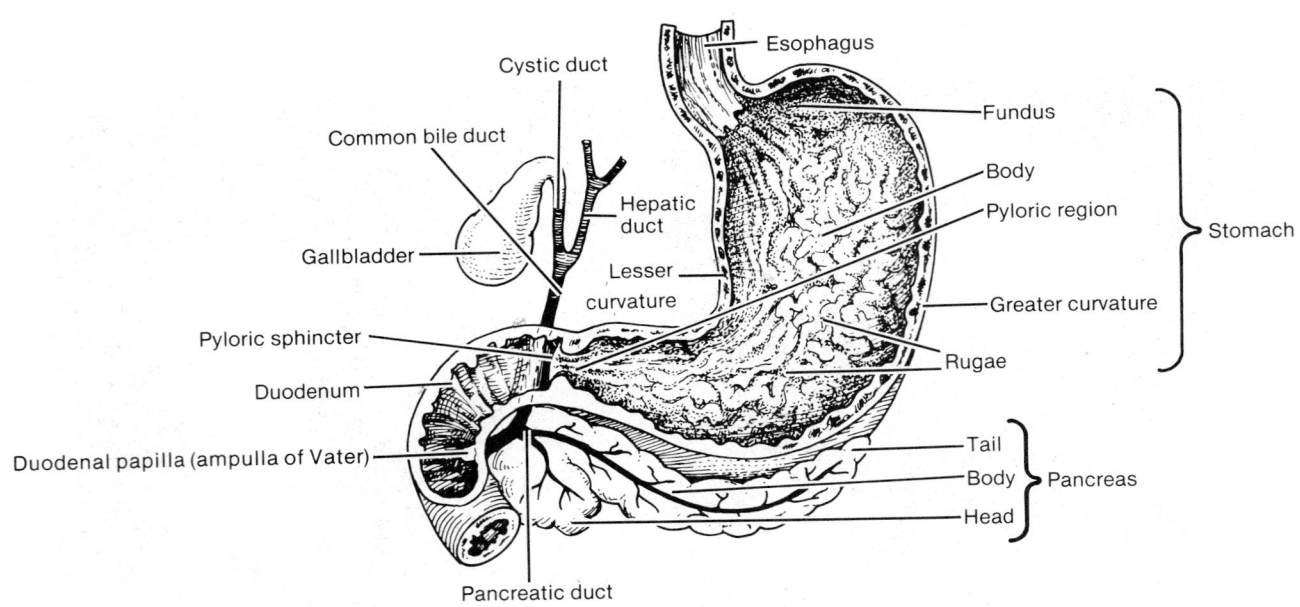

FIGURE 38-10. **Cross section of the upper gastrointestinal tract showing the interior anatomy of the stomach and duodenum and their relationship to the biliary tree and pancreas.**

sification and digestion of fat, and it also increases the activity of pancreatic lipase. Most of the bile in the intestine is reabsorbed in the terminal ileum and recycled *(enterohepatic circulation),* and only a small amount is excreted in the feces.

Liver function can be determined by various laboratory tests and methods of patient assessment. Liver size and position can be assessed by the scratch test, but usually percussion and auscultation are used to more accurately identify the upper and lower borders. Liver tenderness can be assessed with palpation below the lower border of liver dullness.

Altered physiology

Obstruction of the common bile duct by stones, stricture, or carcinoma prevents bile from entering the gut and results in jaundice (Figure 38-11). Lack of bile in the intestine results in impaired absorption of fat soluble vitamins and impaired fat digestion, which results in excess fecal fat and fatty acids *steatorrhea.* The stools will be clay colored because of a lack of bile pigments. Resection of the terminal ileum or impairment of ileal function resulting from disease impairs bile salt reabsorption and causes a bile diarrhea.

PANCREAS

The pancreas embryologically is a foregut derivative (see Figure 38-5), and pancreatic pain is referred to the right epigastrium and to the lower back.

Anatomically, the head of the pancreas lies within the C of the duodenum in the right upper quadrant. The body and tail lie posterior to the stomach in the left upper quadrant (Figure 38-10). The main pancreatic duct usually joins with the common bile duct, and both drain into the second part of the duodenum via the ampulla of Vater. Normally, the pancreas cannot be palpated.

The pancreas has an *endocrine* function, producing the hormones insulin, somatostatin, glucagon, and pancreatic gastrin from various cells in the islets, and an *exocrine* function, producing the enzymes amylase, trypsin, and lipase from the *acini.*

Exocrine secretions, which drain into the duodenum, contain water, enzymes, and electrolytes such as bicarbonate, which is used to neutralize acid in the duodenum.

Pancreatic secretion, about 1500 ml per day in the adult, is under neural (vagus) and hormonal (secretin, pancreozymin) control. Sight, smell, and taste of food release vagally mediated digestive enzymes. The presence of food and acid in the duodenum and upper jejunum cause the release of the hormones pancreozymin and secretin, respectively. Pancreozymin stimulates the production of an enzyme-rich pancreatic secretion, whereas secretin releases a bicarbonate-rich secretion.

The protein-digestive enzymes, trypsin and chymotrypsin, are secreted in their inactive forms, trypsinogen and chymotrypsinogen. Then trypsinogen is

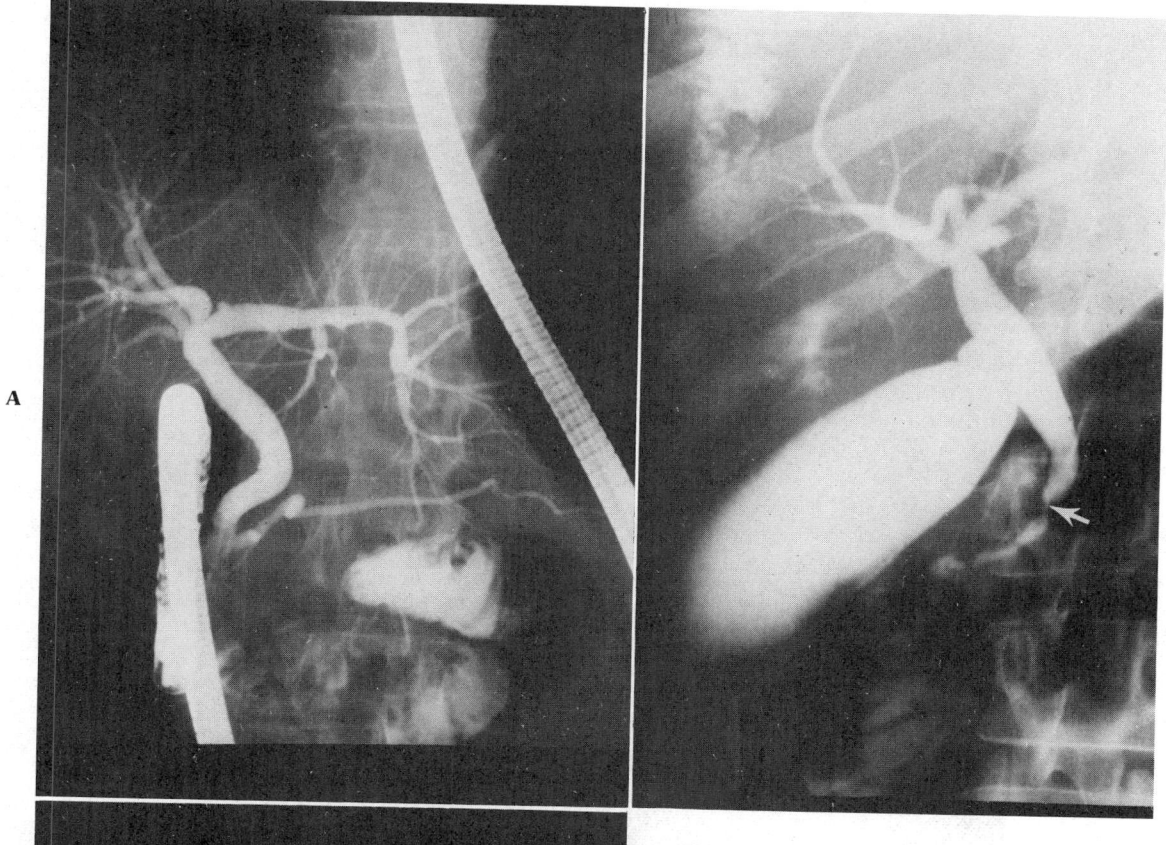

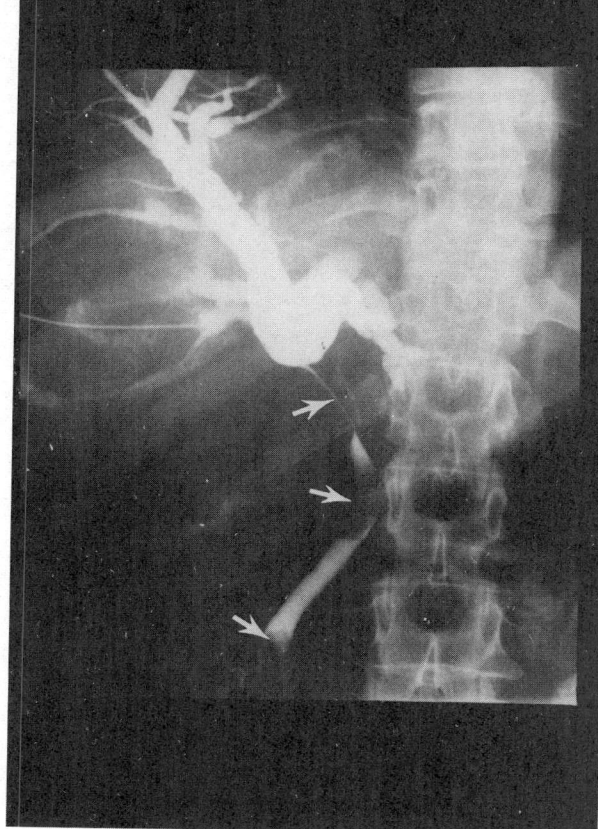

FIGURE 38-11. *A,* Endoscopic retrograde cholangiopancreatography (ERCP) showing a normal common bile duct (vertical) and a normal pancreatic duct (horizontal). The coiled tube is the endoscope. *B,* A benign stricture of the common bile duct. *C,* Dilated intrahepatic bile ducts and compression of the common bile duct by a carcinoma of the gallbladder. The lowermost arrow shows a stone in the common bile duct. (Courtesy Dr. Ann Conrad.)

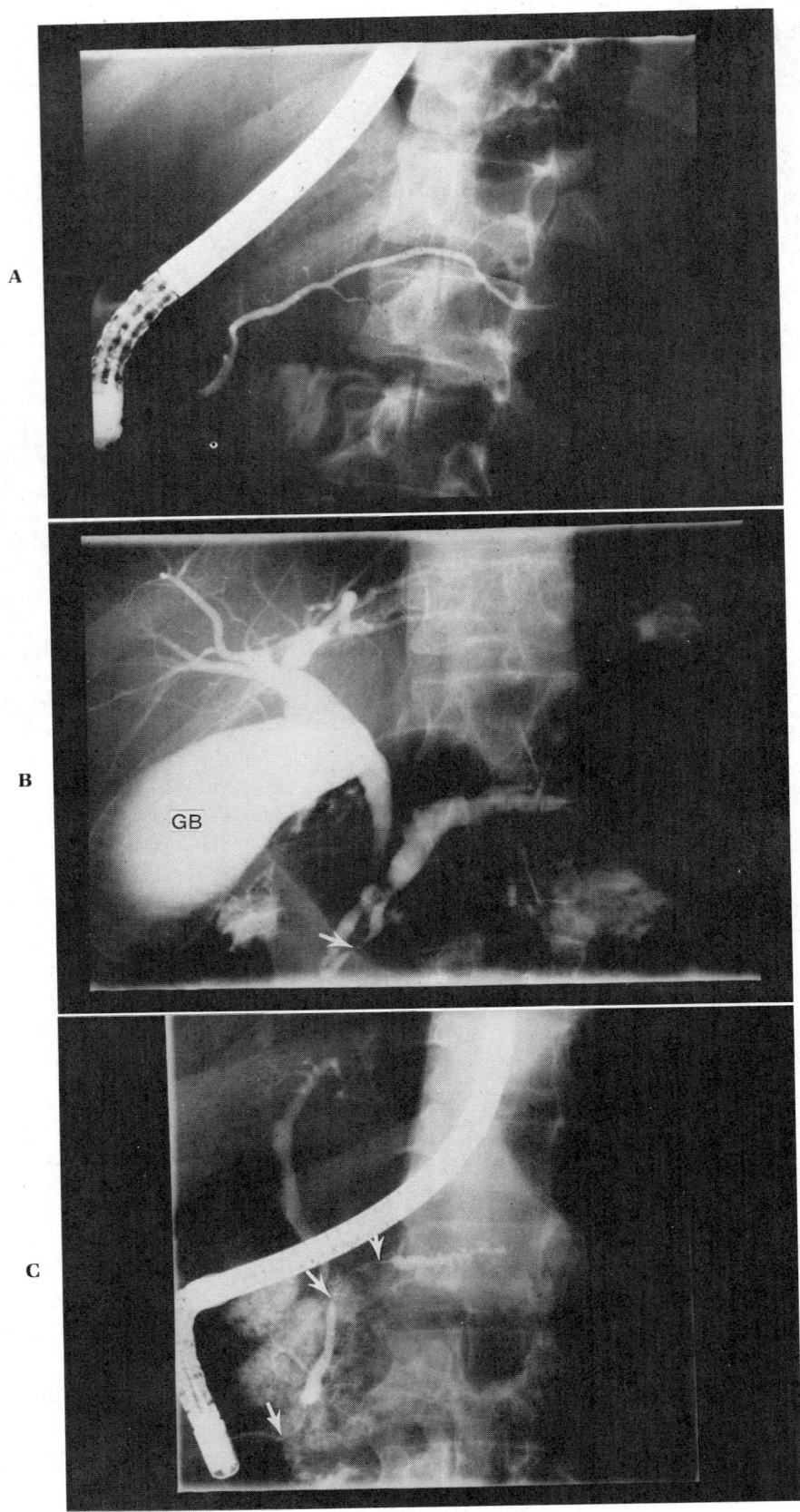

FIGURE 38-12. *A,* ERCP showing a normal pancreatic duct. *B,* The arrow illustrates a stricture of the pancreatic duct. Proximal to the stricture, the pancreatic duct is dilated. GB, Gallbladder. *C,* An ERCP showing a vertical common bile duct and horizontal pancreatic duct. The small arrow illustrates the small cannula used to cannulate the ducts. The two larger arrows show the margins of a tumor extending circumferentially around the main pancreatic duct. (Courtesy Dr. Ann Conrad.)

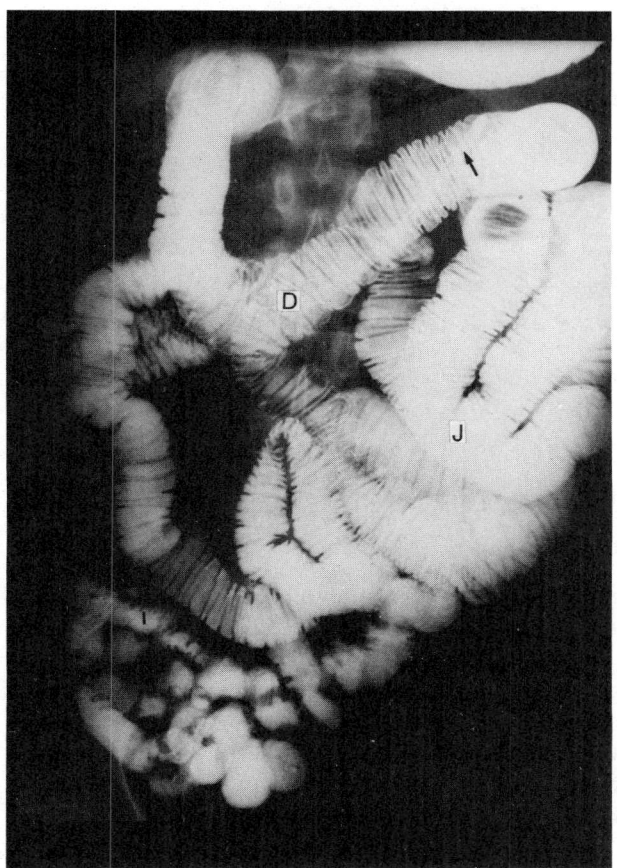

FIGURE 38-13. **This barium study illustrates a normal small bowel study. The arrow shows the radiopaque tube through which the contrast material was injected.** D, **Duodenum;** J, **jejunum;** I, **ileum.** (Courtesy Dr. Ann Conrad.)

Pancreatic amylases continue the carbohydrate breakdown started by salivary amylase. Carbohydrates are broken down to absorbable components disaccharides and monosaccharides.

Altered physiology

The congenital disease, cystic fibrosis, may result in a relative or absolute lack of pancreatic enzymes, with resultant malabsorption of food and steatorrhea.

In the adult, the exocrine pancreatic function may be impaired as a result of recurrent or chronic pancreatitis. Drainage may be obstructed by duct strictures and neoplasms in the head of the pancreas (Figure 38-11). Lack of pancreatic enzymes results in malabsorption syndromes. Lack of lipase in the gut causes diarrhea resulting from the increase in fecal fats and fatty acids (steatorrhea). Oral pancreatic enzymes may be used to treat these pancreatic insufficiencies.

SMALL INTESTINE

Embryologically, except for the first part and a portion of the second part of the duodenum just distal to the insert of the ampulla of Vater (foregut derivatives), the small intestine is a midgut derivative (see Figure 38-5). Small intestinal pain is referred to the periumbilical region.

The small intestine, a muscular tube (Figure 38-13) that includes the duodenum, jejunum, and ileum, empties into the cecum. It is approximately 660 cm long. Its absorption surface from the mucosa is huge, perhaps 200 to 500 square meters, because of mucosal folds, villae, and microvillae (Figures 38-14 and 38-15).

Partly digested food, or *chyme,* enters the duodenum. Bile, pancreatic juice, and small intestinal secretions, including enzymes, are added to and mixed with the chyme. The bulk of digestion or breakdown of food into absorbable *moieties* occurs in the small intestine. These digested foods and some minerals and vitamins are absorbed into the body from the small intestine. In addition, the bulk of 5500 ml of fluid from saliva, gastric secretion, bile and pancreatic juice,

activated in the duodenum and intestine by enterokinase. Trypsin can also activate trypsinogen and chymotrypsinogen. These two enzymes further breakdown proteases and peptones to absorb amino acids.

Lipase is secreted in an active form, but its activity may be aided by bile salts. Lipase and bile salts break down fats into glycerol and fatty acids.

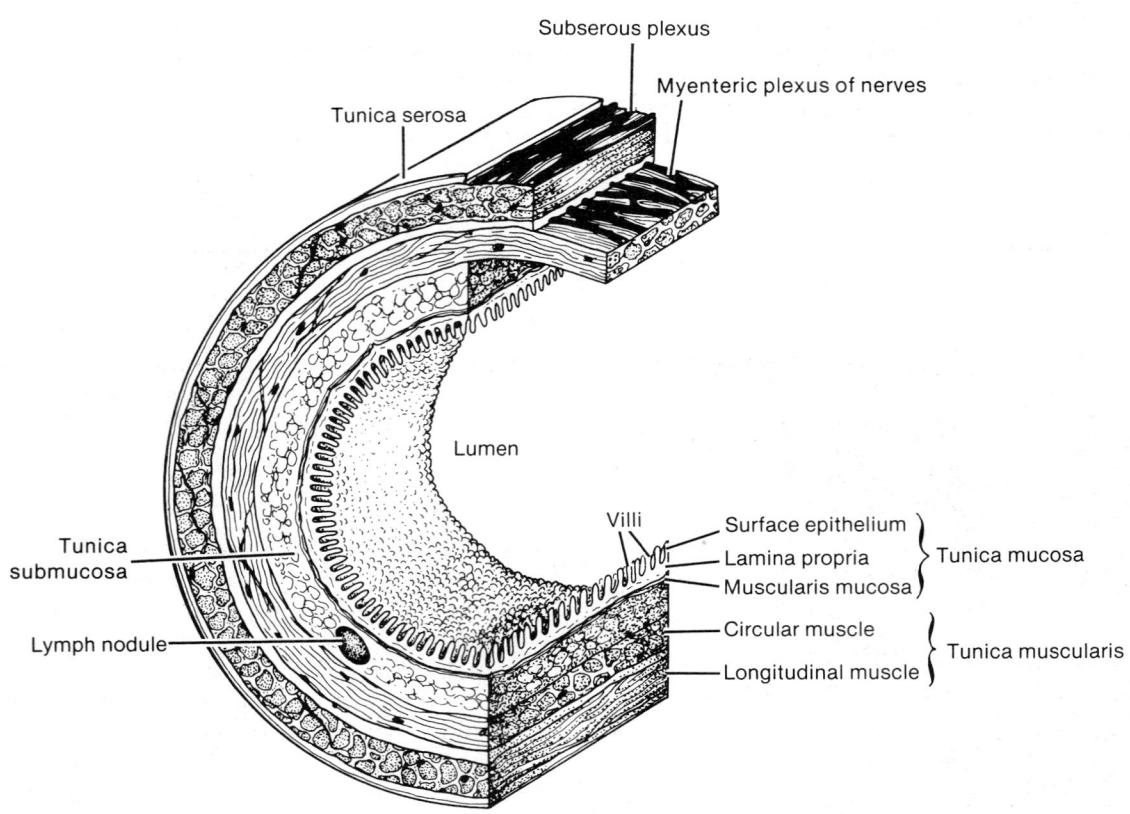

FIGURE 38-14. **Cross section of the small intestine.**

Average volumes of gastrointestinal secretion per day	
Saliva	1500 ml
Gastric juice	1500 ml
Bile	1000 ml
Pancreatic juice	1500 ml
Intestinal juice	2500 ml
	8000 ml

and 2500 ml of intestinal juice are absorbed (see box); 500 to 1000 ml of small intestinal contents enter the cecum per day.

The endocrine function of the small intestine includes the production of previously mentioned hormones: cholecystokinin (pancreozymin), secretin, intestinal gastrin and motolin, and serotonin.

The small intestinal exocrine function includes water, electrolytes, alkaline mucus secretion (especially from the duodenum), and digestive enzymes, which help pancreatic enzymes split carbohydrates, fats, and proteins into absorbable moieties.

Motility of the small intestine appears to be under the influence of the autonomic nervous system and an intrinsic nerve plexus that may be influenced by hormones and drugs. Intestinal movements are caudal. Segmentation helps mix chyme, and peristaltic waves gradually move the food to the cecum.

Altered physiology

Intestinal disease, such as celiac disease, lymphomas, Crohn's disease, and extensive intestinal resection cause malabsorption of food (and colonically directed fluids) with resulting malnutrition and diarrhea.

LARGE INTESTINE

Embryologically, the large intestine proximal to the splenic flexure is of midgut origin, and the splenic flexure to the anus is of hindgut origin (see Figure 38-5). Midgut pain is referred to the periumbilical region and hindgut pain to the suprapubic region.

The large intestine includes the cecum and at-

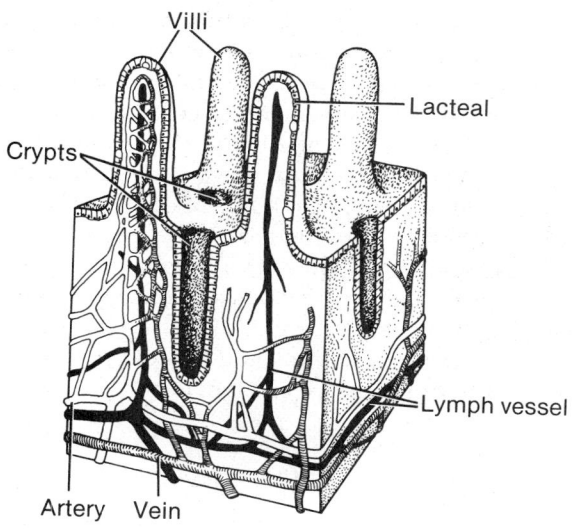

FIGURE 38-15. **Diagram showing villi of the small intestine. These markedly increase the absorptive surface of the small intestine.**

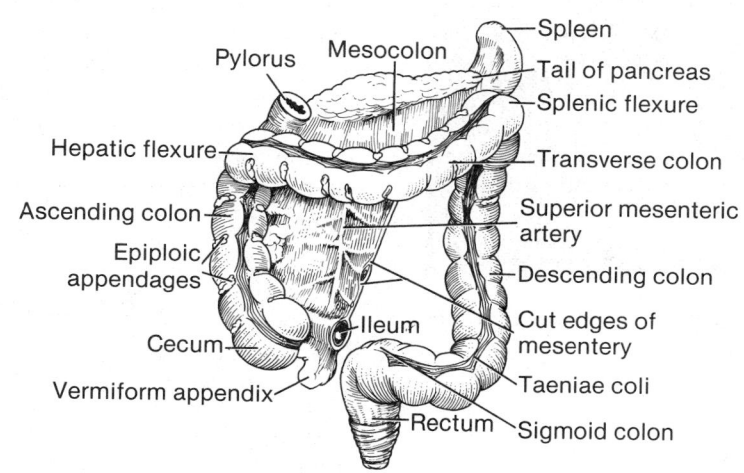

FIGURE 38-16. **The large intestine (colon).**

tached appendix, ascending colon, transverse colon, descending colon, sigmoid portions, and the rectum, parts of which are found in the upper and lower right and left quadrants (Figures 38-16 and 38-17). The outer longitudinal muscles are gathered into three teniae coli and extend from the base of the appendix to the rectum, where they become circumferentially arranged as in the small intestine.

The large intestine or colon receives 500 to 1000 ml of fluid contents from the ileum, from which it absorbs water and electrolytes. The residuum is stored in the colon-rectum and expelled as feces. Mucus, which probably has a lubricating function, is secreted by colonic mucosa. There is no known hormonal production by the colon.

Colonic motility is not well understood, but consists predominantly of segmentation and mass movements. These movements may be influenced by the autonomic nervous system, by hormones, and by drugs such as opiates. Colonic segmentation results in the mixing of colonic contents and allows for better fluid absorption. Mass peristaltic movements tend to occur after meals (gastrocolic reflex) and convey the fecal contents to the rectum. When the rectum becomes distended (150 to 300 ml), a defecation reflex may be voluntarily denied but if conditions are appropriate, defecation can occur.

Assessment of the small and large intestine includes inspection of the abdomen for distention related to fluid, gas, or masses. Auscultation of the abdomen precedes percussion. Normal bowel sounds can be heard at regular or irregular intervals every 5 to 15

cosa; decrease fluid reabsorption; or decrease distensibility of the rectum and perhaps alter motility. All these may be factors in colonic inflammatory diarrhea. Drugs such as opiates increase colonic segmental activity and thus slow colonic transit time and promote fluid reabsorption, which may result in constipation or slow down diarrhea. Causes of constipation are not fully understood, but low-fiber diets (i.e., small volume of bulk) probably allows for more water reabsorption from the fecal matter and possibly slower colonic transit time of the stool. Dehydration, psychologic factors (i.e., stress or depression), and lack of physical activity may also contribute to constipation.

SUMMARY

Most medications (greater than 90%) are taken orally and absorbed from the gastrointestinal tract. Thus a sound knowledge of the anatomy, physiology, and assessment of this system is important in planning and managing drug therapy. Because gastrointestinal irritation is a common side effect of most drugs administered orally, the nurse needs to be able not only to minimize this effect, but also to recognize when symptoms may be indicative of other gastrointestinal problems.

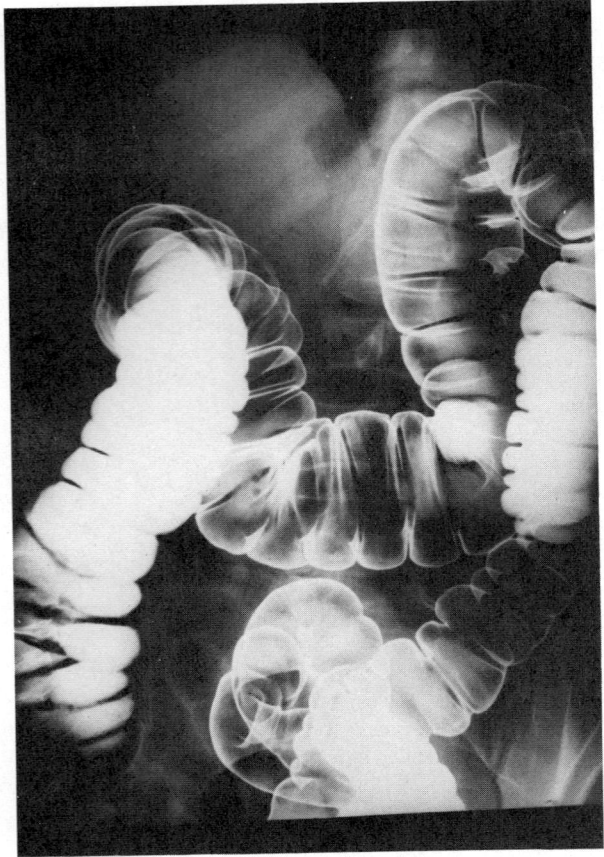

FIGURE 38-17. **Barium enema illustrating a normal colon. (Courtesy Dr. Ann Conrad.)**

seconds, depending on when the last meal was eaten. Absent or soft bowel sounds can be indicative of diminished intestinal motility. Increased bowel sounds with borborygmi may be heard in the presence of pathologic conditions (e.g., intestinal obstruction and gastroenteritis). Percussion of all four quadrants should be completed systematically to identify fluid, gas, or masses and should be followed by light and deep palpation. Deep palpation may produce tenderness over the cecum and sigmoid colon. The cecum, ascending colon, descending colon, and sigmoid colon (when filled with feces) can be palpated as soft rounded masses.

Altered physiology

Increased affluent from the small bowel because of either disease or faster transit time may be beyond the absorptive capacity of the colon, and diarrhea may result. Colonic inflammatory disease may increase exudation or secretion of fluid from the damaged mu-

BIBLIOGRAPHY

Cooke, A.R. Control of gastric emptying and motility. *Gastroenterology*, 1975, *68*, 804-816.

Cooke, A.R. The role of the mucosal barrier in drug induced gastric ulceration and erosions. *American Journal of Digestive Diseases*, 1976, *21*, 155-164.

Cooperman, A.M., & Cook, S.A. Gastric emptying—physiology and measurements. *Surgical Clinics of North America*, 1976, *56*, 1277-1287.

Davenport, H.W. *Physiology of the digestive tract.* Chicago: Year Book Medical Publishers, 1971.

Dozois, R.R., & Kelly, D.A. Gastric secretion and motility in duodenal ulcer: Effect of current vagotomies. *Surgical Clinics of North America*, 1976, *56*, 1267-1276.

Emmelin, N. Secretory mechanisms. In W. Sircus and A.N. Smith (Eds.). *Scientific foundations of gastroenterology.* London: William Heinemann Medical Books, Ltd., 1980.

Fox, S., & Behar, J. Control of lower oesophageal sphincter pressure and acid reflux. *Clinical Gastroenterology*, 1979, *8*, 37-52.

Hogan, W., Viegas, de A., & Winship, D. Ethanol induced acute esophageal motor dysfunction. *Journal of Applied Physiology*, 1972, *32*, 755-760.

Levy, M. Aspirin use in patients with major upper gastrointestinal bleeding and peptic ulcer disease. *New England Journal of Medicine*, 1974, *290*, 1158-1162.

Rodes, J., & Calcraft, B. Aetiology of gastric ulcer with special reference to the roles of reflux and mucosal damage. *Clinical Gastroenterology*, 1973, *2*, 227-243.

Sircus, W., & Smith, A.N. *Scientific foundations of gastroenterology*. London: William Heinemann Medical Books, Ltd., 1980.

Soll, A.H. Three-way interactions between histamine, carbachol, and gastrin on aminopyrine uptake by isolated canine parietal cells. *Gastroenterology*, 1978, *74*, 1146. (Abstract)

Van Thiel, D.H., Gavaler, J.S., Joshi, S.N., Sara, R.K., & Stremple, J. Heartburn of pregnancy. *Gastroenterology*, 1977, *72*, 666-668.

CHAPTER 39

Antacids, Ulcer Medications, and Digestants

Walter W. Yakimets

Medications discussed in this chapter

Antacids
  Aluminum carbonate
  Aluminum hydroxide
  Aluminum phosphate
  Calcium carbonate
  Dihydroxyaluminum
    aminoacetate
  Dihydroxyaluminum so-
    dium carbonate
  Magaldrate
  Magnesium carbonate
  Magnesium hydroxide
  Magnesium oxide
  Magnesium trisilicate
  Sodium bicarbonate

Anticholinergic
  Propantheline
Digestants
  Glutamic acid hydrochlo-
    ride
  Pancreatic enzymes
    Pancreatin
    Pancrelipase
H_2-receptor antagonists
  Cimetidine
  Ranitidine
Miscellaneous
  Metoclopramide
  Simethicone
  Sucralfate

This chapter discusses the use, dose, side effects, and drug interactions associated with antacids, ulcer medications, and digestants. The clinical aspects of diseases treated with these medications are also discussed.

DISEASES TREATED WITH ANTACIDS AND ULCER MEDICATIONS

Medications that neutralize gastric hydrochloric acid, or inhibit gastric secretion, are used for symptomatic relief and for the possible healing of acid peptic disorders. These disorders are usually associated with gastric hypersecretion of hydrochloric acid and pepsin, and include duodenal and gastric ulcers, stress ulcers, erosive gastritis, and *reflux esophagitis* (Figure 39-1).

Duodenal ulcers

A duodenal ulcer is a peptic acid disorder consisting of a defect in the mucosa, usually in the first part of the duodenum, that penetrates to the submucosa (or deeper) and is associated with an inflammatory reaction (Figure 39-2). This is an affliction mainly of young people, but it can affect the elderly as well. Duodenal ulcers are much more common in men, but there are recent suggestions that the incidence in women is increasing. The disease seems to be familial and tends to affect persons in stressful situations. Duodenal ulcers are recurrent, but tend to heal (even without treatment) and may even go into spontaneous remission for long periods of time. The disease appears to be cyclic, with most recurrences in the spring and fall. Although the disease is commonly associated with an increase in gastric acid and pepsin levels, the pathogenesis is not well understood.

The main symptom of duodenal ulcers is an *epigastric* burning discomfort that occurs most commonly when the stomach is empty (e.g., between meals and at night). Ulcer pain is often aggravated by spicy and acid foods, alcohol, and coffee. Relief from pain is obtained by eating, drinking milk, and taking antacids and drugs that block the secretion of acid. On physical examination, midepigastric tenderness to the right of the midline may be present. Diagnosis is usually by history and may be confirmed by x-ray examination and *endoscopy*.

Therapy for duodenal ulcers, except for complications that may require surgical intervention, includes the following:

1. Avoidance of gastric stimulants or irritants such as acidic and spicy foods, alcohol, coffee, tobacco, and aspirin
2. Use of more frequent but smaller meals, which will dilute and *buffer* acid
3. Use of antacids to neutralize and buffer hydrochloric acid
4. Use of histamine 2 (H_2) blockers such as cimetidine or ranitidine
5. Use of sedative-hypnotics such as benzodiaze-

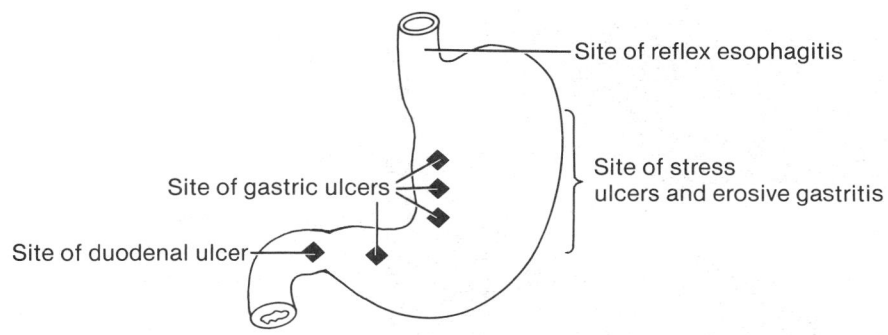

FIGURE 39-1. **Common sites of acid peptic disorders.**

pines (see Chapter 15, "Sedative-Hypnotics") during periods of increased stress

6. Use of anticholinergics (see Chapter 23, "Parasympathomimetics and Parasympatholytics") in the occasional case to prolong the effect of antacids or decrease nocturnal acid secretion

Intensive antacid therapy (e.g., dosing every hour) should be carried out for 2 to 3 weeks followed by a less intensive regimen (e.g., dosing after each meal and at bedtime) for 3 more weeks. Some patients have difficulty following treatment regimens, and some ulcers become resistant to the effects of medication. Such cases are referred to as *intractable*. Indications for surgery in duodenal ulcer disease include intractability, duodenal obstruction, hemorrhage, and perforation of the ulcer.

Gastric ulcers

A gastric ulcer is a defect in the gastric mucosa that extends to the submucosa and is associated with an inflammatory reaction (Figure 39-3). Prepyloric ulcers, like duodenal ulcers, commonly are associated with high gastric acidity. Ulcers in other parts of the stomach may be associated with normal or low acidity. This condition tends to affect middle-aged or older people and is more common in lower socioeconomic groups and in smokers. The etiology of gastric ulcers is unknown, but changes in mucosal resistance and bile reflux may play a role.

Symptoms and signs of gastric ulcers are similar to duodenal ulcers. Diagnosis may be confirmed by x-ray examination (Figure 39-3) or endoscopy. A biopsy of any gastric ulcer that looks like a carcinoma on x-ray examination or endoscopy, or one that does not show significant healing after 6 weeks of adequate therapy, should be done through a *gastroscope*.

Treatment of gastric ulcers, like duodenal ulcers, is initially medical. Antacids provide symptomatic relief,

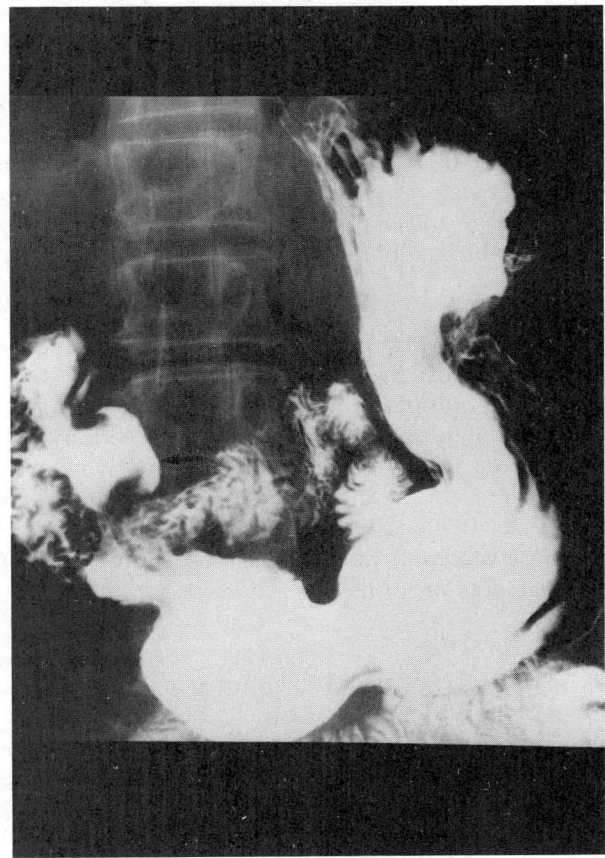

FIGURE 39-2. **Barium meal showing a large duodenal ulcer. Arrow points to an ulcer in the first part of the duodenum. (Courtesy Dr. Ann Conrad.)**

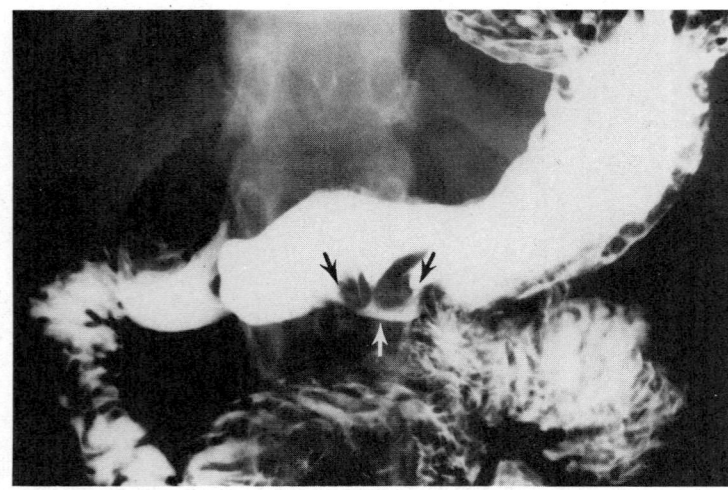

FIGURE 39-3. **Barium meal showing a large gastric ulcer in the greater curve of the antrum. (Courtesy Dr. Ann Conrad.)**

but there is no evidence that they speed healing. In-hospital treatment with cessation of smoking promotes gastric ulcer healing. Outpatient carbenoxolone therapy accelerates gastric ulcer healing, but carbenoxolone given to hospitalized patients does not provide an additional benefit.

Stress ulcers

Superficial gastric ulcers or erosions may occur in persons suffering from extensive burns, sepsis, head injuries, or multiple trauma. These ulcers commonly bleed and may prove to be fatal in the seriously ill. The best treatment is to deal with the underlying medical problem and to prophylactically use antacids or cimetidine. If bleeding occurs despite prophylactic therapy, a *vagotomy* and drainage procedure, or even a total *gastrectomy*, may be required.

Erosive gastritis

The ingestion of alcohol, aspirin, cortisone, and antiinflammatory drugs have been reputed to result in gastric erosions or exacerbation of a duodenal ulcer. Some of these compounds may damage the mucosal barrier, but the exact pathogenesis of gastric erosion is unknown. Symptoms include epigastric burning discomfort and on occasions, nausea. Treatment includes use of antacids or cimetidine (or ranitidine) or both, and occasionally if bleeding is extensive, surgery may be required.

Reflux esophagitis

Reflux esophagitis is caused by a reflux of gastric contents into the esophagus. Examined with an *endoscope* symptomatic patients may show no abnormality, or they may show changes ranging from min-imal redness to frank ulceration. This condition may occur at any age and in either sex. It is commonly seen in infants and young toddlers following drinking from their bottles in a supine position.

Symptoms of esophageal reflux include heartburn, epigastric pain, and regurgitation. Symptoms often become worse when the patient reclines or bends over or for women in the later stages of pregnancy. Foods and other factors that lower esophageal *sphincter* tone, such as alcohol, chocolate, and cigarettes, especially if taken before reclining, tend to aggravate the symptoms. Diagnosis is largely based on symptoms and may be confirmed by *esophageal manometric studies*, barium swallow, and endoscopy.

Initial treatment consists of the following:

1. A diet that avoids foods, liquids, and other products that decrease lower esophageal sphincter (LES) tone or increase gastric acid secretion, such as coffee, alcohol, chocolate, spicy or acidic foods, and tobacco
2. A prohibition of food or liquids from 7 PM until breakfast (for infants, thickened formula is fed in an upright position)
3. An elevation of the head of the patient's bed 15 to 20 cm
4. Weight reduction if overweight
5. Antacids to neutralize and buffer gastric acid
6. Metoclopramide, which increases LES tone and gastric emptying, may be given in addition to antacids
7. Cimetidine or ranitidine, which may be used instead of antacids or metoclopramide, but should be used with caution until further experience is gained with its use

If therapy fails, surgery may be indicated.

ANTACIDS

Antacids neutralize or reduce gastric acid concentration and thereby provide rapid relief of ulcer pain. Controversy still exists as to whether antacids provide only symptomatic relief (i.e., neutralize hydrochloric acid) or help ulcer healing. Recent controlled studies would indicate that duodenal ulcer healing is hastened by antacids. This raises the question, how much reduction of acid concentration is necessary for effective treatment of duodenal ulcers? It has been demonstrated that if the pH of a given amount of gastric juice is raised from 1.3 to 1.6, 50% of the acid is neutralized, and if the pH is raised to 3.3, approximately 99% of the acid is neutralized. If gastric acid is decreased sufficiently (pH of 4.0 or more), pepsinogen activation (and peptic activity) may be impaired or stopped. In addition, the antacid aluminum hydroxide adsorbs pepsin, thus reducing the amount of active pepsin. Calcium carbonate also reduces pepsin activity, but the mechanism is unknown. Simethicone, a defoaming agent, is sometimes added to antacids to help relieve gas. Theoretically it causes gas bubbles to disperse and is relatively nontoxic.

Compliance

Optimal patient use of antacids or patient compliance may be limited by the following:
1. Degree of symptoms
2. Taste of the medication
3. Dosage schedule
4. Dosage form (liquids or tablets)
5. Side effects
6. Motivation to get well

Patients will take medications if they are in pain, but once the symptoms are reasonably well controlled, patient compliance decreases. This occurs despite instructions. Many patients complain of the chalky taste of antacids. Some patients refuse to take antacids because the taste upsets or nauseates them. Many antacids are flavored by peppermint, which tends to reduce LES tone and increase acid production. It is not known if these side effects of peppermint flavoring are significant in the doses used. Fruit-flavored antacids tend to be less *palatable* than those flavored with peppermint.

Dose

The antacid dosage frequently suggested is 15 to 30 ml of liquid antacid hourly. This schedule is based on endoscopic studies of gastric emptying of antacids given to a fasting patient. This regimen is rarely followed, partly because of the frequency of ingestion nuisance and partly because of the side effects from the accumulated daily dose (e.g., diarrhea caused by magnesium hydroxide). A reasonably well accepted, effective dose schedule consists of two tablets, or 15 ml of liquid, 1 and 3 hours after meals and at bedtime (7 doses daily). Studies have shown that the antacid effect is prolonged when given with food—hence the 1-hour-after-food dose. Antacids that tend to cause diarrhea (e.g., magnesium hydroxide) may be alternated with ones that are constipating (e.g., aluminum hydroxide gel).

Liquid antacids are more effective than those in tablet form. However, for the outpatient tablets are easier to carry and use. In hospitals, use of liquid antacids is preferable to tablets.

Side effects

Side effects of antacids, although common, are rarely serious if used judiciously. Diarrhea is a common complication of magnesium-hydroxide combinations. Constipation occurs with aluminum hydroxide. In patients with renal failure, magnesium-containing antacids should be avoided because of risks of hypermagnesemia. Since many antacids contain sodium, they should be carefully screened for sodium content before being given to patients on salt restriction. Sodium bicarbonate, if taken over prolonged periods, may lead to metabolic alkalosis (i.e., milk-alkali syndrome) or acid rebound. Prolonged use of calcium carbonate compounds may cause renal calculi.

Types of antacids

Aluminum hydroxide. Aluminum hydroxide is a moderately effective antacid, but is not as effective as magnesium hydroxide, calcium carbonate, or sodium bicarbonate. It buffers gastric acid to approximately 4.0 without interfering with electrolyte balance, and does not produce *acid rebound*. Systemic absorption is limited so that aluminum toxicity is rarely a problem. It is largely ineffective in tablet form, but the efficacy of the tablets may be improved somewhat by chewing them. Aluminum hydroxide is also mixed with magnesium hydroxide to decrease the diarrheal effect of the latter. In patients who get diarrhea even with the magnesium-aluminum hydroxide mixtures, aluminum hydroxide may be alternated in equal doses.

The usual dose of aluminum hydroxide is 15 ml 1 and 3 hours after meals and at bedtime, followed by sips of water or milk to ensure that the medication gets to the stomach. The main side effect is constipation. In large doses over a prolonged therapy course, phosphate depletion resulting in anorexia, malaise, and muscle weakness may occasionally occur.

Aluminum carbonate. Aluminum carbonate, an aqueous suspension, has properties, uses, and side effects that are similar to aluminum hydroxide gel.

The average adult dose is 4 to 8 ml repeated as necessary. Aluminum carbonate binds one-third more phosphate than aluminum hydroxide and therefore may be used in the management of phosphate renal stones.

Aluminum phosphate. Aluminum phosphate is a slow-acting antacid with properties similar to aluminum hydroxide. Unlike aluminum hydroxide, it does not interfere with phosphate absorption.

The usual dose is 5 to 15 ml as necessary.

Aluminum phosphate use may result in hyperphosphatemia in patients with renal impairment.

Dihydroxyaluminum aminoacetate. Dihydroxyaluminum aminoacetate is an antacid with properties and actions similar to those of aluminum hydroxide gel.

The usual dose is 0.5 to 2.0 gm 1 and 3 hours after meals and at bedtime, or as necessary. Prolonged use of the drug may cause constipation.

Dihydroxyaluminum sodium carbonate. Dihydroxyaluminum sodium carbonate is an antacid that combines the properties of both sodium bicarbonate and aluminum hydroxide.

The average adult dose is 300 to 600 mg as required (1 to 2 tablets). For better acid-neutralizing effect, the tablets should be chewed.

Calcium carbonate. Calcium carbonate readily neutralizes gastric acid and also reduces pepsin activity by binding with it. The drug is inexpensive, effective, readily available, and gives prolonged relief of symptoms. Calcium carbonate should not be used regularly for prolonged periods because of potentially serious renal problems resulting from calcium absorption. Its use should be restricted to the relief of occasional epigastric distress. This medication is readily available in reasonably palatable tablets, which makes it handy for home bedside use or for carrying in the pocket or purse.

The usual dosage is 1 to 2 tablets (300 to 500 mg of calcium carbonate per tablet) chewed as necessary for occasional use. Side effects with prolonged use may include hypercalcemia (which may lead to renal calculi and renal damage), constipation, and occasionally *alkalosis*. Calcium carbonate is contraindicated in patients with renal impairment. Calcium carbonate causes acid rebound and increased serum gastrin. It is unknown whether these side effects are significant.

Magnesium hydroxide (milk of magnesia). Magnesium hydroxide is an excellent hydrochloric acid neutralizer. It neutralizes gastric acid without producing alkalosis and has a demulcent effect. However,

because of its laxative properties, it is rarely used as an antacid. Since any absorbed magnesium ions are rapidly excreted in the urine, magnesium preparations should not be given to patients with renal impairment because of the risks of magnesium toxicity.

The antacid dose of magnesium hydroxide is 5 to 10 ml 1 and 3 hours after meals and at bedtime, mixed with half a glass of water or milk to assure it reaches the stomach. The major side effect is diarrhea.

Magnesium oxide. Magnesium oxide is a potent antacid, but its antacid effect is limited by its laxative properties. Magnesium oxide is converted to magnesium hydroxide in water. Its properties, uses, and side effects are essentially those of magnesium hydroxide.

The dose is 250 to 500 mg 1 and 3 hours after meals and at bedtime, or as necessary. Side effects include diarrhea.

Magnesium-aluminum hydroxide gels. Magnesium-aluminum hydroxide gels are popular especially for use in hospitals. These mixtures are used to counterbalance the laxative properties of magnesium compounds by the constipating effects of aluminum hydroxide. With the magnesium-aluminum gels commonly used, diarrhea may still be a problem in some patients and, therefore, one can alternate equal doses of the mixture with aluminum hydroxide. The buffering effect of the mixture is not as marked as that of magnesium hydroxide, but if a pH of 3.5 is considered adequate, then the magnesium-aluminum mixture is satisfactory. The magnesium-aluminum hydroxide gel is reasonably palatable.

The usual dose is 15 to 30 ml 1 and 3 hours after meals and at bedtime. More frequent doses may be used if the regimen is inadequate. Side effects include diarrhea. Magnesium-aluminum mixtures should not be given to patients with renal impairment because of the risk of magnesium toxicity. These antacids may increase absorption of some oral anticoagulants. These mixtures also impair absorption of drugs such as digitalis and tetracyclines, and may increase the excretion of aspirin.

Magaldrate. Magaldrate is a complex hydroxymagnesium aluminate. It is an effective antacid that can usually maintain a pH between 3.5 and 4.0. The systemic effects are similar to those of magnesium hydroxide.

The usual adult dose is 400 to 800 mg 1 and 3 hours after meals and at bedtime or as necessary.

Magaldrate, because of its low sodium content, may be used in patients on salt restriction, such as those with congestive heart failure, hypertension, toxemia, and renal failure.

Magnesium carbonate. Magnesium carbonate is a weak antacid and mild laxative. It is converted to magnesium chloride and carbon dioxide in the presence of acid in the stomach, and may cause belching.

The usual dose is 250 to 500 mg as necessary. Magnesium carbonate should not be given to patients with renal failure because of the risks of hypermagnesemia.

Magnesium trisilicate. Magnesium trisilicate is a relatively weak antacid. It absorbs pepsin and is said to form an ulcer protective coat of gelatinous silicone dioxide by the reaction of magnesium trisilicate and gastric contents. In high doses it has a laxative effect and can cause hypermagnesemia in patients with renal failure.

The usual dose is 0.5 to 2.0 gm as necessary or 1 and 3 hours after meals, and at bedtime. It should not be used in patients with renal failure. If used over long periods of time, renal stones may form.

Sodium bicarbonate (baking soda). Sodium bicarbonate is a readily available, inexpensive, and effective antacid. It acts rapidly and is readily absorbed but with repeated doses may cause a serious *metabolic alkalosis* or acid rebound. The use of this antacid should, therefore, be limited to the occasional home use.

The usual dose is 2 gm (½ teaspoon) in water, occasionally. Side effects with prolonged use include systemic alkalosis and hypernatremia. Gastric distention may occur because carbon dioxide is released when the sodium bicarbonate reacts with the hydrochloric acid in the stomach, but this is usually relieved by a satisfying belch. Sodium bicarbonate should not be given to salt-restricted patients, or those with problems such as congestive heart failure, renal impairment, or hypertension because sodium causes retention of water in the body, aggravating these conditions.

ULCER MEDICATIONS

Anticholinergics

Anticholinergic drugs (see Chapter 23, "Parasympathomimetics and Parasympatholytics") decrease gastric emptying and secretion. At the present time there is insufficient evidence to show that these drugs alone are effective in the control of duodenal ulcers. However, if ulcer healing or ulcer symptoms, especially night pain, are resistant to antacids or cimetidine and ranitidine, then anticholinergics may be added to the primary drug(s) as a single bedtime dose. Their effectiveness may be associated with decreased emptying of the antacid and decreased secretion of acid. Side effects are minimal with one bedtime dose. If anticholinergics are used every 6 hours, toxic side effects may include visual disturbances, dry mouth, urinary retention, and central nervous system problems, especially in the elderly. Anticholinergics are contrain-

dicated in patients with prostatic hypertrophy, glaucoma, or urinary retention.

Propantheline bromide. Propantheline bromide may be used to decrease acid secretion. The drug comes in 15 mg tablets for oral use. Dosage should not normally exceed one tablet every 6 hours. To decrease nocturnal secretion, one tablet may be given at bedtime with an antacid or cimetidine. Side effects are listed under anticholinergics.

Miscellaneous ulcer medications

Carbenoxolone. This compound, derived from licorice, has been used in Great Britain with some success in the treatment of gastric, and to a lesser extent duodenal, ulcers. Patients with gastric ulcers have frequently been hospitalized, treated with antacids, and prohibited from smoking. In various studies gastric ulcers treated with carbenoxolone did significantly better than control groups. Carbenoxolone-treated outpatients did as well as hospitalized patients. The therapeutic benefit of this drug appears to be an increased secretion of gastric mucoprotein. The dose regimen of carbenoxolone to treat gastric ulcers is one to two 50 mg tablets three times a day after meals. Since carbenoxolone is rapidly absorbed from the stomach, it is not effective in the treatment of duodenal ulcers. Capsules are designed to release the active compound in the pyloric antrum. Several studies have shown significant improvement in duodenal ulcer healing compared with controls. The dosage for duodenal ulcer therapy is a 50 mg time-release capsule (Duogastrone) four times a day. Side effects of carbenoxolone are sodium retention, hypokalemia, and hypertension. Its use should be avoided in the elderly and in patients with heart disease, hypertension, or hepatic and renal impairment. Absorption is impaired if given with antacids.

Cimetidine. Histamine is a potent stimulant of gastric secretion, yet gastric secretion is not inhibited by antihistaminics. It has been demonstrated that two types of histaminic receptors, H_1 (blocked by antihistaminics) and H_2 (blocked by H_2 antagonists), are present. H_2 receptors are located, among other sites, in relation to parietal cells. Cimetidine blocks H_2 receptors, markedly decreasing gastric secretion. It is effective in the healing of duodenal ulcers. Cimetidine is also as effective in ulcer healing and symptom control as antacids are. Its use in gastric ulcers has not been fully evaluated.

The dose commonly used for ulcer and reflux esophagitis therapy is 300 mg given three times a day with meals and at bedtime. Cimetidine is available for intravenous use in doses of 300 mg every 4 to 6 hours. The dosage should be reduced in patients with renal failure. Long-term use of this drug has not been fully evaluated, and it should be used with caution in periods exceeding 4 to 6 weeks. Side effects include gynecomastia, impotence, constipation, diarrhea, mental confusion, and muscular pains. Cardiac dysrhythmias have been reported with intravenous use. Its use in protecting against a recurrence of acid-peptic disorders has not been fully evaluated as yet. There is some suggestion that there is an increased risk of ulcer perforation after discontinuation of cimetidine. Clinical use of cimetidine in children is limited. Cimetidine is of value in the symptomatic treatment of hypersecretion and ulceration that occurs in *Zollinger-Ellison syndrome* (*gastrin*-secreting tumor of the pancreas).

Metoclopramide. Metoclopramide increases gastric emptying and LES tone. Its use has not yet been fully evaluated, but it appears to work fairly well in the treatment of reflux esophagitis. It has a central antiemetic effect, and appears to be of value in the treatment of nausea and vomiting secondary to surgery and radiation therapy.

Metoclopramide may be given orally, intramuscularly, or intravenously in doses of 10 mg three to four times a day ½ hour before meals and at bedtime. Side effects include constipation, diarrhea, extrapyramidal reactions, and drowsiness.

DISEASES TREATED WITH DIGESTANTS

Digestants are medications that replace normally occuring digestive compounds: hydrochloric acid, digestive enzymes, and bile. Bile salts and hydrochloric acid replacement therapy was more popular in the past but is rarely used now. The most commonly used digestants at present are pancreatic enzymes. Disorders causing pancreatic enzyme insufficiency include chronic pancreatitis and cystic fibrosis. In addition the surgical removal of the pancreas and neoplasms obstructing the pancreatic duct can cause a pancreatic enzyme insufficiency. These disorders may be present with *steatorrhea* and malnutrition.

Chronic pancreatitis

Chronic pancreatitis is the most common cause of pancreatic insufficiency in adults and is often a sequela of alcoholism. The mechanism by which alcohol causes pancreatitis is unknown but may be, in part, a result of the direct toxic effect of alcohol on *acinar cells*. Repeated attacks of pancreatitis result in decreased pancreatic *exocrine* and, less commonly, endocrine function. The predominant symptom is severe epigastric pain radiating to the back. Pancreatic exocrine insufficiency may be manifested by patients with steatorrhea and malnutrition. This diagnosis of exo-

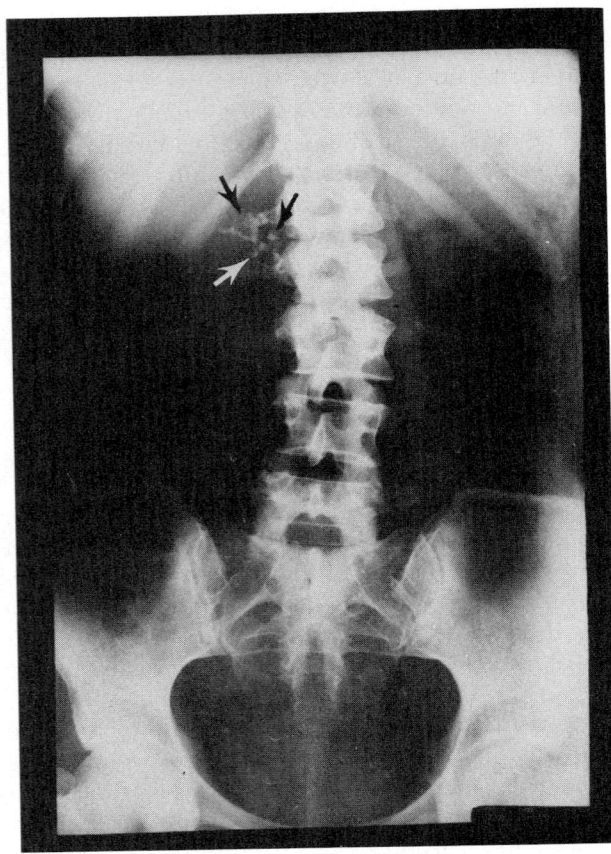

FIGURE 39-4. **Radiograph showing calcification (*arrows*) in head of pancreas. Calcification is indication of chronic pancreatitis. (Courtesy Dr. Ann Conrad.)**

crine insufficiency can be confirmed by 72-hour-fecal-fat studies and the secretion test. Endocrine insufficiency results in diabetes mellitus. X-ray examination may show calcification of the pancreas (Figure 39-4), and endoscopic retrograde pancreatography may show pancreatic duct calculi and strictures.

Therapy for chronic pancreatitis includes the following:

1. Avoidance of alcohol
2. Pancreatic enzyme replacement
3. Surgery
4. Insulin therapy if necessary

Cystic fibrosis

Cystic fibrosis is a genetically transmitted disease that results in impaired mucous gland function, especially increased mucus production in the lungs, and impaired pancreatic function. Pancreatic function is deficient in 80% of patients suffering from this disease. Although the disease is commonly diagnosed in childhood, some cases remain undiagnosed until adolescence. An early manifestation may be the inability to pass *meconium* in the neonate. Children may have steatorrhea, malnutrition, and recurring pulmonary infections. Diagnosis can be confirmed by the sweat test, by measurement of pancreatic enzyme activity on duodenal aspirates, and by 24-hour stool collection. The course of the disease is influenced by pulmonary problems and not by pancreatic insufficiency.

Therapy varies somewhat with the severity of the disease and may include the following:
1. Mucolytic agents to decrease respiratory mucus viscosity and allow secretions to be coughed up
2. Prophylactic antibiotics to minimize pulmonary infections
3. Pancreatic enzyme replacement therapy
4. Low-fat diet
5. Salt replacement, especially during hot weather and febrile episodes
6. Avoidance of drugs containing antihistamines and antitussives, because these can dry secretions and diminish productive coughing
7. Administration of water-soluble miscible vitamin preparations of A, D, E, and K (usually twice the recommended dosage)

Surgical removal of the pancreas

An extensive or complete pancreatectomy may be done for relief of chronic pancreatic pain and for pancreatic neoplasms. These procedures will remove all or a good part of the exocrine and endocrine functions of the pancreas, resulting in steatorrhea, malnutrition, and diabetes mellitus.

Therapy includes the following:
1. Pancreatic enzyme replacement
2. Insulin

Obstruction of pancreatic drainage

Pancreatic duct drainage may be totally obstructed by neoplasms on the head of the pancreas, the ampulla of Vater, and the common bile duct. These patients with neoplasms may have epigastric pain, jaundice, or both. Diagnosis may be confirmed by a barium meal, endoscopy, endoscopic retrograde cholangiopancreatography (ERCP), and at times by *percutaneous transhepatic cholangiography.* Steatorrhea and malnutrition are a result of a lack of pancreatic enzymes.

Therapy may include the following:
1. Surgery if the case is operable
2. Palliative bile duct drainage to the duodenum (or jejunum in surgically incurable cases)
3. Pancreatic enzyme replacement
4. Analgesics

DIGESTANTS
Pancreatic enzymes

Pancreatic enzymes are available in powder form and are derived from the pancreas of pigs and cows. Commercially available pancreatic enzymes vary somewhat in their amylase, trypsin, lipase, and protease content and in their potency. It is, therefore, worthwhile to try several preparations, in case some seem relatively ineffective. These preparations may be in capsules, enteric-coated tablets, and in powders. Gastric acid and pepsin tends to destroy the enzymes. Pancreatic enzyme activity may be preserved by using antacids, cimetidine or anticholinergic drugs.

The dosage of pancreatic enzymes varies with the individual patient and with the preparation (average adult doses range 1 to 2 tablets or capsules per meal or approximately 1 to 6 gm per day, depending on the preparation).

Side effects include allergies (especially to hog pancreatic enzymes), nausea, buccal and perianal soreness (especially in children), and poor control of steatorrhea. The use of hog pancreatic enzymes may result in cultural or religious problems.

Glutamic acid hydrochloride

Glutamic acid hydrochloride is a form of hydrochloric acid available in capsules and is used occasionally to treat achlorhydria. Its effectiveness in the treatment of gastric hypoacidity is debatable. If used, glutamic acid hydrochloride is taken with or immediately following meals.

SUMMARY

Antacids are commonly used medications because of the frequency of acid-peptic symptoms. These symptoms can occur after dietary indiscretions but can also be a part of a more serious acid-peptic disorder, such as duodenal ulcers. The choice of antacids is not always rational and depends on such things as sales promotion and taste, rather than on neutralizing effect. Patients tend to prefer tablets to liquids. In addition to antacids, anticholinergics, H_2 receptor blockers, cimetidine, and ranitidine are also discussed in the treatment of various ulcers.

Digestants are not commonly used, except those that replace pancreatic enzymes. Often one has to try several varieties before an optimum effect is achieved for the patient.

With an understanding of the use, dose, side effects and drug interactions associated with the antacids, ulcer medications, and digestants, the nurse can provide optimal care to patients who require these medications.

ADVERSE/SIDE EFFECTS OF ANTACIDS, ULCER MEDICATIONS, AND DIGESTANTS*

ALLERGIC EFFECTS

Lacrimation
Rash
Sneezing

AUTONOMIC NERVOUS SYSTEM

Anticholinergic effects (dry mouth, urinary retention, and visual disturbances) (propantheline)

CARDIOVASCULAR SYSTEM

Dysrhythmias (occasionally reported with intravenous cimetidine)
Hypertension (may occur with carbenoxolone)

CENTRAL NERVOUS SYSTEM

Drowsiness (metoclopramide)
Mental confusion (cimetidine, metoclopramide)

METABOLIC AND ENDOCRINE SYSTEMS

Alkalosis
Gynecomastia (cimetidine)
Hypercalcemia
Hypermagnesemia
Hypernatremia
Hypokalemia
Hypophosphatemia

GASTROINTESTINAL SYSTEM

Constipation
Diarrhea
Sore mouth and anus (pancreatic enzymes especially in chidren)

NEUROMUSCULAR (EXTRAPYRAMIDAL) SYSTEM

Muscle pains
Parkinsonism symptoms (metoclopramide)

RENAL SYSTEM

Renal calculi
Renal failure

*See Chapter 11, "Drug Toxicity", for an overview of drug toxicity.

CLINICALLY SIGNIFICANT DRUG INTERACTIONS*

Primary drug	Interacting drug	Possible effect(s)	Probable mechanism(s)
All antacids	Lithium	Decreased lithium effect	Increased renal excretion
Aluminum hydroxide	Tetracyclines	Decreased serum level (absorption) of tetracyclines	Chelate polyvalent ions Acid pH necessary for dissolution
Cimetidine	Beta-adrenergic blockers	Increased plasma concentration of beta-adrenergic blockers	Decreased metabolism
Cimetidine	Benzodiazepines	Increased plasma concentration of benzodiazepines	Decreased clearance
Cimetidine	Lidocaine	Increased plasma concentration and resultant toxicity	Decreased clearance
Cimetidine	Phenindione	Prolongation of prothrombin time	Inhibition of hepatic metabolism
Cimetidine	Phenytoin	Increased phenytoin concentration and resultant toxicity	Inhibition of hepatic metabolism
Cimetidine	Procainamide	Increased procainamide half-life	Decreased clearance
Cimetidine	Theophylline	Increased theophylline half-life and toxicity	Inhibition of hepatic metabolism
Cimetidine	Warfarin	Prolongation of prothrombin time	Inhibition of hepatic metabolism
Sodium bicarbonate	Amphetamines	Increased serum level of amphetamines	Decreased urinary excretion
Sodium bicarbonate	Aspirin	Decreased serum level of aspirin	Increased urinary clearance
Sodium bicarbonate	Tetracyclines	Decreased serum level (absorption) of tetracyclines	Chelate polyvalent ions Acid pH necessary for dissolution

*See Chapter 10, "Drug Interactions," for an overview of drug interactions.

Nursing of patients requiring antacids

ASSESSMENT

A complete nursing assessment is essential in establishing a baseline from which to plan and individualize drug therapy regimens and to monitor patient response. Assessment should include a detailed drug history to ascertain contraindications, cautions, potential drug interactions, and individual drug-taking patterns before drug therapy is initiated. In addition, assessment should include detailed baseline data related to the patient's history of hypersecretion, ulcer disease, reflux esophagitis, or indigestion. Familial factors, age, stress management, and the characteristics of epigastric pain (heartburn or indigestion as well as its duration and association to meals, position, bedtime, stressful situations, or relationship to certain foods and beverages), should be identified. Because gastrointestinal pain can be referred and because certain conditions (e.g., gallstones, gastric malignancy, hiatal hernia, and pancreatitis) can mimic indigestion, assessment should be completed carefully. The patient's use of antacids, alcohol, and tobacco also requires careful exploration, and a dietary history should be included to identify foods and liquids that have been found to cause gastrointestinal distress and that should be avoided (e.g., coffee, acidic or spicy foods). It should be identified if the patient has had any hematemesis or melena, and if so, the characteristics should be recorded carefully.

Laboratory data should include a complete blood count, hematocrit, hemoglobin, and coagulation studies, especially if the patient has a history of gastric bleeding. X-ray studies, endoscopy, gastroscopy, and biopsy may be indicated.

Assessment of the patient's general health state and baseline vital signs (including pulse, blood pressure, and respirations) should be recorded, especially if the patient has a history of gastrointestinal bleeding.

CONTRAINDICATIONS AND CAUTIONS

Magnesium salts should be administered with caution to patients with renal failure because hypermagnesemia can result, characterized by lethargy and drowsiness. If magnesium is not excreted and is allowed to accumulate, coma, respiratory failure, and circulatory collapse can result. Calcium carbonate is also contraindicated in the presence of renal failure because hypercalcemia can result, and at higher levels systemic alkalosis and tetany. Patients who are prone to alkalosis or patients who consume large quantities of milk should avoid calcium carbonate as well. In addition, calcium carbonate should be administered with caution to patients with hyperthyroidism or those patients prone to the formation of renal stones. Calcium intake should be monitored closely in these patients.

In patients requiring sodium restriction, such as those patients with congestive heart failure or hypertension, an antacid preparation should be chosen that is low in sodium content (e.g., magaldrate), especially if long-term antacid therapy is indicated.

DRUG INTERACTIONS

Even though antacids are nonprescription medications, they have the ability to interact with a wide variety of both prescription and nonprescription medications. For example, antacids can decrease the absorption and increase the excretion of penicillins, phenylbutazone, and most tetracyclines, thus antagonizing the effects of these medications. When taken concurrently with such medications as amphetamines, narcotic analgesics, quinidine, and theophylline, antacids may increase the absorption of these medications and decrease their excretion by the kidney thus maximizing the effects of these medications (see Clinically Significant Drug Interactions).

Because antacids increase the pH of the stomach, they can cause the enteric coating of coadministered medications (e.g., ferrous sulfate, sodium salicylate, bisacodyl) to dissolve prematurely, releasing the contents into the stomach where they can either cause increased gastrointestinal irritation or be inactivated or degraded in the still relatively acid environment of the stomach. Thus, the coadministration of antacids and enteric-coated medications is contraindicated. Doses of interacting drugs when coadministered should be spaced at least 1 to 2 hours before or after the administration of the antacid.

ADMINISTRATION

Antacids are taken orally in either liquid or tablet form. Frequent administration is required especially during initial therapy because of the frequent emptying of the stomach contents. Liquid preparations are usually available in suspension form. Because they can separate upon standing, they should be shaken thoroughly to ensure an adequate dose. Liquid forms have rapid action and greater neutralizing activity than tablet forms of antacids. However, tablets are usually preferred by the patient because they are convenient to take and are more palatable. The taste of the antacid is an important consideration in assisting patients with long-term antacid therapy.

Liquid antacids

Liquid preparations should be administered with a small amount of water or milk to ensure that the medication reaches the stomach. When liquid antacids are administered through a nasogastric tube, the antacid should be followed with 5 to 15 ml of water to flush the tube. The patency of the nasogastric tube should be ensured before the administration of the medication.

Tablet antacids

Tablets should be taken as directed and must be thoroughly chewed or dissolved in the mouth before swallowing. This increases the surface area of the medication and its effectiveness in neutralizing stomach acid. Patients must be warned not to swallow antacid tablets whole because tablets that do not dissolve completely in the gastrointestinal tract are not only ineffective in controlling stomach acid, but can cause intestinal obstruction.

The frequency of administration is individualized. Therapeutic effect, however, depends on the antacids being taken correctly and at the specified time. Patients should be responsible for self-medication but usually require assistance in following their prescribed therapy, recording antacid use, and monitoring response.

MONITORING PATIENT RESPONSE
Therapeutic response

The effectiveness of antacid therapy can be monitored by a reported de-

Continued.

Nursing of patients requiring antacids—cont'd

Therapeutic response—cont'd

crease in epigastric distress, heartburn, or regurgitation. Diagnostic tests indicate healing of ulcers. When response is monitored, it is important to be alert to signs that may indicate gastric perforation or other complications including sudden intense epigastric pain or referred pain to both shoulders with guarded abdominal muscles. The amount, color, frequency, and consistency of stools, as well as any vomitus or nasogastric suction, should be monitored, especially in patients with a history of ulcer or gastrointestinal bleeding. Black, tarry, or sticky stools are indicative of upper gastrointestinal bleeding, whereas maroon-colored stools may indicate lower gastrointestinal bleeding. Hematochezin, or the rectal evacuation of blood, indicates severe bleeding. Coffee ground emesis or hematemesis occurs with upper gastrointestinal bleeding. Medical assistance should be sought immediately and the patient monitored carefully in the presence of acute bleeding.

Adverse side effects

Side effects should be monitored carefully (see Adverse/Side Effects of Antacids, Ulcer Medications, and Digestants). The most common side effects associated with antacid therapy are diarrhea (especially with magnesium salts) and constipation (especially with aluminum or calcium salts). Elimination patterns should be carefully monitored especially in the elderly, and if diarrhea or constipation becomes severe or bothersome, alternate therapy should be explored, including the use of combination products or the alter-nation of aluminum salt products with magnesium salt products.

Other common side effects include acid rebound and nausea. Electrolyte imbalance can also occur with prolonged use of antacids (e.g., hypermagnesemia with the use of magnesium salts; hypernatremia with sodium salts and other sodium-containing antacid preparations; hypercalcemia with the use of calcium-containing antacids). Alkalosis or milk alkali syndrome can also occur, especially with sodium bicarbonate use or calcium carbonate use over time (particularly if the antacid is consumed with milk).

PATIENT EDUCATION

The patient and family should have a clear understanding of the medication regimen; they should be aware of the exact name of the antacid preparation prescribed, its dosage, storage, administration, and possible side effects. The patient should know how to minimize common side effects such as constipation or diarrhea. The patient and family should be able to identify early signs that indicate that the prescriber should be contacted (e.g., prolonged diarrhea, vomiting blood, passing blood in the stool).

In addition to the monitoring of adverse effects, the patient should monitor therapeutic response and recognize the importance of continuing the antacid therapy as directed even though symptoms are relieved.

Patients should be advised that self-medication without consultation with the health care provider can cause harmful effects because all antacids are not alike. In addition, their use can mask serious conditions that may require immediate treatment.

When antacids are taken for the treatment of ulcers, patients and their families often require assistance in adapting to changes in lifestyle that are often indicated in the treatment of peptic ulcer disease. Patients need to identify aspects of their lifestyle that affect their condition and how these can be changed or modified. Although there is no evidence that any particular diet prevents recurrence of esophageal or peptic ulcers, many patients find that certain foods bother them and thus they should be encouraged to avoid these foods that cause them distress. They should also be encouraged to avoid caffeine; alcohol; spicy foods or other foods that stimulate gastric irritation; and aspirin, cortisone, or other antiinflammatory medications (especially if they have erosive gastritis). Smoking and alcohol use should be stopped because although not a direct cause of the ulcer condition, they can interfere with ulcer healing. In addition, the patient may require assistance with stress management at home or at work, including exploration of a planned exercise program, meditation, psychotherapy, or a change in work responsibility.

Long-term treatment is often difficult for patients and their families, and support is often required. Individualizing therapy to the patient's own pattern of hypersecretion is helpful as well as providing follow-up care and monitoring.

Nursing of patients requiring cimetidine

ASSESSMENT

See previous section, Nursing of Patients Requiring Antacids.

CAUTIONS

Cimetidine should be administered cautiously to patients with a history of renal failure. It has also been associated with hematologic abnormalities because it is related to known hematotoxins.

DRUG INTERACTIONS

Cimetidine can alter the metabolism of various drugs (see Clinically Significant Drug Interactions).

ADMINISTRATION

Cimetidine can be administered by oral, intramuscular, or intravenous routes. Adjustment in dosage is not usually required. Intramuscular injection does not require dilution of the parenteral preparation; however, dilu-tion is required for intravenous bolus injection as well as for intermittent or continuous infusion. Hypotension has been reported in relation to intravenous injection of undiluted medication. Cimetidine can be administered in most common intravenous solutions (e.g., 5% or 10% dextrose, dextrose and sodium chloride, 5% dextrose and lactated Ringer's solution, lactated Ringer's, and sodium chloride 0.9%). (See

Nursing of patients requiring cimetidine—cont'd

ADMINISTRATION—cont'd

Nursing Drug Digest for concentration and infusion rates.)

Cimetidine, given by oral solution, tablets, intramuscular injection, or intravenously, should be administered with meals. Antacids are used with cimetidine for relief of ulcer pain, but should generally not be administered simultaneously with oral cimetidine because they may decrease the oral absorption of cimetidine.

Reduced dosage should be used in the elderly or patients with renal failure.

MONITORING
PATIENT RESPONSE

Monitoring is important because cimetidine is a relatively new drug. It can be used safely with routine monitoring of effects.

See previous section, Nursing of Patients Requiring Antacids.

Therapeutic response

Monitor patients for decreased complaints of gastric pain, heartburn, irritation, or distress related to hypersecretion of stomach acid. A gastric pH of 3.5 or higher is desirable and is monitored when possible.

Adverse side effects

Common side effects include headache, fatigue, dizziness, diarrhea, and constipation. Muscular pain, skin rash, and gynecomastia have also been reported. Central nervous system side effects (e.g., confusion, dizziness) seem to be dose related, and the elderly and those patients with renal failure should be monitored closely for these effects especially when higher doses of cimetidine are given.

Mental confusion, psychosis, and hematologic problems (e.g., leukopenia, thrombocytopenia, agranulocytosis) have also been reported in relation to the use of this medication (see Adverse/Side Effects of Antacids, Ulcer Medications, and Digestants).

PATIENT EDUCATION

See previous section, Nursing of Patients Requiring Antacids, for general patient teaching.

Nursing of patients requiring digestants

ASSESSMENT

A complete nursing assessment is essential in establishing a baseline from which to plan and individualize drug therapy regimens and to monitor patient response. Assessment should include a detailed drug history to ascertain contraindications, cautions, potential drug interactions, and individual drug-taking patterns before drug therapy is initiated. In addition, assessment should include detailed baseline data related to the patient's condition, including pulmonary and nutritional assessment. Dietary history and elimination patterns, including frequency and characteristics of stools, are important in monitoring therapy. Steatorrhea, malnutrition or failure to thrive in infants, flatulence, and anal irritation should be assessed.

Laboratory data will vary on the individual patient's condition and may include sweat tests and fecal fat studies.

Alcohol abuse is associated with pancreatitis, and alcohol use should be assessed. Pain associated with the condition, as well as referred pain, should be assessed and recorded. Urine sugar and acetone and fasting blood sugars are indicated because diabetes mellitus is often associated with this condition.

SENSITIVITY,
CONTRAINDICATIONS,
AND CAUTIONS

See the text material and the Nursing Drug Digest for individual agents.

ADMINISTRATION

Pancreatic enzymes are available in powder form, capsules, or enteric-coated tablets. Antacids or cimetidine may be given with pancreatic enzymes to preserve their action, although this is not common treatment in children with cystic fibrosis. Dosage is highly individualized. Since pancreatic enzymes are different strengths, the type of enzyme is usually determined by the strength needed. The enzymes are not mixed together.

These are general rules for administering digestants to children with cystic fibrosis:

1. Administer in the middle of the meal or preferably before the meal;
2. Do not mix enzymes with hot or warm food, mashed potatoes, or baby fruit containing tapioca;
3. Mix enzymes in a small amount of food, preferably applesauce, immediately before administration.

Enzymes can be increased or decreased according to the amount of fat in the diet, the size of the meal or snack, or the quality of the bowel movement.

MONITORING PATIENT
RESPONSE

Monitor patients for therapeutic and adverse side effects associated with the use of individual agents.

PATIENT EDUCATION

The patient and family should have a clear understanding of the medication regimen; they should be aware of the exact name of the digestant preparation prescribed, its dosage, storage, administration, and possible side effects. The patient should know how to minimize common side effects such as constipation or diarrhea. The patient and family should be able to identify early signs that indicate that the prescriber should be contacted (e.g., anal soreness with pancreatic enzymes).

In addition to the monitoring of adverse effects, the patient should monitor therapeutic response and recognize the importance of continuing the digestant therapy as directed even though symptoms are relieved.

Long-term treatment is often difficult for patients and their families, and support is often required. Individualizing therapy to the patient's own needs is helpful as well as providing follow-up care and monitoring.

GENERAL INSTRUCTIONS FOR DISCHARGE/OUTPATIENTS

ANTACIDS

This medication is an antacid for the treatment of your condition. It should help relieve troublesome symptoms but is not expected to cure your disorder.

Follow the instructions on the label exactly. Do not take a larger or smaller dose of this medication than prescribed unless told to do so by your health care provider. If your symptoms improve, continue to take the medication as directed until you are told you no longer require it.

Antacids may alter absorption of some anticoagulants and antibiotics. Be sure to tell your health care provider if you are taking any other medication including drugs purchased without a prescription so that an appropriate antacid can be prescribed. Because of this do not start or discontinue any medications without checking with your health care provider.

Antacids can cause bothersome side effects including diarrhea, constipation, or nausea. If these persist or become too bothersome, notify your health care provider so that your dosage schedule can be modified or another antacid may be selected. Do not stop taking this medication or change to another antacid yourself without discussing this with your health care provider because all antacids are not alike and can affect you differently.

If you observe any other side effects, report them to your health care provider.

If you suffer from high blood pressure, heart disease, liver disease, or have kidney or bladder problems, please inform your health care provider so that antacids that can aggravate your condition can be avoided.

This medication has been prescribed especially for you. Do not share it with friends or relatives.

Keep this medication and all other medications out of the reach of children.

If you have any questions about your medication regimen or other aspects of your care, contact your health care provider.

CIMETIDINE

This medication is used to treat conditions that result in too much stomach acid, such as gastric and duodenal ulcers. Taken as directed it should help to relieve troublesome symptoms such as heartburn and stomach pain.

Take this medication as directed by your health care provider just before eating or just after eating. If you find that you have stomach pain between meals, let your health care provider know, so that an appropriate antacid can be prescribed or so that your cimetidine dosage can be adjusted.

This medication should be taken for the full length of time as indicated by your health care provider. Try not to miss any doses because this will ensure maximum effectiveness in the treatment of your condition. Remember, it may take several days or weeks before you feel its effectiveness.

If you miss a dose of this medication, do not take the missed dose and do not double your next dose.

Do not start or stop taking any other medications while you are taking cimetidine without first consulting with your health care provider.

This medication can cause bothersome side effects in some people, including headaches, diarrhea, dizziness, confu-

sion, tiredness, skin rash, and breast tenderness (or enlargement in men), which will go away when the medication is discontinued. Most people, however, have few or no side effects. If you develop any of these and if they become severe or continual, notify your health care provider because you may require a change in your medication dosage or regimen. Do not drive or operate dangerous machinery or do jobs that require alertness until you know how this medication effects you. Use care going up and down stairs, and if you should become dizzy, sit or lie down immediately. When you feel better, get up slowly. If you observe any other side effects, report them to your health care provider.

If you are pregnant or breast feeding, do not take this medication unless specifically told to do so by your health care provider.

If you desire to become pregnant while you are taking this medication, discuss this with your health care provider.

This medication has been prescribed especially for you. Do not share or trade this medication with family or friends.

Keep this medication and all other medications out of the reach of children. Store in a dry, dark place. Refrigeration is not necessary.

If you have any questions about your medication regimen or other aspects of your care such as your diet or stress management contact your health care provider.

If you are being treated for an ulcer, notify your health care provider immediately if you notice faintness, weakness, vomiting of blood, or black tarry bowel movements because this may indicate ulcer bleeding.

NURSING DRUG DIGEST

Medication (trade name*)	Indication	Usual dosage and administration	Dosage forms, preparation, and storage	Contraindications, cautions, and comments	Monitoring
ANTACIDS					
★ **Aluminum carbonate** Basaljel*	Duodenal and gastric ulcers, reflux esophagitis, stress ulcers, and erosive gastritis	*Adults:* 500-1000 mg ml PO repeated as necessary usually 1 and 3 hr after meals and q.h.s. Shake suspension thoroughly before administration	Suspension: 400, 1000 mg/5 ml Tablet: 500 mg Capsule: 500 mg Store in airtight containers	Similar to aluminum hydroxide May be used in the treatment of phosphatic nephrolithiasis because of its ability to decrease phosphate absorption The usual dosage for this condition is 40 ml 1 hr before each meal and q.h.s.	Observe for constipation Monitor serum phosphate
Aluminum hydroxide gel Amphojel Amphojel S5* Antacid Powder* B-A* Basaljel* Di-Gel* Flacid* Gelusil* Glycogel* Liquid Antacid Maalox* Magna Gel* Mylanta* Norelac*	Duodenal and gastric ulcers, reflux esophagitis, stress ulcers, and erosive gastritis	*Adults:* 15 ml or 1-2 tablets chewed or dissolved in mouth 1 and 3 hr after meals and q.h.s. with small amount of fluid Shake suspension thoroughly before administration	Suspension: 200, 600 mg/5 ml Tablets: 300, 500, 600 mg Capsule: 500 mg	Low neutralizing capacity May cause nausea and vomiting May cause constipation Tablets are much less effective than liquid Prolonged use may cause hypophosphatemia	Observe for constipation Monitor serum phosphate Monitor for early signs of hypophosphatemia (e.g., anorexia, malaise, and muscle weakness)
★ **Aluminum phosphate** Phosphagel	Duodenal and gastric ulcers, reflux esophagitis, stress ulcers, and erosive gastritis	*Adults:* 15-45 ml or 1-2 tablets chewed or dissolved in mouth repeated as necessary usually 1 and 3 hr after meals and q.h.s. Shake suspension thoroughly before administration	Tablet: 400 mg Suspension: 233 mg/5 ml Avoid freezing; store at temperatures under 30° C	Unlike aluminum hydroxide, aluminum phosphate does *not* interfere with phosphate absorption Low neutralizing capacity	Observe for constipation

Continued.

NOTE: For additional details regarding the individual agents listed in this table, see the text and other tables in this chapter.
*Indicates a multiple active ingredient product. For a complete listing of all active ingredients see the *Drug Reference Guide to Brand Names and Active Ingredients.*
♦ Indicates that the drug is generally available only in Canada.
★ Indicates that the drug is generally available only in the United States.

NURSING DRUG DIGEST—cont'd

Medication (trade name)	Indication	Usual dosage and administration	Dosage forms, preparation, and storage	Contraindications, cautions, and comments	Monitoring
Calcium carbonate Albicon* Alka-2 Chewable Antacid Alkets* Amitone Bisodol* Calcet* Camelox* Chooz* Dicarbosil Equilet Glycate* Glycogel* Gustalac* Krem* Pepto-Bismol* Tums	Duodenal and gastric ulcers, reflux esophagitis, stress ulcers, and erosive gastritis	*Adults:* 300-1000 mg PO occasionally as indicated Tablets should be chewed or dissolved in mouth *Do not* administer with milk, because it may cause "milk-alkali syndrome"	Tablets, chewable: 300, 350, 420, 500, 600, 750 mg	*Contraindicated* in patients with renal failure Prolonged use may cause hypercalcemia, urinary tract calculi, and renal damage May cause acid rebound High neutralizing capacity	Monitor for hypercalcemia with prolonged, frequent use Observe for constipation
Dihydroxy-aluminum aminoacetate Alamino Alglyn Alminate Alzinoy Aspogen Dimothyn Doraximin Prodoxin Robalate	Duodenal and gastric ulcers, reflux esophagitis, stress ulcers, and erosive gastritis	*Adults:* 0.5-2 gm as required 1 and 3 hr after meals and q.h.s. Tablets should be chewed or dissolved in mouth	Tablet, chewable: 500 mg Liquid: 500 mg/5 ml	Prolonged use may cause constipation Neutralizing capacity is low	Monitor serum phosphate Observe for constipation

Drug	Uses	Dosage	Dosage forms	Nursing considerations	
Dihydroxy-aluminum sodium carbonate Rolaids	Duodenal and gastric ulcers, reflux esophagitis, stress ulcers, and erosive gastritis	*Adults*: 300-600 mg PO as required or 1 and 3 hr after meals and q.h.s. Tablets should be chewed or dissolved in mouth before swallowing	Tablet: 300 mg Store in airtight containers	Sodium content may be significant with chronic use (53 mg/tablet)	Observe for constipation Observe for fluid retention
Magaldrate Riopan Riopan Plus*	Duodenal and gastric ulcers, reflux esophagitis, stress ulcers, and erosive gastritis	*Adults*: 400-800 mg PO as necessary or 1 and 3 hr after meals and q.h.s. Tablets should be chewed or dissolved in mouth Shake suspension thoroughly before administration	Suspension: 480 mg/5 ml Tablet, chewable: 480 mg	May cause diarrhea Do *not* use in renal failure because of the risk of magnesium toxicity	Observe for diarrhea
★ **Magnesium carbonate** Albicon* Alkets* Antacid Powder* Anti-Acid No. 1* BiSoDol* DeWitt's Antacid Powder* Di-Gel* Dimacid* Escot Capsules* Estomul-M* Flacid* Formula Magsic* Glycogel* Krem* Kudrox* Marblen* Noralac* Ratio* Silain-Gel* Spastosed*	Duodenal and gastric ulcers, reflux esophagitis, stress ulcers, and erosive gastritis	*Adults*: 250-1000 mg PO as necessary or 1 and 3 hr after meals and q.h.s. followed by 120 ml (4 oz) water	Powder	May cause diarrhea Do *not* use in renal failure because of the risk of magnesium toxicity May cause eructation	Observe for diarrhea

Continued.

NURSING DRUG DIGEST—cont'd

Medication (trade name)	Indication	Usual dosage and administration	Dosage forms, preparation, and storage	Contraindications, cautions, and comments	Monitoring
Magnesium hydroxide Alurex* Alurex No. 2 Aluscop* B-A* Banacid* BiSoDol Antacid* Gelusil Extra Strength Liquid* Haley's M-O* Laxsil* Liquid Antacid* Maalox* Magna Gel* Mylanta* Nutramag*	Duodenal and gastric ulcers, reflux esophagitis, stress ulcers, and erosive gastritis See also Chapter 41, "Laxatives and Antidiarrheals"	*Adults:* 5-10 ml or 1-2 tablets 1 and 3 hr after meals and q.h.s. Tablets should be chewed or dissolved in mouth	Suspension: 390 mg/5 ml Tablet: 325, 650 mg	May cause diarrhea Do *not* use in renal failure because of the risk of magnesium toxicity	Observe for diarrhea
★ **Magnesium oxide** Albicon* Alkets* Aludrox* Aluscop* Beelith* Buffinol* Camalox* Creamalin*	Duodenal and gastric ulcers, reflux esophagitis, stress ulcers, and erosive gastritis See also Chapter 41, "Laxatives and Antidiarrheals"	*Adults:* 250-500 mg as necessary or 1 and 3 hr after meals and q.h.s. Tablets should be chewed or dissolved in mouth and followed by water or milk	Capsules: 140, 400 mg Powder Tablets: 400, 420, 500, 650 mg Store in airtight containers	May cause diarrhea Do *not* use in renal failure because of the risk of magnesium toxicity	Observe for diarrhea

Delcid* Di-Gel* Estomul-M* Gelusil* Kolantyl* Kudrox* Magnatril* Silain-Gel*				Observe for diarrhea
★ **Magnesium trisilicate** A.M.T.* Antacid Powder* Azolid-A* Banacid* Chooz* Dewitt's Antacid Powder* Escot Capsules* Gaviscon Antacid* Gaviscon-2 Antacid* Gelumina* Magnatril* Neutrasil Noralac* Pama* Tri-Sil Trimagel* Trimax Trisogel* Trisomin	Duodenal and gastric ulcers, reflux esophagitis, stress ulcers, and erosive gastritis	*Adults:* 0.5-2 gm PO as necessary *or* 1 and 3 hr after meals and q.h.s. Tablets should be chewed or dissolved in mouth	Powder Tablet: 500 mg	May cause diarrhea Do *not* use in renal failure because of risk of magnesium toxicity May interfere with absorption of tetracyclines and anticholinergics Low neutralizing capacity

Continued.

NURSING DRUG DIGEST—cont'd

Medication (trade name)	Indication	Usual dosage and administration	Dosage forms, preparation, and storage	Contraindications, cautions, and comments	Monitoring
Sodium bicarbonate Alka-Seltzer Effervescent Antacid* Alka-Seltzer Effervescent Pain Reliever and Antacid* Antacid Powder* Bell-Ans BiSoDol* Brioschi Bromo-Seltzer* Ceo-Two Suppositories* Citrocarbonate* Dewitt's Antacid Powder* Diatrol* Eno* Neut Sellymin Soda Mint Syllamelt Effervescent*	Duodenal and gastric ulcers, reflux esophagitis, stress ulcers, and erosive gastritis	*Adults:* 300 mg-2 gm PO occasionally Administer with glassful of water Tablets should be chewed	Powder Tablets: 325, 500, 520, 650 mg	*Contraindicated* in hypertension, heart failure, and renal failure May cause alkalosis and hypernatremia May cause eructation May contribute to kidney stone formation High neutralizing capacity Contains 27% sodium	Monitor intake and output Observe for fluid retention Monitor for signs of alkalosis

	Indications	Dosage	Preparations	Remarks	Nursing Implications
ANTICHOLINERGICS **Propantheline** Banlin Giquel Norpanth Novopro-panthil Pro-Banthine Pro-Banthine with Phe-nobarbital* Propanthel Robantaline Ropanth	Duodenal ulcer	*Adults:* 15 mg PO t.i.d. before meals and q.h.s.	Tablet: 15 mg	*Contraindicated* in glaucoma, prostatism May cause vesical disturbances, dry mouth and urinary retention	Observe for atropine-like side effects (e.g., dry mouth, blurred vision, urinary retention, constipation)
MISCELLANEOUS **Cimetidine** Novo-Cimetine Peptol Tagamet	Duodenal ulcer, stress ulcer, erosive gastritis, reflux esophagitis, gastric ulcer	*Adults:* 300 mg q.i.d. with meals and q.h.s. PO, IM, *or* IV Decrease dose to 300 mg q.8-12h. in severe renal failure (creatinine clearance <10 ml/min) Dilute IV injection to 20 ml and administer *slowly* over 2 min to prevent hypotensive effect	Tablets: 200, 300, 400 mg Solution: 300 mg/5 ml (with 3% alcohol) Injectable: 300 mg/2 ml Injectable form can be added to or diluted with D₅W and NS Diluted solution is stable for 48 hr at room temperature Do *not* refrigerate	Not fully evaluated for use in pregnancy Decrease dose in renal failure Inhibits hepatic microsomal oxidation (metabolism) and may prolong the action of concurrently administered medications, particularly in the elderly Causes prolonged prothrombin time if used with warfarin	Observe for gynecomastia, constipation, diarrhea, mental confusion, muscle and joint pain Observe for cardiac dysrhythmias with renal failure
Metoclopramide Cerucal Maxeran Maxolon Primperan Reglan	Reflux esophagitis, nausea (indication *not* FDA approved)	*Adults:* 10 mg PO t.i.d. 30 min before meals and q.h.s.	Tablet: 10 mg Injectable: 5 mg/ml Syrup: 5 mg/5 ml Protect from light	*Contraindicated* in mechanical obstruction of the GI tract, GI hemorrhage, hypersensitivity, and pheochromocytoma May cause nausea, drowsiness, or extrapyramidal symptoms	Observe for constipation, diarrhea, drowsiness, extrapyramidal signs

Continued.

NURSING DRUG DIGEST—cont'd

Medication (trade name)	Indication	Usual dosage and administration	Dosage forms, preparation, and storage	Contraindications, cautions, and comments	Monitoring
Ranitidine Zantac	Duodenal ulcer, benign gastric ulcer, reflux esophagitis	*Adults:* 150 mg PO b.i.d. AM and h.s. Maintenance: 150 mg PO q.h.s. Decrease dosage (up to 50%) in severe renal impairment	Tablet: 150 mg	Rapidly absorbed after oral administration with approximately 50% bioavailability of an oral dose Primarily eliminated via the kidneys Appears to be more effective and possesses significantly fewer side effects than the other available H_2 blocker, cimetidine Use may mask symptoms of gastric carcinoma Use in children or pregnant or breastfeeding mothers has not yet been fully evaluated	Because experience with this drug is limited, carefully monitor for therapeutic and for any untoward effects
Simethicone DiGel* Flacid* Gax-X Gelusil* Gelusil II* Gelusil M* Laxsil* Maalox Plus* Mylanta II* Mylanta-2 Extra Strength* Mylico Phazyme* Phazyme-PB* Phazyme-9S* Riopan Plus* Sidonna* Silain-Gel* Simeco* Tri-Cone*	Flatulence	*Adults:* 40-100 mg q.i.d. after meals and q.h.s. *Children:* Over 12 years of age, same as adult dose Tablets should be chewed thoroughly	Tablet: 40, 80 mg Drops: 40 mg/0.6 ml Shake drops well before use	Effectiveness is questionable	Monitor for effect

Drug	Use	Dosage/Preparation	Side effects	Nursing implications
Sucralfate Carafate	Duodenal ulcers (short-term therapy)	Adults: 1 gm PO q.i.d. 1 hr before meals and at bedtime for 4-8 weeks NOTE: When indicated, antacids should be administered ½ hr before or after sucralfate; they should not be coadministered	Tablet: 1 gm	Toxicity is reportedly minimal	Monitor for effect
DIGESTANTS **Pancreatic enzymes** Digestalin* Dizyme* Donnazyme* Elzyme 303 Enzypan* Kanolase* Panteric Viakase Zypan*	Pancreatic insufficiency	Adults and children: 1-5 dosage units with meals or snacks; if necessary may be increased to hourly doses if not prevented by nausea or diarrhea In cystic fibrosis dose will depend on the degree of enzyme deficiency and food (fat) intake; thus, dosage will need to be individualized according to patient response Pancreatin should be administered in enteric-coated tablets or capsules (which the patient should be instructed to swallow whole to prevent destruction in the stomach)	Tablets, capsules, granules, powder (available in a wide variety of combination strengths)	*Contraindicated* in hypersensitivity May cause GI distress	Observe for buccal and perianal soreness in children Observe for allergies such as nausea and rash
Pancrelipase Accelerase Cotazym Cotazyme Digestive Enzyme-PXP* Ilozyme Pancrease	Pancreatic insufficiency	Adults and children: 1-5 dosage units with meals or snacks; if necessary may be increased to hourly doses if not prevented by nausea or diarrhea In cystic fibrosis dose will depend on the degree of enzyme deficiency and food (fat) intake; thus, dosage will need to be individualized according to patient response	Tablets, capsules, granules, powder (available in a wide variety of combination strengths)	*Contraindicated* in hypersensitivity May cause GI distress	Observe for buccal and perianal soreness in children Observe for allergies such as nausea and rash

Continued.

NURSING DRUG DIGEST—cont'd

Medication (trade name)	Indication	Usual dosage and administration	Dosage forms, preparation, and storage	Contraindications, cautions, and comments	Monitoring
Glutamic acid hydrochloride Acidogen Acidoride Acidulin Antalka Cerebro-Nicin* Dizyme* Glukor injection* Gutan hydrochloride Hydrionic Kanulase* Magacin* Muriamic Muripsin*	Hypochlorhydria	*Adults:* 300-1000 mg PO t.i.d. before meals	Capsule: 340 mg Tablet: 325 mg	Effectiveness or necessity is questionable 340 mg of glutamic acid hydrochloride provides approximately 1.8 mEq of HCl	

BIBLIOGRAPHY

Austad, W.I. Pancreatitis: The use of pancreatic supplements. *Drugs*, 1979, *17*, 480-487.

Banarer, M., & Ritschel, W.A. Antacid suspensions. A dilemma between acid neutralizing capacity and palatability. *Continuing Pharmacy Practice*, 1982, *5*, 246-249.

Bernstein, J.E., & Kasich, A.M. A double-blind trial of simethicone in functional disease of the upper gastrointestinal tract. *Journal of Clinical Pharmacology*, 1974, *14*, 617-623.

Binder, H.J., Cocco, A., Crossley, R.J., Finkelsteing, W., Font, R., Freidman, G., Droarke, J., Hughes, W., Johnson, A.F., McGuigan, J.E., Summers, R., Vlahcenic, R., Wilson, E.C., & Winship, D.H. Cimetidine in treatment of duodenal ulcer: A multicenter double blind study. *Gastroenterology*, 1978, *74*, 380-388.

Black, J.W., Duncan, W.A.M., Durant, C.J., Ganellin, C.R., & Parsons, E.M. Definition and antagonism of histamine H_2-receptors. *Nature*, 1972, *236*, 385-390.

Butler, M.L., & Gersh, H. Antacid vs placebo in hospitalized gastric ulcer patients: A controlled therapeutic study. *American Journal of Digestive Disease*, 1975, *20*, 803-807.

Cohen, J., Weitman, A.P., Dargie, H.J., & Krikler, D.M. Life threatening arrhythmias and intravenous cimetidine. *British Medical Journal*, 1979, *2*(6193), 768.

Cooke, A.R. The role of the mucosal barrier in drug-induced gastric ulceration and erosions. *American Journal of Digestive Disease*, 1976, *21*, 155-164.

Curtailing a life-threatening crisis—G.I. bleeding. *Nursing 81*, 1981, *11*(4), 71-73.

Davies, W.A. & Reed, P.I. A controlled trial of duogastrone in duodenal ulcer. *Gut*, 1977, *18*, 78-83.

Fox, S., & Behar, J. Control of lower esophageal sphincter pressure and acid reflux. *Clinical Gastroenterology*, 1979, *8*, 37-52.

Green, F.W. Jr., Norton, R.A., & Kaplan, M.M. Pharmacology and clinical use of antacids. *American Journal of Hospital Pharmacy*, 1975, *32*, 425-429.

Piper, D.W., & Kang, J. Which antacid? *Drugs*, 1979, *17*, 124-128.

Hastings, P.R., Skillman, J.J., Bushnell, L.S., & Silen, W. Antacid titration in the prevention of acute gastrointestinal bleeding. *New England Journal of Medicine*, 1978, *298*, 1041-1045.

How innocuous is the white medicine? *British Medical Journal*, 1975, *2*, 405-406.

Ippoliti, A.F., Sturdevant, R.A.L., Isenberg, J.I., Binder, M., Camacho, R., Cano, R., Cooney, C., Kline, M.M., Koretz, R.L., Meyer, J.H., Samloff, I.M., Schwabe, A.D., Strom, E.A., Valenzuila, J.E., & Wintroub, R.H. Cimetidine vs intensive antacid therapy for duodenal ulcer. *Gastroenterology*, 1978, *74*, 393-395.

Isenberg, J.I. Therapy of peptic ulcer. *Journal of the American Medical Association*, 1975, *233*, 540-542.

Ivey, K.J. Anticholinergics: Do they work in peptic ulcer? *Gastroenterology*, 1975, *68*, 154-166.

Kruss, D.M., & Littman, A. Safety of cimetidine. *Gastroenterology*, 1978, *74*, 478-483.

Leny, G., Lampman, T., Kamath, B.L., & Garrettson, K.L. Decreased serum salicylate concentrations in children with rheumatic fever treated with antacids. *New England Journal of Medicine*, 1975, *293*, 323-325.

MacDougall, D.R.B., Bailey, R.J., & Williams, R. H_2-Receptor antagonists and antacids in the prevention of acute gastrointestinal hemorrhage in fulminant hepatic failure: Two controlled trials. *Lancet*, 1977, *i*, 617-619.

Mar, D.D. Antacid therapy. *American Journal of Nursing*, 1981, *81*(4), 788-789.

Nagy, G.S. Evaluation of carbenoxolone sodium in the treatment of duodenal ulcer. *Gastroenterology*, 1978, *74*, 7-10.

Peterson, W.L., Sturdeuant, R.A.L., Frankl, H.D., Richardson, C.T., Isenberg, J.I., Elashoff, J.D., Jones, J.Q., Gross, R.A., McCallum, R.W., & Fordtran, J.S. Healing of duodenal ulcers with an antacid regimen. *New England Journal of Medicine*, 1977, *297*, 341-345.

Petlin, A.M., & Carolan, J.M. How to stop a GI bleed. *RN*, April, 1981, 43-49.

Selekman, J. Cystic fibrosis: What is involved in the home treatment program for these children, adolescents, and young adults. *Pediatric Nursing*, 1977, *3*, 32-35.

Shwachman, H., & Grand, R.J. Cystic fibrosis. In M.H. Sleisenger & J.S. Fordtran (Eds.). *Gastrointestinal disease—pathophysiology, diagnosis, management*. Philadelphia: W.B. Saunders, 1978.

Sturdevant, R.A.L. Epidemiology of peptic ulcer—report of a conference. *American Journal of Epidemiology*, 1976, *104*, 9-14.

Zeldis, J.B., Friedman, L.S., & Isselbacher, K.J. Ranitidine: a new H_2-receptor antagonist. *New England Journal of Medicine*, 1983, *309*, 1368-1373.

Emetics and Antiemetics

Walter W. Yakimets

Medications discussed in this chapter

Antiemetics/antimotion sickness
Anticholinergic
  Scopolamine
Antiemetics, miscellaneous
  Benzquinamide
  Dephenidol
  Domperidone
  Metoclopramide
  Nabilone
  Tetrahydrocannabinol
  Trimethobenzamide
Antihistaminics
  Buclizine
  Cyclizine
  Diphenhydramine
  Dimenhydrinate
  Hydroxyzine

Antihistaminics—cont'd
  Meclizine
Antipsychotic tranquilizers
  Chlorpromazine
  Droperidol
  Haloperidol
  Perphenazine
  Prochlorperazine
  Promethazine
  Thiethylperazine
  Triflupromazine
Central nervous system stimulants
  Dextroamphetamine
  Ephedrine
Emetics
  Apomorphine
  Ipecac syrup

Emetics are drugs that induce vomiting and are usually used in the treatment of poisoning and of drug overdose. Antiemetics are medications that are used to inhibit nausea or vomiting. The central theme to both of these compounds is vomiting.

VOMITING (EMESIS)

Vomiting is an unpleasant act during which gastric contents are forcibly ejected through the esophagus and out of the mouth. Vomiting is usually preceded by nausea and retching.

Emesis, at least in part, is a protective mechanism whereby a variety of compounds, including poisons and drugs that may cause the body harm, are spontaneously evacuated from the stomach. However, it is difficult to perceive a protective function for the nausea and vomiting associated with such conditions as motion sickness, pregnancy, testicular trauma, and migraine headaches.

Vomiting is under the control of the vomiting center located in the medulla (Figure 40-1). The vomiting center may be stimulated by impulses from the gastrointestinal tract. These impulses may occur with distention mediated by the vagus and sympathetic nerves and by impulses from the *vestibular apparatus* (which occur in motion sickness). In addition, the vomiting center may be stimulated by impulses from the chemoreceptor trigger zone (CTZ) also located in the medulla. The CTZ is activated by chemicals and drugs such as anesthetic agents, apomorphine, digoxin, ipecac, and by such diverse events as pregnancy, radiation, and uremia. In experimental animals, if the vomiting center is removed, no emesis occurs when drugs that act on the CTZ are administered. In other words, the CTZ cannot induce vomiting without the vomiting center. Some drugs, such as ipecac, act on both centers by stimulating the CTZ directly and by irritating the gastric mucosa, thus stimulating the vomiting center (mediated by vagus and sympathetic nerves).

The causes of vomiting are summarized in the boxed material, p. 855.

The treatment of vomiting consists of dealing with the underlying cause where possible (e.g., surgery for intestinal obstruction). However, in some cases such as motion sickness or radiation therapy, the treatment may have to be symptomatic, and in certain cases such as poisoning, vomiting may be induced purposely to remove the remaining toxic material from the stomach.

EMETICS

Emetics are drugs that induce vomiting. These drugs are rarely used except in the treatment of poisoning or drug overdose. Two of the effective emetics commonly used are syrup of ipecac and apomorphine. Both of these compounds induce vomiting by acting centrally. Ipecac also has a local gastric irritant effect.

Survival in poisoning and in drug overdose depends on the toxicity of the agents ingested, the amount

854

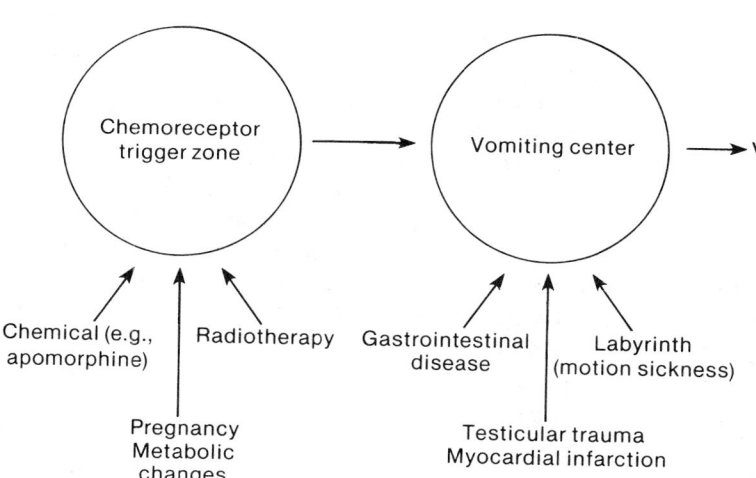

FIGURE 40-1. **Causes of vomiting.**

taken, and the time lapse (absorption time) between ingestion and therapy. This critical information must be acquired in the history, if possible. Furthermore, the patient's condition must be quickly evaluated to determine if immediate vital support of any organ system is necessary.

The mainstays of poisoning or overdose therapy include the following:

1. Urgent vital support of any organ system failure.
2. Removal of as much of the ingested poisons as possible, depending on the material ingested, by inducing emesis or *gastric lavage* (see 5).
3. The prevention of further absorption of poisons, depending on material ingested, by using an adsorbent such as activated charcoal and specific antidotes. *Universal antidote* is *not* advised because certain compounds neutralize each other, and also there is little evidence that it is effective.
4. The increase of excretion of toxins by use of laxatives (rarely effective except with certain poisons) and diuretics (e.g., use of diuretic plus alkalinizing agent to increase excretion of aspirin).
5. Avoidance of further harm (e.g., do not give emetics to patients who have taken corrosive agents).

If the patient's condition permits and time lapse is not more than 2 to 4 hours (or longer with agents that decrease gastric emptying such as aspirin and *anticholinergics*), stomach contents should be emptied. Emetics are more effective than lavage in clearing the stomach. Mechanically induced vomiting is not as effective as vomiting induced by ipecac. Because of side effects of apomorphine, mainly central nervous system depression, ipecac is the preferred emetic for children. Emetics should not be used if the patient is unconscious or has an inadequate *gag reflex* because of the high risk of *aspiration*. In the comatose patient, lavage

---

Causes of vomiting

I. Causes that stimulate vomiting center
   A. Motion sickness
   B. Gastrointestinal diseases such as intestinal obstruction, acute cholecystitis, appendicitis, and *dumping syndrome*
   C. Migraine headache
   D. Labyrinth disorders such as *Ménière's disease*
   E. Increased intracranial pressure as may occur with tumors, trauma, or anoxia
   F. Testicular trauma
   G. Pharyngeal stimulation
   H. *Psychogenic*
   I. Visceral disease such as myocardial infarction and pancreatitis
   J. Cardiac diseases such as inferior wall infarctions
II. Causes that stimulate chemoreceptor trigger zone
   A. Drugs such as anesthetics, anticancer agents, apomorphine, digitalis, and ipecac
   B. Chemicals such as intravenous copper sulfate
   C. Metabolic diseases such as diabetic ketosis and uremia
   D. Pregnancy
   E. Radiotherapy

can be used after the patient has been intubated to prevent aspiration. Emetics should also be avoided where acids or alkalis have been ingested because the return of the offending agent can cause further trauma to the esophagus and pharynx.

Syrup of ipecac

Syrup of ipecac, an oral emetic, is probably the agent of choice in inducing emesis in patients who have ingested poisons or taken an overdose of drugs. It can be used at home or in the hospital. Ipecac induces vomiting by acting centrally on the CTZ and peripherally (reflex) by irritating the gastric mucosa.

Manoguerra and Krenzelok (1978) studied 250 patients treated for overdose or poisoning and showed that ipecac syrup induced emesis in 16.4 minutes (average) in the 81% of patients that vomited after the first dose and in 24.2 minutes (average) in the 96% of patients who had either one or two doses. Ipecac failed to induce vomiting in 3% of their patients, and it was not used in 1% of patients because of side effects resulting from ingested compounds. Similar success rates to induce emesis by ipecac and in similar times have been reported by others. Because children under 1 year of age may have an inadequate gag reflex, ipecac should be used with caution and under medical supervision only.

The dose of syrup of ipecac for children less than 1 year of age is 5 to 10 ml followed by 200 ml of water. This dose may be repeated once after 20 minutes if necessary.

The dose of syrup of ipecac for children 1 to 5 years of age is 15 ml. In children over 5 and in adults the dose given is 30 ml. Since ipecac does not work well on an empty stomach, children 1 to 5 years of age should be given 240 ml of water, and older children and adults should take 360 ml of water. If the first dose is ineffective in 20 minutes, a second dose of 15 ml may be given.

In therapeutic doses the side effects of ipecac are minimal but may include diarrhea and drowsiness. In larger doses side effects may include bradycardia, atrial fibrillation, and hypotension. Deaths have been reported with the ipecac fluid extract, which is 14 times more potent than an equivalent dose of syrup of ipecac.

Ipecac is contraindicated in patients who are comatose, having seizures, in shock, pregnant or who have ingested petroleum distillates, such as gasoline, because of the risk of aspiration of gastric contents and resultant aspiration pneumonitis. Patients who have ingested corrosives, including lye, should not be given an emetic because vomiting of the irritant liquid may further damage the esophagus.

Apomorphine

Apomorphine is a morphine derivative. Its chief use is to induce vomiting in patients who have ingested poisons or taken a drug overdose. Apomorphine acts centrally by stimulating the chemoreceptor trigger zone, which in turn acts on the vomiting center. It induces vomiting promptly (within 10 to 15 minutes) and is almost 100% effective. Oral apomorphine is not a reliable emetic agent, and consequently the drug must be given parenterally. Its use is therefore restricted to hospitals.

The adult dose is 0.1 mg/kg subcutaneously, or alternatively 5 mg as a single dose subcutaneously. If the initial dose is ineffective in inducing vomiting, a second dose should *not* be given. After apomorphine-induced emesis has occured, the patient usually falls into a deep sleep because the drug causes central nervous system depression.

Apomorphine should be given with caution to children, the debilitated, and the inebriant (because of the risks of aspiration), and to those patients with heart disease. Side effects include central nervous system depression, muscle weakness, an irregular and a rapid pulse, decreased blood pressure, and nausea, salivation, and vomiting. Overdosage with apomorphine (and occasionally with therapeutic doses) may cause circulatory and respiratory collapse, coma, and death. The antidote for apomorphine overdosage is the narcotic antagonist, naloxone. For excessive vomiting resulting from apomorphine, chlorpromazine 25 to 50 mg IM may be given.

Apomorphine is contraindicated for patients with central nervous system and respiratory depression because it can exacerbate these effects, and for patients who have ingested corrosive poisons, because vomiting causes further injury to the esophagus.

ANTIEMETICS

Drugs used to inhibit nausea and vomiting are called antiemetics. However, these drugs are not equally effective in all causes of emesis. The causes may be grouped into three broad catagories: (1) motion sickness, (2) chemically induced emesis, and (3) reflexly induced emesis. With the exception of motion sickness, antiemetics, generally, should not be given to children because they may mask symptoms of disease. Similarly, in adults antiemetics should not be used for reflex vomiting, intestinal obstruction, or appendicitis, because the treatment of the emesis, in these cases, is the treatment of the primary problem.

Antiemetics are much more effective if given prophylactically before the nausea and vomiting have started.

Motion sickness

Motion sickness may be induced by any prolonged and vigorous motion. It might occur during land, sea, or air travel or during amusement rides. Some people, especially some children, are more susceptible to motion sickness than others. Motion sickness appears to be a central nervous system response and requires a functional vestibular apparatus (labyrinth). Deaf subjects who have vestibular defects are immune to nausea and vomiting caused by motion sickness. The mechanism by which nausea and vomiting are induced in abnormal motion appears to be stimuli from the vestibular apparatus (labyrinth) acting directly on the vomiting center.

Anticholinergics, antihistaminics, including phenothiazines with antihistaminic properties (e.g., promethazine), and CNS stimulants are drugs that can be used effectively against motion sickness. Anticholinergics and antihistaminics appear to work because of their strong central nervous system anticholinergic effects, and amphetamines appear to work because they activate noradrenalin activity centrally. The action of these drugs appears to be in relationship to the vestibular area. However, the precise mechanism by which anticholinergics and noradrenalin inhibit motion sickness and vomiting is unknown. Amphetamines may be used alone or in combination with anticholinergics and antihistaminics, but the use of amphetamines is limited to certain refractory cases because of their abuse potential.

Antimotion-sickness medications are more effective if given prophylactically.

Anticholinergics. Anticholinergic drugs block parasympathetic nerve transmission by inhibiting acetylcholine at postganglionic receptor sites. However, the exact mechanism of action of anticholinergics in inhibiting the nausea and vomiting of motion sickness is unknown. Their side effects include visual disturbances (i.e., blurred vision), urinary retention, drowsiness, and a dry mouth.

Scopolamine. Scopolamine is an anticholinergic drug that is effective for motion sickness. Its action may be on the cortex or more peripherally on the vestibular apparatus. The exact mechanism of action in unknown. Its use is somewhat limited by its short duration of action and by its side effects.

The usual adult dose for the prevention of motion sickness is one to two 0.3 mg tablets 1 hour before traveling. Its duration of action is about 4 hours, and Wood (1979) recommends its use for short periods of intense motion for susceptible people. If necessary 1 tablet may be given 6 hours after the initial dose and repeated each 6 hours for a maximum of 48 hours. A transdermal delivery system enables dosing once every 3 days. Use of this system merely requires the placement of a small patch behind the ear, calibrated to release 0.5 mg/24 hr to be absorbed through the skin. Toxic side effects include visual disturbances, dry mouth, and drowsiness. Because of its side effects, including agitation, it should be given with caution or not at all to children.

CNS stimulants. Amphetamines appear to inhibit the nausea and vomiting of motion sickness by activating noradrenalin centrally. The exact mechanism of action is unknown. Amphetamines should *not* be widely used because of addiction potential and because safer medications are available.

Dextroamphetamine. This drug, although effective against motion sickness, probably should *not* be used for this purpose because of its addiction potential. The same comment applies to any antiemetic amphetamine combination. Side effects include restlessness, increased blood pressure, and anxiety (see Chapter 20, "Antiparkinsonian Medications and Stimulants").

Ephedrine. Ephedrine, too, is an antimotion-sickness drug but is somewhat less effective than dextroamphetamine. Because of its effect of stimulating the central nervous system, its use for the treatment of motion sickness is *not* recommended.

Antihistamines. Many antihistamines have some antiemetic properties; however, there is *not* a direct correlation between antihistaminic potency and antimotion-sickness effect.

Promethazine. This drug, a phenothiazine with predominant antihistaminic properties, has a potent antimotion-sickness effect. Its mechanism of action, like that of scopolamine, is believed to be the result of its strong central anticholinergic effect, but the exact site of activity and the exact mechanism are unknown. It is also effective against chemically induced nausea and vomiting.

The usual adult dose is 25 mg by mouth ½ hour before traveling, and repeated at 8 hour intervals as necessary. The main side effect is drowsiness. This side effect may be useful especially in children. In children promethazine may be given in divided doses every 12 hours as follows: 5 mg per day for those less than 1 year, 5 to 10 mg per day for those between 1 and 5 years, and 10 to 15 mg per day for those 6 to 10 years of age.

Phenothiazines may increase the effects of central nervous system depressants, such as alcohol, narcotics, tranquilizers, and sedatives. Phenothiazines should be given with caution to patients with liver disease because the liver is the site of metabolism of these agents. Since sedation may occur with these drugs, they should be given with caution to people who drive or work with machinery.

Meclizine. Meclizine appears to be an effective antimotion-sickness medication, and its effect appears to result from depression of labyrinth responsiveness. It is a relatively safe medication and is available over the counter. Meclizine is a long-acting preparation with the duration of action being 12 to 24 hours.

The usual adult dosage is 25 to 50 mg once a day administered 1 hour before traveling. It should not be given to children under the age of 12. Side effects include drowsiness; therefore meclizine should *not* be used by car drivers and operators of machinery. It should not be used in combination with alcohol or tranquilizers, because of the potentiation of CNS depression. Patients with glaucoma should not use meclizine because it makes their condition worse, and *pregnant* women should avoid the drug because of the possibility of fetal abnormalities.

Cyclizine. This antihistaminic, antimotion-sickness preparation also depresses labyrinth responsiveness. It is a fairly safe over-the-counter preparation. The duration of action is 4 to 6 hours.

The usual adult dose is 50 mg orally 30 minutes before traveling and repeated once every 6 hours as necessary. The dose for children (6 to 12 years) is 25 mg by mouth 30 minutes before traveling, repeated every 8 hours as necessary. The main side effect is drowsiness; therefore this medication should be used with caution by machine operators. The drug increases the depressant effect of alcohol and tranquilizers on the central nervous system. Glaucoma patients should not use cyclizine because the drug makes the condition worse. Pregnant women should avoid it because of the possibility of fetal abnormalities.

Dimenhydrinate. Dimenhydrinate is used mainly as an effective antimotion-sickness preparation but also has been used in postoperative vomiting, drug-induced vomiting, and radiation sickness. Its duration of action is 4 to 6 hours.

The usual adult dose is 50 mg every 6 hours as necessary, starting 30 minutes before traveling. The main side effect is drowsiness, and it should be used with caution by machine operators. Anticholinergic side effects may include visual disturbances, dry mouth, and urinary retention. Dimenhydrinate should not be given to patients with glaucoma and prostatism because of possible aggravation of these conditions.

Chemically induced nausea and vomiting

Chemically induced nausea and vomiting may accompany a drug therapy that includes anticancer drugs or anesthetic agents; it may occur with radiotherapy, pregnancy, myocardial infarction, endocrine and metabolic disorders, or with the ingestion of toxic agents. The mechanism of action appears to be the stimulation of the chemoreceptor trigger zone, which in turn stimulates the vomiting center. Phenothiazines are effective in therapy for chemically induced nausea and vomiting, and their action appears to have an inhibitory effect on the CTZ.

Phenothiazines. All members of this group are effective against chemically induced nausea and emesis and, therefore, choice of an agent should take into consideration the minimization of side effects. Phenothiazines exert a direct depressant effect on the CTZ and appear to have some direct effect on the vomiting center.

Phenothiazines are useful in emetic problems related to surgery, radiation therapy, poisoning, and endocrine and metabolic disorders. Their usefulness is less marked in prevention of nausea and vomiting resulting from cytotoxic drugs. Care must be taken in treating nausea and vomiting resulting from drugs such as digitalis because the antiemetics may mask the warning of earlier stages of the toxic problems. In the case of digitalis, an overdose can lead to possible fatal dysrhythmias. Phenothiazines should be given with caution to patients with liver disease because their metabolism may be impaired, and they may further damage an already compromised liver. Phenothiazines may intensify the effects of central nervous system depressants, such as alcohol, opiates, and hypnotics.

Prochlorperazine. This drug is a powerful antiemetic of the phenothiazine group. It is useful in chemically induced emesis, including that caused by opiates, poisoning, and surgery. It can also be given preoperatively to prophylactically control postoperative nausea and vomiting.

The adult dose is 5 to 10 gm, in oral or intramuscular form, every 4 to 6 hours as necessary. Suppositories are in 25 mg size and are given once or twice daily. Oral prochlorperazine may be absorbed slowly because little effect can be detected in 1 hour. However, it appears to be more effective if given 2 hours before traveling.

Doses of prochlorperazine (in base equivalent), syrup, tablet, or suppository, for children are the following: 2.5 mg up to twice daily for those 1 to 5 years of age, 5 mg two or three times daily for those 6 to 12 years of age, 5 mg three to four times daily for those 12 to 16 years of age.

Side effects include extrapyramidal symptoms, which occur more commonly with use of prochlorperazine than with chlorpromazine. However, hypotension and drowsiness are less marked than with chlorpromazine. In children, especially the sick, severe dystonic reactions may occur.

Promethazine. This drug, a phenothiazine with antihistaminic properties, has a potent effect against both motion sickness and chemically induced emesis. The mechanism of action is believed to result from its strong central anticholinergic effect, but the exact site of activity and the exact mechanism are unknown.

The usual adult dose is 25 mg every 8 hours as necessary. The main side effect is drowsiness, which may be useful in children (especially when they are traveling). Promethazine may be given to children in divided doses every 12 hours as follows: 5 mg per day for those less than 1 year, 5 to 10 mg per day for those between 1 and 5 years, and 10 to 15 mg per day for those 6 to 10 years of age.

Phenothiazines may intensify the effects of central nervous system depressants, such as alcohol, narcotics, tranquilizers, and sedatives. They should be given with caution to patients with liver disease because the liver is the site of metabolism of these agents. Since sedation may occur, these drugs should be given with caution to people who drive or who work with machinery.

Triflupromazine. This phenothiazine is effective against chemically induced nausea and vomiting. Like other phenothiazines, triflupromazine is also an antipsychotic drug and may be used for surgical premedication.

The adult dose is a 10 mg tablet two or three times a day. Intramuscularly 5 to 15 mg may be given every 4 hours up to 60 mg per day. Side effects include *extrapyramidal dysfunction* and sedation. These effects are greater with trifluopromazine than with chlorpromazine.

Chlorpromazine. Chlorpromazine has a potent effect on chemically induced nausea and vomiting. It tends to be less popular than the other phenothiazines because of a somewhat higher incidence of side effects, such as sedation, dry mouth, dizziness, and postural hypotension. Prolonged use may cause cholestatic jaundice. Like other phenothiazines it may increase the effects of central nervous system depressants, such as alcohol, sedative-hypnotics, and narcotics. In addition to its antiemetic properties, it is useful in treatment of intractable hiccups. The mechanism by which chlorpromazine may control hiccups is unknown.

The usual adult antiemetic dose is 25 to 50 mg by mouth or intramuscularly three to four times daily. For children over 5 years of age, one-third to one-half the adult dose is given, and for children under 5 years of age the dose is 0.5 to 1.0 mg/kg four times daily. People on this drug should be cautioned about driving or operating dangerous machinery.

Thiethylperazine. This is a potent phenothiazine antiemetic.

Adult dosage is 10 mg orally, rectally, or intramuscularly every 8 to 12 hours as necessary.

Side effects are similar to those of chlorpromazine and include drowsiness. Extrapyramidal effects may occur especially in children and women under 30 years of age.

Perphenazine. Perphenazine, a phenothiazine derivative, is an effective antiemetic agent. It tends to be of value in the prevention or treatment of nausea and vomiting caused by the stimulation of the CTZ.

The usual adult dose for prevention of postoperative nausea and vomiting is 8 mg by mouth or 5 mg intramuscularly before induction of anesthesia. For control of nausea and vomiting the average adult dose is 4 mg by mouth or intramuscularly every 8 hours. This medication probably should not be currently given to children until further studies are performed.

Side effects of perphenazine include extrapyramidal symptoms and sedation. Perphenazine should not be used during pregnancy until further studies on its safety are carried out. It should not be given to patients with liver disease or blood dyscrasias, or to those with central nervous system depression. Perphenazine should not be used by patients driving vehicles or working with machinery.

Miscellaneous agents

Metoclopramide. Metoclopramide, a procaine derivative, has a powerful antiemetic effect. It acts on the chemoreceptor trigger zone, but the exact mechanism of action is unknown. In addition, its antiemetic effect may be enhanced by its ability to increase gastric emptying (increases gastric motility and relaxes the *pylorus*). Metoclopramide is an effective emetic with an antiemetic activity similar to the phenothiazines. It is useful for chemically induced emesis but not for motion sickness. It may be given at the end of an operative procedure to reduce narcotic-induced vomiting.

The adult dosage is 10 mg orally, intramuscularly, or intravenously three to four times a day. Side effects are minimal and may include drowsiness, change of bowel habit (i.e., usually diarrhea but occasionally constipation), and extrapyramidal effects (i.e., restlessness, dystonia, and rigidity). Metoclopramide may intensify the extrapyramidal effects of phenothiazine. Its actions may be decreased by anticholinergics such as atropine. The effects of metoclopramide on the fetus are not fully evaluated as yet. Toxicity seems to occur more commonly in the elderly.

Domperidone. Domperidone, a neuroleptic drug, is currently being evaluated for its antiemetic properties. Early reports are encouraging. Domperidone is a potent peripheral dopamine-blocker devoid of central nervous system activity. Side effects appear to be minimal.

Tetrahydrocannabinol (THC). THC has antiemetic properties that are being investigated at the present time. It seems to be effective in the treatment of nausea and vomiting caused by anticancer drugs, which are resistant to the usual emetics. It must be considered an experimental antiemetic agent at present, but some reports are encouraging.

Trimethobenzamide. Trimethobenzamide, a drug with weak antihistaminic properties, has been used for nausea and vomiting associated with radiation therapy, pregnancy, and Ménière's disease. It is of little value in nausea and vomiting of motion sickness.

The usual adult dose is 100 to 250 mg every 6 to 8 hours by mouth or intramuscularly. The side effects are the same as those for antihistamines.

Haloperidol. Haloperidol, a butyrophenone with clinical effects similar to phenothiazines, is a potent antiemetic, whose action may last up to 24 hours. It may be useful to prevent postoperative nausea and vomiting in the adult with a dose of 1 mg given intramuscularly before induction of anesthesia. Side effects and precautions are similar to those of chlorpromazine, but haloperidol may be given to those patients who are sensitive to the phenothiazines.

Diphenidol. Diphenidol, a drug with antiemetic properties against CTZ or vestibular apparatus stimulation, has significant side effects (e.g., auditory and visual hallucinations, confusion, disorientation). There is little evidence that it is superior to phenothiazines, and its use should, therefore, be limited.

Reflexly induced nausea and vomiting

Nausea and vomiting can occur with the stimulation of the pharynx, myocardial infarction, distention and traction of hollow viscera of the abdomen, testicular trauma, increased intracranial pressure, inflammation of abdominal viscera (such as the pancreas), peritonitis, and chemical irritation of the stomach (such as occurs with the ingestion of copper sulfate). Emesis induced by these means seems to be of a reflex nature. The afferent pathways are the vagal and parasympathetic nerves. The stimuli listed that cause emesis seem to act on the vasomotor center. Vomiting of a reflex nature may be helped by the phenothiazine group of antiemetics, but it must be emphasized that with few exceptions the primary treatment of reflex vomiting is to deal with the primary disease (e.g., treat acute appendicitis). In practice, one would *not* use phenothiazines in the treatment of emesis caused by an acute abdomen for fear of masking important signs and symptoms.

Vomiting during pregnancy. Nausea and vomiting in the first trimester of pregnancy are common and although unpleasant rarely cause serious problems.

The exact cause of vomiting in early pregnancy is unknown, but it appears to parallel the levels of human chorionic gonadotrophin. The mechanism appears to be through stimulation of the CTZ. Vomiting during pregnancy tends to be aggravated by lack of rest and psychologic stress. Often no therapy is required. In more protracted and severe cases improvement follows adequate rest and fairly constant food intake. If vomiting is uncontrolled by conservative measures, dimenhydrinate (previously described in this chapter) is a useful and fairly safe drug.

Vomiting during early pregnancy, in a small number of patients, may be severe (hyperemesis gravidarum) and may lead to dehydration, weight loss, and ketosis. Treatment of hyperemesis gravidarum is hospitalization, intravenous fluid therapy, sedation, and possible parenteral antiemetics, such as dimenhydrinate.

In late pregnancy vomiting may be associated with liver disease or preeclampsia. Both of these conditions may be serious and require prompt therapy.

Vomiting in pregnancy may also be the result of problems that can affect the nonpregnant patient, such as appendicitis and bowel obstruction. Any serious vomiting in pregnancy associated with abdominal pain must be fully evaluated.

Psychologic components. Vomiting, including severe vomiting, may be caused by psychologic disturbances. Psychologic vomiting may occur spontaneously or may be self-induced by the use of fingers, by overeating, or by taking various chemical compounds. The mechanism of spontaneous psychogenic vomiting such as occurs in anorexia nervosa is unknown. The mechanism of self-induced vomiting is more obvious, although the psychologic reasons for such vomiting are more difficult to understand. The treatment of psychogenic vomiting is psychologic counseling.

SUMMARY

Emetics are valuable aids in treating poisoning and drug overdosage. They are more effective in removing gastric contents than lavage. Of the two emetics, ipecac is safer than apomorphine and works nearly as well.

There are basically three different causes of nausea and vomiting. They are motion sickness and chemically and reflexly induced emesis. The basic treatment of reflexly induced emesis is the treatment of the disease. Motion sickness is best treated with an antihistamine. Although antihistamines have side effects, mainly drowsiness, they tend to be safer than scopolamine and amphetamines. The phenothiazines and metoclopramide are effective in treating most of the chemically induced emesis with the exception of the nausea and vomiting caused by anticancer drugs, although they have been used to treat or premedicate for the nausea associated with cisplatin chemother- apy. The specific treatment of the severe nausea and vomiting often associated with cancer chemotherapy is detailed in the Nursing Drug Digest.

ADVERSE/SIDE EFFECTS OF ANTIEMETICS*

ALLERGIC REACTIONS

Contact dermatitis (by personnel handling phenothiazines)
Photosensitivity
Skin rash

AUTONOMIC NERVOUS SYSTEM

Anticholinergic effects (dry mouth, visual disturbances, urinary retention)
Changes in body temperature usually hypothermia
Paralytic ileus

BEHAVIOR

Impaired function because of over- sedation
Uncontrolled restlessness, talkativeness

CARDIOVASCULAR SYSTEM

Dysrhythmias
Bradycardia
Hypotension (may be just postural)

CENTRAL NERVOUS SYSTEM

Drowsiness

HEMATOLOGIC SYSTEM

Agranulocytosis
Anemia (hemolytic)

GASTROINTESTINAL SYSTEM

Constipation
Diarrhea
Nausea
Vomiting

HEPATIC SYSTEM

Cholestatic jaundice

METABOLIC AND ENDOCRINE SYSTEMS

Amenorrhea
Galactorrhea
Gynecomastia
Weight gain

NEUROMUSCULAR (EXTRAPYRAMIDAL) SYSTEM

Akathisia
Dystonia
Muscle weakness
Parkinsonism

OCULAR SYSTEM

Exacerbation of glaucoma

RENAL SYSTEM

Urinary retention

TERATOGENIC EFFECTS

Many of these drugs have not been fully evaulated as to their safety in early pregnancy
Antiemetics should be *contraindicated* in pregnancy

*See Chapter 11, "Drug Toxicity," for an overview of drug toxicity.

CLINICALLY SIGNIFICANT DRUG INTERACTIONS*

Primary drug	*Interacting drug*	*Possible effect(s)*	*Probable mechanism(s)*
Phenothiazines	Alcohol	Drowsiness, lethargy, decreased psychomotor skills, stupor, respiratory collapse, coma, death	Additive or potentiated CNS depression
Phenothiazines	Guanethidine	Decreased guanethidine effect	Block drug uptake at ad- renergic/dopaminergic neuron

*See Chapter 10, "Drug Interactions," for an overview of drug interactions. See also Clinically Significant Drug Interactions in Chapters 18, "Drugs Used to Treat Psychotic Disorders," and 20, "Antiparkinsonian Medications and Stimulants."

Nursing of patients requiring antiemetics

ASSESSMENT

A complete nursing assessment is essential in establishing a baseline from which to plan and individualize antiemetic therapy and to monitor patient response.

Before therapy is initiated, assessment should include a detailed drug history to identify individual sensitivity, possible contraindications to antiemetic therapy, cautions, potential drug interactions, and previous or continuing antiemetic therapy, especially if such therapy is required over a long term.

Assessment data should also include observations and reports of vomiting behavior; associated symptoms, such as abdominal pain or tenderness (record location of pain, intensity, duration, and relation to vomiting if present); and measures used to prevent vomiting. The amount, frequency, appearance, and odor of vomitus, vomiting sensations (salivation, feelings of warmth, headache, nausea, warning or no warning of emesis), and the relationship of vomiting to meals or other factors should be noted.

When vomiting is chronic, prolonged, or persistent (lasting for 24 hours or more), large amounts of fluid and electrolytes can be lost, resulting in severe fluid and electrolyte imbalance. The patient should be assessed for fluid-volume deficit; sodium, potassium, chloride, and magnesium deficits; and metabolic alkalosis, related to the loss of acidic gastric juices containing hydrogen and chloride ions, with bicarbonate being retained to compensate for the lost chloride. The ketosis of starvation may also be present.

Infants, young children, the elderly, and the debilitated are especially prone to fluid and electrolyte deficits related to losses through vomiting. Body weight and serum electrolytes are essential in assessing losses, in monitoring the patient, and in planning nursing care to minimize or prevent possible imbalances. Assessment may also include laboratory analysis of vomitus.

SENSITIVITY

Sensitivity can occur in susceptible individuals, and patients should be monitored for rash or unexpected responses to the medication.

CONTRAINDICATIONS

In the immediate postoperative period antiemetics that may further depress the central nervous system should *not* be used.

CAUTIONS

Antiemetics can obscure signs of underlying pathologic conditions or of overdosage of concomitant drug therapy.

Antiemetics should be administered cautiously to those patients receiving CNS depressants concurrently.

DRUG INTERACTIONS

Antiemetics can potentiate the effects of CNS depressants (see Clinically Significant Drug Interactions).

ADMINISTRATION

Topical medication is indicated for the prevention of motion sickness. Parenteral or suppository forms are indicated in acute vomiting. Oral administration is effective to prevent nausea and vomiting, as well as to control chronic nausea and vomiting.

Suppositories should be inserted gently, and the patient should be informed to avoid having a bowel movement for at least 1 hour so that the medication can be absorbed.

Antiemetics are more effective if taken before nausea and vomiting occur. To enhance the effect of the antiemetic, patients should be encouraged to breathe deeply if nauseated, to limit fluid and food intake, to avoid spicy or fatty foods, and to take small amounts of fluid or food only if tolerated. Some patients may not be allowed to have food or fluid; others may be restricted to clear liquids, a regimen that can be progressed as tolerated.

Other measures that can enhance the effect of the antiemetic should also be implemented. The environment should be well ventilated and cool, and abrupt or undue motion should be avoided. To prevent possible aspiration, patients should be positioned in a semi-Fowler's position with the head elevated on a pillow. An emesis basin should be readily available. Postsurgical patients must be positioned carefully in a side-lying position especially if not fully recovered from anesthesia. If the patient is vomiting, assist him by splinting abdominal wounds or surgical repair sites with a pillow or hands.

After vomiting, patients should be made as comfortable as possible. The vomitus should be removed readily, and soiled garments and linen should be removed and replaced. The amount and character of the vomitus should be noted. Oral care, odor control, control of tension and anxiety, privacy, and reduction of stimuli that may cause vomiting, such as the presence of food—these restrictions and considerations are helpful in controlling nausea and vomiting, thus enhancing the effect of antiemetics.

MONITORING

Therapeutic response

The various classifications of medications used to control nausea and vomiting (antiemetics, antispasmodics, binding agents, and sedatives) act at different times in relation to the route of administration and to individual patient factors. Generally, effect can be noted between 5 and 30 minutes.

Adverse side effects

Drowsiness is a major side effect associated with antiemetics. Patients should be monitored for oversedation, and safety precautions should be implemented as indicated. Aspiration is a major problem associated with vomiting, and patients should be positioned carefully. Ambulation supervision and side rails may be required. Patients should be cautioned against driving or smoking until they know how the medication affects them.

PATIENT EDUCATION

The patient and family should have a clear understanding of the medication regimen, including the exact name of the medication, its action, dosage, storage, administration, and adverse side effects. Patients should know how they will manage these effects. They should also understand how diet, activity, and other measures can be used to enhance the action of their medication and to help control nausea and vomiting. Patients requiring antiemetics for chronic problems with nausea and vomiting often need assistance with maintaining adequate nutrition and bowel elimi-

Nursing of patients requiring antiemetics—cont'd

PATIENT EDUCATION—cont'd

nation. Small frequent meals and the avoidance of foods that tend to slow gastric emptying should be avoided. Hydration and moderate exercise will do much to maintain bowel elimination. Patients requiring antiemetics should be able to identify when their condition indicates that the health care provider should be notified (e.g., persistent vomiting with loss of fluid and electrolytes for more than 24 hours or significant weight loss).

Nursing of patients requiring emetics

ASSESSMENT

A complete nursing assessment is essential in establishing a baseline from which to plan and individualize emetic therapy and monitor patient response because emetics are usually given in cases of poisoning or drug overdose and are contraindicated in certain cases. Before therapy is initiated, assessment should include a specific drug history to identify individual sensitivity to apomorphine or ipecac, what drug or poison was ingested, amount taken, and time lapse between ingestion and treatment. Evaluation of the patient's general condition and vital signs must be done quickly in emergency situations. Emergency equipment should be readily available in case the patient needs respiratory assistance or in case he or she goes into shock or cardiac arrest. The history should also include use of prescription and nonprescription medications, allergies, medical problems, and mental state.

The family and patient require much support and understanding, and measures should be used to prevent undue anxiety and upset, especially in emergency situations. Patient education is better initiated when the patient is stable.

CONTRAINDICATIONS

Although induced vomiting is more effective than gastric lavage, it is contraindicated in patients who are semiconscious, unconscious, comatose, or in sedated states, because of the danger of the aspiration of vomitus resulting from a diminished gag reflex. In addition, emetics are contraindicated in persons who have ingested corrosives because of the potential resultant injury to the esophagus. They are contraindicated in persons who have ingested hydrocarbons because of the possibility of aspiration and lipoid pneumonia. Emetics are also contraindicated in some specific states of poisoning, such as strychnine poisoning, where CNS stimulation can result in convulsions.

CAUTIONS

See administration and monitoring as well as the Nursing Drug Digest.

ADMINISTRATION AND MONITORING

Assess the presence of a gag reflex before administration of emetics.

Ensure administration of the emetic with 100 to 200 ml of water or evaporated milk (milk may delay onset of action) to enhance emetic effect, as well as to decrease the possibility of retching, which can cause gastric or esophageal tears. If the stomach is empty, emesis may not occur.

Walking the patient can also enhance emetic effect. Continuously monitor level of consciousness to prevent possible aspiration.

Vomitus should be assessed in relation to consistency, character, amount, and the presence or absence of ingested material (e.g., tablets). Vomitus should be saved for toxicologic analysis.

Syrup of ipecac

Ensure that the syrup form is administered and *not* the fluid extract, which is 14 times more potent and can result in severe toxicity.

Administer syrup of ipecac by mouth, followed by a glass of water, and monitor for emetic effect, which should occur within 15 to 20 minutes. If vomiting has not occured in 20 minutes, the dose is repeated.

Do not administer more than two doses of syrup of ipecac. Because it is cardiotoxic if absorbed, lavage the stomach to prevent possible cardiotoxic effects if emesis does not occur.

Apomorphine

Apomorphine is administered either subcutaneously or intramuscularly. Only one dose is given. Monitor for emetic effect within 5 minutes. Because it is a narcotic and may cause respiratory depression, its use is contraindicated for patients with respiratory depression. Depressant effects can be countered by the narcotic antagonist, naloxone, as soon as adequate emesis is achieved or in case of accidental overdose.

PATIENT EDUCATION

The patient and family should have a clear understanding of the emergency treatment. Support, empathy, and understanding are essential in situations of overdose as well as accidental ingestion of poisons. Depending on the individual patient, suicide precautions and psychiatric evaluation may be indicated. For childhood poisoning and other poisoning, parent/patient education is aimed at prevention of future poisoning.

The patient and family should do the following:
1. Keep syrup of ipecac in the household in a safe place and be able to describe its use in the event of poisoning.
2. State when syrup of ipecac should *not* be used. Place emergency phone numbers near the telephone.
3. Store household cleaners, gasoline, and medications safely out of the reach of children.
4. Name common plants that can be poisonous, and avoid having these in or around the home.
5. Teach children healthy self-care practices in relation to poison prevention.

GENERAL INSTRUCTIONS FOR DISCHARGE/OUTPATIENTS

ANTIEMETICS

This medication is used to control nausea, vomiting, dizziness and motion sickness.

In some people this drug may cause drowsiness. Do *not* drive a car or operate dangerous machinery or do jobs that require you to be alert until you know how you are going to react to this drug.

Do not drink alcoholic beverages while taking this drug without discussing this with your health care provider.

It is important that you obtain the advise of your health care provider before taking pain relievers, nonprescription drugs, sleeping pills, tranquilizers, or medicine for depression when you are taking this medication.

Most people experience few or no side effects from this drug; however, any medicine can sometimes cause unwanted effects. Notify your health care provider if you develop a skin rash, sore throat, fever, or mouth sores.

If this medicine makes you feel dizzy, be careful going up and down stairs, and change positions slowly. Get out of bed slowly in the morning and dangle your feet over the edge of the bed for a few minutes before standing up. Sit or lie down at the first sign of dizziness.

In addition to the above, if you are taking the following:

Buclizine

These tablets can be taken without water. They can be dissolved in the mouth, chewed, or swallowed whole.

Women who are breast feeding should tell their health care provider before taking this medication.

If your mouth becomes dry, suck on a hard, sugarless candy or ice chips, sip water, or chew sugarless gum. It is important to brush your teeth regularly if you develop a dry mouth.

Chlorpromazine

This medication may make some people more sensitive to sunlight and sun lamps. Avoid getting too much sun and wear protective clothing and sunglasses. A sunscreen may be helpful.

This medication can cause your urine to turn pink, red, or red-brown. This is not unusual, and your urine will return to its normal color when you stop taking this medication.

Be careful not to become overheated or chilled because this medication may make you more sensitive to heat, since it can affect your body's temperature-regulation system.

Take tablets or liquid forms of this medicine with food or with a glass of water. Do not take with antacids or diarrhea medicine. If you must take antacids or diarrhea medicine, take it at least 1 hour before or after taking chlorpromazine.

Store your medicine in a cool dry place, out of the reach of children. Do not get the liquid medication on skin or clothing because a rash can result.

If you have ever had an allergic reaction to a phenothiazine medicine, tell your health care provider before you take any of this medicine.

Women who are pregnant, breast feeding, or planning to become pregnant should tell their health care provider before taking this medication because it may affect nursing infants and unborn babies.

Cyclizine

Notify your health care provider if you notice any changes in your vision or eye pain, fast heartbeat, chest pain, difficulty urinating or if your urine is very dark, or if you notice a yellow color to your skin or eyes.

EMETICS
Syrup of ipecac

This medication is used to cause vomiting. A 30 ml (1-ounce) bottle of syrup of ipecac should be stored for emergency use in a safe place.

In all cases of poisoning by ingestion of chemicals, drugs or other poisons, notify your health care provider, hospital emergency department, or poison control center. The telephone numbers should be placed near your phone for emergencies.

Syrup of ipecac should *not* be given if the person is unconscious, having convulsions, or very drowsy because there is a danger that he or she may choke.

Syrup of ipecac should *not* be given if the substance swallowed was either a strong corrosive substance (such as lye or drain cleaner) or a petroleum product (such as gasoline or kerosene).

Syrup of ipecac should be used as directed on the label. Children under 1 year of age should *not* be given syrup of ipecac. Children over 1 year of age should be given 15 ml (½ ounce). Adults should be given 15 to 30 ml (½ to 1 ounce).

Syrup of ipecac does not work well when the stomach is empty, so follow the dose with ½ to 1 full glass of water.

Vomiting should occur within 20 minutes. Do not waste time waiting for vomiting to occur. Take the person for emergency treatment immediately. Bring the package or container of the poison with label intact.

NURSING DRUG DIGEST

Medication (trade name*)	Indication	Usual dosage and administration	Dosage forms, preparation, and storage	Contraindications, cautions, and comments	Monitoring
ANTIEMETICS/ANTIMOTION-SICKNESS					
★ **Benzquinamide** Emete-Con Quantril	Nausea and vomiting associated with anesthetics and surgery	*Adults:* 50 mg deep IM, followed by another dose in 1 hour; may then be repeated q.3-4h. as needed; 25 mg can also be administered as a single dose by *slow* IV NOTE: IV use may cause hypertension and dysrhythmias and is thus *not* recommended	Injectable: 50 mg/vial Reconstitute with 2.2 ml sterile water for injection Reconstituted solution is stable for 2 weeks at room temperature Store injection before and after reconstitution in a light-resistant container	Safe use in children has not been established	Monitor blood pressure because hypertension or hypotension can occur Observe for drowsiness and observe safety precautions Monitor for antiemetic effect in 15-30 min with duration 3-4 hr
★ **Buclizine** Bucladin-S Equivert Softran Vibazine	Motion sickness Nausea	*Adults:* 50 mg PO ½ hr before travel; may repeat dose in 4 to 6 hr if necessary *Adults:* 50 to 150 mg PO; usual maintenance dose is 50 mg PO b.i.d. Tablets may be dissolved in the mouth, chewed, or swallowed whole	Tablet: 50 mg	May cause drowsiness Safety precautions may be advised Safe use in children or during pregnancy has not been established	Observe for drowsiness

Continued.

NOTE: For additional details regarding the individual agents listed in this table, see the text and other tables in this chapter.
*Indicates a multiple active ingredient product. For a complete listing of all active ingredients see the *Drug Reference Guide to Brand Names and Active Ingredients.*
♣ Indicates that the drug is generally available only in Canada.
★ Indicates that the drug is generally available only in the United States.

NURSING DRUG DIGEST—cont'd

Medication (trade name)	Indication	Usual dosage and administration	Dosage forms, preparation, and storage	Contraindications, cautions, and comments	Monitoring
Chlorpromazine Chlor-Premanyl Chlor-P Z Chlorprom Cromedazine Elmarine Hibanil Largactil Megaphen Promachel Promapar Promosol Psychezine Sonazine Thorazine Tranzine	Nausea and vomiting See also Chapter 18, "Drugs Used to Treat Psychotic Disorders"	*Adults:* 25-50 mg PO or IM t.i.d. to q.i.d. *Children:* 0.5 mg/kg PO q.4-6h. as needed; *or* 0.5 mg/kg IM q6-8h. as needed Tablets may be taken with food or a full glass of water Do not take with antacids or antidiarrheals; space at least 1 hr apart	Tablets: 10, 25, 50 mg Suppository: 25 mg Syrup: 2 mg/ml Protect liquid from light *Discard* dark yellow solution Injectable: 25 mg/ml	*Contraindicated* in coma, jaundice, blood dyscrasias Contact with skin, eyes, clothing should be avoided because contact dermatitis has been reported All phenothiazines potentiate effects of alcohol, sedative-hypnotics, and narcotics May cause dry mouth, urinary retention, postural hypotension All phenothiazines may cause drowsiness; if so, patient should exercise care with machinery use or activities that require alertness Prolonged therapy may cause jaundice May color urine pink, red, or red-brown	Monitor for potential photosensitizing effect Observe for drowsiness
Cyclizine Marezine Marzine Migral* Valoid	Motion sickness See also Chapter 29, "Antihistamines, Antitussives, Decongestants, and Expectorants"	*Adults:* 50 mg PO or IM ½ hr before traveling; repeat q.6h. as necessary *Children:* 6-12 yr, 25 mg PO or IM q.6-8h. starting ½ hr before traveling as necessary May cause pain at the site of injection	Tablet: 50 mg Injectable: 50 mg/1 ml	*Contraindicated* in glaucoma, urinary retention Use with caution or not at all in pregnancy May cause drowsiness May potentiate effect of alcohol, tranquilizers and narcotics Patients should not drive or operate machinery if drowsiness occurs	Observe for drowsiness

Drug	Use	Dosage	How supplied	Precautions/Contraindications	Nursing implications
Dimenhydrinate Dimenest Dramamine Dymenol Eldodram Faston Gravol Nauseal Nauseatol Novodimenate Prevenause Ram Solbrine Trav-Arex Travamine Vertiban	Motion sickness See also Chapter 29, "Antihistamines, Antitussives, Decongestants, Expectorants"	*Adults:* 50-100 mg PO or IM ½ hr before traveling; repeat q.4-6h. as necessary *Children:* 6-8 years, 15-25 mg PO, IM, or PR b.i.d. to t.i.d.; 8-12 years, 25-50 mg PO, PR, or IM b.i.d. to t.i.d. Tablets may be administered with food or a glass of milk if medicine causes stomach upset; tablets should not be broken Capsules should be swallowed whole and should not be taken apart	Tablet: 50 mg Injection: 50 mg/ml Liquid: 12.5 mg/4 ml Suppositories: 50, 100 mg NOTE: Undiluted solution is irritating	*Contraindicated* in glaucoma, urinary retention Use with caution or not at all in pregnancy May cause drowsiness May potentiate effect of alcohol, tranquilizers, and narcotics Patients should not drive or operate machinery if drowsiness occurs	Monitor for drowsiness Safety precautions may be indicated
Diphenhydramine Allerdryl Benadryl Bendylate Benylin Eldadryl Nautamine Standryl SK-Diphenhydramine	Motion sickness See also Chapter 29, "Antihistamines, Antitussives, Decongestants, and Expectorants"	*Adults:* 50 mg PO t.i.d. to q.i.d.; or 10-50 mg IM or IV (maximum 100 mg per injection) *Children:* Over 10 kg, 12.5-25 mg t.i.d. to q.i.d. PO ½ hr before travel and meals; or 5 mg/kg/24 hr IM or IV in 4 divided doses (maximum 300 mg/24 hr)	Tablet: 50 mg Capsules: 25, 50 mg Liquid: 12.5 mg/5 ml Injectable: 10, 50 mg/ml Suppository: 100 mg Elixir: 10 mg/4 ml	May cause drowsiness May mask symptoms of ototoxicity until irreversible harm is done, thus avoid concomitant use of ototoxic drugs (e.g., aminoglycosides) May cause atropine-like side effects (e.g., dry mouth, blurred vision)	Observe for drowsiness Observe for atropine-like effects Monitor hearing
Diphenidol Vontrol	Labyrinth dizziness Nausea and vomiting	*Adults:* 25-50 mg PO q.4h. as needed *Children:* Over 23 kg, 25 mg PO q.4h. as needed Do *not* exceed 5.5 mg/kg/24 hr May need to decrease dose in renal failure because 90% is excreted in the urine	Tablet: 25 mg	*Contraindicated* in psychosis, hypersensitivity, and anuria May cause anticholinergic effects Rarely causes confusion, disorientation, and hallucinations	Observe for CNS adverse effects (e.g., confusion, hallucinations) particularly in the elderly Monitor intake and output Monitor for hypotension
Droperidol Inapsine	Nausea and vomiting Ménière's disease (indication not FDA approved)	*Adults:* 5 mg IM as a single dose to treat an acute attack and suppress associated nausea, nystagmus, vertigo, and vomiting	Injectable: 2.5 mg/ml	*Contraindicated* in hypersensitivity Use with caution in patients with renal or hepatic dysfunction May cause sedation and hypotension May cause extrapyramidal reactions	Monitor vital signs Observe for appearance of extrapyramidal reactions Observe for hypotension, particularly in the elderly and those patients being treated with antihypertensive medications

Continued.

NURSING DRUG DIGEST—cont'd

Medication (trade name)	Indication	Usual dosage and administration	Dosage forms, preparation, and storage	Contraindications, cautions, and comments	Monitoring
Haloperidol Haldol Peridol Serenace	Nausea and vomiting associated with anesthetics and surgery (indication not FDA approved) See also Chapter 18, "Drugs Used to Treat Psychotic Disorders"	*Adults:* 3-9 mg daily in divided doses; *or* 1 mg IM before induction of anesthetic Tablets may be administered with food or water Liquid medicine may be administered in juices, food, milk, or water	Tablets: 0.5, 1, 2, 5 mg Injectable: 5 mg/ml Liquid: 2 mg/ml Preserve in tight, light-resistant containers	Avoid getting liquid on skin or clothing because contact dermatitis has been reported May cause drowsiness May be excreted in breast milk and is thus contraindicated in nursing mothers Use during pregnancy and in children has not been established May potentiate the action of other CNS depressants, including alcohol	Monitor for drowsiness and implement safety precautions as indicated
Hydroxyzine Atarax Equipoise Hy-Pam Marax* Pas Depress Sedaril Vistaril Vistrax*	Nausea and vomiting associated with anesthetics and surgery See also Chapter 29, "Antihistamines, Antitussives, Decongestants, and Expectorants"	*Adults:* 25-100 mg deep IM preoperatively and postoperatively *Children:* 1.1 mg/kg deep IM preoperatively and postoperatively Do *not* administer IV Shake suspension well to ensure accurate dose	Capsules: 10, 25, 50 mg Syrup: 10 mg/5 ml Injectable: 50 mg/ml Suspension: 25 mg/5 ml	*Contraindicated* in hypersensitivity May cause drowsiness May potentiate CNS depression of other medications Safe use during pregnancy not established Inadvertent SC, IV, or intraarterial injection has been associated with pain and induration at injection site, thrombosis, and digital gangrene	Observe for dry mouth Observe for headache Observe for drowsiness and implement safety precautions as indicated Observe for excess CNS depression (particularly if patient is receiving other CNS depressants such as sedatives, narcotics, alcohol, or other psychotherapeutic agents)

Drug	Indications	Dosage	Preparations	Nursing Implications
Meclizine Ancolan Antivert Antivert/25 Bonamine Bonine Vertrol	Motion sickness See also Chapter 29, "Antihistamines, Antitussives, Decongestants, and Expectorants"	*Adults:* 25-50 mg PO daily starting 1 hr before traveling Tablets can be taken without water; place the tablet in the mouth and let it dissolve, chew it, or swallow whole Chewable tablets should be chewed completely before swallowing	Tablets: 12.5, 25 mg Chewable tablets: 25 mg Capsule: 25 mg	*Contraindicated* in glaucoma, urinary retention Use with caution or not at all during pregnancy May cause drowsiness May potentiate effect of alcohol, tranquilizers and narcotics Patients should not drive, or operate machinery if drowsiness occurs Observe for drowsiness and implement safety precautions as indicated
Metoclopramide Cerucal Maxeran Maxolon Primperan Reglan	Nausea and vomiting (indication not FDA approved) Nausea and vomiting associated with cisplatin therapy	*Adults:* 10 mg PO t.i.d. ½ hr before meals and q.h.s. *Adults:* 2 mg/kg slow IV over 15 min, ½ hr before chemotherapy Repeat twice at 2-hr intervals; may repeat additional 3 doses at 3-hr intervals; these doses may be reduced to 1 mg/kg	Tablet: 10 mg Injectable: 5, 10 mg/ml Syrup: 5 mg/ml	*Contraindicated* in patients receiving antipsychotic drugs because of increased incidence of parkinsonism-like effects, GI obstruction, pheochromocytoma, and hypersensitivity May cause drowsiness and dizziness Observe elderly patients in particular for symptoms of movement disorders (e.g., parkinsonism) Watch for constipation, diarrhea, drowsiness, extrapyramidal signs

Continued.

NURSING DRUG DIGEST—cont'd

Medication (trade name)	Indication	Usual dosage and administration	Dosage forms, preparation, and storage	Contraindications, cautions, and comments	Monitoring
Nabilone Cesamet	Severe nausea and vomiting associated with cancer chemotherapy	*Adults:* 1 or 2 mg PO b.i.d. usually at night and 1-3 hr before chemotherapy Maximum: 6 mg daily May need to reduce dosage in presence of hepatic impairment	Capsule: 1 mg	*Contraindicated* in hypersensitivity to marijuana or related products *Contraindicated* in psychosis Peak plasma concentrations occur in approximately 2 hours after oral dosing, with the half-life being approximately 2 hours Because nabilone is a synthetic cannabinoid related to marijuana, it causes similar effects (e.g., impaired mental ability, drowsiness, vertigo, ataxia, anorexia, blurred vision, euphoria, and hallucinations)	Monitor for excess CNS effects (drowsiness, vertigo, ataxia, euphoria, anorexia, hallucinations) Observe for dry mouth Observe for vertigo
Perphenazine Fentazin Phenazine Trilafon	Nausea and vomiting See also Chapter 18, "Drugs Used to Treat Psychotic Disorders"	*Adult:* 4 mg PO or IM q.8h. *Children:* Over 12 years, adult dose; under 12 years of age, 2-4 mg PO q.d. or b.i.d. IV use *not* recommended except to counteract retching or hiccups during surgery Tablets must be swallowed whole; do not crush, chew, or break; do not take at same time with antacids or antidiarrheals; space 1 hr apart Dilute oral concentrate with water, orange juice, milk, or carbonated beverage Color change or precipitation may occur when mixed with cola drinks, black coffee, tea, grape juice, or apple juice	Tablets: 2, 4, 8, 16 mg Injectable: 5 mg/ml Oral concentrate: 16 mg/5 ml Protect solutions from light Discard dark amber or discolored solutions	Avoid contact with skin, clothes, eyes because contact dermatitis has been reported with solutions May cause drowsiness or photosensitivity May color urine pink to reddish brown	Monitor for drowsiness and implement safety precautions as indicated Monitor pulse and blood pressure continuously during IV administration

Drug	Uses	Dosage	Preparations	Nursing considerations
		When IV route is used, monitor blood pressure continuously during IV administration Keep patient in recumbent position because transient dizziness and hypotension have been reported with parenteral use Monitor patient after injection until vital signs are stable Levarterenol should be on hand		
Prochlorperazine Compazine Stemetil Tementil	Nausea and vomiting See also Chapter 18, "Drugs Used to Treat Psychotic Disorders"	*Adults:* 5–10 mg PO, IM, or IV q4–6h. as necessary *Children:* 1–5 years, 2.5 mg PO daily to b.i.d.; 6–12 years, 5 mg PO b.i.d. to t.i.d.; 12–16 years, 5 mg PO t.i.d. to q.i.d. Administer oral concentrate in fruit juice, carbonated drinks or water	Tablets: 5, 10, 25 mg Injectable: 5 mg/ml Syrup: 1 mg/ml Suppositories: 2.5, 5, 25 mg Sustained-release capsules: 10, 15, 30, 75 mg Stored in tightly covered, light-resistant containers	Has greater antiemetic and extrapyramidal effects than most phenothiazines Avoid solution contact with skin, eyes or clothes because of possibility of contact dermatitis Observe for extrapyramidal symptoms in elderly or alcoholic patients and children with dehydration or acute illness Monitor for drowsiness and implement safety precautions as indicated
Promethazine Atosil Fellozine Ganphen Histantil Phenergan Phenergan injection Romsed Zipan-25 & -50	Motion sickness Nausea and vomiting See also Chapter 18, "Drugs Used to Treat Psychotic Disorders"	*Adults:* 25 mg PO q8–12h. as necessary; or 12.5–25 mg q4–12 h. IM or IV as necessary *Children:* Under 1 year, 5 mg/day in 2 divided doses; 1–5 years, 5–10 mg/day in 2 divided doses; 6–10 years, 10–15 mg/day in 2 divided doses Give medication ½ hr before travel Do *not* administer SC	Tablets: 10, 12.5, 25, 50 mg Injectable: 25, 50 mg/ml (50 mg/ml for IM use) Syrup: 6.25, 10, 12.5, and 25 mg in 5 ml Protect liquid from light Do not use injectable if solution darkened or if contains precipitate IV infusion bottle or bag and tubing should be protected from light with foil	May potentiate CNS depressant effects of alcohol, sedative-hypnotics, and narcotics Use with caution in liver disease May cause drowsiness May suppress cough reflex and cause thickening of bronchial secretions Overdosage should be treated with gastric lavage because dystonic reactions of head and neck may result in aspiration Observe for drowsiness, and implement safety precautions as indicated

Continued.

NURSING DRUG DIGEST—cont'd

Medication (trade name)	Indication	Usual dosage and administration	Dosage forms, preparation, and storage	Contraindications, cautions, and comments	Monitoring
Scopolamine Transderm-SCOP Transderm-V Triptone	Motion sickness See also Chapter 23, "Parasympathomimetics and Parasympatholytics"	*Adults:* 0.6 mg PO 1 hr before traveling; may be repeated in 4 hr; or apply transdermal patch to skin area behind ear 4 hr before required antiemetic effect; replace patch q.3 days as required *Children:* 3-7 years, 0.075 to 0.15 mg PO 1 hr before traveling; 7-12 years, 0.15-0.3 mg PO 1 hr before traveling	Tablets: 0.3, 0.4, 0.6 mg Transdermal patch: 1.5 mg (formulated to deliver 0.5 mg/day for 3 days)	*Contraindicated* in hyperthyroidism, cardiac failure, and hypersensitivity Use with caution in glaucoma and enlargement of the prostate Side effects occur more commonly in children Dry mouth, visual disturbances, and drowsiness may occur Wash hands thoroughly after applying transdermal patch to prevent drug from accidentally coming in contact with the eyes	Monitor for disorientation or confusion Implement safety precautions as indicated Monitor for tolerance with prolonged use
Tetrahydro-cannabinol	Nausea and vomiting associated with cancer chemotherapy (indication not FDA approved)	*Adults:* 5-15 mg PO 1 hr before chemotherapy and repeated q.4h. according to protocol NOTE: Experimental use *only* *Elderly:* Start with lower dose	Experimental use only Capsules: 2.5, 5, 10 mg Cigarettes: 2.5, 5, 10 mg	*Contraindicated* in psychosis *Contraindicated* in hypersensitivity to marijuana or its related products Cigarette dosage form should *not* be used by COPD patients May cause tachycardia May cause a variety of CNS effects (e.g., euphoria, hallucinations, anxiety, paranoia) May cause severe drowsiness	Observe for excess CNS activity (see nabilone) Monitor heart rate Observe for drowsiness and monitor for euphoria, hallucinations, and other CNS effects

Drug	Uses	Dosage	Preparations	Nursing Implications
Thiethylperazine Torecan Toresten	Nausea and vomiting See also Chapter 18, "Drugs Used to Treat Psychotic Disorders"	*Adults:* 10 mg PO, IM, or PR q.8-12h. as necessary Do *not* administer by IV route IM injections should be given carefully because inadvertent IV injection of this drug can result in severe hypotension; the patient should be in the recumbent position and should remain in bed for at least 1 hr after the initial injection as indicated, and should be monitored for othostatic hypotension (weakness, faintness); supervise ambulation	Tablet: 10 mg Suppositories: 10 mg Injectable: 5 mg/ml	*Contraindicated* in hypersensitivity to phenothiazines May cause drowsiness Do *not* get on skin because may cause contact dermatitis Observe for extrapyramidal effects which may occur, especially in children and women under 30 Monitor for drowsiness and implement safety precautions as indicated
Triflupromazine Psyquil 25 Siquil Vesprin	Nausea and vomiting See also Chapter 18, "Drugs Used to Treat Psychotic Disorders"	*Adults:* 10 mg PO b.i.d. to t.i.d.; or 5-15 mg IM q.4h. as necessary up to 60 mg/day *Children:* 0.2-0.25 mg/kg PO or IM up to maximum total daily dose of 10 mg *Elderly:* 2.5-15 mg/day IM Shake suspension well to ensure accurate dose Administer oral forms with food or water Do not administer with antacids or antidiarrheals; if necessary, space at least 1 hr apart	Tablets: 10, 25, 50 mg Injectable: 10, 20 mg/ml Suspension: 50 mg/5 ml Stored in light-resistant airtight containers at room temperature Do not use injectable if dark amber or discolored	*Contraindicated* in hypersensitivity to phenothiazines Sedation, antiemetic effects and extrapyramidal symptoms are more marked than with chlorpromazine Do not confuse with trifluoperazine (antipsychotic) Observe for extrapyramidal symptoms and implement safety precautions as indicated

Continued.

NURSING DRUG DIGEST—cont'd

Medication (trade name)	Indication	Usual dosage and administration	Dosage forms, preparation, and storage	Contraindications, cautions, and comments	Monitoring
Trimetho-benzamide Tigan Xametina	Nausea and vomiting	*Adults:* 250 mg PO t.i.d. to q.i.d.; *or* 200 mg IM or PR t.i.d. to q.i.d.; or before and during surgery as indicated Administer IM deeply into dorsogluteal site *Children:* 15-40 kg, 100-200 mg PO or PR t.i.d. to q.i.d. *Not* recommended in children less than 15 kg Do *not* use IM form in children *Elderly:* Start with lower dose	Capsules: 100, 250 mg Suppository: 100, 200 mg Injectable: 100 mg/ml Refrigerate suppositories	*Contraindicated* in hypersensitivity May cause drowsiness Pain, burning and irritation have been reported at IM site Local irritation has occurred following rectal administration	Observe for drowsiness and implement safety precautions as indicated Monitor for skin rash or other signs of hypersensitivity
EMETICS					
★ **Apomorphine**	Poisoning and drug overdose *except* where vomiting is contraindicated (e.g., ingestion of a corrosive)	*Adult:* 0.1 mg/kg SC 1 dose *only*	Tablets, soluble: 6 mg Protect from light Do not use solution that is brown or green or that contains a precipitate	*Contraindicated* in CNS depression Induces vomiting within 5-10 min after injection	Observe for CNS depression Observe for circulatory failure in elderly or debilitated patients Monitor sedative effects after injection, which can persist for 2 hr, and implement safety precautions as indicated Monitor vital signs

Ipecac syrup

Poisoning and Drug overdose *except where vomiting is contraindicated* (e.g., ingestion of a corrosive)

Adults: 15-30 ml PO plus 360 ml water
Children: 1-5 years, 15 ml PO plus 240 ml water; over 5 years of age, 15-30 ml PO plus 240 ml water
NOTE: If no vomiting in 20 min, an additional dose of 15 ml may be given; if the patient still has not vomited, gastric lavage may be indicated; take extreme caution *not* to confuse ipecac syrup with ipecac fluid extract; the fluid extract is approximately 14 times more potent than the syrup, and if inadvertently substituted and administered, may cause *death*

Do *not* administer to semiconscious or unconscious or sedated patients

Syrup: 15, 30 ml

Contraindicated in those with CNS depression, corrosive poisoning, and ingestion of petroleum distillates

Monitor for emetic effect within 15-20 min Observe patient and monitor vital signs; further emergency treatment may be indicated

BIBLIOGRAPHY

Feldman, M., & Fordtran, J.S. Vomiting. In M.H. Sleisenger & J.S. Fordtran (Eds.), *Gastrointestinal disease—pathophysiology, diagnosis, management.* Philadelphia: W.B. Saunders, 1978.

Goulding, R., & Volans, G.N. Emergency treatment of common poisons: Emptying the stomach. *Proceedings of the Royal Society of Medicine,* 1977, *70,* 766-770.

Manoguerra, A.S., & Krenzelok, E.P. Rapid emesis from high-dose ipecac syrup in adults and children intoxicated with antiemetics or other drugs. *American Hospital Pharmacy,* 1978, *35,* 1360-1362.

Reyntijens, A. Domperidone as an antiemetic: Summary of research reports. *Postgraduate Medical Journal,* 1979, *55*(Suppl. 1), 50-54.

Stockman, A., Caron, D., Gallant, J., & Boghaert, A. Postoperative nausea and vomiting treated with domperidone (R 33812): an open and double blind study. *Anesthesisit,* 1978, *27,* 540-543.

Wood, C.D. Antimotion sickness and antiemetic drugs. *Drugs,* 1979, *17,* 471-479.

CHAPTER 41

Laxatives and Antidiarrheals

Walter W. Yakimets

Medications discussed in this chapter

Laxatives
  Bulk-forming laxatives
    Bran
    Methylcellulose
    Plantago seed
  Enemas
    Oil enemas
    Phosphate enemas
    Saline enemas
    Soapsuds enemas
    Tap water enemas
    Total intestinal prepa-
      ration
  Lubricants and fecal soft-
    eners
    Docusate calcium
    Docusate potassium
    Docusate sodium
    Mineral oil
    Poloxamer 188
  Saline laxatives
    Magnesium citrate
    Magnesium hydroxide
    Magnesium sulfate
    Sodium phosphate/so-
      dium biphosphate

Laxatives—cont'd
  Stimulant and irritant
    laxatives
    Bisacodyl
    Cascara sagrada
    Castor oil
    Danthron
    Glycerin
    Phenolphthalein
  Miscellaneous
    Lactulose
    Senna
Antidiarrheals
  Adsorbents
    Cholestyramine
    Kaolin
  Antimicrobials
    See Section X of text
  Hydrophilic agents
    Polycarbophil
    Plantago seed
  Opiates
    Codeine
    Diphenoxylate
    Loperamide
    Paregoric
    Tincture of opium

caused by amebic *dysentery*) are more appropriately treated with a specific antimicrobial agent. It is also important to recognize when caring for individuals with either constipation or diarrhea that both of these conditions can be caused by various medications. For example, constipation is a common side effect related to codeine use, and diarrhea often accompanies the oral use of ampicillin. Careful patient assessment is essential in identifying the cause of the elimination problem and in planning appropriate treatment and nursing care.

Patient demand for laxatives and for antidiarrheals is great, and patient education regarding the prudent use of these agents is essential. Because laxatives are widely used and are probably the most widely sold over-the-counter drug (particularly among the elderly) careful assessment of patients and their use of laxatives is important in preventing abuse and promoting normal bowel function. Although there are definite needs and indications for their use, abuse is common. The unnecessary use of laxatives can result in a laxative habit, fluid and electrolyte imbalances, vitamin and nutrient deficiencies, and physical and psychologic dependence.

CONSTIPATION

Constipation may be defined as infrequent, often difficult, passage of hard and dry stool. The causes, congenital or acquired, include the following:

CONGENITAL

1. Hirschsprung's disease (aganglionic megacolon)

ACQUIRED

1. Dietary deficiencies including lack of bulk and possibly inadequate fluid intake
2. Decreased physical activity caused by aging, hospitalization, injury, lack of exercise

Laxatives are agents that act to promote or facilitate the evacuation of stool from the bowel. *Antidiarrheals* are agents that act to decrease the number and frequency of watery or liquid stools. Laxatives are used in the treatment of *constipation,* and antidiarrheals are used in the treatment of certain types of *diarrhea.* It is important to recognize that not all constipation or diarrhea is appropriately treated with laxatives or antidiarrheals, respectively. Some forms of constipation are caused by obstructions (such as those resulting from colonic carcinoma) that require surgical intervention, and some forms of diarrhea (such as that

877

3. Irregular bowel habits (not taking the time to eliminate completely, ignoring the *defecation reflex*)
4. Emotional upset (stress or depression)
5. Painful perianal diseases
6. Hypothyroidism
7. Pregnancy (possibly because of the smooth muscle relaxant effect of progesterone, the pressure of the growing fetus on the bowel)
8. Long-term abuse of laxatives
9. Side effect of drugs such as aluminum hydroxide, calcium carbonate, opiates, anticholinergics, diuretics
10. Obstructive lesions of the colon (e.g., carcinoma, strictures, *diverticular disease*)
11. Aging with impairment of either rectal sensation or neuromuscular transmission
12. Unknown

The main functions of the colon are dehydration and storage of the bowel contents until there is an appropriate time and place for defecation. Although most of the water in the alimentary tract is absorbed in the small intestine, some 500 to 1000 ml are discharged into the colon. Except for about 100 to 200 ml eliminated in the stool, the colon absorbs most of this water through its large mucosal surface, aided by colonic muscular activity. The passage of intestinal contents through the colon is usually slow. The main propulsive movements, or mass movements, are infrequent. Occuring mainly after meals (gastrocolonic reflex), they allow adequate time for fluid absorption. Segmentation, an important colonic acitivity that allows for greater water absorption, consists of frequent, short segmental contractions of circular muscle. These contractions permit maximal exposure of the colonic contents to the absorptive surface of the mucosa with minimal or no propulsive activity. Thus, if the small intestine delivers less fluid to the colon, if mass movements are fewer, and if segmentation is more vigorous, there may be increased dehydration of the stool. In addition, if the bulk of the stool delivered to the rectum is small (less than 150 to 300 ml necessary to initiate the defecation reflex), the stool may remain for a longer time in the colon and thus become so dehydrated the result is constipation. Likewise, if the defecation reflex is ignored or impaired and bowel movement deferred, an abnormal dehydration of feces can occur. Sometimes the defecation urge is consciously denied (because of painful perianal lesions, such as fissures, or embarrassment in communicating needs that occurs in hospitalized patients on bed rest), and this denial can result in constipation. Children and patients with obstipation or psychogenic megacolon may deliberately withhold bowel movements.

Constipation is a multifactorial problem. For example, if the diet and fluid intake are inadequate (as sometimes occurs in individuals on fad diets or in older people who live on tea and toast or drink small amounts of fluid because of the fear of incontinence), there may be less water delivered to the colon, inadequate food triggering of the gastrocolonic reflex, and inadequate fecal bulk to trigger the defecation reflex for several days. The problem can be compounded if these individuals are taking calcium or aluminum antacids, vitamin preparations containing iron, anticholinergics, opiates, or sedative-hypnotics, which may cause increased dehydration of the stool. Inactivity, stress, or a change in routine may further impair their normal elimination.

Symptoms of constipation tend to be mild. These may include the absence of a bowel movement for 1 to 3 days or a change in usual elimination pattern, abdominal distention, and mild rectal discomfort or fullness. Physical assessment of the abdomen may reveal palpable stool in the colon, and rectal examination may confirm the presence of hard stool in the rectum. Paradoxically, if constipation becomes marked, the hard stool can irritate the rectal mucosa and cause mucus and fluid secretion, resulting in diarrhea around the hard fecal mass.

If constipation is of recent origin or if it is accompanied by alternating diarrhea, abdominal cramps, distention, or melena, colonic evaluation is indicated to exclude serious conditions, such as hypothyroidism, megacolon, or carcinoma. Minimal medical colonic evaluation includes a rectal examination, *sigmoidoscopy*, and *barium enema*. A *colonoscopy* or rectal motility assessment may be indicated. If no obstructive lesion exists, the patient, in addition to increasing dietary bulk, ensuring adequate hydration, and implementing an exercise regimen to promote function and to establish regular bowel habits, may use a laxative to get the bowel working normally.

In addition to the treatment of constipation, laxatives are also used to cleanse the bowel in preparation for colonic surgery and for diagnostic procedures such as barium enema, colonoscopy, and sigmoidoscopy.

LAXATIVES

Laxatives are agents that act to promote and facilitate the evacuation of the bowel. Laxatives should not be given if an obstructive lesion (e.g., carcinoma) or an *acute abdomen* (e.g., *appendicitis* or diverticulitis) is suspected. The choice of a laxative should be based on individual patient need and health status, and those laxatives with minimal side effects should be selected whenever possible.

Laxatives can be conveniently divided into four categories: bulk-forming, lubricant, saline, and stimulant. Bulk forming, lubricant, saline, and stimulant laxatives differ primarily in their mechanisms of action. For example, it is thought that stimulant laxatives act on the nerves innervating the intestines or by local irritation of the intestinal mucosa. Lubricant (or emollient) laxatives are usually oils or wetting agents, which add moisture to the stool bulk and facilitate fecal passage through the intestine. Bulk-forming laxatives increase stool bulk mainly by absorbing water. The increased stool bulk causes pressure on the intestinal walls and thus increased peristaltic action. Saline laxatives add salt to the intestinal contents and cause increased body water to be drawn into the intestinal lumen, thus increasing bulk and lubrication and facilitating fecal passage through the intestine.

Bulk-forming laxatives

The meat and refined cereal diet of the average North American or European contains little natural bulk, and consequently, there is decreased fecal bulk. Intestinal transit time is longer on a low-bulk Western diet than the high-bulk, mainly cereal diet of the developing countries. This slower transit time may allow for more dehydration of the stool. In addition, the small bulk may not be adequate to build up a fecal material. Bulk laxatives, which include bran, plantago seed preparations, and methylcellulose are relatively safe and may be used for prolonged periods of time without serious adverse side effects. Bulk laxatives are not digestible and are not absorbed. Taken as directed with sufficient fluid intake, bulk laxatives absorb water increasing their bulk up to 20 times. The extra bulk increases luminal pressure in the intestine, which in turn stimulates peristalsis and the defecation reflex. The absorbed water also softens the stool and makes it easier to pass. These agents usually act in 12 to 24 hours but may take up to 3 days.

Bulk laxatives such as psyllium preparations and methylcellulose should be stirred into water and followed with adequate water intake. The main complaint associated with bulk laxatives is temporary *flatulence* and *bloating*, symptoms that usually disappear in 2 or 3 weeks with regular use.

Obstruction of the lower two thirds of the esophagus has been reported as a result of taking bulk laxatives in too little water. Because they work by absorbing water, the importance of drinking adequate amounts of water with the preparation cannot be overemphasized. Retrosternal pain after taking a bulk laxative may indicate esophageal impaction. If this occurs, additional water should *not* be taken because it can aggravate the situation by causing the obstruction

to absorb more water and increase in size. There is also risk of aspiration. Although this is a rare complication, the use of these laxatives requires careful patient teaching, and they are contraindicated in cases of dysphagia or in patients with a history of esophageal stenosis. Instances of fecal impaction and intestinal obstruction have also been reported with the use of these laxatives.

In addition to treating constipation, bulk laxatives, because of their ability to absorb water, are also sometimes useful in treating diarrhea.

Bran. Bran is available in breakfast cereals, or it may be bought as miller's or dietary bran in most food or health food stores. Dietary or miller's bran may be used in cooking such foods as muffins, bread, and potatoes. It is palatable and acceptable to most people. There is basically no contraindication to its use except intestinal obstruction, and it has no side effects, except temporary flatulence and bloating. The usual daily dose of bran is provided in one bowl of breakfast cereal or in about 3 tablespoons of bran.

Plantago seed. Plantago (Psyllium) preparations are made from the ground dry seeds of a plant from the Plantago family. These preparations are able to absorb a great deal of water. They are useful as laxatives in that they provide bulk and make the stool softer. Paradoxically because they absorb water, they are also sometimes useful in decreasing the fluidity and number of stools in diarrhea. They are useful after anal surgery and in the treatment of chronic constipation, diverticular disease, *irritable bowel syndrome*, and anal fissures, because the bowel movement, although bulkier, is also softer.

Plantago preparations are available in a variety of mixtures with other compounds. Ground plantago seed may be given two or three times daily (5 to 10 gm) in 240 ml of fruit juice to improve the taste. A palatable *effervescent* preparation is also available that can be mixed with water. The effervescent preparation, available in individual packages, is more expensive, but more acceptable. The usual dose is one package in 240 ml of water two or three times daily. A granular preparation, which can be sprinkled on food or taken directly, is also available.

The main side effects of plantago preparations are temporary flatulence and bloating. Plantago preparations should not be used in patients with intestinal obstruction. Effervescent preparations contain sodium and should not be given to patients on sodium-restricted diets.

Ispaghula, sterculia, and chondrus. These bulk laxative agents currently are not commonly used in North America. Ispaghula preparation, both ground seeds and husk, are derived from a plantago plant, which is similar to the plantago plant from which psyllium seed is derived.

Sterculia, more commonly known as karaya, is a gum obtained from one of the species of Sterculia plant. Powdered sterculia takes up a great deal of water and acts as a bulk laxative. Sterculia or karaya preparations are frequently used in the form of a gum as an adhesive for colostomy or *ileostomy* bags.

Chondrus is derived from dried seaweed.

All of these agents, because they can absorb a great deal of water, act similarly to plantago and have similar indications, contraindications, and side effects.

Methylcellulose. Methylcellulose is a synthetic cellulose derivative that can be used as a bulk laxative. It is able to absorb a great deal of water making the stool bulkier and softer. Increased stool bulk tends to stimulate *peristalsis* and the defecation reflex. Methylcellulose, like other bulk laxatives, is useful in treating diverticular disease, constipation, and painful anal conditions such as fissures, thrombosed *hemorrhoids,* and postoperative trauma. Methylcellulose is also useful in the treatment of diarrhea because it absorbs water.

The dose is 1 to 1.5 gm two to four times daily. Extra water should be taken if this bulk laxative is used to prevent obstruction. Side effects are minimal when taken as directed. Since this agent does not tend to disperse as well as plantago, there is a possibility of bulk or bolus formation.

Carboxymethylcellulose. Carboxymethylcellulose sodium is a synthetic compound that may be used as a bulk laxative. It is believed to be pharmacologically inert. The indications for the use of this compound are similar to those for methylcellulose.

The dosage of carboxymethylcellulose sodium is 4 to 10 gm daily in divided doses. It should be given with adequate fluids to prevent bulk formation.

Lubricant laxatives

There are 3 basic types of lubricant laxatives or stool softeners: mineral oil, the docusates, and poloxamer 188. These agents are chemically dissimilar but all aid bowel evacuation by modest softening of the stool.

Mineral oil. Mineral oil is a mixture of mineral oil hydrocarbons obtained from petroleum crude oils. Mineral oil is nondigestable and only minimally absorbed from the intestine. It apparently softens fecal contents by penetrating and coating them. It may also act by preventing colonic absorption of the water contained in the feces. Mineral oil initially was thought to be a safe compound, but there is sufficient evidence to indicate that its use as a laxative should be stopped, especially in the young and the elderly or debilitated.

The problems with continued use of mineral oil include disturbances in absorption of nutrients and vitamins, especially the fat-soluble vitamins A, D, E, and K; anal seepage of the oil causing anal irritation, discomfort, and annoyance; impaired healing of gastrointestinal surgical wounds; possible carcinogenic effect; aspiration of the oil into the lungs, possibly resulting in lipoid pneumonia; and deposition of small amounts of oil absorbed in the mesenteric lymph nodes, liver, and spleen. Because of these factors use of mineral oil as a laxative is not recommended.

If this preparation must be used, the usual dosage is 30 ml daily by mouth at bedtime. It should not be given with meals, because it may delay gastric emptying and interfere with digestion or absorption of nutrients.

Docusates. Docusates are compounds that act as wetting and dispersing agents. There are three types: sodium, potassium, and calcium salt. These substances facilitate the mixture of aqueous and fatty substances to soften fecal material. Docusates (according to claims) are nonabsorbable, nontoxic, and pharmacologically inert, and do not impair absorption of nutrients.

Docusates are especially useful in softening hard dry fecal material. Because of the risk of liver damage, they should not be used for long periods of time.

Although the main use for these wetting agents is in the treatment of hard, dry stool, they are also used to prevent the formation of firm stool where it may have adverse effects, such as in patients who have cardiac conditions, anorectal surgery, anal fissures, or thrombosed hemorrhoids, and in other patients who should avoid bearing down or straining at the stool. The calcium form is preferred in patients who are on low-sodium diets.

Docusate sodium. Docusate sodium, a wetting agent, can be used to soften hard stool. It produces moderate softening of the fecal mass in 24 to 48 hours.

The recommended adult dose is 50 to 480 mg daily in a single or divided dose. The recommended dose for children under 3 years of age is 10 to 40 mg in a single or divided dose. Because of its bitter taste, it may be given with fruit juices. Larger doses may be given initially. This compound should not be given in conjunction with mineral oil because it increases absorption of the oil. Prolonged use may cause hepatic damage. Because it contains sodium, the preparation should not be used for prolonged periods in patients for whom sodium must be restricted (e.g., those patients with congestive heart failure, renal failure, or hypertension).

Docusate calcium. Docusate calcium is a stool-wetting agent. Its properties and side effects are similar to docusate sodium except that it does not contain sodium and may be safely used for prolonged periods in those patients for whom an excessive sodium intake may cause a problem.

The dose for an adult is 50 to 240 mg in a single or divided dose and 50 to 150 mg daily for children in divided doses. It may occasionally cause abdominal cramps.

Poloxamer 188. Poloxamer 188 is a waxy, nonionic surfactant that may be used as a stool softener.

The dosage is 240 to 750 mg daily, but a course of therapy should not exceed 1 week. A glass of fluid should be taken with each dose. Its stool-softening effect may not be achieved for several days.

Saline laxatives

Saline laxatives, or osmotic agents, are relatively unabsorbed solutes that retain water in the small intestine and thus increase its volume and stimulate peristalsis. They also increase the flow of fluid into the colon. These compounds include sulfate, citrate, phosphate, and tartrate salts of magnesium, sodium, and potassium. Studies suggest that the saline laxatives might act by other than an osmotic effect. They may stimulate motor activities of the intestines. There is also some evidence that they may stimulate the release of cholecystokinin (pancreozymin).

Saline laxatives should not be routinely used. Their adverse effects include electrolyte disturbances, fluid loss, and perhaps interference with digestion and absorption of nutrients. Magnesium saline *cathartics* should not be used in patients with renal failure because of the risk of hypermagnesemia and associated central nervous system toxicity. Sodium salts should be avoided in patients with congestive heart failure or hypertension because of the risk of overloading the vascular system by means of extra sodium retention. Most saline laxatives cause a watery stool 3 to 6 hours or less after administration.

The use of these agents should probably be limited to preparation of the bowel for barium studies, colonoscopy, or surgery and to the occasional treatment of certain cases of constipation. These agents may also be used in evacuating blood from the bowel of patients in hepatic coma, a condition that may occur in cirrhotics who bleed from esophageal varices.

Saline laxatives, like other laxatives, should not be used when intraabdominal inflammation or bowel obstruction is suspected.

Magnesium compounds

Magnesium sulfate (epsom salts). Magnesium sulfate is an osmotic laxative. It is poorly absorbed from the gut and draws water into the lumen, increasing intraluminal bulk and stimulating peristalsis. It also increases the fluid load to the colon. Some of the action of magnesium sulfate may result from the stimulated release of cholecystokinin.

The usual dose in the adult is 15 gm in 250 ml of water by mouth. In children the suggested dose is 100 to 250 mg/kg body weight. The bitter taste may be masked by fruit juice. Side effects at these doses are minimal if used on an occasional basis. Magnesium sulfate is contraindicated in patients with renal failure and in children with intestinal parasitic diseases because of the risk of hypermagnesemia, whose symptoms are flushed skin, thirst, muscle weakness, and feelings of heat.

Magnesium hydroxide (milk of magnesia). Magnesium hydroxide has both antacid and laxative properties. Up to one quarter of the magnesium may be absorbed, and therefore this compound is contraindicated in patients with renal failure. The usual adult dose is 2 to 4 gm in tablet form and 25 to 50 ml in a liquid mixture.

Magnesium citrate. Magnesium citrate solution is used as a laxative. It comes as a palatable effervescent liquid, which can be made even more palatable by administering it chilled or over ice.

The adult dose is 200 ml and usually comes in a bottle of that size. Because of the danger of hypermagnesemia, it should not be used over prolonged periods and should not be used in patients with renal failure.

Sodium compounds

Potassium sodium tartrate. Potassium sodium tartrate is poorly absorbed and is therefore able to draw water into the intestinal lumen. Like other saline laxatives, the increased intestinal fluid causes an increase in peristalsis and evacuation of a fluid stool. Potassium sodium tartrate works in 1 to 2 hours.

The adult dose is 10 gm. It is not toxic in this dose range. Potassium sodium tartrate should not be given to patients with congestive heart failure, hypertension, renal failure, or toxemia because of the risk of sodium retention, which aggravates these conditions.

Sodium sulfate (Glaubers salts). Sodium sulfate may be used as a saline or osmotic laxative. Its taste is unpleasant, and it is not widely used.

The adult dose is 15 gm. Hypernatremia can occur, especially with prolonged use. Like other sodium compounds, sodium sulfate should not be used in patients with hypertension, toxemia, and congestive heart failure because of the risk of the aggravation of these conditions.

Sodium biphosphate. Sodium biphosphate is a saline laxative that is poorly absorbed from the gastrointestinal tract. It causes retention of water in the intestinal lumen and produces a watery stool 1 to 2 hours after ingestion. Sodium biphosphate is also used in enema preparations.

The usual daily dosage is given in the following amounts:

Adults	10 to 20 ml
Children 5 to 10 years	2.5 to 5 ml
Children over 10 years	5 to 10 ml

Hypernatremia may occur with prolonged use.

Sodium phosphate. Sodium phosphate is an osmotic laxative that is fairly pleasant tasting but is somewhat less effective than magnesium or sodium sulfate. It also comes as an effervescent solution.

The average adult dose of sodium phosphate is 4 to 8 gm. For effervescent sodium phosphate it is 10 to 20 gm in water.

Sodium phosphate is contraindicated where sodium and, therefore, extra fluid retention is a problem, such as in toxemia of pregnancy, hypertension, and congestive heart failure. Extraskeletal calcification may also occur.

Stimulant laxatives

Stimulant laxatives include anthraquinone derivatives, diphenylmethane derivatives, castor oil, and glycerin. Their exact mechanism of action is unclear, and it is possible that these laxatives work by several mechanisms. Stimulant laxatives appear to stimulate intestinal peristalsis by stimulating local nerve or muscle fibers in the colon mucosa. In addition, they may interfere with water absorption. These agents are effective and probably the most commonly used laxatives. Some may cause abdominal cramps because of their action. Long-term use should be avoided because they can produce fluid and electrolyte imbalance, and they can also cause a *laxative colon* or *cathartic colon* (i.e., a colon that does not evacuate properly anymore without use of a laxative). In other words, stimulant-laxative abuse may result in the condition that it was used to cure (i.e., constipation). Stimulant laxatives are contraindicated where intestinal obstruction or an acute abdomen is suspected. They are particularly helpful in treating constipation in the elderly, who may lack the necessary physiologic stimulation to their bowels. Dosage is individualized and should start with a minimum dose. The dose may be increased or a stronger drug selected from this group for desired effect.

Anthraquinones. The anthraquinone group of laxatives includes senna, cascara, and aloes and is one of the strongest classes of stimulant laxatives. Aloes

should not be used at all because they are irritating and in large doses may cause nephritis.

Anthraquinones are believed to increase colonic motility and may interfere with normal water reabsorption. Most are effective within 8 to 24 hours, although senna and castor oil are usually effective in 3 to 4 hours. These drugs are excreted in breast milk, and nursing infants can develop diarrhea as a result.

Senna. Senna preparations are reliable and potent laxatives. These compounds do not appear to be absorbed in the small intestine but are changed by colonic bacteria into active compounds. These compounds may act locally on the colon, or they may be absorbed and excreted in the bile (thereby altering the small intestinal function). Basically, senna preparations appear to stimulate colonic motility and may interfere with water and sodium reabsorption. Senna compounds usually work within 8 to 12 hours and occasionally take 24 hours to produce a stool evacuation.

Senna preparations may be found in the milk of lactating mothers, which may cause diarrhea in nursing babies. These preparations may also discolor the urine, making acidic urine yellowish brown and alkaline urine reddish violet. Prolonged use of senna may cause melanosis coli, which is a blackish pigmentation of colonic mucosa.

The adult dose of Senna *fluid extract* is 2 ml. The adult dose of Senna *syrup* is 8 ml. Senna glyosides, Sennosides A and B, which are more stable and reliable than Senna leaf, are usually prescribed in doses of 12 to 36 mg for adults. Side effects are abdominal cramps and discomfort. Fluid and electrolyte disturbances may occur with prolonged use.

Cascara sagrada. Cascara is an anthraquinone cathartic that is somewhat milder and less effective than the senna preparations. It usually takes about 8 hours to work and thus can be given at bedtime. The active ingredients appear to be liberated in the colon. Cascara may stimulate colonic activity and interfere with sodium and water reabsorption. It may be found in the milk of nursing mothers and thus cause diarrhea in nursing babies.

The adult dose of aromatic fluid extract is 5 ml at bedtime, and in children the dose is 1 to 2 ml. The adult dose of cascara sagrada extract tablets is 300 mg. The main side effect is abdominal cramps.

Diphenylmethane laxatives. The two acceptable laxatives of this group are phenolphthalein and bisacodyl. These two compounds act on the colon and take at least 6 hours to produce a fecal evacuation. The exact mechanism of action of these drugs is unknown. Oxyphenisatin was a former member of this group; however, its direct association with hepatic toxicity has caused discontinuation of its use.

Phenolphthalein. Phenolphthalein is a relatively nontoxic laxative of the stimulant laxative group that acts mainly on the colon. The exact mechanism of action is unknown. It is probably the most widely used of all laxatives because it is tasteless and thus lends itself to such forms as laxative candies or gums. In large doses fluid and electrolyte disturbances may occur. Allergies, including severe pruritic pink to purple skin eruptions, have been reported. The incidence of allergies is higher in preparations containing *yellow* phenolphthalein (i.e., unpurified form) as opposed to the *white* or purified form. Phenolphthalein colors alkaline urine pink to red. When used in addition to a soapsuds enema, it may turn stool pink or red.

The adult dose is 60 to 100 mg generally taken at bedtime. Side effects may include abdominal cramps and an allergic rash. Death caused by anaphylactic reactions has been reported, but is rare. Phenolphthalein is ineffective in treating constipation in patients with obstructive jaundice.

Bisacodyl. Bisacodyl, structurally related to phenolphthalein, is administered orally or rectally and is thus available in oral tablet or in rectal suppository forms. It appears to exert its action by stimulating colonic motility. Bisacodyl tablets are *enteric coated* to prevent gastric irritation; thus the tablets should not be chewed, crushed, or taken with antacids, which can destroy the protective coating. The medication is relatively nontoxic, except if taken in large doses.

The adult dose is 10 to 15 mg by mouth or 10 mg by rectal suppository. The dose for children under the age of 2 is 300 µg/kg by mouth or 5 mg by rectal suppository and for children over 2 years of age, 10 mg by rectal suppository. Side effects include abdominal cramps. A rectal burning sensation can occur with the frequent use of the suppository form. Bisacodyl acts within 6 to 12 hours if given orally and within 1 hour if given rectally.

Castor oil. The laxative action of castor oil results from ricinoleic acid. Ricinoleic acid is produced when castor oil is hydrolyzed in the small intestine by pancreatic lipases. Castor oil produces its laxative action by acting on the small intestine, but the precise mechanism of action is unknown. It is possible that castor oil interferes with water and electrolyte reabsorption.

Castor oil should not be used as a routine laxative because of the risks of electrolyte and fluid imbalance. It works well to clear the bowel for x-ray investigation. It acts usually within 2 hours of administration.

The adult dose is 15 to 60 ml, and for children the dose is 5 to 15 ml. As with other stimulant laxatives, castor oil may cause abdominal cramps. It should not be used in patients with intestinal obstruction or in those suspected of inflammatory intestinal problems, including acute appendicitis.

Miscellaneous laxatives

Lactulose. Lactulose is a synthetic disaccharide consisting of one molecule of fructose and one of galactose. Lactulose reaches the colon virtually unchanged, where it is broken down by bacteria to nonabsorbable organic ions, which act as osmotic laxatives. It is used in treatment of constipation and prevention of hepatic encephalopathy by evacuating blood from the gastrointestinal tract following bleeding from esophageal varices in cirrhotic patients. Lactulose works well after surgery and can be used in the treatment of chronic constipation.

The usual adult daily dose of lactulose is 10 to 20 gm, with a larger initial dose and maintenance doses of 6 to 12.5 gm. In the treatment of hepatic encephalopathy one could use 6 to 100 gm per day in three divided doses. In children the average daily dose is 2.5 to 7.5 gm per day according to age.

Lactulose takes several days to work. Lactulose should not be used in patients with galactosemia, and its safety has not been established in pregnancy. Its main side effect is bloating. Lactulose, like other laxatives, should not be used in cases of an acute abdomen or bowel obstruction. Since lactulose may alter colonic flora, prolonged use should be avoided until this aspect has been studied. Caution should also be used when given to diabetics because this drug contains galactose and lactose.

Rectal suppositories

A rectal suppository is a semisolid medicated preparation that is inserted into the rectum where it dissolves and releases its medication (see box, p. 884, left). Several preparations have been incorporated into suppositories to help in the evacuation of the lower bowel. Rectal suppositories are not as effective evacuants of the lower bowel as phosphate, saline, or tap water enemas.

Glycerin suppositories. Glycerin suppositories may be used to clean the lower bowel both in children and adults. These suppositories consist of 70% glycerin dissolved in sodium stearate, which is essentially a soap. The mechanism of action probably results from the hyperosmotic effect of glycerin and the stimulating (irritant) effect of the soap. It is possible that the stimulating effect of suppository insertion and the lubricant property may also be of value in moving the bowel. The success rate of evacuating the bowel is not

---

Administration of rectal suppositories

1. Refrigerate most suppositories because they tend to soften at room temperature.
2. Lubricate suppositories before insertion. Nurse should wear a glove when administering suppository.
3. Administer suppository with patient on left side. Deep breath at time of insertion helps patient relax sphincter.
4. Patient remains on side 20 to 30 minutes after administration of suppository.

Administration of enemas

1. Warm solution to body temperature.
2. Administer with patient lying on left side. Insert lubricated rectal tube as patient takes deep breath to relax anal sphincter.
3. Administer 500 ml of enema fluid.
4. Repeat enemas until patient expels clear fluid if cleansing enemas are required (to clear colon for colonoscopy, surgery, or barium enemas).
5. Cleansing enemas are usually used in conjunction with laxatives.

---

high, but the side effects are minimal with these doses. The usual dose is one to two suppositories daily.

Bisacodyl suppositories. Bisacodyl suppositories stimulate rectal motility shortly after administration. They are more effective than glycerin suppositories, but are not 100% effective.

The dose in children under 2 years of age is one 5 mg suppository and in children over 2 years and in adults it is one 10 mg suppository per day. Side effects include rectal irritation and a burning rectal discomfort in some patients, especially with frequent use.

Enemas

Enemas may not be strictly considered as laxatives, but they fall within the general definition, as do *suppositories,* and are included in conjunction with true laxatives.

Enemas are used usually for the purpose of stimulating defecation. They are also used to help cleanse the bowel for surgery or diagnostic study. In addition they are used, (as are other laxatives) in the establishment of bowel training. Common enemas are tap water, normal saline, and soapsuds, all of which appear to be effective. In certain cases, retention oil enemas, such as olive or mineral oil, may be used to soften and lubricate hard fecal mass.

Lower colonic cleansing is usually adequate for sigmoidoscopic examination, certain cases of constipation, and anal surgery. A tap water, saline, or soapsuds enema (500 ml) at or near body temperature may be administered. Usually one to three such enemas are needed to cleanse the lower bowel (see box, above right). Alternately, a phosphate enema may be used and repeated if necessary.

Total colonic cleansing is necessary for surgery of the colon, colonoscopy, and barium studies of the large intestine. In addition to enemas and laxatives, an adequate quantity of clear fluids taken orally for 24 hours is necessary to ensure a clean bowel. A different enema technique is necessary to clean the whole colon. Instead of a 500 ml enema repeated x times, one can use a single 2000 ml–warmed tap water enema. The 2000 ml enema requires skill in administration (see box, p. 885, left). The nurse must position the patient and make sure that the enema bag is no more than 90 cm above the patient. The risk, as in performing a barium enema, includes a colon rupture. In both cases an adequate history is required to ensure that there is no contraindication, such as inflammatory bowel disease and distal colonic obstruction. For preparing the whole colon, many hospital staffs use a regimen of clear fluids administered orally during the 24 hours before the procedure (a minimum of 1 glass of water hourly for 8 hours), two laxatives: castor oil at noon, and X-prep (a senna preparation), and a 2000 ml–cleansing tap water enema 4 hours later.

The risk of morbidity from enemas in adults is small. Minor rectal mucosal injuries can occur but are probably of no significance. Rectal perforations caused by the enema tube occur occasionally. Fluid and electrolyte disturbances can occur, especially in the elderly, who undergo repeated enemas as preparation for a complete gastrointestinal x-ray examination and then undergo additional enema preparation for surgery.

Tap water and normal saline enemas. Tap water and normal saline enemas may be used for colonic cleansing or for the treatment of certain cases of constipation. They probably act by providing bulk to stimulate the defecation reflex and provide a fluid medium for stool evacuation. Enema fluid may cause cramping if too cold or injury if too warm and should thus be warmed to body temperature. Prolonged use of tap

---

Total colonic cleansing

1. Warm water to body temperature.
2. While patient lies on left side and takes deep breath to help relax anal sphincter, insert lubricated rectal tube.
3. Enema bag should not be more than 90 cm above patient.
4. Do not use in patients with inflammatory bowel disease and distal colonic obstruction.
5. Cleansing enemas are usually used in conjunction with laxatives.

Administration of oil retention enema

1. Oil (e.g., olive oil) should be warmed to body temperature.
2. Administer slowly using small rectal tube. Have patient lie on left side and take deep breath at time of insertion of tube to help relax anal sphincter.
3. Administer oil slowly to minimize peristalsis.
4. Retain oil 30 minutes before evacuation.

---

water or normal saline enemas is not advised because fluid and electrolyte disturbances may occur. Tap water is a basic hypotonic solution and although defecation is usually stimulated before the fluid is absorbed into the body from the bowel, fluid can be readily absorbed in patients who have fluid depletion. Because water enemas can cause rapid fluid shift and fluid overload, they should not be used in infants or children. Normal saline is isotonic and no net water flow occurs, although, sodium absorption can be a problem for patients on sodium-restricted diets or who have fluid-volume excess.

Soapsuds enemas. Soapsuds enemas (castile soap added to either tap water or saline enema solutions) probably stimulate the defecation reflex by providing bulk, by causing irritation to the mucosa wall, and providing a fluid medium for evacuation. The temperature of the enema should be at or near body temperature. Soapsuds enemas may be used for colonic cleansing or for the treatment of constipation, but prolonged use is not advised because they can irritate the mucosa and cause rectal inflammation and colitis.

Oil enemas. Vegetable and mineral oils may be used to soften hard stool. In addition, the 150 to 200 ml of oil may provide bulk to stimulate the defecation reflex. The lubrication effect of mineral oil taken orally may not be of much value because it may pass through the anus without causing the hard stool to be evacuated (see box, above right).

Phosphate enemas. Sodium phosphate and sodium biphosphate enemas are commercially available and easy to administer. They are small-volume enemas (120 ml), which because they are hypertonic draw body fluid into the lumen of the bowel. They probably act in a manner similar to saline laxatives; however, because they are hypertonic and thus draw water into the lumen to irritate the mucosal wall and stimulate the defecation reflex, they can cause fluid-volume deficit especially with frequent or chronic use in children, the elderly, or debilitated. In addition, hypernatremia, hyperphosphatemia, and hypocalcemia have been reported following their use. Phosphate enemas work quickly (within minutes) and generally provide a clean bowel for sigmoidoscopy or for anal surgery.

Total intestinal preparation. Total intestinal preparation is a variant of the enema and is an excellent method of preparing the intestines, especially the colon, for surgery, barium studies, and endoscopy. The day before the scheduled procedure or test, a nasogastric tube is inserted, and 8 to 10 L of Ringer's lactate is infused over an 8-hour period. This preparation is well accepted by most patients and those who have had the laxative-enema cleansing combination prefer the total intestinal preparation. This method of bowel cleansing is contraindicated in patients with bowel obstruction and possibly in acute, fulminant inflammatory bowel disease.

Because 1 to 2 L of the cleansing fluid, which contains sodium, may be retained, total intestinal preparation should not be used in patients with congestive heart failure or sodium restrictions. It should also not be used in the sick and frail elderly.

DIARRHEA

Diarrhea may be defined as an increase in the number and frequency of watery stools. More specifically, diarrhea can be defined as passage of greater than 200 gm of stool per day containing 70% to 90% water. The normal number of stools for any one individual varies, but more than three bowel movements per day is generally considered abnormal for the adult on a Western

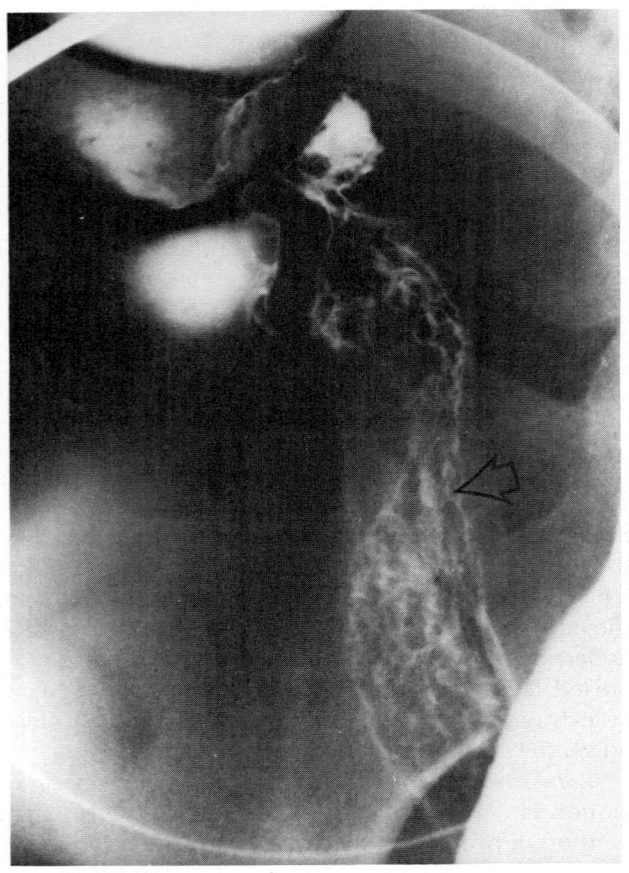

FIGURE 41-1. **Barium enema showing the cecum and terminal ileum. The terminal ileum shows typical changes of Crohn's disease (i.e., limited distention and a cobblestone appearance to the mucosa). (Courtesy Dr. Ann Conrad.)**

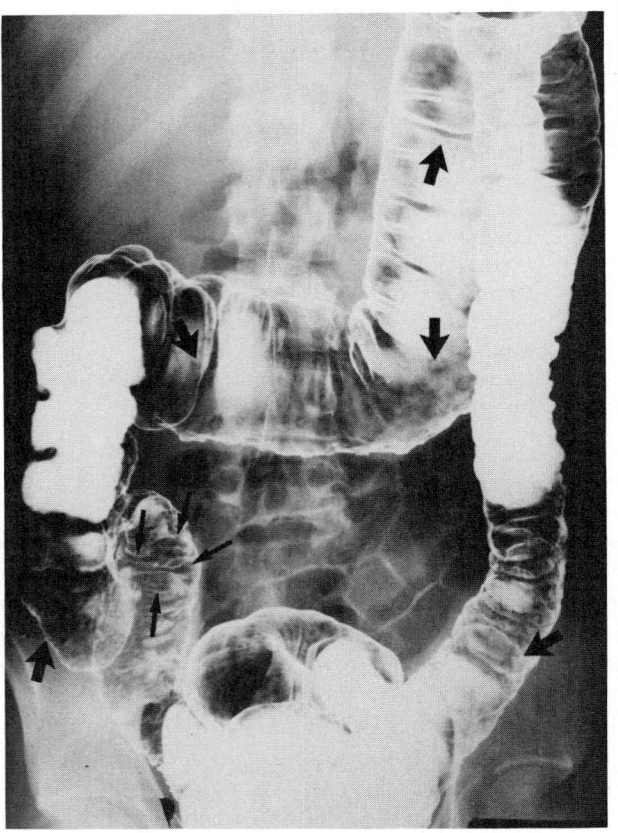

FIGURE 41-2. **Barium enema showing Crohn's disease of the colon. Large arrows point to ulcers in the colon. Small arrows point to ulcers in the terminal ileum.**

diet. Historically diarrhea was thought to be primarily a motility disorder. Although motility alterations may play a role, recent evidence shows that net fluid and electrolyte accumulation is present in most diarrheal disorders. This means that an increase in fluid leaving the small intestine, caused by increased secretion or decreased absorption, may present a fluid load beyond the water absorptive and storage capacities of the colon. In addition to small intestinal causes, diarrhea may be of colonic origin resulting from increased secretion, decreased water absorption, or decreased storage capacity. In certain diseases, such as *Crohn's disease* involving both the large and small intestine (Figures 41-1 and 41-2), diarrhea may be both of small-intestinal and colonic origin.

Diarrhea is a symptom that has many causes. It can be acute, lasting less than 2 weeks, or chronic. The following is a brief outline of the causes grouped under known pathophysiologic changes (modified from Jeejeebhoy (1977) and Fingle and Freston (1979):

I. *Osmotic* retardation of water absorption (mainly in small intestine)
   A. Ingestion of substances that are not absorbed or are poorly absorbed
      1. Artificial sweeteners (e.g., sorbitol)
      2. Lactulose
   B. Dumping associated with abnormal pyloric function
      1. Rapid emptying of hyperosmolar solutions (e.g., carbohydrates) from the stomach as may occur after partial gastrectomy
   C. Malabsorption: presence of certain unabsorbed dietary components in the intestines constitutes an abnormal osmotic load
      1. Enzyme deficiency
         a. Lactose—decreased carbohydrate absorption
         b. Pancreatic lipase—increased fat in colon and its alteration by colonic bacteria

2. Mucosal deficiency (e.g., *sprue*)
3. Gastric acid hypersecretion (e.g., Zollinger-Ellison Syndrome [excess acid impedes ability of jejunum to absorb sodium])
4. Surgical resection of jejunum or ileum (decreased digestive and absorptive capacity)
5. Surgical resection of colon (decreased fluid absorptive capacity)

II. Increased secretion of water and electrolytes
   A. Passive secretion through increased mucosal permeability
      1. Intestinal obstruction
      2. *Inflammatory bowel disease*
      3. *Radiation enteritis*
   B. Active secretion of anions
      1. Bacterial infections
         a. Cholera *enterotoxin*
         b. Perhaps a majority of bacterial infections
      2. Prostaglandins
      3. Bile acids (act on colonic mucosa)
      4. *Vasoactive intestinal peptides*
      5. Increased fatty acid load
      6. *Villous adenoma*
      7. Laxatives
   C. Replacement of absorptive epithelium by crypt epithelium
      1. Viral gastroenteritis

III. Motility disturbances (mechanisms poorly understood or undefined)
   A. Hormonal
      1. Thyrotoxicosis
      2. *Carcinoid* tumors (may secrete hydroxytryptamine)
      3. Prostaglandins
   B. Perhaps inflammatory bowel disease
   C. Perhaps *functional bowel syndrome* (irritable bowel syndrome)

IV. Decreased storage capacity
   A. Inflammatory bowel disease
   B. Subtotal colonic resection

The ileum normally presents about 1000 ml of fluid to the colon daily. The colon absorbs most of the water presented to it, and the daily excretion in the stool is 150 to 300 ml. Normal stools are 60% to 80% water. Colonic absorption takes place through the large surface area of mucosa, aided by the chief colonic movement, segmentation. Segmentation tends to inhibit propulsion of colonic contents toward the anus. Normally the rectum can accommodate about 300 ml of contents before the sensation for a need to defecate is felt.

Current knowledge would indicate that diarrhea occurs as a result of an absolute or relative increase in water presented to or secreted by the colon, and may be associated with motility disturbances and decreased storage capacity of the colon.

Small intestinal water volume may be increased by ingestion of nonabsorbable foods (e.g., sorbitol) or by rapid emptying of hyperosmolar substances (e.g., carbohydrates) from the stomach, a condition that occurs after partial gastrectomy. Malabsorption or inadequate digestion of foods may occur with sprue or *lactase* deficiency, with a resultant inflow of fluid into the intestine. Furthermore, fluid absorption from the small intestine may be impaired (a condition that occurs with gastric acid hypersecretion) because hydrogen ion excess decreases the intestinal mucosa's ability to absorb sodium ions and hence water. Water and anions may be actively secreted into the intestinal lumen by stimulation of cyclic adenosine monophosphate (cyclic AMP), which occurs with intestinal infections such as cholera. Other intestinal infections, such as *Shigella*, also cause active secretion of water and anions, but the exact mechanism(s) of action are not clear yet. In infections with *Shigella dysenteriae I* and *Staphylococcus aureus* there is evidence that damage to intestinal mucosa and inhibition of active absorptive process occurs. Furthermore, the absorptive surface may be reduced (as it is with extensive intestinal resection). With resection of the ileum absorption of fluid is impaired, and absorption of the bile salts, which upon entering the colon stimulate the colonic mucosa to secrete water decreases. Increased volume of contents in the intestine tends to stimulate motility, and by speeding up transit of contents it may further inhibit fluid absorption. Thus through these various mechanisms an increased fluid load is presented to the colon.

The colon can absorb a limited quantity of water, perhaps up to 1000 ml per day. If the ileal outflow is increased beyond the absorptive capacity of the colon, the increased volume will probably stimulate some colonic motility and the defecation reflex. If the ileal outflow increases 300 ml over normal capacity, and the colon cannot adapt to absorb more water, the person may have two or more fluid stools per day.

Diarrhea from increased ileal effluent into the colon becomes worse if the disease process also involves any of the following problems with the colon: colonic absorption decreases, colonic mucosa increases secretion (e.g., pancreatic insufficiency), or colonic motility increases. Even if ileal discharge into the colon is normal, purely colonic diseases (which cause decreased fluid absorption, increase water and electrolyte secretion [e.g., Crohn's colitis, *ulcerative colitis*], increase colonic mass movements, or reduce rectal storage capacity [e.g., Crohn's colitis, ulcerative colitis]), may cause diarrhea. In certain conditions where there is no evident colonic disease, people may get diarrhea because of stress (e.g., stress of exams). Irritable bowel syndrome may also cause diarrhea, but the mechanism of diarrhea is not understood.

In evaluating a patient with diarrhea, the nurse should include in the history the onset and duration of symptoms and any associated symptoms. Diarrhea of sudden onset accompanied by fever, abdominal cramps, nausea, and vomiting is most likely of infectious origin. A history of acute-onset diarrhea should include if other members of the family have similar problems. It should note recent travel and any recent ingestion of drugs including antibiotics (e.g., pseudomembraneous enterocolitis) or laxatives. Longstanding or chronic diarrhea is less likely to be of infectious origin and may be caused by lactose deficiency (e.g., milk intolerance) or inflammatory bowel disease. The presence or absence of blood or mucus in both acute and chronic diarrheas may help in the diagnosis.

Watson (1977) in his article "Clinical Diagnosis of the Cause of Diarrhea" summarizes and clarifies the clinical approach to diarrhea as follows:

I. Acute diarrhea
   A. Noninfectious, without blood or mucus (these are infectious but stool investigations are commonly not helpful)
      1. Viral gastroenteritis
      2. Traveler's diarrhea
      3. Food poisoning
   B. Noninfectious, with blood or mucus
      1. *Salmonella* infections
      2. Cholera
   C. Infectious with blood and mucus
      1. *Bacillary dysentery*
      2. *Amebic dysentery*
II. Chronic diarrhea
   A. Noninfectious, without blood or mucus
      1. Malabsorption
      2. Laxative abuse
      3. Lactose intolerance
      4. Bile salt abnormalities
   B. Noninfectious, with blood and mucus (may be infectious but no organisms have ben isolated as yet)
      1. Crohn's disease
      2. Ulcerative colitis
   C. Noninfectious with mucus
      1. Irritable bowel syndrome

   D. Infectious, without blood or mucus
      1. Blind loop syndromes
      2. Giardiasis
   E. Infectious, with blood and mucus
      1. Amebic dysentery
      2. Schistosomal infection

Physical examination may reveal signs of dehydration, such as loss of skin turgor and increased pulse rate. The temperature may be elevated in infectious diarrheas. Skin changes such as *pyoderma gangrenosum* and *erythema nodosum* may be suggestive of inflammatory bowel disease. Abdominal, perianal, and rectal examination may not be helpful but may indicate a mass (if in right lower quadrant may suggest Crohn's disease) or tenderness (if in left lower quadrant may suggest diverticular disease).

Investigation should include sigmoidoscopy, warm stool for culture and sensitivity and examination for ova and parasites. Stool analysis should be done to exclude some of the malabsorption causes (e.g., steatorrhea). Sigmoidoscopy with mucosal biopsies (and sometimes colonoscopy examinations) is usually part of the investigation of diarrhea. Barium enemas, barium meals, small intestinal barium studies, and small intestinal biopsy (e.g., in sprue) round out the investigation of diarrhea.

Treatment of diarrheas consists of two aspects, one that deals with the causes (e.g., stop laxatives in patients that abuse them) and the other with the symptoms (e.g., opiates to reduce cramps and frequency of stools in traveler's diarrhea, and to correct dehydration and electrolyte imbalance).

ANTIDIARRHEALS

Antidiarrheals include those therapeutic agents that are used to reduce the frequency and fluidity of diarrheal bowel movements. Discussion of antidiarrheal agents does not usually include antibiotics. Antidiarrheals are probably best grouped under their mechanisms of action, which include the following broad categories: (1) agents that absorb water (hydrophilic agents), (2) agents that alter intestinal motility, (3) agents that alter electrolyte transport, and (4) agents that adsorb etiologic factors (*adsorbents*).

Agents that absorb water (hydrophilic agents)

Hydrophilic agents absorb water from the intestinal tract and thereby increase the consistency of stools while decreasing their frequency. These agents cause an increase in the electrolyte and water loss, which can be measured in the ileostomy effluent. The two main hydrophilic agents that have been used in the treatment of diarrhea are plantago seed preparations and polycarbophil.

Plantago seed. Plantago seed preparations are obtained from ground, dried, ripe seeds of the Plantago family of plants. These compounds can absorb a great deal of water, thus making the stool more solid and slowing down the diarrhea. Because of these hydrophilic properties, plantago preparations are also used in treatment of constipation. Plantago preparations appear to be as effective as polycarbophil. The usual dose is 5 to 15 gm in water or fruit juice one to three times daily. Effervescent plantago preparations are more palatable, and the usual dose of the lime-lemon flavored powder is one package one to three times daily in a small amount of water. Effervescent plantago preparations contain sodium and should not be used in patients who are on salt-restricted diets (e.g., patients with congestive heart failure). Although excessive fluid intake should be avoided, because these preparations have been associated with esophageal and bowel obstruction, they should be taken in adequate amounts of water.

Polycarbophil. Polycarbophil is a synthetic resin of the polycarbophilic acid type. Although the granules are pharmacologically inert, they are able to bind about 60 times their weight in water. The average adult dose is 1 to 1.5 gm four times a day. For children, the total daily dose is 0.5 to 1.5 gm for patients between 2 and 5 years of age and 1.5 to 3.0 gm for patients over 5 years of age.

Agents that alter intestinal motility

Opiates. Opiates that are used as antidiarrheal agents include tincture of opium, paregoric, codeine, and synthetic compounds such as diphenoxylate (with atropine added) and loperamide. These compounds appear to inhibit propulsive movements in the small intestine and colon, allowing for more absorption of water and electrolytes. The decrease in the propulsive activity appears to be caused by an increase in the tone and segmenting activity. There also appears to be some evidence that the opiates may stimulate sodium and chloride ion absorption. A further benefit of the opiates, in addition to decreasing the frequency and increasing the consistency of stool, is that they tend to relieve abdominal crampy pain. Water and electrolyte losses in ileostomy effluent are reduced by opiates. Opiates may increase the risk of *toxic megacolon* in patients with fairly fulminant inflammatory bowel disease, especially ulcerative colitis. Opiates are contraindicated in patients with *Shigella* and *Salmonella* infections because they may prolong the symptoms and course of the disease. Opiates should not be used concurrently with other CNS depressants because they can potentiate their effects.

Tincture of opium. Opium tincture is a mixture of opium, alcohol, and water containing 10% of opium (1% of morphine). This medication has analgesic and narcotic properties, and prolonged use may lead to addiction. It is an effective compound to slow down diarrhea and reduce abdominal cramps. The average adult oral dose is 0.6 to 1.5 ml, every 4 to 6 hours (equivalent to 6 to 15 mg of morphine). Oral opium compounds are not well absorbed, and the systemic effects of even 1.5 ml orally are minimal compared with an equivalent dose being administered parenterally. Opium tincture should not be used in fulminant ulcerative colitis because of the risk of toxic megacolon. Tincture of opium should not be confused with camphorated opium tincture or paregoric, which is 25 times as potent.

Paregoric. Paregoric is a camphorated opium tincture that also contains benzoic acid, camphor, and anise oil. It is used alone or in other mixtures as an antidiarrheal.

Paregoric, which is poorly absorbed, may cause addiction with prolonged use. The usual adult dose is 1 to 2 teaspoons or 5 to 10 ml containing 20 mg of powdered opium ever 4 to 6 hours. Paregoric should not be used in conjunction with other CNS depressants because their depressant effects may be potentiated.

Codeine. Codeine is an opium derivative that is fairly well absorbed orally. It is an effective antidiarrheal medication and compares favorably in this regard with diphenoxylate-atropine. The usual adult dose is 15 to 30 mg by mouth every 4 to 6 hours. Prolonged use may cause addiction, but this risk is fairly low. Side effects include nausea, vomiting, and drowsiness. Use is contraindicated in those individuals with a known sensitivity to codeine.

Diphenoxylate-atropine mixture. Diphenoxylate is a meperidine derivative that has constipating properties because of its antiperistaltic effect but does not possess analgesic activities. It is usually sold as a diphenoxylate-atropine mixture (diphenoxylate 2.5 mg and atropine 25 μg per tablet or per 5 ml of solution). Atropine does not appear to decrease the addiction potential of diphenoxylate.

The usual adult dose is 5 mg (2 tablets) every 6 hours (or less). This dosage may be reduced to 2.5 mg every 6 hours as the diarrhea is brought under control.

In children the dose varies with age:

Children 2 to 5 years—2.5 mg twice a day

Children 6 to 8 years—2.5 mg three times daily

Children 9 to 12 years—2.5 mg four times daily

Children over 12 years—5 mg three times daily

Side effects include nausea, vomiting, dizziness, and a dry mouth. This drug should not be used in *Shigella* infections. The atropine component increases toxicity in children especially those with a fluid volume deficit. Diphenoxylate does not appear to have any advantage as an antidiarrheal over codeine. There is a risk of toxic megacolon when diphenoxylate is used as an antidiarrheal in fulminant inflammatory bowel disease.

Loperamide. Loperamide, a synthetic opiate structurally related to diphenoxylate, is an effective antidiarrheal agent. It reduces stool frequency in many diarrheal disorders, including inflammatory bowel disease and irritable bowel syndrome. Loperamide inhibits peristalsis, relieves cramps, and does not cause morphine-like behavioral effects even in high doses. Its duration of action appears to be longer than other opiates.

The adult dose is 4 mg initially, followed by 2 mg after each loose stool to a maximum of 16 mg per day. The average adult dose is 4 to 8 mg per day. The safety of this drug has not been established in pregnant women, nursing mothers, or children. There has been no evidence of tolerance, and incidence of side effects of this drug is low. The reported adverse effects include nausea, abdominal pain, dizziness, and dry mouth.

Antispasmodics

Atropine. Fingle and Freston (1979) point out that from data available there is little evidence that atropine and related antispasmodics play a significant role in the management of diarrhea. In his extensive review of anticholinergics used in treatment of irritable colon syndrome, Ivey (1975) surmises that there is no justification to use these agents in patients with "nervous diarrhea" except perhaps in those with pain as a predominant feature.

Agents that alter electrolyte transport

Agents that alter electrolyte transport are still experimental and are not used routinely for the treatment of diarrhea. Some of the agents that are being evaluated include aspirin, indomethacin, and sulfasalazine.

Adsorbents

The adsorbent antidiarrheals include kaolin, pectin, activated charcoal, aluminum hydroxide, bismuth salts, and attapulgite. Apart from clinical observations of constipation with use of aluminum hydroxide, there is little objective evidence that these agents are effective antidiarrheals. In theory, the adsorbents adsorb enterotoxins, bacteria, viruses, and bile salts; some also have hydrophilic properties.

General adsorbents

Kaolin. Kaolin is a native hydrated aluminum silicate that has been used alone or in combination with other agents in the treatment of diarrhea. This agent is not absorbed by the body. Although it is a commonly used antidiarrheal, there is little objective evidence of its efficacy in medical literature. The usual adult dose is 2 to 30 gm after each bowel movement. In children under 1 year, 1 gm of kaolin may be given 4 to 6 times daily. Kaolin adsorbs such drugs as lincomyin and digoxin and therefore should not be used concurrently with these drugs.

Pectin. Pectin, derived from apples and citrus fruit rinds, is used as an antidiarrheal alone or in combination with kaolin. There is little objective evidence of its efficacy as an antidiarrheal.

Activated charcoal. Activated charcoal is a black, tasteless, odorless powder, prepared from organic material such as peat. It has a high adsorptive capacity. It is difficult to assess how useful charcoal is in the treatment of diarrhea because it is rarely used today. Activated charcoal is capable of adsorbing aspirin, amphetamines, and other drugs and may be used in the treatment of certain drug overdoses.

Attapulgite. Attapulgite is a hydrated magnesium aluminum silicate. Although it is a good adsorbent, its role in the treatment of diarrhea is uncertain.

Aluminum hydroxide. Aluminum hydroxide is commonly used as an antacid, and one of its chief side effects is constipation. As an antidiarrheal it is also used in combination with other compounds, such as kaolin. Its role as an antidiarrheal agent is not well quantitated. The average adult dose is 0.5 to 1 gm, every 2 to 4 hours. The absorption of anticholinergics and tetracyclines may be impaired by aluminum hydroxide which should not be taken concurrently with these drugs.

Bismuth preparations. Bismuth compounds have been used for many gastrointestinal disorders including diarrhea. There is little objective evidence that this drug (probably obsolete) has much use in the treatment of diarrhea.

Ion-exchange resins

Cholestyramine. Cholestyramine is an ion exchange resin that exchanges chloride ions for bile salts and then binds them into an insoluble complex, which is excreted in the feces. Unfortunately, in addition to bile salts, it binds many drugs, such as anticoagulants, digitalis, phenobarbital, and thyroxine. Therefore, it should not be used in combination with these drugs.

Bile salts are absorbed from the intestinal tract, mainly the ileum, and enter into the bile acid pool of the enterohepatic circulation. With ileal resection, an increased amount of bile salts enter the colon and can cause diarrhea by inhibiting multiple transport processes, thereby increasing the net intestinal sodium and water. Fecal bile acid excretion is increased in postvagotomy patients and appears to be the cause of diarrhea in these patients. Diarrhea occuring after ileal resection and after vagotomy is improved with cholestyramine.

The usual adult dose of cholestyramine is 4 gm 3 times a day and at bedtime. The average dose for children over age 6 is 80 mg/kg 3 times a day. Since cholestyramine may bind other drugs, such as anticoagulants and digitalis, these drugs should not be given within 1 hour before or 4 hours after administration of cholestyramine. Side effects of this agent in large doses include steatorrhea, heartburn, and nausea.

ANTIMICROBIALS (TREATMENT OF INFECTIOUS DIARRHEAS)

The discussion of antimicrobial agents is outside the scope of this chapter (see Sections IX, "Antiparasitic Medications," and X, "Antibacterial, Antifungal, and Antiviral Medications"). However, an outline of the antimicrobial agents used in treatment of infectious diarrheas is included.

Infectious diarrheas are caused by a variety of microorganisms including viruses, chlamydia, bacteria, protozoa, helminths, and fungi. Most, if not all, of these diarrheas are associated with a net secretion of fluids and electrolytes.

The usual treatment for infectious diarrheas includes adequate hydration and electrolyte replacement, especially in infants, the elderly, and debilitated; symptomatic use of antidiarrheals; and in many causes a specific antimicrobial agent to deal with the causative organisms.

A summary of infectious organisms and the antimicrobial agents that are effective follows (modified from Edwards, 1977):

Organism	Effective therapeutic agent
Viruses	None
Chlamydia	
Lymphogranuloma venereum	Tetracycline or sulfadiazine
Bacteria	
Staphylococcus aureus (superinfection)	Vancomycin
Salmonella typhi infection	Chloramphenicol
Clostridium botulinum (food poisoning)	Penicillin
Vibrio cholerae	Tetracycline
Shigella	Tetracycline or ampicillin
Mycobacterium tuberculosis	Routine antitubercular drugs
Neisseria gonorrhoeae	Penicillin or tetracycline
Yersinia enterocolitica	Trimethoprim

Organism	Effective therapeutic agent
Protozoa	
Entamoeba histolytica	Metronidazole
Giardia lamblia	Metronidazole
Helminths	
Ascaris lumbricoides	Piperazine citrate
Trichinella spiralis	Piperazine citrate
Strongyloides stercoralis	Thiabendazole
Taenia solium	Niclosamide
Schistosoma mansoni	Niridazole
Schistosoma japonicum	Potassium antimony tartrate
Fasciola hepatica	Emetine hydrochloride
Trichuris trichiura	Mebendazole
Fungi	
Candida albicans	Mycostatin
Histoplasma capsulatum	Amphotericin B
Actinomyces israelii	Penicillin or tetracycline

SUMMARY

Constipation is a condition in which there is infrequent, often difficult passage of hard and dry stool. It has both congenital and acquired causes. Laxatives are used in the symptomatic treatment of constipation or for bowel preparation related to certain diagnostic tests or surgery. They are highly abused by the lay public who may not have adequate knowledge of normal bowel function.

Diarrhea, a condition in which there is an increase in the fluidity and number of stools, is probably associated with an increase in the net secretion of water and electrolytes and with a motility disorder. Most of the antidiarrheals are used in the symptomatic treatment of diarrhea and attempt to decrease the fluidity and number of stools. Many of the over-the-counter antidiarrheals (e.g., kaolin) do not have any objective evidence of their efficacy. Antimicrobial agents act directly on the causative organisms. See Section IX, "Antiparasitic Medications," and Section X, "Antibacterial, Antifungal, and Antiviral Medications," for a discussion of the pharmacology of antimicrobials.

In the community and hospital, the nurse has an important role in helping patients establish and maintain normal bowel function. The identification of those patients prone to elimination problems is essential so that problems can be prevented. Dietary education, pharmacologic intervention, and self-care measures can do much to ensure adequate bowel function.

ADVERSE/SIDE EFFECTS OF LAXATIVES AND ANTIDIARRHEALS*

ALLERGIC REACTIONS

Pigmentation
Pruritus (itching)
Skin rash

AUTONOMIC NERVOUS SYSTEM

Anticholinergic effect (dry mouth,
  urinary retention, visual
  disturbances)
Paralytic ileus

BEHAVIOR

Dependence (addiction)
Impaired function because of
  oversedation

CARDIOVASCULAR SYSTEM

Hypovolemia

CENTRAL NERVOUS SYSTEM

Confusion
Depression
Dizziness
Headache
Insomnia
Restlessness

GASTROINTESTINAL SYSTEM

Anorexia
Bloating
Constipation
Diarrhea
Fecal impaction
Heartburn
Nausea
Melanosis coli
Paralytic ileus
Procititis
Rectal burning discomfort
Steatorrhea
Toxic megacolon
Vomiting

HEPATIC SYSTEM

Cytotoxic effect (docusates)

**METABOLIC AND ENDOCRINE
SYSTEMS**

Dehydration

RENAL SYSTEM

Urinary retention

RESPIRATORY SYSTEM

Depression of respiratory function
Lipid pneumonitis (mineral oil)

*See Chapter 11, "Drug Toxicity," for an overview of drug toxicity.

CLINICALLY SIGNIFICANT DRUG INTERACTIONS*

Primary drug	Interacting drug	Possible effect(s)	Probable mechanism(s)
Bisacodyl	Antacids	Gastric irritation	Increased release of bisacodyl in stomach
Cholestyramine	Anticoagulants	Decreased anticoagulant effect	Decreased absorption
Cholestyramine	Chlorothiazide	Decreased chlorothiazide effect	Decreased absorption
Cholestyramine	Digitalis	Decreased digitalis effect	Decreased absorption
Cholestyramine	Thyroxine	Decreased thyroxine effect	Decreased absorption
Kaolin	Digoxin	Decreased effectiveness digoxin	Decreased absorption
Kaolin	Tetracycline	Decreased effectiveness tetracycline	Decreased absorption
Mineral oil (chronic use)	Fat soluble substances & vitamins	Decreased effectiveness of fat-soluble substances and vitamins	Decreased absorption

*See Chapter 10, "Drug Interactions," for an overview of drug interactions.

GENERAL NURSING IMPLICATIONS

Nursing of patients requiring laxatives

ASSESSMENT

A complete nursing assessment is essential in establishing a baseline from which to plan an individualized laxative therapy regimen and to monitor patient response. Assessment should include a detailed drug history to identify individual sensitivity, possible contraindications to laxative therapy, cautions, potential drug interactions, and individual laxative-taking patterns before therapy is initiated.

Assessment should include detailed baseline data related to the patient's individual bowel and elimination habits and patterns. The frequency and characteristic of usual stool, time of elimination, aids utilized (such as warm drinks in the morning), previous problems with constipation and how these have been treated, and the presence of an ileostomy or colostomy. All these facts should be noted. The current general health state should also be noted.

To identify possible causes of constipation, a dietary history is often indicated to assess the amount of fiber, fluids, and bulk in the diet. Foods that cause constipation should be identified and avoided when possible. The patient's age and developmental stage, self-toileting skills and abilities, attitudes toward elimination practices, and level of knowledge are important considerations in planning laxative therapy. Pregnancy, gastrointestinal disorders, hemorrhoids, or cardiac disease should be noted.

The patient's activity level should also be assessed. Patients who are immobile (including those patients on bed rest and neurologically impaired patients, surgical patients, postanesthesia patients, pregnant and postpartum patients, and the elderly) are especially prone to constipation related to immobility and to weakened abdominal or pelvic floor musculature. These data are important in planning to promote and maintain bowel elimination patterns and to prevent overuse of laxatives.

Physical assessment of the patient should include assessment of the quantity and quality of bowel sounds, the presence of abdominal distention, a rigid abdomen, or abdominal cramps, tenderness, or pain. A digital examination of the rectum may be indicated if an impaction is suspected before laxative therapy is initiated. Because an impaction may be present higher in the colon, if not palpated, further tests may be indicated.

When completing the patient assessment, the nurse should recognize that serious disease conditions, such as intestinal obstruction, diverticulitis, hypothyroidism, megacolon, and cancer or tumors of the rectum or lower bowel, may produce symptoms of constipation. The patient should be carefully questioned regarding the duration and severity of the constipation, other accompanying symptoms, and changes in elimination patterns over time.

A careful drug history is required to assess self-medication behaviors; identify drugs that the patient may be taking that can cause constipation, including aluminum- and calcium- containing antacids, anticholinergics, antihistamines, depressants, diuretics, hormone preparations, muscle relaxants, opium derivatives (codeine and morphine sulfate) and tranquilizers. Potential drug interactions (see Clinically Significant Drug Interactions) and misuse of laxatives should also be explored.

SENSITIVITY

Although laxatives are not usually associated with sensitivity reactions, it must be remembered that any medication has the potential to cause an allergic reaction in a susceptible individual. Phenolphthaleins may occasionally cause hypersensitivity reactions characterized by skin rashes, lupus erythematosus–like syndrome, or Stevens-Johnson syndrome. The yellow unpurified form is more sensitizing in sensitive individuals than the white purified form.

CONTRAINDICATIONS

Laxatives are contraindicated because of the risk of perforation of the bowel in patients with the following: intraabdominal inflammation, obstructive lesions of the bowel, acute abdomen (appendicitis), and intestinal obstructions.

In addition, because certain laxatives (e.g., bisacodyl) are excreted in breast milk, these laxatives are contraindicated in nursing mothers because laxative effects can occur in the infant (see the Nursing Drug Digest for each specific laxative).

CAUTIONS

Habituation (cathartic colon) may occur with chronic use of laxatives (including suppositories) or enemas. If the colon becomes dilated, the defecation reflex can become blunted, thus reinforcing the need for laxatives. Frequent or chronic use of laxatives can also cause fluid and electrolyte imbalances.

DRUG INTERACTIONS

Laxatives can interact with various drugs. For example, laxatives that increase gastrointestinal motility (e.g., bisacodyl) can increase the rate at which drugs pass through the gastrointestinal tract, decreasing their rate of absorption. Other laxatives (e.g., docusates) can enhance the absorption of coadministered drugs (see Clinically Significant Drug Interactions for important drug interactions).

ADMINISTRATION

Laxatives should not be administered to patients with intestinal obstruction, appendicitis, or diverticulitis or intraabdominal inflammation because of the danger of perforation.

Administer laxatives at a time that will not interfere with digestion or absorption of nutrients, rest or sleep, or other activities that cannot be interrupted.

Schedule laxative administration to work in relation to the defecation reflex (e.g., after meals, especially breakfast) (see the Nursing Drug Digest for administration information for each specific laxative). *Continued.*

GENERAL NURSING IMPLICATIONS—cont'd

Nursing of patients requiring laxatives—cont'd

ADMINISTRATION—cont'd

Depending on the patient's condition, a bedpan, commode, or bathroom should be readily accessible. Privacy and odor control should be ensured. The call light should be readily available for patients requiring direct assistance.

MONITORING PATIENT RESPONSE
Therapeutic response

Most laxatives, including enemas and suppositories, take between 15 minutes and 3 days to act, producing individual variation in response. Generally, for simple constipation, a bowel movement should be obtained within 1 week. With planned therapy including the use of diet, fluids, exercise, and other nonpharmacologic interventions, a bowel pattern should be established where the adult patient has two to three formed, soft brown stools per day or 1 to 3 per week, depending on past individual pattern, fluid and food intake, health state, and other factors of daily living. For infants the usual pattern may be from 3 to 5 stools per day. The patient should not have cramping pain or discomfort associated with defecation. If pain or discomfort persists or if a bowel movement has not occured for 1 week or longer, further assessment and treatment are indicated.

Adverse side effects

Laxatives can produce fluid and electrolyte imbalances, cramping, discoloration of the urine and dehydration (see Adverse/Side Effects for common side effects associated with laxatives).

Observe for signs of dehydration and electrolyte imbalance (weakness, loss of skin turgor, dry mucous membranes, dry deep furrowed tongue) especially in the elderly who have had laxatives, including enemas, in preparation for gastrointestinal barium studies and surgery. These deficiencies are corrected by intravenous fluids and electrolytes.

Observe for fluid overload as evidenced by signs of congestive heart failure (shortness of breath, orthopnea) in elderly patients undergoing total bowel preparation. Those patients may retain sodium-containing irrigating solutions, and their cardiovascular system may be unable to compensate for the increased fluid load.

Monitor for marked reversal of symptoms (e.g., patient treated for constipation who has recurrent diarrhea after therapy is initiated).

PATIENT EDUCATION

The patient and family should have a clear understanding of the medication regimen; they should know the exact name of the medication, its action, dosage, storage, administration, and side effects, and what to do to minimize side effects. They should know how to monitor therapeutic effects and be able to identify signs that indicate the health care provider should be contacted. The importance of assisting patients with the maintenance of normal bowel function is extremely important. With careful preparation, the patient should be able to do the following:

1. State the name of the medication.
2. Explain the purpose of the medication.
3. Describe the dosage schedule, including foods or beverages that should be avoided when taking the medication (e.g., avoiding milk or antacids when taking bisacodyl tablets, which can dissolve the enteric coating, resulting in gastric irritation).
4. Describe or demonstrate the method of administration.
5. Describe or demonstrate appropriate storage of the medication.
6. Describe how long the medication should be taken, when it should be discontinued, how to dispose of leftover medication, or how to appropriately obtain more medication as needed.
7. State how common side effects would be recognized.
8. Describe the management of side effects as indicated.
9. Identify when to expect the drug to be effective.
10. State effects that indicate the health care provider should be contacted.
11. Discuss the use of other medications with the health care provider before they are taken with the recognition that laxatives can interact with numerous prescription and nonprescription drugs.

Patient education should also include information about normal bowel function, prevention of constipation, and the dangers associated with the unnecessary use or abuse of laxatives (including laxative habit and cathartic colon). Patients should be aware that certain laxatives with frequent or chronic use can cause fluid and electrolyte imbalances, vitamin deficiencies, and loss of colon muscle tone.

The patient and family members should understand that normal bowel function can be achieved and maintained through a diet that contains high fiber and bulk, including fresh fruits, vegetables, bran, and whole grain cereals. Maintaining an adequate fluid intake of 8 to 10 glasses of water, fruit juices, and liquid foods and exercising regularly can also prevent constipation.

Patients and family members should initiate and maintain regular bowel habits and not ignore the defecation reflex. They should allow time for defecation and maintain a routine time for elimination.

The patient and family should recognize that stress, a change in diet, lack of exercise, and travel can cause constipation that is self-limiting. They should know that simple constipation with symptoms of anorexia, abdominal distention, or discomfort can be treated with a laxative selected in relation to their individual health needs. If the constipation is not relieved with use of the laxative in 1 week, the laxative should be stopped, and the health care provider should be contacted.

Constipation that lasts for 2 weeks, sudden change in bowel patterns, and abdominal pain are reasons for the patient to contact a health care provider before self-medication with laxatives is initiated.

GENERAL NURSING IMPLICATIONS—cont'd

Nursing of patients requiring antidiarrheals

ASSESSMENT

A complete nursing assessment is essential in establishing a baseline from which to plan individualized antidiarrheal therapy regimens and to monitor patient response. Assessment should include a detailed drug history to identify individual sensitivity, possible drug-related causes of diarrhea, contraindications to antidiarrheal therapy, cautions, potential drug interactions, and individual past use of antidiarrheals.

Assessment should also include detailed baseline data related to the patient's overall health state with special attention to fluid and electrolyte status and usual bowel habits and patterns (including the frequency, characteristics, color and amount of diarrhea stool). The onset of diarrhea, its duration and associated symptoms, such as abdominal discomfort, cramping, nausea, and vomiting, should be noted. The presence of rectal bleeding and anal irritation should also be noted. This information is important in planning care and recording therapeutic drug effects.

A dietary history should also be included because certain foods may be associated with the diarrhea.

A careful drug history is required to assess self-medication behaviors and to identify drugs that the patient may be taking that can cause diarrhea including antibiotics (e.g., ampicillin, cephalosporins, clindamycin, neomycin, and tetracyclines), antihypertensives (e.g., guanethedine), antidysrhythmics (e.g., digitalis, propranolol, quinidine), potassium supplements, lactulose, and laxatives. Potential drug interactions can also be identified (see Clinically Significant Drug Interactions).

SENSITIVITY

Although antidiarrheals, other than those containing codeine, are not usually associated with sensitivity reactions, it must be remembered that any medication has the potential to cause an allergic reaction in a susceptible individual.

CONTRAINDICATIONS

Antidiarrheals are contraindicated in patients with known sensitivity to the drug, constipation, impaction, and self-limiting acute diarrhea. Opiates are contraindicated in *Shigella* and *Salmonella* infections because they can prolong symptoms (see the Nursing Drug Digest for each specific antidiarrheal).

CAUTIONS

Addiction may occur with chronic use of antidiarrheals containing opiates (e.g., codeine, paregoric, tincture of opium). In addition, opiates should be used cautiously with concurrent use of other CNS depressants because they can potentiate their effects. Chronic use of antidiarrheals can also result in constipation.

DRUG INTERACTIONS

Antidiarrheals can interact with various drugs. For example, activated charcoal, because of its adsorptive properties, can decrease the effects of aspirin, phenytoin, and other medications. Kaolin can decrease the absorption of anticholinergics, lincomycin, and tetracycline (see Clinically Significant Drug Interactions).

ADMINISTRATION

Antidiarrheals are administered in relation to the number and consistency of diarrhea stools. The dosage is reduced with the control of the frequency and consistency of stool. Some antidiarrheals are administered after each unformed stool, not exceeding a specific amount of drug per day (see the Nursing Drug Digest for administration information for each specific antidiarrheal).

MONITORING PATIENT RESPONSE
Therapeutic response

The various antidiarrheals act at different times, producing individual variation in response. Generally, decrease in the number and fluidity or increased consistency of stools is indicative of therapeutic response. Antidiarrheals that act by decreasing intestinal motility, such as opiates, will also decrease cramping and abdominal pain.

Monitoring of therapeutic response is especially important in the prevention of fluid and electrolyte imbalance that can occur in prolonged diarrheal states, especially in the young, elderly, or ill individual in whom dehydration, potassium deficit, and acidosis can occur. Dosage and administration are often associated with therapeutic response and are important in planning dosage and administration regimens. For example, dosage may be reduced for some antidiarrheals as frequency and fluidity of stools decrease, whereas some antidiarrheals (e.g., diphenoxylate with atropine) are administered after each diarrhea stool not exceeding a total amount per day.

Adverse side effects

Antidiarrheals can produce side or adverse effects related specifically to their active compounds. For example, addiction can occur with prolonged use of opiates. Codeine-containing products can cause nausea, vomiting, and drowsiness. Atropine-containing products can cause dry mouth and other atropine effects, especially in children (see Adverse/Side Effects for general side and adverse effects related to the use of antidiarrheals, and see the Nursing Drug Digest for important side and adverse effects of each specific medication).

Constipation can result from the overuse of antidiarrheals, and the monitoring of elimination is essential (e.g., observe and report if patient treated for diarrhea has not had a bowel movement for 1 to 3 days after therapy is initiated).

PATIENT EDUCATION

The patient and family should have a clear understanding of the medication regimen; they should know the exact name of the medication, its action, dosage, storage, administration, and side effects, and how side effects can be managed or minimized. They should know how to monitor therapeutic response and when the prescriber should be notified in relation to inadequate response to antidiarrheal therapy or sequelae (including fluid and

Continued.

GENERAL NURSING IMPLICATIONS—cont'd

Nursing of patients requiring antidiarrheals—cont'd

PATIENT EDUCATION—cont'd

electrolyte imbalance). Patients should know how to prevent diarrhea from recurring, or if chronic diarrhea is an aspect of their health condition, they should understand how to manage it appropriately.

In general, the patient and family should avoid foods that cause individual problems with diarrhea (e.g., avoid milk and milk products if they have lactose deficiency, avoid sudden increase in the ingestion of fruits and vegetables that can be incompletely digested in the small intestine and metabolized by colonic bacteria, causing osmotic diarrhea and symptoms of gaseousness). They should avoid gas-producing foods, such as beans and cabbage. They should assess water supplies carefully, especially if in mountain areas (i.e., for giardiasis). They should practice handwashing and care in food preparation. Patients should understand how to alter self-care related to self-limiting diarrhea, including the use of clear liquids, weak teas, clear broths, ginger ale, and gelatin to rest the bowel and prevent fluid and electrolyte imbalance, progressing the diet and activity as tolerated. They should also be able to recognize when self-care is ineffective in controlling the condition and when to contact their health care provider. They should understand the importance of and procedure for the collection of specimens to ensure accuracy in collection and prevention of undue anxiety and embarrassment.

GENERAL INSTRUCTIONS FOR DISCHARGE/OUTPATIENTS

LAXATIVES

This medication is a laxative used to treat constipation. Follow the instructions on the label. Read the label carefully and do *not* take more than the recommended dose or more often than recommended because abdominal pain and cramping may occur.

Do *not* take laxatives regularly. Increasing your dietary bulk by eating fresh fruits, vegetables, nuts (especially those with skins), and whole grain cereals can help you maintain normal bowel function. Moderate regular exercise (especially walking) and drinking 8 to 10 glasses of water a day can also help prevent the need for laxatives. Your nurse can help you to maintain normal bowel function.

While you are taking this laxative, check with your health care provider before you start or stop taking any other medications because this laxative can affect how another drug can work. If you have nausea, vomiting, or pain in your stomach or gut, do *not* take this medication. Contact your health care provider.

Notify your health care provider if you have a change in your usual bowel habits that lasts for more than 2 weeks.

Contact your health care provider if this laxative has not relieved your constipation after 1 week of use as directed.

Keep this medication and all other medications out of the reach of children.

Bisacodyl

This drug may be taken in tablet form by mouth or as a suppository rectally.

In addition, if your medication is:

Tablets

The tablets should not be crushed, chewed, or broken before swallowing because they have a special coating that prevents the stomach from being irritated. Milk or antacids can dissolve this coating and should not be taken with the tablet. Swallow the tablet whole with a full glass of water or juice. Store tablets in a dry, dark place. Refrigeration is not necessary.

Suppositories

Suppositories should be stored in the refrigerator. Do not freeze them and be sure they are out of the reach of children. Unwrap the suppository and insert it into the rectum as instructed by your nurse. If you have any questions, be sure to ask your nurse. Also ask for a separate instruction sheet from your nurse or pharmacist on how to insert suppositories correctly.

Cascara or senna laxatives

If while you are taking this laxative as directed you develop severe stomach cramps, contact your health care provider immediately.

Pregnant women or women who are breastfeeding an infant should not use this medication because the medication can affect unborn babies and can be transmitted in breast milk and cause diarrhea in the infant.

This laxative may cause your urine to turn yellow-brown or red. This is a usual effect so do not be alarmed. Do not give this laxative to children unless specifically told to do so by your health care provider.

Mineral oil

This laxative acts by keeping your bowel movements soft. It is best taken on an empty stomach (1 hour before meals or 2 hours after meals). The dose of mineral oil can be mixed in chilled milk or juice. If you have any soreness around your anus or rectum or if you notice any leakage of mineral oil from your rectum, stop taking the mineral oil and contact your health care provider.

GENERAL INSTRUCTIONS FOR DISCHARGE/OUTPATIENTS—cont'd

Mineral oil—cont'd

Do not give this laxative to children under 6 years of age.

Store in the refrigerator out of the reach of children.

Phenolphthalein laxatives

If you develop a skin rash, diarrhea, weakness, difficulty breathing, pain in your stomach, or gut or bone pain, contact your health care provider immediately.

This laxative can cause your urine or your bowel movements to turn pink or red. This discoloration is usual so do not become alarmed. The usual color of your urine or bowel movements will return when you stop taking this medication.

Psyllium hydrophilic muciloid and other bulk-forming laxatives

This laxative comes in powder form. Briskly stir it in at least 240 ml or 8 ounces of water or juice and then drink it immediately. Drink another glass of juice or water after taking each dose of the drug. It is important that you drink lots of water or juice while you are taking this laxative because it works by absorbing water and thus provides more bulk for your bowel movement. Do not be discouraged if your constipation is not relieved immediately after taking this drug. It will be 2 to 3 days before you notice the laxative effect.

Remember you can prevent constipation and promote normal bowel function by doing the following:
1. Eating foods such as whole grain cereals, bran, vegetables, fruits, and nuts, which contain high fiber
2. Exercising moderately every day
3. Drinking 8 to 10 glasses of water a day
4. Emptying your bowels regularly and allowing yourself to be unhurried
5. Always going to the bathroom when you feel the urge to have a bowel movement

ANTIDIARRHEALS

This medication is an antidiarrheal, and it is used for the treatment of diarrhea.

Read the label carefully and do *not* take more than the recommended amount or more often than recommended.

While you are taking this drug, check with your health care provider before taking any other medicines or prescription drugs.

If your diarrhea does not get better within 1 to 3 days, contact your health care provider immediately.

Do not give this medication to anyone else. It has been prescribed especially for you.

Store this medicine in a dry, dark place. Refrigeration is not necessary.

Keep this and all other medicines out of the reach of children.

In addition to these general instructions, if your medication is:

Paregoric

Take this medicine by mixing each dose in a half glass of water.

Be extremely careful when measuring this dose especially for children.

If this medication causes any stomach upset, it may help to take each dose along with some food.

Do not take any other medicine without specifically checking with your health care provider (especially drugs to help you sleep, tranquilizers, pain relievers, and cold or hay fever medications) because of the possibility of harmful side effects.

This medication should not be taken with alcohol because it can cause drowsiness and sleepiness.

This medication may cause daytime drowsiness. You should not drive a car or operate machinery that requires alertness until you know how this medication affects you.

If you have attacks of bronchial asthma, you should notify your health care provider before taking this drug.

Do *not* take this drug if you are allergic to codeine or morphine.

NURSING DRUG DIGEST

Medication (trade name*)	Indication	Usual dosage and administration	Dosage forms, preparation, and storage	Contraindications, cautions, and comments	Monitoring
LAXATIVES					
Bisacodyl Bicol Bisacodyl Bisaco-Lax Bisacolax Dulcodes* Dulcolax Erilax Evac-Q-Kwik* Fleet Bisacodyl Enema Laco Pentalax Rytmil Su-Bisacodyl Theralax	Constipation	*Adults:* 10-15 mg PO; *or* 10 mg PR *Children:* 300 µg/kg PO; *or* 5 mg PR under age 2 and 10 mg PR over age 2 Instruct patients not to chew enteric-coated tablets because this may cause gastric irritation Do *not* administer tablets with milk or antacids because this may dissolve the enteric coating and release irritant drug in stomach Do not break or crush tablets Because action is 6-12 hr, administer tablets at bedtime or before breakfast Administer suppositories after breakfast because they act in 15-60 min	Tablet (enteric coated): 5 mg Suppositories: 5, 10 mg Store suppositories at temperature below 30° C	May cause cramps Suppositories may cause rectal burning discomfort	Monitor fluid and electrolyte status with chronic use Monitor for cramping, nausea, and diarrhea
Bran	Constipation Diverticular disease Fissure-in-ano Hemorrhoids	*Adults:* As breakfast cereal one bowlful daily; as bran, (e.g., miller's bran) 3 tablespoonfuls daily added to cereals or stewed fruits Do *not* administer to patient suspected of having an intraperitoneal pathologic condition	A variety of bulk forms are available	May cause flatulence	

Drug	Uses	Dosage	Preparations	Side effects	Nursing considerations
★ **Cascara sagrada** Amlax Bio-Tab Biolax Biolax SP Caroid Cas-Evac* Casyllium* Kondremul with Cascara Sagrada* Milk of Magnesia-Cascara Suspension* Nature's Remedy Candy Coated* Nature's Remedy Juniors* Nature's Remedy Regular* Oxothatein* Petrogalar* Stimulax*	Constipation Colon cleansing for surgery, colonoscopy, sigmoidoscopy and barium enema	*Adults:* Extract, 5 ml PO at bedtime as needed; tablets, 300 mg PO *Children:* Extract, 1-2 ml PO at bedtime as needed	Extract: aromatic fluid extract Tablets: 120, 200, 300 mg Store in tightly covered light-resistant container Protect from sunlight and excessive heat	May cause cramps May be excreted in mother's milk and result in diarrhea in breastfed babies May color alkaline urine yellow-pink; may turn acid urine yellow-brown; urine darkens to brown or black on standing Large doses may cause enteritis	Monitor fluid and electrolytes with chronic use Monitor for effectiveness in 6-8 hr
Castor oil Alphamul G-W Emulsoil Granulex* Neoloid Ricifruit Unisoil	Constipation Preparation of colon for surgery, colonoscopy, or barium enema	*Adults:* 15-60 ml PO *Children:* Over 2 years, 5-15 ml PO Shake emulsion form well before administration Administer oil by pouring dose into the center of a small glass of cold juice or soft drink, unless contraindicated	Emulsion Oil Store *emulsion* below 5° C (do *not* freeze)	May cause abdominal cramps Prolonged use may cause fluid and electrolyte disturbances Do *not* use in cases of suspected acute abdomen, intestinal obstruction, or inflammatory bowel disease Normal bowel movements may not resume for 1-2 days following complete evacuation of the bowel	Monitor for liquid or semiliquid bowel movement in 2-6 hours in relation to action of drug Monitor for nausea, vomiting, abdominal cramps

Continued.

NOTE: For additional details regarding the individual agents listed in this table, see the text and other tables in this chapter.
*Indicates a multiple active ingredient product. For a complete listing of all active ingredients see the *Drug Reference Guide to Brand Names and Active Ingredients.*
★Indicates that the drug is generally available only in the United States.

NURSING DRUG DIGEST—cont'd

Medication (trade name)	Indication	Usual dosage and administration	Dosage forms, preparation, and storage	Contraindications, cautions, and comments	
Danthron Danivac Damthross* Doctate-P* Dorbane Dorbantyl Dorbantyl Forte* Dorbanty* Doss* Doxan* Doxidan* Istizin Laxatyl* Magcul* Modane Modane-Mild Regulex-D* Roydan Tonelax	Constipation	*Adults:* 37.5-150 mg PO after evening meal *Children:* Same as adult—start with lower doses Administration with fruit juice or soft drink may help mask taste and improve compliance	Tablets: 37.5, 75 mg Solution: 37.5 mg/5 ml (with 5% alcohol)	May color acidic urine brownish May color alkaline urine pink to red	Monitor serum electrolytes with long-term use
Docusate calcium Doxical Doxidan* Surfak	Constipation Preferred laxative in patients who should not strain during defecation (cardiac patients)	*Adults:* 50-240 mg/day PO in single or divided doses *Children:* Over 5 years, 50-150 mg/day PO in divided doses Administer with a glassful of fluid	Capsules: 50, 240 mg Store at 15°-30° C	May cause abdominal cramps Because of possible liver damage should not be used for prolonged periods Do *not* coadminister with mineral oil because systemic absorption of mineral oil may occur	Monitor for mild abdominal cramping Monitor for softened stools with easier passage and no straining 1-5 days after initial dose
★ **Docusate potassium** Dialose Dialose Plus* Rectalad	Constipation Of value in patients where straining during defecation should be avoided	*Adults:* 100-300 mg/day PO in single or divided doses Administer with a glass of water or fruit juice	Capsules: 100, 240 mg	Contains potassium and should be used with caution in patients who are hyperkalemic or who are receiving potassium-sparing diuretics (see Chapter 36, "Diuretics and Antidiuretics")	Monitor for therapeutic effect and for signs of hyperkalemia Monitor potassium serum levels (or probably better to switch to an alternate salt form) in patients at risk for developing hyperkalemia

Docusate sodium Bu-Lax Colace Comfolax Constiban Coprola Correctol* Danthross* Disonate Dual Formula Feen-A-Mint* Extra Gentle Ex-Lax* Feen-A-Mint Pills* Gentlax S* Laxinate Laxinex 100 Molofac Neolax* Sof-Lax Wafers* Stimulax* Trilax*	Constipation Of value in patients where straining during defecation should be avoided	*Adults:* 50–480 mg/day PO in single or divided doses *Children:* 5 mg/kg/day PO in 4 divided doses Bitter taste may be somewhat masked by fruit juices Administer with a glass of water or fruit juice Higher dosage initially tapered to individual response	Capsules: 50, 60, 100, 240, 250, 300 mg Tablets: 50, 60, 100, 300 mg Solution: 10, 50 mg/ml Syrup: 4 mg/ml Drops: 10 mg/ml Store at 15°–30° C Protect liquid and syrup from light Suppositories: 100 mg (*not* recommended)	Do *not* administer in conjunction with mineral oil because it may increase absorption of the oil Contains sodium and should *not* be used in patients on salt-restricted diets, (e.g., congestive heart failure, renal failure)	Monitor for softened stools, with easy passage and no straining 1–3 days after initial dose
Glycerin Agoral* Agoral Plain* Concentrated Milk of Magnesia* Fleet Babylax Glyrol Osmoglyn Rectalad*	Constipation	*Adults:* 1–2 suppositories PR daily *Children:* 1–2 suppositories PR daily	Liquid: 4 ml in rectal applicator Suppositories: Infant and adult preparations	May cause abdominal cramps	

Continued.

NURSING DRUG DIGEST—cont'd

Medication (trade name)	Indication	Usual dosage and administration	Dosage forms, preparation, and storage	Contraindications, cautions, and comments	Monitoring
Lactulose Cephulac Chronulac Duphalac	Constipation Used in treatment and prevention of hepatic encephalopathy	*Adults:* 10-20 gm PO initial dose followed, if necessary, by 6-12.5 gm/day in 3 divided doses *Children:* 2.5-7.5 gm/day PO in 3 divided doses May mask unpleasant taste by dilution with food or fluid such as fruit juice, water or milk	Syrup: 3.3 gm/5 ml Store at room temperature	Use with caution in diabetics because drug contains galactose and lactose Initial dose may cause transient flatulence and intestinal cramps Unpleasant taste May take several days to work May cause nausea and bloating Do *not* use in patients with galactosemia Safety not established in pregnancy Discontinue if diarrhea occurs	Monitor serum electrolytes (K^+, Cl^-, CO_2) periodically in elderly and debilitated who are taking drug for chronic constipation Monitor for production of normal bowel movement within 1-2 days
Magnesium citrate Citrate of Magnesia Citro-Mag Evac-O-Kit* Evac-O-Kwik* National Laxative	Constipation Colonic cleansing for barium enema	*Adults:* 200 ml PO as single dose Avoid chronic use	Solution	*Contraindicated* in renal failure and in children with intestinal parasites because of risk of hypermagnesemia Pleasant taste	Monitor for signs of hypermagnesemia: flushing, thirst, feeling of heat
Magnesium hydroxide Concentrated Milk of Magnesia Haley's M-O* Milk of Magnesia Milk of Magnesia-Cascara Suspension* Phillip's Milk of Magnesia	Constipation Colonic cleansing for barium enema	*Adult:* 15-60 ml/day PO *Children:* 15 ml/day PO Avoid chronic use Suspension: Shake bottle well Follow dose with a glass of water to enhance action at morning or q.h.s	Suspension: 8% by weight Store at room temperature in a tightly covered container	*Contraindicated* in renal failure because absorbed magnesium ions are excreted by the kidney *Contraindicated* in children with intestinal parasites because of risk of hypermagnesemia	With frequent use, monitor for hypermagnesemia (flushing, thirst, feeling of heat) especially in elderly or debilitated patients Monitor for renal dysfunction and electrolyte imbalance Monitor for laxative effect 4-8 hr after dose

Drug	Uses	Dosage/Administration	Form	Contraindications/Cautions	Monitoring
Magnesium sulfate Adlerika Epsom Salt Mag-S	Constipation Colonic cleansing for barium enema	*Adults:* 15 gm in 250 ml water PO in single dose *Children:* 100-250 mg/kg PO as single dose Avoid chronic use	Effervescent granules Mixture: magnesium sulfate 4 gm and magnesium carbonate 500 mg/10 ml	*Contraindicated* in renal failure and in children with intestinal parasites because of risk of hypermagnesemia Bitter taste	Monitor for continued need of medication Monitor for hypermagnesemia (flushing, thirst, feeling of heat)
Methylcellulose Cellothyl Cologel Hydrolose	Constipation Diverticular disease Fissure-in-ano Hemorrhoids	*Adults:* 0.5-2 gm PO b.i.d. to t.i.d. Administer mixed into a glass of liquid Follow dose with another glassful of liquid to ensure dose does not swell in bolus causing esophageal obstruction	Powder Liquid: 450 mg/5 ml (with 5% alcohol)	*Contraindicated* in dysphagia Not systemically absorbed, therefore relatively nontoxic May cause flatulence If esophageal obstruction is suspected, do not follow medication with more water or liquid because obstruction can expand with further fluid absorption; seek medical assistance immediately	Monitor for effect 1-3 days after initial dose Monitor for signs of obstruction Monitor adequate fluid intake
Mineral oil Agoral Plain* Agoral* Fleet Enema Mineral Oil Fleet Enema Oil Retention Haley's M-O* Kondremul with Cascara Sagrada* Kondremul with Phenolphthalein* Kondremul Plain Kondremul* Petro-Syllium No. 1 Plain* Petro-Syllium No. 2 with Phenolphthalein* Petrogalar*	Constipation Fecal impaction	*Adults:* 15-30 ml/day PO at bedtime; place patient in high Fowler's position to prevent aspiration; administer preferably on empty stomach, cold or with orange juice as preferred Delays gastric emptying Do *not* give with food Use *not* recommended	Liquid Store in refrigerator to increase palatability Suspension: 65% Emulsion: 50% *Shake* suspension well before use	Should *not* be used by the young or old May be aspirated and cause pneumonitis May interfere with absorption of fat-soluble vitamins (A, D, E and K)	Monitor for relief of impaction, soft, formed stool without straining in 6-8 hours of initial dose Monitor for anal leakage of mineral oil and irritation. May soil clothing; if noted, use should be discontinued.

Continued.

NURSING DRUG DIGEST—cont'd

Medication (trade name)	Indication	Usual dosage and administration	Dosage forms, preparation, and storage	Contraindications, cautions, and comments	Monitoring
Olive oil enema	Constipation Fecal impaction	*Adults:* 150-200 ml PR Administer warmed, under low pressure to prevent stimulation of the defecation reflex Retain for 60 minutes to overnight to treat impaction	Liquid	May be useful in fecal impaction; repeat enema may be necessary	
Phenolphthalein Agoral* Alophen Amlax* Caroid Laxative Tablets* Correctol* Espotabs Evac-O-Kit* Evac-O-Kwik* Evac-U-Gen Ex-Lax Ex-Lax Pills Extra Gentle Ex-Lax* Feen-A-Lax Feen-A-Mint Feen-A-Mint Gum Feen-A-Mint Pills* Phenolax	Constipation	*Adults:* 30-200 mg PO generally taken at bedtime for morning effect	Tablets: 30, 60, 80, 90, 100 mg Tablets, chewable: 30, 60, 90, 97 mg Powder Mints: 97 mg Liquid: 65 mg	Ineffective as a laxative in presence of obstructive jaundice May cause abdominal cramps and an allergic rash May color urine pink to red-brown	Monitor fluid and electrolyte status with chronic use Monitor for bowel movement 6-8 hours after dose Monitor for skin rash; if observed, discontinue use, notify prescriber

Drug	Uses	Dosage	Preparations	Nursing Implications
Plantago seed Casyllium* Effersyllium Hi-Fibran Hydrocil Fortified* Hydrocil Instant Hydrocil Plain Instant Mix Metamucil* Konsyl L.A. Formula* Metamucil Mucilose Perdiem* Petro-Syllium No. 1 Plain* Plova* Prodiem* Prodiem Plain Senokot with Plantago* Serutan Siblin Sof-Lax Wafers* Syllamalt*	Constipation Diverticular disease Hemorrhoids Anal Fissures	*Adults:* 5-10 gm PO b.i.d. to t.i.d. *Children:* 6-12 years, dosage is half the adult dose For constipation administer powder stirred into 240 ml of water or fruit juice; the granules should be taken, unchewed, and followed with 240 ml of fluid Add liquid to effervescent powder before administration	Powder Packages: effervescent powder Granules: mint flavored	Use with caution in patients with a history of esophageal disorders May cause bloating, which usually improves in 2-3 weeks Do *not* use effervescent powder in patients on salt restriction May reduce appetite if taken before meals Laxative effect usually seen within 24 hours but may be delayed for up to 2-3 days	Monitor for laxative effect 12 hr to 2 days after initial dose
★ **Poloxamer 188** Alaxin Polykol	Constipation	*Adults:* 240 to 750 mg/day PO *Children:* 240 mg/day PO Do *not* give for longer than 1 week Administer a glass of liquid with each dose	Capsules: 240, 250 mg	May require several days of therapy before full stool softening is achieved	Monitor for soft, formed stool 1-3 days after initial dose; discontinue use after effect obtained
Polycarbophil Mitrolan	Constipation	*Adults:* 1-1.5 gm PO q.i.d. *Children:* 2-5 years, 0.5-1.5 gm/24 hr PO in 3-4 divided doses; 5 years and over; 1.5-3 gm/24 hr PO in 3-4 divided doses Administer each dose with 240 ml of water or other liquid Tablets should be thoroughly chewed before swallowing	Tablets, chewable: 500 mg	*Contraindicated* in GI obstruction *Not* systemically absorbed; therefore relatively nontoxic	Monitor for laxative effect

Continued.

NURSING DRUG DIGEST—cont'd

Medication (trade name)	Indication	Usual dosage and administration	Dosage forms, preparation, and storage	Contraindications, cautions, and comments	Monitoring
Saline or tap water enema	Constipation Cleansing of colon for barium studies, surgery or colonoscopy	*Adults:* 500-2000 ml PR Administer warmed Repeat until water returns clear if cleaning colon for surgery, colonoscopy, or barium studies	Solution	Tap water enemas, being hypotonic, are usually not associated with fluid overload; however, in cases of water depletion, enema fluid can be systemically absorbed. This can also occur if repeated enemas are administered as for bowel preparation. *Contraindicated* in patients with CHF or other sodium-retaining conditions *Contraindicated* in cardiac patients as vagal nerve stimulation	Monitor for water intoxication; saline enemas, because they are isotonic, do not usually cause depletion or overload of body water; sodium can be absorbed from the saline enema in certain conditions (i.e., congestive heart failure) and disrupt fluid and electrolyte balance Monitor for water intoxication Monitor enema return For patients with fluid volume depletion receiving tap water enemas monitor for signs of water intoxication (i.e., pallor, weakness, sweating, dizziness, breathing difficulties)
Senna Bekunis Herbal Tea Black Draught Casafru Dr. Caldwell's Senna Fletcher's Castoria Gentlax Gentlax B Gentlax S* Glysennid	Constipation Cleansing of colon for surgery, colonoscopy, sigmoidoscopy, barium enema	*Adults:* 400 mg (tablets *or* syrup) PO at bedtime for constipation; *or* 650 mg (suppository) PR Sennosides 12-36 mg PO Granules 1-2 rounded tsps PO placed in the mouth and swallowed with 240 ml cool beverage followed with additional liquid Granules should not be chewed For relief of constipation administer before breakfast or at bedtime	Powder: 22.5 gm in singledose container Granules Syrup: 220 mg/5 ml (with 7% alcohol) Tablets: 100, 180, 220 mg Suppository: 650 mg Liquid	Combination senna products containing bulk-forming laxative ingredients are *contraindicated* in patients with a history of esophageal disorders because of the risk of obstruction May cause cramps May cause infant diarrhea in lactating mothers	Monitor fluid and electrolyte status with chronic use Monitor for laxative effect 6-24 hours after dose Monitor for flatulence, abdominal cramps If cramping is severe or gripping, dosage may require reduction if to be repeated

Drug	Use	Dosage	Preparation	Comments
Glysennid Norsenna Mucinum-F Norsena Nytilax Perdiem* Prodiem* Senokap DSS* Senokot Senokot with Plantago* Senokot-S* Senolax Swiss Kriss X-Prep		For bowel preparation administer 22.5 gm powder or 75 ml senna extract (X-Prep) on afternoon of day before procedure usually followed with clear liquid diet		May cause acidic urine to turn yellowish brown and alkaline urine to turn reddish violet Prolonged use may cause melanosis coli (black pigmentation of colonic mucosa)
Soapsuds enema	Constipation Colonic cleansing	*Adults:* 500 ml PR Administer warmed Use a solution of 5 ml castile soap per 1 L solution Use is *not* recommended	Mixture of castile soap with water	Use is highly controversial because soap suds enemas can be irritating to intestinal mucosa and are associated with other hazards
Sodium phosphate/sodium biphosphate Fleet Enema* Fleet Pediatric Enema* Phospho-Soda* Saf Tip Phosphate Enema* Vacuetts Adult*	Constipation Fecal impaction Cleansing of colon for sigmoidoscopy	*Adults:* 120 ml PR as retention enema *Children:* Over 2 years, 60 ml PR Avoid chronic use Administer at room temperature to prevent cramping Encourage patient to retain enema until urge to defecate is strongly felt for best results, at least 1 hr	Solution: In commercially prepared 1-dose containers (120 and 128 ml)	*Contraindicated* in patients on salt-restricted diets, (i.e., congestive heart failure, toxemia, renal failure, hypertension) Because these enemas are hypertonic they draw water into the colon; dehydration and electrolyte imbalance can occur with chronic or frequent use Monitor for fluid depletion especially in children, elderly, and debilitated patients or those prone to dehydration
Total intestinal preparation	Colonic cleansing for x-ray examination, surgery, colonoscopy	*Adults:* 8-10 L Ringer's lactate Run through nasogastric tube at about 1 L/hr until rectal evacuation clear of stool	Solution: Prepackaged in liter containers	Risk of water and sodium overload in the elderly Do *not* use in patients who have intestinal obstruction Monitor for fluid overload

Continued.

NURSING DRUG DIGEST—cont'd

Medication (trade name)	Indication	Usual dosage and administration	Dosage forms, preparation, and storage	Contraindications, cautions, and comments	Monitoring
ANTIDIARRHEALS					
Cholestyramine Cuemid Questran	Diarrhea (indication *not* FDA approved) See also Chapter 34, "Vasodilators, Antilipemics, Anticoagulants, and Platelet Aggregation Inhibitors"	*Adults:* 4 gm PO t.i.d. and q.h.s.; dosage based on individual need *Children:* over 8 years of age 80 mg/kg PO t.i.d. Always dissolve in water, carbonated drinks, or applesauce to disguise disagreeable taste and gritty consistency by sprinkling on top of selected fluid; allow to stand 1-2 minutes before stirring Foaming occurs when mixed with carbonated drink because of carbon dioxide release After administration, fill glass and rinse with fluid; have patient drink to ensure adequacy of dose	Powder	May cause steatorrhea, nausea, and heartburn May bind anticoagulants, digitalis, phenobarbital, thyroxine, and decrease their efficacy; anticoagulants and digitalis therefore should not be given within 1 hour before and 4 hours after administration of cholestyramine Dissolve medication before administration because it is irritating to mucous membranes and may cause esophageal impaction if administered in dry form	Monitor for constipation, intestinal impaction, abdominal pain, flatulence, nausea, and vomiting
Codeine	Diarrhea See also Chapter 17, "Analgesics and Narcotic Antagonists"	*Adults:* 15-30 mg PO q.4-6h. as indicated	Tablets: 15, 30, 60 mg	May potentiate the effects of other concurrently taken CNS depressants May cause nausea, vomiting, and drowsiness Prolonged use may cause addiction May be excreted in breast milk	Monitor for signs of abuse or addiction, particularly with chronic use Monitor for constipation
Diphenoxylate Di-Atro* Diaction* Diarsed Lo-Trol* Lofene* Loflo*	Diarrhea	*Adults:* 2.5-5 mg PO q.6h. *Children:* 2-5 years, 2.5 mg PO b.i.d.; 6-8 years, 2.5 mg PO t.i.d.; 9-12 years, 2.5 mg PO q.i.d.; 12 years and over, 5 mg PO t.i.d.	Tablet: 2.5 mg Liquid: 2.5 mg/5 ml	*Contraindicated* in fulminant inflammatory bowel disease because may cause toxic megacolon *Contraindicated* in *Shigella* infections	Monitor for antidiarrheal effect Monitor for atropine-like effects, abdominal discomfort, urinary retention

Drug	Indication	Dosage	Remarks
Lomotil (Canada) Lomotil* (USA) Lonox* Retardin SK-Diphenoxylate*			Atropine content increases risk of toxicity in children May cause nausea, vomiting, dizziness and dry mouth Long-term use may result in physical dependence Excreted in breast milk
Kaolin Amogel PG* Amogel* Bisilad* Diabismul* Donnagel* Donnagel-MB* Donnagel-PG* Kao-Con* Kaodonna* Kaodonna-PG* Kaolin Pectin Suspension* Kaomead* Kaomead w/ Belladonna* Kaopectate* Kaopectate Concentrated* Parepectolin* Pargel* Pecto-Kalin* Pektamalit* Ru-K-N* Woodward's K.P.*	Diarrhea	Suspension *Adults:* 2-30 gm PO after each bowel movement *Children:* under 1 year, 1 gm PO q.4-6h.	Can adsorb lincomycin, pseudoephedrine, and digoxin and thereby decrease their effectiveness May interfere with the absorption of nutrients, especially in the elderly Monitor hydration; withhold in dehydration states especially in children until corrective therapy is initiated to prevent possible toxic effects

Continued.

NURSING DRUG DIGEST—cont'd

Medication (trade name)	Indication	Usual dosage and administration	Dosage forms, preparation, and storage	Contraindications, cautions, and comments	Monitoring
Loperamide Imodium	Diarrhea	*Adult:* 4 mg PO initially, then 2 mg after each loose bowel movement to a maximum 16 mg/day	Capsules: 2 mg Syrup: 2 mg/5 ml	*Contraindicated* in *Salmonella* and *Shigella* infections and other pathogens that penetrate the intestinal smooth muscle wall May cause nausea, dizziness, abdominal pain, and dry mouth Safety not established in *pregnancy,* nursing mothers, and children Should *not* be used in acute pseudomembranous colitis caused by clindamycin, lincomycin, or broadspectrum antibiotics Although this drug is not associated with addiction, it is considered to have potential for abuse Accidental overdose treated with naloxone	Monitor control of diarrhea as dosage may be individualized to one daily dose when improvement in consistency of stools has been established If drug taken to reduce volume of discharge from ileostomy, control of nighttime soiling, drainage control, and ability to maintain daytime hygiene, monitor increased consistency of drainage Monitor for minor transient adverse effects, including dryness of the mouth, fatigue, drowsiness, and dizziness Monitor for signs of overdosage: nausea, vomiting, constipation, and CNS depression
Paregoric Amogel PG* Corrective Mixture with Paragoric* DIA-quel* Kaodonna-PG* Pabizol with Paregoric* Parepectolin* Pecto-Kalin* Ru-K-N*	Diarrhea	*Adults:* 5-10 mg PO b.i.d. to q.i.d. as indicated Administer in water (mixture will be milky) to ensure passage to stomach	Tincture Store at room temperature *Shake* well before use	*Contraindicated* in conjunction with central nervous system depressants Prolonged use may cause addiction May exacerbate respiratory failure Accidental overdose can be treated with Naloxone May cause drowsiness Also known as "camphorated tincture of opium"	Monitor stool frequency and consistency because drug should be discontinued when diarrhea is controlled Observe for drowsiness and implement safety precautions as indicated

Drug	Indications	Dosage	Preparations	Comments	Monitoring
Plantago seed Effersyllium Hi-Fibran Hydrocil Instant Hydrocil Plain Konsyl Metamucil Mucilose Serutan Siblin	Diarrhea (indication not FDA approved)	*Adults:* 5-15 gm PO q.d. to t.i.d. Mix in 1 glass of fluid, and administer promptly before it gels; follow with ½ glass of water	Powder bulk Packages: effervescent preparations	Use with caution in patients with a history of esophageal disorders. Effervescent preparations contain sodium and should *not* be given to patients on salt-restricted diets (i.e., congestive heart failure, renal failure, toxemia, hypertension)	Monitor for fecal impaction
Polycarbophil Mitrolan	Diarrhea (for short term use *only*)	*Adults:* 1-1.5 gm PO q.i.d. *Children:* 2-5 years 0.5-1.5 gm/24 hr PO in 3-4 divided doses; 5 years and over, 1.5-3 gm/24 hr PO in 3-4 divided doses. Administer with *small* amounts of fluids only. Tablets should be thoroughly chewed before swallowing	Tablets; chewable: 500 mg	*Contraindicated* in GI obstruction. *Not* systemically absorbed; therefore relatively nontoxic	Monitor for soft, formed stool
Tincture of opium Dia-Quel Liquid*	Diarrhea	Adults: 0.6-1.5 ml PO b.i.d. to q.i.d. as indicated. NOTE: Do *not* confuse with camphorated tincture of opium (i.e., paregoric); the dose for tincture of opium is one-tenth the dose (by volume) of the camphorated preparation	Tincture: 10% opium (with 18% alcohol) Store at room temperature	*Contraindicated* in patients with central nervous system depression. *Contraindicated* in patients with ulcerative colitis because of risk of toxic megacolon. Prolonged use may cause addiction	Observe for signs of addiction. Monitor for constipation

BIBLIOGRAPHY

Binder, H.J. Net fluid and electrolyte secretion: The patho-physiological basis of diarrhea. *Viewpoints on Digestive Diseases*, 1980, *12*.

Bond, J.H. Office-based management of diarrhea. *Geriatrics*, 1982, *37*, 52-55; 61-64.

Duncombe, V.M., Bolin, T.D., & Davis, A.E., Double-blind trial of cholestyramine in post-vagotomy diarrhea. *Gut*, 1977, *18*, 531-535.

Edwards, L.A. Symposium on diarrhea. 6. Infectious diar-rhea. *Canadian Medical Association Journal*, 1977, *116*, 753-755.

Evans, D.W. Practical advice about a delicate pediatric prob-lem. *RN*, 1978, *41*, 51-52.

Fingl, E. & Freston, J.W. Antidiarrhocal agents and laxatives: Changing concepts. *Clinics in Gastroenterology*, 1979, *8*, 161-185.

Ganinella, T.S. & Bass, P. Laxatives: An update on mechanism of action. *Life Sciences*, 1978, *23*, 1001-1010.

Godding, E.W. Constipation and allied disorders. 3. Thera-peutic agents—Chemical laxatives (section 1). *The Phar-maceutical Journal*, 1975, *215*, 60-62.

Godding, E.W. Constipation and allied disorders. 2. Thera-peutic agents—Hydrophilic bulking agents. *The Phar-maceutical Journal*, 1975, *215*, 34-36.

Godding, E.W. Constipation and allied disorders. 4. Thera-peutic agents—Chemical laxatives (section 2). *The Phar-maceutical Journal*, 1975, *215*, 81-84.

Heel, R.C., Brogden, R.N., Speight, T.M., & Avery, G.S. Loper-amide: A review of its pharmacological properties and therapeutic efficacy in diarrhea. *Drugs*, 1978, *15*, 33-52.

Ivey, K.J. Clinical trends and topics: Are anticholinergics of use in the irritable colon syndrome? *Gastroenterology*, 1975, *68*, 1300-1307.

Jeejeebhoy, K.N. Symposium on diarrhea. 1. Definition and mechanisms of diarrhea. *Canadian Medical Association Journal*, 1977, *116*, 737-739.

Loperamide for diarrhea. *The Medical Letter*, 1977, *19*, 73-75.

Loperamide and other antidiarrheal drugs. *Drug and Ther-apeutics Bulletin*, 1977, *15*, 61-63.

Miller, R.E., Opinion. The cleansing enema. *Radiology*, 1975, *11*, 483-485.

Newton, C.R., The effect of codeine phosphate, lomotil, and isogel on ileostomy function. *Gut*, 1975, *14*, 424-425.

Porter, N. The use of lactulose in post-haemorrhoidectomy patients. *British Journal of Clinical Practice*, 1975, *29*, 235-236.

Rutter, K., & Maxwell, D. Diseases of the alimentary system: Constipation and laxative abuse. *British Medical Journal*, 1976, *2*, 997-1000.

Sandeman, D., Clement, M., & Perrins, E. Oesophageal ob-struction due to hygroscopic gum laxative. *British Medical Journal*, 1980, *1*, 364-365.

Watson, W.C. Symposium on diarrhea. 2. Clinical diagnosis of the cause of diarrhea. *Canadian Medical Association Journal*, 1977, *116*, 739-741.

SECTION IX

ANTIPARASITIC MEDICATIONS

Medications discussed in this section

CHAPTER 42

Antiprotozoals, Antimalarials, and Amebicides

Karin E. Zenk

Medications discussed in this chapter

General antiprotozoals
Co-trimoxazole
Furazolidone
Melarsonyl
Melarsoprol
Metronidazole
Nifurtimox
Pentamidine
Quinacrine
Stibogluconate
Suramin
Tinidazole
Antimalarials
Amodiaquine
Chloroquine

Antimalarials—cont'd
Hydroxychloroquine
Primaquine
Pyrimethamine
Quinine
Amebicides
Carbarsone
Dehydroemetine
Diloxanide furoate
Emetine
Iodoquinol
Metronidazole
Oxytetracycline
Paromomycin

A parasite is an organism that lives upon, within, or at the expense of another organism, the host. Some parasites, *obligatory* parasites, are unable to survive outside a host whereas others, *facultative* parasites, are capable of independent life outside the host. Parasitized animals—reservoir hosts—may serve as a source of infection for humans.

Parasites that cause harm to the host are known as *pathogens*. Harmless or nonpathogenic species of parasites are known as *commensals*. Parasitic diseases involve three basic groups of pathogens: (1) protozoa (single-celled organisms); (2) arthropods (insects and their allies); and (3) helminths (worms). The pharmacologic treatment of the conditions caused by protozoa including amebiasis, trichomoniasis, and malaria is covered in this chapter. The treatment of infestations caused by arthropods, or ectoparasites that live even briefly on the body surface is covered in Chapter 43, "Pediculicides and Scabicides." The treatment of infections caused by helminths, or endoparasites, which live within the body, is discussed in Chapter 44, "Anthelmintics."

Knowledge of the life cycle and the route followed by a parasite from the time and site of entry until its exit from the host is essential in understanding the symptomatology, pathology, and treatment of parasitic diseases.

The treatment of some parasitic diseases requires only a reduction in the number of parasites, whereas the treatment of others requires complete eradication. Since protozoa multiply within the host similar to bacteria, their complete eradication is necessary. Usually laboratory findings are required to establish a diagnosis of parasitic disease because clinical signs and symptoms can be only suggestive of certain conditions. Accurate laboratory diagnosis is essential for drug selection as well as for determining the proper route of administration. Drugs used in the treatment of parasitic diseases should be used only upon positive diagnosis and at the lowest dose possible to treat the disease.

Many patients have multiple parasitic infections. In these patients the order of drug treatment may present a therapeutic problem. Some drugs may be given concurrently to treat multiple parasitic infections but care should be taken that their side effects are not additive. If one of the infections is especially painful or life threatening, it requires treatment first. Successful treatment depends on appropriate dosage, administration, and procedures to prevent reinfection. Bed rest during the acute stages, fever reduction, correction of fluid and electrolyte balance especially in young children, treatment of anemia if present, a bland nutritious diet, prevention of complications, and treatment of intercurrent illnesses are also important.

Parasitic disease may involve the liver, lung, brain, gastrointestinal tract, and other organs and body systems. Prepurgation of the gastrointestinal tract helps to eliminate mucus and fecal debris that protect the parasite in cases of intestinal involvement, but may increase peristalsis and accelerate the passage of the drug through the intestinal tract, thus reducing its absorption or effectiveness. Postpurgation aids in removal of killed or anesthesized parasites from the GI tract and is recommended for certain drugs. Refer to the Nursing Drug Digest of each chapter in this section for instructions regarding the necessity of prepurgation or postpurgation. Purgation should not be used in intestinal obstruction, appendicitis, debilitation, or pregnancy. Some drugs require dosage adjustment or selection of an alternative drug in liver or renal involvement or impairment.

How to obtain unusual antiparasitic drugs. A number of chemotherapeutic agents that are not available commercially or are difficult to obtain are available in the United States through:

> Parasitic Diseases Drug Service
> Parasitic Diseases Branch
> Bureau of Epidemiology
> Centers for Disease Control (CDC)
> Atlanta, Georgia 30333
> Day telephone: (404) 633-3311, extension 3496
> Telephone for nights, weekends, holidays: (404) 633-2176

Some drugs that can be obtained from the CDC are bithionol, nifurtimox, niridazole, pentamidine, and suramin. Information concerning the dosage, contraindications, and side effects of the drugs is sent by the CDC together with the drugs.

> In Canada, contact:
> Health Protection Branch
> Bureau of Human Prescription Drugs
> Ottawa, Ontario
> Day telephone: (613) 993-3660
> Telephone for nights, weekends, holidays: (613) 992-9521

The information in this chapter should be read carefully before administration of any of the antiparasitics in order to be familiar with the drug's parasiticidal action and toxic properties. Some drugs may cover two or more parasites infecting the host in their spectrum of activity. Knowledge of the spectrum of drugs may allow use of single rather than multiple agents. Before treatment is started the parasite should be identified, its location in the host determined, and the intensity of infection and the amount of damage estimated. An agent should be chosen that has the most action on the parasite and the least toxic effect on the host.

ANTIPROTOZOALS

The protozoa are single-celled organisms that cause diseases such as giardiasis, leishmaniasis, *Pneumocystis carinii* pneumonia, trichomoniasis, and trypanosomiasis.

Giardiasis

Giardiasis is caused by the protozoan *Giardia lamblia.* It is transmitted by the ingestion of fecally contaminated food or water. The incubation period is approximately 1 to 2 weeks, but the appearance of symptoms is unpredictable and the period of communicability is indefinite. Giardiasis is diagnosed by specific microscopic identification of the cysts or motile forms of the organism in feces. Stool specimens may not show the organism, and in these cases examination of duodenal fluid, intestinal mucus, or a biopsy specimen from the small intestine may be necessary to reveal the presence of the parasite.

Some clinical features of the disease are diarrhea, abdominal pain, distention, borborygmi, and flatulence. Nausea or epigastric discomfort may be present after meals and may be followed by a diarrheal stool. The diarrhea is not bloody and stools may be pale, bulky, and offensive. There is no eosinophilia in the blood smear. Signs and symptoms of malabsorption may also present. Therapy for this disease is with metronidazole or quinacrine. Additional therapeutic measures include restoration of nutritional status in patients with malabsorption.

Giardiasis is prevented by sanitary disposal of feces as well as careful assessment of water supplies in mountainous areas where animal excrement may pose a problem in rivers and streams. In pregnancy only definite symptomatic infections should be treated since none of the available drugs are free from teratogenic effects. Because giardiasis is frequently a familial infection, it is important to examine and treat other members of the household to prevent reinfection.

Trypanosomiasis

Trypanosomiasis (Chagas' disease, American trypanosomiasis) is caused by *Trypanosoma cruzi,* a protozoal parasite of the blood and tissues of humans and many other vertebrates. One of the essentials of diagnosis is the presence of a hard, edematous, red, and painful cutaneous nodule (chagoma). The patient has intermittent fever, lymphadenitis, hepatomegaly, and signs and symptoms of acute or chronic myocarditis or meningoencephalitis. Trypanosomes can be demonstrated in blood smears or by culture, animal inoculation, or by complement fixation test. In heavily endemic areas the initial infection commonly occurs in childhood. The acute form of the disease may be fatal, particularly in infants and young children. Myocardial damage dominates the chronic form of the disease.

Drugs that are effective against other types of trypanosomiasis, such as the use of suramin against *T. gambiense* and *T. rhodesiense*, may not be effective against *T. cruzi* (Chagas' disease). The drug of choice for the treatment of Chagas' disease is nifurtimox. This drug is useful in destroying the extracellular trypanosomes in the blood, and it may also suppress viable organisms remaining in the chronic phase. In the United States this drug may be obtained from the Center for Disease Control in Atlanta, Georgia.

Trypanosomiasis caused by *T. gambiense* or *T. rhodesiense* is called *African trypanosomiasis*, or sleeping sickness. Suramin, pentamidine, and melarsoprol are drugs used to treat this parasitic disease. Both of these trypanosomes are transmitted by the bites of tsetse flies *(Glossina* sp.). The first sign of infection is a trypanosomal chancre, a local inflammatory reaction that appears about 48 hours after the tsetse fly bite (not all patients have this). The second stage, invasion of the bloodstream and reticuloendothelial system, usually begins several weeks later. Symptoms may appear at once, particularly in *T. rhodesiense* infections, or after several years. An irregular fever pattern with persistent tachycardia is characteristic. Other problems are rashes, delayed sensation to pain, splenomegaly, enlarged lymph nodes, and signs of myocardial involvement. The patient may succumb to myocarditis before signs of central nervous system (CNS) invasion appear. Early CNS changes include personality changes, apathy, and headaches; later changes include tremors, disturbances of speech and gait, mania, somnolence, and anorexia. The patient becomes severely emaciated and finally comatose. Death often results from a secondary infection. In addition to drug treatment, correction of anemia, treatment of concurrent infections, adequate nutrition, and supportive nursing care are essentials in the management of patients with advanced African trypanosomiasis. Without treatment from 25% to 50% of *T. gambiense* infections and over 50% of *T. rhodesiense* infections are fatal. With treatment from 5% to 15% of *T. gambiense* infections and up to 50% of *T. rhodesiense* infections are fatal. If treatment is started before invasion of the CNS occurs, the prognosis is considerably more favorable.

Leishmaniasis

There are three types of leishmaniasis, which are caused by three species of protozoa related to the trypanosomes. These protozoa are transmitted by sandflies (*Phlebotomus* sp.) in which they undergo cyclic development from animal reservoirs (dogs and rodents). Visceral leishmaniasis (kala-azar) is caused by *Leishmania donovani*; cutaneous leishmaniasis (oriental sore) is caused by *L. tropica*; and mu-

cocutaneous or nasooral leishmaniasis (espundia) is caused by *L. braziliensis*. Some signs and symptoms of kala-azar are irregular fever, progressive and marked splenomegaly and hepatomegaly, progressive anemia, leukopenia, and wasting. There may be progressive darkening of the skin, especially on the forehead and hands. Post–kala-azar dermal leishmaniasis may appear 1 to 2 years after apparent cure and may simulate leprosy as multiple hypopigmented macules or nodules develop on preexisting lesions. The lesions tend to heal spontaneously, but secondary infection may lead to gross extension. These lesions may be cleaned, curetted, covered, and left to heal. Antibiotics may be required for the treatment of secondary infection.

Mucocutaneous (nasooral) leishmaniasis is a chronic infection caused by *L. braziliensis*. It is characterized by cutaneous and nasooral involvement, either by direct extension or, more often, metastatically. The anterior part of the cartilaginous septum of the nose is commonly involved, and there may be gross and hideous erosion, including bone. Regional lymphadenitis is common.

Drugs used to treat leishmaniasis include stibogluconate, pentamidine, and topical agents. In patients with few or single lesions that are not cosmetically significant, topical or local treatment may be preferable to the risk of toxicity from systemic antimonial compounds. There is generally no communicable transmission of the disease directly from person to person, although there may be a risk of transmission from person to person with lesions of skin and mucous membranes.

Pneumocystis carinii pneumonia

Pneumocystis carinii pneumonia (interstitial plasma cell pneumonia, *Pneumocystis carinii* infection) is caused by the agent *Pneumocystis carinii*, a protozoan. This organism is ubiquitous in animals, particularly rodents, in many parts of the world. It is probably transmitted through the air. Infection from this agent occurs in persons who are debilitated from other causes or in those with compromised immunologic defenses. Infection occurs in the lungs; clinical features of the disease are fever, cough, dyspnea, and lung infiltrates in a compromised host. Diagnosis can be made by the identification of the organism in sputum, bronchial brushings, or lung biopsy. The drug of choice to treat *Pneumocystis carinii* pneumonia is co-trimoxazole. An alternative drug is pentamidine. Isolation of patients with the disease from an immunologically compromised individual is probably advisable.

Trichomoniasis

Trichomoniasis is a minor protozoal disease. It is a venereal infection caused by *Trichomonas vaginales* and is transmitted by sexual intercourse. It is also believed that spread can occur through towels or other objects. *Trichomonas* is found in 20% to 30% of pregnant patients. Newborn infants of infected mothers have, on occasion, acquired the infection. Symptoms in the female are inflammation and itching or burning of the labia and vagina, and profuse, creamy, yellow, frothy leukorrhea. Symptoms may worsen following menstruation. One third to two thirds of male sexual partners of women with *T. vaginales* infection are also infected, which can involve the urethra and prostate. Trichomoniasis may be asymptomatic. Since the organism is difficult to demonstrate in men, simultaneous treatment of partners of either sex is recommended to reduce the risk of reinfection and to reduce the reservoir of infection.

Trichomoniasis is effectively treated with oral metronidazole, either 250 mg three times a day for 7 days or a single dose of 2 gm with concurrent treatment of sexual partners.

Recent evidence has shown metronidazole to be carcinogenic in some animals, and the urine of patients receiving 750 mg per day of metronidazole has been shown to cause genetic changes in bacteria. Metronidazole has not been shown to be teratogenic, but the manufacturer advises against using it in the first trimester of pregnancy; some experts would not use it in pregnancy at all. AVC cream (aminacrine, sulfanilamide, and allantoin) can be used in pregnant women. Because there are inaccessible foci of trichomonads in the urinary tract of both sexes, a systemic agent is usually indicated, except in pregnancy.

Patients who develop side effects from metronidazole may be treated with antitrichomonal suppositories or AVC cream. Internal menstrual tampons may be utilized to reduce vulvar soiling, pruritus, and odor. Sexual intercourse should be avoided until treatment is completed unless a condom is used. Antipruritic medications are usually not helpful. Occasional warm saline or vinegar douches (60 ml or 4 tablespoons white vinegar per liter of water) may be beneficial in the treatment of leukorrhea.

Since both aerobic and anaerobic bacteria inactivate metronidazole, concomitant bacterial vaginitis could theoretically prevent maintenance of an adequate trichomonicidal concentration of the drug. Strains of trichomonads that are somewhat resistant to metronidazole have recently been isolated, suggesting another possible cause of intractable trichomoniasis. Such disease should be readily treatable since these strains appear to be responsive when the dose is increased. Resistant strains have been documented in only a few cases.

AMEBICIDES

Amebiasis is caused by *Entameba histolytica*. The source of infection is ingestion of fecally contaminated food or water containing the cyst form of the organism. Feces, fingers, food, fluid, fomites, and flies can transmit the disease. Amebiasis can be *intestinal* or *extraintestinal* involving the heart, liver, lungs, and brain. The disease is communicable throughout the duration of the intestinal infection. Amebiasis is diagnosed by the identification of *E. histolytica* in stools or tissue from lesions. Antibiotic therapy within 2 weeks of the culture may cause a false negative stool examination because of a transient reduction in the population of enteric amebas.

There are three forms of amebiasis and treatment is different for each. These are: (1) intestinal asymptomatic (carrier), (2) intestinal symptomatic (amebic dysentery), and (3) extraintestinal (e.g., liver abscess).

The life cycle of *E. histolytica* is simple. The infective cysts, formed in the lumen of the large intestine, pass out in the feces, and after an extracorporeal existence are ingested by a new host. Very few cysts are passed in acute dysentery, but they are passed in chronic infections and carrier states. The mature cysts are resistant to acid in the stomach and pass to the lower part of the small intestine. Here the alkaline digestive juices disintegrate the cyst wall and a four-nucleated melacystic ameba is liberated, which divides into eight small *trophozoites.* These small amebas move down to the large intestine.

In systemic amebiasis the liver is invaded chiefly and other organs less frequently. Dissemination from the primary intestinal focus mainly occurs by way of the bloodstream but may be by direct extension. Extension to the liver, including amebic hepatitis and amebic liver abscess, is the most common and grave complication of intestinal amebiasis.

Treatment includes general supportive measures and specific drug therapy. Patients with severe dysentery should have bed rest and receive a high-protein, bland, high-vitamin diet with adequate fluids and electrolytes. Chemotherapy does several things. It relieves the acute attack, destroys trophozoites in the intestinal lumen and mucosa, and controls secondary bacterial infection.

For intestinal asymptomatic disease iodoquinol or alternatively diloxanide furoate or paromomycin is used. For mild to moderate intestinal disease metronidazole plus iodoquinol or alternatively paromomycin is used. For severe intestinal disease metronidazole plus iodoquinol is used. Alternatively dehydroemetine plus iodoquinol or emetine plus iodoquinol can be given. For hepatic abscess treatment is with metronidazole plus iodoquinol or alternatively dehydroemetine followed by chloroquine phosphate plus iodoquinol. Another regimen for hepatic abscess is emetine followed by chloroquine phosphate plus iodoquinol. Dehydroemetine is probably as effective and less toxic than emetine.

Resolution of liver abscess takes 2 to 12 months. Large abscesses must be drained surgically.

Carriers or "cyst passers" are a dangerous source of infection, and food contamination by them is probably a major source of spread of the disease. Polluted water supplies are responsible for epidemics as are crowded conditions, poor sanitation, and poor personal hygiene where the disease can be spread by direct contact and by flies. Stools of carriers should be examined monthly for 6 months for infective cysts.

ANTIMALARIALS

Malaria is caused by four types of organisms, *Plasmodium vivax*, *P. falciparum*, *P. ovale*, and *P. malariae*. The source of transmission is through infected humans and mosquitoes (*Anopheles* sp.). Malaria is occasionally transmitted by blood transfusion from an infected person or by contaminated syringes and needles. Congenital infections can also occur. The incubation period in humans is from 8 to 37 days, depending on the type of organism and mode of transmission. Shorter incubation periods can occur when infection is caused by blood transfusion. The incubation time in the mosquito from blood meal to capacity to transmit is from 1 week to 1 month. Patients are infective for mosquitoes when gametocytes are circulating in the blood. Diagnosis is made by demonstration of *Plasmodium* parasites in peripheral blood smears (repeated thick and thin smears may be necessary).

Signs and symptoms

P. vivax. No symptoms appear for up to 1 week following the mosquito bite. During this time the parasites are developing in the liver. The merozoites from the preerythrocytic cycle then enter the red cells. The simultaneous rupture of a large number of red blood cells and the liberation of merozoites cause the paroxysms of malaria. With *Plasmodium vivax* the onset of the first paroxysm of the primary attack is characterized by a sudden, shaking chill (cold stage, or rigor)

often lasting for several hours. This is followed by a hot stage. Fever may reach 105° F. Accompanying symptoms persisting for several hours are hot dry skin, flushing of the face, full rapid pulse, headache, backache, nausea, muscle soreness, and convulsions (in children). The patient perspires profusely. The temperature falls and the headache disappears. The patient then usually feels exhausted but fairly good until the next episode. Coinciding with the release of another brood of merozoites in 48 hours, another paroxysm occurs. A series of such paroxysms of diminishing intensity occurs every other day for approximately 2 weeks. After a 2-week latent period a second attack is precipitated, less intense than the primary attack. A series of short-term recurrences may continue for approximately 2 months when a prolonged period of latency follows, indicating that the red blood cell phase has completely died out. Long-term relapses appear in 6 to 9 months.

P. ovale and P. malariae. Malaria caused by *P. ovale* follows a clinical course similar to that of *P. vivax* but is less severe. The clinical course with *P. malariae* is also similar to that of *P. vivax* except that the cycles are every 3 days instead of every 2 days.

P. falciparum. The course of *P. falciparum* is quite different and more severe. Unlike other types of malaria, which of themselves are never fatal, *P. falciparum*, the malignant malaria, can cause death. Red cells are invaded in massive numbers. Old as well as young red cells are involved. Early symptoms include headache, gastrointestinal complaints, malaise, and nausea and may be misdiagnosed as influenza in the early stage. Fever may elevate to 105° F and sometimes to 110° F and may be maintained for many hours. The sweating period is short and overshadowed by the febrile period. With *P. falciparum* one paroxysm may extend to the next with little or no time in between and no relief between episodes for the patient. The patient may become delirious or comatose and die within a few hours. Central nervous system symptoms such as seizures, psychotic tendencies, depression, or excitation may occur. If the patient survives, frequent relapses occur during the first month. After 3 to 5 months, latent periods are longer between attacks until radical cure occurs in about 10 months.

With *P. falciparum* only one exoerythrocytic cycle is developed, whereas with other species the cycle may continue for years so that relapses may occur years after the initial symptoms have subsided.

Congenital malaria. The placenta acts as a barrier to malaria since massive infection of the placenta may occur without infection of the infant. However, if there is a breach in the placenta, congenital infection may occur. The following case illustrates the in utero acquisition of this infection:

A 28-day-old Kampuchean boy was admitted to the hospital with a 2-day history of fever and vomiting. The parents were Kampuchean refugees who arrived in the United States just 2 months before the child's birth. Maternal screen for malaria at that time was negative, and she had no history of malaria symptoms except for unexplained chills before delivery. At birth the infant was well except for prolonged jaundice. On admission he was found to have hepatosplenomegaly, thrombocytopenia, and monocytosis. Blood smears revealed *Plasmodium vivax*. The infant was treated with chloroquine phosphate, which produced a rapid defervescence and clearing of the parasitemia.*

According to this report, treatment of congenital malaria infection caused by *P. vivax* differs from that for infection acquired by mosquito bite; primaquine is unnecessary in treating the former because of the absence of an exoerythrocytic (liver) stage.

Malaria prophylaxis is important in pregnant women since malaria infection is associated with placental infection, a high incidence of low birth weight infants, and congenital infection. Chloroquine is not contraindicated during pregnancy although sulfadoxine-pyrimethamine combination (Fansidar) has been associated with teratogenesis in animals and should therefore not be used in pregnant women until further information is available. Although chloroquine is excreted in breast milk, there is no evidence that breast fed infants are protected. Infants at risk should receive the appropriate dose of chloroquine. Because it is bitter in taste, chloroquine tablets can be crushed and mixed in chocolate or other flavored syrup to improve palatability.

Life cycle. Malaria infection takes place through the bite of an infected female *Anopheles* mosquito.

---

*From Cleary, T.G. Congenital malaria. *Morbidity and Mortality Weekly Report*, Jan. 11, 1980.

The mosquito is the host during the *sexual phase* of the life cycle; humans are the host for the *asexual* developmental stages. After an infective bite, the first stage of development in humans takes place in the liver.

Exoerythrocytic (liver) cycle. The developing parasite becomes a *cryptozoite* in the liver cell of humans. The cryptozoite divides to produce *cryptozoic merozoites*. The liver cell then ruptures and the merozoites are released into the blood. Some reenter the liver and repeat the cycle. Escape from the liver occurs from 5½ to 11 days after the bite.

Erythrocytic cycle. The erythrocytic cycle begins when the cryptozoic merozoites invade the red blood cell. The cryptozoic merozoite then becomes a *trophozoite*, which then becomes a young *schizont*. This schizont splits into merozoites. The red cell ruptures and the merozoites escape into the blood. Some of these then reenter other blood cells to repeat the cycle. The above is the asexual erythrocytic phase.

Some of the merozoites that invade the erythrocytes, instead of developing into schizonts, become *gametocytes* (sexual phase or stage).

This cycle of invasion, multiplication, and red cell rupture may be repeated many times. Symptoms appear after several of the erythrocytic cycles have been completed. With *P. falciparum* multiplication is confined to the red cells after the first cycle in liver cells (the *preerythrocytic stage*). Thus any treatment that eliminates *P. falciparum* parasites from the bloodstream will cure the infection. Without treatment the infection will terminate spontaneously in less than 3 years (usually 10 months). The other three species continue to multiply in liver cells long after the initial bloodstream invasion; therefore *P. vivax*, *P. ovale*, and *P. malariae* infections require treatment aimed not only at parasites in the red cells but also at those in the liver. *P. vivax* and *P. ovale* infections may persist without treatment for as long as 5 years; *P. malariae* infections lasting 40 years have been reported.

Treatment of malaria

Besides supportive treatment such as bed rest, cold sponging, aspirin for fever, and regulation of fluid and electrolytes, treatment of malaria is with chloroquine, amodiaquine, primaquine, quinine, and pyrimethamine. Treatment is divided into several types: suppression or chemoprophylaxis of disease while in an endemic area, prevention of attack after departure from endemic areas, treatment of uncomplicated attack, treatment of severe illness (parenteral dosages), and prevention of relapses ("radical" cure after "clinical" cure). Caution should be exercised in treatment of *P. falciparum* because strains resistant to chloroquine have been recorded. In these cases alternative drugs such as quinine plus pyrimethamine and sulfadiazine must be used.

Because illness is caused by the erythrocytic stages of the parasite, drugs that promptly destroy these forms are indicated. Chloroquine is the drug of choice (except for chloroquine-resistant *P. falciparum*). Primaquine is used to eradicate persisting exoerythrocytic (liver) stages that cause relapses of *P. vivax* malaria. Prophylaxis while in endemic areas should include measures to avoid exposure to night-biting anopheline mosquitoes such as screening, bed nets, and repellants. Weekly doses of chloroquine will suppress clinical activity except if infection is with resistant strains (encountered in Southeast Asia and South America).

Malaria is no longer an unheard of disease in the United States or Canada. Reports of 566 patients who had onset of malaria in the United States and territories from January 1 through June 30, 1980 have been received by the Centers for Disease Control (CDC). This represents a 243% increase over the 165 cases of malaria reported for the same period in 1979. All 1980 cases of malaria have been classified as imported. *Plasmodium vivax* infections were more common (75%) than *P. falciparum* (15%). A contributing factor to the increasing number of malaria cases in the United States is the increased number of refugees (14,000 per month) since August 1979. Canada has also seen an increase in the number of refugees.

P. vivax malaria, endemic in Canada prior to the 20th century, has been forgotten. However, because malaria eradication programs have been threatened by political unrest in many third world countries, and because of the increase in jet travel, malaria is becoming more prevalent in both the United States and Canada. Carrier mosquitoes are becoming increasingly immune to insecticides, and malarial parasites are developing resistance to common antimalarials. Since the problem of chloroquine-resistant and multidrug-resistant *P. falciparum* malaria is becoming more prevalent, the development of longer-acting and more effective drug therapy is becoming paramount. Work on malaria vaccines is being completed, and new classes of antimalarials for *P. falciparum* parasites will soon be available. Health teaching and case finding are important areas that nurses can contribute to in preventing the spread of this disease.

SUMMARY

This chapter has examined the various general and specific antiprotozoal medications. In addition, a brief overview of parasitic infestations has been provided together with the clinically significant details of the life cycles and modes of transmission of the various protozoa. Included was a discussion of the antimalarials and amebicides.

With an understanding of the various individual agents, including their actions and side effects, as well as the mode of transmission of the various infestations, the nurse will be better able to provide optimal care to patients who require these medications. Patient education can be enhanced; adverse drug effects can be anticipated, monitored for, and minimized; and clinically significant drug interactions can be avoided by utilizing the information presented in this chapter.

ADVERSE/SIDE EFFECTS OF THE ANTIPROTOZOALS, ANTIMALARIALS, AND AMEBICIDES*

AUTONOMIC NERVOUS SYSTEM

Anorexia
Nausea and vomiting

CARDIOVASCULAR SYSTEM

Disulfiram-like reaction (nausea, vomiting, headache when alcoholic beverages are consumed while taking certain medications, e.g., metronidazole)
Dysrhythmias
Herxheimer-type reaction
Hypertension
Myocardial damage
Shock
Sudden death with too rapid injection intravenously
Tachycardia

CENTRAL NERVOUS SYSTEM

CNS stimulation progressing to convulsions
Dizziness

Encephalopathy
Headache
Malaise
Paresthesias
Peripheral neuropathy
Sleep disorders
Tremor
Vertigo

CUTANEOUS SYSTEM

Irritation
Morbilliform rash
Pruritus
Reversible pigmentation of palate, nail beds, and skin
Urticaria
Vesicular rash

GENITOURINARY SYSTEM

Kidney damage

HEMATOLOGIC SYSTEM

Agranulocytosis
Aplastic anemia

Blood dyscrasias from folic acid deficiency
Hemolysis in G-6-PD deficiency
Hypoprothrombinemia
Methemoglobinemia
Neutropenia
Thrombocytopenia

HEPATIC SYSTEM

Hepatic failure

METABOLIC EFFECTS

Aggravation of diabetes mellitus
Hypoglycemia

NEUROMUSCULAR SYSTEM

Weakness

OCULAR SYSTEM

Blindness
Disturbances of vision
Photophobia

*See Chapter 11, "Drug Toxicity," for an overview of drug toxicity.

CLINICALLY SIGNIFICANT DRUG INTERACTIONS*

Primary drug	Interacting drug	Possible effect(s)	Probable mechanism(s)
Co-trimoxazole	Methotrexate	Pancytopenia	Synergistic effect on folic acid resulting in severe deficiency
Furazolidone	Insulin	Increased insulin effects (hypoglycemia)	Not established
Furazolidone	Levodopa	Increased levodopa toxicity (flushing, hypertension, tachycardia)	Monoamine oxidase inhibition
Furazolidone	Meperidine	Hypertension, convulsions, coma	Not established
Furazolidone	Sympathomimetics	Hypertensive crisis	Monoamine oxidase inhibition
Metronidazole	Alcohol	Disulfiram-like reaction	Inhibition of activity of aldehyde dehydrogenase
Metronidazole	Oral anticoagulants	Increased anticoagulant effect	Inhibition of hepatic metabolism
Quinine	Digoxin	Increased digoxin serum levels	Decreased digoxin clearance
Quinine	Oral anticoagulants	Increased anticoagulant effect	Decreased vitamin K synthesis

*See Chapter 10, "Drug Interactions," for an overview of drug interactions.

Nursing of patients requiring antiprotozoals and amebicides

ASSESSMENT

A complete nursing assessment is essential in establishing a baseline from which to plan individualized therapy and to monitor patient response. Assessment should include a detailed drug history to identify possible sensitivity, contraindications, cautions, and potential drug interactions before therapy is initiated. A drug history should also include the use of antibiotics within 2 weeks because false negative stool examinations may result especially in relation to intestinal amebicide involvement.

The patient's general condition should also be carefully assessed since fluid and electrolyte imbalance, diarrhea, abdominal pain, malabsorption, fever, skin lesions, hepatomegaly, enlarged lymph nodes, rashes, and behavioral symptoms of CNS involvement may be present depending on the specific parasitic disease being treated. Bed rest, the administration of fluid and electrolyte therapy, dietary therapy, and the prevention of reinfection are important nursing adjuncts to the use of antiprotozoals and amebicides. Isolation or the protection of immunosuppressed patients may also be indicated depending on the causative organism and presenting disease symptoms. Assessment of family or household members may also be indicated.

As with other parasitic conditions, laboratory tests are important in identifying the causative organism to plan appropriate drug therapy and nursing care. Laboratory specimens of stool, blood, duodenal fluid, or vaginal smears may be indicated and must be carefully obtained and sent to the laboratory for analysis. Care must be taken in handling these specimens in order to prevent spreading the parasite, as well as to prevent self-contamination.

SENSITIVITY

Generally antiprotozoals and amebicides have the potential to cause hypersensitivity in susceptible individuals, and patients should be carefully questioned regarding hypersensitivity. If patients have not received the medication before, they require close monitoring especially during the first 24 hours to assess symptoms of hyper-

sensitivity reaction such as skin rashes (e.g., eczema, vesicular rash, morbilliform rash, urticaria).

CONTRAINDICATIONS

Antiprotozoals and amebicides are contraindicated in patients with known hypersensitivity. Some are also contraindicated during pregnancy or in lactating mothers or infants under 1 year of age. (See the Nursing Drug Digest for each specific medication.) Some of these preparations are also contraindicated in patients with *glucose-6-phosphate dehydrogenase (G-6-PD)* deficiency.

DRUG INTERACTIONS

Antiprotozoals and amebicides can interact with some foods, alcoholic beverages, and other medications. For example, furazolidone, when given within 24 hours of alcohol ingestion can produce a disulfiram-like reaction. This drug has also been associated with hypertensive crisis when given with MAO inhibitors, tyramine-containing foods, and indirect-acting sympathomimetic amines. See Clinically Significant Drug Interactions and the Nursing Drug Digest for specific drug information.

ADMINISTRATION

Antiprotozoals and amebicides can be administered orally, although some medications are available in parenteral form as well. The medication should be taken as directed for the full number of days to ensure therapeutic effect. Some amebicides should not be administered intravenously (e.g., dehydroemetine) because of the possibility of severe toxic reactions. See the Nursing Drug Digest for specific information for each medication. Other preparations (e.g., emetine) are irritating to the skin and mucous membranes, and contact with the skin, eyes, or clothing should be avoided.

MONITORING PATIENT RESPONSE
Therapeutic response

Therapeutic response should be noted in respect to laboratory evaluation of stool or other specimens daily or as indicated. The patient's overall condition should show improvement. With intestinal involvement, diarrhea should

diminish. If diarrhea persists or worsens or if adverse side effects are noted, a change in therapy may be indicated. If satisfactory response does not occur within 7 days, the drug should be discontinued. Patients should be on bed rest during acute phases of infection and fluids, stools, and daily weight should be monitored. Fluid and electrolytes should be monitored carefully in the presence of diarrhea in infants, young children, and the elderly or debilitated. With drugs that are excreted slowly (e.g., carbarsone), a rest period of 10 to 14 days may be indicated following each 10-day course of therapy to decrease toxicity.

Stool or other specimens are usually obtained after completion of the treatment for alternate days after initial treatment and at weekly or monthly intervals for 3 or more months. (See the Nursing Drug Digest for each specific medication.) The criterion for cure is the absence of parasites (and their eggs) in laboratory specimens.

Adverse side effects

Various antiprotozoals and amebicides can cause side or adverse effects. These are outlined in Adverse/Side Effects of the Antiprotozoals, Antimalarials, and Amebicides. In addition, overgrowth of nonsusceptible organisms or superinfection has been reported with the use of amebicides (e.g., metronidazole) and patients should be observed for black furry tongue, thick whitish vaginal discharge, and vaginitis.

PATIENT EDUCATION

The patient and family as indicated should have a clear understanding of the importance of the medication regimen as well as related care including the prevention of reinfection. The patient and family should know the exact name of the medication, its action, dosage, method of storage, administration, and adverse effects. They should know how to minimize adverse effects and recognize which effects may indicate that the health care provider should be contacted. The patient and family should understand the length of therapy, and they should know how to monitor therapeutic effects.

Continued.

GENERAL NURSING IMPLICATIONS—cont'd

Nursing of patients requiring antiprotozoals and amebicides—cont'd

PATIENT EDUCATION—cont'd

The patient is usually restricted to bed rest depending on the individual condition or specific medication regimen, and the patient should understand this aspect of care. Isolation is generally not required; however, the meticulous disposal of feces or other contaminated material and the prevention of the spread of infection in relation to the collection and care of specimens should be carefully explained. Patients and family often need assistance with dietary therapy. A low-residue or other diet may be indicated especially with intestinal involvement. Patients need to be aware that foods high in tyramine, such as aged cheese and chianti wine, can produce hypertensive crisis when some antiprotozoals (e.g., furazolidone) are taken for more than 5 days. Other drugs can cause a disulfiram-like reaction (nausea, sweating, fever, flushing, pounding headache, palpitations, dyspnea, dizziness, and a sense of chest constriction that may last up to 24 hours) if alcohol is consumed. Patients should avoid drinking alcohol during the drug therapy and for at least 4 days after therapy is no longer need-ed if they are taking medication such as furazolidone or metronidazole. Patients should be aware that concurrent use of nonprescription medications including nasal sprays, cold and hay fever preparations, and other amine-containing medications can cause hypertensive crisis.

For intestinal involvement, patients must keep the health care provider informed of signs of dehydration and electrolyte imbalance (decreased skin turgor, sunken eyeballs, deeply furrowed tongue, muscle or abdominal cramps) and should be able to monitor stools for mucus or blood and foreign matter. The number, frequency, and other characteristics should be reported to the health care provider. Proper collection and care of stool specimens are necessary to ensure that they are delivered to the laboratory as indicated—(i.e., warm, to facilitate the identification of ameba). Fluid intake and daily weight should also be reported. Screening of family and household members for disease is important. Patients should understand the importance of remaining under the supervision of their health care provider and the need for repeated stool or other specimens for laboratory examination at specific intervals following medication therapy to ensure complete elimination of the parasite.

Patients and family members should be helped to explore the possible sources of infection including contaminated water or food supplies, need for fly control, poor general health or personal hygiene practices, and other sources of contamination to prevent the spread and reinfection. Follow-up of family or household members and suspected contacts may be indicated. For sexually transmitted disease, concurrent treatment of sex partners is important. Women should avoid the use of panty hose, tight underwear, and bubble bath. Cotton underwear is best. Perineal care should be reviewed as indicated. Sexual intercourse should be avoided during treatment or a condom should be used to prevent the spread of infection.

Discharge and outpatient instruction is extremely important in relation to preventing reinfection and to ensure therapeutic response.

Nursing of patients requiring antimalarials

ASSESSMENT

A complete nursing assessment is essential in establishing a baseline from which to plan individualized therapy and to monitor patient response. Assessment should include a detailed drug history to identify possible sensitivity to specific antimalarials, contraindications, cautions, and potential drug interactions before therapy is initiated.

As with other parasitic conditions, prevention and treatment as well as reinfection are major considerations. Planning individualized drug therapy with the patient and family as indicated is essential to enhancing compliance both for persons traveling to endogenous malarial areas and for patients being treated for malaria. Because individuals may require antimalarial therapy for prophylaxis when traveling in malarial areas, prevention of attacks after departure from such areas, treatment of uncomplicated attacks, treatment of severe illness, and/or prevention of relapses ("radical cure"), assessment of the person's general condition should be carefully documented to serve as baseline data to monitor therapy. The indication for antimalarial therapy is important in planning individualized nursing care during attacks such as bed rest, fluid and electrolyte therapy, dietary therapy, and supportive care especially during paroxysms of malaria.

SENSITIVITY

Antimalarials may precipitate acute hemolytic anemia in persons with glucose-6-phosphate dehydrogenase deficiency. A hemolytic reaction including decreased urine output, chills, fever, precordial pain, and cyanosis indicates that the drug should be stopped.

CONTRAINDICATIONS

Antimalarials are contraindicated in patients with known hypersensitivity.

Antimalarials are contraindicated in areas where resistant strains are present.

CAUTIONS

Antimalarials should be used cautiously in pregnant or lactating women, infants and young children, the elderly, and the debilitated or severely ill.

DRUG INTERACTIONS

Quinine may depress prothrombin formation and enhance the effects of anticoagulants. See Clinically Significant Drug Interactions.

GENERAL NURSING IMPLICATIONS—cont'd

Nursing of patients requiring antimalarials—cont'd

ADMINISTRATION

Antimalarials can be administered orally or by intravenous injection depending on the drug, dosage form, and condition of the patient. Administer oral doses with meals to decrease gastrointestinal upset.

When counseling patients regarding chemoprophylaxis, the nurse should stress that the medication should be taken as prescribed for 7 to 14 days before entering malarial areas and should be continued for up to 8 weeks after leaving the area. Chloroquine should be taken once weekly on the same day and at the same time (preferably after a meal). Quinine salts are bitter and when given orally in large doses can cause gastrointestinal distress. Tablets should not be chewed or crushed before swallowing. Because they are protoplasmic, parenteral forms may cause pain, irritation, inflammation, and abscesses at the injection site.

Intravenous administration is contraindicated in the presence of shock, pulmonary edema, cyanosis, severe anemia, or pregnancy. IV administration of the dihydrochloride salt of quinine may produce hypotension and acute circulatory failure. It should be injected slowly and in very dilute solutions, and oral preparation should be substituted as soon as possible.

See the Nursing Drug Digest for specific information regarding the administration of antimalarials.

MONITORING PATIENT RESPONSE
Therapeutic response

Because there is a cumulative action in patients receiving long-term antimalarial therapy, the therapeutic effect may not be observed for several weeks, and a maximum effect may not occur for up to 6 months.

In cases of chemoprophylaxis, the patient should be monitored 1 to 2 weeks following a visit to a malarial area as symptoms of a malaria attack would be observed during this time. In acute attacks patients should be monitored for control of fever and other symptoms. Absence of attack and eradication of parasites from the body in known cases 60 days after the drug is discontinued indicates "therapeutic cure."

Adverse side effects

Antimalarials can cause numerous adverse effects, especially when taken over long periods of time. The usual therapeutic doses of such antimalarials as quinine can produce *cinchonism* (tinnitus, headache, altered auditory acuity, nausea, and blurred vision) but serious adverse effects are rare, although they are related to increased dosage. With prolonged therapy or large doses visual disturbances (disturbed color perception, photophobia, blurred vision, night blindness, diplopia, mydriasis, optic atrophy), fever, sweating, asthma, and angioedema may occur.

Patients receiving long-term therapy should be closely monitored for muscle strength and deep tendon reflexes. Ophthalmic examination including slit lamp, fundoscopy, and visual fields should be done regularly during prolonged therapy. RBC, hemoglobin, and other blood constituents should be carefully monitored. Therapy should be discontinued if weakness, visual or auditory symptoms, or skin eruptions occur.

Quinine overdose

For large amounts of recently ingested quinine lavage is indicated as well as a saline purgative (sodium sulfate, 30 gm in 250 ml water) to enhance peristalsis. Acidifying the urine with ammonium chloride and ensuring adequate fluid balance may assist in elimination of the drug. Emergency supportive measures should be readily available.

Cinchonism, flushed skin, diaphoresis, gastrointestinal disturbances, hypotension, widening QRS complex, ventricular tachycardia, or ventricular fibrillation can occur in severe cases.

Intravascular hemolysis (blackwater fever): hemoglobinuria, azotemia, renal failure, death occurring in 25% to 50%. If evidence of hemolysis appears (darkened urine) quinine should be discontinued immediately.

PATIENT EDUCATION

The patient and family should have a clear understanding of the medication regimen as well as the exact name of the medication, its action, dosage, method of storage, administration, and side effects. They should be assisted in minimizing side effects and should be able to monitor therapeutic response. The patient and family should be able to identify when the health care provider should be notified and what signs indicate that the medication should be stopped. Assisting patients with long-term therapy is extremely important, and patients often need help with planning including care during attacks.

Patients should be advised to take oral doses of antimalarials with meals.

Urine should be examined for changes in color, and the amount voided should be noted. Chills, fever, precordial pain, and cyanosis should be reported to the health care provider.

Red blood cell and hemoglobin determinations, ophthalmic examination, and health assessment are important in the follow-up of the disease as well as in the monitoring of therapy.

The onset of weakness, visual disturbances, or skin eruptions should be reported immediately.

Travelers should be advised to report malaria exposure to their health care provider for up to 5 years after returning from malarious areas. Because carriers can spread disease in blood transfusions, they should *not* volunteer as blood donors. When traveling in malarious areas, other precautions such as dressing with long sleeves and pants, using mosquito nets, and limiting evening travel should be taken. Pregnant women from nonendemic regions should be advised *not* to travel in malarious areas.

GENERAL INSTRUCTIONS FOR DISCHARGE/OUTPATIENTS

ANTIPROTOZOALS

This medication is used for infections such as those caused by intestinal parasites or related organisms.

Follow the instructions on the prescription exactly. Do not take more or less than the prescribed dose.

If you are being treated for diarrhea, monitor your stools and report the number, amount (approximate), odor, and the presence of any mucus, blood, or foreign matter to your health care provider. Household members should also be examined for the infection. If you are being treated for a vaginal infection, monitor your vaginal discharge and let your health provider know if there is any change or increased odor, discharge of whitish material, or itchiness. You should refrain from sexual intercourse during treatment for this condition, and your sex partner should be examined.

Isolation is not required; however, if you are being treated for a gastrointestinal problem, you should not prepare or process foods.

It is important that you remain under the care of your health care provider even after you stop taking this medication. You probably will need to continue to have your stool or other specimens checked by the laboratory. Be sure you understand how specimens should be collected and when. If you have any questions, call your health care provider.

You should take all the tablets as prescribed unless you experience adverse reactions.

Using medications together may cause unfavorable effects. Do not stop or begin taking any other medication without contacting your health care provider.

Do not give this medication to anyone else. It has been prescribed especially for you.

If you are pregnant or think you might be pregnant or are breastfeeding, tell your health care provider before you take this medication.

Some medications can cause unwanted effects in some people. If you notice any unusual or unexpected effects, contact your health care provider.

Keep this and all other medication out of the reach of children.

Metronidazole

If you are taking metronidazole, do not take alcoholic beverages while you are taking this medication because cramps, vomiting, and flushing can occur.

It is possible that skin rashes, nausea, headache, metallic taste, vomiting, diarrhea, furry tongue, nasal congestion, or darkened urine can occur with this medication. If these effects become bothersome or persist, notify your health care provider and stop taking the medication temporarily. Your dosage may need to be changed, or the medication may need to be discontinued.

ANTIMALARIALS

This medication is used to prevent or treat malaria. It may also be used to treat other conditions. If you have any questions about why you require this medication, discuss them with your health care provider.

It is important that you take this medication exactly as directed. Do not take any extra tablets unless you are specifically told to do so by your health care provider.

Take this medication immediately before or after meals or with food to prevent stomach upset.

Try to take this medication at the same time each day. Continue to take this medication for the full treatment as directed by your health care provider.

If you forget or miss a dose of your medication, take it as soon as possible.

GENERAL INSTRUCTIONS FOR DISCHARGE/OUTPATIENTS—cont'd

ANTIMALARIALS—cont'd

If it is almost time for your next scheduled dose do *not* take the missed dose, just continue with your regular dosage. If you have missed more than one dose, contact your health care provider for directions.

If you are pregnant, planning on becoming pregnant, or are breastfeeding, tell your health care provider *before* starting to take this medication because it may affect your unborn or nursing infant.

If you have a medical condition such as eye disease, alcoholism, cirrhosis of the liver, psoriasis, blood disorders, or glucose-6-phosphate-dehydrogenase deficiency, be sure to notify your health care provider before starting this medication.

Keep this and all other medication out of children's reach.

It is important that you check your progress with your health care provider at regular intervals. Keep your appointments.

Most people experience few adverse or unwanted effects from these medications. However, you may experience some unwanted effects. Notify your health care provider.

If you are taking *chloroquine*, notify your health care provider if you notice:
- Bleaching of your hair or unusual hair loss
- Blue-black tinge to the skin, nails, or inside of the mouth
- Blurring of vision or other eye problems including night blindness
- Changes in hearing including ringing or buzzing in the ears
- Fever
- Mood or mental changes
- Unusual sores in your mouth
- Unusual muscle weakness
- Numbness or tingling in the hands or feet
- Skin rash
- Easy bruising or bleeding

If you have had an unusual reaction to any other medications used to treat malaria (such as amodiaquine or hydroxychloroquine) be sure to notify your health care provider before you start taking chloroquine.

Chloroquine can change the color of your urine to rusty-yellow or brown. This is not unusual and your urine will return to normal color when you stop taking this medication.

If your eyes become sensitive to light, sunglasses may help.

If you are taking *quinine*, notify your health care provider if you notice:
- Changes in vision
- Fever
- Skin rash
- Sore throat
- Shortness of breath
- Stomach pain
- Changes in hearing including ringing or buzzing in the ears

If you have ever had an allergic reaction to quinine or quinidine (a heart medication), be sure to notify your health care provider before you start taking quinine.

Be sure to shake the liquid form of this medication well before pouring a dose to ensure that you get the correct dose.

If you are taking *primaquine*, notify your health care provider if you notice:
- Reddening or darkening of your urine
- Chills
- Fever
- Chest pain
- Unusual stomach pain
- Difficulty breathing
- Unusual fatigue
- Passing less urine than normal

If you are taking *pyrimethamine*, notify your health care provider if you notice:
- Skin rash
- Sore throat or tongue
- Unusual diarrhea
- Vomiting

NURSING DRUG DIGEST

Medication (trade name*)	Indication	Usual dosage and administration	Dosage forms, preparation, and storage	Contraindications, cautions, and comments	Monitoring
Amodiaquine Camoquin Flavoquin	Malaria caused by *Plasmodium vivax, P. ovale, P. malariae,* and susceptible strains of *P. falciparum*	*Adults:* Base, 600 mg intiially then 400 mg at 6, 24, and 48 hr PO *Children:* Base, 10 mg/kg initial and 5 mg/kg at 6, 24, and 48 hr PO For prophylaxis of malaria *Adults:* 400 mg weekly on the same day of the week *Children:* Less than 1 year, 50 mg; 2-4 years, 50-100 mg; 5-8 years, 150-200 mg; 9-12 years, 300 mg PO GI disturbances may be minimized by administering with meals Prophylaxis should be started before travel into malarious areas and should be continued for up to 8 weeks after leaving the area	Tablet: 200 mg base	*Contraindicated* in severe liver disease, visual field disorders Causes nausea, vomiting, fatigue, lassitude, vertigo, reversible bluish grey pigmentation of palate, nailbeds, and skin with prolonged use (5 weeks to 6 years of weekly therapy) Overdose quickly results in toxicity Excessive exposure to sun may result in photoallergic dermatitis	Children are especially sensitive to 4-aminoquinoline compounds, and response should be closely monitored
★ **Carbarsone**	Amebiasis (intestinal) *Use not recommended*	*Adults:* 250 mg PO b.i.d. to t.i.d. for 10 days Maximum: 1 gm/day *Children:* 7.5 mg/kg/day PO in 3 divided doses for 10 days Contents of capsules can be mixed with a small amount of food or liquid	Capsule: 250 mg	*Contraindicated* in severe renal or hepatic disease, amebic hepatitis, and hypersensitivity Carbarsone is an organic arsenical May produce skin rash such as urticaria Occasionally causes gastritis and hepatitis Rarely causes severe encephalomyelitis Discontinue at first sign of CNS toxicity or increase in liver function tests This drug is often given with other amebicides	Monitor for signs of arsenic poisoning (i.e., dermatitis, encephalomyelitis, visual disturbances) Monitor liver function tests

Drug	Uses	Dosage	Preparations	Side effects/Notes	Nursing considerations
				Carbarsone is still available for medicinal use, but is *obsolete* as an amebicide because less toxic, more effective drugs are available. Dimercaprol is an antidote for arsenic poisoning	Observe and report skin changes. Observe and report any change in visual acuity. Monitor muscle strength and deep tendon reflexes during long-term therapy; muscle weakness and absence of reflexes indicate therapy should be discontinued
Chloroquine Aralen Avlochlor Quinachlor	Malaria caused by *Plasmodium vivax, P. ovale, P. malariae* and susceptible strains of *P. falciparum*	Suppression while in endemic area. *Adults:* Phosphate salt, 500 mg (300 mg base) PO every week for 6 weeks after last exposure in endemic area; begin treatment 1-2 weeks before exposure; take on the same day at the same time each week. *Children:* Under 1 year: 37.5 mg base; 1-3 years: 75 mg base; 4-6 years: 100 mg base; 7-10 years: 150 mg base; 11-16 years: 225 mg base. Treatment of uncomplicated attack. *Adults:* 1 gm (600 mg base) then 500 mg (300 mg base) in 6 hr, then 500 mg (300 mg base) q.d. for 2 days PO. *Children:* 10 mg base/kg q.d. (maximum 600 mg base) then ½ this dose daily beginning 6 hr later for 2 days PO. Treatment of severe disease. *Adults:* 250 mg (200 mg base) of parenteral form IM q.6h. *Children:* 5 mg/kg base IM q.12h.	Tablet: 250, 500 mg (phosphate salt). Injectable: 50 mg/ml (hydrochloride salt)	*Contraindicated* in severe liver impairment and visual field disorders. Occasionally causes itching, vomiting, headache, confusion, depigmentation of hair or skin, corneal opacity, irreversible retinal injury (usually associated with higher doses), weight loss, partial alopecia, psoriasis, eczema, hemolysis in G-6-PD deficiency (patient should have a screening test for G-6-PD deficiency before this drug is administered). Rarely causes discoloration of nails and mucous membranes of the mouth, nerve deafness (hearing loss), blood dyscrasias (such as agranulocytosis), and photophobia	Monitor for visual disturbances including complaints of night blindness, visual field changes, blurred vision, or difficulty focusing. Ophthalmic examination (slit lamp, fundus, visual fields) should be completed before therapy is initiated and regularly thereafter. Monitor therapeutic response

NOTE: For additional details regarding the individual agents listed in this table, see the text and other tables in this chapter.

*Indicates a multiple active ingredient product. For a complete listing of all active ingredients see the *Drug Reference Guide to Brand Names and Active Ingredients.*

★Indicates that the drug is generally available only in the United States.

Continued.

NURSING DRUG DIGEST—cont'd

Medication (trade name)	Indication	Usual dosage and administration	Dosage forms, preparation, and storage	Contraindications, cautions, and comments	Monitoring
Chloroquine— cont'd	Amebiasis	*Adults:* Phosphate salt, 1 gm (600 mg base) q.d. for 2 days, then 500 mg (300 mg base) q.d. for 2 to 3 weeks PO *Children:* 10 mg base/kg/hr for 21 days (maximum 300 mg base/24 hr)		In falciparum malaria, if patient has not shown a prompt response to conventional doses parasitic resistance to this drug must be considered May cause brown discoloration of urine Minor GI distress or headache usually disappears after a few days Retinopathy is highly unlikely following chemoprophylaxis Inadvertent IV injection may produce quinidine-like effects on cardiac muscle Skeletal muscle weakness and loss of reflexes may occur with prolonged use With long-term use corneal and retinal damage may occur; retinopathy and corneal damage may be irreversible and may progress even after drug is discontinued	
Co-trimoxazole (trimethoprim-sulfamethoxazole) Bactrim Bactrim DS Bactrim IV Eusaprim Septan Septra	*Pneumocystis carinii* pneumonitis See also Chapter 48, "Miscellaneous Antibiotics," and Chapter 49, "Sulfonamides"	*Adults:* 20 mg/kg of trimethoprim and 100 mg/kg of sulfamethoxazole q.d. divided q,6h. for 14 days PO *Children:* 20 mg/kg of trimethoprim and 100 mg/kg of sulfamethoxazole q.d. divided q,6h. for 14 days PO	Suspension: Sulfamethoxazole 200 mg and trimethoprim 40 mg/5 ml Tablet: Sulfamethoxazole 400 mg and trimethoprim 80 mg Double-strength tablet: Sulfamethoxazole 800 mg and trimethoprim 160 mg	*Contraindicated* in megaloblastic anemia because of folate deficiency *Contraindicated* in pregnancy; fetal malformations have occurred in several animal species Reduce dose in renal impairment (see dosage column)	Monitor CBC Observe for sudden appearance of sore throat, fever, pallor, purpura, or jaundice as indications of appearance of a blood dyscrasia Monitor intake and output Monitor for crystalluria

Septra DS
Septra IV
Sulfatrin
Trimetho-
prim-Sulfa

In renal impairment reduce dose to one-half the above if creatinine clearance is between 15 and 30 ml/min; do *not* use if creatinine clearance is below 15 ml/min

Administer on empty stomach to enhance absorption

NOTE: "DS" product indicates double-strength product

May cause blood dyscrasias; periodic blood tests should be done

Patient should maintain adequate fluid intake

May cause crystalluria; soluble at urine pH of 5.5

Infrequently causes renal and liver damage

Monitor urinary pH and ensure alkaline pH by encouraging foods to promote higher pH (milk, nuts, green vegetables, fruit [*not* cranberries, plums, prunes])

★ **Dehydro-
emetine**
Mebadin

Amebiasis (intestinal and extraintestinal)

Injectable: 60 mg/2 ml single-dose ampule

Adults: 1 to 1.5 mg/kg of body weight (maximum 90 mg) q.d. in one dose for up to 5 days IM, SC

Children: 1-1.5 mg/kg of body weight q.d. in 2 divided doses for up to 5 days IM, SC; maximum 90 mg/24 hr

Do *not* administer IV because severe toxic reactions may result

In cases of relapse the course may be repeated after an interval of 14 days; longer periods of treatment may be used in severe cases

Contraindicated in pregnancy because of the severe side effects of this drug and the resultant possible risk to the fetus; toxicity of the drug in the mother may compromise fetal well-being

Contraindicated in patients with organic, cardiac, or renal disease unless benefits outweigh the hazards, such as in hepatic abscess from ameba

Intravenous use is *contraindicated*

Use with caution in elderly patients because of this drug's severe cardiotoxicity and common presence of cardiac disease in the elderly; the result may be greater toxicity in these individuals

Patients receiving dehydroemetine should be hospitalized and remain in bed during treatment

Commonly causes cardiac dysrhythmias, precordial pain, muscle weakness, cellulitis at site of injection

Occasionally causes diarrhea, vomiting, peripheral neuropathy, heart failure

Monitor with daily ECGs while on this drug

Monitor heart rate and blood pressure

Continued.

NURSING DRUG DIGEST—cont'd

Medication (trade name)	Indication	Usual dosage and administration	Dosage forms, preparation, and storage	Contraindications, cautions, and comments	Monitoring
★ Dehydro-emetine —cont'd				Side effects of dehydroemetine are similar to those of emetine, except less severe; since it is eliminated from the body more rapidly, it can be used at higher doses for longer periods, and in cases of relapses, a course can be repeated after a shorter interval, although toxicity is cumulative with this drug also Irritating to eyes and mucous membranes	
★ Diloxanide furoate Furamide	Amebiasis (asymptomatic)	*Adult:* 500 mg t.i.d. for 10 days PO *Children:* 20 mg/kg/24 hr for 10 days PO *Elderly:* Same as adult dose	Tablet: 500 mg	Commonly causes flatulence Occasionally causes urticaria, GI upset with diarrhea	Observe for hivelike pruritic skin rash
★ Emetine	Amebiasis	*Adults:* 1 mg/kg/24 hr (maximum 60 mg/24 hr) for up to 5 days, deep IM or SC *Children:* 1 mg/kg/24 hr in 2 doses (maximum 60 mg/24 hr) for up to 5 days IM or SC Total dose should not exceed 600 mg in adults and 10 mg/kg/course in children A course of emetine should not be repeated more often than every 6 weeks *Do not administer IV*	Injectable: 65 mg/ml	*Contraindicated* in pregnancy because of the severe side effects of this drug and the resultant possible risk to the fetus; toxicity of the drug in the mother may compromise fetal well-being *Contraindicated* in patients with organic, cardiac, or renal disease unless benefits outweigh the hazards, such as in hepatic abscess from amebas *IV use is contraindicated* because it is dangerous and offers *no advantage over IM or SC*	Monitor patient with a cardiac monitor during administration of emetine because of toxic effects on heart; tachycardia is observed especially if patient is allowed to ambulate and may precede ECG change Injections (IM, SC) may cause edema and necrosis; therefore rotate injection sites and monitor sites carefully Monitor intake and output as oliguria has been reported

Record number, frequency, and character of stools; an increase in the number of stools following an improvement in diarrhea may indicate emetine-induced reaction

Monitor ECG before therapy initiated, after the fifth dose, and 1 week later

Monitor pulse (rate and quality) at least t.i.d. and blood pressure q.d.

Monitor neuromuscular function (especially neck and extremities) and report weakness, fatigue, stiffness, pain, or listlessness because they may indicate toxicity

Monitor for any unusual patient response that may indicate toxic reaction

Use caution in elderly patients, because of this drug's severe cardiotoxicity and the common presence of cardiac disease in the elderly; effect may thus be greater toxicity in elderly individuals

Patient should be under close medical supervision during administration

Bed rest is indicated during and after therapy

Toxicity is cumulative

Muscle weakness usually precedes serious signs of toxicity

Many side effects are dose related—large doses have caused acute lesions in the heart, liver, kidney, GI tract, skeletal muscle

Reversible ECG changes may be observed 7 days after discontinuation of drug and may persist for up to 2 months

Emetine is irritating to skin and mucous membranes; avoid contact with skin, eyes or clothing; wash hands well after handling drug

Commonly causes cardiac dysrhythmias, precordial pain, muscle weakness, and cellulitis at site of injection

Occasionally causes diarrhea, vomiting, peripheral neuropathy, and heart failure

Continued.

NURSING DRUG DIGEST—cont'd

Medication (trade name)	Indication	Usual dosage and administration	Dosage forms, preparation, and storage	Contraindications, cautions, and comments	Monitoring
Emetine— cont'd				Irritating to eyes and mucous membranes *Discontinue* drug if tachycardia, fall in blood pressure, muscular or neuromuscular symptoms, or severe GI effects are noted	
★ **Furazolidone** Furoxone	Giardiasis	*Adults:* 100 mg q.i.d. PO *Infants and children:* 6 mg/kg/24 hr in 4 divided doses PO for 7 days Do not use in infants less than 1 month of age because of their immature metabolizing capability	Liquid: 50 mg/15 ml Tablet: 100 mg Store in tight, light-resistant container	Take careful drug history *before* administering this drug May cause nausea and vomiting, vesicular or morbiliform rash, headache, malaise Rarely causes agranulocytosis, acute hemolysis in G-6-PD deficiency Patient should have a screening test for G-6-PD deficiency before starting this drug May cause disulfiram-like reaction if ingested with alcohol or if alcohol is ingested within 4 days after drug is discontinued Do not give with MAO inhibitors Foods high in tyramine may produce hypertensive reaction especially with high doses of drug or therapy longer than 5 days Urine may be discolored brown	Observe for hypersensitivity reactions

Drug	Uses	Dosage	Preparation	Side effects/adverse reactions	Nursing implications
Hydroxy-chloroquine Plaquenil	Malarial attacks caused by *Plasmodium vivax, P. malariae, P. ovale,* and susceptible strains of *P. falciparum*	*Adults:* 620 mg initially followed by 310 mg in 6 hr and 310 mg q.d. for the next 2 days PO *Children:* 10 mg/kg initially followed by 5 mg/kg in 6 hrs and 5 mg/kg q.d. for the next 2 days For malaria prophylaxis *Adults:* 310 mg PO q. week *Children:* 5 mg/kg PO q. week Reduce adverse GI effects by administering with meals	Tablet: 200 mg (equivalent to 155 mg of base) Preserved in tightly closed, light-resistant containers	Hydroxychloroquine has no advantage over chloroquine Occasionally causes itching, vomiting, headache, confusion, depigmentation of hair or skin, hemolysis in G-6-PD deficiency, corneal opacity, irreversible retinal injury, weight loss, partial alopecia, psoriasis, eczema Patient should have screening test for G-6-PD deficiency before administration of this drug Rarely causes discoloration of nails and mucous membranes of the mouth, nerve deafness, tinnitus, hearing loss, agranulocytosis	Observe and report skin changes Observe and report any change in visual acuity, fundus, visual fields Monitor blood cell counts initially before treatment and at least q.3 months
★ **Iodoquinol** Diodoquin Ioquin Moebriquin Yodoxin	Amebiasis (intestinal)	*Adults:* 630 mg PO t.i.d. for 20 days *Children:* 30-40 mg/kg in 3 divided doses q.d. for 20 days (maximum 2 gm/24 hrs) PO *Elderly:* Same as the adult dose	Tablet: 210, 650 mg	*Contraindicated* in those allergic to iodine, since the chemical structure of this drug contains iodine *Contraindicated* in liver disease, since the drug is metabolized in the liver and accumulation of active drug may occur Occasionally causes optic neuropathy Rarely causes rash, acne, slight enlargement of thyroid gland, nausea, abdominal cramps, and pruritus ani Interferes with results of thyroid function tests; interpret thyroid function tests with caution (drug may interfere with these tests for several months)	Observe for signs of decreased visual acuity such as blurred vision Observe for symptoms of iodism (i.e., dermatitis, furunculosis, sore throat)

Continued.

NURSING DRUG DIGEST—cont'd

Medication (trade name)	Indication	Usual dosage and administration	Dosage forms, preparation, and storage	Contraindications, cautions, and comments	Monitoring
Iodoquinol—cont'd				Dosage and duration should not be exceeded because of possibility of optic neuritis	
★ **Melarsonyl** Trimelarsan	Trypanosomiasis	*Adults:* 4 mg/kg/24 hr IM *Children:* 2 mg/kg/24 hr IM May also be administered SC	Injectable for reconstitution; use immediately after preparation	This is a toxic drug Commonly causes Herxheimer-type reaction (which may be minimized by pretreatment with promethazine and a corticosteroid), encephalopathy, peripheral neuritis Side effects are similar to those of melarsoprol Pretreatment with antihistamine and corticosteroids helps minimize patient's discomfort during therapy	Patients on this drug should be hospitalized and observed closely
★ **Melarsoprol** Arsobel Mel-B	African trypanosomiasis; late disease with CNS involvement (sleeping sickness)	*Adults:* 2-3.6 mg/kg/24 hr IV for 3 doses; *after 1 week:* 3.6 mg/kg/24 hr IV for 3 doses; repeat again after 10-21 days *Children:* 18-25 mg/kg total over 1 month; initial dose of 0.36 mg/kg IV increasing gradually to a maximum of 3.6 mg/kg at intervals of 1-5 days for a total of 9-10 doses Use care to avoid extravasation; extremely irritating to tissues	Investigational drug	This is a toxic drug Commonly causes myocardial damage, albuminuria, hypertension, colic Causes Herxheimer-type reaction, encephalopathy (12% of patients), vomiting, peripheral neuropathy Rarely causes shock	Patients receiving this drug should be hospitalized and closely monitored

Drug	Uses	Dosage	Preparations	Remarks	Nursing Management
Metronidazole Flagyl Flagylstatin* Metryl Neo-Tric Novonidazol Protostat Satric Trichazel Trikacide Trikamon	Amebiasis (intestinal, hepatic abscess) Trichomoniasis	Adults: 750 mg t.i.d. for 5-10 days PO Children: 35-50 mg/kg/24 hr in 3 doses for 10 days PO Elderly: Same as adult dose Adults: 250 mg t.i.d. for 7 days PO; or single 2 gm PO dose Sexual partner should be treated concurrently Administer oral dose with meals or with food or milk to decrease GI distress	Tablet: 250, 500 mg Preserved in tightly closed, light-resistant container	*Contraindicated* in first trimester of pregnancy; crosses placenta and appears in breast milk Commonly causes nausea, headache, metallic taste Occasionally causes GI upset, CNS side effects such as vertigo, rash, dark urine Alcohol is contraindicated for 24 hr after administration of drug; may cause disulfiram-like reaction when taken with alcoholic beverages Metronidazole has been found to be carcinogenic in animals May cause flattening of T wave on ECG Advise patient being treated for trichomoniasis that sexual partner should be treated concurrently to avoid reinfection	Monitor for fungal overgrowth (furry tongue, color changes of tongue; curdlike, milky vaginal discharge in women and girls)
★ **Nifurtimox** Bayer 2502 Lampit	*Trypanosoma cruzi* (South American trypanosomiasis) Acute-stage Chagas' disease	Adults: 5 mg/kg/24 hr PO in 4 divided doses increasing by 2 mg/kg/24 hr q. 2 weeks until 15-17 mg/kg/24 hr Children: Dose not available Administration with food or meals may decrease GI distress	Tablet: 100 mg Investigational drug	Commonly causes anorexia, GI distress, weight loss, memory loss, sleep disturbance, tremor; paresthesias, weakening, polyneuritis Rarely causes convulsions	Observe and report CNS symptoms

Continued.

NURSING DRUG DIGEST—cont'd

Medication (trade name)	Indication	Usual dosage and administration	Dosage forms, preparation,	Contraindications, cautions, and comments	Monitoring
Oxytetracycline Abbocin Imperacin Otatryn Oxlopar Oxy-Tetrachel Oxymycin Terramycin Tetramine Urobiotic-250*	Amebiasis (intestinal)	*Adults:* 250 to 500 mg q.6h. for up to 2 weeks PO *Children:* 10 mg/kg of body weight (maximum 600 mg) q.i.d. for 10 days PO, IM, or IV Take oral dose on empty stomach with full glass of water Food may interfere with absorption of oral drug; administer at least 1 hr before or 2 hr after meals; do not administer with milk or give with antacids Check expiration date before administration because outdated drug can be nephrotoxic	Capsule: 125, 250 mg Tablet: 250 mg Syrup: 125 mg/5 ml Injectable: 50, 125 mg/ml (with 2% lidocaine) Protect from heat and light	May cause various skin rashes such as urticaria and exfoliative dermatitis, angioedema, anaphylaxis, pruritus ani, vaginitis, fever, eosinophilia, gastrointestinal irritation Tetracyclines discolor teeth of fetus if given to pregnant women in last trimester; also can discolor teeth in children up to the age of 8 years May cause superinfections with nonsusceptible bacteria and fungi, especially *Candida*	When using tetracyclines in children, check patient's age to be sure child is past completion of tooth formation (8 years) so that tooth discoloration will not occur Monitor for superinfection
★ **Paromomycin** Humagel Humatin	Amebiasis (intestinal)	*Adults and children:* 25-35 mg/kg of body weight daily in 3 divided doses PO Give with meals for 5-10 days Course may be repeated after a 2-week interval Administer with meals to decrease GI upset	Capsule: 250 mg Syrup: 125 mg/5 ml	*Contraindicated* in hypersensitivity and intestinal obstruction Commonly causes nausea, increased GI motility, abdominal pain, and diarrhea Occasionally causes rash, headache, vertigo, and vomiting May cause superinfection with nonsusceptible organisms Use this drug with caution in patients with GI inflammatory disease or ulcerations because absorption may occur If systemically absorbed may cause ototoxicity and nephrotoxicity	Observe for superinfections, especially *Candida* infections during therapy

Drug	Uses	Dosage	Preparations	Side effects/adverse reactions	Nursing considerations
★ **Pentamidine** Lomidine	Trypanosomiasis Leishmaniasis *Pneumocystis carinii* pneumonia	*Adults:* 2-4 mg/kg/24 hr deep IM for 12-14 days May cause pain at injection site followed by abscess formation and tissue necrosis	Investigational drug	May cause vomiting, hypotension, tachycardia, and hypoglycemia May cause impaired renal function and hepatic failure May cause blood dyscrasias May aggravate diabetes mellitus Rarely causes Herxheimer-type reaction	Monitor hepatic and renal function and blood carefully Monitor injection sites
Primaquine	Malaria (*Plasmodium vivax* and *P. ovale*)	*Adults:* 26.3 mg (15 mg base)/day for 14 days PO or 79 mg (45 mg base)/week for 8 weeks *Children:* 0.3 mg/kg base/day for 14 days PO Administer with meals to prevent or relieve GI distress	Tablet: 26.3 mg (equivalent to 15 mg base) Store in tightly closed, light-resistant containers	*Contraindicated* in presence of blood dyscrasias Commonly causes hemolytic anemia in G-6-PD deficiency (most common in blacks, Asian, and Mediterranean peoples) Occasionally causes neutropenia, GI disturbances, methhemoglobinemia in G-6-PD deficiency Patient should be screened for G-6-PD deficiency before administration of this drug Rarely causes CNS symptoms, hypertension, or dysrhythmias Marked darkening of urine suggests hemolytic reaction	Observe and report any change in CNS status, BP, or cardiac rhythm Monitor hemoglobin and erythrocyte counts Monitor intake and output

Continued.

NURSING DRUG DIGEST—cont'd

Medication (trade name)	Indication	Usual dosage and administration	Dosage forms, preparation, and storage	Contraindications, cautions, and comments	Monitoring
Pyrimethamine Daraprim Fansidar*	Malaria (chloroquine resistant *Plasmodium falciparum*) Used in combination with a sulfonamide or quinine Malaria prophylaxis or suppression (chloroquine-resistant *P. falciparum*) Used in combination with sulfonamide	*Adults:* 25 mg b.i.d. for 3 days *Children:* Less than 10 kg, 6.25 mg/day; 10-20 kg, 12.5 mg/day; 20-40 kg, 25 mg/day *Adults:* 25 mg PO once q. week *Children:* 6-11 months, ⅛ tablet; 1-3 years, ¼ tablet; 9-14 years, ¾ tablet weekly Administer drug with meals to decrease GI distress For malaria prophylaxis drug should be started upon entrance to malarious area and should continue for 10 weeks after leaving area	Tablet: 25 mg	Occasionally causes blood dyscrasias, folic acid deficiency If hematologic abnormalities appear, they are usually treated with leucovorin (folinic acid) 3-9 mg IM Rarely causes vomiting, convulsions, shock Administration of leucovorin does not interfere with the antimalarial action Excreted in breast milk	Monitor for blood dyscrasias
Quinacrine Atabrine Tenicridine	Giardiasis	*Adults:* 100 mg t.i.d. PO for 5 days *Children:* 6 mg/kg/24 hr in 3 divided doses after meals for 5 days Maximum: 300 mg/24 hr Administer after meals May need to use NG tube to administer drug directly into duodenum since vomiting is so common; may pretreat patient with an antiemetic; this is especially important in treatment of tapeworm because vomiting can cause migration of segments into stomach and subsequent release of ova Sodium bicarbonate may be prescribed with each dose to decrease GI upset; patient is often placed on a bland, nonfat diet for 24 hr and made to fast on the evening before treatment	Tablet: 100 mg	Use *cautiously* in patients with history of psychosis and those over 60 years because of increased CNS toxicity Vomiting occurs in 25% of patients on this drug Causes yellow staining of skin Commonly causes dizziness and headache Occasionally causes toxic psychosis, insomnia, blood dyscrasias, urticaria, blue and black discoloration of nails, psoriasis-like rash Rarely causes acute liver necrosis, seizures, exfoliative dermatitis, ocular effects	

Drug	Use/Dosage	Preparations	Remarks
Quinine Coco-Quinine Kinine Quine Quinite Strema	Malaria: Use with tetracycline (250 mg q.i.d. for 7 days) or pyrimethamine (25 mg b.i.d. for 3 days) and a sulfonamide (sulfadiazine 500 mg q.i.d. for 5 days) to treat chloroquine-resistant strains of *P. falciparum* (adult doses) *Adults:* 650 mg PO q.8h. for 3 days *Children:* 25 mg/kg q.8h. PO for 3 days *Adults:* 600 mg in 300 ml sodium chloride IV; infuse over at least 1 hr; repeat in 6 to 8 hr (maximum 1.8 gm/24 hr) *Children:* 25 mg/kg IV over at least 1 hr; give ½ dose initially; give other ½ 6-8 hr later Use IV only if PO not tolerated Maximum 1.8 gm/24 hr IV administration can be hazardous; administer *slowly* with constant monitoring of pulse (ECG) and blood pressure to detect dysrhythmia or hypotension Oral route should be used as soon as possible Administer oral dosage after meals to decrease GI distress Do not crush tablets or take capsules apart because drug is extremely bitter	Capsule: 120, 200, 300, 325 mg Tablet: 260, 325 mg Injectable: 500 mg powder for reconstitution Suspension: 110 mg/5 ml	*Postpone use in pregnancy until after delivery because drug crosses the placenta* *Contraindicated in hypersensitivity and pregnancy* *Contraindicated in patients with optic neuritis and tinnitis* Use caution in patients with atrial fibrillation or who show idiosyncrasy in terms of angioedema or visual or auditory symptoms Commonly causes cinchonism Occasionally causes blood dyscrasias, photosensitization, cardiac dysrythmias, hypotension Rarely causes blindness and sudden death if injected too rapidly The name *quinine* is easily confused with the name "quinidine"; use caution in dispensing the correct medication May precipitate asthma in susceptible individuals May cause urticaria or pruritus Patient should be screened for G-6-PD deficiency Oxytocic effect in third trimester of pregnancy Monitor for signs of cinchonism (i.e., blurred vision, GI disturbances, headache, tinnitus) which indicates overdosage

Continued.

NURSING DRUG DIGEST—cont'd

Medication (trade name)	Indication	Usual dosage and administration	Dosage forms, preparation, and storage	Contraindications, cautions, and comments	Monitoring
★ **Stibogluconate** Pentostam	Leishmaniasis	*Adults:* 600 mg/24 hr IM or IV for 6-10 days; may be repeated *Children:* 10 mg/kg/24 hr IM or IV (maximum 600 mg/24 hr) for 6 to 10 days Administer through a fine (25-gauge) needle slowly Avoid leakage into the perivascular tissue because painful inflammation following leakage during IV injection has been noted	Injectable: 190 mg powder for reconstitution	*Contraindicated* in severe hepatic, renal, or cardiac insufficiency Side effects during rapid infusion include cough and vomiting; severe or even fatal reactions such as shock and cardiovascular collapse have occurred Occasionally may cause diarrhea, colic, rash, pruritus, and myocardial damage Rarely causes liver damage, hemolytic anemia, renal damage, shock, sudden death	Monitor vital signs during and after IV infusion Monitor infusion site
Suramin Antrypol Bayer 205 Germanin Naphuride	Trypanosomiasis See also Chapter 44, "Anthelmintics"	*Adults:* 1 gm per dose IV; a 200 mg test dose should be given first to see if patient has a hypersensitivity to the drug Daily 1 gm doses are given on days 7, 14, and 21; weekly doses may be given for another 5 weeks Do *not* repeat the course earlier than 3 months after the first course Total dose should not exceed 5.5 gm in adults because larger doses cause renal toxicity *Children:* 100 mg initial test dose, then 10 to 15 mg/kg of body weight weekly for 5 weeks Suramin may be given IM if IV is impractical Avoid extravasation on IV administration because it causes severe local irritation	Injectable: 1 gm ampule; prepare 10% solution; use only freshly prepared solution because drug deteriorates upon standing after reconstitution Store in a cool place in airtight containers; protect from light	*Contraindicated* in patients with severe renal or ocular disease Commonly causes vomiting, pruritus, urticaria, paresthesias, hyperesthesia of hands and feet, photophobia, peripheral neuropathy Occasionally causes renal damage, blood dyscrasias, shock Patients who are sensitive to suramin may have shock, syncope, acute circulatory failure, and seizures with this drug; it should be administered *only* in the hospital under close supervision	Monitor for symptoms of peripheral neuropathy

★ **Tinidazole** Fasigyn Simplotan	Trichomoniasis	*Adults:* 150 mg b.i.d. PO for 7 days or as a single dose of 2 gm to both men and women	*Contraindicated* in patients with neurologic disease or with blood dyscrasias It should *not* be given to nursing mothers or in the first trimester of pregnancy Advise patient that sexual partner should be treated concurrently to avoid reinfection Commonly causes nausea, dizziness, headache, and dry mouth

BIBLIOGRAPHY

Cleary, T.G. Congenital malaria. *Morbidity and Mortality Weekly Report,* January 11, 1980.

Connor, D.H. Current concepts in parasitology: onchocerciasis. *New England Journal of Medicine,* 1978, *298,* 379-381.

Dyer, R., & Keystone, J. Malaria: a Canadian problem. *Canadian Nurse,* 1981, *77,* 20.

Goldman, P. Metronidazole. *New England Journal of Medicine,* 1980, *21,* 1212-1218.

Knight, R. Giardiasis, isosporiasis and balantidiasis. *Clinics in Gastroenterology,* 1978, *7,* 31-47.

Neva, F. A., & Ottesen, E.A. Current concepts in parasitology: tropical (filarial) eosinophilia. *New England Journal of Medicine,* 1978, *298,* 1129-1131.

Wyler, D.J. Malaria—resurgence, resistance, and research (part 1). *New England Journal of Medicine,* 1983, *308,* 875-878.

Wyler, D.J. Malaria—resurgence, resistance, and research (part 2). *New England Journal of Medicine,* 1983, *308,* 934-940.

CHAPTER 43

Pediculicides and Scabicides

Karin E. Zenk

Medications discussed in this chapter

Pediculicides	Scabicides
Benzyl benzoate	Benzyl benzoate
Lindane	Crotamiton
Malathion	Lindane
Pyrethrins	Sulfur

Pediculosis, or lice infestation in humans, is increasing in epidemic proportions in the United States and Canada in all socioeconomic and cultural groups. School-aged children are especially affected. Scabies is also being seen in pandemic proportions in all age groups and socioeconomic levels.

PEDICULOSIS

Pediculosis involves three types of disease infestation: (1) *Pediculus humanus* var. *capitis* (head lice); (2) *Pediculus humanus* var. *corporis* (body lice); and (3) *Phthirus pubis* (pubic lice or "crabs," so-called because of their appearance).

Human lice are wingless ectoparasites that suck blood from the host. They are whitish gray and are approximately 3 mm long. The bite can cause a sensitivity reaction in some individuals with a wheal developing at the site of the bite usually within 24 hours. Itching results as a reaction to this sensitivity, and scratching can cause excoriation of the skin and secondary infection.

The life span of the louse from the egg or nit stage to death is from 50 to 75 days. Infestation is spread by direct contact with infested individuals or by contact with articles recently contaminated by them. Female head lice firmly attach their nits to the hair shaft close to the skin of the scalp. These lice are most often spread by school children. Body lice infest clothing and can be found in the seams or folds of clothing or underwear where they are in close contact with the body. Eggs are usually deposited in clothing, but in severe infestations may be found attached to body hair. Bites may be found on the skin. Pubic lice infest mainly the pubic area where nits are deposited close to the skin at the base of hair shaft. Nits may also be found deposited in other hairy areas including armpits, eyebrows, or facial hair, especially long or heavy beards.

Head and body lice are spread by personal contact or common use of combs, brushes, clothing (caps, scarves, coats), or bedding. They can also be spread by contact with seats in public places (e.g., buses, theaters). Pubic lice may be spread by sexual contact or by contact with toilet seats, bed linen, or clothing. Diagnosis is made by the identification of pediculi or nits on scalp or body hair, in the seams of clothing, or on skin surfaces. Live adult lice are usually not seen except in cases of severe infestation.

The treatment of pediculosis involves the use of pediculicides including lindane (gamma benzene hexachloride) shampoo, lotion, or cream depending on the type of infestation. Because the shampoo cannot remove nits from the hair shaft, they must be combed out with a fine-toothed comb or removed with a forceps. Disinfecting clothing and other personal items including brushes and combs is indicated to prevent reinfestation. Clothing and bedding should be laundered thoroughly in hot water and machine dried or dry cleaned. Personal hygiene is essential in the prevention and control of lice infestation. Infested homes should be carefully vacuumed. Use of insecticide sprays to fumigate homes, schools, or other infested environments is controversial and is usually not required. Children, however, should be kept home from school and hospital patients isolated until treatment is successful. It is recommended that family members and contacts be examined for infestation and treated as indicated.

Pediculicides should be used carefully because some (e.g., lindane) have been associated with neurotoxicity especially when used frequently or when left on the skin for longer than the recommended period of time. These medications should be used only as directed and use should be limited. (See the Nursing Drug Digest for the appropriate use and duration of contact with skin for each preparation.)

SCABIES

The agent responsible for scabies is the itch mite, *Sarcoptes scabiei*, var. *hom.*, a translucent organism approximately 0.5 mm in length. The impregnated female burrows into the superficial stratum corneum of the epidermis where she deposits eggs and fecal matter. The eggs hatch within a few days. The life span is approximately 1 week from the egg to larval stage followed by another 1 to 3 weeks to adulthood. Females live 2 to 4 weeks longer than males, who die after impregnating the female.

The disease is spread by skin-to-skin contact with infected persons or by contact with their personal effects. Scabies is communicable throughout the duration of the disease. Since symptoms may not appear for as long as 2 months, persons infected with scabies may harbor the mites and be capable of transmitting the disease before lesions or pruritus develop. Skin burrows are difficult to see but may be seen with the assistance of a hand lens as minute, dark wavy lines 1 mm to 1 cm in length. A very small scab may be noted at the open end of the burrow. Specific areas where the eruption occurs include finger webs, hands, wrists, elbows, axillae, the upper thigh and lower buttocks in the crease area, the pigmented area around the nipples in women, and the penis in men.

Scabies does not usually involve the face except in very young children. Itching is intense especially at night and is a major symptom of the disease, although it does not occur for several weeks after the infection when sensitization occurs. The diagnosis is confirmed by microscopic demonstration of the mite from fragments needled from a skin burrow.

There are various scabicides available. The directions for each scabicide are outlined in the Nursing Drug Digest of this chapter and should be followed carefully since these preparations have been associated with toxicity. For example, lindane was found to be neurotoxic in infants and very young children. In one report the blood level of lindane was 17 times greater than expected after a single topical application of a 1% solution of the drug. The infant had seizures and abnormal neurologic function associated with these levels.

In another child significant blood levels were found after repeated application of small amounts to areas of dermatitis and excoriated skin. Thus lindane is a potentially toxic agent that can cause convulsions and even death from therapeutic and accidental overexposure, which can occur when patients apply the drug more frequently or for longer periods of time (weeks or months) than prescribed. A problem that often occurs in relation to misuse of these preparations and resultant toxicity is overtreatment of the condition, which often leads to dermatitis. The patient mistakes the dermatitis for reinfection and resumes treatment. Limiting the quantity of medication available to the patient has been helpful in preventing this problem. Patients should also be encouraged to consult with their health care provider before resuming treatment.

Commonly used alternatives for the treatment of scabies in infants and children include precipitated sulfur in petrolatum and crotamiton. An additional scabicide is benzyl benzoate. One of these alternatives should be chosen to treat children less than 1 year old, children with badly excoriated skin, or pregnant women. Routine retreatment with lindane should be avoided, and the smallest effective dose should be used. In children with excoriated lesions lindane should be washed off after 6 hours rather than after 24 hours to prevent increased absorption of the medication. All of these preparations are irritating to the eyes and should not be used near eyes or on eyelashes. Petrolatum ophthalmic ointment may be used to protect the eyes during application.

The diagnosis of scabies is often missed because it can be confused with numerous other pruritic dermatoses. Some of the most common misdiagnoses include atopic dermatitis, neurodermatitis, contact dermatitis, impetigo, pyoderma, papular urticaria, insect bites, cutaneous larva migrans, and varicella.

Careful instruction to the patient is essential for successful therapy. Treatment can fail if the patient does not follow instructions for medication use or care of clothing. It is important to stress that all areas, not just the eruption, should be covered with medication. One to two ounces (30 to 60 ml) of the lotion should be adequate for an adult. All members of the household and sexual contacts should be treated even if not symptomatic. Clothing should be machine washed in hot water and dried on the hot cycle and ironed. The patient will be 50% better in 48 hours but will still have some itching for days to weeks since the organisms are dead after treatment but are still in the skin. The patient is sensitized to them and will continue to itch until they are gone. The turnover rate of the stratum corneum is 4 days; therefore pruritus can continue for at least this length of time.

The patient should understand how to treat the

infestation, have a prescription for an appropriate amount of medication for the entire family, have an understanding as to why asymptomatic members of the household should participate in the therapy, and should know why itching will continue for awhile.

A nonrefillable prescription should be made out *only* for the amount needed. Because patients tend to apply the drugs more frequently and over longer periods (sometimes weeks or months) than prescribed, limiting the quantity prescribed prevents dermatitis caused by overtreatment, which the patient may mistake for persistence of the scabies. This in turn will minimize percutaneous penetration of the drugs.

Canine scabies

Animal-transmitted scabies is common in the United States. Dogs (usually puppies) are the primary source. Humans are inadvertently infested by direct or indirect contact. Canine-transmitted scabies in humans differs from human scabies in that it has greater ease of transmission, different distribution pattern, absence of burrows, and shorter incubation period. Animal-transmitted scabies is self-limited (several weeks). The animal should be treated by a veterinarian skilled in veterinary dermatology. Symptomatic family members may be treated with supportive measures.

It is not necessary to treat asymptomatic members of the household since the condition is not usually contagious between humans.

Secondary infection

Secondary bacterial infection may complicate scabies. Streptococcal strains that lead to acute glomerulonephritis may colonize scabietic lesions. Associated bacterial infection, especially streptococcal infection, requires appropriate therapy (see Section X, "Antibacterial, Antifungal, and Antiviral Medications").

SUMMARY

This chapter has examined the various types and uses of pediculicides and scabicides. A brief overview of scabies and pediculosis, including the causative organism and mode of transmission, has been presented.

With an understanding of the various individual agents, including their actions and side effects, the nurse will be better able to provide optimal care to patients who require these medications. Patient education can be enhanced; and adverse drug effects can be anticipated, monitored for, and minimized by utilizing the information presented in this chapter.

ADVERSE/SIDE EFFECTS OF THE PEDICULICIDES AND SCABICIDES*

ALLERGIC REACTIONS	**CUTANEOUS SYSTEM**	**HEMATOLOGIC SYSTEM**
Contact dermatitis	Irritant contact dermatitis	Rarely causes aplastic anemia
Eczematous rash	Irritation of denuded skin	
	Irritation of mucous membranes	**OCULAR SYSTEM**
CENTRAL NERVOUS SYSTEM	Stains skin and has unpleasant odor (sulfur)	Eye irritation
CNS stimulation progressing to convulsions		

*See Chapter 11, "Drug Toxicity," for an overview of drug toxicity.

CLINICALLY SIGNIFICANT DRUG INTERACTIONS*

Primary drug	*Interacting drug*	*Possible effect*	*Probable mechanism*
Pediculicides and scabicides	Other topical creams, lotions, or ointments	Reduced effectiveness of pediculicide or scabicide	Dilution or removal of medication

*See Chapter 10, "Drug Interactions," for an overview of drug interactions.

GENERAL NURSING IMPLICATIONS

Nursing of patients requiring pediculicides or scabicides

ASSESSMENT

Assessment should include a detailed drug history to identify possible sensitivity to pediculicides or scabicides. Contraindications to these medications as well as cautions and potential drug interactions should be explored before therapy is initiated.

As with other parasitic disease conditions, a complete nursing assessment is essential to assist in the diagnosis of the causative organism as well as to establish a baseline from which to plan individualized therapy and to monitor patient response.

A general assessment of the skin should be completed and deviations in the usual character of the skin carefully recorded. Inspection, best completed in natural light, and palpation should be utilized to describe the color, shape, and distribution of lesions noted. Subjective complaints of itching, burning, or stinging should also be noted as well as any observations of scratching behavior.

Pediculosis

The diagnosis of pediculosis is made by observation alone. Laboratory verification is *not* needed, although microscopic examination may be used to differentiate between head or body lice and pubic lice. The presence and distribution of lice or nits that can be seen by the naked eye should be recorded carefully. A Wood's lamp may be used for screening large numbers of school children.

The scalp, general body area, and pubic area should be carefully inspected. The back of the head, behind the ears, the upper back, and the nape of the neck as well as the eyelashes are common sites for head lice infestation. The presence of heavy seborrhea, dermatitis, or psoriasis should not be mistaken for nits nor should dandruff, hair roots, or hair spray droplets. The axillae, breasts, finger webs, elbows, and the belt area as well as clothing and bed linen, should be assessed for body lice infestation; the genital area should be inspected for pubic lice. The adult louse is usually not seen but nits can be seen attached to the hair shaft near the scalp or skin surface. The presence of excoriation caused by scratching, secondary infection (pyoderma), and lymphadenopathy should also be assessed and recorded. Erythema, crusting, and oozing of the scalp can be seen in severe infestation where pyoderma has occurred from excessive scratching.

Scabies

Scabies, or mites, cannot be seen with the naked eye; however, burrows or runs may be seen especially in oblique light and with the aid of a hand lens. Microscopic confirmation of the disease is indicated before treatment is initiated because skin lesions are often hard to differentiate. The hands are usually the first areas involved, especially the finger webs and sides of the digits. The flexor surface of the wrist is commonly involved as are the extensor surfaces of the elbows. The infestation is roughly symmetrical, and lesions may be nodular but are usually dry and eczematous. Intertriginous areas and the periumbilical area are also sites of involvement as well as the belt area and lower buttocks. Intense itching, especially at night, is a classic symptom as is the appearance of inflammation and burrows. The patient's general condition and hygiene should also be assessed because nutritional deficiencies can also be present. Bed rest and a nutritious diet are important adjuncts to the use of scabicides. The nursing history should include questions related to the source of infestation (e.g., the presence of domestic animals including dogs or cats). The site(s) of infestation and the character and distribution of lesions should also be recorded. Excoriation of the skin and secondary infection caused by scratching may be present.

The presence of pediculosis or scabies is usually associated with unhygienic environments and poor personal hygiene. This is not always the case because contact with infected individuals or personal items can easily spread these diseases. Because the spread of infestation is by direct contact, isola- tion and care of clothing and linen are indicated. All family members and contacts should be examined for infestation and treated if necessary. In known and suspected cases nurses should protect themselves as well as others from potential infestation. These conditions are often embarrassing to patients and family members, and the nurse's approach to assessment and care must be sensitive and understanding. Assistance in the prevention of reinfestation is extremely important.

SENSITIVITY

Topical medications used in the treatment of pediculosis and scabies are often irritating and can cause sensitivity reactions in certain individuals. Infants and young children as well as those patients with irritated or denuded skin areas should be monitored closely because dermatitis and CNS changes have been reported indicative of local hypersensitivity or toxicity.

CAUTIONS AND CONTRAINDICATIONS

Topical pediculicides and scabicides are contraindicated in patients with known hypersensitivity. The use of these medications is generally contraindicated in infants because of the danger of toxicity. Topical application of some of these medications (e.g., lindane) has resulted in seizures and other abnormal neurologic function. These medications should be used cautiously during pregnancy, and pediculicides and scabicides should be used only as directed. Prolonged use or repeated applications of these medications should be avoided because of the possibility of absorption through the skin resulting in toxicity, which can lead to severe CNS stimulation and death. Oral ingestion of these products has resulted in death. Keep these drugs safely stored out of the reach of children.

DRUG INTERACTIONS

The use of other topical medications can dilute or rub off the topically applied pediculicide or scabicide, thus diminishing its effect. *Continued.*

Nursing of patients requiring pediculicides or scabicides—cont'd

ADMINISTRATION

Pediculicides and scabicides are available in creams and lotions. Shampoo forms are also available for the treatment of head lice. These preparations should be applied topically and used only as directed. Patients can usually be taught how to apply these medications themselves. When assistance is required, nurses should use gloves because these medications can be absorbed through the skin.

These medications should not be allowed to get into the eyes, on eyelashes, or mucous membranes. The ear canal should also be protected especially when shampoos are applied. The eyes can be protected with Vaseline. If any medication comes in contact with the eyes it should be washed away immediately with water.

Shampoos should be applied to the scalp after the hair has been rinsed with warm water. It should be worked into a good lather and left on as directed. The hair should then be rinsed thoroughly and dried with a towel. A fine-toothed comb or forceps should be used to remove nit shells.

Creams and lotions do not have to be applied after bathing but should be applied to dry skin. The smallest effective dose should be used. If denuded areas or lesions are present, it is recommended that the medication be washed off sooner than for intact skin (after 6 hours rather than after 12 to 24 hours). These medications should not be applied to acutely inflamed skin areas.

All infected areas should be covered with a thin coat of the cream or lotion as indicated. The medication should not be rubbed into the skin (see the Nursing Drug Digest). The average adult requires 30 gm (1 ounce) of topical scabicide to cover the trunk and extensor surfaces. Proportionally less is used for children and infants. The scabicide should be applied thinly but thoroughly from the neck downwards to all areas with special attention to the hands, feet, and intertriginous areas.

After treatment of pediculosis or scabies, the patient should bathe or (preferably) shower and cleanse the skin well with soap. Clean clothes and bed linen should be provided to prevent reinfection. See the Nursing Drug Digest for specific information regarding the administration of pediculicides and scabicides.

MONITORING PATIENT RESPONSE
Therapeutic response

Patients treated for pediculosis should be inspected for the presence of new nits 1 to 7 days after treatment. Some practitioners recommend treatment to be repeated after 7 to 10 days because the medication may not be ovicidal, and some lice may not be killed by the initial treatment. Others recommend that patients be retreated only if evidence of continued infestation is found.

Even after effective therapy for scabies, it may take weeks until the signs and symptoms disappear since the hypersensitivity state will not cease immediately upon destruction of the parasite. Itching will continue for some time because the dead organisms are still present in the skin. However, the patient should have less itching and feel better within 48 hours after treatment.

After the infestation has been eradicated, secondary treatment includes measures to alleviate itching and scratching. The topical application of calamine lotion or other soothing lotion may relieve itching and decrease inflammation. Nails should be trimmed short. Elbow restraints may be required especially in children to prevent scratching that can lead to a secondary infection.

Dermatitis may require treatment with corticosteroids, and secondary infections may require treatment with topical antibiotic ointments. Systemic treatment with antibiotics is usually not required.

Patients should be monitored carefully for local irritation caused by the use of the pediculicide or scabicide, secondary infection, or signs of reinfestation.

Adverse side effects

The major adverse effects of pediculicides and scabicides is contact dermatitis, eczematous rash, CNS toxicity, and irritation to mucous membranes, eyes, and denuded skin. Acute toxicity studies show CNS toxicity to be usually related to misuse. Sulfur-containing preparations have an unpleasant odor and can stain the skin.

PATIENT EDUCATION

The patient and family should have a clear understanding of the medication regimen as well as the exact name of the medication, its action, dosage, method of storage, administration, side effects, and what can be done to minimize adverse effects. They should know how to monitor therapeutic effects as well as to identify signs that indicate the medication should be removed immediately and the health care provider contacted.

Patients and family members should be aware that pediculosis or scabies is contagious and spread by direct contact. Isolation is usually indicated in the hospital. Children should be kept home from school until treatment is effective, and clothing and bed linen should be handled separately. The patient and family should know the importance of having family members and other contacts examined for infestation and treated if necessary.

Because these are often embarrassing problems for the patient and family, understanding and assistance in the prevention of reinfestation are extremely important.

Assistance is often needed in identifying the cause of the disease and measures to prevent reinfection. Patients may need a review of personal and environmental hygiene practices including the importance of bathing and wearing clean clothes.

For pediculosis, sheets and clothing can be disinfected by machine washing with hot water and machine drying on the hot cycle for 20 minutes. Ironing should also be done, especially at the seams. Clothes that cannot be washed can be dry cleaned and should be placed in a plastic bag and the cleaner notified.

Temperatures greater than 52° C (125° F) for 5 to 10 minutes kills both lice and nits. Combs and brushes should be soaked in 2% Lysol or a pediculicide shampoo for at least 1 hour or heated in water (65° C) for 5 to 10 minutes.

Fumigation is not necessary, although careful vacuuming is important in controlling lice infestation.

PEDICULICIDES AND SCABICIDES

This medication is used to treat lice infestations or scabies.

Use only as directed and do not use more frequently than prescribed.

Keep this medication away from the eyes, mouth, injured or irritated skin, and out of the ears. If some medication should get into your eyes, flush it away immediately with water.

Notify your health care provider if you notice irritation such as itching or burning after you use this medication that was not present before you used it.

Do not swallow this medication. It is for *external use only*. Keep this medication out of the reach of children as death has resulted from accidental oral ingestion.

This medication has been prescribed especially for you. Do *not* trade or give this medication to any relatives or friends.

Do *not* use other topical medications other than those prescribed while using this medication.

In addition to the above general instructions, if you require this medicated *shampoo* for the treatment of head lice:
- You do *not* need to shave or cut your hair.
- Wet your hair thoroughly with warm water.
- Pour 2 tablespoons (1 ounce, 30 ml) on your palms and apply to your scalp and hair; work into a good lather.
- Rub vigorously in all directions for at least 4 minutes and be sure to cover all hair areas to ensure thorough distribution and contact with the parasite and eggs.
- Allow the shampoo to remain no longer than 10 minutes (A-200).
- Rinse the hair thoroughly with warm water 2 to 3 times, then gently rub dry with a freshly laundered towel.
- Comb the hair with a fine-toothed comb to remove remaining nit shells or eggs.
- If necessary, repeat the same procedure in 24 hours as directed by your health care provider.
- Use this shampoo (lindane, A-200) to clean combs and brushes to prevent the spread of lice or reinfestation. Do not share combs or brushes with other family or household members.
- Do not use this shampoo more frequently than directed because frequent, unnecessary use can cause toxic reactions.
- If you have any questions or notice irritation, nausea, or vomiting, contact your health care provider.

If you require this medication for the treatment of *body lice:*
- Take a hot soapy bath or shower. Use lots of soap to clean your skin.
- Dry off well with a freshly laundered towel.
- Apply this medication (cream or lotion) to the entire area affected as well as the surrounding areas.
- Leave the medication on overnight or for 12 to 24 hours.
- Take another hot soapy bath or shower. Use lots of soap to clean your skin well. Put on freshly laundered or dry-cleaned clothes in order to prevent reinfestation.
- Vacuum your house well. Machine wash and machine dry your clothing and bed linen using the hot cycles to prevent reinfestation. Hot water will kill any lice in your clothes or linen. Clothes that cannot be washed, such as woolens, should be dry cleaned. Bring them in a plastic bag to the cleaners and let them know they may be infested with lice so that the clothing can be handled separately.

If you require this medication for the treatment of *scabies:*
- Take a hot soapy bath or shower using lots of soap to cleanse the skin well.
- Dry the skin well with a freshly laundered towel.
- Apply a thin layer of medication (cream or lotion) over the entire skin surface from the neck down. Be sure to apply the medication in creases or skin folds and under the arms.
- Dress in loosely fitting clothing or pajamas and leave the medication on overnight or for 12 to 24 hours.
- Take another hot soapy bath or shower and use lots of soap to cleanse the skin well.
- Dry the skin well with a freshly laundered towel.
- Put on freshly laundered or dry-cleaned clothes in order to prevent reinfestation with scabies.
- Launder bedclothes and washable clothing in hot water in your washing machine. Machine dry and iron. If clothing cannot be washed, have it dry cleaned.

The itching from the scabies will be improved in 2 days, but you will still have some itching for several days to weeks since the dead organisms may remain in the skin for some time after treatment. Allergy to these organisms causes itching. When the skin layers turn over and slough off, the organisms will be gone and the itching will stop.

All members of your family should be treated for scabies because it is easily passed from one family member to another. If we treat just you, you may be reinfected from another family member.

If necessary, repeat the procedure as directed by your health care provider 7 days after the first treatment. It is important to check with your health care provider before using this medication for a second treatment because many patients mistake irritation caused by the medication as reinfestation and use the medication when it is not necessary. It is best to have your health care provider identify the need for repeated treatment.

NURSING DRUG DIGEST

Medication (trade name*)	Indication	Usual dosage and administration	Dosage forms, preparation, and storage	Contraindications, cautions, and comments	Monitoring
Benzyl benzoate Scabanca Scabiol	Pediculosis capitis and pubis (lice) Scabies (mites)	Adults: Usual required amount is 30 ml per application *Children:* Usual required amount is 20 ml per application Cleanse area with soap and water thoroughly for 10 min Apply an approximately 25% preparation of the drug; when dry reapply; dry Wash off in 24 hr Apply nightly or q.o.d. for 3 treatments *For external use only*	Emulsion: 50% Lotions: 14%, 27%, 50% Cream: 25%	May irritate skin and eyes; may increase itching Avoid contact with eyes, mucous membranes, and urethral meatus Explain instructions for use carefully; make sure patient understands that this is a *topical* medication Do not apply to open or inflamed areas of skin	Observe for hypersensitivity; if observed, wash drug off, discontinue, and notify prescriber
Crotamiton Eurax	Scabies (with antipruritic properties)	Topical; apply to dry skin; bathing before application not necessary; massage a thin layer of cream into the skin of whole body, from chin down, especially body folds, hands, feet, and intertriginous areas, until dry Use approximately 30 gm per application Apply two applications at 24 hr intervals Take cleansing bath 48 hr after last application May repeat in 1 week, if necessary Use gloves to apply *For external use only*	Cream: 10% Lotion: 10%	*Contraindicated* in hypersensitivity; discontinue and wash off drug if sensitivity occurs May cause contact dermatitis and occasional irritant contact dermatitis Explain use of this medication carefully to patient Irritating to denuded skin Avoid contact with eyes, mouth, mucous membranes, and urethral meatus Clothing and bedding should be changed as needed to ensure comfort and before cleansing bath	Observe for irritation or sensitivity

Lindane	Pediculosis (lice)	Cream: 1%	*Adults and older children:* following a soap and warm	*Contraindicated* in hypersensitivity—repeated applications
Gamene	Scabies (mites)	Lotion: 1%	water bath using a soft	may cause dermatitis
gBh		Shampoo: 1%	brush, no more than 20-30	*Caution:* Lindane is absorbed through intact
Gexane			gm of lotion or cream is applied to all parts of the body	skin and is toxic if absorbed in excessive
Kwell			except the face; wash off	amounts
Kwellada			thoroughly in shower or tub	Irritating to skin, eyes,
Scabene			bath after 12 hr	and mucous membranes
			Pediculosis capitis: moisten	Symptoms of toxicity are
			scalp with water; apply up	CNS stimulation progressing to convulsions; can be treated
			to 1 oz of shampoo, lather	with phenobarbital
			for 5 min, rinse, dry; pay	Avoid use in infants
			special attention to areas	Avoid getting on eyelashes
			behind ears and at nape of	May cause eczematous
			neck and back of head; remove nits with fine comb;	rash
			may repeat only once in 1	Rarely causes aplastic
			week if new eggs are seen	anemia
			Combs and brushes should	If lindane irritates the
			also be washed with shampoo to prevent reinfestation	skin, wash off and do not use again
			For external use only	Make sure that patient understands that this is a topical drug
				Patient should understand instructions fully
				Instruct parents to keep this drug out of reach of children
				Clean bedding and clothing should be used after bathing to prevent reinfestation

Continued.

NOTE: For additional details regarding the individual agents listed in this table, see the text and other tables in this chapter.

*Indicates a multiple active ingredient product. For a complete listing of all active ingredients see the *Drug Reference Guide to Brand Names and Active Ingredients.*

♦ Indicates that the drug is generally available only in Canada.

★ Indicates that the drug is generally available only in the United States.

NURSING DRUG DIGEST—cont'd

Medication (trade name)	Indication	Usual dosage and administration	Dosage forms, preparation, and storage	Contraindications, cautions, and comments	Monitoring
Malathion Prioderm	Pediculosis (for head lice and their nits)	*Adults and children:* Sprinkle lotion on hair and gently rub until the scalp is thoroughly moistened; allow hair to dry naturally and for 8-12 hr. Follow with a thorough shampooing and rinsing of the hair and scalp. The dead lice and nits should be removed with a fine-toothed comb. If necessary, may repeat application in 7 days. *For external use only*	Lotion: 0.5%	*Contraindicated* in hypersensitivity. One of the least toxic organophosphate insecticides. Pediculicidal and ovicidal. May cause mild stinging and scalp irritation. Product contains 70% isopropyl alcohol and is *flammable*; patient should be cautioned to avoid open flames and should not use a hair dryer to dry scalp. Atropine (1-4 mg IM or IV) is the antidote for accidental oral poisoning, which may be accompanied by severe respiratory distress. Avoid contact with eyes; flush immediately with water	Monitor for hypersensitivity
Pyrethrins A-200 Pyrinate* Bare* Rid* Rid Liquid Pediculicide* Tisit	Pediculosis (for head, pubic, and body lice and their nits)	*Topical:* Apply sufficient amount to completely wet the hair and scalp or skin of any infested area. Allow application to remain no longer than 10 min. Wash and rinse with plenty of warm water. Remove dead lice and eggs from hair with fine-toothed comb. To restore luster to the hair following scalp applications, follow with a good shampoo. Treatment may be repeated, but not more than twice per 24 hr. *For external use only*	Liquid: 0.18% Gel: 0.18%, 0.3%, 0.33% Shampoo: 0.3% NOTE: Generally found in combination with other pediculicides (e.g., piperonyl butoxide 2%-4% and petroleum distillates)	*Contraindicated* in persons allergic to any of the preparation's ingredients. *Contraindicated* in persons allergic to ragweed. Harmful if swallowed or inhaled. To prevent reinfestation, clothing and bedding should be thoroughly cleaned. Make sure the patient understands that this is a topical drug. Keep away from eyes and mucous membranes because it may cause irritation	

Sulfur	Preferred scabicide for infants, small children, and pregnant women	Following a cleansing scrub, using a soft brush, hot water and soap, skin is dried and sulfur ointment applied Apply nightly for 3 nights May bathe each night before application or once 24 hr after last application *For external use only*	Ointment: 6% (precipitated sulfur in petrolatum); compounding is necessary for prescription; not commercially available	Has staining properties and an unpleasant odor Rarely causes irritation and dermatitis Instruct patient carefully as to proper use Since this medication must be compounded by the pharmacist, allow ample lead time before picking up the prescription Cosmetically less acceptable to most patients than the other medications in this group	If contact with eyes, flush immediately with water Skin irritation may occur from this medication

BIBLIOGRAPHY

Estes, S. Scabies. *Arizona Medicine,* 1978, *35,* 477-479.

Gossel, T., & Wuest, R. Treatment of lice, mite, and tick infestations. *California Pharmacist,* 1977, 20-23.

Hansen, R. Transcutaneous gamma benzene hexachloride absorption and toxicity in infants and children. *Archives of Dermatology,* 1979, *115,* 1224.

Malathion for treatment of head lice. *The Medical Letter,* 1983, *25,* 30-31.

Orkin, M. Scabies in children. *Pediatric Clinics of North America,* 1978, *25,* 371-386.

Orkin, M., and Maibach, H.I. Current concepts in parasitology: this scabies pandemic. *New England Journal of Medicine,* 1978, *298,* 496-498.

Parish, L.C., & Witkowski, J.A. Head lice: epidemic in the schoolroom. *Drug Therapy,* 1980, 145-152.

CHAPTER 44

Anthelmintics

Karin E. Zenk

Medications discussed in this chapter

Anthelmintics	Anthelmintics—cont'd
Bephenium	Piperazine
Bithionol	Praziquantel
Dichlorophen	Pyrantel pamoate
Diethylcarbamazine	Pyrvinium pamoate
Hycanthone	Quinacrine
Mebendazole	Stibophen
Niclosamide	Suramin
Niridazole	Tetrachloroethylene
Oxamniquine	Thiabendazole

This chapter discusses the treatment of helminth infestation. The various major groups of helminths are presented and further broken down into commonly encountered parasitic species. The life cycle of these parasites, including their mode of transmission, is presented as a basis for specific pharmacologic treatment.

The helminths include three major groups: the cestodes (tapeworms), the nematodes (roundworms), and the trematodes (flukes). Infections caused by flukes include schistosomiasis, fascioliasis, paragonimiasis, and clonorchiasis. Cestode infections are caused by five types of tapeworms; nematode, or roundworm, infections are divided into intestinal and tissue types. Infections caused by tissue nematodes include filariasis, loiasis, onchocerciasis, dracunculiasis, and trichinosis. Intestinal nematodes cause ascariasis, enterobiasis (pinworm infection), hookworm disease, trichuriasis (shipworm infection), strongyloidiasis, visceral larva migrans (toxocariasis), and cutaneous larva migrans. Parasitic infections involving helminths are increasing in both the United States and Canada as a result of increasing travel and of increased emigration from Southeast Asia, the Caribbean, and Central and South America. This problem was identified in the resettlement of Indochinese refugees.

In 1979 it was announced that 14,000 Indochinese refugees would be accepted monthly for resettlement in the United States. Canada also accepted large numbers of refugees. Although most of the refugees are free of major contagious diseases, many do have health problems, most frequently tuberculosis and parasitic diseases. Parasitic diseases are particularly common in these refugees. In a survey of 165 Laotian refugees hookworm was found to be the most common intestinal parasite (64%) followed by *Giardia* (18%), *Trichuris* (12%), and *Ascaris* (9%). Many of these infestations are those with which most North American clinicians have had little or no experience.

Refugees infected with intestinal helminths (worms) do not pose a significant public health hazard since adequate sewage disposal interrupts transmission of the helminths, which require several days of incubation in the soil before becoming infective.

As immigration continues, case finding and treatment of parasitic disease is important in the control of these diseases. These infections are treated with anthelmintics.

CESTODE (TAPEWORM) INFESTATIONS

Five species of tapeworm commonly invade humans:

Taenia saginata	Beef tapeworm
Taenia solium	Pork tapeworm
Dipylidium caninum	Dog tapeworm
Diphyllobothrium latum	Fish tapeworm
Hymenolepis nana	Dwarf tapeworm

Of these five species of tapeworm, the beef and pork tapeworms are the most common. All adult tapeworms infecting humans inhabit the small intestine. The adult tapeworm has a head, called a *scolex*, which attaches to the gastrointestinal mucosa; the scolex is followed by the neck region from which a chain of individual segments called *proglottids* arise. Beef and pork tapeworms often exceed 300 cm (approximately 10 feet) in length. Regardless of the total number of the proglottids, it is the scolex that generates new proglottids and will do so even if the rest of the worm has broken off and left the host. Humans become infected by the ingestion of an *encysted* scolex, except in *H. nana* in which the ovum is ingested. Most patients become aware of the infection by seeing proglottides and large segments of worms in their stools. Diagnosis of the infection is made by the identification of proglottids or ova in stool.

Taenia saginata (beef tapeworm)

In *T. saginata*, the most common tapeworm in the United States, eggs are expelled from the proglottids after they pass from the host. The eggs hatch and are ingested by cattle, releasing embryos that encyst in muscles as *cysticerci*. Humans are infected by eating undercooked beef containing live cysticerci. In the human intestine the cysticercus develops into an adult worm. Treatment is with niclosamide.

Taenia solium (pork tapeworm)

With *T. solium* the adult tapeworm causes only intestinal irritation, but the *larvae* go to many parts of the body in the human and encyst as cysticerci. This is called *cysticercosis*. Symptoms of the tapeworm infestation are intestinal irritation. Heavy infestations may occasionally cause weight loss but otherwise no serious symptoms. Large segments can be passed in the stool. If the scolex, or head, is not passed, the worm continues to grow. This can be upsetting to patients who often need much reassurance and support. The cysticerci do cause problems. Most lodge in muscles or connective tissues where they cause muscle pain, weakness, and eosinophilia. They eventually calcify. If they go to the brain they can cause seizures and central nervous system (CNS) changes, such as personality disturbances. Roentgenograms of soft tissues show calcified cysticerci.

For the adult (intestinal) stage treatment is with niclosamide and paromomycin. No specific treatment is available for cysticercosis other than surgical removal of cysticerci in the brain. Anticonvulsants are given for seizures. Because of the poor prognosis it is important to treat *T. solium* thoroughly and early before the larval tapeworms lodge in the CNS.

NEMATODE (ROUNDWORM) INFESTATIONS

Nematode infestations of humans consist of several types and are divided into those involving *tissue* or *intestinal* parasites. Tissue nematodes are those that produce disease by migration through the tissues such as *Dracunculus*, filarial worms, and *Trichinella*.

Those that produce clinical manifestations because of the presence of the adult worm in the gastrointestinal tract are intestinal nematodes and include *Enterobius*, *Trichuris*, *Ascaris*, the *hookworms*, *Strongyloides*, *cutaneous larva migrans* and *Toxocara canis*.

Tissue nematodes

Dracunculiasis. Dracunculiasis is an infection of human connective and subcutaneous tissues by *Dracuncula medinensis* (guinea worm), a parasite indigenous to Africa, southern Asia, northeastern Canada and the United States, and South America. Symptoms are produced when the gravid female discharges her eggs into the skin.

Humans are infected when they swallow water containing the infected *intermediate host*, the *Cyclops*, a crustacean that commonly lives in wells and ponds in the tropics. Larval forms from *Cyclops* are transferred to humans and mature in the connective tissue. After mating, the gravid female, which is one meter in length, moves to the surface of the body. At this time the patient has fever, urticaria, periorbital edema, and wheezing. When the head of the worm reaches the skin a blister develops and ruptures. This is accompanied by intense pain and itching. The worm is usually not visible in the ulcer. The lesion is usually on the feet or ankles. The worm releases all of its larvae, which takes up to 3 weeks. The worm then dies and is either extruded or absorbed. The ulcer heals 4 to 6 weeks from the onset.

General therapy includes bed rest, elevation of the extremity, and control of secondary infection of the ulcer, which is common. Drugs used for this infestation are niridazole or alternatively metronidazole (see Chapter 42, "Antiprotozoals, Antimalarials, and Amebicides"). These drugs may only ameliorate symptoms and may not enhance killing of the worm.

If the worm can be clearly seen or palpated it may sometimes be completely removed by excision or gradually extracted. The gradual extraction may be accomplished by winding a few centimeters of the worm onto a stick each day until it is completely removed.

Dracunculiasis can be prevented by chemical treatment of drinking water.

Filariasis. Filariasis (lymphatic filiariasis) can be caused by *Wuchereria bancrofti* or *Brugia malayia*. Filariasis is widespread in the tropics. Humans are the *definitive host;* the intermediate host is the mosquito. Filariae are threadlike nematodes that invade the lymphatics and the subcutaneous and deep tissues of humans, producing blockage of the lymphatics, acute inflammation, and scarring. *Wuchereria bancrofti* can cause elephantiasis, a massive hypertrophy of the skin and subcutaneous tissues resulting from the lymphatic obstruction. It usually affects the legs, arms, genitalia, or breasts. Other obstructive problems that can occur include hydrocele, scrotal lymphedema, and lymphatic varices. Microfilaria can be seen in the blood. The patient usually has an eosinophilia of 10% to 30%.

Early symptoms of this disease are inflammation of the affected body part; painful, tender vessels; and later obstruction of lymph flow resulting in edema. Abscesses may form at sites of lymphatic inflammation. Episodes may occur for years before obstruction occurs. *Chyluria* may result from the rupture of distended lymphatics into the urinary tract. In early stages of elephantiasis the tissues of the affected part are edematous and soft; later with skin hypertrophy and subcutaneous connective tissue proliferation, the body part becomes hard. As the swelling enlarges, sometimes to enormous size, the skin surface folds and fissures. This gross enlargement, however, does not occur in all patients with the disease and is the exception.

Treatment may be medical or surgical. Moving to a cooler climate reduces the number and severity of acute inflammatory attacks. Diethylcarbamazine is the drug used to treat this disorder. Treatment with diethylcarbamazine is often followed by allergic reactions to the dying parasite. In heavy infestations it may be helpful to pretreat the patient with antihistamines, aspirin, or corticosteroids in order to control allergic symptoms. General supportive care includes bed rest during inflammatory episodes, and antibiotics especially if abscesses are present. Suspension bandages for scrotal lymphedema are helpful. Elevation and use of pressure bandages and support stockings are helpful for edema of the leg. Results from surgical removal of elephantoid breast, scrotum, or vulva are usually satisfactory. Surgery for limb elephantiasis is usually not helpful.

Reassurance of the patient is very important. The prognosis for life is excellent, especially if the patient leaves the endemic area and avoids reinfection. Disease control is accomplished by mass treatment and by mosquito control.

Onchocerciasis. Onchocerciasis is caused by a microfilaria, *Onchocerca volvulus*, and is called "river blindness." This disease is an important world health problem as nearly a half million persons have been blinded by this disease.

This disease is carried by *Simulium* flies (black flies, buffalo gnats). The biting fly introduces infective larvae that develop slowly in the human tissues. Flies are infected in turn by picking up microfilariae while biting.

The microfilariae move around the body and may be found in the skin, subcutaneous tissues, lymphatics, and in the conjunctiva and other structures of the eye. They cause severe itching and local skin color change, either darker or depigmented, probably the result of migrating microfilaria.

Treatment of this disease is with diethylcarbamazine followed by suramin. When the eyes are involved, treatment should be started at a low dose, and antihistamines or corticosteroids should be used to reduce allergic reactions to the disintegration of the microfilariae.

Trichinosis. Trichinosis is primarily a disease of humans and pigs and is caused by *Trichinella spirales*, a tissue and an intestinal nematode. This disease has a relatively high incidence in the United States. Infestation is acquired from eating the inadequately cooked meat of infected pigs, bears, and aquatic mammals such as walrus. Pork may be present in other ground meats, intentionally or by accidental adulteration. Beef hamburger contaminated by a meat grinder also used for pork has resulted in human disease.

The symptoms of trichinosis include diarrhea (early in the course), *myositis*, fever, prostration, periorbital edema, eosinophilia, and myocarditis or encephalitis when larvae migrate to the tissue.

Humans ingest the larval stage, (i.e., encysted in pork muscle). These are liberated in the small intestine where they produce more living larvae, many of which are carried by lacteals and lymphatics to various organs. The larvae penetrate skeletal muscle where they coil up and become encysted. This occurs about 17 days after infestation. From 6 to 18 months later they become calcified.

Treatment of trichinosis is with thiabendazole or mebendazole. Aspirin may give therapeutic response comparable to corticosteroids for severely ill patients. Corticosteroids should not be used because they may prolong the life of the adult worm.

This disease was once more common than now in the United States. In the mid-1950's the practice of feeding uncooked garbage to swine was prohibited. Raw garbage had contained infected pork scraps, which perpetuated the disease. Also responsible for a decrease in incidence is consumer education emphasizing the importance of adequately cooking meat. It is recommended that pork be cooked at a 350° F oven temperature for at least 35 minutes per pound and even longer for a large roast. Smoking, pickling, heavy seasoning, or spicing does not make pork products safe. The governmental meat inspection stamp does *not* pertain to trichinosis and is therefore not a protection against infection. Freezing at 18° C kills larvae within 3 days, and it is recommended that pork meat be frozen before preparation.

Intestinal nematodes

Ascariasis. It is estimated that 25% of the world population, including 4 million Americans, are infested with this nematode. *Ascaris lumbricoides* (roundworm) infects humans from ingestion of infective eggs from soil, contaminated food, toys, dirt, water, or airborne dust. The eggs hatch in the small intestine, release motile larvae that penetrate the wall of the small intestine, and reach the right side of the heart via the mesenteric venules and lymphatics. From the right side of the heart they move to the lung, burrow through the alveolar walls, and migrate up the bronchial tree into the pharynx, down the esophagus, and back to the small intestine. The larvae then mature and lay eggs. The large adult worms, which are 20 to 40 cm long, may live for 1 year or more. Eggs require 3 to 4 weeks in the soil to become infective, then remain so for months to years.

The patient becomes aware of the infection either because of vomiting the worm or through passing one in the stool. When symptomatic, diagnosis is made by microscopic examination of stool.

Treatment is with pyrantel pamoate or mebendazole. An alternative drug is piperazine. Ascariasis, hookworm, and trichuriasis often occur together and may be treated together with mebendazole. Infection is perpetuated by ingestion of ova from the soil. Spread is controlled by treatment of infected persons, good home and community sanitation, and control in use of human feces as fertilizer. There is no danger of direct human-to-human spread. Ascariasis is commonly a household infection of rural areas. Adequate personal hygiene should be stressed and adequate toilet facilities provided.

Signs and symptoms of this infestation may be mild or severe, depending upon the stage of the life cycle and the extent of infestation. In the lung capillary and alveolar system damage with hemorrhage may result as the worms force their way through the tissues. Symptoms include cough and hemoptysis with rales. Eosinophilia occurs at this stage. In the intestinal stage usually there are no symptoms, but with heavy infestation protein deficiency or other nutritional deficiency may result. When the infection is heavy, the worms may migrate (be coughed up, vomited, passed out through the nose, force themselves up the bile duct, the pancreatic duct, appendix, and other sites) if disturbed by fever or certain medication (e.g., tetrachlo-roethylene). This may result in physical blockade and inflammation of the affected duct. With very heavy infestation obstruction of the intestine may occur.

Enterobiasis. Enterobiasis (pinworm, threadworm, seatworm, or oxyuriasis) is one of the more common intestinal infestations and is caused by *Enterobius vermicularis* and is characterized by perianal pruritus. The incidence in North American white children is approximately 40%, whereas blacks show approximately one third that number. Approximately 22 million people are infected in Canada and the United States. In some European communities 80% of the children are infected. The source is infected humans. The eggs are transferred from perianal skin to mouth by contamination of hands, food, *fomites,* or being inhaled and swallowed because the eggs are light in weight and readily conveyed through air. Symptoms of perianal itching are primarily the result of the nocturnal migration of the gravid females to the anal area where they deposit eggs in the perianal folds of the skin and die. The itching may cause the child to be restless, nervous, and irritable, probably from loss of sleep associated with the pruritus ani. Intense scratching may result in secondary infection.

Because neither the adult worms nor ova are commonly found in stool, diagnosis is made with the "Scotch Tape test." Cellophane or transparent tape impressions are taken in the perianal area in the morning before the child has bathed or gone to the toilet (frosted tape should not be used) and a tape slide made. These are less useful done in the doctor's office because the child has usually had a bath before coming to the appointment. Tape slide preparations may be examined at leisure, since eggs remain identifiable for years. At least three tests, on consecutive mornings, should be obtained.

Treatment is with pyrantel pamoate or mebendazole. Alternative drugs are piperazine citrate or pyrvinium pamoate. Treatment of all family members simultaneously should be considered. Treatment may be repeated in 2 weeks to treat possible reinfection from infective eggs not affected by the first treatment.

Hookworm. Hookworm (ancyclostomiasis, necatoriasis) is an intestinal parasitic disease caused by *Necator americanus* or *Ancyclostoma duodenale.* These species are endemic in warm, humid climates. The source of the infection is soil contaminated with feces from infected humans. The eggs in the feces hatch in the soil; the infective *filariform* larvae develop and penetrate the skin (usually bare feet with common bites of invasion being the dorsum of the foot and in between the toes). They migrate to the bloodstream, then to the lungs, trachea, and pharynx. The larvae are then swallowed and attach to the intestinal wall where they develop to maturity. The adult worm resides in the small intestine where females deposit their eggs in the lumen of the intestine. They do not multiply within the host, since the eggs leave the host in the feces. If the feces are deposited where environmental conditions are favorable, eggs will hatch in 24 hours.

Symptoms of hookworm begin with severe itching caused by the development of a kind of dermatitis (i.e., "ground itch") when larvae penetrate the skin. Local erythema, macules, and papules may develop. If considerable numbers of worms migrate through the lung at once, cough, wheezing, bronchitis, or pneumonitis may result. Eosinophila may be present. Hookworm is a chronic infection and there are infrequent symptoms of the adult worm in the intestinal tract. Light infections usually produce no symptoms. With significant infection, symptoms include vague epigastric distress often confused with peptic ulcer disease. Nausea and vomiting are unusual. *Pica* may be present and the appetite is often ravenous except in the later stages of disease. Alterations in bowel habits (constipation) occurs as a result of the change in overall dietary intake. When iron deficiency anemia develops, symptoms occur depending on the worm load, such as weakness, pallor, fatigue, palpitations, and dyspnea associated with hypochromic, microcytic anemia. The mucous membranes and skin become pallid. The worms suck the host's blood and mucosal substances. Blood passes through the worm and hemolyzes 50% of the red blood cells. From 0.03 to 0.26 ml of blood per worm per 24 hours is withdrawn. A light infection of 10 worms could remove as much as 3,500 ml of blood in 5 years from the host. Because the disease is chronic, anemia is the major clinical feature. Anemia is primarily the result of the continuous blood loss. The extent of anemia is proportional to the number of worms and the nutritional intake of the patient. Hypoalbuminemia is the other major clinical manifestation of this disease resulting from chronic blood loss. In children growth and development may be stunted.

Treatment is with pyrantel pamoate or mebendazole. An alternative drug for *Necator americanus* is thiabendazole. If anemia is present, it responds readily to the administration of salts, iron (within several weeks), and a high-protein diet before drug treatment is begun. In severe anemia blood transfusion with packed red cells may be necessary to raise the hemoglobin to 10 gm per 100 ml. In advanced cases it may be necessary to delay drug treatment for 2 to 3 weeks. If ascariasis and hookworm are both present,

mebendazole should be given for the combined infection. Alternatively, piperazine may be given first to eradicate the *Ascaris,* then a drug may be given for the hookworm.

Strongyloidiasis. *Strongyloides stercoralis* is the parasite that causes strongyloidiasis (Cochin-China diarrhea). Moist soil or objects contaminated with human feces contain the infective (filariform) larvae. These larvae can penetrate the skin and are carried to the lungs. Here they develop further, enter alveoli, ascend the trachea to the epiglottis, and are then swallowed. They live imbedded in the mucosa of the small intestine, where the life cycle is completed.

Strongyloides is common in tropical and subtropical areas of the world. In the United States it is prevalent in the southeastern states. Autoinfection is responsible for the persistence of strongyloidiasis in persons who have left endemic areas. The life span of the adult worm may be as long as 5 years. Autoinfection may occur during this time if the larvae are retained in constipated feces or if there is fecal contamination of the perianal region. Such infection may also occur in the presence of diarrhea.

The incubation period from larval penetration of skin to larvae in feces is 2 to 3 weeks. Larvae in feces may be immediately infective. The disease is communicable as long as the person is infected. Some symptoms and signs of *Strongyloides* infestation include pruritic dermatitis at sites of penetration of larvae, malaise, cough, and urticaria. Other symptoms are abdominal colic, flatulence, and diarrhea alternating with constipation. Characteristic larvae can be seen in fresh stool specimens, although the worm is essentially invisible to the naked eye, being less than 2 mm long and transparent.

Treatment of strongyloidiasis is with thiabendazole. In the case of concurrent infestation with *Ascaris* or hookworm, which is not uncommon, these infections are treated first and strongyloidiasis afterward. Side effects of thiabendazole are headache, weakness, nausea, vomiting, vertigo, and decreased mental alertness. *Crystalluria* and leukopenia have been reported.

Trichuriasis. Trichuriasis, commonly called whipworm disease, is widespread in the tropics and subtropics. It is also commonly found in the rural southeastern portion of the United States. It is caused by *Trichuris trichiura.* These small, slender worms, which measure 30 to 50 mm in length, attach themselves to the mucosa of the large intestine. They cause symptoms only when present in very large numbers. The source of the infestation is embryonated eggs from soil contaminated with human feces. New infections are acquired by direct ingestion of infective eggs. The eggs require about 3 weeks in proper soil conditions to embryonate and become infective. There is no direct communicability from person to person.

Light infections are asymptomatic. Heavy to massive infections may cause abdominal pain, distention, nausea, flatulence, diarrhea and occasionally rectal prolapse. Detection of whipworm eggs in the stool is usually required for diagnosis. The patient commonly has an eosinophilia of 5% to 20%. Heavy infections are most often found in malnourished small children.

Treatment is not necessary for light infestations. For heavier infestations mebendazole is used.

Visceral larva migrans. Visceral larva migrans (toxocariasis) is caused by the larvae of certain nematodes such as *Toxocara canis* and *T. cati*, normally found in dogs and cats. The source is soil or fomites contaminated with infective eggs from dog or cat feces. The mode of transmission is ingestion of infective eggs; eggs require several weeks in suitable soil to become infective. Infection usually occurs in young children as a result of eating dirt or close contact with an infected pet. The larvae migrate through the body and lodge in various organs, particularly the lungs, liver, and brain.

Symptoms are fever, cough, hepatomegaly, and nervous symptoms. Other symptoms may occur when such organs as the heart, eyes, and kidneys are invaded. Infections may be asymptomatic. This disease is characterized by an eosinophil count of 30% to 80% and leukocytosis.

Thiabendazole is the drug of choice for treatment of toxocariasis. Corticosteroids, antibiotics, antihistamines, and analgesics may be needed for symptomatic relief. Symptoms may last for months, but the prognosis is good.

TREMATODE (FLUKE) INFECTIONS

Trematode (fluke) infections include schistosomiasis, fascioliasis, paragonimiasis, and clonorchiasis.

Schistosomiasis

Schistosomiasis can be caused by three trematode worms (1) *Schistosoma mansoni*, (2) *S. hematobium*, and (3) *S. japonicum*. The main reservoir for *S. hematobium* and *S. mansoni* is humans, and for *S. japonicum*, a variety of animals. It is not communicable person to person. It is transmitted when the host passes eggs in the stool or urine. The larval stages hatch and infect certain freshwater snails. They multiply in these snails then go out into the water. These larvae *(cercariae)* can penetrate human skin or mucous membranes while swimming or bathing.

Symptoms and signs of infestation with schistosomiasis are a transient erythematous rash that itches. Fever, malaise, urticaria, eosinophilia, and hepatosplenomegaly are also part of the clinical picture. The patient may have diarrhea, gastrointestinal discomfort, weight loss, and ascites. Renal damage with hematuria, urinary frequency, and urethral and bladder pain also occurs.

Drugs used to treat schistosomiasis include niridazole, antimony-containing drugs, (e.g., stibophen), and hycanthone.

Fascioliasis

Fascioliasis (liver rot) is prevalent in sheep-raising countries. The infection is by *Fasciola hepatica*, the sheep liver fluke, which occasionally also infects humans and results from eating the *metacercariae* on raw salads containing watercress or other aquatic vegetables. The metacercariae are passed to these aquatic plants by an intermediate host, the lymneid snails. The infestation causes "liver rot" in sheep, the principal definitive host. Light infections may be asymptomatic, but heavy infection causes fever, eosinophilia, and hepatomegaly. An early clinical symptom is epigastric pain and is related to migration of the larval form within the liver. The adult flukes live in the human biliary tract during the chronic stage and may cause biliary obstruction. The diagnosis is made by finding eggs in the stool. The infestation is treated with bithionol or emetine. In endemic areas (e.g., Algeria, Cuba, France, Great Britain, Hawaii) aquatic plants should not be eaten raw but should be boiled. Washing does not destroy the metacercariae. Safe drinking water should be provided.

Paragonimiasis

Paragonimiasis (pulmonary distomiasis) is mainly confined to the far East (China, Japan, Korea, Philippines) but there are foci throughout the tropics. The agent is *Paragonimus westermani*, called the lung fluke, because the lungs are the organ most often involved in the infestation. The onset is with cough, low-grade fever, and hemoptysis. Pleuritic chest pain is common. Dyspnea, signs of bronchitis and *bronchiectasis*, and weight loss are present in heavy infection.

Humans and many species of domestic and wild animals are host to this infection. Eggs reach the water, penetrate snails, develop, and the emerging cercariae form cysts in crabs and crayfish. When these crabs or crayfish are eaten raw or pickled or when cooking utensils or dinnerware is contaminated, immature flukes are ingested, which form cysts in the small intestine and migrate through the diaphragm and into the lung. Diagnosis is made by the identification of eggs in the sputum and if the sputum is swallowed, also in the stool. Treatment is with bithionol. Paragonimiasis is not directly communicable person to person.

Clonorchiasis

Clonorchiasis is an infection of the biliary passages caused by *Clonorchis sinensis*, the most important liver fluke in humans. This fluke can live in the biliary tract for as long as 50 years. Infection can be acquired in the Far East in countries such as Korea, Taiwan, Japan, Hong Kong, southern China, and Vietnam. The disease may also be acquired by eating infected dried, frozen, or pickled fish imported from the Far East.

The definitive hosts are human, dogs, cats, rats, and pigs. The intermediate host is the freshwater snail. After multiplication and development within the snail, the cercariae are released and penetrate freshwater fish. Humans are usually infected by eating infected raw, dried, salted, or pickled freshwater fish containing encysted metacercariae, although ingestion of cysts in drinking water can also cause the disease. Thorough cooking of freshwater fish prevents infection. This disease is not communicable person to person.

The disease is manifested by liver disease with progressive liver enlargement, tenderness, and right upper quadrant abdominal pain. Chloroquine is used to treat the disease although not always effectively.

SUMMARY

This chapter has examined the various types and uses of the anthelmintics. An overview of the various types of helminths, including their life cycle and mode of transmission, has been presented.

With an understanding of the various individual agents, including their actions and side effects, the nurse will be able to provide optimal care to patients requiring these medications. Patient education can be enhanced, and adverse drug effects can be anticipated, monitored for, and minimized by utilizing the information presented in this chapter.

ADVERSE/SIDE EFFECTS OF THE ANTHELMINTICS*

ALLERGIC REACTIONS

Urticaria

AUTONOMIC NERVOUS SYSTEM

Abdominal pain
Anorexia
Diarrhea
Nausea
Vomiting

CARDIOVASCULAR SYSTEM

Cardiac dysrhythmias
Heart failure
Precordial pain

CENTRAL NERVOUS SYSTEM

Dizziness
Exacerbation of epilepsy
Hallucinations
Headache

CUTANEOUS SYSTEM

Acneiform eruptions
Depigmentation of hair or skin
Discoloration of mucous membranes
 and nails
Rash
Stevens-Johnson syndrome
Yellow discoloration of skin

GENITOURINARY SYSTEM

Crystalluria
Darkening of urine
Urethral burning

HEMATOLOGIC SYSTEM

Hemolysis in G-6-PD deficiency
Leukocyte count decreased

HEPATIC SYSTEM

Liver damage
SGOT elevation

**METABOLIC AND ENDOCRINE
SYSTEMS**

Enlargement of thyroid

NEUROMUSCULAR SYSTEM

Subacute myelo-optic neuropathy
Peripheral neuropathy

OCULAR SYSTEM

Corneal opacity
Optic atrophy
Optic neuritis
Photophobia

*See Chapter 11, "Drug Toxicity" for an overview of drug toxicity.

CLINICALLY SIGNIFICANT DRUG INTERACTIONS*

Primary drug	Interacting drug	Possible effect(s)	Probable mechanism(s)
Tetrachloroethylene	Alcohol	Additive CNS effects	Both alcohol and tetrachloroethylene have CNS effects that are additive when taken together Alcohol should not be taken for 24 hr before or after this drug

*See Chapter 10, "Drug Interactions," for an overview of drug interactions.

GENERAL NURSING IMPLICATIONS

Nursing of patients requiring anthelmintics

ASSESSMENT

A complete nursing assessment is essential in establishing a baseline from which to plan individualized therapy and to monitor patient response. Assessment should include a detailed drug history to identify possible sensitivity, contraindications, cautions, and potential drug interactions before therapy is initiated.

As with other parasitic conditions, assessment of the patient's general condition is important since weight loss, anemia, asthma, lethargy, and other symptoms may present. Parasites may be visible in stool or sputum. Identification of the parasite is important in appropriate drug selection, and stool, urine, or sputum specimens must be carefully obtained to enable accurate diagnosis. Correction of debilitation, anemia, nutritional deficiency, and fluid and electrolyte balance is often indicated before drug therapy is initiated.

The entire family or household may be infected, and a positive diagnosis of infestation in one member warrants examination of others to prevent reinfestation.

A diet history is helpful in planning adequate nutrition, and questions may explore practices in food preparation that may need modification in relation to the prevention of reinfestation.

Infestation often is related to geographic location. The nursing history should include information regarding residence or travel to a foreign country. When completing the assessment, it is helpful to recognize that some parasites are found more commonly in particular groups. For example, *Giardia* is often found in campers, *Enterobius* in children, and *Giardia* and *Amoeba* infections in homosexuals.

Since the patient may be asymptomatic, laboratory examination is required to make specific diagnosis.

SENSITIVITY

Anthelmintics are contraindicated in patients with known sensitivity. Patients who have not received anthelmintics previously should be monitored for urticaria, erythema multiforme, purpura, fever, or arthralgia. Any unusual or new symptoms should be noted that may indicate hypersensitivity.

DRUG INTERACTIONS

See Clinically Significant Drug Interactions.

CAUTIONS AND CONTRAINDICATIONS

Anthelmintics are contraindicated in known hypersensitivity. Some are contraindicated in patients with impaired renal or hepatic function or convulsive disorders. Safe use in pregnancy has not been established.

See the Nursing Drug Digest for specific information regarding each individual agent.

ADMINISTRATION

Anthelmintics should be administered as directed. Some oral forms are bitter tasting and should be mixed with flavored syrup or applesauce, especially when given to children. Others (e.g., pyrvinium) are irritating to the stomach and can cause nausea and vomiting. It is often helpful to administer these medications with food or immediately before or after a meal. Pyrvinium should be administered carefully since suspensions can stain clothing or linen if spilled. Tablets should be swallowed whole and not chewed to avoid staining the teeth and mouth bright red; the patient should be warned that stools will likewise be stained bright red.

For tapeworm infestation, purgation is indicated before therapy to decrease the amount of stool that requires sieving when searching for the scolex. Use of laxatives or enemas before treatment with bephenium, piperazine, or pyrvinium pamoate is not necessary.

In infestations where numerous parasites are involved, the order of treatment and use of various anthelmintics is important. The correction of anemia, fluid and electrolyte balance, and nutritional deficits is indicated before treatment in certain cases.

Continued.

Nursing of patients requiring anthelmintics—cont'd

MONITORING PATIENT RESPONSE

Therapeutic response

After a course of treatment, stools, urine, or sputum specimens should be examined for ova and adult worms at 2 to 5 week intervals to monitor the effectiveness of therapy. If ova are found in the specimen, another course of treatment may be indicated. In severe infections a course of therapy may be repeated after a 1-week interval. Patients should be carefully monitored for an allergic reaction to the dying parasite. For pinworms, patients should be monitored for decreased perianal itching. Symptoms presented by other infestations should also diminish with appropriate treatment. In tapeworm infestation, stools should be carefully sieved to be sure that the scolex is passed.

Many anthelmintics work by paralyzing the worms and thus they are passed alive. This can be frightening and upsetting to patients and their families. Support and understanding during treatment are essential.

Adverse side effects

Various anthelmintics can cause side effects including gastric distress. These medications should be administered with meals. In addition, patients should be monitored for dizziness, and safety precautions should be utilized (e.g., bedrails) as indicated. Piperazine and quinacrine can cause visual changes, and patients should be advised to immediately report any change in visual acuity. Changes in skin color such as yellow staining of the skin can occur with quinacrine; pyrvinium can stain clothing and stool red. Anthelmintics can cause vomiting, diarrhea, and anorexia as well as cardiac abnormalities such as dysrhythmias. Careful monitoring is essential. See Adverse/Side Effects of the Anthelmintics for general side effects of these medications and the Nursing Drug Digest for information about specific medications.

PATIENT EDUCATION

The patient and family should have a clear understanding of the medication regimen as well as the exact name of the medication, its action, dosage, method of storage, administration, and side effects and what can be done to minimize any adverse effects. They should know how to monitor therapeutic effects as well as be able to identify when the health care provider should be contacted and/or the medication stopped.

The infestation and passing of worms through stool or coughing them up in sputum as well as knowledge that they could be in body tissues can be psychologically distressing. Patients and families often worry that health and hygiene care may be seen as inadequate and also worry about giving the condition to family and friends. Patients and their families need much support and understanding. A knowledge of the life cycle of the worm, vectors, and fomites of transmission is helpful in increasing their understanding of how the disease was obtained (e.g., camping, travel, daycare, etc.) as well as what they can do to prevent spread and reinfection. Self-care practices related to personal and environmental hygiene can be reviewed and emphasized including the importance of handwashing after toileting and before food preparation or eating. Nails should be trimmed short and kept clean, and patients should avoid biting them. Hands should be kept away from the face, nose, and mouth. Daily bathing or showering and washing of the perianal area with soap and water should be encouraged. Underwear should be changed daily, and well-fitting cotton underwear should be selected. Clothing and bed linen should be changed daily during treatment and then at regular weekly intervals after effective treatment. Environmental hygiene may need attention since organisms can be spread in the air, especially in heavily contaminated households. Clothing and linen should be machine washed and machine dried on the hot cycles to kill ova.

The hospitalized patient should understand the importance of personal hygiene care and should be provided with his or her own toilet facility. Outpatient or discharge patients should scrub the toilet seat with soap and water after each use until treatment is effective. Pinworms and roundworms are transferred by direct and indirect contact of ova (hands, food, contaminated articles). The patient and family need instruction in personal hygiene, as previously described.

Roundworm infestations can also result from improper disposal of human feces. Sanitary disposal of feces and health education are important to prevent spread and reinfection. In addition, patients traveling to foreign countries, especially underdeveloped areas, may be advised to avoid uncooked foods including salads.

To prevent tapeworm reinfection, patients should be encouraged to store meats properly and to cook them thoroughly. Game meat should be avoided. Fish from fresh lakes and ponds should be carefully inspected for the presence of worms and should be cooked thoroughly.

The patient and family as indicated should be carefully instructed on securing specimens since the quality of the specimen is important in securing accurate diagnosis of the parasitic infestation and in monitoring response to therapy.

Stool specimens

For ova and parasites the specimen should be submitted fresh within 30 to 60 minutes or mixed with a preservative.

For outpatients it is advantageous to collect 3 (e.g., on Monday, Wednesday, and Friday) grape-sized specimens deposited in a vial containing 7 to 9 ml polyvinyl alcohol fixative solution and mixed well. The specimen should not be refrigerated. A purge may be needed to obtain the specimen. If required, saline cathartics (magnesium sulfate) are recommended. Oils, bismuth compounds, barium sulfate, and antibiotics can interfere with the stool examination and should be avoided. The number of stools necessary to rule out parasites depends on the parasite suspected.

In addition to stool examinations, skin, serologic tests, and tests of urine and sputum may also be indicated. The patient should understand why these tests are necessary and how specimens will be obtained.

GENERAL INSTRUCTIONS FOR DISCHARGE/OUTPATIENTS

ANTHELMINTICS

This medication is used to treat worm infections.

It is important that you take this medication exactly as directed. Do not miss any doses, otherwise the infection will not be eliminated. Do not take any more of this medication than directed because it could have some harmful effects. If you have any questions contact your health care provider.

It is not necessary to take a laxative or change your diet unless you have been specifically told to do so by your health care provider.

Most people have few or no side effects from this medication; however, if you should develop itching, a rash or hives, or stomach cramps, call your health care provider.

Personal hygiene is important in preventing reinfection. Be sure to take a shower every morning and wash the anal area well with soap and water to remove eggs that may have appeared during the night.

Try not to scratch the affected area because the area can become inflamed and irritated. Scratching may also increase the chance of reinfection by inadvertently placing the fingers in the mouth or touching food.

Wash your hands frequently during the day, especially after going to the bathroom, before handling food, and before eating.

Keep your hands away from your face, nose, and mouth. Keep your fingernails clean and cut short. Avoid biting your nails.

After taking this medication, change the bed linen, your underwear, and night clothes daily. Wash clothes immediately in the washer and machine dry, both on the hot cycle.

Disinfect the toilet seat and bathtub after use.

Store this medication in a cool dry place.

Keep this medication out of the reach of children.

This medication has been prescribed especially for you. Do not trade or give this medication to any relatives or friends.

If family members are receiving this medication, identify adult and child doses carefully.

SPECIFIC DRUGS

Mebendazole

Chew the tablets well before swallowing and follow with a glass of water.

Piperazine

Dissolve the granules in 2 ounces (60 ml) of water, milk, or fruit juice. Shake the liquid medicine well before pouring it out so that the dose will be mixed well. Follow the medicine with a full glass of water. Notify your health care provider if you notice side effects such as bruising, fever, joint pain, dizziness, blurred vision, trembling, or numbness of the hands and feet.

Pyrantel pamoate

This medication may be taken with milk or fruit juice either with food or on an empty stomach. Shake the liquid medication well before pouring out your dose to be sure it is mixed well. In some people this drug can cause dizziness or drowsiness. Until you know how this medication affects you do not drive or operate dangerous machinery or do jobs that require alertness. If you should become dizzy, sit or lie down right away. Be careful going up or down stairs. Call your health care provider if you develop a headache.

Pyrvinium pamoate

Take before or after meals. Avoid spilling liquid forms of this medication on clothing because it will stain them. Shake liquid medication well. Swallow tablets whole to avoid staining teeth and do not suck, crush, or chew tablets. This medication may cause your stools to turn red. This is not unusual.

Women who are pregnant, breastfeeding, or planning to become pregnant should notify their health care provider before taking this medication.

Quinacrine

This medication may cause the urine and skin to turn yellow. Your skin and urine should return to its usual color within 2 weeks after your treatment is finished. In some people, this medication may cause dizziness. Until you know how this medication affects you, do not drive or operate dangerous machinery or do jobs that require mental alertness. If you should become dizzy, sit or lie down immediately. Go up and down stairs carefully.

Notify your health care provider if you should notice blurred vision, see double, have nightmares, or become depressed.

Thiabendazole

Take this medication with food, preferably after a meal. Shake liquid medication well before pouring out the dose to be sure it is mixed well. Chew tablets before swallowing and follow medication with a glass of water.

This medication may cause your urine to change color. This is not unusual.

This medication may cause you to become dizzy or drowsy. Do not drive or operate dangerous machinery or do jobs that require alertness until you know how this medication affects you.

Call your health care provider if you have fainting spells, notice a yellow color to your skin or eyes, unusual fatigue, or pain in your joints.

OBTAINING STOOL SPECIMENS

Specimens should be collected on separate days—every other day is best.

Do not take the specimen from the toilet bowl or get urine in the sample. Collect the specimen in a wide-mouth container or pan or upon some clean newspapers. Children can be told to use the toilet for a BM only. A large container (old bowl) can be placed under the toilet seat and the child told not to flush.

When three specimens are requested, collect two specimens from normal movements and the third after taking a laxative such as cascara, magnesium sulfate, milk of magnesia, or Fleets phosphosoda. *Do not take mineral or castor oil.* When 6 specimens are required, collect 3 from normal movements and 3 after taking a laxative.

The fresh specimen should be brought to the laboratory as soon as possible after it has been passed in a jar or specimen container, which you can get from your health care provider.

When a preservative (PVA) is used (two bottles are provided):

1. Add stool to the container marked PVA. Liquid or soft part of stool preferred. Fill bottle up to red line or mark only. Mix PVA and stool thoroughly with the enclosed applicator. Keep the bottle at room temperature until you bring it to the laboratory. Write your name and the date on the label.
2. To the empty bottle, add part of the stool (formed part, if possible). The bottle should be no more than half full. Place bottle in a clean paper bag and keep in refrigerator until you bring it to the laboratory.

NURSING DRUG DIGEST

Medication (trade name*)	Indication	Usual dosage and administration	Dosage forms, preparation, and storage	Contraindications, cautions, and comments	Monitoring
★ **Bephenium** Alcopar	Hookworm: *Ascaris lumbricoides, Trichostrongylus orientalis, Ancyclostoma duodenale*	*Adults:* 5 gm in a single dose PO *Children:* Under 23 kg of body weight, 2.5 gm in a single dose PO Give on an empty stomach to prevent vomiting (at least 2 hr after any food); food should not be taken for another 2 hr Taste may be disguised by suspending in a strong sugar solution or carbonated beverage or administer mixed with milk, flavored syrup, or orange juice Since bephenium may cause some vomiting, correct dehydration before administration	Sachets of 5 gm	Safe use in pregnancy not established Use cautiously in hypertension, cardiac, renal, and hepatic disease, and in children under 1 year of age In cases of severe diarrhea from hookworms, may need to give daily for 4 to 7 days No purge is necessary either before or after this drug Side effects are few The drug has a bitter taste and so may cause nausea and vomiting May cause temporary looseness of stools Alcohol may reduce effectiveness of medication; advise patient not to drink alcohol 24 hr before or after medication is taken	If drug used for ascariasis, worms may be present in vomitus; patient should be warned
★ **Bithionol** Actamer Bitin Lorothidol	Flukes: *Fasciola hepatica* (sheep liver fluke), *Paragonimus westermani* (lung fluke)	*Adults:* 30-50 mg/kg every other day for 10-15 doses PO *Children:* Same as adults	Capsule: 500 mg	Warn patient to use *caution* in going out in the sun after taking bithionol May cause photosensitivity reactions, urticaria, and gastrointestinal distress (cramps, diarrhea, vomiting)	

★ **Dichlorophen**
Anthiphen

Tapeworm (*T. saginata, T. solium*)

Adults: 2-3 gm q.8h. PO for 3 doses
Children: 1-2 gm q.8h. PO for 3 doses
Alternatively
Adults: 6 gm PO as a single daily dose for 2 successive days
Children: 2-4 gm PO as a single daily dose for 2 successive days
Give dose early in the day on an empty stomach because it is usually followed in 2-3 hr by intestinal colic and the passing of a few loose stools

Tablet: 500 mg

Contraindicated in impaired liver function and in conditions in which purgation is undesirable, e.g., during the last few months of pregnancy or severe cardiovascular disease
Commonly causes colic, diarrhea, nausea lasting from 4 to 6 hr
Occasionally causes vomiting
Lassitude is another common symptom
Rarely causes urticaria, which disappears without treatment in 24 hr
Has caused jaundice and even death following large doses

★✦ **Diethylcarbamazine**
Barocide
Franocide
Hetrazan

Filarial disease:
Wuchereria bancrofti, Wuchereria malayi, Loa loa, Onchocerca volvulus
Tropical eosinophilia

Adults: 2-4 mg/kg t.i.d. PO; give after meals to help mask sweet taste of drug and minimize GI distress
Children: Same as adults
Adults: 13 mg/kg/day PO for 4-7 days

Tablet: 50 mg
Stable even under conditions of high heat and humidity, such as occurs in the tropics

Use *particular caution* in patients treated for onchocerca, especially on initial treatment, because eye inflammation and other allergic reactions can occur
Common side effects include severe allergic or febrile reactions, because of the filarial infection; GI disturbances
May rarely cause encephalopathy
May also cause headache, general malaise, weakness, joint pains, anorexia
Almost all patients exhibit leukocytosis, first evident on the second day of therapy
Observe for allergy or hypersensitivity

Continued.

NOTE: For additional details regarding the individual agents listed in this table, see the text and other tables in this chapter.
*Indicates a multiple active ingredient product. For a complete listing of all active ingredients see the *Drug Reference Guide to Brand Names and Active Ingredients*.
✦Indicates that the drug is generally available only in Canada.
★Indicates that the drug is generally available only in the United States.

NURSING DRUG DIGEST—cont'd

Medication (trade name)	Indication	Usual dosage and administration	Dosage forms, preparation, and storage	Contraindications, cautions, and comments	Monitoring
★ **Hycanthone** Etrenol	Schistosomiasis	*Adults:* 7.5 mg/kg IM as a single dose; may be repeated in 3 months *Children:* Pediatric dose not available	Injectable: 2 mg/2 ml	*Contraindicated* in liver disease; may cause postnecrotic cirrhosis or death when given to patients with hepatic necrosis or in patients with preexisting liver disease *Contraindicated* in patients with concomitant bacterial or viral infections Assess patient carefully for signs of liver impairment, (e.g., enlarged, tender liver and history of jaundice) May cause pain at the site of injection, nausea, vomiting, anorexia, and dizziness Hycanthone has been shown to be teratogenic, carcinogenic, and mutagenic under experimental conditions Less effective in young children than older children and adults	

Drug	Uses	Preparations	Dosage and administration	Remarks
Mebendazole Telmin Vermox	*Trichuris trichiura*, ascariasis, enterobiasis, and hookworm in single or mixed infestations	Tablet, chewable: 100 mg	*Adults:* Enterobiasis: a single 100 mg dose PO For ascariasis, tricuriasis, and hookworm: 100 mg PO b.i.d. on 3 consecutive days, morning and evening *Children:* Same as adults Tablet should be chewed or swallowed whole	*Contraindicated* in pregnancy or if the patient has exhibited an allergic reaction to the agent Dosage schedule is unusual in that dosing is same for adults and children Mebendazole has not caused systemic toxicity probably because of its poor absorption Clearance of worms from the gastrointestinal tract may not be complete for 3 days after treatment May cause abdominal pain and diarrhea in cases of massive infestation and expulsion of worms
★ **Niclosamide** Niclocide Yomesan	Tapeworms: *Diphytlobothrium latum* (fish tapeworm), *Taenia saginata* (beef tapeworm), *Taenia solium* (pork tapeworm), *Dipylidium caninum* (dog tapeworm) *Hymenolepsis nana,* (dwarf tapeworm)	Tablet, chewable: 0.5 gm	*Adults:* A single daily dose of 4 tablets (2 gm) PO, chewed thoroughly *Children:* 11-34 kg, a single dose of 2 tablets (1 gm) PO, chewed thoroughly; greater than 34 kg, a single dose of 3 tablets (1.5 gm) PO, chewed thoroughly Take on an empty stomach *Adults:* 2 gm/day PO for 7 days *Children:* 11-34 kg, 1 gm PO, followed by 500 mg/day for 6 days; greater than 34 kg, 1.5 gm PO, followed by 1 gm/day for 6 days All tablets must be thoroughly chewed	*Contraindicated* in hypersensitivity Occasional nausea and vomiting Since tapeworm infections are not life threatening, it is recommended that treatment of pregnant women be *postponed* until after delivery

Continued.

NURSING DRUG DIGEST—cont'd

Medication (trade name)	Indication	Usual dosage and administration	Dosage forms, preparation, and storage	Contraindications, cautions, and comments	Monitoring
★ **Niridazole** Ambilhar	*Dracunculus medinensis* (guinea worm) Schistosomiasis: *S. haematobium, S. japonicum,* and *S. mansoni*	Adults and children: 25 mg/kg/ 24 hr PO in 2 divided doses (maximum 1.5 gm/24 hr) for 15 days For schistosomiasis give for 5-10 days	Tablet: 500 mg	*Contraindicated in hepatocellular disease, portal hypertension, or a history of mental disorders or seizures* *Should not be administered during pregnancy since has caused mutagenic effects in bacteria at low doses* Warn patient that drug colors urine and stool dark brown Since it is immunosuppressive, may abolish 48-hr skin test reaction to PPD, mumps, and schistosome antigens for several weeks after therapy is begun Commonly causes immunosuppression, headache, dizziness, vomiting Occasionally causes diarrhea, ECG changes, rash, insomnia, paresthesias Rarely causes convulsions, psychosis, hemolytic anemia in G-6-PD deficiency	Observe for CNS depression Observe for convulsions
Oxamniquine Vansil	Schistosomiasis caused by *Schistosoma mansoni*	*Adults:* 12-15 mg/kg PO as a single dose *Children:* Under 30 kg, 20 mg/ kg PO in 2 equally divided doses administered 2-8 hr apart Administration with food or milk may decrease GI irritation	Capsule: 250 mg	Caution patient about risk of operating hazardous machinery until effects on performance are known May cause dizziness, drowsiness, GI distress	

Drug	Indications	Dosage	Preparations	Side Effects	Nursing Considerations
Piperazine Ancazine Antepar Bryrol Entacyl Multifuge Oxocide Parazine Perin Pincets Pinsirup Verm-X Vermisol Vermizine Veroxil	Alternative drug for treatment of roundworms (*Ascaris lumbricoides*) and pinworms (*Enterobius vermicularis*)	*Adults:* 75 mg/kg (maximum 3.5 gm/day) for 2 days *Pinworm:* 65 mg/kg/24 hr (maximum 2.5 gm/24 hr) for 7 days Repeat after 2 weeks Fasting before treatment is not necessary *Children:* Same as adults	Syrup: 500 mg/5 ml Tablets: 250, 500 mg Store in a tightly closed, light-resistant container	*Contraindicated* in patients with convulsive disorders or with renal or hepatic insufficiency Occasionally causes dizziness and urticaria, nausea, vomiting, and diarrhea Rarely causes exacerbation of epilepsy Visual disturbances (such as blurred vision), ataxia, and hypotonia may occur There have been no harmful effects reported with use of piperazine in pregnancy Possible potentiation of extrapyramidal effects and increased risk of seizures when piperazine is used with phenothiazines It is important to stress the necessity for follow-up treatment for pinworms because the drug does not kill eggs; retreatment after 2 weeks is indicated to kill any pinworms that might have hatched before they start laying more eggs Round worms are passed alive and paralyzed 1-3 days after treatment; a laxative is not needed Pinworms are passed *alive and active* in the first 4 days of therapy Teach prevention of reinfestation May rarely cause convulsions in epileptic patients May cause orange-red discoloration of urine	Monitor for CNS side effects

Continued.

NURSING DRUG DIGEST—cont'd

Medication (trade name)	Indication	Usual dosage and administration	Dosage forms, preparation, and storage	Contraindications, cautions, and comments	Monitoring
Praziquantel Biltricide ★	Schistosomiasis (not for ocular infestation because irreversible damage to the eye may result from parasite destruction)	*Adults:* 60 mg/kg PO divided into 3 equal doses administered on the same day *Children:* Over 4 years of age, same as adults	Tablet: 600 mg	Probably least toxic of the drugs currently available to treat schistosomiasis Appears to be effective for all forms of schistosomiasis May cause GI distress, dizziness, or fever, all of which are usually mild and self-limiting May also be effective for treatment of some tapeworm infections (i.e., cysticercosis).	Monitor for any untoward adverse or side effects because widespread clinical experience with this drug is limited in North America
Pyrantel pamoate Antiminth Combantrin	Ascariasis (roundworm) Enterobiasis (pinworm) Hookworms: *Necator americanus* and *Ancylostoma duodenale*	*Adults:* 11 mg/kg PO as a single dose Maximum 1 gm For pinworms, repeat after 2 weeks *Children:* Same as adults Fasting is not required Shake suspension well to assure accurate dosage May be taken with milk, fruit juice, or food	Suspension: 50 mg/ml Protect from light Store below 30° C	Use *caution* in patients with preexisting liver dysfunction Side effects include anorexia, nausea, vomiting, diarrhea, headache, dizziness, drowsiness, rash, SGOT elevation Safe use in pregnancy has not been determined Family should also be treated for pinworm for best effect Safe use in children under 2 years not established Possibility that piperazine and pyrantel pamoate are mutually antagonistic	

| **Pyrvinium pamoate** Molevac Pamovin Poquil Povan Pyr-Pam Vanquin | Alternate drug for enterobiasis (pinworm) | *Adults:* 5 mg/kg PO as a single dose; repeat in 2 to 3 weeks
Children: Same as adults
Do *not* chew tablets; tablets should be swallowed whole
Administer suspension cautiously so as not to drip on clothing because it stains
Administer before or after meals | Suspension: 10 mg/ml
Tablet: 50 mg
Protect from light | Use with *caution* in children weighing less than 10 kg, and in patients with renal or hepatic disease
Tablets should not be used in patients sensitive to aspirin because of possible cross-sensitivity between tartrazine contained in tablet coating and aspirin; suspension may be used
Occasional vomiting and diarrhea
Rarely causes photosensitivity skin reactions
Drug stains stools bright red and medication will stain clothing if vomited or spilled; stains mouth, lips, and teeth if chewed
It is important to stress the necessity of follow-up treatment for pinworms because the drug does not kill eggs; retreatment after 2 weeks is indicated to kill any pinworms that may have hatched before they start laying more eggs |

Continued.

NURSING DRUG DIGEST—cont'd

Medication (trade name)	Indication	Usual dosage and administration	Dosage forms, preparation, and storage	Contraindications, cautions, and comments	Monitoring
Quinacrine Atabrine Tenicridine	Alternative for tapeworms: *Taenia saginata* (beef tapeworm); *Taenia solium* (pork tapeworm); *Diphyllobothrium latum* (fish tapeworm); *Hymenolepis diminuta*	*Adults:* 800 mg in 2-8 divided doses 10-30 min apart to prevent vomiting *Children:* 18-34 kg, 400 mg in divided doses; 34-45.5 kg, 600 mg in divided doses	Tablet: 100 mg	*Do not use* with alcohol because disulfiram-like reaction has been reported Use *cautiously* in patients with history of psychosis and those over 60 years because of increased CNS toxicity *Postpone* use in pregnancy until after delivery because drug crosses the placenta Frequently causes vomiting (25%), yellow staining of skin and urine, dizziness, headache Occasionally causes toxic psychosis, insomnia, blood dyscrasias, urticaria, blue and black discoloration of nails, ears, and nasal cartilage, psoriasis-like rash Rarely causes acute liver necrosis, seizures, exfoliative dermatitis, ocular effects	A saline purge and cleansing enema may be given before treatment to reduce the amount of stool that must be examined for scolex Entire stool specimen is collected for 48 hours and sieved to find scolex; ultraviolet light may facilitate search because worm becomes fluorescent after absorbing quinacrine; worm is usually passed within 10 hours, alive; it may be in one piece or segmented; cure is presumed when scolex is passed If scolex is not found, stools should be examined periodically for eggs and segments; if these not seen for 3 to 6 months the patient is considered cured
	Hymenolepis nana	*H. nana* infestations may require longer duration			
	Giardiasis	*Adults:* 100 mg t.i.d. for 5 days *Children:* 6 mg/kg/24 hr in 3 divided doses after meals for 5 days; maximum 300 mg/24 hr May need to use NG tube to administer drug directly into duodenum since vomiting is common Give clear liquid diet day before and no food after the evening meal the day before administration An enema may be given to reduce amount of stool to be searched for scolex on following day May pretreat patient with an antiemetic *Elderly:* Use with caution			

| ★ Stibophen
Fuadin | Schistosomiasis | Injectable: 300 mg/5 ml | *Adults:* A total volume of 40 ml is given as follows: 1.5-2.0 ml as a sensitivity test dose on the first day, 3.5 ml on the second, and 5 ml on the third; thereafter, 6 additional doses of 5 ml each are given at 2-3 day intervals; this course should be repeated after 1 or 2 weeks IM
Alternatively, 70 ml may be given in 27 days; in this case, the final 5 ml doses are given q.o.d. for 12 doses
Children: Dose not available
Avoid inadvertent IV injection | *Contraindicated* in severe hepatic, renal, or cardiac insufficiency
Occasionally causes nausea, vomiting, bradycardia, and epigastric pain
With prolonged treatment some damage to hearing and liver may result
Hemolytic anemia has been reported
May cause thrombocytopenia with or without purpura | Observe for bruising or decrease in platelet count; discontinue stibophen if this occurs
Stop treatment in recurrent vomiting, increasing albuminuria, severe and persistent joint pain, or intercurrent febrile illness |
| ★ Suramin
Antrypol
Bayer 205
Germanin | Onchocerciasis
See also Chapter 42, "Antiprotozoals, Antimalarials, and Amebicides" | Injectable: 1 gm ampule; prepare 10% solution
Use only freshly prepared solution
Drug deteriorates upon standing after reconstitution
Store in a cool place in airtight containers; protect from light
Investigational drug | *Adults:* 100-200 mg (test dose) IV then 1 gm at weekly intervals for 5 weeks IV; may be given IM if IV impractical
Total dose should *not* exceed 5.5 gm in adults because larger doses cause renal toxicity
Children: 10-20 mg (test dose) IV then 20 mg/kg IV at weekly intervals for 5 weeks; administer only by *slow IV* injection; may be given IM if IV impractical
Avoid extravasation on IV administration because it causes severe local irritation
Used with diethylcarbamazine | *Contraindicated* in patients with severe renal or ocular disease
Commonly causes vomiting, pruritus, urticaria, paresthesias, hyperesthesia of hands and feet, photophobia, peripheral neuropathy
Occasionally causes renal damage, blood dyscrasias, and shock
Patients who are sensitive to suramin may have shock, syncope, acute circulatory failure, and seizures with this drug
It should only be given in the hospital under close supervision | Monitor for anaphylaxis—resuscitation equipment and emergency drugs should be readily available |

Continued.

NURSING DRUG DIGEST—cont'd

Medication (trade name)	Indication	Usual dosage and administration	Dosage forms, preparation, and storage	Contraindications, cautions, and comments	Monitoring
Tetrachloroethylene Nema (veterinary product)	Hookworm	*Adults:* 0.12 ml/kg PO with a maximum of 5 ml Given as a single dose Retreatment may be required 2 more times at 4-day intervals *Children:* 0.12 ml/kg PO If possible, the diet before administration should be low in fat; the next morning the drug should be given on an empty stomach	Capsules: 0.2, 1.0, 2.5 ml contained in capsules Veterinary preparation is safe and effective used in the proper dose in humans	May cause burning sensation in stomach, abdominal cramps, nausea, and vomiting Because of CNS side effects keep patient on bed rest for 4 hr after administration of the drug CNS effects such as headache, vertigo, inebriation, and rarely, loss of consciousness may occur Severely anemic patients may collapse during therapy Because of its CNS effects, alcohol should not be taken 24 hr before or after administration of tetrachloroethylene	Observe for CNS side effects Monitor RBC counts and fluid status
Thiabendazole Mintezol	Cutaneous larva migrans (creeping eruption) *Strongyloides stercoralis* Visceral larva migrans Useful in patients with multiple worm infestations because it is effective for *Ascaris, Enterobius, Strongyloides,* and *Trichuris*	*Adults:* 25 mg/kg b.i.d. for 2 days PO Maximum 3 gm/24 hr *Children:* Same as adults Tablet should be chewed before swallowing and followed with water Shake suspension well Administration with meals may decrease GI distress	Suspension: 500 mg/5 ml Tablet, chewable: 500 mg	Commonly causes nausea, vomiting, vertigo Occasionally causes leukopenia, crystalluria, rash, hallucinations, olfactory disturbance Rarely causes tinnitus, Stevens-Johnson syndrome, shock Because of its CNS side effects, caution patient not to engage in activities requiring mental alertness	Observe for CNS side effects

Since the drug has hepatic toxicity potential, it should not be used in patients with hepatic disease or decreased hepatic function

Fluid and electrolyte balance should be reestablished and reduction of anemia completed before treatment for hookworm

BIBLIOGRAPHY

Chute, K. Anthelmintics in the treatment of human parasitic infections. *California Pharmacist,* 1977, 14-17.

Drugs for parasitic infections. *The Medical Letter,* 1979, *21,* 105-112.

John, R.L. Giardiasis and amebiasis: symptoms, specimens, the counseling you'll need to do. *RN,* 1981, *44,* 53-57.

Leopold, G., Ungethum, W., Groll, E., Diekmann, H., Nowak, H., & Wegner, D. Clinical pharmacology in normal volunteers of praziquantel, a new drug against schistosomes and cestodes. *European Journal of Clinical Pharmacology,* 1978, *14,* 218-291.

Praziquantel—a new antiparasitic drug. *The Medical Letter,* 1982, *24,* 108-109.

SECTION X

ANTIBACTERIAL, ANTIFUNGAL, AND ANTIVIRAL MEDICATIONS

Medications discussed in this section

Penicillins and Cephalosporins

Don Leach
Philip K. Ng

Medications discussed in this chapter

*Penicillinase-resistant peni-
cillins*
  Cloxacillin
  Dicloxacillin
  Methicillin
  Nafcillin
  Oxacillin
*Penicillinase-susceptible
penicillins*
  Antipseudomonal peni-
    cillins
    Carbenicillin disodium
    Carbenicillin indanyl
      sodium
    Piperacillin
    Ticarcillin
  Nonantipseudomonal
    penicillins
    Amoxicillin
    Ampicillin
    Azlocillin
    Bacampicillin
    Cyclacillin
    Hetacillin
    Mezlocillin

*Penicillinase-susceptible
penicillins—cont'd*
    Penicillin G
    Penicillin G, benza-
      thine
    Penicillin G, procaine
    Penicillin V
Cephalosporins
    Cefaclor
    Cefadroxil
    Cefazolin
    Cefoperazone
    Ceforanide
    Cefotaxime
    Cefuroxime
    Cephalexin
    Cephaloridine
    Cephalothin
    Cephapirin
    Cephradine
Cephamycins
    Cefamandole
    Cefoxitin
Oxacephem
    Moxalactam

PENICILLINS

A substance produced by penicillium molds and first noted to have antibacterial properties in the late nineteenth century was rediscovered in 1928 by Sir Alexander Fleming, who termed the substances *penicillin*. Ten years later, Florey and his colleagues developed a process for producing large quantities of penicillin. Since that time numerous antimicrobial agents have been discovered; however, the penicillin antibiotics continue to be the antibacterial agents of choice for many infections.

Mechanism of action

The penicillins exert a bactericidal effect by altering and inhibiting bacterial cell wall synthesis. They are most effective during the rapid bacterial growth phase when cell wall synthesis is taking place. They alter the formation of peptidoglycan cross-linkages, which normally give strength to the bacterial cell wall of gram-positive organisms. The resulting cell wall is weakened because of defective peptidoglycan synthesis and the bacteria are subsequently destroyed by osmotic lysis. On the other hand, most gram-negative organisms have a fairly strong lipopolysaccharide coat and are less dependent on the integrity of the peptidoglycan cross-linkages for resistance to osmotic lysis. Therefore, gram-positive organisms are more susceptible to the action of penicillins than are gram-negative bacteria (see box, p. 980).

Clinical use

Penicillins are effective against most gram-positive and gram-negative cocci but are usually ineffective against gram-negative bacilli. The sensitivities of microorganisms to penicillins are listed in the box. Although there are many types of penicillins, penicillin G is the penicillin of choice for treating most infections caused by penicillin-sensitive bacteria because of its low toxicity and its high antibacterial efficacy.

Most species of *Streptococcus* are sensitive to penicillin G. Therefore penicillin G is the drug of choice for streptococcal endocarditis, pneumonia, meningitis, bacteremia, and various streptococcal upper respiratory tract infections. Infections caused by *Neisseria meningitidis* and *Neisseria gonorrheae* are also effectively treated with penicillin G.

Some bacteria, such as *Staphylococcus aureus*, produce an enzyme, penicillinase (β-lactamase), which can destroy the antibacterial activity of most penicillin antibiotics. Penicillinase inactivates the penicillin antibiotics by splitting open the β-lactam ring of the antibiotic molecule. The production of penicillinase by bacteria is usually controlled by an extrachromosomal piece of deoxyribonucleic acid (DNA) called a

Microorganisms sensitive to penicillins

Gram-positive cocci

Enterococcus*
Staphylococcus aureus (nonpenicillinase-
   producing)†,‡,§,||
Staphylococcus aureus (penicillinase-
   producing)‡
Staphylococcus epidermidis‡
Streptococcus pyogenes†,‡,§,||
Streptococcus pneumoniae
   (pneumococcus)†,‡,§,||

Gram-negative cocci

Neisseria gonorrheae (gonococcus)†,§
Neisseria meningitidis (meningococcus)†,§

Gram-positive bacilli

Bacillus anthracis†
Corynebacterium diphtheriae†,§
Listeria monocytogenes†,§,||

Gram-negative bacilli

Escherichia coli§,|| (some are resistant)
Enterobacter||
Haemophilus influenzae§ (occasionally
   resistant)
Proteus mirabilis§,|| (some are resistant)
Pseudomonas aeruginosa||
Salmonella§
Shigella§ (not sensitive to amoxicillin and
   cyclacillin)

Anaerobes

Anaerobic cocci†,§,||
Bacteroides fragilis||
Clostridia†,§,||

Actinomyces

Actinomyces israelii†

Spirochetes

Leptospira†
Treponema pallidum†

*Microorganisms sensitive to a combination of a penicillin
   (ampicillin or penicillin G) and an aminoglycoside
   (gentamicin or streptomycin).
†Microorganisms sensitive to penicillin G and penicillin V.
‡Microorganisms sensitive to penicillinase-resistant
   penicillins (cloxacillin, dicloxacillin, methicillin, nafcillin,
   and oxacillin).
§Microorganisms sensitive to amoxicillin, ampicillin, and
   cyclacillin.
||Microorganisms sensitive to carbenicillin and ticarcillin.

plasmid. These bacteria are generally resistant to very high levels of penicillin. As much as 80% of nonhospital-acquired and 90% of hospital-acquired *Staphylococcus* infections are caused by penicillinase-producing *Staphylococcus.* These staphylococcal infections are, therefore, best treated with penicillinase-resistant penicillins such as cloxacillin, dicloxacillin, methicillin, nafcillin, and oxacillin.

The spectrum of activity of amoxicillin, ampicillin, and cyclacillin is similar to that of penicillin G. These penicillins are also active against certain strains of gram-negative bacilli such as *Escherichia coli* and *Haemophilus influenzae.* Hence they are sometimes used to treat infections caused by susceptible gram-negative bacilli. In general, for bacteria sensitive to penicillin G, penicillin G is preferred over these broader (extended) spectrum agents. Ampicillin is commonly used in the initial therapy of bacterial meningitis in infants and children. Bacterial meningitis in these age groups is frequently caused by *Streptococcus pneumoniae, Haemophillus influenzae*, and *Neisseria meningitidis*, all of which are usually sensitive to ampicillin. Because of the recent emergence of ampicillin-resistant *Haemophilus influenzae*, chloramphenicol is used concurrently with ampicillin in the initial treatment of pediatric meningitis until the culture and sensitivity of the causative organism are established. Ampicillin, amoxicillin, and cyclacillin can also be used in treating acute otitis media, upper respiratory tract infections in young children, and urinary tract infections in children and adults.

Carbenicillin and ticarcillin are penicillin analogs with a broader spectrum of activity than ampicillin. They are effective against *Pseudomonas aeruginosa, Enterobacter*, and indole-positive *Proteus.* However, carbenicillin and ticarcillin are used almost exclusively for treating systemic infections caused by *Pseudomonas aeruginosa.* These agents are commonly used with an aminoglycoside antibiotic because this combination is synergistic against *Pseudomonas aeruginosa.*

The oral form of carbenicillin, the indanyl ester, is only used in treating infections of the upper and lower urinary tract and prostatitis because it does not reach adequate serum concentrations at doses that can be tolerated by the GI tract. The oral salt is generally reserved for those infections caused by *Pseudomonas aeruginosa, Enterobacter*, or indole-positive *Proteus.*

Prophylactic therapy

The penicillins have been proved effective in preventing the recurrence of rheumatic fever in chronic prophylactic doses. However, the benefit of penicillin in preventing rheumatic fever after a streptococcal infection has occurred or preventing a poststreptococcal glomerulonephritis has not been established.

For the prevention of recurrences of rheumatic fever in adults and children, benzathine penicillin G (1.2 million units IM every month) appears to be more effective than oral penicillin therapy, possibly because of noncompliance in patients receiving oral therapy. Patients allergic to penicillin should receive erythromycin.

For prophylaxis against bacterial endocarditis, patients with a predisposing cardiac lesion should receive a crystalline and procaine penicillin G mixture intramuscularly or oral penicillin V 1 hour before and 2 days after a dental procedure, and a crystalline and procaine penicillin G mixture and streptomycin intramuscularly 1 hour before and for 2 days after GI or genitourinary tract surgery or instrumentation. Those allergic to penicillin should receive erythromycin for prophylaxis in dental procedures and erythromycin plus streptomycin intramuscularly for prophylaxis in GI or genitourinary tract surgery or instrumentation. Antibiotic prophylaxis should be directed at the most common organism(s) causing the infection in the organ system and the situation for which it is being used. In this case *Streptococcus viridans* are the most common organisms causing endocarditis after oropharyngeal procedures and enterococcus after abdominal and genitourinary procedures.

Pharmacokinetics

Oral absorption. Of an oral dose of penicillin V and amoxicillin, 60% or more is absorbed. Penicillin G, penicillinase-resistant penicillins (e.g., cloxacillin, dicloxacillin, oxacillin), and other broader spectrum penicillins (e.g., ampicillin, indanyl carbenicillin) are absorbed orally to an extent of 50% or less. The poor bioavailability of these agents is partly the result of their acid lability. The presence of food in the stomach reduces the oral absorption of most penicillins except amoxicillin; therefore, they should be taken on an empty stomach (i.e., 1 hour before or 2 hours after meals).

Distribution. Levels of the penicillins are generally adequate in most biologic fluids (e.g., urine, serum, synovial, pleural, pericardial, and ascitic fluids). The penicillins do not penetrate well into the intact CNS, but their cerebrospinal fluid levels are adequate if the meninges are inflamed.

Elimination. Up to 30% of the penicillins is inactivated by the liver and 70% or more is excreted unchanged in the urine by glomerular filtration and active tubular secretion. Because of the rapid excretion of penicillins into the urine, they are eliminated quickly from the body and have short half-lives (e.g., 0.5 to

1.3 hours) in patients with normal renal function. Although most penicillins are excreted by the kidneys, their dosage adjustments are usually unnecessary in patients with moderate renal impairment because of the low toxicity of the penicillins.

Toxicity

Because the major mode of action of the penicillins is the alteration of cell wall synthesis and because mammalian host cells do not have cell walls, penicillins do not generally produce direct dose-related toxicity in humans. However, penicillin G doses of greater than 20 million units per day are occasionally associated with CNS effects that are the result of direct neurotoxic properties. These effects range from slight obtundation and twitching to seizures. Children and patients with renal impairment receiving high doses of penicillins are more prone to these toxicities.

The most important adverse effect of the penicillins is allergy. Allergic reactions are reported to occur in up to 10% of those receiving a penicillin. These adverse effects range from mild rashes to severe urticaria and anaphylaxis. The penicillin and cephalosporin antibiotics have similar chemical structures, but clinically significant cross-allergic reactions to cephalosporins occurs in only 8% to 10% of patients allergic to the penicillins. Hence cephalosporins can be cautiously tried in patients with milder penicillin-related reactions, but should generally be avoided in those with severe urticaria or anaphylaxis caused by the penicillins.

Preparations and routes of administration

Penicillin G (sodium penicillin G, potassium penicillin G, procaine penicillin G, benzathine penicillin G). Penicillin G can be administered both orally and parenterally. An oral dose provides only about 20% of the serum concentration that is achievable with an equivalent dose administered parenterally. Thus, when switching from parenteral doses of penicillin G to oral penicillin G an equivalent oral dose would be 5 times that administered parenterally. If penicillin V were substituted the oral dose would only be twice as great. However, in most clinical situations the conversion from parenteral to oral penicillin G is not a critical factor. The water soluble sodium and potassium salts of penicillin G should be administered intravenously and the water insoluble suspension preparations procaine and benzathine penicillin G must be administered intramuscularly. The intravenous products should be administered every 2 to 4 hours by intermittent intravenous infusion or constant infusion. Aqueous penicillin G contains about 1.7 mEq of potassium or 2.0 mEq of sodium for each 1 million units

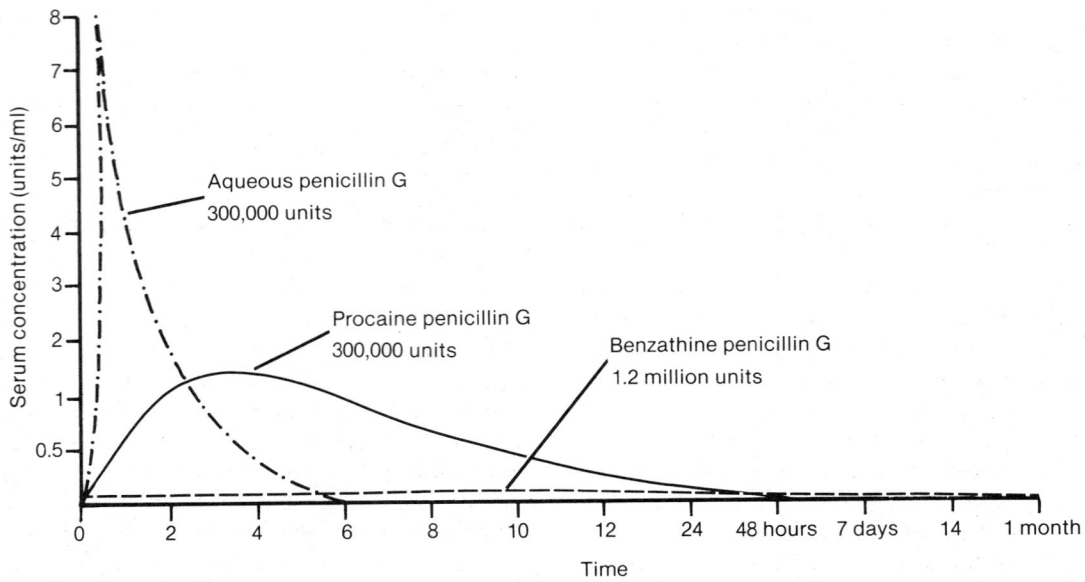

FIGURE 45-1. **Plasma concentrations of intramuscular penicillin G preparations. This chart depicts the various dose response curves for the three forms of penicillin G. (1) Aqueous penicillin G 300,000 units given intramuscularly will produce a peak concentration of 8 units/ml in ½ hour, which will decline to 4 units/ml 1 hour after the injection and 0.1 unit/ml after 5 hours. (2) Procaine penicillin G, 300,000 units given intramuscularly will reach a peak serum concentration of 1.5 units/ml in 1 to 3 hours but will fall to 0.15 units/ml by 24 hours. (3) Benzathine penicillin G, 1.2 million units intramuscularly will reach a peak of 0.15 units/ml on the first day, 0.03 units after 2 weeks, and 0.003 units/ml after 1 month.**

of penicillin, depending on which salt form is used. Therefore, the additional potassium or sodium load must be considered in patients receiving large doses of aqueous penicillin G who are prone to hyperkalemia or hypervolemia (e.g., patients with impaired renal function).

Procaine penicillin G and benzathine penicillin G are repository preparations for intramuscular injection. Intramuscular procaine penicillin G provides a peak serum concentration 1 to 3 hours after administration and declines gradually to about 10% of the peak value over 24 hours. Patients allergic to procaine should not be given procaine penicillin G. Benzathine penicillin G provides antimicrobial activity in the serum for up to 26 days after a single intramuscular injection (Figure 45-1). However, because of the extremely low serum concentrations associated with the use of this product, it should only be used in the prophylaxis of rheumatic fever, in the treatment of streptococcal pharyngitis, or in treating syphilis occurring outside of the CNS.

Acid-stable penicillins (penicillin V). Phenoxymethyl penicillin, or penicillin V, is acid stable and provides approximately twice the oral absorption of penicillin G. Penicillin G and penicillin V have a similar antibacterial efficacy against gram-positive aerobic bacteria (see box, p. 985). However, penicillin V is considerably less effective against other gram-negative and anaerobic bacteria that are sensitive to penicillin G. Therefore, penicillin V may be the oral penicillin of choice for treating infections caused by many aerobic gram-positive organisms sensitive to penicillin G.

Penicillinase-resistant penicillins (cloxacillin, dicloxacillin, methicillin, nafcillin, oxacillin). Methicillin and nafcillin are usually administered intravenously for staphylococcal infections. Nafcillin is metabolized by the liver to a significant extent, and dosage adjustment is therefore not required in patients with impaired renal function. Nafcillin appears to produce a higher incidence of neutropenia and other hematologic complications. However, methicillin has been reported to be associated with a higher incidence of interstitial nephritis. Methicillin-induced interstitial nephritis is a hypersensitivity reaction associated with fever, rash, eosinophilia, and proteinuria, which usually occurs after 1 to 4 weeks of therapy. It has been proposed that this abnormality results from either the deposition of an antigen-antibody complex in the tubular membrane or that a metabolite (dimethoxyphenyl penicilloyl) is bound directly to renal proteins with a resulting immune response. Fortunately, the associated abnormalities and the renal sequelae are reversible in most cases when the drug is discontinued.

Because methicillin and nafcillin given parenterally produce higher and more predictable serum concentrations than the orally administered penicillinase-resistant penicillins, they are used in the more serious staphylococcal infections.

Cloxacillin, dicloxacillin, nafcillin, and oxacillin are available in oral dosage forms. Of these oral penicillins, cloxacillin and dicloxacillin are preferred because of their more predictable oral absorption.

Extended-spectrum penicillins (amoxicillin, ampicillin, bacampicillin cyclacillin, hetacillin). Ampicillin and its analogs have almost identical spectrums of antibacterial activity. Unlike its analogs, ampicillin can be administered both orally and parenterally. The parenteral form is usually administered intravenously, but it can be administered intramuscularly if needed. Ampicillin has been commercially available for a much longer period of time than the other agents, and is currently the most commonly prescribed extended-spectrum penicillin.

Amoxicillin and cyclacillin are two analogs of ampicillin that are better absorbed orally. Serum concentrations obtained with these two extended-spectrum penicillins are 2 to 4 times greater than those obtained with comparable doses of ampicillin. This factor is not important in most respects because therapeutically equivalent oral doses are used. Lower doses of amoxicillin and cyclacillin are used because both of these agents are more completely absorbed from the GI tract. Thus, both drugs produce less diarrhea than ampicillin, especially in children.

Hetacillin, an inactive compound, is converted in vivo to ampicillin after oral absorption. It achieves lower serum concentrations than ampicillin at equivalent doses and theoretically may cause less diarrhea.

Amoxicillin and ampicillin have identical oral indications and can be used interchangeably at therapeutically equivalent doses. Cyclacillin, on the other hand, has not been approved for treating infections caused by *Neisseria gonorrheae, Neisseria meningitidis, Salmonella,* or *Shigella.* Neither cyclacillin nor hetacillin appears to have therapeutic benefits beyond those provided by ampicillin and amoxicillin.

Bacampicillin, like hetacillin, is a prodrug form of ampicillin that is converted in vivo to the parent drug.

Thus the indications and spectrum of activity of bacampicillin are identical to ampicillin. The adverse effects caused by bacampicillin are similar to those of ampicillin, except for diarrhea, skin rash, and nausea, which may occur less often. The major benefit of this prodrug is much more complete absorption with a rapid in vivo conversion to ampicillin. This factor is responsible for serum levels twofold to threefold those attained by equivalent oral doses of ampicillin and results in a recommended dosing interval of 12 hours in most situations. However, currently no evidence exists that bacampicillin has a significant clinical benefit over the less expensive ampicillin or other ampicillin-like agents.

Antipseudomonal penicillins (carbenicillin, carbenicillin indanyl sodium, ticarcillin). Carbenicillin and its congener ticarcillin are primarily used for treating serious systemic infections caused by *Pseudomonas aeruginosa.* They are poorly absorbed when administered orally and must be given parenterally to achieve therapeutic serum concentrations. Because high doses of these agents (e.g., 30 to 40 gm of carbenicillin per day) are used in systemic pseudomonal infections, the intravenous route is preferred over the intramuscular route. Carbenicillin and ticarcillin have an identical spectrum of antibacterial activity. However, on a weight-to-weight basis, ticarcillin is considerably more active than carbenicillin against *Pseudomonas aeruginosa.* Thus, a lower dose of ticarcillin is required to treat pesudomonal infections and fewer dose-dependent adverse effects are encountered. Each gram of carbenicillin and ticarcillin contains about 5 mEq of sodium. The massive doses of these agents required to treat a systemic pseudomonal infection can result in a sodium overload in patients with CHF or renal failure.

These agents also cause a dose-related platelet dysfunction that results in an enhanced bleeding tendency. Thus, patients with a predisposition to bleeding complications may be compromised further with high doses of these agents. Similar to other penicillin antibiotics, carbenicillin and ticarcillin may cause severe allergic reactions and dose-related CNS toxicity.

Pseudomonal infections are commonly treated with an aminoglycoside antibiotic in combination with carbenicillin or ticarcillin. Because of the physical incompatibility between the aminoglycoside antibiotics and carbenicillin or ticarcillin, these agents should not be combined in the same intravenous solution and should be given at different times.

Carbenicillin indanyl sodium was developed to provide an orally absorbable ester of the parent compound. At the upper limit of GI tolerance (i.e., 4 gm/

day) in oral therapy, minimum inhibitory concentrations (MICs) for most susceptible bacteria cannot be reached in the serum, but adequate urinary and prostatic levels are achieved; thus this agent is used solely to treat urinary tract infections and prostatitis.

Newer penicillins

Azlocillin. Azlocillin is a newer broad-spectrum semisynthetic ureidopenicillin with significant activity against many gram-negative and gram-positive aerobic bacteria. Azlocillin has been shown to have greater activity against *Pseudomonas aeruginosa* than ticarcillin and mezlocillin, and is also effective against some *Pseudomonas* strains resistant to carbenicillin.

The majority of the drug is eliminated unchanged by the kidney and exhibits a serum half-life of less than 1 hour in patients with normal renal function. The serum half-life is moderately increased in renal failure to approximately 6½ hours. Extrarenal elimination of azlocillin appears to be biliary.

Clinical studies with azlocillin have been very encouraging, with extremely good antipseudomonal activity in both children and adults for a variety of infection sites.

The adverse effects reported for azlocillin resemble those reported for the other antipseudomonal agents, including GI distress, thrombophlebitis, eosinophilia, and leukopenia.

Mecillinam.* Mecillinam is a penicillin derivative with a unique antibacterial spectrum. It is relatively inactive against gram-positive cocci, but is highly active against *E. Coli, Salmonella, Shigella, Klebsiella, Enterobacter,* and *Citrobacter.* Likewise, mecillinam exerts a bactericidal action by an entirely different mechanism than other penicillins and thus shows significant synergistic antibacterial activity when combined with other β-lactam antibiotics.

Mecillinam is absorbed from the GI tract as the pivoloyl-oxymethyl ester pivmecillinam. The parent compound, which is not absorbed from the GI tract, is absorbed in the ester form and hydrolyzed to mecillinam plus pivalic acid and formaldehyde. Reported adverse effects include hypersensitivity reactions, thrombophlebitis, eosinophilia, pruritus, and elevated serum transaminases.

Mecillinam may be a useful antibiotic because of its unique mechanism of action and its spectrum of antibacterial activity. In clinical tests a combination of amoxicillin and pivmecillinam was found to be better than amoxicillin alone in treating urinary tract infec-

---

*Investigational agent in the United States.

tions. Similar results were found with a combination of cephradine and mecillinam.

Mezlocillin. Mezlocillin is a acylureido-penicillin that is related to carbenicillin in its clinical use. The drug appears to be clinically useful against *Streptococcus faecalis, Bacteroides fragilis, Klebsiella pneumoniae,* and carbenicillin-resistant *Pseudomonas aeruginosa.* Additionally, it has been shown active against *Enterobacter cloacea, Peptostreptococcus, Escherichia coli,* and indole-positive *Proteus.*

The majority of mezlocillin is eliminated renally in unchanged form. A 50% reduction in the dose is recommended if the patient's creatinine clearance is below 25 ml/min and a 67% reduction in the dose is recommended if the creatinine clearance is below 10 ml/min.

The drug is generally administered in an intermittent rapid infusion over 10 to 20 minutes using 5% dextrose in water vehicle. Adults with normal renal function have received a wide range of doses in various trials (e.g., 4 to 20 gms/day) with only mild adverse effects reported. The doses used in children range from 100 to 200 mg/kg/day.

Piperacillin. Piperacillin is a carbenicillin analog with a broad spectrum of activity against gram-positive and gram-negative aerobic and anaerobic bacteria. The agent has notable activity against *Bacteroides, Enterobacter, Klebsiella, Proteus,* and *Pseudomonas* species.

The pharmacokinetic profile of piperacillin is very similar to carbenicillin, with a large majority of the administered agent being excreted unchanged by the kidneys, poor oral absorption, and a dose-dependent serum half-life of 40 to 80 minutes.

Piperacillin acts by inhibiting the cell wall synthesis of susceptible bacteria and exerts a bactericidal action similar to other penicillins.

The antibacterial activity of piperacillin against *Pseudomonas aeruginosa* appears to be significantly greater than the antipseudomonal activity of both ticarcillin and carbenicillin. *Pseudomonas aeruginosa* is inhibited in vitro by piperacillin concentrations from 4 to 16 times lower than the concentration of the other two agents.

Piperacillin appears to offer many of the advantages of the available antipseudomonal agents, including synergistic action against many bacteria when used concomitantly with the aminoglycosides. In addition, increased antipseudomonal activity will allow smaller doses and fewer dose-dependent adverse effects (e.g., salt loading).

Although the preliminary clinical results are very encouraging, the final judgment on the value of this drug cannot be made until further clinical experience has been obtained.

CEPHALOSPORINS

The cephalosporins are a group of antibiotics that were introduced for clinical use in the 1960s. They were first derived from *Cephalosporium acremonium*, a fungus discovered close to a sewer outlet near the Sardinian coast in 1948. These antibiotics are structurally related to the penicillins and have many similar physical characteristics. Likewise, the cephalosporins and the penicillins share a similar mode of antibacterial action and similar types of adverse drug reactions.

Mechanism of action

The cephalosporins are bactericidal to susceptible organisms. They inhibit cell wall synthesis in multiplying bacteria and this results in the destruction of the microorganisms. For a more complete description, please refer to the mechanism of action described for the penicillins.

Clinical use

The spectrum of antibacterial activity of cephalosporins is shown in the box, at right. Most of the cephalosporins, except cefamandole, ceforanide, cefoxitin, and cefuroxime, have a similar spectrum of activity. They are effective against most gram-positive cocci (e.g., *Staphylococcus, Streptococcus*) and some gram-negative bacilli (e.g., *Escherichia coli* and *Klebsiella*). Cefamandole, ceforanide, cefoxitin, and cefuroxime have enhanced activity against *E. coli, P. mirabilis,* and *Klebsiella,* and may be active against indole-positive *Proteus* and *Enterobacter.* In addition, the anaerobic bacteria, *Bacteroides fragilis,* are sensitive to cefoxitin.

Cephalosporins can be used to treat gram-positive and gram-negative infections caused by susceptible bacteria when less expensive agents or agents with narrower spectrums (e.g., dicloxacillin, nafcillin, penicillin G) cannot be used. They are the drugs of choice in a few situations such as with *Staphylococcus aureus* infections (especially in penicillin-allergic patients), infections caused by sensitive strains of *Klebsiella* and hospital-acquired aspiration pneumonia. Cephalosporins are sometimes combined with an aminoglycoside (e.g., gentamicin, tobramycin) for initially treating an undefined bacteremia. Short courses of parenteral cephalosporins are frequently used for prophylaxis in patients undergoing various surgical procedures.

Bacteria sensitive to cephalosporins

Gram-positive cocci*

Staphylococcus aureus
Staphylococcus epidermidis
Streptococcus pneumoniae (pneumococcus)
Streptococcus pyogenes

Gram-negative cocci†

Neisseria gonorrheae (gonococcus)
Neisseria meningitidis (meningococcus)

Gram-positive bacilli

Listeria monocytogenes‡

Gram-negative bacilli

Enterobacter§
Escherichia coli‖
Haemophilus influenzae§
Klebsiella pneumoniae‖
Proteus mirabilis†
Other *Proteus* (indole positive) §,¶
Salmonella†
Shigella†

Anaerobes

Bacteroides fragilis¶
Other anaerobes†

---

*Cephalothin, cefazolin, and cefamandole are more active against gram-positive cocci than cephalexin, cephradine, and cefoxitin.
†Moderately sensitive.
‡Susceptible to cephalothin.
§Susceptible to cefamandole.
‖Cefazolin, cefamandole, and cefoxitin are more active.
¶Susceptible to cefoxitin.

Toxicity

Hypersensitivity reactions are the most common type of adverse effects caused by the cephalosporins. Although cephalosporins are chemically related to the penicillins, clinically significant cross-reactivity to the cephalosporins is present in 8% to 10% of penicillin-allergic patients. Hence cephalosporins may be used cautiously in patients with minor allergic reactions to the penicillins, but should generally be avoided in patients who have a history of severe, immediate penicillin-allergic reactions.

Thrombophlebitis is frequently caused by the intravenous administration of large doses of the cephalosporins because of direct tissue irritation. Minor allergic reactions such as fever, rash, and eosinophilia are also frequently encountered, especially after several days of high dose therapy. A positive direct Coombs' test has been reported in over 3% of the patients receiving cephalosporins, but it is rarely accompanied by hemolytic anemia.

Cephaloridine is the most nephrotoxic cephalosporin and is associated with acute tubular necrosis in patients receiving over 4 grams per day. Cephaloridine has been withdrawn from the U.S. market and is rarely used today because of this toxic potential. The other cephalosporins are rarely implicated as nephrotoxic agents. However, cephalosporins should be used carefully in elderly patients, in patients receiving concomitant therapy with other nephrotoxic agents, and in patients with a preexisting renal disease.

Pharmacokinetics

Oral absorption. All of the parenteral cephalosporins (i.e., cefamandole, cefazolin, ceforanide, cefoxitin, cefuroxime, cephaloridine, cephalothin, cephapirin, cephradine), except cephradine, have poor oral bioavailability and should only be administered by injection. Oral absorption of cefaclor, cefadroxil, cephalexin, and cephradine is usually good; therefore they can be administered orally.

Distribution. The cephalosporins are widely distributed in various tissues and body fluids (e.g., kidney, pericardial, peritoneal, pleural, skin, soft tissues, synovial fluids, and urine). The levels in tissues and body fluids are generally adequate. None of the cephalosporins penetrate the CNS in sufficient quantity to treat CNS infections. Therefore, they should *not* be used in treating bacterial meningitis.

Elimination. All cephalosporins are mainly excreted unchanged in the urine by active tubular secretion and glomerular filtration. About 30% to 40% of cephalothin and cephapirin are metabolized to weakly active metabolites. Thus, cephalosporin dosing must be adjusted when the creatinine clearance is less than 30 ml/min. Hemodialysis will improve the elimination of these drugs in severe renal failure, but will not achieve the normal elimination rate.

Preparations and routes of administration

Parenteral cephalosporins (cefamandole, cefazolin, ceforanide, cefoxitin, cefuroxime, cephaloridine, cephalothin, cephapirin, cephradine). All parenteral cephalosporins can be administered intramuscularly and intravenously. Cephalothin and ceph-

apirin are usually not administered intramuscularly because of the local irritation and severe pain associated with this route of administration. Cefamandole, cefazolin, cefoxitin, and cephaloridine are less painful when given intramuscularly.

In contrast to the other cephalosporins, cefazolin at a similar dose attains significantly higher peak serum concentrations because of a higher degree of plasma protein binding. It also has a twofold longer half-life (i.e., 7.7 hours) than most of the parenteral cephalosporins. Hence it can usually be administered less frequently or in one half of the amount. Likewise, ceforanide is a unique parenteral cephalosporin in terms of its pharmacokinetic characteristics. Because of a serum half-life of 3 hours (i.e., 5 times the half-life of cephalothin), therapeutic serum concentrations of ceforanide can be maintained with twice daily intramuscular or intravenous administration.

Oral cephalosporins (cefaclor, cefadroxil, cephalexin, cephradine). Oral cephalosporins are usually well absorbed orally. Food may delay or reduce the oral absorption of these agents. Hence it seems appropriate to administer these agents orally 1 hour before or 2 hours after meals. Cefadroxil is eliminated by the kidneys more slowly than the other cephalosporins; therefore, it can be given 2 times a day instead of 4 times a day.

All of the oral cephalosporins have an antibacterial spectrum similar to that of cephalothin. However, the enhanced activity of cefaclor against *Haemophilus influenzae* makes it especially useful in treating otitis media and respiratory tract infections in children.

Third-generation cephalosporins

The cephalosporin antibiotics have been introduced for therapeutic use in groups called "generations." The newest group, the "third-generation" cephalosporins, consists of three agents; moxalactam, cefotaxime, and cefoperazone. Although moxalactam is structurally unique and is technically referred to as a 1-oxacephem, the group as a whole has many features similar to existing cephalosporins. The third-generation agents have an identical mechanism of action that is common to the β-lactam antibiotics, are for parenteral use, and have the low adverse reaction potential associated with other cephalosporins. On the other hand, the third-generation cephalosporins do have several characteristics that make them unique among the β-lactam type antibiotics; they are exceptionally resistant to the β-lactamases, including both the penicillinases and the cephalosporinases; they have an enhanced spectrum of activity that includes the *Enterobacteriaceae* and other gram-negative bacteria, and *Bacteroides fragilis;* and they penetrate into

Causes of antibiotic treatment failure

Abscess in the intramuscular injection site or phlebitis in the intravenous injection site

Example: The patient continues to be febrile because of phlebitis caused by a cephalosporin.

Antibiotic not given properly

Example: Noncompliance in an outpatient. Giving an antibiotic (e.g., penicillin G) orally instead of using an IV injection in a patient in shock or with a serious infection.

Appropriate surgery ignored

Example: A patient with an abscess, an infection of necrotic tissue, or an infection behind an obstructed conduit (renal, biliary, intestinal, or respiratory) does not respond to proper antibiotic therapy until appropriate surgery is performed.

Contamination of intravenous equipment

Example: Failure to change the intravenous tubing at frequent intervals.

Defective immune system of the host

Example: Patients with cancer receiving immunosuppressive therapy. Patients with granulocytopenia.

Drug antagonism

Example: Using bacteriostatic (e.g., tetracycline) and bactericidal (e.g., penicillin) agents together. Bacteriostatic agents inhibit the action of bactericidal agents.

Incompatibility of drugs mixed in intravenous fluids

Example: Combining an aminoglycoside (e.g., gentamicin) and a penicillin (e.g., carbenicillin) in the same IV bottle or IV line.

Interference of antibiotic absorption by another drug or food

Example: Administration of penicillin G (an acid labile antibiotic) with orange juice.

Normal variation in clinical course

Example: After the initiation of appropriate antibiotic treatment, marked improvement of a patient with acute pyelonephritis is generally not evident until 3 to 4 days later. A patient with bacterial endocarditis treated with an adequate antibiotic may continue to be febrile into the second or third week of antibiotic therapy.

Poor drug penetration and diffusion to the site of infection

Example: Use of a cephalosporin to treat meningitis even though cephalosporins do not penetrate well into the CNS even with inflamed meninges.

Resistance of the pathogens

Example: Development of pathogen resistance during the course of antibiotic therapy; superinfection.

Wrong diagnosis

Example: Use of antibiotics to treat viral infections (e.g., common cold).

Wrong dose

Example: Too low a dose may not be effective and can induce the development of bacterial resistance.

Wrong dosing interval

Example: Too long a dosing interval can result in the proliferation of bacteria at the end of each dosing interval because of subtherapeutic levels at the end of the dosing interval.

the cerebrospinal fluid in sufficient quantities to be useful theoretically in certain cases of bacterial meningitis.

At recommended doses, moxalactam and cefoperazone produce higher peaks and more slowly declining plateau serum concentrations than does cefotaxime. Whereas cefotaxime has an elimination half-life in patients with good renal function of approximately 1 hour, moxalactam and cefoperazone have an elimination half-life that is twice as great. Thus, they can be administered every 8 to 12 hours in many therapeutic applications, as compared to the usual 4- to 6-hour intervals recommended for most other cephalosporins.

In severe hepatic impairment the elimination half-life of cefoperazone can be significantly increased resulting in a much greater serum concentration. Moxalactam and cefotaxime, on the other hand, are primarily dependent on renal elimination and may accumulate in severe renal failure.

Dosing adjustments should be considered for most antibiotics according to differences in renal or liver function, patient age, bacterial sensitivity testing, and the site of infection. However, because of a low toxic potential, the β-lactam antibiotics need only be adjusted in radically impaired patients.

The incidence of adverse reactions to the third-generation cephalosporins is comparable to other β-lactam antibiotics. The less serious reactions most commonly encountered include skin rash, fever, headache, phlebitis, and diarrhea. More serious problems such as anaphylaxis, granulocytopenia, and other hematologic abnormalities have been reported, but the numbers are low and the incidence will not be reliable until further experience is obtained.

Unlike other available cephalosporins, the third-generation agents sufficiently penetrate into the cerebrospinal fluid to be of potential value in selected cases of bacterial meningitis. However, more experience is needed to define the actual role these agents will play in the treatment of CNS infection. The third-generation cephalosporins have also shown promise in bacteremia and septicemia and in pulmonary, genitourinary, and intraabdominal infections.

CAUSES OF ANTIBIOTIC TREATMENT FAILURE

In addition to carefully monitoring the therapeutic response and adverse effects during antibiotic therapy, it is also important to be able to recognize the causes of failure in antibiotic therapy so their occurrence can be minimized. The common causes of antibiotic treatment failure are listed in the box on p. 987.

SUMMARY

This chapter has examined the various types and uses of penicillins and cephalosporins. The mechanisms of action, clinical use, and pharmacology have been presented for the various agents.

With an understanding of the various individual agents, including their actions and side effects, the nurse will be better able to provide optimal care to patients requiring these medications. Patient education can be enhanced; adverse drug effects can be anticipated, monitored for, and minimized; clinically significant drug interactions can be avoided; and the therapeutic effect monitored for by using the information presented in this chapter.

ADVERSE/SIDE EFFECTS OF PENICILLINS AND CEPHALOSPORINS*

Penicillins

ALLERGIC REACTIONS

Allergic vasculitis
Anaphylactic reactions (about 1:10,000)
Eosinophilia
Rash (more commonly with ampicillin, high incidence in patients with infectious mononucleosis or cytomegalovirus infection and receiving ampicillin)
Serum sickness

CARDIOVASCULAR SYSTEM

Excessive sodium load (carbenicillin and ticarcillin contain 4.7 mEq and 5.2 mEq of sodium ion per gram of antibiotic, respectively; caution in patients with CHF or renal failure)
Hyperkalemia (potassium penicillin G contains 1.7 mEq of potassium ion per 1 million units; caution in patients with renal failure)
Hypokalemia (carbenicillin, piperacillin, ticarcillin)

CENTRAL NERVOUS SYSTEM

Convulsions (with excessively rapid IV injection of high dose of penicillin G, especially in patients with renal failure)

GASTROINTESTINAL SYSTEM

Diarrhea (common with ampicillin, penicillinase-resistant penicillins, and indanyl carbenicillin given orally)
Glossitis

Nausea (more common with indanyl carbenicillin and penicillinase-resistant penicillins)
Pseudomembranous colitis (rare, especially with ampicillin)
Stomatitis

HEMATOLOGIC SYSTEM

Bleeding tendency because of platelet dysfunction (carbenicillin)
Coombs' positive hemolytic anemia (hemolytic anemia is rare but Coombs' test may become positive in some patients receiving penicillins; appears to be a hypersensitivity reaction)
Eosinophilia (allergic reaction)
Neutropenia (especially with carbenicillin and nafcillin)

HEPATIC SYSTEM

Hepatitis (carbenicillin and oxacillin; appears to be a hypersensitivity reaction)

RENAL SYSTEM

Nephritis (most common with methicillin; in the form of interstitial nephritis often with fever, eosinophilia, and abnormal urinary sediment; appears to be a hypersensitivity reaction)

MISCELLANEOUS EFFECTS

Drug fever
Pain at injection sites
Phlebitis
Sterile intramuscular abscess
Superinfection (especially with extended-spectrum penicillins)

Cephalosporins and cephamycins

ALLERGIC REACTIONS

Anaphylaxis
Rash
Serum sickness

GASTROINTESTINAL SYSTEM

Diarrhea
Gastrointestinal upset

HEMATOLOGIC SYSTEM

Bleeding tendency because of thrombocytopenia (moxalactam)
Coombs' positive hemolytic anemia (hemolytic anemia is rare but Coombs' test may become positive in some patients receiving cephalosporins and cephamycins; appears to be a hypersensitivity reaction)
Eosinophilia (allergic reaction)
Neutropenia

HEPATIC SYSTEM

Transient increases in levels of serum liver enzymes (may not be associated with clinically significant liver damage)

RENAL SYSTEM

Nephrotoxicity (especially with cephaloridine)

MISCELLANEOUS EFFECTS

Disulfiram-like effect (moxalactam)
Drug fever
Pain at injection sites
Phlebitis
Sterile intramuscular abscess
Superinfection

*See Chapter 11, "Drug Toxicity," for an overview of drug toxicity.

CLINICALLY SIGNIFICANT DRUG INTERACTIONS*

Primary drug	Interacting drug	Possible effect(s)	Probable mechanism(s)
Cephalosporins (cefamandole, cefoperazone, moxalactam)	Alcohol	Disulfiram-like reaction (nausea, flushing, tachycardia, hypotension)	Not established
Cephalosporins (cephaloridine, cephalothin)	Aminoglycosides	Increased nephrotoxicity	Additive toxic effects on kidneys
Cephalosporins and penicillins	Probenecid	Increased serum level of cephalosporins and penicillins, which may lead to toxicity	Inhibition of renal excretion of cephalosporins and penicillins
Penicillins	Tetracyclines	Decreased penicillin effectiveness	Interference of bactericidal effect of penicillins

*See Chapter 10, "Drug Interactions," for an overview of drug interactions.

GENERAL NURSING IMPLICATIONS

Nursing of patients requiring penicillins

ASSESSMENT

The penicillins are used in preventing and treating various infections. Drug therapy for prophylaxis is directed at the most likely infecting organism and has been shown to lower the incidence of infection after intrusive procedures and operations. The benefits of prophylactic drug therapy must be weighed against the risks of an allergic reaction, toxicity, or the emergence of drug-resistant organisms. The choice of drug depends on the site of the procedure or operation (e.g., orthopedic, cardiac surgery) and the likely infecting organism. Baseline data should include specific information about the patient's condition and general health state. Assessment should be completed carefully so that changes in the condition can be identified readily. For prophylaxis, therapy is started usually just before surgery with a second dose given if surgery is delayed or prolonged. The therapy must be individualized.

When penicillins are used for treating infection, a nursing assessment is particularly important in the diagnosis of the causative organism and thus in the choice of the drug for the treatment of the specific infection. Whenever possible the organism responsible for the infection should be identified *before* the drug therapy is initiated. Thus, the collection of specimens (e.g., blood, sputum, urine, wound drainage), as indicated, should be completed carefully for smear, culture and sensitivity studies. Specimens should be carefully obtained according to hospital or agency procedure and should serve not only in drug selection, but also in monitoring the patient's response to therapy. Sensitivity or susceptibility tests are essential in treating bacterial infections.

Serious infections, such as bacterial meningitis or sepsis (e.g., bacteremia, especially a gram-negative bacilli infection) require prompt treatment. Antimicrobial drugs should *not* be withheld pending laboratory studies for these conditions. Drug selection is made on the probable source of infection and the therapy modified as indicated when laboratory studies are completed. This procedure is also indicated when an infection is suspected or present in patients with immunosuppressive conditions such as patients with granulocytopenic cancer, in which an infection can be a medical emergency.

When an infection is suspected or present, the assessment should include detailed information regarding the patient's general health state, as well as the presence of symptoms indicating an infection, including an elevated temperature of more than 101° F (38.3° C), chills, sweats, redness or pain in an area not previously affected, fatigue, anorexia, weight loss, cough, change in wound character or drainage, change in character or amount of sputum, elevated white blood cell count, or other observations related to the specific infectious condition. Isolation measures should be readily implemented as indicated to prevent the spread of infection to others.

Because the use of penicillins has been associated with serious and fatal hypersensitivity reactions in susceptible patients, in addition to specific baseline data the assessment must include a detailed drug history to identify any possible hypersensitivity before the drug therapy is initiated. Because of the possibility of cross-sensitivity, an allergy to cephalosporins should also be identified. An intravenous sensitivity test or other sensitivity tests are advised before the first dose of penicillin. The drug history should also include information regarding possible contraindications, cautions, potential drug interactions, and drug-taking patterns.

SENSITIVITY

Generally, allergic reactions to penicillins are rare; however, any drug has the potential to cause a hypersensitivity re-

GENERAL NURSING IMPLICATIONS—cont'd

Nursing of patients requiring penicillins—cont'd

SENSITIVITY—cont'd

action in susceptible individuals. Allergic reactions occur in approximately 10% of patients receiving penicillin. Patients should be carefully questioned during the drug history regarding the possibility of hypersensitivity to penicillin. If a history of an allergy to penicillin is identified, the patient should be asked to describe the reaction. It is also important to recognize that cross-sensitivity to cephalosporins occurs in 8% to 10% of patients allergic to penicillins.

Hypersensitivity reactions are also more common in patients who have a history of allergy (e.g., asthma).

Contact dermatitis or hypersensitivity reactions can occur with direct contact with the skin, which should be avoided by nurses with sensitivity to penicillin.

CONTRAINDICATIONS

The use of penicillins is contraindicated in patients with a known hypersensitivity to any of the penicillins or cephalosporins (see the Nursing Drug Digest for additional contraindications to specific agents).

CAUTIONS

Methicillin has been associated with acute interstitial nephritis (AIN), as have other penicillins (e.g., oxacillin). AIN should be suspected in patients with eosinophilia, abnormal urinalysis findings including eosinophiluria, hematuria, proteinuria, fever, and skin rash. Oliguria may or may not present. This condition resolves spontaneously 1 to 3 weeks after the discontinuation of the offending drug. Monitoring is essential because the sooner the drug is stopped the better.

Carbenicillin and ticarcillin have been associated with severe bleeding when administered in high doses. Carbenicillin and ticarcillin can prolong the bleeding time, beginning 12 to 24 hours after the initiation of drug therapy and peaking in 7 to 10 days. Hemorrhage is considered rare, occuring in high doses and with those patients with impaired renal function whose dosage had not been appropriately reduced. Monitor

these patients for bleeding, purpura, bruising, ecchymosis, and petechiae. Bleeding usually subsides 24 to 48 hours after the discontinuation of the drug, because these drugs are rapidly excreted. In severe cases, hemorrhage from incisional wounds, oozing from venipuncture sites, hematemesis, or bloody stools have been noted. Monitor patients for prolonged bleeding time. It is important to note that prothrombin time (PT) and partial thromboplastin time (PTT) usually remain normal.

Excess potassium or sodium, resulting in hyperkalemia or hypernatremia, can occur when penicillins of these salts are administered to patients with impaired renal or cardiac function and should be avoided in these patients. When administered to patients prone to electrolyte imbalance, careful monitoring is required.

Penicillin G, greater than 20 million units per day, has been associated with CNS toxicity resulting from its neurotoxic properties (see The Nursing Drug Digest for additional cautions related to specific drugs).

DRUG INTERACTIONS

Penicillins have the potential to interact with numerous drugs in a variety of mechanisms. The concomitant use of a bactericidal (e.g., penicillin) and a bacteriostatic antibiotic (e.g., tetracycline) results in a decreased effectiveness of the bactericidal antibiotic. Because penicillin is often used with other antibiotics (e.g., aminoglycosides) for synergistic effects in treating various conditions (e.g., endocarditis), check to see that actions are additive or synergistic before combining antibiotics. It is also important to recognize that some antibiotics interfere with each other's absorption or are incompatible when mixed in the same IV solution or syringe (e.g., carbenicillin and gentamicin). Penicillins, when mixed with aminoglycosides for IV administration, generally cause a substantial inactivation of the aminoglycoside. See Clinically Significant Drug Interactions and Appendix IV, "Intravenous Incompatibilities."

ADMINISTRATION

Penicillins are available in various dosage forms for oral, IM, or IV use. Dosage requires adjustment when the routes of administration are changed for some drugs because of the variability in availability and distribution. An oral dose of penicillin G requires 5 times the parenteral dose to obtain equivalent serum concentrations. Two times the parenteral dose of penicillin V is required to obtain equivalent serum concentrations from the oral route.

Dosage is highly individualized according to individual patient factors such as age and the severity of infection. Because of the low range of toxicity associated with the penicillins, dosage adjustments are usually not necessary with moderate renal dysfunction. Dosage is generally reduced in patients with impaired renal function related to creatinine clearance. Because all penicillins, except nafcillin, are excreted mostly unchanged in the urine, excretion is delayed in infants, elderly patients, and in patients with impaired renal function. Nafcillin, being metabolized in the liver, may require dosage adjustment in hepatic failure (see the Nursing Drug Digest for specific information regarding dosage and administration of specific individual agents).

Before administering penicillins, the following should be completed.

Review the hospital protocol for treating anaphylaxis. Be sure that emergency drugs and equipment are readily available in the event of anaphylaxis.

Check with the patient to determine whether there has been a previous allergic reaction to the penicillins or the cephalosporins. Ask for a description of the allergic reaction. This is important because with the stress or anxiety related to admission the patient may have forgotten an allergy, even if asked during the admission history. Record and report any history of allergy to penicillins or cephalosporins. Conspicuously mark the chart, the patient's name wristband, and the patient's bed about the drug(s) that the patient is al-

Continued.

GENERAL NURSING IMPLICATIONS—cont'd

Nursing of patients requiring penicillins—cont'd

ADMINISTRATION—cont'd

lergic to. Specific hospital protocol should be followed. Also instruct the patient not to take the drug(s) in the future unless the prescriber, having reviewed the history of drug allergy, specially instructs the patient to do so.

Obtain samples (e.g., blood, urine, sputum, CSF) as specified by the prescriber for culture and sensitivity tests routinely before the first dose of the antibiotic.

Space the time of antibiotic administration as evenly as possible throughout 24 hours (e.g., q.i.d. means every 6 hours around the clock) to ensure adequate antibiotic blood levels during each dosing interval.

Ensure the order for an antibiotic is reviewed by the prescriber at least every 5 to 7 days or according to hospital policy so that the order is either renewed or canceled.

Oral administration

Penicillins such as ampicillin, cloxacillin, dicloxacillin, hetacillin, nafcillin, oxacillin, penicillin G, penicillin V, amoxicillin, and bacampicillin are available in various oral dosage forms including tablets, suspensions, and capsules. Other penicillins such as azlocillin, carbenicillin, methicillin, mezlocillin, piperacillin, and ticarcillin are poorly absorbed orally and are given parenterally.

It is important to note that ampicillin, cloxacillin, dicloxacillin, hetacillin, nafcillin, oxacillin, penicillin G, and penicillin V are broken down by gastric and duodenal acid and that the presence of food in the stomach interferes with the absorption of most orally administered penicillins. These drugs should be administered 30 minutes to 1 hour before or 2 hours after meals. Amoxacillin and bacampicillin can be taken with food and are absorbed well orally.

When administering oral penicillins, remember to administer oral penicillins and cephalosporins routinely on an empty stomach (i.e., 1 hour before meals or at least 2 hours after meals) to increase absorption.

If the patient is vomiting, withhold the oral medication and notify the prescriber.

Do *not* administer oral medications with fruit juices because this can also decrease absorption. Oral preparations should be taken with a full glass of water.

Shake suspensions well before pouring the dose to ensure an accurate amount of medication is given and not just supernatant liquid.

Parenteral administration

Intramuscular administration

Many of the penicillins can be given parenterally by the IM or IV route (see the Nursing Drug Digest for specific information regarding dosage forms and routes of administration for each agent). It is important to note that IM injections should be made in large healthy muscle such as the dorsogluteal or ventrogluteal muscle in ambulatory older children and adults, or the vastus lateralis in infants and young children. Because quadriceps contracture has been associated with frequent IM injections in the vastus lateralis or rectus femoris muscle in infants, usually associated with antibiotic therapy, special attention should be paid to recording the injection sites and the number of injections given. It has been recommended that injections be followed with warm compresses and passive range of motion exercises to prevent this adverse affect. Adult sites should likewise be monitored and rotated with each injection.

Special attention is required when preparing penicillin preparations for IM injection because suspensions (e.g., procaine penicillin G) require shaking to ensure the adequate mixture of the medication to obtain an accurate medication dosage. Penicillin G benzathine is slowly absorbed after an IM injection, whereas penicillin G procaine is more rapidly absorbed. Injections are often painful, and because of the viscosity of these medications, the injection should be made smoothly to prevent an occlusion of the needle. The site should be gently rubbed after the in-

jection to prevent tissue damage. A Z-track technique or air lock is recommended to prevent the leakage of medication into the subcutaneous tissue layer. Procaine penicillin G should not be administered to patients with a questionable allergy history, because of its prolonged action.

Intravenous administration

Penicillins can be administered by the IV route intermittently or continuously depending on the drug, the indication, and individual patient factors (see the Nursing Drug Digest for specific information regarding the IV administration of specific agents).

It is important to recognize that water insoluble preparations (e.g., procaine penicillin G, benzathine penicillin G) cannot be administered by IV infusion and can *only* be given intramuscularly. Other important considerations include the identification of drug incompatibilities with the IV solution and the length of time a specific drug is stable after reconstitution (see the Nursing Drug Digest and Appendix IV, "Intravenous Incompatibilities").

In addition, the following should be noted.

Do *not* administer long-acting penicillins (e.g., procaine penicillin G and benzathine penicillin G) intravenously, because both long-acting penicillins are in the form of a suspension that can cause an embolism if given intravenously.

Do *not* mix intravenous antibiotics in the same syringe, the same IV line, or the same IV bottle unless incompatibility is clearly not present. Flush infusion sets carefully between the administration of drugs that are not compatible.

Dilute IV antibiotics in compatible IV fluids, which are usually indicated on the labels or in package inserts, for intermittent IV infusion. Also check the stability data of the antibiotics in IV fluids and in the manufacturer's package inserts. Label after reconstitution with diluent, dilution, date, time, and signature.

GENERAL NURSING IMPLICATIONS—cont'd

Nursing of patients requiring penicillins—cont'd

Intravenous administration—cont'd
Note that IV solutions containing multiple vitamin preparations are not to be used to dilute penicillin because they inactivate the penicillins.

MONITORING PATIENT RESPONSE
Therapeutic response

The onset and duration of antibiotic therapy is largely dependent on the dosage form, the route of administration, and individual patient factors. After oral administration, peak blood levels for oral penicillins are usually reached within 1 to 2 hours. Because of the short half-life of all penicillins (30 to 60 minutes), frequent dosing is necessary although some (bacampicillin) can be dosed less frequently. Rapid blood levels are obtained after parenteral administration. The more insoluble procaine and benzathine salts of penicillin G are slowly absorbed from the IM site. The duration of action is also affected by renal function, lasting 3 to 6 hours or longer with increased renal impairment. There is also variation in the clinical course from days to weeks as related to individual patient factors. It is important that patients be made aware of when effects can be expected, and they should know how to monitor for therapeutic effect.

Generally, patients should be monitored for the following: decreased temperature or reduction of fever, decreased WBC count, decreased inflammation or pain, increased appetite, increased energy or sense of wellbeing, or other indications related to the need for penicillin therapy as identified in a baseline assessment within 3 to 5 days of therapy (e.g., clearing of expectoration, change in sputum color, decreased inflammation at site of infection). Patients requiring penicillin for prophylaxis should be monitored for signs indicating the absence of the infectious process.

Monitoring the therapeutic response is especially important because the failure of antibiotic therapy is common, and if the patient is unresponsive to one class of penicillin, another (e.g.,

penicillinase-resistant) may be more beneficial in treating the infection. It is important to note that the drug may be ineffective if the incorrect route of administration is used, host resistance is poor, if the drug cannot reach the infection site, or if the abscess is not adequately drained.

As with other antibiotics, therapy should be guided by bacteriologic studies, susceptibility tests, and clinical response. Thus monitoring the therapeutic response cannot be overemphasized.

Adverse side effects

Adverse side effects vary widely depending on the specific penicillin preparation and its route of administration (see Adverse/Side Effects of Penicillins and Cephalosporins, for a summary of adverse side effects associated with the penicillins).

Major adverse side effects associated with the use of penicillins include gastric distress, such as nausea, vomiting, diarrhea, and an overgrowth of nonsusceptible organisms or superinfections. Generally, penicillins have a low potential for toxicity; however, for very high doses monitor for CNS toxicity (e.g., twitching, seizures), especially in children and patients with renal impairment.

Bleeding associated with carbenicillin and ticarcillin (in high doses) and AIN associated with methicillin and other penicillins should be carefully monitored for.

One of the major adverse effects is anaphylactic shock occurring from hypersensitivity to penicillin administered by any route. Monitor for flushing, generalized pruritus, abdominal cramps, nausea, vomiting, peripheral cyanosis, tachycardia, and hypotension. If these occur, the drug should be discontinued immediately and the patient should receive immediate emergency treatment, including epinephrine, diphenhydramine, hydrocortisone, or other IV corticosteroids to reverse the reaction. Oxygen and airway maintenance with intubation may be indicated, along with other supportive measures.

Because the penicillins are generally excreted by the kidneys, monitor renal function. Penicillins require dosage adjustment in renal impairment to prevent an accumulation of drug in the body, causing possible toxicity.

Because ampicillin sensitivity can lead to the potentially fatal adult respiratory distress syndrome (ARDS), shock lung, or stiff lung, patients with allergic reactions to ampicillin should be warned that life-threatening complications can develop up to 2 weeks after the discontinuation of the antibiotic. Patients should be monitored closely or discharged outpatients should be urged to obtain medical help at the first signs of pulmonary infiltration and congestion. Impaired lung compliance and decreased oxygen transport, despite ventilatory assistance, has also been noted with a drug reaction.

In general, it is important to monitor for allergic reactions such as anaphylactic shock, skin rash, or urticaria in the patient after the administration of the antibiotic. Report the allergic reaction(s) immediately.

Have aqueous epinephrine (1:1000) and oxygen immediately available in case of an allergic reaction.

Monitor for pain or abscess at the site of the IM injection, and rotate the injection sites.

Monitor for redness, edema, pain, and tenderness along the vein into which the drug is administered.

Monitor for diarrhea during the course of oral antibiotic treatment; if severe, notify the prescriber and withhold the drug.

Monitor for superinfection, especially fungal infections (e.g., candida infections of the mouth and vagina).

PATIENT EDUCATION

The patient and the family, as indicated, should be fully informed about the nature of the patient's condition and the treatment plan, and should be involved in the health care planning

Continued.

GENERAL NURSING IMPLICATIONS—cont'd

Nursing of patients requiring penicillins—cont'd

PATIENT EDUCATION—cont'd

whenever possible. The patient and the family should have a clear understanding of the anticipated course of the therapy and the medication regimen, including the exact name of the medication, its general action, purpose, dosage, storage, administration, and adverse side effects, especially if they are to be responsible for the drug therapy. They should know how to monitor the therapeutic response and how to identify common adverse side effects and signs that indicate the health care provider should be notified.

Health teaching with counseling and follow-up is extremely important for such conditions as rheumatic fever, endocarditis, or other conditions requiring penicillin therapy. Discharged patients or outpatients may need help to carry out the daily care and supervision at home. Patients and their families need to understand the major complications associated with infections such as streptococcal infections (e.g., rheumatic fever, acute glomerulonephritis). Assistance is often required with symptomatic measures (e.g., keeping a child out of school, bed rest with acute infections, modified activity or dietary requirements) for home care.

Patient education is a major nursing responsibility and cannot be overemphasized. In addition, some patients require antibiotic therapy intravenously for up to 6 weeks, thus requiring hospitalization for prolonged periods. Nursing attention to minimize the effects of hospitalization, (e.g., immobility, boredom) and to promote family and social functions is often required. An understanding of the therapy regimen and the use of heparin plugs to maintain mobility and independence are important in this regard.

Nursing of patients requiring cephalosporins

ASSESSMENT

Because cephalosporins are broad-spectrum antibiotics, they are active against a variety of aerobic gram-positive and gram-negative microorganisms, especially the third-generation cephalosporins. These drugs are used orally primarily in preventing and treating various infections, including respiratory, skin, genitourinary, and otitis media infections. Parenteral cephlosporins are used in treating osteoarticular infections, septicemia, endocarditis, and other infections. Although the cephalosporins can be used for patients allergic to penicillin, a small percentage of these patients (approximately 10%) subsequently develop allergies (hypersensitivity) to the cephalosporins. When organisms are unknown in serious infections, the cephalosporins may be used therapeutically in combination with other antibiotics (e.g., aminoglycosides). These drugs are often used prophylactically before bowel, cardiac, gynecologic, or orthopedic surgery.

For information regarding patient assessment see the assessment section for the penicillins.

SENSITIVITY

Generally, allergic reactions are rare with the cephalosporins; however, any

drug has the potential to cause a hypersensitivity reaction in susceptible individuals. Patients should be carefully questioned during the drug history regarding the possibility of a hypersensitivity to cephalosporin. If a history of an allergy to the cephalosporins is identified, the patient should be asked to describe the reaction. It is also important to recognize that 8% to 10% of these patients are also allergic to the penicillins.

Although primarily associated with the penicillins, including methicillin, carbenicillin, oxacillin, nafcillin, ampicillin, and amoxicillin, and it seems likely that all of the penicillins have the potential to induce AIN, the cephalosporins have also been associated with this condition. Patients should be carefully monitored, especially those patients on prolonged drug therapy for serious infection, because AIN does not follow a classic pattern and is often difficult to distinguish from other forms of acute renal failure. Patients may manifest a hypersensitivity triad (e.g., rash, fever, eosinophilia) or be asymptomatic to renal failure.

The offending drug should be discontinued immediately and supportive care implemented as indicated. Further use of the cephalosporins or the penicillins should be avoided.

CONTRAINDICATIONS

Cephalosporins are contraindicated in patients with a known hypersensitivity to the cephalosporins. It is important to recognize that approximately 10% of patients with a hypersensitivity to the penicillins have a cross-hypersensitivity to the cephalosporins, and use of the cephalosporins in these patients is contraindicated.

CAUTIONS

Cephalosporins should be generally avoided in those patients with severe urticaria or anaphylaxis associated with the penicillins.

Moxalactam has been associated with hemorrhage, with prolonged bleeding times resulting from an interference with platelet function not dose related. Monitor bleeding times and patients for signs of bleeding, such as epistaxis, oozing from the needle puncture site, or retroperitoneal bleeding. The drug should be discontinued if the bleeding is severe and an alternative antibiotic used. Careful monitoring of patients receiving this medication is essential. Use Tes-Tape to evaluate glycosuria in diabetic patients receiving the cephalosporins, because these drugs can cause false positive results if the Clinitest tablet or Benedict's solution is employed.

GENERAL NURSING IMPLICATIONS—cont'd

Nursing of patients requiring cephalosporins—cont'd

DRUG INTERACTIONS

The cephalosporins have the potential to interact with other drugs (see Clinically Significant Drug Interactions). It is important to note that the cephalosporins (e.g., moxalactam, cefoperazone sodium) can cause disulfiram-like reactions after patients ingest alcohol, resulting in severe nausea, vomiting, or hypotension. Elixirs should not be administered to patients receiving these medications for several days after therapy because even a small amount of alcohol can sometimes trigger the reaction. Discharged patients and outpatients should be cautioned about waiting at least 72 hours to 1 week before ingesting alcoholic beverages.

Administration with the aminoglycosides may increase the risk of nephrotoxicity.

ADMINISTRATION

As with the penicillins, the cephalosporins are available in various oral and parenteral dosage forms. The first-generation cephalosporins are available in various dosage forms for oral, IM, and IV administration. Some of these drugs can be given both parenterally and orally, whereas others cannot (see the Nursing Drug Digest).

The second-generation cephalosporins (e.g., cefoxitin, cefamandole) are available for administration by the IM or IV routes (see the Nursing Drug Digest and package inserts for reconstitution and administration). Others of these drugs (e.g., cefaclor) are available for oral use only.

The third-generation cephalosporins (e.g., cefotaxime) and the fourth-generation cephalosporins (e.g., cefoperazone, moxalactam) are available for IM or IV use. See the Nursing Drug Digest for specific information regarding the dosage forms and administration of each drug.

Oral administration

Although the rate of absorption is decreased by the presence of food in the GI tract and can result in lower and delayed peak blood levels, it does not effect the total amount of the drug absorbed. Some cephalosporins (e.g., cefaclor, cephalexin) are given orally because they are well absorbed from the GI tract, whereas others (e.g., cefazolin, cephalothin, moxalactam) are given parenterally because they are not well absorbed from the GI tract. Some others (e.g., cephradine) can be given by either route.

Before administering the cephalosporins, ask patients if they have an allergy to the cephalosporins or the penicillins. If an allergy is identified, ask the patient to describe the reaction. Monitor the patient carefully if a history of an allergy to the penicillins is present.

See the section on the penicillins regarding points to consider when administering the cephalosporins.

Dosage varies with the severity of the infection and individual patient factors. Some dosage reduction is indicated in renal dysfunction. Do not administer the cephalosporins to patients who have had a recent severe immediate reaction to the penicillins.

Parenteral administration
Intramuscular administration
See the section on the penicillins for general points to remember.

Review the package insert for reconstitution, administration, and storage procedures. Intramuscular injections should be made into large healthy muscle. It is recommended that if greater than 1 gm is to be given the drug should be divided and injected at different sites. No more than 1 gm of the drug should be injected into one site. These drugs are usually well absorbed from the injection site; however, injections are associated with pain and irritation. For some cephalosporins, (e.g., cephamycins, cefoxitin) simultaneous administration of lidocaine (0.5% to 1%) may decrease the pain of the injection without interfering with absorption. Check hospital policy and with the prescriber before administration.

Intravenous administration
Cephalosporins are highly irritating when given intravenously. Whenever possible they should be diluted and infused over 30 minutes. A filter needle should be used when preparing the medication; this has been found to prevent irritation.

Monitor the infusion sites for phlebitis. The sites should be alternated if the therapy exceeds 72 hours or if pain or irritation is noted. Hospital policy and individual patient factors should be followed regarding the care of sites. For many patients, changing the sites every 72 hours is not possible because of the lack of infusion sites or healthy veins. Careful monitoring and meticulous care of equipment and preparation of the medication for infusion is essential.

MONITORING PATIENT RESPONSE
Therapeutic response

The onset and duration of action are dependent on the route of administration and on the individual patient's renal function. The actions of the cephalosporins are bactericidal, being more effective against rapidly dividing organisms. Usually orally administered cephalosporins peak in 1 to 2 hours, intramuscularly administered drugs in 30 minutes to 2 hours, and intravenously administered drugs are dependent on the rate of infusion and occurs when the infusion is completed.

Monitoring for signs that the drug is working is extremely important with all antibiotics. See the section, Monitoring Therapeutic Response, in the section on the penicillins.

Adverse side effects

The major adverse side effects of the cephalosporins are GI disturbances, superinfections, and the most dangerous adverse side effect of nephrotoxicity. Patients should be carefully monitored for nausea, vomiting, stomach upset, and diarrhea. Oral assessment should be completed during the drug therapy for an overgrowth of nonsusceptible organisms or mouth ulcers, and women should be monitored for unusual vaginal discharge, itchiness, or discomfort. This is important so that the superinfection can be treated appropriately. It is extremely important to monitor the renal function, especially in patients who have a history of renal impairment. Although nephrotoxicity is associated with the older cephalosporins, patients receiving the third-

Continued.

GENERAL NURSING IMPLICATIONS—cont'd

Nursing of patients requiring cephalosporins—cont'd

Adverse side effects—cont'd

generation cephalosporins (e.g., cefo-taxime, moxalactam), even though less likely to develop this adverse effect, should have their BUN and serum creatinine levels monitored at least weekly during prolonged therapy. Because high doses of the cephalosporins over 2 weeks or longer can cause leukopenia or eosinophilia, complete blood counts should be monitored during therapy, and the nurse should monitor for signs that indicate changes in these areas.

As with the penicillins, the cephalosporins are also associated with allergic reactions including rash and itching.

It is important to recognize that some cephalosporins (e.g., cephamycins, cefoxitin) interfere with the measurement of creatinine in the urine. They also can cause a false positive reaction for glucose in the urine, and Tes-Tape, as opposed to Clinitest tablets, should be used with diabetic patients, who should be monitored carefully when receiving these medications (see the Nursing Drug Digest for specific agents and Adverse/Side Effects of Penicillins and Cephalosporins, for an outline of the adverse side effects of the cephalosporins).

PATIENT EDUCATION

See the section, Patient Education, in the section on Nursing of Patients Requiring Penicillins.

GENERAL INSTRUCTIONS FOR DISCHARGE/OUTPATIENTS

PENICILLINS

This drug is an antibiotic. It is used to treat or prevent infections. If you do not understand why you require this medication, contact your health care provider.

Important: If you have allergies or are allergic to penicillin or cephalosporin drugs, tell your health care provider *before* taking this medication.

Take this medication exactly as prescribed. If you have any questions, contact your health care provider.

Take the medication on an empty stomach (i.e., 1 hour before meals or 2 hours after meals). Penicillin works best if it is taken on an empty stomach.

Take the medication at evenly-spaced intervals throughout 24 hours if possible (e.g., 3 times a day generally means every 8 hours around the clock).

Take all the medication that is prescribed and complete the entire course of treatment even if you are feeling better. If you do not take the drug as prescribed for the full course of treatment, the infection may return.

Take this medication with a full glass of water. Do not take this medication with fruit juice, food, milk, or antacids, because they can prevent the medication from being absorbed from your stomach and small intestine and you will not get the full effect of the medication.

Be sure to refrigerate oral antibiotic suspensions and shake them well before use.

Store tablets in a dry, dark place. Refrigeration is not necessary.

Store liquid penicillin suspension in the refrigerator only if told to do so on the label of the bottle. Do not freeze.

Store capsules in a dry, dark place. Refrigeration is not necessary.

If you forget to take a dose, take the dose as soon as you realize that you missed a dose, then take the medication at the same time as before.

Any medication can cause unwanted effects or side effects. You may notice some side effects when taking this medication.

Gastrointestinal upset and diarrhea are some side effects that can occur. If these persist or become severe, notify your health care provider.

While you are taking this medication, call your health care provider if you develop an upset stomach, diarrhea, a black, furry-looking tongue, or an unusual vaginal discharge. These may indicate a superinfection. Your health care provider can assist you with these troublesome effects.

Do not take any other prescription or nonprescription drugs without calling your health care provider. Penicillin can interact with other drugs and may cause harmful or unwanted effects.

Stop taking this medication if you develop a rash, itching, hives, difficulty breathing, fever or chills, or joint pain in the ankles, knees, elbows, or wrists. Call your health care provider immediately. If you cannot get your health care provider, call your nearest emergency room and explain you have been taking penicillin and have developed these symptoms. They will be able to tell you what to do next.

GENERAL INSTRUCTIONS FOR DISCHARGE/OUTPATIENTS—cont'd

PENICILLINS—cont'd

Discard any extra antibiotic medication remaining after a course of therapy is completed. Do not save leftover medication for other illnesses.

Do not trade or give this antibiotic to any relatives or friends. This medication was prescribed especially for you.

Keep this and all medications out of children's reach.

In addition to the general instructions, if you are taking *amoxicillin*, you may take this drug with meals.

CEPHALOSPORINS

This drug is an antibiotic like the penicillins and is used to treat or prevent infections. If you do not understand why you require this medication, contact your health care provider.

Important: If you have allergies or are allergic to cephalosporins or penicillins, tell your health care provider *before* taking this medication.

Take this medication exactly as prescribed. If you have any questions, contact your health care provider.

Take your medication with a full glass of water about 1 hour before or 2 hours after meals. Doses should be evenly spaced throughout the day. If this medication upsets your stomach, you can take it with food or a meal.

Be sure to refrigerate oral antibiotic suspensions or liquid medications and shake well before pouring out your dose. This ensures that you are getting the correct amount of medicine.

Store capsules in a dry, dark place. Refrigeration is not necessary.

If you forget to take a dose, take the dose as soon as you remember that you missed a dose, then take the medication at the same time as before.

Any medication can cause unwanted effects or side effects. You may notice some side effects when taking this medication, such as upset stomach, vomiting, anal itching, mild diarrhea, or headache. If these effects persist or become bothersome, contact your health care provider.

While you are taking this medication, call your health care provider immediately if you observe these signs: itching, difficulty breathing, pain in the joints, or hives. If you cannot get your health care provider, call your nearest emergency room and explain you have been taking cephalosporin and have developed these signs. They will be able to tell you what you should do next.

Finish your medication as prescribed, even if you are feeling better, unless told to stop the medication by your health care provider.

Tell other health care providers, including your dentist, that you are taking this medication.

Cephalosporins can interfere with certain blood or urine laboratory tests. If you are having laboratory work done, tell those doing the tests that you are taking this medication.

Some cephalosporins affect certain urine sugar test readings. Some liquid forms may also contain sugar. If you have diabetes, check with your health care provider to see if this medication can affect your tests for urine sugar or if the sugar content in the medication is appropriate for you.

Discard any extra or leftover antibiotic medication after your course of therapy. Do not save leftover medications for use for other illnesses.

Do not trade or give this antibiotic to any relatives or friends. This medication was prescribed especially for you.

Keep this and all medications out of children's reach.

While you are taking this medication, call your health care provider if you develop an upset stomach, black furry-looking tongue, or an unusual vaginal discharge. These signs may indicate an overgrowth of nonsusceptible organisms or a superinfection. Your health care provider can assist you with these effects.

NURSING DRUG DIGEST

Medication (trade name*)	Indication	Usual dosage and administration	Dosage forms, preparation, and storage	Contraindications, cautions, and comments	Monitoring
Amoxicillin Amoxil Larotid Novamoxin Penamox Polymox	Systemic and urinary tract infections caused by susceptible gram-positive and gram-negative bacteria Acute, uncomplicated gonorrhea	*Adults:* 750-1500 mg/24 hr PO in 3 divided doses q.8h. *Children:* 20-40 mg/kg/24 hr PO in 3 divided doses q.8h. *Adults:* 3 gm PO plus 1 gm probenecid PO as single dose Prolong the dosing interval in patients with impaired renal function (e.g., creatinine clearance 50 ml/min or less) Administer with food or milk to decrease GI irritation PO use only	Capsules: 250, 500 mg Suspension: 50 mg/ml, 125 mg/5 ml, 250 mg/5 ml Reconstituted oral suspensions are stable for 1 week at room temperature or for 2 weeks at 2°-8° C Tablets, chewable: 125, 250 mg	Food does not decrease oral absorption	Observe for yeast infections (particularly of the mouth and vagina) Observe for hypersensitivity (anaphylaxis, erythematous maculopapular rash, urticaria)
Ampicillin Acillin Alpen Amcill Ampen Ampicin Ampicin-PRB* Ampilean Amplin Biotal Biosan Fannipen Novoampicillin Omnipen Penbristol Penbrock Pensyn Polycillin Polycillin-PRB*	Systemic and urinary tract infections caused by susceptible gram-positive and gram-negative bacteria	*Adults:* 2-4 gm/24 hr PO in 4 divided doses q.6h.; or 2-12 gm/24 hr IM/IV in 4-6 divided doses given q.4-6h. Administer 1 hr before or 2 hr after meals to increase GI absorption Do *not* administer with acidic fruit juices because these may facilitate decomposition of the ampicillin in the GI tract Chewable tablet should *not* be swallowed whole *Children:* 50-100 mg/kg/24 hr PO in 4 divided doses q.6h.; or 100-200 mg/kg/24 hr up to 400 mg/kg/24 hr IM/IV in 4-6 divided doses given q.4-6h.	Capsules: 250, 500 mg Injectable: 125, 250, 500 mg, 1, 2, 2.5, 4 gm/vial Suspension: 125, 250, 500 mg/5 ml Tablet, chewable: 125 mg Reconstituted oral suspensions are stable for 1 week at room temperature and for 2 weeks at 2°-8° C Reconstituted ampicillin trihydrate for IM administration is stable for 15 days at room temperature Reconstituted ampicillin sodium for IM or IV injection must be used within 1 hr after reconstitution	Avoid giving ampicillin to patients with viral infections (e.g., infectious mononucleosis, cytomegalovirus infection) because of high incidence of skin rashes Too rapid IV administration of high dosage (e.g., 2 gm or more over 10 min) can produce convulsions or muscular irritability	Observe for skin rashes Observe for hypersensitivity (anaphylaxis, erythematous maculopapular rash, urticaria) Observe for yeast infections (particularly of the mouth and vagina)

Drug	Use	Dosage	Supply and Storage	Remarks
Ponocil Principen Probampacin* Probenicillin Supen SK-Ampicillin Totacillin	Acute, uncomplicated gonorrhea	*Adults:* 3.5 gm PO plus 1 gm probenecid PO as a single dose Administer reconstituted ampicillin slowly by IV injection over a period of at least 10-15 min Administer reconstituted ampicillin in compatible IV fluids (50-100 ml) by IV infusion over a period of ½ hr for each dose Change IV site every 48 hr to minimize vein irritation Prolong the dosing interval in patients with severe renal impairment (e.g., creatinine clearance 25 ml/min or less)		
★ **Azlocillin** Azlin	Antipseudomonal penicillin	*Adults:* 200-350 mg/kg/24 hr in 4-6 divided doses by slow IV injection over 5 min or IV infusion over 30 min *Maximum:* 24 gm/24 hr *Children:* 450 mg/kg/24 hr in 6 divided doses by slow IV injection over 5 min or IV infusion over 30 min *Maximum:* 24 gm/24 hr Use in newborns is *not* recommended because of limited experience Reduce dosage in renal impairment	Injectable: 2, 3, 4 gm/vial Store below 30° C Reconstituted to 10-100 mg/ml with NS, D_5W, or lactated Ringer's is stable for 24 hr	Inactive against penicillinase-producing bacteria More active than carbenicillin, ticarcillin, and mezlocillin against *Pseudomonas* and anaerobes Not as active as mezlocillin against other gram-negative bacilli; often combined with an aminoglycoside in life-threatening infections Contains 2.2 mEq (50 mg) sodium per gram
★ **Bacampicillin** Spectrobid	Systemic and urinary tract infections caused by susceptible gram-positive and gram-negative bacteria Acute, uncomplicated urogenital gonorrhea (not pharyngeal)	*Adults:* 400-800 mg PO b.i.d. q.12h. *Children:* 25-50 mg/kg/24 hr PO in 2 divided doses q. 12h. *Adults:* 1600 mg plus 1 gm probenecid PO *Children:* Not suggested for children weighing less than 25 kg Can be given orally without regard to meals	Tablet: 400 mg (equivalent to 280 mg ampicillin) Suspension: 125 mg (equivalent to 87.5 mg ampicillin)/5 ml Shake suspension well before use	Food does not alter absorption significantly

Continued.

NOTE: For additional details regarding the individual agents listed in this table, see the text and other tables in this chapter.
*Indicates a multiple active ingredient product. For a complete listing of all active ingredients see the *Drug Reference Guide to Brand Names and Active Ingredients.*
♣ Indicates that the drug is generally available only in Canada.
★ Indicates that the drug is generally available only in the United States.

NURSING DRUG DIGEST—cont'd

Medication (trade name)	Indication	Usual dosage and administration	Dosage forms, preparation, and storage	Contraindications, cautions, and comments	Monitoring
Carbenicillin (disodium) Geocillin Geopen Geopen Oral Pyopen	Severe systemic infections caused by *Pseudomonas aeruginosa* and other susceptible gram-negative bacteria	*Adults:* 30-40 gm/24 hr IV in 6 divided doses given q.4h. *Children:* 400-600 mg/kg/24 hr IV in 6 divided doses given q.4h. Maximum: 40 gm/24 hr	Injectable: 1, 2, 5 gm/vial; 2, 5, 10 gm/piggyback unit Reconstitute with at least 5 ml sterile water for injection per gm of carbenicillin Reconstituted carbenicillin disodium is stable for 24 hr at room temperature and for 72 hr when refrigerated	Rapid IV infusion of large doses can cause GI disturbances such as nausea, vomiting, and unpleasant taste Neurologic toxicities such as hallucinations, impaired sensorium, neuromuscular irritability, and seizures may occur in patients with renal impairment who are receiving high doses of the antibiotic	Observe for sodium and fluid overload in patients with renal failure or CHF, because 1 gm of carbenicillin disodium contains 4.7 mEq of sodium
	Serious urinary tract infections caused by *Pseudomonas aeruginosa* and other susceptible gram-negative bacteria	*Adults:* 200 mg/kg/24 hr IV in 6 divided doses given q.4h. *Children:* 200 mg/kg/24 hr IV in 6 divided doses given q.4h. Carbenicillin disodium can be given as a single IM injection if the dose is 2 gm or less Administer reconstituted carbenicillin in compatible IV fluids (100-150 ml) by IV infusion over 1-2 hr for each dose Change IV site every 48 hr to minimize vein irritation		*Never mix* carbenicillin and aminoglycoside antibiotics in the same IV bottle or IV line because of rapid inactivation of the aminoglycosides by carbenicillin Carbenicillin should rarely be used alone for severe systemic infections to avoid the development of resistant organisms Should be combined with an aminoglycoside antibiotic for synergistic effect Reduce dosage or prolong dosing interval in renal impairment (e.g., creatinine clearance 50 ml/min or less) May cause bleeding tendencies with high doses Contains 4.7 mEq of sodium per gm of carbenicillin disodium	Observe for easy bruising and bleeding in patients receiving a high dose of carbenicillin, because of platelet dysfunction Monitor serum potassium for hypokalemia

Name	Uses	Dosage	Supplied	Nursing implications
Carbenicillin (indanyl sodium) Geocillin Geopen oral	Urinary tract infections caused by *Pseudomonas aeruginosa* and other susceptible gram-negative bacteria (do *not* use for systemic infections)	*Adults:* 1528-3056 mg/24 hr PO in 4 divided doses q.6h. *Children: Not* recommended for use in children PO use *only*	Tablet: 382 mg Protect from moisture and temperature greater than 30° C	Oral use commonly causes dose-related nausea, diarrhea, and occasional flatulence. Help patient establish good oral care to minimize unpleasant taste. Oral carbenicillin indanyl sodium is strictly used for urinary tract infections only; *not* effective for systemic infections. Observe for yeast infections (particularly of the mouth and vagina)
Cefaclor Ceclor	Systemic and urinary tract infections caused by susceptible gram-positive and gram-negative bacteria	*Adults:* 750-1500 mg/24 hr PO in 3 divided doses q.8h. Maximum: 4 gm/24 hr *Children:* 20-40 mg/kg/24 hr PO in 3 divided doses q.8h.; total daily dose *not* exceeding 1 gm. Shake suspension well before administration. The dosage and dosing interval are usually unchanged in patients with renal function impairment. PO use *only*	Capsules: 250, 500 mg Suspension: 125, 250 mg/5 ml	More effective in otitis media in comparison with other cephalosporins, especially against *Haemophilus influenzae*
Cefadroxil Duricef Ultracef	Systemic and urinary tract infections caused by susceptible gram-positive and gram-negative bacteria	*Adults:* 1-2 gm/24 hr PO in 1-2 divided doses q.12h. *Children:* dosage has not been established. PO use *only*. Prolong the dosing interval in patients with severe impaired renal function (e.g., creatinine clearance 25 ml/min or less)	Capsule: 500 mg Tablet: 1000 mg Suspension: 125, 250, 500 mg/5 ml	Food does not decrease oral absorption

Continued.

NURSING DRUG DIGEST—cont'd

Medication (trade name)	Indication	Usual dosage and administration	Dosage forms, preparation, and storage	Contraindications, cautions, and comments	Monitoring
Cefamandole Mandol	Systemic infections caused by susceptible gram-positive and gram-negative bacteria	*Adults:* 3-12 gm/24 hr IM/IV in 3-6 divided doses given q.4-8h. *Children:* 50-150 mg/kg/24 hr IM/IV in 4 divided doses q.6h. Administer IM dose into a large muscle mass (e.g., gluteal region or lateral aspect of thigh); *or* administer reconstituted cefamandole in compatible IV fluids (1 gm/ 50 ml) by IV infusion over a period of ½-1 hr for each dose; *or* administer reconstituted cefamandole (further dilute each gm with 10-20 ml of compatible diluent) slowly by IV injection over 3-5 min Reduce the dosage or prolong the dosing interval in patients with renal function impairment (e.g., creatinine clearance 80 ml/min or less)	Injectable: 500 mg, 1, 2 gm/ vial Reconstitute with at least 10 ml sterile water for injection per gm of cefamandole Reconstituted cefamandole is stable for 24 hr at room temperature or for 72 hr under refrigeration A solution of 1 gm in 22 ml sterile water for injection is isotonic	Cefamandole is particularly active against *Enterobacteriaceae* and *Haemophilus influenzae* IM injection is *not* as painful as IM cefoxitin Contains 3.3 mEq sodium per gram	
Cefazolin Ancef Kefzol	Systemic infections caused by susceptible gram-positive and gram-negative bacteria	*Adults:* 1-6 gm/24 hr IM/IV in 3-4 divided doses q.6-8h. *Children:* 25-50 mg/kg/24 hr IM/IV in 3-4 divided doses q.6-8h. Administer reconstituted cefazolin (500 mg or 1 gm further diluted with at least 10 ml of sterile water for injection) slowly by IV injection over 3-5 min Inject deeply into a large muscle mass in IM administration	Injectable: 250, 500 mg, 1, 5, 10 gm/vial Reconstituted cefazolin sodium in sterile water for injection is stable for 24 hr at room temperature or for 96 hr at 5° C Protect the vials from light	Better tolerated in IM injection than cephalothin or cephapirin Contains 2 mEq sodium per gram	

Drug	Uses	Dose	Preparations	Remarks
		Prolong the dosing interval in patients with impaired renal function (e.g., creatinine clearance 50 ml/min or less) Administer reconstituted cefazolin in compatible IV fluids (50 to 100 ml) by IV infusion over a period of about ½ hr for each dose		
	Acute, uncomplicated gonorrhea	Adults: 2 gm IM plus 1 gm probenecid PO as a single dose		
Ceforanide Precef	Systemic infections caused by susceptible gram-positive and gram-negative bacteria	Adults: 500-1000 mg IM or IV q.12h. Children: 20-40 mg/kg/24 hr IM or IV in 2 divided doses q.12h.	Injectable: 500 mg, 1 gm	Not as active against gram-positive bacteria as cephalothin or cephapirin Ceforanide can be given q.12h. because its elimination is about 6 times slower than that of cephalothin
Cefotaxime Claforan	Serious systemic infections caused by susceptible gram-positive and gram-negative bacteria	Adults: 3-12 gm/24 hr IM/IV in 3-6 divided doses q.4-8h. Children: dosage has not been established Cefotaxime administration should be reduced in patients with severely impaired renal function Administer 1-2 gm cefotaxime, reconstituted in 10 ml of compatible diluent, slowly by IV over 3-5 min or by IM by injecting 1 gm per deep muscular site Administer cefotaxime reconstituted in compatible IV solution through an IV system over a longer period of time or by addition of a greater quantity of cefotaxime directly into an IV bottle for continuous infusion	Injectable: 500 mg, 1, 2 gm/vial; 1, 2 gm infusion bottle Reconstituted cefotaxime is stable at room temperature for 24 hr; for 10 days when refrigerated, and for at least 13 weeks if frozen	Cefotaxime has a high degree of stability against β-lactamases (penicillinases and cefalosporinases) Contains 2.2 mEq sodium per gram

Continued.

NURSING DRUG DIGEST—cont'd

Medication (trade name)	Indication	Usual dosage and administration	Dosage forms, preparation, and storage	Contraindications, cautions, and comments	Monitoring
Cefoxitin Mefoxin	Systemic infections caused by susceptible gram-positive, gram-negative, and anaerobic bacteria (e.g., *Bacteroides fragilis*)	*Adults:* 3-12 gm/24 hr IM/IV in 3-6 divided doses given q-4-8h. *Children:* 50-200 mg/kg/24 hr IM/IV in 4 divided dose q-4-8h. Reduce the dosage or prolong the dosing interval in patients with renal function impairment (e.g., creatinine clearance 50 ml/min or less) Mix cefoxitin with 0.5% lidocaine (without epinephrine) for IM injection to reduce pain Administer reconstituted cefoxitin in compatible IV fluids (1 gm/50 ml) by IV infusion over a period of ½ hr for each dose; *or* administer reconstituted cefoxitin (1 gm/10 ml) slowly by IV injection over 3-5 min	Injectable: 1, 2 gm/vial; 1, 2 gm infusion bottle Reconstituted cefoxitin is stable for 24 hrs at room temperature or for 1 week under refrigeration Reconstituted solutions are white to light amber in color Store vials and infusion bottles below 30° C	Cefoxitin is particularly effective against indole-positive *Proteus, Serratia,* and *Bacteroides fragilis,* and against cephalothin-resistant gram-negative bacteria IV injection may cause phlebitis and thrombophlebitis Contains 2.3 mEq sodium per gram	
Cefuroxime Zinacef	Systemic infections caused by susceptible gram-positive and gram-negative bacteria	*Adults:* 750 mg IM t.i.d.; or 750-1500 mg IV bolus or infusion over 30 min t.i.d. For IM use, inject suspension into a large muscle with a 21-gauge needle Reduce dosage in severe renal impairment	Injectable: 750, 1500 mg/vial Store below 25° C Reconstitution; for IM use add 3.2 ml water for injection to 750 mg and shake gently; for IV use add 7 ml water for injection to 750 mg or 19 ml to 1500 mg Reconstituted solutions are stable for 6 hr at room temperature and 48 hr if refrigerated	Increased stability to β-lactamase Best of cephalosporins against *Acinetobacter* Less active than cefamandole or cefoxitin against *Staphylococcus aureus, Serratia* and indole-positive *Proteus;* not active against *Bacteroides fragilis* Contains 2.4 mEq sodium per gram	

Cephalexin
Cephorex
Cepor
Keflex
Keforal
Novolexin

Systemic and urinary tract infections caused by susceptible gram-positive and gram-negative bacteria

Adults: 1-4 gm/24 hr PO in 4 divided doses q.6h.
Children: 25-50 mg/kg/24 hr PO in 4 divided doses q.6h.; in severe infections and otitis media, the dosage may be doubled
Prolong the dosing interval only in patients with severe renal impairment (e.g., creatinine clearance 10 ml/min or less)
PO use *only*

Capsules: 250, 500 mg
Tablet: 1 gm
Suspension: 125, 250 mg/5 ml
Pediatric drops: 100 mg/ml
Reconstituted oral suspensions are stable for 14 days at 2°-8° C

Cephaloridine
Ceporan
Loridine

Systemic infections caused by susceptible gram-positive and gram-negative bacteria
Potential for nephrotoxicity is high; hence other parenteral cephalosporins are preferred

Adults: 750 mg-4 gm/24 hr IM/IV in 3-4 divided doses q.6-8h.
Children: 30-50 mg/kg/24 hr up to 100 mg/kg/24 hr but *not* exceeding 4 gm/24 hr IM/IV in 3-4 divided doses q.6-8h.
Reduce dosage or prolong dosing interval in patients with renal impairment (e.g., creatinine clearance 60 ml/min or less)
Administer IM dose into a large muscle mass (e.g., gluteal region or lateral aspect of the thigh); *or* administer reconstituted cephaloridine slowly by IV injection over a period of 3-4 min *or* administer reconstituted cephaloridine in compatible IV fluids by IV infusion over ½-1 hr for each dose

Injectable: 500 mg, 1 gm/vial
Reconstituted cephaloridine is stable for 96 hr under refrigeration
Protect from light
Warming diluent in hand to body temperature during reconstitution will facilitate dissolution of the drug
If recrystallization occurs before injection, warm vial in hand and shake until crystals are dissolved

Contraindicated in patients with renal impairment because cephaloridine's nephrotoxicity may further reduce the renal function
Change IV site every 48 hours to minimize vein irritation
A dosage of more than 4 gm/24 hr of cephaloridine may cause serious nephrotoxic reactions; therefore no more than 4 gm/24 hr should be given to any patient
Observe for nephrotoxic reactions such as decreased urine output, increased BUN, and increased serum creatinine

Continued.

NURSING DRUG DIGEST—cont'd

Medication (trade name)	Indication	Usual dosage and administration	Dosage forms, preparation, and storage	Contraindications, cautions, and comments	Monitoring
Cephalothin Ceporacin Keflin Neutral Keflin Seffin	Systemic infections caused by susceptible gram-positive and gram-negative bacteria	*Adults:* 2-12 gm/24 hr IM/IV in 4-6 divided doses q.4-6h. *Children:* 60-100 mg/kg/24 hr IM/IV in 4-6 divided doses q.4-6h. IM injection is painful and should be avoided if possible Administer IM dose into a large muscle mass (e.g., gluteal muscle region or lateral aspect of the thigh); *or* administer reconstituted cephalothin (1 gm in 10 ml diluent) slowly by IV injection over 3-5 min; *or* administer reconstituted cephalothin in compatible IV fluids (50-100 ml) over a period of about ½ hr for each dose	Injectable: 1, 2, 4, 20 gm/vial Reconstituted cephalothin for IM/IV injection is stable for 12 hr at room temperature or for 96 hr under refrigeration If the vial contents do not completely dissolve, an additional small amount of diluent (e.g., 0.2 to 0.4 ml) may be added and the contents warmed slightly The concentrated solution will darken, especially at room temperature; slight discoloration of the solution is permissible Precipitation may occur in reconstituted vials and can be redissolved by warming to room temperature with constant agitation	Change IV site every 48 hr to minimize vein irritation High incidence of phlebitis (17% to 50%); IV injection of concentrated solution increases incidence of phlebitis Contains 2.8 mEq sodium per gram	Observe for signs of renal impairment Observe for phlebitis
Cephapirin Cefadyl	Systemic infections caused by susceptible gram-positive and gram-negative bacteria	*Adults:* 2-6 gm/24 hr up to a maximum 12 gm/24 hr IM/IV in 4-6 divided doses q.4-6h. *Children:* 40-80 mg/kg/24 hr IM/IV in 4 divided doses q.6h. Prolong the dosing interval in patients with severe renal impairment (e.g., creatinine clearance 10 ml/min or less) Administer reconstituted cephapirin slowly by IV injection over a period of 3-5 min; *or* administer reconstituted cephapirin in compatible IV fluids by IV infusion over a period of ½-1 hr for each dose	Injectable: 500 mg, 1, 2 gm/vial; 4 gm piggyback vial; 20 gm hospital bulk package Reconstituted cephapirin is stable for 12 hr at room temperature and for 10 days at 4° C	Change IV site every 48 hr to minimize vein irritation Contains 2.4 mEq sodium per gram	Observe for signs of renal impairment

				IM injection is painful and should be avoided if possible
Cephradine Anspor Velosef	Systemic infections caused by susceptible gram-positive and gram-negative bacteria	*Adults:* 1-4 gm/24 hr PO in 4 divided doses q.6h.; *or* 2-8 gm/24 hr IM or IV in 4-6 divided doses q.4-6h. *Children:* Over 9 months of age, 25-50 mg/kg/24 hr PO in 4 divided doses q.6h.; *or* 50-100 mg/kg/24 hr IM or IV in 4-6 divided doses q.4-6h. Reduce the dosage or prolong the dosing interval in patients with renal function impairment (e.g., creatinine clearance 50 ml/min or less) Administer IM dose into a large muscle mass to minimize muscle pain and induration (inadvertent SC injection has caused sterile abscesses) Administer reconstituted cephradine (diluted with 5-20 ml of suitable diluent) slowly by IV injection over 3-5 min; *or* administer reconstituted cephradine in compatible IV fluids (50-100 ml) by IV infusion over a period of 30 min for each dose Administer oral forms with food or milk to decrease GI irritation	Tablet: 1 gm Capsules: 250, 500 mg Suspension: 125, 250 mg/5 ml Injectable: 250, 500 mg, 1 gm/vial; 2, 4 gm in 100 ml infusion bottle Reconstituted IM/IV injections may vary in color from straw to yellow, but this does not affect the potency The reconstituted cephradine for IM/IV injection is stable 2 hr at room temperature or for 24 hr at 5° C The reconstituted IV infusion solutions are stable for 10 hr at room temperature or for 48 hr at 5° C Protect from light	IM use is painful Change IV site every 48 hr to minimize vein irritation Food does *not* decrease GI absorption

Continued.

NURSING DRUG DIGEST—cont'd

Medication (trade name)	Indication	Usual dosage and administration	Dosage forms, preparation, and storage	Contraindications, cautions, and comments	Monitoring
Cloxacillin Bactopen Cloxapen Cloxilean Novocloxin Orbenin Tegopen	Systemic infections, caused by penicillinase-producing staphylococci	*Adults:* 2-4 gm/24 hr PO in 4 divided doses q.6h. *Children:* Over 20 kg; 2-4 gm/24 hr; more than 20 kg; 50-100 mg/kg/24 hr PO in 4 divided doses q.6h. No change in dosage or dosing interval in patients with renal function impairment Administer 1 hour before or 2 hours after meals to increase GI absorption Do *not* administer with acidic fruit juices because these may facilitate decomposition of cloxacillin in the GI tract PO use *only*	Capsules: 250, 500 mg Solution: 125 mg/5 ml Refrigerate reconstituted solution and discard unused portion after 14 days		Observe for bacterial and fungal superinfections
★ **Cyclacillin** Cyclapen-W	Systemic and urinary tract infections caused by susceptible gram-positive and gram-negative bacteria	*Adults:* 1-2 gm/24 hr PO in 4 divided doses q.6h. *Children:* Over 2 months of age, 50-100 mg/kg/24 hr PO in 4 divided doses q.6h. Prolong the dosing interval in patients with renal function impairment (e.g., creatinine clearance 50 ml/min or less) PO use *only*	Suspension: 125, 250 mg/5 ml Tablets: 250, 500 mg	Possibly lower incidence of side effects (e.g., diarrhea) in comparison with ampicillin	
Dicloxacillin Diclocil Dycill Dynapen Pathocil Veracillin	Systemic infections caused by penicillinase-producing staphylococci	*Adults:* 1-2 gm/24 hr PO in 4 divided doses q.6h. *Children:* Over 40 kg, 1-2 gm/24 hr; under 40 kg, 25-50 mg/kg/24 hr PO in 4 divided doses q.6h. No change in dosage or dosing interval in patients with renal function impairment Administer 1 hr before or 2 hr after meals to increase GI absorption PO use *only*	Capsules: 125, 250, 500 mg Suspension: 62.5 mg/5 ml Refrigerate reconstituted suspension, and discard unused portion after 14 days	Suspension has an unpleasant taste	Observe for yeast infections (particularly of the mouth and vagina)

★ **Hetacillin**
Natacillin
Penplenum
Verapen-K
Versapen
Versapen-K

Systemic and urinary tract infections caused by susceptible gram-positive and gram-negative bacteria

Adults: 900-1800 mg/24 hr PO in 4 divided doses q.6h.
Children: 22.5-45 mg/kg/24 hr PO in 4 divided doses q.6h.
Administer 1 hr before or 2 hr after meals to increase GI absorption
Do *not* administer with acidic fruit juices because these may facilitate decomposition of the drug in GI tract
Shake suspension well before administration
PO use *only*

Capsules: equivalent to 225, 450 mg ampicillin
Drops: equivalent to 112.5 mg ampicillin/ml
Suspension: equivalent to 112.5, 225 mg ampicillin/5 ml
Refrigerate reconstituted suspension, and discard unused portion after 14 days

Hetacillin is an inactive compound that is hydrolyzed to ampicillin; hence offers no advantage over ampicillin
See Ampicillin

See Ampicillin

Methicillin
Azapen
Celbenin
Dimecillin-RT
Penistaph
Staphcillin
Synticillin

Systemic infections caused by penicillinase-producing staphylococci

Adults: 4-12 gm/24 hr IM/IV in 4-6 divided doses given q.4-6h.
Children: 100-200 mg/kg/24 hr IM/IV in 4-6 divided doses given q.4-6h.
Prolong the dosing interval in patients with severe renal function impairment (e.g., creatinine clearance 10 ml/min or less)
Administer reconstituted methicillin (further dilute each gm with 50 ml) slowly by IV injection at a rate of 10 ml/min; *or* administer reconstituted methicillin (further diluted to 50-100 ml) by IV infusion over 30 min for each dose
Inject deeply IM into large, healthy gluteal muscle (lateral thigh especially in infants and young children)
Methicillin IM injections may often be very painful

Injectable: 1, 4, 6 gm/vial; 1, 2, 6 gm piggyback unit
Reconstituted methicillin is stable for 24 hr at room temperature or for 4 days at 2°-15° C
IV solutions should be used within 8 hr
Protect from heat

Methicillin may be given IM, but this route should be avoided if possible
Change IV site every 48 hours to minimize vein irritation
Methicillin has been associated with acute interstitial nephritis (methicillin nephritis)
Contains 3 mEq sodium per gram

Observe for signs of interstitial nephritis: decreased urine output, increased BUN, increased serum creatinine level, hematuria, and casts in urine

Continued.

NURSING DRUG DIGEST—cont'd

Medication (trade name)	Indication	Usual dosage and administration	Dosage forms, preparation, and storage	Contraindications, cautions, and comments	Monitoring
★ **Mezlocillin** Mezlin	Serious systemic or urinary tract infections caused by susceptible gram-positive and gram-negative bacteria	*Adults:* 200-350 mg/kg/24 hr IM or IV given in 4 to 6 divided doses; the daily dose should *not* exceed 24 gm/24 hr *Children:* 1 month-12 years, 300 mg/kg/24 hr (i.e., 50 mg/kg q.4h.) IM or IV Dosing adjustment is only required with severe renal impairment Infuse IV over 30 min	Injectable: 1, 2, 3, 4 gm/vial; 2, 3, 4 gm infusion bottle Store below 30° C Slight darkening in color does not affect potency	Mezlocillin is much more active against gram-negative bacteria than many of the gram-positive organisms, including *Streptococcus faecalis* (*enterococcus*) Contains 1.85 mEq sodium per gram	
Moxalactam Moxam	Systemic and urinary tract infections caused by susceptible gram-negative and gram-positive organisms	*Adults:* 6-12 gm/24 hr IM or IV in 3 divided doses q.8h. *Children:* Up to 1 week, 50 mg/kg q.12h. IM or IV; 1-4 weeks, 50 mg/kg q.8h.; 4 weeks-12 months, 50 mg/kg q.6h.; over 12 months, 50 mg/kg q.6-8h. Maximum: 200 mg/kg/24 hr for serious infections Loading dose of 100 mg/kg is recommended in gram-negative meningitis before using the above schedule Renal impairment may require adjustment of dosage IM administration requires that each gm of moxalactam be reconstituted with 3 ml of appropriate diluent	Injectable: 1, 2 gm/vial After reconstituted, the vials are stable for 24 hr at room temperature or 96 hr if refrigerated	Current data suggest that moxalactam penetrates the CNS sufficiently to be of use in specific cases of bacterial meningitis Moxalactam is stable in the presence of β-lactamases and may retain activity despite the resistance to other β-lactam antibiotics Contains 3.8 mEq sodium per gram	
Nafcillin Nafcil Nallpen Unipen	Systemic infections caused by penicillinase-producing staphylococci	*Adults:* 2-4 gm/24 hr PO in 4 divided doses q.6h.; *or* 2-12 gm/24 hr IM or IV in 4-6 divided doses q.4-6h. *Children:* 50-100 mg/kg/24 hr PO in 4 divided doses q.6h.; or 100-200 mg/kg/24 hr IM/IV in 4-6 divided doses q.4-6h.	Suspension (oral): 250 mg/5 ml Capsule: 250 mg Tablet: 250 mg Injectable: 500 mg, 1, 2 gm/vial; 1, 2, 4 gm piggyback unit Reconstitute with 1.7 ml sterile water for injection per 500 mg nafcillin	IM injection is painful Change IV site every 48 hr to minimize vein irritation Sterile abscesses and thrombophlebitis occur frequently Contains 2.9 mEq sodium per gram	Observe for yeast infections

No change in the dosage or the dosing interval in patients with renal function impairment
Administer IM dose by deep intragluteal injection
Administer reconstituted nafcillin (further diluted to 15 to 30 ml with suitable diluent) slowly by IV injection over 5 to 10 min; or administer reconstituted nafcillin (further diluted to 100 ml with compatible IV fluids) by IV infusion over 30 min for each dose
Shake suspension well before administration

Reconstituted nafcillin for IM/IV injection is stable for 3 days at room temperature or for 7 days at 2° to 8° C
Unused portion of reconstituted suspension should be discarded after 1 week

Oxacillin
Bactocill
Bristopen
Penstaphe
Prostaphlin
Resistopen

Systemic infections caused by penicillinase-producing staphylococci

Adults: 2-4 gm/24 hr PO in 4 divided doses q.6h.; *or* 2-12 gm/24 hr IM/IV in 4-6 divided doses given q.4-6h.
Children: 50-100 mg/kg/24 hr PO in 4 divided doses given q.6h.; 100-200 mg/kg/24 hr IM/IV in 4-6 divided doses given q.4-6h.
No change in the dosage or the dosing interval in patients with renal function impairment
Administer IM dose by deep intragluteal injection
Administer reconstituted oxacillin (further diluted to 1 gm/25 ml with compatible IV fluids) by IV infusion over 15-30 min for each dose
Administer oral forms with food or milk to decrease GI irritation

Capsules: 250, 500 mg
Suspension (oral): 250 mg/5 ml
Injectable: 1, 2, 4 gm/vial; 1, 2, 4 gm piggyback unit; 4 gm bulk package
Reconstitute with 10.8 ml sterile water for injection per gm of oxacillin
Discard reconstituted solution after 6 hr

IM injection is painful
Change IV site every 48 hr to minimize vein irritation
IV injection may cause thrombophlebitis
Contains 2.8 mEq sodium per gram

Observe for yeast infections

Continued.

NURSING DRUG DIGEST—cont'd

Medication (trade name)	Indication	Usual dosage and administration	Dosage forms, preparation, and storage	Contraindications, cautions, and comments	Monitoring
Penicillin G Avercillin Crystapen Crysticillin 300 A.S. Duracillin Estencilline Falapen Forticillin G-Recillin K-Cillin 250 K-Cillin 500 K-Pen Liquapen Megacillin Neolin Novopen-G Palacillin Penalev Pencitabs Penidural Penidural-500 Penisem Quidpen G Sugracillin Tucillin Wycillin and Probenecid*	Systemic infections caused by susceptible gram-positive (not penicillinase-producing staphylococci), some gram-negative (Meningococcus, Gonococcus), and some anaerobic (clostridia, anaerobic cocci) bacteria	*Adults:* 1.6-3.2 million units/24 hr PO in 4 divided doses q.6h.; *or* 1.2-24 million units/ 24 hr IM/IV in 4-6 divided doses given q.4-6h. *Children:* 25,000-100,000 units/ kg/24 hr PO in 4 divided doses q.6h.; *or* 25,000-300,000 units/kg/24 hr IM/IV in 4-6 divided doses given q.4-6h. Do not administer penicillin G by direct IV injection Administer reconstituted penicillin G (further diluted to 50-100 ml with compatible IV fluids) by IV infusion over a period of ½-1 hr for each dose Administer oral forms 1 hr before or 2 hr after meals to increase absorption Do *not* administer with acidic fruit juices because these may facilitate decomposition of the drug in the GI tract	Tablets: 100,000, 200,000, 250,000, 400,000, 500,000, 800,000 units Solution (oral): 125,000, 200,000, 250,000, 400,000 units/5 ml Injectable: 200,000, 500,000, 1,000,000, 5,000,000, 10,000,000, 20,000,000 units/vial To reconstitute: loosen the powder; hold vial horizontally, rotate it, and add diluent slowly directing the stream against the wall of the vial; then shake vial vigorously Reconstituted penicillin G for IM/IV injection is stable for 7 days under refrigeration Dry powder is stable in room temperature NOTE: 400,000 units = 250 mg	Change IV site every 48 hours to minimize vein irritation Penicillin V is preferred over penicillin G for oral use because of better acid stability and GI absorption of penicillin V Penicillin G IM injection is not recommended because of local pain Penicillin G sodium contains 2.0 mEq of sodium per million units 1 mg of penicillin G is about 1600 units Use penicillin G sodium instead of penicillin G potassium in patients with renal failure because hyperkalemia can occur (penicillin G potassium contains 1.7 mEq of potassium per million units) PO administration with antacids may decrease GI absorption	

Penicillin G Benzathine	Uses	Dosage	Preparations	Remarks
Penicillin G Benzathine Bicillin Bicillin L-A Duapen Megacillin suspension Permapen	Systemic infections caused by susceptible gram-positive bacteria	*Adults:* 1.6-2.4 million units/24 hr PO in 4-6 divided doses q.4-6h.; or 1.2 million units/24 hr IM in a single dose *Children:* Over 12 years, 1.6-2.4 million units/24 hr PO in 4-6 divided doses given q.4-6h.; under 12 years, 25,000-90,000 units/kg/24 hr PO in 3-6 divided doses given q.4-8h.; less than 27 kg 300,000-600,000 units IM in a single dose; over 27 kg 900,000 units IM in a single dose Inject deep into the muscle and do *not* massage injection site Rotate IM injection site	Suspension (oral): 150,000 units/5 ml Tablet: 200,000 units Injectable: 300,000, 600,000 units/ml Shake multiple-dose vial vigorously before withdrawing medication Use a 20-gauge needle, and do not let medication remain in the syringe for long because the needle may become plugged and the syringe frozen	Benzathine is inactive but causes slow absorption of penicillin G from the injection site Inadvertent IV administration has caused death from cardiac arrest
	Prophylaxis for rheumatic fever and glomerulonephritis following an acute attack	*Adults:* 400,000 units/24 hr PO in 2 divided doses q.12h. on a continuous basis; 1.2 million units/month IM in a single dose; or 0.6 million units IM every 2 weeks *Children:* Over 12 years, 400,000 units/24 hr PO in 2 divided doses given q.12h. on a continuous basis; 1.2 million units/month IM in a single dose; or 0.6 million units IM every 2 weeks		
	Early syphilis (first, second, and third stage syphilis of less than 1 year's duration)	2.4 million units IM in a single dose		Fever occurring during the first 6 hr following administration to patients with syphilis may indicate Jarisch-Herxheimer's reaction caused by massive destruction of spirochetes by penicillin
	Syphilis of more than 1 year's duration	2.4 million units IM weekly for 3 successive weeks		
	Congenital syphilis	50,000 units/kg IM in a single dose Do *not* administer IV		

Continued.

NURSING DRUG DIGEST—cont'd

Medication (trade name)	Indication	Usual dosage and administration	Dosage forms, preparation, and storage	Contraindications, cautions, and comments	Monitoring
Penicillin G procaine Ayercillin Crysticillin 300 A.S. Crysticillin 600 A.S. Duracillin A.S. Pfizerpen-AS Wycillin	Systemic infections caused by susceptible gram-positive bacteria	*Adults:* 0.6-1.2 million units/24 hr IM in 1-2 doses given q.12-24h. *Children:* 0.3-1.2 million units/ 24 hr IM in a single dose Warm solution to facilitate injection Do not rub injection site Inject deep into a muscle at a slow steady rate Rotate IM injection site Do *not* administer the drug IV	Injectable: 300,000, 500,000, 600,000 units/ml Note whether the brand used requires refrigeration because same brands should be stored under refrigeration Shake multiple-dose vial vigorously before withdrawing medication Use a 20-gauge needle to aspirate medication from the vial	Procaine causes slow absorption of penicillin from the injection site	
	Prophylaxis against bacterial endocarditis in patients with rheumatic or congenital heart lesions who are to undergo dental or upper respiratory tract surgery or instrumentation	*Adults:* 600,000 units IM the day of the procedure, 600,000 units IM 1-2 hr before procedure, and 600,000 units q.d. for 2 days following the procedure			
	Uncomplicated gonococcal infections	*Adults:* 4.8 million units IM divided into 2 doses and injected at different sites at one visit with 1 gm probenecid PO just before the injection			
	Acute salpingitis (pelvic inflammatory disease) caused by gonococci	*Adults:* 4.8 million units IM divided into 2 doses q.12h. and injected at different sites at one visit with 1 gm probenecid PO just before the injection; follow by ampicillin 500 mg PO in 4 divided doses for 10 days			

	Uses	Dosage	Dosage forms	Remarks
	Early syphilis (first and second stage, and latent of less than 1 year's duration)	*Adults:* 600,000 units/24 hr IM in a single dose for 8 days		
	Syphilis of more than 1 year's duration	*Adults:* 600,000 units/24 hr IM in a single dose for 15 days		
	Congenital syphilis with abnormal spinal fluid	*Children, infants:* 50,000 units/kg/24 hr IM in a single dose for at least 10 days Inject deeply into upper outer quadrant of buttocks in adults and into midlateral thigh in children For IM injection *only*		
Penicillin V Betapen-VK Cecillin-VK Compicillin V Compocillin-VK Deltapen-VK Genecillin-VK-500 Hi-Pen Ledecillin VK LV Penicillin Nadopen-V Novopen-V Novopen-V-500 Pen VK Pen-Vec-K Penapar Penapar VK Penbec-V Robicillin VK Suspen Uticillin-K V-Cil-K V-Cillin-K Veetids "125," "500"	Systemic infections caused by susceptible gram-positive bacteria	*Adults:* 1-2 gm/24 hr PO in 4 divided doses q.6h. *Children:* 0.5-1 gm/24 hr PO in 4 divided doses q.6h. PO use *only*	Chewable wafers: 250 mg Liquid: 125, 250 mg/5 ml Suspension (oral): 125 mg/0.6 ml Tablets: 125, 250, 500 mg NOTE: 125 mg = 200,000 units	Better absorbed orally than penicillin G Observe for yeast infections (particularly of the mouth and vagina)

Continued.

NURSING DRUG DIGEST—cont'd

Medication (trade name)	Indication	Usual dosage and administration	Dosage forms, preparation, and storage	Contraindications, cautions, and comments	Monitoring
Piperacillin (sodium) Pipracil	Systemic and urinary tract infections caused by susceptible gram-positive and gram-negative bacteria Acute, uncomplicated gonococcal urethritis	*Adults:* 12-24 gm/day given in equally divided doses q.4-6h. IM or IV *Children:* doses have not been established for children under 12 years of age Administer IM dose into a large muscle mass; IM dose should not exceed 2 gm per site Administer IV dose slowly over 3 to 5 min; each gm should be reconstituted with at least 5 ml of diluent; if slow infusion is used (i.e., over 30 min) dilute to at least 50 ml once reconstituted Dosing adjustment is not required unless the creatinine clearance is less than 40 ml/min; then the dosing interval should be increased to 8 hr and dose reduced to 9-12 gm/day; if creatinine clearance is less than 20 ml/min, dosing interval is increased to 12 hr and dose reduced to 6-8 gm/day	Injectable: 2, 3, 4 gm vials; 3, 4 gm infusion bottles Store at 15°-30° C	Contains 1.85 mEq sodium per gram	
Ticarcillin Ticar	Severe systemic infections caused by *Pseudomonas* and other susceptible gram-negative bacteria	*Adults:* 300 mg/kg/24 hr IM/IV in 4-6 divided doses given q.4-6h. *Children:* 200-300 mg/kg/24 hr IM/IV in 4-6 divided doses given q.4-6h.	Injectable: 1, 3, 6 gm/vial; 3 gm piggyback bottle Reconstitute with at least 4 ml sterile water for injection per gm of ticarcillin disodium	See carbenicillin disodium IV injection may cause pain at the injection site and phlebitis	See carbenicillin disodium Monitor serum potassium level for hypokalemia

Urinary tract infections caused by *Pseudomonas aeruginosa* and other susceptible gram-negative bacteria	*Adults:* 150-200 mg/kg/24 hr IM/IV in 4 divided doses q.6h. *Children:* 150-200 mg/kg/24 hr IM/IV in 4 divided doses q.6h. Administer IM dose deeply into a large muscle mass *Do not* administer more than 2 gm at each IM injection site Reduce dosage in renal impairment	Reconstituted ticarcillin is stable for 24 hr at room temperature or for 72 hr under refrigeration	Similar to carbenicillin but more active against *Pseudomonas aeruginosa* on a weight basis *Never mix* ticarcillin and the aminoglycoside antibiotics in the same IV bottle or IV line because of rapid inactivation of the aminoglycoside by ticarcillin Ticarcillin disodium contains 5.2 mEq of sodium per gm Lower dose-dependent side effects (e.g., platelet dysfunction, sodium and fluid overload, hypokalemia) than carbenicillin because lower dose of ticarcillin is used Contains 5.2 mEq of sodium per gm	Observe for yeast infections (particularly of the mouth and vagina) Observe for sodium retention and weight gain Observe for signs of platelet dysfunction (e.g., bleeding, ecchymosis, and petechiae)

BIBLIOGRAPHY

Aronoff, G.R., Sloan, R.S., Luft, F.C., Nelson, R.L., Maxwell, D.R., & Kleit, S.A. Mezlocillin pharmacokinetics in renal impairment. *Clinical Pharmacology and Therapeutics*, 1980, *28*(4), 523-528.

Ballentine, R., & Huber, S. Cephalosporins: an update. *American Journal of Internal Therapeutics and Clinical Nutrition*, 1982, April, 17-29.

Barza, M. Antimicrobial spectrum, pharmacology, and therapeutic use of antibiotics. Part 2. Penicillins. In R.R. Miller & D.J. Greenblatt (Eds.). *Drug Therapy Reviews* (vol. 2). New York: Elsevier North Holland, Inc., 1979.

Barza, M. The nephrotoxicity of cephalosporins: an overview. *Journal of Infectious Diseases*, 1978, *137*(Suppl.), S60-S73.

Barza, M, & Miao, P.V.W. Antimicrobial spectrum, pharmacology, and therapeutic use of antibiotics. Part 3. Cephalosporins. In R.R. Miller & D.J. Greenblatt (Eds.). *Drug Therapy Reviews* (vol. 2). New York: Elsevier North Holland, Inc., 1979.

Bennet, W.M., Muther, R.S., Parker, R.A., Feig, P., Morrison, G., Golper, T.A., & Singer, I. Drug therapy in renal failure: dosing guide for adults. *Annals of Internal Medicine*, 1980, *93*, 62-89.

Bergman, H.D. Cefaclor. *Drug Intelligence and Clinical Pharmacy*, 1980, *14*, 11-16.

Border, W.A., Lettman, D.H., Egan, J.D., Sass, H.J., Glode, J.E., & Wilson, C.B. Antitubular basement-membrane antibodies in methicillin-associated interstitial nephritis. *New England Journal of Medicine*, 1978, *291*(8), 381-384.

Burch, K.H., Pohlod, D., Saravolatz, L.D., Madhavan, T., Kiani, D., Quinn, E.L., Del Busto, R., Carenas, J., & Fisher, E.J. Ceforanide: in vitro and clinical evaluation. *Antimicrobial Agents and Chemotherapy*, 1979, *16*(3), 386-391.

Cefamandole (Symposium). *Journal of Infectious Diseases*, 1978, *137*(Suppl.), S1-S194.

Cefoxitin: microbiology, pharmacology, and clinical use (Symposium). *Journal of Antimicrobial Chemotherapy*, 1978, *4*(Suppl.), 1-256.

Coppens, L., & Klastersky, J. Comparative study of anti-pseudomonas activity of azlocillin, mezlocillin and ticarcillin. *Antimicrobial Agents and Chemotherapy*, 1979, *15*(3), 396-399.

Cyclacillin (Cyclapen)—another new penicillin. *The Medical Letter*, 1980, *22*, 13-14.

Davies, M., Morgan, J.R., & Anand, C. Interaction of carbenicillin and ticarcillin with gentamicin. *Antimicrobial Agents and Chemotherapy*, 1975, *7*, 431-434.

Dickinson, G.M., Cleary, T.J., & Hoffman, T.A. Comparative evaluation of piperacillin in vitro. *Antimicrobial Agents and Chemotherapy*, 1978, *14*, 919-921.

Dudley, M., & Barriere, S. Cefotaxime: microbiology, pharmacology, and clinical use. *Clinical Pharmacy*, 1982, March-April, 114.

Ervin, F.R., Bullock, W.E., Jr., & Nuttal, C.E. Inactivation of gentamicin by penicillins in patients with renal failure. *Antimicrobial Agents and Chemotherapy*, 1976, *9*, 1004-1011.

Fu, K.P., & Neu, H.C. Azlocillin and mezlocillin: new ureido penicillins. *Antimicrobial Agents and Chemotherapy*, 1978, *13*(6), 930-938.

Fuji, R. Results of a multicentric clinical study of mezlocillin in Japan. *Arzneim. Hel-Forschung*, 1979, *29*, 2005-2008.

Gardner, P. Reasons for antibiotic-failure. *Hospital Practice*, 1976, *11*, 41-45.

Goldman, P.L., & Petersdorf, R.G. Prophylactic antibiotics: controversies give way to guidelines. *Drug Therapeutics*, 1979, *9*, 57-77.

Hess, J.R., Berman, S.J., Boughton, W.H., Sugihara, J.G., Musgrave, J.E., Wong, E.G., & Siemsen, A.M. Pharmacokinetics of ceforamide in patients with end stage renal disease on hemodialysis. *Antimicrobial Agents and Chemotherapy*, 1980, *17*(2), 251-253.

Leroy, A., Humbert, G., Godin, M., & Filastre, J.P. Pharmacokinetics of azlocillin in subjects with normal and impaired renal function. *Antimicrobial Agents and Chemotherapy*, 1980, *17*(3), 344-349.

Lloyd, C., & Martin, W. A review of the new penicillins: azlocillin, Mezlocillin and piperacillin. *American Journal of Internal Therapeutics and Clinical Nutrition*, 1982, April, 9-16.

Mandel, G.L., & Sande, M.A. Penicillins and cephalosporins. In A.F. Gilman, L.S. Goodman, and A. Gilman (Eds.). *The pharmacological basis of therapeutics* (6th ed.). New York: MacMillan Inc., 1980.

Machey, C., & Hopefl, A.W. Keeping infections down when risks go up. *Nursing 80*, 1980, *10*(6), 17-21.

McGowan, J.D., & Telry, P.A. Susceptibility of gram-negative aerobic bacilli resistant to carbenicillin in a general hospital to piperacillin and ticarcillin. *Antimicrobial Agents and Chemotherapy*, 1979, *15*(1), 132-138.

Menday, A.P., & Marsh, B.T. Preliminary experiences with parenteral mecillinam. *Current Medical Research and Opinion*, 1979, *6*, 221-228.

Meyers, B.R., Hirschman, S.Z., Strougo, L., & Srulevitch, E. Comparative study of piperacillin, ticarcillin, and carbenicillin pharmacokinetics. *Antimicrobial Agents and Chemotherapy*, 1980, *17*(4), 608-611.

Moellering, R.C., & Swartz, M.N. The newer cephalosporins. *New England Journal of Medicine*, 1976, *294*, 24-28.

Neu, H.C. Amoxicillin. *Annals of Internal Medicine*, 1979, *90*, 356-360.

Neu, H.C. Mecillinam, a novel penicillanic acid and derivative with unusual activity against gram-negative bacteria. *Antimicrobial Agents and Chemotherapy*, 1976, *9*, 793-799.

Neu, H.C., & Garvey, G.J. Comparative in vitro activity and clinical pharmacology of ticarcillin and carbenicillin. *Antimicrobial Agents and Chemotherapy*, 1975, *8*, 457-462.

Pancoast, S.J., Jahre, J.A., & Neu, H.C. Mezlocillin in the therapy of serious infections. *American Journal of Medicine*, 1979, *67*, 747-752.

Parry, M.F., & Neu, H.C. Ticarcillin for treatment of serious infection with gram-negative bacteria. *Journal of Infectious Diseases*, 1976, *134*, 476-485.

Penicillin allergy. *The Medical Letter*, 1978, *20*, 498.

Petersdorf, R.G. Antimicrobial prophylaxis of bacterial endocarditis: prudent caution or bacterial overkill? *American Journal of Medicine*, 1978, *65*, 220-223.

Polk, R.E. Moxalactam. *Drug Intelligence and Clinical Pharmacy*, 1982, *16*, 104-112.

Quintiliani, R., & Nightingale, C.H. Cefazolin. *Annals of Internal Medicine*, 1978, *89*(part I), 650-655.

Rahal, J.J., Jr., & Simberkoff, M.S. Adverse reactions to anti-infective agents. *Disease-A-Month*, 1978, 1-67.

Reed, M., Bertino, J., Aronoff, S., et al. Evaluation of moxalactam. *Clinical Pharmacy*, 1982, Mar-Apr, 124-134.

Thadepalli, H., & Rao, B. Clinical evaluation of mezlocillin. *Antimicrobial Agents and Chemotherapy*, 1979, *16*(5), 605-610.

Thompson, R.L. The cephalosporins. *Mayo Clinic Proceedings*, 1977, *52*, 625-630.

Tjandramaga, T.B., Mullie, A., Verbesselt, R., DeSchepper, P.J., & Verbist, L. Piperacillin: human pharmacokinetics after intravenous and intramuscular administration. *Antimicrobial Agents and Chemotherapy*, 1978, *14*, 829-837.

Two new oral cephalosporins. *The Medical Letter*, 1979, *21*, 85-87.

Weinstein, A.J. The cephalosporins: activity and clinical use. *Drugs*, 1980, *19*, 137-154.

Welling, P.G. Influence of food and diet on gastrointestinal drug absorption: a review. *Journal of Pharmacokinetics and Biopharmaceutics*, 1977, *5*, 219-334.

Wilkoswke, C.J. The penicillins. *Mayo Clinic Proceedings*, 1977, *52*, 616-624.

Aminoglycosides

Don Leach

Philip K. Ng

Medications discussed in this chapter

Aminoglycosides	Aminoglycosides—cont'd
Amikacin	Netilmicin
Gentamicin	Paromomycin
Kanamycin	Streptomycin
Neomycin	Tobramycin

Since the introduction of streptomycin in 1944, the aminoglycoside antibiotics have occupied a unique and important role in antimicrobial therapy. Initially, streptomycin was used primarily for its action on the tubercle bacillus, and until 1952 was the sole agent available for the effective treatment of tuberculosis. However, from the introduction of kanamycin in the early 1960s until the present, the primary use of the aminoglycoside antibiotics has been to treat serious infections caused by gram-negative bacilli.

The aminoglycosides, as a group, share a similar chemical structure consisting of a glycoside linkage of various amino sugars. Likewise, they share similar pharmacologic, toxicologic, and microbiologic properties.

MECHANISM OF ACTION

The aminoglycosides are bactericidal agents that alter protein synthesis in sensitive organisms. The drugs enter the bacterial cells through a complex process that involves an aerobically-generated active transport mechanism. Next they attach to the bacterial ribosome and the genetic code is misread. Thus, under the influence of the aminoglycosides, bacteria produce faulty proteins by inappropriately incorporating amino acids in polypeptide chains.

Although the aminoglycosides are known to alter protein synthesis, additional mechanisms of antibacterial action have been postulated to explain their rapid bactericidal effect. It has been postulated that the aminoglycosides induce the detachment of ribosomes from mRNA. It has also been suggested that the drugs are bactericidal because of the changes they cause in the cell wall (Figure 46-1).

BACTERIAL SENSITIVITY AND RESISTANCE

In general, the aminoglycosides are effective against most aerobic gram-negative bacteria, less effective against aerobic gram-positive bacteria, and, ineffective against obligate anaerobes and facultative anaerobic bacteria under anaerobic conditions (see box, p. 1021).

Although the antibacterial spectrum of the aminoglycoside antibiotics is relatively broad, gentamicin, tobramycin, and amikacin are usually reserved for parenteral use against aerobic gram-negative rods. In general, these three agents are active against similar bacteria, but amikacin requires a higher serum concentration than the other two agents to achieve the same antibacterial effect. This difference in potency, however, is clinically insignificant and can be rectified by administering proportionately larger doses of amikacin. Gentamicin and tobramycin are considered to be identical in activity against most gram-negative rods and in many cases can be prescribed interchangeably. One important difference between tobramycin and gentamicin concerns activity against *Pseudomonas aeruginosa*. Tobramycin is 2 to 4 times more active against *Pseudomonas aeruginosa* than is gentamicin. Kanamycin and streptomycin, two other parenterally administered aminoglycosides, have a narrower spectrum of activity than gentamicin, tobramycin, and amikacin. Kanamycin is rarely used in gram-negative bacillary infections and streptomycin is restricted to use in less common infections (e.g., tularemia and plague). Neomycin has a broad spectrum of activity, but is not used systemically because of an intolerable toxicity resulting from therapeutic serum concentrations.

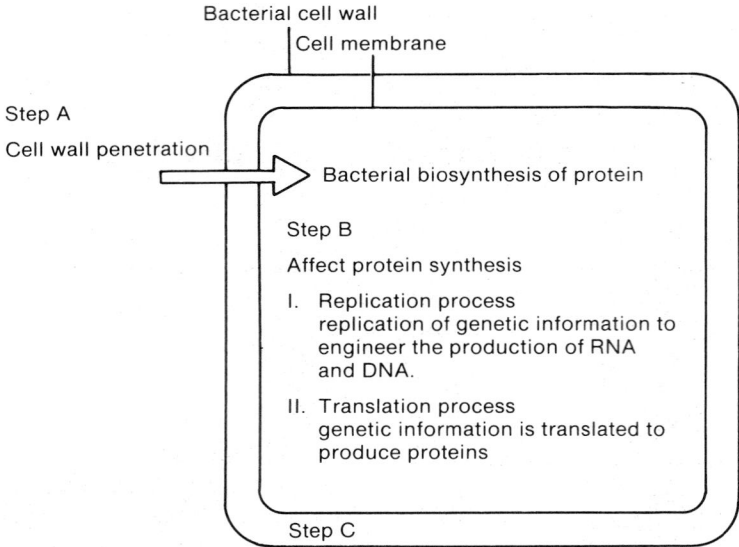

Steps of aminoglycoside action

A. Aminoglycosides penetrate bacteria through a complex process including energy-dependent active transport

B. Aminoglycosides attach to the 30S ribosome and disrupt the synthesis of bacterial proteins by

   1. Causing the genetic code to be misread

   2. Causing abnormal initiation complexes

C. Aminoglycoside may secondarily alter the cell envelope or disrupt required metabolic functions

FIGURE 46-1. **Aminoglycoside antibacterial action.**

Bacterial resistance to antibiotics varies geographically over time and tends to increase with the frequency of use. Streptomycin and kanamycin are the oldest parenterally administered aminoglycosides and have acquired the greatest number of resistant strains of bacteria. Gentamicin and tobramycin have acquired less bacterial resistance than kanamycin and streptomycin, and in most cases the two former agents have similar patterns of resistance. However, an important exception to this involves the extremely pathogenic bacteria *Pseudomonas aeruginosa.* Tobramycin is effective against up to 50% of the *Pseudomonas aeruginosa* that are resistant to gentamicin.

Amikacin is one of the newer aminoglycosides and has the least amount of acquired bacterial resistance. The lack of bacterial resistance to amikacin is not merely the result of its newness, but also to its chemical design, which provides resistance to all except one of the antibiotic-inactivating enzymes produced by bacteria. Bacterial resistance to amikacin is usually caused by the altered penetration of the aminoglycoside and thus usually results in cross-resistance to the other aminoglycosides.

MECHANISM OF BACTERIAL RESISTANCE

Three modes of bacterial resistance are usually associated with the lack of response to the aminoglycoside antibiotics: (1) production of aminoglycoside-inactivating enzymes by the bacteria; (2) altered aminoglycoside receptor or target affinity; and (3) reduced penetration by the aminoglycoside into the bacterial cell.

First, the most clinically significant mechanism of resistance to the aminoglycosides is the production of antibiotic-inactivating enzymes by bacteria. These enzymes are concentrated in the cell membrane and are capable of destroying the antimicrobial action of the antibiotic before it reaches its site of activity. The ability to produce these enzymes is commonly passed from one bacteria to another by the transfer of extra-chromosomal deoxyribonucleic acid (DNA), called

Bacteria sensitive to the aminoglycosides

Gram-negative enteric bacilli (aerobic)

Acinetobacter
Citrobacter
Enterobacter
Escherichia coli
Klebsiella
Proteus
Providencia
Pseudomonas aeruginosa
Serratia

Gram-positive cocci

Staphylococcus aureus
Staphylococcus epidermidis

Other bacteria

Haemophilus influenzae

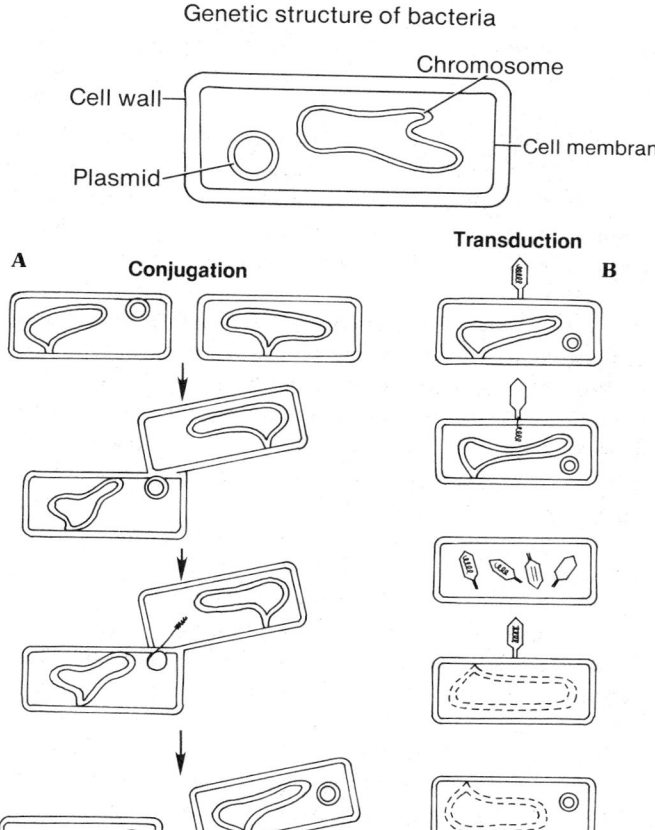

Genetic structure of bacteria

FIGURE 46-2. **Conjugation and transduction transfer of plasmids. A, Bacterial conjugation results in the exchange of DNA material between mating bacteria. This exchange includes the genetic determinants of the plasmid. B, Bacterial viruses (bacteriophages) infect bacteria and reproduce by using the bacterial replication apparatus. The bacteriophage reproduced in a resistant bacterium may acquire the host DNA resistance, which can then be transferred to nonresistant bacteria through the same infectious cycle.**

plasmids or "R" (resistance) factors. The plasmids are passed from one bacteria to another during conjugation (Figure 46-2, *A*). Plasmids are commonly transmitted to bacteria of the same species or to other pathogenic genera. Plasmids may also be passed to bacteria through a vector such as a bacteriophage (Figure 46-2, *B*). The vector introduces a plasmid into the bacteria by transduction along with other genetic material. If the bacteria survive the infection, the extra-genetic material is integrated into its genetic determinants and provides resistance to the antibiotic.

Second, a minor change in the ribosomal structure in the bacteria can reduce the ribosomal binding affinity for the aminoglycoside. Although this mechanism of resistance to the aminoglycosides has been documented in vitro, it does not appear to be significant in vivo.

A third mechanism of resistance is based on the cellular penetration of the antibiotic. Antibiotic penetration will vary not only with the specific bacteria, but also with the environment. Transport of the aminoglycoside into the bacterial cell includes aerobic energy-dependent processes. The effectiveness of the transport is dependent on factors such as oxygen tension, pH, and the concentration of divalent cations (e.g., calcium, magnesium). Therefore, anaerobic and acidic conditions inhibit cellular penetration and result in a low bacterial sensitivity to the aminoglycosides.

PHARMACOKINETICS

The aminoglycosides are polar compounds that are poorly absorbed from the GI tract. Only 0.5% to 5% of an orally administered aminoglycoside will reach the systemic circulation. On the other hand, parenteral administration of the aminoglycosides usually yields reliable and predictable serum concentrations. Subcutaneously and intramuscularly administered aminoglycosides are less reliable in severely debilitated patients, and the drugs should only be given intravenously to the severely ill.

Neomycin and kanamycin are often administered orally and rectally to sterilize the GI tract. In patients with normal renal function, the small amount of these agents absorbed from the GI tract is rapidly excreted. However, in patients with poor renal function, these drugs can accumulate to toxic serum concentrations after multiple doses. In addition, the enhanced absorption of neomycin or kanamycin on instillation into the pleural and peritoneal cavities or during wound irrigation may also lead to toxic serum concentrations, especially in patients with severely impaired renal function.

The aminoglycosides are widely distributed throughout most of the extracellular fluids except for cerebrospinal fluid and the aqueous humor of the eye. The drugs are poorly bound to plasma proteins, with reports ranging up to 20%. After multiple doses, therapeutic concentrations of the aminoglycosides have been found in bronchial secretions, synovial fluid, bile, and pleural fluid. Other tissues, such as muscle, fat, and hard bone, achieve aminoglycoside concentrations well below those in the serum.

The aminoglycosides are completely excreted unchanged in the urine by glomerular filtration. The drugs have a serum half-life of 2 to 3 hours in patients with normal renal function. The half-life varies inversely with the glomerular filtration rate and may be extremely prolonged in patients with renal failure. The drugs are not metabolized by the liver nor are they appreciably excreted in the bile.

TOXICITY

The major adverse effects associated with the use of the aminoglycosides are nephrotoxicity and ototoxicity. All of the aminoglycosides cause these effects, but the prevalence of the reactions vary with the individual agents.

Nephrotoxicity

Sustained high serum concentrations of the aminoglycosides exert a direct toxic effect on the epithelial cells of the kidney's proximal tubules. The aminoglycosides are transported across the membrane of these cells where they uncouple oxidative phosphorylation and inhibit mitochondrial ATP formation. The eventual result of the toxic effect is poor control of Na^+ and K^+ movement, and an osmotic lysis of the involved cells. Damage to the proximal tubule will alter the reabsorptive capability of the kidneys, which leads to a decrease in glomerular filtration and rising serum creatinine concentrations (Figure 46-3, A). Significant damage to a large number of proximal tubule cells must occur before glomerular filtration is altered. A rise in serum creatinine is usually not seen until after

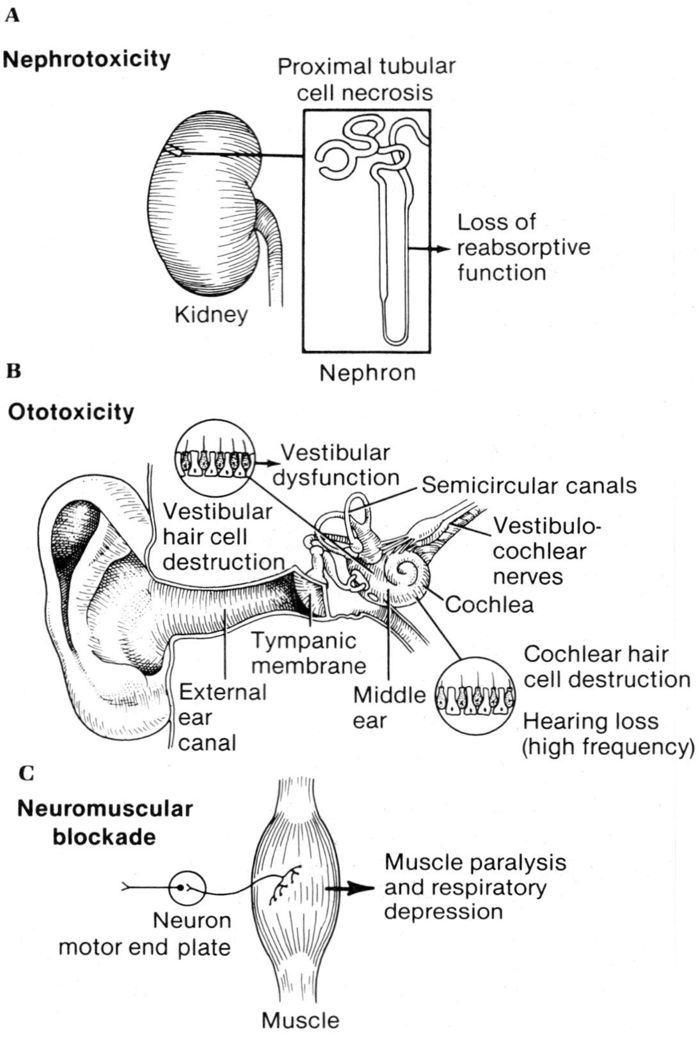

A
Nephrotoxicity

Proximal tubular cell necrosis

Loss of reabsorptive function

Kidney

Nephron

B
Ototoxicity

Vestibular dysfunction
Semicircular canals
Vestibular hair cell destruction
Vestibulo-cochlear nerves
Cochlea
Tympanic membrane
External ear canal
Middle ear
Cochlear hair cell destruction
Hearing loss (high frequency)

C
Neuromuscular blockade

Muscle paralysis and respiratory depression
Neuron motor end plate
Muscle

FIGURE 46-3. **Aminoglycoside toxicity. A, Nephrotoxicity—the aminoglycosides are directly toxic to proximal tubule cells, leading to cell death and renal impairment. B, Ototoxicity—high endolymph concentrations of the aminoglycosides may result in vestibular and cochlear hair cell death and resultant vestibular or auditory damage. C, Neuromuscular blockade—aminoglycosides cause inhibition of acetylcholine release presynaptically and a loss of transmitter sensitivity postsynaptically, which can lead to acute muscular paralysis and apnea.**

more than 5 days of therapy with these drugs. Therefore, serum creatinine and BUN values are not extremely sensitive nor specific indicators of early aminoglycoside nephrotoxicity.

Urinary β_2 microglobulin, urinary casts, and urinary enzyme excretion are all more sensitive indicators of proximal cell damage. These urine tests provide earlier evidence of a problem, but they are not specific for aminoglycoside renal tubular damage and do not aid in excluding other possible causes. Renal tubular damage caused by the aminoglycoside antibiotics is reversible in most cases after the discontinuation of the drug. The renal tubular cells have a regenerative capability and renal function will usually return to pretreatment levels in 20 to 60 days.

Ototoxicity

The aminoglycosides can cause both vestibular and cochlear dysfunction (Figure 46-3, B). Aminoglycoside-induced ototoxicity involves a direct toxic effect on the sensory cells of both the auditory and the vestibular areas of the inner ear. The cells are progressively affected until they are destroyed, and do not regenerate once lost. The extent of the damage is generally related to the number of destroyed cells. Thus, aminoglycoside ototoxicity is cumulative and is most likely noticed in patients who have had previous damage or in elderly patients who may have a compromised reserve of functioning sensory cells. Furthermore, other drugs that cause ototoxicity (e.g., furosemide and ethacrynic acid) may add to the ototoxicity of the aminoglycosides when they are combined.

Auditory dysfunction usually shows up first with a loss of high-frequency perception or tinnitus. Further progression to total deafness can occur suddenly without warning. Vestibular dysfunction usually produces symptoms of vertigo, nausea, and vomiting. However, compensatory mechanisms of balance usually prevent continued functional impairment.

The incidence of aminoglycoside ototoxicity is related to the concentration of the drug in the otic fluid. The half-life of the aminoglycosides in the ear is 5 to 6 times the serum half-life, and thus very high concentrations of the drugs can be reached in the inner ear on multiple dosing.

Miscellaneous

Neuromuscular blockade has been associated with all routes of aminoglycoside administration (Figure 46-3, C). However, it is a dose-related effect that most commonly occurs when high serum concentrations of the agents are achieved. Neomycin and kanamycin are the agents most frequently associated with this effect, but it can be caused by any of the aminoglycosides.

The aminoglycosides may impair neuromuscular transmission by altering the release and receptor interaction of acetylcholine at the neuromuscular junction and may also impair the action of calcium at this site. This adverse effect usually occurs when the aminoglycosides are administered in association with anesthetic agents. Further predisposing factors to

neuromuscular blockade are poor renal function, high aminoglycoside serum concentrations, and previous neuromuscular disease. Neuromuscular blockade often affects the respiratory musculature and can lead to hypoventilation and respiratory paralysis.

The preferred treatment for aminoglycoside-induced neuromuscular blockade is intravenously administered calcium. Cholinesterase inhibitors (e.g., edrophonium and neostigmine) are also used with limited success.

The aminoglycosides rarely cause allergic reactions. However, allergic cross-sensitivity is common in patients who have experienced an allergic reaction to one of the aminoglycosides. Thus, hypersensitivity becomes important when considering the use of neomycin and other aminoglycosides on superficial wounds that could be treated with other agents. Hypersensitivity reactions to topically applied neomycin have been reported to occur in up to 8% of patients. Thus, the use of the aminoglycosides to treat superficial wounds may needlessly cross-sensitize patients to other aminoglycosides and preclude using these antibiotics to treat more serious diseases.

Orally administered aminoglycosides may cause an intestinal malabsorption syndrome that is much like nontropical sprue. The malabsorption syndrome is usually associated with orally administered neomycin at doses above 6 gm per day for an extended period of time.

These drugs may also cause superinfections when given orally. It is common for a yeast overgrowth to develop in an extended course of oral neomycin therapy. Staphylococcal enterocolitis has also been reported with the use of oral neomycin.

CLINICAL USE

The aminoglycosides are often the most effective antibiotics available for treating infections caused by gram-negative bacilli. Despite their effectiveness, the adverse potential of these agents, especially when administered parenterally, requires that they be reserved for relatively serious infections. Furthermore, because there are so few agents that are effective against gram-negative bacilli, the aminoglycosides should be reserved for the serious infections that cannot be treated with other agents. Thus, the indiscriminant use of the aminoglycosides should be avoided, especially when considering the consequences of allergic cross-sensitivity and the emergence of resistant strains. The treatment of superficial infections with an aminoglycoside is usually inappropriate and is not recommended.

Serious gram-negative infections

Gentamicin, tobramycin, and amikacin are the parenteral aminoglycosides of choice for treating serious gram-negative infections such as bacteremias, abdominal abscesses, and gram-negative meningitis. Because of poor CSF penetration, levels depend on both dosage and degree of inflammation of the meninges. The choice between these agents in this type of infection will depend on bacterial sensitivity studies and the origin of the infection. In general, gentamicin or tobramycin are most commonly considered the drugs of first choice, and amikacin is reserved for infections caused by bacteria resistant to the other two agents.

A gram-negative infection of the CNS may be best treated with an aminoglycoside. However, these agents do not effectively penetrate the blood-brain barrier. Therefore, in addition to parenteral administration, they must also be administered directly by intrathecal or intraventricular injection to achieve therapeutic aminoglycoside concentrations in the CNS.

Combination therapy

The aminoglycosides are frequently combined with other antibiotics to cover fully a mixture of infecting organisms or to cover the likely infecting microorganisms before they can be identified. In addition, certain combination therapies involving an aminoglycoside provide synergistic activity against bacteria that are not sensitive to single-agent therapy.

Bacteremias of an unidentified etiology are often treated with a combination of antibiotics, including an aminoglycoside with a penicillin or a cephalosporin. A combination of an aminoglycoside and chloramphenicol or clindamycin is used to treat serious abdominal infections. Commonly, abdominal infections are caused by a mixture of aerobic and anaerobic enteric microorganisms, many of which are not sensitive to the aminoglycosides. Thus, clindamycin or chloramphenicol is combined with an aminoglycoside to cover the presence of anaerobic bacteria, as well as the aminoglycoside-sensitive gram-negative rods.

Serious infections such as pneumonias and bacteremias caused by *Pseudomonas aeruginosa* usually warrant combination antibiotic therapy. A synergistic antibacterial effect is obtained in pseudomonal infections with a combination of ticarcillin or carbenicillin and gentamicin, tobramycin, or amikacin. This combination is, however, chemically incompatible and requires that the agents not be mixed before administration and that they not be administered concurrently at the same injection site.

A combination of gentamicin or streptomycin with penicillin G or ampicillin has been shown to be synergistic for treating enterococcal endocarditis. The mechanism for the enhanced activity of this combination is the improved bacterial cell penetration of the aminoglycosides resulting from penicillin-induced bacterial cell wall damage.

Miscellaneous infections

Streptomycin is currently considered the agent of choice for treating tularemia and plague. It is also recommended for use in combination with tetracycline for treating brucellosis. Streptomycin continues to be used in tuberculosis, but is now reserved for use in resistant or disseminated cases requiring a combination of three or more drugs.

Other uses

Neomycin and kanamycin are occasionally used orally for GI sterilization. Neomycin is the agent most commonly used for this purpose. Gastrointestinal sterilization reduces the chance of infection secondary to bowel surgery and also decreases the intestinal bacterial production of ammonia in hyperammonemia associated with hepatic coma.

Gentamicin and neomycin ophthalmic preparations are also available for treating bacterial infections of the eye and its adnexa. These preparations may be associated with mild irritation, local burning, or stinging.

The dose of gentamicin solution for treating less severe ophthalmic infections is one or two drops in the affected eye every 4 hours. In more severe cases this dose may be increased up to two drops every hour. If gentamicin ointment is used, a small amount should be instilled into the eye up to three times daily.

Various combination ophthalmic preparations containing neomycin are available commercially. The recommended doses, as well as the effectiveness of these preparations, will depend on the combination.

AMINOGLYCOSIDE DOSING

The aminoglycosides can potentially cause severe dose-related ototoxic and nephrotoxic effects. Furthermore, the therapeutic to toxic range of the aminoglycosides is very narrow, requiring extremely careful therapeutic management.

Parenteral administration of the aminoglycosides will initially require a loading dose that is somewhat larger than the maintenance doses. The loading dose is individualized on the basis of the patient's body weight. The maintenance dose is given to replace the amount of drug eliminated during the dosing interval.

Thus, the maintenance dose for the aminoglycosides is based on the renal excretion of the drug. Because the aminoglycosides are eliminated to a large extent by glomerular filtration, creatinine clearance is used to gauge the patient's renal elimination capability.

In the absence of a creatinine clearance value for the patient, the serum creatinine measurement can be used to estimate the clearance of creatinine. Serum creatinine values are the function of endogenous pro-

duction (i.e., related to muscle mass), as well as glomerular filtration. Serum creatinine values can be normal in elderly patients despite a compromised renal function. It becomes important to estimate creatinine clearance in all elderly patients even though they have a serum creatinine in the normal range. An aminoglycoside dosing chart can then be used to select a reasonable maintenance dose for the patient (Table 46-1).

TABLE 46-1

Aminoglycoside dosing chart

1. Select loading dose in mg/kg (IDEAL WEIGHT) to provide peak serum levels in range listed below for desired aminoglycoside

Aminoglycoside	Usual loading doses	Expected peak serum levels
Gentamicin	1.5 to 2.0 mg/kg	4 to 10 µg/ml
Tobramycin	1.5 to 2.0 mg/kg	4 to 10 µg/ml
Amikacin	5.0 to 7.5 mg/kg	15 to 30 µg/ml
Kanamycin	5.0 to 7.5 mg/kg	15 to 30 µg/ml

2. Select maintenance dose (as *percentage* of chosen loading dose) to continue peak serum levels indicated above according to desired dosing interval and the patient's corrected creatinine clearance*

C(c)cr (ml/min)	Half-life† (hr)	Dosage interval		
		8 hr (%)	12 hr (%)	24 hr (%)
90	3.1	84	—	—
80	3.4	80	91	—
70	3.9	76	88	—
60	4.5	71	84	—
50	5.3	65	79	—
40	6.5	57	72	92
30	8.4	48	63	86
25	9.9	43	57	81
20	11.9	37	50	75
17	13.6	33	46	70
15	15.1	31	42	67
12	17.9	27	37	61
10‡	20.4	24	34	56
7	25.9	19	28	47
5	31.5	16	23	41
2	46.8	11	16	30
0	69.3	8	11	21

From Sarubbi, F.A., & Hull, J.H. Amikacin serum concentrations: pharmacokinetic predictions. *Annals of Internal Medicine*, 1978, *89*(Part I), 612-618.

*Calculate corrected creatinine clearance C(c)cr as:

C(c)cr male = 140 − age/serum creatinine

C(c)cr female = 0.85 × C(c)cr male

†Alternatively, one half of the chosen loading dose may be given at an interval approximately equal to the estimated half-life.

‡Dosing for patients with C(c)cr ≤ 10 ml/min must be assisted by measured serum levels.

Serum concentrations

Serum concentrations of the aminoglycosides can be obtained in most urban hospitals, and are an extremely valuable means of guiding therapy with these drugs. Serum peak and trough concentrations should be used to guide dosing. Blood samples for peak serum concentrations should be drawn ½ hour after IV infusion. Trough concentrations should be determined immediately before the next dose.

Desirable peak serum concentrations for gentamicin and tobramycin in seriously ill patients will range from 5 to 10 μg/ml. The trough concentrations of gentamicin and tobramycin in these patients should range from less than 1 to 1.5 μg/ml.

Desirable concentrations for amikacin in seriously ill patients should range from a peak of 20 to 30 μg/ml to a trough concentration of 4 to 8 μg/ml.

If the aminoglycoside is administered intramuscularly, the peak serum concentration should be determined 1 hour after the dose is given and the trough should be determined at the end of the dosing interval.

SPECIFIC AGENTS

Amikacin

Amikacin has the broadest spectrum of activity of the systemically administered aminoglycosides. It is also active against many bacteria that are resistant to the other aminoglycosides. For this reason, the use of amikacin has been restricted in many hospitals to prevent the emergence of resistant strains. Thus, amikacin is the agent usually chosen to treat unidentified bacteremias and nosocomial infections caused by bacteria that are likely to be resistant to other aminoglycosides.

Amikacin is commercially available only in parenteral form. It can be administered intravenously and intramuscularly.

Gentamicin

Gentamicin is the aminoglycoside of choice for treating many serious gram-negative bacillary infections. But because of hospital resistance patterns the use of tobramycin and amikacin in the place of gentamicin continues to increase. Gentamicin is commercially available in parenteral and topical preparations. The parenteral preparations can be administered IM or IV, but IV administration is preferred for severely ill patients. Gentamicin is also available in a 0.1% cream and ointment, and in a 0.3% ophthalmic ointment and solution.

Kanamycin

The use of kanamycin has declined greatly since the release of the other less toxic and more effective aminoglycosides. It has pharmacokinetic and chemical properties similar to amikacin. For systemic therapy kanamycin must be given parenterally, with the IM route being preferred. The maximal daily adult parenteral dose of kanamycin is 1.5 gm and the total recommended dose for a complete course of therapy in adults is 15 gm. Oral therapy with kanamycin has been used for prophylactic bowel preparation in abdominal surgery and for hyperammonemia.

Neomycin

Neomycin is a broad-spectrum aminoglycoside that can be administered orally, topically, or parenterally. However, because of its severe ototoxic and nephrotoxic potential, it is generally restricted to nonparenteral administration. Neomycin is used in combination with polymyxin B and bacitracin in many topical preparations. It is given orally for bowel sterilization procedures in prophylaxis for abdominal surgery and for treating hepatic coma. The doses given orally range from 4 to 12 gm per day for adults. Caution should be exercised in oral therapy to ensure that an adequate renal function is present.

Netilmicin

Netilmicin is chemically related to gentamicin and shares the physical characteristics common to the aminoglycosides. Although it is less active against *Pseudomonas*, the indications for the use of netilmicin will probably be very similar for those of gentamicin and tobramycin. Netilmicin may be effective in treating other bacteria resistant to gentamicin because of its ability to resist enzymatic degradation. Furthermore, animal studies suggest that netilmicin is less nephrotoxic and ototoxic than gentamicin. Further clinical trials are needed to compare the various benefits of this newer agent over the other aminoglycosides currently available.

Paromomycin

Paromomycin is an aminoglycoside antibiotic that has been used to treat intestinal amebiasis, hepatic coma, and various tapeworm infestations. However, it is not currently considered the drug of choice for any of these problems. The drug is chemically similar to the other aminoglycosides and shares many of the same pharmacologic properties. Paromomycin is used only orally for treating GI disease and because it is poorly absorbed from the GI tract, toxic serum concentrations are a problem only in patients with severe renal impairment. The adverse potential of paromomycin is comparable to the other aminoglycosides. The recommended dose for treating intestinal amebiasis in children and adults is 25 to 35 mg/kg per day in three divided doses. The dose should be taken with meals for 5 to 10 days. The recommended dose for managing hepatic coma is 4 gm daily divided into several doses for 5 to 6 days.

Streptomycin

Streptomycin can be administered by a variety of routes, but the preferred parenteral route is by deep IM injection. Although nephrotoxicity is less common with streptomycin than with the other aminoglycosides, streptomycin is ototoxic at the recommended dose when administered for a prolonged period of time.

Tobramycin

Tobramycin is only available commercially in a parenteral form. It can be administered intravenously or intramuscularly, but the IV route is preferred for severely ill patients. The dosage indications, desired serum concentrations, and toxicity are all very similar to those of gentamicin. Tobramycin has been reported to cause less nephrotoxicity than gentamicin at equiv-

alent doses. However, the clinical significance of this difference is as yet unclear. Tobramycin also has a greater activity against *Pseudomonas aeruginosa* than does gentamicin.

SUMMARY

This chapter has examined the various types and uses of the aminoglycoside antibiotics. The mechanism of action, pharmacology, and toxicology for the various agents have been presented. In addition, an overview of the mechanisms of bacterial resistance has been discussed.

With an understanding of the various individual agents, including their actions and side effects, the nurse will be better able to provide optimal care to patients who require these medications. Patient education can be enhanced, adverse drug effects can be anticipated, monitored for, and minimized, clinically significant drug interactions can be avoided, and the therapeutic response appropriately monitored for by using the information presented in this chapter.

ADVERSE/SIDE EFFECTS OF THE AMINOGLYCOSIDES*

ALLERGIC REACTIONS

Allergic dermatitis (topical neomycin)
Anaphylactic reactions (extremely rare)
Drug fever
Eosinophilia

CARDIOVASCULAR SYSTEM

Depression of cardiac function (rapid parenteral administration of streptomycin or kanamycin)

CENTRAL NERVOUS SYSTEM

Acute organic brain syndrome
Blurring of vision
Pain
Paresthesias

GASTROINTESTINAL SYSTEM

Malabsorption syndrome (oral neomycin because of damage to GI mucosa or binding of bile salts)
Superinfection (oral neomycin— infrequent)

HEMATOLOGIC SYSTEM

Agranulocytosis (extremely rare)

HEPATIC SYSTEM

Elevations of serum liver enzyme levels (SGOT, SGPT, and alkaline phosphatase)

NEUROMUSCULAR SYSTEM

Neuromuscular blockade (weakness of skeletal muscles, respiratory depression, and apnea; can be partially or completely reversed by IV administration of calcium salts)

OTOLOGIC SYSTEM

Cochlear toxicity (hearing loss, tinnitus)
Vestibular toxicity (nausea, vomiting, dizziness, vertigo, loss of balance)
(May occur more commonly with certain predisposing factors: high peak or trough serum levels, old age, high cumulative dose, long-

term therapy [more than 10 days], simultaneous administration of other ototoxic drugs such as ethacrynic acid, and furosemide; toxicities are usually irreversible but sometimes are reversible)

RENAL SYSTEM

Nephrotoxicity (acute tubular necrosis; manifested in the form of increased BUN, increased serum creatinine level, presence of protein and tubular cells in urine; may occur more frequently with certain predisposing factors: high peak or trough serum levels, old age, dehydration, high cumulative dose, long-term therapy (more than 10 days, simultaneous administration of other nephrotoxic drugs such as amphotericin B and cephalothin; nephrotoxicity is usually reversible if the drug is discontinued at the first signs of renal dysfunction)

---

*See Chapter 11, "Drug Toxicity," for an overview of drug toxicity.

CLINICALLY SIGNIFICANT DRUG INTERACTIONS*

Primary drug	Interacting drug	Possible effect(s)	Probable mechanism(s)
Aminoglycoside (oral neomycin)	Anticoagulants (oral)	Increased prothrombin time leading to bleeding	Decreased vitamin K production by gut bacteria and impaired vitamin K oral absorption
Aminoglycosides (gentamicin)	Cephalothin	Increased nephrotoxicity	Not established
Aminoglycosides	Ethacrynic acid	Increased ototoxicity	Additive ototoxicity
Aminoglycosides	Furosemide	Increased ototoxicity	Additive ototoxicity
Aminoglycosides	Methoxyflurane	Increased nephrotoxicity	Additive or synergistic nephrotoxicity
Aminoglycosides	Penicillin V	Decreased duration of effect of aminoglycosides	Decreased aminoglycoside half-life
Aminoglycosides	Surgical skeletal muscle relaxants (e.g., succinylcholine, tubocurarine)	Respiratory paralysis	Increased neuromuscular blockade

*See Chapter 10, "Drug Interactions," for an overview of drug interactions.

GENERAL NURSING IMPLICATIONS

Nursing of patients requiring aminoglycosides

ASSESSMENT

The aminoglycosides are used primarily for treating serious gram-negative bacilli infections (e.g., bacteremias). It is important to recognize that these agents are *not* recommended for treating superficial infections. The choice of drug depends on bacterial sensitivity studies. This is important not only in determining if an aminoglycoside is needed or if a less toxic antibiotic (e.g., penicillin) can be used, but also in indicating which specific agent should be used.

The aminoglycosides can be used for prophylaxis or, as in abdominal surgery, for bowel sterilization. Ophthalmic preparations are available for treating eye infections and aminoglycosides can be used topically for treating certain skin infections and for wound or urinary tract irrigations. Specific assessment data related to the purpose of aminoglycoside therapy should be included to serve as a baseline for monitoring patient response.

Baseline data should include specific information about the patient's condition and general health state. Assessment should be completed carefully so that changes in the patient's condition can be identified readily. Laboratory specimens are particularly important in the diagnosis of the causative organism and thus in the choice of drug for the treatment of the specific infection. Whenever possible, the organism responsible for the infection should be identified *before* the drug therapy is initiated. Thus, the collection of specimens (e.g., blood, sputum, urine, wound drainage), as indicated, should be completed carefully for smear and sensitivity studies according to hospital or agency procedure. These assist not only in drug selection, but also in monitoring the patient's response to therapy. Other nursing observations indicative of infectious processes should likewise be reported and documented, including symptoms of infection such as elevated temperature, chills, redness or pain in an area not previously affected, fatigue, change in character or color of sputum or wound drainage, elevated white blood cell count, or other observations related to the specific infectious condition. Isolation measures should be readily implemented as indicated to prevent the spread of infection to others.

Because the aminoglycosides are associated with both nephrotoxicity and ototoxicity, baseline data should include the determination of renal function, as well as hearing and vestibular function, so that patients can be monitored for early signs of these toxicities.

It is recommended that patients be weighed carefully and have baseline renal function studies completed before the therapy is started. The nursing history should also identify if patients have a concurrent renal disease or a history of renal disease or if they have been taking nephrotoxic agents (e.g., cephaloradine and methicillin), because these may increase the nephrotoxic effects of the aminoglycosides. It is also recommended that patients requiring aminoglycosides have a baseline audiogram completed before the initiation of the drug therapy so that ototoxicity can be monitored. It should also be determined if they have been taking other ototoxic drugs (e.g., furosemide) or if they have a history of excessive noise exposure or ear infections, because these can potentiate the ototoxic effects of these medications. Testing for high-frequency hearing loss and renal function should be carefully monitored during therapy.

GENERAL NURSING IMPLICATIONS—cont'd

Nursing of patients requiring aminoglycosides—cont'd

ASSESSMENT—cont'd

The drug history should include, in addition to the use of nephrotoxic or ototoxic medications, a history of any drug allergy to the aminoglycosides, and information regarding possible contraindications, cautions, potential drug interactions, and individual drug-taking patterns before therapy is initiated.

SENSITIVITY

Hypersensitivity, although rare with the aminoglycosides, may occur with virtually any drug and should be monitored for.

It is important to note that cross-sensitivity is common in patients with a history of an allergic reaction to one of the aminoglycosides, including those topically applied. This is another reason why these medications are reserved for treating severe infections. If used for minor infections or for infections that can be treated by a less potent antibiotic, and an allergic reaction develops, the aminoglycosides may not be used when needed for a severe infection when it occurs.

CONTRAINDICATIONS

Aminoglycosides are contraindicated in patients with a known hypersensitivity to any of the aminoglycosides.

CAUTIONS

Aminoglycosides should be used with caution in pregnant women and neonates because the available data are limited. These drugs should be used with caution in patients with neuromuscular diseases such as myasthenia gravis because of the potential neuromuscular blocking activity of the aminoglycosides (See Chapter 26, "Ganglionic and Neuromuscular Stimulants and Blockers"). These drugs should also be used with caution in patients with a compromised renal function or hearing deficits because of the potential of the aminoglycosides to cause nephrotoxicity and ototoxicity.

DRUG INTERACTIONS

Aminoglycosides are often given with other drugs for synergistic effects. It is important to note that many of these drugs are incompatible (e.g., ticarcillin and amikacin), and cannot be administered concomitantly or at the same injection site. The aminoglycosides are often incompatible when mixed with other drugs for parenteral administration, and the same IV infusion line should not be used. See the Nursing Drug Digest and Appendix IV, "Intravenous Incompatibilities," for details regarding specific aminoglycosides.

Aminoglycosides are associated with drug interactions primarily related to synergistic toxicity with other drugs, which also cause ototoxicity, nephrotoxicity, or neuromuscular blockade. See Clinically Significant Drug Interactions for specific interactions involving the aminoglycosides.

ADMINISTRATION

Aminoglycosides are available in various dosage forms for oral, parenteral, and topical administration. Because of their limited GI absorption (less than 5%), the aminoglycosides are administered parenterally for systemic effect and are administered orally for local effect within the GI tract (e.g., sterilization of the bowel before GI surgery, treatment of amebiasis).

Aminoglycosides have also been administered intrathecally and intraventricularly for CNS gram-negative infections because they do not readily cross the blood-brain barrier when given by other routes. Because of the narrow therapeutic index of these medications and the related ototoxicity and nephrotoxicity, extreme care is required in preparing doses. See Table 46-2 for an aminoglycoside dosing chart, especially for elderly patients. Drug dosing should be determined in relation to peak and trough levels.

Serum drug levels are important in determining the drug dose for optimal therapeutic response and minimal toxicity. A loading dose based on the patient's weight, or ideal lean body weight if the patient is obese, because aminoglycosides do not distribute well into body fat, is given to obtain rapid therapeutic serum levels. The maintenance dose varies in relation to the type and severity of the infection, as well as in relation to the patient's age, weight, and renal function. For both loading and maintenance doses, serum drug levels must be obtained at exact times to obtain accurate results. Peak levels must be drawn minutes after the completion of an IV dose and 1 hour after IM administration. Trough levels must be drawn immediately before the next scheduled dose.

When administering aminoglycosides, the following points should be remembered.

Check with patients before administering the prescribed drug to determine whether they have had any allergic reaction to the aminoglycosides.

Obtain samples (e.g., blood, urine, sputum, cerebrospinal fluid) as specified by the prescriber for culture and sensitivity tests routinely *before* the first dose of the antibiotic(s).

Space the time of the antibiotic administration as evenly as possible throughout 24 hrs (e.g., t.i.d. means every 8 hours around the clock).

Ensure that the order for an antibiotic is reviewed by the prescriber at least every 5 to 7 days so that the order is either renewed or canceled.

Oral administration

Aminoglycosides should be taken orally with a full glass of water. Gastrointestinal upset can occur when these medications are taken orally, as well as side effects such as soreness of the mouth or rectal area and diarrhea. Taking the medication with food or meals may minimize the GI distress and will not effect the drug absorption.

Parenteral administration

Intramuscular and IV routes can result in adequate blood levels in relatively healthy patients. The IM route should not be used for debilitated or severely ill patients.

Watch for pain or abscess at the site of the IM injection. Rotate the sites carefully and make the injections into large healthy muscle. If healthy muscle sites are limited, it is recommended to use IV administration. *Continued.*

GENERAL NURSING IMPLICATIONS—cont'd

Nursing of patients requiring aminoglycosides—cont'd

Parenteral administration—cont'd

Observe for redness, edema, and pain along the vein into which the drug is administered. Do not infuse aminoglycosides into inflamed veins or if irritation at the infusion site is noted. The site should be changed if irritation or inflammation is noted.

Do not mix parenteral antibiotics in the same syringe, same IV line, or same IV bottle unless compatibility is clearly present.

Dilute IV antibiotics in compatible IV fluids, which are indicated on the labels or package inserts, for intermittent IV infusion. Also, check the stability data of the antibiotics in IV fluids in the manufacturers' package inserts. Do *not* use outdated medication.

Aminoglycosides such as amikacin, gentamicin, and tobramycin generally should be diluted in 100 ml of 5% dextrose and water or normal saline for IV infusion. The infusion rate should be over 30 minutes and no longer than 45 minutes. A faster infusion rate has been associated with an increased risk of ototoxicity and a slower infusion rate has been associated with decreased effectiveness because it prevents the drug from reaching maximal blood levels.

(See the Nursing Drug Digest for specific information regarding dosage forms and administration.)

MONITORING PATIENT RESPONSE
Therapeutic response

Patients should be carefully monitored according to baseline data obtained before the initiation of therapy in relation to the indication for aminoglycoside therapy, such as a reduction of fever, an increased sense of well-being, and an increased appetite.

In addition, serum concentrations of an aminoglycoside should be monitored in relation to the therapeutic response. Because of the importance in monitoring the therapy, these blood samples need to be drawn carefully in relation to drug administration.

The onset and duration of antibiotic therapy is dependent on the dosage form and route of administration, as well as on individual patient factors. Monitoring the therapeutic response is especially important because if the antibiotic therapy fails another drug or therapy regimen can be implemented readily. This is particularly important in serious infections. As with the other antibiotics, in addition to serum concentrations of the aminoglycoside, the therapy should be guided by bacteriologic studies, susceptibility tests, and clinical response.

Adverse side effects

The major adverse effects associated with the aminoglycosides are nephrotoxicity, ototoxicity, neuromuscular blockade, and an overgrowth of nonsusceptible organisms or superinfections. A malabsorption syndrome after the oral administration of neomycin greater than 6 gm per day has also been reported, as has enterocolitis with oral neomycin.

Monitoring the adverse effects is particularly important with the aminoglycosides because of the severity of the related toxicities and because they can be prevented or minimized with early detection.

Nephrotoxicity

Monitor for signs of nephrotoxicity, including proteinuria, decreased creatinine clearance, elevated BUN, or elevated serum creatinine. Nephrotoxicity is more likely to occur with large doses of the aminoglycosides or when other nephrotoxic drugs such as cephaloridine are administered concurrently. Renal function usually returns to normal following the discontinuation of the aminoglycoside as the renal cells regenerate. It should be noted that neomycin is the most nephrotoxic of the aminoglycosides and is thus only rarely administered parenterally. Streptomycin is the least nephrotoxic. The other aminoglycosides fall roughly in the middle between neomycin and streptomycin in relation to nephrotoxicity.

Monitor weight and renal function and compare with the baseline data. To minimize this adverse effect, maintain hydration and monitor the renal function. Signs of nephrotoxicity include casts in the urine, oliguria, proteinuria, decreased creatinine clearance, and an elevated BUN. The incidence seems greatest with amikacin. Gentamicin and tobramycin are generally less nephrotoxic. Because serum creatinine and BUN are not *early* indicators of nephrotoxicity, in addition monitor urinary β_2 microglobulin, casts, and urinary enzyme excretion, which are indicative of proximal tubule cell damage. When monitoring do not exclude other causes. Monitor patients for 20 to 60 days after the discontinuation of aminoglycoside therapy for pretreatment levels of function, because effects can occur during this time.

Monitor intake and output and report sudden change in urine output.

Ototoxicity

Monitor patients carefully for ototoxicity, including both vestibular and cochlear involvement. This is particularly important because if detected *early* this adverse effect is generally reversible. However, if not monitored for and detected the ototoxicity may become severe and irreversible even after the discontinuation of the drug. Deafness has occurred several weeks after therapy had been discontinued.

Vestibular dysfunction should be monitored, including nausea and vomiting with motion, vertigo, and headache. The symptoms of cochlear damage are tinnitus and loss of hearing. Initially, hearing loss is in the high-frequency range and can only be detected by audiometric examination. Audiometric reassessment during therapy is recommended especially with patients prone to this adverse effect, particularly elderly patients and those patients with either renal impairment on long-term high-dose therapy, or who are receiving other ototoxic drugs (e.g., ethacrynic acid, furosemide).

Supervise ambulation and provide bedside rails as necessary to protect patients with aminoglycoside-induced vestibular dysfunction.

GENERAL NURSING IMPLICATIONS—cont'd

Nursing of patients requiring aminoglycosides—cont'd

Neuromuscular blockade

Neuromuscular blockade is associated with high serum concentrations and especially with the administration of aminoglycosides with anesthetic agents. This effect is associated in particularly with patients with neuromuscular disease.

Observe for respiratory depression and apnea, especially in patients with hypocalcemia, neuromuscular diseases such as myasthenia gravis, and in patients recovering from anesthesia after surgery.

Other adverse side effects

Observe for the overgrowth of nonsusceptible organisms and treat appropriately (e.g., an antifungal for a fungal overgrowth based on culture and sensitivity studies).

See Adverse/Side Effects of the Aminoglycosides for an outline of effects associated with the aminoglycosides.

Remember to monitor ototoxicity and nephrotoxicity closely in patients with certain predisposing factors: old age (greater than 70 years of age), high cumulative dose, prolonged duration of therapy (more than 10 days), high peak or trough serum levels, preexisting renal dysfunction, and concurrent administration of other ototoxic (e.g., ethacrynic acid, furosemide) or nephrotoxic (e.g., amphotericin B, cephalothin) drugs.

PATIENT EDUCATION

The patient and the family, as indicated, should be fully informed about the nature of the patient's condition and the treatment plan, and should be involved in the health care planning whenever possible.

The patient and the family should have a clear understanding of the anticipated course of the therapy and medication regimen including the exact name of the medication, its general action, purpose, dosage, storage, administration, and specific adverse side effects associated with its use, including nephrotoxicity and ototoxicity. The patient and the family should be able to make an informed consent in relation to the use of aminoglycosides for treating serious infections or for use as indicated. It is particularly important that the patient and the family be able to monitor adverse side effects and to recognize how these effects can be minimized (e.g., increasing fluid intake unless contraindicated). Because ototoxicity can be reversed or damage minimized if detected early, it is of special importance that the patient be involved in monitoring effects so that tinnitus, dizziness, or other early signs can be readily detected and reported. The patient and the family should also be able to monitor the therapeutic response, because the therapy can often be over several weeks.

Nursing attention should be directed at assisting patients with preventing infections and at assisting patients with prolonged periods of hospitalization or treatment. Patient and family involvement can do much to minimize the effects of hospitalization and promote therapeutic regimens and family functioning.

GENERAL INSTRUCTIONS FOR DISCHARGE/OUTPATIENTS

AMINOGLYCOSIDES

Follow the instructions on the prescription exactly.

This medication may be taken without regard to meals.

Keep taking this medicine for the full time of treatment and do not skip any doses, even if you are feeling better.

Use a specially marked measuring spoon or other device to measure each dose accurately, because the average household spoon may not hold the right amount of liquid.

Stinging, itching, skin rashes, and different skin reactions are a few side effects that can occur in some patients when topical antibiotics are used. If these persist or become extreme, notify your health care provider.

Gastrointestinal upset, diarrhea, irritation or soreness of the mouth or rectal area can occur when these antibiotics are taken orally. If these persist or become extreme, notify your health care provider.

Report any loss of hearing, ringing sounds, or a feeling of fullness in the ears, unsteadiness, dizziness, or marked decrease in frequency of urination or amount of urine to your health care provider.

Do not trade or give this antibiotic to any relatives or friends. It was prescribed especially for you.

Keep this and all medications out of children's reach.

NURSING DRUG DIGEST

Medication (trade name*)	Indication	Usual dosage and administration	Dosage forms, preparation, and storage	Contraindications, cautions, and comments	Monitoring
Amikacin Amikin	Serious systemic infections caused by susceptible gram-negative bacteria and *Staphylococcus aureus* Uncomplicated lower urinary tract infections caused by susceptible gram-negative bacteria	*Adults:* 15 mg/kg/24 hr IM/IV in 2-3 divided doses q.8-12h. *Children:* 15 mg/kg/24 hr IM/IV in 2-3 divided doses q.8-12h. Total daily dose for adults should *not* exceed 1.5 gm Rotate IM injection sites *Adults:* 500 mg/24 hr IM/IV in 2 divided doses q.12h. Do *not* administer the drug by rapid IV injection Reduce the dosage or prolong the dosing interval in patients with renal function impairment (e.g., creatinine clearance 80 ml/min or less) A loading dose of 7.5 mg/kg can be used in these patients with subsequent doses and dosing intervals adjusted according to serum level and renal function studies Administer amikacin in compatible IV fluids (e.g., 500 mg/200 ml) by intermittent IV infusion over 30-60 min for each dose Use ideal lean body weight of the patient to calculate the dosage if the actual body weight is greater than the ideal lean body weight	Disposable syringe: 500 mg/2 ml Injectable: 100, 500, 1000 mg/vial The injectable is stable at room temperature Pale yellow coloration of the injectable does not indicate a decrease in potency Do not mix carbenicillin or ticarcillin with amikacin in the same IV bottle or same IV line because of rapid inactivation of amikacin	Amikacin is usually reserved for infections caused by gram-negative bacteria resistant to gentamicin and tobramycin Avoid excessively high peak (i.e., >30 μg/ml) or trough level (i.e., >10 μg/ml); incidence of ototoxicity and nephrotoxicity may increase in the presence of persistently high serum levels of the drug Usual duration of treatment is 7-10 days	Assess for hearing loss Monitor renal function Monitor serum peak (blood sample drawn at 30 to 60 min after the end of an IV infusion or at 60 min after an IM injection) and trough (blood sample drawn just before the next dose) amikacin levels

Drug	Uses	Dosage	How Supplied	Remarks
Gentamicin Apogen Bristagen Cidomycin Garamycin Garamycin Ophthalmic Garamycin Otic Genticin	Serious systemic infections caused by susceptible gram-negative bacteria and *Staphylococcus aureus*; serious urinary tract infections caused by susceptible gram-negative bacteria	*Adults:* 3–5 mg/kg/24 hr IM/IV in 3 divided doses q.8h. *Children:* 5–7.5 mg/kg/24 hr IM/IV in 3 divided doses q.8h. Use ideal lean body weight of the patient to calculate the dosage if the actual body weight is greater than the ideal lean body weight Rotate IM injection sites Usual duration of treatment is 7–10 days	Injectable: 20 (pediatric), 80 mg/vial Disposable syringe: 60, 80 mg Ophthalmic ointment: 3 mg/gm Ophthalmic solution: 0.3% Topical cream: 0.1% Topical ointment: 0.1% The injectable is stable at room temperature Do *not* mix carbenicillin or ticarcillin with gentamicin in the same IV bottle or same IV line because of rapid inactivation of gentamicin	Gentamicin and ampicillin in combination is effective against endocarditis caused by group D *Streptococcus* resistant to penicillin and streptomycin combination Avoid excessively high peak (i.e., >10 µg/ml) or trough level (i.e., >2 µg/ml); incidence of ototoxicity and nephrotoxicity may increase in the presence of persistently high serum peak and trough levels of the aminoglycoside and when therapy is continued for longer than 10 days Gentamicin is usually combined with carbenicillin or ticarcillin in the treatment of serious infections caused by *Pseudomonas aeruginosa* Widespread topical use of gentamicin may lead to development of resistant bacteria Monitor renal function Observe for signs of hearing loss Monitor serum peak (blood sample drawn at 30–60 min after the end of an IV infusion or at 60 min after the IM injection) and trough (blood sample drawn just before the next dose) gentamicin levels
	Uncomplicated lower urinary tract infections caused by susceptible gram-negative bacteria	*Adults:* 2 mg/kg/24 hr IM/IV in 1–2 divided doses q.12–24 h. (in patients with normal renal function) Do *not* administer the drug by rapid IV injection Administer gentamicin in compatible IV fluids (diluted to 1 mg/ml) by intermittent IV infusion over 30–60 min for each dose Reduce the dosage or prolong the dosing interval in patients with renal function impairment (e.g., creatinine clearance 80 ml/min or less); a loading dose of 1.5–1.7 mg/kg can be used in these patients with subsequent doses and dosing interval adjusted according to serum level and renal function studies		
	Infections of the eye caused by susceptible bacteria	Ophthalmic solution: apply 1 or 2 drops into the affected eye or eyes q.1–4h. Ophthalmic ointment: place small amount of the ointment in the lower conjunctival sac b.i.d. to t.i.d.		
	Skin infections caused by susceptible bacteria	Cream or ointment: apply to affected area t.i.d. to q.i.d.		

NOTE: For additional details regarding the individual agents listed in this table, see the text and other tables in this chapter.

*Indicates a multiple active ingredient product. For a complete listing of all active ingredients see the *Drug Reference Guide to Brand Names and Active Ingredients*.

★ Indicates that the drug is generally available only in the United States.

Continued.

NURSING DRUG DIGEST—cont'd

Medication (trade name)	Indication	Usual dosage and administration	Dosage forms, preparation, and storage	Contraindications, cautions, and comments	Monitoring
Kanamycin Anamid Kanabristol Kanacidin Kantrex Klebcil	Serious systemic infections caused by susceptible gramnegative bacteria and *Staphylococcus aureus*	*Adults:* 15 mg/kg/24 hr IM/IV in 2-3 divided doses q.8-12h. *Children:* 15 mg/kg/24 hr IM/IV in 2-3 divided doses q.8-12h. Total adult parenteral dose should *not* exceed 1.5 gm daily Use ideal lean body weight of the patient to calculate the dosage if the actual body weight is greater than the ideal lean body weight Inject IM deeply into upper outer quadrant of the gluteal muscle The IM route of administration is preferred, and the IV route should only be used when the IM route is not possible Do *not* administer the drug by rapid IV injection Administer kanamycin in compatible IV fluids (e.g., NS or D₅W 500 mg/200 ml) by IV infusion over 30-60 min for each dose	Injectable: 75, 500 mg; 1000 mg/vial Capsule: 500 mg Some vials may darken during storage, but this does not indicate a loss of potency The injectable is stable at room temperature	Oral use is *contraindicated* in bowel obstruction and is ineffective in the treatment of systemic infection; oral use can produce nausea and vomiting Antimicrobial spectrum of kanamycin is similar to that of gentamicin and tobramycin but it is not active against *Pseudomonas*; hence its parenteral use has decreased Although kanamycin and other aminoglycosides, given orally, are not absorbed well, a significant amount of the drug can still accumulate in patients with poor renal function to produce toxic effects Avoid excessively high peak (i.e., >30 µg/ml) and or trough levels (i.e., >10 µg/ml); incidence of ototoxicity and nephrotoxicity may increase in the presence of high serum peak and trough levels of the aminoglycoside Usual duration of treatment is 7-10 days	Monitor for renal function Assess for hearing loss Monitor kanamycin serum peak (blood sample drawn at 30-60 min after the end of an IV infusion or at 60 min after an IM injection) and trough (blood sample drawn just before the next dose) kanamycin levels
	Uncomplicated lower urinary tract infections caused by susceptible gramnegative bacteria	*Adults:* 500 mg/24 hr IM/IV in 1-2 doses q.12-24h.			
	Adjunctive treatment in hepatic encephalopathy	*Adults:* 8-12 gm/24 hr PO in divided doses			
	Peritonitis and peritoneal contamination resulting from surgery	*Adults:* 500 mg in 20 ml sterile water for injection instilled through a catheter sutured into the wound at closure			
	Preoperative bowel sterilization	*Adults:* 1 gm PO q.h. for 4 doses then q.4h. for 4 doses or 1 gm PO q.h. for 4 doses then q.6h. for 6-12 doses			

Drug	Use	Dosage	Preparations	Nursing considerations
	Wound irrigation	Children: 50 mg/kg/24 hr PO in 4 divided doses q.6h. Up to 2.5 mg/ml in normal saline irrigation solution Rotate IM injection sites Reduce the dosage or prolong the dosing interval in patients with renal function impairment (e.g., creatinine clearance 80 ml/min or less); a loading dose of 7.5 mg/kg can be used in these patients with subsequent doses and dosing interval adjusted according to serum level and renal function studies		
Neomycin Clinicydin* Cordran-N* Cortisporin Cream* Cortisporin Ointment* Cortisporin Ointment Maxitrol Mycifradin Myciguent Mycitracin* Mycolog* Neobiotic Neo-Cort-Dome* Neo-Cortef* Neo-Delta-Cortef* Neo-Deltef* Neo-Hytone* Neo-Polycin* Neobiotic Neocin Neosone Neosporin Neotal NeoDecadron* Otic Neo-Cort-Dome* Otocort Ear Drops* Spectrocin	Adjunctive treatment of hepatic encephalopathy Preoperative bowel sterilization Infectious diarrhea caused by enteropathogenic E. coli Eye infections caused by susceptible bacteria Prophylaxis and treatment of skin infections caused by susceptible bacteria	Adults: 4-12 gm/24 hr PO in 4 divided doses q.6h.; or 200 ml of 1% solution or 100 ml 2% solution as an enema retained for 20-60 min q.6h. Adults: 1 gm PO q.h. for 4 doses, then 1 gm q.4h. for 5 doses Children: 50-100 mg/kg/24 hr PO in 4-6 doses q.4-6h. First dose should be preceded by a saline cathartic Adults: 50 mg/kg/24 hr PO in 4 divided doses q.6h. for 2-3 days Children: 50-100 mg/kg/24 hr PO in 4 divided doses q.6h. for 2-3 days Opthalmic ointment: apply to affected eye or eyes q.d. to t.i.d. Cream and ointment: apply topically to the cleansed affected area q.d. to t.i.d. NOTE: A parenteral dosage form of neomycin is available but should not be used because parenteral neomycin is more ototoxic and nephrotoxic	Injectable: 500 mg/vial Cream: 5 mg/gm Ointment: 5 mg/gm Ophthalmic ointment: 5 mg/gm Tablet: 500 mg Liquid: 125 mg/5 ml	Oral use is contraindicated in bowel obstruction and is ineffective in the treatment of systemic infections Although neomycin and other aminoglycosides, given orally, are not absorbed well, a significant amount of the drug can still accumulate in patients with poor renal function to produce toxic effects PO neomycin may produce a mild laxative effect Observe for allergic dermatitis when neomycin is used topically because it is highly sensitizing Observe for diarrhea and superinfection when neomycin is used orally Monitor renal function

Continued.

NURSING DRUG DIGEST—cont'd

Medication (trade name*)	Indication	Usual dosage and administration	Dosage forms, preparation, and storage	Contraindications, cautions, and comments	Monitoring
Netilmicin Netromycin	Serious systemic infections caused by susceptible gram-negative bacteria and *Staphylococcus aureus*	*Adults:* 4.5 to 7.5 mg/kg/24 hr IM/IV in divided doses q.8h. *Maximum: Do not exceed 6 mg/kg/24 hr for longer than 48 hr* Do *not* administer the drug by rapid IV injection Rotate IM injection sites Administer netilmicin in compatible IV fluids (e.g., 80 mg/50-100 ml) by intermittent IV infusion over 30-60 min for each dose Use ideal lean body weight of the patient to calculate the dosage if the actual body weight is greater than the ideal lean body weight *Children:* 6 mg/kg/24 hr IM/IV in divided doses q.8h. Reduce the dosage or prolong the dosing interval in patients with renal function impairment A loading dose of 2 to 2.5 mg/kg can be used in these patients with subsequent doses and dosing interval adjusted according to serum level and renal function studies	Injectable: 10, 25, 50, 100 mg/ml May be diluted with NS, D₅W, D₁₀W, sterile water for injection, Ringer's solution, or lactated Ringer's solution Stable for 24 hr at room temperature and 48 hr if refrigerated, at a concentration of 3 mg/ml Do *not* mix carbenicillin or ticarcillin with netilmicin in the same IV bottle or same IV line because of rapid inactivation of netilmicin	The spectrum of activity of netilmicin is similar to that of gentamicin, but it is effective against some strains resistant to gentamicin Netilmicin may be less ototoxic than other aminoglycosides	Assess for hearing loss Monitor renal function Monitor serum peak and trough levels
★ **Paromomycin** Humagel Humatin	Hepatic coma See also Chapter 44, "Anthelmintics"	*Adults:* 4 gm/24 hr in 3 divided doses following meals for 5-6 days	Capsule: 250 mg Syrup: 125 mg/5 ml	*Contraindicated* in severe renal impairment	Observe for signs of overgrowth of nonsusceptible organisms

Drug	Uses	Dosage	Availability/Remarks	Nursing Considerations
Streptomycin Isoject-Streptomycin Strepolin Strycin	Tuberculosis	*Adults:* 20 mg/kg/24 hr up to 1 gm/24 hr IM single dose in combination with one or more antitubercular drugs (e.g., isoniazid, ethambutol, or rifampin) up to 3 mo; ultimately streptomycin should be discontinued or reduced in dosage to 1 gm 2 times a week; the total period of treatment is a minimum of 1 year Rotate IM injection sites	Injectable: 1, 5 gm/vial The injectable is stable at room temperature Exposure to light may cause the solutions to darken, but color change does not necessarily indicate a loss of potency	Avoid contact of streptomycin with skin because drug is irritating; if need to prepare often, wear disposable gloves Other aminoglycosides (e.g., amikacin, gentamicin, and tobramycin) are more effective than streptomycin against gram-negative bacteria Major indications of streptomycin are for treatment of tuberculosis and in combination with penicillin for the treatment of endocarditis caused by *Enterococcus* and *Streptococcus viridans* 25% to 75% of patients receiving 1-2 gm/day for 2-4 mo exhibit some vestibular toxicity Administration during the third trimester of pregnancy may result in fetal hearing impairment Streptomycin causes less renal toxicity than the other aminoglycosides	Monitor renal function Assess for hearing loss (especially in patients being treated for longer than 2 mo)
	Endocarditis caused by alpha and nonhemolytic *Streptococcus*	*Adults:* 2 gm/24 hr IM in 2 divided doses q.12h. for the first week and 1 gm/24 hr IM in 2 divided doses q.12h. for the second week *plus* penicillin concurrently			
	Enterococcal endocarditis	*Adults:* 2 gm/24 hr IM in 2 divided doses q.12h. for first 2 weeks and 1 gm/24 hr IM in 2 divided doses q.12h. for another 4 weeks *plus* penicillin concurrently Do *not* administer IV A smaller daily dose should be used in elderly patients according to age, renal function, and cranial nerve VIII function Administer the drug by deep IM injection because superficial injection may cause pain and sterile abscess Reduce the dosage in patients with renal function impairment (e.g., creatinine clearance 50 ml/min or less); loading dose of 15 mg/kg can be used in these patients with the subsequent doses adjusted according to serum level and renal function studies			

Continued.

NURSING DRUG DIGEST—cont'd

Medication (trade name)	Indication	Usual dosage and administration	Dosage forms, preparation, and storage	Contraindications, cautions, and comments	Monitoring
Tobramycin Nebcin Tobrex	Serious systemic infections caused by susceptible gram-negative bacteria and *Staphylococcus aureus;* serious urinary tract infections caused by susceptible gram-negative bacteria Uncomplicated lower urinary tract infections caused by susceptible gram-negative bacteria	*Adults:* 3-5 mg/kg/24 hr IM/IV in 3 divided doses q.8h. *Children:* 3-5 mg/kg/24 hr IM/IV in 3 divided doses q.8h. Use ideal lean body weight of the patient to calculate dosage if the actual body weight is greater than the ideal lean body weight Usual duration of treatment is 7-10 days *Adults:* 2-2.5 mg/kg/24 hr IM/IV in 1-2 divided doses q.12-24h. Do *not* administer the drug by rapid IV injection Administer tobramycin in compatible IV fluids (e.g., NS or D₅W—80 mg/100 ml) by intermittent IV infusion over 20-60 min for each dose Rotate IM injection sites Use deep IM injections Reduce the dosage or prolong the dosing interval in patients with renal function impairment (e.g., creatinine clearance 80 ml/min or less) A loading dose of 1.5-1.7 mg/kg can be used in these patients with subsequent doses and the dosing interval adjusted according to serum level and renal function studies	Injectable: 10 mg/ml (pediatric) Disposable syringe: 60, 80 mg The injectable is stable at room temperature Do not mix carbenicillin or ticarcillin with tobramycin in the same IV bottle or same IV line because of rapid inactivation of tobramycin	The antibacterial activity of tobramycin is similar to that of gentamicin, but tobramycin is slightly more active against *Pseudomonas aeruginosa* Tobramycin may be less nephrotoxic than gentamicin Avoid excessively high peak (i.e., >10 µg/ml) and or trough levels (i.e., >2 µg/ml); incidence of ototoxicity and nephrotoxicity may increase in the presence of persistently high serum peak and trough levels of the aminoglycoside and when therapy is continued for longer than 10 days Tobramycin is usually combined with carbenicillin or ticarcillin in the treatment of serious infections caused by *Pseudomonas aeruginosa*	Monitor renal function Assess for hearing loss Monitor serum peak (blood sample drawn at 30 to 60 min after the end of an IV infusion or at 60 min after an IM injection) and trough (blood sample drawn just before the next dose) tobramycin levels

BIBLIOGRAPHY

Appel, G.B., & Neu, H.C. Gentamicin 1978. *Annals of Internal Medicine*, 1978, *89*, 528-538.

Barza, M., & Scheife, R.T. Antimicrobial spectrum and therapeutic use of antibiotics. *Journal of the Maine Medical Association*, 1977, *68*, 194-210.

Barza, M., & Scheife, R.T. Antimicrobial spectrum, pharmacology, and therapeutic use of antibiotics. Part 4. Aminoglycosides. In R.R. Miller & D.J. Greenblatt (Eds.). *Drug therapy reviews* (vol. 2.). New York: Elsevier North Holland, Inc., 1979.

Brewer, N.S. The aminoglycosides, streptomycin, kanamycin, gentamicin, tobramycin, amikacin, neomycin. *Mayo Clinic Proceedings*, 1977, *52*, 675-679.

Davies, J. & Courvalin, P. Mechanism of resistance to aminoglycosides. *American Journal of Medicine*, 1977, *62*, 868-872.

Dee, T.H., & Kozin, F. Gentamicin and tobramycin penetration into synovial fluids. *Antimicrobial Agents and Chemotherapy*, 1977, *12*, 548-549.

Dikman, S., Bosch, J., Chung, J., & Kahn, T. Gentamicin and netilmicin nephrotoxicity. *Antimicrobial Agents and Chemotherapy*, 1976, *10*, 827-836.

Fee, W.R. Jr., et al. Clinical evaluation of aminoglycoside toxicity: tobramycin versus gentamicin, a preliminary report. *Journal of Antimicrobial Chemotherapy*, 1978, *4*(Suppl A), 31-36.

Finland, et al. Tobramycin. *Journal of Infectious Diseases*, 1976, *134*(Suppl), S1-S234.

Fu, K.P., & Neu, H.C. In vitro study of netilmicin compared with other aminoglycosides. *Antimicrobial Agents and Chemotherapy*, 1976, *10*, 526-534.

Gill, A.A., & Kern, J.W. Altered gentamicin distribution in ascitic patients. *Amercian Journal of Hospital Pharmacy*, 1979, *36*, 1704-1706.

Holloway, B.W., & Asche, L.V. Mechanisms and clinical implications of antibiotic resistance in bacteria. *Drugs*, 1977, *14*, 283-290.

Hull, J.H., & Sarubbi, F.A. Gentamicin serum concentrations: pharmacokinetic predictions. *Annals of Internal Medicine*, 1976, *85*, 183-189.

Igarastti, M., Levy, J.K., & Jarger, J. Comparative toxicity of netilmicin and gentamicin in squirrel monkeys. *Journal of Infectious Diseases*, *1978*, *137*, 476-480.

Kahlmeter, G., et al. Gentamicin and tobramycin in patients with various infections—nephrotoxicity. *Journal of Antimicrobial Chemotherapy*, 1978, *4*(Suppl A), 47-52.

Lanao, J.M., et al. The influence of ascites on the pharmacokinetics of amikacin. *International Journal of Clinical Pharmacology and Therapeutic Toxicology*, 1980, *18*, 57-61.

Langslet, J., & Habel, M.L. The aminoglycoside antibiotics. *American Journal of Nursing*, 1981, *81*(6), 1144-1146.

Masur, H., Whelton, P.K., & Whelton, A. Neomycin toxicity revisited. *Archives of Surgery*, 1976, *111*, 822-825.

Price, K.E., Defuria, M.D., & Pursiano, T.A. Amikacin, an aminoglycoside with marked activity against antibiotic-resistant clinical isolates. *Journal of Infectious Diseases*, 1976, *134*, S249-261.

Sarubbi, F.A., & Hull, J.H. Amikacin serum concentrations: prediction of levels and dosage guidelines. *Annals of Internal Medicine*, 1978, *89*, 612-618.

Schentag, J.J., Gengo, F.M., Plant, M.E., et al. Urinary casts as an indicator of renal tubular damage in patients receiving aminoglycosides. *Antimicrobial Agents and Chemotherapy*, 1979, *16*, 468-474.

Schentag, J.J., Cumbo, T.J., Jusko, W.J., et al. Gentamicin tissue accumulation and nephrotoxic reactions. *Journal of the American Medical Association*, 1978, *240*, 2067-2069.

Schentag, J.J., Plant, M.E., Centra, F.B., et al. Aminoglycosides nephrotoxicity in critically ill surgical patients. *Journal of Surgical Research*, 1979, *26*, 270-279.

Schentag, J.J., Sutfin, T.A., Plaut, M.E., et al. Early detection of aminoglycoside nephrotoxicity with urinary beta-2-microglobulin. *Journal of Medicine*, 1978, *9*, 201-210.

Schentag, J.J., et al. Comparative tissue accumulation of gentamicin and tobramycin in patients. *Antimicrobial Agents and Chemotherapy*. 1978, *4*(Suppl), 23-30.

Smith, C.R., Maxwell, R.P., Edwards, C.Q., et al. Nephrotoxicity induced by gentamicin and amikacin. *Johns Hopkins Medical Journal*, 1978, *142*, 85-90.

Tobramycin (Symposium). *Journal of Infectious Diseases*, 1976, *134*, 51-234.

Tobramycin—comparative toxicity of aminoglycoside antibiotics (Symposium). *Antimicrobial Agents and Chemotherapy*, 1978, *4*(Suppl A), 1-101.

Weinstein, A.J. McHenry, M.C., & Gavan T.L. Systemic absorption of neomycin irrigating solution. *Journal of the American Medical Association*, 1977, *338*, 152.

Wendell, H., et al. Penetration of tobramycin into infected extravascular fluids and its therapeutic effectiveness. *Journal of Infectious Diseases*, 1977, *135*, 957-961.

Tetracyclines

Gerald R. Greene

Medications discussed in this chapter

Tetracyclines
  Chlortetracycline
  Demeclocycline
  Doxycycline
  Methacycline

Tetracyclines—cont'd
  Minocycline
  Oxytetracycline
  Tetracycline

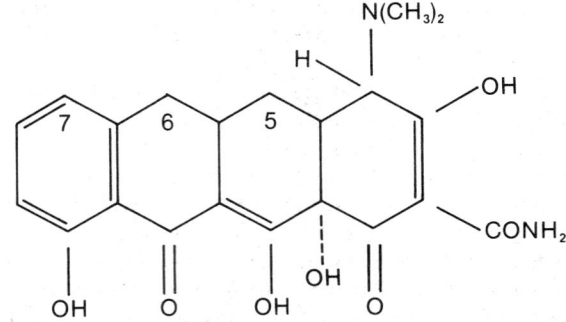

FIGURE 47-1. **General chemical structure of the tetracyclines. Substitutions at positions 5, 6, and 7 determine specific drug.**

The tetracyclines are a closely related group of broad-spectrum antibiotics with a core compound composed of four benzene rings aligned side by side. Substitutions at the 5, 6, and 7 positions create the different analogs, but more extensive chemical changes cause the compound to lose its antibiotic properties (Figure 47-1). Chlortetracycline was introduced by Duggar in 1948 and was the first truly broad-spectrum antibiotic. This first tetracycline was a metabolic byproduct of the fungus *Streptomyces aureofaciens* and was named aureomycin. Two years later, oxytetracycline became available. Tetracycline, introduced in 1952, was created initially by chemically removing one of the chemical radicals from chlortetracycline. Other tetracyclines available in the United States include demeclocycline and methacycline. More recent tetracyclines, doxycycline and minocycline, have a slightly different pharmacology and a broader antimicrobial spectra than the older members of the family.

The tetracyclines are bacteriostatic, and increasing numbers of organisms have become resistant over the years. The tetracyclines are used for treating both human and animal infections and as additives to animal feeds. They may also be used prophylactically in certain situations. In general they are well tolerated; however, because of adverse affects on growing bones and teeth, tetracyclines should *not* be used by children younger than 8 years of age or by pregnant women except in special circumstances.

MECHANISM OF ACTION

The tetracyclines act within microorganisms by blocking the attachment of *transfer-RNA* to ribosomes where essential proteins are made. The organism ceases active metabolism because of a lack of functional essential proteins. The exact mechanism of action of the tetracyclines at the ribosomal level to inhibit or alter protein synthesis is not known. A number of theories have been proposed, none of which have been fully validated. At higher doses the tetracyclines may also damage the cell membrane, causing a loss of vital intracellular components. The tetracyclines can exhibit an *antianabolic* effect on mammalian cells at high doses and may diminish the effect of parenteral nutrition. In vitro studies have shown that the tetracyclines are bacteriostatic (i.e., they inhibit the microorganism's metabolism and reproduction, but in fact do not kill it). There is a resumption of vital activities when the tetracycline is no longer available in effective concentration. Clinically, the tetracyclines have the same effect as bactericidal antibiotics, but they probably should be avoided in situations where the patient is immunosuppressed.

ANTIMICROBIAL SPECTRUM

The tetracyclines act against a broad range of infectious agents. These include aerobic and anaerobic bacteria (e.g., *Mycoplasma, Chlamydia, Spirochetes, Rickettsia*) and some *protozoa*. The tetracyclines are, in general, effective against gram-positive cocci; however, some streptococci, pneumococci, and up to 50% of staphylococci may be resistant. Resistance varies with geographic location. Minocycline may be somewhat more effective, but antibiotics other than tetracycline should be used to treat staphyloccocal infections. The tetracyclines act against a number of gram-negative enteric bacteria such as *E. coli*; however, *pseudomonas* is almost always resistant. The tetracyclines are the drugs of choice in some unusual bacterial infections including plague, brucellosis, tularemia, and rat bite fever. They are effective against most strains of *gonococcus*. Tetracyclines have activity against some anaerobic bacteria. *Bacteroides fragilis* is resistant to all tetracyclines except, occasionally, doxycycline.

Tetracyclines are the antibiotics of choice for treating rickettsial infections such as Rocky Mountain spotted fever, Q fever, and typhus. Chloramphenicol is an alternative drug in rickettsial infections. The tetracyclines are also used to treat chlamydial infections such as psittacosis, genitourinary infections, and trachoma. *Mycoplasma*, which causes atypical pneumonia and genitourinary infections, is susceptible to the tetracyclines. Most of the microorganisms that cause pelvic inflammatory disease in women are susceptible to the tetracyclines. The tetracyclines are effective against the causative agents of most venereal diseases. They are *not* indicated for pneumococcal and streptococcal infections or those caused by *opportunistic* organisms acquired in the hospital.

BACTERIAL RESISTANCE

The exact mechanism by which bacteria become resistant to the tetracyclines is not known. Both *plasmid* and chromosomal mediated resistance has been documented. A number of plasmids that transmit tetracycline resistance have been specifically identified. It is theoretically possible for bacteria to become resistant during therapy, but this is infrequently observed. Some resistant strains demonstrate a decreased accumulation of the drug intracellularly. In other resistant bacteria the tetracyclines are prevented from binding to the bacterial cell membrane, which is necessary before the drug can enter the organism. Still other organisms can cause an increased excretion of tetracycline out of the cell. Resistance to the tetracyclines varies by geographic location and is related, in part, to their use. This suggests that resistant strains can be selected or induced by the excessive use of the tetracyclines.

There is concern that the tetracyclines used in animal feeds as growth promoters can lead to the induction of tetracycline-resistant bacterial flora, which may subsequently infect man. Some ranch hands caring for animals fed tetracycline-containing feeds become colonized with tetracycline-resistant bacterial strains. The controversy surrounding the use of tetracyclines in animal feeds has not been resolved.

PHARMACOKINETICS

The tetracyclines are primarily prescribed for oral use; however, parenteral dosage forms are available for serious infections. Tetracyclines are absorbed well from the gastrointestinal tract after oral administration; however, food and milk will decrease absorption. Divalant and trivalant cations such as calcium and iron bind tetracyclines and prevent absorption. Aluminum- and magnesium-containing antacids will also inhibit tetracycline absorption. The hydrochloride salts are more soluble and thus are better absorbed from the gastrointestinal tract than the parent compounds. Doxycycline and minocycline are absorbed to a greater extent and can be administered with meals. Food may diminish gastrointestinal discomfort accompanying the administration of these newer tetracyclines. After oral administration, peak serum levels of the tetracyclines range from 1 to 4 µg/ml of serum and are achieved 1 to 3 hours after administration. The serum half-life of tetracycline is approximately 8½ hours, and that of doxycycline and minocycline is 18 to 20 hours. Thus, tetracycline and other earlier compounds are administered every 8 hours, whereas minocycline and doxycycline can be given every 12 hours. In some instances doxycycline can be administered in a once-daily dosage regimen.

Although tetracycline is available for intravenous use, it is generally not administered by this route because of thrombophlebitis and hepatotoxicity accompanying intravenous tetracycline use. The intravenous route is used in life-threatening infections or when the patient cannot take oral medication. Doxycycline serum levels are comparable following intravenous and oral administration.

Tissue penetration by the tetracyclines is directly related to their lipid solubility. Tetracycline is the least lipid soluble, with doxycycline 5 times more soluble than tetracycline. Minocycline is 5 times more lipid soluble than doxycycline. Thus minocycline has the best tissue penetration of the tetracyclines. Minocycline is the only tetracycline that is excreted by the salivary glands. Doxycycline and minocycline achieve high tissue levels in the female reproductive organs, in the lung and bronchial wall, and in the kidney and prostate. Minocycline achieves the highest level in cerebrospinal fluid, which is approximately 30% of the serum level.

The tetracyclines are primarily excreted in unchanged form by the kidneys, and the dosage should be reduced or other antibiotics used in patients with renal impairment. Doxycycline does not accumulate in renal failure. To a lesser extent, the tetracyclines are also eliminated in the feces. With the exception of doxycycline, most of the tetracyclines are metabolized to some extent in the liver and excreted in the bile. Doxycycline is also excreted through the bowel wall, and in renal failure most of the drug may be excreted by this route. Hemodialysis may remove 20% to 30% of the tetracycline in the serum; however, peritoneal dialysis has no effect on tetracycline serum levels. Doxycycline and minocycline are not affected by dialysis.

TOXICITY AND SIDE EFFECTS
Gastrointestinal system

The tetracyclines can cause minor gastrointestinal disturbances such as heartburn, nausea, and vomiting, possibly because of an irritant effect on the stomach. Taking minocycline or doxycycline with food may alleviate gastrointestinal discomfort. The tetracyclines may affect normal bowel flora. Diarrhea occasionally occurs and is probably the result of an overgrowth of nonsusceptible organisms after a loss of normal colonic flora, or as the result of a direct irritant effect of the tetracycline. Doxycycline usually does not cause diarrhea. Rarely there may be an overgrowth of *Candida* organisms or staphylococci causing severe colonic infections, particularly in debilitated patients. Antibiotic-associated *pseudomembranous colitis* is also rarely associated with tetracycline use.

Teeth and bones

The tetracyclines have been shown to affect the development of chicken embryos. Although teratogenicity has not been proven for the human fetus, the use of tetracyclines in pregnancy is usually avoided. Tetracyclines slow bone growth in human infants, but there is catch-up growth once the medication is discontinued. The tetracyclines stain and damage (hypoplasia) developing teeth, in direct proportion to the amount used during childhood. Tetracycline forms fluorescent compounds in the teeth and bones that can be demonstrated by ultraviolet light. Adverse effects on teeth and on bones usually contraindicate the use of tetracyclines in children younger than 8 years of age. However, there are still large quantities of the tetracyclines manufactured in pediatric dosage forms and sold in the United States each year. Doxycycline may bind less to teeth than the other tetracyclines.

Toxicity in renal failure

The tetracyclines, except for doxycycline, accumulate in renal failure. This may lead to further renal damage. Accumulation of the tetracyclines may also cause fatty degeneration of the liver leading to hepatic failure. Antianabolic effects may be enhanced in renal failure. Accumulation of minocycline in renal failure may enhance its ototoxicity. The tetracyclines are ordinarily avoided in patients with renal failure or if they must be used, serum levels should be followed carefully.

Renal toxicity

Nephrogenic diabetes insipidus has been reported with the use of demeclocycline, and acute interstitial nephritis (AIN) has rarely been induced by minocycline.

Hepatic toxicity

Excessive doses of the tetracyclines by either the oral or parenteral route can cause hepatic damage. There is an increased incidence of hepatic toxicity when the tetracyclines are administered during pregnancy or to patients in shock or who have renal failure. The pathologic changes include fatty infiltration and hepatocellular degeneration.

Allergic reactions

Allergic reactions such as urticaria and angioneurotic edema have occasionally been reported with the tetracyclines. Anaphylactic reactions to these medications are rare.

Other toxicities

Outdated tetracycline has been associated with the development of Fanconi's syndrome, in which there is damage to the renal tubules with a loss of vital serum constituents into the urine. Photosensitive rashes with erythema and blistering have occurred with tetracycline use, particularly with demeclocycline. The tetracyclines have been associated with the pseudotumor cerebri syndrome, in which there are signs and symptoms of increased intracranial pressure, including bulging fontanel in infants, severe headaches, lethargy, papilledema, and photophobia. These symptoms resolve on discontinuation of the medication. Minocycline causes vertigo and nausea in recipients, which is a troublesome side effect. This has been reported in up to 90% of patients receiving minocycline; however, on the average, approximately 50% to 60% of patients will suffer some dizziness when given this medication.

CLINICAL USE

Respiratory infections

The tetracyclines are used for the ambulatory treatment of respiratory tract infections in adults, particularly for recurrent bronchitis. This condition is ordinarily caused by unencapsulated *Haemophilus influenzae* bacteria. The year-round or seasonal prophylactic use of the tetracyclines may be appropriate for patients with chronic bronchitis. The tetracyclines may be used to treat pneumonia because they are effective against organisms (e.g. *Mycoplasma*) that cause ambulatory or atypical pneumonia. They have an activity against the agent of Legionnaire's disease, but erythromycin would be used if Legionnaire pneumonia was documented. They are not ordinarily used for exudative pharyngitis because group A streptococci may be resistant. Penicillin or erythromycin should be used in known pneumococcal infections because these organisms can also be resistant to tetracycline. Although minocycline achieves high levels in the sputum, the long-term use of this drug would be precluded by its side effects of dizziness and nausea.

Genitourinary infections

The tetracyclines may be used occasionally for urinary tract infections caused by susceptible organisms, and might be effective against organisms found resistant in the laboratory because of the high levels that occur in the urine. The tetracyclines are particularly useful for treating pelvic inflammatory diseases in women. This condition may be caused by gonorrhea, *Chlamydia*, or anaerobic bacteria, all of which are usually susceptible. Prostatitis is usually amenable to therapy with tetracyclines. Tetracycline is also effective in nongonococcal urethritis caused by *Ureaplasma* organisms. Other venereal diseases such as syphilis, chancroid, and lymphogranuloma venereum respond to tetracycline therapy but may require 2 weeks or more of medication. The tetracyclines are usually effective in treating gonorrhea; however, penicillin-resistant strains may not respond to the tetracyclines clinically.

Gastrointestinal infections

The tetracyclines have been shown to diminish the symptoms and shorten the course of cholera. The tet-

racyclines can also be used to treat shigellosis; however, this is ordinarily a self-limited infection. The tetracyclines had been used prophylactically before gastrointestinal surgery to prevent postoperative infections. Other antibiotics are currently used for this purpose. Doxycycline taken once daily, has been shown in controlled trials to be effective in reducing the incidence of traveler's diarrhea in Peace Corps volunteers in Kenya. Doxycycline-resistant strains of enteropathogenic *E. coli*, which is the primary cause of traveler's diarrhea, have been identified in the Far East and in Southeast Asia.

Rickettsial infections

The tetracyclines are the drugs of choice for infections caused by rickettsia. These include typhus (all types), Rocky Mountain spotted fever, and rickettsial pox. The tetracyclines are used to treat Q fever, which is caused by the rickettsia *Coxsiella burnetti*, and will ameliorate, but not ordinarily cure, Q fever endocarditis. Chloramphenicol is also used for rickettsial infections and might be the drug of choice if the patient has renal or hepatic impairment.

Chlamydial infections

The tetracyclines are effective against chlamydial infections such as psitticosis, pneumonia caused by the organism *Chlamydia psittaci*, acquired from birds. Trachoma is a recurrent chlamydial eye infection that is the most common cause of blindness in the world. Trachoma responds to topical tetracycline use. The tetracyclines are also effective in chlamydial genitourinary tract infections such as lymphogranuloma venereum and pelvic inflammatory disease.

Acne

Administered once or twice daily, tetracycline is often effective in treating moderately severe to severe acne. Most patients with acne will show an improvement when taking tetracycline. Tetracycline prescribed in this fashion may be administered for months or years. Because of unproved but possible teratogenic effects, young women taking tetracycline for acne should be warned that the medication may be a danger to the fetus should they become pregnant.

Brucellosis

The tetracyclines are usually administered with streptomycin in the treatment of brucellosis, which is a severe systemic infection caused by organisms usually acquired from animals or from unpasteurized dairy products. Antibiotics are administered 2 to 3 weeks for this infection, and there may be relapses that require further treatment.

Other infections

The tetracyclines are the drugs of first choice in treating unusual but potentially severe bacterial infections, including plague, tularemia, relapsing fever, rat bite fever, and melioidosis. The tetracyclines, in combination with other medications, are effective against chloroquine-resistant falciparum malaria. Minocycline has been shown in controlled trials to eradicate the meningococcal carriage in the upper respiratory tract and was recommended for individuals who had close contact with patients who had meningococcal infections. However, because of the vertigo that accompanies minocycline use, rifampin is now the drug of choice for prophylaxis in this situation.

The tetracyclines should not be used when bacteriostatic antibiotics may result in a disadvantage to the patient. This includes patients who are immunosuppressed as a consequence of a medication or an underlying illness. Infections, such as endocarditis, which are life-threatening and occur in poorly circulated areas of the body, ordinarily will not respond to bacteriostatic antibiotics. Q fever endocarditis is the *only* exception. Infections caused by enteric bacteria, especially those occurring in patients already hospitalized, will probably not respond to the tetracyclines. These organisms include *Pseudomonas*, *Serratia*, and *Klebsiella*. Tetracycline should not be used for known staphylococcal infections because in some areas more than 50% of *Staphylococcus aureus* have been shown to be resistant to the tetracyclines. Central nervous system infections are usually not treated with the tetracyclines.

SUMMARY

The tetracyclines are a group of antibiotics that are closely related chemically and in antimicrobial spectra. They are useful against a wide variety of infectious organisms. Because of their adverse effects on the bones and teeth, the tetracyclines are *not* recommended for children younger than 8 years of age, or for pregnant women, except in special circumstances. The most common side effects of the tetracyclines are mild gastrointestinal disturbances. There may occasionally be diarrhea caused by a pathogen overgrowth. The tetracyclines other than doxycycline may exacerbate renal failure or cause hepatotoxicity in patients with renal impairment. Hepatotoxicity may also be seen when the tetracyclines are used during pregnancy, or for patients in shock. Doxycycline and minocycline have better tissue penetration and longer half-lives than the older compounds. Most use of tetracycline is via the oral route. Tetracycline resistance is generally related to tetracycline use in a given locale and may thus differ from one clinical practice site to another.

ADVERSE/SIDE EFFECTS OF THE TETRACYCLINES*

ALLERGIC REACTIONS

Anaphylaxis (rare)
Rash
Urticaria

CUTANEOUS SYSTEM

Photosensitivity (demeclocycline)

GASTROINTESTINAL SYSTEM

Candidal or staphylococcal colitis
   (rare)
Nausea and vomiting
Overgrowth diarrhea
Pseudomembranous colitis (rare)

RENAL SYSTEM

Fanconi's syndrome (rare; outdated
   tetracycline)
Interstitial nephritis (rare;
   minocycline)
Nephrogenic diabetes insipidus (rare;
   demeclocycline)
Worsening of renal failure

HEPATIC SYSTEM

Hepatic fatty degeneration (when
   used in renal failure, during
   pregnancy, or in shock; from
   overdose)
Jaundice (rare)

TEETH AND BONES

Slowing of bone growth in infants
   (reversible)
Staining of teeth in children
Tooth hypoplasia in children

MISCELLANEOUS EFFECTS

Phlebitis associated with IV use
Pseudotumor cerebri
Vertigo (vestibular; minocycline)

---

*See Chapter 11, "Drug Toxicity," for an overview of drug toxicity.

CLINICALLY SIGNIFICANT DRUG INTERACTIONS*

Primary drug	Interacting drug	Possible effect(s)	Probable mechanism(s)
Tetracyclines	Antacids containing calcium, aluminum, or magnesium	Decreased effectiveness of tetracyclines	Divalent and trivalent cations (e.g., calcium, aluminum, magnesium) bind tetracyclines in the GI tract, thus decreasing absorption
Tetracyclines	Iron salts	Decreased effectiveness of tetracyclines	Bind tetracyclines in the GI tract, thus decreasing absorption
Tetracyclines	Methoxyflurane	Increased nephrotoxicity	Not established
Tetracyclines	Penicillins	Decreased effectiveness of penicillins	Tetracyclines interfere with bactericidal activity of penicillins

*See Chapter 10, "Drug Interactions," for an overview of drug interactions.

GENERAL NURSING IMPLICATIONS

Nursing of patients requiring tetracyclines

ASSESSMENT

The tetracyclines are used to treat various infections caused by gram-positive and gram-negative bacteria, rickettsiae, and other organisms. They are also used to treat chronic bronchitis and acne vulgaris. Baseline data should include specific information about the patient's general condition and health state.

Assessment should be completed carefully so that changes in the patient's condition can be identified readily. Tetracylines are bacteriostatic antibiotics with a broad spectrum of activity. Because of widespread bacterial resistance and because of their bacteriostatic nature, however, their use is generally limited to mixed respiratory infections, various sexually transmitted diseases, and certain specific infections (e.g., bubonic plague, Rocky Mountain spotted fever). See the Nursing Drug Digest for specific conditions treated with individual agents. Whenever possible, the organism responsible for the infection should be identified *before* drug therapy is initiated. Sensitivity tests are essential in the use of tetracyclines because many strains of bacteria have been found to be resistant to the tetracyclines. Culture and sensitivity

studies are recommended to determine the susceptibility of the infecting organisms to the tetracyclines. It is important to carefully collect specimens (e.g., blood, sputum, urine, wound drainage) according to hospital or agency procedures. These data should serve not only in drug selection, but also in monitoring therapeutic response to drug therapy.

Assessment should include detailed information regarding the patient's general health state, as well as renal and hepatic function. The presence of symptoms indicating infection, such as elevated temperature, chills, redness or pain in an area not previously affected, fatigue, anorexia, change in wound or sputum character, elevated white blood cell count, or other observations related to the specific condition being treated should be assessed.

It is also important to determine that female patients are not pregnant before administering tetracyclines.

Isolation measures should be readily implemented as indicated to prevent the spread of the infection to others.

Assessment should also include a detailed drug history to identify a possible

sensitivity to tetracyclines, contraindications, cautions, drug interactions, and individual drug-taking patterns before therapy is initiated.

SENSITIVITY

Hypersensitivity to the tetracyclines does *not* occur to as great an extent as occurs with the penicillins. Patients with a prior history of allergies or asthma appear to be at a higher risk for developing a sensitivity to the tetracyclines. It must be noted, however, that any drug has the potential to cause a hypersensitivity reaction in a susceptible individual. It should also be noted that cross-sensitivity between the various tetracyclines occurs commonly.

CONTRAINDICATIONS

Tetracyclines are contraindicated in patients with a known hypersensitivity to any of the tetracyclines. Tetracyclines are also contraindicated in the following cases: pregnancy or during lactation, unless the potential benefit to the patient outweighs the risk to the fetus or the nursing infant; serious infections (e.g., bacterial endocarditis) in which a bactericidal antibiotic is essential; and severe renal or hepatic impairment.   *Continued.*

Nursing of patients requiring tetracyclines—cont'd

CAUTIONS

Administration of the tetracyclines during the second and third trimester of pregnancy or to children younger than 8 years of age may cause permanent tooth discoloration. It may also inhibit bone growth.

Dosage must generally be reduced in renal impairment (see the Nursing Drug Digest).

Photosensitivity reactions may occur in patients receiving tetracyclines. Such patients should be advised to avoid prolonged exposure to the sun by wearing protective clothing and using chemical sunscreen agents.

Tetracyclines should be used cautiously in patients who are malnourished or debilitated because of their potential antianabolic effect, particularly at high doses.

DRUG INTERACTIONS

Tetracyclines have the potential to interact with a variety of drugs in various mechanisms.

Divalent and trivalent cations (e.g., calcium, iron, magnesium) can bind with orally administered tetracyclines (except for doxycycline) and can thus significantly decrease their gastric absorption.

Bacteriostatic antibiotics (e.g., tetracyclines) can interfere with the action of bactericidal agents (e.g., penicillins). See Clinically Significant Drug Interactions for other clinically significant drug interactions involving tetracyclines.

ADMINISTRATION

Tetracyclines are available in various dosage forms for oral, parenteral, and topical administration. The dosage should be reduced in the presence of renal failure for all of the tetracyclines except for doxycycline and minocycline. These two tetracyclines are metabolized in the liver and generally do not have their half-lives of elimination significantly increased by renal failure; however, blood levels should be monitored in severe renal failure and the dosage modified as necessary.

Always check expiration dates, and never administer any outdated medications. Outdated tetracyclines can cause nephrotoxicity and metabolic acidosis; administration of outdated tetracyclines has resulted in death.

Check that the order for the antibiotic is reviewed at appropriate intervals by the prescriber.

Oral administration

Tetracyclines are usually absorbed well after oral administration. They should be taken with a full glass of water on an empty stomach, 1 hour before or 2 hours after meals. Food and milk, as well as aluminum-, magnesium-, and calcium-containing antacids will decrease their absorption and these should generally not be given concurrently. Iron salts should also be avoided. Bedtime doses should be taken at least 1 hour before retiring to prevent esophagitis.

If nausea, diarrhea, or anorexia is caused by the oral form of tetracycline, the medication can be administered with food (not milk or dairy products) or the dosage may need to be decreased. If these effects persist, the discontinuation of the drug is recommended.

Parenteral administration

Parenterally administered tetracyclines have been associated with severe liver damage, particularly when administered to patients with impaired renal function.

Intramuscular administration

Intramuscular administration of tetracyclines commonly results in pain and irritation at the injection site. Absorption from the intramuscular route is poor and erratic. Thus, the intramuscular route is generally *not* recommended. When this route is used, a preparation containing a local anesthetic is generally better tolerated by the patient. It is important to check for a hypersensitivity to the local anesthetic before the injection. An ice pack placed on the site may also relieve the discomfort. All injections should be made in healthy large muscles. An air-lock or Z-track technique should be used to prevent any leakage of the medication into the subcutaneous fat, which can result in local irritation. If it occurs, the irritation can be relieved with an ice pack.

Intravenous administration

Intravenous administration, as well as intramuscular administration is used when the patient cannot take the medication orally. However, doxycycline and minocycline are usually administered intravenously for life-threatening or serious infections. Tetracyclines should be carefully reconstituted and infused as recommended (see the Nursing Drug Digest for specific information regarding each agent). Tetracyclines should be diluted well to decrease the irritation to the veins and the resulting phlebitis, and administered slowly at a rate not exceeding 20 mg/min preferably over ½ to 1 hour.

Avoid calcium-containing solutions, and protect the infusion from sunlight.

Because tetracyclines are irritating when administered intravenously, monitor the infusion site for local irritation and thrombophlebitis. These adverse effects can be minimized by using dilute solutions of the drug and by avoiding extravasation into surrounding tissues.

MONITORING PATIENT RESPONSE
Therapeutic response

The onset and duration of antibiotic therapy depend on the dosage form, route of administration, individual patient factors, and the severity of the infection being treated. Monitoring the patient's therapeutic response in relation to an improvement in the condition being treated must be done carefully. In addition, bacterial resistance must also be monitored.

Adverse side effects

Major adverse side effects associated with the use of tetracyclines are outlined in Adverse/Side Effects of the Tetracyclines. Generally, monitor for the overgrowth of nonsusceptible organisms, and plan to minimize or prevent this effect. Meticulous oral care and frequent perineal care, especially after bowel movements, is helpful in preventing the overgrowth of nonsusceptible organisms. Patients should be questioned regarding any unusual vaginal discharge or itching, as well as the occurrence of a black, furry tongue. Patients should be aware of these possible effects and report these symptoms immediately so that appropriate treatment for these effects can be implemented.

Gastrointestinal side effects, including nausea and diarrhea are also common following the oral administration of tetracyclines. It is important to differentiate between diarrhea as a direct side effect of the tetracycline or as a result of the overgrowth of nonsusceptible organisms. Cultures and sensitivity tests must be performed to make this differentiation.

Nursing of patients requiring tetracyclines—cont'd

Adverse side effects—cont'd

Because tetracyclines can cause decreased renal function, it is imperative that renal function be monitored, including intake and output. Oliguria should be readily reported. Because of potential renal adverse side effects of the tetracyclines, their use in treating renal infections, even though indicated on the basis of cultures and sensitivity tests, is *not* recommended.

PATIENT EDUCATION

The patient and the family, as indicated, should have a clear understanding of the medication regimen, including the exact name of the medication, its general action, purpose, dosage, storage, administration, adverse side effects, and how these effects can be minimized or prevented. This is particularly important for patients who will be discharged with the medication. They should know how to monitor the expected therapeutic response and to recognize that the medication should be continued even after they are feeling better, up to 72 hours after their temperature has returned to normal or other effects indicate the therapeutic response has occurred. Patients requiring the tetracyclines for a prolonged period (e.g., for treating acne) need to understand clearly their specific medication regimen. Patients should be able to recognize when the health care provider should be notified. They should also recognize the importance of not taking outdated medication, and they should know how to dispose of unused medication. Patient education must be individualized, and the nurse's role in this area cannot be overemphasized (see General Instructions for Discharge/Outpatients for points for discharged outpatient instructions).

GENERAL INSTRUCTIONS FOR DISCHARGE/OUTPATIENTS

TETRACYCLINES

This medication is an antibiotic used to treat or prevent infections. If you do not understand why you require this medication, ask your health care provider.

With the exception of minocycline and doxycycline, tetracyclines should not be taken with food. They work best if taken with a full glass of water on an empty stomach 1 hour before or 2 hours after meals.

Tetracyclines should not be taken with milk or other dairy products, including cheese, cottage cheese, or ice cream, or with antacids or iron preparations because these can prevent the medication from being absorbed.

Take this medication exactly as directed. Follow the instructions on the prescription exactly. If you have any questions contact your health care provider.

Continue to take this medication as directed until the prescription is finished, even though you may be feeling better. If you do not take the full treatment as prescribed, your infection may return.

If you are taking the liquid form of this medication, shake it well before pouring each dose. Use an accurate measuring device for measuring each dose.

Some unwanted side effects can occur in some people when they take this medication, such as a mild stomach upset or mild diarrhea. If these occur they can usually be prevented by taking the medication with a cracker or a small snack, and by avoiding dairy products.

Notify your health care provider if you notice diarrhea, vaginal itching or an unusual vaginal discharge, rectal irritation, white patches in the mouth, a black, furry tongue, or severe stomach upset. Your health care provider can help you with these unwanted effects.

Notify your health care provider if you develop a rash, itching, or hives, which can indicate an allergic reaction to this medication.

Some tetracyclines such as demeclocycline can make you more sensitive to sunlight and make you more sensitive to sunburn. If you are taking demeclocycline, avoid prolonged exposure to the sun and wear protective clothing and sunglasses when in the sun. A chemical sunscreen may be used.

Tetracyclines can cause unwanted effects in the fetus if you are pregnant or become pregnant when taking this medication. If you are pregnant or thinking about becoming pregnant, discuss this with your health care provider before taking this medication.

Tetracyclines can be found in breast milk, and can cause unwanted effects in infants who are breast fed. If you are breastfeeding an infant, do not take this medication without first checking with your health care provider.

Do not take any other medications while you are taking this medication without first checking with your health care provider, because tetracyclines can interact with various other medications and cause harmful or unwanted effects.

If you must take iron or vitamins with iron, always take them 3 hours before or 2 hours after taking this drug because they can prevent the tetracyclines from being absorbed.

If you forget to take a dose of this medication, take your dose as soon as you remember you have missed a dose. Then take your medication as prescribed at the same time as before.

Because this medication can cause permanent tooth discoloration in children it should generally not be given to children under 8 years of age.

If you do not require all of this medication or for some reason your health care provider directs you to stop taking the medication, be sure to flush the unused medication down the toilet. Do not save the medication for another condition. Outdated tetracycline can cause harmful toxic effects and should *not* be used.

Store this medication in a dry, dark place. Refrigeration is not necessary.

Keep this and all other medications out of the reach of children.

This medication is prescribed especially for you. Do not share or trade this medication with your family or friends.

NURSING DRUG DIGEST

Medication (trade name*)	Indication	Usual dosage and administration	Dosage forms, preparation, and storage	Contraindications, cautions, and comments	Monitoring
Chlortetracycline Aureomycin Chrysomysin	Skin infections Superficial ophthalmic infections caused by susceptible organisms	*Adults:* Apply to infected area one or more times daily *Children:* Same as adults *Adults:* Apply to infected eye q.2h. as indicated	Ointment: 3% Ophthalmic ointment: 1%		Observe for overgrowth of nonsusceptible organisms
Demeclocycline Declomycin Declostatin* Demeclor Ledermycin Novociclina Tollerclin	Infections caused by susceptible bacteria (*Rickettsia, Mycoplasma, Spirochetes,* and *Chlamydia*)	*Adults:* 150 mg PO q.i.d. or 300 mg b.i.d. *Children:* Over 8 years, 6-10 mg/kg/24 hr PO in 2 or 4 divided doses Do *not* administer with milk, dairy products, or antacids Reduce dose in renal failure	Capsule: 150 mg Tablets: 150, 300 mg Store away from light and heat	Should *not* be used during pregnancy Drug should be discontinued if rash appears Be aware of photosensitivity Patients should use sunscreen Should not be used in patients with renal impairment Essentially same spectrum as tetracycline	
Doxycycline Doxy-II Doxychel Vibramycin	Serious systemic infections caused by susceptible microorganisms (as with demeclocycline); when oral medication *cannot* be administered Infections caused by susceptible microorganisms	*Adults:* 100-200 mg/24 hr IV in 1-2 doses *Children:* Over 8 years, 1-2 mg/kg/day IV in 1-2 doses Should be infused over 1-4 hr Should *not* be administered IM Switch to oral form when patient is able *Adults:* 200 mg PO first day followed by 100 mg/day in 1-2 divided doses *Children:* Over 8 years, 4 mg/kg PO first day followed by 2 mg/kg/day in 1 or 2 divided doses	Injectable: 100 mg Stable for 12 hr after reconstitution; store away from light Capsules: 50, 100 mg Tablet: 100 mg Syrup: 50 mg/5 ml (after reconstitution) Suspension: 25 mg/5 ml (after reconstitution) Shake suspension well before use Store away from light and heat	Should *not* be used during pregnancy Should not be given with antacids Should be taken a full 10 days to treat a streptococcal infection Phlebitis common Can cause tissue damage if it extravasates Does *not* accumulate in patients with renal impairment May be taken with food to decrease GI distress Overdose may lead to toxic accumulation	Check IV sites

	Uses	Dosage	Availability	Remarks
	Gonorrhea	*Adults:* 200 mg PO stat and 100 mg h.s. followed by 100 mg b.i.d. for 3 days		Has somewhat broader spectrum than tetracycline
	Traveler's diarrhea	*Adults:* 100 mg/day PO		May cause GI distress, particularly when taken on an empty stomach or at bedtime Monitor for diarrhea
★ **Methacycline** Molciclina Rondomycin	Infections caused by susceptible microorganisms	*Adults:* 600 mg/day PO in 2-4 divided doses *Children:* Over 8 years, 6-12 mg/kg/day in 2-4 divided doses	Tablet: 300 mg Store away from light and heat	Should *not* be used during pregnancy Accumulates in renal failure
	Mycoplasma pneumonia	*Adults:* 900 mg/day PO in 2-4 divided doses for 6 days Should be taken on an empty stomach Reduce dose in renal failure; do *not* administer with milk, dairy products, or antacids		Essentially same spectrum as tetracycline Should be used full 10 days to treat a streptococcal infection
Minocycline Minocin Ultramycin Vectrin	Serious systemic infections caused by susceptible microorganisms	*Adults:* 200 mg PO, IV followed by 100 mg q.12h. PO, IV *Children:* Over 8 years, 4 mg/kg PO, IV followed by 2 mg/kg q.12h. PO, IV Should be infused over 1-4 hr Should *not* be infused rapidly Avoid extravasation Change to oral form when patient is able May be taken with food to decrease GI distress Should *not* be given with antacids Reduce dosage in severe renal failure	Injectable: 100 mg vial Reconstitute according to instructions Usually 100 mg is reconstituted with 5 ml sterile water for injection; this can then be further diluted to 100-1000 ml Stable for 24 hr at room temperature after reconstitution Capsules: 50, 100 mg Tablets: 50, 100 mg Suspension: 50 mg/5 ml (5% alcohol) *Shake* suspension well before use Do not freeze suspension Store away from light and heat	Should be avoided during pregnancy Phlebitis common Broader spectrum than tetracycline Commonly causes dizziness (e.g., vestibular toxicity) Check IV sites

Continued.

NOTE: For additional details regarding the individual agents listed in this table see the text and other tables in this chapter.
*Indicates a multiple active ingredient product. For a complete listing of all active ingredients see the *Drug Reference Guide to Brand Names and Active Ingredients.*
★Indicates that the drug is generally available only in the United States.

NURSING DRUG DIGEST—cont'd

Medication (trade name)	Indication	Usual dosage and administration	Dosage forms, preparation, and storage	Contraindications, cautions, and comments	Monitoring
Oxytetracycline Abbocin Imperacin Otetryn Oxlopar Oxymycin Oxy-Tetrachel Terra-Cortril Spray with Polymyxin B Sulfate* Terra-Cortril* Terramycin Terramycin Ointment* Terramycin Ophthalmic Ointment* Terramycin Ophthalmic* Terramycin Otic Ointment* Terramycin with Polymyxin B* Terramycin Topical Ointment* Terramycin Vaginal Tablets* Terrastatin* Tetramine Urobiotic 250*	Serious infections caused by susceptible organisms when oral medication cannot be taken Infections caused by susceptible microorganisms	*Adults:* 250 mg IM q.d. or 300 mg IM daily in 2-3 doses *Children:* Over 8 years, 15-25 mg/kg/day IM in 1-3 divided doses Should be administered as deep IM injection *Adults:* 1-2 gm/day PO in 2-4 divided doses *Children:* Over 8 years, 25-50 mg/day PO in 4 doses Do *not* administer with milk, dairy products, or antacids Should be taken on an empty stomach Decrease dose in renal failure	Injectable: 100, 250 mg/ml Store away from light and heat Capsules: 125, 250 mg Tablets: 125, 250 mg Syrup: 125 mg/5 ml	Accumulates in renal failure Should *not* be used during pregnancy May cause necrosis or abscess at injection site Essentially same spectrum as tetracycline Check dose and expiration date	Monitor injection site Observe for overgrowth of nonsusceptible organisms
Tetracycline Achromycin Cefracycline Comycin* Cyclopar Deycline G-Mycin GT-500 Maytrex	Serious infections caused by susceptible microorganisms when oral medication *cannot* be taken	*Adults:* 250 mg/day IM or 300 mg/day IM in 2-3 doses; *or* 250-500 mg IV q.d. in 2 doses Should not exceed 2 gm/day *Children:* Over 8 years, 15-25 mg/kg/day IM (not to exceed 250 mg/single daily injection) in 1-3 doses; *or* 10-20 mg/kg/day IV in 2 doses	Injectable: 100, 250, 500 mg Reconstituted solutions stable for 12 hr For IM use, reconstitute 100 mg with 2 ml sterile water for injection For IV use, reconstitute 100 mg and 250 mg with 2 ml sterile water for injection	Accumulates in renal failure Phlebitis common IM can cause abscess Should *not* be used during pregnancy May cause photosensitivity	Check IV and IM sites Observe for overgrowth of nonsusceptible organisms

Drug	Indications	Dosing	Preparations	Comments
Muracine Neo-Tetrine Novatetra Panmycin Piracaps Polycycline Retet Ro-Cycline Sumycin Tetracaps Tetrachel Tetracyn	Infections caused by susceptible microorganisms	Usual dose is 12 mg/kg/day IV Deep IM injection into large muscle mass IV should be infused over 1-4 hr Switch to oral form when patient is able Adults: 1-2 gm/day PO in 2-4 doses Children: Over 8 years, 25-50 mg/kg/day PO in 2-4 doses	Reconstitute 500 mg with 10 ml sterile water for injection Reconstituted solutions are diluted to 100-1000 ml in D$_5$W or NS Capsules: 250, 500 mg Tablets: 250, 500 mg Syrup: 125 mg/5 ml Store away from light and heat	Overgrowth of opportunistic organisms may occur
	Gonorrhea	Adults: 1.5 gm PO followed by 500 mg q.6h. for 4 days		
	Syphilis	Adults: 500 mg PO q.i.d. for 10-15 days		
	Brucellosis	Adults: 500 mg PO q.6h. for 3 weeks		
	Acne	Adults: 250 mg PO q.d. to b.i.d. Decrease dose in renal failure Do *not* administer with milk, dairy products, or antacids		

BIBLIOGRAPHY

The choice of antimicrobial drugs. *The Medical Letter*, 1980, *22*, 5-12.

Chopra, I., Howe, G.B., Linton, A.H., et al. The tetracyclines: prospects at the beginning of the 1980's. *Journal of Antimicrobial Chemotherapy*, 1981, *8*, 5-21.

Committee on Drugs. Requiem for tetracyclines. *Pediatrics*, 1975, *55*, 142-143.

Drew, T.M., Altman, R., Black, K., et al. Minocycline for prophylaxis of infection with *Neisseria meningitidis*: high rate of side effects in recipients. *Journal of Infectious Diseases*, 1976, *133*, 194-198.

Eichenwald, H.F., & McCracken, G.H. Antimicrobial therapy in infants and children. Part I. Review of antimicrobial agents. *Pediatrics*, 1978, *93*, 337-356.

Fanning, W.L., & Gump, D.W. Distressing side-effects of minocycline hydrochloride. *Archives of Internal Medicine*, 1976, *136*, 761-762.

Greene, G.R. Tetracycline in pregnancy (letter). *New England Journal of Medicine*, 1976, *295*, 512-513.

Jacobson, J.A., & Daniel, B. Vestibular reactions associated with minocycline. *Antimicrobial Agents and Chemotherapy*, 1975, *8*, 453-456.

Jukes, T.H. Antibiotics in meat production. *Journal of the American Medical Association*, 1975, *232*, 292-293.

Levy, S.B., Fitzgerald, G.B., & Macone, A.B. Changes in intestinal flora on farm personnel after introduction of a tetracycline-supplemented feed on a farm. *New England Journal of Medicine*, 1976, *295*, 583-588.

Ray, W.A., Federspiel, C.F., & Schaffner, W. Prescribing of tetracycline to children less than 8 years old: a two-year epidemiologic study among ambulatory Tennessee medicaid recipients. *Journal of the American Medical Association*, 1977, *237*, 2069-2074.

Roy, I., Bach, V., & Thadepalli, H., The *in vitro* effect of doxycycline against anaerobic bacterial isolates from the female genital tract: doxycycline (Vibramycin) recent investigations and clinical experience. *Excerpta Medica*, 1977, *3*, 21-25.

Sack, D.A., Kaminsky, D.C., Sack, R.B., et al. Prophylactic doxycycline for traveler's diarrhea: results of a prospective double-blind study of Peace Corps volunteers in Kenya. *New England Journal of Medicine*, 1978, *298*, 758-763.

Siegal, D. Tetracyclines: new look at old antibiotic. I. Clinical pharmacology, mechanism of action and untoward effects. *New York State Journal of Medicine*, 1978, *78*, 950-956.

Seigel, D. Tetracyclines: New look at old antibiotic. II. Clinical use. *New York State Journal of Medicine*, 1978, *78*, 1115-1120.

Smith, J.G., Jr., Chalker, D.K., & Wehr, R.F., The effectiveness of topical and oral tetracycline for acne. *Southern Medical Journal*, 1976, *60*, 965-967.

Totterman, L.E., & Saxen, L. Incorporation of tetracycline into human fetal bones after maternal drug ingestion. *Acta Obstetrica et Gynecologica Scandinavica*, 1969, *48*, 542-549.

Walters, B.N., & Gubbay, S.S. Tetracycline and benign intracranial hypertension: report of five cases. *British Medical Journal*, 1981, *1*, 19-20.

CHAPTER 48

Miscellaneous Antibiotics

Louis A. Pagliaro
Ann M. Pagliaro

Medications discussed in this chapter

This chapter covers a number of different miscellaneous antibiotics. These drugs are structurally diverse, but share the common pharmacologic property of having antibacterial activity.

These agents are predominantly *bacteriostatic* and many cause serious adverse effects (e.g., blood dyscrasias, nephrotoxicity, ototoxicity). Therefore they are usually *not* the antibiotics of first choice, but are selected when other, safer antibiotics cannot be used in a particular patient (e.g., when the patient is hypersensitive to the antibiotic of first choice).

Following is a brief discussion of each agent listed in alphabetical order. Further specific details can be found for each agent in the Nursing Drug Digest.

BACITRACIN

Bacitracin is an antibiotic produced from a gram-positive organism of the group *Bacillus subtilis*. It is effective against many gram-positive organisms, but is *ineffective* against most gram-negative organisms. Because of its limited spectrum of activity and its ability to cause severe kidney damage when used systemically (i.e., intramuscularly), bacitracin is most commonly found in combination with other antiinfectives in various topical preparations.

Because of its nephrotoxic effects, the use of systemic bacitracin is limited to treating severe life-threatening infections caused by bacitracin-sensitive organisms that are *not* sensitive to treatment with other less toxic drugs. On rare occasions, bacitracin has been administered intrathecally to treat septic coccal meningitis and brain abscesses caused by sensitive organisms.

Whenever bacitracin is used systemically, baseline renal function, including BUN, creatinine, fluid intake and output, and microscopic urinalysis, should be assessed and periodically monitored during treatment. When bacitracin is administered parenterally, fluids should be forced and the urinary pH kept at 6 or above by the administration of sodium bicarbonate, unless contraindicated. Because the renal damage caused by bacitracin is dose related, any noted change in renal function is a reason for reducing the dosage or discontinuing the drug.

Although the development of bacterial resistance to bacitracin is uncommon, systemic use can result in the overgrowth of nonsusceptible organisms, particularly fungi (e.g., *Monilia*). This should be monitored for and, if observed, appropriately treated.

CHLORAMPHENICOL

Chloramphenicol was originally derived from *Streptomyces venezuelae*, but is now mainly produced synthetically. Chloramphenicol exerts its antibacterial activity by binding to the 50S subunit of the bacterial *ribosomes*, thus inhibiting protein synthesis. Because chloramphenicol, clindamycin, erythromycin, and lincomycin all act at the 50S subunit of the bacterial ribosomes, they may antagonize each other's action and should *not* be used concurrently.

Chloramphenicol is effective against a wide range of both gram-positive and gram-negative bacteria. Inhibition of most sensitive organisms occurs at chloramphenicol blood levels of 5 to 20 μg/ml. Because it is primarily bacteriostatic, the use of chloramphenicol can result in the overgrowth of nonsusceptible organisms, including fungi.

Bacterial resistance to chloramphenicol is usually *plasmid* mediated. Complete resistance is not widespread, but is found among certain bacteria, notably *Acinetobacter*, *Proteus*, *Pseudomonas aeruginosa*, and *S. marcescens*. Some strains of *Haemophilus influenzae* and *Salmonella* have also developed resistance to chloramphenicol.

When it is administered by the intramuscular route, peak chloramphenicol blood levels are lower and occur later than when either the oral or intravenous route is used. Thus, intramuscular use is *not* generally recommended.

Chloramphenicol effectively crosses the blood-brain barrier, achieving concentrations in the cerebrospinal fluid ranging from 35% to 65% of that found in the serum. Thus it is often used to treat meningitis caused by susceptible organisms in infants and children.

The most serious toxicities associated with systemic chloramphenicol use are bone marrow depression and the gray baby syndrome of the newborn.

The bone marrow depression can be differentiated into two types. The first typically manifests itself as *reticulocytopenia* and is the more common of the two types. It is dose related and is usually reversible. The second is much more severe and manifests itself as *aplastic anemia*. It is relatively rare, usually delayed in onset, often sudden in progression, and usually fatal. To minimize the morbidity and mortality associated with these drug-induced blood dyscrasias, it is imperative that appropriate blood studies be periodically performed during treatment. Maintaining the chloramphenicol peak serum levels below 25 μg/ml appears to minimize the occurrence of the reversible form of bone marrow suppression associated with chloramphenicol use.

When systemically administered to newborn infants during the first several days of life, chloramphenicol has caused a syndrome known as the gray baby syndrome. This syndrome appears after several days of treatment and is characterized by abdominal distention, pallid cyanosis, irregular respiration, vasomotor collapse, and death, usually within a few hours after the onset of symptoms. Although blood levels in these reported cases were unusually high (i.e., greater than 90 μg/ml), use of chloramphenicol during the first few days of life is generally contraindicated unless the blood levels are carefully monitored and kept below 25 μg/ml.

The systemic dosage of chloramphenicol should be decreased in the presence of renal or hepatic damage. Monitoring serum levels can assist in this regard.

Topical use of chloramphenicol is usually safe and well tolerated unless the drug is applied over large denuded or abraded areas of skin or is applied for a long period of time, in which case, the absorption can be significant and systemic toxicity may result. It should be noted that the use of chloramphenicol ophthalmic ointments may slow the rate of corneal healing.

CLINDAMYCIN

Clindamycin exerts its antibacterial activity by binding to the 50S subunit of the bacterial ribosomes, thus inhibiting protein synthesis. Because clindamycin, chloramphenicol, erythromycin, and lincomycin all act at the 50S subunit of the bacterial ribosomes, they may antagonize each other's action and should *not* be used concurrently.

Clindamycin is effective against many gram-positive organisms, but is *ineffective* against most gram-negative organisms.

Clindamycin is well absorbed from the gastrointestinal tract and its absorption is not significantly affected by food. Because of its ability to cross biologic membranes, clindamycin can cross the placenta and can also be excreted in breast milk. However, it does not appear to cause any significant toxicity for the developing fetus or the nursing infant. Dosage should be modified in the presence of renal or hepatic impairment. Clindamycin can also be applied topically for treating acne.

The most significant toxicity associated with clindamycin is diarrhea, which has on occasion resulted in colitis. If diarrhea occurs and is significant, the drug should be discontinued and appropriate therapy initiated. Endoscopic evaluation to demonstrate pseudomembrane or ulcer formation may be indicated. A principal cause of clindamycin-associated colitis is thought to be *Clostridium difficile* (which is usually sensitive to vancomycin). Treatment with anticholinergics (e.g., atropine) and antiperistaltics (e.g., codeine, diphenoxylate) is usually ineffective and may actually cause the condition to worsen. Because serious relapses of colitis have occurred up to 1 month following apparently successful treatment, follow-up observation and monitoring are recommended. Patients should be instructed to report any recurrent attacks of diarrhea to their health care provider.

Culture and sensitivity test results should be monitored for the development of resistant strains with prolonged use. *Cross-resistance* between clindamycin and lincomycin can occur and should be kept in mind when changing the patient from one antibiotic to another. The overgrowth of nonsusceptible organisms can occur and should be monitored for.

COLISTIMETHATE

Colistimethate is a *bactericidal* antibiotic derived from colistin. It is administered parenterally by either the intramuscular or intravenous route. Once in the body, colistimethate must undergo chemical hydrolysis (see Chapter 5, "Drug Metabolism and Elimination") to form colistin for antibacterial activation. Because colistimethate is predominantly excreted by the kidneys, renal function *must* be monitored and the dosage adjusted accordingly.

Major toxicities of colistimethate are associated with the renal and neuromuscular systems. Early signs of decreased renal function include diminished urine output, increased BUN, and increased serum creatinine. Colistimethate therapy should be discontinued at the first sign of drug-induced renal impairment.

Use of colistimethate may cause various neurologic disturbances, including dizziness, numbness or tingling in the extremities, and slurring of speech. Potentially more serious is colistimethate's reported ability to interfere with nerve conduction at the neuromuscular junction. Colistimethate, as well as certain other antibiotics (e.g., kanamycin, neomycin, polymyxin, streptomycin), can cause varying degrees of neuromuscular blockade resulting in muscle weakness and, if the respiratory muscles are affected, apnea. Risk of this potentially lethal adverse effect increases in the presence of renal impairment and whenever two or more agents with neuromuscular blocking activity are administered concurrently.

COLISTIN

Colistin is an antibiotic produced from the bacillus *Polymyxa colistinus*. Colistin, which was previously known as polymyxin E, is a polymyxin antibiotic and is closely related to polymyxin B. It acts as a cationic detergent that exerts its bacteriostatic effect by disrupting the cell membrane of various gram-negative organisms, particularly *Pseudomonas aeruginosa*. There is a complete cross-resistance between colistin and polymyxin B.

Colistin is available as a powder (300 mg bottle) that is mixed with distilled water to yield an oral suspension containing 5 mg/ml. This suspension should be shaken well before removing a dose. Any unused sus-

pension should be discarded after 24 hours. Colistin is *not* systemically absorbed following oral administration, but is used for its local effects within the gastrointestinal tract.

CO-TRIMOXAZOLE

Co-trimoxazole is a combination product that contains the antibacterial agents trimethoprim and sulfamethoxazole in a fixed 1:5 ratio.

Trimethoprim selectively inhibits bacterial dihydrofolate reductase, the enzyme that reduces dihydrofolic acid in bacteria to its tetrahydro form. This causes a sufficient reduction in the synthesis of folate coenzymes and a resultant decrease in nucleic acid biosynthesis to provide bacteriostatic activity against a variety of gram-negative and gram-positive organisms.

Trimethoprim is rapidly absorbed following oral administration and is largely (approximately 80%) excreted in unchanged form in the urine. It is primarily metabolized in the liver and has a biologic half-life of approximately 10 hours.

Sulfamethoxazole is structurally related to para-aminobenzoic acid (PABA) (as are the other sulfonamides—see Chapter 49, "Sulfonamides"). This structural similarity enables sulfamethoxazole to function as a competitive antagonist to PABA during the bacterial use of PABA in the production of folic acid. Thus, sulfamethoxazole exerts a bacteriostatic effect against those bacteria that need PABA as a precursor in the production of folic acid.

Sulfamethoxazole is rapidly absorbed following oral administration and is partially (approximately 20%) excreted in unchanged form in the urine. It is metabolized (inactivated) in both the liver and the kidneys and has a biologic half-life of approximately 10 hours.

The use of these two agents, trimethoprim and sulfamethoxazole, together in a fixed combination product takes advantage of their different sequential mechanisms of action. Co-trimoxazole is bactericidal, has a broader spectrum of antibiotic activity, and has a lower frequency of development of bacterial resistance than is observed with the use of either constituent agent alone. Co-trimoxazole is useful in treating a variety of gastrointestinal, genital, respiratory, and urinary tract infections caused by susceptible gram-negative and gram-positive organisms.

The majority of adverse effects from co-trimoxazole involve the cutaneous system, with a wide variety of different rashes (e.g., *morbilliform, purpuric, urticarial*) occurring in up to 6% of treated patients. More serious cutaneous reactions (e.g., *exfoliative dermatitis*, Stevens-Johnson syndrome, toxic epidermal necrosis) may also occur, particularly in elderly patients, but are rare. Common oral and gastric reactions include *glossitis*, nausea, *stomatitis*, and vomiting. Administration of co-trimoxazole with food or milk may help decrease these effects.

Use of co-trimoxazole is *not* recommended in infants under 2 months of age, during pregnancy, or in breastfeeding mothers. In addition, caution should be used in administering co-trimoxazole to patients with a folate deficiency. Hematologic studies should be performed and regularly monitored in these patients. Trimethoprim is also available alone for use in patients who cannot use sulfonamides.

ERYTHROMYCIN

Erythromycin exerts its antibacterial activity by binding to the 50S subunits of the bacterial ribosomes, thus inhibiting protein synthesis. Because erythromycin, chloramphenicol, clindamycin, and lincomycin all act at the 50S subunit of the bacterial ribosomes, they may antagonize each other's action and should *not* be used concurrently.

Depending on the dose used and the sensitivity of the microorganism, erythromycin can be either bacteriostatic or bactericidal. The spectrum of activity for erythromycin is similar to that for penicillin G and it is commonly used as an alternative in patients who are allergic to penicillin.

In addition to the base, several salt forms of erythromycin are available, including the estolate, ethylsuccinate, gluceptate, lactobionate, and stearate. The pharmacology of these various salts is identical to that of erythromycin base, except in relation to the following points.

Erythromycin estolate is an oral preparation that is absorbed from the gastrointestinal tract principally as the propionyl ester. The estolate form of erythromycin is *not* acid labile and can thus be administered with food or acidic fruit juices (e.g., orange juice), whereas the other oral forms of erythromycin are acid labile and should not be administered with food or acidic fruit juices. The estolate salt form of erythromycin is, however, the preparation most commonly associated with the development of cholestatic jaundice, particularly in adults. Erythromycin estolate is thus *contraindicated* in patients with hepatic dysfunction. Large oral doses of the estolate have also been associated with transient auditory impairment and with pyloric stenosis in infants. Because it offers *no* significant therapeutic advantage over the other forms of erythromycin (apart from acid stability), and because it is associated with a significantly higher incidence

of hepatic damage than occurs with the other forms of erythromycin, use of erythromycin estolate is generally *not* recommended.

Erythromycin ethylsuccinate can be administered orally or parenterally by the intramuscular route. The oral preparation is acid labile and should be administered on an empty stomach. Food or acidic fruit juices should not be administered with this preparation because they can cause it to be significantly degraded in the stomach before absorption. The intramuscular route is painful and is generally not recommended. When the intramuscular route is used, erythromycin ethylsuccinate usually includes 2% butyl aminobenzoate as a local anesthetic to help decrease the pain at the injection site. Once absorbed (from the oral or intramuscular route) the ethylsuccinate salt is hydrolyzed to the active base form of erythromycin.

Erythromycin gluceptate is a parenteral form of erythromycin that is available for intravenous administration.

Erythromycin lactobionate is a salt form that is similar to the gluceptate and is also administered by the intravenous route. Transient auditory impairment has been associated with the intravenous administration of large daily doses (greater than 4000 mg) of the lactobionate form.

Erythromycin stearate is administered orally. It dissociates to its erythromycin base in the duodenum before absorption. This oral preparation is acid labile and should be administered on an empty stomach. Skin rashes and urticaria appear to occur more commonly with the stearate form of erythromycin.

Except for the effects previously noted, serious toxicity is only rarely associated with erythromycin. The only general contraindication to its use is in patients with a known hypersensitivity to erythromycin. Caution should be used in administering any erythromycin preparation to patients with preexisting hepatic impairment, and appropriate monitoring should be performed. In addition, *superinfections*, caused by the overgrowth of nonsusceptible organisms (particularly fungi) are rare, but should be monitored for, particularly when patients are on long-term therapy.

The topical application of erythromycin ophthalmic ointment (0.5%) at birth is an effective prophylaxis against neonatal conjunctivitis, including gonococcal ophthalmia neonatorum.

FUSIDIC ACID

Fusidic acid is derived from the bacteria *Fusidium coccineum*. Fusidic acid exerts its antibacterial effect by disrupting the transfer of amino acids to the protein formed on the ribosomes of bacteria. Depending on the dosage administered and the sensitivity of the bacteria, fusidic acid can be either bacteriostatic or bactericidal.

Fusidic acid is effective against gram-positive bacteria, particularly *Staphylococcus aureus.* Bacterial resistance to fusidic acid can develop, but cross-resistance with other antibiotics has not been observed. Caution should be used, however, if fusidic acid is to be used concurrently with either erythromycin or tetracycline, because there is a high incidence of staphylococcal strains that are resistant to erythromycin and tetracycline.

Fusidic acid is highly protein bound (i.e., greater than 97%) and does *not* penetrate the blood-brain barrier. Thus, it is not indicated for treating a brain abscess or meningitis, even when the causative organism is sensitive to it.

Several forms of fusidic acid are available, including diethanolamine fusidate, fusidic acid hemihydrate, and sodium fusidate. Following is a brief discussion of the special qualities of each form of fusidic acid.

Diethanolamine fusidate is the parenteral form of fusidic acid (580 mg of diethanolamine fusidate is equivalent to 482 mg of fusidic acid). This preparation should be administered *only* by IV infusion. Rapid IV infusion can cause venospasm and thrombophlebitis. Diethanolamine fusidate must be diluted and buffered before administration and should be administered *only* by slow IV infusion into a vein with a good blood flow, over a minimum period of 6 hours. The IV solution should be diluted to 250 to 500 ml and administered with NS, D_5W, or plasma. Do *not* infuse with amino acid solutions or with whole blood because hemolysis of the erythrocytes may occur.

Fusidic acid hemihydrate is the oral suspension form of fusidic acid. The suspension is incompletely absorbed (approximately 70%) and must thus be dosed higher than the tablet form to achieve the same therapeutic blood levels. Because of this bioavailability problem (see Chapter 4, "Drug Availability and Distribution"), the suspension is recommended only for infants and for older patients who have difficulty swallowing tablets.

Sodium fusidate is used in the coated tablet form of fusidic acid (250 mg of sodium fusidate is equivalent to 240 mg of fusidic acid). This form is well absorbed from the gastrointestinal tract and is the generally preferred dosage form and route of administration. The principal adverse effect associated with the tablet form of fusidic acid is mild gastrointestinal distress, which can be decreased by administering food or milk with the tablets.

GRAMICIDIN

Gramicidin is derived from the bacteria *Bacillus brevis.* Gramicidin is effective against gram-positive cocci and some *Neisseria* species. It exerts its bactericidal effect by altering the permeability of bacterial membranes, particularly to cations such as potassium.

Gramicidin is a potent hemolytic and is thus *not* administered systemically. It is used topically, usually in combination with other antibacterials, to provide a wider spectrum of activity and to decrease the development of bacterial resistance.

LINCOMYCIN

Lincomycin is derived from the bacteria *Streptomyces lincolnensis.* Lincomycin exerts its antibacterial activity by selectively binding to the 50S subunit of the bacterial ribosomes, thus inhibiting protein synthesis. Because lincomycin, chloramphenicol, clindamycin, and erythromycin all act at the 50S subunit of the bacterial ribosomes, they may antagonize each other's action and should *not* be used concurrently.

Lincomycin is effective against many gram-positive organisms. Its clinical use has been largely replaced, however, by its derivative, clindamycin, which has greater activity and causes fewer adverse effects.

Lincomycin is contraindicated in patients hypersensitive to it or to its derivative, clindamycin. It is also contraindicated in patients with severe monilial infections and in newborn infants.

All IV doses should be diluted and infused over a period of 30 to 120 minutes (see the Nursing Drug Digest for specific details). The rapid administration of large (i.e., greater than 4000 mg), undiluted doses of lincomycin has resulted in cardiopulmonary arrest.

A variety of minor adverse effects (e.g., nausea, rashes) can accompany the use of lincomycin. However, the major adverse effects are severe hypersensitivity reactions and severe persistent diarrhea, which may result in acute colitis. If either of these two severe adverse effects occur, lincomycin should be immediately withdrawn and appropriate corrective measures instituted.

NOVOBIOCIN

Novobiocin is derived from *Streptomyces niveus.* It exerts its bacteriostatic effect by inhibiting protein synthesis and by interfering with the formation of the bacterial cell wall. It is effective against susceptible strains of *Staphylococcus* and *Proteus.*

Novobiocin is well absorbed from the gastrointestinal tract and is administered both orally and parenterally (IM, IV).

Because novobiocin is a potent sensitizing agent that commonly causes urticaria and maculopapular rashes, its use is limited to treating susceptible strains of bacteria that are resistant to other antibiotics or in which the use of other effective antibiotics is contraindicated. Bacterial resistance develops often and rapidly with the use of novobiocin, particularly among staphylococci.

Because novobiocin can adversely affect bilirubin metabolism, causing hyperbilirubinemia, its use in newborn infants is contraindicated. Novobiocin can also occasionally cause jaundice and blood dyscrasias (e.g., anemia, leukopenia). These effects should be monitored for and, if observed, novobiocin therapy should be immediately discontinued.

Novobiocin has been largely replaced by other antibiotics that are less toxic and that possess wider spectrums of activity.

POLYMYXIN B

Polymyxin B is derived from *Bacillus polymyxa*. Polymyxin B acts as a cationic detergent, exerting its bactericidal effect by interacting with and disrupting the cell membranes of various gram-negative bacilli, particularly *Pseudomonas aeruginosa*. Development of bacterial resistance is unusual; however, there is complete cross-resistance between polymyxin B and colistin (polymyxin E).

Absorption following oral administration is poor; thus polymyxin B is usually applied topically or administered parenterally (i.e., IM or IV). The IM route of administration is the preferred parenteral route. Polymyxin B is often combined with a local anesthetic (e.g., procaine hydrochloride 1%) for IM administration; however, the pain following IM administration is usually not significantly decreased by the local anesthetic. Up to 60% of the parenterally administered dose of polymyxin B is eliminated in the urine. Thus, the dosage *must* be reduced in the presence of renal impairment.

Several neurologic or neuromuscular adverse effects can be caused by polymyxin B, including blurred vision, dizziness, generalized weakness, *ptosis*, and slurred speech. Neuromuscular blockade with resultant respiratory paralysis can also occur, particularly when large doses are administered or when other neuromuscular blockers are administered concurrently.

Nephrotoxicity is probably the most significant adverse effect associated with polymyxin B. Renal function must be carefully monitored and the concurrent administration of other potentially nephrotoxic drugs (e.g., the aminoglycosides, cephaloridine) should be done with extreme caution or avoided because they may potentiate the nephrotoxicity caused by polymyxin B. In addition, it should be noted that both the neurotoxicity and the nephrotoxicity of polymyxin B are generally exacerbated in the presence of renal insufficiency.

SPECTINOMYCIN

Spectinomycin is an antibiotic produced by *Streptomyces spectabilis*. It exerts its bacteriostatic effect by binding to the 30S subunit of bacterial ribosomes, thus inhibiting protein synthesis.

Spectinomycin is effective against a wide range of gram-negative bacteria, particularly gonococci. Development of bacterial resistance to spectinomycin as a result of bacterial mutation may occasionally occur and should be monitored for.

Spectinomycin is administered by the intramuscular route *only*. Suspensions for IM use should be stored at room temperature after preparation, and any unused portion should be discarded after 24 hours. It is usually well tolerated, but may occasionally cause minor local (e.g., pain at injection site) or systemic (e.g., chills, dizziness, fever) adverse effects. Neither nephrotoxicity nor ototoxicity have been associated with its use.

Spectinomycin is *not* effective against established or incubating syphilis. Treatment of gonorrhea with spectinomycin may actually mask or delay the appearance of symptoms of incubating syphilis. Thus, appropriate monitoring and follow-up should be established if the diagnosis of syphilis is suspected.

TROLEANDOMYCIN

Troleandomycin is a synthetic derivative of oleandomycin, an antibiotic produced from *Streptomyces antibioticus* (oleandomycin is no longer available for use in North America). Troleandomycin exerts its bacteriostatic effect by inhibiting protein synthesis in sensitive bacteria.

Troleandomycin is effective against various gram-positive organisms, particularly pneumococci (e.g., *Diplococcus pneumoniae*) and streptococci (e.g., *Streptococcus pyogenes*).

Troleandomycin is readily absorbed from the gastrointestinal tract and is administered only by the oral route. Liver function should be monitored because troleandomycin-induced liver changes are usually reversible if promptly recognized and if the drug is immediately discontinued. Use of troleandomycin has been associated with an allergic type of cholestatic hepatitis and with hyperbilirubinemia and jaundice. Extreme caution must therefore be exercised in administering troleandomycin to patients with impaired hepatic function, and if at all possible an alternate appropriate antibiotic should be substituted in these patients.

Prolonged therapy is associated with superinfections caused by the overgrowth of nonsusceptible organisms. Because both erythromycin and troleandomycin belong to the group of macrolide antibiotics, patients hypersensitive to one agent may be hypersensitive to the other.

It is *not* recommended that troleandomycin therapy be continued for longer than 10 days unless a provision is made to frequently monitor liver function tests.

VANCOMYCIN

Vancomycin is an antibiotic derived from *Streptomyces orientalis.* It is effective against many strains of gram-positive bacteria. It exerts its bactericidal effect by binding to cell wall precursors and thus inhibits cell wall synthesis in susceptible organisms.

Vancomycin is poorly absorbed when administered orally and is irritating to tissues when administered intramuscularly. It is, therefore, usually administered intravenously. A large amount (i.e., approximately 80%) of vancomycin is excreted by the kidneys. The dosage *must* be reduced in the presence of renal impairment. Vancomycin can be administered orally if it is to be used for its local effect within the gastrointestinal tract (e.g., to treat antibiotic-associated colitis).

Use of vancomycin can result in the overgrowth of nonsusceptible organisms. This should be monitored for and appropriately treated.

The most prominent and severe adverse effects associated with the use of vancomycin are nephrotoxicity and ototoxicity. These occur with greater frequency and severity in the presence of renal impairment or when large doses are administered. Hearing loss is often permanent and may be preceded by tinnitus. Elderly patients appear to be particularly susceptible to the ototoxic effects of vancomycin. Nephrotoxicity and ototoxicity must be carefully monitored for.

SUMMARY

Although not usually the drugs of first choice for most commonly encountered infections, the group of miscellaneous antibiotics discussed in this chapter offers alternatives to the more commonly used antibiotics. This is of particular use when resistant organisms are encountered that pose a danger to the life of the patient, as well as when the use of the more standard antimicrobials may be contraindicated in a particular patient (e.g., hypersensitivity to the penicillins).

Use of these agents is not without risk because many can cause serious adverse effects, including blood dyscrasias, nephrotoxicity, and neurotoxicity. However, with the careful monitoring of the blood level concentrations of the antibiotics and the careful monitoring of renal and hepatic function these agents can be safely and effectively used.

ADVERSE/SIDE EFFECTS OF MISCELLANEOUS ANTIBIOTICS*

Because of the wide range and diversity of the miscellaneous antibiotics discussed in this chapter, the reader is referred to the discussion of the individual agents in the body of the chapter and to the Nursing Drug Digest for adverse side effects associated with the individual antibiotics.

---

*See Chapter 11, "Drug Toxicity," for an overview of drug toxicity.

CLINICALLY SIGNIFICANT DRUG INTERACTIONS*

Primary drug	Interacting drug	Possible effect(s)	Probable mechanism(s)
Bacitracin	Nondepolarizing muscle relaxants (e.g., pancuronium, tubocurarine)	Increased neuromuscular blockade with possible respiratory depression	Additive or synergistic action
Chloramphenicol	Phenytoin	Increased effect of phenytoin	Inhibition of metabolism
Chloramphenicol	Sulfonylureas	Increased effect of sulfonylureas	Inhibition of metabolism
Clindamycin	Nondepolarizing muscle relaxants (e.g., pancuronium, tubocurarine)	Increased neuromuscular blockade with possible respiratory depression	Additive or synergistic action
Colistimethate	Nondepolarizing muscle relaxants (e.g., pancuronium, tubocurarine)	Increased neuromuscular blockade with possible respiratory depression	Additive or synergistic action
Co-trimoxazole	Phenytoin	Increased effect of phenytoin	Inhibition of metabolism
Erythromycin	Carbamazepine	Increased effect of carbamazepine	Inhibition of metabolism
Erythromycin	Digoxin	Increased effect of digoxin	Increased bioavailability
Erythromycin	Theophyllines	Increased effect of theophyllines	Inhibition of metabolism
Lincomycin	Nondepolarizing muscle relaxants (e.g., pancuronium, tubocurarine)	Increased neuromuscular blockade with possible respiratory depression	Additive or synergistic action
Polymyxin B	Nondepolarizing muscle relaxants (e.g., pancuronium, tubocurarine)	Increased neuromuscular blockade with possible respiratory depression	Additive or synergistic action
Troleandomycin	Carbamazepine	Increased effect of carbamazepine	Inhibition of metabolism
Troleandomycin	Methylprednisolone	Increased effect of methylprednisolone	Inhibition of metabolism
Troleandomycin	Theophyllines	Increased effect of theophyllines	Inhibition of metabolism

*See Chapter 10, "Drug Interactions," for an overview of drug interactions.

GENERAL NURSING IMPLICATIONS

Nursing of patients requiring miscellaneous antibiotics

ASSESSMENT

The miscellaneous antibiotics discussed in this chapter are usually selected when other less toxic antibiotics cannot be used. The choice of drug depends on the site of infection, the infecting organism, and individual patient factors. Baseline assessment data should include specific information about the patient's general health state and the need for antibiotic therapy. Whenever possible, the organism responsible for the infection should be identified *before* the drug therapy is initiated with antibiotics. The collection of specimens (e.g., blood, urine, sputum, wound drainage) should be completed according to hospital procedures for smear, culture, and sensitivity studies. Sensitivity or susceptibility tests are essential in the diagnosis

and treatment of the infection and in monitoring the patient's response. Assessment should include detailed information regarding the presence of symptoms indicating an infection, including elevated temperature, redness or pain in an area not previously affected, fatigue, anorexia, change in wound character, elevated white blood cell count, or other observations relevant to the specific infectious condition. Isolation measures should be readily implemented as indicated to prevent the spread of the infection to others.

Assessment should include a detailed drug history before initiating antibiotic therapy to identify possible hypersensitivity to specific or related agents, contraindications, cautions, drug interactions, and drug-taking patterns.

Baseline renal function tests (BUN, creatinine, urinalysis) are indicated with many of the miscellaneous antibiotics and should be completed and periodically monitored during therapy. Hematologic studies are also indicated for various individual agents.

SENSITIVITY

Generally, with the exception of lincomycin in which a hypersensitivity reaction is a major adverse effect, allergic reactions are rare. However, it is important to note that any drug has the potential to cause a hypersensitivity reaction in susceptible individuals. Patients should be carefully questioned during the drug history and before the administration of the antibiotics regarding the possibility of a hypersen-

Continued.

Nursing of patients requiring miscellaneous antibiotics—cont'd

SENSITIVITY—cont'd

sitivity to the respective agent. If a history of an allergy is identified, the patient should be asked to describe the reaction.

See the Nursing Drug Digest for specific information regarding hypersensitivity related to each agent.

CONTRAINDICATIONS

The use of individual antibiotics is contraindicated in patients with a known hypersensitivity. See the Nursing Drug Digest for contraindications to specific agents.

CAUTIONS

It is important to note that some of the antibiotics discussed in this chapter (e.g., clindamycin) cross the placenta and can also be excreted in breast milk. Although this has not been associated with toxicity in the fetus or the nursing infant, these drugs should be used cautiously during pregnancy and in nursing mothers.

A decrease in the dosage is indicated for many of the antibiotics discussed in this chapter in the presence of renal or hepatic impairment. In addition, the concurrent use of nephrotoxic or hepatotoxic medications should be avoided with these agents.

Cross-resistance can occur (e.g., colistin and polymixyn B, clindamycin and lincomycin), and this should be kept in mind when changing from one antibiotic to another.

See the Nursing Drug Digest for cautions related to each specific agent.

DRUG INTERACTIONS

The antibiotics discussed in this chapter can interact with each other in some cases and with other drugs.

It is important to recognize that bacteriostatic antibiotics can slow down cell growth and therefore may inhibit the action of bactericidal antibiotics.

See Clinically Significant Drug Interactions for specific interactions associated with individual agents.

ADMINISTRATION

The miscellaneous antibiotics discussed in this chapter are available in oral, intramuscular, intravenous, topical, and ophthalmic preparations. Not all are available for administration in these forms, and special attention should be paid to the specific route of administration of each drug. It is especially important to note that various salts of the same drug are given by different routes. These considerations are discussed in the body of the chapter in relation to each drug, and further information regarding the dosage and administration of each drug is provided in the Nursing Drug Digest.

MONITORING PATIENT RESPONSE
Therapeutic response

The onset and duration of antibiotic therapy depend largely on the specific drug, the dosage form, route of administration, individual patient factors, type of infection, and the seriousness of the infection. Generally patients should be monitored for therapeutic effect as related to the baseline assessment data such as decreased temperature, decreased white blood cell count, decreased signs of redness, pain or inflammation at the affected area, increased appetite, increased energy, increased sense of well-being, or other indications as related to the need for antibiotic therapy. Monitoring the therapeutic response is especially important because antibiotic therapy commonly fails, and if the patient is unresponsive to one antibiotic agent another may be selected that can prove more beneficial in treating the infection. As with other antibiotics, the therapy should be guided by bacteriologic studies, susceptibility tests, and clinical response. Thus monitoring the patient's response cannot be overemphasized.

Adverse side effects

Adverse side effects vary widely depending on the specific antibiotic and on its route of administration. Nephrotoxic or ototoxic effects are associated with the use of polymyxin B and vancomycin. Bone marrow depression can be caused by chloramphenicol, in addition to other effects, and diarrhea leading to colitis can occur with the use of clindamycin and lincomycin. Neurologic and neuromuscular adverse effects, including blurred vision, numbness or tingling of the extremities, slurred speech, and muscle weakness, can occur in patients receiving colistimethate or polymyxin B, and rashes are a cutaneous side effect associated with the use of co-trimoxazole or novobiocin.

Generally, all of the miscellaneous antibiotics can cause an overgrowth of nonsusceptible organisms, particularly fungi, and patients should be monitored carefully for this effect and nursing care planned to minimize this effect.

For adverse side effects associated with the use of each specific antibiotic discussed in this chapter, see the Nursing Drug Digest.

PATIENT EDUCATION

The patient and the family, as indicated, should have a clear understanding of the indication for the antibiotic therapy and the course of the therapy, as well as the exact name of the medication, its dosage, action, storage, administration, adverse side effects, and how these can be prevented or minimized. They should understand how to monitor for the therapeutic effect and be able to identify symptoms that indicate the health care provider should be notified. Patients, especially those who are responsible for drug therapy at home, must understand the importance of following the medication plan as prescribed and not discontinuing the medication because they are feeling better. For respective medications, patient education must be carefully individualized. For medications such as clindamycin, a serious relapse of colitis has occurred up to 1 month after the treatment was discontinued. The importance of follow-up cannot be overemphasized, and patients should be instructed to report any recurrent attacks of diarrhea, or other effects related to specific agents, to their health care provider to prevent serious sequelae. Patient education regarding the prevention of infection may also be indicated depending on the indication for antibiotic therapy.

See General Instructions for Discharge/ Outpatients, the text of this chapter, and the Nursing Drug Digest for specific information that should be included in discharge planning or in hospital education as related to the use of each agent.

MISCELLANEOUS ANTIBIOTICS

This drug is an antibiotic. It is used to treat or prevent infections. If you do not understand why you require this medication, contact your health care provider.

Take this medication exactly as prescribed and follow the directions on the prescription label. If you have any questions about how this medication should be taken contact your health care provider.

Some medicines work better if they are taken with a full glass of water on an empty stomach. Other drugs are best taken with meals or a snack to prevent stomach upset. Check with your health care provider regarding how you should take this medication.

Take this medication as directed until it is finished or until your health care provider tells you it is no longer needed. If you have any of the medication left over, flush it down the toilet. Do *not* save it for treating another infection later. Outdated antibiotics can cause harmful and unwanted effects.

If you forget to take a dose, take the dose as soon as you realize that you have missed a dose, then take the medication at the same time as before unless told otherwise by your health care provider.

Any medication can cause unwanted side effects. You may notice some side effects when taking this medication, such as stomach upset or diarrhea. If the side effects persist or become bothersome or severe, contact your health care provider immediately.

While you are taking this medication, call your health care provider if you develop a black, furry appearance to your tongue or white patches in your mouth. Women may notice vaginal itching or an unusual vaginal discharge or anal itching. These signs may indicate an overgrowth of nonsusceptible organisms or a superinfection. Your health care provider can assist you with these troublesome, but treatable, effects.

Do not take any other prescription or nonprescription drugs without calling your health care provider. Antibiotics can interact with other antibiotics or other types of drugs and can cause unwanted or harmful effects.

Stop taking this medication if you develop itching, hives, a skin rash, fever, or chills, and notify your health care provider immediately. If you cannot contact your health care provider, call your nearest emergency department and explain you have been taking this medication and have developed these signs. These signs may indicate an allergic reaction. The emergency personnel will tell you what to do next.

Do not trade this medication with your family or friends or give it to any one else. It was prescribed especially for you.

Store this medication as directed on the label. Keep this and all other medication out of the reach of children.

NURSING DRUG DIGEST

Medication (trade name*)	Indication	Usual dosage and administration	Dosage forms, preparation, and storage	Contraindications, cautions, and comments	Monitoring
Bacitracin Alba-3 Ointment* Baciquent Ointment Baciquent Ophthalmic* Bacitin BPN Ointment* Clinicydin* Cortisporin Ointment* Cortisporin Ointment Ophthalmic* Mycitracin* Neo-Polycin* Neosporin* Polysporin Ophthalmic* Topitracin Triple Antibiotic Ointment*	Topical infections caused by susceptible gram-positive organisms	*Adults:* Apply topically as necessary 1-6 times/day *Children:* Same as adults Do *not* apply to largely denuded areas of skin because systemic absorption and toxicity may result	Injectable: 10,000, 50,000 units/vial Ointment (ophthalmic): 500 units/gm Ointment (topical): 500 units/gm	Hypersensitivity to bacitracin is uncommon even with repeated courses of therapy May cause renal failure the result of tubular and glomerular necrosis with IM use	Monitor for decreased renal function (e.g., increased BUN and serum creatinine, decreased urine output) and for renal toxicity (early signs include slight albuminuria and granular casts in the urine)
	Systemic infections caused by sensitive organisms *not* susceptible to other less toxic drugs NOTE: It is recommended that systemic use be limited to hospitalized infants with staphylococcal pneumonia and empyema	*Children:* 1000 units/kg/24 hr IM in 2-4 divided doses May cause pain at IM injection site Do *not* administer IV	Topical solutions are prepared by dissolving the powder in sterile water for injection or sodium chloride for injection to yield a concentration of 500-1000 units/ml (250 units/ml for ophthalmic use) Parenteral solutions for IM administration are prepared by dissolving the powder in sodium chloride for injection *with 2% procaine* added to yield a concentration of 5000 to 10,000 units/ml Refrigerate reconstituted solution	Use with caution in patients with reduced renal function Maintain adequate fluid intake	Observe for the possibility of superinfection caused by the overgrowth of nonsusceptible organisms, particularly *Monilia*
Chloramphenicol Alficetyn Amphichlor Amphicol Chlomin Chloromycetin Chloromyxin Chloroptic Chloroptic S.O.P.	Topical infections caused by susceptible organisms	*Adults:* Ophthalmic preparations may be applied to the conjunctival sac q.3-4h. as required Otic solutions (2-4 drops) should be instilled into the external ear canal b.i.d. to t.i.d. Topical creams and ointments may be applied t.i.d. to q.i.d. as required *Children:* Same as adults	Ophthalmic ointment: 10 mg/gm Ophthalmic solution: 5 mg/ml Otic solution: 0.5% Topical cream: 1% Topical ointment: 1% Suspension: 125 mg/4 ml Capsules: 50, 100, 250 mg Injectable: 1 gm For parenteral use dissolve contents of one vial (1 gm) in 10 ml of sterile water for injection to yield a concentration of 100 mg/1 ml	*Contraindicated* in hypersensitive patients Topical application to large denuded areas of skin may result in significant systemic absorption and resultant toxicity Use with caution in patients with impaired renal or hepatic function	Monitor for any signs (e.g., vacuolization of the erythroid cells, reduction of reticulocytes, leukopenia) and symptoms of bone marrow depression (e.g., bleeding, fatigue, sore throat), and if any are noted withdraw chloramphenicol immediately and notify the prescriber

Drug	Uses	Dosage	Supplied	Contraindications, Cautions, and Comments	Nursing Considerations
Cylphenicol Econochlor Ophthalmic Elase-Chloromycetin Ointment* Enicol Fenicol Isopto Fenicol Kemicetine Leukomycin Mychel Mycin Nova-Phenicol Ophthalmic Novochlorocap Ophthochlor Pantofenicol Pentamycetin Sopamycetin	Systemic infections caused by susceptible organisms for which chloramphenicol is the drug of choice (*not* for use in trivial infections)	*Adults:* 50-100 mg/kg/24 hr IM or IV in 4 divided doses q.6h. *Children:* Same as adults Decrease dosage in hepatic or renal impairment Monitor blood levels of chloramphenicol and adjust dosage to stay within the optimal therapeutic range of 5-20 μg/ml *Newborn infants:* 25 mg/kg/24 hr IV in 2-4 equally divided doses q.6h. NOTE: after 14 days the full-term infant can receive the normal children's dose See gray syndrome under Contraindications, Cautions, and Comments	Refrigerate reconstituted solution Discard unused solution after 7 days Discard cloudy solutions	The gray syndrome, characterized by abdominal distention, progressive pallid cyanosis, vasomotor collapse, and death has been associated with the administration of chloramphenicol to neonates during the first 48 hours of life; although this syndrome has been linked to excessive chloramphenicol levels in these neonates (>90 μg/ml), it is recommended that this agent generally be *avoided* in premature infants and neonates during the first few days of life May cause aplastic anemia and reversible and irreversible bone marrow depression	Monitor neonates closely for signs of the gray baby syndrome; also monitor blood levels closely to be sure that they remain in the therapeutic range (especially for neonates) Observe for possibility of superinfection caused by the growth of nonsusceptible organisms, including fungi
Clindamycin Cleocin Dalacin C Sobelin	Treatment of serious infections caused by sensitive anaerobic bacteria and in treating serious infections caused by sensitive gram-positive bacteria when other appropriate antibiotics *cannot* be used Topical treatment of acne vulgaris	*Adults:* 150-450 mg PO, IM, IV q.6h. Maximum: 4.8 gm/24 hr IV; or 600 mg single IM injection *Children:* Over 1 month of age, 8-20 mg/kg/24 hr PO in 3-4 equal doses Administer with a glassful of water to avoid possibility of esophageal irritation Administration with food or milk does *not* effect absorption and may decrease GI irritation Apply a thin coat of the topical solution to affected areas b.i.d. The topical solution is for *external* use only	Capsule: 75, 150 mg Injectable: 300 mg/2 ml, 600 mg/4 ml Oral solution: After reconstitution with water each 5 ml of oral solution contains 75 mg clindamycin Reconstituted solution is stable for 14 days at room temperature Do *not* refrigerate reconstituted solution, because it may thicken and become difficult to pour and administer Topical solution: 10 mg/ml	*Contraindicated* in hypersensitivity to clindamycin GI distress may occur in up to 3% of patients May occasionally cause mild to moderate generalized morbilliform-like skin rash May cause severe or persistent diarrhea, which has resulted in colitis Topical solution contains alcohol, which may irritate eyes and mucous membranes	Monitor culture and sensitivity results Observe for diarrhea; if chronic or significant diarrhea is observed clindamycin should be discontinued and the prescriber notified

Continued.

NOTE: For additional details regarding the individual agents listed in this table see the text and other tables in this chapter.

*Indicates a multiple active ingredient product. For a complete listing of all active ingredients see the *Drug Reference Guide to Brand Names and Active Ingredients.*

♣ Indicates that the drug is generally available only in Canada.

★ Indicates that the drug is generally available only in the United States.

NURSING DRUG DIGEST—cont'd

Medication (trade name)	Indication	Usual dosage and administration	Dosage forms, preparation, and storage	Contraindications, cautions, and comments	Monitoring
Colistimethate Coly-Mycin M Parenteral	Infections caused by sensitive gram-negative organisms	*Adults:* 2.5 mg/kg/24 hr IM or IV divided in 2-4 equal doses Maximum: 5 mg/kg/24 hr *Reduce dose* in renal impairment because significant amount is excreted unchanged in the urine *Children:* Same as adults Aerosol use *Adults:* 25-50 mg administered by nebulizer or IPPB b.i.d. to t.i.d. *Children:* 2-15 mg administered by nebulizer or IPPB b.i.d. to q.i.d.	Injectable: 150 mg For IM/IV use, dissolve contents of vial in 2 ml of sterile water for injection After reconstitution each ml contains 75 mg of colistimethate For *aerosol* use dissolve contents of vial in 1-2 ml NS or D₅W *Discard* unused solution after 24 hours	*Contraindicated* in hypersensitivity Use with *extreme* caution in combination with other drugs that may cause neuromuscular blockade, because respiratory arrest may occur Nephrotoxicity may occur and appears to be dose dependent	Monitor renal function for changes that will necessitate a reduction in colistimethate dosage Monitor respiratory status Observe for possibility of superinfection caused by the overgrowth of nonsusceptible organisms
★ **Colistin** Coly-Mycin S Coly-Mycin S Otic*	Gastroenteritis and enterocolitis caused by sensitive organisms, usually including *Escherichia coli* and *Shigella*	*Children:* 5-15 mg/kg/24 hr PO in 3 equally divided doses Reduce dosage in renal impairment	Oral suspension: 300 mg bottle Reconstitute with 37 ml of distilled water to yield 25 mg/5 ml Store reconstituted suspension at room temperature Shake suspension well before withdrawing dose Discard any unused reconstituted suspension after 14 days	*Contraindicated* in hypersensitivity Nephrotoxicity may occur with high doses, particularly in the presence of azotemia Oral dose is *not* significantly absorbed Adverse effects are usually minimal	Observe for possibility of superinfection caused by the overgrowth of nonsusceptible organisms Monitor renal function for changes that will necessitate a reduction in colistin dosage

Co-trimoxazole (trimethoprim and sulfamethoxazole in a 1:5 ratio)
Apo-Sulfatrim
Bactrim
Bactrim-DS
Novotrimel
Protrin
Septra
Septra-DS
Septran
SMZ-TMP
Trib
NOTE: *DS stands for double strength*

Infections caused by susceptible gram-negative and gram-positive organisms

Adults: 2-3 adult tablets PO b.i.d., morning and evening
Children: Under 2 years of age, 2.5 ml pediatric suspension PO b.i.d., morning and evening; 2-5 years of age, 1-2 pediatric tablets PO or 2.5-5 ml pediatric suspension PO b.i.d., morning and evening; 6-12 years of age, 2-4 pediatric tablets PO or 5-10 ml pediatric suspension PO b.i.d., morning and evening; over 12 years of age, same as adult dose
NOTE: Children's dose corresponds to approximately 6 mg/kg/24 hr of trimethoprim and 30 mg/kg/24 hr of sulfamethoxazole
For certain acute infections (e.g., salmonellosis or *P. carinii* pneumonitis) higher pediatric doses on the order of 20 mg/kg/24 hr of trimethoprim and 100 mg/kg/24 hr of sulfamethoxazole may be required
Reduce dosage in renal impairment
Administer with a glassful of water
IV: Used when PO route is contraindicated, as well as in certain specified infections (e.g., *Pneumocystis carinii* pneumonitis)
Administer by IV drip over 60-90 min
Do *not* administer IM

Pediatric suspension: 40 mg trimethoprim and 200 mg sulfamethoxazole/5 ml
Pediatric tablets: 20 mg trimethoprim and 100 mg sulfamethoxazole
Adult tablets: 80 mg trimethoprim and 400 mg sulfamethoxazole
Double strength (DS) tablets: 160 mg trimethoprim and 800 mg sulfamethoxazole
Injectable: 80 mg trimethoprim and 400 mg sulfamethoxazole/5 ml ampule (for IV infusion)
Dilute parenteral form in D₅W, NS, or Ringer's solution (usually 75-150 ml/5 ml ampule) before administration
Store diluted solution at room temperature and start infusion within 1 hour of dilution

Contraindicated in hypersensitivity to either of the two components of co-trimoxazole, severe renal (serum creatinine > 2 mg/100 ml) or hepatic impairment, neonates, and pregnancy
Often causes GI distress
Excreted in breast milk and use should be avoided in nursing mothers
May cause rash and dermatitis

Monitor for neutropenia and thrombocytopenia, particularly in elderly patients
Monitor laboratory culture and sensitivity reports

Continued.

NURSING DRUG DIGEST—cont'd

Medication (trade name)	Indication	Usual dosage and administration	Dosage forms, preparation, and storage	Contraindications, cautions, and comments	Monitoring
Erythromycin Dowmycin E E-Mycin Erymycin Erythrocin Erythrogran Erythroguent Erythromid Ilosone Ilotycin Novorythro Pediamycin Pfizer-E Revrocin Robimycin RP-Mycin SK-Erythromycin Staticin* Wyamycin	Mild to moderate infections caused by susceptible organisms	*Adults:* 250 mg PO q.6h. (1 hr before or 2 hr after meals) In severe infections or when the oral form is not tolerated, 10-20 mg/kg/24 hr may be administered by continuous infusion or in equally divided doses by slow IV (over 20-60 min) q.6h. May cause irritation, pain, and thrombophlebitis at IV injection site *Children:* 30-50 mg/kg/24 hr PO divided in 4 equal doses (1 hr before or 2 hr after meals); parenteral dose is same as adult Do *not* administer PO with acidic fluids (e.g., orange or tomato juice) because erythromycin (except for the estolate salt) may be inactivated in an acidic environment NOTE: Although food decreases the GI absorption of some PO forms (e.g., stearate salt), may need to be administered with meals to reduce GI distress Erythromycin is also applied locally in the treatment of acne vulgaris	Tablets: 250, 500 mg Tablets, chewable: 125, 250 mg Capsules: 125, 250 mg Suspension: 125, 250, 400 mg/5 ml Injectable: 250, 500, 1000 mg/vial For IV use add 10 ml of sterile water for injection (*without* preservatives) to the 250 mg or 500 mg vial (20 ml to the 1000 mg vial) Store the reconstituted solution in the refrigerator Discard any unused reconstituted solution after 7 days For continuous infusion further dilute reconstituted solution with NS or D₅W to yield 1 gm/L The diluted solution is stable for 4 hr	*Contraindicated* in hypersensitivity and severe liver dysfunction or disease Commonly causes GI distress, including abdominal pain, cramping, diarrhea, nausea, and vomiting Various salts and the free base form of erythromycin are available Therapeutically, the different salts are equivalent except for the apparent higher incidence of intrahepatic cholestasis associated with the estolate salt; it is thus recommended that the estolate salt form of erythromycin *not* be used	Observe for possibility of superinfection caused by the over growth of nonsusceptible organisms
Fusidic acid (fusidic acid hemihydrate, sodium fusidate; diethanolamine fusidate) Fucidin	Infections caused by susceptible gram-positive organisms, particularly *Staphylococcus aureus* and *Neisseria* species	*Adults:* 500 mg PO q.8h. or by IV infusion, in a wide-bore vein with good blood flow, over 6-8 hr NOTE: Because of incomplete absorption of the suspension (i.e., 70%), the adult PO dose of the suspension is 15 ml	Tablet: 240 mg (250 mg sodium fusidate) Suspension: 246 mg/5 ml Injectable: 482 mg (580 mg diethanolamine fusidate) Each package of IV vials contains one 50 ml vial containing 482 mg fusidic acid and one vial containing 50 ml sterile phosphate-citrate buffer (pH 7.4-7.6) for use as diluent	*Contraindicated* in hypersensitivity to fusidic acid or its salts Commonly causes GI distress, which is usually mild but may necessitate discontinuation of therapy in up to 2% of patients	Monitor culture and sensitivity test reports for the development of bacterial resistance to fusidic acid Monitor hepatic function regularly, and decrease the dose if *any* impairment is noted

Uses	Dosage	Preparations	Nursing considerations
Topical infections caused by susceptible organisms	Rapid IV administration may result in venospasm and thrombophlebitis Children: 1-5 years of age, 5 ml of suspension PO q.8h.; 6-12 years of age, 10 ml of suspension PO q.8h.; or (for all ages) 20 mg/kg/24 hr IV in 3 divided doses infused over 6-8 hr period Decrease dose in hepatic impairment No dose adjustment is necessary for renal impairment Do not administer IM or SC, because tissue injury may occur Administration of oral preparations with food or milk may decrease GI distress Adults: Apply a small amount of cream or ointment to lesion t.i.d. to q.i.d. as indicated Children: Same as adults	Each reconstituted package should be further diluted with 500 ml of plasma, D$_5$W, D$_{10}$W, or sodium chloride for injection Do not dilute with amino acid solutions or whole blood (because of risk of hemolysis of the erythrocytes) Discard any cloudy or opaque reconstituted solutions Cream: 2% Ointment: 2% Gauze impregnated with ointment (2%)	Fusidic acid is excreted mainly in the bile May need to decrease dose when administered concurrently with other drugs that are also excreted in the bile (e.g., lincomycin, rifampin) Because fusidic acid is highly protein bound (>97%), the dose may need to be reduced when other highly protein-bound drugs (e.g., phenylbutazone) are administered concurrently Use with caution in patients with hepatic dysfunction
Gramicidin Cortisporin Cream* Gramoderm* Kenacomb* Myco Triacet Cream and Ointment* Mycolog* Mytrox* Neosporin-G Cream* Nysolone* Polysporin* Spectrocin* Tricilone NMG* Topical infections caused by susceptible gram-positive organisms	Adults: Apply topically 2-6 times daily as indicated Children: Same as adults Do not apply to large areas of abraded or denuded skin because systemic absorption may occur For external use only	Available in a variety of strengths in cream and ointment formulations, generally in combination products	Contraindicated in hypersensitivity May cause hepatic and renal damage if absorbed from the topical site Usually found in combination antibiotic ointments and creams May cause local irritation or allergic reaction Not for use in nose, ears, eyes, or closed body cavities Because of severe renal and hepatic toxicity if parenterally administered, gramicidin is limited to topical use only Observe for local irritation or allergic reaction

Continued.

NURSING DRUG DIGEST—cont'd

Medication (trade name)	Indication	Usual dosage and administration	Dosage forms, preparation, and storage	Contraindications, cautions, and comments	Monitoring
Lincomycin Cillimycin Lincocin Mycivin	Serious infections caused by susceptible gram-positive organisms when other appropriate antibiotics cannot be used	*Adults:* 500-600 mg PO, IM, IV q.8-12h. NOTE: IV dose should be diluted with a minimum 250 ml D$_5$W or NS and infused over 30-120 min Maximum: 8.4 gms/24 hr *Children:* (over 1 month of age) 10-20 mg/kg/24 hr as single IM injection, *or* IV in 2-3 equally divided doses or IV administered as for adults; *or* 30-60 mg/kg/24 hr PO in 3-4 equally divided doses May need to decrease dose in renal impairment	Capsules: 250, 500 mg Injectable: 300 mg/ml Syrup: 250 mg/5 ml	*Contraindicated* in hypersensitivity, in patients with monilial infections, and in newborns May cause severe and persistent diarrhea, which occasionally results in colitis Not usually a drug of first choice, but it is useful in certain cases when the drug of first choice cannot be used (e.g., penicillin allergy) Rapid IV infusion may cause hypotension	Monitor for severe or persistent diarrhea; if observed, discontinue lincomycin and notify the prescriber Observe for the possibility of superinfection caused by the growth of nonsusceptible organisms Monitor blood pressure for hypotension during parenteral administration
★ **Novobiocin** Albamycin Cardelmycin Cathomycin Inamycin	Serious infections caused by susceptible organisms when safer medications cannot be used	*Adults:* 250-500 mg PO q.6-12h. *Children:* 15-45 mg/kg/24 hr PO in 4 equally divided doses q.6h. Administer with a glassful of water NOTE: Parenteral administration can be used as a *temporary* measure when the oral route cannot be used *Adults:* 500 mg IM or IV infusion q.12h. *Children:* 15-30 mg/kg/24 hr IM or IV infusion in 2 equally divided doses q.12h.	Capsule: 250 mg Syrup: 125 mg/5 ml Injectable: 500 mg/vial with 5 ml diluent For IM use, the 500 mg may be reconstituted with the provided diluent For IV use, the 500 mg may be reconstituted with the provided diluent and then further diluted to 250-3000 ml with sodium chloride solution or Ringer's solution, depending on the rate of administration and the patient's fluid and salt requirements	*Contraindicated* in hypersensitivity and in newborn infants Excreted in breast milk; use should probably be avoided in nursing mothers May cause neonatal hyperbilirubinemia Development of resistant strains of organisms, particularly staphylococci, may occur with prolonged use Often causes allergic reactions, including fever, pruritus, skin rash, and urticaria	Monitor culture and sensitivity test results for the development of bacterial resistance to novobiocin Observe for any allergic reactions Monitor for symptoms of blood dyscrasias (e.g., anemia, bleeding, leukopenia)

Drug	Uses	Dosage	Remarks	Nursing Considerations
		Continuous IV infusion is *preferred*; however, when necessary the 5 ml of reconstituted solution containing 500 mg may be further diluted to a total of 30 ml and administered by slow IV over 10 min Rapid IV administration may cause pain and thrombophlebitis May cause pain at injection site	NOTE: *Do not* use dextrose solutions because they are uncompatible with novobiocin	May cause blood dyscrasias
Polymyxin B Aerosporin Alba-3 Ointment* Clinicydin* Cortisporin Cream* Cortisporin Ointment* Lidosporin Otic Solution* Neo-Polycin* Neosporin* Neosporin-G Cream* Neotal* Otocort Ear Drops* Polysporin* Polysporin Ophthalmic* Terramycin Ointment* Terramycin Ophthalmic* Terramycin Vaginal*	Systemic infections caused by susceptible gram-negative bacilli *P. aeruginosa* meningitis Topical infections caused by susceptible strains of *P. aeruginosa*	*Adults:* 15,000-25,000 units/kg/24 hr in 2 equally divided IV infusions or 4 equally divided IM injections IM use is *not* recommended because of severe pain at the injection site *Children:* Same as adults Intrathecal: 50,000 units/24 hr in a single intrathecal injection for 3-4 days, followed by 50,000 units/24 hr every other day for at least 14 days following negative results of cerebrospinal fluid culture *Children:* Over 2 years of age, same as adults *Adults:* Apply topically as indicated b.i.d. to q.i.d. *Children:* Same as adults	Injectable: 500,000 units/20 ml vial For IV use dissolve 500,000 units polymyxin B in 300-500 ml D₅W For IM use dissolve 500,000 units polymyxin B in 2 ml sterile water for injection, sodium chloride for injection, or 1% procaine hydrochloride solution For intrathecal use dissolve 500,000 units polymyxin B in 10 ml sodium chloride for injection Reconstituted solutions for parenteral use should be refrigerated Discard any unused solution after 72 hr Available in combination form in various creams and ointments	*Contraindicated* in hypersensitivity to any of the polymyxins May cause nephrotoxicity; may cause neurotoxicity Use with caution in patients with myasthenia gravis May cause severe pain at IM injection site Monitor for signs of nephrotoxicity (e.g., albuminuria, azotemia, cylindruria) Monitor for signs of neurotoxicity (e.g., apnea, ataxia, dizziness, fever)

Continued.

NURSING DRUG DIGEST—cont'd

Medication (trade name)	Indication	Usual dosage and administration	Dosage forms, preparation, and storage	Contraindications, cautions, and comments	Monitoring
Spectinomycin Trobicin	Acute penicillin-resistant gonorrheal urethritis, cervicitis, or proctitis, and for the treatment of acute gonorrhea in patients allergic to penicillin Disseminated gonococcal infections caused by penicillinase-producing *Neisseria gonorrhoeae*	*Adults:* Men 2 gm IM as single dose into upper outer quadrant of the gluteal muscle; women 4 gm IM as single dose into upper outer quadrant of the gluteal muscle or equally divided between two gluteal injection sites *Adults:* 2 gm IM b.i.d. for 3 days Do *not* administer IV	Injectable: 2 gm with 3.5 ml ampule of bacteriostatic water for injection; and 4 gm with 6.2 ml ampule of bacteriostatic water for injection When reconstituted, yields a concentration of 400 mg/ml Reconstituted suspension should be stored at room temperature Shake reconstituted suspension well before withdrawing dose Discard any unused suspension after 24 hr	*Contraindicated* in hypersensitivity *Not* effective for treatment of syphilis May mask or delay symptoms of incubating syphilis Discomfort at IM injection site is usually minimal	Observe serologic test results monthly (for 3 months) for symptoms of incubating syphilis
★ **Troleandomycin** Cyclamycin Olicin Tao	Severe infections caused by susceptible strains of *Clostridium*, *Corynebacterium*, pneumococci, staphylococci, and streptococci	*Adults:* 250-500 mg PO q.6h. *Children:* 125-250 mg (6.5-11 mg/kg) PO q.6h. NOTE: Duration of therapy is usually 10 days Administer with a glassful of water May need to decrease dose in hepatic impairment	Capsule: 250 mg Suspension: 125 mg/5 ml	*Contraindicated* in hypersensitivity and in severe hepatic dysfunction May cause hepatic toxicity Commonly causes GI distress	Observe for possible superinfections caused by the overgrowth of nonsusceptible organisms Monitor for signs of hepatic toxicity, including hyperbilirubinemia and jaundice (particularly when therapy continues for more than 10 days); if observed, discontinue the drug and notify the prescriber

| Vancomycin Vancocin | Severe staphylococcal infections *not* treatable with other less toxic antibiotics | *Adults:* 500 mg IV (infused over a period of 20-30 min) *Children:* 45 mg/kg/24 hr IV divided in 4 equal doses *Elderly:* Use reduced dosage Reduce dosage in renal impairment Do *not* administer IM For IV use, dissolve contents of one ampule (500 mg) in 10 ml of sterile water for injection and further dilute with 100-200 ml NS or D$_5$W before infusion | Injectable: 500 mg Powder for oral solution: 10 gm Prepare powder for oral solution by mixing with 115 ml of purified water to yield 500 mg/6 ml Refrigerate reconstituted solution | Monitor for signs of nephrotoxicity (e.g., albuminuria, azotemia), particularly in elderly patients Monitor for signs of ototoxicity (e.g., tinnitus, hearing loss), particularly in elderly patients Observe for possible superinfection caused by the overgrowth of nonsusceptible organisms |
| | Treatment of staphylococcal enterocolitis | *Adults:* 500 mg PO (by mouth or nasogastric tube) q.6h. *Children:* 45 mg/kg/24 hr PO in 4 equally divided doses For PO use, dissolve contents of one ampule (500 mg) in 30 ml of water and administer orally or by nasogastric tube (or use powder for oral solution) | Prepared solution is stable for 1 week under refrigeration | *Contraindicated* in hypersensivity and in severe renal dysfunction Risk of ototoxicity and nephrotoxicity are increased by prolonged use and high blood concentrations May cause pain and thrombophlebitis at IV injection site Rapid IV administration may cause hypotension |

BIBLIOGRAPHY

Bernstein, G., Davis, J., & Katcher, M. Prophylaxis of neonatal conjunctivitis. *Clinical Pediatrics*, 1982, *21*, 545-550.

Kucers, A. Good antimicrobial prescribing: chloramphenicol, erythromycin, vancomycin, tetracyclines. *Lancet*, 1982, *2*, 425-429.

Marks, M.I., & Laferriere, C. Chloramphenicol: recent developments and clinical indications. *Clinical Pharmacy*, 1982, *1*, 315-320.

Newton, M., Gilbert, G.P., & Newton, D.W. Parenteral antibiotics: the hazards to watch for. *RN*, 1981, *44*, 45-51.

Powell, D.A., & Nahata, M.C. Chloramphenicol: new perspectives on an old drug. *Drug Intelligence and Clinical Pharmacy*, 1982, *16*, 295-300.

Schumacher, G.E. Pharmacokinetic and microbiologic evaluation of antibiotic dosage regimens. *Clinical Pharmacy*, 1982, *1*, 66-75.

Schwartz, J., Swanson, L., & Bartle, B. Anti-infective therapy—clinical perspective of erythromycin. *On Continuing Practice*, 1982, *9*, 26-31.

Stiklorius, C. A safe approach to IV antibiotics. *RN*, 1981, *44*, 37-39.

CHAPTER 49

Sulfonamides

Randall A. Prince

Medications discussed in this chapter

Systemically available sulfonamides	Systemically available sulfonamides—cont'd
Short-acting	Long-acting
Sulfacytine	Sulfamerazine
Sulfamethazine	*Special-use sulfonamides*
Sulfamethizole	Topical sulfonamides
Sulfisoxazole	Mafenide
Intermediate-acting	Silver sulfadiazine
Sulfadiazine	Sulfacetamide
Sulfamethoxazole	Miscellaneous
Sulfapyridine	Sulfasalazine

In 1935, Dogmagk discovered the chemotherapeutic value of an azo dye, prontosil. Mice given this compound were protected from developing streptococcal infections. Later it was discovered that prontosil was broken down in vivo to sulfanilamide, the compound responsible for the antibacterial activity of prontosil. These discoveries marked the birth of the first effective antibacterial agent to be used systemically for bacterial infections in humans. Over the years, numerous compounds were developed by modifying the chemical structure of sulfanilamide. These compounds are generally referred to as *sulfonamides.*

MECHANISM OF ACTION

The antibacterial activity of the sulfonamides rests with their ability to compete with para-aminobenzoic acid (PABA) in the folic acid synthesis pathway of certain microorganisms. Only microorganisms that cannot use preformed folic acid are susceptible to the sulfonamides. The structural similarity of PABA and the sulfonamides allows the sulfonamides to act as competitive substrates, thereby blocking the conversion of PABA to folic acid (Figure 49-1). By blocking the production of folic acid, a disruption of chemical pathways ultimately necessary for the synthesis of DNA occurs. The resultant action of the sulfonamides on susceptible microorganisms (i.e., production of folate deficiency) is bacteriostatic.

The sulfonamides act synergistically with several other antibacterials, but most notably with the agent trimethoprim (see Chapter 48, "Miscellaneous Antibiotics"). The combination of a sulfonamide and trimethoprim produces sequential blocks in bacterial folate synthesis (Figure 49-1). The combined effect is bactericidal for many organisms rather than bacteriostatic, as is seen when each agent is used alone. In addition, the sulfonamides may potentiate the antibacterial effects of penicillin and the polymyxins, and the antiprotozoal activity of pyrimethamine.

Purulent drainage and PABA are significant inhibitors of sulfonamide activity. The presence of purines and thymidine in purulent drainage from tissue breakdown lessens the bacterium's need for folic acid precursors, thereby potentially maintaining bacterial growth. The addition of PABA to culture media or clinical specimens will antagonize the antibacterial effect of the sulfonamides. Additionally, the administration of medications that are PABA derivatives, such as certain local anesthetics, may antagonize the sulfonamide effect.

SPECTRUM OF ANTIMICROBIAL ACTIVITY

In vitro susceptibility to the sulfonamides is reliably noted for *Streptococcus pneumoniae, Streptococcus pyogenes, Haemophilus influenzae, Haemophilus ducreyi, Yersinia pestis, Pseudomonas pseudomallei, Escherichia coli, Nocardia* species, *Vibrio cholerae, Chlamydia trachomatis, Corynebacterium diphtheriae, Bacillus anthracis,* and *Actinomyces israelii.* Resistance to the sulfonamides is commonly reported for *Neisseria meningitidis* (serogroups B and C), *Neis-*

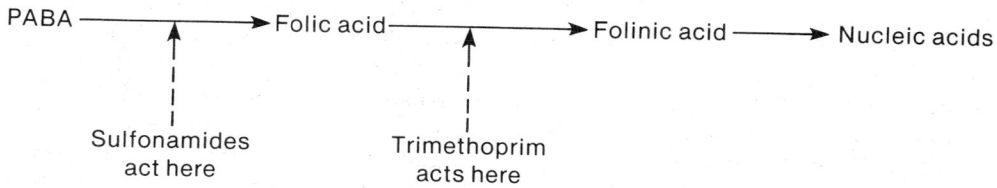

FIGURE 49-1. **Sites of action of sulfonamides and trimethoprim.**

seria gonorrhoeae, Shigella flexneri, and *Shigella sonnei.*

Aside from the organisms able to use preformed folic acid, bacterial resistance develops primarily as a result of increased PABA synthesis by bacteria. The resultant increased production of PABA by the bacteria antagonizes the sulfonamide action. Because this mechanism for *bacterial resistance* is not universally observed, other resistance mechanisms suggesting a change in bacterial enzyme function in some fashion have been proposed. Regardless of the mechanism responsible for the resistance development, the sulfonamides have fallen victim to widespread resistance, thereby limiting their clinical use. If resistance is noted to a particular sulfonamide, resistance is implied for the entire class of the sulfonamides.

CLASSIFICATION

There are a variety of ways in which to classify the systemically available sulfonamides. The simplest and possibly the most relevant way is based on the rate of bodily elimination (i.e., elimination half-life [$T_{1/2}$]). This classification labels the sulfonamides as short acting, intermediate acting, or long acting with corresponding half-lives of 4 to 8 hours, 8 to 16 hours, and greater than 16 hours. The short-acting sulfonamides are sulfisoxazole, sulfacytine, and sulfamethizole; the intermediate-acting are sulfamethoxazole, sulfadiazine, and sulfapyridine. Some clinicians would include an ultrashort and ultralong class as well. Indeed, sulfamethizole is an ultrashort-acting sulfonamide ($T_{1/2} = 2$ hours. Of the sulfonamides used for systemic infections in the United States, all are either short or intermediate acting, with the exception of sulfamerazine, a long-acting sulfonamide present in sulfonamide combination products. In addition to the systemic sulfonamides, there is a category of agents that shall be referred to as special-use sulfonamides.

These agents are mafenide, silver sulfadiazine, sulfasalazine, and sulfacetamide.

SOLUBILITY

It is somewhat unusual that the first sulfonamide, sulfanilamide, was not influenced greatly by pH for solubility; yet the subsequent derivatives depend on pH for solubility. Because of this dependency, some authors classify sulfonamides based on their solubility at a commonly encountered urine pH. Poor urine solubility of a sulfonamide or its metabolites could lead to crystallization and possible renal toxicity. This is likely to occur when the urine concentration of the sulfonamide exceeds the urinary solubility. A poorly soluble sulfonamide, sulfadiazine, has solubilities of 950 μg/ml and 265 μg/ml at pH 7 and 5.5, respectively. Sulfisoxazole, a highly soluble sulfonamide, has solubilities of 4724 μg/ml and 1533 μg/ml at pH 7 and 5.5, respectively. The metabolites of sulfonamides are generally less soluble than the parent compound, with the exception of sulfapyridine and sulfadiazine.

In the early years of sulfonamide therapy, renal complications caused by the poor solubility of available agents were commonly encountered. Attempts at increasing solubility, using alkalinization or increased hydration, were either not commonly instituted or failed to prevent the complication. It was then shown that the sulfonamides could be mixed together while maintaining their individual solubilities. Antibacterial effectiveness was maintained because the individual antibacterial activities are additive. Therefore, the sulfonamide mixtures could possess a therapeutic efficacy with less risk of crystallization. Since the advent of the highly soluble sulfonamides (e.g., sulfisoxazole), mixtures of the sulfonamides are little used today. Most of the available preparations are combinations of sulfadiazine, sulfamerazine, and sulfamethazine, and are referred to as triple sulfonamides.

PROTEIN BINDING

Sulfonamides are weakly bound to albumin to varying degrees. Sulfisoxazole is greater than 85% bound, whereas sulfadiazine is 40% to 60% bound. The bound fraction of the drug is microbiologically inactive; however, the clinical importance of the dynamics between the bound and unbound fractions is controversial. Reduced protein binding may be found in patients with renal failure, thereby increasing the risk of some adverse effects caused by elevated levels of active drug.

PHARMACOKINETICS

Absorption of the sulfonamides is generally rapid and complete. Peak blood levels are usually attained within 2 to 4 hours after oral administration. Almost all of the administered sulfonamide dose can be recovered in the urine as the parent compound and its metabolite.

The sulfonamides are widely distributed to various tissues and fluids of the body. Penetration into saliva, aqueous humor, bile, prostatic tissue and fluid, and lung tissue has been reported. Cerebrospinal fluid (CSF) levels vary considerably with the sulfonamides. Sulfisoxazole CSF concentrations are 10% to 20% of the corresponding serum concentrations, whereas sulfadiazine CSF levels are at least 50% that of serum levels. Various sulfonamides have been shown to readily cross the human placenta. Concentrations in cord blood are usually higher than in the amniotic fluid. Cord levels greater than 50% of the corresponding maternal blood levels have been reported for sulfadiazine and sulfamethoxazole. The passage of the sulfonamides into human milk occurs, with predicted levels of the sulfonamides being at least 50% of the corresponding blood levels. A notable exception is sulfisoxazole, which attains milk levels of less than 10% that of the blood levels. Nursing infants are able to efficiently absorb the sulfonamides, thereby exposing themselves to potential toxicities. Although the sulfonamides should not be administered to nursing mothers, sulfisoxazole would appear to offer little risk in the development of kernicterus to nursing infants beyond the newborn period in healthy, full-term neonates.

Metabolism of the sulfonamides occurs predominantly in the liver. The main pathway of metabolism is acetylation, with glucuronidation being of lesser significance. The acetylated metabolites are considered microbiologically inactive; however, these metabolites are actively involved in producing certain adverse reactions (e.g., crystalluria). Additionally, the acetylation of most of the sulfonamides is genetically determined,

with individuals being classified as either fast or slow acetylators. Aside from being responsible for increases in certain adverse effects, acetylator-type differences have, in part, been responsible for discrepancies in the blood and urine sulfonamide concentrations observed in different pharmacologic studies.

Excretion of the sulfonamides and their metabolites is almost entirely done by the kidneys. Glomerular filtration is the primary mechanism; however, both the parent compound and its acetylated derivative undergo tubular secretion. Serum protein binding and urinary pH greatly influence the way in which the kidney handles the sulfonamides and their metabolites. Also, the sulfonamides are reabsorbed by the renal tubules to varying degrees.

CLINICAL PHARMACOLOGY OF SELECTED AGENTS

Sulfisoxazole

Sulfisoxazole is rapidly and completely absorbed after oral and intramuscular administration. Peak blood levels of 121 to 210 µg/ml usually occur 2 hours after the administration of a 2-gm oral or intramuscular dose. An intravenous 2 gm dose will produce higher blood levels averaging 260 µg/ml. The distribution to tissue compartments is rapid, with a volume of distribution ranging from 13% to 20% of body weight. The elimination from the body is relatively rapid, with a half-life of 4.6 to 7.8 hours. The elimination of the drug occurs exclusively via the kidneys, with an average of 54% of a dose excreted as the parent compound. The remainder of the dose is excreted as the microbiologically inactive acetylated derivative. Approximately 28% to 35% of sulfisoxazole is present in the blood as acetylated derivative. Average urinary concentrations of 1000 µg/ml can be achieved with a typical therapeutic regimen.

Up to 85% of sulfisoxazole has been reported to be protein bound, primarily to albumin. This high degree of protein binding may, in part, be responsible for a limited tissue distribution.

Sulfamethoxazole

Peak blood levels of sulfamethoxazole are usually attained in approximately 4 hours after an oral dose. After an 800 mg oral dose, peak blood levels range from 26 to 63 µg/ml. Approximately 65% of this amount is intact sulfamethoxazole. Sulfamethoxazole's volume of distribution is 12 to 18 L, comparable to sulfisoxazole's restricted volume of distribution. Approximately 66% of the drug is bound to plasma proteins.

Sulfamethoxazole is metabolized by acetylation and

glucuronide conjugation in the liver. Approximately 20% and 60% to 80% of the total sulfamethoxazole concentration present in the blood and urine, respectively, is the acetylated derivative.

Its elimination via the kidneys accounts for 95% of an administered dose. Approximately 30% of the total urinary concentration is intact sulfamethoxazole. Although subject to wide variation, the elimination half-life averages 9 hours. After an 800 mg dose, urine concentrations of total sulfonamide average 300 to 450 μg/ml in individuals with normal renal function.

Sulfadiazine

After oral administration, sulfadiazine produces peak blood levels in about 3 hours. A dose of 500 mg will achieve peak levels of 17 to 19 μg/ml. Approximately 90% of a total sulfadiazine blood level is the parent compound.

Sulfadiazine is about 40% to 60% protein bound. Its volume of distribution averages 36% of body weight. The kidneys eliminate sulfadiazine and its metabolites exclusively. Within a 24-hour period, 50% and 22% of a dose can be recovered in the urine for sulfadiazine and its acetylated metabolite, respectively. Its elimination half-life is highly variable and has been reported to range between 9 and 16 hours.

Sulfacytine

Data on sulfacytine are primarily available from the manufacturer, not the literature. Peak blood levels appear in 2 to 3 hours after an oral dose. After repeated dosing of 1 gm orally per day, mean total sulfacytine levels of about 17 μg/ml are attained. Approximately 86% of sulfacytine is protein bound.

Sulfacytine is metabolized in the liver, undergoing acetylation and glucuronide conjugation. It is rapidly cleared from the body by the kidneys, with a half-life of elimination of 4 hours. Following a single oral dose, 88% of the drug is recovered in 24 hours. About 80% of the urine concentrations are intact sulfacytine, with the remainder being the acetylated and conjugated metabolites. After the recommended therapeutic dosing schedule, the mean urinary concentrations of sulfacytine were 419 μg/ml.

Sulfamethizole

Sulfamethizole achieves peak blood level concentrations within 2 hours after oral administration. Peak blood levels of 10 to 20 μg/ml may be expected after a 500 mg oral dose. The acetylation of sulfamethizole is limited, accounting for 3% or less of the total sulfonamide levels. Its volume of distribution is about 35% of body weight and it is about 85% protein bound.

About 80% to 90% of a dose is excreted by the kidneys as the parent compound. It is cleared rapidly by the kidneys, as evidenced by a short half-life of elimination (i.e., 2 hours).

Sulfasalazine

Sulfasalazine is not used as an antibacterial agent per se; however, it consists, in part, of a systemically available sulfonamide, sulfapyridine. Its use is primarily in ulcerative colitis and Crohn's disease. When sulfasalazine is administered orally, bacteria in the colon split it into its main components, a salicylate moiety and sulfapyridine. Because sulfasalazine's mechanism of action is unknown, either of the components may be regarded as active. The sulfapyridine is rapidly absorbed into the blood and undergoes acetylation. It is approximately 60% protein bound, with a distributive volume of 40% of body weight. The acetylator type greatly influences the concentration of acetylated sulfapyridine present in the blood and the urine. About 30% and 60% of the acetylated metabolite is present in the serum of slow and fast acetylators, respectively. Total sulfapyridine serum levels greater than 50 μg/ml correlate well with adverse effects. The elimination half-life of sulfapyridine varies from 5 to 13 hours. Most of a dose of sulfasalazine is recovered in the urine as sulfapyridine and its metabolites (~60%), sulfasalazine (≤15%), and 5-aminosalicylic acid and its metabolites (≤30%).

ADVERSE EFFECTS

The list of adverse effects attributed to the sulfonamides is impressive. Virtually every organ system of the body has been affected in varying degrees, ranging from mild rashes to life-threatening reactions. Overall incidence figures vary from 1% to 15%. A relatively recent prospective study observed a 3% frequency of adverse reactions requiring medication discontinuation for sulfisoxazole and sulfamethoxazole in a hospitalized population.

Hematologic reactions

Although the occurrences are rare, *agranulocytosis, thrombocytopenia, aplastic anemia,* and *hemolytic anemia* have been associated with sulfonamide administration. On a worldwide basis, the sulfonamides—particularly the combination product of sulfamethoxazole and trimethoprim (i.e., co-trimoxazole)—have been leading causes of these hematologic toxicities.

The sulfonamides appear to have a direct toxic effect on the bone marrow. The development of aplasia of the bone marrow with concomitant *pancytopenia* may have a fatal result.

Thrombocytopenia was one of the earliest recognized hematologic abnormalities associated with sulfonamide therapy. There is uncertainty about the mechanism(s) responsible for the reaction, with both an immunologic and a direct bone marrow toxic mechanism being proposed. The combination product, co-trimoxazole, is the leading cause of thrombocytopenia associated with sulfonamide therapy. One study reported only one case of thrombocytopenia out of 1359 uses of sulfisoxazole and sulfamethoxazole in hospitalized patients. Fortunately, the platelet count will usually return to normal in about 2 weeks following sulfonamide discontinuation.

Data from adverse reaction registry groups show that the sulfonamides are the leading reported cause of agranulocytosis and neutropenia. Sulfasalazine and co-trimoxazole are most often implicated. A direct bone marrow toxic effect and an immunologic mechanism have been proposed. Figures vary about the mortality associated with this hematologic picture, but approximately 20% to 50% of cases may be fatal. Once the offending drug has been discontinued in those patients who survive, bone marrow function returns to normal in 2 weeks, but recovery may occasionally be delayed for several weeks.

Most reports list the sulfonamides as the second most common cause of hemolytic anemia, with methyldopa being the most common cause. Sulfonamide-induced hemolysis is most often seen in individuals with a glucose-6-phosphate dehydrogenase (G-6-PD) deficiency. G-6-PD deficiency is most commonly encountered in blacks and people of Mediterranean origin. Deficiency of the red cell enzyme, G-6-PD, ultimately results in hemolysis when an oxidant drug, such as a sulfonamide, is administered. If hemolysis occurs, discontinuation of the sulfonamide is warranted, with complete recovery being usual.

Hemolysis can also occur with sulfonamide therapy in individuals with a glutathione-peroxidase deficiency and certain hemoglobinopathies (e.g., hemoglobin H or hemoglobin Zürich). These aforementioned conditions are rare.

Eosinophilia is a common hematologic reaction occurring in approximately 1% of sulfonamide uses. Although eosinophilia may occur alone, other findings consistent with hypersensitivity phenomena are often seen concomitantly.

Gastrointestinal reactions

A wide variety of gastrointestinal manifestations have been encountered with sulfonamide therapy. It appears that the different sulfonamides have varying frequencies of gastrointestinal side effects. The prominent side effects seen are nausea, vomiting, and anorexia. Abdominal pain, diarrhea, and gastrointestinal bleeding are uncommon observations. Sulfapyridine commonly causes gastrointestinal complaints, whereas sulfisoxazole and sulfamethoxazole are infrequent offenders.

Allergic reactions

Reactions involving the skin are probably the most common adverse effect caused by sulfonamide therapy. The reactions are considered to be hypersensitivity phenomena. The drug eruptions can be relatively mild (e.g., macular or maculopapular rash), or they can be severe and life-threatening (e.g., *Stevens-Johnson syndrome* and *toxic epidermal necrolysis*). Although the frequency of adverse dermal reactions is sulfonamide specific, the more commonly used sulfonamides (e.g., sulfisoxazole and sulfamethoxazole) will cause untoward dermatologic reactions in 2% of patients. The commonly seen reactions are fixed drug eruptions, *urticaria*, and miscellaneous eruptions such as *erythema multiforme, erythema nodosum, angioneurotic edema*, and pruritic and *petechial* eruptions. Photosensitivity reactions occur uncommonly with select sulfonamides. The severe dermatologic reactions, toxic epidermal necrolysis and Stevens-Johnson syndrome, have been almost exclusively caused by the long-acting sulfonamides, particularly sulfamethoxypyridazine and sulfadimethoxine. The long-acting sulfonamides are no longer commercially available in the United States, in part because of the reports of these severe dermatologic reactions. Fortunately, these severe reactions are rare with the available sulfonamides.

Drug fever with or without other concomitant manifestations such as rash, malaise, and pruritus, occurs in 1% to 3% of patients receiving short-acting sulfonamides. The onset of fever is usually in 1 to 2 weeks, but may be seen early in therapy in a previously sensitized patient. Rarely, the fever is accompanied by joint pain, bronchospasm, *leukopenia*, and urticarial eruptions, thereby mimicking a *serum sickness* syndrome.

Vasculitis has been recognized for a long time as a potential adversity to sulfonamide therapy. Although the vascular lesions resemble *periarteritis nodosa*, this drug-induced vasculitis is self-limiting and should improve with drug discontinuation. Sulfonamides have been considered by some authorities to be activators of episodes of periarteritis and *systemic lupus erythematosus* in susceptible individuals as opposed to a direct cause of the disease process. Sulfathiazole and sulfanilamide were most often associated with these adverse reactions; however, sulfisoxazole and sulfamethoxazole have been implicated on rare occasions.

Generally speaking, a patient who has had an allergic reaction to one sulfonamide should not receive any sulfonamide subsequently. Although *cross-sensitivity* is not an absolute certainty, it is best to observe this generalization when possible.

Hepatic reactions

Liver injury is produced by the sulfonamides by an unknown mechanism(s). Because a typical pattern of hypersensitivity reaction (i.e., fever, rash, and eosinophilia) may often precede the onset of jaundice, many consider the reaction an allergic phenomenon. The pathologic picture may be one of hepatocellular necrosis with or without *cholestasis.* Recovery is usual after drug discontinuation; however, liver damage may progress and death may ensue. This *rare* reaction has been reported with many of the sulfonamides, including sulfamethoxazole and sulfisoxazole.

Urinary tract effects

Sulfonamides may cause serious renal complications by means of a variety of mechanisms. Obstructive nephropathy caused by sulfonamide crystallization is the foremost mechanism. Other mechanisms include hypersensitivity reactions, direct toxic effects, and hemoglobin cast precipitation as a result of sulfonamide-induced hemolysis.

Decreased urinary solubility may lead to the formation of crystalline deposits in the calyces, pelvis, ureters, and bladder. Clinically, a typical patient has *hematuria,* crystalluria, *oliguria,* or *anuria* and is *azotemic.* Decreased solubility may result from a poor state of hydration, high concentrations of the sulfonamide and its metabolite in the urine, or the presence of a more acidic urinary pH. The inherently less soluble sulfonamides such as sulfadiazine, sulfathiazole, and sulfapyradine have been the major causes of obstructive nephropathy. The more highly soluble sulfonamides (e.g., sulfisoxazole) cause crystalluria rarely. A prospective study failed to identify any cases of nephropathy with sulfisoxazole or sulfamethoxazole therapy. Maintenance of adequate hydration and elimination of urinary acidifying agents (e.g., high-dose ascorbic acid) is advocated during sulfonamide therapy. Some clinicians recommend urinary alkalinization with sodium bicarbonate during therapy with sulfadiazine, a poorly soluble sulfonamide.

Development of allergic *interstitial nephritis,* direct tubular toxicity, or *hemoglobinuria* with acute renal failure associated with sulfonamide-induced hemolysis in G-6-PD patients is rare.

Miscellaneous reactions

A variety of neuropsychiatric effects have been associated with sulfonamide therapy on occasion. These effects include restlessness, drowsiness, psychosis, dizziness, and depression. Pancreatitis has rarely been seen with sulfonamides.

The sulfonamides have the potential to displace bilirubin from its albumin-binding sites. The development of *kernicterus* because of sulfonamide administration to premature babies, neonates, and pregnant women near term therefore remains plausible. The risk of kernicterus caused by sulfonamide administration in a pregnant woman resulting in placental transfer of the sulfonamide to the baby is debatable. As a general policy, the sulfonamides should *not* be used in these risk groups.

DRUG INTERACTIONS

The sulfonamides have the potential for many drug-drug interactions, primarily by means of competitive protein-binding. Few interactions, however, have been well documented clinically. The major potential problems appear with the concomitant administration of a sulfonamide with oral anticoagulants, hypoglycemic agents (e.g., tolbutamide and chlorpropamide), and phenytoin. The sulfonamide in each case will augment the clinical effect of the drug, possibly leading to overt toxicity. Although the generic term *sulfonamide* is used here for labeling purposes, sulfonamide drug interactions are caused only by certain sulfonamides. Either sulfisoxazole or sulfamethoxazole have been implicated in the drug interactions mentioned in this section.

Certain laboratory tests may be interfered with by sulfonamide therapy. False positive results for urine glucose may occur when a copper reduction method (e.g., Clinitest) is used. Sulfisoxazole may produce false positive results for urine protein if the sulfosalicylic acid test is employed. Interference with urinary urobilinogen tests (Urobilistix) may occur with sulfisoxazole also.

CLINICAL USES

Sulfonamides no longer occupy a predominant position in combating bacterial infections. Their use is limited, primarily because of the development of widespread bacterial resistance. Their limited use, however, does not diminish their importance in treating a finite group of infections. Of the available sulfonamides, sulfisoxazole is the most widely prescribed and is one of the top 200 prescription products in the United States. The combination product, sulfamethoxazole and trimethoprim, has surpassed sulfisoxazole's usage and is one of the top 100 prescription products in the United States.

Urinary tract infections

Sulfonamides are considered by many authorities to be a treatment of choice in acute, uncomplicated urinary tract infections. The organisms most often causing this type of infection, *E. coli* and *Proteus mirabilis*, are susceptible to the high sulfonamide concentrations achieved in the urine. Additionally, the sulfonamides are relatively inexpensive and carry a low risk of serious adverse reactions. A highly soluble sulfonamide (e.g., sulfisoxazole) is considered to be the sulfonamide of choice for these infections.

Traditionally, the prescribed regimen uses a large initial dose (i.e., loading dose), followed by smaller maintenance doses for up to 1 to 2 weeks of therapy. The loading dose is a carryover from the early sulfonamide era in which the rapid achievement of high blood levels was desired in treating systemic infections. Also, the sulfonamides used at that time were sometimes poorly and erratically absorbed. With the advent of the rapidly and completely absorbed sulfonamides that achieve high urine concentrations quickly, the use of a loading dose for treating urinary tract infections seems unreasonable. A clinical trial addressing this issue has demonstrated that a loading dose of sulfisoxazole was not necessary in treating acute, uncomplicated urinary tract infections. Unfortunately, the official prescribing information for the sulfonamides states that a loading dose should be used. Recently, the issue of how long the therapy should be instituted in acute urinary tract infections has been raised. Several studies have shown that the therapy of acute urinary tract infections, particularly cystitis, is amenable to a single dose of an antibacterial, including sulfonamides. However, the practice of using single-dose therapy has not as of yet become commonplace in the United States.

The treatment of complicated urinary tract infections is usually guided by in vitro sensitivity studies because the infecting organism(s) often has unusual sensitivity patterns. In addition, therapy may be continued for several weeks to be effective or, as in the case of recurrent infection therapy, long-term suppressive therapy may be warranted. Sulfonamides are not used often for complicated urinary tract infections because the infecting organism(s) is not sensitive or there is a fear of resistance development during therapy, as is the case in chronic suppressive therapy for recurrent urinary tract infections. Co-trimoxazole (i.e., trimethoprim-sulfamethoxazole) is commonly used to treat complicated urinary tract infections because it possesses good activity against many of the pathogens encountered and resistance has not been a problem. This combination product has been particularly useful in treating women with recurrent urinary tract infections. Low-dose therapy (20 mg trimethoprim, 200 mg sulfamethoxazole per day) has been effective in preventing reinfections in women when used prophylactically (see Chapter 48, "Miscellaneous Antibiotics").

Nocardiosis

The actinomycete, *Nocardia asteroides*, is the main causative organism of nocardiosis in the United States. The disease process may be localized or disseminated. Usually the *Nocardia* species is acquired through the respiratory tract. Sulfonamides are considered the mainstay of therapy. Some clinicians prefer to combine the sulfonamide with an antibiotic, such as ampicillin, cycloserine, or erythromycin, because of documented in vitro synergy. Although sulfadiazine is the most widely used sulfonamide in this condition, the use of sulfisoxazole or triple sulfonamide products should be equally effective. Sulfonamide blood levels of 80-160 µg/ml are considered therapeutic. Six weeks of therapy is regarded as a minimum, with many months of therapy often being necessary.

Chancroid

This venereal disease is caused by *Haemophilus ducreyi*. It commonly occurs among nonwhite uncircumcised men and uncommonly affects women. The lesion typically begins as a tender *papule* and converts to a painful ulcer. These lesions are most often located on the genitalia or perianal areas. Sulfonamides (i.e., co-trimoxazole), are considered the treatment of choice. Alternative treatments include tetracycline, erythromycin, or streptomycin.

Chlamydia trachomatis infections

Sulfonamides are considered appropriate therapy for many of the clinical manifestations of *Chlamydia trachomatis* infections. In ocular infections (e.g., trachoma and inclusion conjunctivitis), oral sulfonamide or tetracycline therapy with or without concomitant topical therapy is considered the treatment of choice for adults. Topical therapy alone is not advocated because it might not eradicate the organism even though symptoms are suppressed. Oral erythromycin or sulfonamide therapy is considered appropriate in treating infants. The treatment of lymphogranuloma venereum (LGV), a sexually transmitted *C. trachomatis* infection, is amenable to sulfonamide therapy. Therapy is usually for 3 weeks, with either a sulfonamide, tetracycline, or erythromycin being administered. Other genital infections (e.g., urethritis) are usually not treated with a sulfonamide. Either tetracycline or erythromycin therapy for up to 2 weeks is considered most effective for these infections. Finally, sulfisoxazole or erythromycin is considered the treatment of choice for *C. trachomatis* pneumonia in infants. Therapy for 2 to 3 weeks has been advocated.

Streptococcal infections

Sulfonamides are no longer used to treat infections caused by *Streptococcus pyogenes*. In particular, sulfonamides fail to eradicate the streptococci from the pharynx when used to treat pharyngitis. Additionally, the sulfonamide therapy for acute pharyngitis may not prevent the occurrence of late nonsuppurative complications (e.g., rheumatic fever). Penicillin or erythromycin is generally considered the treatment of choice in *S. pyogenes* infections. However, sulfonamides are as effective as oral penicillin as prophylactic agents in the prevention of streptococcal infections and recurrent rheumatic fever episodes in rheumatic patients. Although the duration of prophylactic therapy is controversial, patient compliance with oral regimens is universally poor. Therefore, parenteral benzathine penicillin G is the treatment of choice for prophylaxis with sulfonamide therapy being an alternative, particularly in penicillin-allergic patients. Sulfadiazine or sulfisoxazole at 1 gm per day for adults or 0.5 gm per day for children weighing less than 25 kg is recommended.

Meningococcal infections

Therapy for *Neisseria meningitidis* (meningococcus) meningitis should *not* include sulfonamides because resistance is commonplace. Parenteral sulfonamides may be used in this infection only if the meningococcus has proved to be sensitive to the sulfonamide. Penicillin or chloramphenicol is preferred for the treatment of meningococcal infections.

Close contacts of a patient with meningococcal disease should receive prophylactic therapy. Currently, rifampin is the treatment of choice for meningococcal prophylaxis. However, if the strain is known to be sulfonamide sensitive, sulfisoxazole or sulfadiazine may be preferred. Therapy is for 2 days with oral sulfonamide doses of 2 gm daily for adults, 1 gm daily for children aged 1 to 12 years, and 5 mg/kg daily for children less than 1 year of age. It must be emphasized that only close contacts (e.g., household contacts) should receive prophylaxis, not casual acquaintances.

Melioidosis

This rare disease is caused by *Pseudomonas pseudomallei*. The greatest concentration of cases is in Southeast Asia, with the usual clinical manifestation being a pulmonary infection. Therapy is best directed by sensitivity studies; however, the organism is usually susceptible to sulfisoxazole or co-trimoxazole. The duration of therapy is at least 1 month with high-dose therapy recommended.

Toxoplasmosis

Toxoplasmosis is an infection caused by the protozoon *Toxoplasma gondii*. Although the disease is usually asymptomatic, lymphadenopathy is the most common clinical manifestation. Unfortunately, a variety of serious manifestations may occur, including ocular defects and fulminant multisystem disease. Serious sequelae from congenital toxoplasmosis may take months for presentation. The therapy of choice is the combination of pyrimethamine and a sulfonamide, which has been shown to be synergistic against *T. gondii*. Either sulfadiazine or a triple sulfonamide product may be used. Sulfisoxazole is less active and should not be used. Combined therapy for 30 days is considered adequate.

Dermatitis herpetiformis

Dermatitis herpetiformis is a morbid dermatologic condition of an unknown etiology. It is a chronic process marked by recurrences and intense pruritus. The disease typically produces grouped vesicular lesions covering the extensor surfaces of the body symmetrically. Sulfapyridine in doses of 1 to 1.5 gm daily is considered a treatment of choice. Some clinicians, however, prefer the sulfone, dapsone, to sulfapyradine. Response to either therapy is usually prompt, and the formation of new lesions is arrested after about 2 days of therapy.

Otitis media

Sulfonamide usage has had a resurgence in the treatment of acute otitis media because of a significant percentage of *Haemophilus influenzae* in certain areas of the country that is resistant to ampicillin. In those areas where *H. influenzae* resistance is significant, either one of two combination products may be recommended—erythromycin-sulfisoxazole or co-trimoxazole. Each of these combinations is effective against ampicillin-resistant *H. influenzae* and the other commonly infecting organisms in otitis media. Many clinicians prefer co-trimoxazole because it may be administered only twice daily. The sulfonamides have also been effective in treating recurrent otitis media. One study has shown sulfisoxazole (1 gm daily) to be an effective prophylactic agent in preventing recurrent otitis media in susceptible children.

Burn therapy

Mafenide and silver sulfadiazine play a prominent role in treating burn wounds and in preventing burn wound sepsis. Mafenide, a compound structurally similar to the sulfonamides, was the first of the two agents to be used topically in burn therapy. It has an excellent spectrum of antibacterial activity, including action against *Pseudomonas aeruginosa.* Activity against *Pseudomonas aeruginosa* is important because fatalities caused by burns are most often related to sepsis caused by this organism. Additionally, mafenide is an excellent penetrator of tissue and *eschar* and is absorbed systemically after topical administration. Unfortunately, it does have significant adverse effects associated with its use. The two major drawbacks to its use are painful administration and the potential development of metabolic acidosis resulting from the carbonic anhydrase activity of mafenide and its metabolite. Hypersensitivity phenomena may occur, but whether cross-sensitivity occurs with the sulfonamides is uncertain. Mafenide remains a treatment of choice in second- and third-degree burns.

Silver sulfadiazine is an excellent antibacterial agent with activity against both gram-positive and gram-negative organisms, including *Pseudomonas aeruginosa.* In comparison with mafenide, it is virtually painless but does not penetrate tissue as well. Hypersensitivity reactions (e.g., rashes) may occur, and cross-sensitivity reactions with the other sulfonamides may also occur. Silver sulfadiazine has become an extremely popular agent for second- and third-degree burns because of its low toxicity profile and its effectiveness as an antibacterial.

Ocular infections

Two ophthalmic sulfonamide preparations are available—sulfacetamide sodium and sulfisoxazole diolamine. As discussed previously, they may be used in conjunction with systemic therapy in treating trachoma. Although bacterial resistance patterns have limited their use through the years, they are still used to treat conjunctivitis, corneal ulcers, and superficial ocular infections. Organisms causing these processes should be of a known sensitivity to the sulfonamides. Their use in ocular infections has been associated with a low incidence of side effects; however, hypersensitivity phenomena may occur. A life-threatening reaction (e.g., Stevens-Johnson syndrome) has been associated with sulfacetamide's use. Patient's exhibiting hypersensitivity reactions to the systemic sulfonamides are at the risk of a reaction when the ophthalmic sulfonamides are subsequently administered.

Inflammatory bowel disease

Although its mechanism of action is not fully appreciated, sulfasalazine is a mainstay of treatment for *ulcerative colitis.* It is particularly useful in the mild to moderate forms of the disease. Pharmacotherapy is just one facet of the treatment of this inflammatory bowel disease, because patients with this disease usually require a multifaceted approach to treatment that may include nutritional and psychologic counseling. In the acute phases of this disease, doses of 4 to 8 gm daily may be necessary for remission, with the dose being tapered to 2 to 4 gm daily as maintenance therapy. Maintenance therapy may be lifelong; however, patients with mild disease may be able to discontinue therapy after about 2 symptom-free years.

A trial of sulfasalazine is considered appropriate for treating mild to moderate *Crohn's disease,* particularly first attacks. A national cooperative study has shown that patients may respond well to sulfasalazine therapy after a first attack, especially if the disease is present in the colon. Many clinicians will try sulfasalazine 4 to 6 gm daily for 6 weeks in mild to moderate Crohn's disease, hoping for a positive response, because not all patients will respond to this therapy. Patients who have a relapse or who have severe Crohn's disease invariably require corticosteroid therapy. Unfortunately, sulfasalazine does not appear to be effective in preventing acute flare-ups of Crohn's disease once the patient is in remission.

SUMMARY

This chapter has examined the various types and clinical uses of the sulfonamides. With an understanding of the various individual agents, including their actions and side effects, the nurse will be able to provide optimal care to patients requiring these medications. Patient education can be enhanced, adverse drug effects can be anticipated, monitored for, and minimized, clinically significant drug interactions can be avoided, and the therapeutic response monitored by using the information presented in this chapter.

ADVERSE/SIDE EFFECTS OF THE SULFONAMIDES*

ALLERGIC REACTIONS

Angioneurotic edema
Drug fever
Erythema multiforme
Erythema nodosum
Macular or macular papular rash
Photosensitivity reactions
Pruritic and petechial eruptions
Serum sickness–like syndrome
Stevens-Johnson syndrome
Toxic epidermal necrolysis
Urticaria
Vasculitis

CENTRAL NERVOUS SYSTEM

Depression
Dizziness
Drowsiness
Headache
Psychosis
Restlessness

GASTROINTESTINAL SYSTEM

Abdominal pain
Anorexia
Diarrhea
Gastrointestinal bleeding
Nausea
Vomiting

HEMATOLOGIC SYSTEM

Agranulocytosis
Aplastic anemia
Eosinophilia
Hemolytic anemia in G-6-PD and glu-
    tathione-peroxidase deficiencies
Neutropenia
Thrombocytopenia

HEPATIC SYSTEM

Hepatitis (hepatocellular necrosis
    with or without cholestasis)

RENAL SYSTEM

Acute tubular necrosis
Anuria
Crystalluria
Hematuria
Interstitial nephritis
Obstructive nephropathy
Toxic nephrosis

MISCELLANEOUS EFFECTS

Jaundice
Pancreatitis
Potential for kernicterus

*See Chapter 11, "Drug Toxicity," for an overview of drug toxicity.

CLINICALLY SIGNIFICANT DRUG INTERACTIONS*

Primary drug	Interacting drug	Possible effect(s)	Probable mechanism(s)
Sulfonamides	Hypoglycemic agents (chlorprop-amide and tolbutamide)	Increased hypoglycemic effect	Displacement of the hypoglycemic agent from protein-binding sites and inhibition of metabolism
Sulfonamides	Warfarin	Increase of warfarin's antico-agulant effect	Interference with warfarin metab-olism
Sulfonamides	Phenytoin	Increase of phenytoin activity	Inhibition of phenytoin metabolism

*See Chapter 10, "Drug Interactions," for an overview of drug interactions.

Nursing of patients requiring sulfonamides

ASSESSMENT

The sulfonamides are used to treat and prevent various infections, including urinary tract infections, infections associated with second- and third-degree burns, eye infections, and sexually transmitted diseases. The choice of sulfonamide depends on the site of the infection, the causative organism, the geographical region, and individual patient factors. Baseline data should include information about the patient's general health state and specific information regarding the presence of symptoms indicating the presence or absence of an infection. These symptoms may include an elevated temperature, redness or pain in an area not previously affected, fatigue, anorexia, skin lesions, wound drainage, an elevated white blood cell count, or other observations related to the specific infection or condition being treated.

Whenever possible, the organism responsible for the infection should be identified *before* sulfonamide therapy is initiated. Isolation measures should be implemented as indicated to prevent the spread of the infection to others.

The collection of specimens for culture and sensitivity tests should be obtained carefully according to hospital procedures. This is important not only in drug selection, but also in monitoring the patient's therapeutic response to the selected drug therapy.

Because the use of these medications is associated with hematologic, hepatic, and renal toxicities, baseline hematology and renal and hepatic function should be assessed, including routine laboratory tests (e.g., urinalysis, CBC, electrolytes, BUN, creatinine). In addition, the assessment before initiating sulfonamide therapy must include a detailed drug history to identify any possible hypersensitivity, contraindications, cautions, drug interactions, and individual patient drug-taking patterns.

SENSITIVITY

Generally, allergic reactions to the sulfonamides are more likely to occur with the topically applied sulfonamides. However, any drug has the potential to cause a hypersensitivity reaction in susceptible individuals. It is important to note that cross-sensitivity to the other sulfonamides may occur in approximately 20% of cases.

CONTRAINDICATIONS

Sulfonamides are contraindicated in patients with a known hypersensitivity to a specific sulfonamide.

Sulfonamides are also contraindicated in patients with severe renal or hepatic impairment or porphyria (see the Nursing Drug Digest for contraindications to specific sulfonamides).

CAUTIONS

Adequate fluid intake helps prevent the crystalluria and stone formation associated with the use of the sulfonamides.

See the Nursing Drug Digest for specific cautions related to individual agents.

DRUG INTERACTIONS

The sulfonamides have the potential to interact with many other drugs in a variety of mechanisms. See Clinically Significant Drug Interactions for specific interactions with the sulfonamides.

Some sulfonamides (e.g., sulfisoxazole and sulfamethoxazole) can cause false positive results for urine glucose when Clinitest tablets are used to test urine glucose. They can also interfere with the results of urobilinogen tests with Urobilistix.

Evaluation of the urine for glucose should be done with a glucose-oxidase method (e.g., Clinistix), because sulfonamides may interfere with copper reduction methods (e.g., Clinitest).

ADMINISTRATION

Sulfonamides are available in various dosage forms for oral, intramuscular, intravenous and topical administration, including ophthalmic and vaginal preparations. Dosage is individualized according to individual patient factors such as age, body weight, and the severity of the infection. See the Nursing Drug Digest for specific information regarding the dosage and administration of each sulfonamide. In addition, the following should be noted.

Before administering sulfonamides, ask patients if they are allergic to sulfonamides. If so, ask patients what happened, when did it happen, and with which sulfonamide did the allergic reaction occur.

The allergic history should be recorded in the patient's medical records. Additionally, the outside of the patient's chart and the bed should be appropriately marked indicating the allergy. An allergy alert hospital wrist band should also be applied. Inform patients that they should always indicate to their physician, nurse, and pharmacist that they are allergic to sulfonamides. They should be instructed not to take any sulfonamide medication unless specifically instructed to do so.

Samples obtained for culture and sensitivity tests should be collected before initiating antibacterial therapy.

Administration scheduling should be evenly spaced based on the 24-hour clock (e.g., three times daily should be interpreted as every 8 hours). This type of scheduling ensures consistency in the sulfonamide bodily disposition.

Administer the sulfonamides at the same prescribed times during the day to minimize absorption fluctuations. Preferably, administer the oral sulfonamide on an empty stomach with a full glass of water. See the Nursing Drug Digest for specific information regarding administration by other routes.

MONITORING PATIENT RESPONSE
Therapeutic response

The onset and duration of the sulfonamides is largely dependent on their classification as short-, intermediate-, or long-acting sulfonamides, as well as on the dosage form, the route of administration and individual patient factors. When the sulfonamides are used to treat an infection, it is important to monitor the therapeutic effect in relation to a decreased temperature, decreased white blood cell count, decreased pain or inflammation, increased appetite, increased energy, increased feelings of well-being, or other indications related to the need for the specific agent. Cultures for sensitivity tests should also be used as needed in monitoring the patient's response.

Monitoring the therapeutic response is especially important because antibiotic therapy commonly fails and can result in an increased severity of the infection, which could cause severe sequelae in such conditions as urinary tract infections or burns. If the patient is unre-

Nursing of patients requiring sulfonamides—cont'd

Therapeutic response—cont'd

sponsive to one sulfonamide another may be more beneficial in treating the infection, or another group or combination of antibiotics can be used. If the sulfonamide is being administered for an acute urinary tract infection, the patient's symptoms should be relieved in 3 days. If not, the prescriber should be promptly notified because repeat cultures may be necessary for a reassessment of the infection.

Adverse side effects

Adverse side effects can vary among the various sulfonamides. See Adverse/Side Effects of the Sulfonamides for an outline of common adverse effects of these agents. Because of the severity of some toxicities associated with the use of these drugs, including hematologic reactions and gastrointestinal and urinary tract effects, monitoring is particularly important so that serious effects can be noted readily and the drug therapy discontinued. This is usually associated with a return to the normal or pretreatment function of these systems.

Monitor for signs of Stevens-Johnson syndrome, including bullous lesions on the skin and mucous membranes, fever, malaise, and anorexia.

Monitor for signs of blood dyscrasias (e.g., fever, sore throat, bleeding, malaise), including agranulocytosis and hemolytic anemia, particularly in patients with G-6-PD deficiency.

Observe for the overgrowth of nonsusceptible organisms and the development of bacterial resistance.

Fever must be monitored for and the cause (e.g., drug fever, agranulocytosis, infection) must be differentiated so that appropriate measures can be taken.

A knowledge of the more common and severe adverse effects is important in relation not only to monitoring for their occurrence, but also to planning to prevent or minimize them during therapy when needed. Increasing hydration and increasing the pH of the urine can prevent urinary crystalluria and other untoward affects. Adequate hydration must be maintained to minimize the risk of crystalluria.

Observe the patient frequently for adverse effects, particularly skin reactions. If a problem is encountered, notify the prescriber promptly and stop the administration of the sulfonamide until instructed otherwise.

PATIENT EDUCATION

The patient and the family, as indicated, should have an understanding of the anticipated course of therapy and medication regimen, especially if drug therapy is to be prolonged over weeks or months. They should know the exact name of the drug, its general action, purpose, dosage, storage, administration, and adverse side effects. They should understand how to minimize or prevent unwanted effects and be able to monitor for their occurrence. Because the therapy for some conditions is prolonged, patients may become noncompliant and support and follow-up may be indicated. It is important that patients monitor the signs of the therapeutic effect, as well as signs that indicate the health care provider should be notified.

Health teaching (e.g., with sexually transmitted diseases, urinary tract infections, prevention of burns) may be indicated.

GENERAL INSTRUCTIONS FOR DISCHARGE/OUTPATIENTS

SULFONAMIDES

This medication is an antibiotic used to treat or to prevent infections. If you do not understand why you require this medication, ask your health care provider.

Important: If you have allergies or are allergic to the sulfonamides, tell your health care provider *before* taking this medication.

Take this medication only as directed and continue to take this medication as prescribed until it is used up unless told otherwise by your health care provider. It is important that you do not stop taking this medication even if you feel better, because your infection may not be entirely gone and it may return if you do not take the full course of treatment.

For best results, take this medication as directed on an empty stomach with a full glass of water.

This medication can cause unwanted side effects in some patients. It is important that you notify your health care provider if you develop a sore throat, easy bruising, or sores in your mouth.

Notify your health care provider immediately if you develop a skin rash, severe itching, hives, a swollen face, have difficulty breathing, or have fainting spells. These are uncommon; however, they could indicate you are having an allergic reaction to this medication. If you cannot get in touch with your health care provider, contact your nearest emergency room. The emergency room personnel can tell you what to do next.

This medication when taken by pregnant women can cross the placental barrier to the infant. This medication can also be found in breast milk when taken by nursing mothers. If you are pregnant or thinking about becoming pregnant or are breastfeeding an infant, notify your health care provider *before* taking this medication.

This medication was prescribed especially for you for a specific reason. Do not give it to friends or relatives or save this medicine for another time. Flush away any unused portion of this medicine. Outdated antibiotics can become ineffective or cause unwanted or harmful effects.

Store this medication as directed on the label of the container.

Keep this and all other medications out of the reach of children.

NURSING DRUG DIGEST

Medication (trade name*)	Indication	Usual dosage and administration†	Dosage forms, preparation, and storage	Contraindications, cautions, and comments	Monitoring
Mafenide Marfanil Sulfamylon	Second- and third-degree burns	*Adults:* Topical application over entire burn surface 1/16 of an inch thick q.d. or b.i.d. until healing is progressing well or until the burn site is ready for grafting Apply with sterile gloves using reverse isolation techniques *Children:* Same as adults *External use only*	Cream: 85 mg/gm (8.5%)	*Contraindicated* in hypersensitivity Mafenide is *not* inhibited by pus May cause pain on application	Monitor acid-base balance closely in patients with either impaired renal or pulmonary function because of the inhibition of carbonic anhydrase by mafenide and its metabolite
Silver sulfadiazine Silvadene Flamazine	Second- and third-degree burns	*Adults:* Topical application over entire burn surface 1/16 of an inch thick q.d. to b.i.d. Apply with sterile gloves using reverse isolation techniques *Children:* Same as adults May need to *decrease* dose in renal impairment (particularly in extensive burns because of significant systemic absorption) *External use only*	Cream: 10 mg/gm (1%) *Discard* darkened cream	*Contraindicated* in pregnancy at term, premature infants, and newborn infants during the first month of life Use with extreme caution in patients with a history of a hypersensitivity to sulfonamides Use in extensive burns may result in marked absorption of sulfadiazine and may cause hematologic abnormalities	Monitor sulfonamide serum levels Observe for fungal overgrowth
Sulfacetamide Bleph Bleph-10 Liquifilm Blephamide Ointment* Blephamide Ophthalmic* Blephamide S.O.P.* Cetamide	Conjunctivitis, corneal ulcer, or superficial ocular infections caused by susceptible organisms Adjunct in trachoma therapy	*All age groups:* Instill 1 drop (30%) q.2h. in lower conjunctival sac; 1-2 drops (10%) q.2h.; *or* small amount of ointment q.i.d. and q.h.s. *Adults:* Instill 2 drops (30%) q.2h. *Ophthalmic use only*	Ophthalmic solution: 15%, 30% Ophthalmic ointment: 10% Darkened solutions should be discarded Store in cool place, 8°-15°C	*Contraindicated* in patients with a known or suspected sensitivity to sulfonamides Stinging or burning may be experienced, particularly with 30% solution	Observe for allergic or sensitivity reaction

	Uses	Dosage	Dosage Forms	Precautions	Nursing Considerations
Isopto Cetamide Isopto Ceta-pred* Metimyd* Ophthel-S Op-Sulfa30 Optimyd* Optosulfex Sebizon Sodium Sulamyd Sulamyd Sodium Sulf-10 Sulf-30 Sultrin* Vasosulf*					
★ **Sulfacytine** Renoquid	Acute urinary tract infections caused by susceptible organisms	*Adults:* 500 mg initially, then 250 mg PO q.i.d. for 10 days *Children: Not* recommended for children under 14 years of age	Tablet: 250 mg	*Contraindicated* in patients allergic to sulfonamides, pregnancy at term, and during the nursing period Encourage fluids	Monitor patient for adequate urine output Monitor urine pH Monitor cultures and urinalysis
★ **Sulfadiazine** Codiazine Cremodiazine Eskadiazine Microsulfon Solu-Diazine Sulfadets Sulfonamides Duplex*	Systemic and urinary tract infections caused by susceptible organisms Prevention of recurrent attacks of rheumatic fever	*Adults:* 2-4 gm initially, then 2-4 gm/24 hr in 4 divided doses PO *Children:* Over 2 months of age, 75 mg/kg initially, then 150 mg/kg/24 hr in 4 divided doses PO (maximum 6 gm/24 hr) *Children:* Over 30 kg, 1 gm/24 hr PO; under 30 kg, 0.5 gm/24 hr PO Avoid extravasation	Tablets: 300, 500 mg Injectable: 250 mg/ml Dilute each 250 mg with 4 ml sterile water for injection Protect from light	*Contraindicated* in patients allergic to sulfonamides, pregnancy at term, and during the nursing period Alkalinization of urine with sodium bicarbonate may be necessary to increase urinary solubility Encourage fluids, if possible Medications that acidify urine should be avoided	Monitor urinary output, cultures, and urinalysis Monitor urine pH

NOTE: For additional details regarding the individual agents listed in this table, see the text and other tables in this chapter.

*Indicates a multiple active ingredient product. For a complete listing of all active ingredients see the *Drug Reference Guide to Brand Names and Active Ingredients.*

†Use of sulfonamides in infants younger than 2 months of age is *not* recommended except as adjunctive therapy for congenital toxoplasmosis because of the potential to displace bilirubin from its protein-binding sites and to cause kernicterus.

★Indicates that the drug is generally available only in the United States.

Continued.

NURSING DRUG DIGEST—cont'd

Medication (trade name)	Indication	Usual dosage and administration	Dosage forms, preparation, and storage	Contraindications, cautions, and comments	Monitoring
Sulfamethizole Azo-Sulfstat* Azotrex* Microsul Microsul-A* Proklar Signa Sul-A* Sulfstat Forte Thiosulfil Thiosulfil Duo-Pak* Thiosulfil-A* Thiosulfil-A Forte* Thiosulfil Forte Uremide* Urifon Urolucosil Utrasul	Urinary tract infections caused by susceptible organisms	*Adults:* 0.5-1 gm PO t.i.d. to q.i.d. *Children:* Over 2 months of age, 30-45 mg/kg/24 hr in 4 divided doses PO	Tablets: 250, 500, 1000 mg Suspension: 250, 500 mg/5 ml	*Contraindicated* in patients allergic to sulfonamides, pregnancy at term, and during the nursing period Encourage fluids	Monitor urinary output, cultures, and urinalysis
Sulfamethoxazole Azo Gantanol* Gantanol Sinomin Uro-Gantanol*	Acute, recurrent, or chronic urinary tract infections and systemic infections caused by susceptible organisms	*Adults:* Mild to moderate infection, 2 gm initially, then 1 gm b.i.d.; severe infection, 2 gm initially, then 1 gm PO t.i.d. *Children:* Over 2 months of age, 50-60 mg/kg initially, then 25-30 mg/kg PO b.i.d.; do *not* exceed 75 mg/kg/ 24 hr	Tablets: 500, 1000 mg Suspension: 500 mg/5 ml	*Contraindicated* in patients allergic to sulfonamides, pregnancy at term, and during the nursing period Encourage fluids	Monitor fluid intake, urinary output
Sulfapyridine Dagenan	Dermatitis herpetiformis	*Adults:* Up to 2 gm/day PO in 4 divided doses until improvement, then reduce dose to minimum effective dose Administration with food or milk may decrease GI distress	Tablet: 500 mg	*Contraindicated* in patients allergic to sulfonamides, pregnancy at term, and during the nursing period Often causes GI distress Encourage fluids	Monitor urinary output

Drug	Uses	Dosage forms	Dosage	Nursing considerations
Sulfasalazine Azopyrin Azulfidine Azulfidine En-Tabs Rorasul Salazopyrin SAS-500	Ulcerative colitis Crohn's disease	Tablet: 500 mg Tablet (enteric-coated): 500 mg Suspension: 250 mg/5 ml Enema: 3 gm/100 ml	*Adults:* Initial, 3-4 gm/24 hr PO in evenly divided doses Maintenance, 2 gm/24 hr PO in divided doses; *or* 1 rectal enema q.h.s. *Children:* Over 2 years of age Initial, 40-60 mg/kg/24 hr in evenly divided doses; maintenance, 30 mg/kg/24 hr in evenly divided doses PO *Adults:* 4-6 gm/24 hr in evenly divided doses *Children:* 2-5 years old, 1.5-2 gm/24 hr; over 5 years old, 2-4 gm/24 hr All doses should be evenly divided Administration with food or milk may decrease GI distress; if immediate GI distress is not relieved by food, enteric-coated tablets may be useful	*Contraindicated* in patients allergic to sulfonamides, pregnancy at term, and during the nursing period May cause agranulocytosis or neutropenia GI discomfort may be experienced shortly after medication administration Dosage should be individualized May color alkaline urine orange-yellow Observe for rash, sore throat, or purpura
Sulfisoxazole Azo-Gantrisin* Azo-Soxazole* Azosul* Azo-Sulfisoxazole* Cantri Vaginal Cream* Entusul Gantrisin Gantrisin Cream Gantrisin Ophthalmic Koro-Sulf Novosoxazole Pediazole* Rosoxol SK-Soxazole Suldiazo* Sulfalar Sulfizole Vagilia Cream/Suppositories*	Acute, recurrent, or chronic urinary tract infections and systemic infections caused by susceptible organisms	Tablet: 500 mg Syrup: 500 mg/5 ml Suspension: 500 mg/5 ml Emulsion: 1000 mg/5 ml Injectable: 400 mg/ml (40% solution); use sterile water for injection as diluent; do not use any other diluent because of incompatibility; dilute each 250 mg with 4 ml sterile water for injection	Oral therapy *Adults:* 2-4 gm PO initially, then 4-8 gm/24 hr in 4-6 divided doses *Children:* 75 mg/kg PO initially, then 150 mg/kg/24 hr (4 gm/m²/24 hr) in 4-6 divided doses; *maximum is 6 gm/24 hr* Administration 1 hr before or 2 hr after meals may facilitate absorption Emulsion therapy *Adults:* 4-5 gm emulsion q.12h. *Children:* 60-75 mg/kg emulsion initially, then 60-75 mg/kg b.i.d.; *maximum is 6 gm/24 hr* NOTE: Emulsion dosing is b.i.d. because this product is long acting Parenteral therapy *Adults:* 50 mg/kg (1.125 gm/m²) initially, then 100 mg/kg/24 hr (2.25 gm/m²/24 hr); in 2-4 divided doses SC, IV, or IM *Children:* Same as adults	*Contraindicated* in patients allergic to sulfonamides, pregnancy at term, and during the nursing period May produce false positive urine glucose and urine protein results Encourage fluids Monitor fluid intake urinary output Observe for allergic or sensitivity reaction

Continued.

NURSING DRUG DIGEST—cont'd

Medication (trade name)	Indication	Usual dosage and administration	Dosage forms, preparation, and storage	Contraindications, cautions, and comments	Monitoring
Sulfisoxazole —cont'd		NOTE: Use parenteral therapy when oral dosing is impractical; dilute injection to 5% solution with sterile water for injection for IV and SC administration; IM dose may be administered undiluted			
	Conjunctivitis, corneal ulcer, or superficial ocular infections caused by susceptible organisms; adjunct in trachoma therapy	Solution: Instill 2-3 drops t.i.d. to q.i.d. Ointment: Instill a small amount in the lower conjunctival sac q.d. to t.i.d. and q.h.s. NOTE: Solution and ointment are for ophthalmic use *only*	Ophthalmic solution: 4% Ophthalmic ointment: 4%		
SULFONAMIDE COMBINATIONS					
★ **Sulfadiazine and sulfamerazine** Sulfonamides Duplex	Acute, recurrent, or chronic urinary tract infections and systemic infections caused by susceptible organisms	*Adults:* 2-4 gm initially, then 2-4 gm/24 hr in divided doses PO *Children:* Over 2 months of age, 75 mg/kg initially, then 150 mg/kg/24 hr in divided doses PO	Suspension: 250 mg of each/ 5 ml	*Contraindicated* in patients hypersensitive to sulfonamides, pregnancy at term, and during the nursing period	Observe for allergic or sensitivity reaction
★ **Sulfamerazine, sulfadiazine, and sulfamethazine** Neotrizine Triple Sulfa Terfonyl Trisem	Acute, recurrent, or chronic urinary tract infections and systemic infections caused by susceptible organisms	*Adults:* 2-4 gm initially, then 2-4 gm/24 hr in divided doses PO *Children:* Over 2 months of age, 75 mg/kg initially, then 150 mg/kg/24 hr in divided doses PO Maximum: 6 gm/24 hr	Tablets: 162 or 167 mg of each component Suspension: 167 mg of each/ 5 ml	*Contraindicated* in patients hypersensitive to sulfonamides, pregnancy at term, and during the nursing period	Observe for allergic or sensitivity reaction

BIBLIOGRAPHY

Appel, G.B., & Neu, H.C. The nephrotoxicity of antimicrobial agents. *New England Journal of Medicine*, 1977, *296*, 784-787.

Arneborn, P., & Palmblad, J. Drug-induced neutropenias in the Stockholm region 1976-1977. *Acta Medica Scandinavica*, 1979, *206*, 241-243.

Bailey, R.R. Single dose antibacterial treatment for uncomplicated UTIs. *Drugs*, 1979, *17*, 219-221.

Bergan, T., Brodwall, E.K., Vik-Mo, H., et al. Pharmacokinetics of sulphadiazine, sulphamethoxazole and trimethoprim in patients with varying renal function. *Infection*, 1979, *7*, S382-S387.

Böttiger, L.E., Furhoff, A.K., & Holmberg, L. Drug-induced blood dyscrasias: a ten-year material from the Swedish Adverse Drug Reaction Committee. *Acta Medica Scandinavica*, 1979, *205*, 457-461.

Cohen, A.E. Sulfacytine in uncomplicated urinary tract infections: double-blind comparison with sulfisoxazole. *Urology*, 1976, *7*, 267-271.

Craig, W.A., & Welling, P.G. Protein binding of antimicrobials: clinical pharmacokinetic and therapeutic implications. *Clinical Pharmacokinetics*, 1977, *2*, 252-268.

Das, K.M., & Dubin, R. Clinical pharmacokinetics of sulphasalazine. *Clinical Pharmacokinetics*, 1976, *1*, 406-425.

Gottschalk, H.R., & Stone, O.J. Stevens-Johnson syndrome from ophthalmic sulfonamide. *Archives of Dermatology*, 1976, *112*, 513-514.

Harrison, H.N. Pharmacology of sulfadiazine silver. *Archives of Surgery*, 1979, *114*, 281-285.

Hekster, C.A., & Vree, T.B. Clinical pharmacokinetics of sulphonamides and their N₄-acetyl derivatives (vol. 31). In H. Schönfeld (Ed.). *Antibiotics and chemotherapy.* New York: S. Karger, 1982.

Iravani, A., Richard, G.A., & Baer, H. Treatment of uncomplicated urinary tract infections with trimethoprim versus sulfisoxazole, with special reference to antibody-coated bacteria and fecal flora. *Antimicrobial Agents and Chemotherapy*, 1981, *19*, 842-850.

Kaplan, E.L., Bisno, A.L., Derrick, W., et al. American Heart Association report: prevention of rheumatic fever. *Circulation*, 1977, *55*, S1-S4.

Kauffman, R.E., O'Brien, C., & Gilford, P. Sulfisoxazole secretion into human milk. *Journal of Pediatrics*, 1980, *97*, 839-841.

Lang, P.G. Sulfones and sulfonamides in dermatology today. *American Academy of Dermatology*, 1979, *1*, 479-492.

Meyer, M., Straughn, A.B., Ramachander, G., et al. Bioavailability of sulfadiazine solutions, suspensions, and tablets in humans. *Journal of Pharmaceutical Sciences*, 1978, *67*, 1659-1661.

Parkin, J.L. Antimicrobial treatment of otitis media: penicillins, cephalosporins, sulfonamides. *Otolaryngology and Head and Neck Surgery*, 1981, *89*, 376-380.

Patel, R.B., & Welling, P.G. Clinical pharmacokinetics of cotrimoxazole (trimethoprim-sulphamethoxazole). *Clinical Pharmacokinetics*, 1980, *5*, 405-423.

Prince, R.A., Cassel, D.H., Hepler, C.D., et al. Comparative trial of two sulfisoxazole regimens in acute urinary tract infection. *Drug Intelligence and Clinical Pharmacy*, 1981, *15*, 863-866.

Richards, M.L., Prince, R.A., Kenaley, K.A., et al. Antimicrobial penetration into cerebrospinal fluid. *Drug Intelligence and Clinical Pharmacy*, 1981, *15*, 341-368.

Slywka, G.W., Melikian, A.P., Straughn, A.B., et al. Bioavailability of 11 sulfisoxazole products in humans. *Journal of Pharmaceutical Science*, 1976, *65*, 1494-1498.

Summers, R.W., Switz, D.M., Sessions, J.T., et al. National cooperative Crohn's disease study: results of drug treatment. *Gastroenterology*, 1979, *77*, 847-869.

Van Arsdel, P.P. Allergy and adverse drug reactions. *Journal of the American Academy of Dermatology*, 1982, *6*, 833-845.

Vree, T.B., O'Reilly, W.J., Hekster, Y.A., et al. Determination of the acetylator phenotype and pharmacokinetics of some sulphonamides in man. *Clinical Pharmacokinetics*, 1980, *5*, 274-294.

CHAPTER 50

Drugs Used to Treat Tuberculosis and Leprosy

Jon Auricchio

Medications discussed in this chapter

Antitubercular agents	*Antitubercular agents—cont'd*
Aminosalicylic acid	Rifampin
Capreomycin	Streptomycin
Cycloserine	*Antileprotic agents*
Ethambutol	Clofazimine
Ethionamide	Dapsone
Isoniazid	Rifampin
Pyrazinamide	Sulfoxone

Tuberculosis and leprosy result from an infection by the tubercle bacillus *Mycobacterium tuberculosis* in the case of tuberculosis and *Mycobacterium leprae* in leprosy. Although both diseases result from tissue invasion by mycobacteria, the clinical manifestations and pathophysiology of the two differ markedly. Therefore, each will be discussed as a separate entity.

TUBERCULOSIS

Mycobacterium tuberculosis is a slow-growing organism that requires oxygen for growth. Special staining characteristics make this bacillus unique compared with other bacteria. Its resistance to decolorization by acid alcohol when stained with carbol-fuchsin has resulted in its being referred to as an "acid-fast bacilli," a term commonly encountered in reference to mycobacteria.

Mycobacteria are strict *aerobes*. As a result they tend to find optimum growing conditions in tissues with relatively high oxygen tensions. Any organ in the body is susceptible, but the infection is most common in the lungs (especially the apices), kidneys, the growing ends of long bones, and the central nervous system.

The transmission of tuberculosis is by the inhalation of airborne bacilli contained in infectious units called "droplet nuclei." Sputum contaminated with bacilli is aerosolized during coughing or sneezing and undergoes evaporation, resulting in droplets of varying size. The larger particles become deposited on the surface of the large airways and the nasopharynx and are subsequently cleared from the body by mucociliary mechanisms of the upper respiratory tract (URT). The smaller particles, specifically those 2 to 10 μ in diameter, are infectious. Their small size enables them to traverse the normal defense mechanisms of the URT resulting in bacilli reaching the alveoli where a nidus of infection is set up. Bacilli multiply and are disseminated to other organs of the body via the lymphatic and circulatory systems. Infected individuals are the major reservoir for the dissemination of disease.

Several points are worth noting in relation to the transmission of the disease. First, individuals are infective only if *large* numbers of organisms are present in their sputum. Patients with extrapulmonary tuberculosis are minimum hazards for transmitting the disease and need not be in respiratory isolation. Patients who have positive sputums and have been started on chemotherapy have a reduced infectivity. The exact time a patient becomes noninfectious after being started on chemotherapy is not known, but does occur before the sputum smear or culture becomes negative. Generally, patients put on chemotherapy who show a decline in malaise, fever, cough, night sweats, and numbers of bacilli in their sputum represent a minimal risk of transmitting the disease at 2 weeks, and can resume normal activity.

When dealing with tuberculosis, one must distinguish between an infection by the tubercle bacillus and tuberculous disease. This distinction is important because the choice of treatment differs depending on which one the patient has.

Infection

Infection by the tubercle bacillus basically means that a patient has come in contact with the tubercle bacilli. It has gained entrance into the body, but there is no clinical evidence of a pathologic condition. The body has successfully checked the invasion of the organism. Thus there will be no symptoms present suggestive of tubercular disease, and the patient appears healthy. Indeed, most patients infected with *M. tuberculosis* never go on to develop the disease.

Disease

Tuberculous disease is considered present when clinical signs of tissue invasion or symptoms occur. It is most commonly diagnosed on a routine chest radiograph, but may be suspected in the presence of various symptoms consistent with tuberculosis. Classical symptoms of pulmonary tuberculosis include weight loss, malaise, fatigue, night sweats, chronic productive cough, and *hemoptysis*. It is important to remember that the symptoms may or may not be present, and the key to discovery is in looking for the disease.

Skin tests

Skin testing is based on the observation that when a patient becomes infected with mycobacteria, the immune system becomes sensitized to the bacteria. If the patient is challenged with an extract containing mycobacterial *antigen* (Ag), a reaction mediated by the immune system takes place. If the patient has not been infected, the response fails to develop. The presence or absence of infection is clinically detected by skin testing.

Purified protein derivative (PPD) is used as the skin-testing Ag and is prepared from heat-killed liquid cultures of mycobacteria. Clinically, two strengths are used: the standard intermediate strength containing 5 tuberculin units (TU) per 0.1 ml and a second strength containing 250 TU per 0.1 ml. The intermediate strength PPD is used as a diagnostic test for an infection with *Mycobacterium tuberculosis*; 0.1 ml is injected intradermally and the results are read in 48 and 72 hours. The reading consists of measuring the area of *induration* that develops around the site of the injection. A positive reading is 10 mm or more of induration. An important note is that a positive reaction indicates only that the patient has come in contact with mycobacteria. It provides no information about if the patient has the clinical disease. Specific diagnosis of tuberculous disease depends on isolation and culture of the bacteria in the laboratory.

There are some pitfalls to be aware of regarding skin testing. Both false positive and false negative reactions can occur. False positive reactions may occur as a result of contact with mycobacterial species that have a negligible or limited pathogenicity for humans.

These are referred to as atypical mycobacteria. False negative reactions may occur in patients infected with mycobacteria or in those with the clinical disease. When this occurs, the patient is said to be anergic. There are several well-recognized causes of *anergy*, such as sarcoidosis, viral exanthema, severe malnutrition (commonly seen in chronic alcoholics), advanced age, certain malignant lesions, and treatment with immunosuppressive or steroidal drugs. In addition, several studies have shown that up to 20% of patients in whom active tuberculosis has developed may be anergic. Most patients who fail to react to PPD also fail to react to other commonly encountered antigens. As a result, skin testing with antigens to which most patients have been exposed, as well as PPD, is commonly used to discern if a patient is anergic or merely PPD negative. Antigens commonly employed to detect anergy include streptokinase-streptodornase, mumps, coccidiomycosis, and trichophyton.

Drug therapy

When deciding which drugs to include in the treatment regimen for tuberculosis, one must first ascertain if the patient is merely infected with mycobacteria or has the mycobacterial disease. If an infection is the case, then chemoprophylaxis with a single drug, isoniazid (INH), may be the treatment of choice. If the clinical disease is present, then therapy with a combination of drugs is most appropriate. It is important to remember that cultures for tuberculous bacilli must be obtained *before* initiating chemotherapy. Cultures obtained after instituting therapy have a high probability of being negative, thereby preventing both precise diagnosis and drug sensitivity testing.

Central to every treatment regimen, both for chemoprophylaxis and the active disease, is the use of INH. It is a highly effective bactericidal agent with a low toxicity, making it an ideal agent to be included in most treatment regimens. Therefore, a brief mention of special problems encountered with its use will be made.

Isoniazid is eliminated from the body predominantly by hepatic metabolism, with lesser amounts being excreted renally. Metabolism appears in part to be genetically influenced, because two populations of individuals exist: those who metabolize INH rapidly (i.e., fast acetylators) and those whose metabolism is considerably slower (i.e., slow acetylators). Metabolic degradation of INH follows two pathways, one resulting in isoniazid hydrazone and the other proceeding via acetylation, producing acetylisoniazid. The acetylation pathway is genetically influenced (see Chapter 9, "Genetic Factors Affecting Drug Response").

Differences in acetylator phenotype may have clinical implications. A severe, sometimes fatal hepatotoxicity has been associated with the use of INH. The exact mechanism by which INH hepatocellular dysfunction is unknown, but current evidence favors a toxic metabolite as the offending agent. It has been shown that acetylisoniazid is converted to acetyl hydrazine, which is further metabolized to a highly reactive compound. This reactive metabolite has been shown to produce liver necrosis in animals and is postulated to be the hepatotoxin in humans. One can appreciate that individuals who are fast acetylators produce more acetylisoniazid, which in turn can be converted to the toxic metabolite. If this concept is correct, then patients who are fast acetylators should be more susceptible to hepatic injury than their slow acetylating counterparts. Current evidence indicates that patients who are rapid acetylators are indeed more prone to develop INH hepatitis. However, data refuting the postulate that acetylator status is a risk factor for developing hepatitis are also being reported. This, in conjunction with the fact that the incidence of hepatitis increases with increasing age, suggests factors other than acetylator phenotype may play a role in the development of INH hepatitis.

Another implication of acetylator status concerns the therapeutic consequences of the more rapid degradation of INH, the chemically active form. It has been shown that serum levels of INH are only 30% to 50% that of slow acetylators. A possible consequence of lower serum levels would be a larger number of treatment failures in patients who are rapid acetylators. Clinically, however, there is no evidence supporting a difference in the therapeutic efficacy between the two groups. There are data suggesting that patients who are fast acetylators may do less well in programs where INH is given only once a week.

In contrast to the therapeutic implications for patients who are fast acetylators, patients who are slow acetylators may be more prone to developing the peripheral neuropathy associated with INH use. This toxicity is associated with a deficiency in the levels of pyridoxine (vitamin B_6). In humans, pyridoxine is converted to pyridoxal phosphate by the enzyme pyridoxal kinase. Pyridoxal phosphate functions as a coenzyme in many biochemical reactions involved with nervous system function. INH inhibits the action of pyridoxine kinase by complexing with pyridoxine, thereby preventing the formation of the biologically active pyridoxal phosphate. Patients who are slow acetylators, by maintaining higher serum levels of INH, may be more prone to developing peripheral neuropathy. It has been recommended that patients receiving

INH also be given supplemental doses of pyridoxine to avoid this problem. This was more of a problem when large doses of INH were recommended for treatment. With the present recommended doses of 3 to 5 mg/kg (up to 300 mg) the incidence of peripheral neuritis is quite low (approximately 2%). As a result, the routine administration of pyridoxine is no longer recommended except for those patients who are at a particular risk. These include elderly patients, those with poor nutritional status, patients who are chronic alcoholics, and patients with diabetes.

Active tuberculosis

Drugs used to treat tuberculosis are divided into two groups (Table 50-1). First-line drugs are those that are the most efficacious and the least toxic. These agents are used in the initial treatment regimens. Second-line drugs are those that have a greater toxicity or are less efficacious than the first-line agents. They are *reserved* for use when there is drug resistance or in the event of the development of an adverse drug reaction necessitating a change in drug therapy.

A variety of treatment regimens have been used against tuberculosis, but in general the initial treatment consists of at least two bactericidal drugs against which the organism is sensitive. Usually a three-drug regimen employing INH, rifampin, and ethambutol, or INH, streptomycin, and ethambutol is used. Therapy is continued for periods of 18 to 24 months.

The necessity for multiple drugs and long durations of treatment is based on two observations. First, drug-resistant mutations occur naturally, with an estimated frequency of 1 in 100,000 bacilli for INH and 1 in 1,000,000 bacilli for streptomycin. Thus, when large numbers of bacilli are present, as occurs in cavitary lesions, the likelihood of a drug-resistant mutant is high. By giving the initial chemotherapy with multiple drugs, the probability of drug-resistant bacilli surviving in the bacterial population is extremely small. Second, viable organisms may exist in a latent state, making

TABLE 50-1

Primary and secondary antitubercular drugs

First-line drugs	*Second-line drugs*
Ethambutol	Aminosalicylic acid
Isoniazid	Capreomycin
Rifampin	Cycloserine
Streptomycin	Ethionamide
	Pyrazinamide

them immune to chemotherapy. These organisms may become activated and renew growth after therapy has ceased. Therefore, to ensure adequate treatment, daily chemotherapy for extended periods is employed.

With the discovery of rifampin, the overall treatment of tuberculosis has been greatly improved. Rifampin is a highly effective bactericidal drug. Its inclusion in initial treatment regimens has resulted in a steady decrease in the total length of treatment. Data also show that streptomycin is no longer needed to prevent resistance when rifampin is included in the drug regimen. This has led to the use of a new treatment protocol termed "short-course therapy."

Short-course therapy has several advantages over the standard regimens requiring 18 to 24 months of therapy. Prolonged regimens require patient compliance for 15 to 20 months after clinical recovery to assure that a relapse will not occur. This places a tremendous burden on the most compliant of patients and totally overwhelms the less compliant. In addition, drug toxicity increases in proportion to the duration of the treatment. These considerations, in conjunction with the increased overall cost of prolonged treatment, make shorter treatment protocols desirable.

At present several short-course regimens are being evaluated. However, because of insufficient data or poor results only one regimen is currently recommended by the Center for Disease Control and the American Thoracic Society. This regimen follows.

INH 300 mg plus rifampin 600 mg daily for a period ranging from 2 weeks to 2 months. Therapy is then continued employing either daily (if self-given) or twice weekly (supervised) INH plus rifampin. If the regimen is to be given twice weekly the dosage of INH is increased to 15 mg/kg/dose. If a regimen of daily self-administration is used careful monitoring by use of pill counts, clinic attendance, urine tests, and sputum examination should be done to insure compliance. Treatment is continued for no less than 9 months.

The short-course regimen is an alternative only for adults with uncomplicated pulmonary tuberculosis. A shortened regimen cannot be recommended for patients with extrapulmonary tuberculosis, drug-resistant cases, or patients with complicating medical conditions (see boxed material below left, no. 4).

Chemoprophylaxis

As mentioned previously, patients may be infected with mycobacteria but do not have the disease. Most infected patients do not go on to develop the disease, although they are at risk of doing so throughout their lifetime. The majority of new cases of tuberculosis develop from patients already infected with mycobacteria. As a result, they become the sources of a new infection. Chemoprophylaxis is aimed at preventing these infected patients from developing and subsequently spreading the disease.

Several studies have shown that the daily treatment of infected patients with INH for 1 year can decrease the chances of developing active tuberculosis. The decision to use chemoprophylaxis must be individualized for each patient, considering the risk of developing the clinical disease, adverse drug reactions, the opportunity for infecting others, and the patient's motivation. In general prophylaxis is reserved for patients in whom the chance of developing INH-associated liver disease or other adverse reactions appears to be less than the risk of developing tuberculosis. Several situations warrant chemoprophylaxis; these are listed in the box at left. Certain conditions are associated with an increased risk of developing tuberculosis. These include prolonged therapy with corticosteroids or immunosuppressive drugs, diseases such as leukemia, Hodgkin's disease, silicosis, and diabetes, and after gastrectomy or renal transplantation. The reason for this increased susceptibility is not entirely clear. However, all of these conditions share the problem of immune system dysfunction and when tested with

---

Recommendations for INH prophylaxis in patients who are PPD positive

1. Household members and other close associates of patients with recently diagnosed tuberculosis
2. Patients with findings on the chest roentgenogram consistent with nonprogressive tuberculous disease, in whom there are neither positive bacteriologic findings nor a history of adequate chemotherapy
3. Newly infected patients (e.g., recent PPD converters)
4. Positive PPD reactors in the following situations
   a. Prolonged corticosteroid therapy
   b. Immunosuppressive therapy
   c. Certain reticuloendothelial diseases (e.g., lymphomas, leukemia)
   d. Diabetes
   e. Silicosis
   f. Postgastrectomy patients

PPD and other antigens are usually found to be anergic. The lack of the ability to mount an immune response against the tubercle bacillus favors the development of tuberculous disease. In general, patients younger than 35 years of age who are PPD positive should be treated prophylactically regardless of the absence of risk factors. Patients who are PPD-positive reactors over 35 years of age with no risk factors are not as a group routinely recommended for therapy. If additional risk factors are present and the patient is over 35 years of age, one must weigh the risk versus the benefits of prophylaxis.

The regimen employed for chemoprophylaxis is INH 300 mg per day for 1 year. Although it seems reasonable to assume that other drugs (e.g., rifampin) would be effective for prophylaxis, studies have been done using only INH.

LEPROSY

Leprosy (Hansen's disease) is a chronic, slowly progressive disease resulting from an infection by the acid-fast rod *Mycobacterium leprae*. Unlike other mycobacterial diseases, it predominantly attacks the skin, peripheral nerves, and nasal mucosa. Tissues such as the mucosa of the URT, muscles, and testes may also be involved.

Leprosy tends to be most common in countries with tropical climates. The major prevalence today is in Africa, South and Southeast Asia, and South America. It is also found in the United States in areas such as Texas, California, Hawaii, Louisiana, and Florida, but with a much lower prevalence, and in various refugee and immigrant populations in both the United States and Canada.

The transmission of the disease is not entirely understood, but most likely it is by the shedding of bacteria from ulcerated nasal mucosa. The bacteria may gain entrance to the body through the skin or mucosa of the URT. Once the infection has occurred, a prolonged incubation period of from 2 to 4 years occurs.

The clinical manifestations of leprosy are many and differ depending on which clinical classification one is dealing with; lepromatous, tuberculoid, or borderline.

Lepromatous leprosy

Lepromatous leprosy is characterized by an insidious onset, with the first lesions appearing as bilaterally symmetrical patches with shiny erythematous surfaces. If left untreated, the lesions progress, resulting in skin thickening of the forehead, eyebrows, nose, *malar* surfaces, and earlobes. Gradually destruc-

tion of small peripheral nerves occurs, producing a symmetrical anesthesia of the extensor surfaces of the forearms, hands, legs, and feet with a slow spread to the trunk and face. As the disease continues, the large nerve trunks become involved and a destruction of the nasal mucosa may occur with throat involvement leading to the collapse of the nasal bridge and laryngeal obstruction. Death may result from respiratory obstruction or a secondary infection. Lepromatous leprosy is characterized by an impairment of cell-mediated immunity. As a result large numbers of organisms are present, and this form tends to be more rapidly progressive and severe than other forms.

Tuberculoid leprosy

Tuberculoid leprosy is characterized by fewer skin lesions but has a more pronounced neurologic involvement. Skin lesions tend to be either plaques or have a raised edge with a flat healing center 3 to 30 cm in size. Lesions are asymmetrical, hypopigmented, anesthetic, and dry with well-defined margins. Large peripheral nerves or cutaneous nerves in association with the skin lesions may be involved. There usually is both sensory and motor nerve involvement. In contrast to the lepromatous form no immune deficiency exists and only rarely can organisms be found.

Borderline leprosy

Borderline leprosy combines the clinical features of the previous two types, such as peripheral nerve involvement and symmetrical lesions that tend to be erythematous and hypoesthetic with a waxy surface. Borderline leprosy may change to either the lepromatous or the tuberculoid form.

Drug treatment

Drug treatment of leprosy involves the use of only a limited number of agents. Dapsone is the drug of choice for all forms of leprosy. The dosage of the drug is gradually built up over several weeks to minimize adverse reactions. The World Health Organization recommends a dose of 6-10 mg/kg body weight per week (approximately 50-100 mg/day in adults). The major problem encountered with dapsone is hemolysis, which has an extremely high incidence with doses of 200 to 300 mg per day. Other adverse effects encountered with dapsone include anorexia, nausea, vomiting, headache, and nervousness.

Sulfoxone, another drug of the same class, may be used when patients cannot tolerate the gastrointestinal effects of dapsone. The dosage is somewhat different (see the Nursing Drug Digest), but is gradually increased over several weeks like dapsone.

Certain problems are encountered in treating leprosy. The persistence of bacteria despite adequate therapy may occur. Thus, viable *M. leprae,* still sensitive to dapsone, have been isolated from patients even after 10 years of therapy. This is presumably because some bacteria remain metabolically inactive and are therefore insensitive to the drug.

Drug resistance is also an increasing problem. Evidence has accumulated showing that in certain areas of the world, about 3% of the lepromatous patients under treatment each year develop dapsone resistance. Notwithstanding the problems of persistence and resistance therapy with a single agent, dapsone, for the tuberculoid and borderline forms is appropriate. Patients with the lepromatous form should receive dapsone and at least one other drug to decrease the probability of resistance. Generally the companion drug of choice is rifampin given in doses of 600 mg per day. It has excellent activity against *M. leprae* and rapidly reduces the numbers of viable organisms present in the infected tissue. The duration of treatment for the combined regimen has not been established. Rifampin has been used for periods of 3 to 6 months with a continuation of the dapsone for life.

For patients who develop hypersensitivity reactions to the sulfones, alternate drugs need to be used. The two commonly used alternative agents are clofazimine and rifampin.

Certain reactional states have been reported during treatment of leprosy. Lepra reactions are perhaps the most severe. They tend to occur in patients with the borderline disease and are accompanied by changes in cellular immunity. The precipitation of lepra reactions can result from the initiation or the interruption of antibiotic treatment. Existing lesions become swollen and edematous. The nerves may become exquisitely tender and painful, and fever, malaise, and prostration with a steady deterioration, sometimes ending in death, may occur.

Erythema nodosum lepra usually occurs in patients with the lepromatous form of leprosy and also may be precipitated by treatment. It tends to be characterized by the appearance of dome-shaped, red, painful lesions that may ulcerate. These lesions may last several days before disappearing and commonly are followed by new eruptions. There may be a low-grade fever with *lymphadenopathy* and arthralgias. Other problems include inflammation of the fingers, iritis, and nephritis.

The management of the reactional states varies. The use of antipyretics and analgesics is appropriate for milder forms. Severe forms are usually treated with corticosteroids (60 mg in divided doses). If the problem continues, some therapists switch to clofazimine, which possesses both antibacterial and antiinflammatory properties. Discontinuation of sulfone therapy, as done in the past, is no longer recommended by most leprologists.

Response to treatment

Generally the mucosal lesions respond first to therapy, with lesions of the nasal mucosa, laryngeal nodules, and oropharyngeal area responding more slowly. Skin lesions may require several years to clear, and ocular lesions show little response. Patients with the tuberculoid form generally require treatment for 3 to 5 years. Patients with the lepromatous and borderline forms require longer treatment regimens, up to 10 years for the borderline form and lifetime therapy for the lepromatous form.

SUMMARY

This chapter has examined the various medications used to treat tuberculosis and leprosy. A brief overview of the conditions, including the mode of transmission, has also been presented. With an understanding of the various individual agents used to treat these conditions, including their actions and side effects, the nurse will be better able to provide optimum care to patients who require these medications. Patient education can be enhanced; adverse drug effects can be anticipated, monitored for, and minimized; clinically significant drug interactions can be avoided; and the therapeutic response appropriately monitored for by using the information presented in this chapter.

ADVERSE/SIDE EFFECTS OF ANTITUBERCULAR DRUGS*

ALLERGIC REACTIONS

Anaphylaxis
Arthritis (SLE syndrome occurs predominantly with INH; question patient for signs of weakness, fever, joint pain, and swelling)
Fever (more common with aminosalicylic acid, streptomycin, and cycloserine, and less with INH)
Pruritus
Rash
Urticaria

BEHAVIOR

Depression
Psychosis (excitement, aggression, confusion; predominantly with ethionamide and cycloserine, and rarely with INH)

CENTRAL NERVOUS SYSTEM

Ataxia
Convulsions
Dizziness
Drowsiness and somnolence
Dysarthria
Eighth cranial nerve damage (streptomycin and capreomycin are worst offenders)
Headache
Seizures
Vertigo (predominantly streptomycin and capreomycin)

GASTROINTESTINAL SYSTEM

Anorexia (common with pyrazinamide, aminosalicylic acid, and ethionamide)
Hepatitis (common with INH, less common with pyrazinamide and rifampin)
Nausea (common with pyrazinamide, aminosalicylic acid, and ethionamide)
Vomiting (common with pyrazinamide, aminosalicylic acid, and ethionamide)

HEMATOLOGIC SYSTEM

Hemolysis (major problem with dapsone; monitor for fatigue, dyspnea, pallor and increased heart rate)
Thrombocytopenia (rarely with rifampin and more common with intermittent therapy)

HEPATIC SYSTEM

Hepatitis (isoniazid)
Hepatotoxicity (ethionamide, isoniazid, pyrazinamide, rifampin)

METABOLIC AND ENDOCRINE SYSTEMS

Difficulty in managing diabetes
Gynecomastia
Hyperuricemia (precipitation of acute gout with ethambutol and pyrazinamide)
Hypokalemia

NEUROMUSCULAR SYSTEM

Asthenia
Muscle twitching
Neuromuscular blockade
Tremor

OCULAR SYSTEM

Optic neuritis (ethambutol)

RENAL SYSTEM

Nephrotoxicity (significant problem with streptomycin and capreomycin)

*See Chapter 11, "Drug Toxicity," for an overview of drug toxicity.

CLINICALLY SIGNIFICANT DRUG INTERACTIONS*

Primary drug	Interacting drug	Possible effect(s)	Probable mechanism(s)
Aminosalicylic acid	Isoniazid	Elevated blood levels of isoniazid may increase potential for toxicity	Aminosalicylic acid decreases acetylation of isoniazid resulting in elevated blood level
Isoniazid	Carbamazepine	Increased carbamazepine effect and toxicity	Inhibition of carbamazepine metabolism
Isoniazid	Phenytoin	Increased toxicity of phenytoin	Inhibition of hepatic metabolism
Rifampin	Aminosalicylic acid	Decreased effect of rifampin	Decreased absorption of rifampin
Rifampin	Anticoagulants (oral)	Decreased effect of warfarin	Increased metabolism
Rifampin	Corticosteroids	Decreased effect of corticosteroids	Increased metabolism of corticosteroids
Rifampin	Oral contraceptives	Decreased effect of oral contraceptives	Increased metabolism
Rifampin	Propranolol	Decreased effect of propranolol	Increased metabolism of propranolol
Rifampin	Quinidine	Decreased effect of quinidine	Increased metabolism
Rifampin	Tolbutamide	Diminished hypoglycemic response	Increased metabolism of tolbutamide
Streptomycin	Cephalothin	Increased nephrotoxicity	Not established
Streptomycin	Ethacrynic acid	Increased ototoxicity	Synergistic ototoxic effects
Streptomycin	Furosemide	Increased ototoxicity	Synergistic ototoxic effects

*See Chapter 10, "Drug Interactions," for an overview of drug interactions.

GENERAL NURSING IMPLICATIONS

Nursing of patients requiring antitubercular medication

ASSESSMENT

It is important to ascertain if the patient is being treated for an infection by a tubercle bacillus (patient usually has no symptoms and a healthy appearance) or for tuberculous disease (in which signs of tissue invasion or other symptoms occur such as weight loss, malaise, fatigue, night sweats, chronic productive cough, or hemoptysis). Assessment of the patient's general appearance, present symptoms, and health state should be completed, because this information is important in planning nursing care and in monitoring the patient's response to drug therapy regimens. Assessment usually includes skin tests; however, these must be interpreted carefully because positive skin tests indicate that the patient has come in contact with mycobacteria and does not necessarily indicate the presence of disease. As with other infections, specific laboratory isolation and culture of bacteria from patient secretions or tissue samples are required for the diagnosis of this disease condition.

Cultures for tuberculous bacilli should be obtained before initiating drug therapy.

It is important to note that some patients may require the institution of therapy *before* bacteriologic or histologic studies can be made. Drugs are individually selected in these cases, and changes are made in therapy when studies are completed. Baseline assessment of these patients is particularly important in monitoring their response.

A baseline assessment, including skin tests and roentgenograms, is important in establishing the diagnosis and influences the drug therapy protocols. Prophylaxis may be indicated. An infection requiring chemoprophylaxis is usually treated with one drug (e.g., isoniazid), whereas disease conditions are generally treated with combination drug therapy.

Community follow-up in relation to patient contacts, as well as screening of household members, is indicated in newly diagnosed active cases (see box, p. 1093, for patients who are recent converters). This is important because as tuberculosis cases have fallen over the years, so has the general awareness of the public. It is important to note

that a number of reports have documented diagnostic and therapeutic errors, probably as a result of inadequate assessment, leading to delayed or inadequate treatment exposing others, including health care workers, to infectious cases. Assessment is essential in controlling tuberculosis.

Nurses should be concerned with controlling the disease by case finding and working with other health care workers in making these patients noninfectious, preventing contacts who are infected but who are not ill from becoming infectious, and in preventing persons who are not yet infected from acquiring the infection. Arrangements must be made to minimize the risk of exposure of contacts in the home, especially children and close associates.

Isolation measures should be readily implemented as indicated in relation to individual patient requirements. Because pulmonary tuberculosis is spread by droplet infection, respiratory isolation is usually indicated. However, the use of masks in general is ineffective after a brief time, although the use of the ultra filter mask has been recommended. Usually patients can be taught to cover their mouths when coughing or sneezing and to use tissues and disposable sputum containers. Generally isolation is not indicated. In active cases in which the spread of the disease is a concern, in addition to these measures the patient can be isolated and air control techniques used to minimize the potential spread of the infection until the drug therapy takes effect. The psychologic aspects of the condition, as well as the use of masks and isolation, need specific nursing attention as indicated. Ultraviolet lighting is often used in many hospitals to control airborne infections. This form of intervention is effective for tuberculosis.

In addition to baseline assessment data, the assessment must include a detailed drug history before initiating the drug therapy to identify possible hypersensitivity, contraindications, cautions, potential drug interactions, and individual drug-taking patterns.

It is important to keep in mind that therapy is determined by the extent of the patient's disease, the likelihood of the presence of drug-resistant organisms, additional social and medical

conditions, especially those treated with drugs that may be affected by *antitubercular* drugs (Chapter 10, "Drug Interactions," and Clinically Significant Drug Interactions) that may complicate therapy. A history of previous tuberculosis treatment should be identified. Drug resistance or the potential for drug resistance should be suspected in patients who have undergone several courses of antitubercular therapy or who have become infected in Southeast Asia, Mexico, or the Far East. Problems associated with compliance should be identified so that nursing plans can be better developed to meet patient requirements.

SENSITIVITY

Generally, allergic reactions to antitubercular medications are rare; however, any drug has the potential to cause a hypersensitivity reaction in susceptible individuals.

CONTRAINDICATIONS

The use of antitubercular medications is contraindicated in patients with a known hypersensitivity to a specific drug.

Prophylaxis with isoniazid is contraindicated in patients who have hepatic disease and should be delayed until after delivery in pregnant women (see the Nursing Drug Digest for contraindications to specific agents).

CAUTIONS

Severe, potentially fatal hepatotoxicity (e.g., INH hepatitis) has been associated with the use of INH, especially in patients who are rapid acetylators (rapid metabolizers of the drug). This effect also appears to be associated with increased age. INH should be used with caution in elderly patients and in patients who are rapid acetylators.

Peripheral neuropathy has been reported among patients receiving high doses of INH. The concurrent use of pyridoxine (vitamin B_6) has been recommended to minimize or prevent this effect; however, it is no longer felt to be required except for those patients who may be at a high risk of developing this adverse effect, including elderly patients, patients with a poor nutritional status, patients who are chronic alcoholics, and patients who are diabetic.

Eating certain aged cheese, wines, or
Continued.

GENERAL NURSING IMPLICATIONS

Nursing of patients requiring antitubercular medication—cont'd

CAUTIONS—cont'd

other foods high in tyramine content while taking INH may cause an acute vascular reaction rarely (somewhat similar to that observed with tyramine and monoamine oxidase inhibitors— see Chapter 19, "Drugs Used to Treat Affective Disorders").

Drug resistance can occur with the use of antitubercular medications.

DRUG INTERACTIONS

Antitubercular drugs can interact with other drugs through a variety of mechanisms. Patients receiving multiple drug therapy for other medical conditions can pose a major problem with tuberculosis drug regimens. INH interferes with the metabolism of phenytoin, and the addition of INH to the regimen of a patient stabilized on phenytoin may result in phenytoin toxicity.

Rifampin can increase the hepatic metabolism of certain other drugs, including oral contraceptives, corticosteroids, oral hypoglycemics, and oral anticoagulants. Managing patients who require one or more of these drugs in combination with rifampin can thus be difficult and this situation should be avoided when possible.

It is important to note that women who are taking oral contraceptives and rifampin concurrently should be made aware of the increased risks of pregnancy and assisted with alternate measures of birth control as indicated.

(See Clinically Significant Drug Interactions for specific drug interactions.)

ADMINISTRATION

A variety of treatment regimens (e.g., chemoprophylaxis, short-course therapy, standard regimens, prolonged regimens) have been recommended and depend on the indication for the antituberculosis medication (e.g., prophylaxis, infection, disease) and on individual patient factors. See the Nursing Drug Digest for specific information regarding dosage and administration, as well as the discussion of the individual agents in the text of this chapter.

Antituberculosis medications are primarily administered by the oral route. They should be taken on an empty stomach with a glassful of water when possible, because the presence of food can decrease the peak serum level and the total amount of drug absorbed.

The total daily dose can usually be taken at one time to increase compliance.

Injectable forms of antitubercular medications (e.g., capreomycin) should generally be administered 1 hour after the oral forms when used in combination therapy, so that peak concentrations of both drugs can occur simultaneously.

Because no pediatric formulation for some of these agents are available (e.g., rifampin), capsules can be opened and the contents mixed with applesauce, or jelly before administration (see Chapter 2, "Preparation, Administration, and Monitoring of Medications" and the Nursing Drug Digest). A suspension can also be made up in syrup according to the manufacturer's instructions.

MONITORING PATIENT RESPONSE
Therapeutic response

A patient on chemotherapy generally becomes noninfective before the sputum smear for culture becomes negative. Monitor patients for a decline in malaise, fever, cough, night sweats, and numbers of bacilli in sputum after approximately 2 weeks. At this time the risk of the transmission of the disease generally is minimal and normal activities can usually be resumed.

Monitoring usually includes periodic roentgenograms, sputum cultures, and clinical examination, depending on the indication for antitubercular therapy.

Monitoring the patient's therapeutic response is important because therapeutic failure is commonly associated with errors in drug selection, incorrect use of multiple drugs, failure of the patient to follow the drug regimen as prescribed, cessation of the drug therapy before the infection is adequately treated, and drug resistance.

Adverse side effects

Observe for symptoms of hypersensitivity, such as skin rashes, fever, or pruritus.

Monitor patients for signs of hepatitis or other liver dysfunction: yellow discoloration of the skin or mucous membrane under the tongue, or sclera of the eyes (jaundice). This complication is associated with several antitubercular drugs, including INH, rifampin, ethionamide, and pyrazinamide.

Hepatitis is associated with severe liver damage caused by isoniazid, particularly in patients older than 35 years of age and in those patients who drink alcohol daily. Monitor serum transaminase activity. If it rises to three times the normal range and is accompanied by increased bilirubin or alkaline phosphatase levels, the drug should be discontinued.

Rifampin is hepatotoxic, and because it is a potent enzyme inducer, it may promote the production of the hepatotoxic metabolites of INH. Monitor patients receiving rifampin and INH for signs such as GI distress, rashes, and thrombocytopenia purpura.

Rifampin can also cause the urine or tears to turn red. Warn patients of this reversible (but potentially distressing) effect.

In addition, observe and report any *petechiae, purpura,* or *ecchymoses* in the mouth or on the skin.

Observe and report any visual complaints such as problems in reading fine print and green color discrimination. Problems of green color discrimination may be assessed by daily observations of traffic lights or other means.

Question the patient and report any joint pain, swelling, or numbness.

Question the patient and report any GI symptoms such as anorexia, nausea, vomiting, or abdominal pain or tenderness.

GENERAL NURSING IMPLICATIONS

Nursing of patients requiring antitubercular medication—cont'd

It is important to note that drug toxicity increases over time.

See Adverse/Side Effects, for a summary of adverse effects related to these medications.

PATIENT EDUCATION

Compliance in taking antitubercular medicine is the major determinant of successful treatment. The necessity of prolonged administration without symptoms favors noncompliance, and the patient should be instructed about the importance of regularly taking these medicines. The patient should be made aware of the risks involved (including reinfection or drug resistance) with not taking the drug(s) as prescribed or discontinuing the use of the medication(s) unless told to do so by the health care provider.

The patient and the family, as indicated, should be fully informed about the nature of the disease. Misconceptions should be identified and questions answered honestly. They should be involved readily in care planning because this does much to promote compliance. The patient and the family, as indicated, should have a clear understanding of the anticipated course of therapy and medication regimen, including the exact name of the medication(s), general action, purpose, dosage, storage, administration, and adverse/side effects and how these can be prevented or minimized.

The patient should be able to identify signs that indicate that the health care provider should be notified.

Patients should know how to monitor their therapeutic response and to recognize the importance of following therapy as indicated, especially when it is prolonged.

Patient education regarding diet and other aspects of self-care, as well as preventing the spread of the disease,

should be completed. Patients should be taught to cover their nose and mouth with tissues when coughing or sneezing and to expectorate sputum into tissues or a disposable container. Patients should be encouraged to avoid close contact with others and crowded living conditions. The diagnosis of tuberculosis has many social implications and can be psychologically distressing. Patients require a sound knowledge of their condition, as well as support and assistance in adapting to changes that can occur with this disease.

Patients should be instructed about possible GI upset when taking these medicines. They should be informed that although antitubercular medications work best when taken on an empty stomach, 1 hour before or 2 hours after meals, that if nausea is a problem, the medications can be taken with food or a meal.

Each patient should be counseled concerning the hepatotoxicity of INH and other antituberculars. Patients should be told to contact their nurse or physician if any of the following symptoms develop: abrupt development of loss of appetite, fatigue, weakness, vomiting, diarrhea, joint pain, right upper quadrant pain, fever of 37.7° to 40° C (100° to 104° F), jaundice, and flulike symptoms such as cough, running nose, sore throat, or muscle pain.

Patients requiring INH should be warned to avoid foods containing large amounts of vasoactive compounds (e.g., tyramine or histamine), which can cause an acute vascular reaction including a frontal headache; palpitations; flushing of the face, back, and arms; and an elevated blood pressure (rare).

Foods to be avoided include aged cheeses (Cheshire, Swiss) red wines (e.g., Chianti), or some fish (e.g., tuna, skipjack).

If patients are to be placed on a drug regimen containing rifampin, they should be advised that the urine and tears may become orange-red. Patients should be told not to become alarmed because this is a usual reaction to taking this medication, and they should continue taking the medication. Inform patients *not* to wear *soft* contact lenses while taking rifampin because tear discoloration can permanently stain the lenses.

Multiple drugs requiring daily administration over a long duration of therapy (18 to 24 months with at least two to three bactericidal agents) or the indication for prolonged regimens (15 to 20 months after clinical recovery) require increased patient education, follow-up, and support.

Self-medication or supervised medication regimens may be indicated depending on the patient's self-medication abilities and other factors.

Monitoring of compliance when patients self-medicate, may include tablet counts, as well as monitoring clinic attendance, urine tests, and routine sputum examinations.

Health teaching and counseling are extremely important, as are follow-up and monitoring the therapeutic regimen. Because compliance with prolonged therapy is difficult for many patients, nurses can help patients plan their drug regimen and treatment approaches to ensure the completion of adequate therapy.

After a course of successful therapy, most patients can be discharged from supervision. Patients should be instructed, however, to seek health care assistance if they develop a persistent cough, a persistent fever, or hemoptysis.

GENERAL NURSING IMPLICATIONS—cont'd

Nursing of patients requiring antileprotics

ASSESSMENT

Assessment of the patient's general health state, appearance, distribution of lesions and a history of the infection are important in planning care and in individualizing and monitoring the drug therapy, because lesions are usually characteristic of the type of leprosy (e.g., tuberculoid, lepromatous, borderline). A complete blood count should be obtained before treatment and monitored frequently during therapy (weekly for 1 month, monthly for 6 months, and then twice a year). Laboratory identification of organisms is essential in diagnosing the patient's condition, in drug selection, and in monitoring the patient's response. Surgical intervention is often indicated, along with chemotherapy. In addition to the baseline assessment data, the assessment should also include a detailed drug history before initiating the drug therapy to identify any possible hypersensitivity, contraindications, cautions, potential drug interactions, and individual drug-taking patterns.

SENSITIVITY

Generally, allergic reactions associated with the *antileprotics* are uncommon; however, any drug has the potential to cause a hypersensitivity reaction in susceptible individuals.

Hypersensitivity has been associated with the sulfones resulting in the need for the use of an alternate drug (e.g., clofazimine, rifampin).

Lepra reactions, which can be severe, can occur in borderline types of leprosy associated with the interruption of antibiotic therapy. An erythema nodosum lepra has been associated with the lepromatous form of leprosy. These reactions are usually treated with antipyretics, analgesics, or clofazimine and corticosteroids. Delayed hypersensitivity or reversal reactions associated with tuberculoid types can result in cutaneous ulcerations and peripheral neuropathy.

CONTRAINDICATIONS

The use of antileprotics is contraindicated in patients who have displayed a hypersensitivity reaction to a particular agent.

See the Nursing Drug Digest for specific contraindications to each agent.

CAUTIONS

See the Nursing Drug Digest for cautions associated with the use of these agents.

DRUG INTERACTIONS

Specific drug interactions for these agents are listed in Clinically Significant Drug Interactions.

ADMINISTRATION

A limited number of drugs are used in treating leprosy. They are available in tablets and capsules for oral administration and may cause anorexia, nausea, or vomiting. Do *not* break or crush dapsone tablets or sulfoxone oral enteric-coated tablets.

Dapsone is the drug of choice for all forms of leprosy. The dosage is gradually increased over several weeks to minimize adverse reactions. See the Nursing Drug Digest for specific information regarding the dosage and administration of each agent.

Drug therapy is often indicated for life in treating leprosy. The tuberculoid form requires a minimum 3 to 5 years of treatment and the lepromatous and borderline forms require a minimum 10 years to a lifetime of treatment.

MONITORING
PATIENT RESPONSE
Therapeutic response

Mucosal lesions respond to therapy first, with lesions of the nasal mucosa, the laryngeal nodules, and the oropharyngeal areas responding more slowly to drug therapy. Lesions may require several years to clear, and ocular lesions usually have little response.

Monitor for the persistence of bacteria despite adequate therapy.

Adverse side effects

The major adverse side effect associated with these drugs in general is hemolysis. Observe patients for anorexia, headache, nervousness, nausea, and vomiting.

See the Nursing Drug Digest for adverse effects associated with specific agents.

PATIENT EDUCATION

The patient and the family, as indicated, should be fully informed about the nature of the disease and its specific treatment, including drug regimens, surgical intervention, and the irreversibility of existing damage. They should have a clear understanding of the anticipated course of the therapy and medication regimen, including the exact names of medications, their general actions, dose, storage, administration, common adverse side effects, and how these can be prevented or minimized. They should be able to identify signs that indicate the health care provider should be notified. This is important because much of the therapy is required on an outpatient basis. The importance of following the drug regimens cannot be overemphasized, and patients often need much follow-up and support with long-term therapy regimens. Psychologic support in relation to scarring, body image concerns, and social reactions to this condition are often indicated. General health teaching, including the maintenance of adequate nutrition and the promotion of healthy home environmental conditions, is usually required. Because patients require constant laboratory and clinical supervision, this must be ensured by careful discharge planning and follow-up care.

GENERAL INSTRUCTIONS FOR DISCHARGE/OUTPATIENTS

ANTITUBERCULAR MEDICATIONS

This medication is used to treat tuberculosis. If you do not understand why you require this medication, check with your health care provider.

Follow the instructions on the prescription exactly. Your drug therapy regimen has been planned especially for you. If you have any questions about how to take your medication, contact your health care provider.

It is best to take these medicines on an empty stomach 1 hour before or 2 hours after meals. If nausea develops, do not stop taking your medicine, but take it with meals.

This drug can cause liver problems in some patients. Contact your health care provider if you notice an abrupt change in your appetite, fatigue, weakness, vomiting, diarrhea, joint pain, pain in the upper right side of your abdomen, a fever 37.7° to 40° C (100° to 104° F), flulike symptoms such as a cough, running nose, sore throat, or muscle pain, or if you notice a yellow color to your eyes or skin.

When taking drug regimens including isoniazid, pyrazinamide, or rifampin, avoid drinking alcohol, because of a possible increased risk of developing liver problems.

Notify your health care provider if you start or stop taking any other medications while taking this medication.

Keep this and all other medications out of the reach of children.

Do not trade or give this medication to any friends or relatives. It has been prescribed especially for you.

In addition to these general instructions, if you are taking *isoniazid* (INH), avoid foods such as aged cheeses (Cheshire, Swiss), red wines (Chianti), or tuna or skipjack fish while using this medication. Eating any of these foods while taking isoniazid can result in headache, flushing of your face, arms, and back, increased blood pressure, and a rapid heart beat (rare).

If you are taking *rifampin*, this drug can cause your urine and tears to become orange-red. Do not become alarmed. This is normal when taking this medication. Continue taking your medication as prescribed. Because of this effect, it is important that you not wear *soft* contact lenses because the tear discoloration can permanently stain your lenses. When you no longer require this medication and stop taking it, the color of your urine and tears will return to normal.

ANTILEPROTIC MEDICATIONS

This medication is used to treat leprosy. If you do not understand why you require this medication, check with your health care provider.

Follow the instructions on the prescription exactly. If you have any questions about how this drug should be taken, contact your health care provider.

This drug can cause unwanted effects in some patients, such as an upset stomach. It is helpful to take this medication with food or milk to prevent or decrease this effect. Swallow the tablets whole.

If you notice that you feel more tired than usual or have abdominal pain, diarrhea, a skin rash, or if you notice a yellow color to your skin or eyes, notify your health care provider. Your health care provider will tell you if you should continue to take the medication.

Do not trade or give this medication to relatives or friends. It has been prescribed especially for you.

Keep this and all medication out of the reach of children.

In addition to these general instructions, if your medication is *clofazimine*, this drug can cause your skin to appear reddish. This is a harmless effect. You should continue to take your medication as prescribed.

NURSING DRUG DIGEST

Medication (trade name*)	Indication	Usual dosage and administration	Dosage forms, preparation, and storage	Contraindications, cautions, and comments	Monitoring
Aminosalicylic acid Nemasol Pamisyl Propasa Rezipas	For treatment of pulmonary and extrapulmonary tuberculosis when *combined* with other agents after a failure with the primary drugs	*Adults:* 14-18 gm/24 hr PO in 2-3 divided doses *Children:* 275-400 mg/kg PO in 3-4 divided doses Administer with food to decrease GI upset	Tablets: 0.5, 1 gm; enteric-coated, 0.5 gm Powder: 3, 4, 18 gm packets Aminosalicylic acid may deteriorate rapidly if exposed to heat, sunlight, or water Do not use tablets or powder that are brown or purple	Major problem is GI upset, which leads to poor patient compliance; rarely used The salt form, potassium aminosalicylate, should *not* be administered to patients receiving digitalis, on diuretic therapy, with severe renal impairment, or with hyperkalemia The salt form, sodium aminosalicylate, should *not* be administered to patients with CHF or severe renal impairment The salt form, calcium aminosalicylate, should *not* be administered when calcium is contraindicated (e.g., hypercalcemia)	Observe patient for GI upset Monitor renal and hepatic function
Capreomycin Capastat Caprocin	For treatment of pulmonary and extrapulmonary tuberculosis when *combined* with other agents after a failure with the primary drugs	*Adults:* 15-30 mg/kg/24 hr IM *Children:* Safety for use with children not established Administer by deep IM into a large healthy muscle Maximum: 1 gm/24 hr Do *not* administer by IV route; may cause neuromuscular blockade Decrease dosage in renal impairment	Injectable: 1 gm May reconstitute drug in 2 ml normal saline for injection or sterile water for injection; allow 2-3 min for dissolution Some discoloration of solution may occur, but there is no change in potency Reconstituted solutions are stable for 48 hours at room temperature and 14 days if refrigerated	*Contraindicated* in patients receiving other ototoxic drugs (e.g., streptomycin) May cause eighth cranial nerve or renal toxicity	Monitor creatinine and BUN because drug is nephrotoxic Observe for signs of dizziness, ringing or buzzing in the ears, nausea, vomiting, and unsteadiness Monitor serum potassium because drug may cause hypokalemia

Drug	Use	Dosage	Preparations	Remarks
Clofazimine Lamprene	For treatment of all forms of leprosy when organisms are sulfone resistant	*Adults:* 100 to 300 mg/24 hr PO *Children:* Not established Optimal dosing interval has not been established, but daily to twice weekly is effective This drug is not available commercially; it may be obtained from National Leprosarium, United States Public Health Service Hospital, Carville, La. 70721	Capsule: 100 mg	This drug accumulates as crystals in tissues, imparting a red discoloration to the skin; not an indication to discontinue the drug Drug may accumulate in the GI tract causing abdominal pain, diarrhea, and, rarely, bowel obstruction
★ **Cycloserine** Closine Oxamycin Serociclina Seromycin Tisomycin	For treatment of pulmonary and systemic tuberculosis when *combined* with other agents after a failure with the primary agents	*Adults:* 10-20 mg/kg/24 hr PO *Children:* 5-15 mg/kg/24 hr PO Maximum: 1 gm/24 hr Decrease dosage in renal impairment	Capsule: 250 mg	Use with caution in patients with existing seizure or psychiatric disorders May cause drowsiness; caution against driving or operating equipment Excreted in human breast milk	Observe patients for personality changes Monitor for drowsiness
Dapsone Avlosulfon Disulone Udulac	For treatment of all forms of leprosy	*Adults:* 6-10 mg/kg/week PO (approximately 50-100 mg/24 hr) *Children:* Same as adult Administer with food or milk to decrease GI upset	Tablets: 25, 100 mg	Major problem is hemolysis; may also see GI upset commonly Long-term use may add to the nerve damage associated with leprosy WHO recommends long-term therapy (5-10 + years) to reduce secondary dapsone resistance	Observe for anemia Observe for allergic dermatitis Monitor for GI upset

Continued.

NOTE: For additional details regarding the individual agents listed in this table, see the text and other tables in this chapter.

*Indicates a multiple active ingredient product. For a complete listing of all active ingredients see the *Drug Reference Guide to Brand Names and Active Ingredients.*

★ Indicates that the drug is generally available only in the United States.

NURSING DRUG DIGEST—cont'd

Medication (trade name)	Indication	Usual dosage and administration	Dosage forms, preparation, and storage	Contraindications, cautions, and comments	Monitoring
Ethambutol Etibi Myambutol	Primary treatment of pulmonary and systemic tuberculosis in combination with other agents	Adults: 15 mg/kg/24 hr in single dose PO Retreatment, 25 mg/kg/24 hr PO Children: Not recommended in children younger than 13 years of age; older than 13 years of age, same as adult dose Maximum: 1500 mg/24 hr	Tablets: 100, 400 mg	Contraindicated in optic neuritis Contraindicated in patients with a hypersensitivity to drug May precipitate an acute attack of gout in susceptible patients May cause optic neuritis	Watch for changes in visual acuity and poor red-green color discrimination, especially in doses of 25 mg/kg/24 hr Monitor serum uric acid levels and observe for symptoms of gout
★ **Ethionamide** Trecator Trecator-SC Trescatyl	For treatment of pulmonary and systemic tuberculosis when combined with other agents after a failure with the primary drugs	Adults: 10-20 mg/kg/24 hr in 4 divided doses PO (usual dose 0.5-1 gm/24 hr) Children: Optimum dose is not established Maximum: 1 gm/24 hr Administer with food or milk to decrease GI irritation	Tablet: 250 mg	Contraindicated in patients with severe liver damage May potentiate the toxicity of other tuberculosis medications This drug may cause a peripheral neuropathy and is recommended to be given with pyridoxine Patients may notice a metallic taste	Monitor patients for signs of peripheral neuropathy (e.g., numbness and tingling in extremities)
Isoniazid Armazide Cotinazin Di-Isopacin* Dinacrin Ditubin Double Isopacin* Hyzyd Inapasade-SO* INH Tablets Isolyn Isotamine Laniazid Niconyl Nidaton Nydrazid Panazid	Chemoprophylaxis of tuberculosis (alone) Primary treatment of tuberculosis in combination with other agents	Adults: 5-10 mg/kg/24 hr PO in a single dose Maximum: 300 mg/24 hr Children: 5-10 mg/kg/24 hr Maximum: 500 mg/24 hr If GI upset occurs, may be taken with meals	Tablets: 50, 100, 300 mg Injectable: 100 mg/ml (for IM use) Syrup: 50 mg/5 ml Store at room temperature	Contraindicated in patients with severe liver disease or previous history of isoniazid hepatic injury May be present in human breast milk Administration of pyridoxine, 5 mg/24 hr, can treat the peripheral neuropathy caused by isoniazid and is routinely recommended May cause dizziness, hepatitis, hypersensitivity, lupuslike reaction, peripheral neutropion, or psychosis	Monitor SGOT and SGPT Observe for signs of peripheral neuropathy (numbness and tingling in extremities), especially with higher doses Reverse symptoms of neuropathy with B₆ (pyridoxine)

Drug	Use	Dosage / Forms	Remarks	Nursing Considerations
Pycazide Pyrizidin Rifamate* Rimifon Rolazid Teebaconin Tisin Tyvid			Fast acetylators may be more prone to develop hepatitis	
Pyrazinamide Aldinamide Tebrazid	Second-line drug for treating pulmonary and systemic tuberculosis when *combined* with other agents after a failure with primary agents	*Adults:* 20-35 mg/kg/24 hr in 3 or 4 doses PO Maximum: 3 gm/24 hr Tablet: 500 mg	*Contraindicated* in patients with severe liver damage This drug may cause severe liver damage This drug may precipitate acute gout in predisposed patients Patients with diabetes may be more difficult to manage when started on this drug Use with caution in renal disease	Observe for fever, malaise, dark urine, nausea, and vomiting Observe for signs of arthralgia or gout
Rifampin Rifadin Rifamate Rimactane Rofact	Primary treatment of pulmonary and systemic tuberculosis in *combination* with other agents Probable role in chemoprophylaxis of tuberculosis (alone) Leprosy (in combination with dapsone) (indication *not* FDA approved)	*Adults:* 600 mg/24 hr PO in one dose *Children:* Older than 5 years, 10-15 mg/kg up to 600 mg/24 hr PO; under 5 years, dosage not established If a dose is missed, do *not* double the next dose but resume the normal schedule *Avoid* administration on an irregular basis because side effects may occur more frequently and can be more severe Administer 1 hr before or 2 hr after meals to increase absorption Capsules: 150, 300 mg	*Contraindicated* in a hypersensitivity to the drug May cause jaundice GI disturbances (e.g., cramps, nausea, vomiting, diarrhea) may be severe enough to warrant discontinuation of the drug Use with caution in patients with preexisting hepatic disease Advise patient that the urine, tears, saliva, and sweat may turn reddish orange Advise patient to avoid use of soft contact lenses while taking this drug (may color lenses)	Monitor more closely for hepatic dysfunction when used with INH

Continued.

NURSING DRUG DIGEST—cont'd

Medication (trade name)	Indication	Usual dosage and administration	Dosage forms, preparation, and storage	Contraindications, cautions, and comments	Monitoring
Streptomycin Isoject-Streptomycin Strepolin Streptosol 25* Strycin	Primary treatment of pulmonary and systemic tuberculosis in *combination* with other agents Also indicated in bacterial infections by *susceptible* organisms See also Chapter 46, "Aminoglycosides"	*Adults:* 15 mg/kg/24 hr IM in one dose up to 1 gm maximum NOTE: Dosage must be reduced in elderly patients or patients with impaired renal function *Children:* 20-30 mg/kg IM Maximum: 1 gm/24 hr Administer by IM route *only* Pain and inflammation at the injection site may occur; alternate injection sites and avoid injections greater than 500 mg/ml	*For IM injection only* Injectable: 0.5, 1, 5 gm For reconstitution use NS for injection or sterile water for injection Add 4.2-4.5 ml to each 1 gm vial for 200 mg/ml or 17 ml to 5 gm vial for 250 mg/ml	*Contraindicated* during pregnancy because may cause hearing loss in the fetus *Contraindicated* in patients who have had adverse reactions to other aminoglycosides (e.g., tobramycin, gentamicin, amikacin, neomycin) Adds little to first treatment regimen Secreted into human breast milk May cause renal damage May cause eighth cranial nerve damage	Observe for signs of dizziness, ringing or buzzing in ears, nausea, vomiting, and unsteadiness Monitor renal function
★ **Sulfoxone** Diasone	For treatment of all forms of leprosy	*Adults:* 1st-2nd week, 330 mg PO twice a week; 3rd-4th week, 330 mg PO four times a week; 5th week and beyond, 330 mg PO for 6 days, 1 day off, then repeat Administer with meals to decrease GI upset Have patient swallow tablet whole to decrease GI irritation *Children:* Older than 4 years, ½ the adult dose	Tablet (enteric coated): 165 mg Protect tablets from light	Major problem is GI upset Major use is in patients who cannot tolerate dapsone	Monitor complete blood count Observe for anemia Observe for allergic dermatitis

BIBLIOGRAPHY

Addington, W.W. The treatment of pulmonary tuberculosis: current options. *Archives of Internal Medicine,* 1979, *139,* 1391.

American Thoracic Society. Guidelines for work for patients with tuberculosis: an official statement of the American Thoracic Society. *American Review of Respiratory Disease,* 1973, *108,* 160.

American Thoracic Society. Treatment of tuberculosis in alcoholic patients. *American Review of Respiratory Disease,* 1977, *116,* 559.

Arnold, H.L. Paradoxes and misconceptions in leprosy. *Journal of the American Medical Association,* 1966, *196,* 139.

Banner, A.S. Tuberculosis: clinical aspects and diagnosis. *Archives of Internal Medicine,* 1979, *139,* 1387.

Coleman, D.A. TB: the disease that's not dead yet. *RN,* 1984, *47*(9), 48-57.

Comstock, G.W., Ferebee, S.H., & Hammes, L.M. A controlled trial of community wide isoniazid prophylaxis in Alaska. *American Review of Respiratory Disease,* 1967, *95,* 935.

Decker, E.L. Skin testing for anergy: a review with proposed guidelines. *Hospital Formulary,* 1980, May, 368.

Dickson, D.S., Baily, W.C., & Hirschowitz, B.I. The effect of acetylation status on isoniazid hepatitis. *American Review of Respiratory Disease,* 1977, *115*(Suppl), 395.

Drugs for tuberculosis. *The Medical Letter,* 1982, *24,* 17-19.

Falk, A., & Fuchs, G.F. Prophylaxis with isoniazid in inactive tuberculosis: a Veterans Administration Cooperative Study XII. *Chest,* 1978, *73,* 44-48.

Geppert, E.F., & Leff, A. The pathogenesis of pulmonary and miliary tuberculosis. *Archives of Internal Medicine,* 1979, *137,* 1381.

Glassroth, J., Robins, A.G., & Snider, D.E. Tuberculosis in the 1980's. *New England Journal of Medicine,* 1980, *302*(26), 1441-1448.

Grove, D.I., Warren, K.S., & Mahmoud, A.A.F. Algorithms in the diagnosis and management of exotic diseases. XV. Leprosy. *Journal of Infectious Diseases,* 1976, *134,* 205.

Guidelines for short-course tuberculosis chemotherapy. *Morbidity and Mortality Weekly Report,* 1980, *29*(9), 97-105.

Hauser, M., & Baier, H. Interactions of isoniazid with foods. *Drug Intelligence and Clinical Pharmacy,* 1982, *16,* 617-618.

Lauver, G.L. Current status of the chemotherapy of tuberculosis: parts I and II. *Arizona Medicine,* 1978, *35,* 91.

Leff, A.L., Lester, T.W., & Addington, W.W. Tuberculosis: chemotherapeutic triumph but a persistent socioeconomic problem. *Archives of Internal Medicine,* 1979, *139,* 1375.

Leprosy—an update on recent developments. *Canada Diseases Weekly Report,* 1983, *8,* 13-20.

Mangione, R.A., & Sause, R.B. Antimicrobial Management of pulmonary tuberculosis. *Pharmacy Times,* 1984, *50,* 74-83.

Mitchell, J.R., Zimmerman, H.J., Ishak, K.G., et al. Isoniazid liver injury: clinical spectrum, pathology and probable pathogenesis. *Annals of Internal Medicine,* 1976, *84,* 181.

Reichman, L.B., & McDonald, R.J. Practical management and control of tuberculosis. *Medical Clinics of North America,* 1977, *61,* 1185.

Rooney, J.J., Crocco, J.A., & Kramer, S. Further observations on tuberculin reactions in active tuberculosis. *American Journal of Medicine,* 1976, *60,* 517.

Scheinhorn, D.J., & Angelillo, V.A. Antituberculous therapy in pregnancy. *Western Journal of Medicine,* 1977, *127,* 195.

Snider, D.E., Layde, P.M., Johnson, M.W., et al. Treatment of tuberculosis during pregnancy. *American Review of Respiratory Disease,* 1980, *122,* 65.

Some foods don't mix with isoniazid. *Nurses' Drug Alert,* 1983, March, 21.

Waters, M.F.R. The diagnosis and management of dapsone-resistant leprosy. *Leprosy Review,* 1977, *48,* 95.

World Health Organization. A study of two twice-weekly and a once weekly continuation regimens of tuberculosis chemotherapy including a comparison of two durations of treatment. *Tubercle,* 1977, *58,* 129.

CHAPTER 51

Antifungals and Antivirals

Don Leach
Larry Bettesworth

Medications discussed in this chapter

Antifungal agents	Antifungal agents—cont'd
Acrisorcin	Tolnaftate
Amphotericin B	Triacetin
Candicidin	Undecylenate (calcium,
Ciclopirox	zinc)
Clotrimazole	Undecylenic acid
Econazole	*Antiviral agents*
Flucytosine	Acyclovir
Gentian violet	Amantadine
Griseofulvin	Idoxuridine
Haloprogin	Interferon
Ketoconazole	Ribavirin
Miconazole	Trifluridine
Natamycin	Vidarabine
Nystatin	

Fungal disease can appear in a variety of ways in any mammalian host, including humans. Certain fungi when ingested can produce *mycotoxicoses* or mycetism, a toxic reaction. The presence of a fungal antigen in the body may evoke an allergic or hypersensitivity response from the host. Fungi may also invade living tissue in an infectious process called *mycosis*. Even though it is possible for any of these to occur alone or in combination, mycosis as a single entity is by far the most common fungal disease.

Fungal infections can be conveniently divided into systemic and superficial mycosis. Systemic mycosis is a serious disease and can have an extremely rapid and fulminant course. Superficial mycosis involving the skin, hair, and nails is usually chronic with little associated morbidity.

SYSTEMIC FUNGAL INFECTIONS

Unlike bacterial and viral infections, systemic fungal infections are usually not transmitted between human hosts. Fungi usually gain entrance into the body by inhalation or direct cutaneous inoculation. Infections with these organisms are limited by host exposure to the specific geographic location in which the organisms are found. Some fungi such as species of *Candida* are widely distributed and have been known to cause disease in most parts of the world. Other fungi are only found in specific geographic locations. Coccidiodomycosis is usually encountered in the southwestern United States, Mexico, and in certain countries of Central and South America. Maduromycosis is almost exclusively found in the tropical zones where few people wear shoes. Certain fungal infections may be more common in individuals whose occupations cause frequent contact with specific species of fungus. Sporotrichosis, has a worldwide distribution, but most commonly affects men who are laborers, farmers, or florists, because the fungus is found in soil, peat moss, and decaying vegetation.

Systemic fungal infections occur often in individuals whose host defense mechanisms have been weakened or impaired by disease, trauma, drugs, or various genetic or environmental factors. A break in host defense capability commonly allows *Candida* species, which are normally present in the gastrointestinal tract and the female genital tract, to invade human tissue and infect the host. Systemic candidiasis is becoming an increasingly common complication in hospitalized patients who become immunocompromised by cancer chemotherapy.

The toxic potential of the agents available for treating systemic mycoses requires documentation of the infecting organism. Identification of the organism by microscopy, serology, and culture should be done before initiating drug therapy.

REVIEW OF AGENTS USED IN SYSTEMIC MYCOSES

Amphotericin B

Amphotericin B is an antibiotic produced in fermentation by *Streptomyces nodosus*, a common soil-borne bacterium. It is an extremely water insoluble drug that will precipitate when mixed in electrolyte solutions. Thus the drug should be mixed for intravenous administration in a 5% dextrose in water solution at a concentration that is no greater than 0.1 mg/ml. The drug is poorly absorbed from the GI tract and is usually administered intravenously.

Although amphotericin B is available in a product (Mysteclin-F) that contains both tetracycline and amphotericin B in oral dosage forms (e.g., capsules and syrup) for treating candidal overgrowth that occurs in a large number of patients taking the tetracyclines, its use is *not* recommended. A national research council advisory panel has found that this combination is ineffective and recommends against indiscriminate prophylaxis. Because of these findings and opinions, the *oral* use of amphotericin B is *not* discussed in this text.

Mechanism of action. Amphotericin B is fungicidal when adequate concentrations are achieved in the infected tissue. The drug acts by attaching to sterols (e.g., ergosterol, cholesterol) contained on the plasma membranes of the cells. The presence of amphotericin B damages the osmotic barrier normally provided by the membrane by altering membrane permeability and thus disrupting the normal cellular function. The drug exerts a cytotoxic effect on both fungal organisms and human cells. However, it is more selective for fungal membranes that contain more ergosterol than cholesterol.

In addition, this mechanism can improve the penetration of other antifungal agents given concomitantly with amphotericin B. Flucytosine, combined with amphotericin B, exerts a synergistic antifungal effect because it can more easily penetrate the fungal cell to reach its intracellular site of action. This combination allows a significant reduction in the required daily dose of amphotericin B and in the total duration of treatment, and it appears to have a higher cure rate.

Clinical use. The spectrum of antifungal activity for amphotericin B includes a wide variety of pathogenic fungi. Amphotericin B is the agent of choice either alone or in combination with other antifungal agents for most life-threatening fungal infections. It is effective against *Blastomyces dermatiditis*, *Histoplasma capsulatum*, *Cryptococcus neoformans*, *Coccidioides immitis*, *Sporotrichum schenckii*, species of *Candida*, and certain strains of *Aspergillus*.

Pharmacokinetics. Amphotericin B is largely bound to sterol-containing tissue membranes leaving a small concentration in the serum. The drug penetrates poorly into the cerebrospinal fluid and thus requires intrathecal or intraventricular administration

in meningitis. Amphotericin B is extensively metabolized, and only 5% of the unchanged drug is excreted by the kidneys. It has been reported that amphotericin B is detectable in the urine for 7 to 8 weeks following the discontinuation of therapy. However, because of the low percentage of renal excretion, renal impairment does not significantly alter the dosing requirements of amphotericin B.

Toxicity. Amphotericin B is toxic to human cells, as well as to fungal cells, because of a similar cellular structure. The adverse effects associated with the use of amphotericin B result from both a direct cytotoxic effect and from a less common hypersensitive response.

Chills, fever, and nausea are commonly encountered side effects that may occur immediately after beginning intravenous therapy with amphotericin B. Headache, anorexia, vomiting, thrombophlebitis, and hyperthermia also may be encountered, but usually appear later in the therapy. Hydrocortisone is often administered concomitantly with amphotericin B to decrease the incidence of adverse effects. However, when these effects appear, the severity of the reaction does not appear to be diminished. Further, no controlled studies exist to substantiate the effectiveness of hydrocortisone used in this manner.

Direct nephrotoxicity is perhaps the most serious dose-dependent effect of amphotericin B. The drug causes both proximal and distal tubular damage. It initially appears as cylinduria on urinalysis followed by signs of tubular dysfunction such as a nephrogenic diabetes insipidus, hypokalemia, and hypomagnesemia. The nephrotoxicity occurs to some extent in most patients receiving the recommended dose of 1 mg/kg/day for prolonged periods. The renal damage is reversible in most cases after the discontinuation of the drug. This effect is a direct extension of the desired pharmacologic action and can be prevented clinically by gradually decreasing the total daily dose while observing for renal function improvement by monitoring urinalysis and serum potassium levels.

Anemia may develop over a period of several weeks of therapy. This effect is the result of impaired red cell production and is reversible when the drug is discontinued. *Leukopenia* and thrombocytopenia have also been reported to occur rarely. Hypersensitivity reactions to amphotericin B ranging from anaphylaxis to mild rashes have also been reported and likewise occur infrequently.

Dose and administration. To determine possible sensitivity, a test dose of 1 mg of amphotericin B should be administered. It should be administered by slow intravenous infusion over 20 to 30 minutes. The

Administering amphotericin B for injection

Because amphotericin B for injection is generally restricted for use in patients with progressive or potentially fatal fungal infections and because of the serious adverse side effects associated with the intravenous use of amphotericin B, the following material has been provided to examine its use more closely.

Because of the many precautions and special measures required for the preparation and administration of this drug, the following is outlined. Nurses responsible for administering this drug should also review the manufacturer's package insert.

A variety of dosing schedules exist for administering amphotericin B. These are individualized for the specific patient. The following schedule may be used as indicated.

Day 1: 1 mg test dose infused over 2 to 6 hours
Day 2: 5 mg infused over 6 to 8 hours
Day 3: increase the daily dose by 5 to 10 mg every other day or daily until a total daily dose of 0.5 to 1 mg/kg is reached with a *maximum* daily dose of 1.5 mg/kg

The test dose is a screening measure to determine individual patient response to amphotericin B because of the drug's numerous side effects; usually 1 mg of amphotericin B is diluted in 500 ml of 5% dextrose and water (D_5W) and administered by slow intravenous infusion over 2 to 6 hours. The pulse rate and temperature of the patient should be taken every 15 to 30 minutes for at least 4 hours after the test dose infusion has begun. The patient should also be monitored for other adverse effects.

For intrathecal administration, 0.5 mg of amphotericin B is administered 3 times a week. Each dose is dissolved in at least 5 ml of cerebrospinal fluid. Because the treatment is usually continued for 2 to 4 weeks, an Ommaya reservoir may be surgically placed in the scalp to facilitate the administration of the amphotericin B and to eliminate the need for repeated intrathecal injections.

Amphotericin B is available for reconstitution in powder form. The powder should be stored in the refrigerator and protected from light. The drug is reconstituted with 10 ml of sterile water for injection. The sterile water should be free of preservatives or bacteriostatic agents. The reconstituted medication (5 mg/ml) remains stable for 1 week when stored in the refrigerator and protected from light. Do *not* reconstitute with saline solutions.

To administer reconstituted amphotericin B, the appropriate dose requires further dilution with 250, 500, or 1000 ml of D_5W to produce a concentration for administration not greater than 0.1 mg/ml. For a dose of less than 25 mg, dilute in 250, 500 or 1000 ml of D_5W; for a dose of 25 to 50 mg dilute in 500 or 1000 ml of D_5W.

A dose greater than 50 mg should be diluted in 1000 ml of D_5W.

There is no exact infusion rate (i.e., ml per hour), and generally the entire volume is infused over a minimum 6 to 8 hours to minimize the adverse effects.

Because amphotericin B commonly is associated with adverse reactions involving chills, fever, and nausea, the addition of a corticosteroid (e.g., hydrocortisone sodium succinate or methylprednisolone sodium succinate) is often added to help prevent these reactions. However, this practice has not been confirmed by clinical studies and is not universally recommended. Meperidine may also be indicated for severe chills.

Administering amphotericin B for injection—cont'd

Most inline filters must be avoided when amphotericin B is infused because of the large molecular size of the drug. If used, the active drug may be removed by the filter. A filter should be greater than 1 mµ. A minidrip or Safti-check set may be used to infuse the drug and to regulate the rate of infusion. A Vol-u-trol should *not* be used because of its membrane valve, which has a pore size of 0.8 mµ and may likewise filter out the amphotericin B.

During infusion, because the drug is relatively insoluble, the bottle should be agitated occasionally to prevent precipitation. The infusion bottle should be protected from light by covering with a paper bag (foil is not necessary) because the drug deteriorates when exposed to direct or reflected sunlight. It is not necessary to wrap or protect the IV tubing from light.

With amphotericin B, because it does not contain any preservative or bacteriostatic agent, the potential for sepsis is high, and preparation requires a meticulous *aseptic* technique to prevent infection.

No other medications should be directly added or piggybacked with amphotericin B. This drug is incompatible with most medications, including normal saline and potassium chloride. The following medications can be added and are compatible up to 7 hours when added to an amphotericin B concentration of 0.1 mg/ml D_5W.

    Chlorpheniramine 10 mg
    Diphenhydramine 25 mg
    Hydrocortisone sodium succinate 100 mg
    Methylprednisolone sodium succinate 40 mg
    Heparin 500 units

Common adverse side effects associated with the use of amphotericin B include fever, chills, headache, nausea, and vomiting. The frequency and severity of these effects are associated with the dose and rate of the intravenous infusion. These effects can be minimized by administering an antihistamine, aspirin, meperidine, or corticosteroids before beginning the infusion.

Thrombophlebitis is a complication that can result from the irritating effects of this drug. It can be minimized by administering the drug on alternate days, rotating venipuncture sites, or adding heparin (500 units/L) to the reconstituted amphotericin B solution.

Nephrotoxicity is another adverse effect. Monitor for an inability to concentrate urine, especially in patients who are receiving the drug over a prolonged period. Because of the numerous adverse effects associated with amphotericin B, the following should be monitored:

    Daily dose (should *not* exceed 1.5 mg/kg, or 50 mg)
    Renal function (BUN, serum creatinine, urine output, urinalysis and urinary electrolytes)
    Blood cell count (CBC, hematocrit)
    Electrolyte balance (serum sodium, potassium, chloride levels)
    Vital signs (temperature, heart rate, blood pressure every hour once the infusion is begun and for 2 hours after it is completed)

patient's vital signs should be checked every 30 minutes for 4 hours following the dose. During the first week of therapy the dose should be increased in 5 mg increments up to a daily dose of 0.3 mg/kg given as a slow intravenous infusion over 4 to 6 hours. In the second week an adjustment can be made up to 0.5 to 0.6 mg/kg/day if renal function permits it. In circumstances requiring more rapid increases in dose, the extreme toxic potential of the drug must be judiciously weighed against the potential harm of the disease (see box; pp. 1110-1111).

Flucytosine

Mechanism of action. Flucytosine is a fluorinated pyrimadine that acts as an antimetabolite altering nucleic acid synthesis in susceptible fungi and yeasts. This agent is not active against human cells.

Clinical use. Flucytosine has a much narrower spectrum of activity than amphotericin B. Organisms sensitive to the fungistatic action of flucytosine include *Cryptococcus neoformans*, species of *Candida*, and a few species of *Aspergillus.* Primary and acquired resistance to the drug has been the limiting factor to its clinical usefulness. However, it is used in serious systemic fungal infections individually or commonly in combination with amphotericin B.

Pharmacokinetics. Flucytosine is well absorbed from the gastrointestinal tract and is only commercially available in oral dosage form. However, a parenteral dosage form is currently under investigation.

The drug is widely distributed in the body fluids and tissues with little protein binding. It penetrates the cerebrospinal fluid, reaching concentrations of 65% to 90% of the serum concentration. Therefore, flucytosine is of value for patients with cryptococcal meningitis or disseminated candidiasis who are intolerant of amphotericin B.

Flucytosine is eliminated largely by glomerular filtration, with 80% of the administered dose excreted unchanged in the urine. Because the major pathway of elimination is the kidney, flucytosine must be dosed according to renal function.

Toxicity. The adverse effects caused by flucytosine are mild compared with amphotericin B. Nausea, vomiting, and diarrhea are seen in approximately 25% of the patients receiving therapeutic doses. Bone marrow depression leading to leukopenia, thrombocytopenia, and anemia occur in 8% to 13% of patients. However, white cell, red cell, and platelet counts usually return to normal if the dosage is reduced. In addition, an elevation of hepatic enzymes has been reported in about 25% of patients.

Dose and administration. Flucytosine is administered orally at doses of 100 to 150 mg/kg/day in equally divided doses every 6 hours. Flucytosine is generally administered with another agent such as amphotericin B because of the rapid formation of fungal resistance. In addition, the toxicity of amphotericin B can be minimized when these agents are used together because of reduced dosage requirements.

In renal impairment, the flucytosine dosage should be adjusted to maintain peak serum concentrations below 100 μg/ml. Hemodialysis will remove flucytosine from the serum in clearance rates similar to creatinine. Replacement doses of 25 mg/kg to 50 mg/kg after dialysis will maintain therapeutic serum levels.

Miconazole

Mechanism of action. Miconazole is a fungicidal agent that acts by altering mycotic cell membrane permeability. This action results in the leakage of essential cellular elements.

Clinical use. Miconazole is occasionally used for treating severe systemic mycoses in the parenterally administered form. The drug has a broad spectrum of activity against pathogenic yeasts and fungi, including species of *Cryptococcus, Paracoccidioides, Coccidioides, Petriellioides, Candida,* and *Histoplasma.*

Pharmacokinetics. Miconazole is poorly absorbed from the GI tract and is only administered topically and parenterally. Intravenous doses of miconazole widely distribute to body tissues, with the highest concentrations most likely to occur in the adrenal gland, liver, lungs, and kidneys. However, cerebrospinal fluid penetration is poor with intravenous administration. Thus the drug should be administered intrathecally to treat CNS infections. Miconazole is rapidly metabolized with 1% to 20% of the administered agent being excreted unchanged in the urine.

Toxicity. The adverse effects of intravenous miconazole seem to be less severe than those encountered with amphotericin B. Nausea, vomiting, rash, anemia, pruritus, fever, and hyponatremia have all been reported to occur commonly with high intravenous doses. Central nervous system abnormalities caused by intravenous miconazole include tremors, confusion, dizziness, seizures, and hallucinations, which occur in up to 16% of patients receiving this drug.

Dose and administration. Parenteral doses of miconazole are administered by intermittent intravenous infusion over 30 to 60 minutes. The daily adult dose varies from 200 mg to 3600 mg per day in three equally divided doses. The dose should be diluted in at least 200 ml of normal saline or D_5W. Central venous catheter administration may be used to minimize thrombophlebitis and to avoid multiple venous puncture.

Intrathecal doses of 15 to 20 mg of miconazole should be administered with systemic doses in treating fungal meningitis. This dose should be repeated every 3 to 7 days.

A dilute solution containing 200 mg of miconazole may be directly instilled into the bladder to treat urinary bladder mycoses. The pediatric dose of intravenous miconazole is 20 to 40 mg/kg/day, with a maximum 15 mg/kg per infusion. The drug is not recommended for use in pregnancy.

Miconazole does not appreciably accumulate in renal impairment. Thus, the dose should not be altered on the basis of renal function but on the basis of the therapeutic effect or the appearance of toxic effects.

THERAPY OF SUPERFICIAL FUNGAL INFECTIONS

The superficial mycoses in general are far less serious problems in terms of the overall health of the host than the systemic mycoses. They may be self-limiting, and the individual is often asymptomatic. Tinea pedis, or athlete's foot, is the most common type of superficial fungal infection. The prevalence of tinea pedis is reported to be as high as 65% among groups of young physically active individuals. Another common form of superficial mycosis is caused by a ubiquitous yeastlike organism, *Candida albicans. Candida albicans* is normally present on mucous membranes of the respiratory, gastrointestinal, and vaginal tracts. In situations favoring the growth of this microorganism, it can gain dominance over normal bacterial flora and become either superficially or systemically infective. Candidiasis is commonly induced by antibiotic therapy that destroys the usual dominant bacteria, by agents that impede the normal host defense mechanisms (e.g., immunosuppressive agents), or by diseases such as diabetes mellitus and leukemia where the host defense is compromised by the disease.

AGENTS USED TO TREAT SUPERFICIAL MYCOSES

Griseofulvin

Mechanisms of action and clinical use. Griseofulvin is a *fungistatic* agent that disrupts cell mitosis by altering DNA production. The drug is administered orally for treating fungal infections of the skin, nails, and hair. It is deposited quickly into the new growing keratin layers of the skin. As the keratin layers are shed, those cells containing the drug resist further growth by the organism. Thus therapy with griseofulvin must be continued until all of the infected tissue is shed and replaced with new fungus-free cells.

Species of *Trichophyton, Microsporum,* and *Epidermophyton* are the fungi most often associated with a superficial mycosis called *dermatophytosis.* Griseofulvin is the oral agent of choice for most dermatophytoses, but is ineffective against the organisms causing systemic fungal disease.

Pharmacokinetics and toxicity. Griseofulvin is erratically absorbed from the gastrointestinal tract, and studies have revealed a wide interpatient variability with a given oral dose. The absorption of the drug is reported to be substantially improved when it is taken with a fatty meal. It is metabolized to a large extent in the liver, with less than 1% excreted unchanged in the urine.

Griseofulvin causes few serious adverse effects. Normal doses of griseofulvin may cause low-grade headache, nausea, vomiting, diarrhea, and mental confusion. However, allergic reactions and transient blood dyscrasias, including neutropenia, leukopenia, and monocytosis, have been reported. Because griseofulvin is derived from a species of penicillin, the possibility of cross-sensitivity in patients hypersensitive to penicillin must be considered.

Dose and administration. The length of treatment for dermatophytoses with griseofulvin will depend on the infected tissue. Fungal skin infections open to air will respond completely in 2 to 4 weeks. However, fungal infections of the toenails may require therapy for over 6 months. Because the agent only inhibits the growth of mature fungi, treatment must continue until all of the old tissue is grown out and removed. The dose of griseofulvin in adults is 0.5 to 1 gm, and for children it is 10 mg/kg daily. The dose should be given in one or two equally divided doses. The ultramicrosized or micronized preparation requires only one half of these doses because of better oral absorption.

Nystatin

Nystatin is a chemical congener of amphotericin B. They thus share similar chemical and physical properties. However, unlike amphotericin B, nystatin is used almost exclusively in the topical therapy for superficial *Candida* infections of the mouth, vulvovaginal areas, gastrointestinal tract, and skin. Nystatin is a fungicidal agent that acts by affecting the permeability of fungal cell membranes in a manner similar to amphotericin B.

Toxicity. Few toxic effects are reported with the topical application of nystatin. Large oral doses may cause nausea, vomiting, and diarrhea. Hypersensitivity reactions and systemic toxicity have not been reported with this agent.

Dose and administration. Nystatin is available in a variety of dosage forms, including vaginal tablets, creams, lotions, ointments, oral suspensions, and drops. The oral dose of the drug will vary from 500,000 to 1 million units, three to four times daily. For oral candidiasis, the medication should be kept in contact with the infected tissue for at least several minutes. Both nystatin liquid preparations swished for several minutes before swallowing and nystatin vaginal tablets melted in the mouth provide sufficient contact time for treating oral candidiasis. Nystatin creams and ointments should be applied to the affected areas two to three times daily.

Imidazoles (clotrimazole, miconazole)

The imidazoles, clotrimazole and miconazole, are congeners with similar chemical and pharmacologic properties. The spectrum of activity for these two agents includes most fungi pathogenic to humans. Although miconazole is occasionally used for the parenteral therapy of systemic mycoses, the imidazoles as a group are usually used to treat superficial infections caused by the dermatophytes and by *Candida* species. The imidazoles exert a fungistatic and *fungicidal* effect on susceptible organisms by altering cell membrane permeability.

Toxicity. The adverse effects experienced with the topical use of the imidazoles are minor. Stinging, erythema, desquamation, and pruritus have been reported to occur rarely (see Adverse/Side Effects of the Antifungals and Antivirals).

Dosage and administration. The imidazoles are available in creams, solutions, and vaginal tablets. Clotrimazole is also available in oral troches. The topical application of the creams or solutions to infected skin and nails consists of once or twice daily applications for at least 4 weeks. Vulvovaginal application of the creams and vaginal application of the tablets should be made once daily for 2 weeks.

Tolnaftate

Tolnaftate is the first chemical compound that is topically fungicidal to many organisms causing dermatophytoses. It is effective against species of *Trichophyton*, *Epidermophyton*, and *Microsporum*, but has no activity against *Candida* or bacteria. Tolnaftate rarely causes hypersensitivity reactions, but there are a few reported accounts of mild skin irritation with topical use. Tolnaftate is supplied as a cream, powder, or solution. It should be applied to the skin twice daily for 2 to 4 weeks for most dermatophytoses, but may be required for a longer period of time in treating a long-standing infection.

Haloprogin

Haloprogin is a fungicidal agent used topically to treat the usual causes of dermatophytoses. The agent is poorly absorbed through intact, as well as damaged, skin, and prolonged use is not associated with systemic toxicity. However, local irritation, burning, inflammation, vesicle formation, and pruritus may be encountered, especially when treating seriously infected lesions. Haloprogin is available as a 1% cream or solution and is applied twice daily for 2 to 4 weeks.

Undecylenic acid and salts

Undecylenic acid is a fungistatic agent that is active against most fungi that cause superficial mycoses. However, the activity achieved with usual therapeutic doses is not always effective in eradicating the fungi, and it is estimated to provide a cure rate of only 50%. Undecylenic acid preparations are most commonly used for tinea pedis and have been combined with zinc and calcium to improve their therapeutic action in dermatophytoses. These compounds are available in a variety of concentrations for use on the skin and mucous membranes. These agents should be limited to the chronic control of the minor superficial fungal infections and not for the primary treatment of the acute exacerbation of an infection.

Compound undecylenic acid ointments with 5% undecylenic acid and 20% zinc undecylenate are commonly used in proprietory antifungal preparations. In addition, powders containing 2% undecylenic acid with 20% zinc undecylenate are also commonly used antifungal agents.

Miscellaneous agents

The agents listed in this miscellaneous section are only rarely considered of primary value in treating fungal infections. In most cases they will be used as adjuvant therapy and should be combined with other more effective antifungal agents.

Natamycin. Natamycin is a broad-spectrum antifungal agent that is now rarely used. It is useful in ocular fungal infections such as keratitis. It is also the agent of choice in infections caused by *Fusarium solani*. Natamycin is not irritating to the eye and therefore can be used when other first-line agents are not tolerated. Natamycin is applied topically as a suspension or as an ophthalmic ointment.

Candicidin. Candicidin is another polyene antibiotic like amphotericin B and nystatin that is produced by a soil-borne actinomycete. Like nystatin, candicidin is only used topically to treat vaginal candidiasis. Adverse reactions to candicidin are rare, with only a few reports of local irritation or sensitization to the drug. Candicidin is available in vaginal tablets or ointment and is applied intravaginally twice daily for 14 days.

Acrisorcin. Acrisorcin is an antifungal agent used

to treat tinea versicolor. It is applied to the skin in a 0.2% cream on a twice-daily basis until 6 weeks after the lesions have cleared. The adverse effects caused by topically applied acrisorcin are caused by hypersensitivity reactions or by local irritation. Hives, blisters, burning, stinging, and photosensitivity are the most common complaints.

Gentian violet. Gentian violet is a disinfectant that may be used to treat vaginal candidiasis or tinea pedis. As the crystal violet salt in a 0.1% solution or ointment, it is useful in treating tinea pedis and is applied one or two times daily. It is well tolerated, and adverse effects are rare. Because of the risk of systemic absorption for both the mother and fetus, gentian violet should not be vaginally administered during the third trimester of pregnancy.

ANTIVIRAL THERAPY

Significant progress in the pharmacologic prevention and treatment of viral disease has been slow. The unique life cycle of the virus has proved to be the most confounding aspect in the search for antiviral agents. Unlike bacteria, viruses live and multiply inside a host cell. They use the host cell replication apparatus for their own progenerative process. This life cycle presents the problem of finding an agent that is adequately specific to kill the virus while sparing the host cell.

Most chemicals capable of directly killing viruses would be similarly damaging to the host cell. Therefore, the major thrust of antiviral research has been aimed at finding ways to impair the process of viral replication. Viruses were once believed to use the cellular replication apparatus of the host to perform identical functions. However, significant differences in the replication processes of viruses have now been identified. Isolation and further clarification of these differences will provide points for applying new antiviral therapy in the future.

PROPHYLAXIS AND TREATMENT OF VIRAL DISEASE

Amantadine

Amantadine is an antiviral agent that has been available in the United States since 1966 for the prophylaxis of influenza A.

Mechanism of action. The mechanism of the *virustatic* action of amantadine is not now fully understood. However, it has been postulated that amantadine may interfere with the viral penetration of host cells, as well as block the viral uncoating process and subsequent release of viral nucleic acids into the host cell.

Clinical use. Amantadine is effective in preventing influenza A infection when the drug is taken at least 1 day before exposure to the virus. It is also effective in ameliorating influenza A if taken within 48 hours after the onset of the illness. Amantadine has been reported to significantly decrease the frequency and quantity of viral shedding.

Amantadine is recommended for general prophylactic therapy in patients at a high risk of dying but only during a documented influenza A epidemic. The drug should be used for the prophylaxis and disease amelioration in high-risk patients who have been exposed to the influenza A virus. Amantadine may be used for the prophylaxis and treatment of individuals whose continued services to the community are necessary in an epidemic situation, such as health care workers. However, the benefits of the drug should be carefully considered along with the potential toxicity.

Pharmacokinetics. Amantadine is well absorbed in the gastrointestinal tract and is commercially available only in an oral dosage form. The drug is not metabolized, and the vast majority of the administered drug is excreted unchanged in the urine. Thus, the dose of amantadine must be adjusted on the basis of renal function to prevent drug accumulation.

Toxicity. The incidence of all adverse effects associated with the therapeutic doses of amantadine is reported to be from 5% to 20%. The adverse effects are dose related and most commonly occur in elderly patients and in patients with impaired renal function. Central nervous system disturbances include nervousness, difficulty in thinking and concentrating, and insomnia. The incidence of more serious adverse effects such as hallucinations, seizures, or coma is low.

Dose and administration. The dose of amantadine for adults is 200 mg once daily or 100 mg twice daily. The pediatric dose is 4.4 to 8.8 mg/kg, not to exceed 150 mg per day. The adverse effects of amantadine are well correlated to drug serum concentrations and can usually be decreased by reducing the dose.

For prophylactic administration, amantadine should be given to patients immediately on documentation of the epidemic and continued for the duration. Amantadine may also be used to protect the patient from the influenza A virus until an active immunity can be established. Amantadine should be continued for 2 weeks following the influenza A vaccination.

Vidarabine

Vidarabine is a virustatic agent that acts by inhibiting the replication of DNA viruses. The drug has a proved therapeutic effectiveness against herpes simplex viruses and poxviruses. The sensitivity of the hepatitis B virus to vidarabine is presently under investigation and the results appear encouraging. Currently, vidarabine is recommended for use in herpes simplex encephalitis and *keratoconjunctivitis* and in herpes zoster infections in patients who are immunosuppressed.

Mortality and neurologic sequelae from herpes encephalitis are significantly reduced by the early administration of vidarabine. Whitley, et al (1981) demonstrated a reduction in 1-year mortality from 70% in patients treated with a placebo and less effective therapy to 40% in those patients treated with vidarabine. Likewise, the neurologic sequelae of the disease in those patients treated with vidarabine was significantly reduced.

Pharmacokinetics. Vidarabine is a highly water insoluble compound that is only administered topically (as an ointment) and intravenously. For intravenous injection, vidarabine must be dissolved in a concentration not exceeding 0.45 mg/ml of intravenous fluid or 450 mg of vidarabine per 1000 ml of solution.

The drug is widely distributed in body tissues and moderately penetrates the cerebrospinal fluid. It is metabolized by the liver to active metabolites that are excreted rapidly by the kidneys. A single dose is completely eliminated within 12 hours. Renal impairment requires dosage adjustment to avoid drug accumulation.

Toxicity. The usual side effects occurring with intravenous administration are nausea, vomiting, anorexia, and diarrhea. Although CNS and bone marrow toxicity are seen with high intravenous doses, the toxicities are usually of little practical clinical significance.

Dose and administration. The recommended intravenous daily dose of vidarabine is 15 mg/kg administered by constant infusion over 12 to 24 hours. Acute herpes keratoconjunctivitis and recurrent epithelial keratitis are treated with vidarabine ointment, placed in the conjunctival sac every 3 hours, five times daily. It is recommended that the therapy be changed if there is no improvement after 7 days or if complete reepithelialization has not occurred after 21 days. Because vidarabine in high systemic concentrations may have a mutagenic, teratogenic, and oncogenic potential, it should be used judiciously in all patients, especially pregnant women. As with any therapy, the adverse potential should be carefully compared with the benefit of treatment.

Idoxuridine

Idoxuridine is a halogenated pyrimidine that acts as an antimetabolite in the production of DNA in human and viral cells. Idoxuridine is effective against a wide variety of DNA viruses in vitro, including herpes virus, vaccinia virus, varicella virus, and cytomegalovirus. However, the drug is used almost exclusively for the topical treatment of herpes keratoconjunctivitis.

Toxicity. Local application of idoxuridine to the conjunctiva may cause local irritation, inflammation, pain, and photophobia. Hypersensitivity reactions have also been reported, but are rare.

Dose and administration. Idoxuridine is administered directly into the conjunctival sac in a 0.5% ointment or a 0.1% solution. The ointment is placed into the conjunctival sac five times daily or every 4 hours, with the last dose at bedtime. The ophthalmic solution is instilled into the eye every hour during the day and every 2 hours at night until reepithelialization occurs. Thereafter the interval between doses is increased to 2 hours during the day and 3 to 4 hours at night. Treatment with idoxuridine should be continued 3 to 5 days after the infection clears.

Trifluridine

Trifluridine is a fluorinated pyrimidine nucleoside used topically to treat certain virus infections of the eye. The antiviral mechanism of action of trifluridine is not fully understood, but it does inhibit DNA synthesis in mammalian cell cultures.

The effectiveness of this agent dictates that it be mentioned as an alternative therapy for keratoconjunctivitis and recurrent epithelial keratitis caused by herpes simplex virus and vaccinia virus. However, the adverse potential of this agent has resulted in restricted clinical application. Trifluridine has been associated with mutagenesis in animal studies and is teratogenic to chick embryos when injected directly into the yolk sac. Although the mutagenic and teratogenic effects have not been seen with use in humans, strict adherence to the dosage and frequency of administration is highly recommended. The safe use of trifluridine has not been satisfactorily demonstrated in pregnant and lactating women. The potential benefits of using this drug must be carefully weighed against the potential risks. Other more commonly encountered side effects of this agent are local irritation, palpebral edema, punctate and epithelial keratopathy, hypersensitivity reactions, and stromal edema.

The 0.1% ophthalmic solution of trifluridine is instilled into the affected eye every 2 hours while the patient is awake up to a maximum of nine drops per day. This dose is continued until full reepithelialization occurs, at which time a dose of one drop every 4 hours while the patient is awake with a daily maximum of five drops is recommended for an additional 7 days.

Acyclovir

Acyclovir is an antiviral agent that has demonstrated a high level of activity against herpesvirus infections. The active metabolite of acyclovir, acyclo GTP, has been shown to be 10 to 30 times more effective against herpesvirus-specific DNA polymerase than cellular DNA polymerase. This characteristic of the drug makes it selectively more toxic to the infecting herpesvirus than to the host cells. Furthermore, the active metabolite is generated 30 to 120 times faster in experimental tissues infected with herpesvirus than in uninfected tissue cultures.

Although there is a paucity of pharmacologic data available on this agent, few side effects have so far been demonstrated. Activity against herpes simplex virus Type 1 and Type 2, herpes simiae, varicella zoster virus, and Epstein-Barr virus has been demonstrated.

INVESTIGATIONAL AGENTS

Interferon. Interferon is not commercially available currently, but promises to be a significant form of antiviral therapy in the future. Interferons are endogenous substances produced by mammalian cells when infected by a virus. The interferons are glycoproteins that indirectly cause an inhibition of viral replication. The substance stimulates noninfected cells to produce a polypeptide that blocks the translation or transcription of messenger RNA in the infected cells.

The action of the interferons are species specific, and consequently, human interferon is most effective against viral infections in humans. However, the difficulty of mass production, purification, and distribution of interferon has impeded the study and clinical use of the drug.

The current study of interferon in patients with a wide variety of viral diseases has been encouraging. Hepatitis B virus, herpes zoster virus in patients with cancer who are immunosuppressed, cytomegalovirus in renal transplant recipients, and other viruses have been shown to be sensitive to the antiviral effects of interferon.

The potential for adverse effects in patients receiving low to moderate doses of interferons by subcutaneous, intramuscular or topical routes of administration appears to be negligible. Large doses given parenterally (i.e., greater than 500,000 units/kg/day) may cause fever, fatigue, malaise, and reversible bone marrow depression. It is unclear whether these effects are the result of interferon itself or of product impurities.

Ribavirin. Ribavirin is a triazole nucleoside that is currently under study to determine its potential as an antiviral agent suitable for use in humans. It was first reported to have a broad spectrum of activity against viruses in 1972. Since then many claims have been made regarding its effectiveness against a variety of viruses, including influenza A and B, Type 2 herpes virus hominis, and hepatitis B virus. Although there have been many in vitro studies of the effectiveness of this agent, few well-done in vivo studies have demonstrated the superiority of this agent over other currently available agents. In addition, further evaluation of its adverse potential as a teratogen, mutagen, carcinogen, and as an immunosuppressant must be undertaken before it can be recommended for antiviral use in humans.

SUMMARY

This chapter has examined the various types and uses of the antifungal and antiviral medications. The treatment of fungal and viral infections has been briefly discussed and the pharmacology and pharmacokinetics of the related agents has been presented. With an understanding of the various agents, including their actions and side effects, the nurse will be better able to provide optimum care to patients who require these medications.

ADVERSE/SIDE EFFECTS OF THE ANTIFUNGAL AND ANTIVIRAL AGENTS*

Antifungal agents
ALLERGIC REACTIONS

Erythema
Pruritus (most common with miconazole following IV administration)
Skin rashes
Urticaria

GASTROINTESTINAL SYSTEM

Diarrhea (more commonly associated with systemic administration)
Nausea (more commonly associated with systemic administration)
Vomiting (more commonly associated with systemic administration)

HEMATOLOGIC SYSTEM

Anemia
Leukopenia (rare)
Thrombocytopenia (rare)

HEPATIC SYSTEM

Increased SGOT
Increased alkaline phosphatase

RENAL SYSTEM

Hematuria
Increase in BUN
Nephrotoxicity (occurs in 80% of patients receiving amphotericin B daily)
Proteinuria
Serum potassium depletion

Antiviral agents
ALLERGIC REACTIONS

Pruritus
Skin rash

HEMATOLOGIC SYSTEM

Anemia (lowered hematocrit, hemoglobin)
Bone marrow depression (vidarabine in doses greater than 20 mg/kg can cause bone marrow depression; reversible in 3 to 5 days following termination of IV administration)
Thrombocytopenia (rare)

*See Chapter 11, "Drug Toxicity," for an overview of drug toxicity.

CLINICALLY SIGNIFICANT DRUG INTERACTIONS*

Primary drug	Interacting drug	Possible effect(s)	Probable mechanism(s)
Acyclovir	Probenecid	Increased concentration of acyclovir	Decreased excretion of acyclovir
Amphotericin B	Digitalis glycosides	Digitalis toxicity	Amphotericin B may decrease serum potassium
Griseofulvin	Anticoagulants (warfarin)	Decreased anticoagulant effect	Increased liver metabolism
Griseofulvin	Barbiturates	May decrease griseofulvin effect	Decreased absorption of griseofulvin

*See Chapter 10, "Drug Interactions," for an overview of drug interactions.

GENERAL NURSING IMPLICATIONS

Nursing of patients requiring antifungals

ASSESSMENT

The antifungals are used to treat various systemic and superficial fungal infections. The drug therapy is directed at the causative organism and the type of infection, whether systemic or superficial. Baseline assessment data should include specific information about the patient's general health state and specific condition as related to the need for the antifungal therapy. Careful inspection of the skin, hair, nails, or affected areas such as the mouth or vagina is indicated before initiating therapy for superficial infections. This assessment serves as a baseline from which to monitor the patient's therapeutic response. This is especially important because therapy for superficial infections is usually indicated until the infection has cleared completely.

Because the antifungals used to treat systemic fungal infections can be toxic, adequate identification of the infecting organisms is required *before* initiating the drug therapy. The patient should be prepared adequately and assisted when specimens are collected for microscopy and serology for culture and sensitivity studies. Isolation is usually not required, because systemic fungal infections are generally not transmitted from person to person.

In addition to information regarding the patient's general health state and the need for the antifungal therapy, it is often important, especially with superficial infections, to obtain an occupational history, a record of recent antibiotic therapy, and information regarding general self-care practices and activities. This information is helpful in identifying the cause of the infection and in helping patients prevent a reinfection. For patients requiring systemic treatment it should be ascertained if they have other health conditions such as a history of heart disease, cancer, immunosuppression, trauma, or drug use. Because of the toxicity associated with the systemic antifungals, in addition to culture and sensitivity studies, renal function tests, including urinalysis, are also indicated.

The drug history should be taken before initiating the therapy and should include specific information regarding any possible sensitivity, contraindications, cautions, drug interactions, and individual drug-taking patterns.

SENSITIVITY

Generally, allergic reactions to the antifungal medications are rare; however, any drug has the potential to cause a hypersensitivity reaction in a susceptible individual. Both systemic and superficial agents have been associated with hypersensitivity reactions.

The use of amphotericin B has resulted in hypersensitivity reactions from mild rashes to anaphylaxis. Thus it is recommended that a test dose be given before initiating the full therapy to identify patient sensitivity.

CONTRAINDICATIONS

The use of the antifungals is contraindicated in patients with a known hypersensitivity to a specific agent.

See the Nursing Drug Digest and the text of this chapter for contraindications associated with each agent.

CAUTIONS

The antifungals should be used with caution.

Amphotericin B affects human, as well as fungal, cells and although it is more selective for fungal cells, it can cause toxic effects.

Drug resistance has been associated with the use of flucytosine.

Miconazole is not recommended in pregnancy.

Gentian violet should not be used for treating superficial vaginal infections in pregnant women during the last trimester because it is associated with systemic absorption.

See the text of this chapter and the Nursing Drug Digest for specific cautions related to the use of each agent.

DRUG INTERACTIONS

Certain antifungals can interact with other drugs in a variety of mechanisms. See Clinically Significant Drug Interactions for specific drug interactions.

ADMINISTRATION
Superficial antifungals

The superficial antifungals are administered orally and topically in a variety of dosage forms including vaginal inserts, ophthalmics, solutions, ointments, suppositories, creams, troches, and powders.

Griseofulvin is administered orally. It is usually given with a fatty meal to increase absorption.

Nystatin is available in numerous dosage forms for topical administration, including oral suspension, creams, solutions, and vaginal tablets.

Tolnaftate is available in ointment, solution, and powder forms. Natamycin is available in an ophthalmic solution and an ointment for treating ocular fungal infections.

These should be administered using a medically aseptic technique and, whenever possible, patients should be taught the correct administration and allowed and encouraged to administer their own medication with supervision before discharge. Outpatients must be carefully assessed in relation to their self-medication abilities and their understanding of drug administration (see Chapter 2, "Preparation, Administration, and Monitoring of Medications").

Systemic antifungals

The antifungals can be administered orally or intravenously for treatment of systemic infections. Flucytosine is well absorbed from the gastrointestinal tract and is administered orally, whereas amphotericin B, because it is poorly absorbed from the gastrointestinal tract, is administered by intravenous infusion. The administration of amphotericin B requires special dilution and administration protocols.

Continued.

GENERAL NURSING IMPLICATIONS—cont'd

Nursings of patients requiring antifungals—cont'd

Systemic antifungals—cont'd

Dosing is individualized to the patient and to the need for systemic antifungal therapy. It is important to note that some of the antifungals, (e.g., flucytosine) must be dosed according to renal function because they are nephrotoxic, whereas others (e.g., miconazole) are dosed according to the therapeutic or toxic effect.

The antifungals are often administered concurrently with another antifungal medication. Because of the possibility of drug interactions, they are not administered together at the same time or in the same infusion.

Intrathecal or intraventricular administration of some of the antifungals (e.g., amphotericin B, miconazole) is indicated for treating fungal meningitis infections.

In addition to intermittent intravenous administration, miconazole is also administered topically and as a bladder irrigant. It may be administered by way of a central venous catheter to decrease the thrombophlebitis associated with its use as well as multiple venous punctures that are sometimes required with intermittent intravenous administration because of infiltration or vein damage.

Points to remember

Before administering the antifungals, be sure to:
- Check with patients to determine whether they have had any allergic reactions to any of the antifungal medications.
- Obtain samples (e.g., blood, urine, sputum, cerebrospinal fluid) as specified for culture and sensitivity tests.

When administering antifungals, remember that:
- If an antifungal medication is to be given in divided doses each day, one must space the time of administration as evenly as possible throughout the 24 hours (i.e., b.i.d. means every 12 hours around the clock).
- Ensure that the order for the antifungal medication is reviewed by the prescriber at least every 5 to 7 days so that the order is either renewed or canceled.
- Do not mix parenteral antifungal medications in the same syringe, same IV line, or same IV bottle.
- Dilute intravenous antifungal medications in compatible intravenous fluids, which are indicated in this chapter.

See the Nursing Drug Digest for specific information regarding the dosing and administration of the antifungals.

MONITORING PATIENT RESPONSE
Therapeutic response

The onset of action of antifungal therapy depends largely on the dosage form, the route of administration, the type of infection being treated, and individual patient factors. Generally, patients should be carefully monitored for clearing of lesions associated with superficial infections. Patients being treated for systemic infections should be monitored for decreased temperature, decreased white blood cell counts, increased appetite, increased energy, increased feelings of well-being, and other signs of an improvement in the patient's condition. Specimens should be obtained to monitor the effectiveness of the therapeutic regimen.

Because the treatment must continue until the fungal infection is cleared, monitoring is particularly important.

Adverse side effects

The usual adverse side effects associated with the antifungals when used to treat superficial infections include low-grade headache, diarrhea, mental confusion (griseofulvin), and blood dyscrasias. Toxic effects are usually minor with the topical use of the antifungals and can include local stinging, erythema, desquamation, pruritus, hives, or vesicle formation.

Adverse side effects and toxicities are generally associated with the antifungals when they are used in treating systemic infections, and patients should be monitored carefully. The major adverse effects associated with the antifungals used in treating systemic infections are nephrotoxicity, anemia, and CNS effects.

Nephrotoxicity

Monitor patients for cylindruria (urinalysis indicated), nephrogenic diabetes insipidus, hypokalemia (serum electrolytes indicated), and hypomagnesemia (serum electrolytes indicated).

These effects are usually reversible after the discontinuation of the offending antifungal medication.

Observe and report any changes in kidney function, such as hematuria, proteinuria, increased BUN, increased serum creatinine, or difficulty in urination.

Monitor nephrotoxicity closely in patients receiving amphotericin B with the following predisposing factors: old age (older than 70 years of age), high dose, prolonged duration of therapy (more than 10 days), preexisting renal dysfunction, and the concurrent administration of other nephrotoxic drugs (e.g., the aminoglycosides).

Monitor intake and output in patients receiving amphotericin B or flucytosine, and report any sudden change in urine output.

Anemia and other blood dyscrasias

Monitor complete blood counts, including hematocrit, for anemia, leukopenia, and thrombocytopenia, especially over several weeks of therapy.

CNS effects

Monitor patients for tremors, confusion, delirium, seizures, or hallucinations, especially in relation to miconazole when given in high intravenous doses.

Miscellaneous effects

Observe and report symptoms of hypersensitivity, such as skin rashes, fever, chills, laryngeal edema, or asthma.

Observe and report any changes in skin color or temperature, burning on urination, or other signs or symptoms of infection.

See Adverse/Side Effects of the Antifungals and Antivirals for an outline of ad-

GENERAL NURSING IMPLICATIONS—cont'd

Nursing of patients requiring antifungals—cont'd

Miscellaneous effects—cont'd
verse side effects associated with the use of the antifungals, and the Nursing Drug Digest for adverse effects associated with specific agents.

PATIENT EDUCATION
Superficial infections

Superficial infections can usually be best treated by self-medication by outpatients. Even hospitalized patients should be allowed and encouraged to self-medicate with careful instruction and supervision according to hospital policy. This is especially important because superficial infections may require prolonged therapy after discharge. The patient and the family, as indicated, should have a clear understanding of the medication regimen including the exact name of the medication, its dosage, administration, storage, purpose, general action, potential adverse side effects, and what can be done to minimize these effects. Because the antifungals are required until the infection is cleared, it is particularly important that the patient be able to monitor the therapeutic response. Health teaching and the promotion of

self-care abilities is often indicated to prevent a reinfection and the need for further antifungal therapy. Patients being treated for tinea pedis should be encouraged to wear shoes, wear waterproof sandals in public showers, change stockings daily, especially after exercise, and to wear comfortable and clean footwear. Women being treated for vaginal infections may need to be reminded to wear cotton underwear, review perineal and personal hygiene care, discuss avoiding intercourse until the infection clears, or encourage partners to use condoms.

The medication must be administered correctly to ensure therapeutic response, and patient education in relation to self-medication and follow-up cannot be overemphasized. Patients must be shown how to use the medication and be given step-by-step written instructions, whenever possible, to follow at home.

Whenever possible, patients should be examined by the health care provider to ensure that the therapeutic effect has been accomplished before the medication is discontinued.

Patients should also be taught to use perineal pads when vaginal tablets or creams are used to prevent staining of underwear or clothing. They should be cautioned against using tampons that can absorb the medication or further irritate vaginal tissues.

Systemic infections

The patient and the family, as indicated, should be fully informed about the nature of the patient's condition and the treatment plan and should be involved in the health care planning whenever possible. The patient and the family should understand the course of the therapy and the medication regimens, including the exact name of the medication to be used, its general action, purpose, adverse side effects, administration, and the need for a test dose as an indicator for sensitivity (e.g., for the use of amphotericin B). The need for close monitoring for the toxic effects associated with these medications requires that the patient and the family be able to help monitor the response and to make informed decisions about the treatment plan.

Nursing of patients requiring antivirals

ASSESSMENT

The antivirals can be used for prophylaxis (e.g., amantadine) and for treating various viral infections (e.g., herpes zoster, keratoconjunctivitis). Baseline assessment should include specific information about the patient's general health state and specific condition as related to the need for the antiviral therapy. The assessment serves as a baseline from which to monitor the patient's therapeutic response to the drug therapy. This is particularly important because the drug therapy is usually continued 3 to 7 days after the infection has cleared.

When patients are assessed, it is important to identify if they have concurrent health problems, including cardiac disease, immunosuppression, or a

bacterial infection, and if the viral condition is a recurrent one. Information regarding general self-care practices, especially as related to the indication for therapy (e.g., plantar warts), is helpful in developing a nursing plan to promote self-care to prevent the infection whenever possible. Because of the adverse effects associated with the use of some of the antifungals, it should be ascertained if the patient is pregnant or nursing an infant.

The drug history should be completed before the drug therapy is initiated and should include specific information regarding any possible sensitivity, contraindications, cautions, or drug interactions. Individual drug-taking patterns and abilities should also be identified.

SENSITIVITY

Generally, allergic reactions to the antiviral medications are rare; however, any drug has the potential to cause a hypersensitivity reaction in susceptible individuals.

CONTRAINDICATIONS AND CAUTIONS

The use of the antiviral medications is contraindicated in patients with a known hypersensitivity to the specific agent.

Trifluridine and vidarabine are contraindicated in pregnancy and in nursing mothers, and should be used cautiously in patients because of the mutagenic, teratogenic, and oncogenic effects associated with their use. The risk must be weighed against the ben-

Continued.

GENERAL NURSING IMPLICATIONS—cont'd

Nursing of patients requiring antivirals—cont'd

CONTRAINDICATIONS AND CAUTIONS—cont'd

efits of the therapy (see the Nursing Drug Digest for cautions associated with the use of specific agents).

ADMINISTRATION

The antivirals are available in a variety of dosage forms for oral (e.g., amantadine), parenteral (e.g., interferon), and topical (e.g., idoxuridine, vidarabine) administration. See the Nursing Drug Digest for specific information regarding the dosage and administration of each agent.

It is important to note that a dosage adjustment is required in relation to renal function for amantadine and vidarabine (intravenous).

When the antivirals are used for prophylaxis, they should be given to the patient immediately on documentation of an epidemic and continued for its duration. Influenza vaccine should be used until immunity is established (approximately 2 weeks).

Before administering the antivirals:
- Check with patients to determine whether they have had any allergic reactions to any of the antiviral medications.
- Obtain samples (e.g., blood, urine, sputum, cerebrospinal fluid) as specified for culture and sensitivity tests.

When administering the antivirals, remember the following:
- If an antiviral is to be given in divided doses each day, one must space the time of administration as evenly as possible throughout the 24 hours (i.e., b.i.d. means every 12 hours around the clock).
- Ensure the order for the antiviral medication is reviewed by the prescriber at least every 5 to 7 days so that the order is either renewed or canceled.
- Do not mix the antiviral medications in the same syringe, same IV line, or same IV bottle.
- Dilute intravenous antiviral medications in compatible intravenous solutions, which are indicated in this chapter.

MONITORING PATIENT RESPONSE

Therapeutic response

When the antivirals are administered for influenza prophylaxis, monitor patients for the absence of flulike symptoms or other signs of infection.

When the antiviral ophthalmic preparations (e.g., idoxuridine, vidarabine) are used for treating viral ocular conditions, monitor for reepithelialization.

Monitor the affected site for an improvement in the lesion. This is important because the therapy is usually indicated for 3 to 5 or more days after the infection clears, to prevent a reinfection.

Observe the patient for the appropriate therapeutic response such as reduction of fever, increased sense of well-being, increased appetite, and clearing of the lesions.

Adverse side effects

Adverse side effects are dose related for many of the antivirals (e.g., amantadine) and can be minimized or prevented by decreasing the dose of the medication; therefore, monitoring is essential. It is important to note that adverse effects occur most commonly in elderly patients and in patients with impaired renal function.

Local irritation, pain, inflammation, and photophobia have been associated with the use of the topically administered antivirals (e.g., idoxuridine).

Reversible bone marrow depression and other effects, including nausea, vomiting, anorexia, diarrhea, fever, fatigue, and malaise, have been associated with intravenous administration of some of the antiviral agents (e.g., vidarabine, interferon).

PATIENT EDUCATION

The patient and the family, as indicated, should be fully informed about the nature of the patient's condition and the treatment plan and should be involved in the health care planning whenever possible. The patient and the family should understand the course of the therapy. They should know the exact name of the medication, its general action, purpose, adverse side effects, and how these effects can be minimized. Because the antivirals are required until the infection is cleared, it is particularly important that patients be able to monitor their therapeutic response and understand this concept of care, especially if they are self-medicating on a discharge or outpatient basis.

Health teaching is often indicated in relation to promoting self-care practices to prevent a reinfection whenever possible. Patients requiring treatment for plantar warts should be encouraged to wear shoes, to avoid public showers, and to use sound self-care practices when swimming. The medication must be administered correctly to ensure therapeutic response and patient education in relation to self-medication, and follow-up cannot be overemphasized. Patients must be shown how to use the medication as prescribed and should be given a step-by-step written instruction sheet, whenever possible, to follow at home. This is important even if the patient has demonstrated competence in medication administration with supervision. Whenever possible, patients should be examined by the health care provider to ensure that the therapeutic effect has been accomplished before the medication is discontinued.

Patient education must be individualized to the patient and the individual need for the antiviral therapy. Patients at risk for influenza infection because of age or underlying disease condition (e.g., cardiac or pulmonary disease, immunosuppression, sickle cell anemia, neuromuscular disorders) need to be identified and taught to recognize the importance of seeking prophylaxis. These patients must also be able to self-monitor themselves for early signs indicating an infection.

Other patients (e.g., those requiring ocular therapy for viral infections) need to be aware that most herpes simplex infections may cause corneal ulceration, and that approximately one fourth of the first episodes of keratitis

GENERAL NURSING IMPLICATIONS—cont'd

Nursing of patients requiring antivirals—cont'd

PATIENT EDUCATION—cont'd

are followed by a recurrence within 2 years. Recurrences may eventually cause visual damage in a small percentage of patients. Although corneal transplants have been used to treat severe scarring, monitoring the condition and seeking medical care as indicated are important in preventing irreparable damage. Patients need to be made aware of the possibility of viral resistance that can occur. These patients should be able to monitor for reepithelialization and to avoid overtreatment which can lead to ocular toxicity.

Patients requiring interferon should also be taught about the medication therapy, as with the other antivirals and other medications. Patients have been successfully taught to administer their own intramuscular injections and how to monitor side effects, as well as what to do when adverse side effects are recognized. Many of these patients are taught to use their health care providers via the telephone in maintaining self-medication as outpatients. Patients are usually told to take acetaminophen (Tylenol) for fevers to 39° C (103° F) be-

cause aspirin should be avoided because of its anticoagulant effect, especially if the patient is receiving chemotherapy and has a tendency to bleed.

Patients are told how to monitor their white blood cell counts, and when these are low they are cautioned to avoid exposure to infection. Other areas, including diet and preventing fatigue, are also included in teaching plans along with specific attention to the drug therapy.

GENERAL INSTRUCTIONS FOR DISCHARGE/OUTPATIENTS

ANTIFUNGALS

This drug is used to treat various fungal infections. If you do not understand why you require this medication, check with your health care provider.

Follow the instructions on the prescription exactly.

This medication has been prescribed especially for you. Do not trade or give this medication to any relatives or friends.

Notify your nurse or physician if you start or stop taking any other medications while taking this medication.

Keep this and all medications out of the reach of children.

In addition to the general instructions, if you are taking *griseofulvin,* it should

be taken immediately after meals to decrease the incidence of GI upset and to improve the amount of drug that is absorbed.

Antifungals can be used in various forms depending on the condition being treated. Check with your nurse regarding any questions you have about how you should be taking this medication.

ANTIVIRALS

This drug is used to treat various infections caused by viruses. If you do not understand why you require this medication, check with your health care provider.

Follow the instructions on the prescription exactly.

This medication has been prescribed especially for you. Do not trade or give this medication to any relatives or friends.

Notify your nurse or physician if you start or stop taking any other medications while taking this medication.

Keep this and all medications out of the reach of children.

If you have a viral infection or if your child is being treated for a viral infection, do not take or give aspirin. Aspirin can cause unwanted effects, especially in children who have a viral infection. If you have any questions, check with your health care provider.

NURSING DRUG DIGEST

Medication (trade name*)	Indication	Usual dosage and administration	Dosage forms, preparation, and storage	Contraindications, cautions, and comments	Monitoring
★ **Acrisorcin** Akrinol	Dermatophytosis caused by *Malassezia furfur*; therefore, used in treatment of tinea versicolor	*Adults:* Apply b.i.d. to affected areas Treatment should continue for 6 weeks after the clearing of lesions *Children:* Same as adults	Cream: 0.2%	May cause hives, blisters, and erythematous vesicles May cause burning sensation when applied to eczematous lesions Avoid contact with the eyes May cause photosensitivity	Observe for burning, irritation, or other untoward effects after topical application
Acyclovir Zovirax	Topical treatment of initial herpes genitalis Systemic treatment of initial and recurrent mucosal and cutaneous herpes simplex infections in patients who are immunocompromised, and severe initial episodes of herpes genitalis	*Adults:* Cover all lesions 6 times daily at 3-hr intervals for 7 days Use a fingercot or rubber glove to apply medication to prevent autoinfection or transmission of the infection to others *Adults:* 15 mg/kg/24 hr IV Infuse 5 mg/kg over 1 hr q.8.h. for 7 days *Children:* 750 mg/m²/24 hr IV Infuse 250 mg/m² over 1 hr q.8h. for 7 days Decrease dose in renal impairment Systemic preparation for IV infusion *only; do not* administer by any other parenteral route	Ointment: 5% in polyethylene glycol base Injectable: 500 mg Reconstitute sterile powder for injection (500 mg) with 10 ml of sterile water for injection; this *must be* further diluted within 12 hr with a standard electrolyte or glucose solution to a concentration of 7 mg/ml (or less) *before* administration Discard unused solution 12 hours after dilution Store at room temperature (refrigeration may cause precipitation)	Rapid infusion may cause renal tubular damage Maintain hydration during IV use May cause pain or phlebitis at injection site May cause encephalopathic reactions characterized by agitation, confusion, seizures, or coma Avoid contact with eyes	Monitor renal function Monitor injection site for pain or phlebitis Monitor for encephalopathic reactions (e.g., confusion, seizures)

| Amantadine
Symmetrel
Virofral | Prophylaxis of influenza A virus
Symptomatic treatment for influenza A virus
See also Chapter 20, "Antiparkinsonian Medications and Stimulants" | Adults: 100 mg b.i.d. or 200 mg/day as single dose PO
Children: 1-9 years of age, 4.4-8.8 mg/kg/day in 2 to 3 equally divided doses
Maximum 150 mg/day
Administer 1 hr before or 2 hr after meals to facilitate absorption
Dosage in renal failure
Creatinine clearance 10-50 ml/min
Adults: 100 mg/day
Children: 2.2-4.4 mg/kg/day in 2 to 3 equally divided doses
Creatinine clearance less than 10 ml/min
Adults: 20 mg/day
Children: 0.2-0.45 mg/kg/day in 2 to 3 divided doses | Capsule: 100 mg
Syrup: 50 mg/5 ml
Store capsules in a dry place protected from moisture | Contraindicated in patients with a demonstrated hypersensitivity
Use with caution in elderly patients, patients with renal failure, and patients with epilepsy, because of CNS toxicities
To be effective, therapy must be initiated within first 24-48 hr after onset of symptoms
Excreted in breast milk; use in nursing mothers should be avoided
May cause drowsiness, dizziness, or mental depression
May cause orthostatic hypotension
May cause dry mouth, blurred vision, or urinary retention
May cause photosensitivity reaction
Abrupt discontinuation may exacerbate Parkinson's disease
Livedo reticularis may appear 1 month to 1 year after initiation of therapy; if occurs, discontinue drug | Monitor for seizure activity and report
Monitor for development of CHF
Monitor renal function for required dosage adjustment |

NOTE: For additional details regarding the individual agents listed in this table, see the text and other tables in this chapter.
*Indicates a multiple active ingredient product. For a complete listing of all active ingredients see the *Drug Reference Guide to Brand Names and Active Ingredients.*
★Indicates that the drug is generally available only in the United States.

Continued.

NURSING DRUG DIGEST—cont'd

Medication (trade name)	Indication	Usual dosage and administration	Dosage forms, preparation, and storage	Contraindications, cautions, and comments	Monitoring
Amphotericin B Fungizone	Severe systemic fungal disease, cryptococcosis, blastomycosis, disseminated forms of candidiasis, coccidioidmycosis, and histoplasmosis, mucormycosis, and aspergillosis IV use is generally *restricted* to treating patients with progressive or potentially fatal fungal infections Cutaneous candidal infections	*Adults and children:* Initially 0.25 mg/kg/24 hr IV infusion, increase gradually 5 mg/day as tolerated up to 0.6/mg/kg/day or *alternate* day up to 1 mg/kg/24 hr (daily dosage should *never* exceed 1.5 mg/kg) IV infusion should be mixed at a concentration of 0.1 mg/ml and administered slowly over 6 hr *Children:* Same as adults Protect from light during administration Decrease dose in renal impairment *Adults:* Apply liberally to lesions b.i.d. to q.i.d.	Injectable: 50 mg/vial Store in refrigerator before reconstitution In preparing solution for administration, reconstitute dry powder with sterile water for injection (no preservatives) Do *not* reconstitute with saline solutions Reconstituted solution should be diluted in D₅W to obtain a concentration of 0.1 mg/ml IV infusions (0.1 mg/ml or less) are stable in the presence of light for up to 24 hr after preparation Any precipitated solution should be discarded Protect from light Cream: 3% Lotion: 3% Ointment: 3%	*Contraindicated* in hypersensitivity and in renal failure (serum creatinine 3 mg/dl or greater) Hydrocortisone 25 mg has been added to amphotericin B infusions to decrease the incidence of febrile reactions; the addition of hydrocortisone to the amphotericin B infusion has become common practice in many hospitals; however, no controlled studies have been performed to confirm the use of hydrocortisone for this purpose May cause untoward rise in BUN to greater than 40 mg/dl May often decrease renal function Renal dysfunction induced by amphotericin B is generally reversible, but may be permanent, particularly in patients where the total dosage exceeds 5 gm Adverse effects from *topical* use are rare May have a drying effect and cause minor local irritation *Cream* (more so than ointment or lotion) may cause minor skin staining *Topical* preparations may stain clothing	Monitor BUN at weekly intervals Monitor intake and output Monitor temperature for febrile reaction (may be accompanied by shaking chills, hypotension, nausea, and delirium); if patient develops acute shaking chills, stop infusion; administer IV meperidine 25-50 mg and wait for symptoms to subside—resume infusion at a slower rate Monitor for signs of hypokalemia (e.g., muscle weakness) Monitor for anemia Monitor for signs of renal damage (e.g., granular and hyaline casts in urine, microhematuria) Monitor for therapeutic effect Lesions usually respond in a few days but may take up to 4 weeks

Drug	Uses	Dosage	Preparations	Precautions	Nursing considerations
★ **Candicidin** Candeptin Candimon Vanobid	Vulvovaginal candidiasis	*Adults:* One vaginal tablet/suppository or 5 gm (one applicatorful) of ointment inserted high in the vagina in the morning and at bedtime for 14 days; treatment may be repeated if symptoms persist or reappear	Vaginal tablet: 3 mg Vaginal suppository: 3 mg Vaginal ointment: 3 mg/5 gm	May cause slight local *vaginal irritation* If suppositories are used during pregnancy, they should be inserted digitally; use of vaginal applicator for ointment is contraindicated during pregnancy Instruct patient on use of vaginal applicator	Monitor for vaginal irritation
★ **Ciclopirox** Loprox	*Tinea* infections Candidiasis	*Adults:* Apply b.i.d. morning and evening	Cream: 1%	*Contraindicated* in hypersensitivity Avoid use of occlusive dressings	
Clotrimazole Canesten Gyne-Lotrimin Lotrimin Mycelex Trimysten	Dermatophytoses (fungal infections) of feet, skin, hair, or nails caused by *Trichophyton, Microsporum, Epidermophyton,* and *Candida albicans* Vulvovaginal candidiasis Oropharyngeal candidiasis	*Adults:* Massage into affected and surrounding skin b.i.d. (morning and evening) *Children:* Same as adults *Not* for ophthalmic use *Adults:* One tablet intravaginally q.d. (preferably q.h.s.) *Adults:* Dissolve one troche in mouth 5 times a day for 14 days	Topical solution: 1% Cream: 1% Vaginal tablet: 100 mg Oral troche (uncoated tablet): 10 mg	*Contraindicated* in hypersensitivity. Adverse effects are uncommon Skin rash may occur Instruct patient on use of vaginal applicator Instruct patient to dissolve troche *slowly* in mouth	Observe for skin rash
Econazole Ecostatin	*Tinea* infections Cutaneous candidiasis	*Adults:* Apply b.i.d. morning and evening *Candida* infections should be treated for 2-4 weeks *Children:* Same as adults For *topical* use only (*not* for ophthalmic use)	Cream: 1% Store at room temperature, 15°-25° C	*Contraindicated* in hypersensitivity May cause local skin irritation	Observe for local irritation
Flucytosine Ancobon Ancotil	Serious systemic infections caused by *Candida, Cryptococcus, Torulopsis,* and a few species of *Aspergillus*	*Adults:* 50 to 150 mg/kg/24 hr PO or 1.5-2.25 gm/m²/24 hr in 4 divided doses q.6h. Nausea or vomiting may be reduced if capsules are given a few at a time over 15 min Decrease dose in renal impairment	Capsules: 250, 500 mg Protect from light	Give with caution in patients with impaired renal function or bone marrow depression May caused nausea, vomiting, diarrhea, and bone marrow depression Therapeutic serum levels are generally 20-90 μg/ml Toxicity occurs at serum levels above 100 μg/ml	Monitor for bone marrow depression Closely monitor renal and hepatic function Monitor serum levels

Continued.

NURSING DRUG DIGEST—cont'd

Medication (trade name)	Indication	Usual dosage and administration	Dosage forms, preparation, and storage	Contraindications; cautions, and comments	Monitoring
Gentian violet Genapax GVS GVS Vaginal Hyva Hyva Vaginal	Cutaneous or mucocutaneous infections caused by *Candida albicans*	*Adults:* Topical solution: 0.25% or 0.5% (range 0.02%-1%) Solution applied to lesions with cotton b.i.d. to t.i.d. for 3 days. For instillation in closed cavities reduce concentration to 0.01%	Topical solution: 0.5%, 1%, 2%	Keep infected areas dry and open to air during therapy. May cause irritation or sensitivity reactions and ulceration of mucous membranes (1% and 2% solutions show greatest incidence of irritation)	
	Vulvovaginitis See also Chapter 55, "Antiseptics and Local Anesthetics"	*Adults:* Insert one suppository or tampon high in the vagina q.d. or b.i.d. for 12 days. Alternative: Insert one applicatorful of gentian violet cream intravaginally every other day for 4-6 applications	Tampon: 5 mg Vaginal cream: 1.35% Vaginal suppository: 17.2 mg Vaginal tablet: 2 mg	Avoid prolonged therapy or swallowing of solution because esophagitis or laryngitis may develop. Do not use on facial lesions because permanent discoloration of skin may result. Instruct patient on use of vaginal applicator. Administration during the third trimester of pregnancy can result in systemic absorption and toxicity for both the mother and the fetus; it is, therefore, recommended to avoid vaginal use of gentian violet during the third trimester of pregnancy	

Drug	Uses	Dosage	Dosage forms	Remarks
Griseofulvin Cortussin Dilyn Fulvicin P/G Fulvicin U/F Grifulvin-V Grisactin Grisovin-FP Grisowen Gris-PEG Likuden	Dermatophytosis caused by species of *Trichophyton, Microsporum,* and *Epidermophyton*	Dose—microsize *Adults:* 500 mg/24 hr as single dose or as 2 equal doses PO with food *Children:* 10 mg/kg/24 hr or 300 mg/m²/24 hr with food; widespread lesions—450-600 mg/m²/24 hr PO divided into two to four doses with food Dose—ultramicrosize *Adults:* 250 mg/24 hr with food *Children:* 5 mg/kg/24 hr or 150 mg/m²/24 hr PO divided into two to four doses with food; widespread lesions may require 225-300 mg/m²/24 hr in divided doses Administer after meals to decrease GI upset and enhance absorption	Tablets: 125, 250, 500 mg (microsize); 125, 250 mg (ultramicrosize) Capsules: 125, 250 mg (microsize) Suspension (oral): 25 mg/ml (microsize) *Shake suspension well before use*	*Contraindicated* in patients with porphyria and liver disease May cause headaches, but this effect is usually mild and disappears as therapy progresses Skin and hair infections require 4-6 weeks of therapy Nail infection up to 12 months of treatment Itching is usually relieved within a few days Absorption is directly related to the fat content of coadministered meals Ultramicrosized form is more rapidly and completely absorbed than the microsized form and is thus effective at half the microsized dose May cause photosensitivity reaction Observe for hypersensitivity (e.g., skin rashes, urticaria, angioneurotic edema [rare])
Haloprogin Halotex	Dermatophytosis caused by species of *Tricophyton, Microsporium, Epidermophyton, Malassezia,* and *Candida*	*Adults:* Apply b.i.d. for 2 to 4 weeks *Children:* Same as adults	Cream: 1% Solution: 1%	May cause irritation, pruritus, burning sensations, vesiculation, increased maceration, and sensitization Discontinue therapy if irritation or sensitization occurs Avoid contact with eyes

Continued.

NURSING DRUG DIGEST—cont'd

Medication (trade name)	Indication	Usual dosage and administration	Dosage forms, preparation, and storage	Contraindications, cautions, and comments	Monitoring
Idoxuridine Dandrid Dendrid Herplex Herplex-D Liquiflm Kerecid S.O.P. Stoxil	Herpes simplex keratitis	*Adults:* Solution: One drop instilled in infected eye q.1h. during waking hours and q.2h. during sleeping hours; alternative: one drop instilled every min for 5 min repeated q.4h. Ointment: Apply inside conjunctival sac of infected eye q.4h. while awake and q.h.s. Continue therapy for 5 to 7 days after lesion has healed to minimize recurrence *Children:* Same as adults	Ophthalmic ointment: 0.5% Ophthalmic solution: 0.1% Store solution under refrigeration at 2°-8° C Store ointment under refrigeration at 2°-15° C Protect from light	If reepithelialization has not occurred within 21 days, other forms of therapy should be used Boric acid should *not* be administered during therapy because it may cause irritation in the presence of idoxuridine Do *not* mix with other ophthalmic medications—the stability of idoxuridine may be altered May cause various adverse ophthalmic reactions (e.g., blurred vision, edema, inflammation, irritation, pain, pruritus) Hazy vision that follows application should be of short duration	Monitor patients for vision loss
★ **Ketoconazole** Nizoral	Candidiasis Oral thrush Coccidioidomycosis Histoplasmosis	*Adults:* 200-400 mg/day PO *Children:* Less than 20 kg, 50 mg/day PO; 20-40 kg, 100 mg/day PO; more than 40 kg, 200 mg/day PO	Tablet: 200 mg	*Contraindicated* in hypersensitivity Nausea and vomiting are common Inhibits testosterone and may cause sexual dysfunction or gynecomastia in men May cause liver dysfunction characterized by fatigue, nausea, vomiting, jaundice, dark urine, or pale stools If signs of liver dysfunction are noted, ketoconazole should be discontinued immediately to prevent fatal hepatic necrosis	Monitor liver function

Drug	Uses	Dosage/Route	Preparations	Nursing Considerations
Miconazole Daktarin Micatin Monistat Monistat 3 Monistat 5 Tampons Monistat 7 Vaginal Cream	Severe systemic fungal infections, coccidioidomycosis, candidiasis, cryptococcosis, paracoccidioidomycosis, and chronic mucocutaneous candidiasis	*Adults:* Coccidioidomycosis 1800-3600 mg/24 hr IV in 3 divided infusions; infuse over 30-60 min Cryptococcosis, 1200-2400 mg/24 hr IV in 3 divided infusions; infuse over 30-60 min Candidiasis, 600-1800 mg/24 hr IV in 3 divided infusions; infuse over 30-60 min Paracoccidioidomycosis 200-1200 mg/24 hr IV in 3 divided infusions; infuse over 30-60 min *Children:* 20-40 mg/kg/24 hr in 3 divided infusions (do *not* exceed 15 mg/kg/single infusion) Administer by IV infusion *only* for above indications; infuse over 30-60 min	Injectable: 10 mg/ml Dilute in at least 200 ml of fluid; use sterile NS or D₅W for diluent Store between 15° and 30° C	Use in pregnant or nursing women is not recommended until further information is available Rapid administration of undiluted drug may cause tachycardia May cause anorexia, nausea, vomiting, and diarrhea May cause phlebitis at site of injection May cause fever and chills Cardiorespiratory arrest has occurred with first dose, so a 200 mg test dose with a physician in attendance has been recommended by the manufacturer Administration for prolonged periods may cause itching Hyperlipidemia caused by the vehicle (PEG 40 castor oil), in which miconazole is dissolved may occur Observe for GI side effects and treat accordingly Monitor for signs of hyponatremia
	Fungal meningitis	*Adults:* 20 mg intrathecally (undiluted) q.3-7 days		
	Fungal bladder infection	*Adults:* Instill 200 mg of diluted solution into bladder		
	Vulvovaginal candidiasis	*Adults:* Insert one applicatorful intravaginally q.h.s. for 7 days; *or* insert 1 tampon vaginally q.h.s. for 5 nights (remove every morning)	Vaginal cream: 2% Tampons: 100 mg	May cause local vaginal irritation Instruct patient on use of vaginal applicator
	Dermatophytosis	*Adults:* Apply to affected area b.i.d. morning and evening *Children:* Over 2 years of age, same as adults	Cream: 2% Lotion: 2% Powder: 2%	May cause local irritation
★ **Natamycin** Natacyn	Fungal keratitis, conjunctivitis, and blepharitis caused by *Fusarium, Aspergillus, Cephalosporium, Penicillium,* and *Candida* species	*Adults:* Ophthalmic suspension: instill one drop in conjunctival sac q.1-2h. for 3 days; then, one drop q.3-4h. for 3-4 weeks or until no signs of active disease *Children:* Same as adults For ophthalmic use *only*	Ophthalmic suspension: 5% Ophthalmic ointment: 1% *Shake* suspension well before use	Because of poor penetration it is not used to treat deep corneal mycoses May cause ocular edema or mild irritation

Continued.

NURSING DRUG DIGEST—cont'd

Medication (trade name)	Indication	Usual dosage and administration	Dosage forms, preparation, and storage	Contraindications, cautions, and comments	Monitoring
Nystatin Achrostatin V* Candex* Comycin* Declostatin* Flagylstatin* Kenacomb* Korostatin Vaginal Tablets Moronal Myco Triacet Cream & Ointment* Mycolog* Mycostatin Mytrex* Nadostine Nilstat Nyaderm Nysolone* Nystaform Ointment* O-V Statin Terrastatin* Tetrastatin* Tricilone NNG* Viaderm-N	Dermatophytoses (fungal infections) of skin, nasal, oral, vaginal and anal orifices caused by Candida (Monilia) albicans and other Candida species Intestinal Candida infections	*Adults:* Apply to affected areas b.i.d. to t.i.d. until healing is complete *Children:* Same as adults *Adults:* 1,500,000 to 4,000,000 units/24 hr PO in 4 divided doses *Children:* Premature and full-term newborns, 400,000 units PO in 4 divided doses; older infants and children, 1-2 million units/24 hr PO in 4 divided doses Dissolve one lozenge (oral tablet) in mouth q.4h One tablet (100,000 units) intravaginally q.d. for 2 weeks *Not effective against systemic infections*	Cream: 100,000 units/gm Ointment: 100,000 units/gm Lotion: 100,000 units/gm Powder: 100,000 units/gm Oral tablets: 100,000, 500,000 units Oral suspension: 100,000 units/ml Vaginal tablet: 100,000 units Protect from heat, light and moisture	Treatment should be continued at least 48 hr after clinical cure to prevent relapse Instruct patient on use of vaginal applicator Good oral care should be carried out before each drug treatment Contact time is key to success for monilial infections of the mouth May use vaginal tablets as oral lozenge If suspension is being used, swish and hold suspension in mouth as long as possible before swallowing May cause nausea, vomiting, and diarrhea, especially with large oral doses	
Tolnaftate Aftate Pitrex Sporiline Tinactin Tinaderm Tonoftal	Dermatophytoses (fungal infections) of feet (athlete's foot), skin, hair, or nails caused by Trichophyton, Microsporium, or Epidermophyton	*Adults:* Apply small quantity b.i.d. for 2 to 3 weeks (some cases may require treatment for 4 to 6 weeks) *Children:* Same as adults *For external use only*	Cream: 1% Powder: 1% Powder, aerosol: 1% Solution: 1% Gel: 1% Liquid, aerosol: 1%	Adverse effects are uncommon—mild skin irritation may occur	

Drug	Uses	Dosage	Preparations	Remarks
★ **Triacetin** Enzactin Fungacetin Vanay	Dermatophytoses (fungal infections) of feet (athlete's foot) and skin, caused by species of *Trichophyton, Microsporium,* and *Epidermophyton*	*Adults:* Apply b.i.d. *Children:* Same as adults	Cream: 25% Liquid: 30% Ointment: 25% Powder: 33.3% Topical aerosol: 15%	May cause minor skin irritation Avoid contact with eyes May damage rayon fabrics—cover treated areas with clean light bandage Product should be used for at least 1 week after infection clears
★ **Trifluridine** Viroptic	Epithelial keratitis caused by herpes simplex virus	*Adults:* Instill 1 drop in affected eye q.2h. while awake Maximum: 9 drops per 24 hr *Children:* Same as adults Do *not* use continuously for more than 21 days	Ophthalmic solution: 1% Refrigerate between 2° and 8° C	Observe eye for sensitivity *Contraindicated* in hypersensitivity May cause mild stinging on instillation Prolonged administration may cause epithelial keratopathy
Undecylenic acid, zinc undecylenate, calcium undecylenate Blis-To-Sol* Caldesene Desenex Fungiderm Nuvola Medicated Shampoo Podiaspray* Quinsana Plus Medicated Foot Powder Quisana Plus* Rid-Itch-Cream Solvex Athlete's Foot Spray* Verdefam Cream* Verdefam Solution*	Dermatophytoses (fungal infections) of feet (athlete's foot), skin, and hair caused by species of *Trichophyton, Microsporium,* and *Epidermophyton*	*Adults:* Apply b.i.d. to t.i.d. as indicated *Children:* Same as adults	Ointment: 20% zinc undecylenate, 5% undecylenic acid Soap: 2% undecylenic acid Powder, aerosol: 20% zinc undecylate, 2% undecylenic acid Powder: 10% calcium undecylenate Solution: 10% undecylenic acid Foam: 10% undecylenic acid Cream: 20% zinc undecylenate, 3% undecylenic acid	Infections usually require 2–4 weeks of therapy Undiluted solution may cause stinging when applied to broken skin Avoid contact with eyes and inhalation of powder Do *not* apply to mucous membranes in concentrations greater than 1%

Continued.

NURSING DRUG DIGEST—cont'd

Medication (trade name)	Indication	Usual dosage and administration	Dosage forms, preparation, and storage	Contraindications, cautions, and comments	Monitoring
Vidarabine Ara-A Vira-A	Herpes simplex encephalitis	*Adults:* 15 mg/kg/day IV for 10 days; doses up to 20 mg/kg/day IV have been used in serious infections *Children:* Same as adults Vidarabine should be administered *only* by IV infusion; divide IV doses into 2 equal doses and administer each dose by IV infusion over 12 hr; IV doses must be diluted in appropriate IV solution; rapid or bolus injections should *not* be used; vidarabine should *not* be given IM or SC because of decreased absorption	Injectable: 200 mg/ml Dilute solution before administration IV fluid used to prepare vidarabine solution may be prewarmed to 35°-40° C (95°-100° F) to facilitate dissolution of the drug Final filtration with an inline 0.45 μ filter is necessary Discard unused portion after 48 hr Do *not* refrigerate diluted solution	If reepithelialization of conjunctiva *has not* occurred within 21 days, other forms of therapy should be used	Monitor hepatic and renal function Monitor fluid status for overload
	Acute keratoconjunctivitis and recurrent epithelial keratitis caused by herpes simplex virus	*Adults:* Apply 1.3 cm (½ inch) into lower conjunctival sac 5 times daily q.3h. until reepithelialization occurs, then b.i.d. for 7 days			

BIBLIOGRAPHY

Amantadine: does it have a role in prevention and treatment of influenza? (Symposium). *Annals of Internal Medicine*, 1980, *92*(pt.1), 256-258.

Bryson, E.J., Monhan, C., Pollack, M., & Shields, W.D. A prospective double blind study of the side effects associated with the administration of amantadine for influenza A virus prophylaxis. *Journal of Infectious Diseases*, 1980, *141*, 543-547.

Buchanan, R.A. Advances in antiviral chemotherapy. *Canadian Medical Association Journal*, 1979, *120*, 7-10.

Cartwright, R.Y. Use of antibiotics: antifungals. *British Medical Journal*, 1978, *8*, 108-111.

Comer, J.B. Amphotericin B: ten common questions. *American Journal of Nursing*, 1981, *81*(6), 1166-1167.

Dolan R. Amantadine and influenzae. *American Family Physician*, 1979, *19*, 127-130.

Douglas, J.M., Critchlow, C., Benedetti, J., et al. A double-blind study of oral acyclovir for suppression and recurrences of genital herpes simplex virus infection. *The New England Journal of Medicine*, 1984, *310*(24), 1551-1556.

Drugs for the treatment of systemic fungal infections. *The Medical Letter on Drugs and Therapeutics*, 1984, *26*(658), 36-38.

Elliott J. Consensus on amantadine use in influenza A. *Journal of the American Medical Association*, 1979, *242*, 2383.

Fishaut, M. & Mostow, S.R. Amantadine for severe influenza A pneumonia in infancy. *American Journal of Diseases of Children*, 1980, *134*, 321-323.

Hirsch, M.S., & Swartz, M.N. Antiviral agents. *New England Journal of Medicine*, 1980, *302*, 903-907.

How to minimize side effects with IV amphotericin B. *Reactions*, 1980, July, 11.

Jacobs, P.H. Fungal infections in childhood. *Pediatric Clinics of North America*, 1978, *25*, 357-370.

Jarratt, M. Dermatologic insight herpes simplex. *Journal of Dermatology and Allergy for the Practicing Physician*, 1979.

Jordan, W.M., Bodey, G.P., Rodriquez, V., Ketchel, S.J., & Henney, J. Miconazole therapy for treatment of fungal infections in cancer patients. *Antimicrobial Agents and Chemotherapy*, 1979, *16*, 792-797.

Kaufman, C., & Frame, P.E. Bone marrow toxicity associated with 5-flurocytosine therapy. *Antimicrobial Agents and Chemotherapy*, 1977, *11*, 244-247.

McAdams, C.W. Interferon, the penicillin of the future? *American Journal of Nursing*, 1980, *80*(4), 714-719.

McHenry, M.C., & Ficker, D.D. New antibacterial and antimycotic drugs: critical appraisal. *Medical Clinics of North America*, 1978, *62*(5), 887-897.

Pazin, G.J., Armstrong, J.A., Lam, M.T., Tarr, G.C., Jannetta, P.J., & Ho, M. Prevention of reactivated herpes simplex infection by human leukocyte interferon. *New England Journal of Medicine*, 1979, *301*, 225-230.

Perkins, H.M., & Hanlon, P.R. Epidural injection of local anesthetic and steroids for relief of pain secondary to herpes zoster. *Archives of Surgery*, 1978, *113*, 253-254.

Plotkin, S.A. The clinical significance of cytomegalovirus infection. *Drug Therapy (Hospital)*, 1979, *9*(2), 155-164.

Sidwell, R.W., Huffman, J.H., Khare, G.P., Allen, L.B., Witkowski, J.T., & Robins, R.K. Broad spectrum antiviral activity of virazole; 1-β-D-ribofuranosy − 1, 2, 4- triazole-3-carboxamide. *Science*, 1978, *177*, 705-706.

Sohn, C.A. Evaluation of ketoconazole. *Clinical Pharmacy*, 1982, *1*, 217-224.

Stevens, D.A., Levine, H.B., & Deresinski, S.C. Miconazole in coccidiomycoses: therapeutic and pharmacological studies in man. *American Journal of Medicine*, 1976, *60*, 191-202.

Straus, S.E., Takiff, H.E., Seidlin, M., et al. Suppression of frequently recurring genital herpes: a placebo-controlled double-blind trial of oral acyclovir. *The New England Journal of Medicine*, 1984, *310*(24), 1545-1550.

Sung, J.P., Grindahl, M.A., & Levine, H.B. Intravenous and intrathecal miconazole therapy for systemic mycoses. *Western Journal of Medicine*, 1977, *126*(1), 5-13.

Tamm, I. Antiviral agents. *New York State Journal of Medicine*, 1979, *79*(7), 1001-1004.

Washington, D. Helping the patient with vaginitis. *RN*, 1984, *47*(9), 63-65, 67, 69.

Whitley, R.J., Soong, S.J., Hirsch, M.S., Karchmer, A.W., Dollin, R., Galasso, G., Dunnick, J.K., Alford, C.A., & the NIAID Collaborative Antiviral Study Group. Herpes simplex encephalitis: vidarabine therapy and diagnostic problems. *New England Journal of Medicine*, 1981, *304*(6), 313-318.

ANTINEOPLASTIC MEDICATIONS

Medications discussed in this section

CHAPTER 52

Antimetabolites and Antineoplastic Antibiotics

Branimir Ivan Sikic

Medications discussed in this chapter

Antimetabolites
  Folic acid antagonists
    Methotrexate
  Purine analogues
    Mercaptopurine
    Thioguanine
  Pyrimidine analogues
    Azacitidine
    Cytarabine
    Floxuridine
    Fluorouracil

Antineoplastic antibiotics
  Anthracyclines
    Daunorubicin
    Doxorubicin
  Bleomycin
  Dactinomycin
  Mitomycin
  Plicamycin

Cancer is the second most common cause of death in industrially developed countries, and actually comprises more than 100 different diseases or types of malignancies. Cancer by definition is an uncontrolled and destructive proliferation of cells. *Carcinogenic* chemicals, radiation, viruses, and heredity may all play a role in causing the various cancers, but in most individual cases of cancer, the exact cause is unknown. The nature of the transformation of a normal cell into a malignant or cancer cell is still poorly understood and is the focus of much research. This transformation results in the capability of cancer cells to *invade* and *metastasize*. Invasion means the direct spreading of the cancer cells into the surrounding tissues with the destruction of normal cells. Metastasis is the spread of cancer cells via the bloodstream or lymphatic system to other parts of the body.

The incidence of many cancers is increasing throughout the world. In part, this is the result of increased longevity and decreased mortality from other diseases, but it may also be the result of increased exposure to various carcinogens or cancer-causing agents in the environment. Cigarette smoking and other forms of tobacco use are by far the single most important identified cause of cancer, accounting for the large majority of all lung cancers, and increasing the risk of several other kinds of *malignancies*, including cancers of the head and neck, esophagus, pancreas, and bladder. There have been many advances in the treatment of these cancers through surgery, radiation therapy, and chemotherapy. However, only one third of all patients with cancer are cured, as defined by the disappearance of all evidence of the cancer and the probability of a normal lifespan. Prevention of the disease by such measures as the elimination of cigarette smoking, the identification of carcinogens, and the reduction of exposure to such chemicals remains a major public health priority.

More than 30 drugs are known to be useful in certain kinds of cancers. Several of these drugs may be used together *(combination chemotherapy)*, or in conjunction with surgery and radiation therapy *(combined modality treatment)*. *Chemotherapy* has increased the cure rate to over 50% in 10 kinds of human cancers even when these tumors are widespread or at an advanced stage. These curable tumors are most common in children and young adults and include acute lymphocytic leukemia, Hodgkin's disease, non-Hodgkin's lymphomas, Burkitt's lymphoma, testicular carcinomas, trophoblastic choriocarcinoma, Ewing's sarcoma, retinoblastoma, rhabdomyosarcoma, and Wilms' tumor.

Patients with incurable cancers may benefit from so-called *palliative chemotherapy*, treatment that temporarily shrinks the tumors, prolongs life by several months or a few years, and alleviates the symptoms. These types of tumors include ovarian and breast carcinomas, acute myelocytic leukemia, and oat cell cancer of the lung. Several other cancers are usually resistant to chemotherapy, including melanoma, colorectal and renal carcinomas, and non–oat cell lung cancers.

The concept of *adjuvant chemotherapy* for certain cancers is becoming increasingly important. This involves chemotherapy after the complete surgical removal of a tumor, when there is a low chance of a cure with surgery alone. This approach has been successfully used in treating breast cancers and is being tested in several other types of cancer. The possible benefits of adjuvant chemotherapy after surgery must be carefully weighed against the toxicities of chemotherapy and the risk of dying from a recurrence of the cancer.

TOXICITIES OF ANTICANCER DRUGS

Anticancer drugs act by various mechanisms to inhibit cell proliferation and are usually not selective in their effects; normal cells in the body undergoing cell division are also damaged to some degree. This lack of selectivity between drug effects on cancer cells and drug effects on normal cells is the cause for most of the adverse or toxic side effects of anticancer drugs and is the major limiting factor in the dosage and frequency with which chemotherapy can be administered to patients.

The normal tissues that are the most common sites of toxicity from these agents include the bone marrow stem cells (which produce white blood cells, platelets, and red blood cells), the mucosal lining cells of the gastrointestinal (GI) tract, and the hair follicles. These tissues have a higher proportion of cells that are actively dividing, and therefore are especially susceptible to anticancer drugs. The lowering of white blood cell and platelet counts is usually maximal 10 to 14 days after treatment and recovers by 21 to 28 days. Therefore, the chemotherapy is usually scheduled in cycles every 3 to 4 weeks. During the *nadir*, or low point, of the blood counts, patients may be at an increased risk

for serious infections and hemorrhage, and should be closely monitored. In particular, patients should be instructed to immediately report any fever, cough, discomfort, or other untoward symptom that develops during the few days that their white blood cell and platelet counts are expected to be low.

A common side effect that is distressing psychologically to many patients is hair loss, which may result in complete baldness a few weeks after beginning chemotherapy. It has been reported that this side effect may be diminished or avoided for some drugs by inflating a chemotherapy pressure cuff to slightly above the systolic blood pressure around the scalp during and for a few minutes after drug injection. Alternatively, a specially designed ice pack can be placed over the scalp during this period, but these measures are often not helpful. The use of a wig, attractive scarves, and other head coverings may be important for the patient's body image. The hair regrows usually a few weeks after the cessation of chemotherapy, although occasionally the color or texture may be different after regrowth.

Nausea and vomiting are commonly observed after the administration of anticancer drugs and can be ameliorated to some extent by antinauseants such as the phenothiazines. Marijuana or its active extract tetrahydrocannabinol (THC) are also sometimes useful in reducing nausea after chemotherapy (see Chapter 40, "Emetics and Antiemetics"). Nausea usually begins 2 to 6 hours after treatment and may last up to 1 or 2 days. Decreased appetite, alterations in the sense of taste for food, and weight loss are also commonly as-

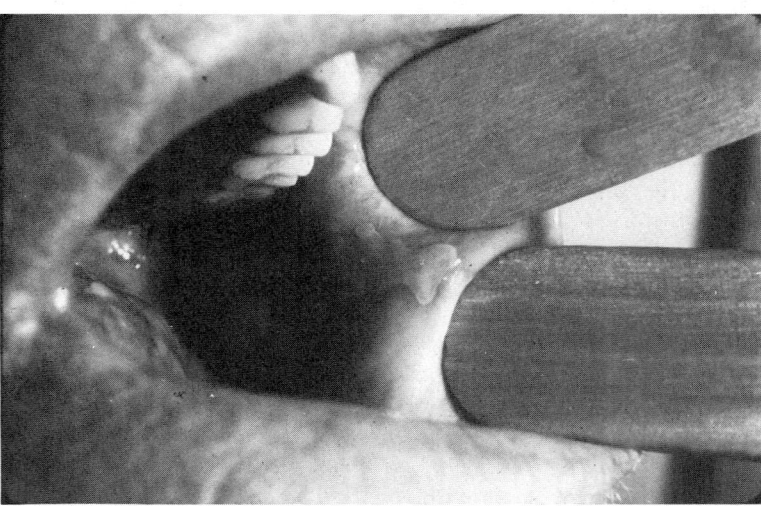

FIGURE 52-1. **Mucositis, or inflammation and erosion, of the lining of the mouth, which may occur 5 to 7 days after administration of antimetabolites or antineoplastic antibiotics.**

sociated with chemotherapy. Toxicity to the GI lining may be manifested by diarrhea and inflammation and ulcerations of the lining of the mouth and tongue *(mucositis)* (Figure 52-1). After several chemotherapy treatments, patients may become psychologically conditioned and actually vomit before their treatment or even at the thought of visiting the hospital or the oncologist's office.

Oral mucositis is a particular problem in patients receiving high doses of *antimetabolites* or anthracyclines, or radiation therapy to the mouth area in addition to chemotherapy. These patients should be instructed in a program of meticulous oral hygiene, including brushing the teeth with a soft toothbrush and correct gentle flossing after each meal or at least twice daily. These should be discontinued, however, if the patient's platelet count falls below 20,000, because of the increased bleeding tendency. An antifungal and antibacterial mouthwash may be prescribed, as well as a topical anesthetic solution, when mucositis occurs. The patient's diet should consist of bland, soft foods and nonacidic liquids during this period. Recovery from mucositis usually occurs within 5 to 7 days.

Some toxicities occur commonly with specific anticancer drugs, such as cardiac damage from doxorubicin, pulmonary fibrosis from bleomycin, peripheral neuropathy (i.e., numbness, weakness) from vin-

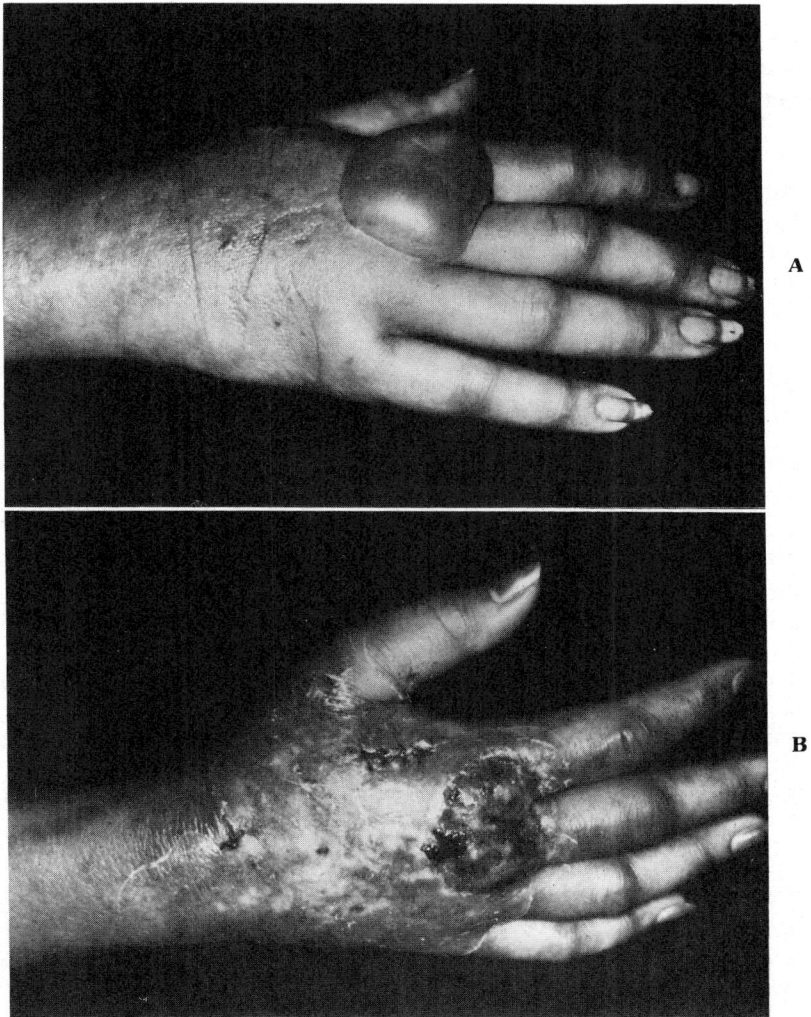

FIGURE 52-2. Extravasation of doxorubicin outside of a vein during injection, producing necrosis of the skin and underlying tissues. *A,* Blistering 1 week after extravasation. *B,* Severe damage evident 3 to 4 weeks after extravasation. This patient required plastic surgery and was left with considerable deformity and loss of function of her hand.

cristine, and bladder irritation (i.e., cystitis) from cyclophosphamide. Infertility and the cessation of menstruation are common side effects, especially of high-dose combination chemotherapy. These drugs depress normal immunologic function, and may thus predispose the patient to certain kinds of infections during the period on chemotherapy.

Less common side effects may affect many organs, including the liver, kidneys, lungs, and skin. Because most of these drugs (especially the alkylating agents) directly affect the structure and function of deoxyribonucleic acid (DNA), they are also potentially carcinogenic and *teratogenic*. The risk for developing a secondary malignancy caused by the chemotherapy is actually small, except for patients treated with combinations of alkylating agents together with radiation therapy, in which there may be 5% to 10% risk of acquiring acute myelocytic leukemia in patients who are cured from their first cancer.

Several anticancer agents (the anthracyclines, carmustine, dacarbazine, the vinca alkaloids, dactinomycin, mechlorethamine, plicamycin, and mitomycin) are potent chemical irritants. These drugs *must* be injected intravenously, and special care must be taken to avoid extravasation out of the vein into the subcutaneous tissues. Such extravasation may cause extensive local tissue necrosis that may require plastic surgery and skin grafting for repair (Figure 52-2). Intravenous injection with these drugs should be performed with special precautions, including the use of a butterfly-type intravenous (IV) needle, frequent checking for venous return, and immediate cessation of the injection if pain or other signs of *extravasation* are produced at the injection site. Pain does not always occur at the injection site with extravasation, and careful monitoring is required.

Many patients have preconceived misconceptions about the toxicities of chemotherapy. Appropriate information and counseling may alleviate fears and improve patients' tolerance for treatment. Most of the side effects of these drugs are reversible (e.g., patients who lose their hair will usually have regrowth of their scalp and body hair after the completion of the chemotherapy). The role of the nurse in the care of the cancer patient receiving chemotherapy extends beyond a mere knowledge of the specific drug side effects and the methods of administration. Every member of the team of professionals caring for the patient with cancer should be aware of the emotional trauma, stresses, and anxieties associated with this illness, not just for the patient but also for the patient's family. Communication with the patient and the family and attention to their concerns and needs are essential aspects of treatment.

There are more than 100 different types of cancers, and knowledge about their clinical patterns and treatments is expanding rapidly. Many patients are candidates for clinical research studies to compare established and promising new therapies, and to develop improved treatments. Such studies have produced remarkable progress in treatment of leukemias, Hodgkin's lymphoma, and testicular carcinoma. The referral of patients for clinical protocols at centers for cancer treatment, or by oncologists affiliated with such centers, is essential if progress is to continue.

ANTIMETABOLITES
Folic acid antagonists

Methotrexate. Methotrexate has a similar structure to the vitamin, folic acid. The drug inhibits the binding of folic acid to the enzyme, dihydrofolate reductase. This blocks the formation of compounds that are essential for DNA synthesis (i.e., thymidylate and purines), thus preventing cell division and causing cell death. Cells are most vulnerable to methotrexate in the *S-phase* of the cell cycle (Figure 52-3).

Methotrexate is an important drug in the cure of acute lymphoblastic *leukemia*, Burkitt's lymphoma, and gestational choriocarcinoma, as well as for adjuvant treatment of breast cancers and the sarcomas. It is also used for the palliation of metastatic breast, head and neck, cervix, lung, and ovarian cancers.

Very high doses of methotrexate are sometimes used with *leucovorin rescue* for osteogenic sarcoma and other tumors. This form of treatment is potentially toxic and should be administered only in specialized situations. Leucovorin is a reduced form of folic acid, and bypasses the metabolic block produced by methotrexate. As an antidote for high doses of methotrexate, leucovorin is administered intravenously or orally, 10 to 25 mg every 6 hours for 2 to 3 days.

Myelosuppression is the major dose-limiting toxicity of methotrexate, with a nadir in blood counts occurring 7 to 14 days after treatment. Methotrexate toxicity often depends on the duration of exposure. High-dose methotrexate may produce severe myelosuppression and GI toxicity in the form of mucositis and diarrhea. Sufficient leucovorin should be given in all treatments using high-dose methotrexate to rescue normal cells. The nurse should be aware of prolonged toxicity and the need for leucovorin rescue.

Methotrexate may also be given *intrathecally* to treat, or in some cases to prevent, meningeal metastases. Methotrexate given intrathecally is first dissolved in Elliott's B solution. Toxicity by this route commonly includes headaches and occasionally more

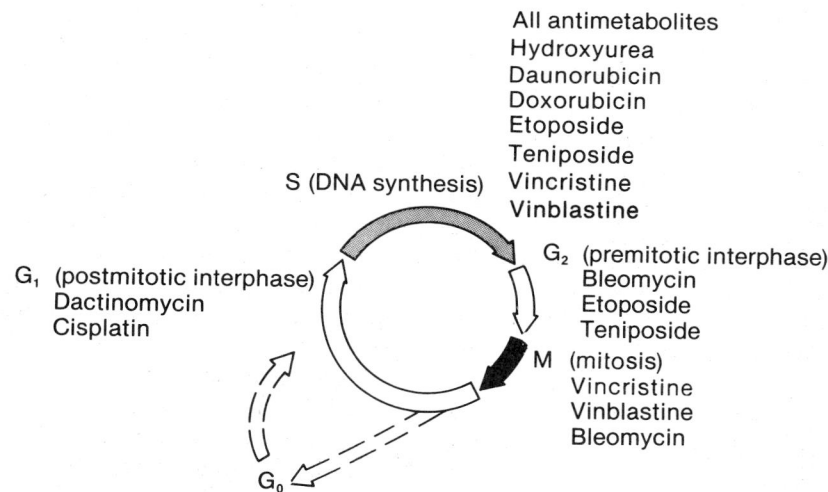

FIGURE 52-3. **Sites of maximal effect of anticancer drugs in the cell cycle. Drugs are listed in the phase of the cycle in which cells are most susceptible. For drugs that are not listed, such as the alkylating agents, there is no phase-specific activity, and in other cases the data are conflicting or incomplete.**

severe neurologic symptoms, including spinal cord damage with numbness and weakness.

Methotrexate is eliminated from the body in the urine, and therefore patients should have adequate kidney function. Renal toxicity may be avoided during high-dose methotrexate therapy by maintaining a high output of alkaline urine, with large volumes (3 to 4 L/day) of IV fluids and sufficient bicarbonate to maintain the urinary pH above 7. The usual dose of IV methotrexate is 20 to 40 mg/m². The drug may also be given IM or PO.

Purine analogues

Mercaptopurine. Mercaptopurine has a structure and mechanism of action similar to thioguanine. It is useful in acute leukemias. The drug should be taken as a single oral dose of 2.5 mg/kg, between meals to facilitate absorption.

In addition to myelosuppression and nausea, hepatic toxicity with jaundice occurs in up to one third of patients and necessitates the discontinuation of treatment with this agent.

Mercaptopurine is metabolically inactivated by the enzyme xanthine oxidase. A dangerous drug interaction may therefore occur between mercaptopurine and allopurinol, which blocks xanthine oxidase and is commonly used to prevent a buildup of uric acid in leukemia. Patients receiving allopurinol should receive only 25% of the usual dose of mercaptopurine.

Thioguanine. Thioguanine is an antimetabolite *analogue* of guanine, a purine used for the synthesis of DNA and ribonucleic acid *(RNA)*. The antimetabolite inhibits the synthesis of normal purines, and itself becomes incorporated into DNAs and RNAs, which cannot then function normally.

Thioguanine is used to treat acute myelogenous leukemia. Its major toxic effects are myelosuppression, mild nausea, vomiting, diarrhea, and occasional *jaundice*. It is administered orally, with the usual dose being 2 mg/kg, taken as a single dose between meals, to assure adequate absorption. Patients should be informed about the importance of having liver function studies performed and to report any changes in the color of the skin or the mucous membranes.

Pyrimidine analogues

Azacitidine. Azacitidine is an analogue of the natural pyrimidine cytidine, and interferes with the production of DNA and RNA. Its use is restricted to the secondary treatment of acute myelogenous leukemia. Toxic side effects include severe nausea, diarrhea, myelosuppression, and occasional liver dysfunction.

The usual dose is 300 to 400 mg/m²/day IV for 5 days.

Cytarabine. Cytarabine is an analogue of the pyrimidine nucleosides cytidine and deoxycytidine. It kills cells in the S-phase of the cell cycle by inhibiting the enzyme DNA polymerase.

The drug is useful in acute leukemias. Its major toxic effect is myelosuppression, but nausea and mucositis may also occur, especially with high doses or with prolonged infusions.

The usual dosage is 100 to 200 mg/m² daily for 5 to 10 days, given IM, IV push, SC, or by continuous IV infusion. It may also be given intrathecally for meningeal leukemia, 25 to 50 mg/m² once or twice weekly.

Floxuridine. Floxuridine is an investigational agent that consists of fluorouracil linked to a deoxyribose sugar. It inhibits thymidylate synthetase, can be incorporated into RNAs, and clinically can be used interchangeably with fluorouracil. It is used in GI cancers as an infusion of 0.1 to 0.5 mg/kg/day for 1 to 2 weeks, either IV or via the hepatic artery for hepatic metastases. Its toxic effects include myelosuppression, nausea, mucositis, darkening of the veins, and occasional CNS toxicities, including unsteadiness of gait (ataxia), blurred vision, depression, and dizziness.

Fluorouracil. Fluorouracil is a pyrimidine analogue that can inhibit DNA synthesis by binding to the enzyme thymidylate synthetase. It can also be incorporated into RNA instead of uridine, thus resulting in fraudulent RNAs.

The drug is used in GI (colorectal) and breast cancers, and is a component of the cyclophosphamide, methotrexate, fluorouracil (CMF) regimen used for the adjuvant therapy of breast cancers. Toxic effects of fluorouracil include myelosuppression, mild nausea, mucositis, skin sensitivity to sunlight, discoloration of the fingernails (dark brown hyperpigmentation), and sclerosis and discoloration of veins used for injection.

The drug is usually administered as either an IV bolus injection or as an IV infusion of 12 mg/kg (300 to 600 mg/m²) per day (maximum 800 mg/24 hr).

Fluorouracil is also available as a cream for the topical treatment of superficial skin cancers. A nonmetal applicator or glove is used to apply the cream. Only a small amount of fluorouracil is absorbed into the circulation from the skin, so the systemic toxicity is minimal. Patients should be instructed to avoid direct sunlight, to use a chemical sunscreen preparation when out in the sun, and to be aware of potential photosensitivity reactions.

ANTINEOPLASTIC ANTIBIOTICS
Anthracyclines

Daunorubicin. Daunorubicin is an anthracycline similar in structure, mechanism, and pharmacologic properties to doxorubicin. It is used primarily in acute leukemias at a dose of 30 to 60 mg/m² IV daily for up to 3 days. Daunorubicin is generally used in combination with cytarabine. The same precautions regarding cardiac toxicity and extravasation apply for daunorubicin as for doxorubicin.

Doxorubicin. Doxorubicin is one of the most useful drugs against a variety of cancers. It is an anthracycline compound produced and isolated from a *Strepto-*

myces fungus. Its exact mechanism of action is in dispute, but it appears to bind tightly to DNA, and kills cells in the S-phase preferentially. It is used in acute leukemias, *lymphomas, sarcomas,* and carcinomas of the breast, ovary, endometrium, stomach, bladder, thyroid, lung, and testis.

The most important toxic effects of doxorubicin are myelosuppression and cardiac toxicity. The cardiac toxicity is cumulative with each dose, and produces CHF in 25% to 30% of patients who have received total cumulative doses greater than 550 mg/m². The risk of cardiac toxicity is greater in patients who have a preexisting heart disease, who are over 70 years of age, or who have had radiation therapy involving the heart. Other toxicities of doxorubicin include nausea, *alopecia,* stomatitis, and recall of previous radiation damage to the skin or esophagus. Radiation recall consists of a severe inflammation of the skin or GI tract, after doxorubicin treatment, in areas previously treated with radiation therapy.

The drug is a potent *vesicant,* and care must be taken to avoid extravasation during IV injection. The usual dose is 60 to 75 mg/m² IV every 3 weeks if used as a single agent, or 30 to 50 mg/m² in combination regimens. The drug should be injected slowly, through a running IV over 10 to 15 minutes, rather than as a rapid bolus.

Some of the drug is excreted in the urine, and will impart a reddish color to the patient's urine for 1 or 2 days after treatment. Because most of the drug is metabolized by the liver and excreted into the bile, doses should be reduced in patients with liver disease or extensive liver metastases.

Bleomycin

Bleomycin is a mixture of glycopeptides produced by a Japanese soil fungus. The drug kills tumor cells by attaching to DNA and generating free radicals from oxygen, which then react with DNA to produce strand breaks and fragmentation. Maximum cell killing occurs in the G₂ and M-phases of the cell cycle.

Bleomycin is especially useful in testicular carcinomas, where it is part of the curative cisplatin (Platinol), vinblastine, bleomycin (PVB) regimen. It is also active against lymphomas and squamous cell carcinomas of the skin, head and neck, and cervix.

The lungs are the major site of bleomycin toxicity, with pulmonary fibrosis developing in 10% to 20% of patients who receive total cumulative doses of greater than 400 units. Pulmonary toxicity may be accompanied by symptoms of a cough and shortness of breath, and is fatal in about 1% of patients who receive bleomycin.

The majority of patients treated with bleomycin develop a low-grade to moderate fever a few hours after treatment. This fever is usually less than 39° C, may be accompanied by chills and sweating, and usually lasts less than 24 hours. Rarely, acute reactions similar to anaphylaxis may occur, with low blood pressure, wheezing, and mental confusion. Because this reaction has occurred in perhaps 1% of patients with lymphomas, the manufacturer recommends that patients be treated with a test dose of 1 to 2 units of bleomycin before beginning treatments with standard doses. Patients should be observed for 2 hours after the test dose, and if there is no fall in blood pressure, or no wheezing, the treatment with standard doses may commence.

The lungs and skin are thought to be particularly sensitive to bleomycin because they lack an enzyme that inactivates the drug. The majority of patients receiving bleomycin will develop a mild to moderate skin toxicity, with increased pigmentation and thickening of the skin, especially over pressure areas such as the knuckles and elbows. A major advantage of bleomycin is its lack of toxicity to the bone marrow. Bleomycin is eliminated from the body by the kidneys, and doses must be reduced or avoided in patients with moderate to severe renal disease (i.e., when the creatinine clearance is less than 25 ml/min).

The usual dose is 10 to 20 units/m² IV, IM, or SC weekly, or by continuous infusion for 3 to 7 days.

Dactinomycin

Dactinomycin is a chromopeptide isolated from *Streptomyces*. It binds to DNA and inhibits RNA and protein synthesis. It is used in the childhood solid tumors (e.g., Wilms' tumor, Ewing's sarcoma, and rhabdomyosarcoma), as well as in other sarcomas, choriocarcinoma, melanoma, and testicular carcinomas. Its major side effects are nausea, vomiting, myelosuppression, alopecia, and mucositis. The exacerbation of radiation-produced injuries may occur. The usual dose is 0.3 to 0.5 mg/m² IV daily for 5 days, or 1 to 1.5 mg/m² IV every 3 to 4 weeks. Extravasation must be avoided because the drug is a potent vesicant.

Mitomycin

Mitomycin is a fungal product that can bind to and cross-link DNA, and is therefore sometimes classified as an alkylating agent. It is used in the palliative treatment of carcinomas of the stomach, pancreas, colon, breast, and cervix.

The major toxic effect of mitomycin is prolonged and cumulative myelosuppression. It also produces nausea and occasional renal and pulmonary toxicity. It is a local vesicant, and may produce severe necrosis of tissues if extravasated outside of a vein. The usual dose is 10 to 20 mg/m² IV administered every 6 weeks.

Plicamycin (Mithramycin)

Plicamycin is a chromomycin produced by a *Streptomyces*. Its major use is to lower the excessive serum calcium levels produced by some *tumors*. The usual dose for this purpose is 25 µg/kg every 3 to 7 days IV. It is also occasionally used in testicular carcinomas. Its major toxic effects are nausea, myelosuppression, a bleeding disorder caused by an impairment of blood clotting, and hypocalcemia. It is also a vesicant, and extravasation outside of a vein must be avoided.

SUMMARY

A general introduction to cancer chemotherapy, including an overview of the various anticancer agents, their mechanisms of action, adverse side effects, and toxicities, has been presented in this chapter. The various antimetabolites and antineoplastic antibiotics have been examined in detail. Alkylating and miscellaneous drugs used to treat cancer are discussed in Chapter 53. By using the information presented in this chapter, the nurse will be able to anticipate adverse side effects, monitor and minimize these effects, avoid clinically significant drug interactions, and enhance patient education regarding individual drug therapy regimens. With an understanding of the antimetabolites and antineoplastic antibiotics, the nurse will be better able to provide optimal care to patients requiring chemotherapy with these agents.

ADVERSE/SIDE EFFECTS OF ANTIMETABOLITES AND ANTINEOPLASTIC ANTIBIOTICS*

Common toxicities

ALOPECIA

Usually begins 2 to 3 weeks after the start of chemotherapy and may be complete at 1 to 2 months. Hair regrows almost always after the completion of the chemotherapy. Some drugs do *not* usually produce hair loss, notably bleomycin.

LOCAL VESICANT EFFECTS: PHLEBITIS

These drugs can cause severe damage to tissues if extravasation occurs during injection: doxorubicin, daunorubicin, mitomycin, plicamycin, and dactinomycin.

MYELOSUPPRESSION

Leukopenia and thrombocytopenia are the major dose-limiting factors for most anticancer drugs, with a nadir in blood counts 7 to 14 days after treatment.

NAUSEA AND VOMITING

Usually this occurs a few hours after treatment, lasting up to 24 hours, and is partially relieved by antiemetics. The most severe nausea is produced by azacitidine, fluorouracil, and mitomycin.

Occasional toxicities

ALLERGIC REACTIONS

Anaphylaxis has been reported, rarely, with bleomycin and doxorubicin. Hives along the vein used for injection may occur with doxorubicin.

CARDIAC SYSTEM

CHF—doxorubicin, daunorubicin.

CUTANEOUS SYSTEM

Dermatitis—methotrexate.
Hyperpigmentation—bleomycin, fluorouracil.
Nailbed discoloration—fluorouracil, daunorubicin, doxorubicin.

GASTROINTESTINAL SYSTEM

Mucositis, diarrhea—methotrexate, bleomycin, or fluorouracil administered by infusion for several days.

HEPATIC SYSTEM

Cirrhosis—methotrexate.
Jaundice—mercaptopurine, azathioprine, thioguanine, azacitidine, plicamycin.

NEUROLOGIC SYSTEM

Methotrexate given intrathecally may cause headaches, weakness, and numbness.
Fluorouracil may cause temporary loss of coordination (ataxia).

RESPIRATORY SYSTEM

Lung damage (fibrosis) is most often produced by bleomycin, related to the total cumulative dose of the drug, but may also occur with mitomycin and methotrexate.

RENAL SYSTEM

Decreased renal function, manifested by increased blood creatinine and BUN concentrations, and decreased creatinine clearance—methotrexate, mitomycin.

Long-term toxicities

CARCINOGENIC EFFECTS

Increased risk of acute leukemia, especially when alkylating agents and radiation are used together.

INFERTILITY

Amenorrhea, azoospermia—full effects in humans for many drugs and combinations are not yet known.

TERATOGENIC EFFECTS

Especially in the first trimester of a pregnancy; high risk for all anticancer agents.

*See Chapter 11, "Drug Toxicity," for an overview of drug toxicity. The incidence and severity of these toxic side effects vary from drug to drug and from patient to patient.

CLINICALLY SIGNIFICANT DRUG INTERACTIONS*

Primary drug	Interacting drug	Possible effect(s)	Probable mechanism(s)
Mercaptopurine	Allopurinol	Increased pharmacologic effects; fatal myelosuppression	Allopurinol blocks the metabolism of mercaptopurine
Methotrexate	Probenecid	Increased methotrexate effect and toxicity	Probenecid inhibits the renal excretion of methotrexate
Methotrexate	Salicylates	Increased methotrexate effect and toxicity	Salicylates decrease renal tubular secretion of methotrexate and also displace methotrexate from protein-binding sites
Methotrexate	Smallpox vaccination	Generalized vaccinia	Impairment by methotrexate of the normal immunologic response to vaccine

*See Chapter 10, "Drug Interactions," for an overview of drug interactions.

GENERAL NURSING IMPLICATIONS

Nursing of patients requiring antimetabolites or antineoplastic antibiotics

ASSESSMENT

Various antimetabolites and antineoplastic antibiotics are used in treating cancer. Drug therapy is individualized and is often a part of a broad therapeutic regimen. A combination of various anticancer drugs (i.e., combination therapy), surgery, or radiation therapy (i.e., combined modality treatment) may be indicated. Treatment can be palliative or curative. A complete nursing assessment is important in relation to planning individualized nursing care. Baseline data should include a general assessment of the patient's overall health with special attention to nutritional status, oral assessment, and elimination patterns. Renal and hepatic function should be identified and hearing assessed, especially when ototoxic drugs are indicated. The identification of family and other support systems should be included in the nursing assessment, as well as the effects the patient's treatment and condition may have on home or employment responsibilities. The patient's knowledge of and response to the diagnosis of cancer should receive careful attention, as well as the patient's readiness for learning and understanding the treatment regimen. Nursing care and patient teaching must be carefully individualized to the patient's and family's coping abilities. Newly diagnosed patients require much support and assistance in relation to the acceptance of their condition and the treatment plan. Nursing care and approaches often require alteration and adaptation to the patient's changing needs.

Patients often need assistance with specimen collection, including blood, urine, and cerebrospinal fluid. If the treatment is palliative, attention should be given to documenting symptoms. Isolation measures should be implemented if the patient is, or is likely to become, immunosuppressed.

Baseline data should include a detailed drug history, including the identification of any possible sensitivity, contraindications, cautions, and drug interactions. The patient's self-medication abilities and drug-taking patterns should be identified. It is important to ascertain if the patient has received any previous chemotherapy. The type and extent of such therapy should be recorded.

SENSITIVITY

Generally, allergic reactions to the antimetabolites and the antineoplastic antibiotics are rare. However, any drug has the potential to cause a hypersensitivity reaction in susceptible individuals. Allergic reactions have been reported with the use of these medications and patients should be made aware of the possibility of the occurrence of an allergic reaction. Patients receiving these medications should be carefully monitored for anaphylaxis, including laryngeal edema, stridor, hoarseness, or respiratory difficulty. Epinephrine, diphenhydramine, hydrocortisone, and resuscitation equipment should be readily available, especially when these medications are administered parenterally, and patients should be monitored carefully for signs of anaphylaxis during the administration and for at least 1 hour after administration.

Continued.

GENERAL NURSING IMPLICATIONS—cont'd

Nursing of patients requiring antimetabolites or antineoplastic antibiotics—cont'd

SENSITIVITY—cont'd

If a serious allergy occurs with the use of one of these agents, another agent should be substituted by the prescriber. In the event that the agent is the drug of choice for the particular patient, desensitization may be indicated.

CONTRAINDICATIONS

The use of the antimetabolite and antineoplastic drugs is contraindicated in patients with a known hypersensitivity to the specific medication. If the medication is the drug of choice for a specific condition, desensitization may be indicated (see the Nursing Drug Digest for contraindications for each specific agent).

CAUTIONS

The antimetabolites and antineoplastic drugs should be used cautiously in patients who are severely debilitated, who have severe leukopenia, anemia, thrombocytopenia, or severe renal or hepatic dysfunction, because of the toxicities associated with these drugs. Anticancer drugs should be used cautiously in pregnancy, especially during the first trimester, because of their association with teratogenesis and fetal death (see the Nursing Drug Digest for specific cautions for each agent).

DRUG INTERACTIONS

The antimetabolites and antineoplastic antibiotics have the potential to interact with other drugs. Mercaptopurine is metabolically inactivated by the enzyme xanthine oxidase and thus a dangerous drug interaction may occur between this drug and the xanthine oxidase inhibitor allopurinol. Patients requiring both medications concurrently should receive only one third to one fourth of the usual dose of mercaptopurine. Failure to reduce the dose will result in increased levels of mercaptopurine with a resultant potential for severe toxicity. See Clinically Significant Drug Interactions and the Nursing Drug Digest for specific information about each agent.

ADMINISTRATION

The antimetabolites and antineoplastic antibiotics are available in various dosage forms for PO, IM, IV, topical or local,

intrathecal and intraventricular administration. For example, mercaptopurine is usually administered orally between meals to enhance absorption. Cytarabine is administered either IM, IV, SC, or intrathecally. Fluorouracil can be administered either by IV infusion or bolus. The dosage and administration are highly individualized and various specific medication regimens or protocols have been developed. Because of the effect these medications generally have on bone marrow, hair follicles, and the mucosal lining of the GI tract, chemotherapy is often scheduled in cycles of 3 to 4 weeks, as indicated in the chemotherapy protocol.

It is important to note that many of these drugs are *not* usually administered by nurses because of their relative toxicity. Some drugs may be administered by nurses when given by one route (e.g., IV infusion) and not another (e.g., intrathecal). Oncology nurse specialists are administering anticancer drugs that have been previously only administered by physicians with a specialty in oncology medicine. It is the responsibility of the professional nurse to observe the limits of practice in relation to the administration of these drugs. The nurse should also be alert to the changing roles of practice and assist the patient and the person administering the medication, as indicated. Thus, an understanding of the administration of these drugs is important in relation to preparing and supporting patients who require chemotherapy and in monitoring adverse effects directly related to administration (e.g., extravasation with IV administration).

It should be noted that many of these drugs have a direct irritant effect on the skin, eyes, and mucous membranes, and should be handled carefully and with special precautions. These drugs have been associated with not only local irritation and allergic reactions, but they have also been associated with mutagenic and carcinogenic effects. Research has shown that nurses handling these drugs have excreted various amounts of the drugs in their urine. It is especially important on oncology units, where nurses are involved fre-

quently with the care, preparation, and administration of these drugs, that these effects be kept in mind and the hospital protocol carefully followed.

Contact with the skin through environmental contamination following spillage should be avoided. It is important to note that contact can occur by means other than direct skin contact with liquid preparations, including the inhalation of aerosolized drug, which can occur when the needle is withdrawn from the vial, when ampules are opened, when air is expelled from the syringe, or when needles or syringes are clipped. Although masks, gloves, and eye protection (e.g., goggles) have been recommended, the use of these is controversial. Research has found that for such drugs as nitrogen mustards (see Chapter 53, "Alkylating and Miscellaneous Drugs Used to Treat Cancer"), only polyvinylchloride gloves were effective or protected against penetration. Rubber gloves or polyethylene gloves did not provide this protection.

Practitioner drug interactions or adverse effects have been reported, including nausea, lightheadedness, dizziness, headache, facial flushing, and nasal sores associated with handling these medications.

Because of these effects, it is recommended that pharmacists prepare anticancer drugs using the appropriate technique and vertical laminar airflow hoods. All health care team members involved in the use of these drugs should work together to formulate guidelines to ensure the practitioner's safety in the preparation and administration of these medications.

If these drugs come in contact with the skin or eyes, the affected areas should be thoroughly washed with water. Leftover drugs should be disposed of carefully according to hospital or health care facility protocols.

In general, before the antimetabolites or antineoplastic antibiotics are administered, the following should be completed.

Become familiar with the package insert for the preparation, administration, dose range, and side effects of

GENERAL NURSING IMPLICATIONS—cont'd

Nursing of patients requiring antimetabolites or antineoplastic antibiotics—cont'd

ADMINISTRATION—cont'd

each drug. Doublecheck the dose of each drug. Check appropriate laboratory test results before administering the drugs (blood counts, kidney and liver function).

Discuss the treatment with the patient. If the patient has had a previous cycle of the same treatment, ask about and report unusual or severe side effects.

Patients on protocol treatments should have signed an informed consent form before the first treatment.

If nausea has been a severe problem with previous cycles, pretreatment with antiemetics should be considered.

Special care should be taken to avoid IV extravasation of doxorubicin, daunorubicin, dactinomycin, plicamycin and mitomycin. These drugs should be generally administered IV as follows.

1. A 23-gauge butterfly or scalp vein needle should be used for IV infusions. Large syringes filled with 0.9% sodium chloride or 5% dextrose should be available to check venous patency and to flush the vein after drug injection.
2. The preferred sites of injection are the easily visible veins of the forearm. If these are not available, veins on the back of the hand may be used, or even less preferable, the antecubital fossa. Damage to the nerves and tendons may be especially severe if extravasation occurs in these latter areas, and these sites are generally *not* recommended.
3. The needle should be lightly taped, with the skin puncture site and vein visible for any sign of extravasation.
4. The patency of the vein should be tested before treating by injection of 10 to 20 ml of 0.9% normal saline. The rate of the injection should be smooth and gentle to avoid rupturing the vein. Flushing of the vein with 10 to 20 ml saline should be done after each drug injection or infusion.
5. Generally, if pain occurs during the administration of these drugs, the injection should be immediately discontinued, the patency of

the vein evaluated, and a different site for the injection of the remaining drug should be considered. Pain is not a reliable sign and vein patency must be evaluated carefully during administration. Generally, the administration is completed by a physician; however, clinical nurse specialists in oncology nursing with special training are administering many of the anticancer drugs.

The physician should be notified immediately of any possible extravasation of the vesicant drugs. Appropriate antidotes (e.g., sodium bicarbonate for doxorubicin and daunorubicin) should be infiltrated at the site and cold compresses applied for 24 hours. The nurse should observe for and the patient should be advised to report any redness (erythema), blistering, or ulceration of the skin. If pain and erythema persist for longer than 1 week after a suspected extravasation, the patient should be referred to a plastic surgeon.

Doxorubicin can cause intense local inflammation and pain, with extravasation resulting in ulcers and an impaired normal range of motion in the affected limb. The ulceration can involve irreversible damage to underlying tendons, nerves, and vessels, with extensive tissue loss. The initial appearance of an inflammation usually does not indicate the deeper erosion and tissue involvement. Treatment of this adverse effect can require surgery, grafting, and extensive physical therapy. The condition, however, should be prevented whenever possible. Monitoring the patient for complaints of stinging, burning, or pain at the injection site immediately on the administration of the drug can indicate extravasation. Extravasation is suspected if swelling and redness are noted at the injection site. It is important to differentiate between signs of extravasation and a local allergic reaction to this drug, usually manifested by itching at the point the drug entered and inflammation extending the length of the vein and into adjacent tissue. Tiny papules or a urticarial rash may appear at the injection site.

Many have found that it is possible to prevent skin necrosis and ulcer formation with local coricosteroid therapy. Contractures and a loss of limb motion may be prevented through immediate nursing intervention by nurses involved in the administration of this medication when careful monitoring is completed and standard extravasation orders are developed enabling nurses to begin immediate treatment.

Various methods have been used to prevent severe pain and tissue damage at the site of extravasation of doxorubicin, including the injection of hydrocortisone sodium succinate via the IV tubing before removing the needle, followed with an ice pack. Another method of treatment that is recommended by oncologist nurses who have completed research in this area is to remove the needle immediately after extravasation occurs or is suspected and to apply an ice pack to the area. Hydrocortisone sodium succinate is injected intradermally and subcutaneously into the involved tissue area with 25-gauge needles. The dosage varies with the size of the infiltration. This can be followed by the application of a thin film of hydrocortisone cream (1%), covered with a sterile gauze dressing and the reapplication of the ice pack for 24 hours. The hydrocortisone cream may be reapplied twice a day if indicated, and patients encouraged to move the extremity involved and to report any pain or skin tension. It has been suggested that this method be applied to the infiltration areas of other anticancer drugs (e.g., vincristine).

MONITORING PATIENT RESPONSE
Therapeutic response

Monitoring the patient's therapeutic response can vary with the type of cancer and the treatment regimen, and may include a change in the tumor size, blood test results, improved organ function, an increased sense of wellbeing, and an ability to resume or maintain activities of daily living. Remission requires specific monitoring as indicated by the patient's individual condition. Patients who have received therapy for the treatment of cancer are

Continued.

GENERAL NURSING IMPLICATIONS—cont'd

Nursing of patients requiring antimetabolites or antineoplastic antibiotics—cont'd

Therapeutic response—cont'd

monitored for the absence of a relapse or metastasis.

Adverse side effects

The major adverse effects associated with the use of the antimetabolites and antineoplastic antibiotics are related to their toxic effects on the bone marrow, GI mucosa, and integument, which have cells with a relatively rapid turnover rate making them more prone to the toxic effects of these medications. Effects on the bone marrow result in leukopenia and thrombocytopenia. Effects on the GI mucosa can cause mucositis, nausea, vomiting, and diarrhea. Effects on the integument can result in various skin lesions and alopecia. Although these are major effects associated with the use of these medications, others can occur (see the Table, Adverse/Side Effects, for an outline of adverse effects associated with the use of these medications). Monitoring is essential, as is planning to minimize these effects, because some can be life-threatening and psychologically distressing.

Effects on bone marrow

Thrombocytopenia. Patients receiving the antimetabolites or antineoplastic antibiotics should have a routine monitoring of platelet counts and be observed for signs of bleeding. Platelet counts begin to fall 4 to 14 days after the chemotherapy is started, depending on the individual agent. Platelet counts are usually at their lowest between 7 and 14 days after the therapy is started. Serious bleeding can occur when the platelet counts are 10,000 or less. Moderate bleeding can occur when the platelet counts are 10,000 to 30,000, and bleeding is relatively low when the platelet counts are 30,000-100,000.

Monitor patients for bruising, petechiae, especially involving the lower extremities, bleeding from the gums or nares, and blood in the urine, stool, sputum, or nasal secretions.

Bleeding can result in anemia and patients should also be monitored for pallor, dizziness, tachycardia, tinnitus, and angina. Laboratory red blood cell counts, hemoglobin levels, and hematocrit should be monitored routinely.

IM injections should be avoided, as should rectal temperatures and the administration of rectal suppositories when the platelet counts are very low or when bleeding is a problem. Intravenous infusion sites should be monitored for the oozing of blood. If IM injections must be given, pressure should be applied for 3 to 5 minutes to the injection site after the injection is given. Laboratory slips should be labeled with "bleeding precautions." It is important to avoid medications that can interfere with platelet function (e.g., aspirin). (See the Patient Education section of this table for information regarding the management of this effect.)

Leukopenia. The lowering of white blood cell counts (less than 5000/mm³) usually is maximal 10 to 14 days after the treatment is started. It is during the nadir that patients are at the greatest risk for contracting an infection related to this adverse effect. Patients should be advised to report immediately any fever, cough, sore throat, or other symptoms suggestive of infection during this period, 10 to 14 days after treatment. A blood count should be performed, and the patient should be examined. Outpatients who develop fever while neutropenic are usually hospitalized for empiric broad-spectrum antibiotic therapy.

Protective isolation should be implemented to prevent the exposure of the patient to infections, including colds, draining wounds, chicken pox, herpes zoster, and measles. Meticulous hygiene care and careful handwashing are important in preventing an infection.

Monitor the patient for fever, cough, lung congestion, mouth ulcers, painful teeth, sore throat, pain on urination, draining wounds, discomfort, or other untoward symptoms that may develop during the few days that white blood cell counts are low. The patient's temperature should be carefully monitored and the use of aspirin or acetaminophen should be avoided, because these drugs can mask the presence of fever. Chest radiographs and specimen cultures (e.g., blood, urine, stool, sputum) should be completed as indicated. A strict aseptic technique is required with all laboratory work and parenteral

infusions. The infections may require immediate treatment with antibiotics or transfusion with granulocytes. Outpatients may require hospitalization if the leukopenia is severe.

The recovery of white blood cell counts usually occurs in 21 to 28 days.

The initial or induction therapy for acute leukemias is more intense than the usual cyclic chemotherapy for other cancers. The goal of the induction treatment is the elimination of leukemic cells from the bone marrow, to enable repopulation with normal cells. The period of leukopenia and thrombocytopenia is therefore more prolonged, usually 3 to 4 weeks. Patients with acute leukemias are hospitalized for this induction period, preferably in a unit designed for the compromised host (i.e., the severely immunosuppressed patient).

Gastrointestinal effects

Patients should be monitored carefully for toxic drug effects on the mucosal lining of the GI system resulting in mucositis, anorexia, nausea, vomiting, taste distortion, and diarrhea. These effects can cause an alteration in nutritional status, fluid and electrolyte imbalance, and dehydration. Routine monitoring of serum electrolytes, intake and output, and daily weights is indicated.

Mucositis. An inflammatory response involving the oral mucosa occurs about 7 days after the start of chemotherapy, often correlating with the lowest white blood cell counts. About 2 or 3 days before the lowest point, the oral mucosa is at its worst. This occurs sooner in children than in adults because their oral mucosa has a higher mitotic index.

The nursing history should include a careful oral assessment for patients admitted for a first or repeat course of chemotherapy. The presence of gingivitis, impacted wisdom teeth, dentures, or other dental prostheses require careful identification, as well as a history of oral problems with any previous chemotherapy. Because major dental work should not be completed while patients are on chemotherapy, dental work should be taken care of whenever possible before the chemotherapy is started. An assessment of the patient's

GENERAL NURSING IMPLICATIONS—cont'd

Nursing of patients requiring antimetabolites or antineoplastic antibiotics—cont'd

Gastrointestinal effects—cont'd

usual oral care habits should also be recorded. This information is particularly important in monitoring changes and planning, as well as in evaluating the effectiveness of oral care measures.

The first signs of oral involvement can appear within 2 to 3 days and begin to reverse gradually and disappear in about 10 days in children and a little later in adults. During this time, assess the mouth at regular intervals at least twice daily. Inspect the lips, tongue, hard and soft palates, tonsillar fossa, gingiva, and oral structures for moisture, color, texture, and the presence of inflammation, infection, bleeding, or debris. Bleeding may be intermittent or oozing.

The presence of thrombocytopenia and leukopenia make the mouth susceptible to bleeding and infection, in addition to the direct effects of the chemotherapy on the oral mucosa epithelial cells. The bleeding can be severe even with minor trauma when the platlet counts are below 20,000/mm³, and gram-negative opportunistic bacterial and fungal infections often occur during periods of leukopenia. These changes require that the oral care be adapted to the individual patient's requirements during the chemotherapy regimen.

Oral care should be completed twice a day with a soft toothbrush and flossing should be completed carefully. Dentures, orthodontic retainers, and bands should be entirely eliminated or removed when possible for at least 8 hours daily. It is important to follow the blood counts and the platelet counts to anticipate any oral problems so that oral care measures can be adapted to the possible effects of thrombocytopenia or leukopenia. Mouth lesions should be cultured to detect any infection. Flossing should not be done when the platelet counts drop to below 20,000, and brushing with a soft toothbrush should be discontinued. The mouth should be gently cleaned with gauze pads soaked in a water and a hydrogen peroxide solution (1 part of hydrogen peroxide to 5 to 6 parts water) or in a prescribed antibacterial or antifungal solution.

Daunorubicin has caused xerostomia resulting in reduced saliva and increased viscosity of saliva. Artifical saliva may be indicated.

Various antifungal and antibacterial mouthwashes have been used and can be prescribed, as well as topical anesthetics (lidocaine viscous), when mucositis is severe.

Nystatin ice cups (made with black cherry concentrate, sterile water, and nystatin powder, frozen and eaten with a spoon) or other mouthwashes can be used. Acetaminophen with codeine elixir can be swished and swallowed for both local and systemic effects.

Lemon glycerine swabs should not be used for oral care because the lemon can decalcify the teeth and the glycerin can absorb water and further dry and irritate the oral mucosa.

Oral rinses may be indicated 3 to 4 times daily or every 2 hours as indicated, or oral irrigation may be required if the mucositis is severe. Suction equipment should be readily available.

The mouth can be rinsed with a solution containing equal parts of cetylpyridinium (e.g., Cepacol) mouthwash, hydrogen peroxide, and water. If this is irritating, a solution of 5 ml sodium bicarbonate in 500 ml normal saline has been recommended.

Oral lesions can be painful and often prevent the patient from eating or drinking adequately. Analgesics are best taken 30 to 60 minutes before meals as prescribed for pain. Diets should be bland, with low sugar and soft foods during periods of mucositis. Liquids should be nonacidic. Recommend liquids or semiliquids such as fruitades, carbonated beverages, ices (e.g., popsicles), and gelatin desserts. Apple and grape juices can aggravate oral lesions, and rough foods or foods with citric acid can cause the ulcers to burn. The temperature of the food should also be carefully monitored to prevent burns. For some patients, nasogastric feedings or total parenteral nutrition may be indicated.

Monitor for recovery of the oral lesions in 5 to 10 days.

Nausea and vomiting. Monitor patients for nausea and vomiting associated with the chemotherapy. Nausea and vomiting can occur 2 to 6 hours after the treatment and can continue for 1 to 2 days. Cisplatin therapy may result in nausea that lasts for several days. A dietary assessment should be completed to identify and eliminate foods that may exacerbate the nausea and vomiting. Antiemetics may be indicated just before the chemotherapy.

When nausea occurs, it is often helpful to administer the medications just before bedtime if possible to prevent this adverse effect. To prevent vomiting, offer cold compresses to the forehead, encourage patients to avoid sudden movement, and keep an emesis basin nearby and empty. It is particularly important to control odors and provide privacy and oral hygiene.

It is important to monitor patients for anticipatory or conditioned nausea and vomiting associated with the chemotherapy treatment before the treatment or a visit to the oncologist's office. Initiation of antiemetic therapy as much as 24 hours before chemotherapy may lessen the intensity of the nausea.

Diarrhea and constipation. Monitor bowel function, including the frequency, consistency, and amount of stool. If diarrhea is noted, rule out constipation especially if the patient is immobile or receiving medications such as analgesics (e.g., codeine) that can cause constipation. Monitor the perianal area for irritation. Sitz baths and ointment, in addition to hygienic measures may be indicated. Constipation may require stool softeners, enemas, and dietary and exercise assessment and modification.

Integument effects

A variety of effects can occur in the integumentary system as a direct result of the chemotherapy on the rapid turnover rate of the epithelial cells, including changes in pigmentation, nail discoloration, alopecia, dandruff, and psoriasis. Patients should be made aware of these effects and be reassured that they will disappear with the discontinuation of therapy. Local tissue irritation and severe necrosis can occur from ex-

Continued.

GENERAL NURSING IMPLICATIONS—cont'd

Nursing of patients requiring antimetabolites or antineoplastic antibiotics—cont'd

Integument effects—cont'd

travasation of the medication into the tissues during IV administration, and this requires careful monitoring. Maintaining adequate venous access for IV infusion may be a major problem with some patients. Allergic reactions and irritation can occur with direct contact with many of these drugs (see Administration section in this Table).

Monitor the integumentary system for these effects, which can be painful and sometimes require medical treatment. The skin should be assessed frequently throughout the day during care. The skin should be kept clean and dryness prevented. Positioning to prevent skin breakdown every 1 to 2 hours is indicated, especially when patients are immobile or debilitated. Excessive sunlight should be avoided. Tepid baths, emollient lotions, ointments, and creams (e.g., Nivea cream, A & D ointment), and topical anesthetics may be indicated. Antihistamines may be required to relieve pruritus.

The adverse effects associated with the integument can cause body image concerns and attention to this is important. Encourage verbalization and reassure patients that the effects are temporary. One of the main adverse effects of chemotherapy that can cause distress is alopecia.

Alopecia. Alopecia (hair loss) can be emotionally distressing for many patients, and they should be forewarned of this adverse effect and assisted with anticipating the loss of hair and its effect on the patient's sense of body image.

Monitor patients for small amounts of hair loss to complete baldness occurring a few weeks after the chemotherapy is started. Hair loss can involve body and pubic hair in addition to scalp hair. Although this effect can occur with most of the antimetabolites or antineoplastic antibiotics, it occurs especially with dactinomycin, daunorubicin, and doxorubicin. Various techniques have been used in an attempt to prevent this effect, including scalp tourniquets, scalp sphygmomanometers, and ice turbans. These have been

generally unsuccessful in preventing hair loss and are contraindicated in certain cancers such as leukemias because it is thought that cancer cells circulating in the scalp may be protected as well.

It is important to monitor for the regrowth of hair a few weeks after the drug is discontinued, although the hair color or texture may be different. It is important to monitor the patient's response to the loss of hair and to any changes in color or texture.

Miscellaneous effects

Pulmonary complications. Bleomycin and methotrexate are known to produce pulmonary toxicity. Monitoring for pulmonary effects is important because the onset of symptoms can vary. The antimetabolites can produce symptoms with an abrupt onset, compared with those of the alkylating agents. Symptoms can begin once the administration of the drug has been completed. Recovery is usually rapid and complete.

A baseline assessment of respiratory function, including rate and depth of respirations, use of accessory muscles, the inspiratory to expiratory ratio, and breath sounds, should have been completed during the initial nursing assessment. During the chemotherapy, monitor respiratory function routinely to detect changes in the patient's respiratory status. Patients who are receiving drugs associated with pulmonary effects, radiation therapy, or patients with lung lesions are at a particular risk for this adverse effect.

Monitor patients for dyspnea, cough, fever, rales, a change in vital signs, or alterations in breathing pattern or level of consciousness.

Cough is an early sign of pulmonary toxicity. Pneumonitis can occur with bleomycin particularly.

Respiratory infections can result from the patient's altered immune system in addition to effects directly associated with the anticancer drugs. It is important to monitor for symptoms of sinus, throat, middle ear, and lung infections. Monitor the sputum for changes in col-

or, amount, and thickness. Cultures should be obtained for sensitivity studies. Careful monitoring is essential to initiate prompt treatment if an infection or pulmonary complications develop.

Cardiac complications. Some anticancer drugs (e.g., doxorubicin and daunorubicin) are directly toxic to the cardiac muscle cells and have the potential for decreasing cardiac output. Monitor cardiac function.

Hepatic complications. Monitor for hepatotoxicity, including liver enlargement, jaundice, lethargy, pain, tenderness over the liver area, dark-colored urine and urobilinogen, liver function studies (monitor routinely), and serum electrolytes (monitor routinely).

Renal complications. Glomerular or tubular toxicities secondary to direct drug effect can also occur. Monitor intake and output, BUN and creatinine clearance, and urine pH to determine the degree of acidity or alkalinity (alkylinization may be needed).

Increasing fluid intake, if not contraindicated, to 2 to 4 L/day before drug treatment and increasing fluids before and during treatment are helpful in minimizing this effect and assist in the elimination of the drug.

Monitor patients for the following, which may indicate hemorrhagic cystitis related to direct drug irritation occurring with bladder instillation of the drug: persistent urge to void, burning or discomfort on urination, hematuria (assess urine for occult blood), and discomfort and spasm (analgesics or antispasmodics may be required).

Inform the patient that within 1 hour after the injection of the medication, the urine may be discolored, and the discoloration may continue intermittently for 24 hours. This will prevent undue concern.

Neurologic complications. Neurologic toxic effects have been associated with the use of many of the anticancer drugs. The first sign of neurotoxicity is decreased deep tendon reflexes followed by foot and wrist drop, numb-

GENERAL NURSING IMPLICATIONS—cont'd

Nursing of patients requiring antimetabolites or antineoplastic antibiotics—cont'd

Miscellaneous effects—cont'd

ness, tingling, and paresthesias. Muscle weakness tends to occur *later*. Constipation may be caused by toxicity to the autonomic nervous system. In addition, monitor patients for ataxia (cerebral dysfunction), lethargy, mood swings, ototoxicity and other sensory alterations, and seizures.

The neurologic effects of these drugs may be difficult to separate from the effects of the diagnosed cancer or resultant CNS involvement. Headache and vertigo can indicate CNS metastasis. A careful initial baseline assessment and monitoring during therapy is important in making this differentiation. The neurologic effects can also affect the patient's sense of self-concept, mobility, and self-care abilities. Nursing assistance is needed in these areas as indicated.

Sexuality complications. Sexual dysfunction has been associated with the use of the anticancer drugs and this effect, like the others, can be quite distressing to patients and requires professional nursing assistance. Many patients may not feel comfortable discussing sexuality and may not share their problems or demonstrate any discomfort when aspects of sexuality are discussed. It is important for the nurse to be sensitive to the individual patient's needs in this area so that assessment and monitoring can be completed and the adverse effects associated with this area minimized.

Monitor patients for changes in menstrual pattern, changes in libido, and premature menopause.

PATIENT EDUCATION

The patient and the family, as indicated, should be fully informed about the nature of the patient's condition and the treatment plan and should be involved in the health care planning whenever possible. The collaboration of health care team members in the care of patients requiring antimetabolite or antineoplastic medications cannot be overemphasized. To prevent undue confusion and anxiety, the health care team should be clear about what the patient understands and how each

member can work to promote the patient's understanding of the condition and treatment.

In general, the patient and the family should have a clear understanding of the anticipated course of the therapy and medication regimen, including the exact name of the medication, its general action, purpose, dosage, storage, administration, and adverse side effects especially, because patients prepared for common and sometimes devastating adverse effects can accept them better and plan to minimize or prevent them. This is especially important if the patient will be self-medicating on a discharged or outpatient basis.

The patient and the family should be able to monitor the patient's therapeutic response, identify and manage common adverse effects and recognize signs that indicate the health care provider should be notified. Discharged or outpatients may require help in carrying out self-care routines at home and usually need follow-up or supervision. Patient education is a major nursing responsibility and cannot be overemphasized.

Course of therapy

The patient and the family should have a clear idea of the course of the therapy. They should know that the chemotherapy may be administered in cycles or in conjunction with surgery or radiation therapy. They should understand the importance of therapy and the need for continued care and follow-up. The diagnosis of cancer is often devastating to the patient and the family and much support is needed. Any questions the patient or the family may have regarding the therapy or progress should be answered honestly. Nursing must be adapted to the patient's psychologic reaction to the diagnosis, the treatment plan, and the grieving process.

The patient and the family should have a realistic view of what to expect in relation to the chemotherapy. Patients often want to know whether they will be cured. The patient's therapeutic response must be explained in relation

to the individual patient's need for the chemotherapy. Remissions and relapses need to be discussed, as well as the possibility of metastasis. Communication between nurses and physicians regarding the patient's expectations and questions is important to avoid conflicting messages.

Adverse side effects

Although the therapeutic effects of anticancer therapy should be emphasized, the patient and the family should be aware of possible adverse side effects. This is important because these effects can be both life-threatening and emotionally upsetting.

Patients and their families should know that the adverse effects usually disappear when the chemotherapy is discontinued. The management of adverse side effects, such as dose reduction, the use of alternative drugs, taking medication before bedtime if able to prevent nausea and vomiting, and other measures, should be explored with the patient and the family as indicated. Patients should understand that they will be assisted with the adverse side effects if they should occur. It is important to acknowledge fear and distress associated with the possible adverse side effects associated with anticancer drugs.

Points for managing common adverse side effects

Thrombocytopenia

For thrombocytopenia, the nurse should encourage the patient to do the following:

- Monitor self for oozing, intermittent bleeding, easy bruising, and rash.
- Ensure a safe environment.
- Avoid trauma (be sure the patient understands the importance of avoiding minor trauma—e.g., avoid straight blades or razors; use an electric razor; file toenails and fingernails; use a soft toothbrush instead of a hard toothbrush).
- Avoid hot baths, sun, or harsh temperature changes.
- Avoid drugs that interfere with platelet function including aspirin.

Continued.

GENERAL NURSING IMPLICATIONS—cont'd

Nursing of patients requiring antimetabolites or antineoplastic antibiotics—cont'd

Thrombocytopenia—cont'd

- Report bleeding in the mouth or nose, reddish urine or dark stool (which could indicate internal bleeding), and drowsiness or mental changes that may indicate bleeding in the CNS.

If anemia is a problem, patients should understand that tiredness may occur. They should set priorities and schedule activities throughout the day to avoid fatigue, maintain good nutritional habits, and take multivitamins with minerals, if needed.

Inform patients that a blood transfusion may be required. It is important that they understand that this does not indicate the therapy is ineffective.

Leukopenia

Patient education in relation to preventing infections is particularly important, as are measures to prevent bleeding. The patient should understand when the risk of an infection is highest.

Teach patients that they are most susceptible to infection when the leukocyte counts are at their lowest. Patients should understand the importance of having blood tests to monitor for this effect.

To minimize the effects of leukopenia, teach and encourage the patient to do the following:

- Use hygienic practices in daily care.
- Use a good handwashing technique, especially before eating.
- Prevent exposure to people with infections, colds, or contagious diseases such as chickenpox or measles.
- Monitor self for early signs of infection, including warm or red skin, tenderness, open lesions, respiratory congestion, elevated temperature, or cough. Both the patient and the family should be taught to monitor the patient's temperature accurately and to report any abnormalities. They should also understand the importance of not using drugs that can mask an elevated temperature, such as aspirin or acetaminophen.

Mucositis

Teach the patient and the family, as indicated, to complete an oral assessment daily and to monitor for signs of inflammation, bleeding, infection, and common changes associated with periods of chemotherapy, leukopenia, and thrombocytopenia. Instruct the patient in meticulous oral care and in the modification of oral care measures as needed during therapy. Instruct the patient to do the following:

- Gently brush the teeth with a soft bristle toothbrush at least twice a day and gently floss the teeth with unwaxed dental floss.
- Discontinue flossing and brushing when the platelet count falls below 20,000 because of possible bleeding tendency and to rinse the mouth as directed (the patient should be taught to avoid commercial mouth washes that can irritate the mucous membranes).
- Report dryness, discomfort, and increased sensitivity to hot or cold foods. The patient should be taught to avoid irritating, spicy, or tart foods, citrus juices, and extremes in food temperature. Patients should be taught to select nutritious ground, pureed, soft, or liquid foods during periods of oral irritation and to avoid rough-textured foods.
- Avoid alcohol and smoking, which can dry and irritate the mucous membranes, and use a lip balm to prevent irritation.
- Report any inflammation and sores to the health care provider.
- Use prescribed antibacterial, antifungal, and analgesic medications as indicated.

Nausea and vomiting

Patient teaching is required to help patients minimize the GI effects of the chemotherapy, including nausea, vomiting, and diarrhea. Other related problems also may include anorexia, taste distortion, and stomatitis. It is important to be positive in presenting information to the patient for the management of these effects and to inform patients that they may not experience these effects.

In general, patients should avoid foods that can cause nausea or vomiting, such as meat, and select appetizing nutritious foods that are usually well tolerated such as chicken, fish, eggs, cottage cheese or other cheeses, cold cuts, sandwiches, and fruit plates. Patient likes and dislikes should be incorporated into meal planning. A full meal before therapy is often helpful to many patients, as is distraction. The severity of nausea or vomiting requires careful assessment, because antiemetics may be indicated before treatments or during the therapy regimen. Hard sugarless candy can be sucked to mask the taste of the medication during the infusion if this is a problem. Tetrahydrocannabinol (THC) has been used by some patients effectively and this may need to be explored along with psychotherapy or meditation. It is important that patients be taught to brush their teeth or rinse their mouth as directed before and after meals as a measure to decrease nausea and vomiting. In addition, the following measures can also be taught to minimize nausea:

- Drink carbonated beverages or tea.
- Eat a dry cracker before becoming active.
- Eat smaller, more frequent meals and chew foods well before swallowing.
- Relax and eat with someone.
- Suck on ice chips at the onset of nausea.
- Avoid overpowering aromas.

For vomiting, control the vomiting with a cool environment, loose clothing, a cold moist towel to the forehead, oral hygiene, and control of odors. Teach the patient to insert rectal suppositories as prescribed to control vomiting.

Diarrhea

For diarrhea, teach patients to avoid roughage in the diet and to maintain specified amounts of fluids and calories per day.

Teach personal hygiene care and the importance of monitoring the weight daily. The patient should be taught to monitor stools, including recording the date, time, consistency, and color of bowel movements, and to report troublesome or persistent diarrhea, weight

GENERAL NURSING IMPLICATIONS—cont'd

Nursing of patients requiring antimetabolites or antineoplastic antibiotics—cont'd

Diarrhea—cont'd

loss, or constipation. If anal irritation occurs, a sitz bath or ointments to the anal area may be indicated. The patient should be taught to apply the ointments as prescribed.

Integument

For integument effects, teach patients to use good hygienic practices and to keep the skin clean and dry. Teach them to assess the skin regularly for breakdown, irritation, discoloration, rashes, itching, psoriasis, dandruff, or discomfort. They should also be taught to inspect the nails for discoloration. The patient should understand the importance of avoiding excessive sunlight and should report unusual observations or excessive itching or discomfort.

Extravasation

Patients receiving IV therapy should understand the importance of keeping the extremities immobilized during the infusion and what they can do to prevent extravasation. They should understand the importance of letting the person administering the drug know if they feel burning, pain, or any other unusual sensation that might indicate extravasation.

Alopecia

Alopecia is emotionally distressing and patients react to this adverse effect individually. The reaction to the potential or actual change in the body image caused by hair loss is related to the value the individual patient places on hair. Patients need support in anticipating and accepting this adverse effect of the chemotherapy and need reassurance that their hair will usually grow back. They also need to realize that the hair color or texture may be different. Assistance with the selection of head coverings, wigs, or hairpieces is often needed. Children, as well as adults, should be involved in making selections. Patients with long hair may prefer to have their hair cut to a shorter length to lessen the effect of the hair loss. Hair can be lost in large clumps with combing or shampooing or be found on the pillow when the patient wakes up in the morning. Patient education is important in preparing them for these effects. Body hair and pubic

hair can also be lost and the patient needs to be made aware of this. The use of makeup, false eyelashes, and eyebrow pencils as indicated can also be explored. Men may be concerned about the loss of their beard or moustache. It is important to correct misconceptions and to offer support and understanding. The patient should understand why the hair loss occurs with the drug therapy and should be encouraged to express feelings regarding this change in their body image.

The patient should understand that the use of permanents, hair coloring, or frequent shampooing or brushing can effect the degree of hair loss. Patients should be encouraged to use a soft hairbrush only as needed for grooming and to wash the hair only as needed.

Patients often have questions regarding available techniques thought to diminish hair loss. These techniques and their results should be discussed with the patient, including scalp tourniquets and ice turbans.

Neurotoxicity

For neurotoxicity, the patient and the family should be taught to report any numbness, tingling, weakness, or change in consciousness.

Urinary tract and renal toxicity

Urinary tract and renal toxicity can occur, and the patient and the family should understand the importance of maintaining fluid intake, especially the importance of increased fluid intake to prevent hemorrhagic cystitis. The patient and the family should be assisted with planning to meet this requirement, and an individualized daily fluid requirement plan should be implemented.

Sexual dysfunction

Sexual dysfunction, including amenorrhea, premature menopause, and sterility have been associated with the use of many of the antimetabolites and antineoplastic antibiotics. Patients and their families should be informed of these adverse effects and assisted with these problems. They should be aware that the menses usually return to normal after the drug is discontinued, and

even with this adverse effect contraception should be continued. It is also important to note that certain of these drugs can cause false positive pap smear results.

The change in libido with chemotherapy can be distressing to the patient and the patient's partner. Encourage the verbalization of this problem and involve the partner as indicated in discussions and teaching.

Pretreatment teaching is important in relation to the potential problem of sterility. The patient may want to explore the possibility of using a sperm bank and should be made aware of this option.

Patients should be referred to sexual dysfunction clinics as indicated.

Self-concept

For self-concept, pretreatment teaching is essential to prepare patients for the possible adverse side effects associated with these drugs. It should be remembered that individual patient response to the diagnosis of cancer must be considered when patients are given information, because they may not be hearing all that is said and may not be able to make informed choices because of the associated distress. This aspect of teaching must be handled carefully and with a health care team approach.

Psychologic problems, including grieving, sleep pattern disturbances, and ineffective coping of the patient and the family, can occur. Support coping mechanisms and develop the coping abilities of the patient and the family. A knowledge of the cancer process, possible drug toxicities, adverse side effects, and how to decrease or minimize these effects greatly assist the patient and the family in maintaining control and coping abilities. Patient education does much to enable the patient and the family to withstand the treatment and to assist in care.

The nurse's role in health promotion includes patient education regarding the early identification of cancer early warning signs, stop-smoking programs, and self-breast or self-testicular examination. Nurses should become active

Continued.

GENERAL NURSING IMPLICATIONS—cont'd

Nursing of patients requiring antimetabolites or antineoplastic antibiotics—cont'd

Self-concept—cont'd

not only in promoting self-care behaviors to decrease the risk of cancer, but also in promoting public policies directed at decreasing environmental risks.

Nurses working with patients requiring the anticancer drugs have developed patient education materials to enhance patient self-medication and an understanding of their condition and treatment. Group teaching has been effective in teaching selected groups of patients. Patients receiving the anticancer drugs as outpatients or who self-medicate as inpatients require information and education that will give them responsibility in their self-care while allowing them to adjust to the demands of the anticancer therapy. Nurses should direct their research and attention to various teaching approaches for various ages of patients with various conditions requiring anticancer drug therapy. A team approach to patient teaching is also an important consideration in planning to meet the education requirements of patients regarding drug therapy.

GENERAL INSTRUCTIONS FOR DISCHARGE/OUTPATIENTS

ANTIMETABOLITES AND ANTINEOPLASTIC ANTIBIOTICS

This medication is primarily used to treat various forms of cancer. It can sometimes be used for the treatment of other conditions. If you do not understand why you require this medication, check with your health care provider.

Follow the instructions on the prescription exactly. If you have any questions about how this medication should be taken, check with your health care provider.

Take this medication with some food or with a meal. It is often helpful to take this medication at bedtime to prevent nausea and vomiting.

Avoid drinking alcoholic beverages while you are taking this medication. This can cause unwanted effects in some patients.

This medication can cause your skin to become more sensitive to sunlight. When you are outside, shade your skin and wear protective clothing or use a sunscreen. Avoid excessive exposure to sunlight.

Notify your health care provider immediately if you notice a sore throat, fever, mouth sores, diarrhea, skin rash, bruising, dark urine, or black bowel movements.

If you are pregnant, thinking about becoming pregnant, or breastfeeding, do not take this medication until you discuss this with your health care provider. The use of this medication has been associated with birth defects or unwanted effects in nursing infants. Your nurse can discuss methods of birth control with you, as well as infant care, if you must take this medication.

Until you learn how this medication affects you, do not drive, operate dangerous machinery, or put yourself in situations where decreased mental alertness may cause harm.

Do not start or stop taking other medications while on this medication without first checking with your health care provider. This medication can cause unwanted effects if taken with other medications.

Store this medication in a dry place and protect from light. Keep this and all medications out of the reach of children by placing them in a locked drawer or a locked medicine cabinet.

Do not trade or give this medication to your family or friends. It has been prescribed especially for you and can cause unwanted effects in people who do not require it.

It is very important that you keep appointments with your health care provider and have blood tests completed as directed. If you have any questions about the need for visits to your clinic, hospital, or laboratory, discuss these with your health care provider.

If you are receiving chemotherapy as an outpatient; whenever possible, bring a family member or friend to accompany you on days when the chemotherapy is administered to you as an outpatient. Do not drive an automobile or perform other tasks requiring mental alertness after taking antinausea medication, which usually causes drowsiness. Immediately report any fever, or other signs of infection or bleeding, which are especially dangerous at the low point in blood counts. The time of the lowest blood counts is usually 1 to 2 weeks after the chemotherapy.

Nomogram for Determination of Body Surface Area in Adults

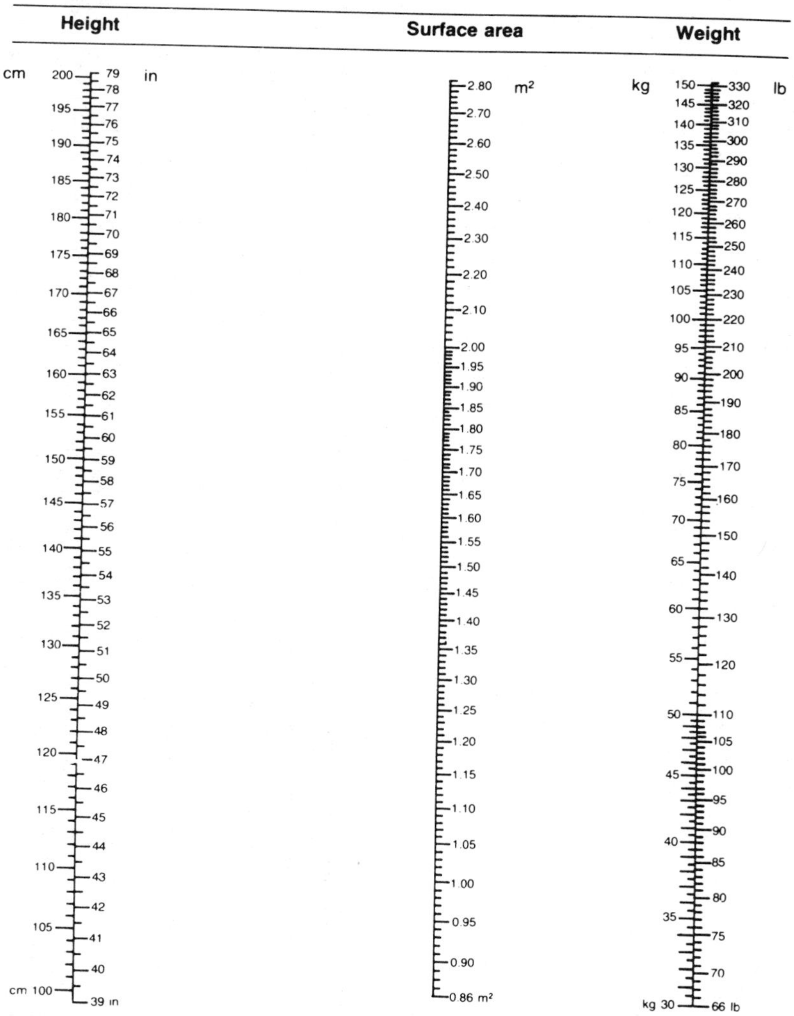

Height	Surface area	Weight

A straightedge placed so that it connects the patient's height in the left column with his weight in the right column will intersect the center column at the point indicating the patient's body surface area.

FIGURE 52-4. Nomogram for determination of body surface area in square meters (m²) for adults. (Reprinted by permission from Dorr, R.T., and Fritz, W.L. *Cancer chemotherapy handbook*, New York: Elsevier, 1980.

Nomogram for Determination of Body Surface Area in Children

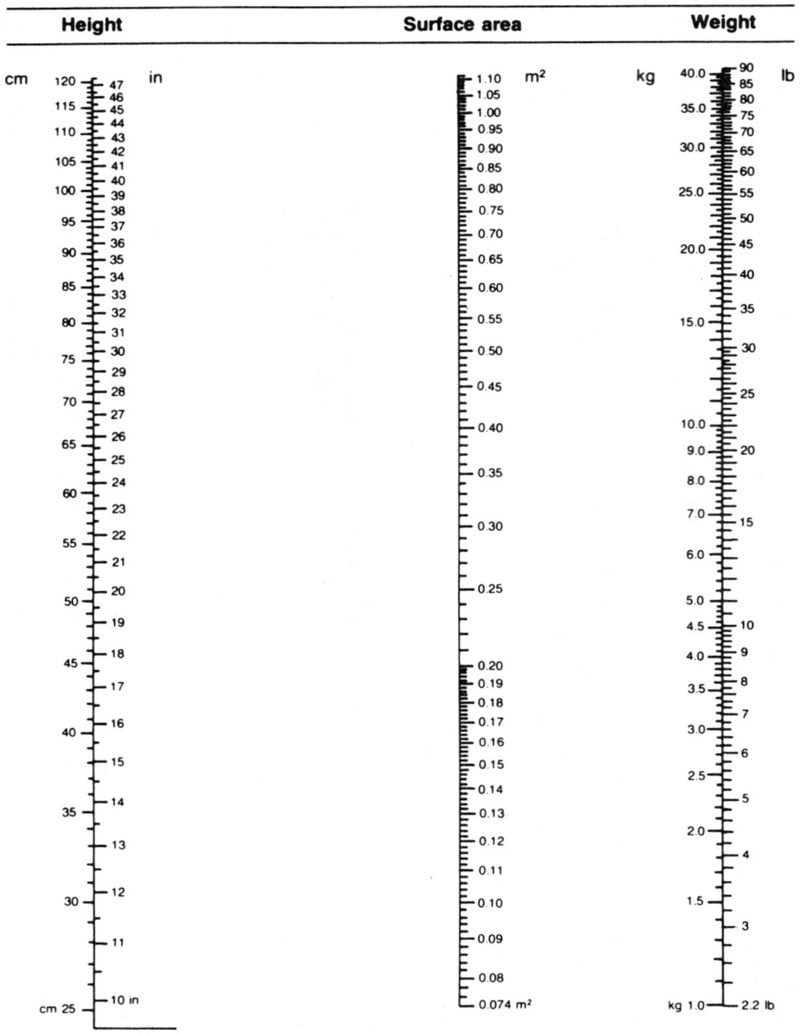

A straightedge placed so that it connects the patient's height in the left column with his weight in the right column will intersect the center column at the point indicating the patient's body surface area.

FIGURE 52-5. **Nomogram for determination of body surface area in square meters (m²) for children. (Reprinted by permission from Dorr, R.T., and Fritz, W.L.** *Cancer chemotherapy handbook,* **New York: Elsevier, 1980.)**

NURSING DRUG DIGEST

Medication (trade name*)	Indication	Usual dosage and administration†	Dosage forms, preparation, and storage	Contraindications, cautions, and comments	Monitoring
Azacitidine (investigational agent)	Acute myelogenous leukemia Chronic myelogenous leukemia	300-400 mg/m² daily IV (investigational) Prepare a new solution q.8h. during continuous infusion Administer *only* by slow continuous infusion	Injectable: 100 mg/vial Reconstitute with 20 ml of sterile water for injection, and dilute further with Ringer's lactate, for infusion at pH 6.2-6.5 to provide optimum pH and stability	Because of occasional severe liver toxicity, azacitidine should be used cautiously in patients with impaired liver function Nausea, vomiting, fever, and hypotension may be profound with rapid IV infusion	Monitor for stomatitis, rash, and hypophosphatemia
Bleomycin Blenoxane	Testicular cancer, lymphomas, Hodgkin's disease, head and neck, cervix, and skin cancers	5-15 units/m² weekly IV, IM, or SC; *or* by continuous IV infusion for 3-5 days IV is generally administered slowly over 10 min Reduce dosage in renal impairment	Injectable: 15 units/vial Reconstitute with 1-5 ml NS, D₅W, or sterile water for injection (use 5-20 ml for IV use) Reconstituted solution is stable for 24 hr at room temperature and 48 hr if refrigerated (2°-8° C)	Relatively *contraindicated* in patients with pulmonary or renal dysfunction Acute anaphylactoid reactions have been reported in 1% of patients with lymphoma; administer a test dose and observe for 2 hr in lymphoma patients Lung toxicity (e.g., pneumonitis, fibrosis) may occur, especially after total cumulative doses of 300 units Fever is a common side effect, occurring a few hours after the injection Fever and chills usually respond to acetaminophen Patients should be instructed to take antipyretics such as acetaminophen if fever occurs Not toxic to bone marrow	Observe for hypersensitivity (wheezing, low blood pressure) with first doses Observe for evidence of pneumonitis (e.g., dyspnea, rales) Monitor for cutaneous toxicities particularly in the second and third weeks of treatment

Continued.

NOTE: For additional details regarding the individual agents listed in this table see the text and other tables in this chapter.
*Indicates a multiple active ingredient product. For a complete listing of all active ingredients see the *Drug Reference Guide to Brand Names and Active Ingredients.*
†The dosages of the anticancer agents apply generally for both adults and children. Doses are usually calculated according to body surface area, m², which may be determined from the nomograms in Figures 52-4 (adults) and 52-5 (children). The doses listed are the ranges used in various protocols, but must be individualized according to the patients' blood counts and hepatic and renal function. Experimental protocols may employ doses and schedules of drug administration that differ from those listed in this table.
★Indicates that the drug is generally available only in the United States.

NURSING DRUG DIGEST—cont'd

Medication (trade name)	Indication	Usual dosage and administration	Dosage forms, preparation, and storage	Contraindications, cautions, and comments	Monitoring
Bleomycin—cont'd				Cutaneous toxicity, including hyperpigmentation and ulceration, may be severe and may require the cessation of bleomycin	
Cytarabine Cytosar Cytosar-U	Acute myelocytic leukemia	100 mg/m² IV or SC twice daily for 5-7 days, or by continuous IV infusion for 5-7 days 25-50 mg/m² intrathecally weekly for meningeal leukemia Rapid IV administration may cause projectile vomiting	Injectable: 100, 500 mg/vial (store refrigerated) Reconstitute with bacteriostatic water for injection (5 or 10 ml for 100 mg and 500 mg vials, respectively) Reconstituted solution is stable for 48 hr at 15°-30° C Discard cloudy solutions For intrathecal use, reconstitute with Elliot's B solution	Relatively *contraindicated* in patients with bone marrow suppression Use with caution in hepatic dysfunction Nausea, diarrhea, and tomatitis are common Solution is *not* compatible with fluorouracil or methotrexate May cause photosensitivity Flulike syndrome (cytarabine syndrome) with anorexia, fever, headache, and malaise is common Bone marrow suppression is major toxicity	Observe for mouth ulcerations Observe IV site during continuous infusions for signs of infection Monitor fluid intake and output Monitor for anemia, leukopenia, and thrombocytopenia
Dactinomycin Cosmegen	Testicular cancer, sarcomas, melanoma, choriocarcinoma, and Wilms' tumor	0.3-0.5 mg/m²/24 hr IV for 5 days; *or* 1-2 mg/m² IV over a period of 1 week and repeated, if warranted, after 3 weeks Avoid extravasation Avoid infusion through cellulose IV filters For IV administration *only*	Injectable: 0.5 mg/vial Reconstitute with 1.1 ml sterile water for injection (without preservatives) Reconstituted solution may be added to infusions of D₅W or NS	*Contraindicated* in chickenpox and herpes zoster infections (because of generalized, potentially life-threatening disease that may result) Potent vesicant; avoid contact with skin Binds to cellulose filters Alopecia occurs commonly, as well as leukopenia and thrombocytopenia May cause acneiform rash, stomatitis, or anorexia Severe radiation recall reactions in skin can occur	Monitor blood cell counts Observe for cutaneous toxicity (e.g., alopecia, skin eruption) Monitor injection sites for any signs of infiltration and resultant tissue necrosis

Drug	Uses	Dosage/Administration	Preparation	Comments	Nursing considerations
Daunorubicin Cerubidine	Acute leukemias	30-60 mg/m²/day IV for 3 days q 3-4 weeks. Dose must be reduced in patients with liver dysfunction (up to 50%-75%). Decrease dose (as much as 50%) in renal impairment (serum creatinine greater than 3 mg/dl). Inject over 5-10 min, checking frequently for venous return. Discontinue injection if pain occurs around IV site. Special care must be taken to avoid extravasation outside of the vein during injection; if extravasation occurs, immediately infiltrate the subcutaneous tissues with 5 ml of 8.4% sodium bicarbonate and 4 mg of dexamethasone or other established agency protocol. *Do not* exceed total cumulative dose of 550 mg/m². For IV administration *only*	Injectable: 20 mg/vial. Incompatible with heparin, hydrocortisone, cephalothin, dexamethasone, or diazepam, and will form a precipitate if mixed in the same IV bottle or line. Reconstitute with 4 ml sterile water for injection. Stable for 24 hr at room temperature (48 hr under refrigeration) after reconstitution. Flush IV line with saline before and after the drug injection	Relatively *contraindicated* in the presence of known cardiac disease. Avoid contact with skin. Patient should be instructed to expect reddish urine for 1 or 2 days after treatment. Bone marrow depression occurs within 7-14 days. Potent vesicant. Cumulative cardiac toxicity, usually at *total* doses above 550 mg/m². Often causes alopecia	Observe for ankle swelling or dyspnea on exertion (cardiac toxicity). Monitor injection site for infiltration and resultant tissue necrosis
Doxorubicin Adriamycin	Breast cancer; sarcomas, lung cancer, ovarian cancer, acute leukemias, lymphomas, Hodgkin's disease, bladder cancer, testicular cancer; endometrial cancer, neuroblastoma, and Wilms' tumor	40-75 mg/m² IV every 3 weeks. Dose must be reduced in patients with liver dysfunction (up to 50%-75%). Inject over 5-10 min, checking frequently for venous return. Discontinue injection if pain occurs around IV site. Special care must be taken to avoid extravasation outside of the vein during injection; if extravasation occurs, immediately infiltrate the subcutaneous tissues with 5 ml of 8.4% sodium bicarbonate and 4 mg of dexamethasone or other established agency protocol. *Do not* exceed total cumulative dose of 550 mg/m². For IV administration *only*	Injectable: 10, 50 mg/vial. Incompatible with heparin and other basic drugs in solutions (may form a precipitate). Reconstitute with 5 ml or 25 ml of NS or sterile water for injection for the 10 and 50 mg vials, respectively. Stable for 24 hr at room temperature (48 hr under refrigeration) after reconstitution. Protect from sunlight	*Contraindicated* in severe myelosuppression. Relatively *contraindicated* in the presence of known cardiac disease. Avoid contact with skin. Flush IV line with saline before and after the drug injection. Patient should be instructed to expect reddish urine for 1 or 2 days after treatment. Bone marrow depression occurs within 7-14 days. Potent vesicant. Cumulative cardiac toxicity, usually at *total* doses above 550 mg/m². Often causes alopecia. Can cause recall reactions in irradiated skin	Observe for ankle swelling or dyspnea on exertion (cardiac toxicity). Monitor injection site for infiltration and resultant tissue necrosis

Continued.

NURSING DRUG DIGEST—cont'd

Medication (trade name)	Indication	Usual dosage and administration†	Dosage forms, preparation, and storage	Contraindications, cautions, and comments	Monitoring
★ **Floxuridine** FUDR	Colorectal and gastric cancers, usually via hepatic artery infusion for liver metastases	0.1-0.5 mg/kg/24 hr as IA infusion for 1-2 weeks For intraarterial (IA) use *only*	Injectable: 500 mg/vial Protect from light Reconstitute with 5 ml sterile water for injection Stable after reconstitution for 14 days at 2°-8° C	*Contraindicated* in severe bone marrow depression and cachexia Rapidly metabolized to fluorouracil Rarely used because it has no advantage over fluorouracil Toxicities are similar to those of fluorouracil given by the same schedule	Observe for mouth ulcerations
Fluorouracil Adrucil Efudex Fluoroplex	Colon, breast, gastric, pancreatic, ovarian, and prostatic cancers	12 mg/kg (300-600 mg/m²) daily for 4 days, followed (in the absence of toxicity) by 6 mg/kg/24 hr IV on days 6, 8, 10, and 12 Maximum: 800 mg/24 hr Flush IV line between administration of fluorouracil and other drugs Can be injected over 1-2 min Decrease dosage in patients with low blood counts or impaired hepatic function	Injectable: 500 mg/vial Protect from light Solution should not be refrigerated because precipitation may occur Dilution before injection is not necessary unless given by continuous infusion Solution: 2%, 5% Cream: 5%	*Contraindicated* in severe bone marrow depression and cachexia Stomatitis and diarrhea may occur with continuous infusion Incompatible with other drugs in solution Skin and nail hyperpigmentation may occur Topical preparations cause local inflammation, which usually progresses to ulceration, but heals following cessation of topical therapy (sometimes not until 2 months) May cause photosensitivity Patients should be warned of increased skin sensitivity to sunlight Wash hands after applying cream or solution Promote oral hygiene	Observe for mouth ulcerations
	Superficial basal cell carcinoma	Apply 5% cream or solution b.i.d to cover lesion; apply with gloved finger or applicator			

Drug	Uses	Dosage	Preparation	Considerations	Assessment
Mercaptopurine Purinethol	Acute leukemias	2.5 mg/kg/24 hr PO Administer as single daily dose between meals, to facilitate absorption Maximum: 5 mg/kg/24 hr	Tablet: 50 mg	Allopurinol inhibits mercaptopurine metabolism; this interaction is potentially fatal, and requires reduction of mercaptopurine dose to 25% of normal Liver toxicity (e.g., jaundice) may occur	Observe for and report jaundice or upper abdominal discomfort Observe for mouth ulcerations
Methotrexate Folex Mexafe	Breast cancer, choriocarcinoma, lymphomas, acute leukemia, cervix cancer, head and neck cancer, sarcomas, and lung cancer	10-40 mg/24 hr IM, IV, PO; or 12 mg/m² intrathecally NOTE: Methotrexate is administered PO, and its sodium salt (methotrexate sodium) is administered parenterally Reduce dosage in renal impairment	Injectable: 5, 20, 25, 50, 100, 250 mg/vial Tablet: 2.5 mg Reconstitute with sterile water for injection (without preservatives) May be used in high IV doses with leucovorin (citrovorum) rescue, alkalinization of urine, and maintenance of good urine output Reconstitute for intrathecal use with Elliot's B solution	*Contraindicated* in patients with renal impairment If leucovorin rescue is used with high-dose methotrexate, patients should be warned to take leucovorin q.6h. as prescribed Myelosuppression and GI side effects (mucositis, diarrhea) are common Should be avoided in pregnancy, because it is a potent teratogen and abortifacient Solution is *not* compatible with cytarabine Maintain urinary pH greater than 6.5 to prevent precipitation Prolonged administration may cause hepatic or pulmonary toxicity	Monitor renal function Monitor fluid intake and output of patients receiving high doses Check urinary pH of hospitalized patients receiving high-dose methotrexate
Mitomycin Mitocin-C Mutamycin	Colon, gastric, breast, cervix, and pancreatic cancer	10 mg/m² IV every 6-8 weeks, in combination chemotherapy 20 mg/m² IV every 6-8 weeks as a single agent Avoid extravasation For IV administration *only*	Injectable: 5, 20 mg/vial Reconstitute the 5 or 20 mg vial with 10 or 40 ml sterile water for injection, respectively Reconstituted solution is stable for 7 days at room temperature and 14 days if refrigerated	Use with caution in presence of renal impairment Potent vesicant Myelosuppression is delayed and may be prolonged for 2-4 weeks Alopecia is common Commonly causes leukopenia or thrombocytopenia Avoid contact with skin	Monitor for leukopenia or thrombocytopenia

Continued.

NURSING DRUG DIGEST—cont'd

Medication (trade name)	Indication	Usual dosage and administration†	Dosage forms, preparation, and storage	Contraindications, cautions, and comments	Monitoring
Plicamycin Mithracin	Hypercalcemia secondary to malignancy, testicular cancer (rarely used)	12.5-25 µg/kg IV every 3-7 days Avoid extravasation Dilute in 1 L of D₅W and administer over 4-6 hr For IV use *only*	Injectable: 2.5 mg/vial Store refrigerated Reconstitute with 5 ml sterile water for injection immediately before use and discard unused portion; dilute with sterile water for injection, NS, or D₅W	*Contraindicated* in severe bone marrow suppression May cause hepatic damage and blood clotting abnormalities Often causes nausea and vomiting Avoid contact with skin	Monitor serum calcium Observe for symptoms of hypocalcemia (muscle cramps, tetany)
Thioguanine Lanvis	Acute leukemias	2 mg/kg/24 hr PO Administer as single daily dose between meals Decrease dosage in patients with impaired renal or hepatic function Maximum: 3 mg/kg/24 hr	Tablet: 40 mg	Liver toxicity (e.g., jaundice) may occur Encourage increased fluid intake May cause bone marrow toxicity (anemia, leukopenia, thrombocytopenia)	Observe for and report jaundice Monitor for anemia, leukopenia, and thrombocytopenia

BIBLIOGRAPHY

Amonsen, S., & Gren, J.E. Relationship between length of time and contamination in open intravenous solutions. *Nursing Research,* 1978, *27*(5), 372-374.

Barlock, A.L., Howser, D.M., & Hubbard, S.M. Nursing management of adriamycin extravasation. *American Journal of Nursing,* 1979, *79*(1), 94-96.

Bender, R.A., Zwelling, L.A., Doroshow, J.H., Locker, G.Y., Hande, K.R., Murinson, D.S., Cohen, M., Myers, C.E., & Chabner, B.A. Antineoplastic drugs: clinical pharmacology and therapeutic use. *Drugs,* 1978, *16,* 46-77.

Bennett, J.M., & Reich, S.D. Bleomycin. *Annals of Internal Medicine,* 1979, *90,* 945-948.

Bleyer, W.A. The clinical pharmacology of methotrexate: new applications of an old drug. *Cancer,* 1981, *41,* 36-51.

Bowers, D.G., & Lynch, J.B. Adriamycin extravasation. *Plastic and Reconstructive Surgery,* 1978, *61,* 86-92.

Bubela, N. Is your client at risk for respiratory complications? *The Canadian Nurse,* 1983, *79,* 46-48.

Chemotherapy and you—a guide to self help during treatment (NIH publication No. 80-1136). U.S. Department of Health and Human Services, National Cancer Institute, Office of Cancer Communications, Building 31, Room 10A18, Bethesda, Md. 20205.

D'Arcy, P.F. Reactions and interactions in handling anticancer drugs. *Drug Intelligence and Clinical Pharmacy,* 1983, *17,* 532-538.

Dean, J.C., Salmon, S.A., & Griffith, K.S. Prevention of doxorubicin-induced hair loss with scalp hypothermia. *New England Journal of Medicine,* 1979, *301,* 1427-1429.

Donehower, R.C., Myers, C.E., & Chabner, B.A. New developments on the mechanism of action of antineoplastic drugs. *Life Sciences,* 1979, *25,* 1-14.

Dorr, R.T., & Fritz, W.L. *Cancer chemotherapy handbook.* New York: Elsevier, 1980.

Fredette, S.L. & Gloriant, F.S. Nursing diagnoses in cancer chemotherapy in theory. *American Journal of Nursing,* 1981, *81*(11), 2013-2019.

Gullo, S. Chemotherapy: What to do about special side effects. *RN,* 1977, *40*(4), 30-32.

Hagan, S.J. Bring help and hope to the patient with Hodgkin's disease. *Nursing 83,* 1983, *13,* 58-64.

Ignoffo, R.J., & Friedman, M.A. Therapy of local toxicities caused by extravasation of cancer chemotherapeutic drugs. *Cancer Treatment Review,* 1980, *7,* 17-27.

Koren, M.E., & Herrman, C.S. Cancer immunotherapy, what, why. *Nursing 81,* 1981, *11,* 34-41.

Kremer, W.B. Cytarabine. *Annals of Internal Medicine,* 1975, *82,* 684-688.

Krumm, S., Vannatta, P., & Sanders, J. Group approaches for cancer patients—a group for teaching chemotherapy. *American Journal of Nursing,* 1979, *79*(5), 916.

Levitt, D.Z. Cancer chemotherapy—those dreaded side effects and what to do about them (part 5). *RN,* 1981, *44*(2), 56-59.

Levitt, D.Z. Cancer chemotherapy—those dreaded side effects and what to do about them (part 6). *RN,* 1981, *44*(3), 69-72.

Lum, J.L., Chase, M., Cole, S.M., Johnson, A., Johnson, J.A., & Link, M.R. Nursing care of oncology patients receiving chemotherapy. *Nursing Research,* 1978, *27*(6), 340-346.

Maxwell, M.B. Scalp tourniquets for chemotherapy-induced alopecia. *American Journal of Nursing,* 1980, *80*(5), 900-903.

McHugh, M.K. Deciphering diagnostic studies: white blood cell tests. *Nursing 82,* 1982, *12*(1), 10-15.

Miller, S.A. Nursing actions in cancer chemotherapy administration. *Oncology Nursing Forum,* 1980, *7,* 8-16.

Ostchega, Y. Preventing . . . and treating . . . cancer chemotherapy's oral complications. *Nursing 80,* 1980, *10*(8), 47-52.

Pinedo, H.M. *Cancer chemotherapy.* New York: Elsevier, yearly from 1979.

Pochedly, C. Acute lymphoid leukemia in children. *American Journal of Nursing,* 1978, *78*(10), 1714-1716.

Pratt, W.B., & Ruddon, R.W. *The anticancer drugs.* New York: Oxford University Press, 1979.

Thomas, N.P., Cloak, M., Crosson, K., & Kwan, J. Preparing cancer patients to administer medication. *Patient Counseling and Health Education,* 1983, *3*(4), 137-143.

Tietze, K.J., & Linkewich, J.A. Adverse reaction reviews—drug-induced pulmonary diseases—part 1: antineoplastic drugs. *Hospital Pharmacy,* 1983, *18,* 627-631.

Von Hoff, D.D., Layard, M.W., Basa, P., Davis, H.L., Jr., Von Hoff, A.L., Rozenoweig, M., & Muggia, F.M. Risk factors for doxorubicin-induced congestive heart failure. *Annals of Internal Medicine,* 1979, *91,* 710-717.

Welch, D., & Lewis, K. Alopecia and chemotherapy. *American Journal of Nursing,* 1980, *80*(5), 903-905.

Wroblewski, S.S., & Wroblewski, S.H. Caring for the patient with chemotherapy-induced thrombocytopenia. *American Journal of Nursing,* 1981, *81*(4), 746-749.

Alkylating Agents and Miscellaneous Drugs Used to Treat Cancer

Branimir Ivan Sikic

Medications discussed in this chapter

Alkylating agents
  Nitrogen mustards and
    related derivatives
    Chlorambucil
    Cyclophosphamide
    Ifosfamide
    Mechlorethamine
    Melphalan
  Alkyl sulfonates
    Busulfan
  Nitrosoureas
    Carmustine
    Lomustine
    Semustine
    Streptozocin
  Ethyleneimines
    Thiotepa
  Triazenes
    Dacarbazine

Vinca alkaloids
  Vinblastine
  Vincristine
  Vindesine
Enzyme
  Asparaginase
Hormonal agent
  Tamoxifen
Miscellaneous agents
  Cisplatin
  Etoposide
  Hexamethylmelamine
  Hydroxyurea
  Interferons
  Mitotane
  Procarbazine
  Teniposide

ALKYLATING AGENTS

Alkylating agents comprise five subgroups of anti-cancer drugs, including alkyl sulfonates, ethyleneimines, nitrogen mustards, nitrosoureas, and triazenes. These drugs kill cells by damaging *DNA*, particularly by reacting with guanine bases to produce DNA strand breakage, cross-linking, and mispairing of bases (Figure 53-1). By definition, alkylating agents are highly *electrophilic* compounds that can therefore react with *nucleophilic* groups on molecules to form covalent bonds. Alkylating agents in general can kill dividing cells in all phases of the cell cycle and some nondividing cells. In addition to killing cancer cells and some normal cells, these drugs can produce genetic

NOTE: A general introduction to cancer chemotherapy is presented at the beginning of Chapter 52.

damage, which accounts for their *mutagenic, carcinogenic,* and *teratogenic* side effects.

Nitrogen mustards

Mechlorethamine. Mechlorethamine is the first modern anticancer drug, discovered in the 1940s to be effective in the treatment of *lymphomas*. Its major current use is in the MOPP regimen (mechlorethamine, vincristine [Oncovin], procarbazine, and prednisone) for Hodgkin's disease. Other, less reactive nitrogen mustards are now preferred for the treatment of non-Hodgkin's lymphomas, *leukemias,* and various other cancers.

Mechlorethamine is highly reactive and unstable in solution. It must therefore be injected intravenously immediately after reconstitution.

The major toxicity of mechlorethamine is *myelosuppression.* The *nadir* of *leukopenia* and *thrombocytopenia* occurs 10 to 14 days after treatment, and blood counts return to normal at 21 to 28 days. Nausea and vomiting occur 1 to 2 hours after injection and may be intense. *Alopecia, mucositis,* and diarrhea may also be produced. *Immunosuppression* may lead to activation of latent herpes-zoster infections. Chronic toxicities of mechlorethamine include amenorrhea and infertility resulting from inhibition of *oogenesis* and *spermatogenesis.*

The usual dosage in the MOPP regimen is 6 mg/m^2 on days 1 and 8 of a 28-day cycle. The drug is a potent *vesicant* and should be injected carefully into the tubing of a rapidly flowing infusion of half-normal to normal saline. Gloves, as specified by agency guidelines, should be used when reconstituting and handling mechlorethamine. If *extravasation* occurs, the subcutaneous tissues should be infiltrated immediately with 4% sodium thiosulfate. This solution should be available in the *chemotherapy* clinic and may be prepared

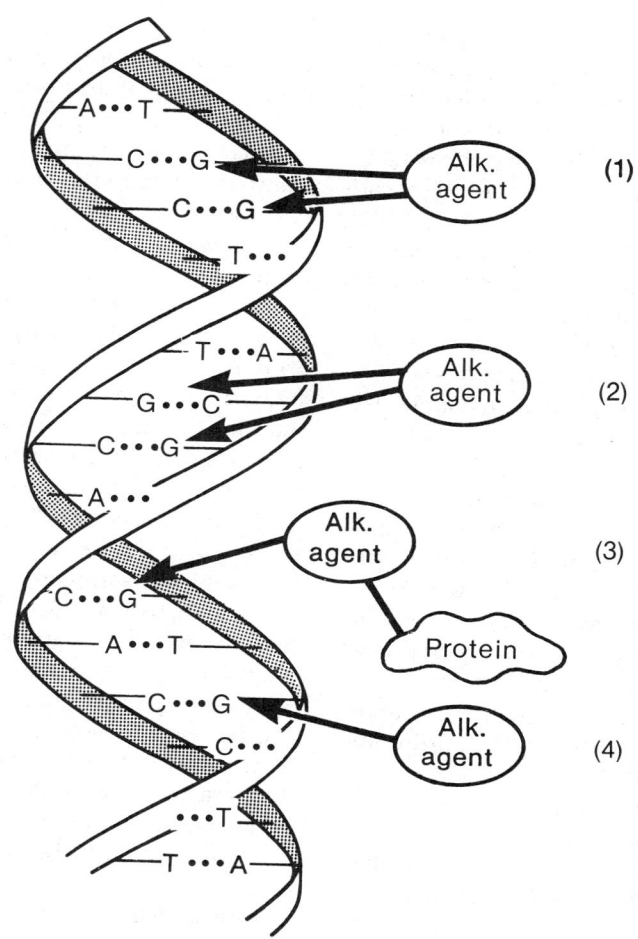

FIGURE 53-1. **Schematic diagram of potential reactions and mechanisms of action of alkylating agents. The electrophilic groups of alkylating agents bond covalently with nucleophiles (oxygen, sulfur, nitrogen, phosphorus) on DNA and proteins within cells. Most alkylating agents are bifunctional (can react at two sites on the drug) and thus can form cross-linkages between adjacent nucleotides on the same DNA strand (1), between the two strands of DNA** (2), **or between DNA and an adjacent protein molecule** (3). **Monofunctional agents (e.g., streptozocin) will bond at only one site** (4).

by diluting 4 ml of 10% sodium thiosulfate injection (USP) with 6 ml of sterile water.

Cyclophosphamide. Cyclophosphamide is the most extensively used nitrogen mustard. The parent drug is inactive, and is enzymatically converted to active forms (i.e., 4-hydroxy-cyclophosphamide and aldophosphamide). The drug can be administered orally, intravenously, or intramuscularly.

Cyclophosphamide is clinically useful in a wide spectrum of cancers, including lymphomas, leukemias, *sarcomas*, and carcinomas of the breast, ovary, and lung. It is also used as an immunosuppressive agent in certain noncancerous diseases, such as Wegener's granulomatosis and childhood nephrosis.

Its major toxicity is myelosuppression. Nausea is less severe than with mechlorethamine, but alopecia is more common than with the other nitrogen mustards. Cyclophosphamide has a unique tendency to cause a chemical cystitis, with symptoms of pain on urination and occasionally bloody urine. The chemical cystitis associated with the use of cyclophosphamide can usually be avoided with adequate hydration by instructing the patient to drink large quantities of fluids (2 to 3 L) for several hours after a treatment. Chronic treatment may result in fibrosis of the bladder and rarely, bladder cancer. Large doses (50 to 75 mg/kg) have produced cardiac toxicity. As with other alkylating agents, amenorrhea, infertility, teratogenesis, and carcinogenesis are potential adverse side effects.

The usual doses of cyclophosphamide are 100 mg/m² orally daily for up to several months, 250 mg orally daily for 5 days, or 500 to 1000 mg/m² intravenously. To avoid cystitis, patients should be advised to take their dose in the morning and drink at least 2 L of liquids during the day.

Melphalan. Melphalan produces less nausea and vomiting than cyclophosphamide and does *not* cause alopecia. The drug is used primarily to provide *palliation* for breast and ovarian cancers and multiple myeloma. Its mode of action and chronic toxicities are similar to the other nitrogen mustards. The usual dosage is 0.1 to 0.2 mg/kg/day taken orally for 5 days, repeated every 4 to 6 weeks.

Chlorambucil. Chlorambucil is intermediate in chemical reactivity between mechlorethamine and melphalan. Its mechanism of action and clinical use are similar to cyclophosphamide and melphalan. Myelosuppression is the major toxicity. Alopecia does *not* occur, and nausea is less severe than with cyclophosphamide. The usual dose is 0.1 to 0.2 mg/kg by mouth.

Ifosfamide. Ifosfamide is a close structural analogue of cyclophosphamide, with similar antitumor activity and toxicities. It is an investigational agent, and therefore has restricted use in the experimental treatment of lymphomas, leukemias, and breast, lung, and testicular cancers. Its toxic effects include nausea, myelosuppression, alopecia, and cystitis. Lethargy, impaired renal function, and transient liver enzyme abnormalities have also been reported.

Several intravenous doses and schedules have been used investigationally, in the range of 3 to 5 gm/m² IV every 3 weeks, either as a single bolus or in divided doses over 3 to 5 days. Maintenance of adequate oral or intravenous hydration, at least 2 L/day during treatment, is important to reduce the risk of hemorrhagic cystitis.

Alkyl sulfonates

Busulfan. Busulfan is an alkylating agent whose only significant clinical use is in the palliation of chronic myelocytic leukemia. Myelosuppression is the major toxic effect. As with several other alkylating agents, lung toxicity (i.e., pulmonary fibrosis) may occur with prolonged treatment, usually 1 to 2 years or more. Increased skin pigmentation may also result from chronic treatment with busulfan. The usual dose is 4 to 8 mg by mouth daily.

Nitrosoureas

Carmustine. The nitrosoureas also alkylate and form cross-links in DNA, although by a different chem-

ical mechanism than the nitrogen mustards. Carmustine is lipid soluble and can thus enter the brain and cerebrospinal fluid, unlike most other anticancer agents. For this reason, it is useful in patients with primary brain tumors. It is also active against lymphomas, melanoma, and lung and gastrointestinal cancers.

The major toxicity of nitrosoureas is delayed and cumulative myelosuppression, with nadirs of leukopenia and thrombocytopenia occurring 4 to 6 weeks after treatment. Severe nausea is commonly produced, so that it is advisable to pretreat patients with an antiemetic. Alopecia, mucositis, and occasional pulmonary and hepatic toxicities may occur. As with other alkylating agents, the nitrosoureas are potentially mutagenic, teratogenic, and carcinogenic.

Carmustine is first dissolved in 3 ml of ethyl alcohol, then in 27 ml of sterile water, and then further diluted for intravenous infusion. The usual dose is 200 mg/m² IV every 6 to 8 weeks. The alcohol used to initially dissolve the drug usually causes burning or pain at the injection site, which can be ameliorated by infusing the drug over 1 to 2 hours. Other techniques that can be used to reduce local pain during infusion include injection of 1% lidocaine solution into the vein (to a maximum of 3 ml), and application of cold compresses over the arm. Extravasation should be avoided, and gloves should be used when reconstituting the drug.

Lomustine. Lomustine is similar to carmustine in its spectrum of action and toxicities. It is administered orally, in doses of 130 mg/m² as a single agent or 60 to 80 mg/m² in combination with other drugs. Because of the delayed myelosuppression, treatment can usually be given only every 6 to 8 weeks.

Semustine. Semustine is a lipid-soluble nitrosourea used primarily for gastrointestinal cancers. It is still an investigational drug in the United States, supplied by the National Cancer Institute. The usual dose is 200 mg/m² taken orally every 6 to 8 weeks. Toxicities are similar to those observed for carmustine and lomustine.

Streptozocin. Unlike the lipid-soluble nitrosoureas, which are chemically synthesized, streptozocin is a water-soluble nitrosourea produced by a *Streptomyces* fungus. It is used specifically for islet cell carcinomas of the pancreas and *malignant* carcinoid *tumors*. Myelosuppression is mild, but most patients develop some renal toxicity as measured by spillage of protein and glucose into the urine, and kidney damage may be severe in 5% to 10% of cases. Almost all patients have nausea and vomiting. The usual dose is 500 mg/m² IV daily for 5 days, or 1.5 gm/m² IV weekly.

Streptozocin may also be infused via the hepatic artery at a dose of 500 mg/m² daily for 5 days, in patients whose major site of disease is liver metastases.

Ethyleneimines

Thiotepa. Thiotepa is an alkylating agent that was synthesized in the early 1950s, but is no longer widely used. It is active in breast and ovarian cancers, and is sometimes instilled directly into the urinary bladder as treatment for multiple superficial bladder tumors. Nausea and myelosuppression are the major toxicities. It is not a vesicant.

The usual dose of thiotepa is 0.2 mg/kg daily for 5 days, IV or IM, and repeated every 4 weeks. For bladder instillation, 60 mg is usually administered in 60 ml of sterile water and retained for 2 hours.

Triazenes

Dacarbazine. Dacarbazine is useful in the treatment of Hodgkin's disease, sarcomas, and melanoma. It can cause severe nausea and vomiting. Myelosuppression is usually mild. Patients may also develop symptoms similar to the flu, with muscle aching and fever after decarbazine treatment. The drug is sensitive to light and should be shielded with aluminum foil, because protection from light during long-term (24-hour) infusion or storage is necessary. Light protection is not necessary for short infusions. The drug is a vesicant, and may cause pain during infusion even without extravasation. The usual dose is 250 mg/m² IV for 5 days, or 800 to 1000 mg/m² IV as a single injection every 3 to 4 weeks. Pain along the vein during infusion may be reduced by further diluting the drug and infusing it slowly, over 4 to 6 hours.

VINCA ALKALOIDS

Vincristine and *vinblastine* are both produced by the leaves of the periwinkle plant, *Vinca rosea*. They are useful agents in acute lymphoblastic leukemia, lymphomas, and several other types of cancers. These drugs kill cells by binding to tubulin, a type of protein that forms the mitotic spindle during cell division. Cells treated with these agents characteristically are arrested in their growth during *mitosis*, or *M*-phase. Although their structure and mechanism of action are similar, there are significant differences between vincristine and vinblastine in their clinical activity and toxicity, so they are discussed separately.

Vincristine

Vincristine is important for the potentially curative combination chemotherapy of Hodgkin's disease (MOPP regimen), non-Hodgkin's lymphomas, and acute lymphoblastic leukemia. It is also used in several childhood cancers, including Wilms' tumor, Ewing's sarcoma, rhabdomyosarcoma, and neuroblastoma. In adults it is also used for cancers of the breast, lung, and cervix and sarcomas.

Vincristine is relatively less myelosuppressive than vinblastine. Both are vesicants and may produce alopecia and nausea. The major toxicity of vincristine is neurologic, with damage to nerves, resulting in numbness, tingling, decreased reflexes, and weakness. Damage to the autonomic nervous system may result in severe constipation. Patients should be advised to take bulk-forming agents and laxatives if necessary to avoid constipation. Neurologic toxicity tends to be more severe in older patients, and commonly requires discontinuation of treatment. Recovery from the neurologic symptoms is not complete even after cessation of therapy with vincristine.

The usual dose is 1.4 mg/m² IV weekly, with a maximum single dose of 2 mg. Higher maximum doses have been used in experimental protocols. The drug is a vesicant, and extravasation should be avoided.

Vinblastine

Vinblastine is especially useful in testicular carcinomas, as part of the curative PVB regimen (cisplatin or Platinol, vinblastine, and bleomycin). It is also useful in Hodgkin's disease and non-Hodgkin's lymphomas, breast cancer, and renal cell carcinoma.

Myelosuppression is the major dose-limiting toxicity of vinblastine, in contrast to vincristine. The blood count nadir occurs at 4 to 7 days after treatment, with recovery by 14 to 21 days. Neurologic toxicity is less severe than with vincristine, but muscle aching is common after high doses.

The usual dose is 0.1 to 0.2 mg/kg IV weekly, with care taken to avoid extravasation. The drug may also be administered as a continuous intravenous infusion of 1.5 to 2.0 mg/m² daily for 5 days, but this mode of administration requires a central catheter because of the risk of extravasation.

Because both vincristine and vinblastine are metabolized and excreted by the liver and biliary systems, doses should be reduced for patients with extensive liver disease or biliary obstruction. A general guideline is to reduce the dose by 50% if the patient's serum bilirubin is greater than 1.5 mg/dl.

Vindesine

Vindesine is an experimental vinca alkaloid synthesized by modifying the chemical structure of vinblastine. Initial studies have shown activity in leukemias, lymphomas and lung and breast cancers. Its major toxicities are myelosuppression and peripheral neuropathy, both of which are intermediate in severity between vinblastine and vincristine.

As with vincristine, the neuropathy may be manifested by numbness, weakness, myalgias, severe constipation, and urinary retention. Other toxicities include nausea, vomiting, diarrhea, alopecia, and phlebitis at the injection site.

Various doses and schedules are being investigated, ranging from 2 to 3 mg/m² weekly by IV bolus injection to 1.0 to 1.5 mg/m² daily for 5 days by continuous IV infusion. Extravasation should be avoided, and a central catheter used if the drug is administered by continuous infusion. Dosages should be reduced in patients with liver impairment.

ENZYMES

Asparaginase

Asparaginase is the only enzyme currently employed as an anticancer drug. It has a specific effect against acute lymphoblastic leukemia cells, which cannot themselves synthesize asparagine. The enzyme reduces the supply of this amino acid to the leukemia cells, leading to inhibition of protein synthesis and cell death. Normal cells contain asparagine synthetase and are unaffected. The treatment is therefore selectively toxic to leukemia cells, which lack asparagine synthetase. Unfortunately, asparaginase is not useful in cancers other than acute lymphoblastic leukemia.

Asparaginase is a protein purified from the bacterium *Escherichia coli,* and various allergic reactions may be produced, including hives or skin rashes in 20% of cases and potentially fatal anaphylactic reactions in 5% to 10%. One third of patients may experience mild fevers, nausea, or loss of appetite. Hepatic toxicity may occur, and especially in adults, neurologic toxicity may be manifested as drowsiness or confusion. Unlike most anticancer agents, asparaginase does not produce myelosuppression or alopecia.

Asparaginase is preferably administered IM, although IV injection is also used. Dosages range from 6000 units/m² daily IM three times weekly for 3 to 4 weeks, to 1000 units/kg daily for 10 to 14 days.

Because of the high incidence of severe allergic reactions, patients should be pretreated with antihistamines and observed for a few hours after treatment. Epinephrine and hydrocortisone should be readily available and administered if wheezing, shortness of breath, or facial swelling is observed. An IV line should be in place. The manufacturer suggests that an intradermal skin test of 2 units should be given before the first full dose and before each treatment that is spaced more than 7 days apart. Patients are observed for 45 minutes after the test dose before injection of the full dose.

HORMONAL AGENTS

Hormones and hormone antagonists are useful in the treatment of cancers of the breast, uterine endometrium, prostate, and kidney, and of lymphomas and *lymphocytic leukemias.* The pharmacology of hormones is discussed in Section XIV of this text. The advantages of hormonal therapy are lack of severe toxicity to normal tissues and occasional prolonged remissions.

One hormonal antagonist, tamoxifen, is especially useful in breast cancer treatment and is discussed here in more detail.

Tamoxifen

Tamoxifen is a synthetic antiestrogen. It binds tightly to estrogen receptor proteins within the cell and prevents normal estrogen activity. Estrogen receptors, or estrogen binding protein, can be measured in biopsies of breast cancers to predict responsiveness to hormonal treatments. The probability of a beneficial response to tamoxifen therapy is as high as 60% to 70% if estrogen receptors are present in a breast cancer and up to 10% if receptors are not detected.

There are few adverse side effects of tamoxifen, primarily hot flashes in 10% to 20% of patients and, less commonly, nausea, vaginal dryness, menstrual irregularities, headaches, and increased bone pain. Premenopausal patients receiving tamoxifen are still at risk for becoming pregnant and should be advised to take appropriate precautions. The usual dose is 10 to 20 mg taken orally twice daily.

MISCELLANEOUS AGENTS

Hydroxyurea

Hydroxyurea inhibits the enzyme ribonucleotide reductase, which is involved in DNA synthesis. The drug is therefore toxic to cells in the *S-phase* of the cell cycle. Its major clinical use is in the treatment of chronic *myelocytic leukemia.* Myelosuppression is the major toxicity. Nausea and skin rashes occur occasionally. The usual dose is 20 to 40 mg/kg daily, taken orally in divided doses, with dose reductions for patients with impaired renal function.

Procarbazine

Procarbazine was originally synthesized as a possible antipsychotic drug and was then found to inhibit some experimental cancers in animals. The drug is thought to damage DNA by producing hydroxyl and perhaps methyl-*free radicals*. Its major clinical uses are in Hodgkin's disease (the MOPP regimen), non-Hodgkin's lymphomas, and small cell lung cancer. Major side effects of procarbazine include nausea, myelosuppression, and neurologic toxicity. Patients may develop mental confusion, depression, agitation, or sedation, and commonly they report nightmares or insomnia while taking procarbazine. Nausea may be ameliorated by taking the full daily dose at bedtime, along with an antiemetic.

Drug interactions of procarbazine with tranquilizers, sedative-hypnotics, and antipsychotics that result in increased sedation, have been reported. Occasional adverse interactions with alcohol may occur as a disulfiram-like reaction characterized by headaches, flushing, and sweating. Patients should be warned *not* to drink or to consume only small amounts of alcoholic beverages during treatment. Patients should also be advised to avoid tyramine-containing foods, such as red wine and aged cheese, and sympathomimetic drugs, while taking procarbazine, since it may act as a monoamine oxidase inhibitor. Use of these agents may provoke severe hypertensive reactions (see monoamine oxidase inhibitors in Chapter 19, "Drugs Used to Treat Affective Disorders").

The usual dose of procarbazine is 100 mg/m² taken by mouth daily for 14 days, repeated every 28 days.

Mitotane

Mitotane is a derivative of the insecticide DDT (chlorophenothane), and produces necrosis of adrenal cortical cells. Its sole use is for palliation of metastatic adrenal cortical carcinoma.

Side effects of mitotane include nausea, anorexia, diarrhea, drowsiness, and skin rash. Because normal cells in the adrenal glands are also affected by the drug, patients should receive corticosteroid replacement therapy. The usual dose of mitotane is 2 to 10 gm daily taken orally, in divided doses, depending on gastrointestinal and neurologic tolerance. Dosages should be reduced in patients with liver impairment.

Hexamethylmelamine

Hexamethylmelamine is chemically similar to some alkylating agents, although its mechanism of action is not known. It is still considered an investigational agent, used in ovarian carcinomas and breast and small cell lung cancers. Its major toxicity is nausea and vomiting, but long-term use may lead to myelosuppression or peripheral neuropathy.

The usual dose is 4 to 12 mg/kg taken by mouth daily, or 100 to 200 mg/m² taken by mouth daily for 7 to 14 days.

Cisplatin

Cisplatin is an inorganic chemical derivative of platinum (cis-diamine-dichloroplatinum). Its action is similar to alkylating agents in that it produces cross-linkages in DNA. It is especially useful in testicular and ovarian carcinomas and is also active against head and neck, lung, bladder, and prostate cancers.

The major toxicities of cisplatin are nausea, vomiting, and damage to the kidneys. The renal toxicity is dose related and cumulative, but may be avoided in most cases by maintaining a high urine flow during treatment with large volumes of oral and intravenous fluids. Nausea and vomiting from cisplatin may be so severe as to require hospitalization to maintain adequate hydration and electrolyte balance.

The drug produces myelosuppression. Anemia occurs with chronic administration and may require transfusions of red blood cells. Other toxicities include hearing loss and tinnitus in 10% to 30% of patients, severe peripheral neuropathy, which appears to be dose related, and magnesium depletion, which can result in muscle cramps and weakness. Alopecia may occur at higher doses.

The usual dose of cisplatin is 40 to 100 mg/m² as an intravenous infusion lasting from 1 to 24 hours. The treatment is usually administered in the hospital. If outpatient treatment is performed, patients should be warned to drink at least 3 L of fluid on the day of treatment, and to report inability to maintain this level of fluid intake if vomiting is produced.

Etoposide and teniposide (epipodophyllotoxins)

Etoposide (VP-16) and teniposide (VM-26) are derived from extracts of the roots of the American Mandrake or May apple. These drugs inhibit DNA synthesis by cells. They are useful in the treatment of small cell lung cancers, testicular carcinomas, Hodgkin's and non-Hodgkin's lymphomas, and acute leukemias. Their clinical toxicity includes mild nausea, alopecia, myelosuppression, and allergic reactions.

The usual dose of etoposide is 50 to 150 mg/m² administered intravenously daily for 3 to 5 days, or 200 to 300 mg/m² weekly, and for teniposide, 50 mg/m² administered intravenously daily for 3 to 5 days, or 100 mg/m² weekly. The drugs are sparingly soluble, and must be reconstituted carefully in 0.9% sodium chloride. The IV infusion should last 30 to 60 minutes. The patient's blood pressure should be checked *every* 15 minutes during the infusion and immediately after the infusion to monitor for hypotension.

Interferons

Interferons are proteins produced by mammalian cells in response to viral infections. In addition to their antiviral effects, interferons have been shown to occasionally inhibit the growth of some animal and human tumors. The mechanisms for this antitumor activity are not known, but may involve both direct inhibition of cellular proliferation and enhancement of the immune system. Until recently, clinical testing was limited by the small amounts of interferons obtainable from cultures of human cells. However, genetic engineering techniques have enabled mass production of human interferons by microorganisms. Several clinical trials are currently ongoing to assess the benefits and toxicities of various types of interferons in cancer patients. Many years of investigation will be required before the significance of interferons in the treatment of various cancers is known.

OTHER INVESTIGATIONAL AGENTS

In the past decade more than 150 potential anticancer drugs have undergone clinical testing sponsored by the National Cancer Institute of the United States. Fewer than 10% of these have shown sufficient benefit in patients to warrant approval for noninvestigational, commercial use. Examples of compounds undergoing current clinical testing include AMSA, cytembena, dibromodulcitol, methyl-GAG, mitoxantrone, and pipobroman. These drugs were selected because of their anticancer effects in laboratory animals and in cultured cells. Other agents that are known to modify or augment the immune system have also undergone clinical studies in cancer patients. They include BCG (bacillus Calmette-Guérin), levamisole, and *Corynebacterium parvum.* The results of these studies

have been largely disappointing, and therefore these "immunotherapeutic" agents will not be discussed here in detail.

Clinical trials of promising new anticancer drugs are generally divided into three phases. Phase I studies are designed to establish a safe dose in patients, to define the toxicities, and to obtain initial clinical pharmacologic data. The purpose of phase II studies is to determine whether a drug is active against various types of cancers in patients. These trials are generally done with patients who have failed standard treatment, or for whom there is no effective noninvestigational therapy. Drugs that appear effective in phase II trials are then tested in phase III trials, which are controlled comparisons of new agents or combinations of drugs with other active drugs or drug combinations. Nurses involved in the care of these patients should be familiar with the investigational protocols. They may contribute valuable observations to the studies and further develop knowledge related to the nursing care of patients requiring these medications.

SUMMARY

Cancer chemotherapy has progressed substantially since the first patients were treated with these drugs in the 1940s. Cures are now possible for some types of cancer with chemotherapy alone or with the combination of chemotherapy plus surgery or radiotherapy. Many other cancers do not respond favorably to the drugs that are currently available. Effective treatment for these tumors will ideally become available as research continues on the nature of these diseases.

ADVERSE/SIDE EFFECTS OF ALKYLATING AGENTS AND MISCELLANEOUS ANTICANCER DRUGS*

Common toxicities

LOCAL VESICANT EFFECTS: PHLEBITIS

These drugs can cause severe damage to tissues if extravasation occurs during injection: carmustine, dacarbazine, mechlorethamine, vinblastine, vincristine, and vindesine

NAUSEA AND VOMITING

Usually this occurs a few hours after treatment, lasts less than 24 hours, and is partially relieved by antiemetics; the most severe nausea is produced by carmustine, cisplatin, dacarbazine, lomustine, mechlorethamine, semustine, and streptozocin

ALOPECIA

Usually begins 2 to 3 weeks after the start of chemotherapy and may be complete at 1 to 2 months; hair regrows normally almost always after completion of chemotherapy (however, it may grow back a different color or a different texture); some drugs do *not* usually produce hair loss—notably, asparaginase, chlorambucil, hormones, interferons, and melphalan

MYELOSUPPRESSION

Leukopenia and thrombocytopenia are the major dose-limiting factors for most anticancer drugs, with a nadir in blood counts 10 to 14 days after treatment; nitrosourea alkylating agents characteristically produce a delayed nadir, 4 to 6 weeks after treatment; drugs that do *not* produce myelosuppression include asparaginase, hormones, and mitotane

Occasional toxicities

ALLERGIC REACTIONS

Severe reactions (i.e., anaphylaxis) are common with asparaginase; a test dose and pretreatment with a corticosteroid and antihistamines are recommended before every treatment; anaphylaxis has been reported rarely with cisplatin, etoposide, mechlorethamine, and teniposide; hives along the vein used for injection may occur with dacarbazine

CARDIOVASCULAR SYSTEM

Congestive heart failure—high-dose cyclophosphamide and ifosfamide

CUTANEOUS SYSTEM

Hyperpigmentation—busulfan
Skin rash—procarbazine

GASTROINTESTINAL SYSTEM

Mucositis, diarrhea—mechlorethamine
Constipation—vincristine, vindesine, vinblastine

GENITOURINARY SYSTEM

Microscopic or hemorrhagic cystitis—cyclophosphamide and ifosfamide

HEPATIC SYSTEM

Elevated serum transaminases, jaundice—asparaginase

NEUROLOGIC SYSTEM

Numbness and tingling, muscle aches, weakness, constipation, and footdrop are common with vincristine and vindesine, and occasionally occur with vinblastine, cisplatin, and hexamethylmelamine
Somnolence and mental confusion may be caused by asparaginase, carmustine, lomustine, mitotane, procarbazine, and semustine

RENAL SYSTEM

Decreased renal function, manifested by azotemia (i.e., increased blood creatinine and urea concentrations)—cisplatin; proteiniura, glycosuria, azotemia—streptozocin

RESPIRATORY SYSTEM

Lung damage (fibrosis) may occur with nitrosoureas and other alkylating agents

Long-term toxicities

CARCINOGENIC EFFECTS

Increased risk of acute leukemia, especially when alkylating agents and radiation therapy are used together

INFERTILITY

Amenorrhea, azoospermia—full effects in humans for many drugs and combinations are not yet known; alkylating agents are implicated as the major cause of gonadal failure in young patients on chemotherapy

TERATOGENIC EFFECTS

Especially in the first trimester of a pregnancy; high risk for all anticancer agents

*See Chapter 11, "Drug Toxicity," for an overview of drug toxicity.

CLINICALLY SIGNIFICANT DRUG INTERACTIONS*

Primary drug	Interacting drug	Possible effect(s)	Probable mechanism(s)
Cisplatin	Aminoglycosides	Increased renal toxicity	Additive effect
Cyclophosphamide	Succinylcholine	Increased succinylcholine effect, respiratory depression	Decreased plasma cholinesterase activity
Procarbazine	Alcohol	Flushing, sweating, hypotension, nausea	Disulfiram-like reaction

*See Chapter 10, "Drug Interactions," for an overview of drug interactions.

GENERAL NURSING IMPLICATIONS

Nursing of patients requiring alkylating agents and miscellaneous drugs used in the treatment of cancer

ASSESSMENT

The alkylating agents and miscellaneous anticancer drugs are used to treat various types of cancers. Some of these drugs, (e.g., nitrogen mustards) can also be used in the treatment of such conditions as childhood nephrosis. It is important that the nurse understand the reason for drug selection and reinforce this with the patient to prevent undue anxiety or fear often associated with the diagnosis of cancer.

A complete nursing assessment is important in planning individualized nursing care for patients requiring these medications. Baseline data should include a general assessment of overall health, with special attention to the indication for drug therapy, nutritional status, oral assessment and elimination patterns. Renal and hepatic function should be noted and a neurologic assessment completed. Audiometric testing should be completed before the initiation of chemotherapy with agents known to be ototoxic (e.g., cisplatin).

When alkylating or miscellaneous anticancer drugs are required for the treatment of cancer, the identification of family and other support systems and the effects the patient's treatment and condition may have on home or employment responsibilities should be included in the nursing assessment.

The patient's knowledge of and response to the diagnosis of cancer and his or her readiness for learning and understanding of the treatment regimen should receive careful attention. Nursing care and patient teaching must be carefully individualized to the patient's and family's coping abilities. Newly diagnosed patients require much support and assistance in relation to the acceptance of their condition and treatment plan. Nursing care often requires alteration and adaptation to the patient's changing needs.

Patients often need assistance and support with specimen collection, including blood, urine, or cerebrospinal fluid. If treatment is palliative, attention should be given to the documentation of symptoms. Isolation measures should be implemented if the patient is, or is likely to become, immunosuppressed.

Baseline data should include a detailed drug history, including the identification of possible sensitivity, contraindications, cautions, and drug interactions. The patient's self-medication abilities and drug-taking patterns should be identified. It is important to ascertain if the patient has received previous chemotherapy. The type and extent of such therapy should be recorded.

SENSITIVITY

Generally, allergic reactions to the alkylating agents and miscellaneous drugs used in the treatment of cancer are rare. However, any drug has the potential to cause a hypersensitivity reaction in a susceptible individual. Allergic reactions, including the appearance of chills, fever, hives, or skin rash, occur in approximately 20% of patients receiving asparaginase (E. coli strain). Potentially fatal anaphylactic reactions occur in approximately 5% to 10% of the patients receiving this medication. It is recommended that an intradermal skin test be completed before the administration of a full dose of this medication before the initial administration of this drug and when a week or more has elapsed between doses. Vital signs and patient monitoring should be carefully completed after administration of the test dose. Antihistamines, epinephrine, hydrocortisone, and resuscitation equipment should be readily available, and an IV should be in place. Patients should be continuously monitored for a few hours after a full dose for wheezing, shortness of breath, facial swelling, or other untoward signs because of the high incidence of allergic reactions associated with this medication (see the Nursing Drug Digest and the body of this chapter for information regarding sensitivity related to specific agents).

CONTRAINDICATIONS

The use of alkylating agents and miscellaneous drugs used in the treatment of cancer are contraindicated in patients with a known hypersensitivity to a particular agent (see the Nursing Drug Digest for information regarding each individual agent).

CAUTIONS

The alkylating agents and miscellaneous anticancer drugs are associated with teratogenic, mutagenic, and carcinogenic effects. These drugs should be used with caution in pregnancy especially during the first trimester be-

GENERAL NURSING IMPLICATIONS—cont'd

Nursing of patients requiring alkylating agents and miscellaneous drugs used in the treatment of cancer—cont'd

CAUTIONS—cont'd

cause of their association with teratogenesis. Increased risk of acute leukemia has been reported with the use of alkylating agents and concurrent radiation therapy (see the Nursing Drug Digest for specific cautions associated with each agent).

DRUG INTERACTIONS

The alkylating agents and miscellaneous anticancer drugs can interact with other medications. For example, procarbazine can interact with tranquilizers, sedative-hypnotics, and antipsychotics resulting in increased sedation. Disulfiram-like reactions have been reported with headache, flushing, and sweating when this drug has been taken with alcohol. Because it may act as an MAOI, procarbazine can cause severe hypertension when tyramine containing foods are taken concurrently (e.g., aged cheese, Chianti wine) (see Clinically Significant Drug Interactions for interactions associated with these medications).

ADMINISTRATION

Alkylating agents and miscellaneous anticancer drugs are available in various dosage forms for oral, intramuscular, intravenous and topical administration. For example, chlorambucil, melphalan, procarbazine, and tamoxifen are administered orally, whereas others (e.g., cyclophosphamide) are administered in oral, intramuscular, or intravenous forms. In addition to intramuscular or intravenous administration, thiotepa can be prepared for bladder instillation. Streptozocin, although usually administered intravenously, can be infused via the hepatic artery to treat liver metastasis. Dosage and administration is highly individualized and various specific medication regimens or protocols have been developed. Mechlorethamine is administered days 1 and 8 of a 28-day cycle because of its extended myelosuppressive effects. It also must be administered readily after reconstitution because it is highly unstable in solution and as with many other anticancer agents must be administered carefully because of its vesicant effects. Carmus-

tine must be dissolved in alcohol and then sterile water and further diluted for intravenous infusion, and dacarbazine must be protected from light when infusion is prolonged. Etoposide requires constant blood-pressure measurement because of its hypotensive effects during and immediately after administration (see the Nursing Drug Digest and the body of this chapter for information regarding the preparation and administration of these medications).

It is important to note that many of these drugs are *not* usually administered by nurses because of their relative toxicity. Some drugs may be administered by nurses when given by one route (e.g., oral, intravenous infusion) and not another (e.g., intrathecal). Oncology nurse specialists are administering anticancer drugs that have been previously only administered by physicians with a specialty in oncology medicine. It is the responsibility of the professional nurse to observe the limits of practice in relation to the administration of these drugs. The nurse should also be alert to the changing roles of practice. The nurse should assist the patient as well as the person administering the medication as indicated. Thus, an understanding of the administration of these drugs is important if the nurse is to prepare and support patients who require chemotherapy and to monitor adverse effects directly related to anticancer drug administration (e.g., extravasation with intravenous administration).

It should be noted that many of these drugs have a direct irritant effect on the skin, eyes, and mucous membranes and should be handled carefully and with special precautions. Not only have these drugs been associated with local irritation and allergic reactions, but they have also been associated with mutagenic and carcinogenic effects. Research has shown that nurses handling these drugs have excreted various amounts of drug in their urine. It is especially important in oncology units where nurses are commonly involved with the care, preparation, and administration of anticancer drugs that these

effects be kept in mind and hospital guidelines or protocols be carefully developed and followed.

Practitioner drug interactions, or adverse effects associated with handling these medications, have been reported, including nausea, lightheadedness, dizziness, headache, facial flushing, and nasal sores.

Contact with skin through environmental contamination following spillage should be avoided. It is important to note that contact can occur by means other than direct skin contact with liquid preparations. Inadvertent contact can occur through inhalation of aerosolized drug when the needle is withdrawn from the vial, when ampules are opened, when air is expelled from the syringe, or when needles or syringes are clipped. Although masks, gloves, and eye protection (glasses or goggles) have been recommended, the use of these is controversial. Research has found that for such drugs as the nitrogen mustards, only polyvinylchloride gloves are effective in protecting against penetration. Rubber gloves or polyethylene gloves do *not* provide this protection.

Because of these effects, it is recommended that pharmacists prepare anticancer drugs using appropriate technique and vertical laminar air-flow hoods. All health care team members involved in the use of these drugs should work together to formulate guidelines to ensure practitioner safety in the preparation and administration of these medications.

In general, before alkylating agents or miscellaneous anticancer drugs are administered, the following should be completed:

1. Become familiar with the package insert for preparation and administration, dose range, and side effects of each drug. Double-check the dose of each drug. Check appropriate laboratory test results before administering drugs (blood counts and kidney and liver function).
2. Discuss the treatment with the patient. If the patient has had a pre-

Continued.

GENERAL NURSING IMPLICATIONS—cont'd

Nursing of patients requiring alkylating agents and miscellaneous drugs used in the treatment of cancer—cont'd

ADMINISTRATION—cont'd

vious cycle of the same treatment, ask about and report unusual or severe side effects.

3. Patients on protocol treatments should have signed an informed consent before the first treatment.
4. If nausea has been a severe problem with previous cycles, pretreatment with antiemetics should be considered.

Special care should be taken to avoid intravenous extravasation of the following drugs because of their vesicant effects: carmustine, dacarbazine, etoposide, mechlorethamine, streptozocin, vinblastine, vincristine, and vindesine. These drugs are generally administered as an IV infusion over 30 to 60 minutes, except for the vinca alkaloids, which may be injected as an IV bolus. The following precautions should be observed:

1. A 23-gauge "butterfly" or scalp vein needle should be used for IV infusions. Large syringes filled with 0.9% sodium chloride for injection or 5% dextrose should be available to check venous patency and to flush the vein after drug infusion; 25-gauge needles should not be used because of their tendency to become occluded.
2. The preferred sites of injection are the easily visible veins of the forearm. If these are not available, veins on the back of the hand may be used, or even less preferable, the antecubital fossa. Damage to nerves and tendons may be especially severe if extravasation occurs in these latter areas; therefore, these sites should be used only when no other venous access is available. They are generally *not* recommended.
3. The needle should be lightly taped, with the skin puncture site and vein visible for any sign of extravasation.
4. The patency of the vein should be tested before treatment by injection of 10 to 20 ml of 0.9% sodium chloride. The rate of injection should be smooth and gentle to avoid rupturing the vein. Flushing

of the vein with 10 to 20 ml 0.9% sodium chloride should be done after each drug injection or infusion.

5. If pain occurs during administration of these drugs or if extravasation is suspected for any other reason, the injection should be immediately discontinued and the patency of the vein evaluated. The physician, if not present, should be notified immediately of any possible extravasation of vesicant drugs. Because it maintains a direct route to the affected area, the needle or catheter should not be removed. Generally, as much of the infiltrate as possible should be aspirated and up to 50 ml of 0.9% normal saline infused to dilute any remaining infiltrated drug. Appropriate antidotes (i.e., sodium thiosulfate for carmustine and mechlorethamine) should be infiltrated at the site, and ice packs or cold compresses applied for 24 hours. These can be followed by warm compresses. The affected extremity should be elevated. The nurse and the patient should watch for and report any redness or erythema, blistering, or ulceration of the skin. If pain and erythema persist for longer than 1 week after a suspected extravasation, deeper tissue damage may be present. The patient should be referred to a plastic surgeon for consultation regarding debridement or skin grafting. In some cases, hydrocortisone may be infused into the area or intradermal and subcutaneous injection of corticosteroid may be injected into the area with a 25-gauge needle immediately after the extravasation to help reduce pain, edema, inflammation, and sequelae. Oncology nurse specialists have found that standing orders for the immediate treatment of extravasation can prevent or minimize patient pain and sequelae, especially with such drugs as doxorubicin (see Chapter 52, "Antimetabolites and Antineoplastic Antibiotics").

6. Hold drug ampules away from the face when opening them. If these drugs come in contact with the skin or eyes, the affected areas should be thoroughly washed with water. Leftover drugs should be flushed down a drain with ample rinsing or disposed of carefully. Drug disposal is controversial. At this time there is *no* standard recommended procedure for discarding anticancer drugs.

MONITORING PATIENT RESPONSE
Therapeutic response

The monitoring of therapeutic response can vary with the type of cancer and treatment regimen and may include a change in tumor size, blood test results, radiographic studies, improved organ function, an increased sense of well-being, and ability to resume or maintain activities of daily living. Remission requires specific monitoring as indicated by the patient's individual condition. Patients who have received therapy for the treatment of cancer are monitored for the absence of relapse or metastasis.

Patients requiring alkylating agents and miscellaneous drugs used in the treatment of cancer for other reasons (e.g., nephrosis) should be monitored for improvement related to the indication for the use of the drug (e.g., decrease in edema and proteinuria or other signs indicative of improvement in nephrosis).

Adverse side effects

The major adverse effects associated with the use of alkylating agents and miscellaneous anticancer drugs are related to their toxic effects on the bone marrow, gastrointestinal mucosa, and integument, which have cells with a relatively rapid turnover rate, making them more prone to the toxic effects of these medications. Effects on bone marrow result in leukopenia and thrombocytopenia. Effects on gastrointestinal mucosa can cause mucositis, nausea, vomiting, and diarrhea. Effects on the integument can result in various skin lesions and alopecia. Although, these are major effects associated with

GENERAL NURSING IMPLICATIONS—cont'd

Nursing of patients requiring alkylating agents and miscellaneous drugs used in the treatment of cancer—cont'd

Adverse side effects—cont'd

the use of these medications, others can occur (see Adverse/Side Effects of Alkylating Agents and Miscellaneous Anticancer Drugs for an outline of adverse effects associated with the use of these medications). Monitoring is essential, as is planning for the minimization of these effects because some can be life threatening and psychologically distressing.

Effects on bone marrow

Myelosuppression is a major adverse effect associated with many of the alkylating agents and miscellaneous anticancer drugs, including mechlorethamine, cyclophosphamide, chlorambucil, and hydroxyurea. This effect can be delayed and cumulative with carmustine. It can occur 4 to 6 weeks after treatment with nitrosoureas. Nadir occurs earlier with vinblastine, usually 4 to 7 days after treatment with recovery in 14 to 21 days. It is particularly important for the nurse to be aware of times for nadir to be expected so that a plan for minimizing this effect and for preventing complications may be implemented.

Thrombocytopenia. Patients should be monitored for signs of bleeding, and *platelet* counts should be monitored routinely when patients are receiving chemotherapy with these medications.

Depending on the individual agent platelet counts begin to fall 4 to 14 days after chemotherapy begins. Platelet counts are usually at their lowest between 7 and 14 days after therapy is started.

Serious bleeding can occur when platelet counts are 20,000 or less, whereas moderate bleeding can occur when platelet counts are 20,000 to 50,000. Bleeding is relatively low when platelet counts are 50,000 to 100,000.

Monitor patients for bruising, petechiae, especially involving the lower extremities, bleeding from the gums, epistaxis, cloudy or red urine, black tarry or bloody stools, unusual vaginal bleeding, hemoptysis, hematemesis, and drowsiness or decreased level of consciousness.

The urine, stool, sputum, or nasal secretions should be monitored regularly for occult blood as indicated.

Anemia can result in patients where bleeding is a problem or as a direct effect of chemotherapy on the production of erythrocytes. Monitor patients for fatigue, pallor, pale conjunctiva, dizziness, dyspnea on exertion, tachycardia, tinnitus, and angina.

Laboratory red blood cell counts, hemoglobin, and hematocrit should be monitored closely. Intramuscular injections should be avoided, as should rectal temperature readings and the use of rectal suppositories when platelet counts are low or when bleeding is a problem. Blood pressure measurement should also be avoided if the platelet count is low (less than 20,000). Blood pressure should be taken only as required. Intravenous infusion sites should be monitored for oozing of blood, and surgical wounds should likewise be monitored if present. If intramuscular injections must be given, pressure should be applied for 5 to 10 minutes at the injection site after the injection is given and the site monitored for hematoma. Laboratory slips should be labeled with "bleeding precautions," and pressure should be applied to sites for 5 to 10 minutes after blood is drawn. Scheduling is important so that as few blood specimens as possible be drawn for various tests. It is important to avoid medications known to interfere with platelet function, including anticoagulants and aspirin.

Leukopenia. The lowering of white blood cell counts (less than 4000/mm³) usually is maximal 10 to 14 days after treatment is started. It is important to monitor patients during this time for early signs of infection and to implement protective isolation measures as indicated because it is during the nadir that patients are at greatest risk for infection related to this adverse effect.

Protective isolation should be implemented to prevent exposure of the patient to infections, including colds, draining wounds, chicken pox, herpes zoster, measles, and other infections.

Meticulous hygiene care and careful handwashing are important in preventing infection.

Monitor patients for red or warm skin, fever, cough, lung congestion, mouth ulcers, open lesions, painful teeth, sore throat, pain on urination, draining wounds or other discharge, discomfort or tenderness, or other untoward symptoms that may develop during the few days that white blood cell counts are low. The temperature should be carefully monitored and the use of aspirin or acetaminophen should be avoided because these drugs can mask the presence of fever. Chest radiographs and specimen cultures (e.g., blood, urine, stool, sputum) should be completed as indicated. Strict aseptic technique is required with all laboratory work and parenteral infusions. Infections may require immediate treatment with antibiotics or transfusion with granulocytes. Outpatients may require hospitalization, if leukopenia is severe.

Recovery of white blood cell counts usually occurs in 21 to 28 days.

Gastrointestinal effects

Patients should be monitored carefully for toxic drug effects on the mucosal lining of the gastrointestinal system that result in mucositis, anorexia, nausea, vomiting, taste distortion, or diarrhea. These effects can cause alteration in nutritional status and fluid and electrolyte balance. Routine monitoring of serum electrolytes, intake and output, and daily weights may be indicated.

Mucositis. An inflammatory response involving the oral mucosa occurs about 7 days after the start of chemotherapy, often correlating with the lowest white blood cell counts. About 2 or 3 days before the lowest point, the oral mucosa is at its worst. This occurs sooner in children than adults because the oral mucosa has a higher mitotic index.

The nursing history should include a careful oral assessment of patients admitted for a first or repeat course of chemotherapy. The presence of gingivitis, impacted wisdom teeth, dentures, or other dental prostheses requires

Continued.

GENERAL NURSING IMPLICATIONS—cont'd

Nursing of patients requiring alkylating agents and miscellaneous drugs used in the treatment of cancer—cont'd

Gastrointestinal effects—cont'd

careful identification; so does a history of oral problems with previous chemotherapy. Because major dental work should not be completed while patients are on chemotherapy, this should be taken care of whenever possible before chemotherapy is started. An assessment of the patient's usual oral care habits should also be recorded. This information is particularly important in monitoring changes and planning effective oral care measures.

The first signs of oral involvement can appear within 2 to 3 days, a condition that begins to reverse gradually and resolves in about 10 days in children or a little later in adults. During this time, assess the mouth at regular intervals, at least twice daily. Inspect lips, tongue, hard and soft palates, tonsillar fossa, gingiva, and oral structures for moisture, color, texture, and the presence of inflammation, infection, bleeding, or debris. Bleeding may be intermittent or oozing. The presence of thrombocytopenia and leukopenia make the mouth susceptible to bleeding and infection in addition to the direct effects of chemotherapy on the oral mucosa epithelial cells. Bleeding can be severe even with minor trauma when platelet counts are less than 20,000 mm^3, and gram-negative opportunistic bacterial and fungal infections often occur during periods of leukopenia. These changes require that oral care be adapted to the individual patient's requirements during chemotherapy.

Oral care should be completed twice a day with a soft toothbrush, and flossing should be conducted carefully. Dentures, orthodontic retainers, and bands should be entirely eliminated or removed when possible for at least 8 hours daily. It is important to follow blood counts and platelet counts to anticipate oral problems so that oral care measures can be adapted to possible effects of thrombocytopenia or leukopenia. Mouth lesions should be cultured to detect infection. Flossing should not be done when the platelet counts drop to less than 20,000, and brushing with a soft toothbrush should be discontinued. The mouth should be gently cleaned with gauze pads soaked in a water and hydrogen peroxide solution (1 part of hydrogen peroxide to 5 to 6 parts water) or in a prescribed antibacterial or antifungal solution.

Various antifungal and antibacterial mouthwashes have been used and can be prescribed, as can topical anesthetics (lidocaine viscous), when mucositis is severe.

Nystatin ice cups (made with black cherry concentrate, sterile water, and nystatin powder, frozen and eaten with a spoon), or other mouthwashes can be used. Acetaminophen with codeine elixir can be swished and swallowed for both local and systemic effects.

Lemon glycerine swabs should not be used for oral care because the lemon can decalcify the teeth, and the glycerine can absorb water and further dry and irritate the oral mucosa.

Oral rinses may be indicated 3 to 4 times daily or every 2 hours as indicated, or oral irrigation may be required if mucositis is severe. Suction equipment should be readily available.

The mouth can be rinsed with a solution containing equal parts of cetylpyridinium (e.g., Cepacol) mouthwash, hydrogen peroxide, and water. If this is irritating, a solution of 5 ml sodium bicarbonate in 500 ml normal saline has been recommended.

Oral lesions can be painful and often prevent the patient from eating or drinking adequately. Analgesics to relieve oral discomfort are best taken 30 to 60 minutes before meals as prescribed. Bland soft diets with low sugar are usually tolerated well during periods of mucositis. Liquids should be nonacidic. Liquids or semiliquids, such as fruit ades, carbonated beverages, ices (e.g., popsicles), and gelatin desserts, should be recommended. Apple and grape juices can aggravate oral lesions, and rough foods or foods with citric acid can cause ulcers to burn. The temperature of food should also be carefully monitored to prevent burns. For some patients, nasogastric feedings or total parenteral nutrition may be indicated.

Monitor for the recovery of oral lesions in 5 to 10 days.

It is important to note that colostomy or ileostomy stomas can also be affected by drug effects on the gastrointestinal mucosa. Stomas should be monitored carefully for irritation and tissue breakdown. Meticulous stoma care is indicated.

Nausea and vomiting. Nausea and vomiting are associated with many of the alkylating agents and miscellaneous anticancer drugs. They can occur 2 hours after mechlorethamine is administered and may be intense. Severe nausea and vomiting may require hospitalization for the correction and maintenance of fluid and electrolyte balance with cisplatin. Nausea can be severe with carmustine and dacarbazine; however, it may be less severe with cyclophosphamide. Patient response may also be individual. Monitor patients for nausea and vomiting, especially as associated with their individual chemotherapy. A dietary assessment should be completed to identify and eliminate foods that cause nausea and vomiting. Antiemetics may be indicated just before chemotherapy or even beginning 24 hours beforehand.

When nausea occurs, it is often helpful to administer medications, just before bedtime if possible, to prevent this adverse effect. For example, the full daily dose of procarbazine can be taken at bedtime to decrease nausea. To prevent vomiting, offer cold compresses to the forehead, encourage patients to avoid sudden movement, and keep the emesis basin nearby and empty. It is particularly important to control odors and provide privacy and oral hygiene. Avoid exposure of the patient to disagreeable sights, sounds, and odors. Room deodorizers, soft music, and other diversions may be helpful. Change patient positions slowly to minimize stimulation of the vestibular process. Discourage oral intake if necessary and plan to meet nutritional and fluid requirements through other means as indicated.

It is important to monitor patients for psychologic nausea and vomiting as-

GENERAL NURSING IMPLICATIONS—cont'd

Nursing of patients requiring alkylating agents and miscellaneous drugs used in the treatment of cancer—cont'd

Gastrointestinal effects—cont'd

sociated with chemotherapy treatment before treatment or a visit to the oncologist's office.

Monitor intake and output, amount and character of emesis, daily weight, hydrational and nutritional status, fluid and electrolyte balance, and factors associated with nausea and vomiting.

Diarrhea or constipation. Monitor patients for changes in elimination patterns associated with the use of chemotherapy. Monitor frequency, color, consistency, and amount of stool. It is important to note that vincristine can affect the autonomic nervous system resulting in constipation, and this is an early sign of neurotoxicity associated with this drug. It should be kept in mind as well that constipation may be related to immobility or the use of medications such as codeine. The anal area should be assessed for irritation, and sitz baths and ointments for the anal area (in addition to hygienic measures) may be indicated when diarrhea occurs as an adverse effect of anticancer drugs. Constipation may require stool softeners, bulk-forming laxatives, enemas, and dietary and activity assessment and adjustment.

Integument effects

A variety of effects can occur in the integumentary system as a direct result of chemotherapy on the rapid turnover rate of the epithelial cells. These effects include changes in skin pigmentation, nail discoloration, alopecia, dandruff, and psoriasis. Patients should be made aware of these effects and be reassured that they will disappear with discontinuation of therapy. Local tissue irritation and severe necrosis can occur from extravasation of medication into the tissues during intravenous administration, and this requires careful monitoring. Maintaining adequate venous access for intravenous infusion may be a major problem with some patients. Allergic reactions and irritation can occur with direct contact with many of these drugs (see section on administration).

Monitor the integumentary system for these effects, which can be painful and

sometimes require medical treatment. The skin should be assessed frequently throughout the day. The skin should be kept clean and dryness prevented. Positioning to prevent skin breakdown every 1 to 2 hours is indicated, especially when patients are immobile or debilitated. Excessive sunlight should be avoided. Tepid baths, emollient lotions, ointments and creams (e.g., nivea cream, A&D ointment), and topical anesthetics may be indicated. Antihistamines may be required to relieve pruritus.

The adverse effects associated with the integument can cause body image concerns, and attention to this is important. Encourage verbalization and reassure patients that the effects are temporary. One of the main adverse effects of chemotherapy that can cause distress is alopecia.

Alopecia. Hair loss can be emotionally distressing for many patients, and they should be forewarned of this adverse effect and assisted with the anticipation of loss of hair and its effect on body image.

Monitor patients for small amounts of hair loss to complete baldness, which occurs a few weeks after chemotherapy is started. Hair loss can involve body and pubic hair in addition to scalp hair. Although this effect can occur with most anticancer drugs, it occurs especially with mechlorethamine, vincristine, and cyclophosphamide. Various techniques have been used in an attempt to prevent this effect, including scalp tourniquets, scalp sphygmomanometers, and ice turbans. These have been generally unsuccessful in preventing hair loss and should probably not be used in certain cancers (leukemias, lymphomas) in which cancer cells may be circulating through the blood vessels of the scalp.

It is important to monitor for regrowth of hair a few weeks after the drug is discontinued, although hair color or texture may be different. It is important to monitor patient response to loss of hair as well as to changes in color or texture.

Certain drugs (e.g., melphalan, asparaginase, low-dose cisplatin, and chlorambucil) do *not* cause alopecia. The patient should be informed of this to prevent undue worry or concern related to this effect.

Miscellaneous effects

Pulmonary complications. Most of the alkylating agents are known occasionally to produce pulmonary toxicity. Monitoring for pulmonary effects is important. Busulfan is associated with pulmonary fibrosis with prolonged treatment from 1 to 2 years. Carmustine is also associated with pulmonary fibrosis. Chlorambucil has been implicated in causing alveolitis, interstitial fibrosis, and other effects. Melphalan can also produce respiratory insufficiency.

A baseline assessment of respiratory function (including rate and depth of respirations, use of accessory muscles, the inspiratory to expiratory ratio, and the quality of breath sounds) should have been completed during the initial nursing assessment. During chemotherapy, monitor respiratory function routinely to detect changes in respiratory status. Patients who are receiving drugs associated with pulmonary effects, radiation therapy, or those patients with lung lesions are at particular risk for this adverse effect.

Monitor patients for dyspnea, cough, fever, rales, a change in vital signs, alterations in breathing pattern or level of consciousness, ineffective airway clearance, and weakness.

Cough is an early sign of pulmonary toxicity.

In addition to effects directly associated with anticancer drugs, respiratory infections can result from the patient's altered immune system. It is important to monitor for symptoms of infection of the sinus, throat, middle ear, and lung. Monitor sputum for changes in color, amount, and thickness. Cultures should be obtained for sensitivity studies. Careful monitoring is essential in order to initiate prompt treatment if infection or pulmonary complications develop. *Continued.*

GENERAL NURSING IMPLICATIONS—cont'd

Nursing of patients requiring alkylating agents and miscellaneous drugs used in the treatment of cancer—cont'd

Miscellaneous effects—cont'd

Cardiac complications. Some anticancer drugs (e.g., high-dose cyclophosphamide) are directly toxic to cardiac muscle cells and have the potential for cardiotoxicity and adverse effects on cardiac output.

Monitor for shortness of breath, chest pain, changes in cardiac rhythm, dyspnea, changes in ECG, and heart failure.

Hepatic complications. Hepatic toxicity occurs occasionally with carmustine and other anticancer drugs. Monitor for liver enlargement, *jaundice,* lethargy, pain, tenderness over the liver area, dark urine and urobilinogen, liver function studies (routinely), serum electrolytes (routinely), and serum bilirubin.

Renal and urinary tract complications. Various anticancer drugs have been associated with renal toxicity and with various adverse effects affecting the urinary tract, including hemorrhagic cystitis and chemical cystitis.

Renal toxicity is dose related with cisplatin. Streptozocin therapy can cause severe renal damage resulting in proteinuria and glucosuria. Renal insufficiency can progress to acute tubular necrosis (ATN). Although these effects are usually dose related and tend to be cummulative, they can occur after a single dose of streptozocin in susceptible individuals. Monitoring of renal function is essential in patients receiving these drugs.

Monitor intake and output, blood urea nitrogen (BUN) and creatinine clearance, oliguria, daily weight, fluid and electrolyte balance, overhydration/underhydration, and urine for proteinuria and glucosuria.

Increasing fluid intake, if not contraindicated, to 2 to 4 L/day before treatment and during treatment helps promote the elimination of the drug. Concurrent infusion of mannitol may be prescribed to increase urinary excretion of cisplatin when administered.

Ifosfamide, when instilled in the bladder, can cause direct drug irritation, resulting in hemorrhagic cystitis. Cyclophosphamide can cause chemical cystitis and has been associated with fibrosis of the bladder with chronic use. Monitoring of patients is essential. Monitor for a persistent urge to void, burning or discomfort on urination, dysuria, hematuria, and spasm (analgesics or antispasmodics may be required).

Adequate hydration, 2 to 3 L of water or fluids for several hours after treatment, can minimize or avoid this effect. Patients taking cyclophosphamide as outpatients should be advised to take their dose in the morning and drink at least 2 to 3 L of fluids during the day.

Neurologic complications. Neurologic toxicities have been associated with the use of many of the anticancer drugs, in particularly vincristine, videsine, asparaginase, and procarbazine. The first signs of neurotoxicity are usually decreased deep tendon reflexes, followed by numbness, tingling, and paresthesias. Neurotoxicity caused by the vinca alkaloids usually, however, starts with constipation and progresses to ataxia, difficulty walking, paresthesia, pain at the fingertips, or other symptoms of neurotoxicity. Constipation results from direct damage to the autonomic nervous system with vincristine in particularly. These effects are usually dose related; however, it is important to note that even with discontinuation of the drug, recovery may not be complete. Ototoxicity can also occur with anticancer drugs, with damage to the eighth cranial nerve (especially in children and the elderly). Hearing loss can be unilateral or bilateral with high-frequency hearing loss. Audiometric assessment should be completed at regular intervals during treatment.

Monitor for numbness, tingling, weakness, ataxia, lethargy, mood swings, mental confusion, depression, agitation, sedation, nightmares, insomnia, ototoxicity, tinnitus, difficulty hearing normal conversation, other sensory alterations, and seizures (seizure precautions may be indicated).

Neurologic effects of drugs may be difficult to separate from the effects of the cancer (e.g., CNS involvement). Headache and vertigo can indicate CNS metastasis. A careful initial baseline assessment and monitoring during therapy are important in this differentiation. Neurologic effects can also effect self concept, mobility, and self-care abilities. Nursing assistance is needed in these areas as indicated.

Sexuality complications. Sexual dysfunction has been associated with the use of anticancer drugs, and this effect can be distressing to patients and can require professional nursing assistance. Many patients may not feel comfortable discussing sexuality and may not share their problems. It is important for the nurse to be sensitive to the individual patient's needs in this area so that assessment and monitoring can be completed and adverse effects minimized.

Monitor for changes in menstrual pattern (amenorrhea), changes in libido, premature menopause, hot flashes (associated with tamoxifen).

Infertility can occur with many of the anticancer drugs.

PATIENT EDUCATION

The patient and family as indicated should be fully informed about the nature of the patient's condition and treatment plan. They should be involved in the health care planning whenever possible. The collaboration of health team members in the care of patients requiring alkylating agents or miscellaneous drugs used in the treatment of cancer cannot be overemphasized. To prevent undue confusion and anxiety, the health care team should be clear on what the patient understands and how each member can work to promote patient understanding of the condition and treatment.

In general, the patient and family should have a clear understanding of the anticipated course of therapy and medication regimen, including the exact name of the medication, its action, purpose, dosage, storage (if they will be self-medicating at home), administration, and adverse side effects associated especially with the specific agent(s). This is important because pa-

GENERAL NURSING IMPLICATIONS—cont'd

Nursing of patients requiring alkylating agents and miscellaneous drugs used in the treatment of cancer—cont'd

PATIENT EDUCATION—cont'd

tients prepared for common and sometimes devastating adverse effects can accept them better and plan to minimize or prevent them when possible.

The patient and family should be able to monitor therapeutic response, identify and manage common adverse effects, and recognize signs that indicate that the health care provider should be notified. Discharge/outpatients may require help in carrying out self-care routines at home and follow-up or supervision. Patient education is a major nursing responsibility.

Course of therapy

The patient and family should have a clear idea of the course of therapy. For example, they should know that chemotherapy may be administered in cycles or in conjunction with surgery or radiation therapy. They should understand the importance of therapy as well as the need for continued care and follow-up. The diagnosis of cancer is often devastating to the patient and family, and much support is needed. Any questions that the patient or family may have regarding therapy or progress should be answered honestly. Nursing must be adapted to the patient's psychologic reaction to the diagnosis and treatment plan. The nurse must relate to the patient's grieving process.

The patient and family should have a realistic view of what to expect in relation to chemotherapy. Patients often want to discuss if they will be cured. Therapeutic response must be explained in relation to individual patient need for chemotherapy. Remissions, relapses, and the possibility of metastasis need to be explained.

Misconceptions should be clarified. Patients and their families should be taught and encouraged to ask questions about therapy as active consumers of health services. Conflicting statements by physicians, nurses, and other members of the health care team can be avoided by communication among them.

Adverse side effects

Although the therapeutic effects of anticancer therapy should be emphasized, the patient and family should be aware of possible adverse side effects. This is important because these effects can be both life threatening and emotionally upsetting.

Patients and their families should know that effects usually disappear when chemotherapy is discontinued. The management of adverse side effects includes dose reduction, use of alternative drugs, administration of medication before bedtime if this prevents nausea and vomiting, and an increase of fluid intake. Other measures should be explored with the patient and family as indicated. Patients should understand that they will be assisted with adverse side effects if they should occur. It is important to acknowledge fear and anxiety associated with the possible adverse side effects of the anticancer drugs.

Thrombocytopenia

Encourage the patient to do the following:

Monitor self for oozing and intermittent bleeding, easy bruising, rash.

Ensure safe environment.

Avoid trauma (be sure patient understands importance of avoiding minor trauma).

Avoid straight blades, razors; use electric razor.

File toenails and fingernails.

Use soft toothbrush as opposed to hard toothbrush.

Avoid hot baths, sun, or harsh temperature changes.

Avoid drugs that interfere with platelet function, including aspirin.

Avoid wearing tight or constricting clothing.

Report bleeding in mouth or nose; rectal bleeding or unusual vaginal bleeding; reddish urine or dark stool, which could indicate internal bleeding; drowsiness or mental status changes that may indicate bleeding in CNS.

If anemia is a problem, patients should understand that tiredness may occur. They should be taught to set priorities

and schedule activities through the day to avoid fatigue, eat a high protein diet to increase erythrocyte production, maintain good nutritional habits, and take multivitamins with minerals, if needed.

Inform patients that blood transfusions may be required. It is important that they understand that this does *not* indicate therapy is ineffective.

Patient education is particularly important if the patient will be at home when the platelet nadir occurs.

Leukopenia

Patient education in relation to the prevention of infection is particularly important as are measures to prevent bleeding. The patient should understand when the risk of infection is highest.

To minimize the effects of leukopenia, teach and encourage the patient to do the following:

Utilize hygienic practices in daily care.

Use good handwashing technique, especially before eating.

Avoid exposure to people with infections, colds, or contagious diseases (such as chickenpox, measles).

Monitor self for early signs of infection including warm or red skin, tenderness, open lesions, cough, respiratory congestion, elevated temperature. (Both the patient and family should be taught to monitor temperature accurately and report abnormalities.)

Understand the importance of not using drugs that can mask an elevated temperature such as aspirin or acetaminophen.

Prepare low-bacteria diet with all foods cooked and with increased calories and protein.

Teach patients that they are most susceptible to infection when leukocyte counts are at their lowest. (The patient should understand the importance of having blood tests to monitor this.)

Continued.

GENERAL NURSING IMPLICATIONS—cont'd

Nursing of patients requiring alkylating agents and miscellaneous drugs used in the treatment of cancer—cont'd

Mucositis

Teach the patient and family to complete an oral assessment daily and to monitor for signs of inflammation, bleeding, infection, and changes associated with periods of chemotherapy, leukopenia, and thrombocytopenia. Instruct the patient in meticulous oral care and in the modification of oral care measures as needed during therapy. Instruct the patient to do the following:

Gently brush teeth with a soft bristle toothbrush at least twice a day.

Gently floss teeth with unwaxed dental floss.

Discontinue flossing and brushing when platelet count falls below 20,000 because of bleeding tendency and to rinse mouth as directed.

Avoid commercial mouth washes, which can irritate mucous membranes.

Report dryness, discomfort, and increased sensitivity to hot or cold foods.

Avoid irritating, spicy, or tart foods, citrus juices, and extremes in food temperature.

Select nutritious ground, pureed, soft or liquid foods during periods of irritation, and avoid rough textured foods.

Avoid alcohol and smoking, which can dry and irritate mucous membranes.

Use lip balm to prevent lip irritation. (Inflammation and sores should be readily reported to the health care provider.)

Use prescribed antibacterial, antifungal, and analgesic medications as indicated.

Nausea and vomiting

Patient teaching is required to help patients minimize gastrointestinal effects of chemotherapy, including nausea, vomiting, constipation, and diarrhea. Other related problems also may include anorexia, taste distortion, and stomatitis. It is important to be positive in presenting patient information for the management of these effects. It is also important to inform patients that they may not experience these effects.

In general, patients should avoid foods that can cause nausea or vomiting (such as meat) and select appetizing nutritious foods that are usually well-tolerated, such as chicken, fish, eggs, cottage cheese or other cheeses, cold cuts, sandwiches, and fruit plates. Patient likes and dislikes should be incorporated into meal planning. A full meal before therapy is often helpful to many patients as is distraction. The severity of nausea or vomiting requires careful assessment because antiemetics may be indicated before treatments or during periods of drug therapy. Hard sugarless candy can be sucked to mask the taste of medication during infusion if this presents a problem. Tetrahydrocannabinol (THC) has been used by some patients effectively, and this may need to be more fully explored along with psychotherapy or meditation. It is important that patients be taught to brush their teeth or rinse their mouth as directed before and after meals as a measure to decrease nausea and vomiting. In addition, the following measures can also be taught to minimize nausea:

Drink carbonated beverages or tea.

Eat a dry cracker before becoming active.

Eat smaller more frequent meals, and chew foods well before swallowing.

Relax and eat with someone.

Suck on ice chips at the onset of nausea

Avoid overpowering aromas.

The following measures can be taught to minimize vomiting:

Control vomiting with a cool environment, loose clothing, a cold moist towel to the forehead, oral hygiene, and control of odors.

Insert rectal suppositories as prescribed to control vomiting.

Diarrhea and constipation

Teach personal hygiene care and the importance of monitoring weight daily and maintaining specified amounts of fluids and calories. The patient should be taught to monitor stools, including the recording of the date, time, consistency, and color of bowel movements.

The patient should report troublesome or persistent diarrhea, weight loss, or constipation. If irritation occurs, a sitz bath or ointments, as prescribed to the anal area, may be indicated. The patient should be taught to apply ointments as needed.

Integument

Teach patients to use good hygienic practices and to keep the skin clean and dry. Teach them to assess the skin regularly for breakdown, irritation, discoloration, rashes, itching, psoriasis, dandruff, or discomfort. They should also be taught to inspect the nails for discoloration. The patient should understand the importance of avoiding excessive sunlight and should report unusual observations or excessive itching or discomfort.

Patients receiving intravenous therapy should understand the importance of keeping extremities immobilized during infusion and what they can do to prevent extravasation. They should understand the importance of letting the person administering the drug know if they feel burning, pain or other sensations that might indicate extravasation.

Alopecia. Alopecia is emotionally distressing, and patients react to this adverse effect individually. The reaction to the potential or actual change in body image caused by hair loss is related to the value the individual patient places on hair. Patients need support in anticipating, as well as accepting, this adverse effect of chemotherapy. They need reassurance that their hair will grow back. They also need to be prepared for the fact that (rarely) hair color or texture may be different. Assistance with the selection of head coverings, wigs, or hairpieces is often needed. Children, as well as adults, should be involved in making selections. Patients with long hair may prefer to have their hair cut to a shorter length to lessen the effect of hair loss. Hair can be lost in large clumps with combing or shampooing or be found on the pillow when the patient wakes up in the morning. Patient education

GENERAL NURSING IMPLICATIONS—cont'd

Nursing of patients requiring alkylating agents and miscellaneous drugs used in the treatment of cancer—cont'd

Integument—cont'd

is important in preparing them for these effects. The use of makeup, false eyelashes, and eyebrow pencil as indicated can also be explored. Men may be concerned about the loss of their beard or mustache. Body hair and pubic hair can also be lost, and the patient needs to be made aware of this. It is important to correct misconceptions and to offer support and understanding. The patient should understand why hair loss occurs with the drug therapy and should be encouraged to express feelings regarding any change in body image.

The patient should understand that frequent shampooing or brushing and the use of permanents or hair coloring can affect the degree of hair loss. Patients should be encouraged to use a soft hairbrush only as needed for grooming and to wash the hair only as needed.

Patients often have questions regarding techniques that are available to diminish hair loss. These techniques, as well as possible results, should be discussed with the patient including scalp tourniquets and ice turbans.

Neurotoxicity

In addition to what symptoms to expect and what symptoms to report to the health-care provider, teach the patient and family seizure precautions.

Patients treated with vinblastine or vincristine should be taught that numbness and tingling of the fingers and toes are common adverse side effects after each dose. Muscle aching and weakness may also occur and should be reported. These agents also commonly produce constipation as a result of autonomic nervous system toxicity, and patients should be educated to anticipate and deal with this effect.

Urinary tract/renal toxicity

The patient and family should understand the importance of maintaining fluid intake (especially the importance of increased fluid intake) to prevent hemorrhagic cystitis or chemical cystitis as related specifically to cyclo-

phosphamide. The patient and family should be assisted in developing and implementing a plan to meet this daily fluid requirement. The patient and family should be able to monitor intake, daily weight and urinary output.

Sexual dysfunction

Sexual dysfunction, including amenorrhea, premature menopause, and sterility, have been associated with the use of many of the alkylating agents and miscellaneous anticancer drugs. Patients and family as indicated should be informed of this adverse affect and assisted with this problem. They should be aware that menses usually return to normal after the drug is discontinued, and that even with this adverse effect, contraception should be continued. Women who are pregnant or planning to become pregnant require counseling and teaching regarding teratogenesis and possible infertility. The change in libido can be distressing to the patient as well as to the patient's partner. Encourage verbalization of this problem and involve the partner as indicated in discussions and teaching. Pretreatment teaching is important in relation to the potential problem of sterility. The patient may want to explore the possibility of sperm banking and should be made aware of this option.

Self-concept

Pretreatment teaching is essential to prepare patients for the possible adverse side effects associated with these drugs. It should be remembered that individual patient response to the diagnosis of cancer must be considered when patients are given information because they may not be hearing all that is said and may not be able to make informed choices as a result of the associated distress. This aspect of teaching must be handled carefully and in relation to a health care team approach.

Psychologic problems, including grieving, sleep pattern disturbance, and ineffective coping of the patient and family, can occur. Support coping mechanisms, and develop the coping abilities of the patient and family. A knowledge of the cancer process, possible toxicities and adverse side effects, and how to decrease or minimize these effects greatly help the patient and family maintain control and coping abilities. Patient education does much to enable the patient and family to better withstand the treatment and assist in health care.

Patients receiving home care or who are being treated as outpatients should be made aware of the possible risks involved in careless handling of anticancer agents and contaminated excreta, such as urine or vomitus. They should be taught to protect themselves and to follow proper procedures as indicated.

Nurses working with patients requiring anticancer drugs have developed patient education materials to aid patient self-medication and the understanding of their condition and treatment. Group teaching has been effective in teaching selected groups of patients. Patients receiving anticancer drugs as outpatients or who self-medicate as inpatients require information and education that will give them responsibility in their self-care while allowing them to adjust to the demands of anticancer therapy. Nurses should direct research and attention to various teaching approaches for patients of different ages or with different conditions requiring anticancer drug therapy. A team approach to patient teaching is also an important consideration.

The nurse's role in health promotion (one that includes patient education regarding early warning signs of cancer, stop-smoking programs, and breast self-examination) is an important area of focus. Nurses should become active not only in the promotion of self-care behaviors to decrease risk of cancer, but also in the promotion of public policy directed at enviromental risks.

GENERAL INSTRUCTIONS FOR DISCHARGE/OUTPATIENTS

ALKYLATING AGENTS AND MISCELLANEOUS DRUGS USED TO TREAT CANCER

This medication is primarily used to treat various forms of cancer. It can sometimes be used for the treatment of other conditions. If you do not understand why you require this medication, check with your health care provider.

Follow the instructions on the prescription exactly. If you have any questions about how this medication should be taken, check with your health care provider.

Take this medication with some food or with a meal. It is often helpful to take this medication at bedtime to prevent nausea and vomiting.

Avoid drinking alcoholic beverages while you are taking this medication. This can cause unwanted effects in some patients.

This medication can cause your skin to become more sensitive to sunlight. When you are outside, shade your skin and wear protective clothing or use a sunscreen. Avoid excessive exposure to sunlight.

Notify your health care provider immediately if you notice a sore throat, fever, mouth sores, diarrhea, skin rash, bruising, or dark urine or black bowel movements.

If you are pregnant, thinking about becoming pregnant, or breastfeeding, do not take this medication until you discuss this with your health care provider. The use of this medication has been associated with birth defects or unwanted effects in nursing infants. Your nurse can discuss methods of birth control with you as well as infant care if you must take this medication.

Until you learn how this medication affects you, do not drive, operate dangerous machinery, or put yourself in situations where decreased mental alertness may cause danger.

Do not start or stop taking medications while on this medication without first checking with your health care provider. This medication can cause unwanted effects if taken with other medications.

Store this medication in a dry place and protect from light. Keep out of the reach of children by placing it in a locked drawer or locked medicine cabinet.

Do not trade or give this medication to family or friends. It has been prescribed especially for you and can cause unwanted effects in people who do not require it.

It is important that you keep appointments with your health care provider and have blood tests and urine tests completed as directed. This is important in managing your therapy. If you have any questions about need for visits to your clinic, hospital or laboratory, discuss these with your health care provider.

If you are receiving chemotherapy as an outpatient:

1. Whenever possible, bring a family member or friend to accompany you on days when chemotherapy is administered.
2. Do not drive an automobile or perform other tasks requiring mental alertness after taking antinausea medication, which usually causes drowsiness.
3. Immediately report any fever, other signs of infection, or bleeding, all of which are especially dangerous at the low point in blood counts. The time of lowest blood counts is usually 1 to 2 weeks after chemotherapy.

NURSING DRUG DIGEST

Medication (trade name*)	Indication	Usual dosage and administration†	Dosage forms, preparation, and storage	Contraindications, cautions, and comments	Monitoring
Asparaginase Elspar Kidrolase	Acute lymphocytic leukemia	6000 units/m² IM 3 times/week; or 1000 units/kg IV q.d. for 10-14 days, by 30-60 minute infusion in NS or D₅W The manufacturer recommends skin testing and desensitization before administration (for skin testing, inject 0.1 ml of a 20 unit/ml solution intradermally)	Injectable: 10,000 units/vial Store refrigerated (2°-8° C) Reconstitute with 5 ml NS or sterile water for injection Stable for 8 hr after reconstitution; discard cloudy solutions Rotate vial gently to mix; do *not* shake	*Contraindicated* in pancreatitis Relatively *contraindicated* in hypersensitivity Patients should be pretreated with antihistamines; epinephrine and hydrocortisone should be readily available Severe allergic reactions including anaphylaxis may occur, especially with subsequent drug doses May cause CNS depression May cause hyperglycemia May cause nausea	Observe for wheezing, shortness of breath, or swelling around eyes and lips Observe for CNS depression Observe for signs of bleeding Monitor serum glucose
Busulfan Myleran	Chronic myelocytic leukemia	2-8 mg/day PO taken q.d. as a chronic maintenance dose	Tablet: 2 mg	Skin darkening and lung toxicity (pulmonary fibrosis) may occur with long-term (1-3 yr) therapy WBC count decreases in second or third week of therapy May cause severe bone marrow suppression	Monitor blood counts Monitor respiratory status

NOTE: For additional details regarding the individual agents listed in this table, see the text and other tables in this chapter.

*Indicates a multiple active ingredient product. For a complete listing of all active ingredients see the *Drug Reference Guide to Brand Names and Active Ingredients.*

†The dosages of the anticancer agents apply generally for both adults and children. Doses are usually calculated according to body surface area (m²), which may be determined from the nomograms in Figures 52-4 (adults) and 52-5 (children). The doses listed are the ranges used in various protocols, but must be individualized according to the patient's blood counts and hepatic and renal function. Investigational protocols may employ doses and schedules of drug administration that differ from those listed in this table.

♦ Indicates that the drug is generally available only in Canada.

★ Indicates that the drug is generally available only in the United States.

NURSING DRUG DIGEST—cont'd

Medication (trade name)	Indication	Usual dosage and administration	Dosage forms, preparation, and storage	Contraindications, cautions, and comments	Monitoring
Carmustine BiCNU	Brain tumors, melanoma, myeloma, Hodgkin's disease, lymphomas	200 mg/m² IV q 6-8 weeks Pain at site of injection may be ameliorated by infusion over 1-2 hr Avoid extravasation Administer an antiemetic at the time of treatment For IV use *only*	Injectable: 100 mg/vial; store refrigerated (2°-8° C) Unstable in solution Reconstitute just before infusion, by dissolving drug in 3 ml alcohol, then adding 27 ml sterile water for injection The resultant solution contains 3.3 mg carmustine per ml Use gloves when reconstituting Refrigerate reconstituted solution and discard unused portion after 24 hr Discard powder that has liquefied or appears oily	Vesicant The nitrosoureas produce delayed myelosuppression (bone marrow toxicity) 4-6 wks after treatment Severe nausea usually occurs 2 hr after injection, and lasts 4-6 hr May cause lethal lung toxicity (pulmonary fibrosis)	Monitor respiratory status Monitor blood counts
Chlorambucil Leukeran	Breast cancer, lymphomas, Hodgkin's disease, ovarian cancer, chronic lymphocytic leukemia	0.1-0.2 mg/kg/day PO taken q.d. between meals, as a chronic maintenance dose	Tablet: 2 mg	Does not produce alopecia Nausea and vomiting are uncommon Myelosuppression is the major toxicity Chlorambucil is teratogenic	Monitor blood counts
Cisplatin Platinol	Testicular, ovarian, head and neck, lung, bladder, and prostate cancer	40-100 mg/m² IV in large volumes of 0.45% to 0.9% sodium chloride Durations of the infusion may range from 15 min to 24 hr, according to various protocols Pretreat the patient with an antiemetic	Injectable: 10, 50 mg/vial Store refrigerated (2°-8° C) Unstable in dextrose solution; should be reconstituted in sterile water for injection (10 or 50 ml, respectively) Reconstituted solutions stable for 12 hr at room temperature; do not refrigerate solution Platinum in cisplatin forms a precipitate if it comes in contact with aluminum	*Contraindicated* in renal dysfunction Encourage fluid intake The risk of renal toxicity can be reduced by hydration before, during, and after treatments Total fluid intake should be 3-5 L on the day of treatment May produce severe nausea and vomiting May cause ototoxicity (e.g., tinnitus, high-frequency hearing loss) May cause neurotoxicity	Monitor renal function Observe for peripheral neuropathy

Drug	Uses	Dosage	Preparation	Side effects/Comments	Nursing considerations
Cyclophosphamide Cytoxan Neosar Procytox	Breast, lung, and ovarian lymphomas, Hodgkin's disease, sarcomas, myeloma	100 mg/m² PO q.d. or 250 mg/m² PO q.d. for 5 days; or 500-1000 mg/m² IV bolus, every 3-4 weeks; Patients should be advised to take their dose in the morning and drink at least 2 L of liquids during the day; Check that drug is completely dissolved before injection	Tablets: 25, 50 mg; Injectable: 100, 200, 500, 1000, 2000 mg/vial; Add 5 ml sterile water for injection and shake to reconstitute; Solutions not used within 4 hr should be discarded	Encourage fluid intake; Hemorrhagic cystitis may occur, particularly without adequate hydration; May cause nausea and vomiting; Alopecia common; Cyclophosphamide is teratogenic	Observe for dysuria and hematuria (urinalysis for microscopic hematuria)
Dacarbazine DTIC-Dome	Melanoma, Hodgkin's disease, sarcomas	250 mg/m² IV q.d. for 5 days; or 800-1000 mg/m² IV, infused over 1-2 hr every 3-4 weeks; Prolong infusion if pain occurs at site of injection; Protect from light during infusion; Avoid extravasation; Premedicate with antiemetics	Injectable: 100, 200 mg/vial; Store refrigerated (2-8° C); Protect from light; Reconstitute with 9.9 ml of sterile water for injection per 100 mg; Reconstituted solutions should be refrigerated and used within 24 hr	Change in color of solution from yellow to pink indicates decomposition; Potent vesicant; Severe nausea and vomiting may occur a few hours after administration; May produce flulike symptoms 5-7 days after administration with myalgias, fatigue, and malaise lasting 1-2 weeks; May cause hepatic necrosis (rarely)	Assess for extravasation; Observe for anorexia, weight loss, nausea, and vomiting
Etoposide VePesid	Testicular tumors	50-150 mg/m² q.d. for 3-5 days IV or 200-300 mg/m² IV weekly; or 100-300 mg/m²/day PO for 3-5 days; IV infusion should be over 30-60 min to avoid fall in blood pressure; do *not* infuse if precipitation forms (cloudy solution)	Injectable: 100 mg/vial; Limited solubility; Observe for and discard cloudy solutions; Dilute with D5W or NS to yield a 0.2 or 0.4 mg/ml concentration; Stable for 48 hr after dilution at room temperature	Commonly causes nausea, vomiting, and reversible alopecia	Check blood pressure every 15 min during infusion; Monitor blood counts
Hexamethylmelamine (Investigational agent)	Ovarian cancer	(Investigational) 100-200 mg/m²/day PO for 7-14 days, monthly in combination therapy; 8-12 mg/kg/day maintenance, if used alone	Capsules: 50, 100 mg	Nausea and vomiting may be dose limiting; if nausea occurs, an antiemetic should be coadministered	

Continued.

NURSING DRUG DIGEST—cont'd

Medication (trade name)	Indication	Usual dosage and administration	Dosage forms, preparation, and storage	Contraindications, cautions, and comments	Monitoring
Hydroxyurea Hydrea	Chronic myelocytic leukemia	20-40 mg/kg/day PO in 2-4 doses Reduce dosage in renal dysfunction	Capsule: 500 mg	*Contraindicated* in severe bone marrow suppression Encourage fluid intake Leukopenia occurs 7-14 days after initiation of treatment Nausea, skin rash, or mucositis may occur at higher doses (60 mg/kg/day)	Monitor blood counts Assess mucous membranes
Ifosfamide (Investigational agent)	Leukemia, lymphoma, lung cancer, breast cancer	Investigational: 3-5 gm/m² IV q. 3-4 weeks, as a single bolus or divided over 3-5 days	Injectable: 1, 3 gm vials Reconstitute 1 gm with 20 ml or 3 gm with 30 ml of NS Administer within 8 hr of reconstitution	Encourage fluid intake Hemorrhagic cystitis may occur, particularly without adequate hydration May cause nausea and vomiting Alopecia is common	Observe for dysuria and hematuria (urinalysis for microscopic hematuria); monitor intake and output
Interferons (various types—e.g., alpha, beta, gamma) (Investigational agent)	Osteosarcoma, metastatic breast cancer, multiple myeloma, nodular lymphoma, malignant melanoma	Investigational: As per experimental protocol Has been administered intralesionally, IM, IV	Injectable: investigational agent	Use with caution in patients with history of dysrhythmias or myocardial infarction May cause high fever, hypotension, chills, malaise and fatigue (may be severe) GI disturbances and myelosuppression may also occur Blood counts return to baseline following discontinuation of therapy	Monitor renal and hepatic function Monitor blood pressure and vital signs every 15 min for first hr, every hr for the next 4 hr, and then according to experimental protocol Monitor mental status Monitor temperature

Drug	Uses	Dosage	Availability	Side effects	Nursing considerations
Lomustine CeeNU	Lymphomas, Hodgkin's disease, brain cancer, myeloma, melanoma, colon cancer, gastric cancer, lung cancer	130 mg/m² PO q 6 weeks as single agent; 60-80 mg/m² PO in combination chemotherapy; Advise patients to take the drug in the evening on an empty stomach and to avoid eating until the following day	Capsules: 10, 40, 100 mg; Protect from excessive heat (over 40° C)	Severe nausea can occur within 2-6 hr after treatment; Delayed myelosuppression occurs 4-6 weeks after treatment	Monitor blood counts
Mechlorethamine Mustargen	Hodgkin's disease, lymphomas, lung cancer	6 mg/m² or 0.1-0.4 mg/kg IV; Maximum: 0.4 mg/kg for a single course of therapy; Avoid any contact with skin or mucous membranes; Reconstitute just before injection into rapidly flowing saline infusion; Check venous patency before, during, and after infusion; If extravasation occurs, immediately infiltrate 4% sodium thiosulfate into the affected tissues and apply ice compresses intermittently for 12 hr	Injectable: 10 mg/vial; Reconstitute with 10 ml sterile water for injection; Unstable in solution; use immediately; Wear rubber gloves to reconstitute drug	Potent vesicant; May cause phlebitis and venous thrombosis; May cause severe nausea and vomiting; offer antiemetic before treatment	Assess for extravasation; Assess for phlebitis and thrombosis
Melphalan Alkeran	Ovarian and breast cancer, multiple myeloma	0.1-0.2 mg/kg/day PO for 5 days, as a single daily dose	Tablet: 2 mg	Does *not* usually produce alopecia or nausea	Monitor blood counts
Mitotane Lysodren	Adrenal cortical carcinoma	2-10 gm/day PO in 3-4 divided doses; Reduce dosage in hepatic dysfunction	Tablet: 500 mg	Commonly causes anorexia and nausea; Suppression of normal adrenal function requires corticosteroid replacement therapy; May cause CNS depression (drowsiness, dizziness)	Observe for CNS depression; Assess for signs of adrenal insufficiency (low blood pressure, hyponatremia, hyperkalemia)

Continued.

NURSING DRUG DIGEST—cont'd

Medication (trade name)	Indication	Usual dosage and administration	Dosage forms, preparation, and storage	Contraindications, cautions, and comments	Monitoring
Procarbazine Matulane Natulan	Hodgkin's disease, lymphomas, lung cancer, brain cancer (especially for MOPP combination for Hodgkin's disease)	100 mg/m² day PO for 7-14 days; or 1-6 mg/kg/day PO The daily dose should be taken q.h.s. with an antiemetic if nausea occurs Reduce doses for liver impairment (bilirubin over 3 mg/dl) or renal dysfunction	Capsule: 50 mg	Commonly causes bone marrow suppression Disulfiram-like adverse reaction may occur if patient consumes alcohol May cause nausea Synergistic with CNS depressants Patients should be advised that procarbazine may produce insomnia, nightmares, depression, or hallucinations Inhibits monoamine oxidase; therefore sympathomimetic drugs and tyramine-containing foods (i.e., cheeses, bananas, red wine) should be avoided; see MAOIs, Chapter 19	Observe for changes in mental status Monitor blood counts
Teniposide Vumon	Acute lymphocytic leukemia, neuroblastoma, non-Hodgkin's lymphoma	Leukemia: 165 mg/m² twice weekly in combination; neuroblastoma: 130-180 mg/m²/day IV once weekly; lymphoma: 50-100 mg/m²/day IV once weekly Intravenous infusion should be over 30-60 min to avoid fall in blood pressure	Injectable: 50 mg/vial Dilute to 0.1-0.2 mg/ml in D₅W or NS before administration Reconstituted solution stable for 4 hr at room temperature Observe for and discard cloudy solutions after reconstitution	*Contraindicated* in hypersensitivity; bone marrow suppression, and severe hepatic or renal impairment Commonly causes GI distress and bone marrow suppression	Monitor blood counts Monitor renal and hepatic function
★ **Thiotepa**	Breast, ovarian, bladder cancer	0.5-1.0 mg/kg IV, IM or SC at 1-4 week intervals; or 0.2 mg/kg/day for 5 days Dose reduction required in renal or hepatic dysfunction A solution of 60 mg in 60 ml sterile water has been used for bladder instillation	Injectable: 15 mg/vial Store refrigerated (2°-8° C) Reconstitute with 1.5 ml sterile water for injection Discard solutions that are hazy or that have a precipitate Reconstituted solutions are stable for 5 days if refrigerated	May produce anorexia or nausea	Monitor blood counts Observe for nausea

Drug	Uses	Dosage	Preparations	Side effects/Precautions	Monitoring
Vinblastine Velban Velbe	Testicular cancer, breast cancer, lymphomas, Hodgkin's disease, choriocarcinoma, renal cancer	0.1-0.2 mg/kg IV push over 1 min; Avoid extravasation (check venous patency before and after injection); Dose must be reduced in patients with liver dysfunction	Injectable: 10 mg/vial; Store refrigerated (2°-8° C); Reconstitute with 10 ml NS or sterile water for injection	*Contraindicated in leukopenia*; Potent vesicant; Less neurotoxicity but more myelosuppression than with vincristine; May cause nausea; Myalgias (muscle aching) common for a few days after injection; May cause alopecia; May cause constipation; Advise patients to avoid constipation by using mild laxatives and stool softeners	Monitor for peripheral neuropathy (i.e., numbness, weakness, constipation)
Vincristine Oncovin	Lymphomas, Hodgkin's disease, breast cancer, acute leukemias, sarcomas, Wilms' tumor, neuroblastoma	1.0-1.4 mg/m² IV push over 1 min; Avoid extravasation; check venous patency before and after injection; Dose must be reduced in patients with liver dysfunction	Injectable: 1, 5 mg/vial; Store refrigerated (2°-8° C); Reconstitute with NS or sterile water for injection	Potent vesicant; Neurotoxicity is common, with numbness and tingling of hands and feet, weakness, and constipation; advise patients to avoid constipation by using mild laxatives and stool softeners; Jaw pain commonly occurs after the first dose, but is less with subsequent doses; May cause alopecia; May cause nausea	Monitor for peripheral neuropathy (i.e., numbness, weakness, constipation)
Vindesine Eldisine	Leukemias, lymphomas, breast and lung cancer	2-3 mg/m² IV weekly; *or* 1.0-1.5 mg/m²/day for 5 days IV by continuous infusion, q. 3 weeks; For children with leukemia: 2 mg/m²/day for 2 days IV repeated weekly for 8 weeks; Administer IV over 1-3 min; For IV use only	Injectable: 5 mg/vial; Store refrigerated (2°-8° C); Reconstitute with 5 ml NS; Store reconstituted drug refrigerated (2°-8° C) and discard after 2 weeks	Potent vesicant; Leukopenia is the major toxicity; Neurotoxicity is common, with numbness and tingling of hands and feet, weakness, and constipation; advise patients to avoid constipation by using mild laxatives and stool softeners; Myalgias are common for a few days after injection; Jaw pain commonly occurs after the first dose, but is less with subsequent doses	Monitor for peripheral neuropathy (i.e., numbness, weakness, constipation); Monitor urinary output; Monitor blood counts

BIBLIOGRAPHY

Bender, R.A., Zwelling, L.A., Doroshow, J.H., Locerk G.Y., Hande, K.R., Murinson, D.S., Cohen, M., Myers, C.E., & Chabner, B.A. Antineoplastic drugs: Clinical pharmacology and therapeutic use. *Drugs,* 1978, *16,* 46-77.

Bubela, N. Is your client at risk for respiratory complications? *The Canadian Nurse,* 1983, *79*(3), 46-48.

Chemotherapy and you—a guide to self-help during treatment. (NIH Publication NO. 80-1136). Bethesda, Md. 20205: U.S. Dept. of Health and Human Services, National Cancer Institute, Office of Cancer Communications, Building 31, Room 10A18.

D'Arcy, P.F. Reactions and interactions in handling anticancer drugs. *Drug Intelligence and Clinical Pharmacy,* 1983, *17,* 532-538.

Dean, J.C., Salmon, S.A., & Griffith, K.S. Prevention of doxorubicin-induced hair loss with scalp hypothermia. *New England Journal of Medicine,* 1979, *301,* 1427-1429.

Donehower, R.C., Myers, C.E., & Chabner, B.A. New developments on the mechanism of action of antineoplastic drugs. *Life Science,* 1979, *25,* 1-14.

Dorr, R.T., & Fritz, W.L. *Cancer Chemotherapy Handbook.* New York: Elsevier, 1980.

Fredette, S.L., & Gloriant, F.S. Nursing diagnoses in cancer chemotherapy in theory. *American Journal of Nursing,* 1981, *81*(11), 2013-2019.

Gullo, S. Chemotherapy: What to do about special side effects. *RN,* 1977, *40*(4), 30-32.

Hagan, S.J. Bring help and hope to the patient with Hodgkin's Disease. *Nursing 83,* 1983, *13*(8), 58-63.

Heel, R.C., Brogden, R.N., Speight, T.M., & Avery, G.S. Tamoxifen: A review of its pharmacological properties and therapeutic use in the treatment of breast cancer. *Drugs,* 1978, *16,* 1-24.

Koren, M.E. Cancer immunotherapy—What, why. *Nursing 81,* 1981, *11*(1), 34-41.

Krim, M. Towards tumor therapy with interferons, Part I. Interferons: Production and properties. *Blood* 1980, *55,* 711-721.

Krim, M. Towards tumor therapy with interferons, Part II. Interferons: *In vivo* effects. *Blood,* 1980, *55,* 875-884.

Krim, M. Towards tumor therapy with interferons, Part I. Interferons: *In vivo* effects. *Blood,* 1980, *55,* 711-721.

Levitt, D.Z. Cancer chemotherapy: those dreaded side effects and what to do about them. (part 5). *RN,* 1981, *44*(2), 56-59.

Levitt, D.Z. Cancer chemotherapy: those dreaded side effects and what to do about them. (part 6). *RN,* 1981, *44*(3), 69-72.

Lum, J.L.J., Chase, M., Cole, S.M., Johnson, A., Johnson, J.A., & Link, M.R. Nursing care of oncology patients receiving chemotherapy. *Nursing Research,* 1978, *27,* 340-346.

Maxwell, M.B. Scalp tourniquets for chemotherapy-induced alopecia. *American Journal of Nursing,* 1980, *80*(5), 900-903.

McAdams, C.W. Interferon the penicillin of the future? *American Journal of Nursing,* 1980, *80*(4), 714-718.

Miller, S.A. Nursing actions in cancer chemotherapy administration. *Oncology Nursing Forum,* 1980, *7,* 8-16.

Ostchega, Y. Preventing . . . and treating . . . cancer chemotherapy's oral complications. *Nursing 80,* 1980, *10*(8), 47-52.

Pinedo, H.M. *Cancer Chemotherapy.* New York: Elsevier, 1979.

Pochedly, C. Acute lymphoid leukemia in children. *American Journal of Nursing,* 1978, *78*(10), 1714-1716.

Pratt, W.B., & Ruddon, R.W. *The Anticancer Drugs.* New York: Oxford University Press, 1979.

Prestayko, A.W., D'Aoust, J.C., Issell, B.F., & Crooke, S.T. Cisplatin (cisdiamminedichloroplatinum II). *Cancer Treatment Review,* 1979, *6,* 17-39.

Rose-Williamson, K. Cisplatin: Delivering a safe infusion. *American Journal of Nursing,* 1981, *81*(2), 320-323.

Rozenczweig, M., von Hoff, D.D., Henney J.E., & Muggia, F.M. VM-26 and VP-16 213: A comparative analysis. *Cancer,* 1977, *40,* 334-342.

Schein, P.S. Nitrosourea antitumor agents. In S.K. Carter, A. Goldin, K. Kuretani, G. Mathe, Y. Sakurai, S. Tsukagasei, & H. Umezawa (Eds.), *Advances in Cancer Chemotherapy.* Baltimore, Md.: University Park Press, 1978.

Thomas, N.P., Cloak, M., Crosson, K., & Kwan, J. Preparing cancer patients to administer medication. *Patient Counseling and Health Education,* 1982, *3*(4), 137-143.

Welch, D., & Lewis, K. Alopecia and chemotherapy. *American Journal of Nursing,* 1980, *80*(5), 903-905.

Wroblewski, S.S., & Wroblewski, S.H. Caring for the patient with chemotherapy-induced thrombocytopenia. *American Journal of Nursing,* 1981, *81*(4), 746-749.

SECTION XII

DERMATOLOGIC MEDICATIONS

Medications discussed in this section

Review of the Anatomy, Physiology, and Assessment of the Cutaneous System

Eric Schloss

The skin, as the largest organ of the body, provides a surface area of approximately 2 m². As a functioning and adapting organ, the skin must meet the everyday stresses and challenges of the environment, which may harbor many potential injurious agents, varying from physical trauma to sun damage. The skin is uniquely designed for this purpose. Knowledge of cutaneous structure and function is essential to fundamental understanding of many major principles of nursing assessment and care because much of common clinical disease is expressed by the skin, whether it be a manifestation of basic emotions (e.g., "white of fright," "red of rage"), an expression of skin disease ranging widely from acne to zoster, or a manifestation of underlying or systemic disease varying from jaundice or cyanosis to specific skin lesions or rashes. The skin is a convenient and common route of therapy. The following chapters of this section are based on topical therapy, stressing particular aspects of the skin structure and function that may be important with respect to treatment concepts.

An awareness of normal skin structure is necessary before its function and behavior in clinical situations can be understood. The importance of regional differences in skin thickness, numbers of skin appendages (e.g., hair follicles, sweat glands, sebaceous glands), or dermal components (e.g., blood or nerve supply) can have great importance on the assessment and monitoring of patients with conditions of the skin that require pharmacologic treatment with various agents. There may be changes with time or age. Newborn skin may present different problems than that of aged skin or clinically sun-damaged skin. Function and treatment considerations may be drastically altered in abnormal or diseased skin. Fundamentally, however, there is a basic uniform structure of skin, with mainly quantitative differences occurring from site to site over the body.

The skin (Figure 54-1) comprises two basic layers, a thinner outer or top layer of epidermis and a thicker, deeper layer of dermis. Traditionally a third layer, the underlying subcutaneous fat, is included in discussion or functional consideration of the skin. The subcutaneous fat layer has many useful purposes, despite the desire of many to be aesthetically rid of it. In microscopic sections, it is noted to comprise lobules of adipose tissue divided by usually thin connective tissue septae, which contain the blood supply. Subcutaneous fat functions as a heat insulator, shock absorber, caloric reserve depot, and as a route for the administration of many medications (including heparin and insulin) offering slow absorption that can be fairly well predicted.

EPIDERMIS

Although the epidermis varies in thickness at different sites from 0.04 mm in eyelid skin to 1.6 mm on the palm or sole, it has a basic uniform composition at all sites (Figure 54-2). It is a squamous epithelium composed of multilayered squamous platelike and polygonal epithelial cells, held together by specialized cell attachments called desmosomes. Desmosomes look like intercellular bridges on routine light microscopy. A single-layered basal cell layer, which is the mitotically active growth layer, comprises cuboidal or columnar cells. The major part of the nucleated cellular epidermis, however, is called the prickle cell, malpighian cell, or keratinocyte layer. The latter designation is perhaps the most appropriate in view of the primary function of the epidermis, which is to form keratin, a unique fibrous protein. This function is absent normally in nonkeratinizing surfaces (e.g., mucous membranes) except under pathologic conditions.

Above the main keratinocyte layer, a distinct granular layer is present, which contains basophilic keratohyalin granules in their cell cytoplasm. The epidermis is capped or topped by a distinctive keratin

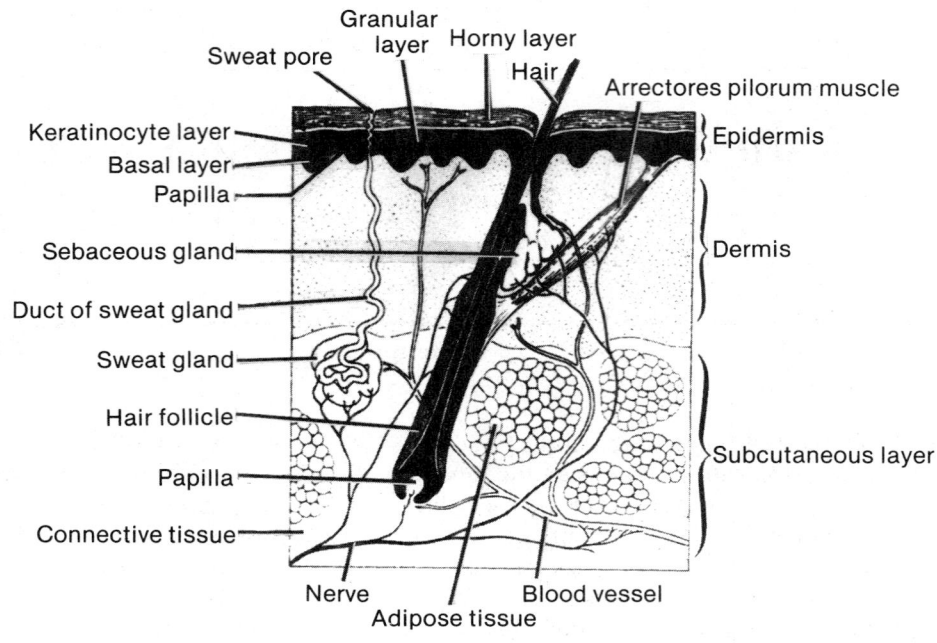

FIGURE 54-1. **Basic layers of skin with essential components.**

FIGURE 54-2. **Normal epidermis showing four distinct layers: (1) basal layer; (2) prickle cell (keratinocyte) layer; (3) granular layer (stratum granulosum); (4) keratin layer (stratum corneum).**

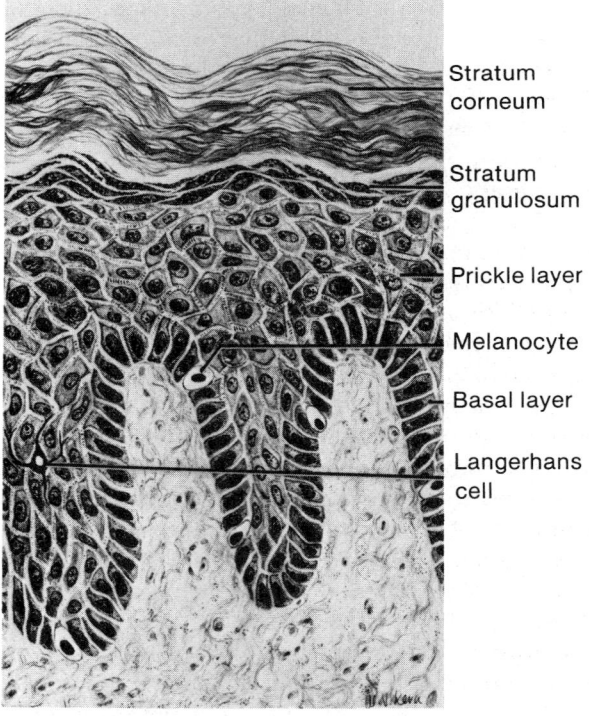

(anucleate) layer, normally varying considerably in thickness at different sites (e.g., thin eyelid versus normally thick palm or sole) but averaging 15 to 40 layers of strata. This keratin, or cornified horny layer, is the major intermediate barrier between the individual and the environment. The barrier function of keratin involves both physical aspects (such as protection from mechanical injury or external trauma, providing weight-bearing and frictional surfaces, and allowing flexibility at other sites) and chemical aspects including impermeability and resistance to corrosives. The keratin functions as a rate-limiting barrier to the absorption of fluid and electrolytes under normal and abnormal environmental conditions. It is concerned with the maintenance of hydration retarding water loss in addition to preventing the entrance of toxins. Keratin also provides a readily accessible route of absorption and a reservoir for topical medications. Its relatively dry surface helps retard the proliferation of microorganisms. Since the barrier function is vital to the understanding of percutaneous absorption, a separate section is devoted to this subject.

Keratinization and growth cycle

The epidermis is continually being renewed in the process of forming a keratinizing surface. The progeny of basal, germinative, mitotically active cells are able to differentiate through malpighian and granular layers to form the end product keratin, which is constantly being exfoliated or shed at the surface in the form of scales by a process not fully understood. Although the normal cell cycle and turnover times in skin are not unanimously agreed on, the average turnover time of stratum corneum is often reported to be 13 to 14 days, with a cell transit time of 12 to 14 days to move from the basal layer to the stratum corneum. These times may vary considerably in the presence of disease states such as psoriasis, where cell mitosis and turnover time are accelerated to greater than 10 times normal. This accelerated cell mitosis and turnover time account for the excess surface scaling observed with psoriasis and are related to the lack of time for normal differentiation and removal.

As cells differentiate, they lose the capacity to reproduce themselves. One basal cell division is thought to produce one new basal cell, along with one migrating cell moving into the malpighian layer. The basal stem cells are the main source of cell renewal. Normal cell cycle time has been reported to be approximately 457 hours, or 19 days, in some studies; however, this may be greatly reduced in the presence of disease states such as psoriasis. The turnover time in psoriasis has been reported (in addition to transit time) to be approximately 7 days.

The regulation of the proliferation of epidermal cells is not clear. Some studies have advocated a chalone or growth regulator (i.e., glycoprotein) as a major influence. However, the role of chalones, cyclic AMP, prostaglandins, and other possible chemical growth mediators is not entirely clear. Therapy in disease states is directed at reducing the rate of epidermal cell proliferation and turnover. Topical corticosteroids act to produce an antimitotic effect in psoriatic epidermis, and other agents such as methotrexate inhibit DNA synthesis (see Chapter 57, "Topical Corticosteroids").

Filamentous material, the major component of cornified cells, may be largely high molecular weight protein. It is possible that tonofilaments are precursors. Keratohyaline granules, which are small basophilic staining granules observed in microscopic sections, are characteristic markers of epidermal keratinization in the granular layer. Their specific role in keratinization, however, is uncertain. The membrane-coating granules (Odland bodies) are also specific markers of keratinization, observed most readily on electron microscopy. Their function is likewise uncertain, but they may play a role in the exfoliation of the keratin layer through their content of lysosomal enzymes. They may also act as an intercellular cement or glue.

The only orifices or pores to penetrate the surface epidermis and tough outer keratin layer are the openings of pilosebaceous follicles. The pilosebaceous follicles are numerous even without visible hairs. They are normally visible in the terminal intraepidermal portion of the eccrine sweat ducts.

Other structures

Several other cells and structures are present in the epidermis. A distinctive melanocytic system of pigmentation is present in variable degree and intensity in different individuals. This is largely governed by hereditary, race, and environmental factors (particularly sun exposure). The melanin-pigment–producing cells are located in the basal layer of the epidermis, with pigment usually prominent microscopically in a supranuclear location (i.e., "sunny side up"). Through pigment transfer (i.e., epidermal-melanin unit), pigment can be transmitted to all levels of the epidermis and thus aids in protection against sun damage because the pigment-laden cells are able to refract, reflect, scatter, and absorb otherwise sun-damaging rays of ultraviolet light. The pigment is produced in intracellular organelles or specialized structures called melanosomes. Normally the melanocyte can be visualized only as a "clear cell" on routine light microscopy and requires electron microscopy or special staining for demonstration.

The epidermal-melanin unit (EMU) is a system of pigment transfer from melanocyte to keratinocyte. One melanocyte can service approximately 36 epidermal cells. The number of EMUs/mm^2 varies in different sites from approximately 2000/mm^2 on the head, forearm, and scrotum to 1000/mm^2 on the rest of the body.

Other cell types may be normally present in epidermis including Langerhans cells. Langerhans cells are seen as higher level "clear cells" on routine light microscopy, but require special staining techniques or electron microscopy for precise demonstration. Their definitive function is not yet known; however, they have more recently been proposed to play an important role in processing antigen in contact with the skin, and thus have a possible role in the regulation of immune function.

DERMIS

The dermis is approximately 15 to 40 times thicker than the epidermis. It is mainly composed of various fibers (e.g., collagen, elastic, reticular), cells (e.g., fibroblasts, tissue macrophages or histiocytes, mast cells), and interstitial ground substances (e.g., mucopolysaccharide). It may be traversed by, and contain, various other structures, including hair follicles, sweat glands, sebaceous glands, blood vessels, lymphatics, and nerves or nerve receptors.

Before these components are discussed, an important region immediately between the epidermis and dermis proper should be emphasized. This is the basal lamina zone or basement membrane zone, more precisely delineated by electron microscopy than light microscopy. The basal lamina is an extracellular dense membrane layer with fine fibrillar material of 200 to 500 Å thickness, separated from the plasma membrane of the epidermal basal cell layer by a clear, less dense, zone called the lamina lucida, of 300 Å thickness. Anchoring fibrils appear to attach basal lamina to the collagen fibers of the dermis.

The basement membrane functions in two major ways: (1) it provides an elastic support through the physical tension of its structure, and (2) it may act as a filtration or diffusion barrier, about which little is known regarding normal physiologic function. A role in epidermal nutrition or percutaneous absorption has been speculated. This zone is an important area for skin disease, because many common dermatoses, such as psoriasis, lichen planus, and a number of blistering processes, seem to have a primary origin at this site. Gaps or duplications in the basement membrane structures may also be seen in relationship to certain skin tumors and other pathologic processes. The epidermal cells may be a major primary source of basal

lamina material, and some pathologic changes may be secondary to proliferative or degenerative changes in the basal cell layer of epidermis. The interaction of the epidermis and the immediate underlying mesenchymal tissue may be important in other respects. Growth and wound repair or healing and epidermal stratification appear to depend on an intact basal lamina. In addition, the reconstruction of the epidermis from keratinocytes of all ectodermally derived structures in the skin demonstrates the pluripotentiality of the basal keratinocyte; thus, healing ulcer sites and burns can regenerate from adjacent hair follicle epithelium and possibly from other similar sources.

The bulk of the dermis by weight comprises the interstitial ground substance, which is not stained routinely on normal light microscopy sections and requires special stains for demonstration. The interstitial ground substance may play a major role in water binding and in the maintenance of tissue hydration and turgor. It is also a vehicle for the diffusion of nutrients to vital structures. The hyaluronic acid content of the interstitial ground substance may be an important barrier to infection by preventing bacterial penetration.

The main cell of the epidermis, the "master" cell or fibroblast, is responsible for the synthesis of the main component fibers (i.e., collagen, elastic, and reticular) or unit collagen fibers, in addition to the ground substance. The initial synthesis takes place intracellularly but is completed extracellularly. The synthetic process is orderly; however, the factors governing it are poorly understood. The major fibrous structure, collagen, represents 90% of the dry weight of the entire dermis. Other cell types in the dermis besides the fibroblasts include the fixed tissue histiocyte (macrophage), which has a phagocytic function, and the mast cell, which is normally present about small blood vessels. The mast cell may well have a role in mediating vascular responses and inflammation through release of chemical mediators such as histamine from secretory granules in its cell cytoplasm.

The biologic functions of the dermis are multiple. Because it is a supple, resilient, protective structure which is resistant to tearing, shearing or other local pressures, its major role is providing protection from external injury. The dermis is normally flexible enough to allow joint movement and stretch while the structure of the fibers and ground substance resists compressive forces. Its role in regulatory interactions with the epidermis is poorly understood. The dermis may also have a major role in providing a barrier to infection, mainly through its hyaluronic acid composition, which may also be important in water binding and storage.

Blood supply

The dermal vasculature comprises two main plexuses that parallel the skin surface in the superficial and deeper dermis and are interconnected by perpendicular communicating vessels. Capillary loops, or arcades, extend into the dermal papillae from the superficial dermis. These may be important in disease states and are particularly prominent in common warts. Capillary loops are also noted to have structural alterations in psoriasis. In addition, there is a rich microcirculation of small vessels supplying the skin appendages (such as hair follicles and sweat glands). Larger vessels may be in the subcutaneous fat; however, the bulk of the vessels in the dermis are of papillary, venular, or arteriole size and are essentially a microcirculation. There may be regional differences in blood supply, for example a prominence of capillaries and venules in the superficial dermis of the lower limbs. A specialized vascular structure known as a glomus represents an arteriovenous anastomosis and is present particularly in acral or digital skin, such as the skin of the fingers or toes. These structures are interposed between an arteriole and venule and are surrounded by oval glomus cells that resemble cells of the smooth muscle type. The structure serves as a sphincter, enabling blood to bypass capillaries. This accelerates blood flow through digital skin. The mechanism is largely controlled by the sympathetic (involuntary, autonomic) nervous system.

Functions of the general blood supply basically include thermal regulation, provision of nutrition for the skin, and a role in response to inflammation.

Thermal regulation. Thermal regulation is a cardinal function of the cutaneous vasculature. Homeostatic temperature is maintained by buffering variation in internal and external environmental temperatures. Blood flow is therefore regulated in relation to the temperature at the central body core and the hypothalamus. Temperature is mediated largely by the autonomic or sympathetic nervous system because blood flow can be controlled through constriction of the arterioles. Pharmacologic mediators such as histamine may also play an important role in the regulation of blood flow. The rate of arteriole inflow and the amount of venous drainage is regulated. Metabolic (heat) energy is transferred to the environment from the cutaneous blood vessels by radiation, convection, and evaporation of sweat, which provides a cooling mechanism. The blood supply provides information to higher nervous system centers allowing adjustments of sweating rates and cutaneous blood flow. There may also be more regional autoregulation of sweating mechanisms.

Provision of nutrition for the skin. The rich blood supply about cutaneous appendages helps supply the increased oxidative requirements of these structures. Essential oxygen, nutrients, and hormones may be transported in the blood to the tissues and carbon dioxide and products of metabolism collected for disposal. The endothelium functions as a semipermeable membrane to water and crystalloids to control permeability and consequent tissue transport.

Role in inflammation. Venules have a particularly prominent role in inflammatory states and basic reactions because many of the events in the inflammatory process are controlled at this level. Histamine appears to affect venules by increasing their permeability. Vascular changes in the upper or papillary dermis in diseased states account for clinical changes such as erythema resulting from vascular dilatation.

Lymphatic vessels.

Less information is known about cutaneous lymphatic vessels. There is an elaborate network of lymphatic vessels in the skin, which parallels the major blood vascular plexuses but is independent of them. One end of a lymphatic vessel terminates in a small vein, whereas the other end is blind. The lymphatic system functions to filter and transport capillary transudate (i.e., lymph) and return it to the venous circulation.

Pilosebaceous follicles

The vast majority of hair follicles on the adult human body are of the pilosebaceous type (Figure 54-3). It is important to recognize that external orifices of the hair follicles provide the main point of direct communication between the external environment and the dermis. These pores are vastly more numerous than the visible hairs. Many represent potential sites of hair growth but this rarely occurs except in certain sites. These follicles are present in all body sites except the palms and soles.

Hair is mainly a cosmetic pellage in humans although in lower animals it has other benefits such as heat conservation. The follicle provides an important pathway for the diffusion or absorption of substances introduced from the skin surface. This is discussed further under percutaneous absorption. It must be noted that the upper infundibulum of the follicle has keratinizing epithelium similar to the epidermal surface and may, along with melanocytes, provide an important source of regeneration of epithelium or pigmentation after injury or with wound healing.

The lower level of the infundibulum is marked by the entrance of the sebaceous duct. Below this level a different form of keratinization in root sheath epithelium, trichilemmal keratinization, occurs, which

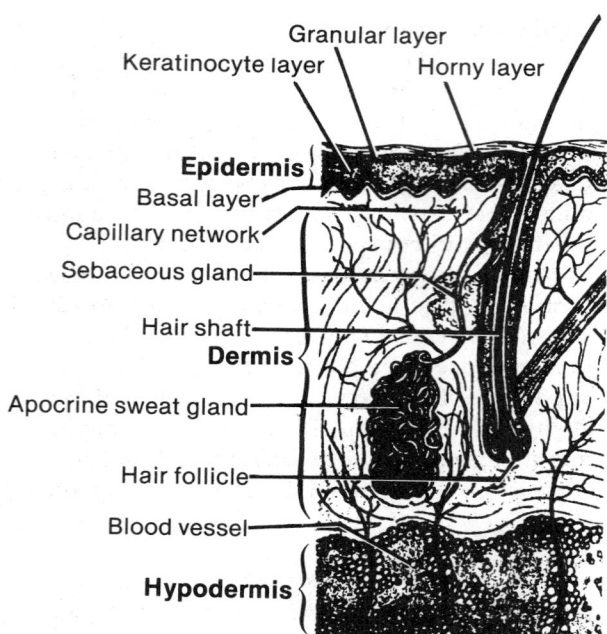

Granular layer
Keratinocyte layer
Horny layer
Epidermis
Basal layer
Capillary network
Sebaceous gland
Hair shaft
Dermis
Apocrine sweat gland
Hair follicle
Blood vessel
Hypodermis

FIGURE 54-4. **Skin adnexal orifices piercing epidermis. Pilosebaceous follicle and eccrine sweat duct unit are the only two structures to normally pierce the epidermis.**

FIGURE 54-3. **Pilosebaceous follicle. Central hair follicle with sebaceous gland attached in center of normal skin. Communication of follicle with external surface is clearly apparent.**

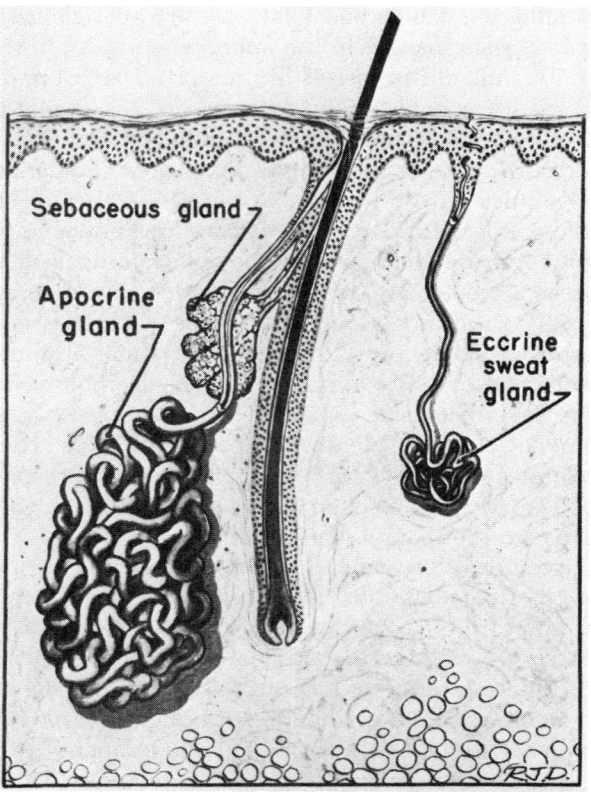

Sebaceous gland
Apocrine gland
Eccrine sweat gland

extends down to the level of the hair erector muscle attachment (arrectores pilorum). This is referred to as the isthmus segment. The smooth muscle, arrectores pilorum, is stimulated to contraction by the autonomic sympathetic nervous system and is responsible for char de poule (goose pimples). The remaining lower portion of the follicle is termed the inferior segment. Hair growth is cyclic and is mainly regulated by androgenic hormonal control. Regional variations of hair growth and cycle are well known.

The majority of sebaceous glands are directly attached to pilosebaceous follicles. Although these glands synthesize lipids, their basic overall function in the skin is unknown. The sebaceous glands are distributed all over the body surface, except for the palms and soles, and are often more numerous on the face and scalp regions.

The sebaceous gland is a holocrine gland under androgenic endocrine regulation. Sebum refers to the composite end product of sebaceous gland secretion and consists of lipids including triglycerides, wax esters, squalene, and cholesterol esters. Acne and other related diseases are disorders of pilosebaceous follicles and not of the sebaceous gland alone. Effective therapy must therefore be directed at the events taking place within the entire follicle, such as obstruction, rather than simple glandular or surface secretion.

Sweat gland units

Eccrine. The other major orifice to pierce the epidermis is the eccrine sweat duct unit, although in contrast to the hair follicle, it cannot be visualized under normal circumstances (Figure 54-4). Approximately 3 million eccrine sweat glands are distributed through the human body (average 143 to 330/cm²). They are present in most sites, except for mucocutaneous junctions, and are absent on the glans penis, clitoris, labia minora, inner surface of the prepuce, and the ears. Eccrine sweat glands are most numerous on the palms, soles, forehead, and axillary region with less density on the arms and legs. They are relatively constant, and no new eccrine sweat gland units are formed after birth.

The eccrine unit comprises a coiled secretory gland, intradermal duct, and a spiral intraepidermal duct (acrosyringium). The gland is innervated by a rich supply of unmyelinated nerve fibers and is most likely under the control of acetylcholine. The main function of the eccrine sweat gland is to make a hypotonic sweat solution that flows to the skin surface for evaporative cooling in times of heat stress.

The concentration of all substances in sweat varies with the rate of perspiration. For example, more sodium is lost at high sweat rates and the concentration of sodium and chloride in sweat is therefore increased. The total sweat can be 2 to 3 L/hour with increased heat stress. Each L of evaporative sweat removes 540 calories of heat from the body. Eccrine sweat is colorless and odorless, and 99% of its weight is water and solutes. It is an acidic secretion with a pH usually ranging from 4.5 to 5.5.

Although sweating may have a poorly understood role in potentiating some forms of skin disease (perhaps by allowing increased absorption of allergens or irritants), its most important physiologic function is in connection with thermal regulation. In this respect, it may flood the surface with its product for evaporative cooling, under primary heat stimuli. The thermostatic mechanism is also under central nervous system hypothalamic control. An increased core or body temperature leads to the stimulation of the hypothalamic centers and increased sweating via cholinergic autonomic nervous system fibers. Exercise will similarly lead to increased sweating. An adaptive role of the sweat gland responses during heat acclimatization is known. In addition, regional heating of the skin can cause an increase in the sweat rate over the heated region, which appears to be a peripheral effect with a possible direct thermal action on the eccrine sweat apparatus. Stimuli other than heat and exercise may also increase sweat responses via nervous system mediation. For example, certain foods increase facial sweating responses (i.e., gustatory response) and quite commonly emotional stress stimulates the sweating response on the palms and soles in addition to the axillary region and other sites.

Apocrine. The less numerous and less important apocrine sweat glands are predominantly concentrated in axillary regions, areolae of the breasts, pubic regions, (e.g., labia, prepuce, scrotum), periumbilical regions, perianal regions, the external ear canal, and the face or scalp regions. The apocrine glands may be free in the dermis or attached to the pilosebaceous follicle by a duct. The apocrine sweat gland apparatus comprises a coiled secretory portion deep in the dermis or subcutaneous fat, and an attached dermal duct portion. The mode of secretion is uncertain; however, it appears to be of decapitation type, with shedding of secretion into the central lumen. The action of bacteria on apocrine secretion reaching the skin surface may account for malodorous body odor; however, the basic physiologic function of the apocrine sweat gland apparatus is unknown.

Nerves

The skin also functions as a major sense organ, a receptor for various stimuli from the environment. The sensations of touch, pressure, temperature, pain, and itch are perceived via skin nerve receptors and pathways. There are millions of microscopic dermal nerve endings throughout the body, particularly prominent in the hairless areas, such as the mucocutaneous regions. Most of these nerve endings are high in the papillary dermis and thus receive stimuli more easily. There is a rich periadenaxal innervation, and hairs may therefore function as sensory structures. Specialized nerve endings, or receptors, may also be present in the dermis or subcutaneous tissue, such as those mediating touch and pressure (i.e., Meissner's or pacinian corpuscles). Most other sensory modalities are thought to be caused by changes in intensity or quality of the stimuli along similar nerve fiber pathways, rather than by other specific receptors.

All nerves supplying the skin come from the spinal cord, except those to the head regions. Transmission to the central nervous system is via the dorsal root ganglia. The autonomic nervous system provides only motor fibers to the skin, with the sympathetic nervous system providing adrenergic influences to control the arterioles and glomus structures of the cutaneous vasculature. These impulses also control the hair erector muscle. Cholinergic fibers appear to mediate eccrine sweating.

Pruritus. Pruritus is a special sensation commonly associated with skin disease, either in a primary or secondary role. Pruritus implies the desire to scratch and has been considered a mild form of pain. Pruritus differs from pain in the speed of impulse transmission or intensity of stimulus. Therapy for pruritus may include the substitution of a competing impulse (such as topical products that impart cooling sensations) or more commonly sedatives or antihistamines, which by their centrally imparted drowsiness effect may inhibit perception of pruritic stimuli and break the scratch-itch cycle.

ASSESSMENT OF THE SKIN
AND APPENDAGES

The skin and appendages are assessed systematically, using inspection and palpation. The skin should be generally inspected in adequate natural light, followed by close inspection and palpation. A regional, cephalocaudal or proximal-distal approach can be used, with comparison between symmetrical parts or areas. Odor and sensory perception should be noted.

Changes in normal skin character can occur as a consequence of such factors as normal aging, exposure to the sun, lack of care, injury, infection, changes in vasculature, disease, and the use of various systemic or topical medications. The skin is an important indicator of overall health and should be assessed carefully.

The skin is assessed for color, temperature, texture, moisture, the presence of lesions or past and present injuries and for any other distinguishing marks, including stains, needle marks, and insect bites. Skin care and grooming of hair and nails should be carefully assessed. Healthy skin should be of normal color, smooth, supple, and resilient. It should be clean and not excessively dry or moist, and free from rashes, bruises, excoriations, lacerations, ulcers, or other abnormal conditions.

Color and pigmentation

Normal skin color ranges from whitish pink to brown or black depending on race. Vascular flush areas (e.g., cheeks, upper chest) and pigment labile areas (e.g., face, axillas, genital area) may vary in color from the general skin color. There is increased pigmentation of areola and genitalia. Alterations in normal patterns of pigmentation should be noted, including hypopigmentation (e.g., complete or partial lack of melanin as occurs in albinism), depigmentation (e.g., vitiligo, which can be localized or generalized), or hyperpigmentation (e.g., tan to brown patchy areas on the forehead, cheeks, and bridge of the nose or other patchy areas that can occur as a result of pregnancy, use of oral contraceptives, phenytoin ingestion, or in such conditions as Addison's disease in which the mucous membranes can also be involved; or lentigines, which are small, flat, light to dark brown lesions on exposed skin occurring at any age but generally associated with aging or chronic sun exposure).

The presence of vascular-related skin discoloration, varicosities and enlarged blood vessels should also be identified. An increased total amount of hemoglobin, an increase in reduced hemoglobin, or capillary stasis can cause the skin to appear red-blue in color. Dusky blue tinged skin, cyanosis, can be observed especially circumorally and at the nail beds. Dark blue tinged skin may indicate inadequate circulation, especially in the extremities. Localized areas of hemorrhagic discoloration may indicate purpura, ecchymosis, or possible underlying hematoma. Jaundice or pallor may also be noted.

Color changes in individuals with dark skin are often difficult to assess. The conjunctiva and sclera, lips, tongue, buccal mucosa, nailbeds, palms, and soles should be inspected for subtle changes in color. Blotchy, uneven color of exposed skin areas in the elderly can be observed as a result of a decrease in the number of melanocytes that occurs with normal aging, giving the skin a faded yellow appearance. This appearance may mask or be mistaken for jaundice. Prolonged skin exposure over many years characteristically produces degeneration of the collagen and elastic tissue in the dermis of sun-exposed areas and imparts a yellowish waxy appearance. This is usually more obvious in individuals with fair complexions. Edema of the skin can cause the skin to appear blanched, puffy, taut, shiny, or distended when compared with surrounding or symmetrical skin areas. It can involve the face, eyes, area of injury, dependent areas, or it can be generalized. Edema can mask the color of melanin and hemoglobin and also obscure the appearance of jaundice.

Temperature

Palpation is used to assess skin temperature, moisture, and texture. Skin temperature is assessed with the back of the hand. Cold or cool skin can be generalized as occurs with shock or localized as a result of loss of circulation to an area. Warm or hot skin can also be generalized as in a fever, or localized indicating inflammation or infection.

Texture

Texture of the skin should be supple, flexible, pliable, and elastic. Skin resilience or turgor should be present. Turgor can be increased in states of tension or decreased in states of dehydration. Turgor is also diminished as a result of normal aging because of the loss of subcutaneous tissue stores, especially in the hands and arms. Because of this, the cheeks or abdomen should be used to assess turgor in the elderly. The thigh or abdomen can be used in infants. Loss of elasticity characteristically occurs in skin damaged by prolonged sun exposure. Loss of elasticity around blood vessels in the dermis leads to more easy bruising with minor trauma and may be a major factor in the common occurrence of senile purpura in the elderly. Dryness of the skin can result from dehydration, aging, decreased environmental temperature and humidity. Skin may appear dry, rough, flaky, and less flexible. Cracking and the development of fissures can be observed. The fineness or coarseness of skin can also be affected by local irritation or trauma as well as by disease state. Skin can be excessively soft and smooth as a result of hyperthyroidism and can be dry and rough as a result of hypothyroidism.

Moisture

The moisture of the skin should be assessed. The skin may be dry, oily, moist, or clammy. Increased skin moisture can occur with increased environmental temperature and humidity, febrile states, or conditions such as shock. Strenuous work or exercise can increase skin moisture. Increased oiliness of skin areas can be related to hormonal changes (particularly during adolescence) or possibly suggest endocrine problems. The general moisture status should be assessed on skin other than the palms, soles, axillary regions, or forehead, which may more commonly be altered in conditions of stress or environmental humidity.

Lesions

Characteristic patterns of lesions can be present at birth (e.g., congenital nevus), or associated more commonly with various age groups. Lesions can be flat or raised, pigmented or nonpigmented, and of various colors. They are described in relation to the pattern of distribution, configuration, symmetry, and morphologic structure. The duration and progression of the lesion should be ascertained and the presence of associated itching, stinging, burning, or other discomfort or sensation. The presence or absence of associated lesions such as mucous membrane involvement may be important in diagnosis.

The distribution of lesions can be localized or generalized. Lesions can occur at pressure sites, intertriginous areas or exposed areas. Certain cutaneous disease states have characteristic patterns or areas of involvement. The configuration of the lesion may be annular, herpetiform, isolated, grouped, linear, polycyclic, reticular, or zosteriform. The morphologic structure can be primary (e.g., macule, papule, nodule, vesicle, bulla, pustule, or wheal) or secondary (e.g., scale, crust, erosion, scar, or fissure). Stages of primary lesions or the presence of various forms of primary and secondary lesions should be identified and measured carefully. It is important to particularly note the change or evolution of lesions with time, and whether the lesions have been modified in appearance by excoriation or therapeutic agents. Self-medication with various topical agents is common and may mask var-

ious essential signs or changes or produce adverse effects. Improper application or noncompliance with prescribed topical therapy, or incorrect diagnosis, may be suspected if lesions worsen with time or do not heal. Because various skin lesions are usually treated topically, it is important that the nurse understand the percutaneous absorption of medications administered by this route.

Hair

The hair should be inspected and palpated carefully because characteristics of quantity, distribution, and quality can indicate much about the patient's health state.

Quantity and distribution. Wide variations in the patterns and amount of hair growth can be observed normally among different individuals and racial groups. Changes characteristically also occur with age and are influenced by hormonal control. Growth of axillary and pubic hair in both sexes and the male beard depends on androgenic hormones, and abnormalities of hair growth in these sites, usually apparent as lack of growth or diffuse loss, can be signs of underlying endocrine disease. Some systemic medications may also influence patterns of hair growth.

Abnormalities of quantity usually present as excessive hair growth (hirsutism) or loss of hair (alopecia). Hirsutism is a term more commonly applied clinically to female patients with excessive hair growth in an adult male pattern of distribution. The beard or upper lip regions are characteristically involved and not uncommonly the limbs and chest area. The majority of these women do not have overt underlying endocrine disease and may be classed as having idiopathic hirsutism. Many of these women have a familial background of hirsutism. Underlying endocrine disease is more suspect if there are other signs of masculinization and major menstrual irregularities.

Alopecia is a term more commonly applied to the scalp and is most characteristically seen at that site. Alopecia is commonly classified into scarring or nonscarring categories of possible cause depending on the status of the involved scalp in the area of hair loss. Most cases of alopecia are nonscarring and are diffuse. These include the common and physiologic male pattern androgenic alopecia—or common male baldness—and the less usual but common female pattern androgenic alopecia. Other causes of diffuse nonscarring alopecia include examples of telogen effluvium, which produce reversible hair loss resulting from sudden changes in the normal hair growth cycle precipitated by severe illness, shock, major operations, or recent pregnancy. Characteristically the hair loss occurs 3 months after the precipitating event and subsequently regrows over the subsequent months. This is in contrast to anagen effluvium induced characteristically by chemotherapeutic agents, which halt hair growth during the growing (anagen) phase and lead to rather quick onset of diffuse alopecia. Other possible causes of diffuse nonscarring alopecia may be systemic drugs (e.g., anticoagulants), endocrine disease, collagen vascular disease, secondary syphilis, and crash diets with marked protein restriction.

Localized areas of nonscarring alopecia may also be present. Alopecia areata is the most common and characteristic entity and produces circumscribed, well-defined, noninflammatory alopecia of the scalp, beard area, eyebrows or eyelashes. It is normally expected to be reversible with time.

Causes of scarring alopecia include discoid lupus erythematosus, lichen planopilaris, and pseudopelade. *Tinea capitis* infection (scalp ringworm), usually seen in children, or excoriations secondary to pediculosis may produce some scarring. Trauma, burns, and tumors of the scalp may also produce localized areas of alopecia. Patches of stubble and broken hairs or hair loss can result from trichitillomania, hair pulling, or excessive scratching of the scalp. Once true scarring has occurred, the hair loss is usually irreversible.

Quality. When hair quality is assessed, the color and texture should be noted. The resiliency and ease of extraction from scalp can also be noted. Many possible abnormalities of the hair shaft structure may occur but are less often of clinical significance. Some of the hair shaft abnormalities, however, may be diagnostic clues to uncommon underlying genetic and metabolic abnormalities, such as Menke's kinky hair syndrome with copper deficiency and neurologic changes. Some of the patients with hair shaft abnormalities fracture the hairs readily, which may lead to varying degrees of alopecia.

Color and texture can be affected by such factors as illness, nutrition, sun exposure, or more specific genetic syndromes such as albinism. Hair dye may be a more obvious cause of color alteration, and various cosmetic procedures or products may affect color or texture. Endocrine disease such as thyroid dysfunction can also affect hair texture. Hypothyroidism may result in increased dryness and coarseness, and hyperthyroidism can cause increased silkiness or fineness of the hair.

Nails

The nail structures, including the nail plate, lateral and posterior folds, cuticle, and underlying nailbed surface, should be carefully inspected and palpated.

The nail plate is usually firm, rectangular, and convex, with the free edge continuous with the cuticle. The nail plate is usually thicker in men than women, and approximately 0.3 to 0.6 mm thick with a smooth and regular surface. The nail plate should be semitransparent presenting the color of the underlying nailbed. The angle between the nail plate and proximal portion of the digit should be 160 degrees. Varying in size, the lunula is usually present, especially on the thumb, but can be absent, especially in the elderly. The lunula may have a bluish hue in darker-skinned patients.

Abnormalities can be noted in nail plate shape, curvature, adhesion to the nailbed, thickness, surface texture, growth rate, and color. The skin folds around the nail plate should also be carefully assessed for the presence of abnormalities.

Shape and curvature. The nail plate can be completely absent in some individuals (anonychia). The missing nail plate is usually a congenital defect, but the loss may be associated with injury or disease. Platyonychia, or flattening of the curvature of the nail plate, may be observed, which can also be hereditary. This can lead to koilonychia, or spoon nail. In this condition, the nail is concave or spoon shaped with the lateral edges turning upward, and may be opaque or white as well. The concave portion is usually fragile. It is a condition associated most characteristically with hypochromic anemia, but may be familial on occasion. Thinning of the nail plate with some curvature may occur with chronic eczema, which often produces a shiny polished appearance to the nails from repeated rubbing or scratching associated with the eczema. Other causes include chronic infection, malnutrition, Raynaud's disease, peripheral vascular disease, or a tumor of the nailbed.

Changes in nail plate adhesion. Separation of the nail plate from the nailbed with an increased free edge can often occur from the nailbed progressing proximally from the free edge (onycholysis), or much less commonly from the roof of the nailbed to the free edge (onychomadesis).

Onycholysis is most commonly caused by trauma, psoriasis, or fungal infection, but it can be congenital. It may also occur on sun exposure in patients receiving oral tetracycline therapy, but the incidence is low.

Changes in nail plate thickness. Thinning can occur as a result of deficient peripheral circulation or nutritional anemias. The nail can also be brittle as a result of nutritional anemias, impaired peripheral circulation, and likely most commonly with prolonged exposure to water or alkaline substances, with dehydration of the nail plate.

Thickening of the nail plate can occur as a result of trauma, defective vascular supply, or as a result of psoriasis or fungal infections. Thickening of the nail plate associated with increased length and curvature is termed onychogryphosis. The cause of this common condition is often uncertain but may be associated with prior injury to the site. Simple overcurvature of the distal nail plate is often induced by improper fitting and cramped footwear. Finger clubbing resulting in an increased angle (often greater than 180 degrees) between the nail and the posterior nailfold can occur in conditions such as chronic obstructive pulmonary disease, lung cancer, cirrhosis, or cardiac disease associated with prolonged hypoxemia. The nail plate thickens, becoming hard and shiny with a curved free end. The matrix atrophies, increasing the angle to 180 degrees, flattening the nail. When palpated, the nailbed feels spongy especially when clubbing is severe. The distal phalanx becomes enlarged with time, and in severe cases there is bony periosteal thickening.

Changes in nail texture and surface. Various degrees of ridging of the nails are common and often unexplained. At times they are secondary to abnormalities of the proximal nail fold and nailbed such as chronic dermatitis. Lesions such as mucous cysts at the proximal nail fold may induce longitudinal grooves or depressions along the length of the nail plate. A common surface alteration is the presence of fine pitting in the nail plate. This is most characteristically seen with psoriatic nail involvement but may be seen with other conditions such as alopecia areata. Subungual hyperkeratosis, in addition to pitting and onycholysis, is also a common sign associated with psoriasis.

Transverse depressions on the nail plate, known as Beau's lines, are caused by temporary interference with nail formation. They are often seen involving all the fingers and toes. They may occur with any severe illness and are particularly common after septic shock. More recently, they have been reported with zinc deficiency. Since a fingernail usually grows at a rate of approximately 1 mm per week, the location of Beau's lines may indicate the approximate date of the preceding severe illness.

Changes in nail color. Various color changes in the nails or nailbed have been described in connection with systemic disease or occasionally systemic drugs. In other instances local factors such as fungus infection (whitish yellow), *Pseudomonas* infection (green or blue-black), psoriasis (yellowish or brown or "oil

droplet" appearance) or local stains or dyes, may produce a color change.

Leukonychia may be seen commonly in varying degrees. Punctate white spots are common and often unexplained. Congenital leukonychia is uncommon. More complete white nail coloration may be seen with cirrhosis of the liver, and crescent-shaped white transverse stripes (Mees-lines) may be seen with chronic arsenic poisoning. Paired narrow white bands parallel to the lunula may be observed with hypoalbuminemia. The nailbed, however, is affected in this instance, not the nail plate, and this may also be true in whitening associated with cirrhosis of the liver.

Some systemic drugs can cause nail color changes. Chloroquine may produce blue-black pigmentation of the nailbeds, and other antimalarial drugs may also cause color changes in the nailbed or nail plate. Fixed drug eruption to phenolphthalein (in some laxatives most commonly) or tetracycline may produce a dark blue or brown coloration.

Other color changes include the "half and half" nail in renal disease with azotemia, with whitening of the proximal nailbed and a change to red, pink, or brown in the distal half. A distinctive yellow coloration may be seen with lymphedema. Azure coloration may be seen with Wilson's disease. Miscellaneous color changes include splinter hemorrhages, which are common and if situated near the distal plate margin are most often of traumatic etiology. They are less often seen as a reliable manifestation of subacute bacterial endocarditis. Tumors of the nailbed may also produce color changes including malignant melanoma, usually with a brown or black longitudinal coloration. Subungual hematoma is a common cause of color change usually producing blackish red coloration.

Skin folds. The skin folds around the nail including the proximal margin and cuticle should be assessed for the presence or absence of skin disease such as eczema or psoriasis, which may also induce changes in the nail plate. The nail folds should be smooth and of the same general color as the skin. Periungual telangiectasia or erythema may be a sign of collagen vascular disease, and the cuticles are often significantly roughened in dermatomyositis. Growths or tumors may be common adjacent to nails. Periungual warts are common and tend to be more persistent and refractory to therapy. Mucous cysts are common at the base of the nail and often cause longitudinal depressions in the nail plate because of pressure on the nail matrix. Inflammatory changes associated with ingrown toenails or paronychial infections are common. This is more common in diabetics with secondary *Candida* infection. Organisms cultured are often mixed flora but may include *Pseudomonas*, staphyloccal, or streptococcal pathogenic bacteria. A history of recurrent erythema and swelling, with or without overt blistering, at the same periungual site may suggest herpetic whitlow caused by herpes simplex virus.

PERCUTANEOUS ABSORPTION

Knowledge of the principles underlying the absorption of ingredients through the skin is necessary for a fundamental understanding of topical drug therapy.

Stratum corneum

The epidermis, or precisely the stratum corneum, as the main barrier to absorption normally fulfills the vital function of limiting free passage of fluid and electrolytes to the outside environment, thus conserving body water. By analogy, the barrier also limits the entry of toxins or chemicals, including those used for therapeutic purposes.

The rate-limiting barrier in the epidermis is the stratum corneum, which is an effective but not complete two-way barrier. The diffusion of molecules through this layer is purely passive. The barrier is not entirely complete, because there is some selective transport of certain molecules. Pharmacologic effectiveness in topical therapy depends on the active therapeutic ingredient being absorbed in sufficient quantity, and without alteration, to exert a therapeutic effect. Once transport across the stratum corneum has taken place, there is little impediment to transport across the remainder of the epidermis into the dermis.

The relative impermeability of the stratum corneum is approximately 1000 times greater than the dermis. This superficial layer averages 15 μ in total thickness, and its component anucleate cells average 30 μ in width and 0.8 μ in depth. The component cells have thicker plasma membranes than their metabolically active nucleated counter parts in the remainder of the epidermis (200 Å versus 75 to 100 Å). The lipoprotein membrane, of approximately 15% lipid, imparts the characteristic of semipermeability. Thus removal of lipids from the membrane destroys its barrier properties.

Normally the stratum corneum permits a continuous controlled transepidermal loss of water by the diffusion of 100 to 150 ml per day under normal environment conditions. There is also 300 to 500 ml lost per day through insensible sweating. This water loss contributes to the hydration of the stratum corneum. The relative humidity of ambient air exposed to the stratum corneum is most important in skin hydration.

Since the water content increases with humidity, it can rise to 70% hydration at 100% humidity, whereas it is only 10% to 20% at 60% humidity. With the increasing humidity the stratum corneum can absorb 6 times its own weight in water and thus increase its thickness from 15 to 45 μ. The hydration and water binding property are related to increasing permeability and diffusion of molecules through the hydrated epidermis.

Transepidermal transport is governed by physical-chemical laws, such as modifications of Fick's law of mass transport expressed as $J = \dfrac{Km \times Dm \times \Delta Cs}{L}$ where J represents the flux or flow, Dm is the diffusion constant, Km is the roughly parallel permeability constant, and ΔCs is the concentration gradient representing the concentration of ingredients on either side of the barrier. L represents the length of the diffusion path, or translated to percutaneous absorption; it represents the thickness of the stratum corneum. The diffusion constant reflects the inherent diffusibility and mobility of a molecule in a membrane and is the opposite of resistance to transport. Km, the partition coefficient, applies to molecules in solution other than water. It describes how many solute molecules are available for diffusion through a membrane and is expressed as the ratio of solubility of a solute in the diffusing membrane and in its solvent. Thus if Km is higher for a given solute, it will leave its solvent (e.g., H_2O) more easily and display more affinity for the diffusing membrane (lipid). The denominator of the equation is perhaps the easiest aspect to understand because flow and overall permeability are thus proportional to the thickness of the stratum corneum. It is therefore easier to understand the simple fact of increased absorption from the thinner skin of the eyelids, face, or skin creases than from the thicker skin of the palms or soles. The entire equation is more reliable at low concentrations and when diffusion has reached a steady state. Other variables may also be important, however, including the electrical forces between molecules, frictional forces, and temperature.

Pathways of transport. There are three possible pathways of transport through the stratum corneum. These include the transcellular path, diffusion through pilosebaceous units and sweat gland orifices, and the intercellular route.

Transcellular path. This route represents the major transport pathway under normal steady state condition and the bulk diffusion through the horny cell layer. Lipid soluble substances penetrate the lipid containing cell membranes and matrix, and polar, water-soluble molecules gain access to the protein fraction of the stratum corneum and cross the lipid barrier between protein molecules. The substances then diffuse through water-logged pores, or openings 10 Å in diameter, which are lined by keratin molecules. These pores or channels enlarge when hydrated and can lead to increased diffusion.

Diffusion through pilosebaceous units and sweat gland orifices. This pathway is occasionally referred to as shunt diffusion as opposed to bulk diffusion of the major transcellular route. Their surface cutaneous openings represent $\frac{1}{1,000}$ to $\frac{1}{10,000}$ of the total surface area of the skin. The stratum corneum invests only the superficial parts of these orifices, and there is little hindrance to transport in the deeper portions of these structures. Only a relatively small number of diffusing molecules are absorbed through this route, but it may be more important in the first 5 minutes of transport before the steady state is reached, mainly because of the more rapid absorption at this time. This route may also be more important in absorption of molecules with low permeability constants, such as polar steroids and larger molecules.

Intercellular route. This potential route is likely of lesser clinical significance but may have a role in electrolyte transport. The potential pathway is between cell substances, such as electrolytes, that are largely insoluble in lipid membranes.

Factors altering transport. There are numerous factors that can alter transport. These include mass or concentration, hydration, choice of vehicle, anatomic site, the nature and severity of the skin condition or disease, local circulation, and other variables.

Mass or concentration. Absorption of molecules applied to the skin is largely proportional to the concentration or mass, but usually only to a critical peak point, after which the relationship is unreliable or ineffective. There is thus a limit to the effective concentration of topical preparations.

Hydration. Maximum hydration of the epidermis is followed by a fivefold increase in permeability. Hydration of the stratum corneum increases the diffusion path and leads to an increased permeability constant of both polar and nonpolar molecules. In addition, occlusion significantly increases the hydration of cornified cells by trapping water of insensible water loss and increasing the skin temperature.

Paradoxically, dehydration also increases absorption by damaging the physical structure of the skin barrier. Thus if the water content of the stratum corneum is less than 10%, it becomes brittle and cracks readily. This occurs particularly at environmental conditions of low temperature and low humidity and is more prone to occur in aging and chronically sun-

damaged skin and with excessive use of soap and water.

Choice of vehicle. The choice of vehicle or solvent may be particularly important in the overall effect on the absorption of topically applied substances. The partition coefficient (Km) or relative partition of molecules between solute and solvent is affected by the nature of the vehicle, as is diffusibility in the membrane and the ease of release of the active ingredient from its contained solvent. The occlusive nature of the vehicle may be critical because it could increase the permeability through increasing hydration; thus there may be greater inherent penetration with ointments than other common vehicles.

Anatomic site (regional variation). The thickness of skin, or particularly stratum corneum may vary significantly in different sites, and absorption is generally inversely proportional to this factor. Thus there is greater ease of absorption in thinner cutaneous sites such as the eyelid, face, and scrotum, and consequently decreased ease of absorption on thicker skin sites such as the palms and soles. In addition, the number of adnexal orifices at different sites may be of importance, particularly where the shunt diffusion route (through pilosebaceous units and sweat gland orifices) of absorption is important. This applies particularly to hairy sites. The ease of application and contact of preparations to such sites may also be of importance. Ointments are generally not used in such areas, whereas gels may have greater application and more effective contact without complications.

Nature and severity of skin disease. Epidermal involvement by skin disease, whether it be psoriasis or dermatitis, may alter barrier function. Thus topical medications, such as topical corticosteroids, may be more effective earlier in the disease with a defective or reduced skin barrier, and less efficient as the barrier heals.

Local circulation. Local hyperemia may contribute to increased absorption by enhancing the removal of diffusing molecules and therefore producing a greater concentration gradient. Both blood supply and the degree of blood flow may vary with anatomic sites, temperature, and other control mechanisms.

Other variables. The stratum corneum barrier may be damaged through the desired therapeutic effect, such as with keratolytic agents. These may enhance absorption through physical damage to the skin barrier. Many compounds, particularly in polar solvents, may chemically alter the horny layer, especially with prolonged use, and therefore increase permeability. Surfactants, such as soaps or detergent formulation in many compounds, bring diffusing substances into closer contact with the stratum corneum; however with prolonged use they may contribute to barrier damage. Added vehicular substances, such as propylene glycol or DMSO, are known to enhance absorption. DMSO is a polar hygroscopic solvent, soluble in both water and lipids, that can function to significantly increase the hydration of the stratum corneum and enhance permeability; however, the in vivo effect may be short lived, and a garlic odor produced on the breath may decrease compliance.

Particle size may be of importance because smaller molecules generally display faster transport. Higher temperature generally enhances absorption through increased molecular motion of diffusing substances. Viscosity is inversely proportional to absorption, and electrical impedance and resistance resides in the stratum corneum; thus factors diminishing this resistance lead to increased permeability.

In addition, the stratum corneum barrier may function as a reservoir for lipid soluble materials such as topical corticosteroids, and continuing release can theoretically significantly affect overall absorption.

TOPICAL THERAPY

The ideal topical agent has been suggested to demonstrate a lack of the three "S's": stench, stain, and sting, in addition to fulfilling the expected therapeutic benefit of the compound.

Many other variables, however, are potentially inherent in the clinical use of the myriad of different topical preparations. Many of these variables are outlined under percutaneous absorption. The ideal vehicle or base has not yet been produced; however, the basic formulation, whether cream, ointment, lotion, gel, or other preparation, may have significant influence on clinical application, compliance, efficacy, and incidence of adverse side effects. The different vehicles or bases, in addition to other additives, stabilizers, and preservatives in the product, may all affect the desired results or influence potential complications. Adequate controlled assessment of the numerous topical products available, either as over-the-counter or prescription items, is generally lacking. In addition, few compounds have been subjected to rigid double-blind controlled studies in situations of clinical use. Reports of benefit are often anecdotal and without valid scientific support. Much of the problem in conducting and assessing these topical therapeutic studies is caused by the number of variables that may have significant effect on such studies. These include particularly compliance, use of other concomitant products, altered environmental conditions, and altered con-

ditions of assessment (including normal versus abnormal skin, presence or absence of occlusion, and other similar factors).

In addition, pharmacokinetic data are greatly limited for topical therapeutic compounds, and there is little reliable information on dosage, particularly in quantitative terms. Absolute dosage equivalents for many preparations are not available, which causes a great deal of empirical therapy, often based largely on clinical experience. In general, dosage requirements are lower in small children because of the greater surface area to volume or weight ratio. Because of this increased ratio, topically applied compounds, as long as they are absorbed efficiently, tend to result in higher concentrations of the ingredients in extracellular fluid; therefore the risk that systemic effects may occur is greater. As the skin barrier is also thinner in infants and children, absorption is not usually hindered.

At the other end of the scale, absorption may be enhanced in aged skin, because of the effects of aging and chronic damage to the skin barrier. Less information is available regarding the precise effects of other variables, such as sundamaged skin and the general physiologic status of the patient.

SUMMARY

The major aspects of cutaneous structure and function have been presented with emphasis on those features influencing topical therapy. Many potential variables may influence topical therapy, particularly as they affect percutaneous absorption. These variables may be mainly patient, skin, or drug related; thus assessment of the skin and factors affecting therapy is essential. An understanding of the basic principles of topical therapy should enable the nurse to make decisions regarding topical care and improve patient care. Although there is a great lack of adequate scientifically controlled data on the many products in current use, through detailed assessment and monitoring, nurses can readily contribute in the development of knowledge for the promotion and maintenance of healthy skin.

BIBLIOGRAPHY

Ackerman, A.B. The structure and function of the skin, I. Development morphology and physiology. In S.L. Mosclella, D.M. Pillsbury, H.J. Hurley (Eds.), *Dermatology* (Vol. 1). Philadelphia: W.B. Saunders Co., 1975.

Braverman, I.M., & Yen, A. Ultrastructure of the human dermal microcirculation: I. The horizontal plexus of the papillary dermis. *Journal of Investigative Dermatology*, 1976, 66, 131-142.

Braverman, I.M., & Yen, A. Ultrastructure of the human dermal microcirculation: II. The capillary loops of the dermal papillae. *Journal of Investigative Dermatology,* 1977, *68,* 44-52.

Brody, N. Ultrastructure of the stratum corneum. *International Journal of Dermatology,* 1977, *16*(4), 245-256.

Fukuyama, K., Inoue, N., Suzuki, H., & Epstein, W.L. Keratinization. *International Journal of Dermatology,* 1976, *15,* 473-487.

Heaphy, M.R., & Winkelmann, R.K. The human cutaneous basement membrane anchoring fibril complex: Preparation and ultrastructure. *Journal of Investigative Dermatology,* 1977, *68,* 177.

Herndon, J.H. Itching: the pathophysiology of pruritus. *International Journal of Dermatology,* 1975, *14,* 465.

Hodge, S.J., & Freeman, R.G. Review: The basal lamina in skin disease. *International Journal of Dermatology,* 1978, *17*(4), 261-279.

Jimbow, K., Quevedo, W.C., Fitzpatrick, T.B., & Szabo, G. Some aspects of melanin biology 1950-1975. *Journal of Investigative Dermatology,* 1976, *67,* 72-89.

Lever, W.F., & Schaumberg-Lever, G. *Histopathology of the Skin* (5th ed.). Philadelphia, Toronto: J.B. Lippincott, 1975.

Matolsky, A.G. Desmosomes, filaments, and keratohyalin granules: their role in the stabilization and keratinization of the epidermis. *Journal of Investigative Dermatology,* 1975, *65,* 127.

Scheuplein, R.J. Mechanism of percutaneous absorption: II. Transient diffusion and the relative importance of various routes of skin penetration. *Journal of Investigative Dermatology,* 1977, *48,* 79-88.

Silberberg-Sinakin, I. On Langerhans cells. Commentary. *International Journal of Dermatology,* 1977, *16*(7), 581-583.

Stingl, G. New aspects of Langerhans cell function. *International Journal of Dermatology,* 1980, *19*(4), 189-213.

Strauss, J.S., Pochi, P.E., & Downing, D.T. The sebaceous gland. *Journal of Investigative Dermatology,* 1976, *67,* 90-97.

Weinstein, G.D. On the cell cycle of psoriasis. *British Journal of Dermatology,* 1975, *92,* 229.

Winthroub, B.V. Inflammation and mediators: review. *International Journal of Dermatology,* 1980, *19*(8), 436-442.

Wright, N. Review: Cell population kinetics in human epidermis. *International Journal of Dermatology,* 1977, *16,* 449-463.

Antiseptics and Local Anesthetics

Eric Schloss

Medications discussed in this chapter

Antiseptics	Local anesthetics
Alcohol	Articaine
Benzalkonium chloride	Bupivacaine
Cetrimide	Chloroprocaine
Chlorhexidine	Dibucaine
Gentian violet	Etidocaine
Hexachlorophene	Lidocaine
Hydrogen peroxide	Mepivacaine
Iodine	Piperocaine
Iodochlorhydroxyquin	Prilocaine
Isopropyl alcohol	Procaine
Mercuric oxide, yellow	Proparacaine
Mercury, ammoniated	Tetracaine
Phenol	
Povidone-iodine	
Silver nitrate	
Thimerosal	

Antiseptics

Antiseptics by definition are chemical compounds applied to tissues to destroy or inhibit the growth of microorganisms. By convention, use of the term *disinfectant* is restricted to substances used on inanimate objects to destroy microorganisms by chemical or physical means. These agents are not discussed in this section, except in the context that some disinfectants may also function as antiseptics in appropriately dilute concentration. Other classes of topical agents used to inhibit or destroy specific infectious agents, such as antibiotics, antifungal agents, scabicides, and pediculicides, are discussed in chapters found in Sections IX and X of this text.

CELLULAR ACTION

Generally antiseptics act on microorganism cells by *coagulation* or denaturation of protoplasmic protein, by cell *lysis* via membrane alteration, or by enzyme inactivation through oxidation or denaturation. The effect may be simply to inhibit microorganism growth or to eradicate irreversibly the unwanted offender. Ideally the latter is desired, and this should be achieved without harming the host's living tissues. However, all antiseptics are general antiprotoplasmic agents, which tend to have a variable and limited range of action. The ideal antiseptic has not yet been developed.

CLINICAL USE

Desirable properties of antiseptics include the following.
1. A microbiologic action spectrum desired for a particular clinical situation
2. Rapidity of onset and sustained action
3. Effectiveness of action (preferably bactericidal rather than bacteriostatic)
4. Ability to resist interference by organic matter (e.g., exudate, blood, and pus) and by other compounds (e.g., soaps)
5. A low surface tension
6. A good therapeutic index (safety margin relating effective concentration and toxicity)
7. The avoidance of allergenicity
8. The esthetic avoidance of the three "S's": sting, stain, and stench
9. Reasonable low cost
10. Stability of the compound in container and on the shelf

There has been a general tendency to limit use of antiseptics to a preventive role on intact skin and mucosa or to a minor role in cleaning wounds. Antiseptics should not be considered as suitable substitutes for proper mechanical cleansing, *debridement*, and irrigation and drainage of obviously contaminated wounds. They do not have a primary positive role in usual wound healing. There is also little evidence to substantiate a principal role for specific topical antiseptics in skin *pyodermas*, including *impetigo*.

VARIABLES

In relation to the desirable properties listed above, the overall effectiveness of antiseptics can be influenced by many factors: the contact time with the organism, pH, temperature, presence of organic matter, and compatibilities with other compounds such as soaps. Pharmacokinetic data are limited for most compounds, and experimental data on effective concentrations and results may not be reliable in clinical situations. Reliable comparison data of various antiseptics are also limited, particularly in relation to specific clinical problems, such as cutaneous infections or impetigo.

ALIPHATIC ALCOHOLS

Ethyl and isopropyl alcohol are most widely used and exert a variable microbiocidal effect roughly in proportion to their lipid solubility. They are often used to reduce local flora before venipuncture or injections via the skin, and also commonly as preoperative washes. Aliphatic alcohols are effective against a broad spectrum of bacteria. The alcohols evaporate quickly and therefore generally have a drying effect on the skin, with negligible *percutaneous absorption* occurring. They are flammable agents, occasionally irritating but nonstaining.

Alcohol (ethyl alcohol)

Alcohol acts quickly with a bactericidal action resulting from a coagulation of protein. It can be used against a reasonably broad spectrum of bacteria, but has relatively low potency and short duration of action because of evaporation. The 70% aqueous solution is often used and appears to reduce the *surface tension* of bacteria better than the undiluted alcohol. Unreliable against fungi or viruses, alcohol is generally avoided in open wounds because of its potential for irritating tissue with consequent stinging or burning pain. Rubbing alcohol, which contains 70% by volume of alcohol, is generally used as a *rubefacient* agent. Denaturing agents are commonly added (e.g., tartar emetic, quinine, or salicylic acid) to minimize toxicity of accidental oral ingestion (by imparting a bitter or undesirable quality to the compound and minimizing potential absorption or tissue exposure), without adversely altering antiseptic action. Occasionally coloring matter is added, such as methylene blue, to additionally minimize risk of accidental ingestion. Other potential complications are dehydration of skin if used in high concentrations, or irritation if left on for prolonged periods. Rarely allergic contact dermatitis occurs.

Isopropyl alcohol

Isopropyl alcohol has a slightly greater bactericidal activity than alcohol (ethyl alcohol) in concentrations greater than 70%, but otherwise has generally a similar effect. It has increased fat-solvent properties, and repeated use leads to more drying action than alcohol. Isopropyl rubbing alcohol is commonly used as a rubefacient.

HALOGENATED COMPOUNDS

Chlorinated compounds

These potent germicidal compounds now have little use as antiseptics because of tissue irritation and have been replaced by better, less toxic compounds. They are still commonly used as disinfectants in the various forms of hypochlorite solution. Elemental chlorine has no medical use.

Preparations

Sodium hypochlorite solution. This compound is prepared under various names, including Dakin's solution, and acts as a potent germicide used to disinfect utensils. The undiluted solution contains 5% sodium hypochlorite.

Sodium hypochlorite solution, dilute. This more dilute hypochlorite solution, known as modified Dakin's solution, contains 0.45% to 0.5% sodium hypochlorite and may be diluted 1:3.

Problems. These solutions are relatively unstable and must be freshly prepared for effective use. They are generally too irritating to skin for use as antiseptics, and also may cause problems by dissolving clots and delaying clotting. There is a toxicity hazard with accidental ingestion, probably more commonly seen with household bleach, which should be properly stored and labeled and kept out of reach of children. The solution is noncorrosive externally, but may be severely irritating and burning to mucous membranes.

Iodine compounds

These compounds comprise (1) solutions containing elemental iodine, (2) iodine-releasing organic compounds (iodophors), and (3) halogenated 8 hydroxyquinolones. The latter compounds are considered separately. Most often iodine solutions or iodophors are used as skin antiseptics on surgical or minor wounds or as preoperative skin preparations.

Elemental iodine is lethal to a broad spectrum of bacteria and is virucidal. It has a potent and rapid action, the mechanism of which results from an iodination of and oxidizing effect on microbial protoplasm. Iodophors are less potent but are also less prone to adverse side effects. All preparations may lose potency with time.

Preparations

Iodine solution. This aqueous solution contains 2% iodine and 2.4% sodium iodide and should not be confused with strong (Lugol's) iodine solution. It is an effective skin antiseptic and is nonirritating. An alcoholic tincture solution is occasionally used but can be irritating to tissue and wounds. The tincture does not confer inherent antibacterial advantages, but may facilitate spread and penetration in tissue of the antiseptic agent.

Povidone-iodine. This organic iodine complex is attached to a carrier or solubilizing agent that liberates free iodine in solution, and the antiseptic activity is proportional to the availability of free iodine. The preparations are available in various forms, including solution and aerosol, as preoperative antiseptic preparations, or as hand scrubs. It is also used as a disinfectant.

Problems. The iodine compounds are reduced in activity by alkaline substances and may be inhibited by organic matter such as pus, blood, and tissue debris. Elemental and inorganic iodide solutions may cause skin staining, but this is generally not seen with the commonly used iodophors. Allergic contact sensitivity may be seen with inorganic compounds or elemental iodine preparations, and there may be a risk of cross reaction with iodized radiographic contrast materials. This is extremely rare with iodophors. Elemental iodine solutions if ingested can be extremely toxic. They have a caustic and corrosive effect on gastrointestinal mucosa. Vomiting, diarrhea, abdominal pain, and occasional rapid death caused by shock have been reported, usually with large amounts (30 to 250 ml) ingested.

Interference with laboratory thyroid function tests is usually not seen with the usual test procedures, but should be considered if the protein-bound iodine (PBI) test is used. The iodine preparations are generally to be avoided if there is a prior history of hypersensitivity reaction to iodine compounds, although such a reaction is extremely uncommon with iodophors.

Halogenated 8 hydroxyquinolones. These iodine-containing synthetic compounds were originally developed as *amebicidal* agents. Although diiodohydroxyquin, containing 64% iodine, has antiseptic action (it is little used topically), the most single important antiseptic agent in this group is iodochlorhydroxyquin, which contains 40% iodine. Iodochlorhydroxyquin was introduced in 1931 as a dusting powder for skin infections and wounds, and has a moderate and rapid action against bacteria, yeast, and fungi. It is more effective against gram-positive organ-

isms, but the basic mechanism of antiseptic action is unknown. Concentration may be important because effective antiseptic action probably requires a concentration of 3% or greater. It is absorbed in minimal degree from skin and mucous membranes. When absorbed from the gastrointestinal tract after oral ingestion, it is metabolized in the liver and excreted via the kidneys. There are many topical iodochlorhydroxyquin preparations, available in various formulations including creams, ointments, and lotions, and in combination with other agents such as corticosteroids or antibiotics. There have been no reports of systemic toxicity from topical iodochlorhydroxyquin. It should not be used in the presence of known iodine sensitivity, and potential cross-reactions with other halogenated hydroxyquinolones may produce systemic contact dermatitis. Iodochlorhydroxyquin uncommonly produces local allergic contact dermatitis but is not a potent sensitizer in usual concentrations or formulations. It can cause direct contact irritation, particularly in concentrations above 3%, and a major cosmetic complication is yellow staining of the skin. If used in the diaper area of infants, it may interfere with the phenylketonuria (PKU) test and produce a false positive reaction.

HEAVY METALS AND THEIR SALTS
Mercurial compounds

All mercury compounds are potentially toxic and have generally been replaced as antiseptics by safer and more effective agents. Their overall weak antiseptic action is probably caused by the inhibition of sulfhydryl enzymes by mercuric ion, but this is reversible, and the antiseptic action is only bacteriostatic. These compounds react readily with the patient's tissue *sulfhydryl* (SH) *groups;* thus they have a low therapeutic index.

Preparations

Inorganic mercury compounds. These compounds, including the oldest used mercuric chloride, are now avoided because of their potential irritation and toxicity and because chronic application can cause systemic mercury intoxication. Suicide attempts resulting in acute poisoning were not rare, and were characterized by gastrointestinal mucosal injury, acute gastritis, colitis, and renal failure. The renal damage was generally irreversible.

Some compounds, more insoluble or metallic mercury preparations, are still used, more often in ointment bases or as oxides of mercury usually in 1% concentration, such as yellow oxide of mercury. Ammoniated mercury ointment has been used in psoriasis therapy and other dermatoses in the past. All of these compounds, however, can produce allergic contact dermatitis. Preferably they should be avoided and replaced by safer agents.

Organic mercury compounds. These compounds are generally less irritating and toxic than inorganic preparations and more bacteriostatic. They have a wide spectrum of action, including both gram-positive and gram-negative organisms, *Candida*, and fungi, but are generally less effective than alcohol. They also penetrate tissue poorly, and the tissues bind the mercury so it becomes limited to the organisms. A variety of proprietary preparations are marketed, including solutions, tinctures, creams, ointments, and suppositories.

MERBROMIN. This preparation has a low therapeutic index. Although commonly used in past years, it should be avoided.

THIMEROSAL. This preparation is perhaps the most commonly used in this group, but is a weak germicide and generally replaced by better and safer agents. Perhaps its main present use is as a preservative in 1:10,000 concentration for biologic products, vaccines, and some blood products. The mercury is tightly bound in the organic complex and acute toxicity is therefore rare; however, chronic use may lead to chronic mercury intoxication, and the compound is also a potential allergic contact sensitizer.

PHENYLMERCURIC NITRATE OR ACETATE. These preparations have been used as skin or mucosa antiseptics and preservatives in ophthalmic solutions but have similar disadvantages, of potential chronic toxicity and contact sensitivity, as other members in this group.

Silver compounds

Most silver preparations have now been replaced by more effective agents as antiseptics. Soluble silver salts are still used but not colloidal preparations, which are less effective because of the reduced availability of free silver. The main mechanism of action of antisepsis is the precipitation of proteins by silver ion. Soluble silver salts also have astringent and caustic actions based on protein precipitation. The inorganic salts such as silver nitrate are highly germicidal in solution at concentrations of 1:1000 or less, but are bacteriostatic in higher dilution. They may be toxic to tissue in bactericidal concentrations. The silver ion penetrates poorly and is precipitated by chloride ions in tissues and body fluids.

Preparations. Silver nitrate may be used in local solutions or solid forms for antiseptic, *astringent,* or caustic actions, depending on concentration used and tissue contact time.

Local solutions. These have been employed in concentrations ranging from 0.01% to 10%. A 1:1000 preparation is strongly bactericidal and destroys most organisms rapidly, but at 1:10,000 is bacteriostatic. Traditionally two drops of a 1% solution are instilled in the conjunctival sac of newborns to prevent ophthalmia neonatorum resulting from gonococcal infection. Aqueous solutions, usually of 0.5% concentration, have been used in second- or third-degree burn dressings because the broad spectrum action is effective against gram-negative organisms, including *Pseudomonas* and *Proteus;* however, complications of electrolyte imbalance resulting from chloride and sodium loss into dressings have limited its usefulness in burn therapy.

Solid forms. Solid or toughened silver nitrate in pencil or stick form is used mainly for a caustic action as a cautery and to treat warts and excessive granulation tissue on minor wounds.

Problems. Toxicity from silver preparations is unusual because of the limited absorption caused by precipitation by chloride ion. It is potentially more of a risk, however, on burn sites or mucous membranes. Oral ingestion of soluble salts in higher concentrations may be corrosive to gastrointestinal mucosa. The chloride precipitation of silver has led to both hypochloremia and hyponatremia resulting from the loss of chloride and sodium ions in burn dressings treated with silver nitrate. *Methemoglobinemia,* although uncommon, is also a theoretical possibility because of excessive absorption of nitrate. A further disadvantage of local applications is the black staining of tissues resulting from deposition of reduced silver exposed to light. *Argyria,* characterized by blue or slate gray pigmentation of the skin and mucous membranes, results from higher concentrations of silver in tissues, and may first be apparent on the conjunctiva. Argyria is a cosmetic problem without tissue or systemic toxicity, but no adequate therapy is available. Potential toxicity of silver salts in other situations can be inhibited by sodium chloride washes. For accidental or intentional oral ingestion, *demulcents* can be used.

Other heavy metals

Zinc salts. Zinc salts have been used as mild antiseptics, astringents, antiperspirants, styptics, and corrosive agents. As with all heavy metals, actions are largely based on precipitation of protein. Various zinc salts have been used, including sulfate, acetate, chloride, and zinc oxide, which is an insoluble compound commonly used in powder, ointment, lotion, or paste form, possessing mild antiseptic and astringent actions. It is a component of calamine lotion and is present in a wide variety of proprietary preparations. Oral ingestion of zinc salt solutions in higher concentrations are irritating to the gastrointestinal tract and induce vomiting; however, more severe toxicity is unusual.

Aluminum salts. The aluminum ion is used mainly for its astringent properties but has mild antiseptic action. This action is based on precipitation of protein in *interstitial* tissue spaces or on cell surfaces, increased because of limited penetrability of the metallic ion. Cell permeability is consequently reduced, and this leads to the drying (astringent) effect. Aluminum salts such as aluminum hydroxide or chlorohydrate are also used as antiperspirants because of the astringent action and because they narrow *eccrine sweat orifices* by way of protein precipitation. One of the more commonly employed aluminum salts, as astringents or mild antiseptics, is aluminum acetate, marketed in various formulations as Burow's solution or other trade name equivalents. They are particularly used in solutions for soaks or compresses applied to infected dermatoses. There is minimal toxicity with the usual topical aluminum preparations. Contact dermatitis can occur, but usually results from additional ingredients in proprietary compounds, such as perfume in antiperspirants.

SURFACE ACTIVE AGENTS

Surface active agents may be defined as substances that alter the energy relations at cell or tissue interfaces. Chemically these compounds have structures balancing *hydrophilic* and *hydrophobic* groups and are classified as *anionic, cationic, nonionic,* and *amphoteric* agents. Anionic agents are those in which the active portion of the molecule carries a negative charge, such as soaps. Cationic agents, in contrast, display a positive charge and are represented by the quaternary ammonium compounds, which are the main true antiinfective or antiseptic detergents in this overall class of compounds. Surface active agents in other categories are either in detergent form or do not have a significant role in clinical antisepsis. Soaps and other detergents cleanse and remove bacteria from skin by essentially mechanical means and are not generally classed as true antiseptics; however, mild antibacterial substances, such as salicylanilides, may be added in some commercial products.

The quaternary ammonium compounds are effective against gram-positive and gram-negative organisms; however, the latter, including *Pseudomonas*, are more resistant and require longer exposure. Spores are resistant, and aqueous solutions are not tuberculocidal. Other actions besides antisepsis include a keratolytic and emulsifier action and a general mechanical detergent action of removing dirt, tissue debris, and bacteria.

The mechanism of antiseptic action is otherwise unknown. These compounds are known to denature protein and lower surface tension, but the antiseptic action does not seem to parallel this. They may have a significant effect on cell membrane permeability, leading to loss of essential cell constituents.

These agents are relatively nonirritating to tissue in usually employed concentrations of 1%, and have a rapid onset of action. They penetrate tissues well, but display relatively low systemic toxicity. Oral poisoning is uncommon. They have a wide industrial use as detergents and sanitizers and are employed as medium all-purpose antiseptics on the skin or mucous membranes or commonly as disinfectants.

Preparations

Benzalkonium chloride. Benzalkonium chloride is the prototype compound. It is freely soluble in water, acetone, and alcohol. Aqueous solutions are slightly alkaline. It has a reasonable broad spectrum of action against microorganisms, except for spores and *tubercle bacilli,* and a rapid onset of action. It may be used to sterilize surgical instruments and other equipment, but it should be monitored for resistant spores. Sodium nitrite is usually added as an antirust agent to prevent corrosion of metal instruments. As antiseptic solutions, a concentration of less than 0.1% is commonly employed, but more concentrated solutions from 2% to 50% are available as disinfectants.

Cetyl trimethyl ammonium bromide (cetrimide). This preparation has been used in topical solution, lotion, powder, or cream formulations as an antiseptic and detergent, commonly in concentrations of 1% or 5%. It has also been used as a disinfectant and is combined with chlorhexidine in one commercial preparation (Savlon).

Miscellaneous compounds. Other quaternary ammonium compounds, such as cetylpyridinium chloride, have been used in lotion, ointment, powder, lozenge, or mouthwash form for topical antisepsis and detergent effect, and a wide number of proprietary preparations are available. Shampoos, such as a Ionil, may also employ quaternary ammonium compounds.

Problems

Quaternary ammonium compounds are inactivated by soaps and other anionic substances, and sites of application should be cleansed of these substances before application. Iodides, bentonite, phenylmercuric nitrate, phenol, alkali hydroxides, and chlorocresol also interfere with effective action. Organic matter such as pus, blood, or tissue debris also hinders action of these compounds. Cotton, cellulose fiber, some plastics, and rubber absorb the compound, and this may hinder disinfection, making its reliability uncertain in cold sterilization of catheters or instruments. These compounds may also be ineffective in *Pseudomonas* outbreaks, and they also lack the ability to kill spores and tubercle bacilli. As antiseptics these compounds have slower onset of action than iodine, and since they are deposited on the skin as an invisible film, the external surface may be sterile while viable bacteria may persist under this film. The compounds, in interaction with keratin, may damage epidermis, especially with chronic use, and may lead to excessive dryness and irritation with time. Accidental contact with concentrated solution either directly or via disinfected fabrics can lead to corrosive lesions, with necrosis and scarring. Allergic contact dermatitis is rare, as is systemic toxicity; however, oral ingestion of concentrated solution will likely lead to irritation or corrosive effects on gastrointestinal mucosa. Systemic toxicity is then possible, and deaths have ensued with paralysis of respiratory muscles.

OXIDIZING AGENTS

Nascent oxygen, which is bactericidal, is the basis of action of oxidizing agents, including peroxides and permanganates. These compounds differ in ease of penetration, rate of oxygen release, effects of the oxygen carrier or other linked compounds, and the mechanism and effect of oxygen release on bacteria.

Preparations

Peroxides. Hydrogen peroxide (H_2O_2) is the most important agent in this group. Benzoyl peroxides are discussed in Chapter 56. H_2O_2 is an unstable compound that, in contact with the enzyme catalase in blood or tissues, rapidly decomposes to oxygen (O_2) and water (H_2O). The liberated oxygen has a germicidal effect, which is brief, lasting only the period of oxygen release. The germicidal effect is largely a mechanical action of liberated oxygen under pressure, which cleans and debrides infected tissue. This effervescence is used to cleanse wounds and has been employed in the past as a gargle, mouthwash, or vaginal douche. The standard preparation is a 3% solution.

Permanganates. Potassium permanganate is the most commonly used and is a vigorous oxidizing agent. Broad-spectrum germicidal activity depends on concentration, and an antifungal action is achieved in usual clinical use. It is commonly employed in dilution greater than 1:5000 to avoid excessive skin irritation and has been dispensed in crystal, solution, or tablet form. In addition to antisepsis, including antifungal action, formation of manganese dioxide in tissue produces an astringent action via the manganese ion,

which helps reduce inflammation by exerting a drying effect to retard exudation. The compound is still occasionally used, particularly in infected dermatoses.

Problems

Hydrogen peroxide is a relatively feeble germicide with a brief action. The release of oxygen on intact skin is slow, and action is better on wounds or mucous membranes. In addition, there is poor tissue penetration. There may be danger of use in closed cavities, such as abscess, because lack of egress of released gas may lead to escape through blood vessels. Reports of air embolism have been recorded. On oral mucosa, excessive use may lead to irritation, and occasionally hairy black tongue has ensued, which is characterized by a brown or black furring of the dorsum of the tongue, associated with excessive accumulation of bacteria and occasionally *Candida* organisms. Hydrogen peroxide may also be damaging to new epithelial cells. Potassium permanganate may be hindered in action in the presence of organic matter. It is irritating to tissues in higher concentrations, and concentrated solutions or contact with dry crystals may be corrosive. The formation of manganese dioxide produces brown staining of tissues, which is only a cosmetic problem. Because of poor absorption there is minimal systemic toxicity risk, and true allergic contact dermatitis is extremely rare.

PHENOLIC COMPOUNDS

The phenolic compounds comprise phenol and a variety of substituted phenols, with structural modifications to the basic chemical structure. All are general protoplasmic poisons, a fact that hampers their routine use as antiseptics because of low therapeutic index and excessive toxicity. Ease of tissue penetration of these compounds also adversely contributes to tissue damage. Even as disinfectants, absorption of the toxic compounds by materials such as rubber or plastics may lead to consequent burns or tissue necrosis on skin contact. Phenol now has limited medical use, and of the substituted phenols, a compound cresol solution is still used mainly as a disinfectant. Resorcinol compounds are present in a wide variety of proprietary antiseborrheic products in low concentration and have little use as straight antiseptics or disinfectants. Parabens (alkyl substituted phenols) are commonly used only as preservatives in a wide variety of commercial preparations, particularly in cream or lotion form. Thymol has limited clinical uses. Of all the phenolic compounds, hexachlorophene (a chlorinated bisphenol) is the most important antiseptic, but has some distinct toxic hazards.

Preparations

Phenol. Phenol has now largely been replaced as a disinfectant or antiseptic by safer and more effective agents. It is most effective in aqueous solution and exerts its action through direct precipitation and denaturation of protein. Phenol is not inactivated by this, however, and continues to penetrate tissue, contributing to increased toxic damage. It was formerly used as a sclerosing agent for hemorrhoid treatment, but the increased tissue penetration can lead to excessive damage to normal structures. Phenol can also produce a local anesthetic action topically and has been used as an antipruritic agent in the past in dilute concentrations of 1:100 or 1:200. The bacterial action spectrum varies with concentration. There is a bactericidal action above 1%, and it is generally bacteriostatic in more dilute concentration. Efficacy is also pH and temperature dependent.

Phenol is absorbed by all routes and can enter the circulation via skin penetration. Excretion is largely via the kidney. Various formulations have been used in the past, and it is perhaps best known in form as carbolic acid. Liquefied phenol has also been available, as have preparations in glycerin and calamine lotion.

Substituted phenols. Many of these compounds are more bactericidal than phenol probably because of the chemical modifications and substitutions increasing lipid solubility and allowing increased penetration of cell membranes. A number of subgroups are important including the following.

1. Cresols (methylated derivatives)
2. Resorcinols (discussed in Chapter 56)
3. Alkyl substituted phenols (parabens)
4. Thymol
5. Halogenated bisphenols (e.g., hexachlorophene)

Cresols. These methyl derivatives have similar toxicity as phenol but are more potent bactericidal agents and are generally less expensive. The action spectrum is relatively wide and includes tubercle bacilli. Medical use is most common as a disinfectant in the form of compound cresol solution, which is composed of 50% cresol in *saponified* linseed oil or other similar oil. In this form it is miscible with water. It is therefore more suitable for use because cresols otherwise have limited solubility in water. It has also been used as a handwash at 2% concentration, and occasionally used in lower concentration in other proprietary cleansers.

Resorcinols. See Chapter 56, "Keratolytics, Antiseborrheics, and Related Medications."

Parabens. These short alkyl esters of *p*-hydroxybenzoic acid are common preservatives in many topical and parenteral preparations. Methyl, ethyl, propyl, and butyl homologues are used, usually in combinations of two or more. They exert a phenol-like precipitant effect and also have an antimetabolic action resulting from the *p*-hydroxybenzoic acid derivation. All are effective in low concentration, such as 0.1% to 0.3%, and at this level have negligible potential systemic toxicity. They may occasionally, however, produce allergic contact dermatitis or *contact urticarial* reactions.

Thymol. Thymol is at least as potent as phenol and may have a wider germicidal action spectrum. It has also been used as an antifungal agent and is not uncommonly employed in 1% or 2% concentration in chloroform to treat *Pseudomonas,* nail infections, or *tinea unguum.* Several proprietary preparations have also been available, but there are no reliable efficacy data for clinical use, and the lower safer concentrations used may not be significantly effective on tissue at practical contact times.

Hexachlorophene. This polychlorinated bisphenol compound has been the most important and useful medicinal phenol. It has been particularly useful as a clinical antiseptic because it is particularly effective against gram-positive organisms, including the common pathogen, *Staphylococcus aureus.* It is less effective against gram-negative bacteria. Hexachlorophene has a high bacteriostatic activity, but usually requires more prolonged contact time to exert a bactericidal effect. It is also fungistatic but has a lesser effect on spores and is less useful as a routine disinfectant.

An important property is accumulation with repeated application, and the residual liquid film left on the skin leads to a steady continuing antibacterial action. If this film is removed with alcohol or thorough soap cleansing, the bacterial flora reestablishes itself promptly. The maximum antibacterial concentration is achieved in 2 to 4 days, and bacterial counts at this time have been reduced by 95% and more if hexachlorophene soap or detergent has been frequently applied. A single scrub with a usual hexachlorophene preparation, however, achieves no greater antibacterial action than normal soap. A further advantage of hexachlorophene is retention of antibacterial action, despite prior or concomitant application of topical vehicles, oils, and soaps. The compound is generally insoluble in water. It has had most common use as a prophylactic scrub or hand antiseptic and skin preparation. There are few reliable efficacy studies of comparison with other agents; however, although iodophors and alcohol may be more effective initially and have a wide spectrum and bactericidal action, hexachlorophene's effect is longer lasting and particularly effective against *Staphylococcus aureus.* In usual form it is also less irritating to skin than many other preparations and does not display the local cutaneous toxicity of other phenolic compounds.

Risk of neurotoxicity, however, has resulted in controversy over its routine use as an infant bath in nurseries, and the compound is known to be absorbed from intact skin, especially with repetitive application. It is now generally used in nurseries only as part of an infection control program, and in April 1972 the American Academy of Pediatrics Committee on Fetus and Newborns suggested that manufacturers state on labels that 3% hexachlorophene is not to be used for routine prophylactic body bathing. Many nurseries have continued with more short-term bathing with adequate rinsing, particularly in normal-sized infants and with *Staphylococcus* outbreaks. Nursery personnel also continue to commonly use hexachlorophene as a hand scrub or wash.

Since December 1971, under FDA order, 3% hexachlorophene must be distributed only by prescription, and over-the-counter proprietary preparations have been discontinued. Hexachlorophene is available as a liquid soap at 0.25% concentration, as a tincture foam at 0.23% concentration, and as an emulsion with 3% hexachlorophene in detergent formulation (pHiso-Hex). The latter is generally considered a more efficient antiseptic than the soap solution. It has also been incorporated in soaps, lotions, creams, ointments, and shampoos. It has not been proved efficacious in acne therapy but continues to be commonly employed in topical treatment of *Staphylococcus* impetigo. It does, however, have reduced efficiency in the presence of organic matter.

Problems

The major problem with the phenolic compounds as a group is toxicity, which can be local or systemic. Phenol, as the prototype compound of this class, is generally considered too irritating for topical use, especially at potentially germicidal concentration greater than 1%. Local toxicity with increased tissue penetration, even from intact skin, can exert corrosive and necrotic damage and red-brown staining of the skin. Even as disinfectants phenolic compounds can be absorbed by fabrics (e.g., rubber, plastics) and may produce contact burns. Other cresols may produce the same effect, and their more common use as disinfectants thus requires close monitoring.

Phenolic compounds, especially phenol, have reduced efficiency at low temperatures and also in alkaline solution, because the phenolate ion is less lipid soluble and thus less able to penetrate cell or tissue barriers. There is potential systemic toxicity even from application to intact skin. The possibility of systemic toxicity is increased, along with excessive local irritation, if phenolic compounds are applied to abraded skin or wounds. Poisoning from oral ingestion leads to corrosive action on oral and gastrointestinal mucosa, and pain, vomiting, shock with renal shutdown, respiratory failure, and rapid death can ensue. Treatment includes passage of a stomach tube and gastric lavage with olive oil, which helps dissolve the phenol compound without absorption. Locally, from skin or mucosa, the phenol can be removed with 5.0% alcohol, glycerin, vegetable oils, sodium bicarbonate solution, or even copious water. Substituted phenols may have similar toxicity. Parabens, as preservatives in clinical preparations, are not considered toxic, but allergic contact dermatitis and increasing reports of contact urticaria have been noted. The incidence of these reactions is considered low with other phenolic compounds. Hexachlorophene has received particular attention because of its frequent and common use and the recent public awareness of its toxicity hazards. Although it is much less irritating locally than phenol and other phenolic compounds, it can lead to similar toxic effects through oral ingestion, and fatalities have been reported as a result of accidental ingestion of hexachlorophene detergent by children.

More recent reports of systemic toxicity after topical application have been stressed, particularly neurotoxicity with diffuse status spongiosis of the brain. It has been observed that hexachlorophene is absorbed from intact skin, especially with repeat application; however, premature infants or infants with abraded or excoriated skin appear particularly at risk, and routine prophylactic body bathing of infants in nurseries with 3% hexachlorophene has thus been discontinued. Other considerations in this regard are discussed previously in this section. Locally, although hexachlorophene is less irritating than other phenolic compounds and many other antiseptics, some burning of the skin and conjunctiva is not uncommon. If exposed, the eye should be rinsed of all suds. Excessively frequent use may produce dryness and irritant dermatitis with time, but allergic contact dermatitis is rare. Because of its more limited antibacterial spectrum and lack of bactericidal action, it has not been used as a routine disinfectant and is ineffective in *Pseudomonas* outbreaks.

MISCELLANEOUS ANTISEPTICS
Chlorhexidine

This bisdiquanide compound has had relatively common medical use as an antiseptic or disinfectant. It has a reasonably broad-spectrum bactericidal action and a continuing antiseptic action on skin. The compound may be less effective for gram-negative organisms, such as *Pseudomonas* and some strains of *Serratia*. Reports of local irritant effects or excessive dryness are relatively uncommon in comparison with iodine or alcohol, but may increase with long-term application. Eye irritation may also result on contact with suds of skin cleanser preparations, and prompt rinsing with water will ameliorate this. Chlorhexidine is not absorbed significantly, and there are few valid reports of systemic toxicity, although accidental swallowing of chlorhexidine solution may be harmful to mucosal surfaces. Chlorhexidine preparations, usually in the form of chlorhexidine gluconate (Hibitane), are available as lotions (commonly in 1% concentration) and antiseptic or disinfectant solutions in 4% or 20% concentrations, which are commonly diluted with deionized or distilled water or 70% alcohol to achieve desired strengths and results, with minimal side effects. A precaution particularly to note is to avoid putting hypochlorite bleaches on clothing fabrics previously in contact with chlorhexidine-containing compounds, because dark stains may develop. If the stain does occur, use of an oxidizing bleach, such as sodium perborate or hydrogen peroxide, should eliminate the chlorine reaction causing the stain.

Chlorhexidine gluconate has also been combined with cetrimide, a quaternary ammonium agent, in at least one commonly used disinfectant preparation (Savlon Hospital Concentrate). It is commonly supplied as a 7.5% v/v (1.5% w/v) concentration of chlorhexidine gluconate, and 15% w/v concentration of cetrimide, in 160 oz plastic containers. Because cork may protect some gramnegative bacteria from antiseptic action, stock solution should be stored in glass- or rubber-stoppered bottles. It is generally diluted to the desired strength with water or 70% alcohol. Sodium nitrite is added to the dilute solution as an antirust agent to prevent corrosion of surgical instruments stored in this solution.

Chlorhexidine-containing throat lozenges are also available as an aid to oral or pharyngeal topical antisepsis. Allergic contact dermatitis to chlorhexidine in any formulation is rarely reported.

Miscellaneous acids

Organic acids with low molecular weights (e.g., trichloracetic, lactic, or formic) and dilute mineral acids (e.g., sulfuric and hydrochloric) can have antiseptic action, but are potentially corrosive and generally limited to other purposes. Several other acids, however, have had use as antiseptics, but have generally been replaced in medical use by safer and more effective compounds.

Boric acid. Boric acid is a weak acid and forms an alkaline sodium salt in solution. It is nonirritating in solutions and was used previously as a corneal rinse

or eyewash and mild topical antiseptic. However, it has a weak mainly bacteriostatic action, and fatalities have been reported with accidental ingestion, so its use has declined with the availability of more effective and safer preparations. The fatal cases ensued from use of common preparations in the household, hospitals, or nurseries, and errors of labeling were encountered, including mistaking boric acid solution for water or boric acid powder for glucose. In addition, boric acid may be absorbed readily in abraded skin and in infants, leading to potential systemic toxicity. It may also slowly accumulate with repeated use because of the relatively slow excretion of the compound. Acute poisoning cases have been characterized by nausea, vomiting, diarrhea, *exfoliative dermatitis*, headache, convulsion, circulatory collapse, renal failure, and shock, generally within 5 days of ingestion. Although their usage should be discouraged, accessible preparations must be clearly labeled as poison. Color is normally added to solutions to further discourage oral ingestion. The topical preparations most commonly used in previous years were available as crystals or granules and prepared as solutions, powders, or ointments in 5% or 10% concentrations. Borax is the sodium salt of tetraboric acid.

Benzoic acid. This relatively weak acid, bacteriostatic in 0.1% concentrations and acid media, is used as a food preservative. It is tasteless, relatively nontoxic, and considered safe to the skin even in higher concentrations. Benzoic acid has also been combined with salicylic acid in topical keratolytic and antifungal agents such as Whitfield's ointment.

Acetic acid. Acetic acid, although not commonly used in commercial preparations is bactericidal to many organisms above 5% concentration. Below this level it is generally bacteriostatic. The compound has clinical effectiveness against *Pseudomonas*, and since it also has activity for *Trichomonas* and *Candida* infection, it has occasionally been employed in vaginal douches for their control.

Dyes

There is little group similarity in basic chemistry or clinical action among the various dyes, and most have been replaced by more effective and cosmetically acceptable antiseptic compounds. Toxicity is limited in usual use, but allergic contact dermatitis is occasionally reported.

Gentian violet. This compound, also known in its pure form as crystal violet, is a *rosaniline dye*. It is effective against gram-positive bacteria, *Candida*, and many fungi; however, gram-negative organisms and acid-fast bacilli are resistant. It has been available in concentrations of 0.02% to 1% for clinical use, as a topical solution or cream. Staining of the skin or mucosa is a major problem, and tattooing can result from application to granulation tissue. It should be particularly avoided on open facial wounds.

Methylene blue. Methylene blue is a weak antiseptic. It is bacteriostatic and is most effective against gram-positive organisms. Because of its possible oxidizing action on hemoglobin iron, high concentrations can potentially lead to methemoglobinemia. There is poor absorption, however, from the gastrointestinal tract with oral ingestion, and toxicity is otherwise limited. Topical preparations have been in the form of powder or aqueous solution, in ampules prepared from dark green crystals. Methylene blue is also used systemically to test renal function, to treat mild genitourinary infections, and to treat drug-induced methemoglobinemia.

Aminacrine. This dye may have weak germicidal effect against gram-positive and gram-negative bacteria, fungi, and *Trichomonas*. It is not inactivated by organic matter. Topical preparations have included a 0.1% powder, 0.2% or 2% cream, and jellies or suppositories of similar strength.

Scarlet red. Because of a presumed action in stimulating tissue proliferation, this compound has had use in wound or ulcer healing. However, reliable effectiveness in this capacity, or as an antiseptic, has not been generally convincing. The compound has been applied as an ointment or oily solution in 4.8% concentration, but as with all the usual dyes, it invariably causes tissue staining. In addition, allergic contact dermatitis has been a common complication. Currently, use is relatively rare.

Aldehydes

Formaldehyde solution and glutaral are the most representative compounds in this category. They have limited use as clinical antiseptics despite bactericidal activity because of tissue toxicity, which can occur even at lower concentration. At higher concentrations they are protein precipitants. They are usually employed, therefore, as disinfectants, or for other uses such as tissue fixation for pathologic study.

Preparations

Formaldehyde solution. Formalin represents 37% by weight of formaldehyde. Methanol is usually added in preparations to retard *polymerization*. It has a wide antiseptic spectrum against bacteria, viruses, and fungi, but action is slow. It is usually used in 2% to 8% concentration as a disinfectant solution, but has also been used as an astringent in concentrations of 20% to 30% to treat hyperhydrosis of the palms and soles.

Glutaral. Glutaral has a similar, but possibly more germicidal, action, which is broad spectrum and effective against spores, viruses, and tubercle bacilli. It has been used more commonly as a therapy for warts and hyperhydrosis.

Problems. Formalin is not used as an antiseptic because of its low therapeutic index and tissue toxicity. Its germicidal action is also too slow for effective clinical use. Alteration of tissue proteins, in addition to local tissue irritation, can lead to allergic contact dermatitis. This is, however, more commonly seen with formalin ester or resin contact, such as in clothing (particularly crease-resistant fabrics) and some shampoos. The compound has a pungent irritating odor, and solution or vapor contact with eyes or other mucous membranes can produce stinging and burning discomfort. Accidental ingestion produces direct irritation of oral and gastrointestinal mucosa, with pain, vomiting, and diarrhea. Significant absorption may produce systemic toxicity, with central nervous system depression and coma. Glutaral has reduced odor and is less irritating to the skin and conjunctiva, but can produce allergic contact dermatitis. A major problem is lack of stability; it loses activity within 2 weeks of preparation. Glutarol is therefore rarely used as a disinfectant. Increased cost may also be a significant factor in its limited use.

SUMMARY

The many types of compounds used as antiseptics have been discussed. They embrace a wide range of products with widely differing chemical structures and modes of action. The ideal antiseptic of effective action without complications—or simply sting, stain, or stench—has not yet been discovered. Some of the compounds covered, such as mercurial compounds, phenol, and boric acid, are potentially too toxic for clinical use and should be replaced by better and safer agents. Many preparations are best restricted to use as disinfectants rather than antiseptics, such as sodium hypochlorite compounds. Common or potential complications of the various products have been particularly stressed, including topical or systemic toxicity and occasional allergic sensitivity (e.g., mercury, iodine). Particular stress on the limitations of hexachlorophene has been emphasized. Some of the more commonly employed antiseptics at present include the aliphatic alcohols (ethyl and isopropyl), iodophors (povidone-iodine), and chlorhexidine. Few controlled valid clinical comparison studies of these preparations have been reported, and often factors such as cost or individual preference determines the choice.

1220

Local anesthetics

Local anesthetics are drugs that block nerve conduction when applied locally to nerve tissue in appropriate concentrations. The following discussion is limited to consideration of anesthetic use in surface and local infiltrative anesthesia. No attempt is made to review other more specialized areas of local anesthesia, such as field or nerve block, epidural, spinal, and regional intravenous methods or routes.

CHEMICAL STRUCTURAL CLASSIFICATION

Drugs normally classified as local anesthetics consist of three fundamental chemical structural parts. These include a hydrophilic amino group and aromatic residue linked by a central intermediate chain. The link between the intermediate group and the aromatic residue is in the form of an amide bond or ester linkage. This important linkage provides a fundamental basis for classification, along with the type of aromatic ring structure, such as para-aminobenzoic acid (PABA) or benzoic acid. Structural alterations in each fundamental group are responsible for new anesthetics, which consequently demonstrate altered intrinsic potency, duration of action, and potential toxicity from the parent or prototype compound.

CELLULAR ACTION

In terms of surface or local infiltrative anesthesia of the skin or mucous membranes, these compounds act locally at the site of application in a circumscribed area on every type of nerve fiber encountered. This action leads to the loss of both sensory and motor activity; however, a major advantage is that the conduction block is essentially reversible.

The fundamental action is the prevention of the initiation and transmission of nerve impulses by stabilizing the nerve cell membranes through a cellular effect on membrane permeability. The precise mechanism is not completely known. Generally, the nerve fibers are blocked sequentially according to size. Small autonomic unmyelinated nerves are blocked first, followed by those mediating pain, temperature, and light touch, and then larger myelinated fibers mediating proprioreception and somatic motor function. Function is recovered in reverse order. However, there may be overlap of these modalities in practice, and with topical or local infiltration little discrimination can be determined under conditions of usual use.

The degree of penetration of the anesthetic depends on several variables including the mode of anesthesia, site, chemical nature of the agent, concen-

---

Classification of local anesthetics	
Esters	*Amides (anilides)*
PABA esters	Lidocaine
Procaine	Mepivacaine
Dibucaine	Prilocaine
Tetracaine	Bupivacaine
Benzoic acid esters	Etidocaine
Cocaine	

---

tration, pH, and volume injected or applied topically. The pH is particularly important to effective action because the water-soluble salts (mainly hydrochlorides) are more stable in acidic solution. This is also true for any added vasoconstrictor material, such as epinephrine. The acid salt is buffered in the tissue and the nonionized weak base liberated, which penetrates the nerve sheath and membranes to produce the anesthetic action. The base forms are soluble in lipid vehicles as formulated in many proprietary anesthetic ointments.

The duration of the block depends on several variables including the intrinsic pharmacologic properties of the agent, the volume and concentration of the solution used, the tissue blood flow, and the presence or absence of vasoconstrictive substances. For most local infiltration procedures the most effective concentration is 0.25% or greater and is commonly given as a 1% or 2% solution of the active ingredient.

Added vasoconstrictive agents (catecholamines, usually epinephrine) prolong and intensify the duration of action by allowing increased contact time of the solution with the nerve. This action is maintained by constriction of local small blood vessels at the site, thus decreasing the absorption of the active anesthetic compound. The vasoconstrictive agent also may reduce toxicity risk by allowing metabolism to keep pace with absorption. Epinephrine itself, however, can be absorbed and occasionally produces systemic effects, such as tachycardia and palpitations. Theoretical local difficulties such as decreased tissue oxygen release and interference with healing are uncommonly encountered in clinical practice, and are usually outweighed by the benefits, including local control of bleeding before and during surgical procedures.

Although of greater clinical importance with more specialized methods of anesthesia, the perineural concentration of the anesthetic, necessary to produce block, is several hundredfold greater than the toxic plasma level, and injection must be limited to the desired site. This will minimize the risk of producing a toxic plasma level from injection into highly vascular sites or exposed open blood vessels. Generally, it is therefore advised for the best therapeutic index to use the least volume of the most dilute solution that is effective.

METABOLISM

The pattern and efficiency of metabolism varies with the type of drug employed and the physiologic status of the patient. Most of the esters are hydrolyzed by plasma cholinesterase at the ester linkage site, and the metabolites are excreted in the urine. Some esters such as cocaine, however, may be largely metabolized by the liver. Amide compounds are metabolized in the liver by microsomal enzymes. The rate of destruction is a major safety factor and may show significant variation in patients. An increased hazard of toxicity could be expected in the presence of liver damage, whereas other patients may have increased tissue binding of the active agent, which may lessen potential risk.

COMPOUNDS

In terms of overall use for both topical and local infiltrative anesthesia, lidocaine, introduced in 1948, is still the predominant agent. Lidocaine has a consistently proved, good therapeutic index with rapid onset and effective duration of action, in usual situations of use, ranging from 90 to 120 minutes. The compound is stable, has a long shelf life, and can be repeatedly autoclaved. A major benefit of lidocaine, in contrast to the nonamide anesthetics, is the absence of risk of allergic contact sensitization reactions.

Other compounds generally have major or potential disadvantages, or fail to confer advantage in clinical usage over lidocaine. A possible exception to this may be some of the newer amide-type longer-acting anesthetics (e.g., bupivacaine, etidocaine) in certain clinical situations. A wide variety of nonamide type bases, used topically in a variety of proprietary products, are readily available. The base form has limited solubility, and little absorption occurs, so the risk of toxicity is negligible. Benzocaine is a common topical form, and most have a PABA ring structure, so the risk of allergic contact sensitization generally outweighs the benefit. Consequently these topical proprietary compounds are generally to be avoided.

Specific compounds

Cocaine. Although limited in usage, as a restricted and controlled drug, cocaine is an example of a natural anesthetic compound, whereas the other local anesthetics are synthetic products. Cocaine is obtained from the leaves of the shrub *Erythroxylon coca* and other species in Peru and Bolivia.

Cocaine is a benzoic acid ester compound and is effective in low concentration. It was formerly used for corneal anesthesia but has now been replaced by safer and more effective agents (i.e., proparacaine, tetracaine). The compound is one of the few local anesthetics with intrinsic vasoconstrictive action. Because of the central nervous system stimulatory effect and common addictive properties, it was confined to surface anesthesia use and is now rigidly controlled.

Procaine. Procaine was the first local anesthetic, synthesized in 1905. It is a PABA ester and can competitively antagonize other compounds with similar structure, such as the sulfonamides. Because structures with the PABA ring are common allergic contact sensitizers, potential cross-reactions with other similarly structured compounds is a risk. The allergenicity, plus the fact that the compound is not efficient topically, has led to a general decline in usage. It has now been largely replaced by more effective and preferred agents, such as lidocaine.

Lidocaine. As outlined previously, lidocaine is the major commonly used local anesthetic agent for both topical and local infiltrative anesthesia. Although it has a good therapeutic index, no significant contact allergenicity, is nonirritating, and stable in both solution and shelf life, an awareness of possible hazards is important before clinical use. Injection or application into vascular areas must be avoided to prevent high and toxic blood levels. Potential side effects include sleepiness and dizziness, although these are uncommon reactions with usual topical or local infiltrative use. There is a potential hazard in patients with liver disease because lidocaine is metabolized mainly by liver enzymes, but this is rarely a contraindication to the usual limited amounts of drug used in uncomplicated local anesthesia for minor procedures.

The usual preparations for local infiltration include ampules, vials, or prefilled syringes of 0.5%, 1% or 2% concentration with or without epinephrine at 1:100,000 or 1:200,000 strengths. Topical compounds are available in 1% or 2% concentrations in aerosol spray and other topical formulations including an ointment (2.5% to 5%), jelly (2%), and viscous lidocaine, which is used commonly for pain relief in diseases of the oral mucosa.

Other amides

The majority of these compounds are *not* effective topically.

Mepivacaine. This compound is similar to lidocaine in potency, duration of action, and toxicity risk. A potential advantage is some intrinsic vasoconstriction properties, and mepivacaine can be used without epinephrine for most procedures. In addition there is no significant drowsiness or lassitude associated with its use. A disadvantage, however, is its lack of topical effectiveness.

Prilocaine. This drug has a slower onset and longer duration of action than lidocaine. It is otherwise similarly effective. Prilocaine may be less toxic because of an enhanced metabolic rate and excretion. Potential side effects include drowsiness and a hazard of methemoglobinemia, particularly in total doses greater than 600 mg. It is not used topically.

Bupivacaine. This newer amide compound has a longer intrinsic duration of action of up to 4 hours, and thus the need for epinephrine is obviated. It may therefore be considered for use particularly for pain relief and for more lengthy procedures requiring local anesthesia. Because of the prolonged action, bupivacaine should be used with caution in ambulatory patients. Toxicity (i.e., shock, respiratory arrest, coma) with vascular injection has been reported, but allergic reaction is apparently unusual. Similar considerations of use would appear also to apply to etidocaine, a similar long-acting agent.

Miscellaneous surface agents

Pramoxine. This topical agent, of differing chemical structure, derived from morphine, has been used for pain relief in oral mucosa and dental procedures, but is excessively irritating locally on application to eye or nasal mucous membrane. It has a claimed low incidence of contact sensitivity, but a potency similar to benzocaine. The drug has been available as a 1% cream or jelly.

Cooling sprays. Various compounds have been used for brief, easily administered local anesthetic effects on tissue in the form of cooling sprays in aerosol containers. Ethyl chloride, the first agent generally used in this form, has been supplanted by various fluorocarbons (fluorochloramethanes) because they are nonflammable. Ethyl chloride, as a flammable compound, is a hazard, and particularly contraindicated for use in conjunction with electrocautery procedures.

The cooling sprays are applied from a distance of about 0.5 m for 3 to 5 seconds, and the application can be repeated several times at usual intervals of 30 seconds. They can be used over wide areas, and there is a wide safety margin.

Other agents. Menthol, camphor, and phenol have all been used topically, more commonly as antipruritic agents than for local anesthesia. The compounds have mainly been used in concentrations less than 1% for this purpose to minimize potential toxicity. The antipruritic effect may result from the substitution of a cooling sensation imparted by these compounds topically. They have been largely replaced as antipruritics by systemic antihistamine or ataractic compounds and topical corticosteroids.

Topical antihistamines may also produce a local anesthetic action, possibly by a depolarizing action at the tissue level. Their use is largely contraindicated because of a general high risk of contact allergic sensitization; however, some compounds, such as diphenhydramine, have been used in solution on oral mucosa for pain relief without significant risk of allergy.

MAJOR ADVERSE REACTIONS

Potential reactions can be manifest systemically or locally. Systemic reactions include toxicity from high plasma concentrations of the local anesthetic agent itself or contained vasoconstrictor. The complication may occur with poor or faulty administration technique, such as direct intravascular injection, or use in contraindicated sites, such as open mucosal wounds or bleeding sites. Excessive concentration and volume may also contribute to toxic plasma levels. Less commonly reduced metabolism may produce toxicity. Signs and symptoms, largely of cardiovascular or central nervous system in nature, may be of slow or rapid onset, reflecting speed of absorption. Coma, cardiovascular collapse, and respiratory arrest may ensue. Rarely is idiosyncratic toxicity encountered without precise relation to dose, concentration, or plasma level. Anaphylaxis is only rarely reported with topical or local infiltrative anesthesia. Generalized allergic hypersensitivity reactions of other types are also unusual. Possible cross-reactions of systemic and topical PABA compounds must be considered in some cases. Possible methemoglobinemia with prilocaine has been discussed previously.

Local reactions (i.e., skin rashes, pruritus) are mainly the result of allergic contact dermatitis to nonamide compounds, particularly of the PABA type. The dermatitis is seen at the site of application initially, but may become generalized and is invariably pruritic. Potential cross-reaction with other systemic or topical PABA compounds must always be considered. Lidocaine is ordinarily free of allergenicity; however, the lidocaine jelly contains parabens as preservatives, which may be an occasional potential source of contact allergy, either as dermatitis or contact urticaria. Allergy to propylene glycol in the lidocaine ointment or aerosol is extremely rare. Topical products, such as the aerosol spray or viscous lidocaine, can interfere with the second stage of the swallowing mechanism, and aspiration is possible if patients are not properly advised regarding limitations of food intake before and following anesthetic use. Occasionally local excess bleeding has ensued from the vasodilator action of lidocaine in the absence of added epinephrine, but this is rarely a major hazard. Conversely, ischemic complications and gangrene have occasionally ensued from improper use of added epinephrine in contraindicated sites, such as terminal digits, the nose, or penis.

PRECAUTIONS

One must be thoroughly familiar with all of the contraindications and risk factors before local anesthetic procedures. Although it is likely that the local anesthetics will have little effect on intact skin, they may easily penetrate open or damaged skin and are absorbed with increased ease from normal mucosal sites. Therefore, as a general rule, approximately one-fourth to one-third of the locally infiltrative dose should be used topically on mucous membranes to diminish the risk of toxicity. It is also important to note that epinephrine does not reduce the risk of toxicity from mucous membrane application. Absolute *contraindications* to topical anesthesia ordinarily include traumatized tissues, open wounds, and open vascular beds (such as posttonsillectomy sites), and sepsis at the application site.

Proper technique with topical spray or injection procedures is necessary. Direct intravascular injection should be avoided and attention given to proper dosage. In general the minimal effective dose and concentration should be employed with slow injection to minimize toxicity. The total 24-hour dose of anesthetic should not exceed 300 mg, or 500 mg if epinephrine is added. Epinephrine is *contraindicated* in sites of end arteries or tight tissue compartments, such as digits, ears, nose, and penis, because ischemia is a potential complication. Epinephrine should also be avoided or minimized in patients with hypertension or cardiac disease and in those taking phenothiazines or monoamine oxidase inhibitors because of potential adverse interactions with catecholamine action.

A prior history of unusual reaction to local anes-

thetic or epinephrine should be noted, and the agents consequently avoided if possible. They should be immediately discontinued with signs of toxicity or hypersensitivity reaction. A prophylactic tray with intravenous medications (i.e., epinephrine 1:1000, hydrocortisone, diphenhydramine) for potential anaphylaxis and ensurance of an adequate oxygen source is a good policy before any local anesthetic procedure. An awareness of the potential risk of increased toxicity in the presence of liver disease is important, but little precise information is available in this regard. If prilocaine is used, a dosage less than 600 mg does not usually produce methemoglobinemia, and this agent is usually avoided in cyanotic patients.

Locally, it is important to note that the anesthetics can be rapidly inactivated by alkali, and the injectable preparation should be an isotonic solution to avoid edema, local irritation, and inflammation. Careful instruction to the patient to avoid food before and after local procedures with topical lidocaine on oral, pharyngeal, or tracheobronchial mucosa to prevent aspiration is clearly a basic requirement. Local anesthetics can cross the placenta, and epinephrine, if used in pregnancy, should be no greater than 1:200,000 concentration because there may be potential danger of vasoconstriction in uterine vessels.

Contact allergy is most clearly preventable by avoidance of use of PABA compound or nonamide anesthetics. This includes avoidance of such preparations in topical base formulations. Significant cross-reactions can occur among the PABA compounds taken by either the topical or systemic route. Sulfonamides, sulfonamide diuretics such as hydrodiuril, sulfonylurea antidiabetic agents, aminosalicylic acid, and many other drugs are included in the potential cross-reactions list. Flares of contact dermatitis or more generalized hypersensitivity reactions have occurred with their use in cases of prior topical PABA contact dermatitis. Other possible cross-reactions with PABA compounds include paraphenylenediamine (present in hair dyes and some proprietary creams), azo and aniline dyes in food or clothing, and other topical PABA products, such as sunscreens. Photocontact dermatitis on sun exposure may also occur with some of these products. Contact dermatitis to lidocaine itself is not reported, but a reaction to added compounds, such as parabens in some preparations, is possible.

SUMMARY

A brief survey of the agents used, their mode of use, and necessary precautions in surface and local infiltrative anesthesia have been presented. Lidocaine has been the predominant preparation employed because of its long-term effectiveness in clinical use and overall low complication rate. This includes a virtual absence of allergic contact sensitivity, which is the main disadvantage of many of the other local anesthetics, particularly those derived from the PABA compounds. Many commercial, topical, over-the-counter preparations contain benzocaine or PABA compound sensitizers and are best avoided.

ADVERSE/SIDE EFFECTS OF ANTISEPTICS AND LOCAL ANESTHETICS*

Antiseptics
ALLERGIC REACTIONS

Allergic contact dermatitis (more common with mercury compounds, iodine solution, and formalin ester; be aware of cross-reacting compounds)
Allergic contact urticaria
Asthma (unusual; occasionally with iodine solution or mercury compounds)
Angioneurotic edema

CARDIOVASCULAR SYSTEM

Air embolism (rare reports with hydrogen peroxide use in closed body cavities)
Cardiac arrest (with systemic toxicity to phenol, formalin, iodine solution, mercury compounds and boric acid)
Cardiovascular collapse

CENTRAL NERVOUS SYSTEM

Coma, convulsions, headache (particularly note potential neurotoxicity of hexachlorophene; otherwise with systemic toxicity usually on accidental or suicidal ingestion of phenol, mercury compounds, boric acid)

CUTANEOUS SYSTEM

Burns (phenol and concentrated solutions; misuse of disinfectants as antiseptics)
Contact dermatitis (allergic; irritation, dryness with most and increased with time)
Exfoliative dermatitis (with systemic toxicity, boric acid, mercury compounds)
Irritancy of mucous membranes—rhinitis, pharyngitis, tracheitis, bronchitis (formaldehyde vapor fumes)
Pigmentation or staining
Local (dyes, silver [black], iodo-chlorhydroxyquin [yellow], phe-nol [brown], potassium permanganate [brown, purple])
Systemic (mercury, silver)

GASTROINTESTINAL SYSTEM

Colitis (mercury compounds)
Corrosive effects, diarrhea, nausea, and vomiting (with accidental or suicidal ingestion of iodine solution, mercury compounds, concentrated benzalkonium chloride, phenol, and other toxic compounds)
Gastritis (more common with formalin or chlorinated compounds)
Pharyngitis
Tongue changes—glossitis, hairy black tongue (with excessive use of hydrogen peroxide in oral cavity)

HEMATOLOGIC SYSTEM

Anemia (unusual, occurs with systemic toxicity)
Delayed clotting (chlorinated compounds)
Leukopenia (unusual, occurs with systemic toxicity)
Methemoglobinemia (rarely with silver nitrate)

METABOLIC AND ENDOCRINE SYSTEMS

Electrolyte imbalance (silver nitrate in burn dressings)
Interference with laboratory tests (iodine and PBI test)

OCULAR SYSTEM

Irritant conjunctivitis (direct topical or vapor fumes [formaldehyde])

RENAL SYSTEM

Nephrotic syndrome (mercury intoxication)
Renal failure—acute or chronic (mercury, phenol, or boric acid toxicity)

WEARING APPAREL

Staining of clothing (use of hypochlorite bleaches on fabrics previously in contact with chlorhexidine compounds)

Local anesthetics
ALLERGIC REACTIONS

Allergic contact dermatitis (to nonamide compounds, especially PABA—be aware of cross-reacting compounds, oral or topical)
Allergic contact urticaria
Anaphylaxis
Angioneurotic edema
Asthma (with PABA compounds)
Photocontact dermatitis

CARDIOVASCULAR SYSTEM

Cardiac arrest (with systemic toxicity)
Ischemic complications (ischemia or gangrene of digits with epinephrine)
Palpitations (to epinephrine or systemic toxicity)
Tachycardia

CENTRAL NERVOUS SYSTEM

Coma, drowsiness, dizziness (with systemic toxicity)

HEMATOLOGIC SYSTEM

Excessive bleeding (uncommonly with local anesthetic without epinephrine)
Methemoglobinemia (with prilocaine)

MISCELLANEOUS EFFECTS

Aspiration
Fire hazards (ethyl chloride spray and cautery)

NOTE: Effects are largely topical and local unless preparation is orally ingested, applied to abraded or denuded areas, or highly toxic.
*See Chapter 11, "Drug Toxicity," for an overview of drug toxicity.

CLINICALLY SIGNIFICANT DRUG INTERACTIONS*

Primary drug	Interacting drug	Possible effect(s)	Probable mechanism(s)
ANTISEPTICS			
Alcohol	Disulfiram	Disulfiram reaction (flushing, headache, hypotension, skin rashes)	Direct pharmacologic effect—desired as an alcohol deterrent
Chlorhexidine	Hypochlorite bleaches	Adverse dark staining of clothing fabric if hypochlorite bleach used on fabric previously in contact with chlorhexidine compound	Chemical dye interaction
Formaldehyde	Formaldehyde resin compounds, wash-and-wear apparel (80% of fabrics containing cotton or rayon). Paper, cosmetics, many shampoos, nail hardeners, industrial materials or chemicals	Allergic contact dermatitis	Type IV cellular hypersensitivity reactions
Iodine compounds (iodine solution)	Iodized radiopaque radiographic contrast materials	Systemic eczematous contact reaction	Generalized dermatitis from systemic administration of a drug cross-reacting with a previous topical sensitizer
Isopropyl alcohol	Dextrostix	False positive blood glucose test if Dextrostix is read with cyetone or dextrometer	Isopropyl alcohol on skin causes falsely elevated readings of blood glucose
Mercury compounds (organic or inorganic)	Metallic, inorganic, or organic, mercury-containing products; mercurial diuretics; calomel (mercurous chloride); mercury amalgams; cosmetic preparations; red (cinnabar) portions of tattoos	Allergic contact dermatitis, systemic eczematous contact-type dermatitis, exfoliative dermatitis	Type IV cellular hypersensitivity reaction; generalized dermatitis from systemic administration of a drug cross-reacting with a previous topical sensitizer (may also be local dermatitis flare in red portion of tattoo with systemic ingestion)
Parabens (present as preservatives in many topical products particularly creams and lotions)	Paraben-containing products; many cosmetics, hair lotions, suntan preparations, soaps and toothpastes, and some adhesives, glues, and shoe dressings	Allergic contact dermatitis, allergic contact urticaria	Type IV cellular hypersensitivity reaction

NOTE: Drug interactions to these compounds are largely limited to contact allergic sensitivity reactions and cross-reactions through topical or systemic administration of a chemically related compound.
*See Chapter 10, "Drug Interactions," for an overview of drug interactions.

Continued.

CLINICALLY SIGNIFICANT DRUG INTERACTIONS—cont'd

Primary drug	Interacting drug	Possible effect(s)	Probable mechanism(s)
LOCAL ANESTHETICS			
Quaternary ammonium compounds (e.g., benzalkonium chloride)	Soaps and anionic detergents; iodides, bentonite, phenol, alkali, hydroxides, and chlorocresol	Prevention of therapeutic effect	Topical inactivation of active quaternary ammonium compound
ANTISEPTICS			
Epinephrine (used in local infiltration anesthetic)	Phenothiazines; tricyclic antidepressants; some antihistamines, diphenhydramine, tripelennamine	Decreased blood pressure, enhanced epinephrine effects	Alpha-adrenergic blockade, decreased uptake of epinephrine at nerve terminals
PABA compounds (procaine, dibucaine, tetracaine, benzocaine)	Many topical products containing benzocaine or PABA anesthetics, paraphenylenediamine, PABA, some PABA-containing azo and aniline dyes, PAS, sulfonamides, diuretics (hydrodiuril), oral hypoglycemics (tolbutamide), artificial sweetening agents (saccharin, Sucaryl)	Allergic contact dermatitis, allergic contact urticaria, photoallergic contact dermatitis, systemic eczematous contact dermatitis	Type IV cellular hypersensitivity reaction; generalized dermatitis from systemic administration of a drug cross-reacting with a previous topical sensitizer
Topical antihistamines	Diphenhydramine	Allergic contact dermatitis, allergic contact urticaria, systemic eczematous contact dermatitis	Type IV cellular hypersensitivity reaction; generalized dermatitis from systemic administration of a drug cross-reacting with a previous topical sensitizer

GENERAL NURSING IMPLICATIONS

Nursing of patients requiring antiseptics

ASSESSMENT

Antiseptics are used in various procedures and treatments including skin preparation for injection of medication and wound care. Antiseptics are selected in relation to their bactericidal or antiseptic activity and to the site to which they will be applied. Nursing assessment should include identification of possible sensitivity, contraindications, cautions, and possible drug interactions before antiseptics are used.

SENSITIVITY

Any drug has the potential to cause a sensitivity reaction in susceptible individuals. With the antiseptics these reactions are primarily localized and confined to the cutaneous system.

CONTRAINDICATIONS

The use of various antiseptics is contraindicated in certain conditions, including known sensitivity. In addition, some preparations may be contraindicated because of incompatibility with a coadministered topical preparation (e.g., benzalkonium and anionic soaps or detergents) (see the Nursing Drug Digest for specific contraindications associated with individual agents).

CAUTIONS

Use antiseptics with caution when applied to large areas of denuded or abraded skin because significant systemic absorption and resultant toxicity may occur.

It is important to note that antiseptics left at the bedside have been inadvertently ingested by patients thinking the antiseptic was an oral medication. Caution is required with the proper handling, labeling, and storage of these preparations (see the Nursing Drug Digest and the body of the chapter for cautions associated with individual agents).

Antiseptics should be clearly labeled for external use only and stored out of the reach of children to prevent inadvertent oral ingestion and resultant toxicity.

DRUG INTERACTIONS

Drug interactions involving the antiseptics are largely limited to contact allergic sensitivity reactions and cross-reactions through topical or systemic administration of a chemically related compound (see Clinically Significant Drug Interactions).

ADMINISTRATION

Antiseptics are available in numerous forms (e.g., solutions, soaps, lotions) for external topical use. They are applied to tissues to destroy and inhibit growth of microorganisms. Administration of the various agents may differ in relation to preparation of the site and duration of contact. It should be remembered that antiseptics are used primarily in the treatment of relatively minor, clean wounds and for the preparation of the skin before incision or injection. Antiseptics should not be considered suitable substitutes for proper mechanical cleansing, debridement, irrigation, and drainage of obviously contaminated wounds.

Generally, before antiseptics are applied, the following should be noted.

1. Familiarization with antiseptics in use, including an awareness of all potential side effects, is important.
2. All compounds should be clearly labeled with appropriate poison labels where indicated and instructions for topical use only.
3. Efficient quality control programs, including bacteriologic surveillance, should be rigidly followed in areas such as hospital operating suites, maternity units, and nurseries in addition to general ward routines. This entails periodic review of antiseptics in use as part of the quality control program, including their efficacy, shelf life, stability, toxicity, and complication rate.
4. It is preferable to restrict the number of antiseptics in use, but to generally avoid using the same compound as both an antiseptic and disinfectant, since concentration and instruction errors could ensue.

5. Solution containers are to be kept out of children's reach, and particular care should be taken to check proper solutions before use with infants and children.
6. Observe and report significant complications (i.e., anaphylaxis, excessive drowsiness). A central registry of such complications is often useful.
7. Check for potential incompatibilities before use, such as soaps or other anionic compounds that can inhibit the action of quaternary ammonium compounds.
8. Instructions of preparation and storage should be clear (i.e., freshness of solution, pH, concentration).
9. Observe and report allergic contact dermatitis and routinely inquire regarding past allergic or hypersensitivity reactions to antiseptic compounds. A patient alert tag or chain should be advised along with appropriate visible notation on patient's chart and bedside.
10. Routinely inquire and check regarding application of proprietary preparations in patient's possession.
11. Have constant awareness of the possibility of accidental or suicidal ingestion, with appropriate emergency procedures, antidotes, and supplies clear and available. Periodic review of emergency procedures is advisable.
12. Avoid if possible mercury compounds, phenol, boric acid, and aldehydes as antiseptics unless specifically indicated.
13. Be familiar with the special regulations and policies regarding use of hexachlorophene, with particular attention to nurseries.

See the Nursing Drug Digest for specific information regarding the use and application of individual antiseptics.

Continued.

GENERAL NURSING IMPLICATIONS—cont'd

Nursing of patients requiring antiseptics—cont'd

MONITORING PATIENT RESPONSE

Therapeutic response

Monitor injection sites, incisions, and wounds for increased healing and absence of signs of infection.

Adverse side effects

Adverse side effects associated with antiseptics are relatively rare and usually consist of minor irritation to the application site. Many preparations have the potential to stain fabric, hair, skin, or nails (see Adverse/Side Effects of Antiseptics and Local Anesthetics).

PATIENT EDUCATION

The patient and family as indicated should have a clear understanding of the use of antiseptics, including the preparation's name, general action, purpose, storage, and adverse side effects. If the patient is to be using the antiseptic at home or as a discharge patient, he or she should understand the correct application. Some antiseptic agents can bleach or stain skin, hair, or fabric, and patients should be advised of these effects.

Because of the potential for serious or fatal overdose if the agent is ingested orally, special attention should be directed at educating the patient about proper storage and handling of these preparations and about what procedure to follow in case of accidental ingestion. The patient should also be made aware that these agents can be irritating to the eyes or mucous membranes and that antiseptics should not be applied to these areas unless specifically advised by a clinician. If antiseptics are accidently applied to the eye, patients should be informed to wash the eye with copious amounts of water and to seek advise from their health care provider if any burning, stinging, or itching persists.

Nursing of patients requiring local anesthetics

ASSESSMENT

Local anesthetics are used in various procedures and treatments, including topical application for local pain relief and for infiltration, nerve, caudal, and epidural block. Therapy and dosage are individualized. A complete nursing assessment should include a detailed drug history identifying possible sensitivity, contraindications, cautions, and drug interactions before therapy is initiated.

SENSITIVITY

Any drug has the potential to cause a hypersensitivity reaction in susceptible individuals, and hypersensitivity to local anesthetics is not a rare occurrence. In addition, cross-hypersensitivity is commonly noted among the various amide-type local anesthetics.

CONTRAINDICATIONS

The use of local anesthetics is contraindicated in patients with known hypersensitivity to a specific or related agent. In addition, local anesthetics are contraindicated in cases of severe shock or heart block. The use of a local anesthetic that contains epinephrine is contraindicated in procedures involving the digits, nose, ears, and penis (see the Nursing Drug Digest for contraindications to specific agents).

CAUTIONS

Local anesthetics should be used cautiously in children, the elderly, debilitated patients, and acutely ill patients. In these individuals, dosage must generally be reduced and adjusted according to patient status and response.

Local anesthetics should be used cautiously during pregnancy. In addition, during paracervical anesthesia, fetal heart rate should be monitored to detect fetal bradycardia, which is particularly likely in the presence of prematurity, toxemia of pregnancy, fetal distress, or with the use of excessive doses.

Use local anesthetics with caution in patients with bradycardia or severe digitalis intoxication and in unconscious patients.

DRUG INTERACTIONS

Drug interactions to local anesthetics are largely limited to contact allergic sensitivity reactions and cross-reactions through topical or systemic administration of a chemically related compound (see Clinically Significant Drug Interactions).

ADMINISTRATION

Local anesthetics are available in various dosage forms for topical and for parenteral administration. The dosage and concentration used depends on the intended use. For parenteral administration, the volume and concentration chosen depend on the general physical state of the patient, the time and extent of the surgical procedure, the duration of anesthesia required, and the degree of muscular relaxation required.

In general, the lowest concentration and smallest dose that will produce the desired therapeutic effect should be administered. Dosage is generally reduced in children, the elderly, and debilitated patients.

Parenteral injections of local anesthetics should be made slowly with frequent aspirations to reduce the possibility of intravascular injection. Inadvertent intravascular injection increases both the incidence of local anesthetic failure and the incidence of systemic adverse effects.

Before administering local anesthetics or assisting with their administration, one should note the following:

1. Familiarization with local anesthetics in use, including an awareness of all potential side effects, is important.
2. It is preferable to limit the num-

GENERAL NURSING IMPLICATIONS—cont'd

Nursing of patients requiring local anesthetics—cont'd

ADMINISTRATION—cont'd

ber of local anesthetics in use to agents such as lidocaine, unless otherwise indicated.

3. A prior history of unusual reaction to local anesthetic or added epinephrine should be noted and the agents avoided.

4. A readily available prophylactic tray with IV medications (i.e., epinephrine 1:1000, hydrocortisone, diphenhydramine) for the treatment of potential anaphylaxis, along with ensurance of adequate oxygen, is a good policy before any local anesthetic procedure.

5. Ensure that epinephrine is not present in local anesthetics administered to sites such as the digits, ears, nose, or penis. Epinephrine should also be avoided in patients receiving phenothiazines or monoamine oxidase inhibitors, unless otherwise indicated.

6. Do not use ethyl chloride spray in the presence of cautery or electrical or flame source because of danger of fire.

7. Follow all recommended procedures for control of restricted drugs, such as cocaine.

8. Be aware of the limits of professional nursing practice as related to the use and administration of local anesthetics.

MONITORING PATIENT RESPONSE

Therapeutic response

Monitor for analgesic and local anesthetic effects. The onset of action is relatively rapid and the duration is rela-

tively short (1 to 2 hours, depending on the preparation used, site of administration, concentration and dosage).

Adverse side effects

Adverse side effects associated with the local anesthetics are largely caused by improper administration. With correct dosage and administration, adverse effects are relatively uncommon. However, both local and systemic adverse effects have been associated with the use of local anesthetics and are predominantly dose related.

Local

Local irritation, burning, itching, or other discomfort can occur with the topical administration of these medications, and patients should be advised of these effects and monitored carefully. Parenteral administration of local anesthetics can also cause transient burning or stinging at the injection site.

Observe and report evidence of local edema or skin rashes of any type. Also report pruritus if present.

Systemic

Systemic effects are more likely to occur with local anesthetics used parenterally or when topical preparations are applied to an area of skin that has been denuded or abraded. Systemic effects are usually dose related and include hypotension, bradycardia, dizziness, apprehension, tremors, convulsions, and respiratory depression.

Observe and report any abnormal cerebral, cardiovascular, or respiratory abnormality following local anesthetic procedures (see Adverse/Side Effects of Antiseptics and Local Anesthetics for an outline of adverse effects related to the local anesthetics).

PATIENT EDUCATION

The patient should have an understanding of the need for the local anesthetic. He or she should know the exact name of the drug, its general action, purpose, and adverse side effects. If the patient is to be self-medicating with a topical local anesthetic, he or she should understand the correct administration and storage of the preparation and activities that should be modified or avoided. For example, patients using an oral viscous preparation of lidocaine should be cautioned against drinking hot beverages, or against the oral ingestion of any food or drug while the oral cavity is anesthetized, to avoid burning, trauma to the oral mucosa and tongue, or aspiration.

Patients should also be advised of the following:

1. Generally avoid topical nonamide (including all PABA) compounds and topical antihistamines to minimize allergic contact reactions. Have prepared lists of potential cross-reacting compounds to avoid, if a history of previous allergic contact reaction exists.

2. Avoid food at least 3 hours before and after local procedures with topical local anesthetic on oral, pharyngeal, or tracheobronchial mucosa to prevent aspiration.

3. Avoid driving or activities requiring alertness because drowsiness can follow a local anesthetic procedure.

GENERAL INSTRUCTIONS FOR DISCHARGE/OUTPATIENTS

ANTISEPTICS

Follow the instructions exactly on all compounds, prescription or nonprescription.

Do not use excessively or for other purposes. Restrict to topical use. Generally avoid eye contact.

Familiarize yourself with conditions of storage, shelf life, and expiration dates where appropriate.

Avoid household remedies or proprietary preparations unless specifically advised or ordered by your health care provider.

Skin rashes or local irritation may develop even if used previously without complication. The onset may be delayed and may begin after discharge even if used without problem in the hospital.

Do not use the same product as an antiseptic and disinfectant.

Consult your health care provider if further information or clarification is required or if complications ensue.

Avoid hypochlorite bleaches on fabrics previously in contact with chlorhexidine compounds to prevent unnecessary staining.

Be aware of possible staining of skin with some compounds.

For external use *only*, unless otherwise directed by your nurse or physician.

This medication has been advised especially for you. Do not trade or give this medication to any relatives or friends.

Keep this and all medications out of children's reach.

LOCAL ANESTHETICS

Avoid food ingestion for 3 hours before and after topical oral procedures or with use of viscous lidocaine.

Report immediately to your nurse or physician any undue reactions, such as wheezing or other breathing problems, excessive dizziness or drowsiness, palpitations or tachycardia, cyanosis, chest pain, or unusual bleeding.

If you have had a previous allergic contact reaction, carefully avoid the potential cross-reacting products named in the list provided to you by the nurse or physician.

Report any skin rashes or pruritus to your nurse or physician.

Do not drive for at least 3 hours following most local anesthetic procedures.

Avoid proprietary (over-the-counter) local anesthetic compounds including "caine" products unless advised by your health care provider.

Keep this medication and all other medication out of the reach of children.

NURSING DRUG DIGEST

Medication (trade name*)	Indication	Usual dosage and administration	Dosage forms, preparation, and storage	Contraindications, cautions, and comments	Monitoring
ANTISEPTICS					
Alcohol Ethanol Ethyl alcohol	Antiseptic For *external* use only	Topical dose not quantitated or standardized Administered usually as 70% aqueous solution	Alcohol USP; Rubbing Alcohol NF Marketed under generic name usually as 70% aqueous solution Check stability and shelf life routinely and discard outdated solutions	Keep room well ventilated Potentially flammable Irritating to mucous membranes or open wounds Drying with excessive use Denaturing agents and coloring added normally to discourage oral use Rarely contact dermatitis May increase local bleeding because of vasodilation Even topical use may cause skin eruptions or systemic manifestations of a disulfiram reaction (i.e., flushing, headaches, hypotension) in patients being treated with disulfiram	Observe skin for dryness

NOTE: For additional details regarding the individual agents listed in this table see the text and other tables in this chapter.
*Indicates a multiple active ingredient product. For a complete listing of all active ingredients see the *Drug Reference Guide to Brand Names and Active Ingredients.*
★Indicates that the drug is generally available only in the United States.

Continued.

NURSING DRUG DIGEST—cont'd

Medication (trade name)	Indication	Usual dosage and administration	Dosage forms, preparation, and storage	Contraindications, cautions, and comments	Monitoring
Benzalkonium chloride Benzachlor-50 Germ-i-Tol Germicin Hyamine 3500 Ice-O-Derm Gel Ionax Medi-Quik* Mediconet* Otic-HC Ear Drops* Pilocar* Sabol Spensomide Theranac Scrub Zephiran Chloride	Antiseptic Disinfectant-detergent For *external* use only	Topical use only Concentrations vary with purpose For preoperative antiseptic 1:2000 to 1:10000 as aqueous antiseptic or wet dressings Aqueous 1:750 with antirust tablets for sterilization of instruments	Aqueous solution: 1:750 Concentrated solution: 21.3% Antirust tablets added to aqueous solution for sterilization of metal instruments as directed Towelettes: moist paper towels impregnated with solution of benzalkonium chloride 1:750, perfume, chlorothymol, alcohol 20% Antiseptic wipes: at least 0.2% concentration Conditions of preparation (i.e., freshness of stock solution, pH, concentration) should be rigidly followed	Inactivated by soaps and anionic compounds, rinse these off carefully before application Action hindered by pus, blood or tissue debris Corrosive and systemic toxicity with accidental ingestion Usually ineffective against *Pseudomonas* May be absorbed by cotton, cellulose, and some plastics, hindering disinfection Accidental contact with concentrated solution directly or via treated fabrics can cause local corrosive skin changes Can be irritating to skin and cause dryness with excess use Rarely causes allergic contact dermatitis Avoid use as both antiseptic and disinfectant using same stock solution Requires regular monitoring of antibacterial effectiveness	Observe for local irritation
Cetrimide Cetavlon Cetril Drapolex Savlon	Antiseptic Detergent For *external* use only	Topical use only Usually employed as 1% solution May use 1% aqueous solution with antirust tablets as cold sterilization solution	Powder: 3 level teaspoons (4.6 gm) dissolved in 450 ml makes a 1% solution Topical solution: 1% Cream: 1% Lotion: 1%	Incompatible with soaps and anionic compounds, iodides, phenylmercuric nitrate, phenol, and chlorocresol; rinse	Observe for local irritation

Drug	Uses	Dosage	Preparation/Strength	Comments
	1:2500 solution can be used as oral mucosal antiseptic, mouth wash, spray, or gargle	Lotion: 1%		these off carefully before use of cetrimide Can cause irritation and dryness with excessive use Can be corrosive and cause systemic toxicity with accidental ingestion
Cetrimide and chlorhexidine Savlon hospital concentrate	Disinfectant Occasional antiseptic For *external* use only	Topical solution as 1:30, 1:100 or 1:200 aqueous solutions or 1:30 alcoholic solution	Supplied as chlorhexidine gluconate 7.5% v/v (1.5% w/v) and cetrimide B.P. 15% w/v Diluted to desired strengths with deionized or distilled water or 70% alcohol or isopropyl alcohol Check stability and expiration date (often require fresh preparation after 2 weeks) Ensure proper storage and limited access	Store stock solutions with glass or rubber stoppers Do not use cork stoppers to prevent gram-negative contamination Avoid use of same stock solution as both antiseptic and disinfectant Add sodium nitrate as antirust agent to prevent corrosion of surgical instruments stored in cetrimide solution Hypochlorite bleach should not be used for laundering garments that have been in contact with cetrimide because a brown stain may develop Sodium perborate may be used as a suitable bleach (2 or 3 oz for a 100-lb load at 80-100° C)

Continued.

NURSING DRUG DIGEST—cont'd

Medication (trade name)	Indication	Usual dosage and administration	Dosage forms, preparation, and storage	Contraindications, cautions, and comments	Monitoring
Chlorhexidine Bactigras Hibicare Hibiclens Hibitane Hibitane Tincture*	Antiseptic Disinfectant For *external* use only	Topical use only Commonly as 1% or 4% solution as antiseptic—dose not standardized (5 ml/application) Apply as directed, 0.5% in 70% alcohol (1:200) common desired concentration for preoperative skin preparations Higher concentrations may be used as disinfectant	Supplied usually as chlorhexidine gluconate in solutions or emulsion of 1%, 4% or 20% concentration, diluted with deionized or distilled water or 70% alcohol to desired strength Check stability and expiration dates	Rinse thoroughly after use Avoid eye contact; rinse promptly with water Dryness or irritation of skin with excessive use Avoid hypochlorite bleaches on fabrics in contact with chlorhexidine to avoid stains If stain occurs, use sodium perborate or hydrogen peroxide Avoid instillation into ear; rinse promptly with water; instillation into middle ear, in case of perforated eardrum, may result in deafness Avoid cork stoppers to minimize risk of gram-negative contamination of stock solvent Avoid use of same stock solutions as both disinfectant and antiseptic to minimize error or confusion Poorly absorbed from GI tract and intact skin; therefore risk of systemic toxicity is minimal	Observe for local irritation Observe skin for dryness

Drug	Action/Use	Administration	Preparations	Precautions	Nursing implications
Gentian violet Genapex GVS GVS Vaginal Hyva Hyva Vaginal	Mild antiseptic Anticandidal Antifungal	Topical use only Topical solution or cream 0.02%-17% concentration Amount per application not standardized For treatment of vulvitis insert vaginally q.d. to b.i.d. until symptoms have resolved Weak antiseptic Best avoided for general use and replaced by more effective and less staining compounds	Cream: 1.35% Gentian violet topical solution, USP contains 1% in 10% alcohol Solution may be diluted to desired concentration with 70% alcohol Vaginal inserts: 0.4% Vaginal tablets: 2.0 mg Tampons: 5 mg	Purple staining of skin or mucosa Tattooing can result from application to granulation tissue Avoid on facial wounds	Observe for skin staining, and inform patient
Hexachlorophene Burdeo* Dermohex Fomac G-11 Gamophen Hexamead-PH Hexaphenyl pHisoHex Soy Dome Cleanser Surgi-Cen WescoHex	Antiseptic Detergent For *external* use only	Topical use *only* Apply as directed and following general policy guidelines, (i.e., hospital and nursing policy guide with particular caution in neonates)	Sudsing emulsion containing entsufon (a synthetic detergent), lanolin, cholesterol, petrolatum and 3% hexachlorophene 0.25% hexachlorophene as liquid soap 0.23% hexachlorophene as tincture foam Also formulated in creams, ointments, lotions, and shampoos	Hazard of neurotoxicity; absorbed from intact skin especially with repeat application Greater risk of toxicity with infants or abraded skin Clearly label preparations and limit use as for policy guidelines 3% hexachlorophene distributed only by prescription (FDA order 1972) Not to be used for routine prophylactic body bathing of infants Can cause local irritation; avoid eye contact; prompt rinsing of suds necessary Excess use may produce dryness or irritation Reduced efficiency in presence of organic matter Rinse thoroughly after use Less effective in *Pseudomonas* outbreaks	Observe for local irritation

Continued.

NURSING DRUG DIGEST—cont'd

Medication (trade name)	Indication	Usual dosage and administration	Dosage forms, preparation, and storage	Contraindications, cautions, and comments	Monitoring
Hexachlorophene—cont'd				Do *not* use on abraded, burned, or denuded skin Do *not* apply vaginally or on other mucous membranes because of increased systemic absorption Can cause systemic toxicity with accidental ingestion; treat with gastric lavage and symptomatic support	
Hydrogen peroxide PerOxyl	Antiseptic	Topical use *only*, 3% solution Irrigation of wounds Amount not standardized	3% solution Check stability and expiration date, and discard if outdated Shaking solution *increases* release of oxygen and decomposition of hydrogen peroxide	Can be corrosive and systemic toxicity with accidental ingestion Hazard with irrigation in closed cavities (rare reports of air embolism) Local mucosal irritation with excessive use Unreliable as primary antiseptic, especially on intact skin Glossitis with excess oral use Hairy black tongue common with prolonged use as an oral mouthwash, but disappears on discontinuance Do not apply to new epithelial cells during the process of wound healing	Observe for glossitis and black hairy tongue

Drug	Action/Use	Dosage	Preparations	Remarks/Cautions	Nursing Considerations
Iodine (tincture of iodine)	Disinfectant Antiseptic For *external* use only	Topical use *only* Applied as 2% solution Amount not standardized or quantitated Avoid use as routine antiseptic	Iodine solution USP contains 2% iodine and 2.4% sodium iodide Iodine tincture USP (above in 50% alcohol)	*Contraindicated* in hypersensitivity to iodines *Do not* confuse with stronger Lugol's iodine, which contains 5% iodine and 10% potassium iodide Can stain tissues or fabrics Bandaging or taping treated areas may cause tissue irritation Can be irritating to wounds Can cause allergic contact dermatitis or hypersensitivity reactions Risk of cross-reaction with iodized radiographic dyes Hazard of accidental ingestion Treat ingestion with gastric lavage using starch solution or 5% sodium thiosulfate to inactivate the iodine May interfere with laboratory test for protein-bound iodide (PBI)	Observe for local irritation Observe for hypersensitivity

Continued.

NURSING DRUG DIGEST—cont'd

Medication (trade name)	Indication	Usual dosage and administration	Dosage forms, preparation, and storage	Contraindications, cautions, and comments	Monitoring
Iodochlor-hydroxyquin Domeform F-E-P Creme* HCV Cream Locacorten-vioform* Myocquin Mystaform Mystaform Ointment* Mystaform-HC* Quin III Quinambicide Quin-O-Creme Tar-Doak Lotion* Vioform Vioform-Hydrocortisone*	Antiseptic	Topical use *only* Usually 3% or less concentrations compounded at prescriber's request	Available in combined proprietary preparations with topical corticosteroids or antibiotics Ointment, cream: 3% Dusting powder: 3% Iodochlorhydroxyquin, hydrocortisone: "regular"—cream and ointment—iodochlorhydroxyquin 3%, hydrocortisone 1%; "mild"—cream and ointment—iodochlorhydroxyquin 3%, hydrocortisone 0.5% Also combined with nystatin for anti-*Candida* yeast topical therapy Check stability, shelf life, and expiration dates	Can commonly cause irritant contact dermatitis Uncommon allergic contact dermatitis Can stain skin, hair, nails, or clothing May interfere with some laboratory tests (i.e., thyroid function) May give false positive ferric chloride test for phenylketonuria (PKU) in infants if present in diaper or urine	Observe for contact dermatitis
Isopropyl alcohol	Antiseptic For *external* use only	Topical dose not quantitated or standardized Applied usually as 70% aqueous solution	Alcohol USP; Rubbing Alcohol NF Marketed under generic name usually as 70% aqueous solution Check stability and shelf life routinely and discard outdated solutions	Keep room well ventilated Potentially flammable Irritating and painful to mucous membranes or open wounds Drying with excessive use Denaturing agents and coloring added normally to discourage oral use Rarely causes contact dermatitis May increase local bleeding because of vasodilation	Observe skin for dryness

Name	Use	Dose	Preparations/Remarks	Adverse Reactions	Nursing Implications
Mercuric oxide, yellow	Antiseptic Antibacterial for treatment of blepharitis and conjunctivitis	Topical use *only* Often as 1% concentration Dose not quantitated or standardized *Avoid* use of mercury products if possible	Ointment: 1%, 2% Protect from light	Even topical use may cause skin eruptions or systemic manifestations of disulfiram reaction (i.e., flushing, headaches, hypotension) in patients being treated with disulfiram Allergic contact dermatitis May be irritating locally Avoid on open wounds Hazard of toxicity with excess use Prolonged ophthalmic use may result in systemic absorption and injury to the eye	Observe for contact dermatitis
Mercury, ammoniated (usually compounded)	Antiseptic Psoriasis scalp therapy For *external* use only	Topical use *only* Dose not standardized Less than 1% concentration is safest *Avoid* use of mercury products if possible	Usually ointment formulations Available as 1% or 5% concentrations before dilution requested	Allergic contact dermatitis May be irritating Avoid on open wounds Hazard of toxicity with excessive use	Observe for contact dermatitis
Phenol (carbolic acid) (usually compounded)	Antiseptic Disinfectant Antipruritic For *external* use only	Topical use *only* Disinfectant solution in greater than 1% concentration Limited topical use in concentration less than 1% Occasional use as topical antipruritic in dilute concentrations of 1:100 or 1:200 Use as antiseptic *not* recommended	Storage solutions, prepare as directed	Irritancy, brown staining or burns common Hazard of toxicity even from topical use (especially greater than 1% concentration) Systemic toxicity with accidental ingestion May cause contact burns even as disinfectants via absorption by rubber and plastics Label as poison and store in locked area Strict avoidance necessary on abraded skin or mucosa	Observe for local irritation

Continued.

NURSING DRUG DIGEST—cont'd

Medication (trade name)	Indication	Usual dosage and administration	Dosage forms, preparation, and storage	Contraindications, cautions, and comments	Monitoring
Phenol— cont'd				Develop clearly posted procedures for topical or systemic complications Locally phenol removal facilitated by 5% alcohol, glycerin, vegetable oil, sodium bicarbonate solution or copious water Ingestion treated early with passage of stomach tube and gastric lavage with olive oil to remove the phenol without absorption	
Povidone-iodine Anbesol Antiseptic Anesthetic* Betadine Bridine Isodine Pharmadine Polydine Solution, Scrub, Ointment Proviodine PVP-Iodine	Antiseptic	Topical use *only* Concentration may vary 0.1-10% Dose not standardized Apply as directed	Available as sudsing skin cleanser, foam solutions, surgical scrub, aerosol spray, ointment, gauze pads, shampoo, and oral and vaginal preparations, with 1%-10% concentration and differing formulations Check expiration date (usually 3 years for solution), and discard outdated stock	*Contraindicated* in hypersensitivity to iodines Rare contact dermatitis or hypersensitivity reaction Protect these products from excessive heat Repeated vaginal application during pregnancy can result in significant systemic absorption of iodine and suppression of the thyroid gland in both mother and fetus Extensive topical application to neonates may cause hypothyroidism To obtain an approximate percentage measure of the iodine content, divide the listed concentration by 10 Nonstaining Treated areas may be bandaged or taped	Observe for contact dermatitis

	Use	Preparation	Dose	Remarks
Silver nitrate				
Silver nitrate ophthalmic solution	Prophylaxis of ophthalmia neonatorum	Silver nitrate ophthalmic solution, USP (1%)	Topical use *only* Two drops of 1% solution to conjunctival sac of newborn	Observe for tissue staining
Silver nitrate solution—prepared	Antiseptic Burn dressings For *external* use only	Also available in topical solutions of 0.01% to 10% concentrations Silver nitrate is light sensitive; keep out of light	Topical use *only* 1:1000 to 1:10000 concentration 0.5% solution generally replaced in burn therapy dressings by safer agents	Hazard in burns because of electrolyte depletion of chloride and sodium Tissue staining or tattooing (black) Argyria possible with excessive use Potential methemoglobinemia with excessive use Avoid accidental ingestion of solution
Thimerosal				
Merthiolate	Antiseptic For *external* use only	Thimerosal NF aqueous solution: 0.1% (1:1000) Tincture-colored alcohol, acetone-water solution of 0.1% thimerosal both available Creams or ointments: 1:1000	Topical use *only* Dose not standardized Applied to skin at 1:1000 (0.1%) concentration or less *Avoid* use of mercury products if possible	Allergic contact dermatitis is rare, but constitutes a *contraindication* to use Incompatible with strong acids, salts, or heavy metals and iodine May be irritating Avoid on open wounds Hazard of toxicity on oral ingestion: solution contains tetraborate ion Observe for contact dermatitis Observe for hypersensitivity to mercury-containing compounds
LOCAL ANESTHETICS				
Articaine Ultracaine D-S* Ultracaine D-S Forte*	Infiltration anesthesia and nerve block anesthesia in *dentistry*	Solution for injection: 4% NOTE: All Ultracaine preparations contain epinephrine	*Adults:* Use lowest dose necessary to provide effective anesthesia	*Contraindicated* in hypersensitivity; severe shock, heart block, severe hypertension, and sepsis near the proposed injection site Resuscitative drugs and equipment should be available May cause methemoglobinemia Overdose may cause CNS excitation and cardiovascular depression Observe for hypersensitivity reactions Usual onset of anesthesia is 1-3 min with a duration of 45-75 min

Continued.

NURSING DRUG DIGEST—cont'd

Medication (trade name)	Indication	Usual dosage and administration	Dosage forms, preparation, and storage	Contraindications, cautions, and comments	Monitoring
Bupivacaine Marcaine Sensorcaine	Local anesthetic	*Adults:* topical and regional and local infiltrative anesthesia (intracutaneous or SC) 2-60 ml of 0.25% solution for local infiltration depending on area and extent of the block Recommended maximum single dose is 150 mg, maximum daily dose is 400 mg in 24 hours *Avoid* intravascular injection *Children:* Over 12 years of age, same as adults *Elderly:* Start with lower doses	Solution for injection: 0.25%, 0.5%, or 0.75% with or without epinephrine 1:200000 Bupivacaine solutions without epinephrine may be autoclaved Routinely check stability, shelf life, and expiration date	*Contraindicated* in obstetrical paracervical block Longer sustained action than lidocaine of up to 4 hr May be useful for pain relief if more prolonged anesthesia required Some intrinsic vasoconstriction activity and can be used without epinephrine Establish general routine policy and registry of complications for local anesthetic procedures (i.e., including errors of dosage or technique, intravascular injection, toxicity, anaphylaxis, aspiration) Be aware of contraindications to local anesthesia in general Routinely inquire and notify prescriber of any previous adverse reaction or complication to local anesthesia	

| ★ **Chloroprocaine**
Nesacaine
Versacaine | Local anesthetic | *Adults:* Infiltration and nerve block, caudal and epidural block
Dose depends on concentration of solution and site to be infiltrated
Use lowest effective dose
Maximum dose 800 mg (1000 mg with epinephrine—1:200,000)
Inject slowly
Avoid intravascular injections
Children: Start with lower doses
Elderly: Start with lower doses | Solution: for injection 1%, 2%, 3%
To prepare 1:200,000 epinephrine-chloroprocaine solution, add 0.15 ml of 1:1000 epinephrine hydrochloride to 30 ml chloroprocaine 2%
Incompatible with caustic alkalis, iodides, iodines, silver salts, and soaps
Discard unused portion | Routinely have available supplies and materials in case of anaphylaxis reaction including tourniquet, ambient oxygen source, IV medications: 1:1000 epinephrine, hydrocortisone, diphenhydramine, syringes, needles, antiseptic
Caution patient regarding drowsiness
Use with caution in severely ill patients
IV regional anesthesia (e.g., Bier's block) and obstetric paracervical block have been associated with cardiac arrest, particularly when the highest concentration (i.e., 0.75%) is used |
| | | | *Contraindicated* in hypersensitivity
Resuscitative equipment and drugs should be available
May cause fetal bradycardia (heart rate less than 120 beats/min for greater than 2 min)
Overdose may cause CNS excitation and cardiovascular depression | Observe for hypersensitivity reactions
Monitor for fetal bradycardia |

Continued.

NURSING DRUG DIGEST—cont'd

Medication (trade name)	Indication	Usual dosage and administration	Dosage forms, preparation, and storage	Contraindications, cautions, and comments	Monitoring
Dibucaine Corticaine Cream* Nupercainal Nupercainal suppositories Nupercaine Nuperlone Otocort Ear Drops*	Local anesthetic	*Adults:* Used parenterally for spinal anesthesia Dosage depends on concentration of solution and site to be anesthetized Maximum: 10 mg Inject *slowly* *Avoid* intravascular injections *Elderly:* Start with lower doses	Ointment: 1% Cream: 0.5% Suppository: 2.5 mg Store below 30° C Solution: 0.5% (for injection) Discard discolored solutions	*Contraindicated* in hypersensitivity Resuscitative equipment and drugs should be available Use caution if applying topical preparation to denuded or abraded areas of skin because systemic absorption may occur Do *not* apply topical preparation to eye	Observe for hypersensitivity
	Topical anesthetic	Apply t.i.d. to q.i.d. sparingly as necessary Topical preparation for *external* use only			
	Rectal suppository for symptomatic relief of hemorrhoids	Insert 1 PR b.i.d.			
Etidocaine Duranest	Local anesthetic	*Adults:* Infiltration and nerve block, caudal and epidural block Dose depends on concentration of solution and site to be infiltrated Use lowest effective dose Maximum: 300 mg (4 mg/kg) (400 mg [5.5 mg/kg] with epinephrine) Inject *slowly* *Avoid* intravascular injections *Children:* Dosage information *not* available; use in children less than 14 years of age is therefore not recommended *Elderly:* Start with lower doses	Solution: for injection 0.5%, 1% (0.5%, 1%, 1.5% are also available with epinephrine 1 :200,000)	*Contraindicated* in known hypersensitivity Use with caution during pregnancy Use preparations containing epinephrine cautiously in patients receiving MAOIs Resuscitative equipment and drugs should be available Overdose may cause CNS excitation and cardiovascular depression	Observe for hypersensitivity reactions

Lidocaine
Anestacon
Bay Caine
Dolicaine
Lida-Mantle
Lidosporin
Otic Solution*
Lidopen Auto-Injector
Medi-Quik*
Nulicaine
Octocaine
Ultracaine
Unguentine Plus*
Xylocaine
Xylocaine Endotracheal Aerosol
Xylocaine Jelly
Xylocaine Ointment
Xylocaine Topical Spray
Xylocaine Viscous
Xylocard

Local anesthetic
See also Chapter 32, "Antidysrhythmics"

Adults: Regional and local infiltrative anesthesia, intracutaneous and SC
Used whenever possible with epinephrine to prolong action, reduce systemic absorption, and decrease bleeding
Avoid intravascular injection
Elderly: Start with lower doses

Lidocaine solutions: 0.5% plain; 0.5% with epinephrine, 1:100000; 0.5% with epinephrine, 1:200000; 1% plain; 1% with epinephrine, 1:100000; 1% with epinephrine, 1:200000; 2% plain; 2% with epinephrine, 1:100,000; 4% plain (topical) tinted
Vials of lidocaine solution containing epinephrine should *not* be autoclaved

Be aware of *contraindications* to local anesthesia in general (i.e., history of previous adverse reaction to the compound)
May be *contraindicated* in presence of open vascular bed or sepsis
Use with epinephrine *contraindicated* in sites of end arteries such as digits and tip of nose
Routinely inquire and notify prescriber of any previous adverse reaction or complication to local anesthesia
Have available supplies and materials in case of anaphylaxis reaction including tourniquet, ambient oxygen source, IV medications: 1:1000 epinephrine, hydrocortisone, diphenhydramine, syringes, needles, antiseptic
Routinely check stability, shelf life and expiration date
Establish general routine policy and registry of complications for local anesthetic procedures (i.e., including errors of dosage or technique, intravascular injection, toxicity, anaphylaxis)
Caution patient regarding drowsiness
Use with caution in severely ill patients

Continued.

NURSING DRUG DIGEST—cont'd

Medication (trade name)	Indication	Usual dosage and administration	Dosage forms, preparation, and storage	Contraindications, cautions, and comments	Monitoring
Lidocaine—cont'd Xylocaine Endotracheal Aerosol	Topical local anesthetic for oropharyngeal and tracheal areas	Physician administration of aerosol spray Each activation of the container delivers 10 mg of lidocaine base	Aerosol container with lidocaine 10 gm w/w, absolute alcohol 18 gm, propylene glycol 11.4 gm and propellants to make 100 gm Available in 50 ml white metered containers with protective plastic cap: single pack: 1 aerosol with nozzle; three pack: 3 aerosols with starter nozzle; nozzle pack, 2 replacement nozzles per pack (8 inch) and 2 nozzles for bronchoscopy Routinely check stability, shelf life, and expiration date	Absolute contraindication if traumatized mucosa, sepsis in area, severe shock, or heart block exist Be aware of contraindications to local anesthesia in general (i.e., history of previous adverse reaction to local anesthetic) Keep out of reach of children and in restricted area with limited access Establish general routine policy and registry of complications for local anesthetic procedures Routinely inquire and notify prescriber of any previous adverse reaction or complication to local anesthesia Routinely have available supplies and materials in case of anaphylaxis reaction May interfere with second stage of swallowing; thus *avoid* administration of food 3 hr before and after use to prevent aspiration	

Xylocaine Jelly	Topical anesthetic	Dose variable: male urethra for cystoscopy apply 10-30 ml; anterior male urethra before catheterization apply 5-10 ml; female urethra 3-5 ml Apply no more than 30 ml/12 hr	Jelly: 2% in sterile viscous aqueous vehicle with sodium carboxymethylcellulose Routinely check stability, shelf life, and expiration date	Possible allergic contact dermatitis to parabens
Xylocaine Ointment	Topical anesthetic	Topical Dose not standardized Use of sterile gauze pad as applicator suggested if applying ointment to denuded skin No more than 30 gm should be applied q.d.	Ointment: 5% lidocaine base Routinely check stability, shelf life, and expiration dates	Use with caution in patients with sepsis at site or severely traumatized mucosa
Xylocaine Topical Spray	Topical local anesthetic	Aerosol spray Each actuation of metered dose valve delivers 10 mg lidocaine base Usually one or two doses adequate	Topical spray: in metered aerosol containers Do not store aerosol container above 48° C	Avoid on traumatized mucosa or if local sepsis at site Do not use on actively bleeding mucosal sites or in presence of open vascular beds (after tonsillectomy) May interfere with second stage of swallowing; thus avoid administration of food 3 hours before and after use to prevent aspiration
Xylocaine Viscous	Topical anesthetic for oral mucosa	Administered orally and held in mouth without swallowing Average dose 15 ml for adults, 5 ml for children Shake bottle before use Dosage should not exceed 20 ml in 6 hr or 120 ml in 24 hours in adults Do not swallow	Viscous: 2% in pink cherry-flavored aqueous solution containing carboxymethylcellulose Routinely check stability, shelf life and expiration dates	Avoid in presence of traumatized mucosa or oral sepsis Keep out of reach of children Accidental oral ingestion may cause seizures and respiratory arrest Avoid administration of food 3 hours before and after use to prevent aspiration

Continued.

NURSING DRUG DIGEST—cont'd

Medication (trade name)	Indication	Usual dosage and administration	Dosage forms, preparation, and storage	Contraindications, cautions, and comments	Monitoring
Mepivacaine Carbocaine Isocaine	Local anesthetic *Not* normally effective for topical use Use is generally restricted to dental procedures	*Adults:* Local and regional infiltration anesthesia May be up to 40 ml of a 1% solution, but varies with site Intracutaneous and SC Avoid intravascular injection Maximum: 400 mg *Children:* Maximum dose for children and adults should *not* exceed 8 mg/kg body weight (optimum 5 to 7 mg/kg) Children less than 3 years of age or 14 kg body weight, use 0.5%-1.5% solutions *only*	Solution for injection: 0.5%, 1%, 1.5%, 2%, 3% Routinely check stability, shelf life, and expiration date	Similar action to lidocaine Be aware of contraindications to local anesthesia in general Mepivacaine has some inherent vasoconstriction activity; thus epinephrine is not usually necessary Establish general routine policy and registry of complications for local anesthetic procedures (i.e., including errors of dosage or technique, intravascular injection, toxicity, anaphylaxis) Routinely inquire and notify prescriber of any previous adverse reaction or complications to local anesthesia Routinely have available supplies and materials in case of anaphylaxis reaction including tourniquet, ambient oxygen source, IV medications: 1:1000 epinephrine, hydrocortisone, diphenhydramine, syringes, needles, antiseptic Caution patient regarding drowsiness	

Drug	Classification	Dosage	Contraindications and Precautions	Nursing Considerations
★ **Piperocaine** Metycaine	Local anesthetic	*Adults:* infiltration (dental and peripheral) and nerve block (caudal in obstetrics) Dose depends on concentration of solution and site to be infiltrated	*Contraindicated* in known hypersensitivity Resuscitative equipment and drugs should be available	Observe for hypersensitivity reactions
		Solution for injection: 0.5%, 1%, 1.5%, 2% Dilute with normal saline Discard unused portion		
★ **Prilocaine** Citanest Xylonest	Local anesthetic	*Adults:* Infiltration and nerve block, caudal and epidural block Dose depends on concentration of solution and site to be infiltrated Maximum single dose 600 mg (8 mg/kg) Inject *slowly* *Avoid* intravascular injections *Children:* Maximum single dose 400 mg (8 mg/kg) *Elderly:* Start with lower doses	*Contraindicated* in hypersensitivity, severe shock, and heart block Resuscitative equipment and drugs should be available Overdose may cause CNS excitation and cardiovascular depression High doses may cause methemoglobinemia	Observe for hypersensitivity reactions Observe for cyanosis
		Solution: for injection 1%, 2%, 3%		
Procaine Glukor* Neocaine Novocain	Local anesthetic	*Adults:* infiltration and nerve block, caudal, and epidural block Dose depends on concentration of solution and site to be infiltrated Maximum dose: 1000 mg Inject *slowly* *Avoid* intravascular injections	*Contraindicated* in known hypersensitivity May cause fetal bradycardia at high doses Resuscitative equipment and drugs should be available	Observe for hypersensitivity reactions Observe for crystallization, cloudiness, or discoloration of solution Observe for fetal bradycardia
		Solution: 1%, 2% Protect from light If necessary to autoclave exterior, use 15 pound pressure at 121° C for 15 min Discard if crystals, cloudiness, or discoloration of solution is noted		
Proparacaine AK-Taine Alcaine Ophthaine Ophthetic	Local anesthetic (for topical ophthalmic use only)	*Adults:* Instill 1-2 drops before procedure	*Contraindicated* in hypersensitivity May cause cycloplegia and conjunctival congestion	Observe for eye irritation
		Ophthalmic solution: 0.5%		
Tetracaine Cetacaine* Minims Pontocaine	Local anesthetic	*Adults:* (Ophthalmic procedures) instill 1-2 drops (0.5%) or ½-1 inch of ointment (0.5%); (local anesthesia) apply cream, ointment, or solution topically as needed; (spinal anesthesia) dose depends on concentration of solution and site to be infiltrated Use lowest effective dose Maximum: 15 mg	*Contraindicated* in hypersensitivity	
		Ophthalmic ointment: 0.5% Ophthalmic solution: 0.5% Ointment: 0.5% Cream: 1% Solution: 2% Injectable: 0.2, 0.3, 1% Store injectable under refrigeration		

BIBLIOGRAPHY

American Academy of Pediatrics Committee on Fetus and Newborn. Hexachlorophene and skin care of newborn infants. *Pediatrics*, 1972, *49*, 625-626.

Cooperman, E.M. Editorial—Hexachlorophene in the nursery. *Canadian Medical Association Journal*, 1977, *117*, 205-206.

Dillon, H.C. Topical and systemic therapy for pyodermas: review. *International Journal of Dermatology*, 1980, *19*(8), 443-451.

Fisher, A.A. *Contact dermatitis* (2nd ed.). Philadelphia: Lea & Febiger, 1975.

Food and Drug Administration Drug Bulletin. *Hexachlorophene and newborns*. U.S. Dept. of Health Education and Welfare, Public Health Service, December 1971.

Franx, D.N., & Perry, R.S. Mechanisms for differential block among single myelinated and non-myelinated axons by procaine. *Journal of Physiology*, 1974, *235*, 193-210.

Henry, J.C., Tschen, E.H., & Becker, L.E. Contact urticaria to parabens. *Archives of Dermatology*, 1979, *115*, 1231-1232.

Hnatko, S.I. Alternatives to hexachlorophene, bathing of newborn infants. *Canadian Medical Association Journal*, 1977, *117*, 223-226.

Horio, T. Photosensitivity reaction to dibucaine. *Archives of Dermatology*, 1979, *115*, 986-987.

Long-acting local anesthetics. *The Medical Letter*, Jan. 14, 1977, *19*(1) (issue 470), 4.

Marshall, J.P., & Schneider, R.P. Systemic argyria secondary to topical silver nitrate. *Archives of Dermatology*, 1977, *113*, 1077-1079.

Mathias, C.G.T., Maibach, H.I., & Epstein, J. Allergic contact photodermatitis to paraminobenzoic acid. *Archives of Dermatology*, 1978, *114*, 1665-1666.

Neldner, K.H. The halogenated 8-hydroxyquinolones: review. *International Journal of Dermatology*, 1977, *16*(4), 267-273.

Shuman, R.M., Leech, R.W., & Alvord, E.C. Neurotoxicity of hexachlorophene in the human. I. A clinico-pathologic study of 248 children. *Pediatrics*, 1974, *54*, 689.

Shuman, R.M., Leech, R.W., & Alvord, E.C. Neurotoxicity of hexachlorophene in the human. II. Actinic-pathologic study of 46 premature infants. *Archives of Neurology*, 1975, *32*, 320.

Tyrala, E.E., Hillman, L.S., Hillman, R.E., & Dodson, W.E. Clinical pharmacology of hexachlorophene in newborns. *Journal of Pediatrics*, 1977, September, 481-486.

Keratolytics, Antiseborrheics, and Related Topical Medications

Eric Schloss

Medications discussed in this chapter

Keratolytics	*Destructive agents—cont'd*
Benzoyl peroxide	Podophyllum resin
Glucuronic acid	Trichloroacetic acid
Lactic acid	*Antiseborrheics*
Propylene glycol	Coal tar
Pyruvic acid	Pyrithione zinc
Salicylic acid	Resorcinol
Sulfur compounds	Salicylic acid
Tretinoin	Selenium sulfide
Urea preparations	Sulfur compounds
Destructive agents	*Miscellaneous agents*
Cantharidin	Anthralin
Fluorouracil, topical	Coal tar
Glacial acetic acid	Methoxsalen

A variety of compounds are discussed in this chapter, many of which have numerous and overlapping properties. The clinical use of many of the various preparations and formulations is often not based on precise scientific information or controlled data, and many of the individual compounds may be used in combination or in differing formulation and concentration for different purposes.

Most of the *keratolytic* agents are intended to produce *desquamation* for *hyperkeratotic* conditions. However, included under this heading, in the context of this chapter, are some agents that have a potentially more destructive and irritant effect on tissue. These latter agents may be used by experienced clinicians for superficial chemotherapy or attempted wart therapy. The effectiveness of these agents must always be balanced against their potential complications. Also included among the keratolytics are some of the more commonly used acne preparations, which may produce desquamation largely through a direct irritant effect. These preparations include topical tretinoin and benzoyl peroxide preparations. These compounds have several other properties. Other compounds, such as salicylic acid, resorcinol, and sulfur, are commonly used topically in proprietary formulations in lower concentrations for *seborrheic dermatitis* and acne, although their specific benefit, apart from a superficial peeling action in acne, is often not clear.

The term *seborrhea* is not a precise one and may have different connotations for different practitioners. Under usual circumstances it refers to the state of skin associated with constitutional seborrheic dermatitis. Although seborrhea is usually thought to refer to oily skin, the abnormality may also be reflected by dry scaling and erythema. Scaling scalp problems, including simple dandruff, true seborrheic dermatitis, and psoriasis, are included here because many of the therapeutic shampoos and other agents may be effective in all of these conditions. Tar preparations are included in this section.

MAINLY KERATOLYTIC AGENTS

Acids

Salicylic acid. Salicylic acid has a long history of use for common dermatologic problems. Many products for common skin conditions, such as warts, calluses, acne, and seborrheic dermatitis, contain salicylic acid. A wide variety of formulations are used, including such vehicles as creams, *ointments, gels, lotions, pastes, shampoos,* and *plasters.*

Cellular action. This acid exerts activity only if applied topically in the form of the free acid and is used predominantly for its keratolytic action. Many variables may influence its therapeutic action, however, particularly the type of vehicle and formulation, and the concentration of salicylic acid employed.

The exact mechanism of desquamation is still uncertain. A concentration greater than 3% appears to be required for this purpose. *Denaturation* or solubilization of the *keratin layer* structural protein may be important in the process, but it has also been suggested that salicylic acid can cause desquamation by dissolution of intercellular cement material.

A number of other actions of salicylic acid are reported and may be largely concentration dependent. Concentrations employed greater than 6% may begin to have a more direct irritant and destructive action on tissue, and concentrations less than 3% are claimed to have more of a keratoplastic effect at least in paste or ointment form. Salicylic acid has a reported broad-spectrum bacteriostatic and antifungal activity even at low concentrations and also has some *photoprotective* action in the near ultraviolet range.

Absorption and metabolism. Percutaneous absorption is normally accomplished relatively easily, with maximum plasma levels occurring 5 to 12 hours after application. Once absorbed, salicylic acid is metabolized, as other salicylates, mainly by liver microsomal enzymes. Most of the absorbed dose can be recovered from the urine because it is largely conjugated to more water-soluble products to facilitate elimination.

Vehicle composition may affect absorption through the skin. Although penetration may be generally increased in ointment form, little conclusive evidence exists for other forms of salicylic acid. Some evidence even suggests a decrease in absorption of salicylic acid from vehicles containing *petrolatum* or polyethylene glycol. The absorption rate is greatly enhanced with increased hydration of the keratin layer, a fact that is particularly applicable under occlusive conditions. The frequency of application, amount, and concentration may also affect the absorption rate; however, valid pharmacokinetic data are unavailable.

Problems. Salicylic acid generally has the favorable quality of lack of odor. It does not stain the skin, although vehicle formulation may influence this. The compound appears to show little evidence of true contact dermatitis, *urticaria*, or other drug hypersensitivity reaction, and no significant cross-reactions have been reported with other salicylate compounds. Problems encountered, however, may be local or systemic in effect. Locally, some of the preparations used, particularly in higher concentrations, may produce irritation, stinging or burning. Particular caution should be exercised in patients with compromised circulation or impaired sensation, such as diabetics, where use of higher concentration preparations (e.g., 40% salicylic acid plasters) may cause excessive tissue injury without early recognition.

The main potential systemic problem is salicylate toxicity, and at least 13 deaths have been reported, predominantly in children. Infants and younger children are more at risk because of their greater ratio of surface area (m^2) to weight (kg). It has been calculated that after the same strength of salicylic acid has been applied to the skin of an infant and an adult, the infant receives 2.7 times the adult's dose in mg/kg. The extracellular space is smaller on a weight and volume basis in infants and children, and consequently higher concentration levels of salicylic acid are produced.

Other risk factors for *salicylism* include the following: greater area of skin involvement, larger amounts and higher concentrations applied, increased frequency of application, application under *occlusive conditions*, and impaired skin barrier function of cutaneous disease states or open wounds. It is also important to realize that salicylate levels in blood may be cumulative with doses from other sources, such as orally administered salicylate compounds or methyl salicylate as used in oil of wintergreen. There are few valid reports of toxicity assessments of the available commercial formulations. However, one evaluation of Keralyt Gel, a preparation containing 6% salicylic acid in a gel comprising 60% propylene glycol and 19.4% ethyl alcohol, showed little potential hazard of systemic toxicity, despite the presence of many of the previously stated risk factors, including routine use (as recommended) under plastic wrap occlusion.

Precautions. Generally, since most of the reported deaths have involved multiple and frequent applications, once-a-day application is recommended. Salicylic acid preparations should not be applied over large areas or for prolonged periods, particularly in the young. On occasion it may be useful to monitor therapy by serum salicylate levels. Other precautions include the recognition of risk in patients with a constricted extracellular fluid compartment (such as infants have and such as occurs in states of dehydration). There is also a potential hazard in patients with impaired hepatic or renal function. If the drug cannot be metabolized or excreted efficiently, higher plasma salicylate levels will result.

As a rough rule of thumb, 1 gm of a 6% salicylic acid preparation will raise the serum salicylate level not more than 0.5 mg/dl plasma in adults under nonocclusive conditions. Patients or parents, and nurses should be aware of and observant for the early signs of salicylism, which in affected children may be manifest with crying, emotional lability, and irritability. Otherwise classic signs of salicylism include thirst, tinnitus, headache, lethargy, confusion, gastrointestinal upset, depression, and disorientation. A blood salicylate level will be confirmatory, and hospitalization for observation and treatment is mandatory. Of course once toxicity is suspected, application of the salicylic acid compound, and all other sources of salicylates, must be discontinued immediately.

Other considerations. Other potential complications of salicylates are rarely reported with topical salicylic acid therapy. These include elevation of serum uric acid levels, effects on platelet function, drug interactions, and interference with laboratory tests. Because of competitive protein binding, psoriatic patients on methotrexate may be at potential risk of methotrexate toxicity, but this appears to be of little significance under usual conditions of therapy and practice. Since salicylates cross the placental barrier, caution with their use during pregnancy is usually advised.

Other α-hydroxy acids. Lactic, pyruvic, or glucuronic acids may be used for similar keratotic clinical conditions as salicylic acid. It is not known if their mechanisms of action differ fundamentally from salicylic acid, and few properties have been recorded with regard to their cutaneous effects. It may be possible, however, that they influence the process of *keratinization* through a mechanism other than direct keratolytic action.

Lactic, pyruvic, or glucuronic acid may be present in various proprietary preparations in a number of different vehicles, mainly marketed for antiwart or callus therapy, and are occasionally formulated in combination with salicylic acid for these purposes. In addition, their use in *ichthyotic skin conditions* has been advocated. The acids are known to be potentially corrosive if accidentally swallowed; however, little documented information is available regarding toxicity of these compounds as topical therapeutic agents.

Miscellaneous acids. Benzoic acid is uncommonly used, but preparations combined with salicylic acid are available including Whitfield's ointment. This preparation has been used as an antifungal agent for superficial *tinea infection* and combines benzoic acid and salicylic acid in *wool fat* (lanolin) and petrolatum. It may exert its antifungal action largely as a keratolytic or desquamating agent, because the fungi are resident in the keratin layer. Some reports of contact dermatitis, possibly because of the wool fat component, have been reported. It has largely been supplanted as a topical fungicide by other agents.

Propylene glycol

Although propylene glycol was first synthesized in 1859, it has found common use in many topical preparations only in recent years. It is a colorless, odorless liquid, *miscible* with water. In topical formulations it is used mainly for its keratolytic action. It is an excellent vehicle because of its hydrating function, its ability to dissolve many organic molecules, and its ability to potentiate release and absorption of the active agent. It has been particularly used in creams, gels, or lotions, but is also found in some antiperspirants.

Cellular action. The precise mode of keratolytic action is uncertain. It is known to denature and increase protein solubility. It may, therefore, exert its effect by direct action on keratin structural protein. The ability to denature protein and remove keratin is similar over the same relatively narrow effective concentration range of 61% to 77%. Acid pH of skin and formulation may also be important for effective action. Another basis for keratolytic action, however, may relate to the fundamental *hydroscopic* ability of the compound. An *osmotic* effect produced may establish a water gradient in the epidermis and also increase desquamation. This osmotic effect may provide the basis for healing fissures in skin or mucous membrane. The hydroscopic quality may also function to hydrate skin by forming a barrier to the evaporation of water from the stratum corneum.

Absorption and metabolism. Propylene glycol is minimally absorbed from intact skin and is considered nontoxic in therapeutic concentrations. The small amount absorbed topically is converted to lactic and pyruvic acid by the liver.

Problems. As a vehicle in many topical preparations, the concentration and formulation must be precise, because small concentration differences can greatly alter drug release from the vehicle by changing the *partition coefficient.*

Although it is nontoxic in usual sites of application, and rarely produces systemic toxicity even with oral ingestion, there is a possible ototoxic effect, and avoidance of use in the ear canal is recommended.

An occasional patient may have irritant contact dermatitis from topical use, especially if undiluted or under occlusion. *Atopic* patients, and others with dermatitis, may be more sensitive to these potential irritant effects, which may be intensified under conditions of lowered humidity or cutaneous dehydration. Occasional cases of allergic contact dermatitis have been reported.

Urea preparations

A number of urea-containing proprietary preparations have been marketed, largely as creams or lotions. They are mainly used as lubricants or emollients in hyperkeratotic or scaling skin disorders (often in concentrations of 10% to 20%). They are proteolytic and solubilize keratin. Little basic clinical evidence is available. Patients may complain of irritation, burning, or stinging if used on inappropriate areas, such as the face or *intertriginous* (crease) regions; however, there is no evidence of allergic contact dermatitis, and toxicity data are not readily available.

DESTRUCTIVE AGENTS

Cantharidin

This irritant crystalline material, prepared from dried insects (i.e., Spanish flies, Russian flies), has limited solubility in water. It is used by some clinicians primarily for wart therapy, particularly in *periungual* locations. Through a direct irritant and vesiculant action, the chemical basis of which is poorly understood, an *intraepidermal vesicle*, which seems to aid in wart resolution, is produced at application sites. As with all destructive wart therapy, however, the wart virus is not killed, and recurrence may still occur. Usually a 0.7% cantharidin concentration in flexible collodion or acetone is used under occlusive bandage for up to 48 hours.

The preparation should be used only by experienced clinicians. Potential complications include pain, secondary infection, or nail damage. The preparation should be particularly avoided in patients with impaired local circulation or neurologic sensation. There is little skin absorption; however, if taken orally, by accident or intent, it is absorbed from the gastrointestinal tract and can lead to toxicity (i.e., vomiting, abdominal pain, cardiovascular collapse) and shock. It is excreted via the kidney. Its false reputation as an aphrodisiac is derived from its irritant effects on the urinary tract.

Podophyllum resin

This compound, most often used for therapy of genital or perianal warts (condylomata accuminata, or venereal warts), is usually prepared as a 20% or 25% dispersed concentration in compound tincture of benzoin, or as an alcoholic solution. Podophyllum resin is obtained from the rhizomes and roots of *Podophyllum peltatum* (mandrake, mayapple) and contains at least 16 different chemicals. Because there are no specific standards for the ratio or concentration of the various chemical ingredients, potency can vary significantly.

Podophyllum resin is a mitotic inhibitor and arrests the cell cycle in metaphase, which may therefore lead to inhibition of wart virus growth and replication. It is also, however, a direct irritant, and patients must be instructed to wash off the preparation within 6 hours of application, or earlier if irritation is noted. The compound should be used only by experienced clinicians, with care to avoid contact with normal skin or mucous membrane, because irritant dermatitis or even chemical burn has ensued from improper application or extravasation. Usually no more than one application weekly is advisable. Systemic toxicity (i.e., nausea, vomiting, anuria, coma, tachycardia) has been reported rarely, and suggestion of the possibility of neurotoxicity (i.e., peripheral toxicity, central nervous system depression) from mucous membrane absorption has been noted. Some practitioners have advocated caution with the treatment of venereal warts during pregnancy with podophyllum resin because of potential toxicity for mother and fetus. It is a safe policy not to allow patients to self-administer podophyllum resin, and the compound should be dispensed for use only by an experienced clinician.

Topical fluorouracil

Although not used specifically as a keratolytic, this topical chemotherapeutic compound may produce a desquamating action on lesions during the course of its action. It is most commonly used for treatment of multiple actinic keratoses on sun-exposed cutaneous sites. There is a selective action against the atypical cells in the epidermis of these potentially premalignant lesions. The enzyme thymidylate synthetase is inhibited by 5-fluorouracil, and this leads to a block in cellular DNA synthesis selectively in the abnormal cells. An inflammatory reaction is produced, confined to lesions, which may progress to vesiculation at its peak intensity. Lesions that may be subclinical, or not readily visible, also respond, and are selectively singled out so that the compound may be applied to the entire affected cutaneous area. Under normal conditions of use, surrounding normal epidermis does not appear to be affected.

Topical fluorouracil is usually applied twice a day to the entire affected area (invariably sun-exposed skin on face, scalp, ears, or dorsa of hands) in 1%, 2%, or 5% solutions or creams, some of which contain propylene glycol. The duration of therapy may vary with the individual, but the inflammatory reaction often peaks around 3 weeks of onset of therapy. Once an intense *erythema* is achieved, topical application is discontinued. Therapy may be accompanied and invariably followed by use of a mild nonfluorinated topical steroid to control the inflammatory reaction. This control does not seem to influence the basic therapeutic efficacy of the fluorouracil compound.

The clinical lesions usually heal rapidly after therapy, although the process may continue at a cellular level for up to 2 months. Patients are usually pleased with the eventual improved cosmetic result; however, lesions tend to recur with time, and repeat courses of therapy may eventually be required. There is little controlled evidence to relate vehicle and concentration to cutaneous localization or efficacy, and all usual preparations appear effective.

Careful instructions to the patients are mandatory, and they should be clearly informed on what to expect, because the erythema, or skin discoloration and burning sensation associated with peak effect, may be distressing to the unwary. Prophylactically it is necessary to avoid sun exposure during therapy, and therapy is often best carried out during winter months (at least in more northern localities). Sun-protection measures (i.e., protective clothing including a brimmed hat and regular topical application of effective sunscreens 1 hour before sun exposure) should be stressed to these patients, because their actinic lesions are a manifestation of their sun sensitivity. There is thus high risk of new lesions with continuing excessive sun exposure or lack of photoprotection.

Pruritus and irritation, although usually limited, are the most common adverse effects of therapy. Care should be taken to avoid inadvertent application of the medication to the eyes. Allergic contact dermatitis is occasionally reported. Otherwise there are few complications reported, and systemic toxicity appears unlikely.

SUPERFICIAL PEELING AGENTS (ACNE PREPARATIONS)

Tretinoin (vitamin A [retinoic] acid)

Topical vitamin A acid preparations in the chemical form of tretinoin (which is the all-transconfiguration), have been employed commonly for a variety of keratinizing problems, but predominantly for *comedonal acne* therapy. It is known to exert an effect on the keratinization process by increasing epidermal cell mitosis and cell turnover, and has been demonstrated to convert abnormal keratinizing lining epithelium in superficial (infundibular) portions of *pilosebaceous follicles* to a more normal state. This aids in the expulsion and prevention of further abnormally adherent keratinous plugs of involved acneiform follicles. The compound is also an irritant, and the superficial peeling action commonly produced may be at least partly on this direct basis. There appears to be a dose-response relationship for irritation, but precise information relating efficacy and pharmacokinetics is limited. An antibacterial effect against the resident organisms (i.e., mainly *Corynebacterium acnes*) in pilosebaceous follicles is also claimed.

Absorption through intact skin is apparently limited, and systemic toxicity from topical preparations in usual therapeutic regimens has not been reported. If used in excessive quantities, irritant dermatitis may ensue; however, true allergic contact dermatitis is rare.

For acne therapy gels or creams are commonly used, most often in concentrations of 0.05% of the active tretinoin ingredient. They are applied generally to an area such as the face on a once-daily or overnight basis, with a gradually increasing time duration schedule (i.e., often commencing with 1 hour and gradually increasing to 8 hours over the course of 1 week).

The patient should avoid contact of preparation with mucous membranes or eyes. Care to observe avoidance of eczematous skin should be taken because contact may aggravate preexisting eczema. Because sunburn may irritate the patient who uses topical tretinoin, it is often applied overnight and sun protection advised. Stinging lotions or perfumes are also best avoided during therapy with the compound.

There is some evidence suggesting enhancement of epidermal penetration by benzoyl peroxide preparation, and combined therapy is often suggested for comedonal acne; however, little evidence of therapeutic effectiveness in established inflammatory lesions of acne has been presented.

Benzoyl peroxide

Numerous commercial benzoyl peroxide preparations are marketed and mainly used in acne therapy, although the compound is also employed in cutaneous ulcer therapy. Benzoyl peroxide is a strong organic oxidizing agent almost insoluble in water. It is potentially explosive in pure form, but appears nonflammable in therapeutic formulation and is nontoxic.

The mechanism of action in acne therapy is unclear; however, several effects are noted, including usual superficial drying and peeling. The relationship of these effects to efficacy is not clearly established on a dose-response basis. By releasing nascent oxygen, benzoyl peroxide has an antimicrobial effect, mainly against anaerobic organisms, and suppression of *Corynebacterium acnes* in the depths of follicles may be a therapeutic factor, but limited microbial data are available.

Little is known about the percutaneous penetration and metabolism of benzoyl peroxide in topical formulation. Systemic toxicity has not been reported. Irritant contact dermatitis is not uncommon if used in excess, and true allergic contact dermatitis can occur in less than 3% of cases.

The quantity applied is carefully limited to minimize excessive irritation, and therapy is usually carried out on a once-daily basis, beginning with gradually increasing time increments of application (i.e., often commencing with 1 hour duration and increasing to 8 hours over the course of a week). Care to avoid contact with the eyes and mucous membranes is necessary, and the preparation may be excessively irritating on areas of thin skin such as the neck. The patient should also be advised that the product may bleach colored fabric on contact. There is some evidence to suggest synergism of action in acne therapy with concomitant use of topical tretinoin.

The usual preparations are used in concentrations of 2.5%, 5%, 10%, and occasionally higher concentration may be employed. Skin type and degree of pigmentation play a role in selection of concentration. The various preparations are usually used as creams, gels, lotions or therapeutic washes, and the products differ mainly in vehicle and base composition. Alcohol, acetone, and water-soluble bases are available, but no definitive data are readily available relating vehicle composition to therapeutic effect.

Pace (1976) has been a particular advocate of benzoyl peroxide for cutaneous ulcer therapy, often in a 20% lotion form but occasionally as a 50% paste. The cellular action may be an oxygen release to facilitate ulcer healing, to compensate for diminished blood supply, and possibly to serve as a cofactor in collagen synthesis.

Resorcinol

Resorcinol is a substituted phenol with mild irritant and keratolytic properties. It is utilized in many proprietary preparations mainly for therapy of acne and seborrheic dermatitis. It is commonly used with other compounds, such as salicylic acid and sulfur, in these preparations, and the action on skin may be difficult to separate from the action of other compounds. Precise information on synergistic action is unavailable. Resorcinol is a colorless material and freely soluble in most solvents.

Many of the local actions of this compound are similar to, but milder than, phenol. It is a protein precipitant, but whether this is the basis of its keratolytic action is uncertain. It also has antiseptic bactericidal and fungicidal action at approximately one-third the effectiveness of phenol.

Most often resorcinol is formulated in ointments or lotions in concentration less than 5%, but an occasional product contains resorcinol in higher concentration, which can be associated with systemic toxicity if swallowed. True allergic contact dermatitis is uncommon, but if it occurs, cross-reaction with other resorcinol compounds, such as hexyl resorcinol, in proprietary preparations (e.g., some scalp lotions, pharyngeal antiseptics, and lozenges) is a potential risk. It is usually advised to dispense resorcinol compounds in dark bottles because discoloration can occur on exposure to sunlight, although potency does not appear significantly altered.

Sulfur

Sulfur has also had long usage in dermatologic conditions, particularly in acne and seborrheic dermatitis. It is often present in combination with other agents, such as resorcinol and salicylic acid in proprietary preparations.

Sulfur has a superficial keratolytic action, but precise data on cellular action are largely unavailable. Its use in acne is controversial because claims of enhancement of *comedogenicity* have been presented, although this is disputed. An antiseptic action is possible, if oxidation to pentathionic acid takes place, but it is not clear if this has therapeutic importance.

Sulfur exists in various forms; however, it is largely colloidal sulfur used in acne and antiseborrheic products. This is elemental sulfur in stable aqueous colloidal solution, often employed in concentrations of 5% or less in the various products. The relationship of concentration to therapeutic efficacy is unclear.

A problem of cosmetic concern, particularly with frequent application, is yellow staining of the skin. Obnoxious odor, such as the proverbial rotten egg, is not a problem with usual proprietary preparations. Although the unusual complication of sulfhemoglobinemia is possible from oral ingestion, other toxicity appears limited and has not been reported with topical application.

Occasionally other sulfur compounds, such as sodium thiosulfate, are used for various skin conditions, including *tinea versicolor*, and in some acne products. Thiosulfates generate free sulfur, especially in acid solution, and have been used in concentrations ranging from 0.5% to 8%. Precipitated sulfur in ointment form is a continuing antiscabetic therapy in concentrations of 10% or less.

ANTISEBORRHEICS

Salicylic acid, resorcinol, and sulfur in low concentration

Salicylic acid, resorcinol, and sulfur, in low concentrations and various combinations and formulations, are some of the most commonly used antiseborrheic preparations. These are discussed in previous sections, and their mode of action as specific antiseborrheic agents is largely unknown.

Selenium sulfide

This compound in detergent suspension is mainly used topically in shampoo form for control of scaling scalp problems, such as simple *dandruff* or seborrheic dermatitis, but is also effective therapy for tinea versicolor.

The basic compound is a bright orange insoluble

powder, which appears to have little toxicity in usual shampoo formulation on intact skin. There is little absorption under usual circumstances, but, absorption may be increased, with a consequent potential toxicity risk if the compound is used on damaged or ulcerated skin.

The compound has an antimitotic effect on epidermis, which may explain control of scaling: cell turnover time is reduced. However, reliable kinetic data are lacking. The compound may be more efficacious because of its substantivity property, which implies a continuing adherence and therapeutic action on the hair and scalp after shampoo and rinse. As with most so-called "dandruff" shampoos, increased frequency of application usually leads to better control, but precise pharmacokinetic data on dose-response relations regarding frequency and amount are limited. It is uncertain whether the detergent vehicle may not also provide significant therapeutic action in itself by its mechanical cleansing action.

The shampoo is usually formulated as a 2.5% suspension in a detergent vehicle, but is also available as a 1% suspension. It is normally recommended to allow lather to remain on the scalp 3 to 5 minutes before rinsing thoroughly. Careful rinsing and washing of the hands are necessary to avoid potential irritancy of the compound, which may be increased by prolonged skin contact. Avoidance of eye contact is particularly stressed because irritant conjunctivitis or keratitis is possible. Because of excessive irritancy or potential toxicity, selenium sulfide should not be used on excessively inflamed, or denuded skin. It is also recommended that heavy metal compounds, such as mercury ointments, be avoided before use because of adverse interaction (i.e., inactivation of the selenium compound and occasional staining of hair have been reported).

Other potential problems are yellow or orange staining of skin and graying of hair with prolonged contact. Although true allergic contact dermatitis caused by the active ingredient is not reported, possible reactions to the scented preparations or vehicles may occur, and as with most sensitivity reactions to shampoos, can be seen on the ears, neck, and face, rather than on the central scalp.

Accidental oral ingestion may lead to gastrointestinal upset, but serious toxicity appears unusual; however, an offensive garlic odor on the breath may result. Selenium sulfide compounds have been reported not to be carcinogenic when applied topically.

Pyrithione zinc

This insoluble organic compound is used in several proprietary shampoo formulations to control dandruff or seborrheic dermatitis of the scalp. Zinc pyrithione can exert an antimitotic effect on the epidermis and has the similar property of substantivity as selenium sulfide. This should allow for persisting therapeutic effect after rinsing.

Limited data are available, but, there is apparently little risk of absorption or toxicity on application to normal scalp in the usual formulations. Caution is usually necessary to avoid irritation of the eye from contact with the solution.

Benzalkonium chloride

Quaternary ammonium compounds, although primarily classified as antiseptics, have also been claimed to have an effective therapeutic action for scaling scalp conditions. Some of these preparations contain additional compounds, such as salicylic acid in low concentration. The benzalkonium chloride is ordinarily used in 2% concentration. Soaps and other detergents are recommended to be avoided before or after use of these shampoos because of potential inactivation of the active ingredient. Eye contact should be avoided because irritation can result.

The detergent action may explain the efficacy of these products. All effective detergent shampoos have a surface active mechanical action to remove scale, dirt, and debris. This action washes the hair, cleanses the scalp, and tends to relieve pruritus, which is a common symptom of many of these scalp problems. Whether benzalkonium chloride has other more specific actions as an antiseborrheic is unclear. No significant toxicity is reported, and true allergic contact dermatitis is rare.

Miscellaneous preparations

Miscellaneous shampoos and cleansers. Other cleansing agents or antiseptics are used in detergent vehicles for shampoos or skin cleansers and may also be effective antiseborrheic agents. These include compounds such as salicylanilides or carbanilides. Sulfur, salicylic acid, and resorcinol are also used in low concentrations. The main therapeutic action may also be caused by a mechanical detergent effect.

These compounds, as therapeutically formulated, have little recorded toxicity data. Irritation or excessive drying may occur with all these detergent compounds if used in excess or for prolonged periods on facial or glabrous skin. Irritation may also be produced on eye contact and should be avoided. True allergic contact dermatitis is uncommon.

Other shampoos, as detergent formulations, may also be effective in simple dandruff or minor scalp scaling. Allergic contact dermatitis caused by added ingredients such as formalin ester, balsam of Peru, perfume, and possibly nickel compounds may occasionally occur.

Tar preparations. By-products of the destructive distillation of woods, or more often bituminous coal, are used topically in many different formulations and strengths for various skin and scalp problems, including seborrheic dermatitis of the scalp and *psoriasis.* At least 300 different products can be derived from this distillation process, and the precise therapeutically active ingredients in coal tar have not yet been defined.

Crude coal tar, as used most commonly for psoriatic skin involvement, is thought to produce suppression of DNA synthesis in the epidermis and diminish cell turnover. It also improves normal keratinization in the usual concentration of 10% or less and may therefore lead to diminished scaling via this effect. Tars also have an antiseptic action, but the importance of this in practice is likely limited.

Tar preparations must be used properly to avoid many potential problems. They have a tendency to exert a direct irritant effect, especially in higher concentration, on thinner and noninvolved skin, eye, and mucous membranes. Tars are inherently insoluble in water and in more common preparations, such as ointment vehicles, it is not uncommon that they induce *folliculitis* or acneiform eruption, especially in hairy areas. As a group they tend to have an objectionable odor and are commonly capable of skin, hair, and fabric staining. Although allergic contact dermatitis is unusual, some of the coal tar fractions are *photosensitizers.* For this reason application is more common at night, with careful removal before sun exposure, which also should be limited.

Many different coal tar commercial preparations are used, particularly as tar distillates or extracts, in a variety of formulations including creams, gels, ointments, lotions, emulsions, soaps, and shampoos. They are also combined with other therapeutic ingredients, such as corticosteroids.

The commonly employed tar shampoos are therapeutically effective, in concentrations ranging from 0.5% to 3%, for the usual scaling scalp problems including seborrheic dermatitis and psoriasis. Their mode of action, however, is not defined well, and efficacy data and valid comparisons of the various products are limited. The contribution of detergent vehicle and other additives to therapeutic effect is also unclear. There is little reliable information on substantivity, and clinical benefit often appears to bear a direct relationship to the frequency of application.

As common potential irritants, care should be taken to avoid use of tars on abraded skin. Contact with the eye should be prevented. The shampoos are capable of staining hair (particularly blonde, bleached, or gray) and should be rinsed carefully. Few valid reports are available on examples of allergic contact dermatitis or photodermatitis with the therapeutic tar shampoos, and there are no valid data to suggest carcinogenicity.

Anthralin. Anthralin is a synthetic organic tarlike substance with greater stability than related parent chrysarobin compound. It has been used in psoriasis therapy in paste, cream, ointment, or solution form or as a scalp pomade, in concentrations ranging from 0.01% to 1%. The precise mode of action is uncertain; however, it may inactivate key enzymes important in cell renewal and inhibit DNA synthesis.

Anthralin is a known direct irritant, usually used only by clinicians experienced with the compound. It should be avoided on abraded or acutely inflamed skin or scalp and also on uninvolved skin and mucous membranes, including the eyes. Besides irritancy, a strong disadvantage is yellow or red-brown staining of skin and clothing fabric. Hair may also be stained by the preparation. Anthralin is not water soluble. It is removed with oils such as warm mineral oil. The stain is difficult to remove and will often remain after the affected area is resolved.

Anthralin-containing preparations should be avoided in patients with renal disease. Anthralin is absorbed from the skin and partly excreted in the urine as chrysophanic acid; however, an unoxidized portion may cause renal irritation and proteinuria with other abnormal urinalysis findings, such as the presence of casts on microscopic examination.

Allergic contact dermatitis is unusual, and systemic toxicity is limited. If inadvertently swallowed, anthralin apparently has a cathartic action (but it is not recommended for this purpose). It is not known to be carcinogenic.

SUMMARY

A wide variety of topical compounds are discussed from acne preparations to destructive agents used for wart therapy or superficial skin tumor chemotherapy. Many compounds have multiple therapeutic uses, and variables such as concentration and formulation may have great influence on clinical application. The mode of action, conditions of application, potential adverse side effects, and precautions required in clinical use are emphasized.

ADVERSE/SIDE EFFECTS OF KERATOLYTICS, ANTISEBORRHEICS, AND RELATED AGENTS*

ALLERGIC REACTIONS

Allergic contact dermatitis
Allergic contact urticaria
Allergic photocontact dermatitis
Asthma (unusual)
Angioneurotic edema

BEHAVIOR

Altered behavior (may be early sign of salicylism, especially in infants; crying, emotional lability, irritability)

CARDIOVASCULAR SYSTEM

Cardiac arrest (unusual; possible with ingestion of corrosive agents or salicylate toxicity)
Cardiovascular collapse and shock (unusual; possible with ingestion of corrosive agents or salicylate toxicity)

CENTRAL NERVOUS SYSTEM

Coma (with oral toxicity)
Convulsions
Depression (with salicylism)
Disorientation (rare reports of podophyllin neurotoxicity)

CUTANEOUS SYSTEM

Burns (contact with corrosive agents)
Folliculitis (with coal tar preparations or ointments on hairy areas)
Irritant contact dermatitis or irritancy, stinging or burning of skin and mucous membranes
Staining (skin, hair and clothing)
Ulceration (salicylic acid plasters in sites of vascular or neurologic impairment, such as the sole of the foot in diabetic patients)

GASTROINTESTINAL SYSTEM

Gastrointestinal upsets (with ingestion of corrosive agents or salicylism)

METABOLIC SYSTEM

Electrolyte imbalance (with salicylism)
Thirst

OCULAR SYSTEM

Irritant conjunctivitis
Keratitis

MISCELLANEOUS EFFECTS

Fetal-maternal complications, stillbirth, respiratory distress, muscular weakness (reported with use of podophyllin in pregnancy)
Ototoxicity (benzoyl peroxide; tinnitus with salicylism)
Renal damage (anthralin compounds)

NOTE: Effects are largely topical and local unless ingested or the compound used is more toxic.
*See Chapter 11, "Drug Toxicity," for an overview of drug toxicity.

CLINICALLY SIGNIFICANT DRUG INTERACTIONS*

Primary drug	Interacting drug	Possible effect(s)	Probable mechanism(s)
Benzalkonium chloride (quaternary ammonium compound present in several common shampoos, lotions and cleansers [e.g., Ionil])	Soaps and anionic detergents	Prevention of therapeutic effect	Inactivation of active quaternary ammonium compound
Resorcinol	Hexyl resorcinol topical or systemic (present in some scalp lotions, throat lozenges [Sucrets], oral troches [Listerine], and some oral anthelmintics)	Allergic contact dermatitis; systemic eczematous contact dermatitis	Type IV cellular hypersensitivity reaction; generalized dermatitis from systemic administration of a drug cross-reacting with a previous topical sensitizer
Salicylic acid	Other salicylate compounds; methyl salicylate (oil of wintergreen); oral salicylates	Salicylate toxicity (salicylism)	Blood levels of salicylate from all sources can be additive

NOTE: Drug interactions involving these topical products include contact allergic sensitivity reactions and cross reactions through topical or systemic administration of chemically related compounds.
*See Chapter 10, "Drug Interactions," for an overview of drug interactions.

GENERAL NURSING IMPLICATIONS

Nursing of patients requiring keratolytics, antiseborrheics, and related topical medications

ASSESSMENT

There are various keratolytics, antiseborrheics, and related topical medications used in the treatment of such conditions as acne, psoriasis, seborrhea, and warts. Drug therapy is individualized and can be a part of a broader therapeutic regimen, including use of ultraviolet light or other treatment measures. These medications can be used singly or in combination depending on the individual patient's needs.

A complete nursing assessment is important in relation to planning individualized nursing care. Baseline data should include a general health assessment, with special attention to the appearance and distribution of lesions. It is important to note that skin lesions can cause psychologic effects related to changes in body image, fear of disfigurement, or contagion. For various reasons, many people consider skin eruptions revolting or infectious and may avoid individuals with observable lesions. This is distressing to many patients, and assessment of the patient's self-concept including self-esteem, body image, and feelings regarding the presenting condition cannot be overemphasized. The nurse's response to the patient's condition, receptiveness to discussing patient concerns, and patient involvement in therapy does much to promote psychologic well-being and therapeutic management of the condition.

Baseline data should include a detailed drug history, especially when the cause of the patient's condition is unknown, because many drugs can cause sensitivity or irritant reactions involving the skin. It is important to ascertain if the patient has been self-medicating with a topical medication or if he or she has been misusing medication prescribed specifically for a diagnosed condition. Patients with exacerbations or flare-ups of skin conditions for which they are being treated may have caused such a condition from incorrectly applying topical medication or from overuse of the topical medication. If applied incorrectly or used more frequently than indicated, many topical medications can cause irritation, inflammation, or a worsening of the condition. Before topical therapy is initiated, possible sensitivity to a specific agent, contraindications, cautions, or drug interactions should be identified. The patient's self-medication abilities and individual drug-taking patterns should be identified to plan individualized care.

SENSITIVITY

Generally, allergic reactions to keratolytics, antiseborrheics, and related topical medications are rare. However, any drug has the potential to cause a hypersensitivity reaction in a susceptible individual. Allergic reactions have occurred with these medications, and patients should be made aware of the possibility of the occurrence of an allergic reaction.

Resorcinol has been associated with cross-sensitivity, and coal tar preparations have been associated with photocontact dermatitis.

Monitor patients for urticaria, erythema, or other local reaction to the application of topical medications.

A trial on a small area of the patient's body is indicated to evaluate the patient's response before the medication is applied generally.

CONTRAINDICATIONS

The use of keratolytics, antiseborrheics, and related topical medications are contraindicated in patients with known hypersensitivity to a specific agent or products that can cause cross-sensitivity (e.g., resorcinol).

See the Nursing Drug Digest for specific contraindications associated with individual agents.

CAUTIONS

Keratolytics and destructive agents should be used cautiously in patients with compromised circulation or impaired sensation (e.g., diabetics). Salicylates should be used cautiously in patients with renal or hepatic dysfunction, decreased extracellular volume, or dehydration and in infants and young children because of the risk of salicylate toxicity. Because they cross the placental barrier, salicylates should be used cautiously in pregnancy. All acids are corrosive if swallowed. Propylene glycol, because it can produce possible ototoxic effects, should not be applied to the ear canal (see the Nursing Drug Digest for specific cautions related to each agent).

DRUG INTERACTIONS

Keratolytics, antiseborrheics, and related topical medications can interact with other drugs

See Clinically Significant Drug Interactions.

ADMINISTRATION

Keratolytics, antiseborrheics, and related topical medications are available in various dosage forms for topical administration, including creams, ointments, gels, lotions, pastes, shampoos, powders, pomades, and plasters. These are available in various percentage preparations and are selected for the specific condition being treated, absorption and penetration qualities, and patient comfort. For example, weeping areas generally respond more readily to the drying effects of an aqueous preparation than to a greasy base medication, whereas dry scaling or pruritic lesions and cracked rash areas generally respond better to the lubricating effect of a petrolatum base medication.

Creams evaporate and cool and dry with an antipruritic effect. They are best used on acute, wet lesions. Ointments hydrate and leave an oily film on the skin as they dry. They are indicated for chronic or dry scaling skin conditions and cracked rash areas. Solutions should be avoided in the treatment of dry lesions because of their tendency to cause further drying, scaling, or itching.

Ointments may be more effective than creams because of their increased occlusiveness, but creams are washable and less greasy and thus are more cosmetically accepted by many patients.

GENERAL NURSING IMPLICATIONS—cont'd

Nursing of patients requiring keratolytics, antiseborrheics, and related topical medications—cont'd

ADMINISTRATION—cont'd

Gels, although they are less occlusive than creams or ointments, allow better skin contact. Gels containing alcohol evaporate and leave the drug and some gelling agent on the skin. Gels and lotions are especially suited to the scalp and hairy areas. Ointments are contraindicated in hairy areas because of their association with folliculitis. Gels, lotions, or solutions containing alcohol or a propylene glycol base can cause burning, stinging, or discomfort, especially if applied to denuded skin areas or the perineal area.

The prescribed amount of the preparation should be applied to the area as indicated. It is important to note that certain topical preparations (e.g., ointments) should *not* be used on intertriginous areas.

When topical medication is administered, gloves are indicated to protect the nurse from irritant effects of medication, staining, or absorbing the medication. If lesions are infected, gloves are indicated to prevent the spread of infection. Sterile application of medication would require the use of sterile gloves and sterile technique. The use of gloves has been controversial because their use can communicate to the patient that he or she is unclean, contagious, or that the nurse is uncomfortable touching the patient. In deciding whether to use gloves in the administration of topical medications, one must consider patient preference, the presence of draining lesions, the use of irritating or staining preparations, and the necessity of guarding against inadvertent absorption of medication. Tongue blades are also commonly used to apply various topical medications, but sometimes application by this method is uncomfortable for the patient. It is important to note that some medications require removal from jars or containers with non-metal applicators (e.g., fluorouracil), and tongue blades or sterile blades can be used for removing the preparations.

Patient privacy should be assured during treatment, and the nurse must be sensitive to the patient's feelings about his or her condition. Nonverbal and verbal behavior is important in communicating acceptance and understanding of the patient's condition.

Creams, lotions, solutions, and ointments should be applied in specific amounts as ordered. A small amount of the prescribed medication should be rubbed into the lesion gently, leaving a thin film. When applying lotions to larger areas, the nurse should use a firm stroke rather than a dabbing motion because it is less irritating to pruritic skin and provides a thin even coat. If large areas are to be treated, they should be treated progressively.

It is important to incorporate patient teaching during application of the medication. The patient and family as indicated should be allowed and encouraged to participate in the application of the medication to enhance understanding of the regimen and self-medication abilities. This is particularly important if the patient or family member will be applying the medication at home.

Generally apply topical medication as directed with ungloved hands (unless gloves are indicated), using a clean, nonsterile technique unless a sterile technique is indicated because of specific patient factors. Touching the skin directly communicates acceptance of the patient's condition and allows assessment of the character of the skin areas and identification of changes in skin temperature and texture. Hands should be washed thoroughly after application of the medication to prevent absorption.

Preparation of the skin should be completed before the medication is applied. Skin lesions should be gently washed with nonirritating soap and warm water unless contraindicated. Inflamed skin should be rinsed with warm water only. Crusts should be softened and removed with treatment baths or normal saline soaks, or they should be washed gently to permit adequate contact of the medication. Depending on the specific condition being treated, other treatments may be indicated.

Nonocclusive or open technique

Creams, ointments, thick lotions

Place approximately 15 ml of cream, ointment, or oil-based lotion on the palms and rub the medication between the hands until it is softened and smooth in consistency. Apply the medication evenly using the palms. Patting or rubbing the skin should be avoided. Use long, even strokes following the direction of hair growth to prevent folliculitis. Creams and ointments should be applied sparingly to affected areas 2 to 3 times daily or as indicated. The cream should be gently massaged into the area until the medication disappears.

Thin lotions

Water- or alcohol-based lotions that are more liquid than oil-based lotions should be applied by dripping the lotion directly onto the affected area and gently stroking it in.

Suspensions

Suspensions require shaking before application to ensure adequate mixture of the medication. Suspensions should be applied with gauze pledgets. Cotton should not be used because it has a tendency to adhere to the skin area being treated. Smooth strokes following the direction of hair growth should be used when applying suspensions. These preparations have a tendency to crack and flake off when dry, and reapplication may be indicated more frequently.

Solutions

Solutions can be applied by the drop when supplied in plastic squeeze bottles. It should be noted that small quantities are adequate. The solution should be gently rubbed into the affected area. If treatment involves hairy sites, the hair should be parted and the solution dropped onto the affected area to allow direct contact with the lesion.

Aerosols

Aerosols (after shaking as directed) should be sprayed directly toward the affected area from 6 to 12 inches and only for as long as specified (usually 1 to 2 seconds). A watch should be used to time the application of the medication. *Continued.*

GENERAL NURSING IMPLICATIONS—cont'd

Nursing of patients requiring keratolytics, antiseborrheics, and related topical medications—cont'd

Powders

Powders should be applied to thoroughly dry skin as directed to minimize caking or crusting. Skin folds should be spread gently to expose the affected area fully during application. The shaker dispenser provides a fine thin layer of powder over the area being treated.

The patient's eyes, nose, ears, and mouth should be protected to prevent inhalation or indirect application of medication to these areas when either aerosols or powders are applied. Inhalation of the medication should be avoided by the nurse.

Treatment of face, ears, scalp

Facial lesions

When treating facial lesions, place a small amount of medication on the fingertips and gently smear it in a thin even layer over the affected area. The eyes, mouth, and nasal folds should be avoided to prevent irritation.

Lesions on the ears

A cotton-tip applicator can be coated with a small amount of medication, and the medication gently applied with a rolling technique if the external ear canal requires treatment.

Scalp

The scalp should be dampened and the hair parted so that liquid preparations can be dribbled directly onto the lesion. Creams or thicker lotions can be applied with the fingertips. The medication should be massaged in well. If a larger area or the total scalp is to be treated, the hair should be parted approximately 1 cm from the original site and the medication applied. This procedure should be continued down the side of the scalp and around the back of the head. The ears and hairline should be treated if indicated. If an irritating preparation is used, petrolatum may be applied over the ears to protect them from the irritant effects of the medication. A paper cap can be used to prevent smearing of medication into the eyes or mucous membranes, especially during the night.

Shampoos should be applied as directed. They are usually left on after lathering for 2 to 5 minutes for maximum effects. The eyes and ears should be protected especially from medicated shampoos, and the shampoo should not be allowed to enter the ear canal. After the recommended treatment, the hair and scalp should be rinsed well with warm water and dried carefully.

Occlusive dressing technique

Occlusive dressings cause increased hydration of the occluded area and increased temperature, thus increasing absorption or penetration of the medication. It is important to note that absorption is increased over denuded areas and can cause local and systemic adverse side effects.

Occlusive dressings should generally not be applied if there is an elevation in body temperature.

Generally, the medication is applied to a clean skin surface as prescribed and covered with a light gauze dressing. The dressing is covered with impermeable plastic, such as plastic wrap, and the edges sealed with tape or other means (e.g., stockinette, gauze wrap). The dressing is left in place for 1 to 3 days and the procedure repeated 3 to 4 times as needed. Patient response is usually rapid, and improvement can be seen after 1 to 3 days. Monitoring is essential because folliculitis can occur under the dressing requiring removal of the dressing.

A plastic shower cap can be used as an occlusive dressing over the scalp when treated to increase penetration and to protect the eyes and mucous membranes from medication smearing.

Points to remember

Generally, before administering topical medications:

Ensure familiarity with the basic compounds and the more commonly used preparations.

Be sure all compounds are clearly labeled with appropriate poison labels where indicated and with instructions for topical use only.

Keep containers and preparations out of the reach of children.

Document instructions of preparation and storage with regular checks as part of general policy.

Establish a regular review policy on the removal of outdated compounds with continuing information on shelf life and stability of both established and newer compounds.

Recheck safety and toxicity of compounds (e.g., corrosive acids), and ensure proper dose and concentration where applicable.

Regularly review potential and recorded adverse side effects of any compound.

Be aware that certain preparations (e.g., podophyllin) should be ordered and administered only by an experienced clinician.

Ensure appropriate vehicles or formulations are used for the proper sites (e.g., avoid ointments and tars in hairy areas). If uncertain, check with the prescribing clinician.

Check for presence or prior use of other topical preparations used on the skin.

Check previous history of adverse side effects of a compound, including topical irritant or allergic contact dermatitis or other hypersensitivity reactions. A patient alert tag or chain should be advised along with appropriate visible notation on the patient's chart and bedside.

Have prepared lists available of potential cross-reacting compounds, either topical or oral.

Be cognizant of contraindications to various products (e.g., podophyllin use in pregnancy).

Be aware of special precautions and considerations of topical salicylic acid especially in infants. Observe and report the early signs of salicylism. Check possible additive effect from other sources of salicylates (oil of wintergreen, oral salicylate compounds).

GENERAL NURSING IMPLICATIONS—cont'd

Nursing of patients requiring keratolytics, antiseborrheics, and related topical medications—cont'd

Points to remember—cont'd

Be aware of possibility of accidental or suicidal ingestion. Ensure appropriate emergency procedures, antidotes, and supplies are available.

MONITORING PATIENT RESPONSE

Therapeutic response

Monitor for effects depending on the indication for therapy. Generally, monitor for improvement in skin lesions and a decrease in inflammation, pruritus, dry scaling, or erythema. It is important to note that erythema is expected with the use of some preparations (e.g., fluorouracil), and once it is achieved, after up to 3 or 4 weeks of treatment, topical application is discontinued. It is important to monitor response so that drug therapy can be modified as indicated to enhance continued healing of lesions.

Adverse side effects

Adverse side effects associated with the topical medications discussed in this chapter most likely result from improper administration. With correct application and use, adverse effects are rare. However, both local and systemic adverse side effects can occur with the use of these medications.

Local

Local irritation, erythema, burning, stinging, itching, or other discomfort can occur with the application of these medications, and patients should be advised of these effects. They should be monitored carefully, especially when higher concentrations or medications associated with irritant effects are used. In addition, monitor for staining of skin, hair, or fabric and for excessive drying.

Systemic

Systemic effects are rare but can occur with application of topical medication to denuded skin areas when large amounts or higher concentrations of drug are used, when frequency of application is increased, or when occlusive dressings are also used.

To prevent salicylate toxicity (associated with the use of salicylic acids), monitor for thirst, tinnitus, headache, lethargy, confusion, gastric upset, depression, disorientation, hyperventilation, and dimness of vision (classic symptoms); EEG abnormalities, acidosis, delirium, hallucinations, convulsions, and coma (if severe).

Infants and young children should be monitored for crying, irritability, and emotional lability.

Monitor salicylate levels, especially if the patient is receiving other sources of the drug. The drug should not be used if salicylism is suspected. Dehydrated patients, those with renal or hepatic dysfunction, and children are at risk and require careful monitoring.

When podophyllum resin is administered, monitor for nausea, vomiting, anuria, coma, and tachycardia.

See Adverse/Side Effects of Keratolytics, Antiseborrheics, and Related Agents for an outline of adverse side effects occurring with keratolytics, antiseborrheics, and related agents, and the Nursing Drug Digest for specific agents.

PATIENT EDUCATION

The patient and family as indicated should have a clear understanding of the patient's condition and need for topical therapy. They should have an understanding of the anticipated course of therapy, especially if the patient has a chronic condition requiring long-term treatment.

The patient and family should know the exact name of the preparation, its dosage form, concentration, its general action, purpose, storage, and adverse side effects. It is particularly important that patients understand how to correctly apply topical preparations and that overuse of these preparations, instead of producing additional therapeutic effect, may produce toxicity. They should understand that topical preparations are for external use only and that overuse can lead to tachyphylaxis.

The patient and family should be able to monitor therapeutic response and recognize common and more serious adverse side effects that indicate the health care provider should be notified. Patients should understand the importance of follow-up care as indicated.

It is particularly important that application and misuse are carefully explained to the patient. He or she should understand how to store medication and the importance of not sharing it with family and friends.

Patient education should include care of normal skin and explanation of effects of aging, diet, sun, and other damaging elements as indicated. Patients should be warned about overexposure to sun and to avoid sun exposure during therapy (especially with topical fluorouracil therapy). They should be advised about the use of sunscreens and protective clothing. If the skin condition is caused by or is exacerbated by wool fibers or other allergens, the patient should be encouraged to avoid these. If itching is a problem, patients should be taught to keep their nails short and clean and to avoid scratching to prevent possible scarring or secondary infections. The use of mitts at night, socks, or restraints may be indicated. Patients should be taught to apply restraints correctly if required.

GENERAL INSTRUCTIONS FOR DISCHARGE/OUTPATIENTS

KERATOLYTICS, ANTISEBORRHEICS, AND RELATED TOPICAL MEDICATIONS

This medication is primarily used to treat various skin conditions. If you do not understand why you require this medication, check with your health care provider.

Follow the instructions exactly as prescribed. If you have any questions about how this medication should be applied, check with your health care provider. This medication is for *topical* or *external* use only.

Apply this medication sparingly in a light coating to the affected areas and rub in gently. Avoid excessive use.

Avoid contact with the eyes unless you are treating an eye condition and have been specifically told to apply the medication to the eye. If you inadvertently get this medication in the eye, rinse it out immediately with water.

Familiarize yourself with conditions of storage, shelf life, and expiration dates where appropriate.

Avoid household remedies or proprietary preparations other than those specifically prescribed or recommended by your health care provider.

The treated area should not be bandaged, covered, or wrapped with plastic wrap unless you are specifically advised to do so by your health care provider because this can cause unwanted effects.

Avoid diapers or plastic pants if applying this medication as prescribed to an affected diaper area of an infant.

Report the development of new skin rashes or changes, itch, eye problems, or failure of therapy to your health care provider.

Do not start or stop taking medications while on this medication without first checking with your health care provider. This medication can cause unwanted effects if used with some other medications.

If you are pregnant, thinking about becoming pregnant, or breastfeeding, do *not* use this medication until you discuss this with your health care provider. The use of this medication during pregnancy or with women nursing infants has not been fully evaluated.

If you have had a previous allergic contact dermatitis or hypersensitivity reaction, carefully avoid the potential cross-reacting products named in the list provided to you by the nurse or physician (e.g., hexylresorcinol compounds, in many proprietary antiseborrheic lotions and scalp preparations cross-react with products such as Sucrets throat lozenges or Listerine oral mouthwash).

Skin rashes or local irritation may develop even if this medication was used previously without any complications. The onset may also be delayed and begin after hospital discharge even if used without a problem in the hospital.

If topical salicylic acid therapy is used, be particularly aware of signs of salicylism and report development of these changes to your nurse or physician immediately.

Be aware of possible staining of skin, hair, or clothing fabric with some compounds.

Observe precautions with sun exposure with some compounds as directed.

Consult your health care provider if further information or clarification is required or if complications ensue.

This medication has been prescribed especially for you. Do not trade or give this medication to any relatives or friends.

Keep this and all medications out of children's reach.

Ensure return appointments with your health care provider particularly if on long-term therapy. This is important in managing your therapy. If you have any questions about your treatment discuss these with your health care provider.

In addition to the general instructions, if you require *fluorouracil solution:*

Apply this medication with a nonmetal applicator, or wear gloves and apply it with the fingertips as prescribed. Wash your hands thoroughly after applying the solution.

This drug can cause temporary redness of the skin. This is expected, so do not become alarmed.

While you are using this medication on your skin, avoid exposing the treated areas of your skin to sunlight. The sun can cause further irritation and make the areas appear redder.

Call your health care provider if this medication causes extreme pain, itching, burning, or discoloration of the skin after use.

Do not become discouraged if you do not see improvement in your skin condition right away. Healing of the skin can take up to 2 months after stopping the medication.

NURSING DRUG DIGEST

Medication (trade name*)	Indication	Usual dosage and administration	Dosage forms, preparation, and storage	Contraindications, cautions, and comments	Monitoring
Anthralin Anthera Anthra-Derm Anthra-Derm Oil Anthraforte Lasan	Psoriasis therapy	Topical ointment or pomade Apply as directed in thin layer Amount not quantitated or standardized Wash hands thoroughly after use Remove ointment with warm oil and bath in morning after overnight use Remove pomade with shampoo in morning after overnight use Apply with a wooden or plastic spatula or plastic gloves; metal should not be used because it will oxidize the anthralin rendering it ineffective Anthralin is an irritant and should *not* be applied with the hands because it may lodge under the nails and irritate; it will also discolor the skin For *external* use only	Ointment: 0.1%, 0.2% (in Lassar's paste—zinc oxide, corn starch, and white petrolatum) Scalp-pomade: 0.8% (in cetyl alcohol-mineral oil ointment base) Oil: 0.25% Anthralin is light sensitive, and the bottle must be capped immediately after use and stored protected from light in a cool, dark area Ensure limited access Ensure clearly visible label Check stability, shelf life, and expiration dates One sign that drug has lost its effectiveness is a change to a purple-brown color	Avoid in patients with renal disease Avoid on acutely inflamed, abraded skin Avoid eye contact because may cause conjunctivitis, corneal opacity, keratitis Avoid application to normal skin or mucosa Accidental ingestion produces catharsis May stain skin, hair, and clothing fabrics Avoid ointment on hairy sites Discontinue use if irritancy develops Avoid if possible on face, genital region, and body creases or fold regions Excessive amounts may be irritating A paper cap should be worn at night when anthralin pomade is applied to the scalp because it melts and may smear onto the pillow and irritate the face or drip onto the neck or behind the ears; plain white petrolatum may be used around the hairline and behind the ears for further protection	Monitor for irritancy, marked erythema, pustules Monitor for renal irritation

NOTE: For additional details regarding the individual agents listed in this table see the text and other tables listed in this chapter.
*Indicates a multiple active ingredient product. For a complete listing of all active ingredients see the *Drug Reference Guide to Brand Names and Active Ingredients.*

Continued.

NURSING DRUG DIGEST—cont'd

Medication (trade name)	Indication	Usual dosage and administration	Dosage forms, preparation, and storage	Contraindications, cautions, and comments	Monitoring
Benzoyl peroxide Acetoxyl Benoxyl Benzac Benzagel Dermodex 5 & 10 Gel Dermoxyl Desquam-X Dry and Clear Epi-Clear* Fostex BPO 5% Loroxide Acne Lotion* Loroxide-HC Lotion* Oxy Wash Oxy-10 Oxy-5 Oxyderm Panoxyl Persadox Persa-Gel Perso-Gel Stri-Dex B.P. Sulfoxyl Lotion Regular & Strong* Teen 5 & 10 Lotion Topex Acne Clearing Medication	Acne therapy	Topical One application daily or nightly Dose not standardized or quantitated, but 2 mm diameter drop sufficient for entire face usually Apply sparingly and with caution on neck, perioral region or other sensitive sites Institute therapy with slowly increasing time increments (i.e., start with 1 hr application and increase to 8 hr over the course of a week and then maintain with daily 8 hr application) More effective if site washed or moistened before benzoyl peroxide applied Usually used with other acne medications (topical or systemic) For *external* use only	Store in cool place Gel: 2.5%, 5%, 10%, 15%, 20% Lotion: 5%, 10%, 20% Wash: 4%, 5%, 10% Check stability, and expiration dates routinely	May take several weeks before beneficial effects noted May cause irritant contact reaction particularly if excessive amounts applied Avoid eye and mucosal contact Less effective on chest and back than face for acne therapy Occasionally causes staining and capable of bleaching fabric or hair Rarely causes allergic contact dermatitis	Monitor for irritant effect
Cantharidin Canthacur Cantharone	Wart therapy (often periungual) Vesiculant	Topical 0.7% concentration of cantharidin; for use by *only* experienced clinicians	0.7% cantharidin in flexible collodion, acetone, alcohol, and ether Clearly label and restrict access	If accidentally applied to eyes or mucous membranes, flush with water for 15 minutes	Monitor for pain, skin irritation, or nail damage

Drug	Uses	Administration	Preparations/Dosage	Cautions	Monitoring
(continued)		Applied under occlusive bandage for up to 48 hr. Unwrapped and inspected by clinician at 48 hr, repeat treatments only under direction of prescriber. For *external* use only	Check stability, shelf life, and expiration date	If accidentally applied to normal skin, immediately remove with acetone or alcohol. Experienced clinician use *only*. *Not to be dispensed*. May cause pain, skin or nail damage. With proper use leaves no scar. Avoid use in patients with local impaired circulation or sensation. Hazard with accidental ingestion (i.e., vomiting, abdominal pain, shock). Avoid contact with eyes or mucous membranes	Monitor for skin irritancy
Coal tar A.T.S.*, Balnetar*, DHS Tar Shampoo*, Estar, L.C.D., Lavatar, Neutratar, Pentrax Tar Shampoo, Psorigel, Racet LCD, Sebutone*, Tar Distillate "Doak", Tar-Doak Lotion*, Targel, Targel S.A., Tersa-Tar, Ultra Clear Medicated Shampoo, Zetar, Zetar Emulsion, Zetar Shampoo*	Psoriasis therapy Antiseborrheic Keratolytic	Topical. Do not leave on long periods. Applied as directed in thin layer to affected skin site, usually q.d. to t.i.d.; may use disposable plastic gloves to apply. Dose not quantitated or standardized. For shampoo, massage lather into scalp for 5 minutes before rinsing thoroughly. Coal-tar extract 2% (equivalent to crude coal tar 5%). Crude coal tar should always be applied in a downward motion in the direction of hair growth to prevent folliculitis. For *external* use only	Used in varying concentrations and usually compounded in ointment (petrolatum) bases. Some preparations contain additional types of tar (i.e., Polytar—0.5%, 1.0% blend of coal tar; juniper tar, and pine tar). Cream, gel, lotion, ointment, paste, shampoo: 0.5%, 1%, 2%, 3%, 4%, 5%, 10%. Emulsion, solution, suspension: 5%, 10%, 20%, 30%. Bath emulsion: 50%. Routinely check stability, shelf life, and expiration dates	Avoid eye and mucous membrane contact. Can produce direct irritancy particularly in higher concentration. Avoid sun or ultraviolet light exposure during treatment periods apart from prescribed use for psoriasis therapy. Not water soluble. Compliance may be a problem because of cosmetic and odor objections. May be photosensitizer. Capable of staining skin, hair, and clothing fabrics. Avoid application to abraded or highly inflamed skin and hairy sites. May be too drying or potential irritant with excessive application or amount. Discontinue if contact allergic dermatitis occurs	

Continued.

NURSING DRUG DIGEST—cont'd

Medication (trade name)	Indication	Usual dosage and administration	Dosage forms, preparation, and storage	Contraindications, cautions, and comments	Monitoring
Fluorouracil Efudex Fluoroplex	Topical chemotherapy (antineoplastic), particularly for actinic keratoses See also Chapter 52, "Antimetabolites and Antineoplastic Antibiotics"	Topical Applied twice daily until peak erythema reaction for approximately 3 weeks Cream preferably applied with glove or nonmetal applicator, but if fingertips are used, hands must be washed *immediately* afterward Total skin area treated should *not* exceed approximately 23 cm × 23 cm area Application is best during winter or nonsunny periods Sun should be avoided during treatment period For *external* use only	Cream: 1%, 5% Solution: 1%, 2%, 5% Check stability and expiration dates routinely	May cause pain, itch, hyperpigmentation, burning, or blistering at the application site The patients should be familiarized with the expected erythema reaction Eye contact should be avoided Complete healing may not occur for 1 or 2 months following therapy May cause allergic contact dermatitis Accidental ingestion may produce toxicity Risk uncertain with use in pregnancy, since the drug is a known cell growth inhibitor, although no confirmed reports of toxicity or teratogenicity reported after topical application May cause photosensitivity Wash hands immediately after handling medication	Monitor for erythema reaction

Lactic acid, pyruvic acid, glucuronic acid combination	Keratolytic Wart therapy	Topical Amount not standardized Applied as directed in thin layer to affected skin site q.d. to t.i.d. May use plastic gloves for application Lotions or fluid solutions applied as 2 drops to site and in wart therapy often covered by tape occlusion for up to 24 hr and repeated q.d. for several weeks Avoid excessive amount or frequency of application For *external* use only	Compounded or available in cream, ointment, lotion, gel, and other formulations (usually compounded in 3%-10% concentration range, but available in some keratolytic or antiwart preparations as 17.5%, 20% or 25% concentrations) Check stability, shelf life, and expiration dates	May be direct irritant in higher concentration or excessive use Caution with use in sites of impaired circulation or sensation Hazard of corrosion with accidental ingestion
Methoxsalen Oxsoralen Soloxsalen	Topical repigmentation in vitiligo in conjunction with controlled doses of ultraviolet light (320-400 nm) or sunlight	*Adults:* Apply to affected lesions in a clinical setting followed by appropriate exposure to ultraviolet light A (UVA) *Children:* Use in children less than 12 years of age is *not* recommended	Lotion: 1%	*Contraindicated* in hypersensitivity, melanoma, invasive skin carcinoma, and photosensitivity diseases May cause severe burns if improperly used *Avoid* concomitant use of other photosensitizing drugs (e.g., coal tar, griseofulvin, phenothiazines, sulfonamides, tetracyclines) Protective clothing or sunscreens *must* be used Observe for photosensitivity

Continued.

NURSING DRUG DIGEST—cont'd

Medication (trade name)	Indication	Usual dosage and administration	Dosage forms, preparation, and storage	Contraindications, cautions, and comments	Monitoring
Podophyllum resin Podoben	Wart therapy (especially venereal warts)	Topical Usually 20%-25% concentration and applied directly by clinician with applicator or cotton swab: usually with protection to surrounding skin and washed off within 6 hours May require repeat application at 1 week intervals For *external* use only	20%-25% podophyllum in tincture of benzoin or alcoholic solution Clearly label and restrict access Check stability, shelf life, and expiration date	Clinician use and application only Can be direct irritant to skin or mucous membrane Occasional contact burns with excess use or extravasation on normal skin or mucosa Carefully rinse off within 6 hr or sooner if irritating *Not* to be dispensed to patient Potential hazard with use in pregnancy to mother and fetus because application to genital warts during pregnancy may lead to increased absorption or direct fetal exposure If systemically absorbed, may cause peripheral neuropathy Petrolatum may be used to provide protection to surrounding skin	Monitor for irritant effects, extravasation
Propylene glycol Aerolone* Barsed Thera-Spray* Buf Foot-Care Lotion* Decubitex*	Keratolytic Lubricant Cutaneous absorption accelerant Healing fissures	Topical Dose not quantitated or standardized Applied as directed in thin layer q.d. to t.i.d. to affected site Often may apply with fingers in usual formulation For *external* use only	Ingredient of many formulations and differing active ingredients; usually gel, cream, or lotion form Not generally used in ointments Commonly 60%-80% concentration employed Check stability, shelf life, and expiration dates routinely	May be more risk from increased absorption of active ingredient(s) Occasional irritant contact dermatitis especially undiluted or under occlusion True allergic contact dermatitis is rare Avoid use in ear canal if possible	

Pyrithione zinc Danex Head and Shoulders Ionil* Ionil-T* Zincon	Antiseborrheic shampoo	Do not use soap or detergent before or after applications of Ionil as the contained benzalkonium chloride may be inactivated Usually directly applied to scalp once daily Leave in lather at least 2-3 min before rinsing thoroughly For *external* use only	Shampoo: 2% (in detergent base) Shampoo: 0.2% Some preparations contain additional ingredients (i.e., Ionil—2% salicylic acid; Ionil-T—2% salicylic acid and 4.5% coal tar)	Avoid eye contact No known significant toxicity or allergic reactions reported when applied to normal skin and hair Has property of substantivity
Resorcinol and sulfur combination Acnomel Rezamid	Acne therapy Antiseborrheic	Topical Cleanse site gently before application Amount not standardized or quantitated Usually applied q.d. in thin layer to affected area with fingertips For *external* use only	Cake: 1% resorcinol, 4% sulfur Cream: 2% resorcinol, 8% sulfur Lotion: 2% resorcinol, 5% sulfur Resorcinol compounds dispensed in dark bottles to avoid discoloration on exposure to light Check stability and expiration dates	Avoid eye contact Considered a mild surface acne treatment Rarely hypersensitivity to compound ingredients is evidenced Cross-reactivity of resorcinol and other substitute phenols including hexyl resorcinol compounds is possible Some available with color blender for cosmetic use Often used with other agents for acne (topical or systemic) Accidental ingestion may produce toxicity (i.e., nausea, vomiting, abdominal pain)

Continued.

NURSING DRUG DIGEST—cont'd

Medication (trade name)	Indication	Usual dosage and administration	Dosage forms, preparation, and storage	Contraindications, cautions, and comments	Monitoring
Salicylic acid Acnaveen* Acne-Dome Medicated Cleanser* Acnesarb Clearasil Medicated Cleanser Compound W* Derma Soft Cream Dry and Clear Acne Cream* Drytex Duofilm* Exzit Medicated Cleanser* Fomac Foam Fostex Cake* Freezone* Keralyt Komed HC* Pernox* Saligel Sebucare Sebulex* Sebutone* Stri-Dex Medicated Pads Therac Therapads* Tinver* Wart-Off Xseb Shampoo	Keratolytic Antiseborrheic Wart therapy Acne	Topical Concentrations in various preparations vary from approximately 1% to 40% Amount not standardized Usually administered no more than once daily Applied as directed (i.e., first hydrate skin and then preparation applied with disposable gloves in thin layer to affected site, often at night and washed off in morning; some keratolytics, such as Keralyt, require plastic wrap occlusion of area during overnight application. Duofilm is applied as 2 or 3 drops with preparation applicator nightly and the wart kept under tape occlusion) Limit to one application daily and smaller amounts applied to minimize toxicity risk Caution with use of higher concentration on sites of impaired circulation or sensation (sole of foot in diabetics) Children less than 12 years of age should have no more than 30 gm applied topically in any 24-hr period. For external use only	Compounded or available in gel, cream, ointment, paste, lotion, shampoo, soap, or plaster formulation in 1%-40% concentration May be component of other products, such as topical corticosteroids and numerous acne and antiseborrheic preparations in combination with sulfur or resorcinol Check stability and expiration dates	Contraindicated in hypersensitivity Formulate general policies regarding topical salicylic acid therapy in risk patients (especially infants) May cause local irritation with higher concentration or excessive use Hazard of systemic salicylate toxicity with percutaneous absorption with greater risk in infants and dehydration Salicylate blood levels may be cumulative with other sources Caution with use during pregnancy No odor or staining normally unless additional ingredients Extremely rare for contact allergy and no significant cross reactions with other salicylate compounds For wart therapy limit compound to wart, and avoid surrounding skin contact if possible	Be aware of and report early signs of salicylate toxicity (i.e., crying, irritability, thirst, headache, tinnitus, lethargy, confusion)

Drug	Uses	Administration	Preparations	Nursing considerations
Salicylic acid and sulfur combination Buf-Acne-Cleansing Bar* Pernox Sebulex	Antiseborrheic shampoo Acne therapy	For acne therapy apply thin layer q.d. to b.i.d. to affected sites Moisten site before application Leave Sebulex shampoo lather on 5 min before rinsing thoroughly For *external* use only	Sulfur 2%, salicylic acid 2%, in a surface active combination of soapless cleansers and wetting agent Ensure clearly visible labeling Check shelf life, stability, and expiration dates	Avoid eye contact Toxicity uncommon
Selenium sulfide Exsel Losel 250 Sebusan Selsun Selsun Blue Sul-Blue	Seborrheic dermatitis scalp Dandruff Tinea versicolor	Shampoo Frequency not standardized; commonly 2-3 times weekly for control Leave on at least 2-3 min before rinsing thoroughly Applied to affected sites on chest and arms for tinea versicolor usually q.d. for 10 min for 1 week, then weekly for 1 month Apply with gloves to prevent absorption through openings in the skin For *external* use only	Shampoo: 1%, 2.5%	May cause orange staining of hair, skin, or clothing fabric Avoid eye contact; may cause chemical conjunctivitis Contact dermatitis uncommon Accidental oral ingestion may be toxic Claimed to have substantivity (shampoo action persists) Pigmentation alterations of tinea versicolor may persist for long periods despite successful therapy Often in a detergent base formulation Rinse hair thoroughly to avoid hair staining and minimize contact dermatitis Wash hands thoroughly after use Selenium sulfide when ingested by infants and young children is extremely toxic This medication can be absorbed through openings in the skin and if used for a prolonged period can be toxic; a sign of toxicity is the smell of garlic on the breath

Continued.

NURSING DRUG DIGEST—cont'd

Medication (trade name)	Indication	Usual dosage and administration	Dosage forms, preparation, and storage	Contraindications, cautions, and comments	Monitoring
Sulfur Cuticura Dry and Clear Acne Cream Epi-Clear* Exzit Medicated Cleanser* Fostex Cake* Fostex CM Klaron* Liquimat Pernox* Postacne Sulfacet Sulfoil Transact	Acne therapy Antiseborrheic	Amount not standardized or quantitated Usually applied q.d. to moistened affected sites with fingertips For *external* use only	Cream: 2% sulfur Lotion: 5% colloidal sulfur in propylene glycol vehicle Check stability and expiration dates Ensure clearly visible labeling	Avoid eye contact Considered milder surface acne treatment Some available with color or blender for cosmetic use Often used with other agents for acne (topical or systemic)	
Tretinoin Aberel Aquasol A Cream Retin-A StieVAA Vitamin A Acid Gel	Acne therapy Occasional flat wart treatment Occasional keratolytic or peeling agent	Topical Applied q.d. or q.h.s. and left on skin for up to 8-10 hr Amount not standardized or quantitated, but 2 mm diameter drop sufficient for entire face Institute therapy with slowly increasing time increments Should *not* be applied in areas of sunburn or active dermatitis	Cream: 0.05%, 0.1% Gel: 0.01%, 0.025%, 0.05% Liquid (topical): 0.05% Check stability and expiration dates routinely	May take several weeks before beneficial effects noted May cause contact irritant reaction particularly if excessive amounts applied Less effective on chest and back than face for acne therapy	

Drug	Category	Directions	Remarks
		Usually used with other acne medications (topical or systemic) For *external* use only	*Reduce* sun exposure during therapy because tretinoin makes skin more susceptible to sunburn Ensure regular follow-up while on therapy Most effective for comedonal acne therapy
Trichloroacetic acid, Glacial acetic acid combination	Topical chemosurgery Corrosive	Topical Applied *only* by experienced clinician Concentration may vary: 10%-25% or more For *external* use only	Physician use only Clearly label as poison Hazard of corrosion and chemical burns on accidental contact Hazard of accidental ingestion, severe corrosion, and toxicity Aqueous solutions Diluted to desired concentration Keep in restricted area with limited access Ensure clear labeling, including poison labels Check stability and storage life
Urea Amino-Cerv Calmurid Carmol Carmol 10 Lotion Kerid Ear Drop* Lowila Cake* Nutraplus Panafil Ointment* Panafil-White Ointment* Uremol Uremol HC* Uretex Uresec Velvelan	Emollient Keratolytic	Topical 10%-20% or 50% concentration, dose not standardized Usually applied t.i.d. to q.i.d. For *external* use only	Cream or lotion most common formulations Usually 10% or 20% concentrations Check stability, shelf life, and expiration dates Protect products from excessive heat May cause stinging or burning or irritant contact dermatitis, especially on abraded areas, thin skin, or face Avoid eye contact Avoid use on face if possible True contact allergy unlikely

BIBLIOGRAPHY

Anders, J.E., & Moeller, P.J. Topicals a welter of options calls for refined application techniques. *RN*, 1982, *45*(9), 33-42.

Anders, J.E., & Leach, E. Sun versus skin. *American Journal of Nursing*, 1983, *83*(7), 1015-1020.

Breza, T., Taylor, V.R., & Eaglestein, W.H. Noninflammatory destruction of actinic keratoses by fluorouracil. *Archives of Dermatology*, 1976, *112*, 1256-1258.

Davies, M., & Marks, R. Studies of salicylic acid on normal skin. *British Journal of Dermatology*, 1976, *95*, 187.

Fisher, A.A. Propylene glycol dermatitis. *Cutis*, 1978, *21*, 166.

Goette, D.K., & Odom, R.B. Allergic contact dermatitis to topical fluorouracil. *Archives of Dermatology*, 1977, *113*, 1058-1061.

Goldsmith, L.A. Propylene glycol. *International Journal of Dermatology*, 1978, *17*, 703-705.

Goldsmith, L.A. Salicylic acid—Review. *International Journal of Dermatology*, 1979, *18*, 32-36.

Hurwitz, S. The combined effect of vitamin A acid and benzoyl peroxide in the treatment of acne. *Cutis*, 1976, *17*, 505-590.

Kaidbey, K.H., & Kligman, A.M. Clinical and histologic study of coal tar phototoxicity in humans. *Archives of Dermatology*, 1977, *113*, 592-595.

Millikan, L.E. Editorial: The safety of selenium sulfide and other news from Washington. *Journal of the American Academy of Dermatology*, 1980, *3*, 430.

Muller, S.A., Belcher, R.W., Easterly, N.B., et al. Keratinizing dermatoses. *Archives of Dermatology*, 1977, *113*, 1052-1054.

Pace, W.E. Treatment of cutaneous ulcers with benzoyl peroxide. *Canadian Medical Association Journal*, 1976, *115*, 1101-1106.

Rasmussen, J.E. Percutaneous absorption in children. In Year Book of Dermatology. Chicago, London: Year Book Medical Publishers Inc., 1979.

Taylor, J.R., & Halprin, K.M. Percutaneous absorption of salicylic acid. *Archives of Dermatology*, 1975, *111*, 740.

Weirich, E.G. Dermatopharmacology of salicylic acid. I. Range of dermatotherapeutic effects of salicylic acid. *Dermatologica*, 1975, *151*, 321.

Young, C.J. Salicylate intoxication from cutaneous absorption of salicylic acid. *Southern Medical Journal*, 1975, *45*, 1075.

CHAPTER 57

Topical Corticosteroids

Eric Schloss

Medications discussed in this chapter

Topical corticosteroids
Amcinonide
Beclomethasone dipro-
    prionate
Betamethasone dipro-
    prionate
Betamethasone valerate
Clobetasol
Clobetasone
Clocortolone
Desonide
Desoximetasone
Dexamethasone
Diflorasone
Flumethasone
Fluocinolone
Fluocinonide
Fluorometholone
Flurandrenolide
Halcinonide
Hydrocortisone
Methylprednisolone
Prednisolone
Triamcinolone acetonide
Triamcinolone acetonide
    in orabase

Topical corticosteroid/
antibiotic combinations
Betamethasone valerate
    with gentamicin
Flumethasone with iodo-
    chlorhydroxyquin
Hydrocortisone with
    iodochlorhydroxyquin
Hydrocortisone with nys-
    tatin and iodochlorhy-
    droxyquin
Methylprednisolone with
    neomycin
Methylprednisolone with
    neomycin and alumi-
    num chlorohydrate
Methylprednisolone with
    sulfur and aluminum
    chlorohydrate
Triamcinolone acetonide
    with neomycin, grami-
    cidin and nystatin

Topical corticosteroids are commonly used for a wide variety of dermatoses, but many variables are inherent in their application to clinical skin disease. A wide number of preparations are available, but only the major categories of topical corticosteroids will be discussed. The basic principles governing their pharmacologic action, conditions of use, and potential adverse side effects may be similar to all in nature if not in degree.

BASIC ACTION

The corticosteroids can have a potentially wide variety of effects on cellular activities including an-
tiinflammatory, immunosuppressive, antiproliferative, and antisynthetic effects. The precise mechanism of action at the cell level is uncertain; however, they are thought to initiate effects mainly through induction of new protein synthesis in target cells. Although not initially described in the skin, the model basically envisages binding of the corticosteroid to receptor sites in target cell cytoplasm, and subsequent *translocation* of the complex to the nucleus, where there is an interaction with high affinity nuclear binding sites. Subsequently, *messenger ribonucleic acid* (mRNA) *transcription* and structural protein and enzyme synthesis proceed.

STRUCTURE-ACTIVITY RELATIONSHIP (SAR)

The mechanism of action, relative potencies, and biologic activity of corticosteroids can be correlated with chemical modification of their basic structure. The basic nucleus common to all steroids is shown in Figure 57-1. Cortisone is inactive topically, because the necessary conversion of the ketone structure at the carbon No. 11 position to the hydroxyl group does not take place in the skin (with oral medication this conversion takes place in the liver). Thus all topical preparations are basic modifications of hydrocortisone. The structure therefore requires a carbon No. 11 hydroxyl group, along with a carbon No. 17 side chain, and a ketone group at carbon No. 20 position. Alterations to any portion of the structure may modify its intrinsic potency, presumably by modifying the ability of the topical corticosteroid to interact (bind) with receptors in the skin. Extrinsic activities (i.e., solubility, penetrability, diffusion, and vehicle compatibility), which may alter cellular effects, can also change with structural modification.

Modification in synthetic compounds affecting intrinsic activity include *fluorination* at the carbon No. 6 or No. 9 positions, which may increase antiinflammatory effects eightfold, and the addition of a double

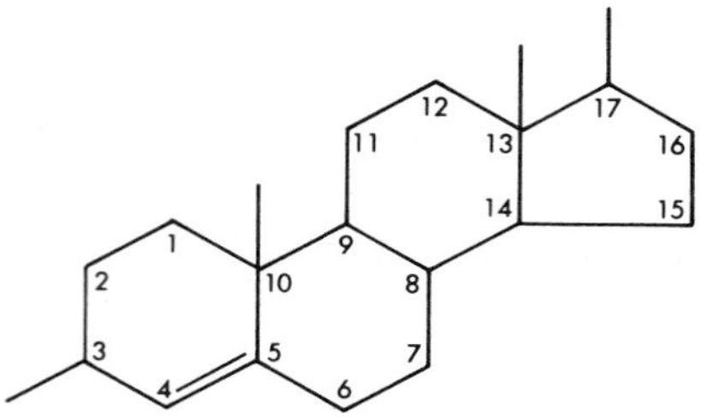

FIGURE 57-1. **Basic nucleus common to all steroids.**

bond between carbons No. 1 and No. 2, which can increase the antiinflammatory effects fourfold. Along with other modifications, such as hydroxylation or methylation at carbon No. 16 and methylation at carbon No. 6, this has led to the development of clinically used compounds, such as triamcinolone, dexamethasone, and betamethasone. These structural changes have also reduced unwanted mineralocorticoid (salt-retaining) properties of the corticosteroids.

Inherent potency varies considerably, and the compounds are usually graded or ranked according to results of the vasoconstrictor assay as developed by Stoughton and McKenzie (1962) (Table 57-1). This standardized in vivo assay measures the effects of topical corticosteroid preparations on human forearm skin, and the blanching (vasoconstriction) produced is usually proportional to clinical antiinflammatory activity with most of the compounds tested. There are claimed exceptions, however, and absolute equivalents of topical corticosteroids have not been established. The vasoconstriction assay has reported a 2000-fold greater effect of clobetasol butyrate over basic hydrocortisone. Unfortunately undesirable cutaneous and systemic adverse side effects also tend to parallel potency rankings, and reports of suppression of the *hypothalamus-pituitary-adrenal (HPA) axis* in clinical use have been recorded with clobetasol butyrate. Some exceptions, however, are also claimed, as clobetasone butyrate also achieves high ranking by *vasoconstrictor* assay, but has been stated to be free of systemic side effects.

Extrinsic activities affecting important variables in clinical use can also be altered by structural modifications. Some of these modifications enhance the *hydrophobic* character of the compounds and increase lipid solubility, allowing increased release from its carrier or vehicle, and enhanced availability of the active compound at the cutaneous site of action. This has been achieved by removing or masking *hydroxyl* (OH⁻) *groups* with insertion of long carbon side chains. For example, fluocinolone acetonide contains an *aceton-*

TABLE 57-1

General potency ranking of topical corticosteroids

Potency	Drug
Extremely potent	Clobetasol
Very potent	Clobetasone
	Halcinonide
Potent	Amcinonide
	Betamethasone diproprionate
	Fluocinonide
Moderately potent	Beclomethasone diproprionate
	Betamethasone valerate
	Desoximetasone
	Fluocinolone
	Flurandrenolide
	Triamcinolone acetonide
Mildly potent	Desonide
	Flumethasone
	Hydrocortisone valerate
Weak	Hydrocortisone
	Methylprednisolone

ide grouping at carbon No. 16-17 position, which masks the hydroxyl groups, and similarly the hydroxyl group at carbon No. 17 is masked by *esterification* with fatty acid, producing betamethasone valerate.

Both of these compounds are commonly used, intermediate or medium strength corticosteroids as shown by vasoconstrictor assay. Changes enhancing structural affinity of the corticosteroid and its tissue receptor may also alter cellular effect. The fluorine group at carbon No. 9 position enables better binding of the carbon No. 11 hydroxyl group with the receptor, likely via an electron withdrawing effect, which favors the carbon No. 11 hydroxyl binding over the *ketone grouping*. It may also help retard metabolic destruction of the compound and enhance and sustain the clinical effect.

MAJOR ACTIONS

Antiinflammation

The basis of the major antiinflammatory action of corticosteroids may have some overlap with immunosuppressive function; however, it is at least partly the result of vasoconstrictive action. The precise basis of this effect is uncertain. It may be a direct effect or produced indirectly via catecholamines, prostaglandins, or histamine reduction at target cell sites. Although many variables are present in topical corticosteroid use, and the vasoconstrictor assay ranking does not always parallel clinical action, it has proved to be a reasonably reliable guide to both intrinsic potency and antiinflammatory activity and can provide an assessment of the variable of vehicle formulation on clinical effects.

Other known antiinflammatory effects include interference with *diapedesis* of polymorphonuclear leukocytes and decreased adherence of white blood cells to *endothelium* of small blood vessels at inflammatory sites. These effects can impede the development of the basic inflammatory reaction. It is uncertain if *lysosome* stabilization occurs in vivo, although there is some in vitro evidence of this. Corticosteroids may also decrease prostaglandin production by inhibiting release of precursors via enzyme inhibition. Other cellular effects are also related to immunosuppressive activity and include impairment of lymphocyte and macrophage function perhaps via interference with local antigen processing in the skin and inhibition of *lymphokine* action on target cells.

In general, the antiinflammatory action is nonspecific in the sense that all types of inflammatory reactions are suppressed regardless of etiology. Other actions that may be important are reduction of membrane permeability, inhibition of toxin or lysosomal enzyme release, and impairment of release or action of other chemical mediators of inflammation.

Antiproliferation

Topical corticosteroids stronger than hydrocortisone exert an antiproliferative action on cells of epidermis and dermal *fibroblasts*. Several effects are noted in the epidermis, particularly *antimitotic* action. Decreased ribonucleic acid (RNA) transcription and consequent reduction of deoxyribonucleic acid (DNA) synthesis occurs, which probably hinders the rate of cell repair. In addition, the topical corticosteroids may have a more specific role in the reformation of the granular layer in *psoriatic* skin. The antisynthetic action also affects the fibroblasts in the dermis, with consequent reduction of collagen and elastin synthesis, and decreased production of *interstitial* acid mucopolysaccharide ground substance.

PERCUTANEOUS ABSORPTION

Percutaneous absorption of topical corticosteroids tends to follow the expression of Fick's law under steady state conditions, and occurs largely by passive diffusion. Fick's law is expressed as $J = \dfrac{Km \times Dm \times \Delta Cs}{L}$, as previously discussed in Chapter 54, "Review of the Anatomy, Physiology, and Assessment of the Cutaneous System."

Absorption is a major variable in topical corticosteroid therapy, as it must occur effectively in order to produce a clinical effect on target tissue. Low steroid permeabilities arise primarily from intrinsically small *diffusion constants* (Dm) in stratum corneum of skin, not decreased solubility per se. The diffusion constant is reduced by addition of *polar groups* to the steroid molecule. Skin appendage sites such as pilosebaceous and eccrine sweat duct orifices may be important diffusion shunts in topical corticosteroid therapy, as diffusion constants are low for polar corticosteroids and they may be diverted to the shunt sites. The inherent structure of the corticosteroid is therefore important in absorption, but there are other important variables, particularly in relation to the vehicle.

The rate of penetration through the stratum corneum depends on the relative water/lipid solubility of the corticosteroid, and its stability and solubility in the carrier *vehicle*. The solubility of the vehicle in the stratum corneum is also an important variable. The addition of substances such as propylene glycol, as in many corticosteroid creams or gels, increases penetration of the compound through the stratum corneum, which is the major barrier to percutaneous absorption. Formulation may be very important, and although few reliable studies of comparisons of cream, ointment, gel, lotion, or other formulations have been performed, this variable must be given serious consideration. Some studies have proposed that ointments generally may be more effective hydrators than creams. However, other considerations such as the increased cosmetic acceptability of creams often play a role in vehicle choice, and additives such as propylene glycol or application under *occlusion* may affect comparison studies. Experimental models have not been precise in predicting efficiency and potential adverse side effects, although the vasoconstrictor assay allows rough assessment of vehicle reliability.

OTHER VARIABLES

Amount

There is no valid correlation of amount of topical corticosteroid applied and effective penetration. Only 1% of an applied dose of hydrocortisone was measurably absorbed; the corollary, of course, is that 99% was wasted. This has led to a general recommendation to apply corticosteroid creams sparingly since there is no apparent benefit from additional amount, and it is also wasteful and uneconomic. Since no absolute equivalents have been established, the precise amounts recommended have remained empirical. A

TABLE 57-2

Amount of topical corticosteroid required for a single daily application to specific body areas

Body area	Approximate amount in grams
Head (not scalp)	1–2
Trunk (anterior or posterior)	3–6
Arms (each)	1–2
Genitoanal area	1–2
Total body	15–30

TABLE 57-3

Hydrocortisone absorption: effect of anatomic region

Anatomic region	Absorption
Forearm	1 × (approximately 1%)
Plantar foot	0.14 ×
Lateral ankle	0.42 ×
Palm	0.83 ×
Back	1.7 ×
Axillae, scalp	3.5 ×
Forehead	6.0 ×
Jaw angle	12.0 ×
Scrotum	42.0 ×

rough guide to amounts required is presented in Table 57-2.

Concentration

There is a rough dose-response relation to concentration, but this may not be appreciated clinically, and a plateau often occurs in practice, particularly as the treated abnormal skin heals. It is generally considered advisable to use the minimal effective concentration in an attempt to lower or minimize the incidence of adverse side effects.

Site

The cutaneous application site thickness is an important variable. As confirmed by inspection of Fick's equation, absorption is inversely proportional to the length of the diffusion path or skin thickness (L). Increased absorption is consequently expected from sites such as the scrotum, face, intertriginous (crease) areas, and scalp, as is reflected in Table 57-3 showing the effect of anatomic region on hydrocortisone absorption. Lower dose and intrinsic potency, along with avoidance of occlusion, is therefore the rule in thinner sites, and the reverse may be more valid in thick cutaneous sites.

Tachyphylaxis (acute tolerance)

Du Vivier has demonstrated tachyphylaxis—a rapid diminution of pharmacologic response with repeated administration of a drug—to topical corticosteroid therapy. The tolerance was demonstrated for antiinflammatory, vasoconstrictive, and antimitotic effects after 6 weeks, and normal actions resumed after a rest period. This raises the possibility that intermittent courses of application may be preferable to continuous applications.

Frequency of application

The optimum frequency of application has not been established. Although tachyphylaxis suggests intermittent application may be preferable, requirements may change with time, particularly as the treated site heals; and with control of a cutaneous disease it is generally felt advisable to use the least amount and lowest concentration necessary for continued healing. Eaglestein et al. (1974) have recorded results with a patient trial using triamcinolone acetonide and concluded six applications a day were no more effective than three. Other data, however, indicate that absorption may increase with long-term administration (at least with hydrocortisone), and there may be more absorption from a single large dose than from the same amount spread out over time.

Type of disease

There are little reliable data to relate the many variables of dose, concentration, frequency of applications, and choice of corticosteroid and vehicle to specific disease entities, although clinical experience is a useful guide. There is perhaps more reliable correlation with comparison of normal versus abnormal skin, because absorption is known to be increased from abraded skin or cutaneous lesions with defective barrier function, particularly where there is loss of stratum corneum.

Occlusion

The variable of occlusion, whether the result of skin folds or extrinsic use of polyethylene wrap, can considerably increase the penetration of topical corticosteroids. The increase has been measured as up to more than tenfold. Occlusion increases hydration of the stratum corneum and local temperature, and may also produce undesired adverse side effects such as *miliaria, folliculitis,* and occasionally cutaneous infection. There is also a greater hazard of local and systemic corticosteroid adverse side effects, particularly with the stronger agents. The incidence of adverse side effects is proportional to the duration of occlusion. One study has shown the persistence of vasoconstriction up to 24 hours after the polyethylene wrap was removed.

Reservoir

A reservoir for applied topical corticosteroid in skin has been demonstrated and the active compound may continue to be released for some time from binding sites in epidermis. The significance of this on optimum frequency of application and other therapy considerations is still uncertain.

Metabolism

Little is known regarding this potential variable. There may be differences in disposal of polar and nonpolar compounds, but the significance in relation to clinical practice is not established.

Vehicle and formulation

Important considerations influencing partition coefficient and overall penetration include:

1. Solubility and stability of the active corticosteroid compound in the vehicle
2. Rate of release of corticosteroid from the vehicle
3. Ability of the vehicle to hydrate the stratum corneum
4. Chemical and physical interactions of vehicle, stratum corneum, and the corticosteroid molecule
5. Influence of additives as penetrants, stabilizers, or therapeutic ingredients

Little clinically applicable data are available regarding the effect on corticosteroid absorption and efficacy of added ingredients such as antibiotics. Additives such as propylene glycol in gels or creams act as accelerants to improve hydration of keratin and increase absorption. Surface-active agents, such as sodium lauryl sulfate, change *partition coefficients* of corticosteroids and tend to produce better release of corticosteroid into target sites in the skin. It has been claimed that ointment bases are more effective than other vehicles in releasing active corticosteroid into applied sites with 10% further spread. However, newer formulations of creams and gels and ingredients such as propylene glycol likely diminish possible differences, and little reliable clinical comparison data of vehicles in specific disease states are available. Generally, lotions are less effective clinically than other more commonly used formulations. Gels are less occlusive than creams or ointments and allow better skin contact. They are comprised of liquids and a gelling agent, and as the gel shears off it leaves the active solution on the skin. They are particularly useful in hairy areas where ointments are generally contraindicated because of the risk of folliculitis.

Cost

In choosing a topical corticosteroid cost may prove a particularly significant factor, and compliance may be affected if costs are too high. Costs may change with time as may comparison prices of different topical corticosteroids. In general, the higher strength preparations tend to be costlier. If a patient requires long-term topical corticosteroid therapy, such as in chronic dermatoses including psoriasis or *atopic dermatitis*, adequate amounts need to be prescribed with refill approval (where not contraindicated) for reliable patients. Dispensing in larger amounts often leads to cost saving with time, particularly in patients with chronic dermatoses.

Cosmetic appearance

This variable cannot be considered lightly because compliance can be a significant problem if the patient dislikes the preparations for cosmetic reasons. Generally, creams have better cosmetic acceptance than ointments since they are easily water washable and often impart a more acceptable sensory sensation to the skin. They are considered less greasy by patients and it is easier to camouflage their use. Gels are considered elegant vehicles with high cosmetic acceptance also, and are often the vehicle of choice in hairy sites. However, they may produce more stinging and burning than creams.

ADVERSE REACTIONS

A wide variety of adverse side effects are possible, and this has led to a continuing search for improved effective preparations to minimize these undesired effects. A vast majority of the adverse reactions result from improper clinical application, and these effects are largely reversible.

Catabolic effects

Atrophy. There may be both epidermal (Figure 57-2) and dermal thinning, and atrophic change can also be manifest as *striae, telangiectasia,* wasting of subcutaneous fat or muscle, bruising or *purpura,* and enhanced fragility, particularly to trauma. The mechanisms of atrophic change are poorly understood, and

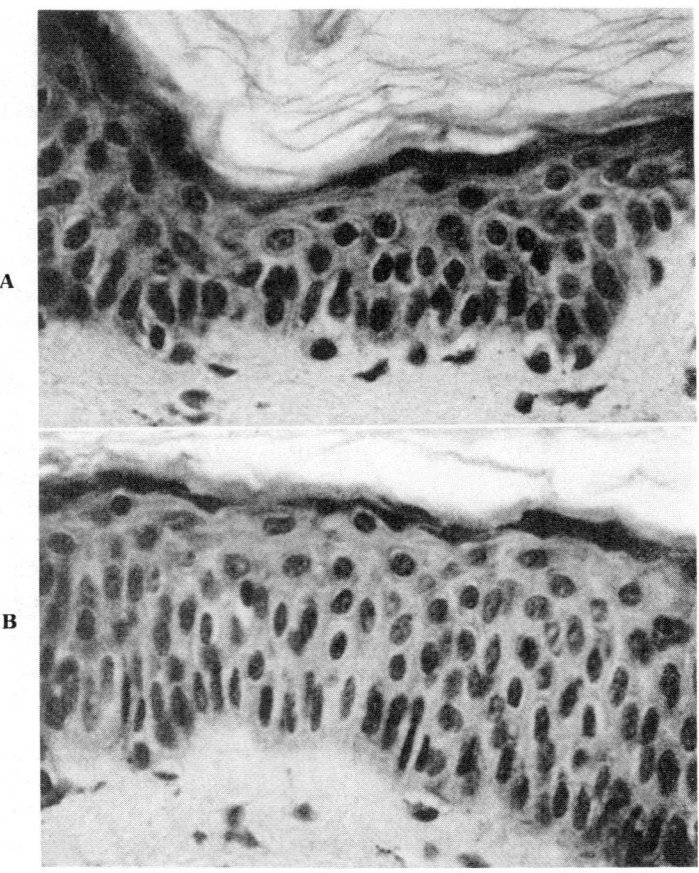

FIGURE 57-2. **Epidermal atrophy.** *A,* **Atrophic (thin) epidermis;** *B,* **normal epidermis.**

there is little precise information on dose—*atrophic* response relationships with various corticosteroid preparations, particularly with long-term use. Many variables may affect the ease of development of atrophic change including skin thickness, the state of the skin barrier, and the effects of occlusion, in addition to the class and concentration of the topical corticosteroid used and the duration of therapy. Atrophic change is most common with potent corticosteroids, especially in crease areas.

The *catabolic* effects are thought to result largely from the antiproliferative and antisynthetic actions of the corticosteroids on both epidermal basal cells and dermal cells, fibers, and tissues. In addition to decreased synthesis by fibroblasts, there may be increased degradation of collagen and ground substance. The loss of tissue support for blood vessels accounts for their increased prominence (telangiectasia) (Figure 57-3) and the bruising tendency (increased fragility). Striae, often more prominent in skin

creases, tend to be more irreversible than other atrophic changes, although the initial red-purple color may fade with time. The atrophic changes are difficult to quantitate, but microscopically there is often thinning of both epidermis and dermis, and the latter shows dilated blood vessels, with separated, small, distorted, collagen fibers, fragmentation, and eventual loss of elastic tissue.

Facial skin eruptions

Steroid rosacea (Figure 57-4). This has become a more frequent complication from improper use of fluorinated topical steroids on the face. It is more common in patients with preexisting *acne rosacea* or with a tendency to ease of blush or flush reactions. However, it is frequently seen in any situation where there is overuse of fluorinated corticosteroids on the face, often for the treatment of initial minor skin conditions such as common acne, rosacea, and seborrheic dermatitis. The eruption may vary from increased *ery-*

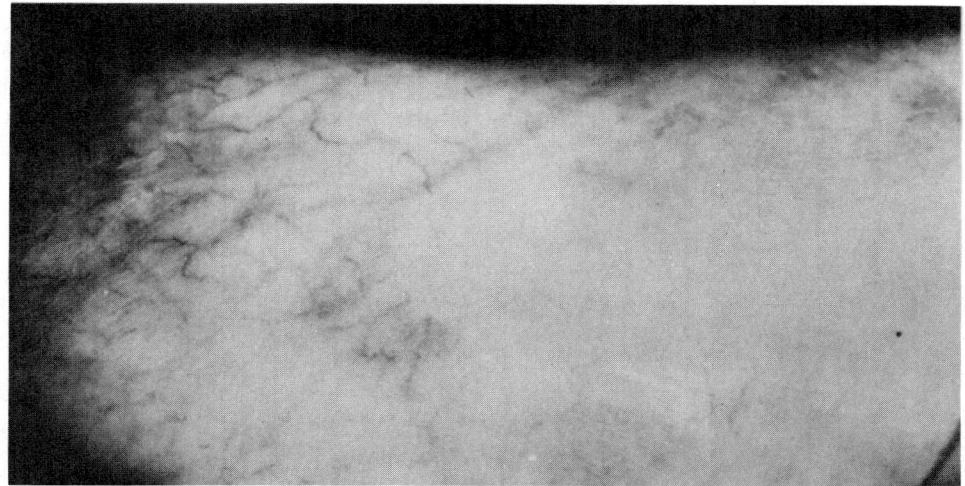

FIGURE 57-3. **Skin atrophy. Thinning, translucence, and telangiectasia prominent.**

thema (redness) to *papulopustular lesions.* It may occur at any age but is more frequently seen in adults. Steroid rosacea may be an example of true "addiction" or rebound effect where patients continue to apply more and more corticosteroid in the misguided belief it will be of increased benefit. A vicious circle may be established as the skin eruption flares on initial discontinuation of the fluorinated corticosteroid preparations and thus the drug is continued, and often in increasing dose.

Perioral dermatitis (Figure 57-5). This erythematous papular facial eruption is more commonly perioral, but may occur at perinasal or other facial sites. Many cases may be examples of steroid rosacea that result from the improper use of topical fluorinated preparations. Perioral dermatitis and corticosteroid rosacea have been increasingly encountered when patients obtain fluorinated corticosteroids from their friends or relatives, or use these agents for other than the prescribed indication. The incidence of true *iatrogenic* disease should be lowered in the future with better awareness of these complications and better patient education. Nonfluorinated topical corticosteroids such as hydrocortisone preparations or desonide appear to be free of these adverse effects.

Modification of local response

Tinea and scabies. The tissue reaction pattern of tinea or scabies may be modified by topical corticosteroids, despite the persistence of the skin infection because of the inhibition of normal tissue response to infection by the antiinflammatory actions of the corticosteroids. Characteristic signs such as the prom-

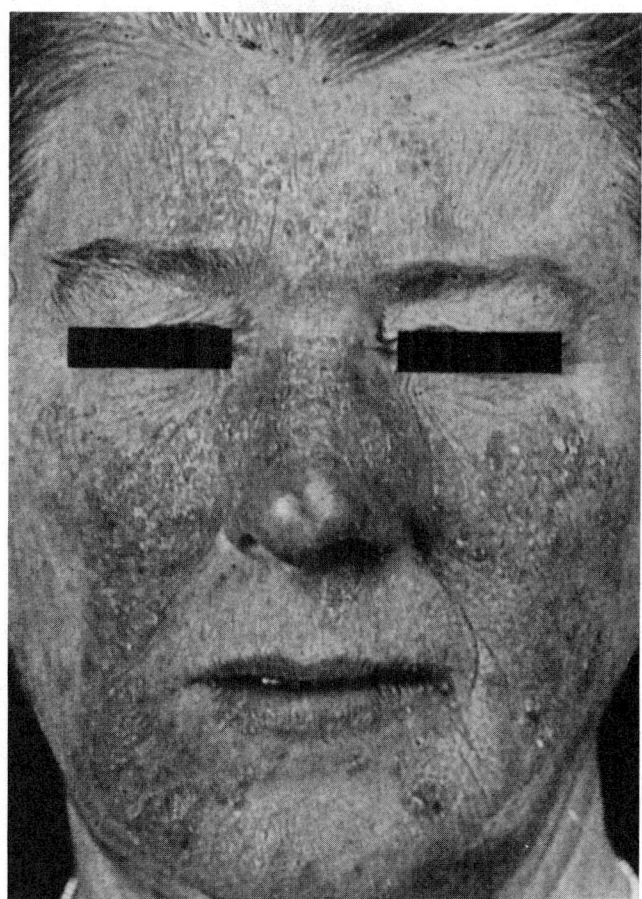

FIGURE 57-4. **Steroid rosacea. Erythema scaling and papulopustular eruption of central face due to misuse of fluorinated topical corticosteroids.**

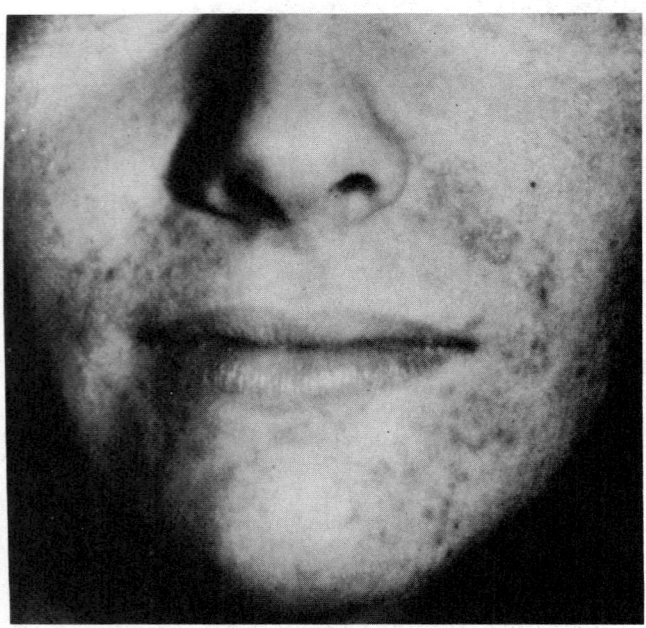

FIGURE 57-5. **Perioral dermatitis. Erythematous papular eruption usually in perioral distribution.**

inent inflammatory border of tinea may be obscured and the diagnosis may therefore be masked and mistaken for a peculiar dermatitis.

Other infections. Indiscriminate use of topical steroids may contribute to floral changes in skin and lead to superinfection or impetigo. In addition to bacterial infections such as with *Staphylococcus aureus,* yeast infections *(Candida)* may also occur. Topical corticosteroids may also aggravate cutaneous or mucosal viral infections such as herpes simplex.

Impairment of wound healing. Topical corticosteroid preparations should not be applied directly to clean or infected wounds since the antiinflammatory and antisynthetic properties may compromise wound healing by directly impairing normal tissue responses of repair and elimination of infection. Normal wound healing is therefore more likely to be delayed and less effective.

Acneiform eruptions or folliculitis. These may result from improper choice of vehicle for the corticosteroid preparation, such as use of ointments in hairy sites. Occlusion, in conjunction with topical application, may also contribute to these reactions. True corticosteroid acne is more commonly seen with oral corticosteroid therapy.

Miscellaneous. Altered pigmentation may be noted at topical corticosteroid treated sites. This can be secondary to postinflammatory effects of the treated skin disease; however, a corticosteroid effect on melanocytes may be operative, and the changes may be more pronounced in atrophic areas. Occasionally fine lanugo hair growth is more prominent in corticosteroid-treated sites.

Ocular effects

Glaucoma and cataracts have been reported particularly after chronic overuse of topical corticosteroids in orbital regions. This may be more common with direct application in the conjunctival sac or cornea. There is a greater risk of glaucoma in genetically predisposed patients or in those with diabetes mellitus and a high degree of myopia. Cataracts are posterior and subcapsular, and children are more susceptible. Topical corticosteroids may also predispose to fungal keratitis, and perforation could result from improper use in the presence of herpes simplex corneal involvement.

Systemic effects

Systemic absorption of topically applied corticosteroids can theoretically lead to *hypothalamic-pituitary-adrenal (HPA) axis* suppression; however, this is not commonly encountered in clinical practice. There have been validated reports of systemic effects particularly with high potency preparations such as clobetasol butyrate, and infrequent reports with other preparations in children or with prolonged use in situations of impaired skin barrier function. The unusual complication may present as Cushing's syndrome with moon facies, truncal obesity and striae, or signs of adrenal failure such as weakness, lethargy, hypotension, and hyperpigmentation. Since small children have a higher surface area to volume ratio with reduced skin and barrier thickness, milder preparations are generally advocated for pediatric dermatoses.

Allergic contact dermatitis

True allergic contact dermatitis is rare to the active topical corticosteroid; however, there may be contact sensitivity to the vehicle or added compounds in some formulations. Clinically this has been most frequent with topical antibiotic or antifungal and corticosteroid combinations such as Mycolog, Kenacomb, and similar products. These contain the known potential sensitizer ethylenediamine as a preservative. Neomycin is also a relatively common allergic sensitizer, particularly in ointment form. Cross reactions may also be seen with structurally related compounds administered topically or systemically. For example, ethylenediamine can cross react with aminophylline, and dermatitis may thus flare during treatment of bronchial asthma. Neomycin may cross react with other antibiotics of the aminoglycoside type. Contact dermatitis to paraben preservatives has also been reported along with *contact urticaria*, and propylene glycol may also be blamed for an allergic contact reaction.

Preparations

A wide variety of active topical corticosteroids in differing formulations are marketed including ointments, creams, gels, lotions, and tapes. Scalp lotions such as Valisone or Synalar are available, and milder corticosteroids such as methylprednisolone in Medrol (with colloidal sulfur and aluminum chlorohydrate) or Neomedrol lotion (with colloidal sulfur, aluminum chlorohydrate and neomycin) are occasionally used in acne therapy. Corticosteroid-coated tapes such as Drenison may also be used in certain clinical situations. Some mucosal preparations are applied in adhesive bases, such as Kenalog in orabase.

Many corticosteroid-antibiotic combination preparations are marketed, such as Neomedrol (methylprednisolone, neomycin), Kenacomb (triamcinolone, neomycin, gramicidin, and nystatin), Valisone G (betamethasone, gentamicin), Locacorten-Vioform (iodochlorhydroxyquin-flumethasone), and Nystaform HC (nystatin, iodochlorhydroxyquin, hydrocortisone). The need for such preparations is often inversely proportional to the reliability of clinical diagnosis, and many combination preparations have a higher potential for causing contact dermatitis.

Formulation may be particularly important; for example, neomycin is a more common sensitizer in ointment form, and additives such as ethylenediamine (in Kenacomb) may be potent allergens. Parabens, commonly used as preservatives, particularly in corticosteroid creams, can also produce allergic contact dermatitis. Many of the variables inherent in the selection of particular formulations have been previously discussed. Dermatologists often select one or two preparations from each category of corticosteroid potency for use in differing clinical situations. The topical corticosteroids are generally prescription drugs; however, topical hydrocortisone 0.5% is available without a prescription in the United States.

Precautions

Adverse side effects are generally avoided if the right preparation and formulation for a particular site and disease state are selected. Particular care is necessary in small children, areas of thin skin, and sites of impaired barrier conditions. In addition, usage is generally limited in the eye region to avoid potential ophthalmic complications. Topical corticosteroids are also usually avoided at sites of cutaneous tuberculosis and fungal or active viral infections such as vaccinia, varicella, herpes zoster, or herpes simplex to prevent local complications such as scarring or perforation and possible dissemination of infection. Fluorinated corticosteroids, which comprise the vast majority of available preparations, are generally to be avoided for routine use on facial skin and minimized in skin crease areas. Compliance may have to be more closely monitored and self-medication without consultation discouraged. This problem has led to common adverse side effects such as corticosteroid rosacea because of the ease of access of these preparations from relatives or friends in addition to unwary nurses and physicians.

Common allergic contact sensitizers are better avoided and replaced by safer effective preparations, and the use of combination products should be minimized. A thorough inquiry regarding application of other topical and systemic drugs may be necessary to avoid hidden sensitizers, such as ethylenediamine or neomycin, and cross-reacting compounds.

SUMMARY

An ever-increasing number of topical corticosteroid preparations are being marketed in an attempt to find preparations with enhanced potency and minimum adverse side effects. The basic principles common to them have been stressed, including structure-activity relationship, mode of action, conditions of clinical use, variables of formulation, and potential adverse side effects.

Few reliable, controlled, clinical comparison studies of the many products are available, and no absolute equivalents have been established to provide more precise dose-response information. The vasoconstrictor potency ranking is a rough guide, but clinical experience, in the face of frequent variables, whether predominantly patient, skin, or drug related, has provided such useful information. Continued research is required.

An understanding of the many possible variables that may influence therapeutic effectiveness is particularly important for patient care. Frequent iatrogenic disorders, such as corticosteroid rosacea from improper use of fluorinated corticosteroids on the face, or contact dermatitis resulting from known common allergic sensitizers in the formulation, should be avoided with a better understanding of the principles of use and knowledge of the ingredients of the various preparations.

ADVERSE/SIDE EFFECTS OF TOPICAL CORTICOSTEROIDS*

ALLERGIC REACTIONS

Allergic contact dermatitis (more common to vehicle ingredients or additives, particularly neomycin and ethylenediamine; occasionally parabens and uncommonly propylene glycol; be aware of cross-reacting compounds, topical or systemic)

Allergic contact urticaria

CUTANEOUS SYSTEM

Acneiform eruptions or folliculitis (more common with improper vehicle or administration such as ointments on hairy sites or with occlusion)

Atrophy (more common with improper use of higher potency fluorinated corticosteroids in areas of thinner skin)

Bacterial impetigo (may predispose or potentiate these infections with indiscriminate use of topical corticosteroids)

Bruising or purpura

Candidiasis (may predispose or potentiate these infections with indiscriminate use of topical corticosteroids)

Fragility

Masking of infections or infestations such as scabies or tinea (tissue reaction may be modified and errors in diagnosis result with improper use of topical corticosteroids)

Perioral dermatitis (extremely common; most often caused by improper use of fluorinated corticosteroids on face)

Pigmentation (may be altered at corticosteroid-treated sites)

Steroid rosacea (extremely common; most often caused by improper use of fluorinated corticosteroids on face)

Striae

Telangiectasia

Viral infections (may predispose or potentiate these infections with indiscriminate use of topical corticosteroids)

Wasting of muscle or subcutaneous fat

METABOLIC AND ENDOCRINE SYSTEMS

Adrenal failure (uncommon reports of increased absorption of more potent topical compounds causing hypothalamic-pituitary-adrenal axis suppression; greater hazard in infants)

Cushing's syndrome (uncommon reports with increased absorption of more potent topical corticosteroids)

OCULAR SYSTEM

Cataracts (posterior and subcapsular; children more susceptible)

Glaucoma (greater risk in diabetic patients, patients with myopia, or in those patients with genetic predisposition)

Keratitis and perforation (fungi or herpesvirus infection)

*See Chapter 11, "Drug Toxicity," for an overview of drug toxicity.

CLINICALLY SIGNIFICANT DRUG INTERACTIONS*

Primary drug	Interacting drug	Possible effect(s)	Probable mechanism(s)
Ethylenediamine (present as stabilizer in some topical corticosteroid creams, such as Kenacomb or Mycolog)	Aminophylline, systemic (combination of theophylline and ethylenediamine bronchodilator) Ethylenediamine-related antihistamines, topical or systemic promethazine (Phenergan) Tripelennamine (Pyribenzamine) Antazoline hydrochloride (Antasan) ophthalmic solution Edetate disodium (EDTA) preservative common in ophthalmic solution	Allergic contact dermatitis Allergic contact urticaria Systemic eczematous contact-type dermatitis	Type IV cellular hypersensitivity reaction Generalized dermatitis from systemic administration of a drug cross-reacting with previous topical sensitizer
Neomycin sulfate (present in several topical corticosteroid antibiotic combination preparations such as Kenacomb and Neosynalar)	Antibiotics, systemic or topical Streptomycin Kanamycin Paromomycin Framycetin Also high coincidental increased sensitivity incidence with bacitracin and gentamicin	Allergic contact dermatitis (more common with ointment form) Allergic contact urticaria Systemic eczematous contact-type dermatitis	Type IV cellular hypersensitivity reaction Generalized dermatitis from systemic administration of a drug cross-reacting with previous topical sensitizer
Parabens (present as preservatives in many topical corticosteroid preparations, particularly creams; Valisone, Aristocort and Lidex are examples of paraben-free creams; most corticosteroid ointments are paraben free)	Paraben-containing products (many cosmetics, hair lotions, suntan preparations, soaps, toothpastes, some adhesives, glues, shoe dressings)	Allergic contact dermatitis Allergic contact urticaria	Type IV cellular hypersensitivity reaction

NOTE: Drug interactions for topical corticosteroids are generally limited to contact allergic sensitivity reactions and cross-reactions through topical or systemic administration of a chemically related compound.

*See Chapter 10, "Drug Interactions," for an overview of drug interactions.

GENERAL NURSING IMPLICATIONS

Nursing of patients requiring topical corticosteroids

ASSESSMENT

Topical corticosteroids are used in the treatment of many skin conditions including pruritus, inflammation (e.g., psoriasis, atopic dermatitis, eczematous dermatitis, seborrheic dermatitis, and contact dermatitis) responsive to topical corticosteroids. Drug therapy is individualized. A complete nursing assessment is important in relation to planning individualized nursing care. Baseline data should include the identification of factors associated with the skin condition with special attention to the appearance and distribution of lesions. Assessment should also include identification of the patient's and family's feelings about the condition. Skin conditions can be distressing to most patients and their families, and assessment of the patient's feelings regarding self-concept including self-esteem and body image cannot be overemphasized.

Assessment should identify factors that are associated with the skin condition (e.g., a history of allergy, emotional tension, or exposure to irritating substance). It should be ascertained if the patient has had the condition before, if he or she is being treated for exacerbation of a chronic condition, or if the patient has been using prescription or nonprescription medications in the treatment of the condition. Self-medication practices should be explored to identify possible effects associated with incorrect application or use. A detailed drug history including other drugs the patient may be taking or has taken should be completed to identify medications that could be associated with the skin condition. The drug history should also include identification of possible sensitivity, contraindications, cautions, and drug interactions before therapy is initiated with topical corticosteroids.

SENSITIVITY

True allergic dermatitis is rare with the use of topical corticosteroids, although contact sensitivity to the base vehicle or to the added compounds present in some formulations (e.g., topical antibiotic or antifungal corticosteroid com-

binations) can occur. It should be noted that any drug has the potential to cause a hypersensitivity reaction in susceptible individuals. Cross-reactions may occur with structurally related compounds.

CONTRAINDICATIONS

The use of topical corticosteroid preparations is contraindicated in patients with known hypersensitivity to a specific or related agent. Topical corticosteroids are contraindicated in active fungal or viral infections or cutaneous tuberculosis.

High-potency corticosteroid products should not be used on infants or children or if the diagnosis is not known. High-potency products should not be used on the face, groin area, or axillas.

See the Nursing Drug Digest for contraindications to specific agents.

CAUTIONS

Topical corticosteroid preparations should be used cautiously on infants and small children because of their proportionately greater body surface area, on patients with skin conditions associated with impaired circulation (e.g., stasis dermatitis), on areas of thin skin (e.g., axillas, groin); and on sites with impaired barrier conditions.

Combination products containing antibiotics or antifungals should be used cautiously and on a limited basis for a short time.

Corticosteroids should be used with caution during pregnancy and with women who are breastfeeding.

Corticosteroid preparations not specifically formulated for ophthalmic use should be used cautiously in the periocular area. Fluorinated corticosteroids should be avoided in routine use on facial skin and minimized in skin crease areas. Combination products should be used minimally.

DRUG INTERACTIONS

Topical corticosteroids can interact with other drugs. These interactions often involve vehicle additives used in the various preparations of topical products (see Clinically Significant Drug Interactions).

ADMINISTRATION

Topical corticosteroids are available in various forms including creams, lotions, ointments, gels, powders, solutions, aerosol sprays, and preparations for specific ophthalmic use. The type of preparation selected depends on the site, the skin condition being treated, and patient preference or cosmetic effect.

Acute tolerance, or tachyphylaxis, can occur with the use of topical corticosteroids. It is recommended that an intermittent course of therapy be used as opposed to continuous treatment for chronic conditions. It has also been found that absorption may increase with long-term treatment. Dosage and administration are highly individualized and should be adjusted to healing of skin areas during the course of treatment if long term. It is generally recommended that the least amount and lowest concentration of medication necessary for healing be used.

Creams evaporate and cool as they dry with an antipruritic effect. They are best used on acute, wet lesions. Ointments hydrate and leave an oily film on the skin as they dry. They are indicated for chronic or dry, scaling skin conditions and cracked rash areas. Solutions should be avoided in the treatment of dry lesions because of their tendency to cause further drying, scaling, or itching. When applied to perineal areas, they may cause burning or stinging.

Ointments may be more effective than creams because of their increased occlusiveness. Creams, because they are washable and less greasy, are more cosmetically accepted by many patients. Gels are less occlusive than creams or ointments and allow better skin contact. Gels containing alcohol evaporate and leave the drug and some gelling agent on the skin. Gels and lotions are especially suited to the scalp and hairy areas. Ointments are contraindicated in hairy areas because of their association with folliculitis. Gels as well as lotions and solutions containing alcohol or a propylene glycol base can cause burning, stinging, or discomfort especially if applied to denuded skin areas or the perineal areas.

GENERAL NURSING IMPLICATIONS—cont'd

Nursing of patients requiring topical corticosteroids—cont'd

Application of topical corticosteroids

Nonocclusive or open technique

Apply medication as directed with ungloved hands using a clean, nonsterile technique unless a sterile technique is specifically indicated. Touching the skin directly communicates acceptance of the patient's condition and allows assessment of the character of the skin areas and the identification of changes in temperature and texture. Hands should be washed thoroughly after application of the medication to prevent absorption. It is important to incorporate patient teaching during application of the medication. The patient or family as indicated should be allowed and encouraged to participate in the application of the medication to enhance understanding of the regimen and self-medication abilities. This is particularly important if the patient or a family member will be applying the medication at home.

Preparation of the skin before application of the medication should be completed first. Treatment baths or soaks may be indicated depending on the individual condition. Skin lesions should be gently washed with nonirritating soap and warm water unless contraindicated. If skin is inflamed, it should be rinsed with warm water only. Normal saline compresses may be used to soften crusts so that they can be removed before application of the medication, or treatment with other solutions (e.g., Burow's solution) may be indicated.

Creams, lotions, solutions, and ointments should be applied in specific amounts as ordered. A small amount of the prescribed medication should be rubbed into the lesion gently, leaving a thin film. When applying lotions to larger areas, firm strokes rather than a dabbing motion should be used, which is less irritating to pruritic skin and provides a thin, even coat. If large areas are to be treated, they should be treated progressively.

Creams and ointments should be applied sparingly to affected areas 2 to 3 times daily or as indicated. The cream should be gently massaged into the area until the medication disappears.

Solutions can be applied by the drop when supplied in plastic squeeze bottles. It should be noted that small quantities are adequate. The solution should be gently rubbed into the affected area. If treatment involves hairy sites, the hair should be parted and the solution dropped onto the affected area to allow direct contact with the lesion.

Aerosols (after shaking as directed) should be sprayed directly toward the affected area from 6 to 12 inches and only for as long as specified (usually 1 to 2 seconds). A watch should be used to time the administration of the specified amount of medication.

Powders should be applied to thoroughly dry skin as directed to minimize caking or crusting. Skin folds should be spread gently to expose the affected area fully during application. The patient's eyes, nose, ears, and mouth should be protected to prevent inhalation or indirect application of medication to these areas when aerosols or powders are applied. Inhalation of the medication should be avoided by the nurse.

Patient privacy should be assured during treatment, and the nurse must be sensitive to the patient's feelings about the condition. Nonverbal and verbal behavior is important in communicating acceptance and understanding of the patient's condition.

Occlusive dressing technique

Occlusive dressings cause increased hydration of the occluded area and increased temperature thus increasing absorption or penetration of the medication. It is important to note that absorption is increased over denuded areas and can cause local as well as systemic adverse side effects.

Occlusive dressings should generally not be applied if there is an elevation in body temperature. Occlusion is rarely necessary with topical corticosteroids.

In treating some cutaneous conditions (e.g., refractory psoriasis, hypertrophic lichen planus, or recalcitrant pustular eruptions on the palms and soles) use of an occlusive dressing may provide additional hydration of the skin and facilitate the therapeutic response to the

topical corticosteroid. The occlusive dressing technique may require modification according to the condition treated and specific formulation.

Generally, the medication is applied to a clean skin surface as prescribed and covered with a light gauze dressing. The dressing is covered with impermeable plastic such as plastic wrap and the edges are sealed with tape or by other means (e.g., stockinette, gauze wrap). The dressing is left in place for 1 to 3 days and the procedure repeated 3 to 4 times as needed. Patient response is usually rapid with improvement seen after 1 to 3 days. Monitoring is essential because folliculitis can occur under the dressing requiring removal of the dressing.

It is also important to monitor for miliaria, cutaneous infection, and increased local and systemic corticosteroid adverse side effects.

Patients receiving occlusive dressing therapy with corticosteroids for prolonged periods should be monitored in addition for hypothalamic-pituitary-adrenal axis suppression with urinary free cortisone and ACTH stimulation tests as well as for Cushing's syndrome, glycosuria, and hyperglycemia.

Points to remember

Before the administration of topical corticosteroids, the following should be noted:

Become familiar with the commonly employed preparations, the available and appropriate vehicles, general guidelines of use, and potential complications.

Avoid compounds known to be more common allergic sensitizers unless ordered by a physician and specifically indicated.

Routinely inquire into prior allergic reactions, and have readily available lists of potential cross-reacting compounds. Ensure that an appropriate notation is readily visible on the chart and bedside.

Check presence or prior use of other topical preparations on the skin.

Routinely check on possible unsuspected use of nonprescribed corticosteroid preparations especially in the presence of skin rash or unusual facial eruption.

Continued.

GENERAL NURSING IMPLICATIONS—cont'd

Nursing of patients requiring topical corticosteroids—cont'd

Points to remember—cont'd

Ensure that more potent preparations are not applied to infants unless specifically indicated and ordered by a physician. Report Cushing's syndrome changes or failure to thrive immediately.

Avoid use of ointments on hairy sites because they may aggravate or cause folliculitis.

Increased absorption of corticosteroid preparations occurs in areas of thin skin including the face, scrotum, and scalp, and intertriginous areas. Generally avoid occlusive dressings in these areas, and generally use lower dose and potency preparations on these sites (see Table 57-3).

Monitor the affected site especially during reapplication of occlusive dressings and during reapplication of medication.

Avoid use of occlusion unless specifically indicated and ordered by the physician. Monitor and report possible complications of occlusion, such as folliculitis.

Observe and report skin rashes; pruritus; atrophic changes of skin, fat, or muscle; purpura; or unusual ocular symptoms or signs.

Report immediately the development or spread of infection, such as suspected impetigo, fungus, yeast, or herpes infections.

Ensure patient understanding of corticosteroid therapy and proper methods of self-medication.

See General Nursing Implications, Monitoring Patient Response.

MONITORING PATIENT RESPONSE

Therapeutic response

Monitor for antiinflammatory effects depending on the indication for topical corticosteroid therapy. Generally, monitor for improvement in skin lesions and a decrease in inflammation, pruritus, swelling, and erythema. It is important to monitor response so that drug therapy can be modified as indicated to enhance continued healing.

Adverse side effects

Adverse side effects associated with the topical corticosteroids are largely the result of improper administration. With correct application and use, adverse effects are rare. However, both local and systemic adverse effects have been associated with the use of topical corticosteroids.

Local

Local irritation, burning, itching, or other discomfort can occur with the application of these medications, and patients should be advised of these effects and monitored carefully. In addition, monitor for:

1. Catabolic effects including atrophy
   a. Epidermal or dermal thinning
   b. Red-purple or silver striae especially in skin creases
   c. Telangiectasia
   d. Wasting of subcutaneous fat or muscle
   e. Enhanced fragility especially to trauma caused by loss of tissue support (bruising, purpura)
2. Facial skin eruptions
   a. Steroid rosacea (increased erythema to papulopustular lesions)
   b. Perioral dermatitis or perinasal dermatitis
3. Modification of local response (infections)
   a. Floral skin changes causing superinfections (bacterial or yeast infections or impetigo)
   b. Impairment of wound healing
   c. Acne eruptions
   d. Folliculitis
4. Miscellaneous adverse effects
   a. Altered pigmentation
   b. Fine lanugo hair growth
   c. Ocular effects (cataracts, glaucoma; occur when drug used in orbital regions or with excessive use of ophthalmic corticosteroid preparations)

Systemic

Systemic effects are rare but can occur with application to impaired skin barrier. Monitor the patient for hypothalamic-pituitary-adrenal axis suppression evidenced by Cushing's syndrome: moon facies, truncal obesity and striae, and adrenal failure (weakness, lethargy, hypotension, hyperpigmentation).

PATIENT EDUCATION

The patient and family as indicated should have a clear understanding of the patient's condition and need for topical corticosteroid therapy. They should have an understanding of the anticipated course of therapy especially if the patient has a chronic condition requiring long-term treatment or treatment as an outpatient. The patient and family should know the exact name of the preparation, its dosage form, concentration, its general action, purpose, method of storage, and adverse side effects. It is particularly important that patients understand how to correctly apply topical corticosteroids and they should also understand that overuse of these preparations may produce toxicity rather than additional therapeutic effect. The patient should understand that topical preparations are for *external* use only, and that overuse can lead to tachyphylaxis.

The patient and family should be able to monitor therapeutic response as well as recognize common and more serious adverse side effects that indicate the health care provider should be notified. Patients should understand the importance of follow-up care as indicated. Although corticosteroid preparations are usually dispensed in small quantities, they can sometimes be dispensed in larger amounts to minimize cost. When this is indicated, it is particularly important that methods of application are carefully explained to the patient to prevent misuse. Proper storage and the importance of not sharing medication with family and friends should also be stressed.

Patient education should also include care of normal skin as well as effects of aging, diet, sun, and other damaging elements as indicated. If the skin condition is caused by or is exacerbated by wool fibers or other allergens, the patient should be encouraged to avoid these. If itching is a problem, patients should be taught to keep their nails short and clean and to avoid scratching to prevent possible scarring or secondary infections. The use of mitts at night, socks, or other restraints may be indicated. Patients should be taught to apply restraints correctly if required.

GENERAL INSTRUCTIONS FOR DISCHARGE/OUTPATIENTS

TOPICAL CORTICOSTEROIDS

This medication is primarily used to treat various skin conditions. If you do not understand why you require this medication, check with your health care provider.

Follow the instructions exactly as prescribed. If in doubt check with your nurse or physician. Do not use this medication for other purposes or new skin rashes.

This medication is for external use only. Avoid contact with the eyes unless you are treating an eye condition with a specific ophthalmic preparation, because this medication has been associated with unwanted effects such as glaucoma. If you inadvertently get this medication in your eyes, rinse out immediately with water.

Apply this medication sparingly in a light coating to affected areas and rub in gently.

Treated areas should not be bandaged, covered, or wrapped with plastic wrap unless specifically prescribed by your health care provider because this can cause unwanted effects.

Avoid diapers or plastic pants on infants if applying this medication as prescribed to an affected diaper area.

Report the development of new skin rashes or changes, itch, eye problems, or failure of therapy to your health care provider.

Do not start or stop taking medications while using this medication without first checking with your health care provider. This medication can cause unwanted effects if taken with other agents.

Familiarize yourself with and avoid possible cross-reacting compounds as provided on the list from your health care provider.

If you are pregnant, thinking about becoming pregnant, or are breastfeeding, do not use this medication until you discuss this with your health care provider. The use of this medication during pregnancy or while nursing infants has not been fully evaluated.

This medication has been prescribed specifically for you. Do not share or give it to relatives or friends. Do not use other people's prescription compounds and do not apply corticosteroid creams to the face unless specifically directed by your health care provider.

Store this medication in a dry place. Check possible outdating period and shelf life times.

Keep this and all medications out of children's reach.

Ensure return appointments with your nurse or physician particularly if you are on long-term therapy. This is important in managing your therapy. If you have any questions about your treatment, discuss these with your health care provider.

NURSING DRUG DIGEST

Medication (trade name*)	Indication	Usual dosage and administration	Dosage forms, preparation, and storage	Contraindications, cautions, and comments	Monitoring
Amcinonide Cyclocort	Antiinflammatory and other topical corticosteroid effects	Topical Applied as directed in thin layer t.i.d. or q.i.d. Amount not quantitated or standardized	Cream: 0.1% Ointment: 0.1%	*Contraindicated* on sites of active viral, fungal, or tuberculous skin lesions Should not be used in the eyes Avoid face or areas of thin skin unless specifically ordered by physician Avoid ointments on hairy sites Ensure patient compliance Be familiar with general guidelines of use and complications of topical corticosteroids Routinely check shelf life, stability, and expiration dates Establish routine check on order renewal for long-term use Report skin atrophy or other complications at earliest sign Routinely check, record, and notify physician of other topical medication in patient's use Be familiar with potential side effects (i.e., maceration, atrophy, miliaria, folliculitis, and [rarely] systemic adrenal axis suppression) of plastic wrap occlusion	

| Beclometha-sone dipro-prionate Propaderm Vanceril | Antiinflammatory and other topical corticosteroid effects (see also Chapter 65, "Corticosteroids and Adrenal Steroid Inhibitors") | Topical Apply as directed in thin layer t.i.d. or q.i.d. Amount not quantitated or standardized | Cream, ointment, and lotion: 0.025% Also available as Propaderm-C cream and ointment containing 3% iodochlor-hydroxyquin | *Contraindicated* on sites of active viral, fungal or tuberculous skin lesions Should not be used in the eyes Avoid face or areas of thin skin unless specifically ordered by physician Avoid ointments on hairy sites Be familiar with general guidelines of use and complications of topical corticosteroids Routinely check shelf life, stability, and expiration dates Establish routine check on order renewal for long-term use Report skin atrophy or other complications at earliest sign Routinely check, record, and notify physician of other topical medication in patient's use Be familiar with potential side effects (i.e., maceration, atrophy, miliaria, folliculitis, and [rarely] systemic adrenal axis suppression) of plastic wrap occlusion |

NOTE: For additional details regarding the individual agents listed in this table see the text and other tables in this chapter.
*Indicates a multiple active ingredient product. For a complete listing of all active ingredients see the *Drug Reference Guide to Brand Names and Active Ingredients.*
★Indicates that the drug is generally available only in the United States.

Continued.

NURSING DRUG DIGEST—cont'd

Medication (trade name)	Indication	Usual dosage and administration	Dosage forms, preparation, and storage	Contraindications, cautions, and comments	Monitoring
Betamethasone dipropionate Diprosone	Antiinflammatory and other topical corticosteroid effects	Topical Apply as directed in thin layer t.i.d. or q.i.d. Amount not quantitated or standardized	Cream, ointment, and lotion: 0.64 mg/gm equivalent to betamethasone alcohol 0.5 mg (0.05%) Aerosol: 0.1%	*Contraindicated* on sites of active viral, fungal, or tuberculous skin lesions	Should not be used in the eyes

Should not be used in the eyes

Avoid face or areas of thin skin unless specifically ordered by clinician

Avoid ointments on hairy sites

Be familiar with general guidelines of use and complications of topical corticosteroids

Routinely check shelf life, stability, and expiration dates

Establish routine check on order renewal for long-term use

Ensure patient compliance

Report skin atrophy and other complications at earliest sign

Routinely check, record, and notify physician of other topical medication in patient's use

Be familiar with potential side effects (i.e., maceration, atrophy, miliaria, folliculitis, and [rarely] systemic adrenal axis suppression) of plastic wrap occlusion

| Betamethasone valerate Betnovate Celestoderm Celestoderm-V Celestone Valisone Valisone Scalp Lotion | Antiinflammatory and other topical corticosteroid effects | Topical Apply as directed in thin layer t.i.d. or q.i.d. Amount not quantitated or standardized | Creams and ointments: regular 0.1% or ½ strength 0.05% concentrations Lotions: 0.1% or 0.05% Valisone scalp lotion: 1.22 mg/ml betamethasone valerate (equivalent to 1 mg betamethasone) Celestoderm V: 1.22 mg/gm of betamethasone valerate (equivalent to 1 mg of betamethasone) Celestoderm V/2: 0.61 mg/ gm betamethasone valerate (equivalent to 0.5 mg betamethasone) | *Contraindicated* on sites of active viral, fungal, or tuberculous skin lesions Should not be used in the eyes Avoid face or areas of thin skin unless specifically ordered by physician Avoid ointments on hairy sites Be familiar with general guidelines of use and complications of topical corticosteroids Routinely check shelf life, stability, and expiration dates Establish routine check on order renewal for long-term use Ensure patient compliance Report skin atrophy or other complications at earliest sign Routinely check, record, and notify physician of other topical medication in patient's use Be familiar with potential side effects (i.e., maceration, atrophy, miliaria, folliculitis, and [rarely] systemic adrenal axis suppression) of plastic wrap occlusion |

Continued.

NURSING DRUG DIGEST—cont'd

Medication (trade name)	Indication	Usual dosage and administration	Dosage forms, preparation, and storage	Contraindications, cautions, and comments	Monitoring
Betamethasone valerate and gentamicin sulfate Valisone-G	Antiinflammatory and other topical corticosteroid effects with antibacterial combination	Topical Apply as directed in thin layer t.i.d. or q.i.d. Amount not quantitated or standardized	Cream, ointment: each gram contains 1.22 mg betamethasone valerate (equivalent to 1 mg betamethasone), and 1.67 mg gentamicin sulfate (equivalent to 1 mg gentamicin)	*Contraindicated* on sites of active viral, fungal, or tuberculous skin lesions. Should not be used in the eyes. Avoid face or areas of thin skin unless specifically ordered by physician. Avoid ointments on hairy sites. Be familiar with general guidelines of use and complications of topical corticosteroids. Routinely check shelf life, stability and expiration dates. Establish routine check on order renewal for long-term use. Report skin atrophy and other complications at earliest sign. Routinely check, record, and notify physician of other topical medication in patient's use. Be familiar with potential side effects (i.e., maceration, atrophy, miliaria, folliculitis, and [rarely] systemic adrenal axis suppression) of plastic wrap occlusion	

| Clobetasol Dermovate | Antiinflammatory and other topical corticosteroid effects | Topical Apply as directed in thin layer t.i.d. or q.i.d. Amount not quantitated or standardized Normally avoided in infants *Not* ordinarily used under tape occlusion Total dose applied weekly should not exceed 50 gm Usually used for limited time; not long-term use | Cream or ointment: 0.05% Store at room temperature | *Contraindicated* on sites of active viral, fungal, or tuberculous skin lesions Should not be used in the eyes Avoid face or areas of thin skin Avoid ointments on hairy sites Extremely potent topical steroid Some reports of absorption with adrenal suppression Ensure patient compliance Be familiar with general guidelines of use and complications of topical corticosteroids Routinely check shelf life, stability, and expiration dates Establish routine check on order renewal for long-term use Report local or systemic signs of adverse effects immediately |

Continued.

NURSING DRUG DIGEST—cont'd

Medication (trade name)	Indication	Usual dosage and administration	Dosage forms, preparation, and storage	Contraindications, cautions, and comments	Monitoring
Clobetasone Eumovate	Antiinflammatory and other topical corticosteroid effects	Topical Apply as directed in thin layer t.i.d. or q.i.d. Amount not quantitated or standardized	Cream or ointment: 0.05%	*Contraindicated* on sites of active viral, fungal, or tuberculous skin lesions Should not be used in the eyes Avoid face or areas of thin skin unless specifically ordered by physician Avoid ointments on hairy sites Be familiar with general guidelines of use and complications of topical corticosteroids Routinely check shelf life, stability, and expiration dates Establish routine check on order renewal for long-term use Report skin atrophy and other complications at earliest sign Routinely check, record, and notify physician of other topical medication in patient's use Be familiar with potential side effects (i.e., maceration, atrophy, miliaria, folliculitis, and [rarely] systemic adrenal axis suppression) of plastic wrap occlusion	
Clocortolone Cloderm	Corticosteroid-responsive dermatoses	*Adults:* Apply a small amount to affected area b.i.d. to t.i.d.	Cream: 0.1%	*Contraindicated* in bacterial, fungal, and viral skin infections	Observe skin for atrophy or local irritation

		Children: Same as adults For *topical* use only *Not* for ophthalmic use	*Contraindicated* in hypersensitivity to the active ingredient or to any of the components of the vehicle May cause local skin reactions such as dryness, itching, folliculitis, and striae Avoid contact with eyes	Observe for signs of infection Observe for systemic corticosteroid effects with prolonged chronic use and when used with an occlusive dressing
Desonide Tridesilon	Antiinflammatory and other topical corticosteroid effects Acne rosacea and seborrheic dermatitis	Topical Apply as directed in thin layer t.i.d. or q.i.d. Amount not quantitated or standardized	Cream and ointment: 0.05%	*Contraindicated* on sites of active viral, fungal, or tuberculous skin lesions Should not be used in the eyes Avoid face or areas of thin skin unless specifically ordered by physician Avoid ointments on hairy sites Can be used in crease areas and face with less risk of corticosteroid side effects Be familiar with general guidelines of use and complications of topical corticosteroids Routinely check shelf life, stability, and expiration dates Establish routine check on order renewal for long-term use Report skin atrophy and other complications at earliest sign Routinely check, record, and notify physician of other topical medication in patient's use Be familiar with potential side effects (i.e., maceration, atrophy, miliaria, folliculitis, and [rarely] systemic adrenal axis suppression) of plastic wrap occlusion

Continued.

NURSING DRUG DIGEST—cont'd

Medication (trade name)	Indication	Usual dosage and administration	Dosage forms, preparation, and storage	Contraindications, cautions, and comments	Monitoring
Desoximetasone Aubason Topicort Topisolon	Antiinflammatory and other topical corticosteroid effects	Topical Apply as directed in thin layer t.i.d. or q.i.d. Amount not quantitated or standardized	Cream: 0.05%, 0.25% Gel: 0.05%	*Contraindicated* on sites of active viral, fungal, or tuberculous skin lesions Should not be used in the eyes Avoid face or areas of thin skin Avoid ointments on hairy sites Be familiar with general guidelines of use and complications of topical corticosteroids Routinely check shelf life, stability, and expiration dates Establish routine check on order renewal for long-term use Report skin atrophy and other complications at earliest sign Routinely check, record, and notify physician of other topical medication in patient's use Be familiar with potential side effects (i.e., maceration, atrophy, miliaria, folliculitis, and [rarely] systemic adrenal axis suppression) of plastic wrap occlusion	

Drug	Action	Administration	Dosage Forms	Contraindications/Cautions	Nursing Considerations
Dexamethasone Aeroseb-Dex Decaspray	Antiinflammatory and other topical corticosteroid effects (see also Chapter 65, "Corticosteroids and Adrenal Steroid Inhibitors")	Topical Spray affected area from approximately 6 inches above the surface for 1-3 seconds, t.i.d. or q.i.d. as indicated	Aerosol spray: 0.01%	*Contraindicated* in hypersensitivity *Contraindicated* in active viral, fungal, or tuberculous skin lesions Avoid spraying in eyes or nose Do *not* apply to perforated eardrum Can be applied to hairy areas with aerosol spray	Monitor for local irritation Observe for signs of local infection
Diflorasone Florone Flutone Maxiflor	Antiinflammatory and other topical corticosteroid effects	Topical Apply a small amount to affected skin area, q.d. to q.i.d. as indicated	Cream: 0.05% Ointment: 0.05% Store between 15° and 30° C	*Contraindicated* in hypersensitivity *Contraindicated* in active viral, fungal, or tuberculous skin lesions *Not* for ophthalmic use Use with caution on lesions close to eyes Use with caution in patients with stasis dermatitis	Monitor for local irritation
Flumethasone Locacorten	Antiinflammatory or other topical corticosteroid effects	Topical Apply a small amount to affected skin area q.d. to t.i.d. as indicated	Cream: 0.03% Ointment: 0.03% Store between 15° and 30° C	*Contraindicated* in hypersensitivity *Contraindicated* in active viral, fungal, or tuberculous skin lesions Do *not* apply to the conjunctiva Use with caution on lesions close to the eyes	Monitor for local irritation

Continued.

NURSING DRUG DIGEST—cont'd

Medication (trade name)	Indication	Usual dosage and administration	Dosage forms, preparation, and storage	Contraindications, cautions, and comments	Monitoring
Flumethasone, iodochlorhydroxyquin Locacorten- Vioform	Topical corticosteroid with antifungal, antibacterial combination	Topical Apply as directed in thin layer t.i.d. or q.i.d. Amount not quantitated or standardized	Cream and ointment: flumethasone 0.02% and iodochlorhydroxyquin 3%	*Contraindicated* on sites of active viral, fungal, or tuberculous skin lesions Should not be used in the eyes Avoid face or areas of thin skin Avoid ointments on hairy sites May cause contact irritation occasionally Rarely causes allergic contact dermatitis Be familiar with general guidelines of use and complications of topical corticosteroids Routinely check shelf life, stability and expiration dates Establish routine check on order renewal for long-term use Report skin atrophy and other complications at earliest sign Routinely check, record, and notify physician of other topical medication in patient's use Be familiar with potential side effects (i.e., maceration, atrophy, miliaria, folliculitis, and [rarely] systemic adrenal axis suppression) of plastic wrap occlusion	

| **Fluocinolone** Dermalar Fluocin Cream Fluoderm Fluonid Neo-Synalar* Synadone Synalar Synalar-HP Synamol Viaderm-F.A. | Antiinflammatory and other topical corticosteroid effects | Topical Apply as directed in thin layer t.i.d. or q.i.d. Amount not quantitated or standardized | Cream (ointment, or solution): 0.025% (regular) or 0.01% (mild) Cream: 0.2% (high-potency) Solution: 0.01% | *Contraindicated* on sites of active viral, fungal, or tuberculous skin lesions Should not be used in the eyes Avoid face or areas of thin skin Avoid ointments on hairy sites Be familiar with general guidelines of use and complications of topical corticosteroids Routinely check shelf life, stability, and expiration dates Establish routine check on order renewal for long-term use Report skin atrophy and other complications at earliest sign Routinely check, record, and notify physician of other topical medication in patient's use Be familiar with potential side effects (i.e., maceration, atrophy, miliaria, folliculitis, and [rarely] systemic adrenal axis suppression) of plastic wrap occlusion |

Continued.

NURSING DRUG DIGEST—cont'd

Medication (trade name)	Indication	Usual dosage and administration	Dosage forms, preparation, and storage	Contraindications, cautions, and comments	Monitoring
Fluocinonide Lidemol Lidex Lyderm Metosyn Topsyn Gel	Antiinflammatory and other topical corticosteroid effects	Topical Apply as directed in thin layer t.i.d. or q.i.d. Amount not quantitated or standardized	Cream or ointment: 0.01% 0.05% Gel: 0.05% Solution: 0.05%	*Contraindicated* on sites of active viral, fungal, or tuberculous skin lesions Should not be used in the eyes Avoid face or areas of thin skin Avoid ointments on hairy sites Gel form permits increased ease of application on hairy areas such as the scalp Be familiar with general guidelines of use and complications of topical corticosteroids Routinely check shelf life, stability, and expiration dates Establish routine check on order renewal for long-term use Report skin atrophy and other complications at earliest sign Routinely check, record, and notify physician of other topical medication in patient's use Be familiar with potential side effects (i.e., maceration, atrophy, miliaria, folliculitis, and [rarely] systemic adrenal axis suppression) of plastic wrap occlusion	

Fluorometholone FML Liquifilm Oxylone	Antiinflammatory or other topical corticosteroid effects	Topical Apply a small amount to affected skin area q.d. to t.i.d. as indicated	Cream: 0.025% Ophthalmic suspension: 0.1%	*Contraindicated* in hypersensitivity *Contraindicated* in active viral, fungal, or tuberculous skin lesions Use cream with caution on lesions close to the eyes Use care when applying ophthalmic suspension to avoid contamination	Monitor for local irritation
Flurandrenolide Cordran Dreniform* Drenison Drocort Haldrone-F	Antiinflammatory and other topical corticosteroid effects	Topical Apply as directed in thin layer t.i.d. or q.i.d. Amount not quantitated or standardized Tape may be left in place up to 24 hr if good adherence and no irritation or complications occur	Cream: 0.0125%, 0.025%, 0.05% Ointments: 0.0125%, 0.025%, 0.05% Tape: flexible, elastic transparent tape made of thin matte-finish polyethylene film containing 4 μg/cm² uniformly distributed in the adhesive layer of synthetic copolymer of acrylate ester and acrylic acid; adhesive surface is covered by the protective paper liner to permit handling and trimming before application Lotion: 0.05%	*Contraindicated* on sites of active viral, fungal, or tuberculous skin lesions Should not be used in the eyes Avoid face or areas of thin skin Avoid ointments on hairy sites Be familiar with general guidelines of use and complications of topical corticosteroids Routinely check shelf life, stability, and expiration dates Establish routine check on order renewal for long-term use Report skin atrophy and other complications at earliest sign Routinely check, record, and notify physician of other topical medication in patient's use Be familiar with potential side effects (i.e., maceration, atrophy, miliaria, folliculitis, and rarely systemic adrenal axis suppression) of plastic wrap occlusion	

Continued.

NURSING DRUG DIGEST—cont'd

Medication (trade name)	Indication	Usual dosage and administration	Dosage forms, preparation, and storage	Contraindications, cautions, and comments	Monitoring
Halcinonide Halog	Antiinflammatory and other topical corticosteroid effects	Topical Apply as directed in thin layer t.i.d. or q.i.d. Amount not quantitated or standardized	Cream: 0.025%, 0.1% Ointment: 0.025%, 0.1% Solution: 0.1%	*Contraindicated* on sites of active viral, fungal, or tubercular skin lesions Should not be used in the eyes Avoid face or areas of thin skin Avoid ointments on hairy sites Be familiar with general guidelines of use and complications of topical corticosteroids Routinely check shelf life, stability, and expiration dates Establish routine check on order renewal for long-term use Report skin atrophy and other complications at earliest sign Routinely check, record, and notify physician of other topical medication in patient's use Be familiar with potential side effects (i.e., maceration, atrophy, miliaria, folliculitis, and [rarely] systemic adrenal axis suppression) of plastic wrap occlusion	

Drug	Uses	Administration	Preparations/Strengths	Nursing Implications
Hydrocortisone Aeroseb-HC Alphaderm Barseb-HC Cortaid Cortamed Cort-Dome Cortef Cortenema Corticreme Cortisporin Cream* Cortisporin Ointment* Cortisporin Otic Suspension* Cortispray Cortril Derma Medicone-HC Ointment* Dermacort Eldecort Heb-Cort Hydro-Cortilean Hydrocortone Hytone Iodocort Cream* Komed HC Lanacort Microcort Neo-Cort-Dome* Rectacort Texacort Unicort Westcort	Antiinflammatory and other topical corticosteroid effects Acne rosacea and seborrheic dermatitis	Topical Apply as directed in thin layer t.i.d. or q.i.d. Amount not quantitated or standardized	Usually compounded in cream form often in emollient base Cream: 0.125%, 0.25%, 0.5%, 1%, 2.5% Ointment: 0.2%, 0.5%, 1%, 2.5% Lotion: 0.125%, 0.25%, 0.5% 1%, 2.5% Gel: 1% Aerosol: 0.5%, 1%	Extremely rare to cause local or systemic corticosteroid side effects Can be used in crease areas and face with safety Be familiar with general guidelines of use and complications of topical corticosteroids Routinely check shelf life, stability, and expiration dates Establish routine check on order renewal for long-term use Report skin atrophy and other complications at earliest sign Routinely check, record, and notify physician of other topical medication in patient's use Be familiar with potential side effects (i.e., maceration, atrophy, miliaria, folliculitis, and [rarely] systemic adrenal axis suppression) of plastic wrap occlusion

Continued.

NURSING DRUG DIGEST—cont'd

Medication (trade name)	Indication	Usual dosage and administration	Dosage forms, preparation, and storage	Contraindications, cautions, and comments	Monitoring
Hydrocortisone, iodochlorhydroxyquin Vioform-Hydrocortisone	Antiinflammatory and other topical corticosteroid effects with antibacterial combination	Topical Apply as directed in thin layer t.i.d. or q.i.d. Amount not quantitated or standardized	Cream and ointment: hydrocortisone, 1% (regular) or hydrocortisone, 0.5% (mild) and iodochlorhydroxyquin 3%	May cause contact irritation occasionally Rarely causes allergic contact dermatitis Iodochlorhydroxyquin may cause yellow staining of skin or fabrics Extremely rare to cause topical or systemic corticosteroid complications Be familiar with general guidelines of use and complications of topical corticosteroids Routinely check shelf life, stability, and expiration dates Establish routine check on order renewal for long-term use Report skin atrophy and other complications at earliest sign Routinely check, record, and notify physician of other topical medication in patient's use Be familiar with potential side effects (i.e., maceration, atrophy, miliaria, folliculitis, and [rarely] systemic adrenal axis suppression) of plastic wrap occlusion	

Hydrocortisone, nystatin, iodochlorhydroxyquin Nystaform-HC	Topical corticosteroid with antifungal or anticandidal combination	Topical Apply as directed in thin layer t.i.d. or q.i.d. Amount not quantitated or standardized	Cream, lotion: hydrocortisone, 0.5%; nystatin, 100,000 units/gm; iodochlorhydroxyquin, 3%	May cause occasional allergic contact dermatitis Extremely rare to cause topical or systemic corticosteroid complications May cause yellow staining of skin or fabric from iodochlorhydroxyquin Be familiar with general guidelines of use and complications of topical corticosteroids Routinely check shelf life, stability, and expiration dates Establish routine check on order renewal for long-term use Report skin atrophy and other complications at earliest sign Routinely check, record, and notify physician of other topical medication in patient's use Be familiar with potential side effects (i.e., maceration, atrophy, miliaria, folliculitis, and [rarely] systemic adrenal axis suppression) of plastic wrap occlusion

Continued.

NURSING DRUG DIGEST—cont'd

Medication (trade name)	Indication	Usual dosage and administration	Dosage forms, preparation, and storage	Contraindications, cautions, and comments	Monitoring
Methylprednisolone Medrol	Antiinflammatory and other topical corticosteroid effects (see also Chapter 65, "Corticosteroids and Adrenal Steroid Inhibitors")	Topical Apply as directed in thin layer t.i.d. or q.i.d. Amount not quantitated or standardized	Ointment: 0.25%, 1%	*Contraindicated* on sites of active viral, fungal, or tuberculous skin lesions Should not be used in the eyes Avoid face or areas of thin skin unless specifically ordered by physician Avoid ointments on hairy sites May cause occasional allergic contact dermatitis to methyl paraben preservative Be familiar with general guidelines of use and complications of topical corticosteroids Routinely check shelf life, stability, and expiration dates Establish routine check on order renewal for long-term use Report signs of skin atrophy and record and notify physician of other topical medication in patient's use Be familiar with potential side effects (i.e., maceration, atrophy, miliaria, folliculitis, and [rarely] systemic adrenal axis suppression) of plastic wrap occlusion	

Methylpred-nisolone, neomycin Neomedrol	Topical corticosteroid with antibiotic combination	Ointment: each gm contains methylprednisolone, 2.5 mg (0.25%); neomycin sulfate, 5 mg (equivalent to 3.5 mg neomycin base)	Topical Apply as directed in thin layer t.i.d. or q.i.d. Amount not quantitated or standardized	*Contraindicated* on sites of active viral, fungal, or tuberculous skin lesions
				Should not be used in the eyes
				Avoid face or areas of thin skin
				Avoid ointments on hairy sites
				May cause allergic contact dermatitis
				Possible neomycin cross sensitivities must be considered
				Be familiar with general guidelines of use and complications of topical corticosteroids
				Routinely check shelf life, stability, and expiration dates
				Establish routine check on order renewal for long-term use
				Report signs of skin atrophy and record and notify physician of other topical medication in patient's use
				Be familiar with potential side effects (i.e., maceration, atrophy, miliaria, folliculitis, and [rarely] systemic adrenal axis suppression) of plastic wrap occlusion

Continued.

NURSING DRUG DIGEST—cont'd

Medication (trade name)	Indication	Usual dosage and administration	Dosage forms, preparation, and storage	Contraindications, cautions, and comments	Monitoring
Methylprednisolone, neomycin, aluminum chlorohydrate Neomedrol Acne Lotion	Acne therapy Occasionally used for seborrheic dermatitis or acne rosacea	Topical application usually q.d. to face, chest, or back Amount not standardized but thin layer advised	Lotion: each ml contains methylprednisolone, 2.5 mg; neomycin, 2.5 mg; aluminum chlorohydrate, 100 mg	Will have drying action Can cause excessive dryness or irritation with excess amount Allergy to neomycin in this formulation unlikely Topical or systemic corticosteroid complications unlikely Be familiar with general guidelines of use and complications of topical corticosteroids Routinely check shelf life, stability, and expiration dates Establish routine check on order renewal for long-term use Report skin atrophy and other complications at earliest sign Routinely check, record, and notify physician of other topical medication in patient's use Be familiar with potential side effects (i.e., maceration, atrophy, miliaria, folliculitis, and [rarely] systemic adrenal axis suppression) of plastic wrap occlusion	

Methylpred-nisolone, alu-minum chlo-rohydrate Medrol Acne Lotion	Acne therapy Occasionally used for seborrheic dermatitis and acne rosacea	Topical application usually once a day to face, chest, or back Skin usually washed or moist-ened before application	Lotion: each ml contains methylprednisolone, 2.5 mg; sulfur, 50 mg; and aluminum chlorohydrate, 100 mg	Will normally have drying effect May cause excessive dryness or irritation with excess use Topical or systemic cor-ticosteroid complica-tions are unlikely Be familiar with general guidelines of use and complications of topi-cal corticosteroids Routinely check shelf life, stability, and expi-ration dates Establish routine check on order renewal for long-term use Report skin atrophy and other complications at earliest sign Routinely check, record, and notify physician of other topical medi-cation in patient's use Be familiar with poten-tial side effects (i.e., maceration, atrophy, miliaria, folliculitis, and [rarely] systemic adrenal axis suppres-sion) of plastic wrap occlusion
Prednisolone Inflamase Inflamase Forte Meti-Derm Pred Forte Pred Mild	Antiinflammatory and other corti-costeroid effects (see also Chap-ter 65, "Cortico-steroids and Adrenal Steroid Inhibitors")	Instill 1-2 drops in affected eye q.d. to q.i.d. as indicated Solution for *ophthalmic use only* Apply a small amount of cream to affected area t.i.d. to q.i.d.	Solution, ophthalmic: 0.1, 1% Cream: 0.5% Store between 15° and 30° C Protect from light	*Contraindicated* in hy-persensitivity *Contraindicated* in ac-tive viral or fungal in-fections Use care when applying topical ophthalmic so-lution to avoid con-tamination Use cream with caution on lesions close to eyes Observe for corneal ul-ceration Monitor for glaucoma Monitor for local irrita-tion

Continued.

NURSING DRUG DIGEST—cont'd

Medication (trade name)	Indication	Usual dosage and administration	Dosage forms, preparation, and storage	Contraindications, cautions, and comments	Monitoring
Triamcinolone acetonide Aristocort Aristoderm Aristogel Flutone Kenalog Kenalog E Tramacin	Antiinflammatory and other topical corticosteroid effects (see Chapter 65, "Corticosteroids and Adrenal Steroid Inhibitors")	Topical Apply as directed in thin layer t.i.d. or q.i.d. Amount not quantitated or standardized	Creams or ointment: 0.025% (dilute), 0.1% (regular), 0.5% Lotion: 0.025%, 0.1%	*Contraindicated* on sites of active viral, fungal, or tuberculous skin lesions Should not be used in the eyes Avoid face or areas of thin skin Avoid ointments on hairy sites Be familiar with general guidelines of use and complications of topical corticosteroids Routinely check shelf life, stability, and expiration dates Establish routine check on order renewal for long-term use Report skin atrophy or other complications at earliest sign Routinely check, record, and notify physician of other topical medications in patient's use Be familiar with potential side effects (i.e., maceration, atrophy, miliaria, folliculitis, and [rarely] systemic adrenal axis suppression) of plastic wrap occlusion Ensure patient compliance	
Triamcinolone acetonide in orabase Kenalog in Orabase	Oral mucosal or dental topical corticosteroid	Adhesive paste Apply by pressing a small dab (approx ¼ inch) to the affected area until a thin film develops May need larger quantity for some lesions Amount and frequency not standardized	0.1% in Orabase, a protective emollient vehicle containing gelatin, pectin and sodium carboxymethyl cellulose in Plastibase (plasticized hydrocarbon gel)	Restrict to oral mucosal use Oral candidiasis may be a complication Review use routinely with prescriber after 1-2 weeks	

| **Triamcinolone acetonide, neomycin, gramicidin, nystatin** Kenacomb Mycolog Myco Triacet Nysolone Tricilone NNG | Antiinflammatory and other topical corticosteroid effects | Topical Apply as directed in thin layer t.i.d. or q.i.d. Amount not quantitated or standardized | Cream and ointment: each gm contains triamcinolone acetonide, 1 mg (0.1%); neomycin, 2.5 mg; gramicidin, 0.25 mg; nystatin, 100,000 units | *Contraindicated* in hypersensitivity to any of the components *Contraindicated* on sites of active viral, fungal, or tuberculous skin lesions Should not be used in the eyes Avoid face or areas of thin skin unless specifically ordered by physician Avoid ointments on hairy sites *Allergic contact dermatitis* may be main complication; may cross-react with aminophylline, neomycin, and other aminoglycoside agents given topically or systemically Best to avoid for routine use Be familiar with general guidelines of use and complications of topical corticosteroids Routinely check shelf life, stability, and expiration dates Establish routine check on order renewal for long-term use Report skin atrophy and other complications at earliest sign Routinely check, record, and notify physician of other topical medication in patient's use Be familiar with potential side effects (i.e., maceration, atrophy, miliaria, folliculitis, and [rarely] systemic adrenal axis suppression) of plastic wrap occlusion Be aware of allergy risk and potential cross reactions |

BIBLIOGRAPHY

Anders, J.E. Topicals—a welter of options calls for refined application techniques. *RN*, 1982, *45*(9), 33-42.

Arnold, V. & Rose, S. Photochemotherapy for psoriasis. *American Journal of Nursing*, 1979, *79*(3), 466-468.

Axelrod, L. Glucocorticoid therapy. *Medicine*, 1976, *55*(1), 39-65.

Ayres, P.J.W., & Hooper, G. Assessment of the skin penetration properties of different carrier vehicles for topically applied cortisol. *British Journal of Dermatology*, 1978, *99*(3), 307-317.

Du Vivier, A. Tachyphylaxis to topically applied steroids. *Archives of Dermatology*, 1976, *112*(9), 1245-1248.

Du Vivier, A., Marshall, R.C., & Brookes, L.G. An animal model for evaluating the local and systemic effects of topically applied corticosteroids on epidermal DNA synthesis. *British Journal of Dermatology*, 1978, *98*, 209.

Dykes, P.J., & Marks, R. An appraisal of the methods used in the assessment of atrophy from topical corticosteroids. *British Journal of Dermatology*, 1979, *101*, 599-609.

Eaglestein, W.H., Farzad, A., & Capland, L. Topical corticosteroid therapy: efficacy of frequent application. *Archives of Dermatology*, 1974, *110*, 955.

Henry, J.C., Tschen, E.H., and Becker, L.E. Contact urticaria to parabens. *Archives of Dermatology*, 1979, *115*(10), 1231-1232.

Howell, J.B. Editorial: Eye diseases induced by topically applied steroids. *Archives of Dermatology*, 1976, *112*, 1529-1530.

Kligman, A.M., & Frosch, P.J. Steroid addiction. *International Journal of Dermatology*, 1979, *18*(1), 23-31.

McKenzie, A.W., & Stoughton, R.G. A method for comparing the percutaneous absorption of steroids. *Archives of Dermatology*, 1962, *86*, 608.

Munro, D.D. The effect of percutaneously absorbed steroids on hypothalamic-pituitary-adrenal function and intensive use in in-patients. *British Journal of Dermatology*, 1976, *94*(Suppl. 12), 67.

O'Malley, B. Mechanisms of steroid hormone action. *Journal of Investigative Dermatology*, 1977, *68*, 1-4.

Ortega, E., Burdick, K.A., & Segre, E.J. Adrenal suppression by clobetasol proprionate. *Lancet*, 1975, *1*, 1200.

Phillips, G.H. Locally active corticosteroids: structure-activity relationships. In L.C. Wilson & R. Marks (Eds.), *Mechanisms of topical corticosteroid activity*. Edinburgh: Churchill Livingstone, 1976.

Polano, M.K., & Ponec, M. Dependence of corticosteroid penetration on the vehicle. *Archives of Dermatology*, 1976, *112*, 675.

Priestley, G.C., & Brown, J.C. Effects of corticosteroids on the proliferation of normal and abnormal human connective tissue cells. *British Journal of Dermatology*, 1980, *102*, 35.

Rasmussen, J.E. Percutaneous absorption of topically applied triamcinolone in children. *Archives of Dermatology*, 1978, *114*, 1165.

Smith, J.G., Sihr, R.F., & Chalker, D.K. Corticosteroid induced atrophy and telangiectasia. *Archives of Dermatology*, 1976, *112*, 115.

Sneddon, I.B. Atrophy of the skin. The clinical problem. *British Journal of Dermatology*, 1976, *94*(Suppl. 12), 121.

Wester, R.C., Noonan, P.K., & Maibach, H.I. Frequency of application on percutaneous absorption of hydrocortisone. *Archives of Dermatology*, 1977, *113*(5), 620-622.

Wester, R.C., Noonan, P.K., and Maibach, H.I. Percutaneous absorption of hydrocortisone increases with long-term administration. *Archives of Dermatology*, 1980, *116*, 186-188.

Wilkinson, D.S., Kirton, V., & Wilkinson, J.D. Perioral dermatitis: a 12 year review. *British Journal of Dermatology*, 1979, *101*(3), 245-257.

ANTIINFLAMMATORY MEDICATIONS

Medications discussed in this section

CHAPTER 58

Nonsteroidal Antiinflammatory Drugs

Frederick G. Pfeiffer

Medications discussed in this chapter

Nonsteroidal antiinflammatory drugs
  Fenamates
    Meclofenamate
    Mefenamic acid
  Indole acetic acid derivatives
    Indomethacin
    Sulindac
    Tolmetin
  Oxicams
    Piroxicam
  Phenylacetic acids
    Alclofenac
    Diclofenac
  Propionic acid derivatives
    Fenoprofen
    Ibuprofen
    Ketoprofen
    Naproxen

Nonsteroidal antiinflammatory drugs—cont'd
  Pyrazolons
    Oxyphenbutazone
    Phenylbutazone
  Salicylates
    Aspirin
    Choline and magnesium trisalicylate
    Choline salicylate
    Magnesium salicylate
    Salsalate
    Sodium salicylate
  Miscellaneous agents
    Benoxaprofen
    Diflunisal
    Zomepirac

A wide selection of drugs is available for the management of rheumatoid arthritis (RA) and other rheumatic diseases including osteoarthritis (degenerative joint disease [DJD]) and gout. Only drugs that have been proved in well-controlled double-blind studies are discussed in this chapter and in Chapter 59, "Remittive and Miscellaneous Agents Used to Treat Rheumatic Diseases and Gout." Basically, there are two groups of drugs used in the treatment of rheumatic disorders: (1) the nonsteroidal antiinflammatory drugs that are effective in reducing pain and inflammation and (2) the disease-modifying or remittive agents such as gold, penicillamine, and azathioprine. The nonsteroidal antiinflammatory drugs are discussed in this chapter and the remittive agents are discussed in Chapter 59.

Generally, rheumatoid arthritis is managed in relation to a pyramidal treatment plan (Figure 58-1).

Nondrug therapy is used to relieve pain, reduce inflammation, and preserve functional capacity of joints and adjoining muscles (Figures 58-2 and 58-3). Therapy often includes patient education, counseling, diet, rest, exercise, use of heat or paraffin dips, occupational and physical therapy, and follow-up. Local and systemic analgesics may be used to relieve pain. When drug therapy is indicated, a stepped approach is often used beginning with aspirin or other salicylates, followed by other nonsteroidal antiinflammatory drugs (NSAIDs) as indicated. Remittive agents are usually reserved for patients who fail to respond to the NSAIDs. Corticosteroids and investigational drugs are usually reserved for patients who are either refractory to the other drugs or who cannot tolerate their associated toxicity or adverse side effects.

SALICYLATES

Aspirin

Pharmacodynamics. Aspirin is an effective analgesic, antipyretic, and, at plasma levels of 15 to 30 mg/dl, antiinflammatory. Acetaminophen has equal analgesic effect compared with aspirin, but has no clinically significant effects on inflammation. At lower doses, aspirin inhibits the effect of cyclooxygenase on the platelet reducing the formation of thromboxane and thus can also be used in the treatment of transient ischemic attacks. Thromboxane inhibition results in less platelet adhesiveness and thus lessens the chance for transient ischemic attacks in the predisposed patient. Aspirin, in usual analgesic doses, raises serum urate levels by inhibiting the renal tubular secretion of uric acid. At doses of 1.9 to 3.9 gm (from 6 to 12 regular-strength [325 mg] tablets), there is usually no change in serum urate levels. At doses above 3.9 gm (12 regular-strength tablets), the serum urate level can be decreased because of a combination of inhibiting both tubular secretion and renal tubular reabsorption

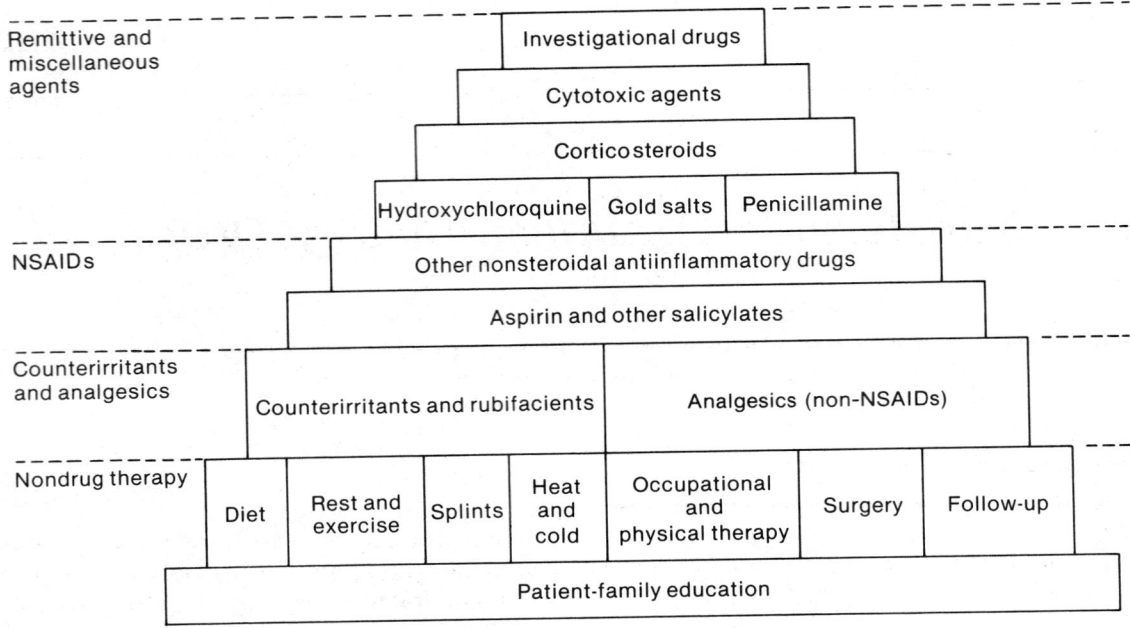

FIGURE 58-1. **Pyramidal treatment plan.**

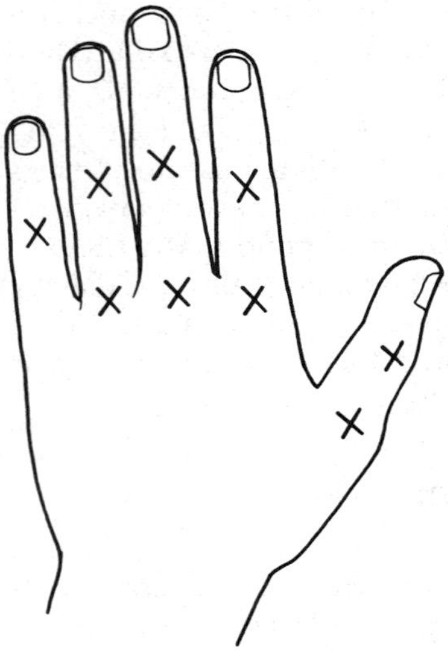

FIGURE 58-2. **Hand joints typically affected by rheumatoid arthritis.**

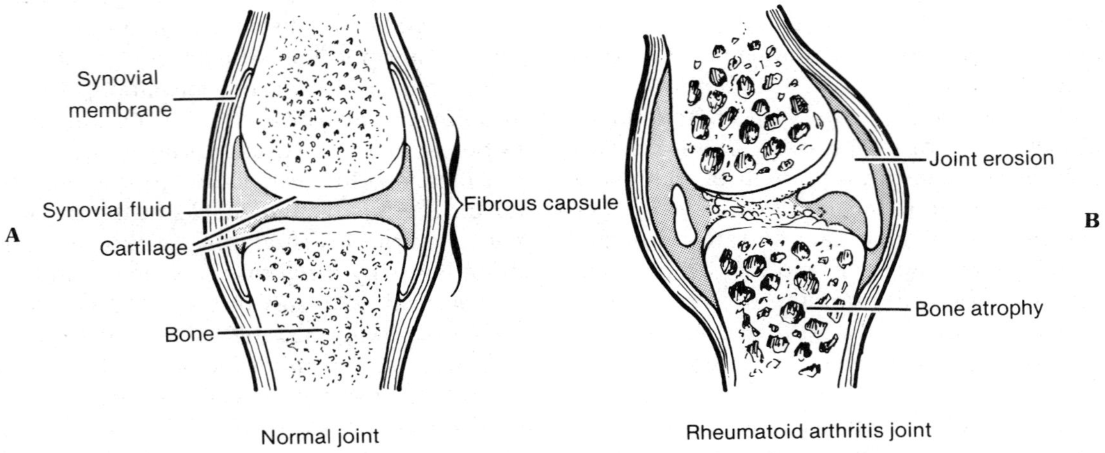

Synovial membrane

Synovial fluid

Cartilage

Bone

Fibrous capsule

Joint erosion

Bone atrophy

A

B

Normal joint

Rheumatoid arthritis joint

FIGURE 58-3. **Joint changes associated with rheumatoid arthritis.** *A,* Normal joint; *B,* rheumatoid arthritis joint.

of uric acid. At plasma levels of 15 to 30 mg/dl hyperventilation may occur from direct stimulation of the medullary respiratory center.

Pharmacokinetics. Aspirin is hydrolyzed into acetic acid and salicylic acid. Even though aspirin is an acidic medication, the duodenum is still the major site for gastrointestinal (GI) absorption because of its larger surface area. Concurrent use of antacids increases the rate of dissolution, but apparently does not change absorption to a clinically significant extent. With usual analgesic doses aspirin attains peak blood levels within 1 to 2 hours after oral administration. The apparent elimination half-life of aspirin depends on plasma levels. At a plasma level (Cp) of 25 mg/dl, the half-life may be up to 10 to 12 hours, whereas at lower levels (5 to 10 mg/dl) the half-life is about 1½ to 2 hours. In the treatment of arthritis the serum half-life may not be as relevant as the half-life in the synovial fluid. There is complex renal excretion and saturable metabolism (i.e., dose-dependent kinetics). The latter phenomenon causes the Cp to rise at a disproportionate rate relative to the daily dose especially with higher doses (more than 10 tablets daily). Renal elimination includes glomerular filtration, proximal tubular secretion, and distal tubular reabsorption. Finally, it is important to remember the influence of urinary pH on aspirin elimination. Raising the pH from 6 to 7 can reduce the Cp by about 50%.

Adverse reactions. Dyspepsia, or heartburn, occurs in about 5% of all patients taking aspirin, but may be more common in pregnant patients or those with parkinsonism. Dyspepsia occurs with oral administration. This common side effect is probably related to peak plasma levels. Therefore, managing this reaction involves reducing the amount of the individual dose. Another alternative is to substitute acetaminophen for the aspirin when reduction of inflammation is not necessary.

Bronchospasm or asthma can be precipitated or exacerbated in the patient with nasal polyps, history of asthma, or chronic obstructive pulmonary disease (COPD). This reaction occurs in about 10% of these patients after doses as small as 120 mg of aspirin. The onset of wheezing, chest tightness, and reduced FEV_1 may occur within 30 to 120 minutes of administration. Managing this problem is difficult since other NSAIDs including indomethacin have been reported to cause bronchospasm also. Sodium salicylate may cause less trouble in asthmatics but is less effective as an antiinflammatory agent than is aspirin.

Hepatotoxicity caused by high doses of aspirin is manifested by cellular damage and cholestatic jaundice. The development of tinnitus or dyspepsia should not be considered a *prodrome* to the liver damage. Thus, increasing the dosage until the patient experiences tinnitus and then reducing the dose by one or two tablets is generally no longer recommended. When the patient is symptomatic, the manifestations include anorexia, nausea, right upper quadrant (RUQ) abdominal pain, jaundice, fever (usually not above 101° F or 38.5° C), clay-colored stools, and cola-colored urine. Some patients, however, are *anicteric* or even completely asymptomatic; therefore the only monitoring parameter may be elevated liver function tests. Elevations of SGOT, SGPT, alkaline phosphatase, and gamma glutamyl transpeptidase occur when the patient has both cellular damage and cholestasis. Finally, in contrast to early data, there is no apparent relationship to either dose or plasma level of aspirin regarding hepatotoxicity.

Management of aspirin-induced hepatitis is similar to viral hepatitis and includes support for the patient and discontinuing the aspirin. There have been no reports of chronic active hepatitis from aspirin.

Drug interactions. Aspirin appears to potentiate the gastritis induced by alcohol. Ammonium chloride or high doses of ascorbic acid may acidify the urine leading to more tubular reabsorption of aspirin. Corticosteroids such as prednisone have been shown to reduce the plasma level of salicylates resulting from increased renal elimination. Low doses of aspirin may raise serum urate levels and attenuate or block the therapeutic effect of sulfinpyrazone or probenecid.

Dosage regimen and comments. Aspirin is usually given at a dose of 2.4 gm (8 tablets) daily in 3 to 4 doses initially in the patient with arthritis. In the elderly, the dose should be reduced somewhat. The maximum daily dose is determined by monitoring the plasma level. For reduction of inflammation, a Cp of 15 to 30 mg/dl is the goal of therapy. The usual patient requires 12 to 20 tablets (3.9 to 6 gm) daily to achieve this goal. Because of saturation kinetics, a change of 2 tablets per day can cause toxicity resulting from the disproportionate use in blood level relative to dose. For example, a patient may have 13 mg/dl plasma level while taking 12 tablets daily (3.9 gm) but the level may be increased to 34 mg/dl with an increase of a single 325 mg tablet!

Local GI irritation is managed by having the patient take each dose of aspirin with a full glass of water and with meals or by switching to an enteric-coated preparation. Tinnitus may not occur in the elderly patient with a hearing deficit. Since aspirin is hydrolyzed to acetic acid, a strong odor of vinegar indicates tablet decomposition. Signs and symptoms of hepatitis need to be explained to the patient. When observed, these signs and symptoms should be reported to the prescriber as soon as possible. Strict compliance to the prescribed regimen of aspirin should be adhered to by the patient when antiinflammatory doses are taken (3.9 to 6 gm/day). Patients need to recognize that aspirin is a potent, effective medicine not just a "safe" over-the-counter drug. There are about 300 products that contain a therapeutic amount of aspirin, and most of these do not require a prescription for purchase. Patients should also recognize that there are no definitive data to substantiate the idea that generic aspirin is inferior to any of the well-known brand names.

Other salicylate products

Choline magnesium trisalicylate and salsalate are salicylate products that can be used in place of aspirin. Since these drugs do not have "acetyl groups," there seems to be no antiplatelet effects. The doses of these products are again governed by monitoring plasma levels. There are some data to indicate that these drugs cause less GI irritation when compared with aspirin.

PYRAZOLONS
Phenylbutazone and oxyphenbutazone

Pharmacodynamics. Phenylbutazone is almost completely metabolized to oxyphenbutazone so that the following statements apply to both drugs. Phenylbutazone is an analgesic and potent antiinflammatory drug, although it apparently is inferior to aspirin and acetaminophen, as an antipyretic. Phenylbutazone reduces platelet adhesiveness, similar to aspirin qualitatively but probably not quantitatively. In addition to prostaglandin inhibition, phenylbutazone may reduce the accumulation of white blood cells (WBCs) and *lysozymes* in the synovial fluid, therefore further helping reduce inflammation.

Pharmacokinetics. Phenylbutazone is absorbed to a variable extent in different patients. The apparent serum half-life is about 72 hours, and the drug is about 99% protein bound, mainly to albumin. Phenylbutazone is eliminated through hepatic metabolism and oxyphenbutazone levels are therapeutic at 5 to 15 μg/ml. Fetal levels of oxyphenbutazone are about 50% of the corresponding maternal blood levels when taken during pregnancy.

Adverse reactions. Dyspepsia is common during the first week of therapy and may be related to the total daily dose of this drug. Using the product with a subtherapeutic amount of antacid plus phenylbutazone (e.g., Azolid-A or Butazolidin-Alka) does not appear to be beneficial in managing dyspepsia. For this reason these preparations were withdrawn from the market.

Hematologic adverse side effects from phenylbutazone are the main reason for limiting the use of this drug to short-term administration in the management of arthritis. Two different syndromes have been described. First, there is bone marrow depression, or *aplastic anemia.* This is more common in elderly patients and may be heralded by neutropenia. The pathogenesis of this is still not exactly known at this time. Second, *agranulocytosis* appears to be more common in younger patients and usually occurs within the first 4 weeks of therapy. The patient may have unexplained fever, sore throat, and lymphadenopathy; these findings are probably better monitoring parameters than the WBC count. Agranulocytosis is not usually heralded by neutropenia in contrast to bone marrow suppression.

Similar to other NSAIDs, there are several reports of sodium and water retention especially in elderly patients. This may induce dependent peripheral edema and exacerbate heart failure in predisposed patients. The sodium retention can also exacerbate preexisting hypertension.

Drug interactions. Phenylbutazone and oral anticoagulants are an extremely dangerous combination. Usually the adverse result is hemorrhage, but the complex nature of this interaction requires close monitoring. Phenylbutazone has an antiplatelet effect that can potentiate the hypoprothrombinemia of oral anticoagulants. The concurrent use of chlorpropamide with phenylbutazone may cause severe, prolonged hypoglycemia. Data regarding other sulfonylurea oral hypoglycemics are less clear but this combination still warrants close monitoring.

Dosage regimen and comments. In elderly patients the long-term use of phenylbutazone for arthritis is inappropriate in almost every instance. An initial dose of 600 to 800 mg per day in 3 or 4 doses is used as a loading dose. In the treatment of acute gout, the daily dose may be even higher. The maximum dose is mainly limited by adverse side effects. For maintenance therapy a daily dose of 400 mg in divided doses has been recommended. Probably the most important aspect of phenylbutazone dosage regimens is the duration of therapy rather than the total daily dose.

Occasionally, taking phenylbutazone with food or milk may help reduce some of the dyspepsia. Phenylbutazone may precipitate or exacerbate hypothyroidism by inhibiting the pituitary release of thyroid-stimulating hormone (TSH). Routine WBC counts seem to be inappropriate in monitoring for the development of agranulocytosis.

ACETIC ACID DERIVATIVES

Indomethacin and sulindac are indole acetic acid products. Tolmetin is a pyrole acetic acid derivative. Indomethacin is the oldest product of the three; therefore data are more complete than with the other two.

Indomethacin

Pharmacodynamics. Indomethacin has analgesic properties independent of its effect on inflammation. It has also been shown to have antipyretic and antiplatelet effects. The antiplatelet effects are not as consistent or persistent as those of aspirin. Similar to phenylbutazone, indomethacin may reduce WBC transfer into joints.

Pharmacokinetics. Indomethacin is well absorbed after oral administration. Its apparent plasma half-life is about 4 hours (range 2 to 6 hours) and reaches a peak Cp of 4 µg/ml 2 hours after administration. The major route of elimination is hepatic metabolism, but no active metabolites have been identified. When indomethacin is taken after meals, the peak plasma level is delayed, but the total amount absorbed is not affected by food.

Adverse reactions. Dyspepsia is probably the most common adverse GI effect. It is probably related to high peak blood levels and appears to be more common during the first several months of therapy. Patients at highest risk for this problem seem to be those with a history of reflux esophagitis. Managing this common perplexing problem may involve instructing the patient to take each dose with a glass of water close to mealtime. If these measures fail, a reduction in the individual dose can be tried. For example, if the patient is taking 50 mg twice daily the regimen may be changed to 25 mg four times a day to reduce the peak blood level.

Central nervous system (CNS) effects include headache, light-headedness, dizziness, and emotional lability. The most common presentation for mood changes is depression with anorexia, sleep disturbances, guilt, and *anhedonia*. Depression may be insidious and more common in elderly patients. In most cases the depression will resolve over weeks to months after the indomethacin is stopped.

Headache from indomethacin is usually a throbbing sensation, which may be frontal or temporal. Many patients also notice dizziness or vertigo during the headache. The exact mechanism for the headache is not known, but apparently it is more common with large incremental dose changes and during the first several months of therapy. Headache from indomethacin may be more common in patients using hydralazine or nitrates concomitantly. Management for this

consists of: (1) slow upward titration of dose, (2) reducing the peak Cp by reducing the amount of an individual dose; and (3) substituting another NSAID at a low initial dose.

Although rare, various blood dyscrasias, including *agranulocytosis*, aplastic anemia, hemolytic anemia, leukopenia, and thrombocytopenia, can occur with indomethacin use and should be monitored for, particularly in patients receiving long-term therapy.

Drug interactions. Indomethacin taken concurrently with the oral anticoagulants (e.g., warfarin) may increase the frequency and severity of hemorrhage. There is still controversy about the precise mechanism and the predictability of this interaction. However, it would seem prudent to monitor for signs of bleeding in a patient receiving both drugs. The diuretic effect of furosemide appears to be significantly diminished in some patients using indomethacin. Captopril's antihypertensive effect can be blocked by concurrent use of indomethacin.

Dosage regimen and comments. Initial doses of indomethacin for rheumatoid arthritis are much lower than those used for treating acute gout. A reasonable starting point is 25 mg two or three times a day. This may be increased by 50 mg per day every 7 to 10 days to a maximum of 150 to 200 mg daily. Elderly patients may receive lower total daily doses. Doubling the dose at bedtime (e.g., 25 mg twice daily plus 50 mg at bedtime) is sometimes helpful in a patient with severe morning stiffness.

Patients with arthritis may not achieve maximum therapeutic benefit for 10 to 14 days on a given dose. In some patients headache may be transient. There are a few case reports that indomethacin may reduce the antihypertensive effects of propranolol. If there is a positive personal or family history of primary depression, the patient must be monitored closely; this is especially important in the elderly.

Sulindac

Pharmacodynamics. Sulindac sulfide is apparently the active principle of sulindac. This metabolite is an effective analgesic independent of its antiinflammatory properties. Similar to aspirin, sulindac sulfide is an effective antipyretic.

Pharmacokinetics. This drug is well absorbed after oral administration, but the exact site and extent are unknown at present. Sulindac is metabolized to its active metabolite, sulindac sulfide. After a 200 mg dose, a peak plasma level of 3 µg/ml is found after 2 hours.

Adverse reactions. Gastrointestinal reactions consist primarily of dyspepsia and nausea. It appears that these effects occur less commonly than with indomethacin. Dyspepsia is probably dose related especially during the first few weeks of therapy. Managing these adverse side effects involves slow upward dose titration and reduction of total daily dose. Disconcerting are some case reports of hepatitis and pancreatitis that have appeared.

CNS effects are qualitatively similar to indomethacin. Both headache and dizziness occur and appear to be dose related. Headache usually occurs 1 to 2 hours after a dose and is apparently more common with large increments in dosage. Management is similar to that for indomethacin. Aseptic meningitis and toxic psychosis have been associated with the use of sulindac.

Another interesting difference among sulindac and the other NSAIDs is the apparent lack of any adverse effect on renal function. There have been reported reductions in renal blood flow and creatinine clearance with drugs such as naproxen or ibuprofen. Thus sulindac may become the drug of choice in patients with azotemia or chronic renal failure.

Drug interactions. At present there are no documented significant adverse drug interactions with sulindac. However, since sulindac has antiplatelet effects, there is always the increased chance of hemorrhage when this drug is combined with an anticoagulant (i.e., heparin or warfarin).

Dosage regimen and comments. Initially, 100 mg twice daily is used in almost all patients. The recommended maximum dose is 200 mg twice daily, which is attained within 2 weeks after the initial dose.

Compliance may be better with sulindac than with naproxen since it may be given twice daily. Food reduces peak plasma levels and delays the time to reach peak levels. A reasonable therapeutic trial with sulindac is 3 weeks at maximum dosage.

Tolmetin

Pharmacodynamics. Tolmetin has antipyretic and analgesic properties similar to aspirin and acetaminophen. Tolmetin is slightly different from indomethacin or sulindac in that it is a pyrole acetic acid derivative. Tolmetin is an antiinflammatory drug and has some antiplatelet effects also. Unlike aspirin, tolmetin does not acetylate platelet cyclooxygenase irreversibly.

Pharmacokinetics. Tolmetin is almost completely absorbed after oral doses and is about 99% protein bound. The major route of elimination is hepatic metabolism with only 10% to 20% being excreted unchanged in the urine. The apparent plasma half-life is about 1 hour.

Adverse reactions. Nausea and dyspepsia are the most common GI effects. Apparently, this occurs less

commonly with tolmetin than with aspirin or indomethacin. These effects appear to be related to the total daily dose or peak plasma levels. Managing these effects is similar to those measures used with indomethacin.

CNS side effects apparently occur less commonly than with indomethacin. Headache and dizziness seem to be less common or severe with tolmetin than with indomethacin. These seem to be related to the total daily dose or peak plasma levels. Managing the CNS effects is usually accomplished by reducing the total daily dose or by substituting another antiprostaglandin drug. It is important to reassure the patient about the benign nature of the headache.

Drug interactions. There have been no consistent adverse drug interactions associated with tolmetin. However, it is prudent to closely monitor for hemorrhage when a patient is using anticoagulants concomitantly.

Dosage regimen and comments. An initial dose of 200 mg three times a day is used for most adults. Increases of 600 mg daily every 1 to 2 weeks is appropriate. A maximum daily dose of 1800 mg administered in two or three divided doses is recommended.

GI side effects are minimized or eliminated by instructing patients to take each dose with food or a full glass of water. The antiplatelet effects of tolmetin are much less significant than those of aspirin. It is interesting to note that tolmetin has been evaluated in its potential for interacting adversely with sulfonylurea hypoglycemics and warfarin with no significant adverse results.

PROPIONIC ACID DERIVATIVES
Ibuprofen

Pharmacodynamics. Similar to the acetic acid derivatives, ibuprofen is an effective analgesic, antipyretic, and antiinflammatory agent. Ibuprofen also reduces platelet adhesiveness qualitatively similar to aspirin.

Pharmacokinetics. Ibuprofen is absorbed after oral administration and reaches peak C_p in 1 to 2 hours. After a 600 mg dose, the C_p reaches 25 μg/dl. When ibuprofen is taken on a long-term basis, the concentration in the joint fluid is greater than the plasma level. The primary route of elimination is hepatic metabolism with only 10% being excreted unchanged by the kidney. Unlike sulindac, there are no known active metabolites of ibuprofen.

Adverse reactions. GI effects include dyspepsia and nausea. The frequency of these effects appears to be less than with the pyrazolon derivatives. With antiinflammatory doses these side effects are dose related. The usual onset of these symptoms is within the first 4 to 6 weeks of therapy and may recur with each dosage increase. Management centers on giving each dose with food or a full glass of water. Substituting tolmetin or sulindac may result in fewer GI complaints. Increasing the dose of ibuprofen gradually also appears to help in some instances.

Adverse CNS reactions are less common with this drug than with indomethacin. These appear to be dose related and consist of drowsiness and dizziness.

Exacerbation or precipitation of dependent edema occurs in some patients. At highest risk are patients with heart failure or chronic renal failure. This adverse effect is probably the result of inhibiting prostaglandins, which mediate natriuresis. Treating this sodium and water retention may involve substituting another NSAID or restricting sodium intake. In recalcitrant cases diuretics may be needed to reverse this adverse reaction.

Drug interactions. It is prudent to monitor for hemorrhage when a patient is taking anticoagulants and ibuprofen concurrently. This may be more necessary with higher doses of ibuprofen.

Dosage regimen and comments. A starting dose of ibuprofen is usually 400 mg four times a day to reduce inflammation. Incremental changes to 2.4 gm per day and then 3.2 gm per day are used every 7 to 10 days. With long-term use taking the drug three times a day may be useful in some patients to improve compliance. The recommended maximum daily dose for the elderly has not been established.

Patients with heart failure, nephrotic syndrome, and cirrhosis of the liver are more likely to develop sodium and water retention from ibuprofen. In patients with known aspirin allergy causing bronchospasm, ibuprofen may cause a similar reaction. The analgesic effect of ibuprofen appears to be independent of its antiinflammatory properties. When ibuprofen is taken with meals, the peak blood level is reduced, but the actual amount of drug absorbed may not be changed.

Naproxen

Pharmacodynamics. Naproxen reduces pain and fever and ameliorates inflammation similar to all of the other NSAIDs. Naproxen also reduces platelet adhesiveness, but the duration of this effect is less than with aspirin. By inhibiting prostaglandin synthesis, naproxen has also been effective in treating primary dysmenorrhea.

Pharmacokinetics. At the usual therapeutic plasma levels, naproxen is about 99% protein bound. After oral administration the drug is well absorbed with a peak level being reached within about 4 hours. Compared with the other propionic acids, naproxen has the longest plasma half life of 12 to 15 hours. It is now apparent that naproxen crosses the placenta easily, but the clinical significance of this is unknown.

Adverse reactions. Nausea, epigastric distress, and dyspepsia are the most commonly reported gastrointestinal effects. These appear to be related to either peak Cp or total daily dose. It is more common to see these effects during the initiation of therapy or an increase in dosage. Management is directed toward reducing the peak Cp and local irritation by giving the drug with food and adequate water.

Adverse CNS reactions include drowsiness and dizziness. These effects occur less commonly than the GI complaints and appear to be related to the total daily dose of naproxen. They may be more common in the elderly.

Drug interactions. Naproxen is known to interact with antacids. There is an interesting difference depending on the particular antacid that is given. Giving sodium bicarbonate with naproxen increases its absorption; using magnesium hydroxide with naproxen has the opposite effect. Other drug interactions also occur. Probenecid increases the plasma level of naproxen, but this interaction is not dose related. It is important to note that oral hypoglycemics and warfarin have been documented in not causing any consistent adverse drug interaction.

Dosage regimen and comments. An initial dose of 250 mg twice daily is usually given with a suggested increase of 250 mg per day every 7 to 14 days. The maximum therapeutic dose appears to be 1 gm per day. In some patients with severe morning stiffness the regimen may be 250 mg in the afternoon and 500 mg at bedtime. A specific dosage regimen for elderly patients has not been established at present.

Naproxen has recently been shown to be effective in the treatment of acute gouty arthritis. Because it is eliminated unchanged in the urine, patients with renal insufficiency need to be monitored closely when large doses are being administered. Naproxen sodium (e.g., Anaprox) is more rapidly absorbed from the GI tract; 275 mg of naproxen sodium is equivalent to 250 mg naproxen. Since naproxen has a longer half-life than the other propionic acids, it may take 7 to 10 days to get the full therapeutic benefit.

Fenoprofen

Pharmacodynamics. Fenoprofen is another propionic acid derivative that is an effective analgesic and antiinflammatory agent. Analgesia occurs at lower doses than those needed to reduce inflammation. The antiplatelet effects of fenoprofen have not been well documented at present.

Pharmacokinetics. Fenoprofen is almost completely absorbed from the GI tract with peak Cp attained within about 1 hour. The apparent plasma half-life is about 2.5 hours, but the half-life in synovial fluid is probably more important. Taking fenoprofen with meals reduces the peak Cp but does not reduce the total amount that is absorbed.

Adverse reactions. Like the other propionic acid derivatives, GI complaints include nausea and dyspepsia. Alcohol can exacerbate GI irritation. It appears to be more common during the first few weeks of therapy and is probably related to peak Cp.

Adverse CNS effects include drowsiness and headache. The headache is usually less severe with fenoprofen than with indomethacin. Management of these effects consists of slow upward titration of the dose and reducing the total daily dose.

Drug interactions. Phenobarbital may accelerate the hepatic metabolism of fenoprofen resulting in less than optimal benefit from a given dose. Aspirin apparently reduces the absorption of fenoprofen from the GI tract.

Dosage regimen and comments. An initial dose of 300 mg four times a day is commonly used with increments of 600 to 1200 mg per day each week. The maximum dose recommended is 3200-3600 mg per day given in four doses. A specific dose for the elderly has not been established.

Fenoprofen's peak Cp is reduced by both food and antacids, but the total amount absorbed is not affected. Drowsiness from fenoprofen may be potentiated by alcohol or antihistamines. There is still controversy about the concurrent use of therapeutic doses of aspirin and fenoprofen since both drugs will reduce pain and inflammation.

Ketoprofen

Pharmacodynamics. Ketoprofen is an analgesic and antipyretic in addition to an antiinflammatory agent. Similar to the other NSAIDs, ketoprofen inhibits cyclooxygenase and therefore the synthesis of prostaglandins.

Pharmacokinetics. Ketoprofen is well absorbed from the GI tract with an apparent plasma half-life of 2 to 4 hours. Peak Cp is attained within 1 hour in most patients. The primary route of elimination is through hepatic metabolism.

Adverse reactions. Gastrointestinal effects from ketoprofen are usually dyspepsia and nausea. These seem to be dose related especially in patients receiving triamterene concurrently. Most commonly these occur during the first 2 to 4 weeks of therapy. Treating the GI effects consists of taking each dose with food or reducing the daily dose.

CNS symptoms appear to be mainly dizziness and headache. These seem to be dose related and best managed by dose reduction.

Drug interactions. No known adverse drug interactions have been reported. A prudent note of caution is necessary when a patient is taking warfarin concurrently with ketoprofen. Monitoring the patient for bleeding is necessary when these two drugs are used together.

Dosage regimen. Initially a dose of 50 mg three times a day is used with a suggested maximum of 300 mg daily. No specific dose recommendations have been established for the elderly. A suppository formulation may also be used in selected patients.

Ketoprofen seems to have analgesic effects independent of its effect on inflammation. It appears to reduce platelet adhesiveness but not to the extent of aspirin. Ketoprofen appears to be another alternative for the patient unresponsive to other NSAIDs.

OXICAMS

Piroxicam

Pharmacodynamics. Piroxicam is an effective analgesic and antiinflammatory agent. At this time piroxicam is the only one of its class available for general use. It reduces platelet adhesiveness qualitatively similar to aspirin.

Pharmacokinetics. Piroxicam is rapidly absorbed from the GI tract reaching a peak Cp in 1 to 2 hours. The apparent plasma half-life is about 40 hours in contrast to most of the other NSAIDs. Concentrations in the synovial fluid usually attain from 40% to 50% of the corresponding plasma level. Only about 10% is eliminated unchanged in the urine with no active metabolites found. At steady state, plasma levels are 5 to 7 μg/ml after the usual adult dosage regimen.

Adverse reactions. Adverse GI effects mainly consist of dyspepsia and nausea. Apparently this is related to either the total daily dose or peak Cp. Managing these effects is usually accomplished by changing to another drug or giving each dose with food.

Adverse CNS effects seem to be primarily drowsiness and dizziness. These effects may be more common in elderly patients. No data are available about any relationship to dose. Treating these symptoms is usually attempted by changing to a propionic acid derivative. Simple analgesics such as acetaminophen are occasionally helpful.

Drug interactions. Piroxicam taken with lithium carbonate may lead to lithium toxicity. This interaction is an apparent paradox since conditions that lead to sodium loss usually raise lithium levels. Piroxicam may occasionally cause sodium retention, which should lead to a decrease in serum lithium levels. Also, it is important to realize that this interaction may persist after the piroxicam is stopped because of its long half-life.

Dosage regimen and comments. Piroxicam is given in daily doses of 20 mg. A reasonable therapeutic trial is 4 weeks before determining therapeutic benefit. A specific dosage regimen for elderly patients has not been established.

Therapeutic doses of aspirin may reduce plasma levels of piroxicam, and there appears to be no benefit to adding antiinflammatory doses of aspirin. Because of piroxicam's long half-life, it may take up to 2 weeks for maximum therapeutic benefit. Therapy for acute gouty arthritis requires higher doses of piroxicam than that used for osteoarthritis or rheumatoid arthritis.

FENAMATES

Meclofenamate

Pharmacodynamics. Meclofenamate is an effective analgesic and antiinflammatory agent. Similar to the other NSAIDs, meclofenamate inhibits cyclooxygenase, which inhibits synthesis of prostaglandins. Unlike the previously mentioned group, meclofenamate appears to compete with prostaglandins at the receptor site, reducing their physiologic effects. Meclofenamate seems to reduce platelet adhesiveness but not to the extent that aspirin does.

Pharmacokinetics. Meclofenamate is rapidly absorbed from the GI tract with peak Cp being attained within 60 minutes. When meclofenamate is taken with meals, the peak Cp is reduced, but the total amount absorbed probably is not. This drug is about 99% protein bound to albumin and its apparent plasma half-life is 3 hours. Meclofenamate is metabolized to an active product, and little is excreted unchanged in the urine.

Adverse reactions. Adverse GI effects are common with meclofenamate including diarrhea, nausea, and epigastric distress. Diarrhea may be severe enough to cause electrolyte disturbances. Diarrhea appears to be related to the total daily dose and may be more common in patients taking quinidine or oral ampicillin concomitantly. In order to manage the diarrhea, meclofenamate usually needs to be discontinued.

Adverse CNS reactions include headache and dizziness and may be related to peak Cp. Apparently these effects occur more commonly in the elderly. Treating the CNS effects by giving more doses per day (i.e., reducing the dosing interval) is sometimes successful. Also changing to piroxicam or a propionic acid derivative may be helpful clinically.

Drug interactions. Meclofenamate taken with war-farin increases the anticoagulant effect of the latter, requiring close monitoring of the prothrombin time. Aspirin may reduce the plasma level of meclofenamate when they are taken concurrently.

Dosage regimen and comments. A beginning dose of 50 mg three times a day is increased by 100 mg per day every 4 to 7 days. The recommended maximum dose is 400 mg daily in 3 to 4 doses. Two to three weeks is needed to assess the optimal benefit from meclofenamate.

Diarrhea may be the dose-limiting parameter of therapy with meclofenamate. Unlike the pyrazolons, meclofenamate has no uricosuric effects. Concurrent administration of antacids does not appear to alter absorption of meclofenamate. Tinnitus has been reported, but its frequency and severity appear to be less than with aspirin. Each 100 mg of meclofenamate contains 0.3 mEq sodium, which may be important in patients needing severe sodium restriction. Because of the severe GI effects, the manufacturer recommends that meclofenamate *not* be the initial drug in the treatment of arthritis.

Mefenamic acid

Pharmacodynamics. This drug relieves the pain and inflammation of arthritis. Mefenamic acid, similar to meclofenamate, appears to compete for prostaglandins at the receptor site. By inhibiting prostaglandin synthesis, its mechanism is similar to all the other NSAIDs or antiprostaglandins. Mefenamic acid reduces elevated body temperature similar to aspirin or naproxen.

Pharmacokinetics. After oral administration, mefenamic acid is rapidly absorbed reaching peak Cp of 10 μg/ml in about 3 hours. The apparent plasma half-life is about 2 hours. Mefenamic acid is eliminated primarily by hepatic metabolism with a small amount eliminated unchanged in the urine.

Adverse reactions. Gastrointestinal side effects are similar to those caused by meclofenamate. Diarrhea, nausea, and epigastric distress appear to be dose related and are more common in the elderly. The diarrhea may be severe enough to cause electrolyte abnormalities. Administering mefenamic acid with meals may help in some patients. Reducing the daily dose by 33% or more may be needed to control the diarrhea.

Adverse CNS effects consist of dizziness, drowsiness, and insomnia. There are no data about any relationship to dose, duration, or plasma levels. These effects may be more common in the elderly. Managing these usually means discontinuing the drug and substituting another NSAID.

Drug interactions. When mefenamic acid is used concurrently with warfarin, there is an increased tendency toward bleeding. This interaction requires close monitoring for prolonged prothrombin times. Also it would seem prudent to monitor for hypoglycemia in patients using both sulfonylurea oral hypoglycemics and mefenamic acid.

Dosage regimen and comments. Few clinicians still use mefenamic acid for its antiinflammatory effects in arthritis. It is used primarily for pain relief on an acute basis. The initial dose is a 500 mg loading dose, followed by 250 mg every 6 to 8 hours to a maximum of 1 to 1.25 gm per day.

This drug appears to compete with prostaglandins for binding at their receptor sites. Mefenamic acid has been used successfully to reduce excess blood loss in patients with moderate to severe *menorrhagia.* Use of mefenamic acid during the third trimester of pregnancy may prolong gestation. Apparently mefenamic acid is not removed by dialysis. There have been reports of reversible hemolytic anemia when mefenamic acid has been used continuously for 12 months or more. There are some data to suggest that dehydration or diuretics may enhance the possible nephrotoxicity of this drug.

PHENYLACETIC ACIDS
Diclofenac

Pharmacodynamics. Diclofenac is an effective antiinflammatory and analgesic. This drug appears to reduce platelet adhesiveness qualitatively similar to aspirin. Diclofenac also reduces fever by a mechanism similar to aspirin.

Pharmacokinetics. Absorption of diclofenac from the GI tract is almost complete. After administration of the enteric-coated tablets, peak Cp of 900 ng/ml is reached in about 4 hours. About 55% is eliminated unchanged by the kidney with no known active metabolites.

Adverse reactions. Gastrointestinal symptoms include epigastric pain, nausea, and diarrhea. These effects may be related to the total daily dose, but the data are unclear at present. No high-risk patients have been identified to date. Managing these symptoms includes taking each dose with food and a full glass of water.

Adverse CNS effects also occur commonly. Dizziness and headache seem to be the most prominent complaints. To date there are no data to support a relationship to either peak Cp or total daily dose. Treating the dizziness appears to be difficult at best, usually requiring a dose reduction or discontinuation of the drug.

Drug interactions. It is of considerable interest that diclofenac does not adversely interact with oral hypoglycemics or warfarin. However, since diclofenac inhibits platelet adhesiveness it is wise to closely monitor patients for signs of bleeding. Aspirin in antiinflammatory doses will lower the Cp of diclofenac.

Dosage regimen and comments. An initial dose of 25 mg three times daily appears to be useful clinically. The suggested maximum is 50 mg three times daily. There is no specific dosage regimen defined for elderly patients.

The analgesic effect of diclofenac appears to be independent of its effect on inflammation. Enterohepatic recirculation seems to occur only in animals not humans. Synovial fluid concentrations appear to exceed the Cp after chronic administration. The manufacturer recommends that diclofenac not be given to patients with nasal polyps, asthma, and aspirin sensitivity.

Alclofenac

Pharmacodynamics. This drug is an effective analgesic and antiinflammatory agent. Alclofenac seems to inhibit cyclooxygenase similar to most of the other NSAIDs. It appears to reduce platelet adhesiveness also. Similar to the fenamates, alclofenac may compete for prostaglandin receptor sites, thereby reducing the effect of already formed prostaglandins.

Pharmacokinetics. Alclofenac is variably absorbed from the GI tract after oral use. Peak Cp is reached within 2 to 4 hours. There may be some variation in these values depending on the formulation of the product (capsules or tablets). Alclofenac is about 99% bound to plasma proteins with an apparent plasma half-life of 3 to 5 hours. About 50% of alclofenac is eliminated unchanged in the urine with no known active metabolites.

Adverse reactions. Dermatologic reactions seem to be more common than with diclofenac. Morbilliform and macular rashes have often led to discontinuation of diclofenac. The usual onset of skin reactions is within the first 6 weeks of therapy. There is no information regarding any relationship to dose or peak Cp in patients exhibiting these rashes. Treating these symptoms includes symptomatic treatment and discontinuing the alclofenac.

Adverse GI side effects include epigastric pain, nausea, and constipation. These appear to be related to the total daily dose. No high-risk patients have been identified to date. Management usually consists of giving each dose with food and sufficient water. If this is unsuccessful, alclofenac is usually discontinued.

Drug interactions. Preliminary data indicate that alclofenac may adversely interact with warfarin. The patient needs to be monitored closely for bleeding episodes. Alclofenac reduces platelet adhesiveness and may cause bleeding problems.

Dosage regimen and comments. A reasonable initial dose is 500 mg three times daily. The recommended maximum dose is 1 gm three times a day. There has been no specific dosage regimen established for the elderly.

Alclofenac's analgesic effects appear to be independent of its effect on inflammation. It appears that alclofenac is better tolerated than equivalent doses of indomethacin. The product formulation of this drug appears to determine the frequency or severity of adverse reactions.

MISCELLANEOUS AGENTS

Benoxaprofen

Pharmacodynamics. Benoxaprofen is an effective analgesic, antipyretic, and antiinflammatory agent. Unlike some of the other NSAIDs, benoxaprofen inhibits lipoxygenase and slightly inhibits cyclooxygenase. Inhibition of the former enzyme reduces the formation of leukotrienes, another mediator of inflammation. It appears that benoxaprofen reduces platelet adhesiveness less than aspirin and some of the other NSAIDs.

Pharmacokinetics. After oral administration absorption is almost complete with peak Cp occurring in about 3 hours. The apparent plasma half-life is about 30 hours and even longer in the elderly. Food reduces the peak blood level but does not affect the total amount absorbed. The major route of elimination is hepatic metabolism with no known active metabolites. Only 10% is renally excreted as the parent drug. Benoxaprofen is not cleared to any clinically significant extent by hemodialysis.

Adverse reactions. Phototoxicity appears to be from ultraviolet light exposure; symptoms include exaggerated sunburn and pruritus. Usually this reaction occurs within the first week of therapy and does not appear to be related to plasma levels of benoxaprofen. Patients known to sunburn easily appear to be at a higher risk for this adverse reaction. Management is best accomplished by prevention through patient education. Sunscreens containing PABA or PABA esters are helpful in preventing this effect in some patients. Once benoxaprofen has been discontinued it appears that the risk for this side effect is markedly reduced after 2 to 4 days.

Another unique adverse drug reaction to benoxaprofen is *onycholysis.* Pain or burning sensation appears to be a prodrome for this adverse effect. Occasionally a patient will experience both phototoxicity and onycholysis. Using nail polish with a PABA sunscreen may prevent this adverse reaction but does not reverse it once onycholysis has occurred.

The most serious adverse side effects are hepatotoxicity and nephrotoxicity. Fatal cholestatic jaundice with elevated alkaline phosphatase and severe abdominal pain has occurred. Nephrotoxicity with elevated serum creatinine levels and decreased creatinine clearance was often associated with the hepatotoxicity. Most of the fatalities occurred in women with an average age of 70 years. Because of these adverse reactions it is unclear whether benoxaprofen will be returned to the market worldwide.

Drug interactions. Probenecid prolongs the plasma half-life of benoxaprofen about twofold; this appears to be more common with larger doses of probenecid. An important absence is the lack of data concerning adverse interactions with digoxin and prednisolone.

Dosage regimen and comments. A beginning dose of benoxaprofen appears to be 300 mg daily with a reduced amount in the elderly. Increases of 150 to 300 mg per day are used every 7 to 10 days. The recommended maximum dose is 900 mg daily. In patients with renal insufficiency daily doses need to be reduced significantly.

The clinical significance of inhibiting lipoxygenase may be important in preventing the production of bronchospasm in the asthmatic patient. Benoxaprofen was marketed in Great Britain for several years before hepatotoxicity was identified. This drug was available for only about 6 months in North America before its removal due to fatal reactions associated with its use.

Zomepirac

Pharmacodynamics. This drug is another acetic acid derivative that was marketed as an analgesic. Zomepirac appears to have antipyretic and antiinflammatory effects also. It inhibits cyclooxygenase thereby interfering with prostaglandin synthesis. Similar to the other acetic acid derivatives, zomepirac inhibits platelet adhesiveness.

Pharmacokinetics. The GI absorption of zomepirac appears to be complete with peak Cp of 4.5 μg/ml being reached in about 1½ hours. The apparent plasma half-life is longer after long-term use, increasing up to about 10 hours. Less than 20% of zomepirac is eliminated unchanged by the kidney. Most of the drug is metabolized with no known active metabolites.

Adverse reactions. Gastrointestinal effects include epigastric distress, dyspepsia, and nausea. These appear to be related to the total daily dose or peak Cp. Managing these adverse side effects involves patient reassurance and administering each dose with food.

Adverse CNS effects usually consist of dizziness and insomnia. There are no data to establish a relationship to dose or duration of therapy. Managing these effects is difficult and may require discontinuation of therapy.

Zomepirac has been removed from the market in North America. The reason for voluntary withdrawal of the drug appears to be allergic reactions and bronchospasm in patients with known aspirin sensitivity. The manufacturers plan to remarket zomepirac with stronger cautions.

Drug interactions. Concurrent administration of aspirin with zomepirac may reduce the effectiveness of zomepirac by reducing its plasma level. Since zomepirac inhibits platelet adhesiveness, prudence dictates monitoring for bleeding when this drug is used with warfarin.

Dosage regimen and comments. For pain relief 50 to 100 mg is given every 4 to 6 hours. In the elderly patient the dose is usually reduced. A specific regimen for reducing inflammation in patients with rheumatoid arthritis has not been established at present.

This drug is chemically and pharmacologically similar to tolmetin. Dizziness and drowsiness may occur during the first week of therapy. When taken with food, zomepirac's absorption is both delayed and decreased. In contrast to aspirin, its effect on platelets returns to baseline values within 48 hours after stopping the medication.

Diflunisal

Pharmacodynamics. Diflunisal is an effective analgesic, antipyretic, and antiinflammatory agent. Since this medication does not have an acetyl group, it probably does not reduce platelet adhesiveness. Apparently diflunisal inhibits cyclooxygenase, one of the enzymes responsible for prostaglandin synthesis.

Pharmacokinetics. After oral administration of 500 mg, diflunisal gives peak Cp of 80 μg/ml. The plasma half-life of diflunisal is longer with increasing doses. Diflunisal is about 98% protein bound at therapeutic concentrations. Apparently, the major route of elimination is hepatic metabolism with less than 10% of the parent drug being excreted in the urine.

Adverse reactions. Gastrointestinal side effects appear to be the most common adverse effects. These include epigastric pain, dyspepsia, and nausea. These effects are probably related to peak Cp rather than total dose. Managing these effects is the same as for aspirin.

Adverse CNS effects include headache and dizziness. The exact mechanism for these effects is unknown. There are no data to support a relationship to dose or plasma level. Managing these effects usually involves discontinuing diflunisal.

Drug interactions. Concomitant use of diflunisal and warfarin has produced increased free warfarin plasma levels. The clinical significance of this interaction is uncertain at present. Diflunisal plus furosemide inhibits the usual rise in serum urate caused by the latter. It is important to note that the diuretic effect of furosemide is not blunted by diflunisal. Concurrent administration of indomethacin and diflunisal is not recommended since the plasma levels of the former are increased dramatically.

Dosage regimen and comments. The initial dose is 500 mg followed by 250 mg every 12 hours. The suggested maximum dosage is a 1 gm loading dose with a maintenance dose of 500 mg twice daily.

Since diflunisal does not affect platelet adhesiveness, it would not be a suitable alternative to aspirin in the treatment of transient ischemic attacks. Hemodialysis is not effective in removing this drug. Diflunisal appears to be superior to propoxyphene as an analgesic and does not have propoxyphene's dependence liability. The antipyretic effect of this drug appears to be less than with comparable doses of aspirin. Diflunisal appears to have a significant uricosuric effect in daily doses between 500 and 1500 mg.

SUMMARY

The various NSAIDs have been discussed in relation to their major indication for arthritic conditions. Although these drugs do not effect cure of the various arthritic conditions, they assist in the relief of pain and inflammation and are used as the first steps in drug therapy for these conditions along with various nonpharmacologic treatment modalities. With an understanding of these agents as well as their contraindications, cautions, drug interactions, administration, and monitoring, the nurse will be better able to assist patients who require these medications and to increase their self-medication and self-care abilities.

ADVERSE/SIDE EFFECTS OF NONSTEROIDAL ANTIINFLAMMATORY DRUGS*

ALLERGIC REACTIONS

Anaphylaxis
Angioedema
Erythema multiforme
Exacerbation of asthma
Hives
Lacrimation
Urticaria

CARDIOVASCULAR SYSTEM

Dependent edema
Dyspnea on exertion
Exacerbation of heart failure
Hyperkalemia
Hypertension
Palpitations
Pleural effusion (mainly with phenylbutazone)
Pulmonary edema
Shortness of breath
Sinus tachycardia
Sodium retention

CENTRAL NERVOUS SYSTEM

Agitation
Ataxia
Confusion
Dizziness
Drowsiness
Fatigue
Hallucinations
Headache
Insomnia
Lethargy
Malaise
Nervousness
Nightmares
Seizures
Toxic psychosis
Tremor
Vertigo
Weakness

CUTANEOUS SYSTEM

Eczema
Erythema nodosum
Exacerbation of psoriasis
Pruritus

GASTROINTESTINAL SYSTEM

Anorexia
Bloating
Constipation
Diarrhea
Dry mouth
Dyspepsia
Epigastric pain
Exacerbation of reflux esophagitis
Exacerbation of ulcer
Flatulence
Gastric ulcer (documented with aspirin)
Gastritis
Gingivitis
Hematemesis
Nausea
Occult bleeding
Overt bleeding
Stomatitis
Vomiting

HEMATOLOGIC SYSTEM

Agranulocytosis
Aplastic anemia
Bone marrow depression
Eosinopenia
Eosinophilia
Hematomas
Hemolysis
Leukocytosis (with salicylate overdose)
Leukopenia
Macrocytic, megaloblastic anemia
Pancytopenia
Purpura
Reduced platelet adhesiveness
Shortened RBC life span
Thrombopenia

HEPATIC SYSTEM

Abdominal pain
Cholestasis
Hepatocellular damage
Jaundice
Right upper quadrant pain

OCULAR AND OTIC SYSTEMS

Amblyopia
Blurred vision
Conjunctivitis
Corneal deposits
Diplopia
Loss of color vision (reversible)
Loss of hearing (reversible)
Macular edema
Mydriasis
Photophobia
Retinopathy
Scotomas
Tinnitus

RENAL SYSTEM

Albuminuria
Creatinine clearance, decreased
Dysuria
Hematuria
Interstitial nephritis
Membranous glomerulonephritis
Nephrotic syndrome
Oliguria
Papillary necrosis
Proteinuria
RBC casts in urine
RBC in urine
Sodium retention
WBC casts in urine
WBC in urine

RESPIRATORY SYSTEM

Alveolitis
Exacerbation of asthma
Pneumonitis
Pulmonary fibrosis

*See Chapter 11, "Drug Toxicity," for an overview of drug toxicity.

CLINICALLY SIGNIFICANT DRUG INTERACTIONS*

Primary drug	Interacting drug	Possible effect(s)	Probable mechanism(s)
Aspirin†	Alcohol	Increased GI bleeding	Additive effect
Aspirin†	Heparin	Hemorrhage	Additive effect
Aspirin†	Oral anticoagulants	Hemorrhage	Additive effect
Indomethacin	β-Adrenergic blockers	Decreased antihypertensive effect	Prostaglandin inhibition
Indomethacin	Lithium	Increased lithium serum levels (toxicity)	Decreased renal excretion caused by prostaglandin inhibition
Oxyphenbutazone	Acetohexamide	Increased hypoglycemic effect	Inhibition of metabolism
Oxyphenbutazone	Chlorpropamide	Increased hypoglycemic effect	Inhibition of metabolism
Oxyphenbutazone	Oral anticoagulants	Increased anticoagulant effect	Displacement from protein binding sites; inhibition of metabolism
Oxyphenbutazone	Phenytoin	Increased phenytoin serum levels (toxicity)	Displacement from protein binding sites; inhibition of metabolism
Oxyphenbutazone	Tolbutamide	Increased hypoglycemic effect	Inhibition of metabolism
Phenylbutazone	Acetohexamide	Increased hypoglycemic effect	Inhibition of metabolism
Phenylbutazone	Chlorpropamide	Increased hypoglycemic effect	Inhibition of metabolism
Phenylbutazone	Oral anticoagulants	Increased anticoagulant effect	Displacement from protein binding sites; inhibition of metabolism
Phenylbutazone	Phenytoin	Increased phenytoin serum levels (toxicity)	Displacement from protein binding sites; inhibition of metabolism
Phenylbutazone	Tolbutamide	Increased hypoglycemic effect	Inhibition of metabolism
Salicylates (including aspirin, choline salicylate, magnesium salicylate, salsalate)	Acetohexamide	Hypoglycemia	Mechanism not established
Salicylates	Chlorpropamide	Hypoglycemia	Mechanism not established
Salicylates	Methotrexate	Increased methotrexate serum levels (toxicity)	Decreased renal excretion; displacement from protein binding sites
Salicylates	Probenecid	Decreased uricosuric effect of probenecid	Competitive antagonism
Salicylates	Tolbutamide	Hypoglycemia	Mechanism not established
Salicylates	Urinary alkalinizers	Decreased salicylate effect	Increased renal excretion

*See Chapter 10, "Drug Interactions," for an overview of drug interactions.
†See also Salicylates.

GENERAL NURSING IMPLICATIONS

Nursing of patients requiring nonsteroidal antiinflammatory drugs

ASSESSMENT

Drug therapy should be initiated only after a complete assessment of the patient has been made and the benefits of drug therapy have been determined. The intial data base should include assessment of the patient's ability to perform self-care tasks. Loss of independence in self-care activities can be psychologically upsetting to patients especially those with progressive degenerative changes in their conditions. Assessment of self-concept including self-esteem and body image is particularly important. Depression may also be present and should be identified so that an individualized nursing care plan can be developed.

Assessment of the patient's symptoms should be completed to serve as a baseline for the monitoring of therapy as well as to individualize nursing care. The patient should be assessed for symmetrical involvement of the joints, particularly of the hands, feet, knees, shoulders, hips, elbows, and ankles. The appearance of affected and unaffected areas should be documented including the presence of pain, inflammation (heat, redness, swelling), morning stiffness, nocturnal pain, limitation of motion, weakness of muscles, atrophy of muscles, muscle strength including grips, and the degree of self-care ability or disability.

Changes in symptoms in relation to time of day or activity should be explored. For example, patients with degenerative joint disease may complain of achiness or increased feelings of tiredness through the day with increased use of the affected joints. Patients with rheumatoid arthritis may complain of morning stiffness that decreases as the day progresses.

Patients should be assisted with the preparation for laboratory and roentgenogram studies often indicated for the medical diagnosis or monitoring of the various types of arthritis. Erythrocyte sedimentation rate, rheumatoid factor, complete blood counts (anemia is associated with rheumatic conditions), and serum electrolytes as well as radiographic examination to determine bone and joint destruction are often indicated in addition to other tests or diagnostic procedures.

Drug therapy is directed at the reduction of pain, inflammation, and deformities associated with the arthritic condition. The first agent of choice is aspirin followed by other salicylates and then the other NSAIDs. These drugs have antiinflammatory and analgesic effects that can vary from patient to patient, and it is not unusual for patients to require a trial of various agents before a suitable drug is found. The nursing history should identify previous hospitalizations, past successes with nondrug therapy (e.g., diet, rest, exercise, heat and cold, occupational or physical therapy), and past successes or failures with specific drug regimens.

Initial assessment should include a detailed drug history to identify possible sensitivity, contraindications, cautions, potential drug interactions, and individual drug-taking patterns and abilities before drug therapy is initiated.

SENSITIVITY

Allergic reactions to aspirin and the other NSAIDs can occur with some degree of regularity, producing hives, asthma, rhinitis, rash, or anaphylaxis, which can be fatal. Hypersensitivity reactions are more commonly encountered in patients with nasal polyps, a history of asthma, or COPD.

CONTRAINDICATIONS

NSAIDs including aspirin are contraindicated in patients with known hypersensitivity to a specific agent or to related compounds as well as in active peptic ulcer disease. It is important to note that nonaspirin NSAIDs are generally contraindicated in patients allergic to aspirin.

See the Nursing Drug Digest for contraindications associated with specific agents.

CAUTIONS

These drugs should be used with caution in patients receiving anticoagulant therapy with coumarin-like medications. They should also be used with caution during pregnancy because prostaglandins may be reduced by the NSAIDs thus affecting uterine contractions. Their use in women who are breastfeeding has not been fully evaluated.

Patients, especially the elderly, with concurrent renal or hepatic dysfunction should be closely monitored with newer NSAIDs.

See the Nursing Drug Digest for specific cautions associated with each agent.

DRUG INTERACTIONS

Because NSAIDs are generally highly bound to serum albumin, they can interact with other highly protein bound drugs (e.g., coumarin-type anticoagulants, phenytoin, oral hypoglycemic agents). NSAIDs can displace or be displaced by one another or by other drugs.

In addition, many of these drugs can inhibit platelet adhesiveness and thus can potentiate the effects of anticoagulants.

See Clinically Significant Drug Interactions.

ADMINISTRATION

Virtually all of the NSAIDs are administered orally in either tablet, capsule, or solution form. Some agents, however, (e.g., aspirin and indomethacin) are also available in rectal suppositories. Oral agents should be taken with meals and a full glass of water to reduce gastric irritation. They should never be taken on an empty stomach. It is important to note that enteric-coated tablets should not be taken with antacids or milk because the coating can be destroyed.

NSAIDs are usually administered three or four times a day. An advantage of agents with a long half-life (e.g., naproxen, piroxicam, sulindac) is that they can be used less frequently, usually twice a day. The dosage of a particular NSAID must be individualized for each patient with the initial dose being at the lower end of the average dose range with incremented increases tailored to the individual patient's response.

Continued.

GENERAL NURSING IMPLICATIONS—cont'd

Nursing of patients requiring nonsteroidal antiinflammatory drugs—cont'd

ADMINISTRATION—cont'd

Although newer NSAIDs can be administered concomitantly with aspirin, a reduction in levels of a number of these agents has been reported with concurrent use of aspirin, although it is unclear if this is associated with reduced effectiveness. Other agents (e.g., indomethacin, ketoprofen) can be administered in suppository form for relief of morning stiffness or nocturnal pain. Phenylbutazone is indicated for conditions with limited duration (e.g., gouty arthritis) and is often discontinued after 1 week of treatment because of its association with sodium and fluid retention and bone marrow depression.

See the Nursing Drug Digest for specific information regarding the administration of individual agents.

MONITORING PATIENT RESPONSE
Therapeutic response

Monitor patients for reduction of pain and inflammation, duration of morning stiffness, onset of fatigue, number and degree of joint involvement, bilateral grip strength, range of motion of joints, number of clinically active joints, ring size of involved hand joints, time required to walk 50 feet, and other effects as associated with the need for NSAID therapy. Monitoring is important because drug efficacy can vary in individual patients, and patients may require a trial of various agents before the most suitable agent is found. If response is poor, the drug is discontinued and another drug is tried. It is important to note that usually 3 to 4 weeks of therapy is required to assess benefit and potential of a specific agent for long-term use. Indomethacin may not achieve maximum therapeutic benefit for arthritis for 10 to 14 days on a given dose; naproxen may take 7 to 10 days for full therapeutic benefit. Aspirin's initial effect is seen in 48 to 72 hours after the first dose. When an aspirin dosage change is made, 3 to 4 days is often required before a change in effect can be noted because the half-life is usually prolonged at doses greater than 3 gm per day.

It is important to note that suppression is usually incomplete with these agents, and true remission or retardation or halting of progressive joint damage cannot usually be anticipated.

Monitoring should include comparison to baseline laboratory data. Radiographic changes should be followed, as should the history of the amount of NSAID and analgesics ingested because this can indicate effectiveness of therapy.

Exacerbations and remission should be carefully documented along with the patient's classification of functional capability in self-care.

Adverse side effects

The use of NSAIDs is associated with gastrointestinal, hematologic, renal, hepatic, and CNS effects and with various sensitivity reactions. Other effects are outlined in Adverse/Side Effects of Nonsteroidal Antiinflammatory Drugs. It is important that patients be monitored for these effects as well as assisted in the management of troublesome effects, especially when long-term therapy is indicated.

Gastrointestinal effects

Monitor patients for gastric irritation, nausea, dyspepsia, vomiting, diarrhea, and constipation.

Gastrointestinal effects can be minimized by administering NSAIDs with food and a full glass of water, milk, or antacids unless contraindicated. Various oral dosage forms are available; thus monitoring is important in relation to the selection of dosage forms tolerated best by the patient (e.g., capsules, enteric-coated tablets, chewable tablets, time-sustained tablets). Patients should be encouraged to avoid alcohol and to report troublesome gastric upset to the health care provider.

Hematologic effects

Monitor CBC, hemoglobin, and hematocrit, and observe for prolonged bleeding time and blood dyscrasias.

Monitor for bleeding associated with decreased platelet counts associated with the use of many NSAIDs: bruising, petechiae, bleeding gums, prolonged clotting time after minor injury, and frank gastrointestinal bleeding (black tarry stool, melena, hematemesis).

Other hematologic effects occurring with some NSAIDs (e.g., phenylbutazone) include bone marrow depression, aplastic anemia (especially in the elderly), and agranulocytosis (especially in younger patients). Monitor for pallor, unexplained fever, sore throat, lymphadenopathy, mouth sores, and other signs of blood dyscrasias.

All of the newer NSAIDs can cause prolongation of prothrombin time, but clinically significant bleeding is uncommon. These effects still require careful monitoring.

Renal effects

NSAIDs or their metabolites are excreted mainly by the kidneys. Because acute renal failure has been associated with prostaglandin inhibition in the kidney caused by these agents the nurse should monitor for oliguria, proteinuria, and elevated creatinine levels and BUN.

Debilitated and elderly patients or patients with congestive heart failure, cirrhosis, chronic renal failure, or systemic lupus erythematosus or patients using diuretics appear more likely to develop acute renal failure associated with the use of NSAIDs.

In addition, these drugs (e.g., phenylbutazone, ibuprofen) are associated with sodium and water retention, which can lead to congestive heart failure. Therefore the nurse should monitor serum electrolytes, edema, and blood pressure. Adequate fluid intake must be maintained and salt intake reduced.

Patients receiving NSAIDs for prolonged periods of time require periodic monitoring of renal function.

Hepatic effects

The NSAIDs have been associated with hepatotoxicity. Monitor for anorexia, nausea, right upper quadrant pain, jaundice, fever, clay-colored stools, cola-colored urine, and elevated liver

GENERAL NURSING IMPLICATIONS—cont'd

Nursing of patients requiring nonsteroidal antiinflammatory drugs—cont'd

Hepatic effects—cont'd

function tests: SGOT, SGPT, alkaline phosphatase, gamma glutamyl transpeptidase, and bilirubin. Because patients may be asymptomatic, monitoring of liver function tests is important.

Monitoring of serum drug levels is important in preventing hepatic toxicity. If observed, NSAIDs should be discontinued.

Central nervous system effects

Various NSAIDs can cause adverse effects affecting the CNS. Monitor for headache (throbbing pain, which can be frontal or temporal), light-headedness or dizziness, emotional lability, depression, sleep disturbances, drowsiness, guilt, and anhedonia.

Reassure patients that the headache is benign. Sometimes a decrease in total daily dose of the NSAID or the substitution of another drug may be indicated. Decreased mental functioning in the elderly may require discontinuation of the drug; thus monitoring is essential. It is helpful to some patients to take their medication at bedtime if possible. Adverse CNS effects are not unusual during initial therapy and may be temporary in some patients.

PATIENT EDUCATION

The patient and family as indicated should be fully informed about the nature of the patient's condition and treatment plan and should be involved in health care planning whenever possible. The patient and family should have an understanding of the anticipated course of therapy and medication regimen including nondrug therapy. When NSAIDs are indicated, they should know the exact name of the medication, its general action, purpose, dosage, administration, and adverse side effects, and how common adverse effects can be minimized or avoided. They should be able to monitor therapeutic response and identify signs that indicate that the health care provider should be notified.

The patient and family should understand that a trial of various agents may be required to find the most suitable agent for the patient's condition. They

should understand that achieving a therapeutic response can take up to 3 weeks with some agents and that failure to achieve a therapeutic response from one agent does not necessarily mean that another agent will not be effective. It is important that the patient understand that there is no cure for rheumatoid arthritis and that drug therapy is indicated to alleviate symptoms. Patients may require continued therapy for life to keep symptoms under control.

Because drug therapy is often used concurrently with other therapeutic treatment modalities including rest, exercise, splints, heat and cold applications, paraffin treatments, and diet, patients and their families need to understand the importance of following these therapeutic regimens along with drug therapy.

Rest is important to reduce strain on joints, and exercise prevents muscle atrophy and maintains function. Patients should understand that rest and exercise need to be balanced. Too much rest can further joint stiffness and swelling in rheumatoid arthritis, too much exercise can cause pain, flaring of symptoms, and exhaustion.

Splints may be indicated to immobilize joints, relieve muscle spasms, and maintain anatomic position especially at night.

Diet should be discussed, especially if anorexia or other gastrointestinal problems are present, so that adequate nutrition can be maintained and promoted and nutritional deficiencies prevented.

Misconceptions should be clarified and patients and families should be advised regarding alternative treatments. Pain, frustration, and lack of knowledge of fraudulent devices (which are costly) can prevent patients from seeking more effective health care. These factors should be readily discussed so that patients can make informed decisions regarding therapy. Patients should be advised to avoid self-treatment with unproved remedies sold over the counter or through the mail and to discuss the desire to try such

treatments with their health care provider. This is important because early diagnosis and proper treatment are more effective in preventing irreversible pain and disability.

Patients requiring NSAIDs need much psychologic support and often require assistance with the maintenance of self-care. When self-care abilities are affected by dysfunction associated with arthritic conditions, assistance in adapting to these changes in independence is required. The nurse should explore the use of self-help devices in promoting and maintaining self-care abilities. Physical therapy programs or referral to occupational therapy may be indicated. The Arthritis Foundation may be helpful in identifying resources and support groups. Self-esteem and autonomy as well as change in body image and loss of independence can cause depression, and assistance directed at these areas is essential. Psychologic counseling may be needed and referral should be explored as necessary.

Self-care should be assessed and monitored carefully in relation to the following classification system:

1. Complete function—the patient has the ability to perform normal self-care functions without assistance
2. Restricted function—the patient is able to function at most activities
3. Severe restriction—the patient is able to function minimally in the performance of self-care
4. Inability to perform self-care measures—the patient is confined to bed or a wheelchair

Patients requiring NSAIDs, particularly aspirin, need to understand the importance of adherence to their drug regimen and maintaining blood levels for therapeutic response. Patients must also understand the importance of laboratory appointments for the monitoring of blood levels of drugs when treatment is being titrated. Follow-up with the health care provider for monitoring of drug therapy and disease condition is also important.

GENERAL INSTRUCTIONS FOR DISCHARGE/OUTPATIENTS

NONSTEROIDAL ANTIINFLAMMATORY DRUGS

This drug is a nonsteroidal antiinflammatory agent used to reduce pain and swelling associated with arthritic conditions. This medication will not cure your condition but will help you control it as long as you continue to take the medication as directed.

Take this medication as prescribed with food (a snack), milk, or a full glass of water. An antacid (low sodium) can also be taken with this medication to help prevent stomach irritation and upset. If stomach upset or indigestion persists or becomes troublesome even when these measures are taken, notify your health care provider.

If you are using a suppository form of this medication, be sure to ask your nurse to assist you with its proper insertion. Obtain a separate instruction sheet to refer to when needed.

Store capsules, tablets, and solutions of this medication in a dark dry place. Refrigeration is not necessary.

Store suppositories in the refrigerator out of the reach of children.

Before taking this medication, notify your health care provider if you have bleeding problems, heart disease, kidney problems, or stomach ulcers.

This medication can take up to 2 to 3 weeks before you notice its effect. This is usual. Do not become discouraged and do not stop taking the drug or increase the dosage or take it more often than recommended. This can cause harmful effects.

Some drugs can cause unwanted or side effects in some patients. Notify your health care provider if you notice blurred vision, swelling in the legs or ankles, a skin rash, ringing in the ears, shortness of breath, redness of the face or arms, swelling of the neck, black bowel movements, unusual bleeding, fever, sore throat, or sores in the mouth.

Do not take this drug with alcohol because stomach irritation can occur.

This drug can cause some patients to become dizzy or light-headed or have headaches. Do not drive or operate machinery requiring alertness until you know how this drug affects you. If these effects occur, they usually disappear after you have been taking the drug for a while. If they persist or become severe, contact your health care provider immediately.

This medication can cause unwanted effects if taken with certain other medications. Do not start or stop taking any medications without first checking with your health care provider.

Do not take this medication if you are taking blood thinners or anticoagulants, antidiabetic drugs, or antiepileptic drugs. This drug can interact with these medications and cause unwanted effects.

If you are pregnant or intend to become pregnant while taking this medication or if you are nursing an infant, notify your health care provider before taking this medication. This drug may cause unwanted effects in unborn babies or nursing infants.

If you are taking this drug once a day and miss a dose, take it as soon as you remember then go back to your regular dosing schedule. If it is within 6 hours of your next dose, do not take this missed dose at all and do not double the next one. Resume your regular dosing schedule. If you have any questions, contact your health care provider.

If you are taking this drug twice a day and miss a dose within 2 hours, take it right away then go back to your regular dosing schedule. If you do not remember until later, do not take the missed dose at all and do not double the next dose. Just continue on your regular dosing schedule.

This medication was prescribed especially for you. Do not share this medication or give it to anyone else.

Keep this medication and all other medication out of the reach of children.

Because your condition will require long-term treatment, you will be required to take this medication for a long time. You will need to keep follow-up appointments with your health care provider so that your therapy can be monitored. You may also require periodic laboratory tests to check blood levels of your medication or blood counts because some of these medications can affect your blood. See your health care provider on a regular basis as indicated.

In addition to the General Instructions, if you are taking:

Naproxen

It is particularly important that you do *not* take this drug with alcohol because it can make you very drowsy.

Indomethacin

This drug can cause your urine or bowel movements to be green. Do not become alarmed; this is a usual effect of this drug.

Notify your health care provider before obtaining a smallpox vaccination.

Aspirin

Avoid over-the-counter medications. These can contain aspirin and may cause your blood level of aspirin to increase rapidly or even reach toxic levels. Always check with your health care provider before taking any other medication.

Do not take aspirin that has a strong vinegar smell. This indicates that the aspirin has decomposed into acetic acid (vinegar) and salicylic acid. Discard the medication down the toilet and obtain a fresh supply.

Do not take milk or antacids within 1 hour of enteric-coated tablets.

NURSING DRUG DIGEST

Medication (trade name)*	Indication	Usual dosage and administration	Dosage forms, preparation, and storage	Contraindications, cautions, and comments	Monitoring
★ **Alclofenac** Mervan	Rheumatoid arthritis Osteoarthritis	*Adults:* 500 mg PO t.i.d. Maximum: 3 gm/day	Tablet: 500 mg	May cause skin rashes (morbilliform, macular) May cause GI distress (epigastric pain, nausea, constipation)	Observe for skin rashes Monitor for GI distress
Aspirin Acetophen Anacin* Apo-Asen A.S.A. Bayer Bufferin* Easprin Ecotrin Encaprin Measurin Novasen Riphen-10 Zorprin	Rheumatoid arthritis Juvenile rheumatoid arthritis Osteoarthritis See also Chapter 17, "Analgesics and Narcotic Antagonists"	*Adults:* For inflammation: 2.4-6.0 gm/day PO in 4-6 divided doses Maximum: 10 gm/day Maintain blood levels between 15-30 mg/dl Chewable tablets may be swallowed whole *Children:* 60-125 mg/kg/day in 4-6 divided doses Do *not* administer milk or antacids within 1 hr of enteric-coated tablets	Capsule: 325 mg Tablet: 325, 650, 975 mg Chewable tablet: 65, 81, 150 mg Enteric-coated tablet: 325, 650 mg Suppository: 65, 130, 195, 325, 625 mg; 1 gm	*Contraindicated* in hemophilia, active ulcer disease, known exacerbation of asthma, thrombopenia, vitamin K deficiency, hypersensitivity May cause GI distress, tinnitus, and hearing loss	Observe for tinnitus and hearing loss Monitor for GI distress/ulcers Monitor for bleeding tendencies
Benoxaprofen Oraflex	Rheumatoid arthritis (*not* currently FDA approved—see Contraindications, Cautions, and Comments)	*Adults:* 400-600 mg/day PO Maximum: 1 gm/day *Elderly:* 300-400 mg/day PO Decrease dosage in impaired renal function	Tablet: 400, 600 mg	*Contraindicated* in patients allergic to aspirin *Removed* from market in August 1982 because of association with fatal hepatitis May cause GI ulceration May cause photosensitivity May cause onycholysis Commonly causes GI distress May cause hepatic toxicity, particularly in the elderly when high doses are used	Observe skin and nails for changes

Continued.

NOTE: For additional details regarding the individual agents listed in this table, see the text and other tables in this chapter.
*Indicates a multiple active ingredient product. For a complete listing of all active ingredients see the *Drug Reference Guide to Brand Names and Active Ingredients.*
★ Indicates that the drug is generally available only in Canada.
★ Indicates that the drug is generally available only in the United States.

NURSING DRUG DIGEST—cont'd

Medication (trade name)	Indication	Usual dosage and administration	Dosage forms, preparation, and storage	Contraindications, cautions, and comments	Monitoring
Choline and magnesium trisalicylate Trilisate	Rheumatoid arthritis Osteoarthritis	*Adults:* For pain: 0.5-1.5 gm per dose PO Maximum: 3 gm/day Maintain serum salicylate levels at 15-30 mg/dl Solution may be mixed with fruit juice before administration	Tablet: 500, 750 mg Solution: 500 mg/5 ml	*Contraindicated* in hypersensitivity to *non-*acetylated salicylates No significant platelet effects Generally well tolerated Use with caution in patients with chronic renal insufficiency and those with active ulcer disease	Observe for tinnitus, which indicates that the dose should be lowered
★ **Choline salicylate** Arthropan	Rheumatoid arthritis Osteoarthritis	*Adults:* For inflammation: 2-4 gm/day PO in single or divided doses Liquid dosage form can be mixed with fruit juices before administration Children: Over 12 years of age, same as adults	Solution: 500, 870 mg/5 ml Tablet: 500, 750 mg	*Contraindicated* in hypersensitivity to salicylates Generally well tolerated No significant effect on platelet adhesiveness	
❦ **Diclofenac** Voltaren	Rheumatoid arthritis Osteoarthritis	*Adults:* 75-150 mg daily PO in 3 divided doses administered with food Maintenance: 25 mg PO t.i.d. with food *Children:* Use *not* recommended because of limited information Do not administer milk or antacids within 1 hr of enteric-coated tablets	Enteric-coated tablet: 25, 50 mg Store at room temperature Protect from humidity	*Contraindicated* in hypersensitivity to diclofenac or any other NSAID and in patients with active ulcer disease May cause a variety of adverse effects including GI irritation, nausea, dizziness, headache, palpitation, angina, skin rashes, and edema	Observe for edema Observe for skin rashes
Diflunisal Dolobid	Mild to moderate pain Osteoarthritis	*Adults:* For pain: 1 gm initially, then 500 mg q.12h. PO For osteoarthritis: 250-500 mg PO b.i.d. with water, milk, or meals Maximum: 1500 mg/day Tablets should be swallowed whole May need to decrease dose in renal impairment	Tablet: 250, 500 mg	*Contraindicated* in hypersensitivity to any NSAID Highly protein bound (>99%) Use with caution in patients with active ulcer disease Eliminated primarily by renal excretion	

Drug (Trade names)	Uses	Dosage	Preparations	Adverse Reactions / Nursing Implications
Fenoprofen — Fenopron, Nalfon, Nalgesic	Rheumatoid arthritis; Osteoarthritis; Mild to moderate pain; Bursitis; Tendinitis	*Adults:* 300-600 mg PO t.i.d. or q.i.d. Downward titration of dose is possible when in remission. Maximum: 3200 mg/day. May be administered with food or milk to decrease GI distress	Capsule: 200, 300 mg; Tablet: 600 mg	*Contraindicated* in hypersensitivity to any NSAID. *Contraindicated* in severe renal failure. May cause dysuria, hematuria, interstitial nephritis, and nephrotic syndrome. May cause elevation of hepatic function tests. Use with caution in hepatic impairment. Common adverse effects include dyspepsia, nausea, vomiting, constipation, dizziness, pruritus, palpitations, and nervousness. GI distress is the most commonly encountered adverse effect. Inhibits platelet function, but to a lesser degree than does aspirin. May cause a variety of adverse effects including nausea, vomiting, diarrhea, dizziness, tinnitus, headache, and edema. Monitor renal function. Monitor hepatic function
Ibuprofen — Advil, Amersol, Motrin, Nuprin, Rufen	Rheumatoid arthritis; Osteoarthritis; Mild to moderate pain; Bursitis; Tendinitis	*Adults:* 300-600 mg PO t.i.d. or q.i.d. Maximum: 2400 mg/day. May be administered with food or milk to decrease GI distress	Tablet: 300, 400, 600 mg	*Contraindicated* in hypersensitivity to any NSAID. Use with caution in patients with active ulcer disease. Inhibits platelet function, but to a lesser degree than does aspirin

Continued.

NURSING DRUG DIGEST—cont'd

Medication (trade name)	Indication	Usual dosage and administration	Dosage forms, preparation, and storage	Contraindications, cautions, and comments	Monitoring
Indomethacin Indocid Indocin	Rheumatoid arthritis Osteoarthritis Ankylosing spondylitis Acute gout	*Adults:* For gout: 150-200 mg PO daily for 3-5 days For rheumatoid arthritis: 25-50 mg PO b.i.d. or t.i.d. NOTE: Doses greater than 200 mg/day generally do *not* increase therapeutic effect, but may significantly increase toxicity *Children:* Safe and effective dose not established *Elderly:* Start with lower doses	Capsule: 25, 50 mg Extended-release capsule: 75 mg Suppository: 100 mg	*Contraindicated* in hypersensitivity to any NSAID May exacerbate ischemic coronary disease May mask the typical signs of infection Commonly causes dyspepsia, nausea, headache, and dizziness Excreted in human breast milk Use with caution in patients with active ulcer disease May aggravate mental depression May cause retinal or corneal changes Use with *caution* in patients with impaired renal function	Observe for corneal or retinal changes Monitor for severe GI distress
🍁 **Ketoprofen** Orudis	Rheumatoid arthritis Osteoarthritis Ankylosing spondylitis	*Adults:* 100-200 mg PO daily in 3-4 divided doses; *or* 100 mg PR AM and PM Maximum: 300 mg/day *Children:* Safe and effective dose not established	Capsule: 50 mg Suppository: 100 mg Store suppositories below 30° C	*Contraindicated* in hypersensitivity to any NSAID *Contraindicated* in active peptic ulcers and active GI inflammatory diseases May mask signs of infection Commonly causes dyspepsia, nausea, vomiting, constipation, headache, fatigue, and skin rashes	

Drug	Uses	Dosage	Preparations	Contraindications/Cautions	Nursing considerations
★ **Magnesium salicylate** Analate Magan	Rheumatoid arthritis Osteoarthritis	*Adults:* 500-1200 mg PO b.i.d. or t.i.d. Maintain salicylate blood levels between 15-30 mg/dl *Children:* Safe and effective dose not established	Tablet: 325, 500, 600, 650 mg Store at room temperature Protect from light	*Contraindicated* in severe renal impairment No significant antiplatelet effects Use with caution in patients with impaired hepatic function or active ulcer disease Magnesium salicylate is less irritating to the GI tract than is aspirin	Observe for GI distress Monitor hemoglobin and hematocrit periodically
★ **Meclofenamate** Meclomen	Rheumatoid arthritis Osteoarthritis	*Adults:* 100-400 mg PO daily in 3-4 divided doses *Children:* Safe and effective dose not established	Capsule: 50, 100 mg Store at room temperature Protect from moisture and light	*Contraindicated* in hypersensitivity to meclofenamate or any other NSAID and in patients with active ulcer disease *Not* recommended by manufacturer as initial therapy because of GI side effects Commonly causes dyspepsia, nausea, vomiting, diarrhea, flatulence, skin rash, headache, and dizziness	
Mefenamic acid Ponstan Ponstel	Mild to moderate pain	*Adults:* 500 mg PO initially, followed by 250 mg PO q.6h. PRN for up to 7 days Decrease dose in renal failure *Children:* Safe and effective dose not established *Elderly:* Start with lower doses	Capsule: 250 mg	*Contraindicated* in hypersensitivity to any NSAID *Contraindicated* in ulceration or chronic inflammation of the GI tract Commonly causes diarrhea, which can be so severe as to necessitate stopping the drug Use with caution in patients with preexisting renal disease	

Continued.

NURSING DRUG DIGEST—cont'd

Medication (trade name)	Indication	Usual dosage and administration	Dosage forms, preparation, and storage	Contraindications, cautions, and comments	Monitoring
Naproxen Anaprox Naprosyn Novonaprox	Rheumatoid arthritis Osteoarthritis Ankylosing spondylitis Juvenile rheumatoid arthritis Mild to moderate pain Bursitis Tendinitis Acute gouty arthritis	*Adults:* For arthritis: 250-375 mg PO AM and PM Maximum: 1000 mg/day For pain: 250-1250 mg daily For gout: 750 mg PO initially, then 250 mg q.8h. *Children:* For juvenile arthritis: 10 mg/kg/day PO in 2 divided doses	Tablet: 250, 275, 375, 500 mg Store at room temperature in light-resistant containers	*Contraindicated* in hypersensitivity to any NSAID Use with caution in active ulcer disease Excreted in human breast milk Commonly causes constipation, dyspepsia, nausea, headache, dizziness, drowsiness, itching, skin rashes, edema, and tinnitus	Observe for sore throat, fever, and oral lesions, which may indicate blood dyscrasias
Oxyphenbutazone Oxalid Oxybutazone Tandearil	Moderately severe rheumatoid arthritis Acute therapy for severe osteoarthritis Ankylosing spondylitis Acute gout Acute arthritis of shoulder Bursitis	*Adults:* For gout: 400 mg PO initially, then 100 mg q.4h. For arthritis: 300-600 mg/day PO in 3-4 divided doses for initial therapy Maintenance: 100-400 mg/day PO Maximum: 400 mg/day Administer with food or milk to decrease GI distress *Children:* Safe and effective dose not established *Elderly:* Start with lower doses	Tablet: 100 mg	*Contraindicated* in patients hypersensitive to oxyphenbutazone or phenylbutazone *Contraindicated* in blood dyscrasias, active ulcer disease, and active inflammatory disease of the GI tract *Not* indicated for initial therapy because of severe toxicity Should *not* be used as simple pain reliever Highly protein bound (>98%)	Observe for anemia and black tarry stools, which may indicate GI bleeding Monitor hematologic tests for indications of bleeding or dyscrasias

Drug	Uses	Dosage	Preparations	Contraindications/Side effects	Nursing considerations
Phenylbutazone Azolid Butagesic Butazolidin Butone Malgesic Neo-Zoline Novobutazone Phenbutazone	Moderately severe rheumatoid arthritis Acute therapy for severe osteoarthritis Ankylosing spondylitis Acute gout Acute arthritis of shoulder Bursitis	*Adults:* For arthritis: 300–600 mg/day PO in 3–4 divided doses for initial therapy Maintenance: 100–400 mg/day PO For gout: 400 mg PO initially, then 100 mg q.4h. (for maximum of 7 days) *Children:* Safe and effective dose not established *Elderly:* Start with lower doses Administer with food or milk to decrease GI distress	Tablet: 100 mg Capsule: 100 mg Store in tight, light-resistant container	*Contraindicated* in patients hypersensitive to phenylbutazone or oxyphenbutazone *Contraindicated* in blood dyscrasias, active ulcer disease, and active inflammatory disease of the GI tract *Not* indicated for initial therapy because of severe toxicity Should *not* be used as a simple pain reliever Highly protein bound (>98%)	Observe for sore throat, fever, and oral lesions, which may indicate blood dyscrasias Observe for anemia and black tarry stools, which may indicate GI bleeding Monitor hematologic tests for indications of bleeding or dyscrasias
Piroxicam Feldene	Rheumatoid arthritis Osteoarthritis	*Adults:* 20 mg/day PO *Children:* Safe and effective dose not established	Capsule: 10, 20 mg	*Contraindicated* in hypersensitivity to any NSAID Commonly causes gastric distress, nausea, decreased hemoglobin, and decreased hematocrit	Observe for signs of anemia
★ **Salsalate** Arthra-G Disalcid Duragesic Mono-Gesic	Rheumatoid arthritis Osteoarthritis	*Adults:* 3000 mg/day PO in 2–3 divided doses Maintain salicylate blood levels between 15–30 mg/dl *Children:* Safe and effective dose not established	Capsule: 500 mg Tablet: 325, 500, 750 mg	*Contraindicated* in hypersensitivity *No* significant antiplatelet effects Salicylic acid, salsalate's primary metabolite, is excreted in human breast milk Can cause GI disturbance and hearing loss Can be used with caution in aspirin-sensitive patients	

Continued.

NURSING DRUG DIGEST—cont'd

Medication (trade name)	Indication	Usual dosage and administration	Dosage forms, preparation, and storage	Contraindications, cautions, and comments	Monitoring
Sodium salicylate Alysine Entrosalyl S-60 Uracel 5	Mild to moderate pain	*Adults:* 325-975 mg PO t.i.d. or q.i.d. Maintain salicylate blood levels between 15-30 mg/dl *Children:* Safe and effective dose not established Do *not* administer milk or antacids within 1 hr of enteric-coated tablets	Tablet: 325, 650 mg Enteric-coated tablet: 325, 650 mg Store at room temperature Injectable: 1000 mg	*Contraindicated* in hypersensitivity to salicylates, active ulcer disease, severe hepatic disorders, severe renal disorders, and severe vitamin K deficiency *Not* recommended for use with patients on sodium restriction Each 325 mg tablet contains 46 mg of sodium No reports of bronchospasm Excreted in human breast milk May cause GI distress and edema	Monitor for fluid retention Observe for tinnitus and hearing loss Monitor for GI distress and ulcers Monitor for bleeding tendencies
Sulindac Clinoril	Rheumatoid arthritis Osteoarthritis Ankylosing spondylitis Acute painful shoulder Acute gouty arthritis	*Adults:* 150-200 mg PO b.i.d. with food Maximum: 400 mg/day *Children:* Safe and effective dose not established	Tablet: 150, 200 mg	*Contraindicated* in hypersensitivity to any NSAID Use with caution in history of active ulcer disease Only NSAID that does *not* affect renal prostaglandins Sulfide metabolite appears to be the active principle Commonly causes gastric pain, dyspepsia, nausea, diarrhea, constipation, skin rash, dizziness, and headache	
Tolmetin Tolectin Tolectin DS	Rheumatoid arthritis Osteoarthritis Juvenile rheumatoid arthritis	*Adults:* 400 mg PO t.i.d. or q.i.d. Maximum: 2000 mg/day *Children:* 15-30 mg/kg/day PO in 3-4 divided doses May be administered with food or milk to decrease GI distress	Tablet: 200 mg Capsule: 400 mg	*Contraindicated* in hypersensitivity to any NSAID Use with caution in patients with active ulcer disease False positive test for proteinuria	Observe for fluid retention

Zomepirac Zomax	Mild to moderately severe pain (orthopedic pain, osteoarthritis pain) (*not* currently FDA approved—see Contraindications, Cautions, and Comments)	*Adults:* 50-100 mg PO q.4-6h. PRN	Tablet: 100 mg	*Contraindicated* in patients allergic to aspirin *Removed* from market March 1983 because of anaphylactoid reactions, including several reported fatal reactions Commonly causes GI distress May cause tinnitus and hearing loss	Each tablet contains 18 mg sodium and each capsule 36 mg sodium May prolong bleeding time May cause edema Commonly causes nausea, dyspepsia, GI distress, diarrhea, abdominal pain, flatulence, vomiting, headache, hypertension, and dizziness Monitor for GI distress Observe for hearing loss

BIBLIOGRAPHY

Arthritis: an overview of current treatment. *About Your Medicines*, 1983, *3*(4), 1-2.

Arthritis comes in many forms. *About Your Medicines*, 1983, *3*(3), 5-6.

Clive, D.M., & Stoff, J.S. Renal syndromes associated with nonsteroidal antiinflammatory drugs. *New England Journal of Medicine*, 1984, *310*, 563-572.

Ehrlich, G.E. Other NSAIDs of choice for rheumatoid arthritis. *Drug Intelligence and Clinical Pharmacy*, 1984, *18*, 39-41.

Hadler, N.M. The argument for aspirin as the NSAID of choice in the management of rheumatoid arthritis. *Drug Intelligence and Clinical Pharmacy*, 1984, *18*, 34-38.

Hodge, N.A. Management of degenerative joint disease and rheumatoid arthritis. Parts I & II. *Drug Store News*, January 1984, Lesson 679-401-84-01.

Hodge, N.A. A review of drug treatment modalities for the arthritic patient: Part II. *Drug Store News*, January 1984, Lesson 679-401-84-02.

Markenson, J.A. Antiarthritic drugs: a comparative overview. *Drug Therapy*, January 1981, 45-57.

McDuffie, F.C., & Benzaia, D. Arthritis update for pharmacists. *Pharmacy Times*, December 1980, 30-37.

Miller, D.R. Combination use of nonsteroidal antiinflammatory drugs. *Drug Intelligence and Clinical Pharmacy*, 1981, *15*, 3-7.

Miller, S.B. NSAIDs: examining therapeutic alternatives. *Geriatrics*, 1982, *37*(3), 70-78.

Parker, W.A. Pharmacotherapy of rheumatoid arthritis. *Canadian Pharmaceutical Journal*, November 1981, 411-417.

Pfeiffer, F.G. Drug treatment of rheumatoid arthritis. Part I. *Drug Store News*, 1982, Lesson 679-401-82-03.

Pfeiffer, F.G. Drug treatment of rheumatoid arthritis. Part II. *Drug Store News*, 1982, Lesson 679-401-82-04.

Poirier, T.I. Reversible renal failure associated with ibuprofen: case report and review of the literature. *Drug Intelligence and Clinical Pharmacy*, 1984, *18*, 27-32.

Porter, R.S. Factors determining efficacy of NSAIDs. *Drug Intelligence and Clinical Pharmacy*, 1984, *18*, 42-51.

Pritchard, R. The pharmacist as adviser to the arthritic patient. *Drug Merchandising*, December 1982, *28*, 30, 64.

Strand, C.V., & Clark, S.R. Adult arthritis, drugs and remedies. *American Journal of Nursing*, 1983, *83*(2), 266-269.

Toxicity of nonsteroidal anti-inflammatory drugs. *The Medical Letter*, 1983, *25*(Issue 628), 15-16.

Remittive and Miscellaneous Agents Used to Treat Rheumatic Diseases and Gout

Frederick G. Pfeiffer

Medications discussed in this chapter

Remittive agents
  Aurothioglucose
  Azathioprine
  Cyclophosphamide
  Dimethyl sulfoxide
  Gold sodium thiomalate
  Hydroxychloroquine
  Penicillamine

Miscellaneous agents (corticosteroids)
  Dexamethasone
  Methylprednisolone
  Prednisone
Agents used to treat gout
  Allopurinol
  Colchicine
  Probenecid
  Sulfinpyrazone

The remittive agents including gold, penicillamine, and hydroxychloroquine; cytotoxic agents; and corticosteroids are a second line of drugs used in the treatment of arthritic conditions nonresponsive to the nonsteroidal antiinflammatory drugs (NSAIDs) or other treatment modalities. Gout is primarily treated with the uricosuric agents (e.g., probenecid, sulfinpyrazone) and the xanthine oxidase inhibitor allopurinol, which inhibits uric acid production. Gouty arthritis is also treated with the various NSAIDs, which are discussed in the body of this chapter as well as more specifically in Chapter 58.

REMITTIVE AGENTS

Gold salts (aurothioglucose and gold sodium thiomalate)

Pharmacodynamics. Each product contains 50% elemental gold, therefore the similarities of the two are much greater than their differences. Aurothioglucose is a suspension in oil whereas thiomalate is water soluble. Gold salts are not true analgesics independent of reducing joint inflammation. The exact cellular mechanism for reducing inflammation is not known at present, although possible mechanisms include (1) inhibition of lysosomal enzymes, (2) inhibition of phagocytosis by white blood cells (WBCs), (3) suppression of cellular immunity reaction of lymphocytes, (4) prevention of synthesis of prostaglandins, and (5) reduction of immunoglobulin concentration in the synovial fluid. Gold's antiinflammatory response is more consistent when the patient has active arthritis progressing to ultimate joint damage.

Pharmacokinetics. Gold salts are poorly and inconsistently absorbed from the GI tract when given orally. The aqueous product is absorbed more rapidly when given IM in contrast to aurothioglucose. After intramuscular administration, gold reaches peak plasma levels (Cp) in about 4 hours, and gold salts are 95% bound to serum albumin. The half-life is extremely long and related to the cumulative dose. The apparent plasma half-life is 7 days after 2 to 3 injections, whereas after 4 months of therapy, the half-life is about 3 months. About 75% of a dose is eliminated by the kidney, although with long-term use renal elimination is slow.

Adverse reactions. Dermatologic reactions consist of skin rashes and exfoliative dermatitis. Skin rash can be exacerbated by sun exposure. Usually the less serious rashes are transient, improving within 48 to 72 hours even with continued therapy. Exfoliative dermatitis usually is heralded by pruritus or stomatitis. This more serious reaction requires a 33% to 50% dose reduction and may need to be treated with systemic corticosteroids. In general, dermatologic reactions occur most often after a cumulative dose of 300 mg or more.

Nephrotoxicity from gold salts can be manifested by mild proteinuria or frank nephrotic syndrome. Usually the patient will be asymptomatic. This effect is not dose related or related to plasma levels of gold.

Appropriate monitoring parameters from the urinalysis include presence of (1) red blood cell (RBC) casts, (2) RBCs, and (3) protein in excess of 5 mg/dl. Fortunately, actual nephrotic syndrome resulting from gold salts is rare. Managing these renal signs and symptoms involves discontinuing the gold if the patient excretes more than 2 gm in 24 hours. The gold salt regimen may be restarted when the urine is clear. Reinstitution of gold therapy is usually at about 50% of the previous dose.

Hematologic side effects include *thrombocytopenia* or neutropenia. Thrombocytopenia is usually defined as a platelet count of less than 100,000/mm³. It appears that the onset of this may be delayed for several months after starting therapy. The proposed mechanism for the thrombocytopenia is shortened platelet survival time rather than direct bone marrow suppression. The patient may also complain of stomatitis or metallic taste. Treating thrombocytopenia includes close monitoring of platelet counts and stopping the gold therapy. Some patients may require 60 mg daily of prednisone or its equivalent.

Neutropenia, which is defined as a neutrophil count of less than 1500, can also result from gold salt therapy. Data are contradictory regarding any dose relationship. Symptoms of unexplained pharyngitis, fever, or lymphadenopathy may occur, especially if the decrease in white blood cell count is rapid. Managing neutropenia clinically requires discontinuation of gold therapy; in some severe cases lithium carbonate may help raise the white blood cell count.

Drug interactions. Penicillamine, a chelating agent, can mobilize gold from the synovial fluid thus reducing its effectiveness. This interaction may be more important if the patient is taking higher doses of penicillamine. Since phenylbutazone can also cause bone marrow suppression, concomitant gold therapy can cause additive toxicity.

Dosage regimen and comments. An initial test dose is 10 mg IM. The following week the patient undergoes a usual predose complete blood count (CBC) and urinalysis, then is given a 25 mg dose IM. The patient receives 50 mg weekly after the CBC and urinalysis until (1) toxicity occurs, (2) a total dose of 800 to 1000 mg is reached, or (3) there is remission of symptoms. Once remission has occurred, the interval between doses is lengthened. Fifty milligrams is given every 2 weeks for 4 to 6 doses, then 50 mg every 3 weeks for 4 to 6 doses. A maintenance schedule is usually 50 mg every month or every 6 weeks as the final step in the dose titration. When the patient has a flare-up of rheumatoid arthritis, the regimen is started back at 50 mg weekly until the next remission. Some clinicians discontinue the gold after an arbitrary period of time, such as 12 to 18 months.

Even after gold salts are stopped, there can be thrombocytopenia or leukopenia because of the drug's long half-life. The possible immunosuppression caused by gold can mask some signs or symptoms of infection. Gold salts can cause a *nitritoid reaction* (i.e., flushing, syncope, fever, giddiness) during the first few months of therapy. If a patient is taking tolmetin concurrently with this drug, the sulfosalicylic acid test for *proteinuria* can be falsely positive. Gold therapy requires patience and compliance since the therapeutic benefit may not be apparent for several months after therapy is started. If the vial of gold is cloudy or discolored beyond pale yellow, it should be discarded.

Auranofin

Pharmacodynamics. Oral *chrysotherapy* from auranofin may provide an alternative to parenteral gold therapy. It appears that auranofin affects immunoglobulins and lysosomes similar to parenteral gold.

Pharmacokinetics. Auranofin is absorbed from the GI tract after oral administration. At steady state, the plasma level of gold is about 0.6 µg/ml and the auranofin is about 50% protein bound. The apparent plasma half-life ranges from 17 to 25 days. The major route of elimination for auranofin is fecal elimination in contrast to 75% renal elimination of parenteral gold.

Adverse effects. Gastrointestinal effects appear to be the most common adverse effects. Diarrhea and nausea with vomiting are the main symptoms. Diarrhea from auranofin may resolve with continued therapy. There are no data regarding a plasma level or dose relationship at present. If the diarrhea is severe or persistent, the patient may require loperamide or diphenoxylate to prevent fluid and electrolyte losses. If this is unsuccessful, the auranofin may have to be stopped.

It appears that hematologic toxicity and nephrotoxicity are much less common with auranofin than with parenteral gold. More data, however, are needed to determine a true comparison.

Drug interactions. Apparently penicillamine can bind oral gold in a similar manner to parenteral gold. Diarrhea from the fenamates may be potentiated with concurrent auranofin therapy.

Dosage regimen and comments. An initial dose of 3 mg twice daily appears to be reasonable. The recommended maximum dose will probably be 9 mg per day in divided doses. No specific monitoring parameters have been established at present. Monthly CBC and urinalysis would seem prudent until the spectrum of adverse side effects is better delineated.

If the lack of toxicity continues, auranofin may replace parenteral gold in the treatment of most patients with rheumatoid arthritis. Diarrhea from auranofin is probably not related to the total daily dose, but this is still unclear. Actual parameters for stopping auranofin have not been established at this time.

Penicillamine

Pharmacodynamics. Penicillamine is not an analgesic or antipyretic and has no effect on platelet adhesiveness. The exact mechanism of penicillamine in relation to rheumatoid arthritis is not known. Possibilities include (1) reduction of immunoglobulins, (2) stabilization of lysosomal membranes, and (3) interruption of WBC chemotactic stimuli.

Pharmacokinetics. Little is known about the metabolic fate of penicillamine in humans. After oral administration, penicillamine achieves peak Cp in 1 to 2 hours and is about 80% bound to plasma proteins. Apparently, the major route of excretion is by the kidneys.

Adverse reactions. Similar to parenteral gold therapy, penicillamine can cause various dermatologic reactions. There are two distinct skin rashes, an early and a late skin rash that may occur from this drug. The early rash is so-named because it usually occurs in the first 2 months of therapy. Its appearance is typically a pruritic, maculopapular rash resembling a classic penicillin rash. Treating this usually involves antihistamines, topical corticosteroids, or only observation. This rash is an indication to temporarily suspend therapy and reinstitute it with a smaller dose. The late rash is characterized by a scaly, severely pruritic reaction resembling eczema or psoriasis. The onset of this rash is usually after 4 to 6 months of therapy and may be related to frequent large increments in dosage. Because its appearance may be delayed for several years after starting penicillamine, it is easily confused with other conditions. This late rash responds to discontinuing the penicillamine and restarting the drug at a lower dose.

Nephrotoxicity from penicillamine has a similar presentation to that from parenteral gold. Usually the onset of the proteinuria is within the first 18 months of therapy. It appears to be more common when the patient is taking 750 mg per day or more for longer than 6 months. Urinalysis for protein is usually monitored weekly for the first 2 to 3 months and monthly thereafter. Some clinicians believe that proteinuria may be prevented if the total daily dose is 300 mg or less. Fortunately, the nephrotic syndrome caused by penicillamine is rare. Managing the proteinuria involves a 24-hour urine collection for protein; if this exceeds 2 gm/24 hours the penicillamine needs to be stopped. Finding RBC casts is another indication for discontinuing the penicillamine therapy.

Thrombocytopenia from penicillamine may be mild or severe. The onset of decreased platelet levels is typically unpredictable. The onset may occur in the first 4 weeks or may not occur until after years of therapy. Apparently it is related neither to a cumulative dose nor to a particular daily dose. Complete blood counts with platelet counts are usually monitored weekly for the first 2 to 4 months of therapy and then less frequently. Unexplained bleeding or easy bruising is an indication for a platelet count. If the platelet count is less than 75,000 to 100,000/mm^3, the penicillamine therapy needs to be stopped. Resolution usually occurs within 7 to 10 days after the drug is discontinued.

Drug interactions. See section under parenteral gold.

Dosage regimen and comments. Initially a dose of 125 mg daily is given. Increases of 125 mg per day are attempted every 8 to 12 weeks. Probably the dose at which no further benefit can be displayed is 1.5 gm daily, but because of serious adverse effects some clinicians consider the ceiling to be 375 to 500 mg daily. It is necessary to give penicillamine a 3 to 4 month therapeutic trial to determine the presence or the lack of therapeutic benefit.

Strict compliance is extremely important with this drug since it has a narrow therapeutic index. Loss of taste is not an indication for the patient to stop taking penicillamine. Zinc sulfate usually is effective in helping restore taste, but as little as 5 mg of zinc may inhibit the drug's effectiveness in rheumatoid arthritis. When assessing studies with penicillamine, be careful to consider only those in which the drug was used for at least several months. Some patients with proteinuria undergoing renal biopsy show immune complex nephritis. Some clinicians believe that penicillamine can directly increase serum cholesterol by an unknown mechanism. Similar to gold, this drug has no intrinsic analgesic activity; thus it usually needs to be used concomitantly with an NSAID.

Hydroxychloroquine

Pharmacodynamics. Hydroxychloroquine, an antimalarial, is not an analgesic or antipyretic per se but it reduces inflammation in patients with arthritis. Proposed mechanisms are stabilization of lysosomal membranes and inhibition of lymphocyte responsiveness in synovial fluid.

Pharmacokinetics. After oral administration hydroxychloroquine is almost completely absorbed from the GI tract. The major route of elimination is by the kidney with about 60% being excreted as unchanged parent drug. The apparent plasma half-life is from 5 to 7 days with an unknown half-life in synovial fluid.

Adverse reactions. Gastrointestinal adverse side effects are primarily bloating, flatulence, and diarrhea alternating with constipation and nausea. Bloating and constipation with nausea probably result from decreased smooth muscle contractions of the GI tract. These may be more common in the elderly and are probably related to excessive peak Cp. Management of these may involve only reassurance since these symptoms may subside over 1 to 2 weeks with continued therapy. Reducing the peak Cp by giving more doses per day is also helpful in most cases.

Ophthalmologic side effects are of two major types—corneal keratopathy and *retinopathy*. The former is not related to the latter and does not result in blindness. Keratopathy is not an indication to stop hydroxychloroquine therapy. It is still unknown whether this is related to cumulative dose, blood level, or total daily dose. Treating keratopathy involves reassurance of the patient that keratopathy does not lead to blindness.

On the other hand, retinopathy may cause blindness. Symptomatic patients may have blurred vision, night blindness, and scotomas. Apparently this adverse side effect is related to elevated Cp and total daily dose. The onset of the retinopathy is usually after at least 6 months of therapy and may be reversible if it is found in the early stages. Several high-risk factors have been identified, including (1) renal insufficiency, (2) concurrent administration of thioridazine, and (3) old age. Prevention appears to be the only form of management available at present. Prevention measures consist of (1) using dark sunglasses, (2) regular eye examinations every 4 to 6 months, (3) monitoring urinary pH to avoid an alkaline urine since hydroxychloroquine is reabsorbed in a basic urine and (4) patient education and follow-up to assure strict compliance to the prescribed regimen.

Pigmentary changes of the skin may be associated with both the cumulative dose and peak Cp. There may also be bleaching or graying of scalp hair. Managing this effect is through reassurance of the patient, but the resolution can be extremely slow after hydroxychloroquine is stopped.

Drug interactions. There are no adverse drug interactions documented at present.

Dosage regimen and comments. An initial dose of 2 mg/kg daily is based on *ideal body weight*. Increases of 1 mg/kg per day are given every 3 to 4 weeks up to a maximum of 4 to 6 mg/kg daily. It is important

to note the lack of a loading dose recommendation. When hydroxychloroquine therapy is stopped the dosages should probably be tapered. Compliance can be improved in most patients by giving the drug once daily.

Similar to both gold and penicillamine, hydroxychloroquine is slow to induce remission. It may take 8 weeks before any significant subjective improvement is noted in rheumatoid arthritis. It may even take 3 to 4 months for any objective improvement.

In contrast to previous information, the presence of psoriasis is not an absolute contraindication to the use of hydroxychloroquine. A family history for retinitis pigmentosa is a contraindication to antimalarial therapy. Two hundred milligrams of hydroxychloroquine is roughly equivalent to 250 mg of chloroquine but hydroxychloroquine is the only antimalarial approved for rheumatoid arthritis by the FDA.

Doses of 25 mg/kg in the pediatric patient have been lethal since there is no known antidote successful in overdose management. Compliance with the exact prescribed dose is mandatory to reduce the chance of serious adverse reactions, including retinopathy.

Azathioprine

Pharmacodynamics. Azathioprine is an immunosuppressive agent used in recalcitrant rheumatoid arthritis. This drug has no intrinsic analgesic or antipyretic effects. Proposed mechanisms of action include a reduction of lymphocyte responsiveness in synovial fluid. Also there is evidence that azathioprine reduces WBC chemotaxis and migration into synovial fluid. Unlike the NSAIDs, this drug does not reduce platelet adhesiveness.

Pharmacokinetics. After oral administration absorption of azathioprine is almost complete with peak Cp being reached in about 2 hours. The apparent plasma half-life of this drug is short since red blood cells and the liver convert azathioprine into its active metabolite, 6-mercaptopurine. There are no established data to correlate azathioprine Cp with either toxicity or therapeutic response.

Adverse reactions. Adverse GI side effects include vomiting and diarrhea and are probably related to the total daily dose. Stomatitis and unusual taste may be associated symptoms. Managing these effects are difficult, but they may respond to reducing the total dose by 25% to 33% per day.

Hepatotoxicity from azathioprine usually consists primarily of cholestatic jaundice. The most appropriate monitoring parameters are abdominal pain, pruritus, jaundice, and elevated levels of alkaline phosphatase and gamma glutamyl transpeptidase (GGT).

High-risk patients appear to be alcoholics and those concurrently taking chlorpromazine. It is still unclear whether this effect is dose related or simply a hypersensitivity reaction. Some patients have *eosinophilia* with a skin rash also. Treating this usually requires discontinuation of the azathioprine at least temporarily.

Hematologic adverse reactions are usually leukopenia and thrombocytopenia. The former reaction appears to be more common. The proposed mechanism is direct bone marrow suppression rather than a decrease in platelet survival. No high-risk patients have been identified at present except for patients receiving immunosuppressives concurrently in cancer chemotherapy. Indications for suspending therapy are a white blood cell count less than 3000 or a platelet count of less than 75,000.

Drug interactions. Allopurinol inhibits the metabolism of azathioprine, requiring a 65% to 75% reduction in the dose of the latter. This seems to be preventable and related to the doses of both drugs.

Dosage regimen and comments. A beginning dose of 0.5 mg/kg daily is recommended for severe rheumatoid arthritis. Increments of 1 mg/kg daily every 7 to 10 days are used clinically. A recommended maximum daily dose is 3 mg/kg based on ideal body weight.

Strict contraception should be practiced during and for 4 to 6 months after stopping azathioprine therapy. If a patient has an abrupt decrease in urinary output, the plasma level of 6-mercaptopurine can increase dramatically. Because of immunosuppression, signs and symptoms of infection can be reduced or masked in some patients. Weekly CBC with platelet counts need to be monitored for the first 3 to 6 months and monthly thereafter. Leukopenia occurs more frequently than thrombocytopenia, and this may be heralded by stomatitis and *eosinophilia.*

Cyclophosphamide

Pharmacodynamics. Cyclophosphamide is an alkylating agent used primarily in cancer chemotherapy. It has no intrinsic analgesic or antiinflammatory action. Cyclophosphamide inhibits mitosis in WBCs and is a general immunosuppressant. This medication may be beneficial in rheumatoid arthritis because of its reduction of WBC chemotaxis in synovial fluid.

Pharmacokinetics. Cyclophosphamide is well absorbed after oral administration with peak Cp being reached in about 1 hour. Hepatic metabolism is the major route of elimination. Cyclophosphamide is excreted in human breast milk. From 20% to 25% of this drug is eliminated unchanged in the urine.

Adverse effects. Gastrointestinal side effects are extremely common. These include nausea, vomiting, diarrhea, and anorexia. These effects appear to be dose related or caused by high peak Cp. No high-risk patients have been identified. Management of these effects is difficult, although reducing the daily dose by 25% is sometimes helpful.

Alopecia is another distressing adverse side effect that appears to be more common with cyclophosphamide than with azathioprine. This effect appears to be associated with large daily doses. Loss of body hair may also accompany the loss of scalp hair. Nothing has been found successful in the management of this problem.

Anovulation, azoospermia, and menstrual disturbances also may occur with cyclophosphamide. Patients using higher doses have a higher frequency of these adverse reactions. These effects are uncommon or rare with azathioprine in comparison with cyclophosphamide. No high-risk patients have been demonstrated to date. Treating these effects in a couple desiring pregnancy involves discontinuation of the cyclophosphamide therapy. These effects are usually reversible after stopping the drug in the majority of patients using it for rheumatoid arthritis.

Hemorrhagic cystitis is another serious adverse reaction to cyclophosphamide. This may result from a toxic metabolite rather than the parent drug. There are no data describing a relationship to cumulative dose, but it may be related to high peak Cp concentrating in the bladder. Managing this reaction involves prevention through patient education. Methods used to prevent this adverse effect include: (1) maintaining a urinary pH above 6.5; (2) drinking 1 to 2 L of water daily; (3) voiding before bedtime; and (4) taking the total dose in the morning to prevent accumulation during sleep.

Drug interactions. Concurrent administration of phenobarbital increases the formation of cyclophosphamide metabolites, which may increase the frequency or severity of hemorrhagic cystitis. Cyclophosphamide may antagonize the *uricosuric* effects of probenecid or sulfinpyrazone.

Dosage regimen and comments. There are two dosage regimens used. The high-dose regimen has an initial dose of 1.5 mg/kg daily based on ideal body weight. The maintenance dose for this first regimen is the same or slightly less. In the low-dose regimen the initial dose is 1 mg/kg per day with a back titration to 0.5 mg/kg daily for maintenance therapy. Weekly CBC and urinalysis need to be monitored for the first 3 to 4 months of therapy and then less frequently. Leukopenia is more common than thrombocytopenia.

Some patients also need an antiemetic before each dose of cyclophosphamide to reduce severe nausea and vomiting.

Hemodialysis will remove cyclophosphamide from the body. Strict contraception needs to be practiced during and for at least 6 months after cyclophosphamide is stopped. Amenorrhea may last for several months after discontinuing the drug. Reversible pigmentation of the skin and fingernails may occur with chronic therapy. Chronic alcohol use may increase the chance of hepatotoxic reactions from this drug. Infections may not present classically because of immunosuppression from this medication. The nadir of WBC usually occurs within 2 to 3 days of a dose, but may be delayed for up to 3 to 4 weeks when a patient is receiving long-term therapy.

Levamisole

Pharmacodynamics. This investigational drug was originally synthesized as an antiparasitic agent and is still used as such. Levamisole does not appear to have any intrinsic analgesic, antipyretic, or antiinflammatory effects, although it may reduce inflammation by stimulating the release of cortisol from the adrenal gland. Apparently, levamisole can improve WBC phagocytosis and T-lymphocyte responsiveness in patients with rheumatoid arthritis.

Pharmacokinetics. After an oral dose of 150 mg, a peak Cp of 700 µg/ml is reached in about 2 hours. The major route of elimination of levamisole is by hepatic metabolism. No active metabolites have been identified.

Adverse effects. Loss of taste and smell occurs often with levamisole. These effects may be related to the total weekly dose of the drug and may be a source of noncompliance for some patients. No high-risk patients have been identified. Stomatitis may also occur. It is not preceded by a metallic taste in all patients, but it does need to be assessed at routine intervals.

Hematologic reactions include *agranulocytosis* and leukopenia. The former is potentially the most dangerous adverse reaction. High-risk patients include women and patients with high rheumatoid factor titers. Apparently there is a specific effect on the bone marrow called maturation arrest. Managing the agranulocytosis includes monitoring the WBC count and differential and discontinuing therapy if the WBC count is less than 3000/mm³.

Another interesting adverse effect is the development of a flulike syndrome. Patients complain of myalgia, nausea, fever, and malaise. Because this syndrome can be the prodrome of agranulocytosis, the patient needs to be alert to these symptoms. Apparently this is a hypersensitivity reaction that is not dose related. When this reaction continues for several days, levamisole therapy should be stopped.

Drug interactions. High doses of prednisone may increase the risk of infection when given concurrently with levamisole. This appears to be related to the daily dose of the prednisone.

Dosage regimen and comments. An initial dose of 150 mg weekly (given in a single dose) is given for 4 to 6 months. Increasing the daily dose beyond 150 mg is not recommended. If after 4 to 6 months there is not sufficient response, 150 mg daily is given 2 days a week (i.e., Monday and Thursday) for 3 to 4 months. The recommended maximum dose is 150 mg daily given 3 days per week; the drug is not given on two consecutive days. The exact duration of therapy is yet to be determined. A differential WBC count needs to be monitored 10 to 12 hours after each dose for the first 3 to 6 months of levamisole therapy. In contrast to gold or penicillamine, there appears to be no need for periodic urinalysis.

If the exact mechanism of levamisole is discovered, the cause of rheumatoid arthritis may be the same. It is impossible to predict which patients will respond to levamisole.

MISCELLANEOUS AGENTS

Corticosteroids (prednisone, dexamethasone, methylprednisolone)

Pharmacodynamics. Prednisone is the prototype for these drugs. It is not a true remission-inducing drug for rheumatoid arthritis in contrast to gold salts, penicillamine, hydroxychloroquine, and perhaps azathioprine. Prednisone has no intrinsic analgesic or antipyretic activity.

Pharmacokinetics. Prednisone needs to be metabolized to prednisolone to be active for reducing inflammation. It is absorbed orally and reaches peak Cp about 3 hours after it is metabolized. The apparent plasma half-life for prednisolone is about 18 hours, allowing for once-daily dosing in most patients. The major route of elimination is by hepatic metabolism.

Adverse reactions. Cushing's syndrome is a major adverse effect associated with the corticosteroids and consists of "buffalo hump," moon-face, hirsutism, and adrenal insufficiency. This effect is related to the duration of pharmacologic doses of systemic corticosteroids (i.e., 15 mg prednisone; 2.5 mg dexamethasone or its equivalent). Alternate-day therapy may reduce the severity and frequency of this syndrome.

Osteopenia or osteoporosis occurs even with alternate-day therapy. Pathologic fractures appear to be the major sequelae of this adverse reaction. Several high-risk factors have been identified. These include post-menopausal women, cumulative dose of 3 gm of prednisone or more, and patients aged 50 years or older. Attempts at managing osteopenia consist of the administration of sodium fluoride, calcium, and vitamin D with increased exercise.

Corticosteroid-induced ulcers were historically described as "silent, easily perforated, and recurrent." It has now been established that there are no definitive data to support a direct cause-and-effect relationship between corticosteroid use and ulcers. From 6% to 8% of patients with rheumatoid arthritis have an associated peptic ulcer disease regardless of the drug therapy for arthritis. It appears to be more common for a patient to have a current ulcer *diathesis* exacerbated rather than an ulcer produced de novo. Antacids are not indicated for prophylaxis.

Subcapsular cataracts from corticosteroids are related to both daily dose and duration of therapy. No high-risk patients have been identified at present except for possibly the elderly. Eye examinations need to be performed every 4 to 6 months to detect the appearance of cataracts. Growth of cataracts can be slowed when corticosteroids are discontinued. Cataract formation appears to be irreversible in most patients.

Hypothalamic-pituitary-adrenal (HPA) axis suppression occurs with long-term use of systemic corticosteroids. Manifestations of this include (1) hypotension, (2) anorexia, (3) fatigue, (4) myalgia, and (5) emotional depression. Supplemental doses of corticosteroids for patients undergoing surgery are usually needed (hydrocortisone, 100 mg the night before; 100 mg every 8 hours the day of surgery; and 100 mg for the first postoperative day). Preventing HPA axis suppression is attempted by using one daily dose at 8 AM and using an appropriate tapering schedule when the corticosteroids are stopped. Dexamethasone has such a long half-life that even alternate-day therapy will not prevent HPA axis suppression.

Drug interactions. Barbiturates increase the metabolism of corticosteroids similar to that with phenytoin. Therapeutic doses of aspirin increase the renal elimination of corticosteroids, thereby reducing their efficacy.

Dosage regimen and comments. Prednisone (5 mg daily) is given orally for 2 to 3 weeks. Increases up to a daily maximum of 10 mg are usually used for patients with rheumatoid arthritis. In the treatment of rheumatoid arthritis, alternate-day therapy is not always successful.

Cortisone, like prednisone, is a prodrug that needs to be metabolized to its active metabolites. Acute therapy for less than 7 days usually does not cause any hyperglycemia, cataracts, or osteopenia. Divided daily doses of systemic corticosteroids lead to more adrenal suppression even when the total daily doses are the same. Intraarticular injections of corticosteroids appear to cause fewer systemic side effects when these doses are limited to fewer than four injections annually. (See Chapter 65, "Corticosteroids and Adrenal Steroid Inhibitors.")

MEDICATIONS USED FOR GOUTY ARTHRITIS

For treating acute attacks of *gout* several medications have been shown to be useful. These include colchicine, phenylbutazone, indomethacin, naproxen, ibuprofen, and sulindac. Acute gouty attacks respond better if the patient takes the medication within 24 hours of the onset of the characteristic pain. The pain will cease whether the patient uses medication or not, but the pain-free intervals become much shorter than with no effective therapy.

Hyperuricemia is not a prerequisite for the development of acute gout, and in fact many patients have asymptomatic hyperuricemia caused by diuretics. A disturbance in the equilibrium between synovial fluid urate and serum uric acid levels appears to be important in the precipitation of an acute attack. This correctly implies that even a reduction in serum urate levels can induce acute gouty arthritis. With appropriate therapy, an attack of gout should begin to resolve in 48 hours. For purposes of discussion of drugs that treat both gout and rheumatoid arthritis, only the dosage regimen may be different; therefore refer to the chapter discussing each drug at length.

Colchicine

Pharmacodynamics. Colchicine has no intrinsic analgesic or antipyretic activity. It does not change either serum uric acid or urinary uric acid levels. Colchicine is not a classical uricosuric or NSAID; rather it is a cellular toxin that disrupts cellular mitosis and reduces mobility of WBCs. The drug is able to inhibit WBC phagocytosis and chemotaxis in synovial fluid. Also it may reduce degranulation of lysosomal membranes preventing this enzyme from damaging the joint.

Pharmacokinetics. After oral administration colchicine is rapidly absorbed from the GI tract. With a 1 mg dose a peak Cp of 320 ng/ml is attained within 30 to 60 minutes. Enterohepatic recirculation causes a second peak about 3 hours after administration. Intracellular WBC concentrations may be 20 times the plasma level after several days of therapy. The major route of elimination is fecal, with only about 10% eliminated unchanged in the urine.

Adverse reactions. Gastrointestinal adverse effects are usually vomiting, nausea, and anorexia. These are so predictable that they can be used as the end-point in determining the dosage of colchicine. These effects appear to be related to the cumulative dose and may be more common in patients using triamterene concomitantly. In patients using colchicine for an acute attack, vomiting is an end-point of therapy. It is unusual for a patient using a prophylactic dose of 1 to 1.5 mg daily to have vomiting, nausea, or anorexia.

Hematologic effects include thrombocytopenia and leukopenia. These appear to be dose related in most instances. Elderly patients may be at a higher risk for these effects. Monitoring CBC's at 2 to 4 week intervals is the best form of management during the first 2 to 3 months of long-term therapy.

Alopecia may occur from long-term use of colchicine. Apparently this is related to the cumulative dose rather than the daily dose. No high-risk patients have been identified. In the majority of cases alopecia is reversible within 3 months after the drug is stopped.

Megaloblastic anemia may occur because of the malabsorption of vitamin B_{12}. Monitoring parameters include anemia, elevated mean corpuscular volume (MCV), and mental confusion. It appears to be more common in the elderly and patients using 2.5 mg or more of colchicine daily. Managing this syndrome is similar to treating vitamin B_{12} deficiency with replacing the stores of this vitamin through IM injections of vitamin B_{12} (cyanocobalamin).

Drug interactions. No adverse drug interactions are known at present.

Dosage regimen and comments. For an *acute attack* an initial dose of 2 mg IV is used. This dose needs to be diluted in at least 20 ml of normal saline when given IV. Following the initial dose, 0.5 mg is given every 6 hours to a maximum of 4 mg IV in 24 hours or until relief occurs or toxicity results. Giving colchicine IV seems to cause less severe vomiting. When colchicine is used orally, a dose of 0.5 mg is given every 1 to 2 hours to a maximum of 4 mg in 24 hours or until relief or toxicity occurs. If the patient has responded to this drug previously, one half of the total dose needed in previous attacks is a reasonable starting point, with 0.5 mg increments every 1 to 2 hours.

As *prophylaxis* of an acute attack colchicine is given orally 0.5 mg two or three times daily for 2 to 6 months

while the patient is being started on allopurinol or a uricosuric. Some clinicians give 0.5 to 2 mg daily or every other day for extended periods of time. This dosage schedule is still unapproved and controversial.

Colchicine is less effective if the patient starts taking it 24 hours or longer after the onset of an attack. Effective response means that colchicine reduces signs and symptoms of inflammation within 24 hours and the patient has complete relief in 3 to 4 days. Apparently colchicine can lower the seizure threshold in patients with a seizure history. When a gout patient undergoes surgery, colchicine needs to be given 72 hours before the procedure and for 3 to 5 days postoperatively. An acute attack can even be prevented if the patient recognizes a prodrome. Prodromal signs include (1) mood changes, (2) local pruritus over the joint, and (3) unexplained diffuse discomfort around the joint. Colchicine may falsely elevate SGOT and SGPT values, which are commonly used liver function tests. If IV colchicine extravasates, nerve and tissue damage can be severe. Unexplained sore throat, fever, and lymphadenopathy may indicate agranulocytosis from colchicine.

Phenylbutazone in acute gout

Dosage regimen. Beginning with 300 mg orally followed by 100 to 200 mg four times daily, phenylbutazone is effective in most patients with acute gout. About 80% of patients will respond if the acute attack has begun within 72 hours. Subsequent doses are 100 mg three or four times daily for 24 to 48 hours; then phenylbutazone is abruptly stopped (see Chapter 58, "Nonsteroidal Antiinflammatory Drugs").

Indomethacin in acute gout

Dosage regimen. An initial dose of 50 mg followed by 50 mg three or four times daily is usually given the first day. Following the initial dose, 50 mg is given three times daily until relief occurs, up to a maximum of 4 more days of therapy. This drug is more effective when it is started within 72 hours of the onset of pain. Indomethacin can be given with food if GI side effects are intolerable (see Chapter 58, "Nonsteroidal Antiinflammatory Drugs").

Ibuprofen in acute gout

Dosage regimen. An initial dose of 1800 to 2400 mg is used in most patients. The following day and daily thereafter a dose of 1200 mg every 8 hours is given. The recommended maximum duration of therapy is 3 to 4 days at 3200 to 3600 mg per day (see Chapter 58, "Nonsteroidal Antiinflammatory Drugs").

Naproxen for acute gout

Dosage regimen. An initial loading dose of 750 mg orally is used clinically. On subsequent days 250 mg three times daily is used. Relief of the acute attack usually occurs within 3 days of beginning naproxen therapy. The recommended maximum number of days used in the acute attack has not been determined (see Chapter 58, "Nonsteroidal Antiinflammatory Drugs").

Fenoprofen for acute gout

Dosage regimen. An initial dose of 800 mg every 6 hours is given on the first day. Subsequent doses used are 300 to 400 mg every 6 hours until relief or up to an arbitrary maximum of 3 days of therapy (see Chapter 58, "Nonsteroidal Antiinflammatory Drugs").

Sulindac for acute gouty arthritis

Dosage regimen. The dosage for sulindac is 200 mg twice daily for 3 to 7 days until relief occurs. The initial and maximum dose are the same. No loading dose is necessary (see Chapter 58, "Nonsteroidal Antiinflammatory Drugs").

Piroxicam for acute gout

Dosage regimen. A dose of 40 mg once daily is given initially. Subsequent daily doses of 40 mg may be used for an arbitrary maximum of 5 days. The initial and maximum dose of piroxicam are the same (see Chapter 58, "Nonsteroidal Antiinflammatory Drugs").

MANAGEMENT OF CHRONIC GOUT

Drugs effective in the prophylaxis of chronic gout include probenecid, sulfinpyrazone, and allopurinol. These drugs reduce serum uric acid levels and can prevent the development of *tophaceous gout.* By disturbing the equilibrium between serum urate and synovial fluid urate, however, these drugs are capable of precipitating an acute attack during the first few weeks of therapy.

Allopurinol

Pharmacodynamics. Allopurinol is an effective xanthine oxidase inhibitor, which directly reduces the formation of uric acid. There are several specific indications for the use of this medication including (1) overproduction of uric acid (defined as 24 hour urinary urate levels of greater than 800 mg), (2) tophaceous gout, (3) renal insufficiency, and (4) history of kidney stones. Allopurinol reduces both serum and urinary uric acid levels. This drug has no intrinsic analgesic or antiinflammatory effects.

Pharmacokinetics. Allopurinol is well absorbed from the GI tract and reaches peak Cp in about 4 hours after oral administration. It is rapidly metabolized in the liver to oxypurinol, which is also a xanthine oxidase inhibitor. A unique feature of both of these drugs is that they are not protein bound at therapeutic doses. Oxypurinol has a serum half-life of 28 hours allowing for once daily dosing.

Adverse reactions. Cholestatic jaundice from allopurinol is probably not related to the duration of therapy but to drug plasma levels. Patients at highest risk include the elderly and those with renal insufficiency. The best monitoring parameters for this adverse effect are elevated alkaline phophatase, elevated GGT, jaundice, pruritus, and abdominal pain. The best form of management of this effect is by prevention and the close monitoring of the high-risk patient. Usually the dose of allopurinol needs to be reduced by 50% when this adverse effect occurs, but sometimes the drug must be stopped.

Skin rashes from allopurinol can assume many forms. The most serious is toxic epidermal necrolysis. This can be fatal and appears to be more common in patients using thiazide diuretics concurrently. If this serious effect occurs, the allopurinol must be discontinued.

Allopurinol is also capable of inducing an acute attack of gout. This is more common in patients who have had an acute attack in the last 6 months. This appears to be related to the total daily dose of allopurinol. Prevention of this involves giving colchicine prophylactically.

Drug interactions. When taken concurrently with allopurinol, the doses of azathioprine and mercaptopurine must be reduced by 75%. Allopurinol plus oral anticoagulants has produced hemorrhage because the metabolism of the oral anticoagulants is reduced.

Dosage regimen and comments. In the average adult an initial dose of 300 mg once daily is used. In the patient with renal insufficiency and in the elderly, the beginning dose is usually 200 mg daily. The goal of therapy is a serum urate level of less than 7 mg/dl. In practice, the maximum dose is usually no more than 600 mg per day.

In severe tophaceous gout allopurinol can be given in combination with maximum doses of a uricosuric such as probenecid.

Metallic taste is common, with or without nausea, but is not a reason for stopping allopurinol. Management of asymptomatic hyperuricemia with allopurinol must be weighed against the risks of long-term adverse side effects. Women who are pregnant or who intend to become pregnant need to alert their health care provider since the teratogenic potential of this medication is unknown. In order to dissolve *tophi,* 6 months of therapy is the minimum therapeutic trial. Patients taking ampicillin concurrently with allopurinol have a higher incidence of ampicillin rash.

Probenecid

Pharmacodynamics. Probenecid is an effective uricosuric that promotes renal tubular excretion of uric acid. This is not a classic antiinflammatory and has no intrinsic analgesic effects. Apparently probenecid also reduces the protein binding of urate, which promotes renal excretion. Several patients have noticed a slight to moderate diuresis during the first few days of therapy. The mechanism for this diuretic effect may be an increase in cortical renal blood flow.

Pharmacokinetics. Probenecid is completely absorbed from the GI tract. The apparent plasma half-life is about 8 hours with about 85% bound to plasma proteins. The plasma half-life increases as the dose increases and when allopurinol is given concurrently. Less than 5% is eliminated unchanged in the urine. Alkalinization of the urine beyond pH 6.5 increases the renal elimination of this drug.

Adverse reactions. Epigastric pain, nausea, and vomiting are the most common GI adverse side effects. These appear to be related to the daily dose of probenecid. The onset of these symptoms is usually within the first 2 weeks of therapy. It is important to differentiate these effects from those caused by colchicine, when colchicine and probenecid are taken together. Simply taking the doses 2 to 3 hours apart will help determine this. No high-risk patients have been identified. Managing these effects involves giving probenecid with a full glass of liquid or with meals. If this is not successful, the daily dose may be reduced by 25% in an attempt to alleviate these problems.

Precipitation of acute gout can occur in patients started on probenecid. The onset of this is more likely during the first 4 to 6 weeks of any dosage and in patients who have had an acute attack in the past 6 months. Apparently this is not dose related in terms of frequency, but may be related to the severity of the patient's condition. Managing this adverse effect is mainly directed at prevention with concurrent administration of colchicine. With each dosage change of probenecid the possibility of this adverse effect recurs.

Since probenecid promotes renal elimination of uric acid, patients may develop urate kidney stones *(urolithiasis)*. Apparently this effect is related to the daily dose of this drug. Patients with a personal or strong family history of urolithiasis probably should *not* receive any uricosuric, including probenecid.

Drug interactions. Probenecid decreases the renal elimination of indomethacin, penicillins, cephalothin,

and acetazolamide. The increase in plasma level of penicillin is used for benefit in the treatment of gonorrhea. Chlorpropamide taken concurrently with probenecid increases the hypoglycemic effect of the former. Aspirin, in doses of less than 2 gm daily, will raise serum urate levels in some patients, thereby antagonizing the therapeutic benefit of probenecid.

Dosage regimen and comments. An initial dose of 250 mg twice daily is used for the first 4 to 7 days of therapy. Increases of 500 mg per day every 10 to 14 days are given to a maximum of 1.5 gm twice daily. The goal of therapy is to reduce serum urate levels to 7 mg/dl or less without intolerable adverse side effects. Colchicine is given concomitantly, 0.5 mg twice daily, for the first 2 to 3 months to avoid an acute attack of gout.

Intermittent use of probenecid is likely to precipitate an acute attack of gout. Acidic urine (pH less than 6) promotes uric acid stone development. Probenecid is especially useful in underexcretors of uric acid determined by a 24-hour urine urate level of less than 600 mg. If a patient has been asymptomatic for a year, a careful back titration of 500 mg per day may be attempted. If this decrease in dosage is attempted, colchicine should be given concurrently to avoid an acute attack of gout. Back titration needs to be slow (i.e., 500 mg per day every 6 to 9 months). If a patient needs an analgesic while using probenecid, acetaminophen appears to be more acceptable than low doses of aspirin. In the patient with transient ischemic attacks, using dipyridamole alone is preferred to low doses of aspirin when probenecid is used concurrently.

Sulfinpyrazone

Pharmacodynamics. Sulfinpyrazone is an effective uricosuric facilitating renal tubular secretion of urate. Apparently sulfinpyrazone is not an analgesic and it is not effective for acute gouty arthritis. Although it is chemically related to phenylbutazone, it is not an effective antiinflammatory drug. Sulfinpyrazone reduces platelet adhesiveness and prolongs platelet survival, thus it is effective in the prevention of transient ischemic attacks.

Pharmacokinetics. After oral administration a peak Cp is reached in about 90 minutes. This medication is about 98% protein bound at therapeutic doses. The major route of elimination is through hepatic metabolism with about 30% being eliminated as the parent drug in the urine.

Adverse reactions. Gastrointestinal reactions include nausea, epigastric distress, and vomiting. These appear to be related to the daily dose. No high-risk patients have been identified at present. Managing these effects includes preventive measures and a dose reduction by about 25%.

Urolithiasis, the result of urinary accumulation of urate, occurs often and is probably dose related. Patients with a personal or strong family history of renal stones are not good candidates for sulfinpyrazone therapy.

Sulfinpyrazone may precipitate an acute attack of gout. The same information applies to this drug as to probenecid.

Drug interactions. Concurrent administration of colchicine and sulfinpyrazone may cause more thrombocytopenia in a dose-related manner. Managing this interaction involves separating the administration of these two drugs by at least 3 hours. Concurrent administration of tolbutamide and sulfinpyrazone may lead to serious hypoglycemia because of reduced metabolism of the oral hypoglycemic.

Dosage regimen and comments. An initial dose of 50 mg twice daily is given for 4 to 5 days. Increments of 100 mg per day are used every 7 to 10 days up to a suggested maximum of 800 mg daily. The goal of therapy is the same as that for probenecid. For most patients the usual maintenance dose is 300 to 400 mg daily. In the elderly patient the dose is decreased by 25% to 50% in most situations.

Strict compliance to the dose is important since the therapeutic index is narrow. Colchicine taken prophylactically will prevent precipitation of an acute attack of gout. Fluid intake may need to be changed in the patient with heart failure since this drug may cause fluid retention in these patients.

SUMMARY

Inflammatory arthritis refractory to nonsteroidal antiinflammatory drugs can be treated with one of several of the remittive agents discussed in this chapter. When therapeutic response is limited, miscellaneous agents including systemic corticosteroids can be used to treat the various arthritic conditions. When these are ineffective in controlling the disease condition, cytotoxic or investigational drugs may be required. Gout can be treated with various NSAIDs as well as uricosurics and the xanthine oxidase inhibitor allopurinol. With an understanding of the actions of the drugs used in the treatment of arthritic conditions and gout, as well as their more serious adverse side effects and potential for drug interactions, the nurse can better assist patients with their drug therapy regimens and monitor effects. The nurse will also be able to better plan individualized patient education programs in order to promote self-medication and self-monitoring abilities, which are especially important when patients are treated on an outpatient basis.

ADVERSE/SIDE EFFECTS OF REMITTIVE AND MISCELLANEOUS AGENTS USED TO TREAT RHEUMATIC DISEASES AND GOUT*

ALLERGIC REACTIONS

Anaphylaxis
Bronchial spasm (penicillamine)
Lupuslike reaction (penicillamine)
Nitritoid reaction (i.e., flushing, syncope [gold salts])
Rashes
Urticaria

CARDIOVASCULAR SYSTEM

Hypertension (corticosteroids)
Hypotension (gold salts, withdrawal of corticosteroids)

CENTRAL NERVOUS SYSTEM

Fatigue
Headache (hydroxychloroquine)
Myasthenia gravis (penicillamine)
Peripheral neuropathy (penicillamine)
Psychiatric changes (corticosteroids)

CUTANEOUS SYSTEM

Acne (corticosteroids)
Alopecia (azathioprine, colchicine, cyclophosphamide)
Bleaching of the scalp hair and eyebrows (hydroxychloroquine)
Eczema
Erythema nodosum
Exfoliative dermatitis (gold salts)
Pigmentation (cyclophosphamide, gold salts)
Pemphigus (penicillamine)
Pruritus
Rashes

GASTROINTESTINAL SYSTEM

Abdominal pain
Anorexia
Bleeding
Bloating
Colitis (gold salts)
Constipation
Diarrhea
Dyspepsia
Flatulence
Gastritis
Impaired taste—dysgeusia (penicillamine)
Metallic taste (gold salts)
Stomatitis
Vomiting
Ulceration

---

*See Chapter 11, "Drug Toxicity," for an overview of drug toxicity.

ADVERSE/SIDE EFFECTS OF REMITTIVE AND MISCELLANEOUS AGENTS USED TO TREAT RHEUMATIC DISEASES AND GOUT—cont'd

HEMATOLOGIC SYSTEM

Agranulocytosis
Aplastic anemia
Bone marrow depression
Eosinophilia
Leukopenia
Neutropenia
Pancytopenia
Reduced platelet adhesiveness
Shortened red blood cell life span
Thrombocytopenia

IMMUNE SYSTEM

Immunosuppression (azathioprine,
 cyclophosphamide, corticosteroids)

MUSCULOSKELETAL SYSTEM

Arthralgia (gold salts)
Aseptic bone necrosis
 (corticosteroids)
Compression fractures
 (corticosteroids)
Myalgia

Proximal muscle wasting
 (hydroxychloroquine)
Transient stiffness

METABOLIC AND ENDOCRINE SYSTEMS (corticosteroids)

Adrenal insufficiency
Cushing's syndrome
Hyperglycemia
Growth retardation in children
Impaired carbohydrate metabolism

OPHTHALMIC SYSTEM

Blurred vision
Cataracts (corticosteroids)
Corneal deposits
Corneal keratopathy
Photophobia
Retinopathy (hydroxychloroquine)
Reversible loss of red color vision
 (hydroxychloroquine)
Scotomas (hydroxychloroquine)

RENAL SYSTEM

Albuminuria
Decreased creatinine clearance
Hematuria
Hemorrhagic cystitis
 (cyclophosphamide)
Membranous glomerulonephritis
Nephrotic syndrome
Proteinuria
Red blood cell casts in urine
White blood cell casts in urine
White blood cells in urine

REPRODUCTIVE SYSTEM

Amenorrhea (cyclophosphamide)
Sterility (azathioprine,
 cyclophosphamide)
Vaginitis (gold salts)

CLINICALLY SIGNIFICANT DRUG INTERACTIONS*

Primary drug	Interacting drug	Possible effect(s)	Probable mechanism(s)
Allopurinol	Azathioprine	Increased azathioprine levels; possible bone marrow depression	Decreased metabolism
Allopurinol	Mercaptopurine	Increased mercaptopurine levels; possible bone marrow depression	Decreased metabolism
Allopurinol	Oral anticoagulants	Increased oral anticoagulant levels; possible bleeding	Decreased metabolism
Azathioprine	Allopurinol	Increased azathioprine levels; possible bone marrow depression	Decreased metabolism
Cyclophosphamide	Succinylcholine	Increased neuromuscular blockade	Decreased plasma cholinesterase activity
Corticosteroids (dexamethasone, methylprednisolone, prednisone)	Barbiturates	Decreased corticosteroid effect	Increased metabolism
Corticosteroids	Phenytoin	Decreased corticosteroid effect	Increased metabolism
Corticosteroids	Rifampin	Decreased corticosteroid effect	Increased metabolism
Probenecid	Dyphylline	Increased dyphylline levels	Decreased renal excretion
Probenecid	Methotrexate	Increased methotrexate levels	Decreased excretion
Probenecid	Penicillins	Increased penicillin levels	Decreased excretion
Sulfinpyrazone	Oral anticoagulants	Increased oral anticoagulant levels	Decreased metabolism
Sulfinpyrazone	Tolbutamide	Increased tolbutamide levels	Decreased metabolism

*See Chapter 10, "Drug Interactions," for an overview of drug interactions.

GENERAL NURSING IMPLICATIONS

Nursing of patients requiring remittive or miscellaneous agents used in the treatment of arthritis or gout

ASSESSMENT

Drug therapy should be initiated only after a complete assessment of the patient has been made and the benefits of drug therapy with the remittive or miscellaneous agents have been determined. The initial data base should include assessment of the patient's general health state, extent of arthritis or gout, and ability to perform self-care tasks. Loss of independence in self-care activities can be psychologically upsetting to patients, especially those who have progressive degenerative changes in their conditions. Assessment of self-concept including self-esteem and body image is particularly important. Depression may also be present and should be identified so that an individualized nursing care plan can be developed.

Assessment of the patient's present symptoms should be completed to serve as a baseline for the monitoring of therapy as well as to individualize nursing care. The patient should be assessed for symmetrical involvement of the joints, particularly the joints of the hands, feet, knees, shoulders, hips, elbows, and ankles. The appearance of affected areas should be documented including the presence of pain, inflammation (heat, redness, swelling), morning stiffness, nocturnal pain, limitation of motion, and muscle strength including grip and attention to weakness and atrophy of muscles.

Joint involvement should be identified and joints evaluated including range of motion and the presence of contractures. The degree of synovitis should be assessed as well as the presence of rheumatoid nodules. Joints should be palpated for tenderness and tenderness recorded on a scale of 0 to 3+. Ulnar deviation should be noted. A nutritional assessment should also be completed including body weight.

Patients should be carefully questioned regarding the history of adverse reactions to other medications including aspirin, the presence of tinnitus, gastrointestinal upset, history of gastric ul-

cer disease, the presence of visual changes, and characteristics of remissions or flares in condition. Patients should be generally inspected for signs of bruising, ecchymosis, skin rashes, scratches, erythema, and oral lesions. Dentures, if present, should be removed for oral assessment to inspect the palate for ulcers or sores. Psychosocial problems and sexual concerns should be assessed as well as coping abilities and emotional status.

Changes in symptoms in relation to time of day or activity should be explored. For example, patients with degenerative joint disease may complain of achiness or increased feelings of tiredness through the day with increased use of the affected joints. Patients with rheumatoid arthritis may complain of morning stiffness that decreases as the day progresses.

Patients should be assisted with the preparation for the laboratory and roentgenogram studies often indicated for the monitoring of the various types of arthritis. Erythrocyte sedimentation rate, rheumatoid factor, complete blood counts (anemia is associated with rheumatic conditions), and serum electrolytes as well as radiographic examination to determine bone and joint destruction are often indicated in addition to other tests or diagnostic procedures.

Because of the severity of the adverse side effects associated with the remittive and miscellaneous agents, specific baseline data are often indicated and should be obtained before drug therapy is started. For example, before gold or penicillamine treatment, baseline CBC with platelet counts and urinalysis are essential to monitor the serious adverse effects associated with these drugs including hematologic and renal toxicities. Baseline ophthalmologic studies are mandatory *before* the initiation of hydroxychloroquine therapy.

Drug therapy is directed at the reduction of pain, inflammation, and the progression of bone and joint degeneration. The nursing history should iden-

tify previous hospitalizations, past successes with nondrug therapy (e.g., diet, rest, exercise, heat and cold, occupational therapy, physical therapy) and past successes or failures with specific drug regimens including NSAIDs and remittive agents.

Initial assessment should include a detailed drug history to identify possible sensitivity, contraindications, cautions, potential drug interactions, and individual drug-taking patterns and abilities before drug therapy is initiated.

SENSITIVITY

Hypersensitivity reactions have been reported with the use of various remittive agents. It is important to note that sensitivity reactions can occur in any susceptible individual, and patients receiving any medication for the first time should be carefully monitored. It is important to note that penicillamine is associated with serious adverse effects and sensitivity reactions and that any interruption of therapy can result in renewal of an initial sensitivity reaction when therapy is resumed (see the Nursing Drug Digest for sensitivity reactions associated with specific agents).

CONTRAINDICATIONS

Remittive and miscellaneous agents are contraindicated in patients with known hypersensitivity to a specific agent (see the Nursing Drug Digest for contraindications to specific agents).

CAUTIONS

The remittive agents have been associated with serious gastrointestinal, renal, hematologic, and dermatologic toxicities. In addition, their use has not been fully evaluated in pregnant or nursing women. Thus these agents should be used with caution in patients with renal dysfunction, heart disease, blood dyscrasias, gastrointestinal disorders, and in the elderly as well as in pregnant or nursing women (see the Nursing Drug Digest for specific cautions associated with the use of each agent).

GENERAL NURSING IMPLICATIONS—cont'd

Nursing of patients requiring remittive or miscellaneous agents used in the treatment of arthritis or gout—cont'd

DRUG INTERACTIONS

The remittive and miscellaneous agents can interact with other drugs as well as with each other. For example, penicillamine can interfere with the absorption of pyridoxine (vitamin B_6) requiring the administration of supplemental pyridoxine to prevent neuropathies. Penicillamine can also cause gold to be mobilized from the synovial tissues resulting in a significant reduction in the therapeutic effect of the gold. Therefore these drugs should not be administered concomitantly.

A potentially lethal drug interaction is possible with the concomitant use of allopurinol and azathioprine. Allopurinol is a xanthine oxidase inhibitor and azathioprine requires xanthine oxidase for metabolism. Because of this effect, allopurinol can cause the accumulation of toxic levels of azathioprine necessitating a dose reduction of azathioprine *to 25%* of the original dose.

Barbiturates can increase the metabolism and clearance of corticosteroids after several days of concomitant therapy. Corticosteroids can also increase renal excretion of aspirin by increasing the glomerular filtration rate. Other drug interactions can also occur (see Clinically Significant Drug Interactions for interactions associated with the agents discussed in this chapter).

ADMINISTRATION

The remittive and miscellaneous agents are available in various dosage forms. Some drugs (e.g., penicillamine) are administered orally whereas others (e.g., gold) are administered intramuscularly. Corticosteroids can be administered orally, intramuscularly, or intraarticularly depending on the dosage form (see the Nursing Drug Digest for specific information regarding administration of these agents).

Dosage is also highly individualized, and various dosage regimens have been developed for specific agents. For example, gold is administered weekly after a test dose until therapeutic response or toxicities are noted. Once remission is achieved, intervals between injections are gradually lengthened.

Penicillamine is best taken orally on an empty stomach. Because it decreases pyridoxine absorption, daily administration of oral pyridoxine is also indicated.

Hydroxychloroquine can be administered once or twice daily depending on individual patient factors.

Corticosteroids can be administered orally, parenterally or intraarticularly. Intraarticular administration results in effects that are largely localized and mildly systemic. It is important to note that, although effective as adjunctive therapy in inflammatory arthritis, intraarticular injections should be restricted to 3 to 4 per year in any one joint and that patients should be encouraged to avoid overuse of a joint that has been injected. Because of their immunosuppressive effects, corticosteroids should *not* be injected into a previously infected joint.

Generally, because of the toxicities associated with these agents, administration should be completed *only* with careful monitoring of renal, hematologic, and gastrointestinal function.

See the Nursing Drug Digest as well as the body of the chapter for specific information regarding the administration of these agents.

It is important to note that investigational agents as well as cytotoxic agents (e.g., cyclophosphamide) should *not* be administered without a signed consent for drug treatment by the patient or legal guardian.

MONITORING PATIENT RESPONSE

Therapeutic response

Arthritic conditions

The therapeutic effects of remittive agents may not be apparent for several weeks (e.g., azathioprine) or months (e.g., hydroxychloroquine, gold, penicillamine) although serious adverse effects may occur at any time after therapy is initiated. Close monitoring is essential over this time so that therapy can be evaluated.

Although repair of damage done or cure does not occur with these agents,

remission is associated with the prevention of further joint destruction and reparative processes within and around the affected joint. Monitor for remission of active disease condition or flare-up:

- Decreased synovitis
- Decreased pain
- Decreased stiffness
- Decreased inflammation
- Decreased erythrocyte sedimentation rate
- Correction of associated anemia
- Decreased rheumatoid factor titer
- Regression of presenting rheumatoid nodules

Gout

Monitor for prompt termination of the acute attack and prevention of recurrent attacks, complications resulting from the deposition of urate crystals in joints or kidneys, and formation of uric acid renal stones.

Adverse effects

The use of remittive and miscellaneous agents in the treatment of arthritic conditions and gout is associated with serious adverse effects requiring careful monitoring. These effects mainly include gastrointestinal, hematologic, and renal toxicities.

Gastrointestinal effects

Monitor patients for nausea, vomiting, anorexia, diarrhea, constipation, and changes in taste (metallic taste associated with gold therapy, loss of sweet and salty taste associated with penicillamine).

Plan to prevent fluid and electrolyte imbalance or nutritional deficiencies associated with these effects, and plan to meet elimination requirements.

Hematologic effects

The use of the remittive agents and other miscellaneous agents is associated with serious hematologic effects including anemias, thrombocytopenia, leukopenia, and neutropenia associated with bone marrow depression. Monitor CBC and platelet count, and observe patients for pharyngitis, fever, lymphadenopathy, unusual bleeding, bruising, petechiae, pallor, and fatigue.

Continued.

GENERAL NURSING IMPLICATIONS—cont'd

Nursing of patients requiring remittive or miscellaneous agents used in the treatment of arthritis or gout—cont'd

Hematologic effects—cont'd

Monitor patients before therapy and at least every 1 to 2 weeks during therapy. Monitoring can be less frequent once response is established.

Renal effects

Nephrotoxicity is a serious adverse effect associated with the use of these agents.

Monitor urinalysis (proteinuria, RBC casts, hematuria), and observe patients for glomerulonephritis, and nephrotic syndrome.

Urine should be examined routinely and before each injection of gold. The elderly or patients with renal dysfunction should be monitored especially carefully.

Other effects

The remittive agents are also associated with various dermatologic toxicities including various skin rashes, exfoliative dermatitis, and alopecia. Skin rashes associated with gold therapy can be exacerbated by sun exposure. Penicillamine use has been associated with an early rash, which is a pruritic maculopapular rash resembling a classic penicillin hypersensitivity rash, and a late rash, which is a scaly pruritic rash resembling eczema or psoriasis. Hyperpigmentation or other pigmentation changes involving the skin and fingernails occurs with cyclophosphamide. Bleaching of the scalp hair or eyebrows can occur with hydroxychloroquine. Patients taking cyclophosphamide or azathioprine should be warned about hair loss and monitored for scalp as well as body hair loss.

Serious ophthalmic effects are also associated with the use of many of the remittive agents. Patients should be monitored for retinopathy, hyperpigmentation of the retina, and loss of vision for red objects, early signs of toxicity associated with hydroxychloroquine. These effects can be irreversible if not identified early and can progress even with discontinuation of the drug as a result of its prolonged half-life. Because patients are usually asymptom-

atic, ophthalmic examinations every 2 to 3 months during therapy are essential. It is also important to plan to minimize this effect by monitoring dosage regimens (adverse effects are associated with prolonged use at high doses) and encouraging patients to use dark glasses in bright sunlight since deposits of drug in the eye seem to impair the normal retinal defense mechanisms against bright light. In addition, monitor patients for complaints of visual glare and seeing fuzzy backgrounds, and halos around light. These symptoms are associated with corneal keratopathy, which is a reversible effect—unlike the retinopathy associated with this drug, which can lead to blindness.

Because of the seriousness of these adverse effects, careful monitoring is essential so that dosage regimens can be modified or the drug discontinued as indicated.

See Adverse/Side Effects of Remittive and Miscellaneous Agents Used to Treat Rheumatic Diseases and Gout in addition to the body of the chapter and the Nursing Drug Digest.

PATIENT EDUCATION

The patient and family as indicated should be fully informed about the nature of the patient's condition and treatment plan and should be involved in health care planning whenever possible. The patient and family should have an understanding of the anticipated course of therapy and medication regimen including nondrug therapy. They should know the exact name of the medication, its general action, purpose, dosage, administration, and adverse side effects and how common and less serious adverse effects can be minimized or avoided. They should be able to monitor for therapeutic response and for more serious adverse effects that indicate that the health care provider should be notified.

Course of therapy

The patient and family should understand the specific drug therapy regimen. They should understand that

therapeutic response can take from weeks to months with some agents. Patients often need much support to continue therapy because adverse effects can readily occur.

It is important that the patient understand that there is no cure for rheumatoid arthritis and that drug therapy is indicated to obtain remission and to minimize joint damage. It is important that the patient and family understand that continued therapy is required to keep symptoms under control.

Because drug therapy is often used concurrently with other therapeutic treatment modalities including rest, exercise, splints, heat and cold applications, paraffin treatments, and diet, patients and their families need to understand the importance of following these therapeutic regimens along with drug therapy.

Rest is important to reduce strain on joints, and exercise prevents muscle atrophy and maintains function. Patients should understand that rest and exercise need to be balanced. Too much rest can further joint stiffness and swelling in rheumatoid arthritis and too much exercise can cause pain, flaring of symptoms, and exhaustion.

Splints may be indicated to immobilize joints, relieve muscle spasms, and maintain anatomic position especially at night.

Diet should be discussed, especially if anorexia or other gastrointestinal problems are present so that adequate nutrition can be maintained and promoted and nutritional deficiencies prevented.

Patients with gout may require assistance in planning a diet to correct obesity, hypertriglyceridemia, and hypertension. They should understand the importance of maintaining adequate hydration in relation to the promotion of renal function as well as a well balanced diet devoid of purine-rich foods.

Misconceptions should be clarified and patients and families should be advised regarding alternative treatments

GENERAL NURSING IMPLICATIONS—cont'd

Nursing of patients requiring remittive or miscellaneous agents used in the treatment of arthritis or gout—cont'd

Course of therapy—cont'd

including investigational treatments (e.g., thoracic duct drainage, plasma pheresis). Pain, frustration, and lack of knowledge of fraudulent devices (which are costly) can prevent patients from seeking more effective health care. These areas should be readily discussed so that patients can make informed decisions regarding therapy. Patients should be advised to avoid self-treatment with unproved remedies sold over the counter or through the mail and to discuss the desire to try such treatments with their health care provider. This is important because proper treatment is more effective in preventing progressive damage and disability.

Patients using remittive and miscellaneous agents require much psychologic support and often require assistance with the maintenance of self-care. When self-care abilities are affected by dysfunction associated with arthritic conditions, assistance in adapting to these changes in independence is required. The nurse should explore the use of self-help devices in promoting and maintaining self-care abilities. Physical therapy programs or referral to occupational therapy may be indicated. The Arthritis Foundation may be helpful in identifying resources and support groups. Self-esteem and autonomy as well as change in body image and loss of independence can cause depression; assistance directed at these areas is essential. Psychologic counseling may be needed and referral should be explored as necessary. Because of the cost of frequent and long-term therapy as well as the cost of many of these drugs (e.g., gold salts), referral to social services may also be indicated.

Self-care should be assessed and monitored carefully in relation to:

1. Complete function—the patient has the ability to perform normal self-care functions without assistance

2. Restricted function—the patient is able to function at most activities

3. Severe restriction—the patient is able to function minimally in the performance of self-care

4. Inability to perform self-care measures—the patient is confined to bed or a wheelchair

Patients requiring remittive agents need to understand the importance of adherence to their drug regimen. They also need to recognize the importance of maintaining appointments with their health care provider for the monitoring of adverse effects. Patients must understand the importance of keeping laboratory appointments for the monitoring of blood and urine or appointments for eye examinations and the need for follow-up with the health care provider for monitoring of their disease condition.

GENERAL INSTRUCTIONS FOR DISCHARGE/OUTPATIENTS

REMITTIVE AND MISCELLANEOUS AGENTS USED IN THE TREATMENT OF RHEUMATOID ARTHRITIS AND GOUT

This drug is a remittive or miscellaneous agent used to treat arthritic conditions or gout.

This medication will not cure your condition but will help you control it as long as you continue to take the medication as directed. If you do *not* understand why you require this medication, check with your health care provider.

Take this medication as prescribed with food (a snack), milk, or a full glass of water (unless otherwise directed) to help prevent stomach irritation and upset. If stomach upset or indigestion persists or becomes troublesome even when these measures are taken, notify your health care provider.

Before taking this medication, notify your health care provider if you have bleeding problems, heart disease, kidney problems, or stomach ulcers.

If you are pregnant or intend to become pregnant or if you are nursing an infant, notify your health care provider before taking this medication. This drug may cause unwanted effects in unborn babies or nursing infants.

If you are taking this drug *once a day* and miss a dose, take it as soon as you remember then go back to your regular dosing schedule. If it is within 6 hours of your next dose, do *not* take the missed dose at all and do *not* double the next one. Resume your regular dosing schedule. If you have any questions, contact your health care provider.

If you are taking this drug *twice a day* and miss a dose within 2 hours, take it right away then go back to your regular dosing schedule. If you do not remember until later, do *not* take the missed dose at all and do *not* double the next dose. Just continue on your regular dosing schedule.

Because your condition will require long-term treatment, you will be required to take this medication for a long time. You will need to keep follow-up appointments with your health care provider so that your therapy can be monitored.

Continued.

GENERAL INSTRUCTIONS FOR DISCHARGE/OUTPATIENTS—cont'd

REMITTIVE AND MISCELLANEOUS AGENTS USED IN THE TREATMENT OF RHEUMATOID ARTHRITIS AND GOUT—cont'd

This medication was prescribed especially for you. Do not share this medication or give it to anyone else.

Serious unwanted affects can occur with the use of this medication. Notify your health care provider immediately if you notice a sore throat and flu-like symptoms, easy bruising, unusual bleeding, a rash, or other troublesome effects. These signs may indicate that your dosage or medication may need adjustment by your health care provider.

Because this medication can cause some unwanted effects on the blood and kidneys, it is important that you keep appointments with the laboratory or health care provider for regular urine and blood tests.

It can take weeks to months before you notice any effect from taking this medication. This is usual. Do not become discouraged and do not stop taking the drug or increase the dosage or take it more often than recommended. This can cause harmful effects.

This medication can cause unwanted effects if taken with certain other medications. Do not start or stop taking any medications without first checking with your health care provider. This drug can interact with these medications and cause unwanted effects.

Store this medication in a dark dry place. Refrigeration is not necessary.

Keep this medication and all other medications out of the reach of children.

In addition to the "General Instructions," if you are taking:

Gold

Exposure to sunlight or sunburn can cause a skin rash or make a skin rash associated with this drug worse. Avoid unnecessary exposure to direct sun, and use a sunscreen and wear protective clothing.

It is important to follow your weekly injection therapy as directed as well as plan to meet laboratory appointments for monitoring your blood and urine. This is particularly important to prevent serious toxicities related to this drug and to improve your response.

Penicillamine

Taste may be affected by this drug. You may notice a change in your ability to taste sweet or salty foods. Do *not* be alarmed. This is a usual effect of this drug. Do not stop taking your medication because of this effect. If this is bothersome it is often helpful to take your medication before meals. If this does not help, check with your health care provider.

Hydroxychloroquine

It is important that you follow your medication schedule exactly. This drug can cause unwanted or toxic effects particularly in relation to your vision. Report fuzzy vision, seeing halos around lights, or unusual glare to your health care provider. It is mandatory that you keep appointments with your ophthalmologist so that your eyes can be checked regularly.

Temporary hair loss may be noticed over the scalp and body. This is *not* permanent.

Prednisone, dexamethasone, or methylprednisolone

Gastric irritation or upset is not unusual with this medication. It is helpful to take each dose with a full glass of water and with breakfast. Taking the dose in the morning at breakfast around 8 AM helps decrease the severity of some adverse side effects.

Take this medication exactly as prescribed. Abrupt withdrawal of this medication can cause worsening of your symptoms or other unwanted effects. If you have any questions about how this drug should be taken, check with your health care provider.

NURSING DRUG DIGEST

Medication (trade name*)	Indication	Usual dosage and administration	Dosage forms, preparation, and storage	Contraindications, cautions, and comments	Monitoring
Allopurinol Alloprin Bloxanth Lopurin Novopurol Purinol Zyloprim	Chronic gout Severe tophaceous gout Prophylaxis of hyperuricemia Uric acid nephropathy (Use in children is generally *restricted* to treatment of hyperuricemia secondary to malignancy)	*Adult:* 200-600 mg/day PO Doses less than 300 mg can be administered once daily; higher doses should be administered in 2-3 divided doses Maximum: 800 mg/day *Children:* 6-10 years, 300 mg/day (or 10 mg/kg/day) in 1-3 divided doses Reduce dosage in renal impairment Maintain adequate fluid intake to ensure a daily urinary output of at least 2 L	Tablet: 100, 200, 300 mg	*Contraindicated* in hypersensitivity Inhibits uric acid formation, thus decreasing both serum and urinary levels	Observe for skin rash Monitor fluid intake and output
★ **Aurothioglucose** Solganol	Rheumatoid arthritis	*Adults:* 1st dose 10 mg IM; 2nd dose 25 mg IM; 3rd dose 25 mg IM; 4th and subsequent doses, 50 mg IM Interval between doses is *1 week* 50 mg dose is continued at weekly intervals until a total of 1 gm has been administered (unless toxicity warrants discontinuation) If the patient has improved and exhibits no signs of toxicity, the 50 mg dose can be further continued at monthly intervals *Children:* 6-12 years, ¼ the adult dose, *not to exceed 25 mg/dose IM* For *IM injection only*	Injectable: 5% (50 mg/ml) suspension containing approximately 50% gold Shake vial well in *horizontal* position before using Use a dry needle and syringe to withdraw the suspension Store between 0° and 30° C Protect from light	*Contraindicated* in hypersensitivity, renal disease, diabetes mellitus, blood dyscrasias, severe hypertension, and congestive heart failure Dermatitis is the most common adverse reaction Stomatitis occurs commonly May cause nephrotic syndrome May cause various blood dyscrasias (e.g., agranulocytosis, aplastic anemia, leukopenia)	Observe patient for at least 15 min following each IM injection Observe for pruritus Observe buccal membranes for shallow ulcers Monitor renal function Monitor blood counts

Continued.

NOTE: For additional details regarding the individual agents listed in this table, see the text and other tables in this chapter.
*Indicates a multiple active ingredient product. For a complete listing of all active ingredients see the *Drug Reference Guide to Brand Names and Active Ingredients.*
★Indicates that the drug is generally available only in the United States.

NURSING DRUG DIGEST—cont'd

Medication (trade name)	Indication	Usual dosage and administration	Dosage forms, preparation, and storage	Contraindications, cautions, and comments	Monitoring
Azathioprine Imuran	Severe rheumatoid arthritis that is unresponsive to less toxic agents	*Adults:* 1-2.5 mg/kg/day PO in a single or 2 divided doses Maintenance: lowest effective daily dose Reduce dosage in renal impairment Coadministration of allopurinol decreases azathioprine metabolism and necessitates a dose *reduction* to ⅓ to ¼ the usual dose *Children:* Use is *not* recommended	Tablets: 25, 50 mg	*Contraindicated* in hypersensitivity and pregnancy Chronic use of this agent increases the risk of developing infection and/or neoplasia May cause GI distress Leukopenia and/or thrombocytopenia appear to be dose related	Observe for signs of infection Monitor for leukopenia
Colchicine ColBenemid* Novocolchine	Gout	*Adults:* At the first warning of an acute attack 1.0-1.2 mg PO (or 2 mg IV over 2-5 min), followed by 0.5-0.6 mg PO q.2h. until pain is relieved or toxicity (i.e., nausea, vomiting, diarrhea) appears Maximum: 4 mg/24 hr Interval treatment: 0.5-0.6 mg PO q.d. to once weekly as needed	Tablets: 0.5, 0.6 mg Injectable: 1 mg/2 ml Injectable can be diluted with NS (*without* a bacteriostatic) Do *not* dilute with D_5W Discard cloudy solutions	*Contraindicated* in hypersensitivity Use with caution in elderly, pregnancy, severe renal disease, severe heart disease, and serious GI disorders Has *no* effect on uric acid metabolism or excretion Adverse effects appear to be dose related Most prominent adverse effects are nausea, vomiting, and diarrhea Prolonged administration may cause bone marrow depression Extravasation may cause severe local irritation	Monitor for initial signs of toxicity (i.e., nausea, vomiting, diarrhea)

Drug	Uses	Dosage	Preparations	Contraindications/Precautions	Nursing Actions
Cyclophosphamide Cytoxan Endoxan Procytox	Rheumatoid arthritis (indication *not* FDA approved) See also Chapter 53, "Alkylating and Miscellaneous Drugs Used to Treat Cancer"	*Experimental use only*	Tablets: 25, 50 mg Injectable: 100, 200, 500, 1000, 2000 mg/vial Store below 30° C	*Contraindicated* in hypersensitivity, severe leukopenia, thrombocytopenia, hepatic dysfunction, and renal dysfunction Use with caution in patients with systemic bacterial, fungal, and viral infections, adrenalectomized patients, pregnancy, and blood dyscrasias Commonly causes anorexia, nausea, vomiting, and leukopenia May cause sterile hemorrhagic cystitis	Observe for signs of infection Monitor for leukopenia Monitor for cystitis
Dexamethasone Decadron Deronil Dexasone Hexadrol	Psoriatic arthritis Rheumatoid arthritis Juvenile arthritis Acute gouty arthritis Ankylosing spondylitis Bursitis Tenosynovitis See also Chapter 65, "Corticosteroids and Adrenal Steroid Inhibitors"	*Adults:* 0.5-4 mg/day PO in 2-4 divided doses Maintenance: use smallest effective dose Intraarticular injections: 2-4 mg into large joints (e.g., knee joint); and 0.8-1.0 mg into small joints (e.g., interphalangeal) Repeat injections at intervals ranging from every 3-5 days to every 2-3 weeks based on patient response Do *not* inject into unstable joints *Children:* Start with lower doses	Tablets: 0.25, 0.5, 0.75, 1.5, 4, 6 mg Injectable: 4 mg/ml Protect injectable from freezing Do *not* autoclave Injectable may be diluted with NS, D_5W, or compatible blood for transfusion Discard unused injectable 24 hr after reconstitution	*Contraindicated* in hypersensitivity, systemic bacterial, fungal, or viral infections, and vaccinia Use with caution in pregnancy, in the presence of infection, peptic ulcer, osteoporosis, tuberculosis, and renal insufficiency Excreted in human breast milk May cause sodium and fluid retention, muscle weakness, peptic ulcer, impaired wound healing, and hypokalemia	Monitor for infection Observe for fluid retention Monitor potassium levels

Continued.

NURSING DRUG DIGEST—cont'd

Medication (trade name)	Indication	Usual dosage and administration	Dosage forms, preparation, and storage	Contraindications, cautions, and comments	Monitoring
Dimethyl sulfoxide DMSO Kemsol Rimso-50	Rheumatoid arthritis (indication *not* FDA approved)	*Experimental use only* *For topical use only*	Solutions, topical: 50%, 70% Store at 20° to 30° C Protect from light Combustible at high temperatures; do *not* autoclave Do *not* use unless solution is clear	*Contraindicated* in hypersensitivity May cause hypersensitivity Patient may develop a garliclike taste that may last several months Experience with systemic use is limited May cause changes in the lens of the eye	Observe for changes in refractive index or appearance of lens Monitor hepatic and renal function periodically Observe for any untoward reactions
Gold sodium thiomalate Myochrysine	Active rheumatoid arthritis in *combination* with other effective agents	*Adults:* Weekly IM injections; first injection, 10 mg; second injection, 25 mg; third and subsequent injections, 25-50 mg until toxicity or a total cumulative dose of 1 gm is administered *Children:* Weekly IM injections; first injection, 10 mg; second and subsequent injections, 1 mg/kg (*not* to exceed 50 mg) Administer with patient in a recumbent position and keep patient recumbent for 10 min following each injection For IM use *only*	Injectable: 10, 25, 50, 100 mg/ml Do *not* use preparations that have darkened (more than pale yellow) or that contain any particulate matter	*Contraindicated* in hypersensitivity, gold toxicity, systemic lupus erythematosus, and severe debilitated states Use with caution in patients with a history of blood dyscrasias, severe hypertension, severe cardiovascular disease, or severe hepatic disease Excreted in human breast milk Dermatitis and pruritus occur commonly; dermatitis may be aggravated by exposure to sunlight May cause nephrotic syndrome May cause stomatitis Do *not* use concomitantly with penicillamine	Monitor CBC Monitor urine for protein and sediment Observe for persistent diarrhea Observe for skin eruptions and pruritus Observe for buccal ulcers

Drug	Uses	Dosage	Preparations	Contraindications and Precautions	Nursing Implications
Hydroxy-chloroquine Plaquenil	Rheumatoid arthritis that is unresponsive to more conventional therapy See also Chapter 42, "Antiprotozoals, Antimalarials, and Amebicides"	*Adults:* 400–600 mg/day PO in a single or 2–3 divided doses with food or milk Maintenance: approximately ½ initial dosage If objective improvement is not noted within 6 months, the drug should be discontinued	Tablet: 200 mg	*Contraindicated* in hypersensitivity, visual changes, and chronic pediatric therapy May cause retinopathy Commonly causes GI irritation, nausea, skin rashes May cause lightened scalp hair and eyebrows, particularly with chronic use Use with caution in pregnancy and in G-6-PD deficiency	Monitor for visual changes Monitor blood cell counts periodically during long-term therapy
Methylpred-nisolone Medrol	Psoriatic arthritis Rheumatoid arthritis Juvenile arthritis Acute gouty arthritis Ankylosing spondylitis Bursitis Tenosynovitis Osteoarthritis See also Chapter 65, "Corticosteroids and Adrenal Steroid Inhibitors"	*Adults:* 4–32 mg/day PO in 4 divided doses Maintenance: Use smallest effective dose *Children:* Start with lower dose Alternate-day therapy: administer total 48 hr requirement PO every *other* day at 8 AM (i.e., the time of minimal endogenous adrenocortical activity)	Tablets: 2, 4, 8, 16, 24, 32 mg	*Contraindicated* in hypersensitivity, systemic bacterial, fungal, or viral infections, and vaccinia Use with caution in pregnancy, in the presence of infection, peptic ulcer, osteoporosis, tuberculosis, and renal insufficiency May cause sodium and fluid retention, muscle weakness, peptic ulcer; impaired wound healing, and hypokalemia	Monitor for infection Observe for fluid retention Monitor potassium levels

Continued.

NURSING DRUG DIGEST—cont'd

Medication (trade name)	Indication	Usual dosage and administration	Dosage forms, preparation, and storage	Contraindications, cautions, and comments	Monitoring
Penicillamine Cuprimine Depen Titra-tabs	Rheumatoid arthritis unresponsive to more conventional therapy	*Adults:* Initially, 125-250 mg/ day PO Increase by 125-250 mg/day at monthly intervals Doses in excess of 500 mg/day should be administered in divided doses Maximum: 1500 mg/day Maintenance: 250-750 mg/day PO Administer all doses on an *empty* stomach at least 1 hr before meals, any other food, milk, or drugs in order to maximize absorption	Capsules: 125, 250 mg Tablet: 250 mg	*Contraindicated* in pregnancy, renal insufficiency, and patients with a history of penicillamine-related agranulocytosis or aplastic anemia Commonly causes generalized pruritus, GI distress, decreased taste perception, thrombocytopenia, and proteinuria May cause various blood dyscrasias (i.e., agranulocytosis, aplastic anemia, granulocytopenia, leukopenia, thrombocytopenia) May cause nephrotic syndrome Do *not* coadminister with any of the other agents used for remission except the corticosteroids Clinical response may not become apparent until 2-3 months after the start of therapy	Monitor hematologic and renal studies Observe for chills, bruising, bleeding, fever, and sore throat (symptoms of thrombocytopenia)

Drug	Uses	Dosage	Dosage Forms	Contraindications/Precautions	Nursing Considerations
Prednisone Apo-Prednisone Deltacortisone Deltasone Meticorten Novo-prednisone Orasone Winpred	Psoriatic arthritis Rheumatoid arthritis Juvenile arthritis Acute gouty arthritis Ankylosing spondylitis Bursitis Tenosynovitis See also Chapter 65, "Corticosteroids and Adrenal Steroid Inhibitors"	*Adults:* 20-30 mg/day PO *Children:* start with lower doses Alternate-day therapy: administer total 48 hr requirement PO every *other* day at 8 AM (i.e., the time of minimal endogenous adrenal cortical activity)	Tablets: 2.5, 5, 10, 20, 50 mg Liquid: 5 mg/5 ml	*Contraindicated* in hypersensitivity, systemic bacterial, fungal, or viral infections Use with caution in pregnancy, in the presence of infection, peptic ulcer, osteoporosis, tuberculosis, and renal insufficiency May cause sodium and fluid retention, muscle weakness, peptic ulcer; impaired wound healing, and hypokalemia	Monitor for infection Observe for fluid retention Monitor potassium levels
Probenecid Benemid Benuryl ColBenemid* Ro-Benecid	Chronic gout Gouty arthritis Hyperuricemia	*Adults:* 250-500 mg b.i.d. PO Maximum: 2000 mg/day Unless contraindicated, maintain liberal fluid intake and sufficient sodium bicarbonate (3-8 gm/day) to maintain an alkaline urine in order to help prevent uric acid deposits in the kidneys *Children:* 2-14 years of age, 25-40 mg/kg/day PO in 4 divided doses	Tablet: 500 mg	*Contraindicated* in hypersensitivity, history of urate kidney stones, and children less than 2 years of age Use with caution in pregnancy, peptic ulcers, and chronic renal insufficiency May cause headache and GI distress	Monitor urinary output and pH Observe for GI distress
Sulfinpyrazone Antazone Anturan Anturane Novopyrazone Zynol	Chronic gouty arthritis Intermittent gouty arthritis	*Adults:* Initially, 200-400 mg/day in 2 divided doses with meals or milk for 7 days Maintenance: 200-800 mg/day PO with food or milk to decrease GI distress Maintain adequate hydration	Capsule: 200 mg Tablet: 100 mg	*Contraindicated* in patients with blood dyscrasias, active peptic ulcers, and hypersensitivity to sulfinpyrazone or phenylbutazone Commonly causes GI distress	Observe for GI distress

BIBLIOGRAPHY

Arthritis: An overview of current treatment. *About Your Medicines*, 1983, *3*(4), 1-2.

Arthritis comes in many forms. *About Your Medicines*, 1983, *3*(3), 5-6.

Garcia, C. Gold therapy in arthritis treatment. *Nurse Practitioner*, 1981, *6*(1), 35, 38, 49.

Hodge, N.A. Management of degenerative joint disease and rheumatoid arthritis: Parts I & II. *Drug Store News*, January 1984, Lesson 679-401-84-01.

Hodge, N.A. A review of drug treatment modalities for the arthritic patient: Part II. *Drug Store News*, January 1984, Lesson 679-401-84-02.

Markenson, J.A. Antiarthritic drugs: a comparative overview. *Drug Therapy*, January 1981, 45-57.

McDuffie, F.C., & Benzaia, D. Arthritis update for pharmacists. *Pharmacy Times*, December 1980, 30-37.

Parker, W.A. Pharmacotherapy of rheumatoid arthritis. *Canadian Pharmaceutical Journal*, November 1981, 411-417.

Pfeiffer, F.G. Drug treatment of rheumatoid arthritis. Part I. *Drug Store News*, 1982, Lesson 679-401-82-03.

Pfeiffer, F.G. Drug treatment of rheumatoid arthritis. Part II. *Drug Store News*, 1982, Lesson 679-401-82-04.

Pritchard, R. The pharmacist as adviser to the arthritic patient. *Drug Merchandising*, December 1982, *28*, 30, 64.

Strand, C.V. & Clark, S.R. Adult arthritis, drugs and remedies. *American Journal of Nursing*, 1983, *83*(2), 266-269.

HORMONES AND HORMONE ANTAGONISTS

Medications discussed in this section

Insulin and Related Medications

Stuart A. Ross

Medications discussed in this chapter

Sulfonylureas
  Acetohexamide
  Chlorpropamide
  Glipizide
  Glyburide
  Tolazamide
  Tolbutamide
Biguanides
  Metformin

Insulins
  Insulin, human biosynthetic
  Insulin, globin zinc
  Insulin injection
  Insulin, isophane
  Insulin, protamine zinc
  Insulin, zinc
  Insulin zinc, extended
  Insulin zinc, prompt
Insulin antagonists
  Diazoxide
  Glucagon

Diabetes is a major health problem in North America. It is recognized as the third leading cause of death in adults after heart disease and cancer and is the leading cause of blindness in young people. The many complications of this condition have far-reaching effects on the individual's personal and family life. Recent evidence suggests that the achievement of ideal control of blood glucose in the diabetic person will delay or even prevent the onset of the complications associated with diabetes, including retinopathy, nephropathy, and neuropathy. The key methods of treatment available for diabetics involve the use of diet alone, diet with oral *hypoglycemic* agents, or diet with insulin.

In terms of etiology, pathogenesis, clinical presentation, and management there are two distinct groups of diabetic conditions: (1) *insulin-dependent diabetes mellitus* (IDDM); and (2) *non–insulin-dependent diabetes mellitus* (NIDDM), according to a classification provided by the National Diabetes Data Group. IDDM generally occurs in a younger age group, often with rapid onset of *hyperglycemia* and ketosis. These patients are more prone to the serious complications of diabetes mellitus, and insulin is the only treatment

available. NIDDM is more commonly found in the older age group and is usually associated with obesity. The onset of diabetic complications is less common than that seen in the insulin-dependent diabetic patient. Diet is the key form of treatment; more rarely oral hypoglycemic agents are used to stimulate insulin release from the pancreas.

ORAL HYPOGLYCEMIC AGENTS
Historical background

The concept of the oral hypoglycemic agent is not new. As early as 1918 it had been reported that administration of guanidine would result in a lowering of blood glucose levels. However, because of the severe toxic neurologic side effects associated with its use, this drug was abandoned. In 1942 the observations of Janbon and later Loubatieres indicated that sulfonamides possessed a hypoglycemic effect. In 1955 it was noted that an antimicrobial sulfonamide, carbutamide, could lower the blood glucose level with no apparent toxic side effects. Later, the first sulfonylurea with hypoglycemic activity, tolbutamide, was released for use in the treatment of diabetes mellitus. Since then other first generation sulfonylurea drugs (e.g., chlorpropamide, acetohexamide, tolazamide) and, more recently, second generation sulfonylurea drugs (e.g., glyburide and glipizide) have been released.

The other group of hypoglycemic agents, the biguanides, were developed from the initial work by Watanabe in 1918 on guanidine. Two compounds were distributed for use in clinical practice—phenformin and metformin. Phenformin has now been removed from the market because of its ability to cause severe lactic acidosis, particularly in the elderly, resulting in death.

Mechanism of action

The sulfonylureas lower blood glucose levels by stimulating the pancreatic islet tissue to secrete in-

TABLE 60-1

Characteristics of oral hypoglycemic agents

Medication	Duration of activity (hr)	Percent excreted in urine
Acetohexamide	Intermediate (12-16)	60%; metabolites are far more potent than original drug
Chlorpropamide	Long (36+)	Initially 60%, but later virtually all of the drug will be excreted in urine
Glipizide	Short (3-6) but larger doses may result in prolonged activity 24+	90%
Glyburide	Short (4-6) but larger doses may have effects at 24+	50% excreted in bile, 50% excreted in urine
Metformin	Short (3-6)	100%
Tolazamide	Intermediate (8-12)	85% excreted in urine; has multiple metabolites, some of which have hypoglycemic activity
Tolbutamide	Short (6-8)	100% after initial carboxylation in liver

sulin. Sulfonylureas augment insulin secretion in response to elevated levels of plasma glucose or amino acids. The sulfonylureas do not need to penetrate the insulin-secreting β-cell but rather derive their effect by sensitizing the β-cell to other insulin-secreting substrates. The sulfonylureas may also have extrapancreatic actions by producing a reduction in the hepatic uptake of endogenous insulin and by increasing insulin receptor–site activity by increasing the number of available insulin receptors.

The sulfonylureas are absorbed rapidly from the gastrointestinal tract and are loosely bound to albumin with about 5% remaining free in the circulation. All of the sulfonylureas have similar pharmacokinetic properties; their main differences are in their duration of action. Each of the sulfonylureas undergoes a variable degree of metabolism and is excreted via the liver or kidney (Table 60-1).

Primary failure

Approximately 3% of all persons given sulfonylurea agents will show a poor response or no response at all in terms of increased insulin secretion and control of the blood glucose level. The most common cause of the primary failure of sulfonylureas is the inappropriate use of the drug in individuals who are in fact insulin-dependent diabetics.

Secondary failure

Those individuals who originally show a positive response to sulfonylurea therapy but after a short period on the drug appear to become *refractory* are referred to as demonstrating secondary sulfonylurea failure. Frequently these patients contribute to secondary failure because they do not follow the instructions for their drug therapy or because they have de-

veloped an infection that is leading to increased insulin resistance. When secondary failure has developed to one sulfonylurea, the change to another may result in an improved therapeutic response.

Available sulfonylureas

Tolbutamide. This drug was the first of the sulfonylureas released for the treatment of diabetes and is still one of the most widely used. Tolbutamide is rapidly metabolized in the liver and its metabolites are all excreted in the urine. Its half-life is 4 to 6 hours; duration of action is 6 to 8 hours. Because of its short action it must be given at least every 12 hours at a dose range of between 500 and 2000 mg per day.

Acetohexamide. This sulfonylurea has a slightly longer action than that of tolbutamide with a duration of action of 12 to 14 hours. It is metabolized in the liver, and the metabolite has more hypoglycemic properties than does the original drug. Acetohexamide is excreted in the urine. The daily dose range is between 250 and 1500 mg and is usually taken in divided doses.

Chlorpropamide. This drug has the longest duration of action of all the sulfonylureas with a half-life of 36 hours and a duration of action of up to 60 hours. It is taken once a day in a dose of between 100 and 250 mg. Virtually all the chlorpropamide is excreted unchanged in the urine. Because of its long duration of action, it is potentially dangerous in those patients who have become ill and have decreased their food intake but continue to take the drug. This is especially so in the elderly person with diabetes who may develop severe and often fatal hypoglycemia. Thus the drug should be used with extreme caution in all elderly diabetic patients.

Chlorpropamide also has an unusual antidiuretic effect and is believed to augment the action of antidiuretic hormone (ADH). It is commonly used in patients with partial diabetes insipidus, who need to be observed closely for hypoglycemia.

Tolazamide. This drug has a slightly longer action than tolbutamide with a duration of action of between 12 and 16 hours. It can be given once or twice daily in a dose of 250 to 1000 mg per day. The drug is metabolized to a number of hypoglycemic agents that are largely excreted by the kidney.

Glyburide. This drug is one of the new so-called second generation sulfonylureas. These drugs are far more powerful than the first generation drugs and are used at much lower dosages. The drug is excreted in equal amounts in urine and bile. The duration of action appears to be short—4 to 6 hours—however, the drug may be detected 24 hours after a single dose. Severe hypoglycemia may result if the drug is taken when food is reduced or stopped because of illness. The effective dose is between 1.25 and 20 mg per day.

Glipizide. This is another of the second generation sulfonylurea drugs. It is more potent than the first generation drugs and is used at much lower doses. The half-life of glipizide is 3 hours, although it can be detected 24 hours after initial administration. The drug is metabolized in the liver, and the majority is excreted as inactive metabolites in the urine. It can be given once or twice daily in a range of 5 to 40 mg per day.

Biguanides

Metformin. Metformin is a biguanide derivative that, like the sulfonylureas, will have an antihyperglycemic effect only when there is insulin secretion. Metformin has no effect on the pancreatic β-cell, and the mode of action is not fully understood. It has been postulated that metformin potentiates the effect of insulin, or it may enhance the effect of insulin on peripheral receptor sites or perhaps inhibit the absorption of food. Metformin is rapidly absorbed, and most of the drug is excreted unchanged in the urine within 24 hours. The drug is not in widespread use because of the fear of lactic acidosis as occurred with phenformin. However, the incidence of lactic acidosis does not seem to be as great in metformin, although there are a few case reports indicating that elderly patients with renal failure receiving this drug may develop lactic acidosis because of impaired renal excretion. The use of the other biguanide, phenformin, has been banned in North America because of the high incidence of lactic acidosis and the associated mortality.

INSULIN RECEPTOR

The identification of a receptor located in the membrane of peripheral cells specific for insulin has led to a greater understanding of the mechanics of insulin action and, in particular, the insulin resistance observed in obesity. In obesity and in the non–insulin-dependent diabetic patient, the cause of insulin resistance is found in the peripheral tissue. The obese patient demonstrates a down-regulation of the number of receptors on target cells, and the decreased number of insulin receptors results in increased insulin resistance and hyperglycemia. In more severe insulin resistance, also associated with obesity, the decreased insulin responsiveness appears to result from a combined receptor and postreceptor defect. Correction of the obesity will commonly lead to an increased sensitivity to insulin and a return to the *euglycemic* state.

Many persons who have been criticized for not losing weight more effectively demonstrate rapid weight loss when their oral hypoglycemic therapy is withdrawn. Although the oral hypoglycemic agents appear to have some effect on increasing the number of available receptors, these agents will also lead to the release of insulin, a hormone that will contribute to obesity. Thus the diabetic patient receiving oral agents is being provided with more insulin and possibly more receptors leading to improved storage of food. Eventually, the number of receptors will become less and the patient more obese, with the result that the patient remains both hyperglycemic and overweight.

These observations emphasize the importance of providing the patient with an individualized diet plan and an education program to promote understanding of the diet and thus achieve an ideal weight. Oral hypoglycemic agents should not be used in obese patients until the dietary maneuvers have been fully used.

UNIVERSITY GROUP DIABETES PROGRAM (UGDP)

The UGDP study was initiated to examine various treatment modalities including diet alone, insulin, and the oral hypoglycemic agents tolbutamide and phenformin. Its goal was to study the effect of these various treatments to determine if blood glucose control could help control or delay the vascular complications of diabetes. After an 8-year period of observation it was concluded that treatment with either tolbutamide or phenformin may, in fact, lead to increased risk of cardiovascular mortality, although the pathologic mechanism behind these changes remains unknown.

Since the publication of the UGDP report there has been considerable controversy over its findings. Statisticians have questioned the statistics applied to achieve the findings, and other researchers have questioned the original data and the means by which they were used to support the final conclusions. No agreement has been reached by the various proponents and opponents of the UGDP study, and it is likely that the debate will never be completely resolved. Perhaps the greatest benefit of this discussion has been the realization that on many occasions the oral hypoglycemic agents have been used inappropriately, especially in the obese diabetic patient. The study has provided health care providers the reminder of the importance of dietary management and weight reduction in diabetic patients before the oral hypoglycemic agents are employed in the therapeutic regimen.

INSULIN

Historical background

The isolation of insulin provided one of the most dramatic developments in modern medicine. In 1921 and 1922 Frederick Banting and Charles Best, working in Toronto, extracted insulin from the bovine pancreas and proved its effect, initially in diabetic dogs and then in a 14-year-old boy, Leonard Thompson. With the discovery of insulin the inevitable early death of the insulin-dependent diabetic patient was averted and prospects of a more normal life could be contemplated. Also with the discovery of insulin came the realization that diabetes was a complex condition,

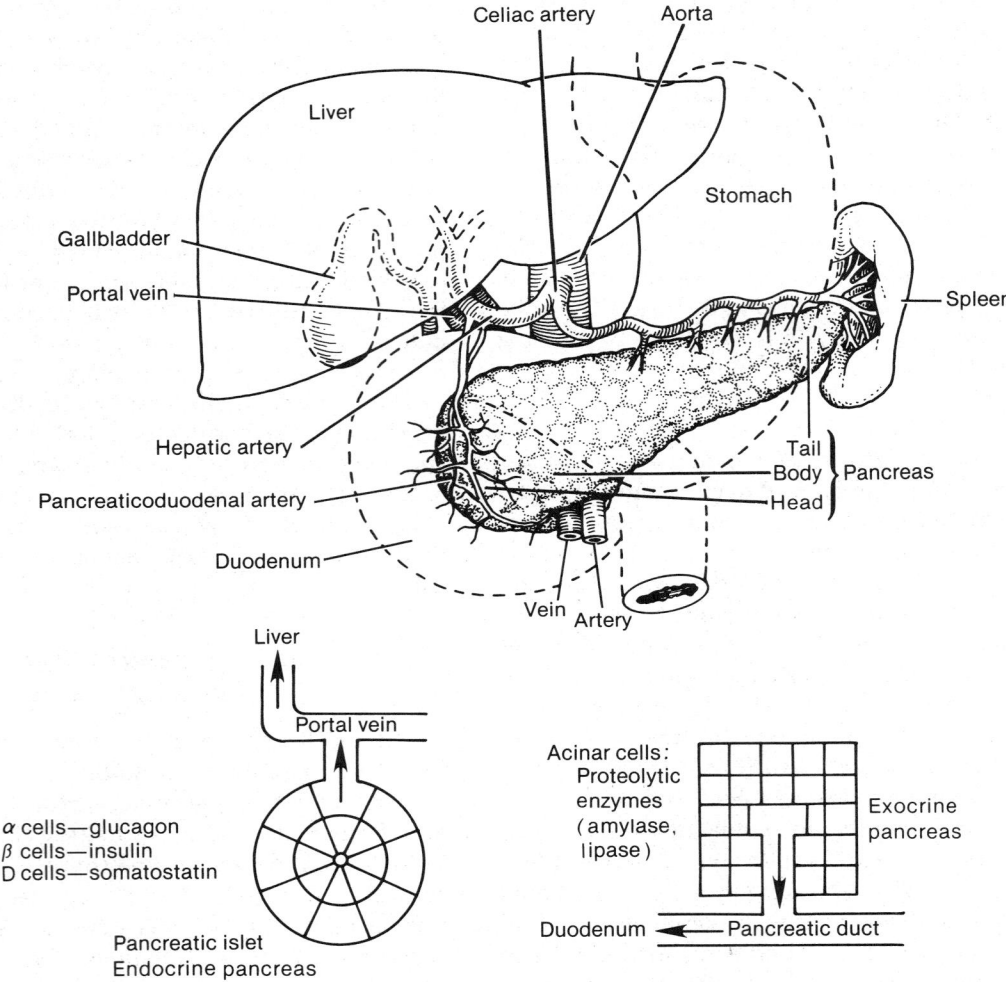

FIGURE 60-1. **The pancreas is located in the abdominal cavity lying just below the liver and stomach. The head of the pancreas is intimately associated with the duodenum, and the tail with the spleen. The pancreas has two major functions, exocrine and endocrine. The exocrine acinar cells constitute the majority of cells in the pancreas and are responsible for producing pancreatic juice. The endocrine islet cells release hormones into a network of veins that drain into the portal vein and then pass to the liver.**

both in terms of etiology and its effect on the metabolism of carbohydrates, proteins, and fats. Insulin is a protein and cannot be taken orally because of its immediate destruction in the stomach. Throughout the years many attempts have been made to devise new techniques of administering insulin to avoid the necessity of a daily injection. The concepts of constant infusion insulin pumps, computerized glucose sensor devices, and subcutaneous insulin reservoirs are still undergoing extensive research.

Endocrine function of the pancreas

Both the exocrine and endocrine portions of the pancreas develop from cells of the duodenal and hepatic diverticulum. The endocrine islets develop separately from the duct system at approximately the twelfth week of gestation. The pancreas is supplied by the splenic, hepatic, and superior mesenteric arteries; the blood supply eventually drains into the portal vein. The islets are composed of at least three types of cells: the α-cell, which secretes glucagon; the β-cell, which secretes insulin; and the D cell, which secretes *somatostatin*. Tiny communication passages between the α- and β-cells, so-called gap junctions, have been identified by electron microscopy. It is thought that insulin, glucagon, and somatostatin interact possibly by local or paracrine action (Figure 60-1).

Structure and biosynthesis

Insulin consists of two chains of amino acids joined together by disulfide bonds and has a molecular weight of about 6000. The two chains are referred to as A (for acidic) and B (for basic), and the complete amino acid structure of insulin is now known.

Insulin is manufactured in the β-cell located in the islets of Langerhans in the pancreas. It is initially formed as a large molecule, preproinsulin, in the rough endoplasmic reticulum. There it is converted to a large, single-chain precursor of insulin termed proinsulin. The proinsulin is then transferred to the Golgi complex where it is concentrated as immature granules. Within these granules conversion of proinsulin to insulin takes place by the cleavage of the connecting peptide between the A and B chains, the so-called C-Peptide, and the removal of four amino acids. The granules will later release their stored insulin and equimolar concentrations of C-Peptide into the circulation (Figures 60-2 and 60-3).

Regulation of insulin secretion

The principal stimulus to insulin secretion is glucose, but amino acids and possibly fatty acids provide a minor stimulus. Gastrointestinal hormones, partic-

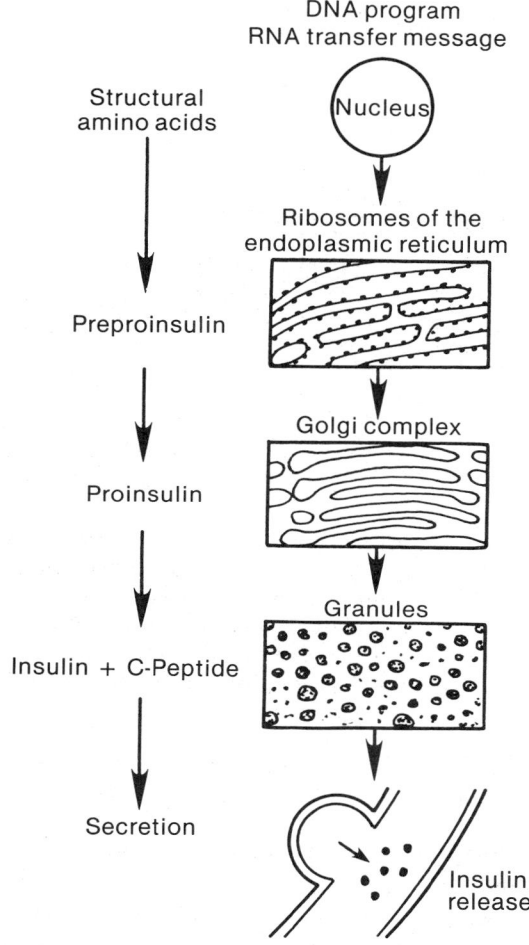

FIGURE 60-2. **Production of insulin will take place within the β-cell, as the result of genetic programming by nuclear DNA and the chemical information transferred by messenger RNA. Amino acids are joined in a specific sequence resulting in the production of a single long chain of amino acids known as preproinsulin. A portion of this chain is then split off to leave the proinsulin molecule, which is then transferred to the Golgi complex where it is packaged into granules; the process of removal of the connecting C-Peptide chain is thus begun. The folding of the insulin molecule also takes place in the Golgi complex. Then insulin and its C-Peptide are stored in granules within the cytoplasm where they are held ready for release into the circulation in response to appropriate stimuli.**

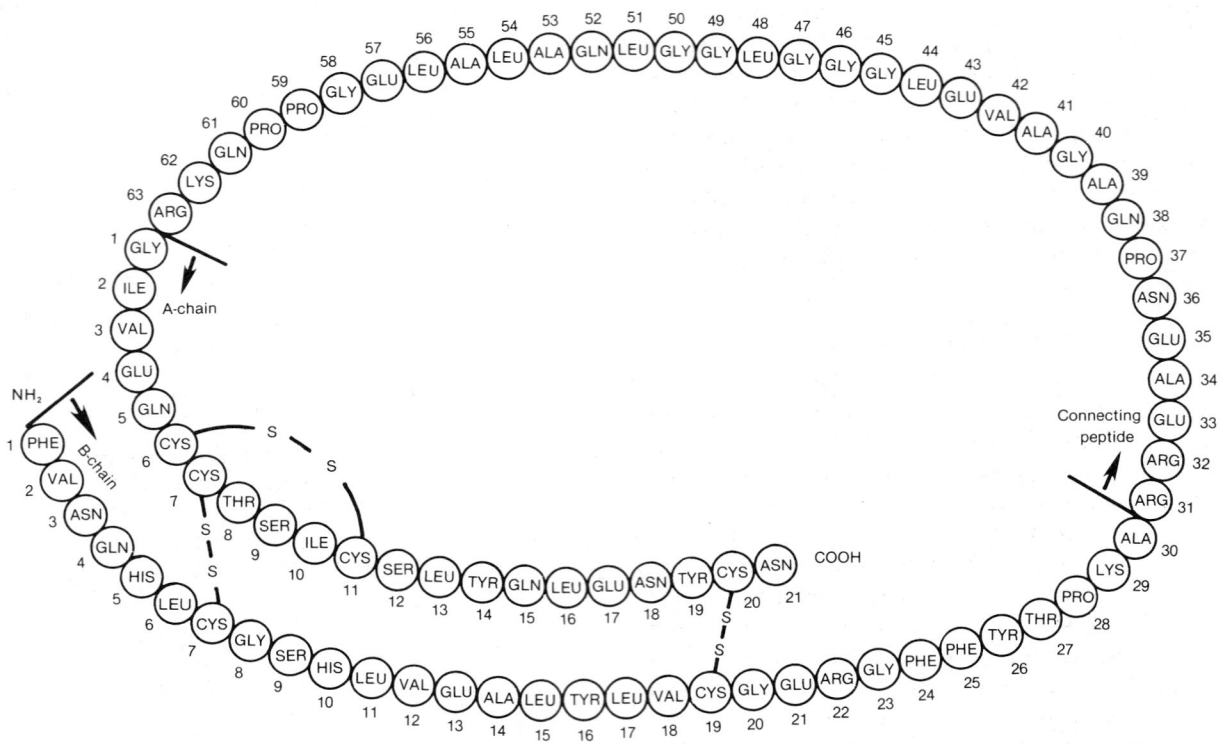

FIGURE 60-3. **Human proinsulin and its conversion to insulin. Insulin has a molecular weight of approximately 6000 and is made up of two chains of amino acids joined together by disulfide bonds. Insulin is formed from a single-chain precursor, proinsulin, which itself was formed from an even larger molecule, preproinsulin. By a process of proteolytic cleavage, four amino acids (31, 32, 64, 65) and the connecting peptide, C-Peptide, are removed, and the proinsulin molecule is converted to insulin.**

ularly gastric inhibitory polypeptide, augment insulin release after the ingestion of glucose or fat.

Effect of other hormones on secretion of insulin

Glucagon, secreted by the pancreatic α cells, will also lead to the stimulation of insulin. Norepinephrine and epinephrine will inhibit insulin secretion by mediation through the α-adrenergic receptors. However, epinephrine will also stimulate the β-adrenergic receptors, which will lead to stimulation of insulin secretion. Parasympathomimetic drugs and possibly vagal nerve stimulation will lead to enhanced insulin secretion.

Somatostatin

Somatostatin is a tetradecapeptide that was first isolated from sheep hypothalamus and received its name because of its inhibitory effect on growth hormone secretion. Somatostatin has now been clearly identified in many other areas particularly in the gas-

trointestinal tract and the pancreas. Somatostatin is known to be secreted by the D cells of the pancreatic islets. It has a potent inhibitory effect on the release of insulin, glucagon, and many other polypeptide hormones. Because of its effect on suppression of insulin secretion, somatostatin infusion will lead to a decrease in glucose tolerance.

Metabolism of insulin

Insulin is carried in the circulation as the free hormone, and only a small portion is associated with plasma proteins. The plasma half-life of insulin is less than 9 minutes; the majority of insulin is destroyed during the first passage through the liver with the remainder largely destroyed in the kidney. Only a small quantity of insulin is inactivated in peripheral tissue such as muscle and fat.

Sources of exogenous insulin

Insulin has been extracted from several animals for human use but the most commonly used sources are

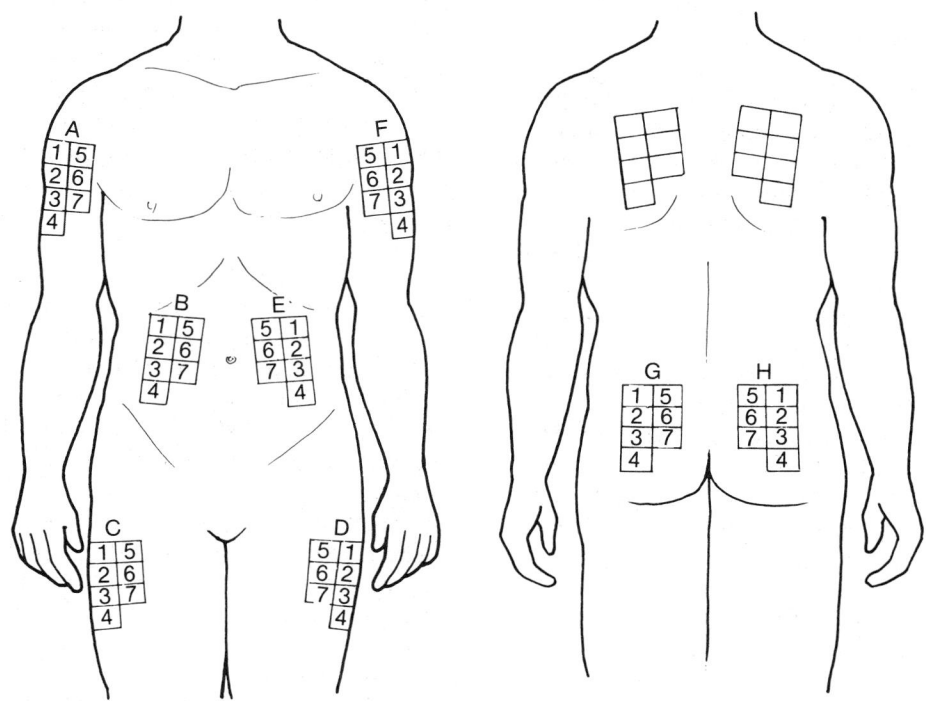

FIGURE 60-4. **Rotation of injection sites. This demonstrates how areas of the body can be divided into small squares, and the patient can commence injecting insulin in each No. 1 square rotating from *A* to *F*. The patient then commences on square No. 2 rotating from *A* to *F* so that each site is used only once every 6 days. This allows a large number of different places to be used for injection, and it will take over 6 weeks before a site is used for a second time.**

pork (porcine) and beef (bovine) insulins. Porcine insulin is the most similar to human insulin and differs only by the substitution of one amino acid at the end of the B chain. Initially, the purified insulins extracted from the animal pancreas contained many contaminants including pancreatic proteins and hormones unrelated to insulin. In 1971 purer forms of insulin were released and further advances have been made in the purification of insulin. The term *single peak* is used to describe insulin that has been purified on *gel chromatography,* yielding a profile consisting of a single peak. A substantial amount of the higher molecular weight materials are purged from the insulin so that the remaining preparation consists of 99% insulin and less than 1% of noninsulin materials. Virtually all insulins available on the commercial market today are single peak preparations. The term *single* or *mono* component signifies single peak insulin that has been further purified by the use of ion exchange chromatography. It also contains 99% insulin and virtually no other contaminants. Single component

and mono component insulin are produced by the Eli Lilly Company, Novo Laboratories, and Nordisk Laboratories.

Antigenicity

Before the production of the more purified insulins, antibody production to exogenous insulin was commonly observed. Those patients demonstrating *antigenicity* would require increasing quantities of insulin before the metabolic effects of insulin could be observed. The antibodies were suspected to be formed because of the multiple exposure to foreign insulin from beef or mixed beef-pork origins. The development of the more highly purified insulins has led to the hope that there will be a marked reduction in the immunogenicity of these insulins. It is now becoming increasingly rare to observe severe insulin resistance because of the development of insulin antibodies, although researchers have demonstrated that the single peak insulins may not produce a natural fall in insulin-antibody titers.

Lipodystrophy

The subcutaneous injection of insulin may result in either hypertrophy (i.e., *lipohypertrophy*) or atrophy (i.e., *lipoatrophy*) of adipose tissue in certain susceptible patients. Hypertrophy takes the appearance of a soft swelling in the area of insulin administration and is believed to result from the synthesis of lipids in local fat cells under the action of insulin. Lipoatrophy, characterized by a loss of fat at the site of the injection of insulin, results in a marked depression or hollowing of the skin. On occasion lipoatrophy may be seen in sites distal to the site of injection. The cause of the atrophy is unknown but may in part be the result of impurities in the injected insulin. The use of single peak pork insulin has led to a reduction of the incidence of lipoatrophy; in fact, an improvement in previous lipoatrophy sites has been noted when the single peak insulins are injected directly into the lipoatrophy site. It is presumed that the insulin is stimulating synthesis of lipids in that region.

Rotation of insulin injection sites

To help prevent the problems of lipodystrophy the patient taking insulin is instructed how to rotate injection sites throughout all four limbs and, commonly, the abdomen, back, or buttocks also. A checklist is often provided to the patient so that he or she may, on a daily basis, know where each injection has been given. This commonly will prevent lipodystrophy or infection in injection sites (Figure 60-4).

Allergy

Insulin allergy can occur in two main forms—local and systemic (delayed). The local allergic response is probably mediated by IgE, and the delayed allergic response is mediated by IgG antibodies. The local response will be immediate (i.e., 2 hours after the injection of insulin) and is characterized by the development of hard, indurated lumps over the injection site. A systemic or delayed reaction may occur many hours after the injection of the insulin and can range from localized areas of itching to the more serious presentation of anaphylaxis. The introduction of the purified insulins has decreased this problem, but some patients are still recognized as having severe insulin allergy. Most of these patients can be successfully desensitized with the use of insulin allergy desensitization kits provided by Eli Lilly and Co. The cause of the allergy may be the animal source of the insulin or some of the carrier materials in the commercial preparation of the insulin, particularly zinc.

Action of insulin

The prime role of insulin is to provide enhanced transport of glucose across certain cell membranes.

Insulin also has an important role in the metabolism of protein and fat and can be considered the key metabolic hormone. In the liver insulin will promote the storage of glucose and the formation of triglycerides and proteins. In the *adipocyte* insulin will enhance the uptake of glucose and its transformation to fat or glycogen. Similarly, in the muscle cell, the insulin will accelerate the transfer of glucose and increase the incorporation of amino acids into protein. In the absence of insulin there will be a marked reduction in the rate of transport of glucose into cells, a decreased activity of the enzyme systems that allow the conversion of glucose to glycogen, an increase in the rate of conversion of protein to glucose, and an increase in the rate of breakdown of stored triglyceride to free fatty acids. The high concentration of free fatty acids observed in the plasma of the diabetic patient is a result of the increased mobilization from the peripheral fat stores where insulin normally inhibits the hormone-sensitive lipase that will allow hydrolysis of the stored triglycerides. The source of the ketone bodies, observed in the severely hyperglycemic diabetic patient, is from the liver where the large quantities of free fatty acids that have been liberated are converted to the ketone bodies—acetoacetic acid, acetone, and β-hydroxybutyrate. The production of large quantities of these ketones, which are strong acids, causes the acidosis observed during insulin deficiency (Figure 60-5).

Insulin preparations

All commercial insulin preparations undergo a bioassay before their distribution to determine their physiologic activity. The potency of the insulin is expressed in USP units against a specific insulin standard. Potency of each insulin preparation is indicated on the label and the more pure preparations now available have potencies of up to 30 units/mg. Insulins are now generally marketed as the U-100 dosage form (100 units/ml) for use with U-100 insulin syringes, which allows greater ease in measuring the exact number of units required for the patient. The insulins are supplied close to a neutral pH, and this permits different types of insulin to be mixed together in the same syringe. Also, it offers greater stability of the hormone so that while the patient is using a particular vial of insulin the vial does not need to be stored in a refrigerator. It is important, however, to protect insulin from extremes of heat and cold.

The insulins can be divided into three main catagories according to their onset and duration of action. These are the short-acting, intermediate-acting and the long-acting insulins (Table 60-2).

Insulin injection (e.g., Regular, Crystalline Zinc) is prepared by the precipitation of insulin with zinc chlo-

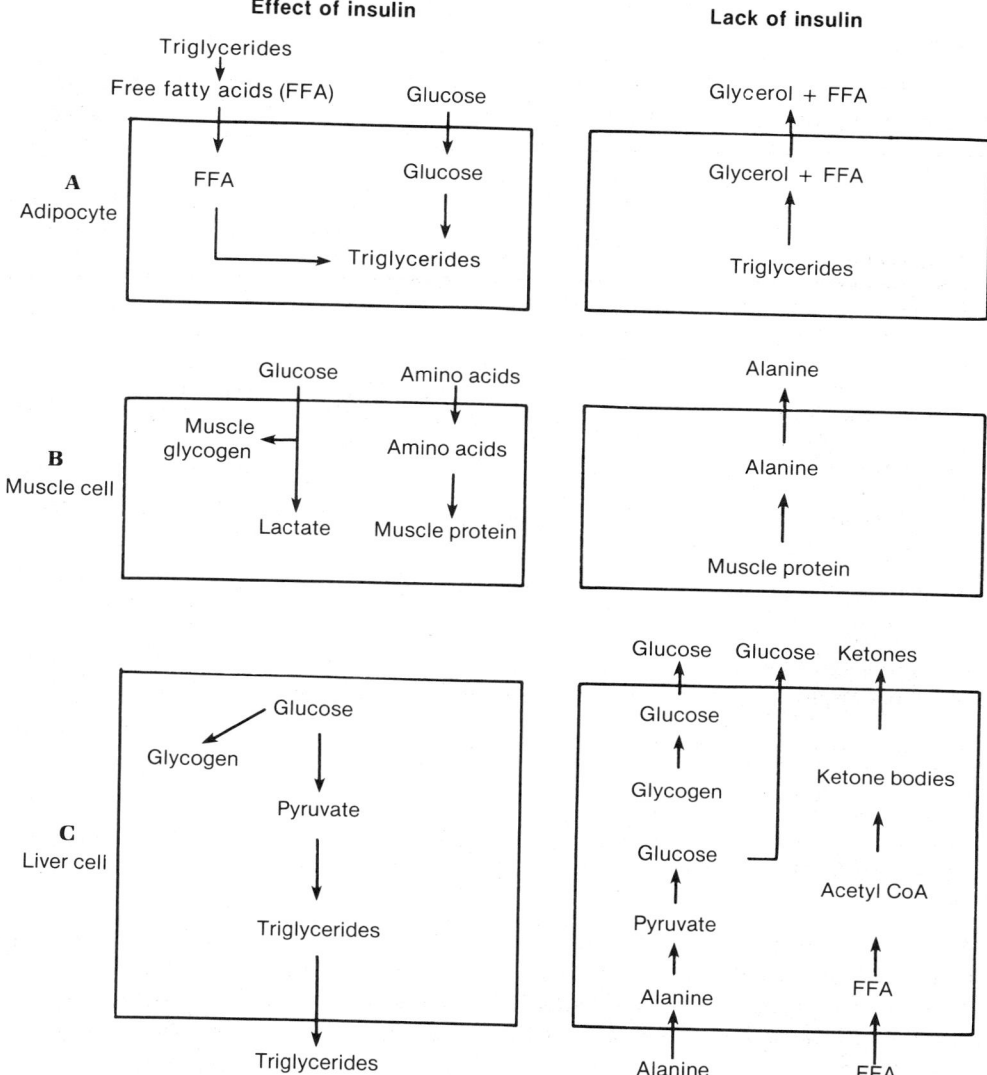

FIGURE 60-5. **Insulin is the key anabolic hormone and will result in the storage of glucose and substrates within the cell.** *A,* **The adipocyte. Under the action of insulin, circulating triglycerides, after being broken into constituent free fatty acids at the cell membrane, will be taken into the adipocyte and reconstituted into triglyceride. Under the action of insulin, glucose also will be transferred into the cell and stored as triglyceride. In the absence of insulin, triglyceride catabolism will take place with the release of glycerol and free fatty acids into the circulation.** *B,* **Insulin will promote the uptake of glucose and amino acids into the muscle cell. Glucose will be stored as muscle glycogen and will form lactate, and amino acids will provide the building block for muscle protein. In the absence of insulin muscle protein will be broken down to the amino acid alanine, which will be released into the circulation and later taken up by the liver for new glucose formation.** *C,* **Liver cell. Insulin is not required for the uptake of glucose into the liver cell, but insulin will promote the formation of glycogen and triglycerides. If a large quantity of glucose is present, large quantities of triglyceride will also be released into the circulation. In the absence of insulin glycogen will be broken down into glucose, particularly under the influence of glucagon and cortisol, and glucose will be released into the circulation. Large quantities of alanine, released from muscle cells, will be metabolized by the liver cells to form new glucose and eventually released into the circulation. Similarly, free fatty acids released from the adipocyte will be metabolized to ketone bodies such as acetoacetic acid, acetone, and β-hydroxybutyrate and released into the circulation.**

TABLE 60-2

Characteristics of the insulin preparations

Duration of action	Preparation	Source	Appearance	Protein content	Onset of action (hr)	Peak action (hr)	Approximate duration of action (hr)
Short-acting	Insulin injection (e.g., Crystalline Zinc, Humulin-R, Regular)	Beef, beef-pork, pork, human*	Clear	Nil	1	2-3	1-6
	Insulin zinc, prompt (e.g., Semilente, Semitard)	Beef-pork	Cloudy	Nil	1	4-8	1-14
Intermediate-acting	Insulin isophane (e.g., Humulin-N, NPH)	Beef, beef-pork, pork, human*	Cloudy	Protamine	2	10-18	2-24
	Insulin zinc (e.g., Lentard, Lente, Monotard)	Beef-pork	Cloudy	Nil	2	10-18	2-24
	Insulin globin zinc	Beef	Clear	Globin	2	10-18	2-18
Long-acting	Insulin, protamine zinc (e.g., PZI)	Beef-pork	Cloudy	Protamine	7	15-22	7-36
	Insulin zinc, extended (e.g., Ultralente, Ultratard)	Beef-pork	Cloudy	Nil	7	16-24	7-36

*The human insulins are actually biosynthetic in origin and are produced by recombinant DNA technology.

ride. No protein carrier is added, and the insulin is clear. Insulin injection will have a rapid onset of action.

A delay in the action of the insulin can be achieved by increasing the size of the insulin crystals and increasing the content of zinc.

Insulin zinc extended suspension (e.g., Ultralente) is an insulin preparation containing larger crystals and higher zinc content than insulin injection, which will allow for slower absorption after subcutaneous injection and thus longer duration of action.

Insulin zinc prompt suspension (e.g., Semilente) is an amorphous complex insulin made with zinc, which will have a rapid onset and a duration slightly longer than that of insulin injection.

Insulin zinc suspension (e.g., Lente, Monotard) is a mixture of insulin zinc prompt suspension and insulin zinc extended suspension to provide an intermediate-action insulin.

Insulin protamine zinc suspension (PZI) is one of the original insulins designed to provide longer action. Delay in the action of the insulin is achieved by the addition of the protein protamine. This insulin is now used only rarely because when the rapid-acting insulin injection (e.g., Crystalline Zinc Insulin) is combined with insulin protamine zinc, the overall effect of the combination is different from what would occur if the same doses of insulin had been administered by separate injection. This has resulted in considerable confusion for patients when trying to adjust insulin regimens. More stable solutions of insulin now have been developed.

Insulin isophane suspension (e.g., NPH—the N refers to a neutral solution, P to the protamine zinc content, and the H identifies the initial preparation of this insulin in the laboratory of Hagedorn) is a crystalline complex of insulin with zinc and a balanced quantity of protamine. Insulin isophane suspension is an intermediate-acting insulin and can be easily mixed with insulin injection (e.g., Regular, Crystalline Zinc Insulin) to achieve steady insulin levels throughout the day.

Insulin sulfated is a chemically modified insulin available specifically for the treatment of patients with resistance to insulin antibodies. The insulin is chemically modified with concentrated sulfuric acid providing an insulin with a short action of 2 to 7 hours, thus requiring twice-a-day administration.

See also biosynthetic human insulin (p. 1391).

TABLE 60-3

Comparison of urine tests for glucose and ketones*

Test	Advantages	Disadvantages	Drugs that may affect test result
Acetest	Provides reasonable quantitation	Inconvenient	Alcohol—false positive Levodopa—false positive Paraldehyde—false positive Salicylates (moderate to high doses)—false positive
Clinistix	Convenient Short time between test and reading result	Scale does not provide good differentiation of glucose concentration Scale colors hard to read	Methyldopa—false negative Salicylates (moderate-high doses)—false negative
Clinitest	Provides best quantitation No false negative results	Least convenient Many false positive results	Ascorbic acid—false positive Cephalosporins—false positive Chloramphenicol—false positive Methyldopa—false positive Salicylates (moderate to high doses)—false positive Sulfonamides—false positive Tetracyclines—false positive
Diastix	Easy to read No false positive results Convenient	Slightly less accurate than Clinitest Suppression of glucose reading can occur when high ketones present	
Ketostix	Convenient Provides reasonable quantitation	Does not measure all ketones, particularly β-hydroxybutyrate	Levodopa—false positive Salicylates (moderate to high doses)—false positive
Tes-Tape	Convenient No false positive results	Difficult to read glucose ranges; can underestimate high values; false negative results can occur Time between urine test and result is longer Instructions to patients can be confusing	Ascorbic acid—false negative Methyldopa—false negative Salicylates (moderate to high doses)—false negative

*Patients should be instructed to report all urine tests as a percentage (e.g., 1%, 2%, 3%, 4%) rather than by the older technique of using "pluses" (e.g., 1+, 2+, 3+, 4+). All urine testing materials should be kept dry in a tight sealed container while not in use. Patients and family should be carefully instructed in the techniques for testing urine and the daily routines that should be followed and should also be aware of the times when testing for ketones should take place. Patients should be instructed so that they may interpret the results of the urine tests in terms of the control of their diabetes.

Therapeutic use of insulin

The correct use of insulin depends on knowledge of the type of insulin to be used and its duration of action. No firm criteria can be laid down as to the exact dosage required by diabetic patients; each individual will need to have the dosage tailored to his or her needs. In general, most patients will be controlled by insulin isophane suspension (e.g., NPH) or insulin zinc in combination with insulin injection (e.g., Regular Insulin). Many patients will be controlled on a single dose of insulin in the morning, but there appear to be advantages in terms of blood glucose control by using multiple injections of insulin throughout the day. On rare occasions patients may obtain some benefit from the use of insulin zinc prompt, insulin zinc extended, or insulin protamine zinc (PZI).

Where possible, the insulin dose is arranged in a 2:1 ratio of long-acting to insulin injection (e.g., Regular Insulin). If patients are on a twice-a-day regimen, a 2:1 ratio of total insulin between the morning and presupper dose will commonly provide adequate control. The dose of insulin must be adjusted to take into account the patient's activities and meal times. Patients are encouraged to make minor adjustments to their insulin regimen according to their urine glucose results or with the use of home blood glucose monitoring systems (e.g., Ames Dextrometer, Chemstrip bG, or glucometer).

The longer-acting insulins can be mixed freely with insulin injection (e.g., Regular Insulin) in the same syringe, and it is generally recommended that the patient learn to draw up the insulin injection first, because contamination of insulin injection with the longer-acting insulin may have profound effects on blood glucose control throughout the day.

Urine testing for glucose

When the concentration of blood glucose rises to a certain level, the kidney will begin to excrete glucose. The exact blood level at which glucose appears in the urine is referred to as the renal threshold, and this value can vary among individuals. Not uncommonly, pregnant diabetic women will display a low renal threshold, whereas elderly patients may have a higher renal threshold. Exact renal threshold can be determined by coincident measurement of urine glucose and blood glucose on several occasions.

Several techniques are available for the measurement of urine glucose, and all readings should be recorded as a percentage of glucose in the urine so that if different techniques are employed, the results will always be comparable.

The Clinitest tablet measures the presence of glucose in the urine by changing to various shades of color depending on the concentration of glucose present. This technique depends on the reducing powers of glucose to effect the color change in the tablet. Thus any reducing substance such as other sugars (e.g., galactose or lactose) or drugs with reducing properties (e.g., ascorbic acid) may indicate the presence of glucose when, in fact, it is absent. This is referred to as a false positive reading. The Clinitest tablets provide the best method of quantitating glucose and are thus valuable in the younger and more unstable diabetic patient. The test is available in two forms: a 5-drop technique that will quantitate glucose up to 2% or a 2-drop method that is more sensitive, allowing quantitation up to 5% of glucose.

The urine test-tape employs a specific glucose oxidase impregnated on the tape and thus will measure only glucose. Some drugs may interfere with the action of specific glucose stick methods (Tes-Tape), giving rise to a false negative result (Table 60-3), and Diastix tape can be inhibited by the presence of high ketone levels in the urine.

The presence of ketones in the urine can be reliably detected by a tablet (Acetest) or a tape technique (Ketostix). Ketodiastix measures both ketones and glucose.

Urine testing should be done before the main meals and before bedtime. If at all possible, the patient should empty the bladder approximately ½ hour be-fore the urine test so that the urine measurement will more accurately reflect the current blood glucose level. This is referred to as a double void technique.

TREATMENT OF DIABETIC EMERGENCIES

Diabetic ketoacidosis (DKA)

Ketoacidosis is precipitated by a marked reduction in insulin action. This may be the result of total lack of insulin or increased resistance to insulin, particularly when infection occurs in an insulin-dependent diabetic patient. Associated with the decrease in insulin action are increases in catecholamines, cortisol, and glucagon, all of which will promote a rise in blood glucose levels.

In the absence of insulin there will be breakdown of stored triglyceride *(lipolysis)* with the release of large quantities of free fatty acids into the circulation where they will eventually be taken up by the liver and transformed into ketone bodies. The main ketones are acetoacetic acid, acetone, and β-hydroxybutyrate. Acetone will be excreted by the lungs and kidneys and therefore can be detected on the breath, or in the urine by the Acetest tablets or Ketostix. However, up to 50% of all ketone bodies are in the form of β-hydroxybutyrate and will not be detected by normal laboratory techniques. Thus quantitation of the acidosis cannot be accurately made by measuring the amount of ketones using the simple ketone-detection techniques.

In *ketoacidosis* there is a generalized decrease in the uptake of glucose and amino acids by muscle. Severe hyperglycemia will result from the excess production of glucose, occurring mainly in the liver, and from the decrease in its uptake by peripheral tissue. With the rise in blood glucose levels an osmotic diuresis will take place with a loss of electrolytes, particularly sodium, potassium, and phosphate. Eventually cellular dehydration and hypovolemia will occur, and severe metabolic acidosis may be present.

The patient may initially have nausea, vomiting, abdominal tenderness, and a smell of acetone on the breath. As the degree of acidosis intensifies the patient will have deep-sighing respirations, referred to as *Kussmaul respiration.* This is a clear indicator of severe metabolic acidosis. There may be signs of severe dehydration, and cardiac dysrythmias may develop as a result of severe hypokalemia. The patient will gradually become comatose and death will occur shortly afterward.

The treatment of diabetic ketoacidosis requires insulin, careful fluid replacement, correction of the electrolyte inbalance, and occasionally the administration of bicarbonate therapy to correct the metabolic acidosis. The precipitating cause of the ketoacidosis

Management of diabetic ketoacidosis (DKA)

Basic principles

Successful treatment depends in large measure on

1. Individualization of therapy rather than rigid adherence to a predetermined regimen
2. Careful and continuous monitoring of clinical and laboratory data

Treatment

A. Emergency treatment
   1. Diagnosis
      a. Urine test for glucose and ketones (catheterize only comatose patients), Dextrostix or Clinitest tablets
      b. Laboratory test for glucose, CO_2, and electrolytes
      c. Arterial blood gases (if urine strongly positive for glucose and ketones)
   2. Assessment of vital signs
      a. Assure adequate airway
      b. Maintain blood pressure
      c. Assure adequate urine flow
      d. Eliminate danger of aspiration (insert nasogastric tube if necessary)
   3. Search for precipitating causes (e.g., infection, myocardial infarction, pancreatitis)
B. Insulin injection (e.g., Regular Insulin, Crystalline Zinc Insulin)
   1. Continuous intravenous infusion of insulin
      a. 5 to 10 units bolus as loading dose
      b. 4 to 6 units per hour as continuous infusion
      c. Insulin can be placed in IV bag or given by piggy-back infusion as indicated from constant-infusion pump
   2. Intramuscular insulin
      a. 5 to 10 units IM initially
      b. 4 to 6 units IM hourly
C. Fluids
   1. First hour: use normal saline particularly if patient appears to be in shock (low blood pressure, inadequate urine output); consider the use of plasma or volume expanders if severe shock is present
   2. Change to 0.45% NaCl with added K^+ in second or third hour of fluid replacement provided blood pressure and urine output are maintained; if bicarbonate is to be used, add to 0.45% NaCl
      a. Assess fluid deficit
      b. Plan replacement of 75% deficit in first 24 hours and 50% to 75% of this deficit in first 8 hours (i.e., $\frac{1}{2}$ to $\frac{3}{4}$ of 75% in first 8 hours)
      c. Add maintenance fluids to total volume
      d. Allow for continuing losses, and add to total volume to be infused
D. Potassium
   1. If hypokalemia is already established at start of therapy, (e.g., by ECG or serum potassium), commence potassium replacement at 10 to 20 mEq in the first hour
   2. If potassium value is unknown, commence potassium replacement in second hour of treatment at 10 mEq/hour
      a. Be prepared to adjust rate of input according to ECG and serum potassium
      b. Ensure adequate urine output *before* commencing potassium replacement
      c. Preferably use potassium phosphate initially rather than potassium chloride
E. Bicarbonate (The need for bicarbonate is not so critical in the younger patient and is *not* recommended in many therapeutic regimens for the treatment of ketoacidosis. If used, bicarbonate must be administered slowly to allow equilibration of pH between cerebrospinal fluid [CSF] and plasma)
   1. Add bicarbonate if
      a. pH <7.1
      b. bicarbonate <10 mmole/L
   2. Administration
      a. Add 2 ampules (88 mEq) to 1 L 0.45% NaCl and infuse in first hour
      b. Give third ampule (44 mEq) in 0.45% NaCl plus potassium in second hour
F. Glucose
   1. When glucose is less than 250 mg/dl, infuse glucose as $\frac{2}{3}$-$\frac{1}{3}$ dextrose-saline solution plus insulin and added K^+

should also be identified if at all possible. (See boxed material, p. 1385.)

Insulin therapy is the key to the management of diabetic ketoacidosis, and in recent years the concept of low-dose infusion of insulin has proved successful. In this technique insulin injection (e.g., Regular Insulin) is placed in the intravenous fluid being administered to the patient. Thus the insulin is received by the patient on a continuous basis until the blood glucose level and the metabolic abnormality have returned to normal. Various regimens have been proposed, and a representative insulin schedule requires the administration of 5 to 10 units of insulin injection given as an intravenous bolus followed by 4 to 6 units of insulin injection throughout each hour. If there has been no improvement in the metabolic situation of the patient within 4 hours of treatment, higher doses of insulin may be required or a further search for the cause of the metabolic abnormality should be made.

When insulin injection (Regular Insulin) is placed in the IV bag containing the intravenous fluid, adsorption of the insulin will take place in the walls of the container and tubing so that some insulin will be lost. However, once the initial adsorption has occurred, there will be no further loss of insulin and a steady quantity of insulin will be delivered to the patient. Therefore no materials need to be added to the IV delivery system to prevent adsorption of the insulin.

Correction of the metabolic abnormalities in diabetic ketoacidosis is usually achieved within 12 to 24 hours of the commencement of therapy. Insulin isophane or insulin zinc should be restarted the same time the intravenous therapy is being discontinued.

Hyperglycemic hyperosmolar nonketotic coma (HHNK)

A major distinction has been made previously between HHNK and ketoacidosis, but in reality there are marked similarities between both disorders. In HHNK there is a relative lack of action of insulin leading to extremely high levels of blood glucose, which causes the hyperosmolar situation. However, in contrast to ketoacidosis, ketosis is not a major feature of HHNK. The exact reasons for this are not known but it is possibly because there is sufficient insulin present to prevent severe lipolysis but not to prevent hyperglycemia. Patients with HHNK have been described as being more sensitive to insulin than patients with ketoacidosis, but once again the low-dose insulin regimens allow easy management of the hyperglycemia and the same dosage schedule can be followed as for the patient in ketoacidosis. Because of the hyperosmolar situation, hypotonic saline is commonly required and in much larger quantities. Electrolyte disturbances can occur, as in ketoacidosis, and potassium supplements will nearly always be required. Potassium supplements, however, should *not* be used until renal function and hydration are evaluated.

Hypoglycemia

Both insulin and the oral hypoglycemic agents are capable of lowering the blood glucose to levels beneath that required for normal metabolism of the nervous tissue, particularly the brain. As the blood glucose level falls, the patient will commonly become aware of a specific series of symptoms heralding the impending hypoglycemic event. These symptoms are precipitated by the simultaneous secretion of epinephrine, which occurs at the onset of the hypoglycemia. The patient will notice a feeling of weakness, hunger, palpitations and tachycardia, sweating, tingling of the lips and the fingers, and headache. If the blood glucose level falls to low levels, the patient will develop diplopia, confusion and disorientation, slurred speech, and eventually lapse into coma and may suffer epileptic-like seizures.

In the early stages of hypoglycemia, the ingestion of carbohydrates will commonly abort the attack, but if hypoglycemia is severe, intravenous glucose is often required. Oral glucose should be administered with great care if the patient is semiconscious, because the risk of aspiration into the lungs will be high. In the unconscious patient, where intravenous equipment is not easily available, glucagon hydrochloride can be used intravenously, intramuscularly, or subcutaneously in a dose of 1 mg. Return to consciousness should be observed within 20 to 30 minutes; otherwise intravenous glucose should be administered as soon as possible (Table 60-4).

Of particular concern is the patient who has been placed on β-blockers, such as propranolol, which will block the epinephrine-induced symptoms of hypoglycemia but not prevent the hypoglycemia itself. The use of β-blockers with insulin is contraindicated.

Management of the diabetic patient during surgery

Surgery can be considered a stress situation and as such will have profound metabolic responses in the patient. The degree of the metabolic disturbance is closely related to the severity of the operation. The key stress hormones are glucagon, cortisol, and the catecholamines, all of which will oppose the actions of insulin.

Glucagon will increase the breakdown of glycogen to glucose (glycogenolysis), increase the rate of pro-

TABLE 60-4

Differentiation of hypoglycemia from hyperglycemia

	Hypoglycemia	Hyperglycemia
Clinical features	Headache Hunger Increased perspiration Blurred vision Tingling in extremities and lips Palpitations Irritability Irrational behavior Tremor Coma Convulsions	Thirst Excess urination Weight loss Nausea, vomiting Abdominal pain Dehydration Acetone on breath "Sighing" respiration (Kussmaul's breathing) Confusion Coma
Laboratory features		
Urine (mandatory first test*; do *not* catheterize patient unless in coma)	Negative glucose and ketones	High glucose and eventually ketones
Plasma glucose	<50 mg/dl	>200 mg/dl Ketoacidosis >300 mg/dl
Etiology	Excessive use of insulin or oral hypoglycemic agents Excessive strenuous exercise without increased food intake	Pancreatic failure Insufficient insulin; associated with increased food intake, decreased exercise, infection, emotional or surgical stress
Treatment	Oral glucose (candy, juice, cola, biscuit) 1 mg glucagon SC; if no response in 15-20 min, give 50% glucose IV	Insulin injection (e.g., Regular Insulin) Fluids and electrolytes Search for precipitating cause

*Because of the increased renal threshold of glucose in the elderly, plasma glucose may be the more appropriate test in this age group.

duction of new glucose (*gluconeogenesis*), and may enhance the breakdown of triglycerides in the periphery (lipolysis). Catecholamines will also increase lipolysis and the breakdown of glycogen. Cortisol will augment the action of glucagon in the liver and cause the breakdown of protein in the peripheral tissues, thereby allowing an increase in the production of glucose precursors for the liver.

During surgery there is increased secretion of the stress hormones, and the resulting increase in blood glucose concentration appears to be proportional to the severity and extent of the operation. Associated with the increase of blood glucose concentration and the release of the stress hormones there is inhibition of insulin secretion. The suppression of insulin secretion during surgery is presumed to result from inhibition by catecholamines.

The aim of treatment of the diabetic patient during surgery is to prevent the occurrence of problems related to the metabolic disturbance associated with the surgery, such as hypoglycemia, infections, and ketoacidosis. It is preferable to admit all diabetic patients requiring elective surgery to the hospital for assessment and stabilization of the diabetes 24 to 48 hours before surgery. The therapeutic regimens will vary according to whether the patient is non–insulin dependent or insulin dependent.

Non–insulin-dependent diabetic. If only minor surgery is contemplated and the patient is well controlled on diet alone, no extra therapy is usually required. The patient should have an assessment of blood sugar control before surgery and immediately postoperatively to ensure that the blood glucose levels have not risen too high.

For the patient on oral hypoglycemic therapy, more care must be taken with therapy during surgery. Because the metabolic response to the surgery is predictable, it can be anticipated that there will be a significant rise in blood glucose during surgery. If, in the 48 hour preoperative assessment, it is established that the patient is not under adequate control on oral hypoglycemic therapy, or if major surgery is contemplated, the oral hypoglycemic agents should be withdrawn and the patient stabilized on insulin before

TABLE 60-5

Management of the diabetic patient requiring surgery

Type of diabetic patient	Management features
All diabetic patients	Admit patient to hospital 24-48 hours before surgery for stabilization
	If patient is not already on insulin, establish whether insulin will be required for the operative period and stabilize patient before surgery
	Provide rapid measurement of blood glucose during surgery and postoperatively (e.g., Dextrostix, Dextrometer)
	Plan surgery in early morning to allow for easy stabilization of diabetes in the postoperative period
Non–insulin-dependent diabetic patients	
Patient controlled on diet alone	*Preoperatively:* maintain patient on diet
	Postoperatively: resume normal diet and monitor blood glucose to check for hyperglycemia
Patient controlled on oral hypoglycemic agents	If patient is poorly controlled or major surgery is planned, stabilize patient on insulin before surgery and control blood glucose during surgery and postoperatively with insulin
Patient on long-acting sulfonylureas (e.g., chlorpropamide)	Stop drug 1 week before surgery and stabilize patient on short-acting sulfonylurea (e.g., tolbutamide, glyburide) or stabilize patient on insulin
Patient on short-acting sulfonylureas (e.g., tolbutamide, glyburide)	Stop drug on morning of operation and reintroduce with first meal in the postoperative period; if major surgery is contemplated, stabilize patient on insulin before surgery
Insulin-dependent diabetic patients	*Preoperatively:* stabilize patient on insulin b.i.d. before surgery
	During surgery: give ⅓ to ½ of total daily insulin as intermediate-acting insulin (e.g., insulin isophane, insulin zinc) immediately preoperatively; commence IV infusion of glucose/electrolyte solution with added K^+. Add insulin injection (e.g., Regular Insulin) to infusion bag to deliver ½-1 unit/ml/hr
	Monitor glucose q.2h. to keep glucose between 90-120 mg/dl
	Postoperatively: continue IV glucose/electrolyte/K^+ and added insulin injection (e.g., Regular Insulin) until patient can resume normal eating; if normal eating pattern is delayed greater than 24 hours, give ⅓ to ½ of the total preoperative daily insulin and continue IV fluids and insulin as above; once patient resumes normal eating pattern, resume normal insulin regimen adjusting according to food intake and mobility of patient
	Monitor patient closely for presence of postoperative infection and treat vigorously while maintaining normoglycemia

surgery and the insulin regimen outlined above used.

All patients on the long-acting hypoglycemic agents such as chlorpropamide should stop taking the agent 36 hours before surgery and be stabilized on insulin.

For those patients who are undergoing minor surgery and are well controlled on the shorter-acting hypoglycemic agents such as tolbutamide or glyburide, the sulfonylurea will be stopped on the day of surgery. Following the operation the sulfonylurea can be reintroduced with the first meal (Table 60-5).

Insulin-dependent diabetic. Many regimens exist for the management of the insulin-dependent diabetic undergoing surgery. The key aspects of therapy include careful management of fluid and electrolytes,

particularly potassium, and the administration of insulin, which will control the elevation of blood glucose and oppose the catabolic actions of the stress hormones.

Insulin regimen

Two regimens are commonly employed as the basis for the management of the diabetic undergoing surgery. In one protocol the stabilized diabetic patient will receive intermediate-acting insulin plus intravenous insulin injection (e.g., Regular Insulin) in the other protocol only intravenous insulin injection is given.

As an example of the first protocol, the stabilized

diabetic patient will receive one third to one half of the total daily dose of insulin, to be given as either insulin isophane or insulin zinc (e.g., if a patient receives 30 units of insulin isophane and 8 units of insulin injection in the morning and 10 units insulin isophane and 4 units of insulin injection in the evening [a total of 52 units], the patient would receive 18 to 26 units of insulin isophane on the morning before surgery). Depending on the duration and severity of the surgery, intravenous insulin administered at a low infusion rate of 0.5 to 1 unit per hour can be used to maintain *normoglycemia* in the operative and immediate postoperative period. This regimen can be repeated daily until the patient is able to resume a normal meal routine, at which time the preoperative insulin regimen can be resumed.

The second procedure is to use intravenous insulin only on the day of surgery. The intravenous insulin can be placed in the glucose-electrolyte intravenous fluid and will be administered from the time immediately before the surgery until the patient has resumed normal eating habits.

In both protocols the insulin is infused simultaneously with the glucose-electrolyte solution at a rate of approximately 0.5 to 1 unit per milliliter per hour.

Monitoring of blood glucose

The key to the control of diabetes is to know the metabolic status of the patient. The blood glucose level should be known immediately before surgery and should be rechecked every 2 hours during surgery and every 3 to 4 hours in the postoperative period. In the past the use of the urine sliding scale to determine the quantity of insulin to be administered resulted in many complex insulin regimens being employed. However, the concept of using the sliding scale is invalid because urine samples will reflect changes in blood glucose level that may have occurred several hours before; the values do not anticipate future changes in the blood glucose level. Blood glucose can now be measured quickly and accurately using such techniques as the Ames glucose monitoring systems, in which blood glucose can be measured within 1 minute. It is essential that staff using this type of equipment receive full training in its usage. Knowledge of the blood glucose level allows one to adjust the rate of administration of insulin to maintain normoglycemia and to prevent the extremes of hypoglycemia and hyperglycemia.

Postoperative complications

Many diabetic patients already have major organ damage, and particular care must be taken with fluid and electrolyte balance to prevent unnecessary car-

diac stress and to maintain adequate renal function. Hypertension should be treated carefully and the blood pressure monitored frequently after surgery. The appearance of infection in the diabetic patient will lead to insulin resistance and elevation of blood glucose levels. Both the infection and blood glucose elevation must be treated adequately. A regimen for the management of the insulin-dependent diabetic is outlined in Table 60-5.

COMPLICATIONS OF DIABETES

The complications of diabetes are numerous and provide some difficult problems. Diabetes will affect virtually all systems in the body giving rise to serious symptoms and deterioration of quality of life. The etiologic factors behind the onset and progression of diabetic complications remain unknown. The controversy as to whether "control" of diabetes will prevent the onset or delay of diabetic complications still persists; however, more recent clinical and experimental data clearly demonstrate that ideal control of glucose is of benefit. The major complications of diabetes are listed in Table 60-6.

As well as advocating ideal blood glucose control, the National Diabetes Advisory Board made specific recommendations to lessen the impact of several of the major complications of diabetes—blindness, nephropathy, foot lesions, perinatal morbidity, and diabetic ketoacidosis. The Advisory Board has suggested the following areas of clinical awareness that could be undertaken in each of these areas.

Foot complications in the diabetic patient result ultimately from peripheral vascular disease, peripheral neuropathy, and eventually infection. These abnormalities can lead to prolonged periods of imposed bed rest and even amputation of the infected limb. It is recommended that the nurse:

1. Instruct the patient in the means of careful daily examination of the feet
2. Ensure that all patients have their feet examined by a professional at least four times every year
3. Encourage use of specialized therapeutic shoes or orthopedic appliances if necessary
4. Identify resources for rapid rehabilitation for the diabetic patient who has had an amputation

Because *diabetic ketoacidosis* can be prevented, the patient should be aware of the clinical features of diabetic ketoacidosis. Appropriate intervention is required to prevent the serious metabolic sequelae of diabetic ketoacidosis.

Perinatal morbidity and mortality can be reduced by ensuring that pregnant diabetic women are cared for by a team of perinatologists, diabetologists, neo-

TABLE 60-6

Complications of diabetes mellitus

System	Complication	System	Complication
Ocular system (diabetic eye disease)		Renal system (nephropathy)	Glomerular lesions
Diabetic retinopathy (highest cause of blindness in younger age group)	Background retinopathy		Nodular
	Vascular lesions		Diffuse
	Capillary dilatation		Exudative
	Aneurysms		Hyalinization
	Arterial dilation		Thickening capillary basement membrane
	Extravascular lesions		Accumulation of basement membrane–like material within the mesangium
	Hemorrhages		
	Cotton wool spots		
	Hard exudates		Fibrin deposition
	Proliferative retinopathy		Clinical presentation
	New vessel formation		Proteinuria
	Fibrous retinitis proliferans		Hypertension
	Vitreous hemorrhage		Progressive renal failure
Lens abnormality	Cataracts	Cardiovascular system	Coronary artery disease
Nervous system (neuropathy)	Cranial nerves		Cerebrovascular disease
	III and VI (diplopia)		Peripheral vascular disease
	VII (facial weakness, rare)	Miscellaneous	Infections
	Autonomic nervous system		More prone to yeast and fungal infections
	Gastric stasis		Urinary tract infections are more frequently seen in diabetics as a result of increased incidence of catheterization, hospitalization, and high glucose concentration in urine
	Diarrhea		
	Urinary retention		
	Postural hypotension		
	Impotence (males)		
	Peripheral nerves		
	Sensory loss		
	Burning, tingling, motor loss		
	Amyotrophy/mononeuropathy		
	Asymmetrical lower leg muscle wasting		
	Pain		
	Minor sensory loss		
	Weakness		

natologists, and specially prepared nurses who have experience in the care of diabetic women during pregnancy and after delivery. Perfect control of the diabetic woman during pregnancy under the supervision of a combined health team results in an improved outcome of the pregnancy.

Diabetic retinopathy is now the leading cause of blindness in young people and the Diabetic Retinopathy Study Research Group has clearly identified the importance of early detection of eye disease and the advocacy of photocoagulation at an early stage of the disease.

Diabetic nephropathy has become one of the most serious of the life-threatening complications of diabetes. The nurse and other health professionals can help lessen the impact of serious diabetic kidney disease by (1) measurement of blood pressure of all diabetic patients at least once a year; (2) vigorous management of hypertension when it occurs; (3) careful adherance to a salt-restricted diet; (4) regular analysis of the urine for protein, serum creatinine, and blood urea nitrogen; (5) early referral of patients with a serum creatinine level equal to or greater than 3 mg/dl to a specialist experienced in diabetic nephropathy; (6) consideration of renal transplantation when the serum creatinine level is greater than 5 mg/dl; and (7) assistance to the diabetic patient after transplantation particularly concerning diabetic retinopathy, diet, and care of the limbs.

The success of the management of the diabetic patient will depend very much on the success of the health care team, including the nurse, physician, dietitian, podiatrist, social worker, and others who care for and advise the diabetic patient.

NEW ADVANCES IN THE TREATMENT OF DIABETES

In recent years the development of newer tests to assess the long-term blood glucose levels of diabetic patients, the production of biosynthetic human insulin (BHI), and various forms of the artificial pancreas would suggest that some of the more traditional means of treating and monitoring the diabetic patient are changing.

Glycosylated hemoglobins

During the formation of the red blood cells, glucose derivatives are continuously formed within the cell and are referred to as glycohemoglobins. When the blood glucose remains elevated for long periods of time, as in uncontrolled diabetes, the levels of glycohemoglobins rise and can be detected by laboratory techniques. Because the life span of the red blood cell is close to 120 days, the extent of the glycosylation can be used as an index of long-term blood glucose control. The incorporation of the glucose to the hemoglobin molecule results in a change in the charge of the molecule, which allows chromatographic separation of various hemoglobin species. The most common measurement made is of HbAlC or HbAl. An elevation of above 9% of total hemoglobin and glycohemoglobin is considered abnormal and represents long-term elevation of the blood glucose.

Biosynthetic human insulin (BHI)

Insulin was one of the first hormones to benefit from the exciting new techniques of recombinant DNA technology. The genetic material of the A and B chains of human insulin is inserted into the genetic material of the bacteria *Escherichia coli,* thereby allowing the production of the two chains of human insulin. Following a purification step the two chains are joined together in the correct manner with disulfide bonds. It appears that this insulin is chemically, biologically, and immunologically identical to pancreatic human insulin. Biosynthetic human insulin is devoid of all pancreatic protein contaminants. It is available in both short-acting (e.g., Humulin-R) and intermediate-acting (e.g., Humulin-N) forms.

Artificial pancreas

The ideal artificial pancreas would be able to sense the blood glucose level and "instruct" a pump system to deliver the required quantity of insulin. Although experimental devices are being used that would meet these requirements, the greatest experience has been achieved using continuous subcutaneous insulin infusion delivered by small pumps that can be programmed to allow for variation in eating and activity. Many studies have now described the metabolic changes that take place in patients receiving long-term subcutaneous insulin infusion. There is no question that these devices provide an exciting future for the insulin-dependent diabetic patient. One day the patient may be relieved of the need to inject insulin every day for life.

Pancreatic transplantation

Pancreatic transplantation has been tried in experimental animals and in some human subjects, and generally two techniques have been utilized: (1) transplantation of sections of a whole pancreas from a donor and (2) injection of viable pancreatic islets into either the peritoneal cavity, portal vein, or liver. The greatest problem with this technique is that of rejection of the transplant by the host and the need for special antilymphocytic serums and immunosuppressive drugs, which may be harmful to the patient. Considerable research has been undertaken to examine these problems, and this technique may yet hold considerable hope for the diabetic patient.

SUMMARY

The oral hypoglycemic agents and insulin have been discussed in relation to the treatment of non–insulin-dependent diabetes mellitus and insulin-dependent diabetes mellitus. An understanding of the indication for these agents as well as their actions, adverse effects, preparation, administration, and potential drug interactions will enable the nurse to plan individualized programs to assist patients with the management of diabetes and to minimize the complications associated with this condition.

ADVERSE/SIDE EFFECTS OF THE ORAL HYPOGLYCEMIC AGENTS AND INSULIN*

Oral hypoglycemic agents
ALLERGIC REACTIONS

Morbilliform or maculopapular
  eruptions
Porphyria cutanea tarda
Photosensitivity reactions
Pruritus
Urticaria

GASTROINTESTINAL SYSTEM

Diarrhea
Epigastric fullness and heartburn
Jaundice
Nausea
Vomiting

HEMATOLOGIC SYSTEM

Agranulocytosis
Aplastic anemia
Leukopenia
Thrombocytopenia

METABOLIC SYSTEM

Hepatic porphyria
Hypoglycemia
Inappropriate antidiuretic hormone
  action

Insulin
ALLERGIC REACTIONS

Allergic urticaria
Anaphylactic reactions
Angioedema
Local inflammatory response

CENTRAL NERVOUS SYSTEM

Blurred vision
Coma
Confusion
Diplopia
Epileptic seizure
Headache
Hunger
Nervousness
Palpitations
Sweating

METABOLIC SYSTEM

Hypoglycemia
Lipoatrophy

*See Chapter 11, "Drug Toxicity," for an overview of drug toxicity.

CLINICALLY SIGNIFICANT DRUG INTERACTIONS*

Primary drug	Interacting drug	Possible effect(s)	Probable mechanism(s)
Diazoxide	Phenytoin	Decreased phenytoin levels	Increased metabolism
Diazoxide	Sulfonylureas	Decreased effect of both drugs on blood sugar	Pharmacologic antagonism
Glucagon	Warfarin	Hemorrhage	Not established
Insulin	Alcohol	Hypoglycemia	Additive effect
Insulin	Fenfluramine	Hypoglycemia	Additive effect
Insulin	Monoamine oxidase inhibitors	Hypoglycemia	Not established
Insulin	Propranolol	Hypoglycemia (often with masked or obscured symptoms)	Additive effect
Sulfonylureas (acetohexamide, chlorpropamide, glipizide, glyburide, tolazamide, tolbutamide)	Alcohol	Hypoglycemia (acute alcohol ingestion) / Hyperglycemia (chronic alcohol ingestion)	Additive alcohol hypoglycemic effect / Increased metabolism of sulfonylureas
Sulfonylureas	Diazoxide	Decreased effect of both drugs on blood sugar	Pharmacologic antagonism
Sulfonylureas	Dicumarol	Hypoglycemia	Decreased metabolism
Sulfonylureas	Fenfluramine	Hypoglycemia	Additive effect
Sulfonylureas	Monoamine oxidase inhibitors	Hypoglycemia	Not established
Sulfonylureas	Phenylbutazone	Hypoglycemia	Decreased metabolism and decreased renal excretion
Sulfonylureas	Salicylates (more than 2 gm/day)	Hypoglycemia	Additive effect
Sulfonylureas	Sulfinpyrazone	Hypoglycemia	Decreased metabolism
Sulfonylureas	Sulfonamides	Hypoglycemia	Decreased metabolism and displacement from plasma proteins

*See Chapter 10, "Drug Interactions," for an overview of drug interactions.

GENERAL NURSING IMPLICATIONS

Nursing of patients requiring oral hypoglycemics or insulin

ASSESSMENT

Patients requiring oral hypoglycemics or insulin require a thorough history and physical examination including laboratory evaluations of blood and urine. It must be identified if the patient is insulin dependent or non–insulin dependent. It is important during initial assessment to identify if the patient has newly diagnosed diabetes or how long the patient has had diagnosed diabetes and how the condition has been treated. Other important data include the age of onset of the condition, previous hospitalizations, self-care abilities in relation to the management of diabetes, and effects of the condition on lifestyle, mental well-being, and family interactions.

Initial nursing assessment should include the results of recent urine testing. It should be ascertained if the specimen was a single- or double-void specimen, if testing was done accurately, and if consistently high readings were obtained for 2 or more days. Ketonuria should be identified, indicating that control has deteriorated and immediate treatment with insulin is necessary, or if the patient has had an insulin reaction within the last 24 hours. A glucagon order should be obtained if the patient has a history of insulin shock. Insulin shock and ketoacidosis are the most common acute problems associated with diabetes, and patients may have either of these conditions. Family or friends may be required to assist with the gathering of data depending on the patient's general condition. Recent periods of inactivity, illness, mental stress, or change in usual diet or activity pattern should also be identified.

The patient's general health state, height, weight, blood pressure, and other vital signs should be assessed. Any history of renal, cardiac, or hepatic disease should be identified. Women of childbearing age should be questioned regarding pregnancy. Patients should also be carefully assessed for the presence of common complications associated with diabetes including neuropathy, nephropathy, retinopathy, or cardiovascular or dermatologic com-

plications and for the presence of any infection. A smoking history should be included in the initial assessment because smoking has been found to affect insulin absorption, and a change in smoking habits can lead to fluctuations in glucose control.

Fasting blood sugar (FBS), serum electrolytes, serum acetone, and other laboratory tests are usually indicated, and are important baseline data for planning individualized therapy. Patients should be assisted with these tests as needed. It is important to note that urine tests for glucose in the elderly may be misleading because the renal threshold for glucose rises with age. The older person may be hyperglycemic without glycosuria. The FBS may fail to detect diabetes in persons whose FBS levels are normal but who are hyperglycemic after meals. A glucose tolerance test is a better test for diagnosing diabetes in the elderly.

The relationship of family members should be assessed to identify sources of emotional support and assistance as well as problems so that individualized care can be planned. The patient's developmental needs, previous patterns of coping with stress, and general reaction to diabetes should be carefully assessed. Patients can be fearful, angry, and concerned about associated health care costs, occurrence of physical impairment, or effects of diabetes on the job and other aspects of lifestyle. Patients often have multiple concerns that require careful exploration, which should be identified during the initial assessment or as soon as possible.

It is also important to assess knowledge and self-care skills to identify learning needs so that individualized teaching can be planned and implemented. Patients who have been managing their diabetes themselves should, when possible, demonstrate urine testing and medication administration so that an accurate assessment can be made of their urine testing and self-medication abilities. This is important because many diabetics become careless with techniques especially over long-term treatment, often resulting in problems with the optimum management of this condition. They also require reinforce-

ment for maintaining accurate self-care practices. In addition, because knowledge and technology are ever changing, this gives the patient the opportunity to learn about new aspects of treatment and care and gives the patient the opportunity to have any developing deficits assessed including effects of such conditions as arthritis, yellowing of the lens, or other age-related changes that can affect self-care management. These deficits as well as other deficits identified with newly diagnosed diabetic patients, should be incorporated into care planning.

In addition to these baseline data, initial assessment should include a detailed drug history to identify sensitivity, contraindications, cautions, potential drug interactions, and drug-taking patterns *before* insulin or oral hypoglycemic therapy is initiated.

SENSITIVITY

Generally, allergic reactions to insulin or oral hypoglycemics are rare; however, any drug has the potential to cause a hypersensitivity reaction in susceptible individuals. Allergic reactions have been reported including both local and systemic reactions to insulin. With the purified insulin preparations allergic reactions are less prevalent including the incidence of (1) local insulin allergy (redness, wheal or firm induration at injection site), (2) systemic insulin allergy (anaphylaxis, urticaria), (3) insulin resistance, and (4) lipodystrophy (lipoatrophy, lipohypertrophy). Desensitization with an insulin allergy desensitization kit may be indicated.

CONTRAINDICATIONS

The use of insulin or oral hypoglycemics is contraindicated in patients with known hypersensitivity to the specific agent.

The use of β-blockers is contraindicated in insulin-dependent diabetic patients because they can block the epinephrine-induced symptoms of hypoglycemia.

See the Nursing Drug Digest for contraindications associated with specific agents.

Continued.

GENERAL NURSING IMPLICATIONS—cont'd

Nursing of patients requiring oral hypoglycemics or insulin—cont'd

CAUTIONS

Oral hypoglycemics with prolonged action (e.g., chlorpropamide) should be used with caution in the elderly, in non–insulin-dependent diabetic patients during illness, or when intake is reduced, because fatal hypoglycemia can occur with continued administration of the drug.

Second generation sulfonylureas are more potent than other sulfonylureas and are used in smaller doses; thus they should be used cautiously.

See the Nursing Drug Digest for cautions associated with specific agents.

DRUG INTERACTIONS

The oral hypoglycemics and insulin have the potential to interact with other drugs in a variety of mechanisms (see Clinically Significant Drug Interactions).

ADMINISTRATION
Oral hypoglycemics

The oral sulfonylureas are dosed according to the half-life and duration of action of each drug. For example, acetohexamide is taken in divided doses through the day; chlorpropamide and tolazamide are taken once per day. Tolazamide dosage is easily adjusted because it is intermediate-acting in duration. Chlorpropamide, because it is long acting, makes dosage adjustments more difficult.

Sulfonylureas should be given immediately before meals with a full glass of water according to the dosage schedule. If the patient is unwell or may not take regular meals, the oral hypoglycemic agent dosage should be reduced or eliminated.

Insulin

Although insulin is usually required on a daily basis over a prolonged period of time, it can also be required intermittently in the treatment of hyperkalemia, during hyperalimentation, or for non–insulin-dependent diabetic patients during pregnancy, surgery, or acute illness. Insulin is usually administered subcutaneously; however, insulin injection (e.g., Regular Insulin) can also be administered intravenously or by insulin pump. Depending on the duration of action and dosage, insulin is given once a day or more frequently. To more closely follow the body's insulin secretion pattern, the trend toward multiple daily doses of intermediate- or long-acting insulin with multiple doses of short-acting insulin before meals is becoming more common. Dosage and administration are highly individualized to the patient's needs.

Insulin is available in various concentrations including U-40 and U-100; U-80 was previously available. The concentration refers to the number of units of insulin per milliliter in a syringe. It is important to use only U-40 syringes with U-40 insulin and U-100 syringes with U-100 insulin to ensure that the correct amount of insulin is administered.

Subcutaneous injection

Insulin is generally administered using sterile technique subcutaneously (see Chapter 2, "Preparation, Administration, and Monitoring of Medications"). The injection site is determined by the condition of the skin and underlying subcutaneous tissue as well as the patient's personal preferences, manual dexterity, and ability to reach sites for safe injection.

The preferred sites of injection are the lateral surfaces of the upper arms, the abdominal tissue along the rib cage, the anterolateral surfaces of the thighs, and the back. The buttocks and the abdomen (between the belt line and symphysis pubis) may be used if the fatty layer is not too extensive and the tissue can be gently pulled up away from the underlying muscle. The shoulders can also be used if enough fatty tissue can be gently pinched up to make the injection (Figure 60-4).

Injection sites should be carefully inspected and palpated for lipodystrophy, scar tissue, nevi, moles, or other deviations. Sites with deviations should *not* be used, nor should areas of inflammation, injury, or local reaction (e.g., wheal with itching). The belt line, skin creases or body folds, joints, and an area 2.5 cm (1 inch) from the umbilicus should likewise *not* be used. Skin areas under prosthesis straps should not be used.

Injections should be made into healthy tissue free from large blood vessels and nerves.

It is important to note that injured or hypertrophied tissue can interfere with insulin absorption. If a site is being used for the first time, absorption can be increased leading to the possibility of an insulin reaction.

The same injection spot should not be used for 6 to 8 weeks. Sites should be rotated to prevent changes in subcutaneous tissue and infection. Injections should be carefully recorded on an injection record.

An individualized rotation schedule should be planned with the patient. The patient's established plan should be followed and adapted as necessary. Although nurses can use all recommended sites as long as tissue is healthy, it is important to recognize that patients may not be able to use all sites realistically. This should be taken into consideration when planning rotation schedules. For example, it may be necessary to delete the dominant arm from the rotation schedule until dexterity is sufficient to use this site. The sites on the back or buttocks may also need to be deleted from the rotation schedule. When individualized rotation schedules are developed with patients, it is important to recognize that absorption can vary from site to site as well as be affected by exercise (e.g., jogging, which would particularly affect the thigh sites).

Rotating insulin injection sites within the same anatomic region (see Figure 60-4) rather than between different regions may help reduce excessive day-to-day variations in blood glucose levels in the insulin-dependent diabetic. It is important to also note that absorption from the different regions varies. For example, absorption is 86% greater from the abdominal site than from the leg sites and 30% greater than from the arm sites. It may be necessary to adjust insulin dosage according to level of absorption at the newly selected region.

GENERAL NURSING IMPLICATIONS—cont'd

Nursing of patients requiring oral hypoglycemics or insulin—cont'd

Subcutaneous injection—cont'd

Insulin is stored in the refrigerator. Patients can keep the vial in use at room temperature without any problems, but for prolonged storage insulin should be refrigerated. Always check the expiration date and read the label carefully to ensure the correct type of insulin is administered. Many manufacturers are color-coding the various insulins as well as matching U-100 to U-100 syringes in packaging. Always be sure that the correct insulin syringe is selected for the concentration of insulin, and be sure needle selection is made in relation to individual patient factors and site of administration.

Because insulin suspensions can settle to the bottom of the multidose vial they should be gently rolled between the palms to mix thoroughly and to prevent the occurrence of bubbles so that the exact dosage is administered. To withdraw insulin, the same amount of air as number of units of insulin to be administered is injected into the vial to prevent a vacuum and the exact amount of insulin withdrawn. It is particularly important that the syringe be checked for the presence of any air bubbles. It is generally accepted practice that insulin be double-checked by another registered nurse in acute care settings before administration. If two types of insulin are to be drawn up in the same syringe, air is first injected into the modified insulin (being careful not to touch the medication) and the needle is then carefully withdrawn. The exact amount of air to displace the insulin as ordered is injected into the vial of insulin injection (e.g., Regular Insulin) and the medication withdrawn. The modified insulin is then withdrawn carefully. It is important to note that the needle should be changed before the modified insulin is drawn up. This procedure helps prevent contaminating insulin in one vial with insulin from another. However, newer insulin syringes have been developed as one-piece units to minimize the amount of dead space and increase accuracy of injections. Thus changing the needle may not always be possible. Because the newer insulin syringes also have microfine needles (26-27.5 gauge), there is a tendency for the needles to become plugged after being inserted into the multidose vial rubber stoppers. It is important that needles be carefully inserted into multidose vials with the bevel up to prevent the occurrence of plugs as well as to prevent dulling or bending of the needle.

The site is grasped between the thumb and fingers and the tissue pinched-up into a pocket in which the insulin is injected. This procedure has been associated with less pain, less lipodystrophy, and more complete absorption. As with other injections, sterile technique is used and the site is cleaned with an alcohol pledget before injection. The needle is withdrawn slowly in the direction it was inserted to prevent the leakage of insulin. The use of the air-lock technique is not recommended for the administration of insulin. The site can be gently wiped with an alcohol pledget; however, it should *not* be massaged after the injection is made. When administering insulin, keep the following points in mind:

1. Ensure that the correct insulin has been drawn up in the syringe in the prescribed proportions for the patient. Check the results of urine glucose and ketone measurements, because adjustment of insulin dosage may be required on a day-to-day or hour-to-hour basis according to the urine test results.
2. Rotate each insulin injection site in the recommended pattern (see Figure 60-4).
3. Clean the skin thoroughly before the injection.
4. After injection through the skin aspirate to ensure that the needle is not in a blood vessel. Check current and previous injection sites for signs of infection, allergic response to the insulin and for signs of lipodystrophy.
5. Continue to check urine for glucose and ketones so that the maximum amount of information is obtained before the next insulin order. Check for other drug administration, particularly β-blockers, which may mask symptoms of hypoglycemia.

MONITORING PATIENT RESPONSE
Therapeutic response

The onset and duration of the hypoglycemic effect of the oral hypoglycemics and insulin largely depend on the individual agent. (See Table 60-2 for onset, peak, and duration of action of each specific agent.) Therapeutic response can also be affected by individual patient factors and the site of insulin administration.

It is important to note that an absence of therapeutic response may be a result of not taking medication as directed or because the patient has developed an infection or illness. If the patient is receiving a sulfonylurea, a change to another sulfonylurea may improve therapeutic response.

Monitor non–insulin-dependent diabetic patients receiving oral hypoglycemics for (1) weight loss if overweight, (2) weight control, and (3) the achievement of ideal blood glucose levels.

Monitor insulin-dependent diabetic patients receiving insulin for (1) normal growth and development and (2) achievement of ideal control of blood glucose.

In the acute care setting or clinic various laboratory tests can be completed in relation to evaluating hypoglycemic response, including the monitoring of 24-hour urinary glucose and glycosylated hemoglobins for assessing quantitative control of diabetes. Various relatively simple and accurate products are available for testing urine for ketonuria and glycosuria as well as for monitoring blood glucose levels (see Table 60-3).

Record the results of these tests on diabetic monitoring records, particularly for observation and reference in relation to long-term therapy. These records are also helpful aids for discussion with the patient and family members regarding therapeutic response to therapy.

Skin preparation with isopropyl alcohol has been associated with false results when blood glucose is monitored

Continued.

GENERAL NURSING IMPLICATIONS—cont'd

Nursing of patients requiring oral hypoglycemics or insulin—cont'd

Therapeutic response—cont'd

with Dextrostix. Therefore it is recommended that the skin be wiped dry with a sterile gauze after the site has been prepared with the alcohol. Following puncture with a lance, blot up the first drop of blood to eliminate the possibility of isopropyl alcohol contamination and then collect the specimen to be analyzed. The sides of the fingers or toes should be used because the capillary blood supply is richer, and these sites have decreased sensation and are thus less painful than the pads of the fingers or toes. The earlobes can also be used as sites for obtaining blood for this test.

Adverse side effects

Adverse effects associated with the oral hypoglycemics and insulin are interrelated generally with the condition and management of diabetes, although some adverse effects are specifically drug related. For example, patients receiving high doses of long-acting oral hypoglycemics such as chlorpropamide should be monitored for drug-induced red blood cell aplasia. Complete blood cell counts should be monitored.

If the patient is on chlorpropamide, watch for signs of increased fluid retention since this may indicate increased antidiuretic hormone action. Check urine regularly for the presence of glucose and ketones; this would indicate that the oral hypoglycemic agents are being used inappropriately and that insulin is probably required.

Observe and report symptoms of hypersensitivity such as skin rashes or fever.

Generally, patients requiring oral hypoglycemics or insulin should be monitored for hypoglycemia, diabetic ketoacidosis (DKA), and HHNK:

1. Hypoglycemia can result from too much insulin or oral hypoglycemic, omission or delay in eating meals, or excessive strenuous exercise without increasing food intake. Hospitalization may be required for patients with hypoglycemia particularly those taking long-acting oral hypoglycemics or insulins.

2. DKA usually requires hospitalization and occurs primarily in diabetic patients as a result of omission of insulin, uncontrolled diabetes, infections, acute illness, pregnancy, trauma, surgery, or emotional stress.

3. HHNK is manifested by extreme, sustained hyperglycemia with severe dehydration. This condition is serious—mortality has been reported as high as 50%. At risk are the elderly who have NIDDM controlled either by diet alone or by diet and oral hypoglycemics. This effect has also been associated with pancreatic disease, glucocorticoid therapy, and the use of total parenteral nutrition, which can often impair glucose tolerance as well as other conditions. The blood glucose level is high (600 to over 2,000 mg/dl), and ketonemia is absent, thus differentiating this condition from DKA. Treatment is directed at establishing and maintaining fluid and electrolyte balance. Low-dose insulin therapy may be indicated to correct hyperglycemia as well as the use of heparin to prevent the development of arterial and venous thrombosis secondary to dehydration and circulatory stasis.

Monitor patients for signs of:

1. Hypoglycemia (see Table 60-4 for a comparison of hypoglycemia and hyperglycemia)
2. Diabetic ketoacidosis (DKA)
   Abdominal tenderness
   Polyuria
   Nocturia
   Enuresis
   Polydipsia
   Headache
   Listlessness, weakness
   Nausea
   Vomiting (may be coffee ground)
   Warm, flushed, dry skin
   Marked dehydration
   Ketonuria
   Glycosuria
   Hyperglycemia
   Ketonemia
   Acidosis
   Kussmaul's breathing
   Acetone breath
   Hypokalemia
   Hyponatremia
   Hypophosphatemia
   Dysrhythmias
   Coma
   Death
3. Hyperglycemic hyperosmolar nonketonic coma (HHNK) (osmotic dehydration)
   Warm skin; elevated body temperature
   Flushed skin
   Dry, loose skin
   Soft eyeballs
   Deeply furrowed tongue
   Lethargy
   Weakness
   Disorientation, confusion, sleepiness (initial); coma (late)
   Hypernatremia or hyponatremia
   Thirst
   Hypokalemia
   Rapid, weak pulse
   Shallow respirations; absence of acetone on breath
   Dry mucous membranes
   Diminished reflexes
   Weight loss
   Polyuria (urine output high)
   Glycosuria (high)
   Serum acetone, negative
   Grand mal seizures
   Hemiparesis
   Positive Babinski reflexes

PATIENT EDUCATION

The patient and family should undergo an education program concerning diabetes so that they are fully aware of the key aspects of treatment, particularly in the use of diet, exercise, and medication. They should be taught the key features of hypoglycemia, hyperglycemia, and DKA so that these extremes of diabetes can be avoided or treated quickly (see Table 60-4). They should understand the complications related to diabetes so that these can be looked for on a regular basis by both the patient and health care provider and treated appropriately.

Patient education is vital in the management of diabetes and must be highly individualized and contain essential information regarding the importance of the control of blood glucose levels. It is important to evaluate the patient's current knowledge of diabetes and re-

GENERAL NURSING IMPLICATIONS—cont'd

Nursing of patients requiring oral hypoglycemics or insulin—cont'd

PATIENT EDUCATION—cont'd

sources of information (e.g., family, friends, books, articles, personal experiences) as well as to clarify misinformation. Knowledge of diabetes and its control helps the patient to maintain independence and control over body, activities, and the future.

The patient and family should know the exact name of the hypoglycemic drug or type and concentration of insulin, its general action, purpose, dosage, method of storage, administration, and adverse side effects. The patient should know how to monitor therapeutic response and be able to identify signs that indicate that the health care provider should be contacted. Because the management of diabetes involves the modification of lifestyle (including personal hygiene, diet, and exercise) as well as drug therapy, the patient must understand these aspects of care in the maintenance of normal blood glucose levels and general health.

It is helpful to outline topics to be covered in teaching sessions and to sequence presentations in relation to the patient's expressed interest to reduce anxiety. Usually the nurse, physician, dietitian, social worker, psychiatrist, or other health workers are involved in teaching programs.

Quizzes and return demonstrations are helpful in assessing progress. Nurses in various settings have developed diabetic teaching care plans. Information packets and other materials are also available through various diabetes associations. Clinical nurse specialists in diabetic care and nurse practitioners are becoming increasingly independent in providing essential care to diabetic patients and can also be used as resources.

Discharge information sheets should be provided for patients to refer to when at home.

Although patient education does take time, a comprehensive program can do much to promote quality of life and increase control with fewer hospitalizations, adverse effects, and reduced complications associated with diabetes. Patients can be assisted to prevent or decrease problems often encoun-

tered in the daily management of this condition. Diabetic day care programs have been used to help patients adapt to insulin requirements allowing them to maintain more usual patterns in daily living so that insulin requirements can be better estimated. These programs also reduce the cost of the associated hospitalization.

Follow-up is particularly important and patients should understand the necessity of keeping appointments with health care providers. The patient should know to telephone the clinic or hospital to report glucose or ketones in the urine, nausea and vomiting, or insulin reaction, or if he or she has any questions about care. Home follow-up should be completed to assess equipment care and the patient's adjustment to the condition. Referral may be indicated to social services for help with social problems.

Monthly group meetings have been helpful to patients and their families to discuss diabetes and to share experiences regarding coping with the condition on a day-to-day basis.

Outline for teaching sessions

I. Diabetes and its control
   A. Nature of condition
   B. Cause
   C. Treatment
   D. Need for continued health care and follow-up
II. Administration of oral hypoglycemics or insulin
   A. Dosage schedules
   B. Storage of medication and equipment; care of equipment
   C. Disposal of outdated medication and used equipment
   D. Insulin injection sites
   E. Insulin administration
   F. Adjusting insulin according to illness or other stress

NOTE: Research has shown that disposable syringes and needles can be safely reused three or four times if they are carefully wiped with alcohol after use and refrigerated. Because the needle is dulled after three or four injections, further use is *not* recommended. Disposable equipment should *not* be reused in a clinic or hospital setting because of the increased risk of infection.

Patients with arthritis, vision problems, or hemiparesis require special approaches to care so that self-medication abilities can be maintained whenever possible. Various measurement aids and modified equipment and techniques can be explored. Prefilled syringes can be used for patients who have difficulty measuring insulin accurately. These are probably safe for 2 to 3 weeks when refrigerated.

III. Balancing diet
   A. Timing and patterns of meals
   B. Exchange groups
   C. Meal planning
   D. Food selection and preparation
   E. Caloric requirements with age, activity, illness, exercise
   F. Weight management, especially with history of obesity

NOTE: Self-care should be maintained as much as possible. Family members or neighbors can assist with shopping or meal preparation if possible. Explore the use of social services including Meals on Wheels as indicated.

IV. Testing
   A. Urine and blood
   B. Frequency
   C. Interpretation/recording/reporting tests accurately

NOTE: When testing urine glucose levels, the elderly may have difficulty differentiating blue-green shades because of age-associated yellowing of the lens.

Self-monitoring of blood glucose is indicated for patients who are pregnant, those with an altered renal glucose threshold, and patients treated with insulin pumps. These patients require instruction in modification of diabetic management because of condition as well as treatment.

VI. Modification of lifestyle or self-care practices
   A. Exercise
   B. Skin care
   C. Foot care and exercises
   D. Dental care
   E. Driving/travel
   F. Bathing (water temperature)
   G. Clothing (leather, well-fitting shoes; avoidance of tight-fitting garments, garters)

Continued.

GENERAL NURSING IMPLICATIONS—cont'd

Nursing of patients requiring oral hypoglycemics or insulin—cont'd

Outline for teaching sessions— cont'd

VII. Prevention and immediate treatment of hypoglycemia, hyperglycemia, and ketoacidosis

NOTE: Patients should be able to prevent hypoglycemia. Patients should be able to recognize signs that indicate an insulin reaction when they occur and know how to treat this effect. Patients should carry simple sugar or nontempting candy to treat a reaction. Family members should be aware of signs indicating an insulin reaction and know how to give the patient orange juice, simple sugar, or a snack as indicated. Family or friends should be taught to administer glucagon for emergency treatment of this condition.

VIII. Prevention of urinary tract infections (common in diabetic patients)
    A. Urogenic bladder and retention
    B. Change in usual voiding pattern
    C. Change in usual urine output
    D. Feeling of bladder fullness after voiding
    E. Loss of urine when laughing or coughing
    F. Burning or discomfort with urination
    G. Cloudy, foul-smelling urine

IX. Complications
    A. Retinopathy
    B. Neuropathy
    C. Cardiovascular changes
    D. Nephropathy

NOTE: These complications can be discussed in relation to prevention and the modification of self-care practices as indicated.

Because up to 50% of patients with IDDM can develop renal dysfunction, the importance of routine monitoring of renal function including laboratory evaluation for proteinuria, blood urea nitrogen, and creatinine level should be discussed. They should have an understanding of normal renal function and be able to recognize signs indicating a change in function including signs of uremia (creatinine clearance below 10 ml/min):
    Progressive loss of appetite
    Meats taking on an offensive odor or taste
    Persistent bad taste in the mouth
    Urinelike odor on breath
    Muscle cramps, especially in legs
    Generalized itching
    Nausea and vomiting that is worse in the morning

GENERAL INSTRUCTIONS FOR DISCHARGE/OUTPATIENTS

ORAL HYPOGLYCEMICS

This medication is used to treat your diabetes and will help you control your blood glucose levels. It works best if taken exactly as directed. If you do not understand why you need this medication, check with your health care provider.

Take this medication as directed before a meal at the same time each day. This will help you to remember to take your medication. This will also help prevent stomach upset and enable the medication to work better.

Take this medication exactly as prescribed. Do not miss any doses. This is important in the control of your diabetes. If you miss a dose, take it as soon as you remember. If it is almost time for your next dose, do *not* take the dose you missed. Continue with your regular dosage schedule. If you are worried or have any questions about whether or not to take the missed dose, contact your health care provider.

If you are pregnant or considering pregnancy or if you are breastfeeding an infant, discuss this with your health care provider before taking this medication. This drug could cause unwanted effects in your unborn baby or nursing infant.

This medication can sometimes cause unwanted effects in some individuals taking it. Notify your health care provider if you notice a skin rash; sore throat; fever; mouth sores; dark-colored urine; yellowish color to the skin or eyes; easy bleeding or bruising; unusual tiredness; diarrhea or light-colored bowel movements; swelling of the face, hands, or legs; muscle cramps; seizures; or sensitivity to sunlight and sunburn.

Test your urine for glucose at least once a day. Test it about 2 hours after your largest meal during the day. Your urine should check negative. Test your urine four times a day if it shows 1% or 2% glucose. Monitor yourself for excessive thirst, frequent urination, and fatigue especially if you have been under mental stress, have a cold or flu, or physical stress. Call your health care provider if your urine tests were previously negative and show 2% glucose for 1 to 2 days.

Remember to monitor your urine glucose once a day while taking this medication to check control of your diabetes. You need to check your urine ketones only if you are showing glucose in your urine test. If you have any questions, check with your health care provider.

GENERAL INSTRUCTIONS FOR DISCHARGE/OUTPATIENTS—cont'd

ORAL HYPOGLYCEMICS—cont'd

Because it is important to balance your diet and exercise with your medication, be alert to maintaining usual activity and diet schedules. Continue to take your medication when ill. Carry nontempting hard candy (e.g., Lifesavers) with you at all times in case you have a hypoglycemic reaction.

Do not take any other medication unless specifically told to do so by your health care provider. This includes both nonprescription and prescription medication. This medication can interact with some other medications and cause harmful or unwanted effects. It is important to recognize that some medications such as cough and cold medicines have a high sugar content and can interfere with your control of diabetes. Other medicines such as aspirin can affect your urine test results.

Avoid alcohol because it can cause low blood sugar, a pounding headache, flushing, upset stomach, dizziness, or sweating.

Carry an identification card and wear a diabetic medical alert bracelet indicating that you have diabetes and that you are taking this medication.

Do not give this medication to family or friends. It is prescribed especially for you.

Store this medication tightly closed in a dry, cool place.

Keep this medication and all other medications out of the reach of children.

INSULIN

This medication is used to treat your diabetes and will help you control your blood glucose or sugar levels. It works best if taken exactly as directed. If you do not understand why you need this medication, check with your health care provider.

Be sure you use the correct type and concentration of insulin prescribed for you. Be sure you use the correct type of insulin syringe for this concentration of insulin. (For example, a U-100 syringe must be used for U-100 insulin; a U-40 syringe must be used for U-40 insulin.) This is important in the management of your diabetes.

Various insulin preparations and syringes can differ from manufacturer to manufacturer. Avoid changing brands of insulin or syringes because this can affect the management of your condition.

Care for your insulin syringe and insulin as taught by your health care provider. If you find you have questions, contact your health care provider.

Always check the expiration date on the insulin label before using the insulin. Do *not* use outdated insulin.

Store unopened insulin in the refrigerator. Do *not* freeze. The vial you are using can be stored at room temperature for up to 1 month. If any insulin is left after a month's time it should be discarded and *not* used.

If you mix two types of insulin for management of blood glucose levels, always mix the two insulins in the same order to prevent mistakes. Always measure your insulin in a well-lighted area.

Monitor your diet, exercise, and insulin as taught by your health care provider. Remember to continue to take insulin when you are ill and to eat small meals and drink clear liquids. Test your urine or blood glucose more frequently when ill. If you are vomiting or are unable to maintain self-care, notify your health care provider immediately.

Monitor yourself for hypoglycemia. If you have signs of low blood sugar, take a simple fast-acting sugar such as 120 ml or 4 ounces (½ cup) of orange juice or a soft drink (be sure it contains sugar and is not a diet, or sugar-free, soft drink), sugar cubes, or hard candy such as 5 to 7 Lifesavers. Wait 10 to 15 minutes for effect. Repeat if necessary. If this is not effective, notify your health care provider immediately.

It is important that your family or friends know how to tell if you are hypoglycemic and what to do to help you. A family member or friend should know how to administer glucagon in an emergency.

Monitor yourself for hyperglycemia. If you are unsure if you are hyperglycemic or hypoglycemic, treat yourself for hypoglycemia.

Test your urine for glucose four times daily—before breakfast, lunch, dinner, and at bedtime. Use the first-voided or double-voided method as taught by your health care provider.

Do not take any other medication unless specifically told to do so by your health care provider. Some medications such as cough and cold remedies contain high amounts of sugar and can interfere with the control of your diabetes. Other medicines such as aspirin can affect urine test results.

Avoid drinking alcoholic beverages. Alcohol can cause low blood sugar, a pounding headache, flushing, upset stomach, dizziness, or sweating.

Be sure to wear a diabetic medical alert bracelet and carry an identification card stating that you are a diabetic and require insulin.

Follow your management plan as taught by your health care provider. Check for acetone only when urine sugars are elevated. Check your urine four times a day if you are ill to monitor control. Keep a careful record of your urine testing.

Be sure you understand how to adjust your insulin requirement for stress, illness, and increased exercise. If you have any questions, check with your health care provider. It is not unusual to have to supplement your daily insulin dose with short-acting insulin injection (e.g., Regular Insulin) if urine sugars and acetone levels are elevated.

Remember to balance your diet, exercise, and rest. Food must be taken in similar quantities when you are taking insulin and at about the same time each day if control is to be achieved.

Rotate your injection sites and check the sites for irritation, infection, or other unusual signs such as swelling at the injection site, loss of fat at or distal to the injection site, or marked depression or hollowing of the skin. Keep a careful record of your injection site rotation.

When traveling, do *not* pack your insulin. Carry your insulin with you.

When driving for prolonged periods, always stop for a rest and snack every 2 hours. Be especially alert to monitoring yourself for hypoglycemic reactions.

Keep insulin and all other medications out of the reach of children.

NURSING DRUG DIGEST

Medication (trade name*)	Indication	Usual dosage and administration	Dosage forms, preparation, and storage	Contraindications, cautions, and comments	Monitoring
ORAL HYPOGLYCEMICS					
Acetohexamide Dimelor Dymelor	Non–insulin-dependent diabetes mellitus	*Adults:* 250-1500 mg PO/24 hr as single or 2 divided doses before breakfast and before evening meal Maximum: 1500 mg/day Administration with food or milk may decrease GI irritation	Tablets: 250, 500 mg	*Contraindicated* in hyperglycemia associated with primary renal disease (use insulin) May cause drowsiness Should not be used in patients with chronic hepatic or renal failure	Urine should be checked regularly for glucose and ketones
Chlorpropamide Chloromide Chloronase Diabeteral Diabinese Insulase Novo-propamide Stabinol	Non–insulin-dependent diabetes mellitus	*Adults:* 100-500 mg PO/24 hr as single dose in AM Administration with breakfast may decrease GI irritation Maximum: 750 mg/day	Tablets: 100, 250 mg	May cause severe GI distress and diarrhea Prolonged half-life up to 36 hr can cause severe hypoglycemia in the elderly particularly if a secondary illness results in impaired intake of food Where possible, switch to a shorter-acting drug such as tolbutamide Administration during the third trimester of pregnancy may cause neonatal hypoglycemia	Check urine regularly
★ **Glipizide** Glucotrol	Non–insulin-dependent diabetes mellitus	*Adults:* 5-15 mg/24 hr PO as single or divided dose (generally 30 min before a meal) Maximum: 40 mg/day Administration with food or milk may decrease GI irritation	Tablets: 5 mg, 10 mg	More powerful than the other oral hypoglycemic agents and can cause severe hypoglycemia particularly in large doses Patients who are not taking food because of illness should have the drug withdrawn	Urine should be checked regularly for glucose and ketones

Drug	Indication	Preparations	Dosage	Precautions	Monitoring
Glyburide DiaBeta Euglucon Micronase	Non-insulin-dependent diabetes mellitus	Tablets: 1.25, 2.5, 5 mg	*Adults:* 1.25–5 mg PO/24 hr as single or divided dose Maximum: 20 mg/24 hr Dose is generally increased by 1.25–2.5 mg weekly Administration with food or milk may decrease GI irritation	More powerful than the other oral hypoglycemic agents and can cause severe hypoglycemia particularly in large doses Patients who are *not* taking food because of illness should have the drug withdrawn	Urine should be checked regularly for glucose and ketones
✿ **Metformin** Diabexyl Glucophage	Non-insulin-dependent diabetes mellitus	Tablet: 500 mg	*Adults:* 500 mg PO t.i.d. *Maximum:* 2500 mg/24 hr Administration with food or milk may decrease GI irritation	*Contraindicated* in hypersensitivity and history of ketoacidosis Still under investigation for the possibility of inducing lactic acidosis Should *not* be used in patients with impaired renal function	Urine should be checked regularly for glucose and ketones
★ **Tolazamide** Tolinase	Non-insulin-dependent diabetes mellitus	Tablets: 100, 250, 500 mg	*Adults:* 100–250 mg/24 hr PO as single dose Maximum: 1000 mg/24 hr (in 2 divided doses) Administration with food or milk may decrease GI irritation	Metabolized to a number of hypoglycemic metabolic substances that are largely excreted by the kidney; should *not* be used in chronic renal failure Use with caution in hepatic dysfunction	Urine should be checked regularly for glucose and ketones
Tolbutamide Neo-Dibetic Novobutamide Oramide Orinase Tolbutone	Non-insulin-dependent diabetes mellitus	Tablets: 250, 500 mg	*Adults:* 500–2000 mg/24 hr PO in divided doses Administration with food or milk may decrease GI irritation Maximum: 3000 mg/24 hr *Elderly:* Start with lower doses	May aggravate peptic ulcers *Not* to be used in obese diabetics who have not had adequate diet therapy Should not be taken if patient is not eating regular meals because of illness	Urine should be checked regularly for glucose and ketones

Continued.

NOTE: For additional details regarding the individual agents listed in this table see the text and other tables in this chapter.
*Indicates a multiple active ingredient product. For a complete listing of all active ingredients see the *Drug Reference Guide to Brand Names and Active Ingredients.*
†See the Insulin entry for general details and information.
✿ Indicates that the drug is generally available only in Canada.
★ Indicates that the drug is generally available only in the United States.

NURSING DRUG DIGEST—cont'd

Medication (trade name)	Indication	Usual dosage and administration	Dosage forms, preparation, and storage	Contraindications, cautions, and comments	Monitoring
INSULIN	Insulin-dependent diabetes mellitus	*Adults:* Dose is variable depending on condition and response—see text Take care drawing up the correct insulin and particularly noting strength of insulin being used Where possible, use a 40-U insulin syringe for low doses of insulin and a 100-U insulin syringe for high doses of insulin Aspirate syringe before injecting insulin *Children:* Same as adults	Injectable: 40, 100 units/ml Insulin should be stored in a cool place, preferably a refrigerator and at *no* time should it be frozen Vials in use do *not* need to be kept in a refrigerator provided they are kept in a cool area and not exposed to extremes of heat and cold	All diabetic patients taking insulin should carry an identification card containing the essential medical information Change in the source of insulin (beef-pork); type (lente, regular, NPH) may need a change in the insulin dosage The number of daily insulin injections, the quantity of insulin, and the time of administration require direct medical supervision and integration with diet and exercise Prompt recognition of hypoglycemia and diabetic ketoacidosis are essential for effective control of diabetes mellitus Local and allergic reactions to the insulins may be seen; rarely hyposensitization may be required Areas of fat atrophy and hypertrophy occur if older insulin preparations are used Insulin requirements may need to be increased at times of stress; infection, surgery and drugs may interfere with the action of insulin and mask hypoglycemia (see Table 60-4)	Monitor blood sugar Monitor urine for ketones Observe for signs or symptoms of hypoglycemia or hyperglycemia

Insulin injection† Crystalline zinc Humulin-R Regular Toronto	Short-term control of elevated blood glucose For use in ketoacidosis	SC or IV; this is the *only* insulin that may be given IV Should be drawn up first when combination insulins are being administered in the one syringe	Bottle should be discarded if the insulin is cloudy, suggesting contamination	Will cause hypoglycemia if used in excessive amount; needs to be balanced with an intermediate insulin
Insulin isophane† Humulin-N NPH Iletin NPH Insulin Protophane NPH	To provide therapeutic levels of insulin throughout the day	SC in single or divided doses Should be given with insulin injection to provide smooth blood glucose control throughout the day Should *not* be given IV		Can cause hypoglycemia 12 to 24 hr after administration
Insulin zinc† Iletin Lente Lente Iletin Lente Insulin Lentard Monotard	To provide therapeutic levels of insulin throughout the day	SC in single or divided doses Should be given with insulin injection to provide smooth blood glucose control throughout the day Should *not* be given IV		Can cause hypoglycemia 12-24 hr after administration
Insulin zinc, prompt† Iletin Semilente Insulin Semilente Semilente Iletin Semilente Semitard	To achieve blood glucose control during the middle of the day and early afternoon	SC with insulin isophane/insulin zinc		Provides early onset of action of insulin, which can be better achieved with a combination of insulin injection and insulin isophane/insulin zinc
Insulin protamine zinc (PZI)†	To provide therapeutic levels of insulin throughout the day	SC NOTE: Mixture of PZI with insulin injection will lead to conversion of a large percentage of insulin injection to the PZI form; thus insulin injection must be drawn into the syringe first before drawing PZI insulin		Rarely used now; better results achieved with insulin isophane/insulin zinc Can be combined with insulin injection Contamination of PZI in the insulin injection vial will lead to a clouding of the normally clear insulin injection

Continued.

NURSING DRUG DIGEST—cont'd

Medication (trade name)	Indication	Usual dosage and administration	Dosage forms, preparation, and storage	Contraindications, cautions, and comments	Monitoring
Insulin zinc, extended† Iletin Ultralente Insulin Ultralente Ultralente Iletin Ultralente Insulin Ultratard	To provide insulin concentrations longer than 24 hr after the administration of the insulin	SC		This insulin has a long action and when used with insulin injection and lente insulin, it may be difficult to determine which insulin is responsible for reactions occurring at certain times of the day	
INSULIN ANTAGONISTS					
Diazoxide Hyperstat Proglycem	Inoperable insulin-secreting tumors See also Chapter 33, "Antihypertensives"	*Adults:* 3-8 mg/kg/day PO divided into 2-3 equal doses *Children:* same as adults *Newborns and infants:* 8-15 mg/kg/day PO divided into 3 equal doses	Capsules: 50, 100 mg Injectable: 300 mg/20 ml (for IV use *only*) Suspension: 50 mg/ml (chocolate-mint flavored) Shake suspension well before use Protect from light	*Contraindicated* in hypersensitivity to diazoxide or thiazides May cause anorexia, nausea, vomiting, or diarrhea May cause hirsutism that subsides on discontinuation Thrombocytopenia may necessitate discontinuation Can cause hypotension and may aggravate diabetic control temporarily Can be used on a long-term basis to inhibit secretion in a patient with an insulinoma	Monitor blood glucose
Glucagon	Treatment of insulin-induced hypoglycemia when glucose solutions are *not* available	*Adults:* 1 mg IV, IM, or SC (1 mg = 1 unit)	Injectable: dispensed as a dry powder in 1 mg and 10 mg ampules packaged with sufficient diluent to make a 1 mg/ml solution Keep refrigerated Stable for 3 months after reconstitution if refrigerated Decomposes at room temperature	*Contraindicated* in hypersensitivity Nausea and vomiting may occur shortly after administration, and this effect will be accentuated by prolonged use May have minimal effect when prolonged hypoglycemia has occurred with depletion of liver glycogen stores	When given SC for hypoglycemic coma induced by either insulin or oral hypoglycemic agents, the patient should return to consciousness within 20 min If this does *not* occur, IV glucose *must* be administered as soon as possible to avoid irreversible damage

BIBLIOGRAPHY

Alberti, K.G.M.M., & Thomas, D.J.B. The management of diabetes during surgery. *British Journal of Anaesthesiology*, 1979, *51*, 693-710.

Assam, R. Metformin-induced lactic acidosis in the presence of acute renal failure. *Diabetologia*, 1977, *13*, 211-217.

Brown, J. Conference on pancreas transplantation. *Diabetes*, 1980, *29*(suppl. 1), 1-128.

Bunn, H.F., Gabbay, K.H., & Gallop, P.M. The glycosylation of hemoglobin: relevance to diabetes mellitus. *Science*, 1978, *200*, 21-27.

Cahill, G.F. Jr., Etzwiler, D.D., & Freinkel, N. Blood glucose control in diabetes. *Diabetes*, 1976, *25*, 237-245.

Cahill, G.F., Jr., Etzwiler, D.D., & Freinkel, N. Control and diabetes. *New England Journal of Medicine*, 1976, *294*, 1004-1005.

Cerasi, E. Insulin secretion: mechanism of the stimulation by glucose. *Quarterly Reviews of Biophysics*, 1975, *8*, 1-41.

Chambers, J.K. Save your diabetic patient from early kidney damage. *Nursing 83*, 1983, *13*(5), 58-63.

Chance, R.E., Enzmann, F.H., Galloway, J.A., Glynne, A., & Marsden, J.H. Introduction: symposium on biosynthetic human insulin. *Diabetes Care*, 1981, *4*, 139.

Champion, M.C., Shepherd, G.A.A., Rodger, N.W., & Dupre, J. Continuous subcutaneous infusion of insulin in the management of diabetes mellitus. *Diabetes*, 1980, *29*, 206-212.

Crea, R., Kraszewski, A., Tadaaki, H., & Itakura, K. Chemical synthesis of genes for human insulin. *Proceedings of the National Academy of Science* USA, 1978, *75*, 5765-5769.

Crofford, O. *Reports to Congress of the National Commission on Diabetes* (DHEW Publication No. [NIH] 76-1018). Washington, D.C.: Government Printing Office, 1975.

D'Arcy, P.F. Tobacco smoking and drugs: clinically important interaction? *Drug Intelligence and Clinical Pharmacology*, 1984, *18*, 302-307.

Diabetic Retinopathy Study Research Group. Four risk factors for severe visual loss in diabetic retinopathy. The third report from the Diabetic Retinopathy Study. *Archives of Ophthalmology*, 1979, *97*, 654-655.

Diabetic Retinopathy Study Research Group. Photocoagulation treatment of proliferative diabetic retinopathy. The second report of Diabetic Retinopathy Study. *Ophthalmology*, 1978, *85*, 82-105.

Diabetic Retinopathy Study Research Group. Preliminary report on effects of photocoagulation therapy. *American Journal of Ophthalmology*, 1976, *81*, 383-396.

Eliopoulus, C.E. Diagnosis and management of diabetes in the elderly. *American Journal of Nursing*, 1978, *78*(5), 884-886.

Fisher, J.N., Shahshahani, N., & Kitabchi, A.E. Diabetic ketoacidosis: low dose insulin therapy by various routes. *New England Journal of Medicine*, 1977, *297*, 238-241.

Fonville, A.M. Teaching patients to rotate injection sites. *American Journal of Nursing*, 1978, *78*(5), 880-883.

Franke, H., & Fuchs, J. Eine neues antidiabetisches Prinzip. Ergenbnisse klinischer Utersuchungen. *Deutsche Medizinische Wochenschrft*, 1955, *80*, 1449.

Gabbay, K.H., Hasty, K., Breslow, J.L., & others. Glycosylated hemoglobins and long-term blood glucose control in diabetes mellitus. *Journal of Clinical Endocrinology and Metabolism*, 1977, *44*, 859-864.

Galloway, J.A., & Bressler, R. Insulin treatment in diabetes. *Medical Clinics of North America*, 1978, *62*(4), 663-680.

Genuth, S., & Martin, P. Control of hyperglycemia in adult diabetics by pulsed insulin delivery. *Diabetes*, 1977, *26*, 571-581.

Gill, M., Ratliff, D., & Harding, K. Hypoglycemic coma, jaundice, and pure RBC aplasia following chlorpropamide therapy. *Archives of Internal Medicine*, 1980, *140*, 714-715.

Goeddel, D.V., Kleid, D.G., Bolivar, F., & others. Expression in *Escherichia coli* of chemically synthesized genes for human insulin. *Proceedings of the National Academy of Science* USA, 1979, *76*, 106-110.

Grazaitis, D., & Sexson, W. Erroneously high Dextrostix values caused by isopropyl alcohol. *Pediatrics*, 1980, *66*, 221-223.

Guthrie, D. Helping the diabetic manage his self-care. *Nursing 80*, 1980, *10*(2), 57-64.

Hayes, M.A., & Brandt, R.L. Carbohydrate metabolism in the immediate post-operative period. *Surgery*, 1952, *32*, 819.

Hodge, R., et al. Multiple use of disposable insulin syringe-needle units. *Journal of the American Medical Association*, 1980, *244*, 266-267.

Itakura, K., Hirose, T., Crea, R., & others. Expression in *Escherichia coli* of a chemically synthesized gene for the hormone somatostatin. *Science*, 1977, 198, 1056-1063.

Janbon, M., Chaptal, J., Vedel, A., & Schaap, J. Accidents hypoglycemiques graves par un sulfamidothiazol. *Montpelier Medicine*, 1942, *441*, 21-22.

Johnson, R.B. Daily management of the diabetic-1983. *Drug Store News*, 1983, Lesson 679-401-83-14, October 17, 1983.

Johnston, D.G., & Alberti, K.G. Diabetic emergencies: practical aspects of the management of diabetic ketoacidosis and diabetes during surgery. *Journal of Clinical Endocrinology and Metabolism*, 1980, *9*, 437-460.

Klemp, P., et al. Smoking reduces insulin absorption from subcutaneous tissue. *British Medical Journal*, 1982, *284*, 237.

Klimt, C.R., Knatterud, G.L., Meinert, C.L., & Prout, T.E. The University Group Diabetes Program: A study of the effects of hypoglycemic agents on vascular complications in patients with adult-onset diabetes. Part I. Design, methods and baseline characteristics. *Diabetes*, 1970, *19*(2), 747.

Klimt, C.R., Knatterud, G.L., Meinert, C.L., & Prout, T.E.: The University Group Diabetes Program: A study of the effects of hypoglycemic agents on vascular complications in patients with adult-onset diabetes. Part II. Mortality results. *Diabetes*, 1970, *19*(2), 789-830.

Kovisto, V., & Felig, P. Alterations in insulin absorption and in blood glucose control associated with varying insulin injection sites in diabetic patients. *Annals of Internal Medicine*, 1980, *92*, 59-61.

Loubatieres, A. The hypoglycemic sulfonamides: history and development of the problem from 1942 to 1955. *Annals of the New York Academy of Science*, 1957, *71*, 4-11.

Lundin, D.V. Reporting urine test results: switch from + to %. *American Journal of Nursing,* 1978, *78*(5), 878-879.

Matthes, M.L. . . . beyond the hospital—diabetic day care. *American Journal of Nursing,* 1979, *79*(1), 105-106.

National Diabetes Data Group. Classification and diagnosis of diabetes mellitus and other categories of glucose and tolerance. *Diabetes,* 1979, *28,* 1039-1057.

Olefsky, J.M., & Kolterman, O.G. Mechanisms of insulin resistance in obesity and noninsulin-dependent diabetes. *American Journal of Medicine,* 1981, *70,* 151-168.

Olefsky, J.M., and Reaven, G.N. Effects of sulfonylurea therapy on insulin binding to mononuclear leukocytes of diabetic patients. *American Journal of Medicine,* 1976, *60,* 89-95.

Pelczynski, L., & Reilly, A. Helping your diabetic patients help themselves a plan for inpatient education. *Nursing 81,* 1981, *11*(5), 24-29.

Pickup, J.C., Keen, H., Parsons, J.A., & Alberti, K.G.M.M. Continuous subcutaneous insulin infusion: an approach to achieving normoglycaemia. *British Medical Journal,* 1978, *1,* 204-207.

Pirart, J. Diabetes mellitus and its degenerative complications: a perspective study of 4,400 patients observed between 1947 and 1973. *Diabetes Care,* 1978, *1,* 168-188.

Planas, A., et al. Chlorpropamide-induced pure RBC aplasia. *Archives of Internal Medicine,* 1980, *140,* 707-708.

Rizza, R.A., Gerich, J.E., Haymond, M.W., & others. Control of blood sugar in insulin-dependent diabetes: comparison of an artificial endocrine pancreas, continuous subcutaneous insulin infusion, and intensified conventional insulin therapy. *New England Journal of Medicine,* 1980, *303,* 1313-1318.

Ross, S.A., & Dupre, J. Effects of ingestion of triglyceride or galactose on secretion of gastric inhibitory polypeptide and on responses to intravenous glucose in normal and diabetic subjects. *Diabetes,* 1978, *27,* 327-333.

Rotter, J.I., & Rimoin, D.L. The genetics of the glucose tolerance disorders. *American Journal of Medicine,* 1981, *70,* 116-126.

Slama, G., Buv, K.N.P., Tchobroutsky, G., & others. Plasma insulin and C-peptide levels during subcutaneous insulin infusion. *Diabetes Care,* 1979, *2,* 251-255.

Slater, N.L. Insulin reactions vs. ketoacidosis: guidelines for diagnosis and intervention. *American Journal of Nursing,* 1978, *78*(5), 875-877.

Small, D. A patient education program. *American Journal of Nursing,* 1978, *78*(5), 889-890.

Smith, P.H., Porte, D., Jr., & Robertson, R.P. Neural regulation of the endocrine pancreas. In J. Pierluissi (Ed.). *Proceedings of the First International Symposium on the Endocrinology of Pancreas and Diabetes.* Excerpta Medica International Congress Series. Amsterdam: Elsevier Publishing Company, 1979.

Sosenko, J.M., Flückiger, R., Platt, O.S., & Gabbay, K.H. Glycosylation of variant hemoglobins in normal and diabetic subjects. *Diabetes Care,* 1980, *3,* 590-593.

Stock-Barkman, P. Confusing concepts is it diabetic shock or diabetic coma? *Nursing 83,* 1983, *13*(6), 33-41.

Smokvina, G.J., & Givens, R.M. Hyperglycemia in the aged. *Journal of Gerontological Nursing,* 1983, *9*(8), 449-451, 462.

Taitelman, U., Reece, E.A., & Bessman, A.N. Insulin in the management of the diabetic surgical patient. Continuous intravenous infusion versus subcutaneous administration. *Journal of the American Medical Association,* 1977, *237,* 658-660.

Todd, B. Drugs and the elderly-insulin update. *Geriatric Nursing,* 1983, September-October, 321-323.

Unger, R.H., Ipp, E., Schusdziarra, & Orci, L. Hypothesis: physiological role of pancreatic somatostatin and the contribution of D cell disorders to diabetes mellitus. *Life Science,* 1977, *20,* 2081-2086.

Waldhausl, W., Bratusch-Marrain, P., Dudczak, R., & Deutsch, E. The diabetogenic action of somatostatin in healthy subjects and maturity onset diabetics. *Journal of Clinical Endocrinology and Metabolism,* 1977, *44*(5), 876-883.

Walesky, M.E. Diabetic ketoacidosis. *American Journal of Nursing,* 1978, *78*(5), 872-874.

Watanabe, C.K. Studies in the metabolic changes induced by administration of guanidine bases. Influence of injected guanidine hydrochloride upon blood sugar content. *Journal of Biological Chemistry,* 1918, *33,* 253.

Welk, D.S. Preventing insulin-induced lipodystrophies. *Nursing 79,* 1979, *9*(12), 42-45.

White, N.E., & Miller, B. Glycohemoglobin a new test to help the diabetic stay in control. *Nursing 83,* 1983, *13*(8), 55-57.

Yue, D.K., & Turtle, J.R. New forms of insulin and their use in the treatment of diabetes. *Diabetes,* 1977, *26,* 341-345.

CHAPTER 61

Thyroid and Antithyroid Medications

David M. Fawcett

Medications discussed in this chapter

Antithyroid medications	Thyroid hormones
Iodine	Levothyroxine (T$_4$)
Methimazole	Liothyronine (T$_3$)
Propranolol	Liotrix (T$_4$ and T$_3$)
Propylthiouracil	Thyroglobulin
Radioactive iodine	Thyroid, desiccated
	Thyroid-stimulating hormone
	Thyrotropin

The function of the thyroid has been compared with that of a thermostat because of the essential central role that this gland plays in regulating normal metabolic activity. The total metabolic system is extremely complex. It includes not only the thyroid gland and its hormones (i.e., triiodothyronine and thyroxine), but also several thyroregulatory factors. Two of these factors are hormones, one secreted by the hypothalamus (i.e., thyrotropin-releasing hormone) and the other by the anterior pituitary gland (i.e., thyrotropin). Other regulatory factors are nonhormonal components found in the blood, including iodide and thyroid hormone–binding proteins. The system also encompasses the nuclear receptors for thyroid hormones that are distributed widely throughout the body in responsive cells. Finally, numerous control points exist in the thyroid system at which interactions with other endocrine components and with the autonomic nervous system may occur. The total system, through sensitive feedback mechanisms, monitors and regulates its own activity and the metabolic activity of all responsive tissues in the body. The result, when each component is behaving normally, is a totally coordinated organism in which all of the body tissues are functioning at an appropriate level of metabolic activity.

An abnormal thyroid function may be the result of a primary disease of the thyroid gland, or it may arise secondarily from the malfunction of one of the other components of the total system. The result, in either case, will be an inappropriate level of cellular metabolic activity. If this level is too high, the patient has *hyperthyroidism* and clinically will exhibit a characteristic group of signs and symptoms caused by the elevated metabolic rate of the affected organs. Conversely, an inappropriately low activity of the system results in *hypothyroidism;* the clinical features associated with the low thyroid function again are characteristic, and, in general, are opposite to those found in hyperthyroidism.

Abnormal and normal thyroid function (and the metabolic activity associated with these states) may be placed on a continuous spectrum. At the two extremes of the continuum are life-threatening disorders: thyroid storm and *myxedema* coma, caused by hyperthyroidism and hypothyroidism, respectively. At the center of the spectrum is found the normal metabolic state. All degrees of thyroid overactivity and underactivity may be found between the central point and the extremes. It is often difficult to define where an abnormality begins. Minimal degrees of thyroid dysfunction can be identified only by using special techniques.

Except in two situations, malignant disease of the thyroid and *goiter* that develops in a patient who is clinically *euthyroid,* the therapy of thyroid disorders is aimed at restoring the normal metabolic activity within the peripheral organ systems. The successful treatment of hyperthyroidism requires reducing the thyroid hormone action at the cellular level. This can be accomplished by several techniques that lower the rate of the secretion of thyroid hormones from the gland, or by blocking the action of the hormones at the periphery. The therapy for hypothyroidism is equally straightforward in principle: deficient thyroid hormone is replaced by the oral administration of an active hormone preparation.

Fully developed thyroid dysfunction, whether it be hyperthyroidism or hypothyroidism, is not difficult to diagnose clinically. However, more subtle forms of thyroid disease are mimicked by many nonthyroidal disorders and must be carefully distinguished from them. The list of such disorders is long, and includes emotional illnesses, other endocrine or metabolic disorders, and diseases of the cardiovascular, respiratory, gastrointestinal, genitourinary, and nervous systems. In many such cases, the clinician must rely on laboratory investigations when confirming a diagnosis of thyroid disease. If the results from the tests are misinterpreted, and this occurs more frequently than it should, patients who are euthyroid may be labeled incorrectly as having thyroid disease and placed on inappropriate long-term therapy.

THYROID ANATOMY AND PHYSIOLOGY

The thyroid gland is located in the neck. It consists of two lateral lobes connected by an isthmus of tissue that crosses the trachea at the level of the second to fourth rings. In the adult human, the gland is approximately 15 to 20 gm. Thyroid tissue, which is lobular in structure, is richly supplied with blood vessels (Figure 61-1). Assessment of the thyroid gland is usually completed with the examination of the head and neck.

The basic unit of the thyroid gland is the *follicle*, which is a small spherical structure consisting of a single layer of epithelial cells surrounding a central cavity. The height of the cells varies with the activity of the gland, being flatter when the gland is relatively inactive. The cavity of the follicle is filled with *colloid*, a homogeneous viscous fluid that contains a high concentration of *thyroglobulin*. Thyroglobulin is a large *glycoprotein* (molecular weight approximately 660,000) that plays a key role in the synthesis and storage of the thyroid hormones. The follicular cells of the thyroid contain the complete biosynthetic machinery required both for the synthesis of thyroglobulin and the thyroid hormones and for hormone secretion.

The thyroid hormones are two iodine-containing amino acids: thyroxine (T_4) and liothyronine (T_3). They are synthesized by the follicular cells of the thyroid and are stored within the gland as part of the thyroglobulin molecule. A sufficient supply of iodine is required for their formation. Because the availability of dietary iodine may vary greatly, the thyroid system has developed a number of control mechanisms that ensure the conservation of this potentially scarce element, and that allow the gland to alter its synthetic pathways to make the most efficient use of the iodine available. On the other hand, if the gland is exposed to levels of iodine that are excessively high, iodide transport into the gland and hormone synthesis are reduced or abolished by other aspects of the same control system.

The process of hormone synthesis begins with the active transport of inorganic iodide from the blood into the thyroid cells (Figure 61-2). The iodide in the blood is usually derived from ingested iodide or other iodine-containing substances. Iodine-containing substances must be reduced to inorganic iodide before the iodine is available to the gland. Most likely this is accomplished by bacterial action in the gut. The level of inorganic iodide in the blood is proportional to the amount of the element ingested, and so is an indirect measure of its availability in the diet.

Apart from the thyroid, the kidney removes significant amounts of iodide from the blood. Although most of the iodide filtered by the renal glomeruli is returned to the blood by tubular reabsorption, a fraction is lost daily in the urine. Under normal circumstances, the concentration of iodide in the urine is inversely related to the activity of the thyroid gland and directly related to the iodide levels in the diet.

The synthesis of the thyroid hormones comprises two distinct processes. First, thyroglobulin is synthesized on ribosomes of the endoplasmic reticulum of the thyroid cells. The synthesis proceeds in a stepwise fashion from unlinked peptide chains to a final, highly structured, carbohydrate-containing protein. The second process is the iodination of tyrosyl residues that are part of the thyroglobulin molecule, and the coupling of the intermediates, monoiodotyrosine (MIT) and diiodotyrosine (DIT), to active iodothyronines (i.e., T_3 and T_4). Both the iodination and the coupling are catalyzed by thyroid peroxidase, an enzyme associated with the *apical* membrane of the thyroid cells.

The iodinated amino acids are released from thyroglobulin by the action of proteolytic enzymes as a mixture of active hormones (T_4 and T_3) and inactive precursors (MIT and DIT). The iodotyrosines do not leave the thyroid cells but are deiodinated by a specific enzyme system. The iodide formed by deiodination is conserved by the gland and most is available for reincorporation into thyroglobulin; a variable amount of iodide leaks from the thyroid cells into the blood. Before secretion, a part of the T_4 may be deiodinated to T_3.

The hormones T_4 and T_3 are secreted from the gland into the blood where they circulate throughout the body. In peripheral cells, particularly those of the liver and the kidneys, a major portion of the T_4 present in

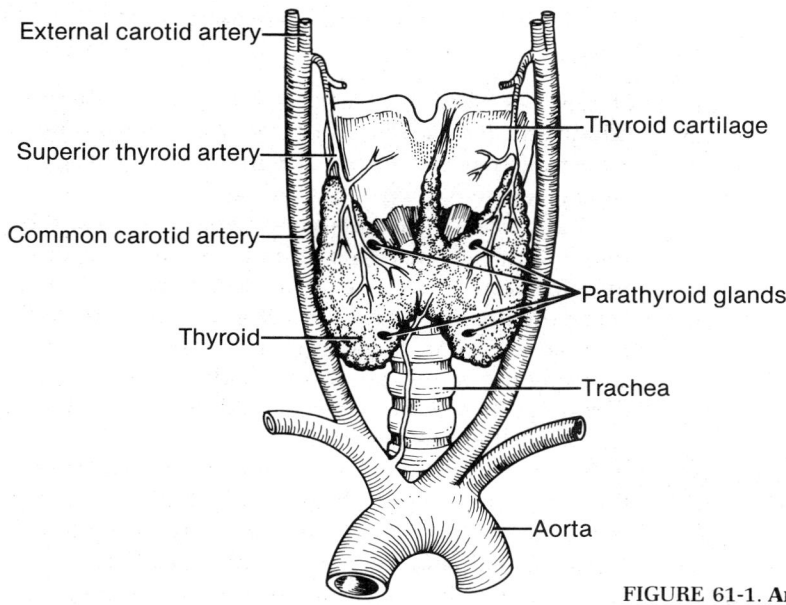

FIGURE 61-1. **Anatomy of the thyroid and parathyroid glands.**

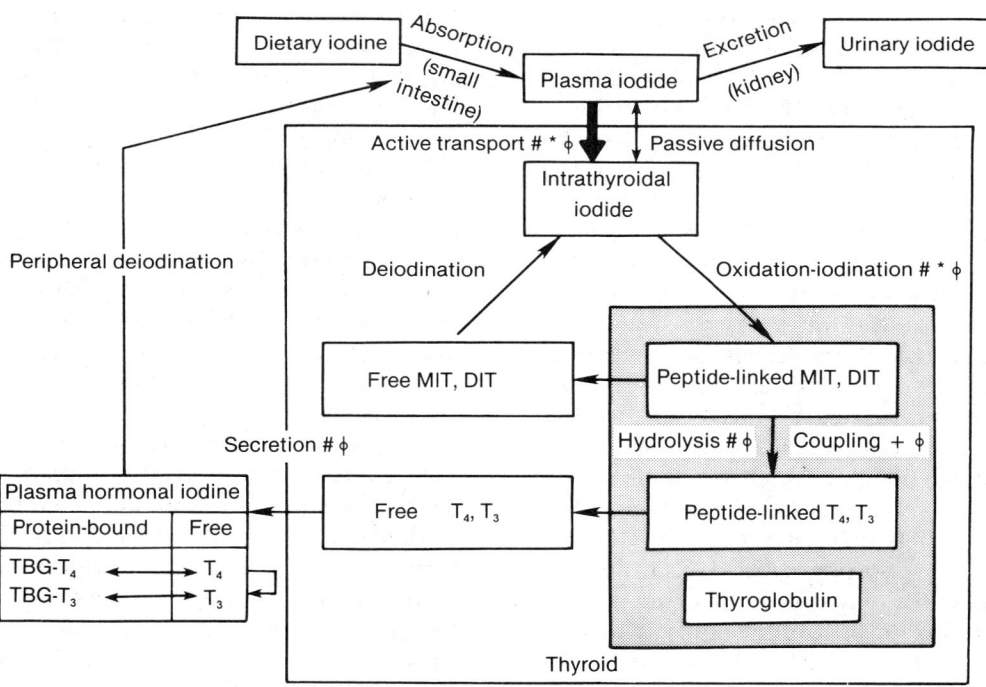

FIGURE 61-2. **Metabolism of iodine. A schematic diagram illustrating the formation, secretion, blood transport, and peripheral metabolism of the thyroid hormones. The largest rectangle represents the follicular cells of the thyroid gland; the smaller rectangle to the left represents the circulating thyroid hormones. The pathway for the nonthyroidal formation of T_3 from T_4 is depicted by the bent arrow to the right of the circulating hormones. A discussion of the events illustrated in the diagram is provided in the text. φ, Stimulated by TSH; *, inhibited by perchlorate, thiocyanate; +, inhibited by propylthiouracil; #, inhibited by excess iodide.**

the blood is converted to T_3. Approximately 80% of the circulating T_3 is derived from T_4 in this manner. All but a small fraction of both circulating hormones are bound to plasma proteins. The most important protein involved in hormone transport is thyroxine-binding globulin (TBG), a glycoprotein; TBG binds reversibly both T_4 and T_3 with a high affinity. The concentration of TBG is low compared with many plasma proteins, with the result being that the available binding sites on TBG become saturated when the concentration of TBG-bound T_4 reaches approximately 20 µg/dl of serum.

Thyroxine (T_4) also binds to another serum protein, thyroxine-binding prealbumin, whereas both T_4 and T_3 bind to serum albumin. However, under normal conditions these interactions are of little significance because nearly 75% of each hormone is bound to TBG; fluctuations in the concentration of that protein will directly affect the total concentrations of the hormones in the blood.

A small but important fraction of each hormone remains free or nonprotein–bound in equilibrium with the bound hormones. The free iodothyronines are the physiologically active circulating hormones. In patients who are euthyroid who have normal levels of thyroxine-binding globulin, the portion of the total serum hormones in the free form is less than 0.05% for T_4 and less than 0.3% for T_3. The absolute concentrations of the free hormones in the blood do not depend on the concentration of TBG. In fact, wide variations in the levels of this protein may be found in patients who are euthyroid.

TBG is synthesized in the liver by a system that is sensitive to the action of steroid hormones. Estrogenic steroids increase the synthesis of TBG so that in pregnancy, or in patients receiving synthetic estrogens (e.g., the oral contraceptives), the TBG levels are elevated. Androgenic steroids and glucocorticoids in large doses decrease the TBG levels. A wide variety of diseases, including hepatitis, cirrhosis of the liver, myeloma, nephrotic syndrome, and in fact, any major illness, may lead to alterations in the concentration of TBG. Furthermore, healthy individuals who are receiving no medications may be found to have abnormal levels of TBG on a genetic basis. Families have been described whose members have either high TBG levels or low TBG levels apparently inherited as an X chromosome–linked characteristic.

The actions of the thyroid hormones are generalized and diffuse; in all but a few tissues (e.g., brain, spleen, gonads), the hormones are concentrated and initiate increases in oxygen consumption and heat production. They stimulate the rate of the metabolism of proteins, fats, and carbohydrates in these tissues. Administration of thyroid hormone is followed by an increase in cardiac output and in the irritability of the nervous system.

The thyroid is essential for normal growth and development. Although the generalized actions of the thyroid hormones have been recognized for many years, the precise, primary mechanism of action at the cellular level has been unclear. Progress in understanding hormone action was made when the nuclei of responsive cells were discovered to contain binding sites for triiodothyronine.

It is believed that thyroid hormones readily enter the cytoplasm of peripheral cells. Much of the T_4 is converted to T_3, which then binds specifically to low-capacity, high-affinity sites in the nuclei. The interaction of T_3 with these nuclear receptors initiates a series of events in which the synthesis of specific control proteins is stimulated through the formation of the appropriate messenger-RNA sequences by the nuclei. Triiodothyronine is postulated to be the principal thyroid hormone with activity at the peripheral sites. Nevertheless, thyroxine acts not only as a prohormone or percursor for T_3, but also has been shown to possess significant inherent activity of its own following binding to nuclear sites. The affinity of these sites for T_4 is lower than for T_3.

Thyroid function is maintained at an appropriate level by a complex system of feedback controls. The principal regulator of thyroid activity is thyrotropin (TSH), a glycoprotein secreted by the anterior pituitary gland. Like two other pituitary hormones, luteinizing hormone (LH) and follicle-stimulating hormone (FSH), TSH consists of two peptide chains designated α and β. The α-chains of LH, FSH, and TSH are similar in structure. The biologic specificity of each hormone resides in its unique β-chain. TSH binds to specific membrane receptors on the thyroid cells. The interaction leads to the activation of membrane-bound adenylate cyclase and the formation of 3′, 5′-cyclic AMP, which acts as a mediator of hormone action.

TSH stimulates most aspects of the thyroid function. It rapidly increases hormone secretion and synthesis and, following a short inhibitory phase, it augments the active transport of iodide into the gland. More generally, thyrotropin stimulation leads to increased protein synthesis and cellularity of the gland. The secretion of TSH by the pituitary is inhibited by the thyroid hormone. Circulating, unbound T_3 and T_4 bind to nuclear receptors of the TSH-producing cells. It is believed this interaction stimulates the formation of an inhibitory protein that decreases TSH secretion and formation. In this way, the blood level of the physiologically active thyroid hormone is maintained at an appropriate level by a process that is independent of the extent of the binding of T_4 and T_3 by plasma proteins such as TBG. In the steady state, as the hormone leaves the circulation to enter the peripheral cells, it is replaced by an equal quantity of the hormone secreted by the gland.

The anterior pituitary cells that produce TSH require tonic stimulation by a hypothalmic factor, thyrotropin-releasing hormone (TRH). TRH is a modified tripeptide that reaches its target cells through the portal system of blood vessels that connects the hypothalamus and the pituitary. TRH stimulates the secretion and synthesis of TSH. Its action is not specific. It also affects the release of other pituitary hormones, including prolactin. The stimulatory action of TRH and the inhibitory effect of the thyroid hormones on the pituitary are in opposition to each other. For any given level of TRH, there is a corresponding level of thyroid hormone required to inhibit TSH secretion. Thus, TRH determines the setpoint sensitivity of the pituitary toward thyroid hormone.

The synthesis and secretion of thyroid hormone are regulated not only through the hypothalamic–pituitary system, but also by an autonomous mechanism involving iodide that is independent of thyrotropin. Thyroidal uptake of iodide is reduced if the blood levels of the element are abnormally high; in fact, the active transport of iodide may be completely abolished. At the same time, elevated levels of intrathyroidal iodide block hormone synthesis and secretion. The advantage of these alterations in thyroid function is taken when iodide is used therapeutically as an *antithyroid* agent to reduce hormone release from the thyrotoxic gland.

In addition to iodide, the activity of the thyroid gland is modified by a large number of substances capable of inhibiting some aspect of the thyroid function. Mention already has been made of the effect of monovalent anions of the group that includes perchlorate and thiocyanate. Such anions block the active transport of iodide into the gland and hence secondarily reduce hormone synthesis and ultimately hormone secretion. A much wider chemical group of substances blocks hormone synthesis at the level of thyroid peroxidase. Many of these are sulfur-containing organic compounds belonging to the class known as thionamides or thiourylenes. Prototypes of this group are thiourea and thiouracil. Their precise mechanism of action remains unclear. Because the inhibitors are metabolized by the gland, they may compete with the iodide as substrates for thyroid peroxidase. Alternately, they may inactivate the oxidized form of the iodide

produced by the peroxidase so that the iodination of thyroglobulin is prevented.

A number of substances belonging to this group of thyroid inhibitors have been employed widely as clinical antithyroid drugs to reduce thyroid activity in patients who are hyperthyroid. The most commonly used drugs of this type are the thioamides: propylthiouracil, methimazole, and carbimazole. Propylthiouracil, unlike the other two, has an additional antithyroid action: it blocks the peripheral and thyroidal conversion of T_4 to T_3, further reducing the concentration of the more active T_3 in the blood and peripheral cells.

A completely unrelated drug, lithium carbonate, used clinically as an antidepressant, also reduces the thyroid function, primarily by inhibiting the secretion of the thyroid hormones. Some investigators have taken advantage of the antithyroid activity of lithium, but it has not been used extensively for this purpose because of a relatively high incidence of undesirable adverse side effects (e.g., tremor, fatigue, thirst, polyuria, GI irritation, and leukocytosis).

Although many other drugs and chemicals are known to exhibit antithyroid activity, only one is of general clinical importance, the β-adrenergic blocker propranolol. Like propylthiouracil, propranolol inhibits the peripheral conversion of T_4 to T_3. However, its main beneficial effect in the treatment of hyperthyroidism is not primarily related to this action; rather, it is the activity of propranolol in blocking β-adrenergic receptors that is helpful to the patient. In *thyrotoxicosis* the high circulating level of thyroid hormones leads to an increased sensitivity of tissues to the catecholamines. Many of the characteristic symptoms of hyperthyroidism are related to this augmented susceptibility. Propranolol, by blocking the β-adrenergic receptors reduces the corresponding symptoms caused indirectly by the elevated thyroid function.

LABORATORY ASSESSMENT OF THYROID FUNCTION

Tests of thyroid function are readily available procedures. They are frequently ordered by clinicians as part of routine patient investigation. Currently, blood tests that measure the circulating levels of the thyroid hormones (T_4 and T_3) by *radioimmunoassay* are the procedures of choice. These tests are sensitive, specific, and much more reliable than older tests such as the basal metabolic rate (BMR) and serum protein-bound iodine (PBI) tests. However, care must be taken in their interpretation. The procedures are most helpful when their limitations are understood. Any factor that alters the level of the binding of the serum hormones to thyroxine-binding globulin (TBG) will proportionately alter the blood levels of total T_4 and T_3 without affecting the concentrations of the free hormones in the circulation. Misinterpretation of these thyroid function tests can be minimized if each result is converted to an index (free T_4 index or free T_3 index). The indices are calculated by multiplying the concentration of T_4 (or T_3) by the value obtained concurrently from the T_3 uptake test. The T_3 uptake test provides an estimate of the degree of the binding of thyroid hormone by the patient's TBG.

Because of the complexity of thyroid hormone metabolism, no single function test will be completely reliable in all circumstances. Careful clinical assessment of the patient must remain the most important part of the investigation of thyroid disorders. The following recommendations are intended as a general guide for the laboratory assessment of thyroid function.

First, thyroid assessment is completed with a careful clinical history and physical examination of the patient. The free thyroxine index (FT_4I) as the initial laboratory test is measured. It is the single most reliable procedure. In most situations, it will be the only thyroid test required.

Later, if necessary, the free triiodothyronine index (FT_3I) is measured to confirm a diagnosis of hyperthyroidism in equivocal cases, *or* the serum thyrotropin (TSH) is measured to confirm a diagnosis of primary hypothyroidism.

Do not rely on serum T_4 levels alone if the patient is receiving medications, is pregnant, or is known to have a familial alteration in serum TBG (instead, the FT_4I should be used). The T_3-uptake (T_3U) test should never be used by itself. It should be ordered only in conjunction with a serum T_4 or a serum T_3 test so that the corresponding index may be calculated. The measurement of serum T_3 should be limited to the confirmation of a diagnosis of hyperthyroidism. Serum T_3 levels as a measure of thyroid function are unreliable in hypothyroidism, and commonly are low in patients who are euthyroid if they are suffering from a nonspecific, nonthyroid condition.

DISEASES OF THE THYROID GLAND AND THEIR TREATMENT

The diseases of the thyroid gland discussed in this chapter are limited to the following two broad categories: (1) hyperthyroidism and (2) hypothyroidism. Because general principles of therapy usually can be applied to all components of a group, all comments with regard to treatment are presented together at the end of each section.

Hyperthyroidism

Hyperthyroidism may be defined as the clinical response that occurs when excessive quantities of active (unbound) thyroid hormones are presented to the peripheral cells of the body. It is a generalized response, because all sensitive tissues are affected. It is usually characterized by elevated circulating levels of T_3 and T_4. Patients who are hyperthyroid have varying general manifestations of an elevated metabolic rate, including increased oxygen consumption, increased heat production, and increased protein catabolism. In addition, the effect of the elevated hormone levels lead to characteristic signs and symptoms related to specific tissues.

Clinical hyperthyroidism may have several causes, some much more common than others. These include the following.

1. Graves' disease (toxic diffuse goiter)
2. Toxic adenoma
3. Toxic multinodular goiter
4. Early subacute *thyroiditis* (transient)
5. Excessive intake of exogenous thyroid hormone (thyrotoxicosis factitia)
6. Trophoblastic tumors secreting high levels of a thyroid-stimulating factor
7. Struma ovarii
8. Pituitary tumor secreting TSH
9. Metastatic thyroid carcinoma producing thyroid hormone
10. Thyroid storm

Graves' disease is the most common form of the condition, followed by toxic multinodular goiter, subacute thyroiditis, and thyroid storm. The other conditions are uncommon or rare.

Graves' disease. Patients with Graves' disease may have all three of the following features or just one or two:

1. Hyperthyroidism associated with diffuse enlargement of the thyroid gland
2. Infiltrative ophthalmopathy
3. Pretibial myxedema (infiltrative dermopathy)

The three entities, although associated, may emerge and subside independently, and may be manifest with differing severity. Some patients will suffer from all three components of the disease, others with two, and some with only one. When infiltrative ophthalmopathy, with or without pretibial myxedema, occurs in the absence of hyperthyroidism, the patient is said to have euthyroid Graves' disease.

Graves' disease, like two other disorders of the thyroid (e.g., Hashimoto's thyroiditis and idiopathic primary atrophy of the gland) is classified as an *autoimmune* disease. There is a strong familial aggregation of these three thyroid disorders, not only within the category of thyroid disease itself, but also within the broader framework of autoimmune disorders in general (including pernicious anemia, myasthenia gravis, and idiopathic Addison's disease). Circulating organ-specific *autoantibodies* have been demonstrated in the various types of thyroid disorders believed to be of autoimmune origin. More than one type of circulating antithyroid antibody may be found associated with Graves' disease, including antithyroglobulin and antimicrosomal antibodies. However, the most interesting class of thyroid *autoantibodies* that has been described in patients with Graves' disease is a group of immunoglobulins (i.e., of the IgG type) that has the property of binding to one or more sites on the cell membrane of the thyroid follicular cells. The binding sites may be identical, or closely associated, with the binding sites for TSH on the same membranes. The thyroid autoantibodies of this class have been described under a variety of names: long-acting thyroid stimulator (LATS), LATS-protector, and human thyroid-stimulating immunoglobulin (HTSI). HTSI will compete with TSH for the binding sites, which is used in one type of assay for detecting the abnormal thyroid stimulators. The binding of HTSI to the thyroid membranes is followed by the stimulation of the pathways sensitive to TSH, including the activation of membrane-bound adenylate cyclase. It seems probable that the uncontrolled stimulation of the thyroid gland found in patients who are hyperthyroid with Graves' disease is related to the binding of HTSI to the thyroid cells.

It is likely that not only the hyperthyroidism and thyroid enlargement of Graves' disease, but also the ophthalmopathy and dermopathy are of autoimmune origin. However, because the three components of the disorder may occur independently, it has been proposed that a different species of abnormal immunoglobulin is responsible for each entity. An inherited defect in immune tolerance, which may be expressed as one or more clinical disorders, would be consistent with most features of this autoimmune disease.

Graves' disease appears with the highest frequency during the third and fourth decades of life. It is approximately 4 to 5 times more common in women than in men. The most usual feature is a fairly rapid diffuse enlargement of the thyroid gland associated with the onset of the signs and symptoms of hyperthyroidism. These include nervousness, weight loss without a loss of appetite, heat intolerance with increased perspiration, a rapid pulse rate with palpitations, a fine tremor of the outstretched fingers and tongue, muscle weakness and shortness of breath with the patient having difficulty in climbing stairs, diarrhea, restlessness, difficulty in sleeping, and menstrual irregularities. In addition, characteristic eye changes are common. These are of two types, the one group related to the increased tone of the sympathetic nervous system caused by the hyperthyroidism, and the other to the infiltrative ophthalmopathy of autoimmune origin.

Under the first category would be included eyelid retraction with lid lag that produces a distinctive staring expression. Of more potential seriousness to the patient are the infiltrative eye changes that are the result of the accumulation of an inflammatory exudate (lymphocytes and fluid rich in mucopolysaccharides) in the retroorbital spaces, as well as throughout the interstitial spaces of the subcutaneous tissues of the eyelids, conjunctiva, and extraocular muscles. Because the bony orbit is a rigid structure, the accumulation of the exudates within the orbit pushes the eye forward leading to *proptosis (exophthalmos)*. If the protrusion of the eye is progressive, the patient may be unable to completely close the eyelids, a condition that, if untreated, leads to damage through the drying of the corneal surface of the eye. Severe exophthalmos may also cause permanent damage to the optic nerve, with a serious impairment of vision. The involvement of the extraocular muscles by the inflammatory process may produce varying degrees of muscle weakness or paralysis with associated problems such as an inability to elevate the eyes, to converge the eyes, or to coordinate bilateral eye movements, leading to diplopia.

Patients suffering from the eye changes of Graves' disease may complain early of irritation of the eyes with a gritty sensation; increased tearing and photophobia are also common components. Fortunately, the severe, progressive eye changes are relatively rare and the usual course is for the eye disease to regress, or at least stabilize, when the patient is restored to a euthyroid state. Occasionally, the eye changes are much more prominent on one side, so they must be carefully distinguished from other causes of unilateral proptosis, such as tumor.

Pretibial myxedema, although pathognomonic of Graves' disease, is a relatively rare complication of the disorder. The dermopathy almost always is bilateral and is of a characteristic appearance. The skin over the anterior aspect of the lower legs is thickened and discolored. Hair growth over the area is usually increased relative to other nonaffected areas. Enlarged hair follicles give the surface the texture of an orange peel. The patient may complain of itchiness. Pretibial myxedema rarely occurs in patients who do not have significant clinical ophthalmopathy. The thickened skin is infiltrated with an exudate similar to the ocular exudate.

Although Graves' disease occurs most commonly in young adult women, it can affect any age and either sex. Affected men may have severe forms of the disease, with serious eye changes or progressive muscle wasting leading to profound incapacitation. In elderly patients the disease may be much less flamboyant than in younger patients because of less obvious eye changes and fewer complaints of heat intolerance, nervousness, and generalized disability. Nonetheless, hyperthyroidism, with its increased stimulation of the heart, may produce a dangerous decompensation of the cardiovascular system in elderly patients unless it is recognized and treated. A cardiac dysrhythmia may be the only sign elicited on the physical examination.

Graves' disease in newborn infants is rarely the result of a primary dysfunction occurring in the baby. Most often it is related to the transfer across the placenta during intrauterine life of the abnormal stimulator, HTSI, from the maternal circulation. There will be a history of current or recent Graves' disease in the mother. Neonatal Graves' disease can be associated with most of the common signs and symptoms of the adult disorder, including goiter, hyperthyroidism, and exophthalmos. The condition is self-limited; as the HTSI disappears from the baby's circulation, the manifestations of the disease disappear. If the infant can be successfully supported through the first critical days or weeks following birth, no serious sequelae are likely.

Toxic nodular goiter. Hyperthyroidism may arise in a patient with a long-standing nodular enlargement of the thyroid. For reasons that have not been explained the nodular areas have a tendency to become autonomous. Many patients with nodular goiter never become hyperthyroid. However, if thyrotoxicosis does develop, the eye and skin changes so characteristic of Graves' disease usually are completely absent. The patients most commonly are middle aged to elderly. Cardiac symptoms may predominate; an examination of the cardiovascular system in any elderly patient with an enlarged thyroid may reveal a previously undiagnosed atrial fibrillation or other cardiac dysrhythmias.

Subacute (de Quervain's) granulomatous thyroiditis. Subacute (de Quervain's) granulomatous thyroiditis is a self-limited viral inflammation of the thyroid. The gland becomes tender and enlarged; symptoms of generalized malaise are common, sometimes accompanied by a mild transient hyperthyroidism. No specific therapy is required. Low-dose corticosteroids are useful for reducing the severity of the symptoms in selected patients.

Thyroid storm. The most severe form of hyperthyroidism is called thyroid storm (crisis). It is a life-threatening disorder and a medical emergency. Fortunately, it has become rare because of a better understanding of the condition and its prevention. Thyroid storm produces an extreme degree of hypermetabolism that places a critical demand on the organ systems of the body. Organ failure may result because of the severe stress. Dysfunction of the cardiovascular, renal, gastrointestinal, hepatic, and central nervous systems is common. Thyroid crisis usually develops in patients with a previously diagnosed, but uncontrolled, hyperthyroidism when they are exposed to a stressful situation such as surgery or an infection. All of the usual signs and symptoms of hyperthyroidism may be present in an exaggerated form, including an extremely rapid pulse rate. Fever is common. Laboratory findings are not unique; markedly elevated serum levels of T_3 and T_4 are not the rule. The early diagnosis and adequate therapy of hyperthyroidism should prevent the onset of thyroid storm except in unusual circumstances involving unpredictable severe stress to the patient.

Treatment of hyperthyroidism. The goal for the treatment of hyperthyroidism is to restore permanently a normal or eumetabolic state in the patient. Most forms of hyperthyroidism are caused by an uncontrolled secretion of thyroid hormone by the gland. To achieve the goal of therapy in these cases, the thyroid output of T_4 and T_3 must be reduced to a normal level on a lasting basis.

Two definitive forms of therapy are available to the patient, each of which carries a high probability of a permanent *remission* of the hyperthyroid state. These involve the destruction or removal of a portion of the functioning gland by either (1) radioiodine or (2) surgery (subtotal thyroidectomy).

With either form of treatment, the clinician or surgeon attempts to reduce the amount of the functioning thyroid tissue to a level at which sufficient follicular cells remain to provide normal levels of the thyroid hormones. The failure to destroy adequate amounts of tissue is followed by a continuation or exacerbation of the hyperthyroidism. If too much glandular tissue is removed or destroyed, the patient will become permanently hypothyroid.

The long-term remission of hyperthyroidism also may be effected in some patients by administering antithyroid medication over a period of weeks, months, or years. However, a euthyroid state can be achieved in the majority of patients who are hyperthyroid only during the time they receive the antithyroid drugs. Following the discontinuation of the therapy, patients may remain euthyroid for indefinite periods, but in many cases the hyperthyroidism returns and a permanent cure can be obtained only by using radioiodine or surgery. Antithyroid drugs play a significant role in the short-term management of patients who are hyperthyroid, and commonly are used to rapidly restore a normal metabolic state in patients before initiating a more definitive therapy.

Drug therapy of hyperthyroidism. Three types of drugs are available for managing the patient who is hyperthyroid: (1) the thioamides, (2) iodine, and (3) β-adrenergic blocking drugs.

Thioamide drugs. The thioamide drugs are a group of compounds that inhibit the synthesis of the thyroid hormone. They are active at the level of thyroid peroxidase. Three drugs belonging to this group are widely used clinically: propylthiouracil, methimazole, and carbimazole. The first two drugs are most commonly employed in North America, whereas carbimazole is more popular in Europe. Carbimazole is converted to methimazole in the blood, so the two drugs are equivalent. Propylthiouracil has an additional antithyroid action not shared by methimazole or carbimazole it inhibits the peripheral conversion of T_4 to T_3. Occasionally, other thioamide drugs such as methylthiouracil will be substituted for the more common medications.

The thioamide drugs may be selected to control hyperthyroidism, either for a short period until more definite therapy becomes effective (radioiodine or surgery), or for the long-term management of the disease with the hope that a remission will be sustained when the treatment is terminated. The initial and maintenance dosages of the drugs will be similar in either case, and will vary somewhat from patient to patient. Initially, a loading dose is given using a standard amount of the drug. The dosage can then be gradually increased if necessary until the patient is rendered euthyroid as judged by clinical examination. Later, in most patients, the dosage may be reduced to a maintenance level that is found to control the symptoms of the disease. The three following situations are important to avoid during therapy.

1. Insufficient drug that fails to control the hyperthyroidism; the patient will continue to be disabled. In such situations, the complications of the disease become more prevalent. When the drugs are used as a part of preparing a patient who is hyperthyroid for surgery, it is essential that undermedication be avoided because of the risk of thyroid storm at the time of the operation.

2. Excessive drug that blocks hormone production to a degree where serum T_4 and T_3 levels fall below normal. Before treatment, the secretion of TSH by the anterior pituitary will have been blocked completely by the elevated circulating concentrations of the thyroid hormones. If the antithyroid medication leads to low thyroid hormone secretion, then TSH levels will begin to rise and increased stimulation of the gland will ensue. This situation may be suspected if the goiter of a patient who is hyperthyroid begins to increase in size during antithyroid medication. The dosage of the drug should then be reduced, or else small amounts of oral thyroxine may be added to the treatment to suppress the endogenous secretion of TSH.

3. The onset of symptoms and signs suggestive of adverse reactions to the antithyroid drug (discussed later). If this happens the drug should be stopped and replaced by one of the other available medications.

The potency of methimazole or carbimazole is approximately 10 times greater than propylthiouracil. The recommended initial dosages of the drugs for the average patient are propylthiouracil, 300 mg daily, and methimazole or carbimazole, 30 mg daily.

It is customary to give the drugs in three equally divided doses every 8 hours. The blood levels of the drug are maintained at an adequate therapeutic concentration by this protocol; the duration of action of the drugs is relatively short (6 to 8 hours). Some report that their patients respond well to a single daily dose equal to the total recommended amount. These investigators feel that patient compliance is better with the single dose, and also that the patients benefit from a regimen that permits long uninterrupted nighttime periods for sleep. However, the divided dose protocol remains the most prevalent. A total of 300 mg of propylthiouracil daily (or 30 mg of methimazole) will be insufficient to control the hyperthyroidism in some patients. Incremental increases in the drug to an effective level should then be instigated. Total dosages exceeding 600 mg are rarely required, although 800 mg or even more sometimes may be necessary. If the patient has severe symptoms, starting doses of 150 or 200 mg of propylthiouracil every 8 hours can be used.

With propylthiouracil or methimazole a euthyroid state can be achieved in most patients within 4 to 6 weeks. For the long-term management of hyperthyroidism, the total duration of the treatment required remains controversial and varies greatly from center to center. Many attempts have been made to devise a reliable method for identifying those patients who are most likely to have a permanent remission of their hyperthyroidism following the cessation of the antithyroid therapy. This is of importance because, unfortunately, the majority of patients (60% to 85%) have a recurrence of their symptoms when the drugs are stopped, often within 3 months.

The administration of T_3, along with the antithyroid drug, has been advocated as a means of separating the two groups. Subjects whose early thyroid uptake of ^{131}I is suppressed while receiving the combination drugs are likely to have a permanent remission. An alternate method has been reported from laboratories with reliable methods for measuring HTSI. Those patients in whom the HTSI levels fall significantly, or disappear, while the antithyroid medication is being given are those in whom a permanent remission is probable. A continuing high level of HTSI at the end of the treatment period would suggest that the hyperthyroidism is still active and symptoms will recur when the therapy is discontinued.

Based on reports from many centers, there is a general agreement that for the long-term management of hyperthyroidism, the initial period of the antithyroid drug treatment should last 6 months to 1 year. If the hyperthyroidism recurs after that time, more definitive forms of therapy (radioiodine or surgery) should be considered because the probability of a complete remission following further treatment is small.

Reports have appeared in the literature describing a permanent remission after long-term antithyroid therapy, but most recommend surgery as a more practical and cost-efficient form of treatment rather than extended periods of drug administration. Even with laboratory aids it is difficult to predict in advance which patients are most likely to obtain a permanent remission of hyperthyroidism with the antithyroid therapy.

In general, however, those patients with a severe infiltrative ophthalmopathy or dermopathy, and those with large thyroid glands, belong to the group least likely to remain euthyroid when the drug administration is stopped. Also, any patient who has had a previous relapse of the disease falls into the same category. It has been reported that the recurrence of hyperthyroidism may be precipitated if the patient receives excessive amounts of iodine in the period when they are off of antithyroid medication. For this reason such patients should avoid medications or diagnostic procedures that would expose them to high levels of iodine.

Patients receiving thioamide drugs should be carefully monitored, especially during the early stages of treatment. A variety of mild to severe side effects have been reported with these agents. Mild side effects such as skin rash, pruritus, or arthralgia often subside after a short period even if the drugs are continued. If they fail to disappear, the patient can be switched to a different drug; this usually results in a remission of the unpleasant symptoms. The use of antihistamines may also be helpful.

Nephrotic syndrome has been reported as another adverse effect associated with thioamide drugs. However, the adverse reaction of most serious importance is *granulocytopenia*, which can proceed to *agranulocytosis*. Hypocalcemia may accompany the agranulocytosis. Most patients who develop this rare complication have been on the drugs for relatively short periods of time, so newly treated patients must be instructed to report immediately the development of new symptoms, especially any that are suggestive of an infection. When granulocytopenia is discovered, the drug should be stopped promptly. With few exceptions, a complete recovery can be expected.

Iodine. The antithyroid action of excess iodine has been the subject of many investigations. The mechanism of this activity remains uncertain, although it is apparent that the effect of iodine is exerted at various control points involved in thyroid hormone production. Exposure of the thyroid to elevated levels of iodine leads to the decreased active transport of iodide, the decreased synthesis of T_3 and T_4, and the diminished secretion of the hormones into the blood. The hyperthyroid gland is especially sensitive to the inhibitory properties of excess iodine. For that reason the chemical is established as a valuable and reliable therapeutic adjunct. It has been used universally as part of the preoperative preparation of patients with hyperthyroidism who require surgery. The iodine is administered daily for approximately 1 week before surgery, usually in addition to a thioamide drug (the thioamide drug is started several weeks earlier to achieve a euthyroid state by the time the iodine is first administered). The combination of antithyroid medications will prevent the onset of thyroid storm and will reduce the vascularity of the gland.

Two iodine preparations are available: (1) Lugol's iodine (which contains 100 mg potassium iodide plus 50 mg iodine as I_2 per ml) and (2) saturated potassium iodide (KI), (which contains 750 mg per ml of the compound).

The recommended daily dose of the preparations (0.5 to 1 ml of Lugol's iodine or 5 to 10 drops of saturated KI) provides blood levels of iodide that are much greater than the minimum required to inhibit the thyroid. The thyrotoxic gland is more sensitive to the antithyroid effects of iodine than is the normal thyroid. A characteristic feature of the iodine effect is the tendency for the inhibitory action to decrease with time; the gland is said to escape from the influence of the excess iodine. At least part of the escape phenomenon is caused by the inherent ability of the normal gland to shut down the active transport of iodide under these circumstances. The long-term treatment of hyperthyroidism with excess iodine is not usually satisfactory for this reason, even though the hyperactive gland is more resistant to escape than is normal tissue.

β-Adrenergic receptor blocking drugs. The excess circulating levels of the thyroid hormones that are characteristic of active hyperthyroidism lead to the stimulation of the sympathetic nervous system. Many of the common symptoms of thyrotoxicosis appear to be the result of this interaction, especially cardiovascular and vasomotor changes (e.g., rapid heart rate, increased systolic blood pressure, sweating, heat intolerance), as well as tremor and anxiety. If the β-adrenergic receptors that mediate these effects are blocked by appropriate drugs, the signs and symptoms of hyperthyroidism are lessened significantly.

The β-adrenergic blocker propranolol has been used widely in patients with hyperthyroidism with general success. The drug has no recognized direct action on the thyroid gland, although it has been shown to inhibit the peripheral conversion of T_4 to T_3. Patients placed on propranolol can be expected to have a rapid reduction in the severity of the signs and symptoms already listed. The dosage of propranolol required to control the hyperthyroid response varies from patient to patient. Administration of as little as 10 mg every 8 hours may be sufficient in some patients with mild disease, whereas a few with severe manifestations may need doses as high as 80 mg three to four times daily. The average dose is 30 to 40 mg every 6 to 8 hours.

The use of either propranolol or some alternate β-adrenergic blocking drug has reduced the frequency with which other antithyroid agents are used for the short-term management of thyrotoxicosis. Even the presurgical preparation of patients selected for subtotal *thyroidectomy* can be achieved solely by using propranolol for 1 to 4 weeks, although the combination of propranolol with the more conventional antithyroid agents is preferred by many. When propranolol is given before surgery, the anesthesiologist should be aware of the medication because of the activity that the drug exerts on the cardiovascular system.

Propranolol is a safe drug when given to patients who are thyrotoxic. There are few contraindications to its use. It should not be given to patients subject to bronchospasm, and caution is required if significant cardiovascular disease is present. There have been reported cases in which a permanent remission of hyperthyroidism was achieved by the long-term administration of propranolol. In general, however, the results have not been encouraging, so it cannot be recommended for the extended management of the disease.

Subtotal thyroidectomy. The surgical removal of a portion of a hyperactive thyroid gland is a well-established method for treating hyperthyroidism. Before the availability of radioiodine as a mode of treatment, surgery was the most widely used procedure. Following the advent of therapy with radioactive iodine, there was a marked decline in the incidence of thyroid surgery. Later there was a trend for some to recommend surgery again because of a concern about the high rates of postradiation hypothyroidism being reported. It was subsequently recognized that the rate of development of late hypothyroidism was no greater following radioiodine therapy than after surgery, so the trend toward increased surgical treatment again leveled off.

In the hands of an experienced surgeon, and with adequate preoperative preparation of the patient with antithyroid medication, surgery is a safe procedure with few complications in carefully selected patients. The most serious complications of thyroid surgery are permanent hypoparathyroidism and recurrent laryngeal nerve damage. In addition, there will be patients in whom either recurrent hyperthyroidism or hypothyroidism will develop after a subtotal thyroidectomy. The incidence of the various complications of surgery vary greatly from center to center. In general the serious complications can be virtually prevented if the surgery is performed only by surgeons with experience in the field. The short-term administration of T_3 may help prevent temporary hypothyroidism following surgery, but recurrent hyperthyroidism and permanent hypothyroidism probably cannot be completely avoided. The more care taken to prevent the one will lead to an increased incidence of the other.

Surgical therapy for hyperthyroidism as an alternative to radioactive iodine has been advocated as the treatment of choice for children, young adults (especially women in the reproductive years), pregnant women, and for patients with large nodular goiters. For many years the arbitrary cutoff age for using radioiodine was 40 years of age. Because there has been little evidence to suggest that therapy with radioactive iodine increases the risk of the later development of a thyroid malignancy or leukemia, many centers have decreased the age at which radioactive iodine can be used.

Surgery still is advocated by most for the definitive treatment in children if long-term antithyroid drug administration does not produce a permanent remission. Surgery can be safely performed during pregnancy, especially in the second trimester, but many prefer to treat hyperthyroidism in pregnancy with antithyroid drugs using as low a dosage as possible to control the symptoms.

Surgery is not recommended for the management of hyperthyroidism that recurs following a subtotal thyroidectomy (the results generally are unsatisfactory), or in patients who are poor surgical risks (including patients who cannot be prepared adequately because of an intolerance to the antithyroid drugs).

Radioactive iodine. If radioactive iodine is given orally to a patient, the radioisotope is accumulated within the follicular cells of the thyroid. The radiation damages or destroys the involved cells, and if the dose of the radioactivity is sufficiently high, the activity of the gland will be reduced.

Radioactive iodine has been used for several decades with great success as a means for treating hyperthyroidism. The therapy is simple to administer, reliable, and, with one exception, is relatively free from important complications or side effects.

The significant complication of the treatment of thyrotoxicosis with radioactive iodine, as with surgery, is permanent hypothyroidism. Hypothyroidism may develop early (within the first 6 to 12 months) at a rate that depends on the dose of radioiodine given. In some patients, at least, this early hypothyroidism is transient. Hypothyroidism also may develop later—in fact, many years after the treatment. The rate of the development of late hypothyroidism is 1% to 2% per year; the rate does not decrease with time, so patients treated by either radioactive iodine or surgery are at a risk for the remainder of their lives, and should be seen by a health care provider at regular intervals.

Two isotopes of iodine (^{131}I and ^{125}I) have been used for treating hyperthyroidism. Most experience has been with ^{131}I. Studies with ^{125}I have failed to find a decreased incidence of hypothyroidism after its use compared with ^{131}I, so it is not widely employed. It is now accepted generally that long-term hypothyroidism cannot be avoided in these patients and probably is a result in part to the natural progression of the disease (patients who received no definitive therapy for Graves' disease other than antithyroid drugs and who ultimately became hypothyroid have been reported).

The incidence of short-term hypothyroidism has been decreased since a reduction in the dose of radioiodine was recommended. The lower dose poses no problems to the patient if it is combined with the extended administration of the antithyroid drugs or propranolol to control symptoms until the effect of the radioactive iodine becomes manifest.

The usual dose of ^{131}I administered orally for the treatment of Graves' disease is 3000 to 4000 rad, approximately one half of the level recommended during the first years of its use. The patient is reexamined at regular intervals after the radioactive material is given. If the hyperthyroidism is not controlled by 6 months, a second dose of radioiodine is administered.

Much larger doses of radioactive iodine are necessary to treat patients with hyperthyroidism who have large, multinodular goiters than for those patients with diffusely enlarged glands. The risk of permanent hypothyroidism is less in the group with nodular glands, so there is less concern with them about the long-term effect of the higher levels of radioactivity. The mean age of the group in which multinodular goiters occur is higher than for the diffuse hyperthyroid group. This favors a more energetic level of treatment for two reasons: (1) a more rapid control of hyperthyroidism is desirable (to avoid cardiovascular complications) and (2) the possibility of long-term complications is not a major problem.

There is no clear-cut answer to the question of which age groups, if any, should be excluded from therapy with radioiodine. Certainly the use of the radioisotope during pregnancy or lactation is contraindicated. However, many feel that patients of any age can be treated safely and efficiently by this means and recommend it as the therapy of choice.

Thyroid storm. Thyroid storm is a medical emergency, and requires prompt and energetic treatment. The patient needs a specific therapy directed against both the hyperthyroidism and the precipitating event, which may be some unrelated illness or infection.

General supportive measures must be applied to deal with the myriad of problems that often result from the severe hypermetabolic state, including administering fluids and electrolytes to achieve adequate hydration, and measures such as hypothermic blankets to reduce fever (aspirin is contraindicated). The appropriate control of CHF, cardiac dysrhythmias, hyperglycemia, and hypercalcemia must be attempted when necessary. The specific treatment of an infection, if present, should be included in the regimen. The use of systemic corticosteroids in thyroid storm is controversial.

The hyperthyroidism is brought under control as

rapidly as possible by the combined use of several antithyroid agents. Large initial doses of propylthiouracil (up to 1200 mg orally) followed by lower quantities (400 to 800 mg daily) are given to block both the thyroid synthesis of the thyroid hormones and the peripheral conversion of T_4 to T_3. Iodine, as Lugol's solution (30 drops daily) or saturated potassium iodide (15 drops daily), is administered to block the secretion of the hormones from the thyroid gland. The iodide may be given intravenously when necessary. Propranolol is beneficial for controlling many of the severe manifestations of the crisis. It can be administered either orally (20 to 80 mg every 4 hours) or intravenously (approximately 2 mg every 4 hours).

Hyperthyroidism in pregnancy. The treatment of a pregnant woman with hyperthyroidism requires special precautions because the placenta is freely permeable to several of the agents that may be administered. Radioiodine should not be given to a pregnant patient, either for the diagnosis or the treatment of thyrotoxicosis. The danger of damage to the fetal thyroid is potentially great. Stable iodide given to the mother will also reach the fetus. The fetal thyroid appears to be especially sensitive to the antithyroid properties of excess iodine. The inhibition of the fetal thyroid function by the iodide leads to increased levels of TSH, which can produce significant increases in the size of the fetal gland. Iodide-induced goiter can cause mechanical difficulties during the delivery of the baby, and also may be the origin of a hypothyroid state at birth. The decreased thyroid function and goiter both disappear within a short period after delivery because the gland is no longer exposed to the excess iodide levels.

Hyperthyroidism in pregnancy can be treated successfully by either surgery combined with antithyroid agents, or by antithyroid agents alone. When surgery is selected, it is usually performed during the second trimester when the risk factors are lowest. However, there is some danger that surgery at this time will induce premature labor.

Antithyroid drugs, such as propylthiouracil, cross the placenta. Fortunately, when low doses of the agents are administered to the mother, there appears to be little risk to the fetus. It has been suggested that the effect of the antithyroid drugs on the fetal thyroid may be counteracted in part by the action of the abnormal thyroid stimulator (HTSI), which also crosses the placenta from the maternal circulation. Low-dose antithyroid therapy (150 to 300 mg propylthiouracil daily in divided doses) will control most cases of hyperthyroidism in pregnant women.

To minimize the potential risk of the drugs to the fetus, the lowest dose that controls the symptoms and keeps the serum level of free thyroxine near the upper limit of normal is recommended. The thyroid hormones (T_4 and T_3) cross the placenta with difficulty, especially in the direction from the mother to the fetus. It is not helpful, therefore, to supplement the antithyroid drugs with T_4 to protect the fetal thyroid (an active analogue of T_4 that does cross the placenta has been described: 3, 5-dimethyl-3'-isopropyl-1-thyroxine may be useful for this purpose).

The thyroid status of both the mother and the baby should be reassessed 1 to 2 weeks after the delivery. If the maternal hyperthyroidism developed for the first time during the pregnancy, a remission can occur postpartum without requiring surgery or radioiodine. However, if the antithyroid medication is stopped too soon after the delivery, a recurrence of the thyrotoxicosis can take place; the drugs should be continued for several months in most patients.

The baby will be euthyroid at delivery in most cases. There is a small risk, however, of either hypothyroidism (from the antithyroid drugs), or hyperthyroidism (from exposure to HTSI). Both conditions are self-limited, but should be recognized so appropriate short-term measures to protect the baby can be taken when necessary.

Although the antithyroid drugs are excreted in the breast milk, their concentration is low; breastfeeding of infants by mothers on the drugs may not be contraindicated.

Hypothyroidism

Hypothyroidism is the clinical response that results when deficient amounts of the thyroid hormones (in the form of free, active T_3 and T_4) are available to the peripheral cells of the body. Like hyperthyroidism, it is a generalized response to abnormal hormone levels. Most tissues of the body will be affected. It is characterized by decreased circulating levels of T_4, but not necessarily T_3. Patients with hypothyroidism have a variety of general manifestations of the low metabolic rate, including decreased oxygen consumption, decreased heat production, and the decreased metabolic clearance of carbohydrates, fats, and proteins. The signs and symptoms of hypothyroidism reflect the multisystem involvement.

Clinical hypothyroidism may have several causes. There is the potential for development of hypothyroidism when any factor damages the thyroid cells, interferes with the hormone synthesis or secretion, reduces the normal stimulation of the gland by TSH, or blocks the peripheral action of the hormones. If the thyroid feedback system that includes the anterior pituitary and the hypothalamus is functioning normally, there is always an increase in thyroid stimulation (by TSH) whenever deficient circulating levels of T_3 and T_4 are present. Whether clinical hypothyroidism will result from a condition that compromises the thyroid function will depend on whether the gland can respond to the increased stimulation by TSH with a significant augmentation of thyroid hormone production. If the response is adequate and hypothyroidism is prevented, the effect of the detrimental factor has been compensated (in such cases, the reserve of the gland to compensate for the further impairment of function is decreased; elevated serum levels of TSH in a patient who is euthyroid should alert the health care provider to this situation). On the other hand, if the elevated TSH fails to stimulate the thyroid to an adequate degree, clinical hypothyroidism ensues. The factors that may produce a deficient thyroid function include the following.

1. Autoimmune disease of the thyroid
2. Administration of radioiodine for the therapy of hyperthyroidism
3. Subtotal thyroidectomy
4. Total thyroidectomy for thyroid cancer
5. Failure of the gland to develop normally during intrauterine life
6. Iodine deficiency
7. Inhibition of the hormone synthesis by antithyroid compounds administered as drugs or as iodine compounds given during radiologic diagnostic procedures, or ingested as naturally occurring goitrogens in foodstuffs or water supplies
8. Inherited deficiencies of key enzymes required for hormone synthesis
9. Pituitary dysfunction resulting in a deficient secretion by TSH
10. Hypothalamic dysfunction resulting in a deficient secretion of TRH and hence TSH
11. Peripheral resistance to thyroid hormones

Clinical features of hypothyroidism. The clinical syndrome of hypothyroidism includes a characteristic group of signs and symptoms. When fully developed, the condition can be diagnosed rapidly by an experienced clinician without requiring the assistance of the laboratory; even a casual inspection of the patient may be all that is required to recognize the distinctive features. On the other hand, the hypothyroidism may be so minimal that the diagnosis requires the aid of special laboratory procedures such as the measurement of serum TSH levels before and after the administration of TRH. Early diagnosis, before the effects of the decreased metabolism have become profound, is desirable.

A patient in whom hypothyroidism has become well established will have the following features to some degree: cold intolerance; dry, coarse skin and hair; fatigue; impaired memory; lethargy and sleepiness; slow speech with hoarseness; weight gain; constipation; muscle cramps; shortness of breath on exertion; and personality changes. In addition, there is a characteristic infiltration of the skin and interstitial tissues with mucopolysaccharide, leading to the peculiar nonpitting edema known as myxedema (in fact, the term *myxedema* commonly is used synonymously with hypothyroidism). The infiltration of the facial skin, especially about the eyes, leads to the distinctive puffy, coarsened appearance of the face that can be diagnostic of the condition. In addition to the features just listed, a slowing of the relaxation phase of the deep tendon reflexes, a slow pulse rate, and an enlarged tongue may be found. The laboratory investigation may show the presence of anemia and elevated serum cholesterol levels. The serum T_4 will be low. If the hypothyroidism is caused by the primary dysfunction of the thyroid, the serum TSH will be elevated.

Hypothyroidism that appears during intrauterine life, or during infancy and early childhood, in addition to the features just listed, will lead to a marked retardation in physical growth and development, and a slowing of mental development. The slowed mental development may become permanent if the hypothyroidism arises before birth and is not treated until the baby is several months old.

The following section discusses the salient features of the more common forms of hypothyroidism.

Autoimmune thyroiditis. The most common cause of spontaneous hypothyroidism developing after birth is an autoimmune disease of the thyroid. Other terms that commonly are used to identify the condition are Hashimoto's thyroiditis and lymphocytic thyroiditis. The incidence of the disease is greatest in middle-aged women (40 to 50 years of age) but it can occur at any age. In fact, it is recognized as the most common form of thyroid disease in both children and adults.

Autoimmune thyroiditis is a slowly progressive disease with an insidious onset. The thyroid gland becomes diffusely infiltrated with lymphocytes and plasma cells, with a loss of normal follicular architecture (in classical Hashimoto's disease, enlarged epithelial cells with oxyphilic cytoplasm may be found; they are called Askanazy cells). Circulating antithyroid antibodies directed against thyroglobulin or thyroid microsomes are characteristically present in high titer.

The thyroid response to the autoimmune disease is of two types. In one, the gland becomes diffusely enlarged and firm (this clinical form is the one usually implied when the term *thyroiditis* is employed). In the other, the atrophy of the normal glandular tissue with lymphocytic infiltration and fibrosis is the prominent change. Goiter is not present (this variant, commonly known as primary or idiopathic atrophy of the gland, is the form commonly associated with classical clinical myxedema).

Autoimmune disease of the thyroid produces changes that decrease the reserve capacity of the gland for hormone production, although overt hypothyroidism may not develop for many years, if ever. Minimally elevated serum levels of TSH in a patient who is euthyroid with a goiter testify to a diminished thyroid reserve.

Autoimmune thyroiditis, whether it occurs as Hashimoto's lymphocytic thyroiditis or as idiopathic thyroid atrophy, is related genetically to other autoimmune disorders, including Graves' disease, pernicious anemia, idiopathic Addison's disease, and hypoparathyroidism. The disorders appear in family aggregations. Nonaffected relatives, as well as patients with the overt disease, may be found to have demonstrable levels of circulating autoantibodies to thyroid, gastric mucosal, or adrenal components.

Hypothyroidism developing after surgical or radioiodine therapy for hyperthyroidism. Any patient who has been treated for hyperthyroidism either by the administration of radioactive iodine or by subtotal thyroidectomy is at risk for developing permanent hypothyroidism (for a fuller discussion of this topic see the earlier section on the therapy for hyperthyroidism). All such patients should be examined on a regular basis so that the appropriate treatment can be started before profound hypothyroidism develops. Thyroid failure may appear many years after the therapeutic procedure, so lifelong surveillance is necessary.

Congenital hypothyroidism. Hypothyroidism present in the newborn infant is an important cause of mental and physical retardation. It occurs with a frequency of approximately 1:5000 to 1:8500 live births. Although most aspects of the disease respond well to therapy, the mental deficiency may be permanent. The best prognosis for normal mental development is found in the group of infants with hypothyroidism who are diagnosed and treated before they are 3 months of age.

Some forms of congenital hypothyroidism are transient, caused by the exposure of the baby to antithyroid agents (including excess iodine) during intrauterine life by the transplacental passage of the agent from the maternal circulation. Because the condition is self-limited, no specific therapy is required.

Permanent congenital hypothyroidism may be caused by the following.

1. The failure of the thyroid to develop normally. In these babies, little, if any, normal tissue can be found on examination. Occasionally, ineffectual remnants of the thyroid tissue are located in the neck, along the tract of the thyroglossal tract, or at the base of the tongue.
2. An inherited deficiency of one key thyroidal enzyme required for the normal biosynthesis of T_4 and T_3. Several variants of this disorder have been described, including the following.
   a. Absence of the active transport system for iodide
   b. Deficiency of thyroid peroxidase
   c. Deficiency of the iodotyrosine coupling enzyme
   d. Deficiency of thyroidal iodotyrosine deiodinase
   e. Formation of an abnormal iodoprotein by the thyroid, rather than normal thyroglobulin
3. Severe iodine deficiency during intrauterine life or in the newborn infant. The most common form of this disorder is *endemic* cretinism that is found in regions of the world where iodine is deficient in the soil and water. Affected children, if untreated, are severely retarded both physically and mentally and also may exhibit characteristic neurologic abnormalities.

Patients with congenital hypothyroidism associated with inherited enzyme defects or with iodine deficiency have enlarged thyroid glands. They are classified as having goitrous hypothyroidism, in contrast to the first group in which the gland fails to develop.

Myxedema coma. The most severe clinical form of hypothyroidism is myxedema coma. Like thyroid crisis it is a medical emergency. Characteristically, it develops in a patient (usually elderly) with an untreated, long-standing thyroid deficiency. It may progress insidiously and be unrecognized until it becomes severe. The profound degree of hypothyroidism leads to a depression of respiration, cardiac output, and blood flow, so that oxygen transport to the CNS is inadequate. *Hypothermia* and neurologic abnormalities develop. Myxedema coma is most common during the winter months, so exposure to cold probably can be a precipitating factor. Other stressful events such as infection may initiate the condition.

Treatment of hypothyroidism. The principal goal of treatment of hypothyroidism is to restore a normal, eumetabolic state to the patient by providing appropriate cellular levels of thyroid hormone through the oral administration of thyroxine or triiodothyronine. The dose of the hormone given must be such that the signs and symptoms of hypothyroidism are abolished without producing hyperthyroidism.

Several oral preparations containing thyroid hormones are available, including the following.

1. Desiccated thyroid prepared from animal sources
2. Thyroglobulin partially purified from animal sources (both desiccated thyroid and thyroglobulin *cannot* be absorbed directly from the GI tract into the blood, but must undergo partial proteolysis by digestive enzymes; they are prepared so that they contain approximately 0.2% iodine by weight)
3. Synthetic L-thyroxine (T_4) (levothyroxine)
4. Synthetic L-triiodothyronine (T_3) (liothyronine)
5. Synthetic T_4 and T_3 in combination (liotrix)

The GI absorption of the synthetic hormones is more predictable than for the desiccated thyroid or thyroglobulin, although as much as 50% of the oral T_4 may not be absorbed.

When the diagnosis of hypothyroidism is established, and before the therapy is begun, the patient must be instructed carefully about the medication. The patient should be told that the drug will be required for life. The risks of undermedication and overmedication should be explained and the common symptoms associated with improper dosage outlined so that the health care provider will be consulted when necessary. At the time the therapy is started for a newly diagnosed patient, the initial dose of the thyroid preparation is usually well below the anticipated final dose. There is some risk, especially in elderly patients, that serious cardiovascular complications (e.g., angina pectoris, cardiac decompensation, or dysrhythmias) will be precipitated by giving the patient too much of the thyroid hormone initially. The dose is increased by increments every 4 to 6 weeks until the final maintenance level is achieved. Less caution is required in younger patients without cardiovascular disease.

The therapy is monitored by a regular clinical examination supplemented by a laboratory assessment. The earliest clinical sign of a restoration of the thyroid status toward normal usually is a diuresis occurring 1 to 2 weeks after starting the hormone. There may also be an increased pulse rate by this time, and the patient may report an increased sense of well-being and an improved energy level. The full restoration of a eumetabolic state requires several months of therapy. However, most of the signs and symptoms of hypothyroidism will have disappeared approximately 6 to 8 weeks after starting the treatment unless low doses are given initially. In patients with primary thyroid disease the elevated serum level of TSH will have returned to normal by this time.

Any of the preparations previously listed can be used successfully for therapy. Levothyroxine has certain advantages over the other medications that make it the treatment of choice. Some of the problems reported with the other agents include the following.

1. The thyroid preparations prepared from animal sources may have variable concentrations of thyroid hormone even when standardized to a constant iodine level.
2. The desiccated thyroid may lose a part of its potency on storage, and can differ in activity from one lot to another.
3. The blood levels of T_3 oscillate widely over a period of 24 hours when T_3 is administered. The patient may be exposed to hormone levels in the hyperthyroid range at times soon after the drug is ingested, whereas at other periods the hormone levels may be low.
4. The laboratory monitoring of thyroid function is difficult with patients receiving T_3 alone or in combination, because the serum T_4 concentration will not reflect the thyroid status of the patient. If the patient receives T_3 alone, the serum T_4 will remain in the hypothyroid range. If combined preparations containing both T_4 and T_3 are administered, the use of the serum T_4 to monitor the therapy can lead to an overdose because it does not accurately assess the total hormone activity.

When synthetic levothyroxine is selected for therapy, there are advantages for both the patient and prescriber. The patient is assured of a drug of constant potency that maintains the blood levels of both T_4 and T_3 in the normal ranges (all T_3 is derived by the peripheral deiodination of T_4 with this drug, so there are no major fluctuations over a 24-hour period). The prescriber is able to use standard laboratory tests (FT_4I) to monitor the therapy. An overdose is less likely to occur. Because the potency of the brand name preparations of T_4 may differ slightly, it has been recommended that the best results are obtained when the patient always receives the same brand.

Some years ago, the recommended doses for the thyroid preparations were revised downward when it was recognized that serum T_3 is derived largely from T_4. Before that time, higher doses of T_4 had been advocated because it was assumed that the serum T_3 levels would remain lower than normal when only the T_4 was given, and hence more exogenous hormone would be required to compensate for an assumed deficiency of T_3.

The potency of desiccated thyroid is 1000 times less than levothyroxine on a weight basis. The recommended daily adult doses for the various thyroid preparations follow: desiccated thyroid, 60 to 180 mg; thyroglobulin, 60 to 180 mg; levothyroxine, 0.10 to 0.20

mg; liothyronine, 0.025 to 0.075 mg; and mixed synthetic T_4 and T_3 (liotrix), 0.10 mg T_4 + 0.025 mg of T_3.

The patient probably should be maintained on the lowest dose that controls the hypothyroidism; for many patients this will be found to correspond to the lower figure quoted in the ranges just listed. Patients with hypothyroidism who are also receiving barbiturate drugs on a regular basis may require higher levels of the thyroid hormones, because the barbiturates increase the thyroid hormone turnover through an increase in hepatocellular binding. The greatest problem with long-term therapy is a relatively high failure of patient compliance. Every attempt should be made to help the patient understand the need for lifelong therapy.

Hypothyroidism in infants and children. The treatment of a thyroid deficiency in adults can be introduced cautiously and conservatively without the risk of a permanent disability (except in the case of myxedema coma). However, this does not apply to infants and children. The danger of permanent mental or physical retardation is great in untreated or undertreated patients. For this reason, comparatively larger doses of levothyroxine are advocated for these patients so that the circulating hormone levels are maintained in the upper normal range for their age group. This corresponds to approximately 0.1 mg of T_4 daily for infants and 0.15 mg of T_4 for older children. The patients should be reassessed on a regular basis to ensure an adequate response in growth and development. Evidence exists that many premature infants are relatively deficient in thyroid hormones at birth. The mortality in this group has been reported to be decreased if the infants are given thyroid hormones for a short time.

Myxedema coma. The prognosis for a patient with untreated myxedema coma is extremely poor. Unless the condition is recognized and treated aggressively, there is little chance the patient will survive. Treatment should be started as soon as a presumptive diagnosis has been made. Confirmatory laboratory tests (T_4 and TSH) should be ordered before therapy is begun, but it may not be judicious to delay the specific management until the results of the tests are known. Thyroid hormone is given initially as a single large dose intravenously (0.3 to 0.5 mg of T_4). Then further hormone is administered, orally or intravenously, at a level of 0.05 to 0.1 mg of T_4 daily. Many favor an IV route for all hormone therapy (until the crisis is under control) because of the unpredictable absorption of the hormone from the GI tract.

Hypothermia is a common clinical feature of myxedema coma. Heat loss can be minimized with light, thermal blankets, but rewarming the patient with hot water or heating blankets is unwise because sudden vasodilation can precipitate a vascular collapse. The administration of corticosteroids is recommended because the adrenocortical function may be decreased by the profound hypothyroid state. This is especially probable if the serum TSH levels are found to be low, suggesting a pituitary dysfunction; in such cases, ACTH secretion also may be deficient and cortisol production may be low. Corticosteroids, in the form of hydrocortisone, are given (100 mg intravenously every 8 hours for 1 week).

The general management of a patient with myxedema coma is not to be overlooked. Any infection or other intercurrent illness must be treated. The cardiovascular status of the patient should be monitored. The fluid replacement must be done with caution because of the considerable danger of fluid retention. The amelioration of the hypothyroid state is slow, although the improvement in the pulse rate, body temperature, blood pressure, and level of consciousness may occur within 24 to 48 hours. Aggressive therapy is continued until the patient is considered out of danger. Therapy with thyroid hormone must be continued for the rest of the patient's life.

SUMMARY

The anatomy and physiology of the thyroid have been presented, as well as the assessment of thyroid function. The causes of thyroid dysfunction, including conditions causing hyperthyroidism and hypothyroidism, have been discussed along with their treatment and management. Drugs used in treating these conditions have been described with attention paid to the mechanisms of action, adverse side effects, and management. With a knowledge of these agents, the nurse will be better able to assist patients with their specific drug therapy regimens. This is particularly important when long-term or lifelong management is indicated.

ADVERSE/SIDE EFFECTS OF THYROID AND ANTITHYROID MEDICATIONS*

Thioamide antithyroids
ALLERGIC REACTIONS

Alopecia
Arthralgia
Edema
Fever
Periarteritis (change medication to a
    different thioamide)
Pruritus
Skin rash
Urticaria

CENTRAL NERVOUS SYSTEM

Drowsiness
Vertigo

GASTROINTESTINAL SYSTEM

Epigastric distress
Nausea
Vomiting

HEMATOLOGIC SYSTEM

Agranulocytosis
Granulocytopenia (discontinue medi-
    cation)

Hypoprothrombinemia
Pancytopenia

HEPATIC SYSTEM

Hepatitis
Jaundice

METABOLIC AND ENDOCRINE SYSTEMS

Cold intolerance
Constipation
Drowsiness
Dry skin and hair (reduce dosage of
    drug)
Edema
Fatigue
Hair loss
Hoarseness
Periorbital edema
Weight gain

NEUROMUSCULAR SYSTEM

Headaches
Myalgia
Neuritis
Paresthesias

OCULAR SYSTEM

Visual disturbances

Thyroid hormones
CARDIOVASCULAR SYSTEM

Angina pectoris
Cardiac dysrhythmias
Hypertension
Palpitations
Tachycardia

CENTRAL NERVOUS SYSTEM

Headache
Insomnia
Nervousness
Tremors

METABOLIC AND ENDOCRINE SYSTEMS

Fever
Heat intolerance (reduce dosage of
    drug)
Weight loss

*See Chapter 11, "Drug Toxicity," for an overview of drug toxicity.

CLINICALLY SIGNIFICANT DRUG INTERACTIONS*

Primary drug	*Interacting drug*	*Possible effect(s)*	*Probable mechanism(s)*
Thioamides (e.g., carbimazole, methimazole, propylthiouracil)	Digitalis glycosides	Digitalis toxicity	Not established
Thioamides	Oral anticoagulants	Decreased anticoagulant effect	Not established
Thioamides	Propranolol	Increased propranolol effect	Increased bioavailability probably because of decreased first-pass effect
Thyroid hormones (e.g., levothyroxine; liothyronine; liotrix; thyroglobulin; thyroid, desiccated)	Digitalis glycosides	Decreased digitalis effect	Not established
Thyroid hormones	Oral anticoagulants	Increased anticoagulant effect	Not established
Thyroid hormones	Propranolol	Decreased propranolol effect	Decreased bioavailability probably because of increased first-pass effect

*See Chapter 10, "Drug Interactions," for an overview of drug interactions.

GENERAL NURSING IMPLICATIONS

Nursing of patients requiring antithyroid agents or thyroid hormones

ASSESSMENT

Patients with symptoms of hyperthyroidism or hypothyroidism require a thorough history and physical examination, including a laboratory evaluation of the blood and urine to ensure an accurate diagnosis, because symptoms of these conditions can be mimicked by many other conditions. The patient's general appearance should be recorded with special attention paid to any symptoms of thyroid dysfunction. Record the symptoms caused by pressure from an enlarged thyroid gland, such as hoarseness, difficulty in swallowing, or shortness of breath. A family history of thyroid dysfunction or other disease conditions should also be obtained. The initial data should also include specific information related to any previous hospitalization or treatment for thyroid dysfunction, as well as a detailed drug history before initiating the drug therapy to identify any possible sensitivity, contraindications, cautions, potential drug interactions, and drug-taking patterns.

These baseline data are important in planning to assist patients with their drug therapy regimens and in monitoring their response.

SENSITIVITY

Generally, allergic reactions to the thyroid hormones are rare; however, any drug has the potential to cause a hypersensitivity reaction in susceptible individuals.

Hypersensitivity reactions are more likely to occur with the antithyroid medications (e.g., methimazole, propylthiouracil).

CONTRAINDICATIONS

The use of the antithyroid medications is contraindicated in patients with a hypersensitivity to a specific agent and in nursing mothers.

The use of the thyroid hormones is contraindicated in patients with acute myocardial infarction, thyrotoxicosis, or an uncorrected adrenal insufficiency.

CAUTIONS

Use the antithyroid medications with caution in pregnancy.

Use the thyroid hormones with caution in patients with hypertension, cardiac disease, adrenal insufficiency, or diabetes mellitus.

DRUG INTERACTIONS

Clinically significant drug interactions involving the antithyroid medications or the thyroid hormones are relatively rare. See Clinically Significant Drug Interactions for specific interactions.

It should be noted that even though interactions directly involving these agents are relatively rare, hyperthyroidism or hypothyroidism induced by these medications can affect the metabolism and clearance of a number of drugs.

ADMINISTRATION

Generally the antithyroid medications and the thyroid hormones are administered orally. The treatment is individualized based on a laboratory evaluation and the clinical status of the patient. See the Nursing Drug Digest for specific information regarding the administration of the various agents discussed in this chapter.

MONITORING PATIENT RESPONSE
Therapeutic response

Generally the therapy is aimed at restoring normal metabolic activity and maintaining normal growth and development. Monitor for the euthyroid state, which in the treatment of hyperthyroidism can be achieved in approximately 4 to 6 weeks. Monitor patients with hypothyroidism for decreased signs and symptoms of this condition.

Generally observe and report symptoms of increased thyroid function (e.g., increased pulse rate at rest; elevated blood pressure; weight loss; fatigue; heat intolerance; palpitations; moist, hot skin; tremor; agitation) or decreased thyroid function (e.g., dry, coarse, cool skin; dry, coarse hair; periorbital edema; lethargy; fatigue; cold intolerance; swelling of hands, feet, and ankles; husky voice).

Measure the pulse rate, the blood pressure, and the body weight at regular intervals during the early phase of therapy when the drug dosage is being adjusted.

Adverse side effects
Antithyroid medications
Monitor patients for signs of hypersensitivity, including skin rashes, fever, urticaria, pruritus, and arthralgia.

Patients receiving thioamide drugs should be carefully monitored for granulocytopenia, which can lead to agranulocytosis manifested by sore throat, skin eruptions, fever, general malaise, and headache.

Also, monitor patients for drug fever and severe skin rashes.

Thyroid hormones
Monitor patients for the following signs of adverse effects that are usually associated with overdose and thus resemble the symptoms of hyperthyroidism: angina pectoris, abdominal cramps, cardiac dysrhythmias, diarrhea, fever, headache, insomnia, nervousness, palpitations, sweating, and weight loss.

Observe and report changes in vision (e.g., blurring of vision, diplopia, decreased visual acuity) or in the appearance of the eyes (e.g., protrusion of the eyes, edema of the periorbital tissues and eyelids, redness of the orbital tissues, limitation of eye movements).

See Adverse/Side Effects of Thyroid and Antithyroid Medications for an outline of adverse effects associated with the use of these medications.

PATIENT EDUCATION

The patient and the family, as indicated, should be fully informed about the patient's condition and treatment plan. They should be involved in care planning whenever possible. The patient and the family should have an understanding of the anticipated course of the therapy and the medication regimen. This is important because the medication may be required for lengthy periods of time with the antithyroid drugs or for the lifetime of the patient as is required with thyroid hormone therapy. Patient education to enhance patient self-medication abilities is essential.

Patients should know the exact name of the medication, its general action, purpose, dosage, storage, administration, and adverse effects. They should know how to monitor the therapeutic response and be able to identify the signs that indicate the health care provider should be notified.

GENERAL INSTRUCTIONS FOR DISCHARGE/OUTPATIENTS

THYROID MEDICATIONS

This medication is used for treating thyroid conditions. If you do not understand why you require this medication, contact your health care provider.

Follow the instructions on the prescription exactly. If you have any questions, contact your health care provider.

Make appointments to see your health care provider at regular intervals as instructed. The dose of the drug may have to be adjusted periodically to ensure the best results.

Report immediately to your health care provider any new symptoms that appear while you are taking the drug, especially fever, sore throat, skin rashes, and changes in vision.

The symptoms that have been troubling you because your thyroid has not been functioning at a normal level should begin to improve slowly as you take the drug. However, it may take several weeks before the improvement is complete. Do not stop taking the medicine unless you are *instructed to do so by your health care provider.*

Inform your health care provider immediately if you are considering becoming pregnant while taking this drug.

This medication has been prescribed especially for you. Do not trade or give this medication to any relatives or friends.

Keep this and all medications out of children's reach.

NURSING DRUG DIGEST

Medication (trade name*)	Indication	Usual dosage and administration	Dosage forms, preparation, and storage	Contraindications, cautions, and comments	Monitoring
Iodine Lugol's solution: 5% iodine + 10% potassium iodide Potassium iodide, saturated solution, USP Sodium iodide, saturated solution, USP	Preparation for thyroid surgery in hyperthyroidism Thyroid crisis	*Adults or children:* 0.5-1.0 ml Lugol's solution *or* 5-10 drops saturated potassium (or sodium) iodide/24 hr PO in water in 3 divided doses for 2-3 weeks before surgery *Adults or children:* 1.0-2.0 ml Lugol's solution *or* 10-20 drops saturated potassium (or sodium) iodide/24 hr PO in water in 3 divided doses, administered with other antithyroid drugs May be given IV as 250-500 mg sodium iodide as a slow infusion over 24 hr	Protect solutions from light	*Contraindicated* in iodide hypersensitivity, tuberculosis, and laryngeal swelling Patient should avoid meals that contain a high content of starch Discoloration of teeth can be minimized by using drinking straw IV administration reserved for patients who cannot take iodine PO because of vomiting or gastric irritation	Observe for signs of iodide sensitivity (e.g., periorbital edema, mucous membrane ulceration, skin rash)
Levothyroxine (T₄) Eltroxin Letter Levoid Levothroid LTS Noroxine Synthroid	Hypothyroidism Cretinism	*Adults:* initial, 0.025-0.10 mg/24 hr PO Increase daily dose by 0.025-0.05 mg every 4-6 weeks until euthyroid *Adults:* Maintenance, 0.1-0.2 mg/24 hr PO *Children:* initial, 0.003-0.005 mg/kg/24 hr PO Increase daily dose by 0.003-0.005 mg/kg every 4 weeks until euthyroid Maintenance, not less than 0.1 mg/24 hr PO in infants Usual maintenance dose in children older than 1 year, 0.1-0.2 mg/24 hr PO	Tablets: 0.005, 0.025, 0.05, 0.075, 0.1, 0.125, 0.15, 0.175, 0.2, 0.3 mg Protect from light and moisture Injectable: 100, 200, 500 mg/vial Prepare IV solution (100 µg/ml) immediately before use by dissolving powder in NS Discard any unused portion of IV solution	*Contraindicated* in acute myocardial infarction, thyrotoxicosis, and uncorrected adrenal insufficiency	Monitor pulse and blood pressure Observe for signs of hyperthyroidism (e.g., diarrhea, nervousness, palpitations) Monitor patients on anticoagulant therapy closely for signs of toxicity (dose of anticoagulant often must be modified)

Continued.

NOTE: For additional details regarding the individual agents listed in this table see the text and other tables in this chapter.
*Indicates a multiple active ingredient product. For a complete listing of all active ingredients see the *Drug Reference Guide to Brand Names and Active Ingredients.*

NURSING DRUG DIGEST—cont'd

Medication (trade name)	Indication	Usual dosage and administration	Dosage forms, preparation, and storage	Contraindications, cautions, and comments	Monitoring
Levothyroxine (T$_4$)—cont'd	Myxedematous coma	*Adults:* 200-500 μg IV first day; 100-300 μg IV second day (if necessary); then full maintenance dose (as above) PO Administer at same time each day (morning dose may prevent insomnia) NOTE: 0.1 mg levothyroxine is approximately equivalent to 65 mg thyroid			
Liothyronine (T$_3$) Cytomel Cytomine Tertroxin	Hypothyroidism	*Adults:* initial, 5-25 μg/24 hr PO; increase daily dose by 5-25 μg every 1-2 weeks until euthyroid. Maintenance, 25-75 μg/24 hr PO	Tablets: 5, 25, 50 μg. Protect from light and moisture. Prepare IV solution (25 μg/ml) immediately before use by dissolving powder in NS. Discard any unused portion of IV solution	*Contraindicated* in acute myocardial infarction, thyrotoxicosis, and uncorrected adrenal insufficiency. Rapid onset and short duration of action. Therapy *cannot* be monitored by measurement of serum levels of T$_4$	Monitor pulse and blood pressure. Observe for signs of hyperthyroidism (e.g., diarrhea, nervousness, palpitations). Monitor patients on anticoagulant therapy closely for signs of overdose (dose of anticoagulant often must be modified)
	Cretinism	*Children:* initial, 5 μg/24 hr PO; increase daily dose by 5 μg every 3-4 days until euthyroid. Maintenance, 25-50 μg/24 hr PO			
	Myxedematous coma	*Adults:* 50-125 μg IV first day; 25-75 μg IV second day (if necessary); then full maintenance dose (as above) PO Administer at same time each day (morning dose may prevent insomnia) NOTE: 25 μg liothyronine is approximately equivalent to 65 mg thyroid			
Liotrix (T$_4$ and T$_3$) Euthroid Thyrolar	Hypothyroidism	*Adults:* initial, 1 tablet (25 μg T$_4$ and 6.25 μg T$_3$) *or* 1 tablet (30 μg T$_4$ and 7.5 μg T$_3$)/24 hr PO	Euthroid Tablets: 30 μg T$_4$ and 7.5 μg T$_3$, 60 μg T$_4$ and 15 μg T$_3$, 120 μg T$_4$ and 30 μg T$_3$, 180 μg T$_4$ and 45 μg T$_3$	*Contraindicated* in acute myocardial infarction, thyrotoxicosis, and uncorrected adrenal insufficiency	Monitor pulse and blood pressure. Observe for signs of hyperthyroidism (e.g., diarrhea, nervousness, palpitations)

Drug	Use	Dosage	Preparations	Nursing Implications
		Increase daily dose by 1 tablet of same potency every 1-2 weeks until euthyroid. Maintenance, 1 tablet/24 hr PO ([50 μg T_4 and 12.5 μg T_3] to [120 μg T_4 and 30 μg T_3]) as required to maintain euthyroid state. Administer at same time each day (morning dose may prevent insomnia). NOTE: 60 μg T_4 and 15 μg T_3 (or 50 μg T_4 and 12.5 μg T_3) is approximately equivalent to 65 mg thyroid	Thyrolar. Tablets: 25 μg T_4 and 6.25 μg T_3, 50 μg T_4 and 12.5 μg T_3, 100 μg T_4 and 25 μg T_3, 150 μg T_4 and 37.5 μg T_3. Protect from light and moisture. *Note that the two commercial preparations of liotrix are of different potencies and should not be used interchangeably*	Monitor patients on anticoagulant therapy closely for signs of overdose (dose of anticoagulant often must be modified)
Methimazole Tapazole Mercazole	Hyperthyroidism	*Adults:* initial, mild cases, 15 mg/24 hr PO in 3 divided doses. Average cases, 30 mg/24 hr PO in 3 divided doses. Severe cases, 40-45 mg/24 hr PO in 3-4 divided doses. Maintenance, 5-15 mg/24 hr PO in 3 divided doses. *Children:* initial, 0.4 mg/kg/24 hr PO in 3 divided doses. Maintenance, 0.2 mg/kg/24 hr PO in 3 divided doses. Administer with food or milk to decrease GI irritation	Tablets: 5, 10 mg. Protect from light	A rare cause of depression of the bone marrow (agranulocytosis, granulocytopenia). Efficacy is less consistent than that seen with propylthiouracil. Administration during pregnancy may cause neonatal (congenital) goiter. Observe for signs of agranulocytosis (e.g., fever, sore throat, skin rashes). Observe for signs of hypothyroidism (e.g., cold intolerance, mental depression)
Propranolol Inderal Novopranol Panolol	Hyperthyroidism (for treatment of sympathetic nervous system effects) (indication *not* FDA approved) See also Chapter 33, "Antihypertensives"	*Adults:* mild cases, 30 mg/24 hr PO in 3 divided doses. Average cases, 90-120 mg/24 hr PO in 3 divided doses. Severe cases, 240 mg/24 hr PO in 3-4 divided doses	Tablets: 10, 20, 40, 60, 80, 90, 120 mg	*Contraindicated* in bronchial asthma, CHF, greater than first-degree heart block. Has *no* direct effect on thyroid gland. Avoid abrupt withdrawal of drug in patients with angina pectoris. Crosses the placenta and may cause bradycardia or hypoglycemia in the neonate if administered during the third trimester of pregnancy. Monitor for cardiovascular effects

Continued.

NURSING DRUG DIGEST—cont'd

Medication (trade name)	Indication	Usual dosage and administration	Dosage forms, preparation, and storage	Contraindications, cautions, and comments	Monitoring
Propyl-thiouracil Propyl-thyra-cil	Hyperthyroidism	*Adults:* initial, mild cases, 150 mg/24 hr PO in 3 divided doses Average cases, 300 mg/24 hr PO in 3 divided doses Severe cases, 400-600 mg/24 hr PO in 3 divided doses Maintenance, 50-150 mg/24 hr PO in 3 divided doses *Children:* initial, 50-150 mg/24 hr PO in 3 divided doses Maintenance, 25-75 mg/24 hr PO in 3 divided doses Administer with food or milk to decrease GI distress	Tablets: 50, 100 mg Protect from light	A rare cause of depression of the bone marrow (agranulocytosis, granulocytopenia) Administration during pregnancy may cause neonatal (congenital) goiter	Observe for signs of agranulocytosis (e.g., fever, sore throat, skin rashes) Observe for signs of hypothyroidism (e.g., cold intolerance, mental depression)
Radioactive iodine I^{131} Iodotope	Hyperthyroidism	*Adults:* 2-10 millicuries (mCi) PO Dose for individual patient based on size of gland, presence or absence of nodularity, and rate of uptake of I^{131} by thyroid Treatment may be repeated in 4-8 weeks if hyperthyroidism persists Radioiodine therapy for hyperthyroidism most commonly reserved for adults over 25 years of age; however, policies regarding age vary from center to center	Capsules: 1-50 mCi Oral solution: 7 mCi/ml Aqueous solution of sodium iodide-I^{131} prepared from stock solution as required for each patient Radioactive material must be stored with adequate shielding and ventilation Protect from heat and light	*Contraindicated* in pregnancy and lactation All antithyroid drugs should be stopped 1 week before administration of radioactive iodine Propranolol may be administered following radioiodine therapy to control symptoms of hyperthyroidism associated with overactivity of sympathetic nervous system Patients must be followed for life because of risk of permanent hypothyroidism	Observe for persistent signs of hyperthyroidism (e.g., heat intolerance, palpitations, nervousness, tremor) Observe at regular intervals (q. 3-6 months for 1-2 years, then once a year for life) for signs of hypothyroidism (e.g., cold intolerance, lethargy, fatigue, dry skin and hair, facial puffiness)

Drug	Uses	Dosage	Remarks	Nursing Considerations
Thyroglobulin (Proloid) (contains T₃ and T₄ in a ratio of 1:2.5)	Hypothyroidism Cretinism	*Adults:* Initial, 15-60 mg/24 hr PO Increase daily dose by 15-60 mg every 4-6 weeks until euthyroid Maintenance, 60-200 mg/24 hr PO *Children:* Initial, 15-30 mg/24 hr PO Increase dose by 15-30 mg/24 hr every 2 weeks until euthyroid Maintenance, 30-200 mg/24 hr PO Administer at same time each day (morning dose may prevent insomnia)	Tablets: 16, 32, 65, 100, 130, 200, 300 mg Deteriorates on exposure to moisture or light	*Contraindicated* in acute myocardial infarction, thyrotoxicosis, and uncorrected adrenal insufficiency Slow onset of action No clinical advantage over thyroid (desiccated)	Monitor patients on anticoagulant therapy closely for signs of overdose (dosage of anticoagulant often must be modified) Observe for signs of hyperthyroidism (e.g., diarrhea, nervousness, palpitations)
Thyroid, desiccated (Dathroid, Delcoid, S-P-T, Thyrar, Thyro-teric)	Hypothyroidism Cretinism	*Adults:* Initial, 15-60 mg/24 hr PO Increase daily dose by 15-60 mg every 4-6 weeks until euthyroid Maintenance, 60-195 mg/24 hr PO *Children:* Initial, 15-30 mg/24 hr PO Increase dose by 15-30 mg/24 hr every 2 weeks until euthyroid Maintenance, 30-195 mg/24 hr PO Administer at same time each day (morning dose may prevent insomnia)	Tablets: 16, 32, 64, 100, 130, 300 mg Deteriorates on exposure to moisture or light	*Contraindicated* in acute myocardial infarction, thyrotoxicosis, and uncorrected adrenal insufficiency Slow onset of action	Monitor patients on anticoagulant therapy closely for signs of overdose (dosage of anticoagulant often must be modified) Observe for signs of hyperthyroidism (e.g., diarrhea, nervousness, palpitations)
Thyrotropin (Thyrotron, Thytropar)	Investigation of hypothyroidism (to distinguish between primary and secondary dysfunction)	*Adults:* 10 IU IM given as a single injection, or repeated daily for 3 days (final injection is given 18 hr before ¹³¹I iodide for thyroid uptake measurement) *Children:* Safe and effective dose not established The test is *not* recommended	Injectable: 10 IU/vial lyophilized thyrotropic hormone Reconstitute in sterile 5% glucose to give 5 IU/ml (solvent supplied in separate ampules) Refrigeration (2°-8° C) required before and after reconstitution Use within 1 week of reconstitution	*Contraindicated* in coronary thrombosis, adrenal insufficiency, and hypersensitivity to thyrotropin Anaphylactic reactions have been reported The use of thyrotropin as a diagnostic test is *no longer necessary* because of the availability of precise laboratory measurements of serum TSH	Monitor patient for signs of hypersensitivity (e.g., urticaria, tachycardia, transitory hypotension, fever)

ACKNOWLEDGMENT

Sincere appreciation is extended by the author to Jan Isaac and Marjorie Mathias for typing the manuscript for this chapter.

BIBLIOGRAPHY

Anderberg, B., Kagedal, B., Nilsson, O.R., Smeds, S., Tegler, L., & Gillquist, J. Propranolol and thyroid resection for hyperthyroidism. *Acta Chirurgica Scandinavica*, 1979, *145*, 297-303.

Beta-blockers in thyrotoxicosis. (Editorial). *Lancet*, 1980, *1*, 184-186.

Bjorkman, U., Ekholm, R., & Ericson, L.E. Effects of thyrotropin on thyroglobulin exocytosis and iodination in the rat thyroid gland. *Endocrinology*, 1978, *102*, 460-470.

Capiferri, R., & Evered, D. Investigation and treatment of hypothyroidism. *Clinics in Endocrinology and Metabolism*, 1979, *8*, 39-48.

Chopra, I.J., Hershmann, J.M., & Hornabrook, R.W. Serum thyroid hormone and thyrotropin levels in subjects from endemic goiter regions of New Guinea. *Journal of Clinical Endocrinology and Metabolism*, 1975, *40*, 326-333.

Comite, F., Burrow, G.N., & Jorgensen, E.C. Thyroid hormone analogs and fetal goiter. *Endocrinology*, 1978, *102*, 1670-1674.

Davidson, B., Soodak, M., Neary, J.T., Strout, H.V., Kieffer, J.D., Mover, H., & Maloof, F. The irreversible inactivation of thyroid peroxidase by methylmercaptoimidazole, thiouracil and propylthiouracil in vitro and its relationship to in vivo findings. *Endocrinology*, 1978, *103*, 871-882.

Davidson, B., Soodak, M., Strout, H.V., Neary, J.T., Nakamura, C., & Maloof, F. Thiourea and cyanamide as inhibitors of thyroid peroxidase: the role of iodide. *Endocrinology*, 1979, *104*, 919-924.

Di Stefano III, J.J., & Mak, P.H. On model and data requirements for determining the bioavailability of oral therapeutic agents: application to gut absorption of thyroid hormones. *American Journal of Physiology*, 1979, *236*, R137-R141.

Edwards, O.M. The management of thyroid disease in pregnancy. *Postgraduate Medical Journal*, 1979, *55*, 340-342.

Emerson, C.H., Anderson, A.J., Howard, W.J., & Utiger, R.D. Serum thyroxine and triiodothyronine concentrations during iodide treatment of hyperthyroidism. *Journal of Clinical Endocrinology and Metabolism*, 1975, *40*, 33-36.

Etling, N., Gehin-Fouque, F., Vielh, J.P., & Gautray, J.P. The iodine content of amniotic fluid and placental transfer of iodinated drugs. *Obstetrics and Gynecology*, 1979, *53*, 376-380.

Feely, J., Isles, T.E., Ratcliffe, W.A., & Crooks, J. Propranolol, triiodothyronine, reverse triiodothyronine, and thyroid disease. *Journal of Clinical Endocrinology*, 1979, *10*, 531-538.

Fenzi, G., Hashizume, K., Roudebush, C.P., & De Groot, L.J. Changes in thyroid-stimulating immunoglobulins during antithyroid therapy. *Journal of Clinical Endocrinology and Metabolism*, 1979, *48*, 572-576.

Field, J.B. Thyroid-stimulating hormone and cyclic adenosine 3', 5'-monophosphate in the regulation of thyroid gland function. *Metabolism*, 1975, *24*, 381-393.

Goswami, A., & Rosenberg, I.N. Studies on a soluble iodotyrosine deiodinase. *Endocrinology*, 1977, *101*, 331-341.

Hoffbrand, B.I. Barbiturate thyroid hormone interaction. *Lancet*, 1979, *2*, 903-904.

Jacobson, J.M., Ramos-Gabatin, A., Young, R.L., Watkins, S.C., & Brown, M.L. Nonequality of brand name T_4 preparations. *Journal of the American Medical Association*, 1980, *243*, 733.

Jefferson, J.W. Lithium carbonate-induced hypothyroidism: its many faces. *Journal of the American Medical Association*, 1979, *242*, 271-272.

Kuzuya, N., Chiu, S.C., Ikeda, H., Uchimura, H., Ito, K., & Nagataki, S. Correlation between thyroid stimulators and triiodothyronine suppressibility in patients during treatment for hyperthyroidism with thionamide drugs: comparison of assays by thyroid-stimulating and thyrotropin-displacing activities. *Journal of Clinical Endocrinology and Metabolism*, 1979, *48*, 706-711.

Laurberg, P. Selective inhibition of the secretion of triiodothyronines from the perfused canine thyroid by propylthiouracil. *Endocrinology*, 1978, *103*, 900-905.

Low, L.C.K., Lang, J., & Alexander, W.D. Excretion of carbimazole and propylthiouracil in breast milk. *Lancet*, 1979, *2*, 1011.

McGuire, R.A., & Berman, M. Maternal, fetal, and amniotic fluid transport of thyroxine, triiodothyronine, and iodide in sheep: a kinetic model. *Endocrinology*, 1978, *103*, 567-576.

McKenzie, J.M., & Zakarija, M. LATS in Graves' disease. *Recent Progress in Hormone Research*, 1977, *33*, 29-57.

McLaren, E.H., & Alexander, W.D. Goitrogens. *Clinics in Endocrinology and Metabolism*, 1979, *8*, 129-144.

Morillo, E., & Gardner, L.I. Hypertriiodothyroninemia in hypothyroidism treated with thyroglobulin. *American Journal of Diseases of Children*, 1979, *133*, 71-72.

Murphy, D. Iodide—an rx for radiation accident. *American Journal of Nursing*, 1982, *82*, 96-98.

Nakashima, T., & Taurog, A. Rapid conversion of carbimazole to methimazole in serum; evidence for an enzymatic mechanism. *Clinical Endocrinology (Oxf)*, 1979, *10*, 637-648.

Oppenheimer, J.H. Thyroid hormone action at the cellular level. *Science*, 1979, *203*, 971-979.

Oppenheimer, J.H., Dillmann, W.H., Schwarz, H.L., & Towle, H.C. Nuclear receptors and thyroid hormone action: a progress report. *Federation Proceedings*, 1979, *38*, 2154-2161.

Penny, R., & Frasier, S.D. Elevated serum concentrations of triiodothyronine in hypothyroid patients: values for patients receiving USP thyroid. *American Journal of Diseases of Children*, 1980, *134*, 16-18.

Querido, A., Bleichrodt, N., & Djokomoeljanto, R. Thyroid hormones and human mental development. *Progress in Brain Research*, 1978, *48*, 337-346.

Rees-Jones, R.W., Rolla, A.R., & Larsen, P.R. Hormonal content of thyroid replacement preparations. *Journal of the American Medical Association,* 1980, *243,* 549-550.

Reynolds, L.R., & Bhathena, D. Nephrotic syndrome associated with methimazole therapy. *Archives of Internal Medicine,* 1979, *139,* 236-237.

Reynolds, L.R., & Kotchen, T.A. Antithyroid drugs and radioactive iodine: fifteen years experience with Graves' disease. *Archives of Internal Medicine,* 1979, *139,* 651-653.

Rezvani, I., Di George, A.M., & Verna, A. Reassessment of the dose of oral thyroxine (T_4) for replacement therapy in hypothyroid children. *Clinical Research,* 1975, *23,* 574A.

Sawers, J.S.A., Toft, A.D., Irvine, W.J., Brown, N.S., & Seth, J. Transient hypothyroidism after iodine-131 treatment of thyrotoxicosis. *Journal of Clinical Endocrinology and Metabolism,* 1980, *50,* 226-229.

Sawin, C.T., Hershman, J.M., Fernandez-Garcia, R., Ghazvinian, S., Ganda, O.P., & Azukizawa, M. A comparison of thyroxine and desiccated thyroid in patients with primary hypothyroidism. *Metabolism,* 1978, *27,* 1518-1525.

Schonberger, W., Grimm, W., Emmrich, P., & Gempp, W. Thyroid administration lowers mortality in premature infants. *Lancet,* 1979, *2,* 1181.

Shambaugh III, G.E., Khoury, N., Zonschein, J., & Sizemore, G.W. Hypocalcemia accompanying agranulocytosis during propylthiouracil therapy. *Annals of Internal Medicine,* 1979, *91,* 576-577.

Slingerland, D.W., & Burrows, B.A. Long-term antithyroid treatment in hyperthyroidism. *Journal of the American Medical Association,* 1979, *242,* 2408-2410.

Taurog, A. The mechanism of action of the thioureylene antithyroid drugs. *Endocrinology,* 1976, *98,* 1031-1046.

Teng, C.S., & Yeung, R.T.T. Changes in thyroid-stimulating antibody activity (TSAb) in Graves' disease treated with antithyroid drug and its relationship to relapse: a prospective study. *Journal of Clinical Endocrinology and Metabolism,* 1980, *50,* 144-147.

Tevaarwerk, G.J.M., & Boyd, D. Propranolol in thyrotoxicosis. II. Serum thyroid hormone concentrations during subtotal thyroidectomy. *Canadian Journal of Surgery,* 1979, *22,* 264-266.

Urbanic, R.C., & Mazzaferri, E.L. Thyrotoxic crisis and myxedema coma. *Heart and Lung,* 1978, *7,* 435-447.

Volpé, R. Subacute (de Quervain's) thyroiditis. *Clinics in Endocrinology and Metabolism,* 1979, *8,* 81-95.

Wilkin, T.J., Gunn, A., Isles, T.E., Crooks, J., & Beck, J.S. Short-term triiodothyronine in prevention of temporary hypothyroidism after subtotal thyroidectomy for Graves' disease. *Lancet,* 1979, *2,* 63-66.

Williams, J.A., & Malayan, S.A. Effects of TSH on iodide transport by mouse thyroid lobes in vitro. *Endocrinology,* 1975, *97,* 162-168.

Wood, L.C., & Ingbar, S.H. Hypothyroidism as a late sequela in patients with Graves' disease treated with antithyroid agents. *Journal of Clinical Investigation,* 1979, *64,* 1429-1436.

Yamamoto, M., Igarashi, T., Kimura, S., Tsukamoto, S., Togawa, K., & Ogata, E. Thyroid suppression test and outcome of hyperthyroidism treated with antithyroid drugs and T_3. *Journal of Clinical Endocrinology and Metabolism,* 1979, *48,* 72-77.

Zonszein, J., Santangelo, R.P., Mackin, J.F., Lee, T.C., Coffey, R.J., & Canary, J.J. Propranolol therapy in thyrotoxicosis: a review of 84 patients undergoing surgery. *American Journal of Medicine,* 1979, *66,* 411-416.

CHAPTER 62

Parathyroid Hormone, Calcitonin, and Related Medications

Loren W. Kline

Medications discussed in this chapter

Hormones	Vitamins
Calcitonin	Calcitriol
Hypocalcemic agents	Dihydrotachysterol
Etidronate	Vitamin D

The hormonal regulation of calcium within narrow limits of concentration is essential for normal functioning of many different biochemical and physiologic processes. Three different hormones are used by the body to accomplish this regulation: parathyroid hormone, calcitonin, and vitamin D. Parathyroid hormone and calcitonin are typical polypeptide hormones. Although not a classic hormone, vitamin D and its biologically potent metabolites are now considered hormones. This classification is made primarily because of the elaborate regulation and control systems affecting the synthesis of the active form of vitamin D.

ANATOMY AND PHYSIOLOGY

Parathyroid glands

The parathyroid (PT) glands were first recognized as distinct anatomic entities in the nineteenth century; however, no particular function was assigned to them. The PT glands are small, yellow-brown, oval bodies, usually intimately connected with the middle posterior surface of the thyroid gland or embedded within this region of the thyroid (Figure 62-1). Usually four or five glands are seen, but as many as 12 have been reported. Histologically the glands consist of densely packed masses and irregular cords of epithelial cells which are supplied with a rich capillary network. Two types of epithelial cells make up most of the glands: the chief, or principal, cells and the oxyphil cells (Fig-

ures 62-2 and 62-3). The chief cells are more abundant and are considered to be the cells responsible for the production of parathyroid hormone (PTH). The function of the oxyphil cells is uncertain. The synthesis of PTH begins with a protein of 115 amino acids called preproparathyroid hormone. This molecule is converted to proparathyroid hormone (pro-PTH) by removal of 25 amino acids as it leaves the ribosomes. Pro-PTH is transported to the golgi apparatus where another six amino acids are removed. The resulting PTH, of 84 amino acids, is stored in secretory granules until released by exocytosis into the blood.

PTH secretion is regulated by the circulating levels of blood calcium. Low levels of calcium stimulate an increase in the circulating PTH levels directly; high levels have a reverse effect. Although high and low blood calcium levels stimulate changes in the circulating levels of PTH, some hormone is continuously present at blood levels of 10^{-11} gm/ml.

Ion metabolism

Calcium is important in many physiologic processes. At the molecular level calcium interacts with a variety of proteins to alter their conformation and function. This interaction includes enzymes that require calcium for activation. Normal physiologic levels of calcium permit maximal activation of these enzymes. *Amylase* and *lipase* are examples of enzymes using calcium for activation. Calcium is essential for contraction of all three muscle types: skeletal, cardiac, and smooth muscle.

In the case of skeletal muscle calcium ions are involved in the excitation-contraction coupling (i.e., calcium acts as a trigger to initiate a series of biochemical reactions between the contractile proteins *actin* and *myosin*, which leads to a mechanical change in length) (Figure 62-4). In cardiac muscle calcium affects the mechanical properties of muscle as well as its excit-

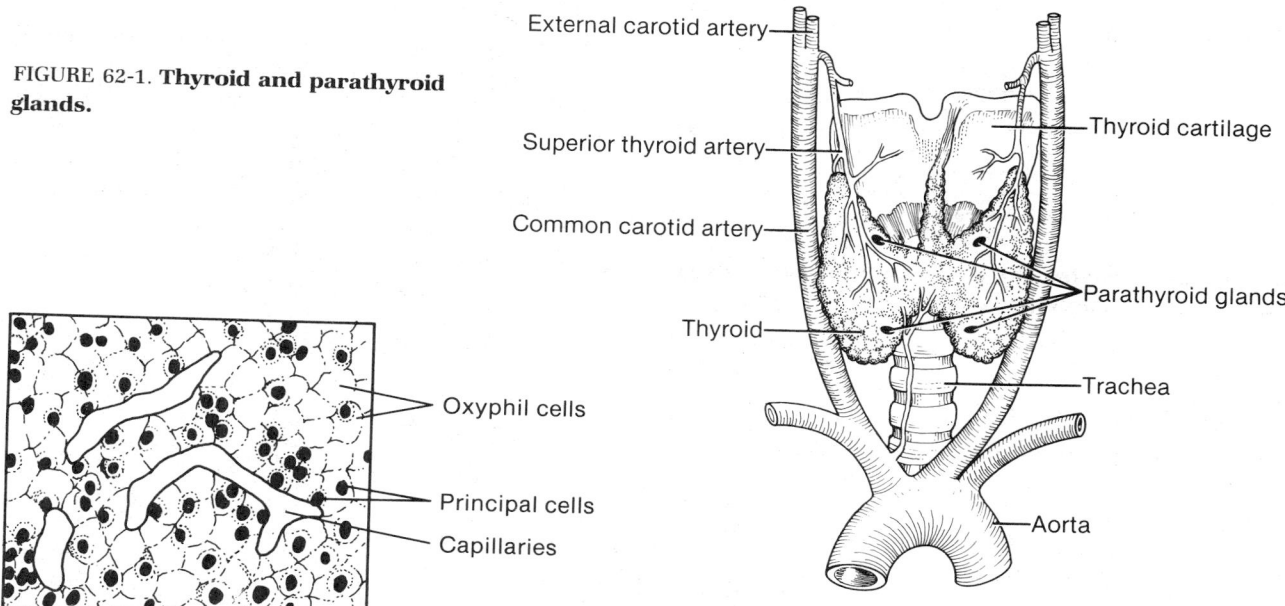

FIGURE 62-1. **Thyroid and parathyroid glands.**

FIGURE 62-2. **Histology of the parathyroid glands.**

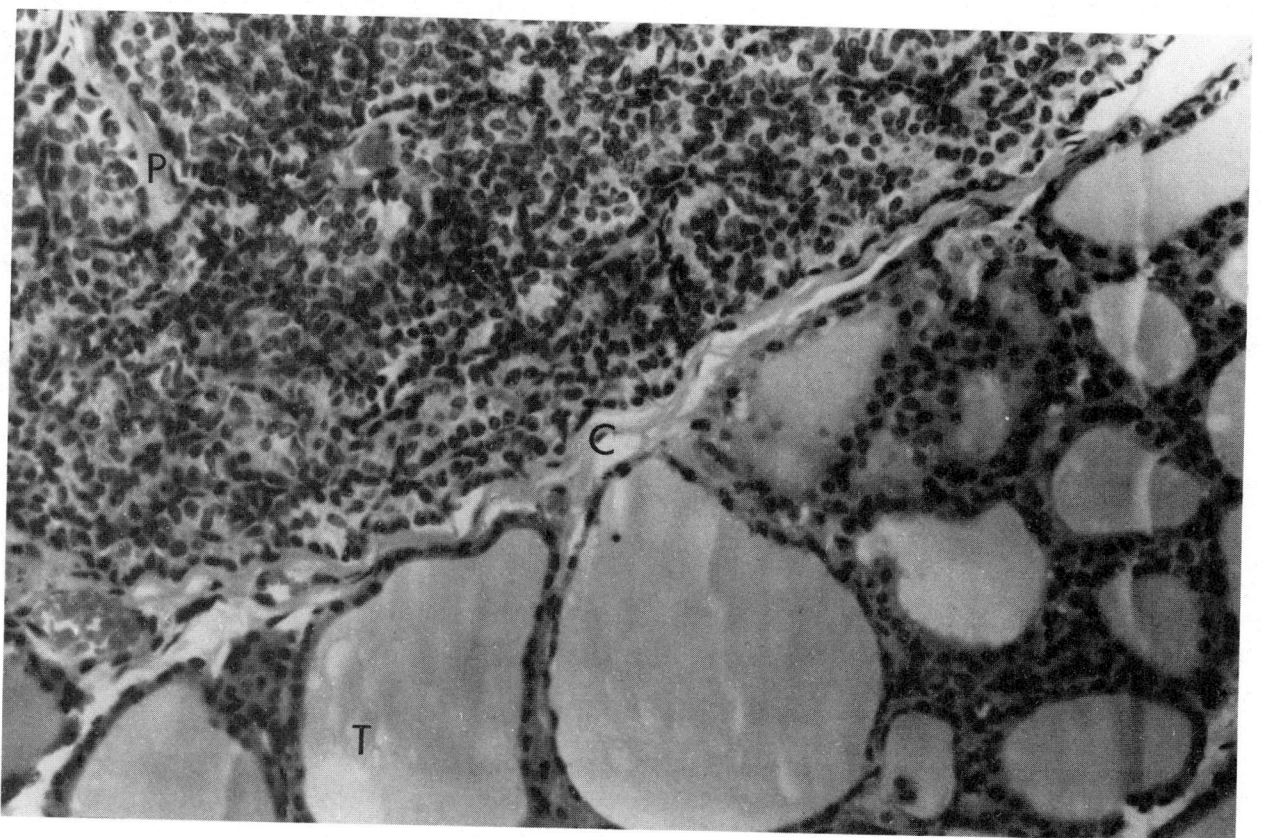

FIGURE 62-3. **Parathyroid gland** (P) **and thyroid gland** (T) **from the rat separated by capsule** (C). **(400 × .)**

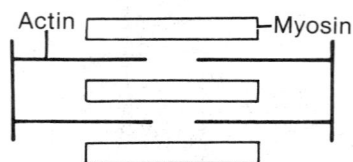

FIGURE 62-4. **Schematic of skeletal muscle showing the location of actin and myosin filaments.**

ability. Contraction of cardiac muscle is associated with an influx of calcium into the muscle cell. The force of contraction is correlated with the extracellular concentration of calcium. The rate and magnitude of interaction between the actin and myosin of the cardiac muscle, which in turn determine the rate and magnitude of the force developed, is positively correlated with the concentration of calcium present. In addition, at low levels of extracellular calcium membrane excitation fails to elicit a contraction.

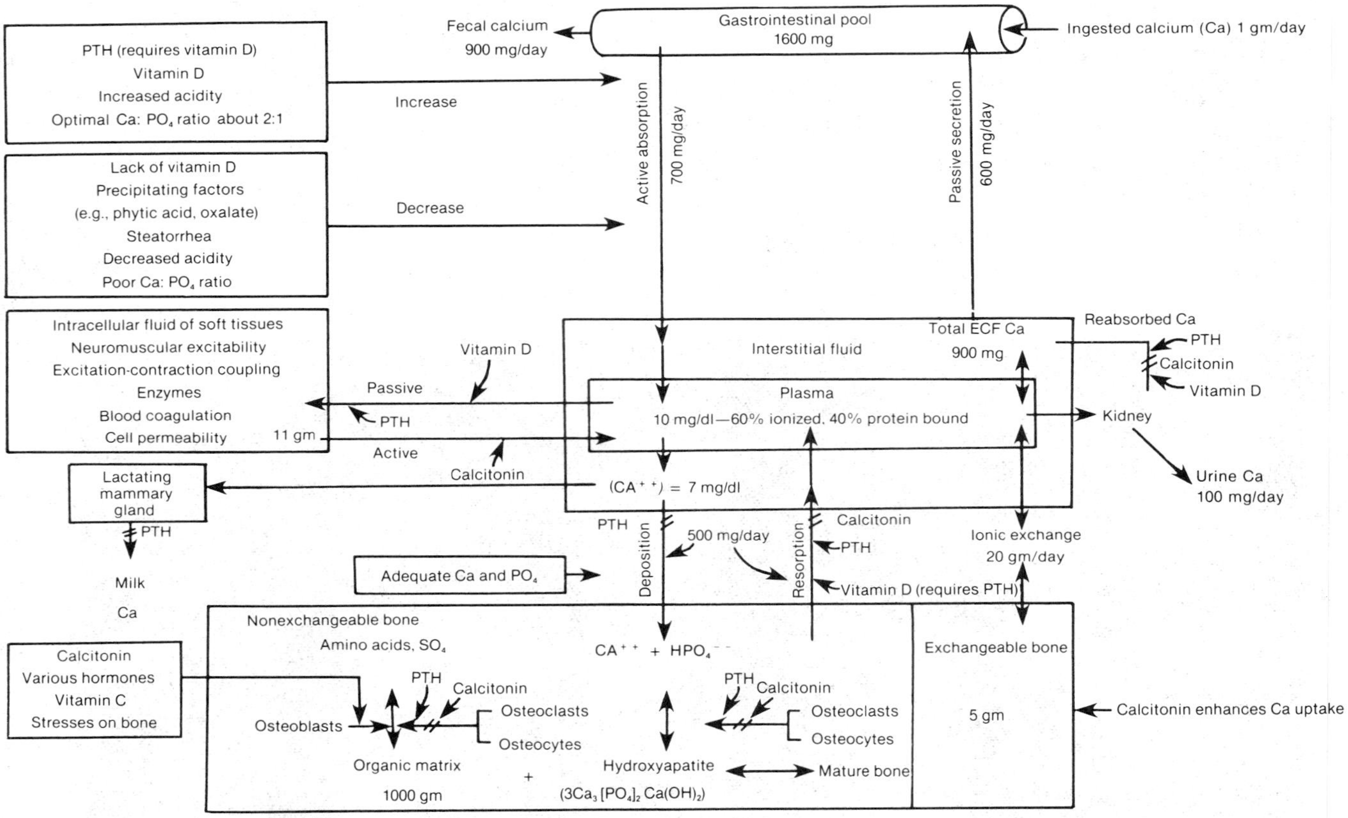

FIGURE 62-5. **Absorption, distribution, metabolism, and excretion of calcium as affected by parathyroid hormone, vitamin D, calcitonin, and various dietary factors. The numerical values inside the blocks representing the various body compartments are the total amounts or concentrations of calcium in that compartment of a 70 kg man. The values on the arrows represent the amount of calcium transferred into or out of the compartment in 1 day. The effects of parathyroid hormone (PTH), calcitonin, and vitamin D (1,25-[OH]$_2$D$_3$) are depicted either by curved arrows, which indicate an *increased effect or stimulation* of the process pointed to by the arrow, or *double wavy lines*, which interrupt the arrows going between the various compartments or biochemical processes and indicate a *decreased effect or depression* of the process. (Modified from Woodbury, D.M. Parathyroid hormone and calcitonin. In L.S. Goodman and A. Gilman [Eds.], *The pharmacological basis of therapeutics* [5th ed.]. New York: Macmillan Publishing Co., 1975).**

Ionic calcium is also essential to normal membrane permeability, nervous irritability, and CNS function. Calcium is also important in regulating hormone release. The secretion of insulin in basal as well as in stimulated states increases in direct proportion to calcium concentration.

The average adult body contains approximately 1100 gm of calcium, 99% of which is found in bone. Intake occurs by the active absorption of the ion from the gut into the extracellular fluids (i.e., plasma and interstitial fluid). The kidneys filter 5000 to 8500 mg of calcium per day. Urinary calcium levels usually range from 100 to 300 mg per day; thus 90% to 95% of the filtered calcium is reabsorbed by the renal tubules.

Calcium is also exchanged with bone. Bone, since it contains over 99% of body calcium, serves as the major reservoir in the maintenance of calcium homeostasis. Bone is constantly turning over, (i.e., continuously being resorbed and formed, which constitute the process of bone remodeling).

Calcium is also contained in the various digestive juices secreted to digest a meal. Some is lost via the feces. In the adult about 1 gm of calcium per day will keep all gains and losses in balance (Figure 62-5).

Hormonal effects

The classic descriptions of the physiologic actions of PTH were based largely on observing the results of administering massive doses of PTH or studies on overt clinical cases of hyperparathyroidism. Both approaches emphasized the view of PTH as primarily an agent of bone destruction. More recent studies indicate that the circulating levels of PTH must be about two orders of magnitude above normal levels before significant *osteolysis* occurs. To understand the role of PTH, the amount of hormone present in the circulation must be considered.

The principal function of PTH is the maintenance of calcium levels within the extracellular fluids, and thereby the prevention of *hypocalcemia.* This function is performed by PTH action on several target organs: the kidney, gut, and bone.

PTH affects the renal handling of various electrolytes. PTH increases phosphate excretion. This excretion results in phosphaturia, or phosphate loss in the urine. The reabsorption of sodium, calcium, and bicarbonate in the proximal renal tubule is reduced by PTH. Most of the sodium and calcium are reabsorbed by the distal tubule. The reabsorption of calcium by the distal renal tubule is markedly enhanced by PTH, and it is this effect that predominates. The significance of this response is not well understood. As calcium is mobilized from bone, phosphate is also liberated. The

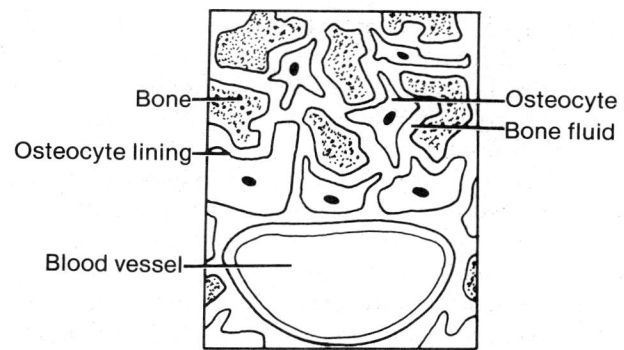

FIGURE 62-6. **Schematic of arrangement of bone cells, bone fluid-storage compartment, and osteocyte lining controlling calcium fluxes.**

phosphate excretion by the kidney removes this excess, leaving the calcium in the blood.

An increase in the circulating levels of PTH has been shown to stimulate the absorption of calcium from the gut. This effect is not the result of a direct action of PTH. The increased levels of PTH stimulate the kidneys to produce a particular metabolite of vitamin D (i.e., 1,25 dihydroxy vitamin D_3 [1,25-$(OH)_2D_3$]) from 25 hydroxy vitamin D_3 usually present in the plasma. This metabolite then stimulates the increased intestinal calcium absorption.

The best known action of PTH is the stimulation of bone resorption. This action has been divided into two components: a fast component, which depends on the activation of the existing cellular apparatus; and a slow component, which involves enzyme synthesis and cellular proliferation. This slow phase can lead to the destruction of all bone constituents, including the organic matrix.

The rapid liberation of calcium after PTH administration involves the movement of preexisting dissolved calcium. This calcium is stored in an extracellular bone fluid compartment. This calcium is in a labile form that is kept from being transformed to *hydroxyapatite* crystals by a mineralization inhibitor (Figure 62-6).

The slow component of PTH action involves complex cellular change within bone. Existing *osteoclasts* are activated within 1½ hours after PTH administration. At 15 to 20 hours increased proliferation of the preosteoclast population of bone is observed. The number of osteoclasts then increases, and the rate of bone resorption is accelerated.

PTH has another effect on bone that is controversial. This effect is the promotion of bone formation. This *anabolic effect* is thought to be a direct cellular response. Two actions of PTH, those of increasing calcium absorption and of retention by the body, are capable of providing the extra mineral required for increasing bone formation. It has been demonstrated that the continuous administration of small doses of PTH cause a hypercalcemia independent of a significant increase in bone resorption. These small doses of PTH seem to stimulate an increase in the number of active *osteoblasts*, together with increased maturation of cartilage and osteoid formation. The effects of these minute continuous doses of PTH tend to support the view that the constant presence of low circulating levels of PTH promote bone formation. High blood concentrations of PTH elicit the *catabolic response*. The catabolic effects may be viewed as an emergency response to a hypocalcemic challenge to the body, whereas the anabolic effects, a long-term maintenance of the bone.

Disorders

Pathologic conditions may occur within any endocrine system. These conditions may in part be characterized by either an oversecretion or undersecretion of a hormone.

Hyperparathyroidism is a condition characterized by abnormally increased activity (i.e., secretion) of the PT glands. This increase often results from tumor formation. The increased levels of PTH favor the catabolic effects of PTH, resulting in the loss of calcium from the bones. Pain and tenderness in the bones may also be present. Spontaneous fractures, especially in the mandible, caused by the weakened condition of the bones and muscular weakness caused by the high circulating levels of calcium are experienced. In addition, abdominal cramps, osteitis fibrosa cystica, excess fibrous tissue and cyst formation in the bone, and hypercalcemia are other symptoms of this condition.

Primary hyperparathyroidism is observed most commonly between the third and sixth decades, but is seen occasionally in both young children and the elderly. The reported incidence of the condition is two to three times higher in women than men. The true incidence, however, is difficult to estimate because many hyperparathyroid patients are asymptomatic. When these patients are diagnosed, the usual treatment is removal of the affected PT gland.

Secondary hyperparathyroidism is defined as hypertrophy of the PT glands and a consequent excessive secretion of PTH. Unlike primary hyperparathyroidism, no tumor is involved; instead the biologic actions of PTH are resisted in the bone, kidney, and intestine. This resistance prevents the body from mobilizing calcium stores when needed; consequently, the condition is marked by hypocalcemia. The glands hypertrophy in response to the body's need for calcium. The pathogenesis of the condition results from progressive renal disease. The kidney fails to excrete phosphate normally. The resulting increase in plasma phosphate levels (i.e., hyperphosphatemia) causes hypocalcemia. The hyperphosphatemia also inhibits the enzymatic conversion of 25-hydroxycholecalciferol, a relatively inactive metabolite of vitamin D normally in the blood, to 1, 25-dihydroxycholecalciferol, the most biologically active form of vitamin D. The result of these renal insufficiencies is secondary hyperparathyroidism.

Several conditions have been described that result from too little PTH. Hypoparathyroidism may be divided into three categories: surgical and idiopathic hypoparathyroidism and pseudohypoparathyroidism.

Surgical hypoparathyroidism is the most common variety. The increased usage of radiopharmaceuticals, especially the radioactive isotope ^{131}I, in the treatment of hyperthyroidism has reduced the number of thyroid operations. This decrease has reduced the number of centers with surgical expertise in thyroid surgery. The need for thyroid surgery for other conditions is still high; however, because of the reduced centers of expertise, the possibility of trauma or damage to the PT glands during thyroid surgery has increased. In addition, because of the intimate anatomic connection between the thyroid and PT glands, the ^{131}I used for hyperthyroidism may cause irradiation damage to the PT glands. This damage is usually transient, but it may be permanent.

Idiopathic hypoparathyroidism is the result of disease or damage to the PT glands. Many of these conditions are congenital. Isolated persistent neonatal hypoparathyroidism is caused by a congenital absence of the PT glands. Branchial dysembryogenesis is also caused by a congenital absence of the PT glands; however, the thymus is also absent. As a result the patient is at risk to repeated severe infections from depressed cell mediated immunity.

Pseudohypoparathyroidism is a rare genetic disorder that appears similar to hypoparathyroidism, in which the target organs do not respond to PTH, despite adequate concentrations of the hormone in the blood. In fact, pseudohypoparathyroidism is characterized by excessive secretion of PTH and hyperplasia of the glands, a response to the resistance to hormone action at the target tissues.

In all varieties of hypoparathyroidism hypocalcemia and its associated symptoms are encountered clinically. The earliest prodromal symptom of hypocalcemia is paresthesia in the extremities. Tetany, consisting of muscle spasm, especially carpopedal spasm and laryngospasm, follows. Eventually generalized convulsions and other CNS manifestations occur. Smooth muscle may also be affected. Hypocalcemia may be followed by spasm of the iris, ciliary muscle, intestine, esophagus, urinary bladder, and bronchi. Hypocalcemia causes changes in the normal electrocardiogram. Prolongation of the QT interval occurs because of prolongation of the ST segment without distortion of the T wave. A long flat ST segment is followed by a T wave of normal amplitude and duration. Tachycardia may also be observed. In chronic hypoparathyroidism ectodermal changes, consisting of hair loss, grooved and brittle fingernails, defects in the dental enamel and tooth root formation, and cataracts, are encountered. Psychiatric symptoms such as emotional lability, anxiety, depression, and delusions are often present.

Hypoparathyroidism is treated primarily with vitamin D with or without supplemental calcium. The vitamin D will elevate circulating calcium levels by several mechanisms discussed later. The oral calcium supplement further helps raise plasma calcium levels. Hypoparathyroidism was previously treated with commercially available parathyroid hormone (i.e., Para-Thor-Mone, Paroidin); however, parathyroid hormone is no longer available commercially or used for this purpose in North America.

CALCITONIN

Calcitonin is a polypeptide hormone synthesized and secreted by cells located in the thyroid gland. These cells are nonfollicular, located between the follicles and not a part of them (Figure 62-7). They have a different embryologic origin than the follicular cells of the thyroid. The calcitonin-secreting cells are referred to as parafollicular cells, C cells, light cells, or argyrophilic cells. The C cells are derived embryologically from the last two pharyngeal pouches of the primitive foregut and are of neural crest origin. The cells metabolize amine precursors through both up-

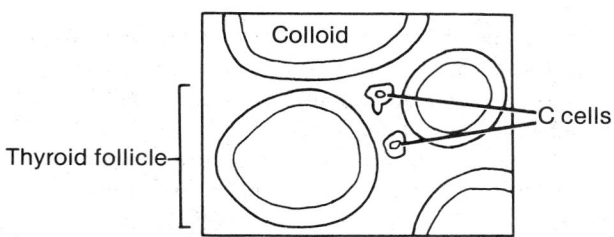

FIGURE 62-7. **Schematic of calcitonin-secreting cells.**

take and decarboxylation. In nonmammalian species the C cells are contained in a distinct organ, the ultimobranchial body. In mammals the C cells are distributed throughout the thyroid.

Radioimmunoassay, immunofluorescence, and immunoperoxidase techniques show calcitonin-like immunoreactivity in the pituitary gland, cerebrospinal fluid, lung, thymus, gut (especially the jejunum), urinary bladder, and the liver. In the CNS the areas with the highest calcitonin or calcitonin-like concentrations are the posterior hypothalamus, the median eminence, and the pituitary gland. Lesser amounts are observed in the substantia nigra, the anterior hypothalamus, the globus pallidus, and the inferior colliculus. The techniques demonstrating the presence of a calcitonin-like material do not prove that the material located is identical to thyroidal calcitonin—only that a similar molecule has been located.

Like PTH, calcitonin has been shown to be continuously present in normal blood. The concentration levels are low, between 5 to 100 pg/ml. As more sensitive techniques are developed, the circulating levels will be determined to a narrower range.

Calcitonin has been termed a hypocalcemic hormone. Injection of large doses of calcitonin into rats produces a dramatic lowering, 20% to 50%, of the plasma calcium levels. This decrease reaches its maximum effect in ½ to 3 hours. Calcitonin produces a similar hypocalcemic effect in all mammals tested.

High plasma calcium levels directly stimulate the secretion of calcitonin. This increase is proportional to the increase in calcium levels. Recent evidence also indicates other factors may stimulate calcitonin secretion. Several gastrointestinal hormones—gastrin, pancreozymin, and glucagon—increase the liberation of calcitonin.

The rapid hypocalcemic response stimulated is caused by a rapid inhibition on osteolysis. Calcitonin almost completely inhibits the actions of osteoclasts. Loss of the reabsorbing surfaces of osteoclasts may occur as early as 15 minutes, after administration and this is quantitatively important by 1 hour. In the long term calcitonin may reduce the number of osteoclasts present in bone. Calcitonin may decrease calcium efflux from the pool of labile bone calcium by lowering cytosolic calcium concentrations in bone cells. The result is an inhibition of bone resorption. Associated with the decrease in osteoclasts is a shift in the cell population to an increase in the number of osteoblasts on calcitonin administration. Calcitonin can also reverse PTH stimulated osteolysis and the associated calcium release.

Calcitonin's action on bone is age dependent. Young

animals, having a high turnover of bone, are more sensitive to calcitonin levels than the adult, in whom the skeletal turnover is lower. In both sexes a progressive decrease in plasma calcitonin is also seen with age.

The principal target organ of calcitonin is bone, but it has other target organs such as the kidney. Calcitonin decreases renal tubular absorption of calcium, phosphate, potassium, magnesium, and sodium, which leads to natriuresis. Calcitonin has not been shown to have any effect on the intestinal absorption of calcium.

The role of calcitonin in the normal functioning of the body is not clearly defined. Because calcitonin inhibits calcium loss from the skeleton, it may protect the skeleton from loss of calcium during periods of calcium stress such as pregnancy and lactation or prolonged calcium deprivation. Circulating levels of calcitonin increase in pregnant and lactating women. In addition, calcitonin may control hypercalcemia after a meal, especially in young animals fed a high-calcium diet, such as milk. Since hormones released in response to the ingestion of a meal stimulate calcitonin secretion, especially gastrin, an increase in circulating calcitonin may anticipate an elevation in plasma calcium levels. The calcitonin released stimulates the rapid storage of absorbed calcium in bone fluid in a readily available form. This calcium is then gradually returned to the extracellular fluid after the digestion and absorption of the meal have ceased and calcitonin levels fallen to resting levels (Figure 62-5). This process decreases *postprandial* calcium loss in the urine and supplies calcium to maintain plasma concentrations during fasting periods. In addition, this slow release of calcium reduces the need for PTH secretion to maintain the fasting calcium levels and thereby minimizes the need for bone resorption.

Recent experiments have shown that calcitonin has effects on tissues other than bone. Administration of calcitonin either subcutaneously, intracerebroventricularly, or parenterally has been shown to reduce feeding in humans, monkeys, and rats. This reduction in feeding may last from 24 hours to 5 days, depending on the dose given. It has been suggested that calcitonin acts as a hormone mediator of the satiety reflex. Calcium ions play an important role in neuronal excitability, neurotransmission, and cerebral function. Calcitonin is known to alter CNS function. Calcitonin could thus exert its influence either through its effects on calcium metabolism or by a direct action on the central nervous system as a neurotransmitter.

Calcitonin has another effect, that of analgesia in humans. This effect was observed when calcitonin was administered either into the cerebrospinal fluid or intravenously. This analgesic effect is similar to that of morphine, but does not involve opiate receptors (i.e., it is not reversed by naloxone). The effect does not exhibit tolerance and probably involves a direct receptor activation. The effect is also independent of endorphin. The analgesic action started within 5 minutes, but reached full effect in 15 minutes. The amelioration of pain lasted 48 hours in some patients and as much as 5 days for others. The mechanism of action is not fully understood.

Therapeutically calcitonin is effective in diminishing hypercalcemia and decreasing plasma phosphate concentrations in patients with hyperparathyroidism, idiopathic hypercalcemia of infancy, vitamin D intoxication, and osteolytic bone metastases. However, long-term use of calcitonin is not recommended because immunologic sensitivity occurs.

Calcitonin has proved to be effective in diseases characterized by increasing skeletal remodeling, bone resorption, and bone formation, such as occurs in Paget's disease. Calcitonin given on a long-term basis in cases of Paget's disease produces symptomatic relief and reduction in alkaline phosphatase activity, urinary hydroxyproline, increased blood flow through the affected area, and a decrease in the osteoclastic population and activity. Calcitonin alone or with oral phosphate is the treatment of choice for Paget's disease.

Medullary carcinoma of the thyroid differs from other thyroid carcinomas because this tumor is derived from the parafollicular, or C, cells. The most important distinguishing characteristic of this carcinoma is that an increased production of calcitonin occurs. Circulating levels of 12,000 to 275,000 pmol/L are observed. The amount of calcitonin in the tumor is correlated to the concentration of calcitonin in the serum. The serum calcitonin level provides an estimate of the severity of the condition as well as the efficacy of a given treatment.

About 30% of patients with medullary carcinoma have diarrhea. The diarrhea is correlated to the secretion of one or more substances in the tumor tissue; thus the diarrhea is also considered dependent on the amount of tumor tissue.

Nonthyroidal tumors have been shown to involve an increase in calcitonin secretion. Both breast and pulmonary carcinomas may be accompanied by such an increase. The calcitonin levels are much lower, 300 to 3000 pmol/L, than in cases of medullary carcinoma of the thyroid. High serum calcitonin levels, 16,000 pmol/L, in patients with small-cell anaplastic pulmonary carcinoma have been reported.

The treatment of choice for medullary carcinoma

of the thyroid is a total thyroidectomy to eliminate all foci of tumor cells. These foci are often situated in both lobes of the thyroid.

Alternative treatments include high-voltage irradiation and chemotherapy. Neither of these measures has been shown to have consistently successful results.

Calcitonin deficiency, from either thyroid agenesis or surgical removal, seems to have little effect on calcium homeostasis. The organism adapts to the absence of calcitonin. No evidence exists that the extrathyroidal calcitonin-like substances assume the calcium-regulating function.

VITAMIN D

The natural form of vitamin D was first isolated in 1937. The deficiency state, rickets in children or osteomalacia in adults, has been known and described since 1645. Although the disease has been plaguing the human race for 300 years, rickets was not associated with a nutritional deficiency until 1919. Great strides in the knowledge of the actions and synthesis of vitamin D have been made since its isolation.

If humans receive sufficient exposure to ultraviolet light, they do not require dietary sources of vitamin D. However, in the colder temperature zones, particularly considering modern living habits, the skin has limited exposure to ultraviolet light. This situation leads to a reduction in the ability to synthesize vitamin D. Thus in the winter months people depend on dietary sources of vitamin D.

The skin is able to synthesize 7-dehydrocholesterol, a precursor of vitamin D. This compound is found in the epidermis, a site to which ultraviolet light can penetrate easily. When exposed to ultraviolet light of 280 to 320 nm, 7-dehydrocholesterol will undergo photolysis and form a substance known as previtamin D_3. Previtamin D_3 undergoes a spontaneous conversion to vitamin D_3, or cholecalciferol.

Vitamin D is not widely distributed. Dietary sources are primarily restricted to the livers of certain fish, sharks, and other marine animals. Vitamin D is not found to a significant extent in vegetable matter.

Dietary vitamin D, either in its natural state or as a food supplement (a plant sterol called ergosterol, which is converted by ultraviolet light to vitamin D_2 or ergocalciferol), is absorbed from the upper end of the small intestine. Bile salts are required; thus vitamin D is absorbed in a manner similar to all lipids. Vitamin D enters the lymphatic system and the bloodstream at the level of the thoracic duct. Vitamin D is stored in the liver and in the adipose tissue of the body. The plasma half-life of the vitamin is short, only a few

hours; however, in the tissues its life span may be a period of months.

It is now known that dietary vitamin D_3 must first be metabolically activated before it can perform its hormonal function on its target tissues, intestines and skeleton. The major form of vitamin D_3 present in the blood is 25-hydroxycholecalciferol (25-OHD$_3$). The vitamin undergoes enzymatic hydroxylation within the liver. This metabolite (25-OHD$_3$) does not act directly on target tissues when present at physiologic concentrations (e.g., 5×10^{-8}m). It must be further hydroxylated in the kidney to 1,25 dihydroxycholecalciferol [1,25-(OH)$_2$D$_3$], the biologically active form of the vitamin. The probable site for this conversion is in the proximal convoluted tubules of the kidney. The renal synthesis of 1,25-(OH)$_2$D$_3$ is regulated by a feedback mechanism that involves serum calcium and phosphate, PTH, and vitamin D itself.

The main action of vitamin D is to aid in the absorption of ingested calcium from the gastrointestinal tract. By increasing the circulatory levels of calcium vitamin D ensures that adequate amounts of the essential elements for bone formation are present. Furthermore, as plasma calcium levels fall, this decrease is detected by the PT glands, which then secrete PTH. PTH, in turn, stimulates 1,25-(OH)$_2$D$_3$ synthesis in the kidney. The actions of 1,25-(OH)$_2$D$_3$ promote calcium absorption in the gastrointestinal tract and mobilize calcium from bone to raise the plasma calcium concentration. The increase in plasma calcium inhibits parathyroid secretion to complete the feedback loop.

The mechanism by which 1,25-(OH)$_2$D$_3$ increases calcium absorption from the gut utilizes a vitamin D–dependent calcium-binding protein. The intestinal production of this protein is inversely proportional to the circulating calcium levels. The protein is secreted into the intestinal lumen to become associated with the mucus layer lining the gut. The protein readily binds free calcium (four calcium ions per molecule). The complex associates with the microvillar brush border of the absorptive cell. The calcium enters the cell and the serosa via passive diffusion or facilitated diffusion.

Vitamin D has two important physiologic functions. It is required for normal mineralization of bone, and it plays an essential role in the homeostatic regulation of plasma calcium concentration.

Neither vitamin D nor any of its metabolites have been shown to have any direct effect on the mineralization of bone. The primary way by which vitamin D promotes normal mineralization of bone is by providing adequate supplies of calcium and phosphate to bone by means of its action to stimulate intestinal absorption of calcium and phosphate. The hypercalcemic effect of vitamin D requires the presence of PTH unless extremely high doses of $1,25-(OH)_2D_3$ are given. The source of this calcium is old bone; thus, the calcium and phosphate contribution to the plasma pool may participate in mineralization sites of new bone formation. This ability to increase plasma calcium serves to maintain plasma calcium at levels required for normal neuromuscular and other functions.

SUMMARY

The various drugs involved in the hormonal regulation of calcium, including parathyroid hormone, calcitonin, and other miscellaneous agents, are discussed. With an understanding of the indications for these medications as well as their action, adverse effects, and administration, the nurse will be better able to assist patients with their individual drug therapy regimens and to prevent untoward effects.

ADVERSE/SIDE EFFECTS OF CALCITONIN AND RELATED MEDICATIONS*

Calcitonin

CENTRAL NERVOUS SYSTEM

Headache
Tingling of hands
Unpleasant taste sensation (metallic)

GASTROINTESTINAL SYSTEM

Diarrhea
Transient nausea, with or without vomiting (especially when treatment is first initiated; tends to decrease or disappear with continued administration)

HEMATOLOGIC SYSTEM

Hypocalcemia

RENAL SYSTEM

Transient diuresis

MISCELLANEOUS EFFECTS

Facial flushing
Inflammation at injection site

Vitamin D

ALLERGIC REACTIONS

Sensitivity to toxic effects

CENTRAL NERVOUS SYSTEM

Anorexia
Convulsions
Extreme thirst
Headache
Mental retardation
Vague aches and stiffness
Vertigo

GASTROINTESTINAL SYSTEM

Constipation
Diarrhea
Nausea
Polydipsia
Vomiting
Weight loss

HEMATOLOGIC SYSTEM

Anemia
Hypercalcemia
Hypervitaminosis D
Mild acidosis

RENAL SYSTEM

Albuminuria
Decreased renal function
Hypertension
Irreversible renal insufficiency
Nephrocalcinosis
Nocturia
Polyuria
Reversible azotemia
Urinary casts

SKELETAL SYSTEM

Decline in rate of linear growth in infants and children
Osteoporosis (adults)

MISCELLANEOUS EFFECTS

Lassitude
Widespread calcification of soft tissues, including heart, blood vessels, renal tubules, and lungs

Calcitriol

CARDIOVASCULAR SYSTEM

Cardiac dysrhythmias

CENTRAL NERVOUS SYSTEM

Headache
Hyperthermia
Somnolence

GASTROINTESTINAL SYSTEM

Anorexia
Constipation
Dry mouth
Nausea
Polydipsia
Vomiting

HEMATOLOGIC SYSTEM

Hypercalcemia

MUSCULOSKELETAL SYSTEM

Bone and muscle pain
Weakness

RENAL SYSTEM

Polyuria

MISCELLANEOUS EFFECTS

Conjunctivitis
Photophobia
Rhinorrhea

*See Chapter 11, "Drug Toxicity," for an overview of drug toxicity.

ADVERSE/SIDE EFFECTS OF CALCITONIN AND RELATED MEDICATIONS—cont'd

Dihydrotachysterol

CENTRAL NERVOUS SYSTEM

Headache
Languor
Somnolence
Tinnitus
Vertigo

GASTROINTESTINAL SYSTEM

Anorexia
Diarrhea

Nausea
Vomiting

HEMATOLOGIC SYSTEM

Hypercalcemia

SKELETAL SYSTEM

Osteoporosis

Etidronate disodium

GASTROINTESTINAL SYSTEM

Diarrhea
Nausea

HEMATOLOGIC SYSTEM

Elevated serum phosphate

SKELETAL SYSTEM

Recurrent bone pain at pagetic sites
Spontaneous fracture

CLINICALLY SIGNIFICANT DRUG INTERACTIONS*

Primary drug	Interacting drug	Possible effect(s)	Probable mechanism(s)
Calcitriol	Cholestyramine	Decreased effect of calcitriol	Decreased absorption of calcitriol
Dihydrotachysterol	Thiazide diuretics	Hypercalcemia	Additive effect
Vitamin D	Mineral oil	Decreased effect of vitamin D	Decreased absorption of vitamin D
Vitamin D	Rifampin	Decreased effect of vitamin D	Increased metabolism of vitamin D
Vitamin D	Thiazide diuretics	Hypercalcemia	Additive effect

NOTE: No clinically significant drug interactions have been associated with the agents discussed in this chapter; however, potentially important interactions are noted.

*See Chapter 10, "Drug Interactions," for an overview of drug interactions.

GENERAL NURSING IMPLICATIONS

Nursing of patients requiring calcitonin and related medications

ASSESSMENT

Patients requiring calcitonin or vitamin D should have a thorough history and physical examination, including laboratory evaluation of blood and urine and roentgenogram or histologic studies. The nursing assessment should include assessment of general health state. A detailed nutritional assessment should be completed, including caffeine intake and special attention to the daily intake of dairy products and high-protein foods such as meat. It is important to note sociocultural aspects associated with diet as well as seasonal variation.

A thorough musculoskeletal assessment is indicated. For example, complaints of aches and pain in the bones, including the vertebrae and ends of long bones, should be identified. Kyphosis in the elderly and loss of height should be noted. Children should have their heights and weights plotted on growth curves. The patient's exercise and activity pattern should also be assessed.

Although laboratory evaluation of blood and urine can confirm hypocalcemia or hypercalcemia, patient manifestations of these conditions should be noted.

Serum phosphorus, alkaline phosphatase, and 24 hour urinary calcium and phosphorus levels are also indicated as well as an electrocardiogram.

Baseline assessment should include specific data related to the patient's presenting condition (e.g., rickets in children, osteomalacia in adults, history of thyroid disease or thyroidectomy) as well as a detailed drug history to identify possible sensitivity, contraindications, cautions, potential drug interactions, and drug-taking patterns before drug therapy with calcitonin or vitamin D is initiated.

Continued.

GENERAL NURSING IMPLICATIONS—cont'd

Nursing of patients requiring calcitonin and related medications—cont'd

SENSITIVITY

Generally, allergic reactions to calcitonin or vitamin D are rare; however, any drug has the potential to cause a hypersensitivity reaction in susceptible individuals.

Calcitonin

Skin tests should be performed before use of calcitonin to check for sensitization.

Because of the protein nature of this hormone, an anaphylactic reaction is possible, and epinephrine should be available when calcitonin is administered.

Vitamin D

Hypersensitivity may be an etiologic factor in infants with idiopathic hypercalcemia. In these patients vitamin D must be severely restricted.

CONTRAINDICATIONS

The use of calcitonin and the miscellaneous agents is contraindicated in patients with a known history of hypersensitivity. In addition, the following should be noted.

Calcitonin

Calcitonin is contraindicated in patients hypersensitive to vitamin D.

Calcitriol

Because calcitriol elevates blood calcium, it is contraindicated in hypercalcemia or vitamin D toxicity. *No* forms of vitamin D should be given to patients taking calcitriol. Calcitriol is not recommended for lactating mothers.

Vitamin D

Vitamin D is contraindicated in hypercalcemia or vitamin D toxicity.

Dihydrotachysterol

Because dihydrotachysterol elevates plasma calcium levels by mobilizing renal reabsorption of calcium, it is contraindicated in hypercalcemia, hypo-calcemia associated with renal insufficiency and hyperphosphatemia, renal stones, hypersensitivity to vitamin D, or in lactating mothers.

See the Nursing Drug Digest for contraindications to specific agents.

CAUTIONS

Calcitonin

Because calcitonin decreases plasma calcium levels, avoid use in women who are or may become pregnant or during lactation. Safe use in children has not been established.

Calcitriol

Since calcitriol elevates blood calcium, use cautiously in patients on digitalis; hypercalcemia may precipitate cardiac dysrhythmias.

Because of calcitriol's narrow therapeutic index, monitor serum calcium, magnesium, phosphorus, alkaline phosphate, as well as urinary calcium and phosphorus levels.

Vitamin D

Use vitamin D cautiously in patients taking digitalis because hypercalcemia may trigger cardiac dysrhythmias.

Avoid use of excess vitamin D during pregnancy.

Be alert that many nonprescription vitamin preparations contain vitamin D, and use of these preparations concurrently may cause vitamin D toxicity.

Etidronate disodium

Do not use in pregnant women unless use is clearly indicated.

Use cautiously in patients with enterocolitis or impaired renal function; frequent bowel movements and diarrhea may occur.

Restrict therapy to not more than 6 months. Do not give longer than 3 months at doses above 10 mg/kg of body weight/day.

DRUG INTERACTIONS

Calcitonin and vitamin D as well as other miscellaneous agents discussed in this chapter are not generally involved in clinically significant drug interactions. See Cautions as well as Clinically Significant Drug Interactions for a list of potential drug interactions.

ADMINISTRATION
Calcitonin

Usually calcitonin is administered subcutaneously or intramuscularly.

Once prepared, the solution should be refrigerated.

Hypocalcemic tetany is possible; be prepared to give parenteral calcium during the first several administrations.

Facial flushing and warmth occur in 20% to 30% of all patients within minutes of injection; usually this condition lasts 1 hour. Reassure patient of the transient nature of this effect.

Calcitriol

Administer orally with a full glass of water. Keep patient strictly on regulated diet and calcium supplement. Individualized teaching and support are important in helping patient maintain drug and diet regimen.

Store drug protected from heat and light.

Vitamin D

Vitamin D is available in various dosage forms for oral use, including capsules and drops. Administer capsules with a full glass of milk. Administer drops in milk, ensuring that the total amount of medication is taken.

Vitamin D is usually administered on a once-a-day or alternate-day dosing schedule. Dosage is highly individualized.

Monitor serum calcium at least weekly during initial period of dosage adjustment.

GENERAL NURSING IMPLICATIONS—cont'd

Nursing of patients requiring calcitonin and related medications—cont'd

Vitamin D—cont'd

Readjust therapeutic dosage as soon as clinical improvement occurs.

When high therapeutic dosages are used, follow progress with frequent serum and urinary calcium levels (Sulkowitch test) and potassium and urea determinations.

In the treatment of hypoparathyroidism calcium or dihydrotachysterol may be required. Mineral oil interferes with absorption of fat-soluble vitamins.

Dihydrotachysterol

Because dihydrotachysterol elevates plasma calcium levels by mobilizing renal reabsorption of calcium, supplementary oral calcium may be required.

Avoid use of thiazide drugs with hypoparathyroid patients because they may cause hypercalcemia.

Etidronate disodium

Tablets are administered as a once-daily dose 2 hours before eating. Do not administer drug with food, milk, or antacids because this could reduce absorption.

Treatment should not exceed 6 months. With doses of greater than 10 mg/kg/day treatment should not exceed 3 months. Doses greater than 20 mg/kg/day are not recommended (see the Nursing Drug Digest for dosing schedules).

MONITORING PATIENT RESPONSE
Therapeutic response
Calcitonin

Because calcitonin decreases plasma calcium levels, rapidly reaching a plateau in a few hours, monitor response by the following.

Evaluate drug effect by periodic serum alkaline phosphatase and 24-hour urinary hydroxyproline levels.

Monitor radiologic and histologic bone changes toward normal.

Monitor patients for relief of bone pain, lowered skin temperature over involved bone, decreased excessive cardiac output, and stabilized hearing if it had been affected.

Calcitriol

Because calcitriol elevates blood calcium, monitor serum calcium level twice weekly; serum calcium level times serum phosphate level should not exceed 70.

Vitamin D

Monitor serum calcium at least weekly during the initial period of dosage adjustment.

Dihydrotachysterol

Dihydrotachysterol elevates plasma calcium levels by mobilizing renal reabsorption of calcium.

Etidronate disodium

Monitor for lowering of serum calcium levels.

Monitor renal function before and during therapy.

Monitor drug effect by serum alkaline phosphatase and urinary hydroxyproline levels because both decrease if the drug is effective.

In the treatment of Paget's disease monitor for decreased bone pain, normal cardiac output (if cardiac output had been abnormally elevated), decreased temperature over superficially located pagetic lesions, and decreased vascularity of bone.

Improvement may not be noted for up to 3 months, and effect can continue for months after the drug is discontinued.

Adverse side effects
Calcitonin

Monitor serum calcium levels closely. Watch for signs of hypercalcemic relapse: bone pain, renal calculi, polyuria, anorexia, nausea, vomiting, thirst, con-

stipation, lethargy, bradycardia, muscle hypotonicity, pathologic fracture, psychosis, and coma.

Periodic examination for urine sediment is recommended.

Calcitriol

Monitor for vitamin D excess and hypercalcemia.

Dihydrotachysterol

Monitor serum and urinary calcium levels; report hypercalcemia immediately.

Etidronate disodium

Monitor for bone pain and possible fractures.

Observe for diarrhea.

Increased dosage theoretically can cause hypocalcemia.

Drug should be discontinued in presence of pathologic fracture.

PATIENT EDUCATION

The patient and family should be fully informed about the nature of the patient's condition and treatment plan and should be involved in health care planning. The patient and family should have a clear understanding of the anticipated course of therapy and medication regimen, including the exact name of the medication, its general action, purpose, dosage, storage, administration, and adverse side effects. They should know how to monitor therapeutic response, prevent common adverse effects, and identify signs that indicate that the health care provider should be notified. Because of the association of diet to the treatment of many conditions requiring these medications, special attention should be given to teaching healthy nutritional practices.

GENERAL INSTRUCTIONS FOR DISCHARGE/OUTPATIENTS

CALCITONIN AND RELATED MEDICATIONS

This medication is used to help maintain normal calcium levels in the body. If you do not understand why you require this medication, check with your health care provider.

Take this medication exactly as prescribed and try not to miss any doses. If you have any questions about how this medication should be taken, check with your health care provider.

This medication can sometimes cause unwanted effects in unborn babies or nursing infants. Notify your health care provider if you are pregnant, considering pregnancy, or are breastfeeding an infant before taking this medication.

If you have been placed on a special calcium diet, follow it closely and check with your health care provider if you have any questions.

This medication has been prescribed especially for you. Do *not* trade or give this medication to any relatives or friends.

Store this medication in a dry, dark place. Refrigeration is not necessary.

Keep this and all medications out of children's reach.

In addition to the general instructions, following is specific information about your medication.

Calcitonin

Follow a well-balanced diet as directed, especially in relation to dairy products and calcium supplements. If you have any questions about your diet or if you have any difficulty following it or taking your calcium supplements, notify your health care provider.

Do not take your medication with any antacids containing magnesium or use mineral oil while taking this medication. These drugs can affect the amount of calcitonin absorbed.

Calcitriol

Calcitriol is a type of vitamin D used to help maintain normal calcium levels in the body.

If you are allergic to vitamin D, do *not* take this medication. Notify your health care provider immediately.

Take this medicine as directed with a full glass of water at the same time every day. Do *not* take extra medication because a danger exists that you can get too much vitamin D. Because of this danger, it is important that you do *not* take any other vitamin products that contain vitamin D unless directed to do so by your health care provider.

Notify your health care provider if you notice any of the following: anorexia, constipation or diarrhea, dry mouth, excessive thirst, headache, irregular heartbeat, muscle or bone pain, nausea or vomiting, metallic taste in the mouth, unusual weakness, or vague aches or stiffness.

Etidronate disodium

Take tablets once a day as directed at least 2 hours before eating. Food, especially food high in calcium, should *not* be eaten for 2 hours after taking this drug because its absorption can be reduced.

Maintain a well-balanced diet, and pay special attention to your calcium and vitamin D intake.

If your diet is restricted in calcium and vitamin D, you may be sensitive to drugs affecting calcium balance and should be carefully monitored by your health care provider while taking this medication. Follow-up with your health care provider is important. Keep appointments and notify your health care provider if you have any questions about your care.

Improvement may not occur for up to 3 months but may continue for months after the drug is stopped.

Calcium supplements

If you must take a calcium supplement to maintain calcium levels in your body, remember the following.

Take tablets and capsules 1 hour to 1½ hours after a meal with a full glass of water.

Dissolve effervescent tablets in a glass of water and drink completely after they have dissolved.

Do not eat unusually large amounts of bran, whole-grain cereals, milk, or dairy products while you are taking this medicine because this practice can cause constipation.

Notify your health care provider if you notice troublesome diarrhea or constipation.

NURSING DRUG DIGEST

Medication (trade name*)	Indication	Usual dosage and administration	Dosage forms, preparation, and storage	Contraindications, cautions, and comments	Monitoring
Calcitonin, salmon Calcimar	Paget's disease of bone Hypercalcemia	*Adults:* 100 IU/day SC or IM; maintenance: 50-100 IU/day or every other day *Adults:* 100-400 IU SC or IM q.d. or b.i.d. *Children:* Safe and effective dose *not* established	Injectable: 200 units/ml Sterile, lyophilized powder; 400 IU/vial with 20 mg hydrolyzed gelatin Store at 15°-30° C Solubilization in the gelatin diluent requires 2-3 min of gentle agitation; reconstituted hormone stable for 2 weeks in refrigerator	*Contraindicated* in hypersensitivity Overdose symptoms include anorexia, vomiting, constipation, muscular weakness, bradycardia, and psychosis Hypersensitivity may occur because of protein nature of the hormone Salmon calcitonin is considerably more potent in humans than porcine or human calcitonins, presumably because of its slower circulatory clearance Have epinephrine ready to treat severe hypersensitivity reactions	Monitor renal function Monitor calcium levels Check for hypersensitivity (skin test) before administration
Calcitriol Rocaltrol	Hypocalcemia in patients undergoing chronic dialysis	*Adults:* initially 0.25 µg daily; dosage may be increased by 0.25 µg/day at 2-4 week intervals Maintenance: 0.25 µg on alternate days up to 0.5-1.25 µg/day	Capsules: 0.25, 0.5 µg	*Contraindicated* in hypercalcemia Calcium intake must be adequate (1 gm daily)	Measure serum calcium levels b.i.d. during dosage titration
Dihydrotachysterol AT 10 DHT Hytakerol Tachystin	Hypocalcemia associated with hypoparathyroidism and in pseudohypoparathyroidism	*Adults:* Initial—0.8-2.4 mg; maintenance—0.2-1 mg daily	Capsule: 0.125 mg Solution: 0.25 mg/ml Tablets: 0.125, 0.2, 0.4 mg Store in a dark, dry place	*Contraindicated* in hypercalcemia and hypervitaminosis D Maintain serum calcium levels at 9-10 mg/dl Dose is often supplemented with 10-15 gm of calcium gluconate daily	Monitor serum calcium levels to avoid hypercalcemia

Continued.

NOTE: For additional details regarding the individual agents listed in this table see the text and other tables in this chapter.
*Indicates a multiple active ingredient product. For a complete listing of all active ingredients see the *Drug Reference Guide to Brand Names and Active Ingredients.*

NURSING DRUG DIGEST—cont'd

Medication (trade name)	Indication	Usual dosage and administration	Dosage forms, preparation, and storage	Contraindications, cautions, and comments	Monitoring
Etidronate disodium Didronel	Paget's disease of bone	*Adults:* 5 mg/kg/day, not to exceed a period of 6 months; give oral dose 2 hr before meals with either water or fruit juice; 10 mg/kg/day may be given in severe cases for a 3 month period Maximum: 20 mg/kg/day Food reduces absorption; therefore, administer 1 hr before or 2 hr after meals *Children:* Safe and effective dose has *not* been established	Tablet: 200 mg	Improvement may take up to 3 months to occur Maintain adequate nutritional status (i.e., especially adequate intake of calcium and vitamin D)	Monitor renal function during therapy Monitor urinary hydroxyproline and serum alkaline phosphatase levels Monitor bone scans for improvement of lesions
Vitamin D (contains either cholicalciferol or ergocalciferol) Alphanettes* Andoin* Aquasol A and D* Calciferol Cal-M* Deltalin Drisdol Hyalex* Ostoforte Radiostal Scott's Emulsion* Tri-Vi-Flor 0.25 mg with Iron Drops* Tri-Vi-Flor* Tri-Vi-Sol Vitamin Drops with Iron* Tri-Vi-Sol* Vi-Daylin ADC Drops*	Refactory rickets Hypoparathyroidism See also Chapter 66, "Vitamins, Minerals, and Trace Elements"	*Adults and children:*12,000-500,000 IU daily *Adults and children:*50,000-200,000 IU daily plus 4 gm calcium lactate q.4h. Dosage individualized under close medical supervision	Capsules: 25,000, 50,000 IU Tablets: 50,000 IU Injectable: 500,000 IU/ml Solution: 8000 IU/ml Drops: 200 IU/drop Protect from light	*Contraindicated* in hypercalcemia and hypervitaminosis D Calcium intake must be adequate Serum calcium levels should be maintained at 9-10 mg/dl	Blood calcium, phosphate, and urea levels must be determined every 2 weeks (or more frequently as indicated) The bones should be radiographed monthly until condition under treatment is corrected and stabilized

BIBLIOGRAPHY

Austin, L.A., & Heath, H. Calcitonin: Physiology and Pathophysiology. *New England Journal of Medicine*, 1981, *304*, 269-278.

Deftos, L.J., Weisman, M.H., Williams, G.W., Karpf, D.B., Fruman, A.M., Davidson, B.J., Parthemore, J.G., & Judd, H.L. Influence of age and sex on plasma calcitonin in human beings. *New England Journal of Medicine*, 1980, *302*, 1351-1353.

DeLuca, H.F. *Vitamin D metabolism and function*. New York: Springer-Verlag, 1979.

Didronel. *American Journal of Nursing*, 1979, *79*, 135-137.

Doepfner, W.E. Pharmacologic effects of calcitonin. *Triangle*, 1983, *22*, 57-68.

Drugs for postmenopausal osteoporosis. *The Medical Letter*, 1980, *22*, 45-46.

Kline, L.W. A hypocalcemic response to synthetic salmon calcitonin in the green iguana, *Iguana iguana. General and Comparative Endocrinology*, 1981, *44*, 476-479.

MacIntyre, I. The physiological actions of calcitonin. *Triangle*, 1983, *22*, 69-74.

Mann, J.L. Calcitriol. *On Continuing Practice*, 1980, *7*, 18-19.

Parfait, A.M. The actions of parathyroid hormone on bone: relation to bone remodeling and turnover, calcium homeostasis, and metabolic bone disease. *Metabolism*, 1976, *25*, 809-844, 909-955, 1033-1069, 1157-1188.

Putkey, J., & Norman, A.W. Hormonal regulation of calcium homeostasis I: Vitamin D. In L.J. Anghileri and A.M. Tuffet-Anghileri, (Eds.). *The Role of Calcium in Biological Systems*. Boca Raton, Florida: CRC Press Inc., 1982, 171-202.

Ramp, W.K., & Waite, L.C. Hormonal regulation of calcium homeostasis II: Parathyroid hormone, calcitonin, and summary. In L.J. Anghileri and A.M. Tuffet-Anghileri, (Eds.). *The Role of Calcium in Biological Systems*, Boca Raton, Florida: CRC Press Inc., 1982, 203-215.

Talmage, R.V., Grubb, S.A., Norimatusu, H., & Vander-Wiel, C.J. Evidence for an important physiological role for calcitonin. *Proceedings of the National Academy of Science*, 1980, *77*, 609-613.

CHAPTER 63

Estrogens, Progestins, and Antiestrogens

Louis A. Pagliaro
Ann M. Pagliaro

Medications discussed in this chapter

Estrogens	Progestins
Chlorotrianisene	Hydroxyprogesterone
Dienestrol	Medroxyprogesterone
Diethylstilbestrol	Megestrol
Estradiol	Norethindrone
Estrogens, conjugated	Norethynodrel
Estrogens, esterified	Norgestrel
Estrone	Progesterone
Estropipate	*Antiestrogens*
Ethinyl estradiol	Clomiphene
Mestranol	Tamoxifen
Quinestrol	

This chapter discusses the estrogens, progestins, and antiestrogens. Although these compounds share some structural similarities and indications for use, they differ in their mechanisms of action and in their adverse side effects. The estrogens and the progestins are properly defined as hormones and are responsible for sexual development and reproductive organ function in women. Natural and synthetic forms of these compounds are used therapeutically. The antiestrogens are synthetic compounds that inhibit estrogen effects by competitively binding to estrogen receptor sites (see Chapter 3, "Mechanisms of Drug Action").

ESTROGENS

The estrogens, or female sex hormones, are responsible for the growth and development of the fallopian tubes, ovaries, uterus, and external genitalia, as well as for the development of secondary sexual characteristics in women. They are primarily responsible for the normal cyclic changes that occur to the endometrium of the vagina and uterus during the menstrual cycle. Estradiol is the major naturally occurring estrogen and is produced by the ovaries. Some estrogens are metabolically produced in the liver.

Various natural and synthetic estrogen preparations have been developed and are available for oral, parenteral, and topical administration. They are generally well absorbed from both the mucous membranes of the genital tract and the gastrointestinal tract.* They may also be absorbed through intact skin and thus cause systemic effects when applied topically. Approximate dosing equivalents for the commonly used estrogens are listed in the box on, p. 1451.

The estrogens are used therapeutically in treating several conditions in women, including conception control, endometriosis, hypogonadism, hypermenorrhea, menopause, and abnormal uterine bleeding. In men, they are used for the palliative treatment of inoperable prostatic cancer.

The prophylactic use of the estrogens to prevent postpartum breast pain and engorement in nonnursing mothers is *not* generally recommended because of the inherent and significantly increased risk of puerperal thromboembolism. Postpartum breast pain and engorement can generally be safely and effectively treated with analgesics and proper supportive nursing care (see also Chapter 64, "Androgens and Anabolic Steroids").

PROGESTINS

The progestins are hormones that are naturally produced primarily by the corpus luteum and the placenta. They play a major role in reproduction by preparing the estrogen-primed uterine endometrium for the implantation of the fertilized ovum, and following implantation, by assisting (together with estrogen) in the development and functioning of the mammary glands. In addition to their progestational effects, some synthetic progestins also possess anabolic, androgenic, or estrogenic activity (usually mild).

Progesterone is the major naturally occurring progestin. In addition to its important hormonal effects,

Approximate dosing equivalents for the estrogens*

Diethylstilbestrol 1 mg
Estradiol 0.5 mg
Estrogens, conjugated 5 mg
Estrogens, esterified 5 mg
Mestranol 0.8 mg

*For example, 1 mg of diethylstilbestrol will provide approximately the same amount of estrogenic response as 5 mg of estrogens, conjugated.

progesterone also serves as a precursor in the production of various endogenous androgens, corticosteroids, and estrogens (Figure 63-1).

Various natural and synthetic progestin preparations are available for oral and intramuscular administration. An intrauterine depot form has also been developed. The progestins are primarily metabolized in the liver, and their metabolites are excreted in the urine. A significant amount of metabolism of the progestins also occurs in the uterus.

The progestins are used therapeutically for several indications, including amenorrhea, conception control, endometriosis, hypermenorrhea, and progestin-responsive carcinomas. It should be noted that estrogen is usually involved as a cofactor or mediating factor in eliciting optimal progestin effects. Although the progestins do not appear to be able to have as significant an action when administered alone, it is interesting to note that their withdrawal is integrally involved in the initiation of several physiologic events, including lactation, menstruation, parturition, and postpartum mental depression.

The use of progestins during the first trimester of pregnancy to prevent habitual or threatened abortion is generally *not* recommended because of (1) a lack of clearly demonstrated efficacy of these agents for this indication, (2) the ability of these agents to cause masculinization of the female fetus, and (3) fetal heart and limb defects that are associated with the use of these agents during the first 4 months of pregnancy.

ORAL CONTRACEPTIVES
Menstrual cycle

To properly understand the actions of the oral contraceptives, it is necessary to briefly review the normal phases of the menstrual cycle, particularly in relation

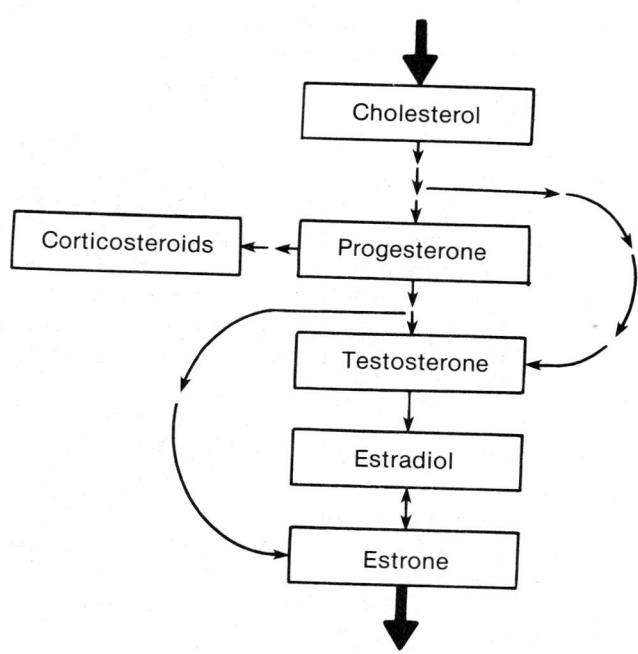

FIGURE 63-1. **Metabolic relationship between various endogenous steroids.**

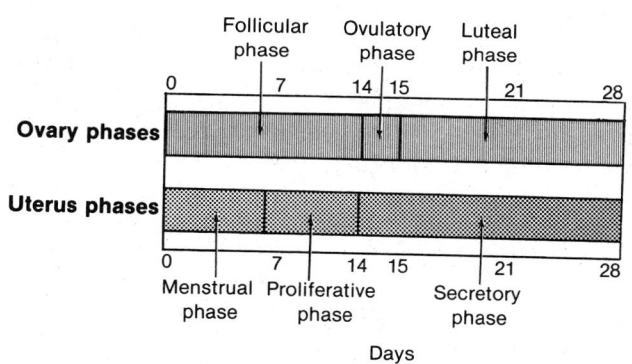

FIGURE 63-2. **A comparison of the phases of the menstrual cycle in relation to effects on the ovaries and uterus.**

to the effects on the ovaries and the uterus (Figure 63-2).

The normal menstrual cycle lasts, on the average, 28 days and is divided into three phases in relation to the effect on both the ovaries and the uterus.

Those phases defined according to their effect on the *ovaries* include the (1) follicular phase, (2) ovulatory phase, and (3) luteal phase. The follicular phase occurs over the first 14 days of the menstrual cycle. During this phase the follicles—which contain oocytes—develop and enlarge, and eventually one, the Graafian follicle, ruptures. The rupture of the Graafian follicle and the consequent release of the enclosed oocyte (ovum) is referred to as ovulation. The ovulatory phase generally occurs on days 13 to 15 of the menstrual cycle. At this time, progesterone secretion begins. The luteal phase (days 15 to 28) follows. During the luteal phase, the ruptured follicle undergoes a change to form the corpus luteum, which in turn maintains estrogen and progestin production during the remainder of the cycle. If pregnancy does *not* occur, the corpus luteum begins to degenerate and ceases hormone production. This decrease in estrogen and progestin production results in the shedding of the endometrial lining of the uterus (i.e., menstruation) and the beginning of a new cycle.

Those phases of the menstrual cycle defined according to their effects on the *uterus* include the (1) menstrual phase, (2) proliferative phase, and (3) secretory phase. The menstrual phase begins on day 1 of the menstrual cycle and lasts for 3 to 6 days. The total discharge of blood and fluid from the vagina during the menses varies but is generally less than 60 ml. This is followed by the proliferative phase (days 6 to 14) during which the endometrial lining of the uterus and the uterine glands and vessels grow in response to the stimulation by the estrogens. The final uterine phase is the secretory phase (days 14 to 28) during which the endometrial lining becomes thicker and the uterine glands begin to secrete. This last phase is primarily under the control of progesterone.

Types of oral contraceptives

Three basic types of oral contraceptives have been developed and are currently available in North America: (1) combination estrogen and progestin, (2) mini or progestin only, and (3) postcoital or estrogen only.

These preparations prevent pregnancy by inhibiting ovulation* and by making the endometrial lining of the uterus unsuitable for implantation by the fertilized ovum (blastocyst).†

One additional type of oral contraceptive, the sequential, was previously available, but has since been withdrawn from use in North America. In the sequential form, estrogen alone was taken for 14 to 16 days of the menstrual cycle (usually beginning on day 5), followed by a combination of estrogen and progestin for an additional 5 to 6 days. Because these products relied primarily on the estrogen

component for conception control, they generally contained higher amounts of estrogen per dose than the currently available combination products and were thus associated with a higher incidence of serious estrogen-related adverse effects (e.g., thromboembolic disorders). In addition, they had a lower rate of protection from pregnancy (i.e., 98% to 99%) in comparison with the combination oral contraceptives.

Combination oral contraceptives. Three general types or formulations of combination oral contraceptives have been developed, including the (1) monophasic, (2) biphasic, and (3) triphasic. These formulations afford close to 100% protection from pregnancy when taken as directed; however, they are also associated with significant morbidity, particularly in women who smoke one or more packages of cigarettes daily.

Monophasic oral contraceptives. The monophasic oral contraceptives use an estrogen and progestin in a fixed ratio that is taken daily for 21 days of the normal menstrual cycle. These agents block ovulation by suppressing the endogenous estrogen and progestin levels. The original formulations generally contained high doses of hormone and were thus associated with increased adverse effects. Most of these preparations have been reformulated as lower dose fixed combinations; however, use of the newer biphasic or triphasic oral contraceptives, which more closely simulate the normal hormonal levels during the menstrual cycle, is generally recommended.

Biphasic oral contraceptives. The biphasic oral contraceptives supply varying amounts of hormone during the first and second halves of the menstrual cycle. Relatively low levels of estrogen and progestin are administered in the follicular phase of the menstrual cycle and increased in the luteal phase. One drawback to these formulations is their association with the inconsistent inhibition of ovulation and an irregular menstruation pattern.

Triphasic oral contraceptives. The triphasic is the most recently developed form of oral contraception and most closely mimics the normal pattern of estrogen and progesterone levels observed during the menstrual cycle in the absence of any exogenous hormones. This approach provides low doses of estrogen and progestin during the follicular phase, with increases in progestin during both the midcycle ovulatory and luteal phases, to mimic more closely the naturally occurring endogenous hormone levels* (Fig-

---

*This is primarily an estrogen effect; however, it can also be caused by progestins.
†This is primarily a progestin effect.

---

*Note that in some preparations the dose of progestin again declines toward the middle to end of the luteal phase.

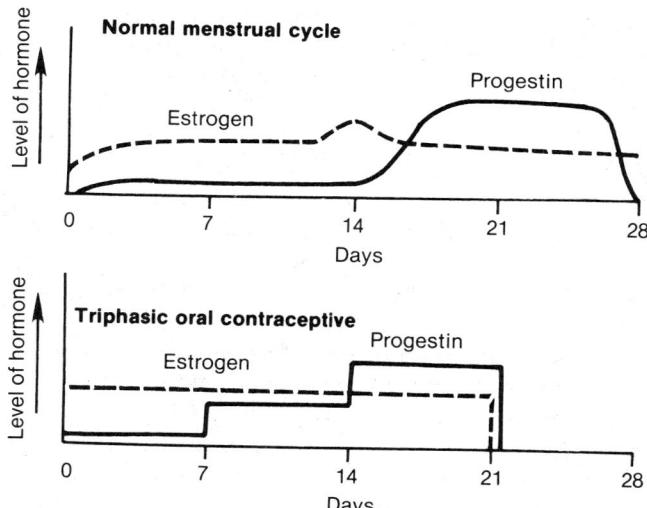

FIGURE 63-3. **Comparison of estrogen and progestin levels during the normal menstrual cycle and while taking triphasic oral contraceptives.**

ure 63-3). The triphasic oral contraceptives achieve conception control with the lowest total hormone intake per cycle and are thus associated with a lower incidence and severity of adverse effects than observed with either the monophasic or biphasic forms.

Because the dose of estrogen is kept at a constant low level throughout the 21-day oral contraceptive dosing period,* preparations that use the triphasic form are commonly referred to as low-dose pills.

Mini pill or progestin only oral contraceptives. The mini pill or progestin only oral contraceptives are dosed once daily for all 28 days of the menstrual cycle. When taken as directed, these drugs offer approximately 97% protection from pregnancy. Because they do not contain an estrogen, use of these preparations is generally associated with a higher incidence of breakthrough bleeding and spotting. Although these preparations possess these minor adverse effects and are slightly less efficacious than the combination products, they do not cause the generally more serious toxicities associated with the use of the estrogens.

Postcoital or estrogen only oral contraceptives. Diethylstilbestrol is the only estrogen currently used as a postcoital or estrogen only oral contraceptive. This preparation is sometimes referred to as the "morning after pill." Use of this preparation is generally unpleasant (it usually causes nausea and vomiting) and possesses the potential for serious estrogen side effects. Therefore, diethylstilbestrol is recommended for con-

---

*Note that in some triphasic preparations the estrogen dose is raised slightly during the second or ovulatory phase.

ception control *only* in cases of emergency (e.g., cases involving incest or rape).

Oral contraceptives and thromboembolic disorders

The most serious adverse effect directly associated with the use of oral contraceptives is the significant increase in thromboembolic disorders, including thrombophlebitis, thromboembolism, and thrombosis (cerebral and coronary).

Although much of this information is based on poorly controlled retrospective studies and generally does not take into consideration the increased incidence of thromboembolic disorders associated with pregnancy, the following points appear to be clear.

Estrogen dose. The incidence of thromboembolic disorders among women taking oral contraceptives is *greater* in those women whose preparation contains a *higher dose of estrogen.*

Age. The risk of thromboembolic disorders related to the use of oral contraceptives *increases with age* beginning at about 30 years of age and increases even more significantly after 40 years of age. In addition, women in this age group who discontinue long-term oral contraceptive use also have a higher incidence of thromboembolic complications.

Tobacco smoking. Women using oral contraceptives, who also *smoke* 15 or more cigarettes per day have a 500% (fivefold) increased risk of having a fatal myocardial infarction, in comparison with women who are also taking oral contraceptives but who do not smoke. In addition, these women, who are taking oral contraceptives and who also smoke, have a 1000% to 1200% (tenfold to twelvefold) increased risk of having a fatal myocardial infarction, in comparison with women who neither use oral contraceptives nor smoke.

Duration of use. Women who use oral contraceptives for *5 or more years* have a 1000% (tenfold) increased risk of death from thromboembolic disorders, in comparison with women who have not used oral contraceptives. The overwhelming majority of deaths in this group occur in women over 35 years of age, so age may be a confounding variable to be considered here.

Even if these incidences have been overestimated, the potential for significant morbidity and mortality associated with the use of oral contraceptives cannot be denied.

The primary risk factors involved appear to be (1) the estrogen dose, (2) the age of the patient, (3) tobacco smoking, and (4) the duration of therapy. Since the more risk factors a patient possesses the greater the probability and danger of thromboembolic complications, patients should be carefully and fully informed and educated regarding oral contraceptive use, and the various risk factors reduced or eliminated whenever possible (see General Nursing Implications and General Instructions for Discharge/Outpatients).

ANTIESTROGENS

The antiestrogens, clomiphene and tamoxifen, are structurally related and appear to act by competitively binding to the estrogen receptor. However, the two drugs are currently used for different indications.

Clomiphene is used to induce ovulation in the treatment of infertility in women. It acts by stimulating the ovaries. Major side effects related to its mechanism of action include the development of ovarian cysts and multiple pregnancy.

Tamoxifen is used for the palliative treatment of advanced, inoperable breast cancer in postmenopausal women. By competitively binding to the estrogen receptor, it impairs estrogen-dependent tumor growth. Major side effects include bone pain and possible visual impairment with long-term use.

SUMMARY

The various estrogens, progestins, and antiestrogens have been discussed. These agents are used for a variety of conditions in women such as conception control, dysmenorrhea, and endometriosis. They are also used to treat various responsive carcinomas in both men and women. Use of these agents must be accompanied by close and careful monitoring because they can cause serious adverse effects (e.g., endometrial carcinoma, thromboembolic disorders).

With an understanding of these various agents, including their indications for use, contraindications, cautions, administration, drug interactions, and monitoring, the nurse will be able to provide optimal therapy and counseling to patients who require these medications.

ADVERSE/SIDE EFFECTS OF ESTROGENS, PROGESTINS, AND ANTIESTROGENS*

CARDIOVASCULAR SYSTEM

Blood clot formation, including cerebral thrombosis, myocardial infarction, pulmonary embolism, and thrombophlebitis
Increased blood pressure

CENTRAL NERVOUS SYSTEM

Dizziness
Headache
Insomnia
Lightheadedness
Mental depression
Nervousness
Visual disturbances, including blurring of vision, flashes, scintillating scotomas, and spots (clomiphene, progestin)

CUTANEOUS SYSTEM

Allergic dermatitis (clomiphene)
Brown blotchy spots on exposed skin
Loss of some scalp hair
Photosensitivity
Skin rash
Urticaria

ENDOCRINE SYSTEM

Acne (progestin)
Breast lumps
Breast swelling and increased tenderness (men or women)
Increased body or facial hair (progestin)
Libido changes—decreased in men, increased in women
Menstrual irregularities, including change in usual pattern of menses, irregular cycle time, breakthrough bleeding, spotting, and absence of menses
Ovarian enlargement (clomiphene)
Ovarian pain, midcycle (clomiphene)
Salt and fluid retention, edema
Unusual tiredness, weakness
Vasomotor symptoms resembling menopausal hot flushes (clomiphene)

GASTROINTESTINAL SYSTEM

Abdominal distention (clomiphene)
Abdominal pain or cramping (clomiphene)
Anorexia

Diarrhea
Nausea
Vomiting

GENITOURINARY SYSTEM

Cervical cancer
Change in vaginal discharge (thick, white, curdlike vaginal candidiasis)
Endometrial cancer
Polyuria (clomiphene)

HEPATIC SYSTEM

Benign liver tumors
Gall bladder obstruction or disease
Hepatitis
Jaundice

RESPIRATORY SYSTEM

Pulmonary embolism (chest pain, shortness of breath)

MISCELLANEOUS EFFECTS

Breast cancer
Melanoma
Pituitary tumors

---

*See Chapter 11, "Drug Toxicity," for an overview of drug toxicity.

CLINICALLY SIGNIFICANT DRUG INTERACTIONS*

Primary drug	Interacting drug	Possible effect(s)	Probable mechanism(s)
Estrogens	Antihypertensives	Decreased antihypertensive effect	Antagonistic pharmacologic effects
Estrogens	Oral anticoagulants	Decreased anticoagulant effect	Antagonistic pharmacologic effects
Estrogens	Rifampin	Decreased estrogen effect	Increased hepatic metabolism
Norethindrone	Rifampin	Decreased norethindrone effect	Increased hepatic metabolism

*See Chapter 10, "Drug Interactions," for an overview of drug interactions.

GENERAL NURSING IMPLICATIONS

Nursing of patients requiring estrogens, progestins, or antiestrogens

ASSESSMENT

Estrogens, progestins, and antiestrogens are used to treat a variety of conditions, including atrophic vaginitis, female hypogonadism, primary ovarian failure, abnormal uterine bleeding caused by a hormonal imbalance, dysmenorrhea, and vasomotor symptoms associated with menopause. The major use of estrogens and progestins, which are sometimes combined, is oral contraception, whereas antiestrogens are primarily used to treat infertility. Estrogen can be used as adjunctive therapy in treating osteoporosis and certain types of cancer (e.g., breast carcinoma, prostatic carcinoma). Progestin can be used to treat endometrial carcinoma.

Assessment should include detailed information regarding the indication for estrogen, antiestrogen, or progestin therapy. In addition, because of the importance of specific information in planning drug therapy and nursing care, a general assessment should include paying careful attention to information such as the patient's age, race, sex, and indication for use. A patient or family history of diabetes, renal or hepatic dysfunction, hematologic disorders (e.g., clotting disorders, anemias), heart disease, lipidemia, endocrine disorders, gallbladder disease, hypertension, or other medical conditions associated with a high risk of complications with estrogen, progestin, or antiestrogen therapy should be carefully explored with each patient.

The general health assessment should also include a sexual history. Urogenital assessment should include the identification of the presence or history of any urogenital anomaly, ovarian mass, vaginal infection, previous urogenital surgery, endometriosis, or pelvic inflammatory disease, including any sexually transmitted disease. A baseline assessment of the abdomen, breasts, and pelvic organs should be completed as indicated. Female patients should be questioned regarding infertility, parity, and past obstetric history (e.g., abortion, any significant problems during labor or the postpartum period such as hemorrhage or thrombophlebitis, and the health of the infant). Previous hormone use, including the use of oral contraceptives or a history of the mother's use of oral contraceptives, should also be determined. The frequency and results of Papanicolaou (Pap) tests and a menstrual history identifying the last normal menstrual period (LNMP) and the presence of menstrual disorders (e.g., amenorrhea, bleeding since the last normal menstrual period) should be explored. Any abnormal bleeding requires full diagnostic measures before the use of these agents is initiated. A pregnancy test (e.g., HCG presence in urine or serum) should be completed as needed.

Baseline hepatic tests are indicated as is a baseline blood pressure determination before initiating therapy. In addition, other tests may be indicated, such as vaginal smears to estimate the levels of endogenous estrogen, an endometrial biopsy to detect the presence of neoplastic lesions, an assay of urinary estrogen, or a test for bleeding in response to progesterone. Because of the association of thromboembolic disease with smoking, a careful smoking history should also be completed for individuals requiring estrogens. The assessment before initiating the therapy should include a detailed drug history to identify any possible hypersensitivity, contraindications, cautions, drug interactions, and drug-taking patterns.

SENSITIVITY

Generally, hypersensitivity to the estrogens, antiestrogens and progestins is rare; however, it is important to note that any drug has the potential to cause a hypersensitivity reaction in susceptible individuals. Because some of the injectables of these agents are made with various oils (e.g., castor oil, corn oil, cottonseed oil, peanut oil, sesame oil, vegetable oil), which differ according to the manufacturer, it is important to question patients carefully regarding the possibility of a hypersensitivity to the particular oil vehicle or to related substances (e.g., peanuts). If a history of an allergy is identified, the patient should be asked to describe the reaction and the prescriber should be consulted.

It is important to note that tartrazine (FDC Yellow No. 5), an orange-yellow azo dye used to color foods, soft drinks, and various drug products, including some antiestrogen products (e.g., Clomid) has caused sensitivity reactions in susceptible individuals. A history of any sensitivity to tartrazine should be ascertained before administering drugs containing this dye. Monitor patients receiving tartrazine-colored preparations for acute asthma, anaphylactic shock, anaphylactoid purpura, blurred vision, hot flushes, general weakness, nonthrombocytopenic purpura, palpitations, rhinitis, rhinorrhea, and urticaria.

Continued.

GENERAL NURSING IMPLICATIONS—cont'd

Nursing of patients requiring estrogens, progestins, or antiestrogens—cont'd

CONTRAINDICATIONS

The use of these agents is contraindicated in patients with a known hypersensitivity.

In addition, the *estrogens* are contraindicated in patients with abnormal vaginal bleeding, breast cancer (except responsive metastatic disease in postmenopausal women), estrogen-dependent cancers, a history of cholestatic jaundice, or thromboembolitic disorders.

The estrogens are also contraindicated in pregnancy, because of their association with congenital malformations, and in lactating mothers because they are excreted in the breast milk and tend to inhibit lactation. Potential adverse effects in the nursing infant are not predictable.

Antiestrogens are contraindicated in patients with abnormal undiagnosed bleeding, liver dysfunction, or a history of ovarian cysts. Antiestrogens are also contraindicated in pregnancy.

Progestins are contraindicated in patients with breast cancer, abnormal undiagnosed bleeding, missed abortion, liver dysfunction, thromboembolic disorders, and thrombophlebitis.

CAUTIONS

Estrogens should be used with caution in patients with asthma, benign breast disease, cardiac insufficiency, cerebrovascular disease, coronary artery disease, diabetes mellitus, endometriosis, epilepsy, gallbladder disease, hepatic dysfunction, hypercalcemia associated with tumors, hypertension, mental depression, migraine headaches, renal dysfunction, and uterine fibroids.

Antiestrogens should be used cautiously because their use has been associated with ovarian cyst formation, multiple pregnancy, birth defects, cataract formation, and other visual disturbances, including blurring of vision or seeing spots and flashes.

Patients should be advised of the visual disturbances that may occur with the use of the antiestrogens and to use caution when operating dangerous machinery or when driving until they know how they are affected by these agents. They should be informed of the importance of an ophthalmologic evaluation in the event of the occurrence of visual symptoms.

Patients should likewise be advised to obtain a pelvic examination at least 3 weeks after starting each course of therapy for infertility.

Progestins should be used with caution during pregnancy because the use of these agents can cause masculinization of the female fetus and birth defects if taken during the first trimester. These agents should also be used with caution in lactating mothers because they can be excreted in the breast milk. Their effects on the nursing infant have not been established, however. It is important to note that the progestins have been associated with decreased glucose tolerance, especially in relation to their use with the estrogens. Progestins should be used with caution in diabetic patients.

It is important to note that sudden loss of vision, diplopia, papilledema, proptosis, or the occurrence of migraine or psychic depression indicates that progestins should be discontinued and the patient further evaluated.

DRUG INTERACTIONS

Concurrent use of the estrogens with anticoagulants can reduce the effect of the anticoagulants. If concurrent use is necessary, an increase in the anticoagulant dose may be required.

Rifampin, as well as other antibiotics including tetracycline, may significantly reduce estrogenic effects because of the accelerated metabolism caused by the induction of hepatic enzymes. Contraceptive failure has been reported with the concurrent use of estrogens with rifampin, tetracycline, ampicillin, and other broad-spectrum antibiotics. Patients requiring these medications, or other medications that may induce hepatic microsomal enzymes, should be advised to use alternative contraceptive precautions, particularly if they are using low-dose oral contraceptive products.

It is important to note that the estrogens can affect various laboratory tests, including glucose tolerance (impaired), metyrapone (reduced response), norepinephrine-induced platelet aggregability (increased), serum triglyceride (increased), sulfobromophthalein (BSP) (increased), and thyroid-binding globulin and protein-bound iodide (increased).

Progestins may affect pregnanediol determination. See Clinically Significant Drug Interactions for other interactions associated with the use of estrogens, antiestrogens, and progestins.

ADMINISTRATION

The estrogens, antiestrogens, and progestins are available in various oral, parenteral, topical, intravaginal, and implantable forms.

The various estrogens are available in capsule or tablet forms and in forms for IM injection and IV infusion. Vaginal creams and suppositories are also available, as well as subcutaneous pellets for implantation.

Antiestrogens are available only in an oral tablet form. Progestins are available in oral and parenteral forms, often in combination with estrogens. Progestasert, a dosage form that is inserted into the uterus, has been developed and requires annual replacement.

Various strengths of these preparations are available. Their dosage and administration varies with the indication for use and according to individual patient factors. The estrogens, antiestrogens, and progestins are generally administered at the lowest effective dose for the shortest possible time to minimize the possibility of adverse effects, including ovarian overstimulation. The estrogens are usually administered on a cyclical schedule to approximate the normal menses and to avoid the overstimulation of estrogen-activated tissue. The antiestrogens are administered in relation to the menstrual cycle for the treatment of infertility and menstrual disorders and are repeated monthly as needed. The oral contraceptives are available in three types of preparations, including combination, mini pill, and estrogen only forms.

The combination products contain estrogen and progestin in various ratios.

GENERAL NURSING IMPLICATIONS—cont'd

Nursing of patients requiring estrogens, progestins, or antiestrogens—cont'd

ADMINISTRATION—cont'd

These forms are generally taken daily for 21 days beginning on day 5 of the menstrual cycle. Menstrual bleeding occurs 1 to 4 days after the hormone has been discontinued and the preparation is resumed 7 days after the last pill. Products are available that have 7 placebo tablets so that the preparation can be taken every day. The mini pill, consisting of progestin alone, is taken for 28 consecutive days. The progestin alone preparation may be used by lactating women or patients who are unable to tolerate estrogen.

It is important to note that estrogen, when administered vaginally or topically, can be absorbed and systemic effects may be noted. Male gynecomastia has been reported in an individual whose wife used vaginal estrogen cream as a lubricant during intercourse two to three times per week.

Before administering any estrogen form, it is important to be sure that the patient is informed about the risks involved with estrogen therapy. By law, the patient must be given a patient package insert (PPI). In addition, it is an important nursing function to assess the patient's understanding of this material and to explain or answer questions that the patient may have. It should be noted that research has shown that some patients do not read the PPI completely, and others do not understand what they have read. Collaboration with the prescriber in planning the therapy with the patient is essential to ensure optimum drug therapy.

Oral administration

Patients should be encouraged to take tablets or capsules with a full glass of water and to swallow them whole without chewing or breaking the tablet or taking the capsule apart. It is important that enteric-coated tablets, which are available for some drugs, are *not* taken with milk or antacids or crushed or broken before administration. Estrogen therapy may cause nausea, especially in the morning with oral or parenteral dosage forms. Their administration with meals or food can reduce this adverse effect.

Intramuscular administration

Intramuscular injections should be made into a large healthy muscle such as the dorsal gluteal or ventrogluteal. The injection should be administered slowly and deeply. A dry syringe and needle of at least 21 gauge should be used for oil vehicle preparations. Frequent injections can be avoided by using long-acting preparations, recognizing that the onset and duration of action are gradual and can be uncertain. This form of administration is useful in patients requiring long-term therapy (e.g., those patients with cancer).

Intravenous administration

Intravenous forms should be diluted and administered according to manufacturer recommendations and infused slowly to decrease flushing and other untoward effects (see the Nursing Drug Digest for specific information regarding the administration of these agents).

MONITORING PATIENT RESPONSE
Therapeutic response

The onset and duration of estrogen, antiestrogen, or progestin therapy depend largely on the specific agent, the dosage form, the route of administration, and on specific patient factors and the indication for therapy. Generally, patients should be monitored for therapeutic effect as related to the baseline assessment data associated with the indication for drug therapy (e.g., monitor patients requiring estrogens for postmenopausal symptoms for relief of original symptoms including vasomotor and other symptoms).

Adverse side effects
Estrogens and progestins

The major adverse side effects associated with the use of the estrogens and the progestins are thromboembolic disorders (e.g., cerebrovascular accident, myocardial infarction, thrombophlebitis) and tumorigenic effects, especially in women over 35 years of age who smoke.

Monitor patients carefully for *more severe effects*, including thrombophlebitis (warmth or pain in calf, Homan's sign [dorsiflexion of the foot with the legs extended elicits Homan's sign, in-dicative of thrombophlebitis]), changes in blood clotting factors (e.g., serum antithrombin levels and platelet aggregation), myocardial infarction (angina), cerebrovascular accident (neurologic changes) and tumorigenic effects, including vaginal and uterine carcinoma, benign hepatomas, and breast tumors. Monitor Pap smear routinely. Breast assessment should be completed regularly.

Monitor for *less severe effects*, including breast tenderness and fullness, dizziness, and edema. Palpate ankles and the pretibial areas for edema and inspect the face and hands for edema formation. Monitor blood pressure. Monitor for GI effects, including anorexia, nausea, vomiting, and diarrhea, and monitor for headache.

Antiestrogens

Patients receiving *antiestrogens* should be monitored for complaints of pelvic pain after therapy is initiated. Pain is associated with enlargement of the ovary, indicating that additional therapy is not indicated and that the dose or duration of the next course should be reduced. The patient should be reassured that the ovarian enlargement is reversible. Patients requiring antiestrogens should also be monitored for other common adverse effects, including ovarian cysts, gastric upset, skin rashes, reversible hair loss, heavier menses, and visual disturbances, which are generally reversible on discontinuation of the drug.

Oral contraceptives

Milder adverse effects associated with oral contraceptives are related to the formulation and generally require approximately 3 months for the body to adjust. Support is often needed at this time. Monitoring response is especially helpful in identifying if the adverse effect experienced is associated with *excess* or *deficient* estrogen or progestin in the individual patient taking combination preparations. Spotting and bleeding in the first part of the cycle can indicate an estrogen deficiency. A change to a product that is estrogen dominant or a balanced hormone preparation could best meet the patient's

Continued.

GENERAL NURSING IMPLICATIONS—cont'd

Nursing of patients requiring estrogens, progestins, or antiestrogens—cont'd

Oral contraceptives—cont'd

individual needs when oral contraception is desired. Nausea, vomiting (especially in the morning), edema, and breast discomfort can also be associated with estrogen effects. Other mild effects such as breast tenderness, depression, fatigue, and lack of initiative can be associated with progestin. Thus most of the adverse side effects associated with the use of oral contraceptives can be reduced or eliminated by monitoring the adverse side effects associated with excesses and deficits and changing to a preparation that more closely approximates the individual patient's hormonal cycle. Monitoring the estrogenic or progestogenic effects can help individualize drug therapy in relation to the selection of an oral contraceptive that provides contraception with the fewest adverse side effects. These hormonal imbalances include effects associated with estrogen excess that mimics pregnancy, estrogen deficiency that mimics menopause, progestin excess that can mimic androgenic changes, and progestin deficiency (see boxed material, p. 1459).

PATIENT EDUCATION

The patient and family, as indicated, should have a clear understanding of the indication for estrogen, antiestrogen, or progestin therapy, the course of the therapy, the exact name of the drug, its dosage, action, storage, administration, adverse side effects, and how these effects can be prevented or minimized. They should be able to monitor for the therapeutic effect and be able to identify symptoms that indicate that the health care provider should be notified. Patients, especially those who are responsible for their drug therapy at home, must understand the importance of following the drug therapy regimen as planned and should not stop taking the medication abruptly. They should understand that the use of these medications generally requires slow changes in dosage and gradual discontinuation. Because of the range of indications for these medications and because of individual patient factors, patient education must be carefully individualized.

Estrogens

When estrogens are used on a short-term basis to retard the progression of estrogen-deficient osteoporosis, patients may need assistance with other aspects of therapy including diet, calcium supplements, physiotherapy, and general health care practices. Patient education should emphasize the importance of regular visits to the primary health care provider to monitor progress.

Patients should understand the importance of not taking estrogen during the first trimester of pregnancy.

Postmenopausal patients requiring estrogen should understand its association with endometrial cancer.

In addition, see General Instructions for Discharge/Outpatients, and the section on oral contraceptive counseling for specific information for discharge/outpatients requiring estrogens.

Progestins

Progestins can have some estrogenic effects, and thus patients should be cautioned regarding these effects. (See the section on oral contraceptive counseling and General Instructions for Discharge/Outpatients.)

Antiestrogens

Patients requiring antiestrogens for the induction of ovulation should understand the potential for ovarian cyst formation, multiple pregnancy, and birth defects before the therapy is initiated. They should understand the importance of follow-up with the health care provider to monitor therapy.

In addition, see General Instructions for Discharge/Outpatients for specific information that should be included in discharge planning and patient teaching.

Oral contraceptive counseling

Patients requiring oral contraceptives should be carefully counseled regarding the adverse effects associated with the use of oral contraceptives. Various alternative contraceptive methods should be explored so that the patient can make an informed decision. It is important to include the patient's partner, as indicated, in counseling sessions and discussions. When oral contraceptives are selected, it is important that the patient understand the various types of preparations available, including estrogen-progestin combination products and the progestin-only preparations (mini pill). The risk-benefit ratio should be discussed carefully with each patient.

Patients should be able to recognize the type of preparation they are using so they can discuss questions with the health care provider accurately and should keep a record themselves of the length of time they have been taking specific oral contraceptives. Patients should understand the relationship of their specific preparation to the days of the menstrual cycle, especially in relation to the problem of a missed dose and what to do if this should occur.

Nutritional assessment and counseling should be included, as indicated, because the use of oral contraceptives can cause a deficiency in pyridoxine (vitamin B_6), vitamin B_{12}, and folic acid. However, these vitamin deficiencies are generally not clinically significant in well-nourished patients. Iron supplements are not usually indicated for healthy women because the oral contraceptives generally lead to a reduced blood loss during the menses and a resultant rise in the serum iron concentration.

Patient education should include self-breast examination (SBE) and information regarding the importance of semiannual Pap tests. It is important that diabetic patients or patients with a history of diabetes understand that the use of the oral contraceptives, including estrogen-progestin combinations, containing higher doses of estrogens can cause an altered glucose tolerance, and that insulin requirements may require adjustment.

It is important to note that patients requiring estrogens, antiestrogens, and progestins and their families as indicated require support during the therapy and assistance in coping with such conditions as cancer, infertility, and menopause. The nurse's role in assisting patients requiring these agents cannot be overemphasized.

Signs of estrogen excess

Abdominal distention
Breast tenderness
Cervical enlargement
Cervical eversion
Cervical mucorrhea, polyposis
Clear vaginal discharge
Cystic breasts
Dizziness, vertigo
Dysmenorrhea
Edema
Fibroid growth
Headache
Hypermenorrhea (profuse and frequent
  menstruation)
Hyperpigmentation (cholasma or mask of
  pregnancy)
Hypertension
Increased breast size (ductal and fatty tissue)
Irritability
Leg cramps
Leukorrhea
Migraine headache
Mucorrhea
Nausea
Nervousness
Syncope
Uterine cramping
Uterine enlargement
Vascular headache
Vomiting
Weight gain, cyclic (fluid retention; increased
  female fat deposition)

Signs of progestin excess

Acne
Alopecia, mild
Amenorrhea (postpill)
Breast tenderness
Change in libido
Decreased duration of menstrual flow
Depression
Dilated leg veins
Fatigue, tiredness
Hirsutism
Hypomenorrhea
Increased appetite
Increased breast size (alveolar tissue)
Oily skin and scalp
Pelvic congestion
Pruritus
Rash
Vaginal infections, *Monilia (Candida)*
Weight gain, persistent, noncyclic

Signs of progestin deficit

Amenorrhea
Decreased breast size
Delayed withdrawal bleeding
Dysmenorrhea
Excessive bleeding
Hypermenorrhea
Spotting and breakthrough bleeding late in cycle
  (days 15 to 21)
Weight loss

Signs of estrogen deficit

Amenorrhea
Atrophic vaginitis
Absence of bleeding
Breakthrough bleeding midcycle
Cystocele, rectocele
Dyspareunia
Hypomenorrhea
Irritability
Malaise
Nervousness
Pelvic relaxation
Small uterus
Spotting, on days 1 to 14 of cycle
Vasomotor symptoms

ESTROGENS, PROGESTINS, OR ANTIESTROGENS

This drug is a hormone used to treat various conditions. If you do not know why you require this medication, contact your health care provider.

Take this medication exactly as prescribed. If you have any questions about how this medication should be taken, contact your health care provider.

Take the tablet or capsule form of this medication with a full glass of water and with some food to prevent stomach upset. Do *not* crush or chew these tablets or capsules.

If you forget to take a dose of this medication, take the dose as soon as you realize that you missed a dose, then take the medication at the same time as before. If you remember just before your next dose is due, take your regular dose and skip the missed dose. Do not double your dose. Notify your health care provider about any changes in your dosing routine.

Inform your dentist and other health care providers that you are taking this medication, because it can be affected by other drugs.

This medication can make your skin more sensitive to sunlight. You may need to wear protective clothing and use a sunscreen on exposed areas when out in the sun.

Keep appointments with your health care provider as indicated so that your progress can be monitored.

If you suspect that you are pregnant, stop taking this medication and contact your health care provider immediately. This medication can cause some unwanted effects on the unborn baby.

Any medication can cause unwanted effects or side effects. You may notice some side effects when taking this medication, such as stomach upset or diarrhea. If the side effects persist, or become bothersome or severe, contact your health care provider immediately.

While you are taking this medication, call your health care provider if you notice any of the following: dizziness; loss of coordination; pain in the chest, groin, or legs, especially the calves of the legs; pains in the stomach, side, or abdomen; pelvic pain; shortness of breath; severe or sudden headache; slurred speech; swelling of the ankles or feet or a sudden weight gain; thick, white, curdlike vaginal discharge or other unusual vaginal discharge; vision changes; or yellowing of the eyes or skin.

Read the patient package insert carefully before taking this medication. Check with your health care provider if you have any questions.

Do not take any other prescription or nonprescription medication while taking this medication without first checking with your health care provider. Hormones can interact with other medications and cause unwanted or harmful effects. Do not start or stop taking any other medication while taking this medication.

Use caution while driving or performing any task that requires complete alertness until you know how this medication affects you.

Do not trade or give this medication to your family or friends. It was prescribed especially for you.

Store this medication as directed on the label.

Keep this and all other medications out of the reach of children.

ORAL CONTRACEPTIVES

This drug is an oral contraceptive used to prevent pregnancy.

Any medication can cause unwanted or side effects. Read your patient package insert carefully and discuss any questions you may have with your health care provider.

Take this medication exactly as prescribed and follow the directions on the prescription carefully.

Take the tablet with a full glass of water or with some food to prevent stomach upset.

It may take about 1 week for the medication to begin to work fully, so it is important that an alternate method of contraception be used during this time.

If you forget to take your pill, take it as soon as you remember. If you miss two consecutive pills, take two pills a day for the next two days. If you miss three or more consecutive pills, stop taking this medication and use another form of contraception for the remainder of your cycle. Consult with your health care provider for further directions before resuming oral contraception.

Take tablets in the sequence order indicated in the package because they may contain different hormone ratios patterned after the natural menstrual cycle. If you miss taking a tablet or if you take them out of order, you may disrupt this cycle and reduce the contraceptive effect.

Take the tablet as indicated at the same time every day. This will help you remember to take your tablet and will also maintain the hormones at a more constant and natural level.

If you stop taking the pill for any reason, use an alternate method of contraception.

While taking this medication, notify your health care provider if you notice any of the following: calf pain, dizziness, headache, nausea, or swelling of the feet or ankles.

The use of this medication can increase your chance of vaginal infections. Notify your health care provider if you notice any unusual vaginal discharge, itching, burning, odor, or pain.

While taking this medication, do not start or stop taking any other medication without consulting with your health care provider. Oral contraceptives can interact with other medications and cause unwanted or harmful effects. It is important to note that some antibiotics, such as tetracycline, can reduce the effect of the oral contraceptive, which has resulted in pregnancy.

Schedule a Pap test semiannually and have a complete physical examination yearly.

Notify your health care provider if you miss a menstrual period. If you have not had a menstrual period for 60 days, discontinue the use of this medication and consult with your health care provider immediately.

If you want to discontinue the use of this medication, check with your health care provider. Hormones should be discontinued gradually. In addition, it is sometimes recommended that if pregnancy is desired, this should be planned 2 or more months after discontinuing the use of the oral contraceptive.

This medication has been prescribed especially for you. Do not give this medication to anyone else.

Keep this medication and all other medications out of the reach of children.

NURSING DRUG DIGEST

Medication (trade name*)	Indication	Usual dosage and administration	Dosage forms, preparation, and storage	Contraindications, cautions, and comments	Monitoring
Chlorotrianisene Tace	Prevention of postpartum breast engorgement in non-nursing mothers (use *not* generally recommended because of questionable efficacy and risk of thrombus formation)	*Adults:* 12 mg PO q.i.d. for 7 days, *or* 50 mg PO q.6h. for 6 doses, *or* 72 mg PO b.i.d. for 2 days	Capsules: 12, 25, 72 mg	*Contraindicated* in undiagnosed vaginal bleeding, pregnancy, puerperal women, breast cancer; thromboembolic disorders, and estrogen-sensitive cancers	Observe for uterine bleeding in women Observe for gynecomastia in men Monitor for thromboembolic complications Monitor for jaundice
				May cause gynecomastia in men May predispose patient to thromboembolic disease	
	Inoperable progressing prostatic carcinoma	*Adults:* 12-25 mg/24 hr PO		May cause increased incidence of gallbladder disease	
	Estrogen replacement for menopausal syndrome	*Adults:* 12-25 mg/24 hr PO for 30 days			
	Atrophic vaginitis Kraurosis vulvae Female hypogonadism	*Adults:* 12-25 mg/24 hr PO for 21 days, followed by a 7-day rest period			
Clomiphene Clomid Dyneric Serophene	Induction of ovulation	*Adults:* 50 mg/24 hr PO for 5 days (if necessary may repeat with 100 mg/24 hr PO for 5 days, *after* at least 30 days rest period) Maximum: 100 mg/24 hr	Tablet: 50 mg	*Contraindicated* in abnormal uterine bleeding, severe liver dysfunction, patients with ovarian cysts, and pregnancy	Monitor for abdominal discomfort Observe for hot flashes Observe for visual disturbances
				May cause multiple pregnancy in approximately 11% of patients; however, over 90% of these are twins Commonly causes abdominal discomfort, visual disturbances, and hot flashes	

Continued.

NOTE: For additional details regarding the individual agents listed in this table, see the text and other tables in this chapter.

*Indicates a multiple active ingredient product. For a complete listing of all active ingredients see the *Drug Reference Guide to Brand Names and Active Ingredients.*

★Indicates that the drug is generally available only in the United States.

NURSING DRUG DIGEST—cont'd

Medication (trade name)	Indication	Usual dosage and administration	Dosage forms, preparation, and storage	Contraindications, cautions, and comments	Monitoring
Dienestrol AVC with Dienestrol* DV Cream/Suppositories Estraguard Ortho Dienestrol Cream Synestrol Wilinestrol	Atrophic vaginitis Kraurosis vulvae	*Adults:* 600 µg vaginal cream (one applicatorful) intravaginally once or twice daily for 7-14 days, then halve the dose for an additional 7-14 days; *or* 1-2 vaginal suppositories intravaginally once or twice daily for 7-14 days, then halve the dose for an additional 7-14 days Maintenance: Generally, 300-600 µg vaginal cream (or 1 vaginal suppository) intravaginally 1-3 times a week For vaginal use *only*	Vaginal cream: 0.01% (100 µg/gm) Store between 15° and 30° C Vaginal suppositories: 0.7 mg Store between 8° and 15° C	*Contraindicated* in pregnancy, thromboembolic disease, breast cancer, and undiagnosed vaginal bleeding May cause fluid retention	Monitor for edema Monitor for unusual vaginal discharge
Diethylstilbestrol A.T.V. DV Estrosyn Honvol Makarol Micrest Prins V/S Stilbetin Stibilium Stilphostrol Tylosterone*	Palliative therapy of inoperable prostatic cancer	*Adults:* 50-200 mg PO t.i.d., gradually reduce to lowest maintenance dose; *or* 500 mg/24 hr by slow IV injection for 5-10 days, followed by 250 mg/24 hr by slow IV injection for 10-20 days Infuse at a rate of 1-2 ml/min for the first 10-15 min, adjusting the rate to administer the remaining daily dose within 1 hr; initial injectable doses are followed by maintenance doses of 250-500 mg by slow IV 3-4 times a week for 1-2 months, followed by 250-500 mg slow IV 2 times a week for 2-4 months, and then 250 mg a week (or longer) thereafter	Tablets, enteric-coated: 0.1, 0.25, 0.5, 1.5 mg Tablets: 0.1, 0.25, 0.5, 1.5, 25, 50, 100 mg Vaginal suppositories: 0.1, 0.5, 1 mg Store vaginal suppositories between 8° and 30° C Injectable: 250 mg/5 ml *Dilute* total daily dose of injectable with 250 ml D₅W, NS, or sterile water for injection *before* administration Store injectable below 20° C Do *not* freeze	*Contraindicated* in hepatic dysfunction, breast cancer, pregnancy, cerebrovascular disease, and thromboembolic disease May cause fluid retention May cause thromboembolic disease Administration during pregnancy has resulted in a significant incidence of nonmalignant genital changes, as well as cervical and adenocarcinoma in female offspring and testicular tumors in male offspring	Monitor serum phosphatases in patients with prostatic cancer (decreases signify drug effectiveness) Monitor for signs of endometrial carcinoma in patients with an intact uterus

Drug	Use	Dosage	Preparations	Nursing considerations
	Palliative therapy for progressive, inoperable, metastatic breast cancer	*Adults:* (selected men and postmenopausal women) 15 mg/24 hr PO		
	Atrophic vaginitis, female hypogonadism, kraurosis vulvae, menopausal symptoms, ovariectomy, and primary ovarian failure	*Adults:* 0.2-0.5 mg/24 hr for 21 days, followed by a 7-day rest period; or 100-500 µg vaginal suppositories q.d. to b.i.d. for 10-14 days		
	Conception control (recommended for emergency treatment only)	*Adults:* 25 mg PO b.i.d. for 5 days; first dose should be administered *within 72 hr after coitus*		
Estradiol Aquadiol Delestrogen Depo-Testadiol* Dimenformon Diogyn Diogynets Di-Ovocylin E-Cypionate Estrace Estraldine Femogen CYP Femogex Hormonin* Mal-D-Fem CYP Menaval-10 Ovocylin Progynon Progynon B Progynova Testaval 90/4* Test-Estrin*	Symptomatic relief of menopausal symptoms, estrogenic supplement	*Adults:* 1-2 mg/24 hr PO for 21 days, followed by a 7-day rest period, *or* 1-5 mg (cypionate salt) IM every 3-4 weeks, *or* 10-20 mg (valerate salt) IM every 4 weeks	Tablets: 1, 2 mg Injectable: 1, 2, 5 mg/ml (cypionate salt); 10, 20, 40 mg/ml (valerate salt) Store between 15° and 30° C	*Contraindicated* in hepatic dysfunction, breast cancer, pregnancy, cerebrovascular disease, endometrial hyperplasia, and undiagnosed vaginal bleeding May cause fluid retention and GI distress Monitor for abnormal vaginal bleeding Monitor for visual changes Observe for edema Monitor weight Monitor for nausea or gastric distress
	Palliative therapy for inoperable prostatic cancer	*Adults:* 1-2 mg PO t.i.d., *or* 30 mg IM every 1-2 weeks		
	Palliative therapy for progressive, inoperable breast cancer	*Adults:* (selected men and postmenopausal women) 10 mg PO t.i.d. (for at least 3 months)		
	Female hypogonadism Primary ovarian failure	*Adults:* 1.5-2 mg (cypionate salt) IM every 4 weeks, *or* 10-20 mg (valerate salt) IM every 4 weeks		

Continued.

NURSING DRUG DIGEST—cont'd

Medication (trade name)	Indication	Usual dosage and administration	Dosage forms, preparation, and storage	Contraindications, cautions, and comments	Monitoring
Estrogens, conjugated C.E.S. Evestrone Kestrin Menotab Oestrilin Oestrilin with Methyltestosterone* Ovest Premarin Premarin with M.T.* Sodestrin Sodestrin H	Symptomatic relief of menopausal symptoms Treatment of postmenopausal estrogen deficiency Palliative therapy for inoperable prostatic cancer Atrophic vaginitis Kraurosis vulvae Palliative therapy for progressive, inoperable breast cancer Abnormal uterine bleeding caused by a hormonal imbalance	*Adults:* 1.25 mg/24 hr PO for 21 days, followed by a 7-day rest period *Adults:* 0.3-1.25 mg/24 hr PO for 21 days, followed by a 7-day rest period *Adults:* 1.25-2.5 mg PO t.i.d. *Adults:* Apply 2-4 gm/24 hr topically or intravaginally (and/or 0.3-1.25 mg/24 hr PO), as indicated, for 21 days, followed by a 7-day rest period *Adults:* (women at least 5 years *postmenopause*) 10 mg PO t.i.d. (for at least 3 months) *Adults:* 25 mg IM or *slow IV,* may be repeated in 6-12 hr if necessary	Tablets: 0.3, 0.625, 1.25, 2.5 mg Cream: 0.0625% (0.625 mg/gm) Injectable: 25 mg/vial (with 5 ml of sterile diluent) Store injectable between 2° and 8° C Injectable is stable for 60 days after reconstitution Reconstituted solution is compatible with NS and dextrose solutions *Discard* injectable solutions that have darkened or that contain a precipitate	*Contraindicated* in hepatic dysfunction, breast cancer (except for those patients selected for palliative therapy of progressive, inoperable breast cancer), pregnancy, cerebrovascular disease, thromboembolic disease, endometrial hyperplasia, and undiagnosed vaginal bleeding May cause fluid retention and GI distress A Pap smear should be taken from female patients *before* initiating therapy Contains 50%-65% of sodium estrone sulfate and 20%-35% of sodium equilin sulfate	Monitor blood pressure Observe breast and pelvic organs periodically for signs of cancer (e.g., periodic Pap smear) Observe for thromboembolic complications Serum phosphatase values are helpful in monitoring the status of prostatic cancer Observe for edema Observe for nausea or other GI distress
Estrogens, esterified Amnestrogen Climestrone Estabs Estratabs Estromed Evex Menest Menotrol Neo-Estrone	Symptomatic relief of menopausal symptoms Treatment of postmenopausal estrogen deficiency Palliative therapy of inoperable prostatic cancer Palliative therapy for progressive, inoperable breast cancer	*Adults:* 0.3-1.25 mg/24 hr PO for 21 days, followed by a 7-day rest period *Adults:* 0.3-1.25 mg/24 hr PO for 21 days, followed by a 7-day rest period *Adults:* 1.25-2.5 mg PO t.i.d. *Adults:* (women at least 5 years *postmenopause*) 10 mg PO t.i.d. (for at least 3 months)	Tablets: 0.3, 0.625, 1.25, 2.5 mg	*Contraindicated* in hepatic dysfunction, breast cancer (except for those patients selected for palliative therapy of progressive, inoperable breast cancer), pregnancy, cerebrovascular disease, thromboembolic disease, endometrial hyperplasia, and undiagnosed vaginal bleeding May cause fluid retention and GI distress	Monitor blood pressure Observe breast and pelvic organs periodically for signs of cancer (e.g., periodic Pap smear) Observe for thromboembolic complications Serum phosphatase values are helpful in monitoring the status of prostatic cancer Observe for edema

SECTION XIV
HORMONES AND HORMONE ANTAGONISTS

Name	Uses	Dosage	Available forms	Nursing considerations
(continued)				A Pap smear should be taken from female patients *before* initiating therapy Contains 75%-85% of sodium estrone sulfate and 6.5%-15% of equilin sodium sulfate, such that the total of these two components is *not* less than 90% of the total esterified estrogens
Estrone Bestrone Di-Genik* Duogen* Estronol Estrusol Femogen Hormestrin Hormonin* Kestrone-5 Menformon A Spanestrin P Theelin	Palliative therapy for inoperable prostatic cancer Atrophic vaginitis Kraurosis vulvae Menopausal symptoms Female hypogonadism Ovariectomy Primary ovarian failure	*Adults:* 2-4 mg IM 2-3 times a week *Adults:* 0.1-0.5 mg IM 2-3 times a week *Adults:* 0.1-2 mg/week IM Administer IM *only*	Injectable: 1, 2, 5 mg/ml	*Contraindicated* in hepatic dysfunction, breast cancer, pregnancy, cerebrovascular disease, thromboembolic disease, endometrial hyperplasia, and undiagnosed vaginal bleeding May cause fluid retention and GI distress A Pap smear should be taken from female patients *before* initiating therapy Monitor blood pressure Observe breast and pelvic organs periodically for signs of cancer (e.g., periodic Pap smear) Observe for thromboembolic complications Serum phosphatase values are of assistance in monitoring the status of prostatic cancer Monitor for edema
Estropipate Ogen Sulesfrex	Atrophic vaginitis Kraurosis vulvae Menopausal symptoms Female hypogonadism Ovariectomy Primary ovarian failure	*Adults:* Apply 2-4 gm/24 hr topically or intravaginally (and/or 0.75-6 mg/24 hr PO) for 21 days, followed by a 7-day rest period *Adults:* 1.5-9 mg/24 hr PO for 21 days, followed by an 8-10-day rest period NOTE: Dosage indicated above is in milligrams of estropipate; use of some brands requires a conversion (e.g., Ogen 0.625 mg is equivalent to 0.75 mg of estropipate; Ogen 1.25 is equivalent to 1.5 mg of estropipate; Ogen 2.5 is equivalent to 3 mg of estropipate; Ogen 5 is equivalent to 6 mg of estropipate)	Tablets: 0.75, 1.5, 3, 6 mg Vaginal cream: 1.5 mg/gm	*Contraindicated* in hepatic dysfunction, breast cancer, pregnancy, cerebrovascular disease, thromboembolic disease, endometrial hypoplasia, and undiagnosed vaginal bleeding May cause fluid retention and GI distress A Pap smear should be taken from female patients *before* initiating therapy Monitor blood pressure Observe breast and pelvic organs periodically for signs of cancer (e.g., periodic Pap smear) Observe for thromboembolic complications Observe for edema Observe for nausea and other GI distress

Continued.

NURSING DRUG DIGEST—cont'd

Medication (trade name)	Indication	Usual dosage and administration	Dosage forms, preparation, and storage	Contraindications, cautions, and comments	Monitoring
Ethinyl estradiol Brevicon* Demulen* Demulen 1/35* Demulen-28* Diogyn E Estinyl Ethinoral Eticylol Feminone Gynetone* Halodrin* Inestra Loestrin* Lo/Ovral* Lynoral Mepilin* Modicon* Nordette* Norlestrin* Nylestin Ortho-Novum 10/11* Ovcon* Ovral* Tri-Norinyl* Zorane*	Symptomatic relief of menopausal symptoms Palliative therapy for progressive, inoperable breast cancer Functional uterine bleeding Conception control Female hypogonadism	*Adults:* 20-50 µg/24 hr PO for 21 days, followed by a 7-day rest period *Adults:* (postmenopausal women) 1000 µg PO t.i.d. *Adults:* 500 µg q.d. to b.i.d. PO until bleeding stops, then 50 µg q.d. to t.i.d. PO for the first 14 days of the menstrual cycle, followed by progesterone for 5 days (may repeat the cyclic dosage 2 additional times as indicated) *Adults:* Used as one of the ingredients in *combination* oral contraceptives Dosage varies according to the formulation, but is generally in the 20-50 µg (ethinyl estradiol) range *Adults:* 150-2000 µg/24 hr PO *Adults:* 50 µg q.d. to t.i.d. for 14 days, followed by a progestin for 14 days; this sequence may be repeated to establish a normal menses NOTE: Dose is in *micrograms*	Tablets: 20, 50, 500 µg	*Contraindicated* in hepatic dysfunction, breast cancer (except for those patients selected for palliative therapy of progressive inoperable breast cancer), pregnancy, cerebrovascular disease, thromboembolic disease, endometrial hyperplasia, and undiagnosed vaginal bleeding May cause fluid retention and GI distress A Pap smear should be taken from female patients *before* initiating therapy Approximately 20 times as potent as diethylstilbestrol	Monitor blood pressure Observe breast and pelvic organs periodically for signs of cancer (e.g., periodic Pap smear) Observe for thromboembolic complications Serum phosphatase values are helpful in monitoring the status of prostatic cancer Observe for edema Observe for nausea and other GI distress
Hydroxyprogesterone Delalutin Deprolutin Duralutin Gesterol L.A. Hylutin	Palliative, *adjunctive* therapy for advanced adenocarcinoma of the uterine corpus (stage III or IV) in nonpregnant women	*Adults:* 1-7 gm/week IM in single or divided doses for 12 weeks *or* until relapse (or toxicity) occurs NOTE: Dose is in grams	Injectable: 125, 250 mg/ml Store at room temperature; if crystals form because of cooling they may be readily dissolved by heating the vial in boiling water	*Contraindicated* in hepatic dysfunction, breast cancer, pregnancy, cerebrovascular disease, thromboembolic disease, endometrial hyperplasia, and undiagnosed vaginal bleeding	Monitor blood pressure Observe for edema Observe breast and pelvic organs periodically for signs of cancer (e.g., periodic Pap smear)

Drug	Uses	Dosage	Availability	Side effects	Nursing implications
	Amenorrhea, functional uterine bleeding	*Adults:* 375 mg IM every 4 weeks Administer IM *only*	Use of a wet needle or syringe may cause the solution to become cloudy; however, the potency is *not* affected	May cause fluid retention and GI distress A Pap smear should be taken from female patients *before* initiating therapy May cause masculinization of the female fetus Fetal heart and limb defects are associated with use during the first 4 months of pregnancy	Observe for thromboembolic complications
Medroxypro-gesterone Amen Curretab Depo-Provera Gesinal Oragest Provera	Palliative therapy for advanced endometrial carcinoma Conception control Endometriosis in *nonpregnant* women Functional uterine bleeding Secondary amenorrhea	*Adults:* 20-400 mg/24 hr PO; *or* 400-1000 mg/week IM (results should be noted within 2-3 months or the therapy should then be discontinued) *Adults:* 150 mg IM every 3 months *Adults:* 50 mg/week IM, or 100 mg every 2 weeks IM *Adults:* 5-10 mg/24 hr PO for 5-10 days beginning on the calculated or assumed 16th-21st day of the menstrual cycle Injectable is for IM use *only* NOTE: A maximum 5 ml IM per injection site is generally well tolerated	Injectable: 50, 100, 400 mg/ml Tablets: 2.5, 5, 10 mg Store between 15° and 30° C	*Contraindicated* in hepatic dysfunction, thromboembolic disease, breast cancer, undiagnosed vaginal bleeding, and hypersensitivity May cause masculinization of the female fetus Fetal heart and limb defects are associated with use during the first 4 months of pregnancy May cause edema, breast tenderness, menstrual irregularities, skin sensitivity reactions (including rashes and acne), and mental depression (occasionally) Amenorrhea and infertility may persist for 18 months (or longer) following treatment with repeated IM injections of medroxyprogesterone	Observe for fluid retention Monitor eyesight for any change in vision Observe for thromboembolic complications

Continued.

NURSING DRUG DIGEST—cont'd

Medication (trade name)	Indication	Usual dosage and administration	Dosage forms, preparation, and storage	Contraindications, cautions, and comments	Monitoring
Megestrol Megace Ovaban Pallace	Palliative or adjunctive therapy for inoperable, metastatic breast carcinoma	*Adults:* 160 mg/24 hr PO in 4 equally divided doses	Tablets: 20, 40 mg	*Contraindicated* in hypersensitivity Use with caution in patients with thromboembolic disorders Generally well tolerated with few adverse effects *Not* to be used as a diagnostic test for pregnancy Use during the first 4 months of pregnancy may be associated with an increased risk of fetal heart and limb defects	
	Palliative or adjunctive therapy for inoperable, metastatic endometrial carcinoma	*Adults:* 80-160 mg/24 hr PO in 4 equally divided doses Maximum: 800 mg/24 hr Decrease dosage in renal failure			
Mestranol Enovid* Enovid-E* Enovid-E 21* Norinyl- 1 + 50* Norinyl- 1 + 80* Norinyl-1 Fe* Norinyl 2* Ortho Novum 1/50* Ortho Novum 1/80* Ortho Novum 2* Ovulen* Ovulen-21* Ovulen-28*	Conception control	*Adults:* Used as one of the ingredients in *combination* oral contraceptives Dose varies according to the formulation, but is generally in the 50-150 μg (mestranol) range	Tablets: 50, 75, 80, 100, 150 μg (*only* available in combination products)	*Contraindicated* in hepatic dysfunction, breast cancer, pregnancy, cerebrovascular disease, thromboembolic disease, endometrial hyperplasia, and undiagnosed vaginal bleeding May cause fluid retention and GI distress A Pap smear should be taken from patients *before* initiating therapy	Monitor blood pressure Observe breast and pelvic organs periodically for signs of cancer (e.g., periodic Pap smear) Observe for thromboembolic complications Observe for edema Observe for nausea and other GI distress

Drug	Uses	Dosage		Remarks
Norethindrone Agestin Brevicon* Lestrin* Micronor Modicon* Noriday Norinyl* Norlestrin* Norlutate Norlutin Nor-Q.D. Ortho-Novum* Ortho-Novum 10/11* Ovcon* Zorane*	Conception control Endometriosis Amenorrhea, functional uterine bleeding	*Adults:* 0.35 mg/24 hr PO starting on the first day of the menstrual cycle; *or* used as one of the ingredients in *combination* oral contraceptives Dose varies according to the formulation, but is generally in the 0.5-2.5 mg (norethindrone or norethindrone acetate) range *Adults:* 10 mg/24 hr PO for 14 days; increase at 14-day intervals by 5 mg/24 hr, which is administered for 6-9 months (maximum: 30 mg/24 hr) *Adults:* 5-20 mg/24 hr PO on days 5-25 of the menstrual cycle, then adjusted as necessary NOTE: The potency of norethindrone acetate is twice that of norethindrone	Tablets: 0.35, 5 mg	*Contraindicated* in hepatic dysfunction, cerebrovascular disease, thromboembolic disease, breast cancer, undiagnosed vaginal bleeding, pregnancy, and migraine Use with caution in patients with hypertension May cause GI disturbances, edema, menstrual irregularities, weight change, and mental depression May cause masculinization of the female fetus Norethindrone is approximately twice as potent as progesterone Monitor blood pressure Observe breast and pelvic organs periodically for signs of cancer (e.g., periodic Pap smear) Observe for thromboembolic complications Observe for edema Observe for nausea and other GI distress
Norethynodrel Enovid* Enovid-E* Enovid-E 21*	Conception control	*Adults:* Used as one of the ingredients in *combination* oral contraceptives Dose varies according to the formulation, but is generally in the 2.5-10 mg (norethynodrel) range	Tablets: 2.5, 5, 10 mg (*only* available in combination products)	*Contraindicated* in hepatic dysfunction, cerebrovascular disease, thromboembolic disease, breast cancer, undiagnosed vaginal bleeding, pregnancy, and migraine Use with caution in patients with hypertension May cause GI disturbances, edema, menstrual irregularities, weight change, and mental depression May cause masculinization of the female fetus Monitor blood pressure Observe breast and pelvic organs periodically for signs of cancer (e.g., periodic Pap smear) Observe for thromboembolic complications Observe for edema Observe for nausea and other GI distress

Continued.

NURSING DRUG DIGEST—cont'd

Medication (trade name)	Indication	Usual dosage and administration	Dosage forms, preparation, and storage	Contraindications, cautions, and comments	Monitoring
Norgestrel Lo/Ovral* Microlut Min-Ovral* Ovral* Ovrette	Conception control	*Adults:* 75 µg/24 hr PO, *or* used as one of the ingredients in *combination* oral contraceptives Dose in combination products varies according to the formulation, but is generally in the 150-500 µg (norgestrel) range	Tablet: 75 µg (also available in various strength combination products)	*Contraindicated* in hepatic dysfunction, cerebrovascular disease, thromboembolic disease, breast cancer, missed abortion, undiagnosed vaginal bleeding, and pregnancy May cause edema, menstrual irregularities, changes in weight, and mental depression May cause thromboembolic or cardiovascular disease, particularly in women who smoke cigarettes heavily	Monitor for fluid retention Monitor for menstrual irregularities Monitor for visual changes Monitor for thromboembolic effects
Progesterone Colprosterone Gesterol Lingusorbs Lipo-Lutin Lucorteum Luteinol Lutocylin Lutromone Membrettes Nalutron Progestasert Progesterol Progestilin Progestin Proluton Syngesterone Syngestrets	Amenorrhea Functional (abnormal) uterine bleeding caused by hormonal imbalance in the absence of organic pathologic condition (e.g., uterine cancer) Conception control	*Adults:* 5-10 mg/24 hr IM for 6-8 days *Adults:* 5-10 mg/24 hr IM for 6 days, *or* single IM dose of 50-100 mg *Adults:* Insert (replace) 1 Progestasert system into the uterine cavity once each year	Injectable: 25, 50, 100 mg/ml (available in both aqueous and oil injectable forms) Store between 15° and 30° C Progestasert: contains 38 mg of progesterone and releases approximately 65 µg/24 hr for 1 year	*Contraindicated* in hypersensitivity, hepatic dysfunction, thromboembolic disease, breast cancer; undiagnosed vaginal bleeding and missed abortion Progestasert is also *contraindicated* in pregnancy, previous pelvic surgery, and previous ectopic pregnancy May cause edema, menstrual irregularities, changes in weight, and mental depression May cause masculinization of the female fetus	Monitor for visual changes Monitor blood pressure Observe breast and pelvic organs periodically for signs of cancer (e.g., periodic Pap smear) Observe for thromboembolic complications Observe for edema

Adverse effects from progesterone are generally mild and uncommon

May cause pain or irritation at the IM injection site

The Progestasert system may cause local inflammatory reactions and perforation of the cervix or uterus

Insertion of the Progestasert may be accompanied by severe pain, bradycardia, and syncope

---

★ **Quinestrol**
Estrovis

Female hypogonadism
Menopausal symptoms
Ovariectomy
Primary ovarian failure

Adults: 100 µg/24 hr for 7 days, followed by a 7-day rest period
Maintenance: 100–200 µg/week PO
NOTE: Dosage is in *micrograms*

Tablet: 100 µg

Contraindicated in hepatic dysfunction, breast cancer; pregnancy, cerebrovascular disease, thromboembolic disease, endometrial hyperplasia, and undiagnosed vaginal bleeding

May cause fluid retention and GI distress

A Pap smear should be taken from female patients *before* initiating therapy

Metabolized to ethinyl estradiol

Monitor blood pressure
Observe breast and pelvic organs periodically for signs of cancer (e.g., periodic Pap smear)
Observe for thromboembolic complications
Observe for edema
Observe for nausea and other GI distress

Tamoxifen
Nolvadex

Palliative treatment of advanced inoperable breast cancer in postmenopausal women

Adults: 10–20 mg PO b.i.d., AM and PM

Tablet: 10 mg
Store tablets protected from heat and light

Contraindicated in hypersensitivity and pregnancy

Commonly causes hot flashes, nausea, and vomiting

May cause visual changes, particularly with long-term, high-dose therapy

Bone pain requiring the use of analgesics may occur

Monitor serum calcium
Monitor for visual changes, particularly with long-term, high-dose therapy
Monitor for hot flashes, nausea, and vomiting
Observe for bone pain

BIBLIOGRAPHY

Aladin, F. Interactions with oral contraceptives. *On Continuing Practice,* 1983, *10*(1), 19-21.

Dickerson, J. The pill, a closer look. *American Journal of Nursing,* 1983, *83*(10), 1392-1398.

DiRaimondo, C.V., et al. Gynecomastia from exposure to vaginal estrogen cream. *New England Journal of Medicine,* 1980, *302,* 1089.

Drug interactions with low dose OCs may increase the risk of pregnancy. *Reactions,* 1980, July, Number 13, 1.

Iazzetta, J. Low-dose oral contraceptives. *On Continuing Practice,* 1980, *7*(4), 11-12.

Kennedy, D.L.C. Estrogens and endometrial cancer. *Drug Intelligence and Clinical Pharmacy,* 1980, *14,* 406-411.

Malkasian, G.D. Exogenous estrogens: a continuing controversy. *Geriatrics,* 1982, *37*(3), 79-88.

Maser, J. Triphasic oral contraceptives. *On Continuing Practice,* 1983, *10*(2), 7-9.

Redmond, M.A. Couple-directed contraceptive counseling. *The Canadian Nurse,* 1982, *78*(8), 38-39.

Sands, C.D., Robinson, J.D., & Orlando, J.B. The oral contraceptive PPI: its effect on patient knowledge, feelings and behavior. *Drug Intelligence and Clinical Pharmacy,* 1984, *18,* 730-735.

Stadel, B.V. Oral contraceptives and cardiovascular disease. *The New England Journal of Medicine,* 1981, *305*(11), 612-618.

Stockley, I.H. Antibiotics and oral contraceptive failure: an update. *The Pharmaceutical Journal,* 1982, November 6, 525-528.

Tartrazine proves a yellow hazard to sensitive patients. *Reactions,* 1980, Number 13, 1-2.

Two triphasic oral contraceptives now marketed. *Clinical Pharmacy,* 1984, *3,* 342-343.

Weinstein, M.C. Estrogen use in postmenopausal women—costs, risks, and benefits. *The New England Journal of Medicine,* 1980, *303*(6), 308-316.

CHAPTER 64

Androgens and Anabolic Steroids

Louis A. Pagliaro

Ann M. Pagliaro

Medications discussed in this chapter

Androgens
  Danazol
  Methyltestosterone
  Testosterone
Anabolic steroids
  Dromostanolone
  Ethylestrenol
  Fluoxymesterone

Anabolic steroids—cont'd
  Methandriol
  Nandrolone
  Oxandrolone
  Oxymetholone
  Stanozolol
  Testolactone

This chapter discusses the male sex hormones, or androgens, and the closely related compounds known as anabolic steroids. Both groups of drugs possess androgenic and anabolic activity. The major difference between the two groups is in the relative proportion of activity they possess. The androgens possess relatively equal amounts of androgenic and anabolic activity, whereas anabolic steroids possess relatively more anabolic than androgenic activity. Because of their closely related spectrum of activity, these two groups of drugs share many similarities in their indications for use and in their adverse side effects.

ANDROGENS

Androgens are hormones naturally produced by the testes, ovaries, and adrenal cortex. They are necessary for the development of male sexual organs and play a role in producing a positive anabolic effect. Androgens are also responsible for the development of secondary male sex characteristics, including enlargement of the larynx, growth of facial and body hair, lowering of the pitch (deepening) of the voice, recession of hair growth at the temples and baldness, and skeletal muscle formation, particularly affecting the shoulder area. Whether androgens directly contribute to male aggressiveness has not yet been clearly established.

In addition, androgens are responsible for the higher hematocrit normally found in men as compared with women. This is because of a direct stimulation of erythrocyte production caused by the androgens. This stimulation is primarily mediated by means of enhanced renal production of erythropoietic stimulating factor (ESF), also known as erythropoietin.

Indications

Androgens are used primarily to treat males who are unable to produce enough endogenous testosterone on their own (e.g., to treat hypogonadal or eunuchoid conditions). Natural and synthetic androgens have been developed and used to treat androgen-responsive, inoperable, metastatic breast cancer in postmenopausal women. Other uses in women include the treatment of endometriosis, the treatment of postpartum breast engorgement and pain in women who do *not* intend to breastfeed their infants, and as adjunctive therapy in the treatment of osteoporosis in postmenopausal women.

Androgens have been used by athletes, primarily male athletes, to increase muscle size and strength. Although muscle size may increase, if protein intake is sufficient, because of the positive anabolic effect of the androgens, there is *no* well-controlled evidence of any increased strength. Indeed, it appears that if the male athlete were to increase protein intake in conjunction with an active strenuous workout program, the same increase in strength often attributed to the androgens would occur even in the absence of the exogenous androgens. This has clinical significance because the use of androgens is associated with toxicity and thus needless use is unwarranted. These comments also apply to the use of anabolic steroids by athletes.

Administration, absorption, and elimination

The androgens are available in both oral and parenteral forms. A pellet form for subcutaneous implantation is also available. The selection of the dosage form depends on the indication for use, the length of therapy, and patient compliance (e.g., for some patients requiring long-term therapy compliance may be increased significantly by using once-monthly injections or subcutaneous implantation).

It should be noted that although testosterone is well absorbed from the gastrointestinal tract, it is rapidly inactivated when administered by the oral route. Thus, testosterone is only available for therapeutic use in parenteral or subcutaneous pellet implantation forms.

Androgens are highly protein bound and are metabolized to inactive metabolites primarily in the liver. The urine is the main route of elimination of these metabolites from the body.

Toxicity

The use of androgens in women can cause varying degrees of masculinization, including deepening of the voice, growth of body and facial hair, menstrual irregularities, and a receding hairline. Other noted effects include acne and sodium retention (with resultant edema).

The use of androgens in prepubertal boys, such as for the treatment of hypogonadism, may result in priapism, acne, and sodium retention. The priapism generally resolves itself with continued use; however, dose reduction may be necessary. Secondary sexual characteristics also develop; however, these are generally desired consequences of therapy. Because premature epiphyseal closure may occur, these patients should be monitored closely for any interference with normal growth (see General Nursing Implications).

In addition, because male athletes often take the androgens at several times the physiologic dose for extended periods of time, endogenous testosterone production may be suppressed or stopped completely and some of the excess exogenous testosterone may be converted to a female sex hormone such as estradiol (see Figure 63-1). The end result of these effects is that the testicles of these male athletes, because of estradiol production, may atrophy with a resultant decrease in sperm counts and a decrease in libido. Gynecomastia, caused by the production of the female sex hormones, may also occur under these circumstances.

The androgens that contain a chemical group (substitution) in the 17-alpha position (Figure 64-1) (e.g., danazol, methyltestosterone), can cause various adverse hepatic effects, including interference with hepatic function tests (e.g., decreased sulfobromophthalein elimination), cholestatic jaundice, and hepatic adenocarcinoma (particularly with prolonged administration over 1 to 7 years).

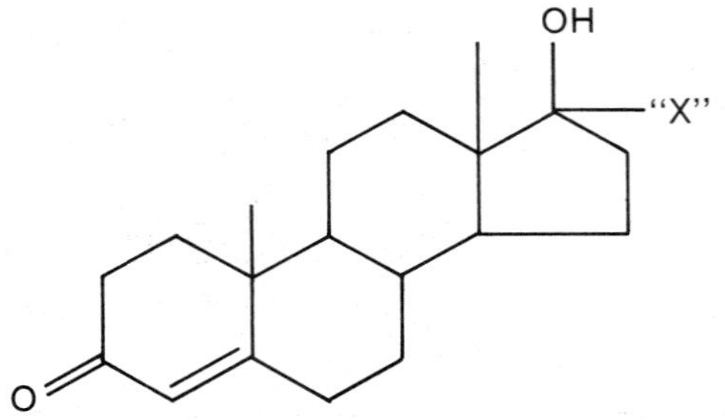

FIGURE 64-1. **General chemical structure of the androgens and the anabolic steroids. The "X" group indicates the location of 17-alpha substitution. Androgens and anabolic steroids with a chemical substitution in this position are more likely to be associated with hepatic toxicity.**

ANABOLIC STEROIDS

The anabolic steroids closely resemble the androgens not only in chemical structure, but also in terms of their actions, administration, absorption, and toxicity. Thus, the general comments previously made about the androgens also apply to the anabolic steroids, *except* that these agents generally possess a relatively stronger anabolic activity and a relatively weaker androgenic activity. Therefore, the anabolic steroids are not indicated for treating hypogonadal function in males, but are indicated for treating various conditions in which a positive anabolic effect is desired.

The anabolic steroids stimulate general body growth by promoting a positive nitrogen balance and calcium retention with a resultant increase in muscle mass, a stimulation of skeletal growth, and an acceleration of epiphyseal closure. They also stimulate erythropoiesis.

The weight gain, perception of well-being or strength, and increase in muscle mass* associated with the use of anabolic steroids, as well as their weaker androgenic effect in comparison with the androgens, have contributed to the high incidence of use or abuse of these agents by both amateur and professional athletes. This widespread use has been uniformly condemned by numerous sports associations; however, the high degree of competition in sports has led many athletes and coaches to continue to use anabolic steroids.

Short-term use has been associated with several adverse effects, including acne, baldness, clitoral enlargement in females, deepening of the voice, edema,

---

*There is considerable evidence to suggest that much of the weight gain associated with the use of anabolic steroids is caused by fluid retention and not by increased muscle mass.

and gynecomastia in males. These short-term adverse effects are usually reversible on the discontinuation of the drug; however, some of these effects, such as clitoral enlargement in females may be irreversible. Long-term use has been associated with additional adverse effects, including hepatitis and hepatic carcinoma. Both of these conditions are potentially fatal and the use of anabolic steroids has been definitely linked to a number of deaths. It appears that these adverse effects can also occur with short-term use in susceptible individuals.

Because anabolic steroids have not been clearly demonstrated to have a positive effect on athletic performance in males except perhaps for a possible psychologic effect, and because the toxicity of these agents has been clearly demonstrated, the use of anabolic steroids to improve athletic performance is *not* recommended (see also the related discussion in the section on androgens).

Because all of the anabolic steroids possess varying degrees of androgenic activity, their use can result in the masculinization of women, fetuses, and children. In addition, their use in children can result in dimin-

ished height because of a premature closing of the epiphyses.

SUMMARY

The various androgens and anabolic steroids have been discussed. These agents are used to treat hypogonadal function in the male and for their positive anabolic effects in both males and females. The androgens are also used in women to treat various androgen-responsive conditions (e.g., endometriosis). A widespread use of the androgens and anabolic steroids involves a desired increase in performance by male athletes. This action of these agents has not been substantiated, and the use of the androgens and the anabolic steroids for this purpose is *not* recommended.

With an understanding of these various agents, including their indications for use, contraindications, cautions, administration, drug interactions, and monitoring, the nurse will be able to provide optimal therapy and assistance to patients who require these medications.

ADVERSE/SIDE EFFECTS OF THE ANDROGENS AND ANABOLIC STEROIDS*

CARDIOVASCULAR SYSTEM

Edema
Elevated blood pressure

CENTRAL NERVOUS SYSTEM

Chills
Dizziness
Excitation
Fatigue
Headache
Irritability
Lethargy
Mental depression
Paresthesias
Sleep disorders
Tremor
Visual disturbances

ENDOCRINE SYSTEM

Decrease in breast size
Decreased ejaculatory volume
Epididymitis
Gynecomastia
Hypercalcemia
Impotence
Male-pattern baldness

Oligospermia
Prepubertal male phallic enlargement
Testicular atrophy
Menstrual irregularities (postpubertal females)

Androgenic effects

(Virilization postpubertal women—both androgens and anabolic steroids)
Acne
Clitoral enlargement
Changes in libido
Emotional lability
Flushing
Hirsutism
Hoarseness
Hypoestrogenic effects
Nervousness
Oiliness of skin or hair
Sweating
Vaginitis (itching, dryness, burning, vaginal bleeding)

GASTROINTESTINAL SYSTEM

Change in appetite
Constipation
Diarrhea

Gastric irritation
Nausea
Vomiting

HEPATIC SYSTEM

Cholestatic jaundice
Hepatic adenocarcinoma (prolonged high-dose therapy with 17-alpha substituted androgens)
Hepatic hypertrophy
Hepatitis

MUSCULOSKELETAL SYSTEM

Muscle cramps
Muscle spasms
Prepubertal premature epiphyseal closure in boys

URINARY SYSTEM

Bladder irritability (anabolic steroids)
Hematuria (androgens)
Urinary obstruction

MISCELLANEOUS EFFECTS

Steroid fever

*See Chapter 11, "Drug Toxicity," for an overview of drug toxicity.

CLINICALLY SIGNIFICANT DRUG INTERACTIONS*

Primary drug	Interacting drug	Possible effect(s)	Probable mechanism(s)
Danazol	Oral anticoagulants	Increased anticoagulant effect	Not yet clearly established
Oxymetholone	Oral anticoagulants	Increased anticoagulant effect	Not yet clearly established
Methyltestosterone	Oral anticoagulants	Increased anticoagulant effect	Not yet clearly established

*See Chapter 10, "Drug Interactions," for an overview of drug interactions.

GENERAL NURSING IMPLICATIONS

Nursing of patients requiring androgens or anabolic steroids

ASSESSMENT

Androgens are used for a variety of conditions, including the treatment of endometriosis, fibrocystic breast disease, hypogonadism (delayed puberty), impotence caused by testicular deficiency, palliation of breast cancer in women 1 to 5 years postmenopause, postpartum breast engorgement of non-breastfeeding mothers, eunuchoidism and eunuchism, male climacteric symptoms, and postpubertal cryptorchidism. Anabolic steroids are sometimes used to treat catabolic effects resulting from corticosteroid therapy (see Chapter 65, "Corticosteroids and Adrenal Steroid Inhibitors"), to treat severe maturational delay when growth hormone is unavailable, to promote weight gain, and to combat tissue depletion. Both androgens and anabolic steroids have been used to treat osteoporosis, anemias, and debilitated states. The baseline assessment data should include specific information about the patient's general health state and the need for androgen or anabolic steroid therapy. The baseline data are particularly important in monitoring the individual patient's response to drug therapy. For example, quantitative urinary and serum calcium level determinations before and during therapy are indicated for patients prone to hypercalcemia (e.g., patients with metastatic breast cancer).

Androgen or anabolic steroid therapy should be preceded by a roentgenogram examination of the wristbone to establish the level of bone maturation in children, because bone maturation may proceed more rapidly than linear growth during treatment, requiring intermittent therapy and periodic roentgenologic examinations.

The nursing assessment should also include a sexual history. Urogenital assessment should include identification of the presence or history of any urogenital anomaly, mass, infection, previous urogenital surgery, or sexually transmitted disease. Baseline assessment of genital development and secondary sex characteristics is indicated in patients with an androgenic deficiency. Baseline assessment of the breasts in postpartum mothers requiring lactation suppression should be completed.

The initial assessment should include information regarding a history of diabetes or the use of anticoagulants, because these conditions can be affected by the use of androgens. Serum cholesterol levels should be determined and monitored in patients with a history of coronary artery disease. In addition, anabolic steroids can alter many laboratory studies during therapy and for 2 to 3 weeks after therapy is discontinued. The assessment should include a detailed drug history before initiating the therapy to identify any possible hypersensitivity to specific agents, contraindications, cautions, drug interactions, and drug-taking patterns.

SENSITIVITY

Generally, allergic reactions to androgens and anabolic steroids are rare. However, it is important to note that any drug has the potential to cause a hypersensitivity reaction in susceptible individuals. Patients should be carefully questioned regarding sensitivity during the drug history and before the administration of these drugs.

CONTRAINDICATIONS

The use of individual androgens or anabolic steroids is contraindicated in patients with a known hypersensitivity to a particular agent.

In addition, androgens and anabolic steroids are contraindicated in patients with carcinoma of the male breast; conditions aggravated by fluid retention (e.g., heart failure, hypertension, renal disease); impaired renal, hepatic, or cardiac function; hypercalcemia; hypertension; prostatic cancer; prostatic hypertrophy with obstruction; and undiagnosed abnormal genital bleeding.

In addition, the androgens are contraindicated in pregnancy (because masculinization of the female fetus can occur) and in elderly asthenic men who may react adversely to androgen overstimulation.

Androgens and anabolic steroids are contraindicated in premature infants and neonates.

See the Nursing Drug Digest for specific information regarding the contraindications to each agent.

CAUTIONS

Androgens should be used cautiously in patients who have a history of coronary artery disease (including myocardial infarction), epilepsy, or migraine headaches.

Androgens should be used with caution in prepubertal boys.

Anabolic steroids should be used cautiously in prepubertal boys, patients with diabetes, patients with a history of coronary artery disease, including myocardial infarction and arteriosclerosis, because serum cholesterol levels can be increased, and patients receiving anticoagulants, antidiabetics, or corticosteroids.

Nursing of patients requiring androgens or anabolic steroids—cont'd

CAUTIONS—cont'd

Anabolic steroids may alter laboratory studies during therapy and for 2 to 3 weeks after the therapy is stopped.

See the Nursing Drug Digest for cautions associated with each individual agent.

DRUG INTERACTIONS

Anabolic steroids can interact with anticoagulants. Patients receiving concurrent anticoagulant therapy should be carefully monitored for increased prothrombin time and potential hemorrhagic complications.

See Clinically Significant Drug Interactions, for specific interactions associated with individual agents.

ADMINISTRATION

The various androgens and anabolic steroids discussed in this chapter are available for administration by the oral, buccal, intramuscular, and subcutaneous pellet routes. Not all are available for administration in these forms, and special attention should be paid to the specific route of administration of each drug. It should be noted that various combination products are also available, including preparations containing other hormones.

Oral

Oral preparations generally should be taken with a full glass of water either before or with meals to minimize gastrointestinal distress or irritation.

Buccal

The buccal tablet should be placed in the pouch of the cheek, a different area used for each dose, and the patient should be encouraged to avoid swallowing until the medication taste disappears. Smoking, eating, or drinking should also be avoided immediately after the administration of the buccal preparation. Oral hygiene is important and should be encouraged to decrease the possibility of irritation from the buccal tablet.

Intramuscular

Preparations for intramuscular administration should be injected deeply into the gluteal muscle in adults.

Pellet implantation

Pellet implantation is usually completed by the physician and is a minor surgical procedure. It is important to monitor patients for irritation and sloughing at the site of implantation.

See the Nursing Drug Digest for specific information regarding the dosage and administration of specific agents.

MONITORING PATIENT RESPONSE

Therapeutic response

The onset and duration of therapy depend largely on the specific agent, the dosage form, the route of administration, and on individual patient factors, including the type of condition being treated.

The duration of action depends on the dosage form and the vehicle. Nandrolone decanoate, when administered intramuscularly, has a 3- to 4-week duration, whereas nandrolone phenpropionate after intramuscular injection has a 1- to 2-week duration. Whereas testosterone proprionate has a 2- to 3-day duration, testosterone cypronate and enanthate have a duration of 4 weeks. Subcutaneous implants of testosterone pellets have a prolonged duration of 3-6 months. Generally, patients should be monitored during therapy for the desired therapeutic effect as related to the baseline assessment data associated with the indication for androgen or anabolic steroid therapy. The onset of effects for the androgens and anabolic steroids is often difficult to determine because individual response varies in relation to specific patient variables and the condition being treated. For example, the therapeutic response in patients with breast cancer is usually apparent within 3 months. It may also take up to 3 months for hematologic and other objective responses to be noted. The therapy should be discontinued if signs of disease progression are noted.

Androgens

Androgen-deficient males should be monitored for their response associated with the presenting condition, such as hypogonadism, gonadotropin deficiencies (e.g., eunuchoidism), oligospermia, or impotence, as indicated. Non-breastfeeding mothers should be monitored for the prevention of postpartum breast pain and engorgement.

Anabolic steroids

Monitor for anabolic effects, including the reversal of tissue-depleting processes, tissue building, and weight gain.

The duration of action and the therapeutic response vary as with the androgens. For example, oxymetholone, when administered for the treatment of anemia, requires 3 to 6 months for a response to occur. The response when oxymetholone is administered for osteoporosis is usually observed in 4 to 6 weeks.

Monitor patients who are underweight because of predisposing catabolic states for weight gain. It is important to note that the provision of an adequate dietary regimen is required to maximize the anabolic effect of these agents.

Anabolic steroids may be effective in senile and postmenopausal osteoporosis and in refractory anemias associated with chronic disease. Monitor laboratory blood work.

Adverse side effects

Adverse side effects are affected by both the age and the sex of the patient, and monitoring these effects is extremely important in relation to managing the therapeutic regimen. Monitor female patients receiving either androgen or anabolic steroid therapy for virilization, especially when large doses are administered for prolonged periods.

Women receiving anabolic steroid therapy should be monitored carefully for menstrual irregularities, and, if observed, the therapy should be discontinued.

It is important to monitor prepubertal boys (i.e., younger than 7 years of age) for precocious development of male sexual characteristics. Children should have a periodic roentgenologic examination of bone growth during therapy because bone maturation may proceed more rapidly than linear growth.

Monitor patients receiving anticoagulant therapy who are also receiving androgens for the following signs indi-

Continued.

Nursing of patients requiring androgens or anabolic steroids—cont'd

Adverse side effects—cont'd

cating increased anticoagulant effects: ecchymotic areas, increased prothrombin time, petechiae, and unusual bleeding.

Monitor diabetic patients for symptoms of hypoglycemia. The dosage of the antidiabetic drug may require adjustment because androgens and anabolic steroids can enhance hypoglycemia. Anabolic steroids can lower the fasting blood sugar (FBS) in both diabetic and nondiabetic patients. Monitor patients receiving anabolic steroids for the development of edema and weight gain associated with these agents. It is important to weigh patients routinely. A sodium-restricted diet or diuretics may be indicated during therapy.

Monitor for symptoms of jaundice, including yellowing of the skin or eyes and darkening of the urine. Dose adjustment may reverse these symptoms when observed. Periodic liver function tests are recommended for patients receiving either androgens or anabolic steroids.

Monitor male patients for priapism, reports of reduced ejaculatory volume, and gynecomastia, because these symptoms indicate that the drug should be withdrawn.

See Adverse/Side Effects of the Androgens and Anabolic Steroids for an outline of the general adverse side effects associated with the use of these agents, as well as the Nursing Drug Digest for each specific agent.

PATIENT EDUCATION

The patient and the family, as indicated, should have a clear understanding of the indication for the androgen or anabolic steroid therapy and the anticipated course of therapy. They should know the exact name of the medication, its dosage, action, storage, administration, adverse side effects, and how these effects can be monitored and minimized. They should be able to monitor for the therapeutic response and be able to recognize symptoms that indicate the health care provider should be notified.

Patients responsible for drug therapy at home must understand the importance of following the medication plan as prescribed and the need to take the medication exactly as indicated. The importance of follow-up cannot be overemphasized, nor can the danger of sharing or giving these medications to anyone else. The use of anabolic steroids has erroneously been thought to enhance athletic ability in males. The nurse has an important role in increasing patient understanding regarding the proper use of these preparations.

Androgens

Women receiving long-term androgen therapy should understand the importance of monitoring their menstrual cycle and be taught to report any menstrual irregularity, because this is indicative that the drug should be discontinued. The patient should also understand that virilization effects may not be reversible on discontinuing the drug.

Emotional support is important during teaching sessions and during therapy. The patient should be taught to report any androgenic effects immediately, because the discontinuation of the drug can prevent further changes. Women should be taught to prevent the risk of vaginitis by wearing cotton underwear and by showering or bathing after intercourse.

Children requiring androgen therapy (and their parents) should be carefully prepared for the precocious development of secondary sex characteristics associated with the use of these agents. They should also be informed of the importance of monitoring bone growth during therapy.

Women requiring androgen therapy for postpartum suppression of lactation should be taught measures to promote postpartum breast comfort and to enhance drug response. These measures include the reduction of nipple stimulation (the breasts should be gently washed once daily during the bath with tepid water and gently patted dry with a soft towel or exposed to the air; avoidance of artificial emptying of the breasts, wearing a bra that provides adequate support), relaxation, ensurance of adequate nutritional intake, restriction of fluids late in the evening and the avoidance of warm fluids during engorgement, delay of sexual intercourse for at least 3 weeks postpartum when lactation should be completely suppressed, and the administration of oral lactation suppressants in the evening (when indicated).

Anabolic steroids

Patients should understand how to monitor for edema associated with anabolic steroid therapy. They should understand other aspects of therapy, as indicated, such as a sodium-restricted diet or the use of diuretics. They should carefully monitor their weight and look for rapid weight gain associated with water retention as opposed to the weight gain caused by the anabolic effects of the drug.

Patients should also be taught to recognize the signs of jaundice, including yellowing of the skin or the eyes, or darkening of the urine, that may indicate untoward drug effects on the liver. They should understand the importance of periodic liver function tests as recommended and the need for follow-up to monitor their response.

Diabetic patients need to be taught to monitor for signs of hypoglycemia, because the various androgens can enhance this effect. When noted, hypoglycemia should be reported immediately to the health care provider so that changes in therapy can be made as indicated.

Because of the various available forms of medication, it is particularly important that patients understand the administration and care of their specific medication. It is important to note that buccal tablets of methyltestosterone, for example, are twice as potent as oral tablets. Patients should also understand the importance of not eating, drinking, chewing, or smoking while the buccal tablet is in place to enhance the absorption of the medication. They should understand that buccal tablets are *not* to be swallowed and may take up to 1 hour to dissolve. Patients receiving buccal tablets should be taught to change or rotate the site of placement with each dose to enhance drug absorption and to minimize buccal irritation.

GENERAL INSTRUCTIONS FOR DISCHARGE/OUTPATIENTS

ANDROGENS AND ANABOLIC STEROIDS

This drug is a hormone used to treat various conditions. If you do not understand why you need this medication, check with your health care provider.

Take this medication exactly as prescribed. If you have any questions about how this medication should be taken, check with your health care provider.

This medication can cause stomach upset in some people. It is helpful to take this medication after meals or with a snack to prevent stomach upset.

If you are pregnant, breastfeeding an infant, or considering pregnancy, check with your health care provider before taking this medication, because this medication can cause unwanted effects in unborn babies or nursing infants.

Some medications can cause some unwanted effects in some people. Notify your health care provider if you notice unusual loss of scalp hair or increased facial hair; blood in your urine; blurred vision; dark-colored urine; edema or swelling of your hands, legs, or ankles; unusual weight gain; hoarseness or deepening of the voice; severe vomiting; unusual restlessness; vaginal itching, dryness, burning, or unusual bleeding; or a yellow color to your skin or eyes.

If you have diabetes, this medication may affect your blood sugar levels. Check your urine glucose regularly and report any abnormal results to your health care provider.

Notify your dentist or other health care providers that you are taking this medication.

This medication has been prescribed especially for you. Do not trade or give this medication to anyone else.

Keep this medication and all other medications *out of the reach of children.*

In addition to these general instructions, if you are taking *methyltestosterone buccal tablets*, place the tablet in the pouch of the cheek and let the tablet dissolve. Do *not* swallow until the tablet has dissolved and the taste of the drug has disappeared. Avoid eating, drinking, or smoking immediately after using the tablet. Change the place in the cheek where you place the tablet with each dose.

If you are taking oral tablets, swallow the tablet whole. Do not crush, chew, or break the tablet into pieces. Take the tablet with a full glass of water.

NURSING DRUG DIGEST

Medication (trade name*)	Indication	Usual dosage and administration	Dosage forms, preparation, and storage	Contraindications, cautions, and comments	Monitoring
Danazol Cyclomen Danocrine	Endometriosis	*Adults:* 200-800 mg/24 hr PO in 2 divided doses for 3-9 months	Capsules: 50, 100, 200 mg	*Contraindicated* in severe cardiac, hepatic, or renal impairment	Monitor for signs of virilization Observe for fluid retention
	Fibrocystic breast disease	*Adults:* 100-400 mg/24 hr PO in 2 divided doses for up to 6 months		*Contraindicated* in abnormal, undiagnosed genital bleeding and in carcinoma of the breast	
	Hereditary angioneurotic edema	*Adults:* 200 mg PO q.d. to t.i.d. Decrease dose in renal failure For women it is recommended to initiate the dosage during menstruation to ensure that the patient is *not* pregnant		May cause fluid retention Acne, edema, flushing, increased hair growth, and weight gain are common Administration during pregnancy may cause virilization of the fetus May cause menstrual irregularities	
★ **Dromostanolone** Drolban Masterone Masterid Masteril	Palliative treatment of postmenopausal women with advanced, androgen-responsive, inoperable, metastatic breast cancer	*Adults:* 100 mg IM 3 times/week	Injectable: 50 mg/ml Store below 40° C Do *not* freeze Do *not* refrigerate Protect from light	*Contraindicated* in nephrosis; severe cardiac, hepatic, or renal dysfunction; men with carcinoma; women with androgen-*non*-responsive operable breast cancer; and premenopausal women May cause virilization, change in libido, and edema Androgenic effects are significantly less than those associated with testosterone	Monitor for virilization Monitor liver function tests Observe for fluid retention Observe for menstrual irregularities

Drug	Uses	Dosage	Preparations/Storage	Contraindications/Precautions	Nursing Considerations
Ethylestrenol Maxibolin	Anabolic effect	*Adults:* 0.1 mg/kg/24 hr PO (usual adult dose is 4 mg/24 hr) for 6 weeks followed by 4 weeks *off* of drug *Children:* Same as adult (usual children's dose is 2 mg/24 hr)	Tablet: 2 mg Elixir: 2 mg/5 ml (10% alcohol)	*Contraindicated* in severe cardiac, hepatic, or renal dysfunction; men with carcinoma; and women with androgen-*non*responsive operable breast cancer May cause virilization, change in libido, and edema	Observe for fluid retention Observe for virilization Observe for menstrual irregularities Monitor bone growth in children
Fluoxymesterone Android-F Halodrin* Halotestin Oratestin Ora-Testryl Ultandren	Anabolic effect Androgen deficiency Delayed puberty in boys Palliative treatment of postmenopausal women with advanced, androgen-responsive, inoperable, metastatic breast cancer Postpartum breast pain and engorgement	*Adults:* 5-10 mg/24 hr PO *Adults:* 2-10 mg/24 hr PO *Adults:* 5-10 mg PO t.i.d. *Adults:* 2.5 mg PO at start of active labor; then 5-10 mg/24 hr PO for 3-5 days postpartum Administration with food or milk may decrease GI distress	Tablets: 2, 5, 10 mg Store between 15° and 30° C Protect from light	*Contraindicated* in nephrosis, hypersensitivity, men with carcinoma, women with androgen-*non*responsive operable breast cancer, and pregnancy May cause virilization, change in libido, and edema	Monitor for hypercalcemia, particularly in women with disseminated breast cancer Monitor for virilization Observe for menstrual irregularities Observe for fluid retention Monitor bone growth in boys treated for delayed puberty
★ **Methandriol** Cellubolic Cytobolin Methostan Stenediol	*Adjunctive* therapy in osteoporosis (senile and postmenopausal) (possibly effective—use is *not* recommended)	*Adults:* 10-40 mg (aqueous preparation) IM/24 hr, or 50-100 mg (oil preparation) IM 1-2 times/week Administer *IM* only	Injectable: 50 mg/ml (both aqueous and oil forms)	*Contraindicated* in hypersensitivity; severe cardiac, hepatic, or renal impairment; and carcinoma of the prostate or breast Proper diet, calcium balance, activity, and vitamin D are probably of *greater* value in treating osteoporosis than the use of methandriol May cause virilization, change in libido, and edema	Monitor serum calcium levels Observe for fluid retention Monitor for virilization

Continued.

NOTE: For additional details regarding the individual agents listed in this table, see the text and other tables in this chapter.
*Indicates a multiple active ingredient product. For a complete listing of all active ingredients see the *Drug Reference Guide to Brand Names and Active Ingredients.*
★Indicates that the drug is generally available only in the United States.

NURSING DRUG DIGEST—cont'd

Medication (trade name)	Indication	Usual dosage and administration	Dosage forms, preparation, and storage	Contraindications, cautions, and comments	Monitoring
Methyltestosterone Android Destrilin with Methyltestosterone* Formatrix* Gynetone* Mediatric* Metandren Neo-Hombreol Metandren Oraviron Orchiste-rone-M Oreton Methyl Premarin with Methyltestosterone* Synandrets Synandrotabs Testaform Testora Testred Virilon	Postpartum breast pain and engorgement Male hypogonadism, eunuchoidism Female breast cancer	*Adults:* 10 mg q.i.d. SL for 3-5 days, *or* 20 mg q.i.d. PO for 3-5 days *Postpubertal:* 5 mg q.d. to q.i.d. SL, *or* 10 mg q.d. to q.i.d. PO Between 1-5 years postmenopausal: Initial, 25 mg q.i.d. SL for 2-4 weeks *or* 50 mg q.i.d. PO for 2-4 weeks Maintenance, half the initial dose if response was obtained NOTE: Dosage must be *individualized* Administration with food or milk may decrease GI distress Sublingual tablets must be allowed to dissolve in the oral cavity and should *not* be swallowed whole	Tablets: 10, 25 mg Sublingual (buccal) tablets: 5, 10, 25 mg Capsules: 10 mg Store in tight, light-resistant containers	*Contraindicated* in severe cardiac, hepatic, or renal dysfunction *Contraindicated* in hypersensitivity, prostatic carcinoma, prepubertal boys, and pregnancy May cause virilization, change in libido, and edema More likely than testosterone to cause liver damage (jaundice) The buccal (or sublingual) tablets are approximately *twice* as potent as the oral tablets	Monitor liver function tests Observe for virilization (in women—deepening of voice, hirsutism, acne, enlargement of clitoris, menstrual irregularities) Observe for fluid retention Monitor for hypercalcemia, particularly in patients with breast cancer
Nandrolone Deca-Durabolin Durabolin Kabolin Nandrobolic LA	Anabolic effect, *adjunctive* therapy in senile and postmenopausal osteoporosis Palliative treatment of postmenopausal women with advanced, androgen-responsive, inoperable, metastatic breast cancer	*Adults:* 50-100 mg (decanoate salt) IM q.3-4 weeks (for up to 12 weeks followed by a 4-week period off the drug *Adults:* 25-100 mg IM/week (phenpropionate salt) Administer deeply into gluteal muscle Administer *IM* only	Injectable: 50, 100, 200 mg/ml (nandrolone decanoate); 25, 50 mg/ml (nandrolone phenpropionate) Store between 15° and 30° C Do *not* freeze	*Contraindicated* in severe cardiac, hepatic, or renal dysfunction, men with carcinoma, and women with androgen-*nonresponsive*, operable breast cancer May cause virilization, change in libido, and edema	Observe for fluid retention Observe for virilization Observe for menstrual irregularities Monitor for hypercalcemia, particularly in patients with breast cancer Observe IM injection site for irritation

Drug		Dosage	Preparations	Remarks	Nursing considerations
★ **Oxandrolone** Anavar Lonavar Protivar Vasorome Kowa	Anabolic effect, *adjunctive therapy* in osteoporosis	*Adults:* 2.5 mg PO b.i.d.-q.i.d. *Children:* 0.25 mg/kg/24 hr PO Decrease dose in renal impairment	Tablet: 2.5 mg	*Contraindicated* in severe cardiac, hepatic, or renal dysfunction, pregnancy, hypercalcemia, and carcinoma of the prostate or breast May cause virilization, change in libido, and edema May help relieve bone pain and restore weight gain and strength when used as an *adjunct* in the treatment of osteoporosis Oxandrolone does *not* replace other treatments for osteoporosis	Observe for fluid retention Observe for virilization Observe for menstrual irregularities Monitor bone growth in children
Oxymetholone Adroyd Anadrol Anadrol-50 Anadroyd Anapolon 50	Severe refractory anemias caused by deficient red blood cell production	*Adults:* 1-5 mg/kg/24 hr PO until remission (3-6 months) *Children:* Same as adults Dosage may be decreased or stopped following remission (NOTE: In cases of congenital aplastic anemia continuous maintenance therapy may be required) Dosage must be *individualized*	Tablets: 5, 10, 50 mg	*Contraindicated* in hypersensitivity, carcinoma of the prostate or breast, pregnancy, nephrosis, and severe hepatic impairment May cause virilization, change in libido, and edema Dosage recommended for treatment of life-threatening refractory anemia is associated with a definite hepatotoxicity; however, this hepatotoxicity is reversible following the discontinuation of the drug or by decreasing the total daily dose	Observe for virilization Observe for fluid retention Monitor liver function tests Monitor serum iron and iron-binding capacity Monitor serum calcium for hypercalcemia Monitor bone growth in children

Continued.

NURSING DRUG DIGEST—cont'd

Medication (trade name)	Indication	Usual dosage and administration	Dosage forms, preparation, and storage	Contraindications, cautions, and comments	Monitoring
Stanozolol Stromba Winstrol	Anabolic effect, aplastic anemia	*Adults:* 2 mg PO b.i.d.-t.i.d. *Children:* Younger than 6 years of age, 1 mg PO b.i.d.; older than 6 years of age, same as adults Administration with food or milk may decrease GI distress	Tablet: 2 mg	*Contraindicated* in hypersensitivity, prostatic carcinoma, mammary carcinoma, pregnancy, and nephrosis May cause masculinization of the human fetus May cause virilization, change in libido, and edema May cause menstrual irregularities	Observe for virilization Observe for fluid retention Observe for menstrual irregularities Monitor liver function tests Monitor bone growth in children
★ **Testolactone** Fludestrin Teslac	Palliative treatment of postmenopausal women with advanced, androgen-responsive, inoperable, metastatic breast cancer	*Adults:* 250 mg PO q.i.d., *or* 100 mg IM 3 times/week Administer IM by deep injection Decrease dose in renal failure	Tablets: 50, 250 mg Injectable: 100 mg/ml Shake suspension well before drawing up dose Store between 15° and 30° C	*Contraindicated* in men with breast cancer; severe cardiac or renal disease, premenopausal women, and hypercalcemia May cause peripheral neuropathy	Monitor serum calcium levels Observe for numbness or tingling sensation in the extremities

Drug	Indications	Dosage	Remarks	Contraindications	Nursing Implications
Testosterone Andrusol Delatestryl Depo-Testa-diol* Depo-Testos-terone Di-Genik* Duogen* Malogen Malogex Mertestate Orchiste-rone-P Oreton Oreton Pellets Perandren Synandrol F Test-Estrin* Testaval 90/4* Testex Testosteroid Testrone Virosterone	Anabolic effect Eunuchoidism Female metastatic, inoperable breast cancer	*Adults:* 10-25 mg IM daily or every other day; *or* 200-400 mg (cypionate or enanthate salt) IM every 4 weeks; *or* 5-10 mg (propionate salt) IM q.d. *Postpubertal:* 10-50 mg IM 3 times/week; *or* 100-200 mg (cypionate or enanthate salt) IM q.1-4 weeks; *or* 10-25 mg IM (propionate salt) 2-4 times/week *Adults:* 100 mg IM 3 times/week; *or* 200-400 mg IM (cypionate or enanthate salt) every 2-4 weeks; *or* 50-100 mg (propionate salt) IM 3 times/week Administer injectable *IM* only NOTE: Based on *established* PO or IM dosage, pellets may be implanted SC q.3-4 months (usual dosage is 150-450 mg—i.e., 2-6 pellets)	Injectable: Testosterone 25, 50 mg/ml; cypionate salt, 50, 100, 200 mg/ml; enanthate salt, 100, 200 mg/ml; proprionate salt, 25, 50, 100 mg/ml Store at 15°-30° C *Shake* suspension *well* before drawing up dose A wet needle or syringe will turn the enanthate salt cloudy, but does *not* affect potency Pellets for SC implantation: 75 mg	*Contraindicated* in severe cardiac, hepatic, or renal dysfunction *Contraindicated* in hypersensitivity, prostatic carcinoma, prepubertal boys, and pregnancy May cause change in libido, virilization, and edema	Monitor liver function tests Observe for virilization Observe for fluid retention Observe for menstrual irregularities

BIBLIOGRAPHY

Angier, N. The case against steroids. *Discover,* 1983, November, 98-101.

Evens, R.P., & Amerson, A.B. Androgens and erythropoiesis. *Journal of Clinical Pharmacology,* 1974, February-March, 94-101.

Mines, A. Suppressing lactation in the non-nursing mother safely, comfortably and knowledgeably. *The Canadian Nurse,* 1982, *78*(5), 42-46.

Rule out pregnancy before using danazol. *Nurses' Drug Alert,* 1983, *7,* 10.

Smith, M.C. Drugs and sports. *U.S. Pharmacist,* 1977, May, 75-76.

Wentz, A. Adverse effects of danazol in pregnancy. *Annals of Internal Medicine,* 1982, *96,* 672-673.

Corticosteroids and Adrenal Steroid Inhibitors

Louis A. Pagliaro

Ann M. Pagliaro

Medications discussed in this chapter

Corticosteroids
- Amcinonide
- Beclomethasone
- Betamethasone
- Clobetasol
- Clobetasone
- Clocortolone
- Corticotropin
- Cortisone
- Cosyntropin
- Desonide
- Desoximetasone
- Desoxycorticosterone
- Dexamethasone
- Diflorasone
- Fludrocortisone
- Flumethasone
- Flunisolide

Corticosteroids—cont'd
- Fluocinolone
- Fluocinonide
- Fluorometholone
- Fluprednisolone
- Flurandrenolide
- Halcinonide
- Hydrocortisone
- Medrysone
- Methylprednisolone
- Paramethasone
- Prednisolone
- Prednisone
- Triamcinolone

Adrenal steroid inhibitors
- Aminoglutethimide
- Metyrapone
- Mitotane

Corticosteroids are drugs that are derived from or related to a group of naturally occurring hormones produced by the adrenal cortex. These drugs can be conveniently divided, on the basis of their physiologic and pharmacologic actions, into three groups: (1) *glucocorticoids*, (2) *mineralocorticoids*, and (3) mixed glucocorticoid/mineralocorticoids.

The glucocorticoids are primarily involved in carbohydrate, fat, and protein metabolism and possess antiinflammatory and immunosuppressive activities. The major naturally occurring glucocorticoid is hydrocortisone (cortisol).* The mineralocorticoids are primarily involved in regulating fluid and electrolyte balance and extracellular fluid volume. The major naturally occurring mineralocorticoid is aldosterone.

---

*Hydrocortisone also possesses some weak mineralocorticoid activity. For a classification of the various corticosteroids according to activity see the boxed material on p. 1489, right.

Many synthetic compounds structurally related to the natural corticosteroids and possessing glucocorticoid or mineralocorticoid activity have been developed for treating adrenocortical disorders and a variety of other conditions amenable to corticosteroid therapy (see boxes, pp. 1487-1489 for corticosteroid-responsive conditions). A knowledge of the actions, dosage, administration, and monitoring of these agents is essential for planning optimum nursing care for patients who require these agents.

Before proceeding, it may be helpful to clarify a common cause of confusion related to the various terms used for the corticosteroids. Depending on the primary focus and perspective, various writers have referred to the drugs discussed in this chapter as adrenalcorticosteroids, adrenocorticosteroids, or corticosteroids.* Any or all of these terms can be used and, except for some slight semantic differences, they all mean the same thing. However, for the sake of clarity and consistency the term *corticosteroid* is used in this chapter.

CORTICOSTEROIDS

Action

Corticotropin. Corticotropin (adrenocorticotropic hormone) is primarily responsible for stimulating the synthesis and, to a lesser extent, the release of en-

---

*The terms *adrenocorticoid* and *corticoid* are also used frequently as being synonymous with corticosteroid; however, this usage is not precise and should be discouraged. Adrenocorticoid or corticoid refers more precisely not only to the corticosteroids that are released from the cortex of the adrenal gland, but also to the other steroids, such as dehydroepiandrosterone and the precursors of the various estrogens and progestins, which are also released from the cortex of the adrenal gland. An even less precise term is *steroid*, which applies not only to the corticosteroids, but also to several hundred other compounds.

Indications for corticosteroid use

This list, arranged according to body systems, is comprehensive yet *not* all-inclusive. It is meant to provide the nurse with a list of indications generally responsive to corticosteroid therapy and for which the corticosteroids have been used therapeutically as sole *or* adjunctive agents (see also boxes, pp. 1488-1489).

Cardiovascular system

Acute rheumatic carditis

Cutaneous system

Atopic dermatitis
Certain poisonous bites
Contact dermatitis, acute
Dermatomyositis, active
Drug eruptions, severe
Eczema
Erythema multiforme
Exfoliative dermatitis
Multiple bee or wasp stings
Pemphigus
Periarteritis nodosa
Polymyositis
Psoriasis, severe
Pustular psoriasis, acute
Pyoderma gangrenosum
Rheumatoid arthritis
Scleroderma
Seborrheic dermatitis, severe
Stevens-Johnson syndrome
Systemic lupus erythematosus
Urticaria of known etiology, acute
(See also box, p. 1488, right)

Endocrine system

Adrenocortical insufficiency
Congenital adrenal hyperplasia
Hashimoto's thyroiditis
Hypercalcemia associated with cancer

Gastrointestinal system

Intractable sprue, acute
Regional enteritis (Crohn's disease), acute
Ulcerative colitis, acute

Hematologic system

Acquired hemolytic anemia
Congenital hypoplastic anemia
Erythroblastopenia
Idiopathic thrombocytopenia
Leukemias
Serum sickness

Hepatic system

Cirrhosis of the liver with refractory ascites

Lymphatic system

Leukemias
Lymphoma

Neurologic system

Brain tumors
Cerebral edema
Increased intracranial pressure
Myasthenia gravis

Ophthalmic system

Chorioretinitis
Iridocyclitis
Iritis
Optic neuritis
Sympathetic ophthalmia
(See also box, p. 1489, left, for topical ophthalmic use)

Renal system

Nephrotic syndrome

Respiratory system

Aspiration pneumonitis
Berylliosis
Bronchial asthma
Pulmonary emphysema
Symptomatic sarcoidosis
Tuberculosis, fulminating or disseminated pulmonary

Miscellaneous

Trichinosis with myocardial or neurologic involvement
Various miscellaneous and allergic conditions

General guidelines for corticosteroid dosage and administration

Individualize dosage according to the severity of the condition being treated and the patient response.

For children, the dosage is based primarily on the severity of the condition being treated and the patient's response as opposed to age or body weight.

Once the therapeutic response is obtained, or following several days of therapy, the dosage should be reduced gradually to the minimum dose that affords a therapeutic response.

When possible, the dosage should be gradually reduced until discontinued.

Oral dosages should generally be administered in four equally divided doses except for those corticosteroids and conditions that are amenable to single- or alternate-day dosing.

For many conditions, the corticosteroids afford palliative relief or adjunctive therapy. In these conditions conventional therapy *must* be used concomitantly as indicated.

Routine monitoring for both therapeutic and toxic effects must accompany and guide the use of the corticosteroids (see General Nursing Implications).

Systemic dosing equivalents for corticosteroids based on glucocorticoid activity*

Betamethasone 0.6 mg
Cortisone 25 mg
Dexamethasone 0.75 mg
Fluprednisolone 1.5 mg
Hydrocortisone 20 mg
Methylprednisolone 4 mg
Paramethasone 2 mg
Prednisolone 5 mg
Prednisone 5 mg
Triamcinolone 4 mg

*For example, 0.75 mg of dexamethasone will provide approximately the same amount of glucocorticoid response as 5 mg of prednisone.

Corticosteroid-responsive dermatoses*

Atopic dermatitis
Contact dermatitis
Eczematous dermatitis
Exfoliative dermatitis
Intertrigo
Intertriginous psoriasis
Lichen planus
Lichen simplex chronicus
Nummular (discoid) eczema
Otitis externa
Postanal surgery
Pruritus ani
Pruritus vulvae
Psoriasis
Seborrheic dermatitis
Stasis dermatitis

*See Chapter 57, "Topical Corticosteroids," for details regarding the dosage and administration of the corticosteroids in treating these conditions.

dogenous corticosteroids. Endogenous corticosteroid release in the body is regulated by a complex interaction of control factors that can be activated by several variables, the most prominent of which is stress (physical or psychologic).

As noted, corticotropin stimulates the synthesis and release of endogenous corticosteroids. Thus its action can be thought of in a manner similar to the oral hypoglycemic agents that stimulate the release of endogenous insulin. Because reliance on endogenous corticosteroid synthesis and release stimulated by corticotropin administration is less predictable and less accurate than the administration of an exogenous corticosteroid, it is recommended that corticotropin and its synthetic derivative, cosyntropin, be used *only* for diagnostic purposes (see the Nursing Drug Digest).

Glucocorticoids

The synthetic glucocorticoids generally produce antiinflammatory, immunosuppressive, and metabolic effects.

Antiinflammatory effects. The glucocorticoids elicit an antiinflammatory response by a number of coordinated mechanisms. The glucocorticoids stabilize cell membranes, inhibit the release of proteolytic enzymes, block plasma exudation, inhibit the migration of polymorphonuclear leukocytes, inhibit phago-

Topical corticosteroid–responsive ophthalmic conditions

Topically applied ophthalmic corticosteroid preparations are rapidly effective. The relief of pain and photophobia are a result of their antiinflammatory action. Topical ophthalmic corticosteroids are indicated for the following.
Acne rosacea keratitis
Allergic conjunctivitis
Anterior uveitis
Blepharitis
Corneal lesions
Episcleritis
Nonspecific superficial keratitis
Phlyctenular keratoconjunctivitis
Sclerokeratitis
Traumatic keratitis
Symblepharon formation may be prevented in the cases of chemical or thermal burns because of the inhibition of fibroblastic proliferation. Because of the decreased scar and new blood vessel formation, clearer corneas may also result with the topical ophthalmic application of the corticosteroids in treating chemical or thermal burns.
NOTE: *Only* topical corticosteroid preparations specifically formulated for ophthalmic use should be used for topical ophthalmic indications in or near the eyes. See box, p. 1487 for systemic ophthalmic corticosteroid use.

Classification of corticosteroids

Glucocorticoids

Betamethasone
Dexamethasone
Fluprednisolone
Methylprednisolone
Paramethasone
Triamcinolone

Mineralocorticoids

Desoxycorticosterone
Fludrocortisone

Combined glucocorticoids and mineralocorticoids

Cortisone
Hydrocortisone
Prednisolone
Prednisone

cytosis, and suppress antibody formation in injured or infected tissue. These effects in turn prevent or decrease the normal inflammatory response and suppress the development of the classic signs of inflammation (i.e., redness, warmth, swelling, and pain), which are usually observable at the site of the injury or infection. Their metabolic effect on carbohydrate metabolism also appears to play a role in the antiinflammatory action of these agents. The glucocorticoids interfere with histamine synthesis, fibroblast formation, collagen disposition, capillary proliferation, microvascular dilation, and increased capillary permeability in response to tissue injury.

Immunosuppressive effects. The glucocorticoids suppress the immune system by a mechanism of action not yet fully elucidated in humans. However, this effect appears to be mediated by means of a cytotoxic action on the thymus gland and lymphoid tissue, re-

sulting in a decreased number of lymphocytes. In addition, the glucocorticoids disrupt the production of antibody-producing plasma cells. Except for polymorphonuclear (PMN) leukocytes, which increase, other white blood cells (i.e., basophils, eosinophils, lymphocytes, monocytes) decrease in response to glucocorticoid administration.

Metabolic effects. The glucocorticoids affect lipid, protein, and carbohydrate metabolism.

Glucocorticoids affect lipid metabolism by enhancing the mobilization of peripheral fat deposits. When given in high doses, these agents can cause fat redistribution with a loss of fat from the extremities and an accumulation in the cheeks ("moon-face"), back, and neck areas ("buffalo hump").

In pharmacologic doses the glucocorticoids increase protein catabolism. These agents decrease the use of amino acids for protein synthesis and instead convert them to glucose. The resultant protein breakdown may lead to muscle wasting and weakness. This catabolism also reduces the bone protein matrix and the lymphatic tissue and thus interferes with wound healing, arrests growth, causes osteoporosis, and suppresses the immune response.

Glucocorticoids affect carbohydrate metabolism by increasing the conversion of amino acids to glucose (i.e., gluconeogenesis), decreasing the peripheral use of glucose, and increasing *glycogenesis.* These combined actions may cause a hyperglycemic effect and resultant insulin release. Long-term glucocorticoid therapy may thus produce diabetes mellitus in susceptible patients, as well as necessitate the adjustment of insulin or oral hypoglycemic dosage or diet in patients with controlled diabetes.

Miscellaneous effects. In addition to the antiinflammatory, immunosuppressive, and metabolic effects, therapeutic doses of the glucocorticoids cause a number of other miscellaneous effects. These effects include an increase in hemoglobin and red blood cell concentration, an inhibition of epiphyseal cartilage and related growth in children, decreased serum calcium levels (decreased GI absorption and increased renal elimination), and CNS behavioral disturbances ranging from elevation of mood and anxiousness to psychosis.

Mineralocorticoids

The synthetic mineralocorticoids produce sodium and fluid retention, as well as hydrogen and potassium excretion. The mineralocorticoids affect the kidney's control of fluid and electrolyte balance. These agents can increase sodium reabsorption and potassium and hydrogen secretion at the distal segment of the renal tubules. Water is retained in association with sodium retention resulting in increased plasma volume and elevated blood pressure. The excretion of hydrogen and potassium, if not corrected, may result in hypokalemic alkalosis (see Chapter 67, "Fluids and Electrolytes").

Mixed glucocorticoid/mineralocorticoids

The combination products possess varying degrees of combined glucocorticoid and mineralocorticoid activity (see General Nursing Implications).

Dosage

The dosage of the corticosteroids is highly individualized and based, even for children, primarily on the clinical condition and the response of the patient instead of a set dosage. The minimum effective dose should always be used for as short a period as possible to minimize adrenal suppression and other associated toxicities. When clinically feasible and appropriate, the daily dose of the corticosteroids is generally administered orally in four equally divided doses. Exceptions include those preparations and conditions that are amenable to single or alternate-day (morning) dosing. It is important to note that various glucocorticoids can be classified as either short-acting, intermediate-acting, or long-acting (see box, above right). Long-acting preparations should not be used in alternate-day dosing regimens (see also box, p. 1488, top left).

> ## *Duration of biologic action of various systemic corticosteroids*
>
> ### *Short-acting agents (8 to 12 hours)*
> Cortisone
> Hydrocortisone
>
> ### *Intermediate-acting agents (18 to 36 hours)*
> Methylprednisolone
> Prednisolone
> Prednisone
> Triamcinolone
>
> ### *Long-acting agents (36 to 54 hours)*
> Betamethasone
> Dexamethasone
> Fluprednisolone
> Paramethasone

Administration and absorption

Most of the systemic corticosteroids* and related drugs are absorbed well from the GI tract after oral administration. Some (e.g., corticotropin, cosyntropin, desoxycorticosterone), because they are poorly absorbed orally, are best administered parenterally. Corticotropin is administered intravenously, whereas cosyntropin and desoxycorticosterone are both administered intramuscularly. Water-soluble preparations are absorbed readily from IM sites, whereas aqueous suspensions and solutions in oil are slowly absorbed after IM injection, resulting in prolonged blood levels lasting days to weeks. Aqueous solutions administered intravenously have a rapid onset of action. Implanted subcutaneous pellets provide 6 to 8 months of therapy.

Toxicity

Just as the corticosteroids can have a therapeutic effect on virtually every organ system in the body, so too can they cause equally widespread toxic effects. The antiinflammatory and immunosuppressive effects of these drugs can often delay the detection of a serious infection and can severely compromise resistance. The effect of the corticosteroids on calcium absorption and excretion and their inhibiting effect on osteoblast activity can result in growth suppression in

---

*For a discussion of the *topical corticosteroids* see Chapter 57, "Topical Corticosteroids."

children, as well as osteoporosis and resultant bone fractures in both children and adults (particularly in immobilized patients, postmenopausal women, and the elderly). This potential adverse effect should be monitored for by physical examination, questioning of the patient regarding rib or vertebral pain, and periodic spinal radiographs for individuals on long-term, chronic, corticosteroid therapy.

Other major adverse effects associated with the use of corticosteroids include the following: behavioral disturbances ranging from nervousness and insomnia to psychosis; fluid and electrolyte disturbances, including edema and hypokalemic alkalosis; myopathy, particularly affecting the extremities; peptic ulceration with a high degree of perforation; and posterior subcapsular cataract formation, in both children and adults, particularly in patients with rheumatoid arthritis receiving long-term chronic corticosteroid therapy.

In addition, cushingoid features, including acne, buffalo hump, hirsutism, moon-face, striae, and truncal obesity, commonly occur with long-term chronic or high-dose therapy. Although these effects are not particularly physically disabling, they can cause profound psychologic concern and disability for the patient (see General Nursing Implications and General Instructions for Discharge/Outpatients).

Corticosteroid-induced toxicity can also occur on the withdrawal or following the discontinuation of the drug. Rapid withdrawal may be associated with symptoms of hypothalamic-pituitary-adrenal (HPA) axis suppression (e.g., anorexia, arthalgia, lethargy, weakness) and an exacerbation of the condition being treated. In addition, the ability of the adrenal cortex to synthesize and release endogenous corticosteroids in response to stress may be severely compromised for a period of up to 1 year following the discontinuation of long-term chronic corticosteroid therapy. These potential postexposure toxicities must be anticipated and carefully monitored for whenever long-term chronic or high-dose corticosteroid therapy is discontinued (see General Nursing Implications).

ADRENAL STEROID INHIBITORS

Three adrenal steroid inhibitors are available for clinical use in North America: aminoglutethimide, metyrapone, and mitotane. Although these agents are functionally related, they are structurally distinct and are used for different clinical indications.

Aminoglutethimide

Aminoglutethimide decreases the *endogenous* production of both aldosterone and hydrocortisone. This is accomplished by the selective inhibition of the enzymatic conversion of cholesterol to delta-5-pregnenolone, which is a necessary precursor of both aldosterone and hydrocortisone. Aminoglutethimide is thus of clinical use in conditions associated with the hypersecretion of aldosterone and hydrocortisone from the adrenal cortex (e.g., *Cushing's syndrome*).

Aminoglutethimide is predominantly excreted in unchanged form in the urine, and thus the dosage may need to be decreased in renal failure. Use of this agent is contraindicated in patients with a known hypersensitivity to either aminoglutethimide or to the structurally closely related sedative-hypnotic glutethimide.

The dosage of aminoglutethimide must be carefully titrated against plasma cortisol (hydrocortisone) levels, and patients must be closely monitored for signs of *hypoadrenocortical* function. In some cases replacement therapy with either a glucocorticoid (e.g., hydrocortisone) or a mineralocorticoid (e.g., fludrocortisone) may be indicated.

Aminoglutethimide also inhibits the peripheral tissue conversion of androgens into estrogens and as such may be of some use in the treatment of breast cancer in postmenopausal women. See the Nursing Drug Digest for additional information.

Metyrapone

Metyrapone decreases the *endogenous* production of hydrocortisone by selectively inhibiting the chemical β-hydroxylation reactions in the adrenal cortex. This effect is accompanied by a compensatory increase in corticotropin secretion in normal individuals and a resultant increase in the urinary excretion of 17-hydroxycorticosteroids. The increased urinary excretion of the 17-hydroxycorticosteroids is the basis for metyrapone's use as a diagnostic test. For the proper performance and interpretation of this test, as well as to prevent metyrapone-induced acute adrenal insufficiency, corticotropin's ability to stimulate the adrenal cortex should be determined *before* the administration of metyrapone. See the Nursing Drug Digest for additional information.

Mitotane

Mitotane is cytotoxic to adrenal tissue and inhibits adrenal function, reducing the endogenous corticosteroid levels. Mitotane's action makes it useful in treating inoperable adrenal cortical carcinoma.

Because mitotane can induce the production of hepatic microsomal enzymes, which are responsible for the metabolism of a wide range of different drugs (see Chapter 5, "Drug Metabolism and Elimination"), the dosage of other concomitantly administered drugs should be monitored and may need to be modified whenever mitotane therapy is initiated or discontinued. See the Nursing Drug Digest for additional information.

SUMMARY

The various corticosteroids and adrenal steroid inhibitors have been discussed. These agents are used to treat a wide variety of conditions affecting virtually every organ system in the body. They likewise have the potential to cause toxicity in as many different organ systems, and their use must thus be carefully monitored. Properly used, these agents can provide dramatic and often lifesaving therapy for seriously ill patients.

With an understanding of these various agents, including their indications for use, contraindications, cautions, administration, drug interactions, and monitoring, the nurse will be able to provide optimal therapy and assistance to patients who require these medications.

ADVERSE/SIDE EFFECTS OF CORTICOSTEROIDS*

CARDIOVASCULAR SYSTEM

Atherosclerosis
Capillary fragility
Edema
Embolism
Hypercoagulability
Hypertension
Petechiae
Thromboembolism
Thrombophlebitis

CENTRAL NERVOUS SYSTEM

Behavioral changes (depression, euphoria, insomnia, mood swings, nervousness, personality changes, and psychoses)
Cerebral edema
Convulsions
Dependence (psychologic and physical)
Increased intracranial pressure
Increased seizure activity in patients with epilepsy
Pseudotumor cerebri

CUTANEOUS SYSTEM

Acne
Ecchymosis
Hirsutism
Hypertrichosis
Impaired wound healing
Keratosis pilaris
Purpura
Striae
Thin, fragile skin

ENDOCRINE SYSTEM

Diabetes mellitus
Glucose intolerance
Growth suppression in children
Hyperglycemic hyperosmolar nonketotic coma (HHNK)
Hyperlipidemia
Hypothalamic-pituitary-axis suppression
Menstrual irregularities
Truncal obesity

GASTROINTESTINAL SYSTEM

Intestinal perforation
Pancreatitis
Peptic ulcer

IMMUNE SYSTEM

Decreased lymphocyte and monocyte function
Impaired immune response
Increased susceptibility to infections

METABOLIC SYSTEM

Changes in lipid, protein, and carbohydrate metabolism
Cushing's syndrome
Hypercholesterolemia
Protein catabolism

MUSCULOSKELETAL SYSTEM

Aseptic necrosis of bone
Fractures
Muscle wasting
Myopathy
Osteoporosis

OPHTHALMIC SYSTEM

Cataracts, posterior subcapsular
Glaucoma

---

*See Chapter 11, "Drug Toxicity," for an overview of drug toxicity.

CLINICALLY SIGNIFICANT DRUG INTERACTIONS*

Primary drug	Interacting drug	Possible effect(s)	Probable mechanism(s)
Corticosteroids	Barbiturates	Decreased corticosteroid effect	Increased hepatic metabolism
Corticosteroids	Diuretics, potassium depleting	Increased incidence or severity of hypokalemia	Additive effect
Corticosteroids	Erythromycin	Increased corticosteroid effect	Decreased hepatic metabolism
Corticosteroids	Phenytoin	Decreased corticosteroid effect	Increased hepatic metabolism
Corticosteroids	Rifampin	Decreased corticosteroid effect	Increased corticosteroid metabolism
Corticosteroids	Troleandomycin	Increased corticosteroid effect	Decreased hepatic metabolism

*See Chapter 10, "Drug Interactions," for an overview of drug interactions.

GENERAL NURSING IMPLICATIONS

Nursing of patients requiring corticosteroids*

ASSESSMENT

The corticosteroids are used to treat many conditions (see boxes, pp. 1487-1489). Thus, patients requiring corticosteroids should be carefully assessed in relation to the specific indication for corticosteroid use so that individualized and optimal drug therapy and nursing care can be planned and monitored. The initial data base should include an assessment of the patient's general health state, paying particular attention to the patient's present height and weight, especially in children, and blood pressure. A laboratory evaluation, including red blood cell counts, white blood cell counts, serum electrolytes, and urinalysis, should also be completed before initiating the drug therapy. In addition, fasting blood sugar and urine glucose determinations are indicated for children, patients who are diabetic or prediabetic, and patients with a familial history of diabetes mellitus. Although current available evidence indicates that the incidence of corticosteroid-induced or associated psychosis is not higher in patients with a previous history of mental illness, the nursing history should nevertheless include identifying any familial or past mental illness. This baseline data is essential in planning and monitoring therapy. The assessment should also include a detailed drug history before corticosteroid therapy is initiated to identify previous corticosteroid use, any possible hypersensitivity, contraindications, cautions, potential drug interactions, and drug-taking patterns.

SENSITIVITY

Generally, hypersensitivity reactions to the corticosteroids are rare; however, any drug has the potential to cause a hypersensitivity reaction in susceptible individuals. Patients should be questioned carefully regarding a history of a hypersensitivity to corticosteroids and asked to describe the reaction. If a hypersensitivity is identified, the prescriber should be consulted before initiating corticosteroid therapy.

Although rare, hypersensitivity has been reported to corticotropin, which is generally derived from a porcine source. Its synthetic derivative, cosyntropin, causes fewer such reactions and can generally be used with caution in patients who are hypersensitive to corticotropin.

CONTRAINDICATIONS

The corticosteroids are generally contraindicated in patients with Cushing's syndrome, fungal infections (severe systemic or untreated), a known hypersensitivity to corticosteroids, psychoses (acute), tuberculosis (active or untreated), and viral infections (severe).

In addition, the corticosteroids are contraindicated in patients who have received live virus vaccines (e.g., smallpox).

It is important to note that prednisone is generally contraindicated in patients with severe hepatic dysfunction because it must be metabolically activated in the liver to prednisolone. An alternate corticosteroid (e.g., prednisolone) should be used in these patients.

CAUTIONS

The corticosteroids should be used with caution in patients with cardiac disease, cirrhosis, CHF, diabetes mellitus, diverticulitis, emotional problems or a history of psychosis, fungal infections, gastritis, glaucoma, hepatic dysfunction, herpes simplex of the eye, hyperlipidemia, hypertension, hypothyroidism, metastatic carcinoma, myasthenia gravis, osteoporosis, peptic ulcer disease, renal dysfunction, tartrazine sensitivity,† thromboembolic tendencies, toxic megacolon, tuberculosis (positive skin test, latent, or a history of), and ulcerative colitis with infection (possible perforation).

---

*For information regarding the adrenal steroid inhibitors, see the discussion in the chapter and the Nursing Drug Digest.

†Tartrazine is found as a coloring agent in some corticosteroid tablet formulations. This differs from manufacturer to manufacturer and from dosage formulation design to dosage formulation design. If the patient is sensitive to tartrazine, the manufacturer's current package insert should be checked before any oral dosages are administered.

Continued.

GENERAL NURSING IMPLICATIONS—cont'd

Nursing of patients requiring corticosteroids—cont'd

CAUTIONS—cont'd

In addition, the corticosteroids should be used cautiously in pregnancy, because they can cross the placental barrier causing unwanted effects in the fetus. In addition, it is important to note that infants born to mothers who have received substantial doses of corticosteroids during pregnancy should be monitored carefully for signs of hypoadrenalism.

The corticosteroids should be used cautiously in women who are breast feeding, because they can be excreted in the breast milk and can cause unwanted effects in the infant, including growth suppression and the inhibition of endogenous corticosteroid production.

The corticosteroids should also be used cautiously in children, because prolonged use may cause suppressed growth and development.

It is important to note that the rectal forms of the corticosteroids, as well as the inhalation, otic, ophthalmic, and topical preparations, although given for local effects, should be used with caution because they can be absorbed systemically.

DRUG INTERACTIONS

The corticosteroids can interact with other drugs causing unwanted effects (e.g., hypokalemia when given with potassium-depleting diuretics) or diminished effects (e.g., the effect of corticosteroids is generally diminished by phenytoin or phenobarbital).

See Clinically Significant Drug Interactions for specific interactions.

ADMINISTRATION

The corticosteroids are available in many dosage forms, including oral, rectal, topical, inhalation, ophthalmic, otic, nasal, and parenteral. The dosage and the vehicle can vary in relation to the various preparations, and paying attention to the concentration of each preparation is essential. The dosage and preparation are selected in relation to the specific indication for the corticosteroid therapy. It is also important to note that the various preparations

are short-acting (8 to 12 hours), intermediate-acting (18 to 36 hours), or long-acting (36 to 54 hours) (see box, p. 1490). The duration of action of these preparations is affected by the dosage form, the route of administration, and individual patient factors.

The corticosteroids should be administered at the lowest dosage possible (see box, p. 1488, top left).

Short-term oral therapy

For short-term oral therapy (2 weeks or less), it is generally recommended that the daily dose be administered in four equally divided doses or that a single daily oral dose be given before 8:00 AM, as indicated, according to the condition being treated. These dosing schedules are recommended to minimize HPA axis suppression and adverse side effects. Short-term, low-dose therapy generally does not require tapering off on the discontinuation of corticosteroid therapy.

Long-term oral therapy

Therapy that is indicated for more than 1 month should be generally dosed on alternate-day schedules.

Patients with an intact HPA axis should take corticosteroid preparations when their serum cortisol (hydrocortisone) levels are normally low to minimize the suppression of endogenous hormone secretion and the development of cushingoid features. Patients who do not have an intact HPA axis (e.g., post-hypophysectomy patients) will mimic normal diurnal cycles of secretion on this schedule. This dosing schedule is recommended so that the HPA axis is minimally suppressed and adverse side effects minimized. This is particularly important in elderly patients, postmenopausal women, and immobilized patients.

To change from a daily dose schedule to an alternate-day dose schedule, the daily dose is usually doubled for the "on" medication day and dropped to zero for the "off" medication day. However, if the daily dose has been long term, the "off" medication day dose should be gradually tapered off as indicated.

An alternate-day schedule of the intermediate-acting preparations lessens the HPA suppression and the development of cushingoid features, allowing endogenous HPA activity to occur on the "off" medication day. If exacerbation of symptoms occurs on the "off" medication day, the medication schedule may have to be changed (see the Nursing Drug Digest for specific information regarding each drug).

For the administration of topical corticosteroids see Chapter 57, "Topical Corticosteroids."

MONITORING PATIENT RESPONSE

Generally, monitor patients requiring the *glucocorticoids* for antiinflammatory effects, immunosuppressant effects, and metabolic effects.

Generally, monitor patients requiring the *mineralocorticoids* for potassium depletion effects, and sodium and fluid retention effects.

Generally, monitor patients requiring *combination glucocorticoids/mineralocorticoids* for antiinflammatory effects, immunosuppressant effects, metabolic effects, potassium depletion effects, and sodium and fluid retention effects.

Therapeutic response

Monitoring the therapeutic response is important in relation to evaluating treatment and adjusting the drug therapy regimen. Once the condition being treated is controlled, the corticosteroids are usually withdrawn. This must often be done gradually to prevent a withdrawal syndrome (e.g., arthralgias, fatigue, fever, malaise, myalgias, weakness, and weight loss). Reduction of the dose depends on the individual patient's clinical response.

Adverse side effects

All patients requiring corticosteroids should be carefully monitored for adverse side effects.

Patients receiving the corticosteroids for prolonged periods in particular require close monitoring during hospitalization and frequent follow-up evaluation after discharge.

GENERAL NURSING IMPLICATIONS—cont'd

Nursing of patients requiring corticosteroids—cont'd

Short-term administration (for acute conditions)

In short-term administration, monitor patients for edema, GI distress, hypersensitivity, and local reactions to the medication.

Long-term administration (for chronic conditions)

In long-term administration, monitor patients for the following adverse effects.

Cushingoid features

Observe patients carefully for acne, buffalo hump, ecchymosis, delayed wound healing, hirsutism, moon-face, pendulous abdomen, red cheeks, reddish purple abdominal striae, supraclavicular fat pads, thin skin and subcutaneous tissue, thin extremities with muscle atrophy, truncal obesity, and weight gain.

Fluid and electrolyte imbalance

Also monitor patients for fluid and electrolyte imbalance including hypernatremia, hypokalemia, and hypocalcemia.

Hypernatremia. Monitor the blood pressure regularly during hospitalization and at each follow-up visit to the health care provider.

Monitor, if indicated, diuretic therapy or antihypertensive therapy.

Monitor the diet for foods high in sodium and delete as indicated, including canned soups and vegetables, prepared luncheon meats, processed cheeses, salted crackers, and salted snack foods.

Hypokalemia. Monitor patients for the following signs of hypokalemia: anorexia, cardiac dysrhythmias, depression, drowsiness, flaccid paralysis, hypotension (postural), muscle weakness, nausea, paresthesias, polydipsia, polyuria, and tetany.

Monitor serum potassium levels regularly during hospitalization and during follow-up.

Monitor the patient's diet for foods high in potassium as indicated, including avocados, bananas, and citrus fruits and juices.

Hypocalcemia. Monitor patients for the following signs of hypocalcemia: carpopedal spasms, cramps, muscle twitching, a positive Chvostek sign, and a positive Trousseau sign.

Gastrointestinal effects

Monitor for GI effects, including the following signs that indicate possible irritation and ulceration of the GI tract: coffee ground vomitus, epigastric pain (usually occurring 1 to 3 hours after meals and relieved by food or antacids), hematemesis, melena, nausea, and vomiting.

Monitor the patient's hematocrit and hemoglobin levels regularly. Periodically monitor stool specimens for occult blood during hospitalization and follow-up visits.

Increased susceptibility to infection

Monitor for increased susceptibility to infection, including a decrease in the number of leukocytes, delayed wound healing, or infection.

It is important to note that corticosteroids can mask the usual manifestations of an infection, including the cardinal signs of inflammation and elevated temperature. Monitor white blood cell counts during hospitalization and regularly at follow-up visits. It is also important to use meticulous care for all wounds and to use protective isolation as indicated.

Because the reactivation of previously encapsulated dormant tubercle bacilli can occur with the use of the corticosteroids, monitor the chest films of patients with a positive PPD or monitor the tuberculin skin tests for patients with a negative PPD.

Prophylactic administration of antituberculin medication (e.g., isoniazid) may be indicated.

Mental and emotional effects

Monitor for mental and emotional effects, including depression, euphoria, insomnia, manic depressive manifestations, nervousness, and psychosis.

Monitor for any mental or emotional changes and observe severely depressed patients for suicidal tendencies. Suicide precautions may be indicated.

If noted, a mental or emotional disturbance generally indicates the need to terminate the corticosteroid therapy. These relatively common effects can be dangerous.

Metabolic effects

Monitor for metabolic effects, including diabetes mellitus (adrenal diabetes) and hyperglycemia.

For patients with no previous history of diabetes mellitus, monitor fasting blood sugar levels regularly and test the urine for glycosuria during hospitalization and at each follow-up visit to the hospital or clinic. Patients should be taught to monitor their urine as indicated.

For patients with diabetes, monitor fasting blood sugar levels regularly and test the urine for glycosuria during hospitalization and at each follow-up visit to the hospital or clinic. Monitor for symptoms of hyperglycemia, including polyuria, polydipsia, and polyphagia. Monitor patients for decreased or blurred vision.

Myopathy

To monitor for myopathy, evaluate muscle strength and question the patient for subjective feelings of weakness.

Osteoporosis

Chronic corticosteroid use may result in decreased intestinal absorption of calcium, the demineralization of bone, a fracture of the vertebral body and associated neurologic damage, increased calcium excretion in the urine, increased protein catabolism, and a lack of bone matrix formation.

Monitoring for corticosteroid-induced osteoporosis is particularly important in postmenopausal women, the elderly, and immobilized patients.

Monitor patients for complaints of bone or radicular pain secondary to vertebral body collapse.

Monitor bone changes with regular radiographic evaluation.

Monitor activity and avoid immobility.

Continued.

GENERAL NURSING IMPLICATIONS—cont'd

Nursing of patients requiring corticosteroids—cont'd

Corticosteroid dependence

For corticosteroid dependence, monitor patients for a flare-up of the condition for which the drug was originally prescribed, signs of adrenal insufficiency, symptoms of withdrawal (physical or psychologic dependence on corticosteroids in patients with adrenal sufficiency and no recurrence of underlying condition), including anorexia, arthralgia, fever, headache, lethargy, myalgia, nausea, skin sloughing, weakness, and weight loss.

Monitor patient stress (e.g., acute infections, surgery), which may necessitate an adjustment in the corticosteroid dose.

Patients receiving long-term corticosteroid therapy should be monitored for the following signs of adrenal insufficiency (hypoadrenalism) that can develop over weeks or months after the therapy has been discontinued: anorexia, anxiety, decreased endurance, dehydration, depression, diarrhea, dizziness, fatigue, GI distress, hyperkalemia, hyperpigmentation of the skin and mucous membranes, hypoglycemia, hyponatremia, nausea, vomiting, weakness, and weight loss.

Miscellaneous adverse effects

Although less common than those effects just listed, it is important to monitor patients for other complications associated with corticosteroid therapy. See Adverse/Side Effects for an outline of adverse side effects associated with the use of the corticosteroids.

PATIENT EDUCATION

The patient and the family, as indicated, should have a clear understanding of the reason for the corticosteroid therapy, the planned course of the therapy, and the risks associated with the use of these medications. Patients, particularly those who will be self-medicating on a long-term basis, should be able to state the exact name of the drug, its dosage, general action, storage, administration, and adverse side effects. In addition, patients should be able to describe how common adverse side effects can be prevented or minimized. The patient and the family should be able to monitor for the therapeutic effect and be able to identify symptoms that indicate that the health care provider should be notified.

Patients should understand the importance of taking the corticosteroid medication at the same time every day to promote the therapeutic effect (e.g., a single daily oral dose should be taken early in the morning around 8 AM; for twice-daily doses, the second dose should be taken no later than 4 PM). Patients should be encouraged to keep a medication calendar as a useful reminder and record of therapy.

To decrease gastric irritation, patients should be taught to take oral corticosteroid preparations with food, milk, or an antacid, although the use of antacids for the prevention of ulcerogenic effects is controversial. The patient may need to be advised to avoid alcohol, caffeine, cigarette smoking, and aspirin or aspirin-containing medications to decrease the risk of ulceration. Patients should recognize the importance of reporting epigastric burning, gastric upset, hematemesis, or melena promptly and to monitor stools for occult blood as indicated. They should also be made aware of the importance of a laboratory assessment of hemoglobin and hematocrit as indicated.

Patients should recognize the importance of notifying the health care provider if they are unable to take their medication because of vomiting. Patients and family members, as indicated, may require instruction on the IM injection of the corticosteroids when the oral route cannot be used.

Patients requiring long-term therapy should be advised of the importance of not abruptly stopping the use of this medication and the importance of gradually decreasing the dosage when the corticosteroids are no longer required, to allow the HPA axis to return to its full function without the development of adrenal insufficiency. The patient should understand that decreased energy levels, depression, or other symptoms may occur on the discontinuation of the therapy and that the return of the HPA axis function is variable.

Patients and their families should be able to identify the symptoms of adrenal insufficiency and understand the importance of notifying the health care provider if these symptoms are noted, especially in relation to a stress state, because the dosage may need to be increased. Individual patients may require a protocol for dosage changes according to preestablished guidelines in the event of this occurrence.

Patients requiring long-term therapy should understand the importance of not waiting until they have less than a 10-day supply of the medication left before they have their prescription refilled. They should also understand the importance of taking extra medication with them when they travel in case they are delayed, and they should carry their medication with them and not pack it in luggage. If they are planning an extensive trip, they should secure an extra prescription for the corticosteroid preparation and carry it with them. Patients should be encouraged to carry medical identification indicating that they are or have been taking a specific corticosteroid preparation, and should continue to carry this identification with them for at least 6 months to 1 year after the therapy has been discontinued. Patients should be taught the importance of informing all health care providers in the event of an injury or accident, as well as for dental or medical procedures, that corticosteroids are or have been taken.

Patients should be fully advised of the long-term effects of corticosteroid therapy, including delayed wound healing and an increased susceptibility to infection and bruising because of capillary fragility. Assistance in planning alterations in foot care and other self-care practices to prevent skin injury should be given, as well as information on the care of minor injuries.

Another area of importance to discuss with patients during patient education sessions is the management of stress while taking corticosteroids. Patients should understand that taking large doses of the corticosteroids can suppress the body's ability to respond to severe physical or psychologic stress

GENERAL NURSING IMPLICATIONS—cont'd

Nursing of patients requiring corticosteroids—cont'd

PATIENT EDUCATION—cont'd

states. The patient needs to know that this medication can mask the symptoms of an infection, such as elevated temperature. Patients should be encouraged to notify their health care provider if a fever occurs lasting more than 24 hours or if any other symptom of infection is noted.

Patients should understand the importance of having blood tests for monitoring the white blood cells and the importance of avoiding people with infections, particularly of the respiratory tract. Patients should be able to monitor injuries for delayed healing and should understand the importance of the follow-up monitoring of tuberculin tests or chest films.

Patients should be encouraged to keep mobile and to eat a diet that includes protein, vitamins, and calcium. Assistance with meal planning to meet the individual patient's requirements should be completed carefully. Patients should be taught to take potassium supplements or to include foods high in potassium as indicated. They should also be taught to have their blood pressure monitored and to use antihypertensives, diuretics, and a sodium-restricted diet as indicated. The importance of maintaining activity balance in avoiding osteoporosis and the importance of radiographic follow-up for the monitoring of bone status should be emphasized. Patients should

also be encouraged to report changes in muscle strength and size and the development of muscle weakness. Because corticosteroids can affect the fluid and electrolyte balance and metabolism, patients should be able to demonstrate an ability to weigh themselves and should be encouraged to monitor their weight several times during the week. Weight changes of 5 pounds or more, dizziness, an irregular heart rate, weakness, or undue fatigue should be readily reported. Assistance with meal planning for low-sodium or high-potassium diets and for other diet regimens as indicated may be required. Patients should be taught to report epigastric pain especially if it occurs 1 to 3 hours after meals and is relieved by food or antacids and to report the vomiting of coffee ground material or blood, black tarry stools, or blood in the stools.

Patients requiring long-term corticosteroid therapy should be carefully prepared for the possibility of changes in body image, including truncal obesity, hirsutism, moon-face, and acne. Emotional support is essential as is a reassurance that a return to normal usually occurs on the discontinuation of the drug. Children and their families may need to be prepared for growth retardation. Children who have received corticosteroids and have retarded growth should be treated individually according to their mental age and condition.

The cost of the corticosteroid therapy may also present a concern for the patient and the family. Assistance with concerns in this area, as well as referral for social assistance as indicated, should be completed.

Both patients and their families should be alert to changes in emotional behavior and to report changes so that the medication dosage or schedule can be adjusted as indicated.

Patients with diabetes should be aware that the corticosteroids can increase the blood glucose, and they should monitor their blood glucose and urine tests carefully. Other patients may also have the hyperglycemic effects of these drugs and should be taught to report symptoms of hyperglycemia, including increased thirst, increased urination, and fatigue. Patients with diabetes should be taught to adjust the dosage, administration, and effects of insulin or other hypoglycemics as indicated.

Patients requiring corticosteroid therapy for the long-term treatment of specific conditions must understand the risks of long-term therapy, including cataracts, glaucoma, hypertension, peptic ulcers, Cushing's syndrome, susceptibility to infection, convulsions, and psychosis. They should be aware of the potential for dependence and the importance of limiting the corticosteroid dosage and use.

GENERAL INSTRUCTIONS FOR DISCHARGE/OUTPATIENTS

CORTICOSTEROIDS

This medication is a corticosteroid and is used to decrease inflammation and to lessen pain, redness, or swelling of inflamed tissues. This medication can be used to treat allergic reactions and helps relieve itching. It can also be used to treat various conditions such as skin problems, asthma, and arthritis. If you do not understand the reason why you require this medication check with your health care provider.

This medication has been prescribed especially for you. Do not trade or give this medication to other family members or friends.

Take this medication exactly as directed. If you have any questions about how this medication should be taken, check with your health care provider. Do not use more or less of this medication than directed, and do not use it for longer than the time prescribed, because this can cause unwanted or harmful effects.

If you miss a dose of this drug and you are taking it every other day, take the missed dose as soon as you remember the same morning. If you do not remember the missed dose until later, take it the following morning, then skip a day and start your regular dosing schedule.

If you are taking this medication once a day, take the missed dose as soon as you remember you missed the dose, then go back to your regular dosing

Continued.

GENERAL INSTRUCTIONS FOR DISCHARGE/OUTPATIENTS—cont'd

CORTICOSTEROIDS—cont'd

schedule. If you do not remember until the next day, do not take the missed dose at all and do not double the next one. Instead, resume your regular dosing schedule.

If you take this medication several times a day, take the missed dose as soon as you remember and then go back to your regular dosing schedule. If you do not remember until the next dose is due, double the next dose and then go back to your regular dosing schedule.

If you have any questions about what to do when you miss a dose of this medication, check with your health care provider immediately.

Be sure to keep appointments with your health care provider so that your progress can be monitored. This is important even after you stop taking this medication because some of its effects can continue.

Do not stop taking this medication without first checking with your health care provider. Often the dose of this medication is reduced gradually before completely stopping it.

Before taking this medication, notify your health care provider if you are pregnant, intend to become pregnant, or are breastfeeding an infant. This medication can cause unwanted effects in unborn babies and nursing infants.

Some patients who require this medication may also require a low-salt diet, as well as a potassium-rich diet. Check with your health care provider if you have any questions about your diet.

It is important that you notify all health care providers that you are taking this medication, especially if you are receiving a vaccination or other immunization or skin test, if you are having any type of surgery (including dental surgery or emergency treatment), or if you have a serious infection or injury.

If you have diabetes, this medication may cause your blood sugar levels to rise. Notify your health care provider if you notice a change in the results of your urine or blood sugar test or if you have any questions.

This medication can cause some unwanted effects in some individuals. Notify your health care provider if you notice the following: bloody or black tarry stools, blurred vision, depression, frequent urination, increased thirst, insomnia, menstrual changes, muscle cramps or pains, nausea or vomiting, rounding of the face, skin rash, sore throat and fever, swelling of the feet or lower legs, unusual tiredness, vomiting, or wounds that will not heal.

After stopping this medication, check with your health care provider if you notice the following: dizziness or fainting, loss of appetite, muscle or joint pain, shortness of breath, stomach or back pain, unusual tiredness, or unusual weight loss.

This medication can be taken by various routes of administration such as by mouth, by injection, rectally, by inhalation, by eye drops and ear drops, or by direct application to the skin in cream or ointment form, depending on the condition being treated.

Oral administration

If you are taking this medication *orally*, take this medication with a full glass of water and with some food to prevent stomach upset unless told to do otherwise by your health care provider. If stomach upset becomes severe or bothersome, check with your health care provider.

Stomach problems are more likely to occur if you drink alcoholic beverages or take aspirin-containing products while you are being treated with this medication.

Do not drink alcoholic beverages while taking this medication unless you have first checked with your health care provider. If you smoke, you may also have to decrease your tobacco smoking. Check with your health care provider.

Inhalation

If you take this medication by *inhalation*, read your package directions carefully and discuss any questions you have with your health care provider. Use the special inhaler provided with this medication. Store your medication away from heat or direct sunlight. Do not puncture or burn the container, because this may cause it to explode.

Notify your health care provider if you notice any signs of infection in your mouth, throat, or respiratory tract.

Gargle or rinse your mouth after each dose to prevent hoarseness and irritation.

Rectal administration

If you are using the *rectal* form of this medication, read the package instructions carefully and discuss any questions you may have with your health care provider.

The enema form of this medication works best after a bowel movement. Shake the bottle, unless otherwise directed, before administration. Lie on your left side and gently insert the rectal tip of the enema. Each bottle contains a single dose. Use it all, unless otherwise directed by your health care provider. Stay on your side for at least 30 minutes so the medicine can work. If possible, retain the enema overnight unless otherwise directed by your health care provider.

The rectal foam aerosol is administered with a special applicator. Do *not* insert any part of the aerosol container into the rectum. Store the container away from heat or direct sunlight and do not puncture or burn it.

Notify your health care provider immediately if you notice rectal bleeding, unusual pain, burning, itching, or other rectal irritation not present when you started using this medication.

Injection (intraarticular)

If you are having this medication *injected* into a joint (e.g., to treat arthritis), do not put too much strain or stress on the joint even though it feels much better. Check with your health care provider regarding how much you should use the joint while it is healing. Notify your health care provider if you notice redness or swelling at the place of the injection.

NURSING DRUG DIGEST

Medication (trade name*)	Indication	Usual dosage and administration	Dosage forms, preparation, and storage	Contraindications, cautions, and comments	Monitoring
Amcinonide	See Chapter 57, "Topical Corticosteroids"				
Aminoglutethimide Cytadren	Cushing's syndrome Metastatic breast cancer	*Adults:* 250 mg PO q.6h. Maximum: 2000 mg/24 hr *Adults:* Postmenopausal women, 250 mg PO b.i.d. for 7 days, followed by 250 mg PO t.i.d. for 7 days, and then 250 mg PO q.i.d. Maximum: 2000 mg/24 hr To achieve optimal therapeutic effects with minimal side effects, administer aminoglutethimide with hydrocortisone 100 mg/24 hr PO) and 60 mg h.s. (i.e., hydrocortisone 100 mg/24 hr PO) for 14 days, followed by 20 mg AM and 20 mg PM (i.e., 40 mg/24 hr PO)	Tablet: 250 mg	*Contraindicated in* hypersensitivity and premenopausal women with metastatic breast cancer May cause adrenocortical insufficiency Commonly causes CNS depression, lethargy, ataxia, skin rash, and GI distress (particularly nausea and vomiting) The skin rash associated with use of this drug typically is a maculopapular generalized or urticarial type, which appears around day 10 of the therapy and should subside by day 16 May also cause dizziness and fever May suppress endogenous aldosterone production Fludrocortisone (100 µg/24 hr PO) has been used to treat aminoglutethimide-induced hypoaldosteronemia Hydrocortisone (40 mg/24 hr PO) has been used to treat aminoglutethimide-induced adrenal insufficiency	Monitor for possible signs of hypoaldosteronemia (e.g., dizziness, hyponatremia, hypotension) Monitor for possible signs of adrenal insufficiency

Continued.

NOTE: For additional details regarding the individual agents listed in this table, see the text and other tables in this chapter.
*Indicates a multiple active ingredient product. For a complete listing of all active ingredients see the *Drug Reference Guide to Brand Names and Active Ingredients.*
★ Indicates that the drug is generally available only in Canada.
★ Indicates that the drug is generally available only in the United States.

NURSING DRUG DIGEST—cont'd

Medication (trade name)	Indication	Usual dosage and administration	Dosage forms, preparation, and storage	Contraindications, cautions, and comments	Monitoring
Beclomethasone Aldecin Inhaler Beclovent Inhaler Beconase Becotide Inhaler Propaderm Propaderm C* Propaderm Vancenase Nasal Inhaler Vanceril Vanceril Oral Inhaler	Corticosteroid-responsive asthma Allergic rhinitis unresponsive to conventional treatment See also Chapter 57, "Topical Corticosteroids"	*Adults:* 2-4 inhalations t.i.d. to q.i.d. Maximum: 20 inhalations (1 mg) a day *Children:* 3-5 years of age, 1 inhalation b.i.d. to t.i.d; 6-14 years of age, 2 inhalations b.i.d. to t.i.d. Maximum: 10 inhalations (500 μg) a day *Adults:* 1 application into each nostril t.i.d. to q.i.d. Maximum: 20 applications (1 mg) a day *Children:* Same as adults Maximum: 10 applications (500 μg) a day Do *not* use in children under 6 years of age	Oral metered-dose aerosol: 50 μg/puff (inhalation) Intranasal metered-dose aerosol: 50 μg/depression of valve	*Contraindicated* in active or untreated tuberculosis; and untreated or severe bacterial, fungal, or viral infections Do *not* use the oral aerosol in the treatment of status asthmaticus or severe bronchiectasis Candidiasis is associated with the use of the oral aerosol form Gargling and rinsing the mouth with water after each use may decrease the incidence of candidiasis Intranasal preparation may cause local irritation and sneezing	Observe for the development of oral candidiasis with the oral metered-dose aerosol Observe for adrenal insufficiency, particularly when patients are switched from systemic corticosteroids to beclomethasone aerosol
Betamethasone	See Chapter 57, "Topical Corticosteroids"				
✦ **Clobetasol**	See Chapter 57, "Topical Corticosteroids"				
✦ **Clobetasone**	See Chapter 57, "Topical Corticosteroids"				
★ **Clocortolone**	See Chapter 57, "Topical Corticosteroids"				

Drug	Indications	Dosage	Preparations/Administration	Cautions/Contraindications	Nursing Considerations
Corticotropin Actest Acthar ACTH Cortrophin Cortrophin-Zinc Depo-Acth Duracton H.P. Acthar Gel	Diagnostic test of adrenocortical function (to determine or rule out insufficiency) NOTE: Corticotropin may be administered for conditions that are responsive to corticosteroid therapy; however, it has been noted to have limited value and is *not* recommended in lieu of the corticosteroids	*Adults:* 10-25 units by slow IV infusion over 8 hr	Injectable: 25, 40, 80 IU/ml Reconstitute with 1-2 ml sterile water or NS for injection Stable for 24 hr after reconstitution if refrigerated *Dilute* IV dose in 500 ml D₅W *before* infusion A repository gel form of corticotropin injection is available for IM or SC administration in doses of 40-80 units every 1-3 days; however, use of this preparation is *not* recommended (see Indications)	*Contraindicated* in active or untreated tuberculosis, untreated or severe bacterial, fungal, or viral infections, acute psychoses, Cushing's syndrome, and active peptic ulcers May mask signs of infection May delay wound healing May suppress pituitary adrenal function Use with caution in patients with CHF, diabetes mellitus, hypertension, infectious disease, osteoporosis, and pregnancy May cause fluid and electrolyte disturbances, such as sodium retention, potassium loss, calcium loss, fluid retention, and alkalosis Use with caution in patients with cirrhosis or hypothyroidism	Observe for cushingoid symptoms (moon-face, buffalo hump, muscle wasting, fluid retention, hirsutism, and mental changes) Observe children for growth suppression Monitor fluid and electrolyte status, particularly in elderly patients Observe for signs of GI ulcers
Cortisone Cortelan Cortistab Cortogen Cortone Neosone*	Conditions responsive to corticosteroid therapy (see box, p. 1487) Acute, nonfatal conditions (e.g., severe seasonal asthma) Chronic, nonfatal conditions (e.g., chronic bronchial asthma, chronic rheumatoid arthritis)	Use minimum effective dose, particularly in chronic conditions (see box, p. 1488, top left) *Adults:* 75-150 mg/24 hr PO or IM *Adults:* 25-75 mg/24 hr PO or IM	Tablets: 5, 10, 25 mg Injectable: 25, 50 mg/ml	*Contraindicated* in active or untreated tuberculosis, untreated or severe bacterial, fungal, or viral infections, acute psychoses, Cushing's syndrome; and active peptic ulcers May mask signs of infection May delay wound healing May suppress pituitary adrenal function	Observe for cushingoid symptoms (moon-face, buffalo hump, muscle wasting, fluid retention, hirsutism, and mental changes) Observe children for growth suppression Monitor fluid and electrolyte status, particularly in elderly patients Observe for signs of GI ulcers

Continued.

NURSING DRUG DIGEST—cont'd

Medication (trade name)	Indication	Usual dosage and administration	Dosage forms, preparation, and storage	Contraindications, cautions, and comments	Monitoring
Cortisone—cont'd	Acute, potentially fatal conditions (e.g., acute rheumatic carditis, systemic lupus erythematosus crisis)	*Adults:* 125-300 mg/24 hr PO or IM in 4 divided doses		May cause hypersensitivity reaction; further use is *contraindicated* in these patients	Monitor for changes in mood, personality, or mentation
				Use with caution in patients with CHF, diabetes mellitus, hypertension, infectious disease, osteoporosis, and pregnancy	Monitor vision for cataract formation, particularly with prolonged administration
	Chronic, potentially fatal conditions (e.g., nephrotic syndrome)	*Adults:* 75-150 mg/24 hr PO or IM		May cause fluid and electrolyte disturbances, such as sodium retention, potassium loss, calcium loss, fluid retention, and alkalosis	
	Adrenal insufficiency (e.g., Addison's disease)	*Adults:* 10-25 mg/24 hr PO or IM (administer together with 4-6 gm of sodium chloride PO)		Use with caution in patients with cirrhosis or hypothyroidism	
	Congenital adrenal hyperplasia	*Children:* 15-50 mg/24 hr PO or IM		Do *not* administer smallpox vaccination while patient is receiving corticosteroid therapy	
		Do *not* administer IV		May cause or aggravate neurotic or psychotic behavior	
				Prolonged administration may result in posterior subcapsular cataract formation	
				Cortisone is available as the acetate salt, a synthetic corticosteroid possessing basic glucocorticoid activity	
Cosyntropin Cortrosyn Synacthen	Diagnostic test of adrenocorticol function (to determine or rule out deficiency)	*Adults:* 250-750 µg (usually 250 µg) slow IV infusion over 4-8 hr (40 µg/hr for 6 hr when 250 µg dose is used), *or* 250 µg (in 2-3 ml NS) IM *Children: younger than 2* years of age, 125 µg (in 1-2 ml NS) IM	Injectable: 250 µg/vial Reconstitute with glucose or saline solutions Do *not* add to blood or plasma because the cosyntropin may become inactivated	*Contraindicated* in hypersensitivity May cause hypersensitivity reactions (rarely) May cause irritation or pain at injection site	Observe for signs of hypersensitivity

Drug	Indications	Preparations and dosages	Clinical considerations	Nursing considerations
		Cosyntropin is a synthetic derivative of corticotropin; 250 µg of cosyntropin causes maximal stimulation of the adrenal cortex to the same extent as does 25 units of corticotropin		
Desonide	See Chapter 57, "Topical Corticoids"			
Desoximetasone	See Chapter 57, "Topical Corticosteroids"			
Desoxycorticosterone ★ Cortate Decostrate Decotone Descotone Doca Acetate Dorcostrin Doxatone Percorten Percorten Acetate Syncortin	Addison's disease, adrenogenital syndrome (salt losing)	*Adults:* 1-5 mg/24 hr IM (acetate salt), *or* 25 mg (for each 1 mg of acetate salt) IM every 4 weeks, *or* 125 mg (for each 1 mg of acetate salt) implanted subcutaneously every 8-12 months. *Children:* Same as adults (except dosage for pellet implantation has *not* yet been established)	Injectable: 5 mg/ml (acetate salt), 25 mg/ml (pivalate salt). Store between 15° and 30° C. Protect from light. Shake pivalate suspension well before withdrawing dose. Pellet (for subcutaneous implantation): 125 mg	*Contraindicated* in active or untreated tuberculosis; untreated or severe bacterial, fungal, or viral infections; acute psychoses; Cushing's syndrome; and active peptic ulcers. May mask signs of infection. May delay wound healing. May suppress pituitary adrenal function. Use with caution in patients with CHF, diabetes mellitus, hypertension, infectious disease, osteoporosis, and pregnancy. May cause fluid and electrolyte disturbances, such as sodium retention, potassium loss, calcium loss, fluid retention, and alkalosis. Use with caution in patients with cirrhosis or hypothyroidism. *Do not* administer smallpox vaccination while patient is receiving corticosteroid therapy	Observe for cushingoid symptoms (moonface, buffalo hump, muscle wasting, fluid retention, hirsutism, and mental changes). Monitor fluid and electrolyte status, particularly in elderly patients. Observe for signs of GI ulcers. Monitor for changes in mood, personality, or mentation. Monitor vision for cataract formation, particularly with prolonged administration

Continued.

NURSING DRUG DIGEST—cont'd

Medication (trade name)	Indication	Usual dosage and administration	Dosage forms, preparation, and storage	Contraindications, cautions, and comments	Monitoring
★ Desoxycorticosterone—cont'd				May cause or aggravate neurotic or psychotic behavior Prolonged administration may result in posterior subcapsular cataract formation Possesses high levels of mineralocorticoid activity with *no* glucocorticoid activity	
Dexamethasone Aeroseb-Dex Decaderm Decadron Decadron Decadron Eye-Ear Solution Decadron Phosphate Resphaler Decaspray Delladec Deronil Dexameth Dexasone Dexone Gammacorten Hexadrol Maxidex Maxidex Ophthalmic NeoDecadron* Novadex Optomethasone SK-Dexamethasone Turbinaire Decadron Phosphate	Conditions responsive to corticosteroid therapy (see box, p. 1487) Acute, nonfatal conditions (e.g., severe seasonal asthma) Chronic, nonfatal conditions (e.g., chronic bronchial asthma, rheumatoid arthritis) Acute, potentially fatal conditions (e.g., acute rheumatic carditis, systemic lupus erythematosus crisis) Chronic, potentially fatal conditions (e.g., pemphigus, systemic lupus erythematosus)	Use minimum effective dose, particularly in chronic conditions (see box, p. 1488, top left) *Adults:* 2-3 mg/24 hr PO; *or* (for acute inflammed joint *not* caused by infection) for small joints (e.g., interphalangeal): 0.5-1 mg intraarticular every 3-21 days; for large joints (e.g., knee): 2-4 mg intraarticular every 3-21 days *Adults:* 0.5-2 mg/24 hr PO in single or equally divided doses *Adults:* 4-10 mg/24 hr PO in 4 divided doses *Adults:* 2-5 mg/24 hr PO in 2-4 divided doses	Tablets: 0.25, 0.5, 0.75, 1.5, 4 mg Elixir: 0.5 mg/5 ml Injectable: 4, 8, 20 mg/ml Do *not* freeze If injectable form becomes frozen, it should be *discarded* Metered-dose inhaler: 0.1 mg/spray *Shake* inhaler well before use	*Contraindicated* in active or untreated tuberculosis; untreated or severe bacterial, fungal, or viral infections; acute psychoses; Cushing's syndrome; and active peptic ulcers May mask signs of infection May delay wound healing May suppress pituitary adrenal function Use with caution in patients with CHF, diabetes mellitus, hypertension, infectious disease, osteoporosis, and pregnancy May cause fluid and electrolyte disturbances, such as sodium retention, potassium loss, calcium loss, fluid retention, and alkalosis Use with caution in patients with cirrhosis or hypothyroidism	Observe for cushingoid symptoms (moonface, buffalo hump, muscle wasting, fluid retention, hirsutism, and mental changes) Observe children for growth suppression Monitor fluid and electrolyte status, particularly in elderly patients Observe for signs of GI ulcers Monitor for changes in mood, personality, or mentation Monitor vision for cataract formation, particularly with prolonged administration

Adrenogenital syndrome, congenital adrenal hyperplasia	Children: 0.5-1.5 mg/24 hr PO	Do *not* administer smallpox vaccination while patient is receiving corticosteroid therapy
Croup as an *adjunct* to conventional therapy with suitable antibiotics	Children: 2-5 mg PO as a single dose	May cause or aggravate neurotic or psychotic behavior
Cerebral edema	Adults: 10 mg IV followed by 4 mg q.6h. IM or IV until symptoms subside and dosage is gradually reduced over a period of 5-7 days, *or* (for *life-threatening* cerebral edema) 1.5 mg/kg IV, followed by 1.5 mg/kg/24 hr IV for 5 days, and then dosage is gradually reduced over 5 days	Prolonged administration may result in posterior subcapsular cataract formation
		Causes relatively *less* sodium and water retention than other corticosteroids
	Maintenance: For inoperable cases of cerebral edema, 2 mg b.i.d. to t.i.d. PO, IM, or IV	
	Children: 0.2 mg/kg/24 hr PO or IV in divided doses, *or* (for *life-threatening* cerebral edema) 1.5 mg/kg IV, followed by 1.5 mg/kg/24 hr IV for 5 days, and then dosage is gradually reduced over 5 days	
Test for Cushing's syndrome	Adults: 0.5 mg PO q.6h. for 48 hr, *or* 1 mg PO at 11 PM and determine plasma cortisol at 8 AM the following morning	
Test to distinguish adrenal tumor from hyperplasia	Adults: 2 mg PO q.6h. for 48 hr	
See also Chapter 57, "Topical Corticosteroids"	Administration of oral forms of dexamethasone with food or meals may decrease GI distress	

Continued.

NURSING DRUG DIGEST—cont'd

Medication (trade name)	Indication	Usual dosage and administration	Dosage forms, preparation, and storage	Contraindications, cautions, and comments	Monitoring
Diflorasone	See Chapter 57, "Topical Corticosteroids"				
Fludrocortisone Alflorone Cortef-F Florinef Fludrocortone	Addison's disease Adrenogenital syndrome (salt-losing)	*Adults:* 50-200 µg/24 hr PO (usual dose is 100 µg/24 hr) *Adults:* 100-200 µg/24 hr PO *Children:* Same as adults	Tablet: 100 µg	*Contraindicated* in active or untreated tuberculosis; untreated or severe bacterial, fungal, or viral infections; acute psychoses: Cushing's syndrome; and active peptic ulcers May mask signs of infection May delay wound healing May suppress pituitary adrenal function May cause hypersensitivity reaction; further use is *contraindicated* in these patients Use with caution in patients with CHF, diabetes mellitus, hypertension, infectious disease, osteoporosis, and pregnancy May cause fluid and electrolyte disturbances, such as sodium retention, potassium loss, calcium loss, fluid retention, and alkalosis Use with caution in patients with cirrhosis or hypothyroidism Do *not* administer smallpox vaccination while patient is receiving corticosteroid therapy	Observe for cushingoid symptoms (moonface, buffalo hump, muscle wasting, fluid retention, hirsutism, and mental changes) Observe children for growth suppression Monitor fluid and electrolyte status, particularly in elderly patients Observe for signs of GI ulcers Monitor for changes in mood, personality, or mentation Monitor vision for cataract formation, particularly with prolonged administration Monitor blood pressure

Drug	Use	Dosage	Preparations	Nursing Considerations
Flumethasone	See Chapter 57, "Topical Corticosteroids"			May cause or aggravate neurotic or psychotic behavior Prolonged administration may result in posterior subcapsular cataract formation Causes relatively *greater* sodium and fluid retention than hydrocortisone, although other physiologic effects are similar Salt-retaining action is of benefit in the treatment of salt-losing adrenogenital syndrome
Flunisolide Rhinalar Syntaris	Allergic rhinitis unresponsive to conventional treatment	*Adults:* 2 sprays in each nostril b.i.d. to t.i.d. Maximum: 6 sprays in each nostril a day *Children:* Under 6 years of age, *not recommended;* 6-14 years of age, 1 spray in each nostril q.d. to t.i.d. Maximum: 3 sprays in each nostril a day Lowest effective dose should be used	Metered nasal spray: 25 µg/spray	*Contraindicated* in active or untreated bacterial, fungal, or viral infections *Contraindicated* in hypersensitivity to the active ingredient or to any of the components of the vehicle May take several days (up to 1 week) before effectiveness of therapy is noted May cause nasal or throat irritation Observe for severe or persistent irritation of nose or throat Observe for systemic corticosteroid effects with prolonged chronic use
Fluocinolone	See Chapter 57, "Topical Corticosteroids"			
Fluocinonide	See Chapter 57, "Topical Corticosteroids"			
Fluorometholone	See Chapter 57, "Topical Corticosteroids"			

Continued.

NURSING DRUG DIGEST—cont'd

Medication (trade name)	Indication	Usual dosage and administration	Dosage forms, preparation, and storage	Contraindications, cautions, and comments	Monitoring
★ **Fluprednisolone** Alphadrol	Conditions responsive to corticosteroid therapy (see box, p. 1487)	Use minimum effective dose, particularly in chronic conditions (see box, p. 1488, top left) *Adults:* 3-30 mg/24 hr PO in single or divided doses *Children:* 0.25-1 mg/kg/24 hr PO in 3-4 divided doses	Tablet: 1.5 mg	*Contraindicated* in active or untreated tuberculosis; untreated or severe bacterial, fungal, or viral infections; acute psychoses; Cushing's syndrome; and active peptic ulcers May mask signs of infection May delay wound healing May suppress pituitary adrenal function Use with caution in patients with CHF, diabetes mellitus, hypertension, infectious disease, osteoporosis, and pregnancy May cause fluid and electrolyte disturbances, such as sodium retention, potassium loss, calcium loss, fluid retention, and alkalosis Use with caution in patients with cirrhosis or hypothyroidism Do *not* administer smallpox vaccination while patient is receiving corticosteroid therapy May cause or aggravate neurotic or psychotic behavior Prolonged administration may result in posterior subcapsular cataract formation	Observe for cushingoid symptoms (moonface, buffalo hump, muscle wasting, fluid retention, hirsutism, and mental changes) Observe children for growth suppression Monitor fluid and electrolyte status, particularly in elderly patients Observe for signs of GI ulcers Monitor for changes in mood, personality, or mentation Monitor vision for cataract formation, particularly with prolonged administration
Flurandrenolide	See Chapter 57, "Topical Corticosteroids"				
Halcinonide	See Chapter 57, "Topical Corticosteroids"				

| **Hydrocortisone** A-hydroCort Cortef Cortenema Cortisol Hydrocortone Solu-Cortef Texacort Unicort Westcort | Conditions responsive to corticosteroid therapy (see box, p. 1487)

Acute, nonfatal conditions (e.g., severe seasonal asthma)

Chronic, nonfatal conditions (e.g., bronchial asthma, rheumatoid arthritis)

Acute, potentially fatal conditions (e.g., acute rheumatic carditis, systemic lupus erythematosus crisis)

Chronic, potentially fatal conditions (e.g., nephrotic syndrome)

Adrenal insufficiency (e.g., Addison's disease)

Prophylaxis against inflammation for dental surgical procedures

See also Chapter 57, "Topical Corticosteroids" | Use minimum effective dose, particularly in chronic conditions (see box, p. 1488, top left)

Adults: 60-120 mg/24 hr PO; or (for acute inflamed joint *not* caused by infection), for small joints (e.g., interphalangeal): 10-25 mg intraarticular every 14-21 days; for large joints (e.g., knee): 25-37.5 mg intraarticular every 14-21 days

Adults: 20-60 mg/24 hr PO

Adults: 100-240 mg/24 hr PO in 4 divided doses

Adults: 60-120 mg/24 hr PO

Adults: 8-20 mg/24 hr PO (administer together with 4-6 gm of sodium chloride PO)

Adults: 20-40 mg PO t.i.d. starting 2 hr before procedure and continuing for 2-3 days | Injectable: 25, 50 mg/ml Tablets: 5, 10, 20 mg Rectal enema: 100 mg/60 ml Rectal foam: 10% (90 mg applicator) Shake rectal enema and foam forms well before use Rectal suppositories: 15, 25 mg | *Contraindicated* in active or untreated tuberculosis; untreated or severe bacterial, fungal, or viral infections; acute psychoses; Cushing's syndrome; and active peptic ulcers

May mask signs of infection

May delay wound healing

May suppress pituitary adrenal function

May cause hypersensitivity reaction; further use is *contraindicated* in these patients

Use with caution in patients with CHF, diabetes mellitus, hypertension, infectious disease, osteoporosis, and pregnancy

May cause fluid and electrolyte disturbances, such as sodium retention, potassium loss, calcium loss, fluid retention, and alkalosis

Use with caution in patients with cirrhosis or hypothyroidism

Do *not* administer smallpox vaccination while patient is receiving corticosteroid therapy

May cause or aggravate neurotic or psychotic behavior

Prolonged administration may result in posterior subcapsular cataract formation | Observe for cushingoid symptoms (moon face, buffalo hump, muscle wasting, fluid retention, hirsutism, and mental changes) Observe children for growth suppression Monitor fluid and electrolyte status, particularly in elderly patients Observe for signs of GI ulcers Monitor for changes in mood, personality, or mentation Monitor vision for cataract formation, particularly with prolonged administration |

Continued.

NURSING DRUG DIGEST—cont'd

Medication (trade name)	Indication	Usual dosage and administration	Dosage forms, preparation, and storage	Contraindications, cautions, and comments	Monitoring
Medrysone HMS Liquifilm Medrocort Visudrisone	Corticosteroid-responsive ophthalmic conditions (see box, p. 1489, left)	*Adults:* Initially, if indicated, 1-2 drops in conjunctival sac of affected eye(s) q.1h. during day and q.2h. during evening Following initial improvement, 1 drop t.i.d. to q.i.d. *Children:* 1 drop in conjunctival sac of affected eye(s) up to q.4h. (usually t.i.d. to q.i.d.)	Ophthalmic suspension: 1% *Do not* freeze	*Contraindicated* in hypersensitivity to medrysone or any of the components of the ophthalmic suspension *Contraindicated* in fungal or viral diseases of the eye or related structures, ocular tuberculosis, and herpes simplex keratitis Prolonged use may result in ocular damage, including glaucoma and posterior subcapsular cataract formation	Observe for adverse ocular effects Monitor for systemic effects, particularly with prolonged use
Methylprednisolone Depo-Medrol Depo-Predate 80 Medrate Medrol Medrol Acetate Medrol Acne Lotion* Medrol Topical Medrone Mepred 40 & 80 Metastab Neo-Medrol* Neomedrol Acne Lotion* Solu-Medrol Urbason Wyacort	Conditions responsive to corticosteroid therapy (see box, p. 1487) Acute, nonfatal conditions (e.g., allergic conditions) Chronic, nonfatal conditions (e.g., rheumatoid arthritis)	Use minimum effective dose, particularly in chronic conditions (see box, p. 1488, top left) Because the adrenal suppressive activity of methylprednisolone is short-acting, it is an appropriate drug for alternate-day therapy; when this regimen is used, the total 48-hr appropriate drug requirement is administered every other day at 8 AM *Adults:* 12-40 mg/24 hr PO; *or* (for acute inflamed joint *not* caused by infection) for small joints (e.g., interphalangeal): 4-10 mg intraarticular every 1-5 *weeks;* for large joints (e.g., knee): 20-80 mg intraarticular every 1-5 *weeks* *Adults:* 8-16 mg/24 hr PO in 4 equally divided doses for 3-7 days Maintenance: 4-12 mg/24 hr PO in 4 equally divided doses	Tablets: 2, 4, 8, 16, 24, 32 mg Injectable: 40, 125, 500, 1000 mg/vial (methylprednisolone sodium succinate); 20, 40, 80 mg/ml (methylprednisolone acetate) Lotion: 2.5 mg/ml (in combination with sulfur) Ophthalmic solution: 1 mg/ml Otic solution: 1 mg/ml Ophthalmic ointment: 1 mg/gm (0.1%) Ointment: 2.5 mg/gm (0.25%) NOTE: For the injectable salts of methylprednisolone: the *sodium succinate salt* form should be administered by slow IV infusion, whereas the *acetate salt* form should be administered by either the IM or intraarticular routes; the acetate salt can also be administered directly (20-60 mg) into a dermatologic lesion	*Contraindicated* in active or untreated tuberculosis; untreated or severe bacterial, fungal, or viral infections; acute psychoses; Cushing's syndrome; and active peptic ulcers May mask signs of infection May delay wound healing May suppress pituitary adrenal function May cause hypersensitivity reaction; further use is *contraindicated* in these patients Use with caution in patients with CHF, diabetes mellitus, hypertension, infectious disease, osteoporosis, and pregnancy	Observe for cushingoid symptoms (moonface, buffalo hump, muscle wasting, fluid retention, hirsutism, and mental changes) Observe children for growth suppression Monitor fluid and electrolyte status, particularly in elderly patients Observe for signs of GI ulcers Monitor for changes in mood, personality, or mentation Monitor vision for cataract formation, particularly with prolonged administration Observe for local irritation with topical preparations

Continued.

Uses	Dosage	Remarks
Chronic, potentially fatal conditions (e.g., nephrotic syndrome)	*Children:* 6-10 mg/24 hr PO in 4 equally divided doses for 3-7 days Maintenance: 2-8 mg/24 hr PO in 4 equally divided doses *Adults:* 20-80 mg/24 hr PO in 4 equally divided doses for 10-14 days (until diuresis) Decrease dose by 1-2 mg/week until maintenance dose is achieved Maintenance: 12-40 mg PO for the first 3 days of each week for 6-12 months	May cause fluid and electrolyte disturbances, such as sodium retention, potassium loss, calcium loss, fluid retention, and alkalosis Use with caution in patients with cirrhosis or hypothyroidism Do *not* administer smallpox vaccination while patient is receiving corticosteroid therapy May cause or aggravate neurotic or psychotic behavior Prolonged administration may result in posterior subcapsular cataract formation Methylprednisolone causes relatively *little* sodium retention Use *only* ophthalmic preparations in or near the eye Topical skin preparations may cause local reactions, such as dryness, folliculitis, irritation, itching, pigmentary changes, and striae Rapid IV administration of large doses may cause cardiovascular collapse
Corticosteroid-responsive dermatoses (see box, p. 1488, right)	*Adults:* Apply a small amount to affected area q.d. to t.i.d. *Children:* Same as adults	
Corticosteroid-responsive ophthalmic conditions (see box, p. 1489, left)	*Adults:* Initially, 1-2 drops of ophthalmic solution (or a small amount of *ophthalmic* ointment) in the conjunctival sac of affected eye(s) q.1h. during day and q.2h. during evening; following initial improvement, 1 drop (or a small amount of the *ophthalmic* ointment) t.i.d. to q.i.d.	
Otitis, external (contact, noninfective eczematoid, or seborrheic dermatitis of the external ear canal)	*Adults:* 2-3 drops of *otic* solution in the external canal of the affected ear(s) t.i.d. to q.i.d.	The sodium succinate salt is compatible for infusion with D$_5$W and NS solutions (also compatible with plasma and whole blood)
Prevention or treatment of transplant organ rejection	*Adults:* 500-2000 mg q.24-48h. by slow IV over at least 10 min	
Adjunct in the treatment of severe shock	*Adults:* 500-1500 mg/24 hr IV in single or divided doses; the initial dose should be administered by slow IV over a period of at least 10 min	
Adjunct in the treatment of ulcerative colitis See also Chapter 57, "Topical Corticosteroids"	*Adults:* 40-120 mg (of the sodium succinate salt dissolved in 30-300 ml water) administered as a retention enema 3-7 times a week for 2 or more weeks	

NURSING DRUG DIGEST—cont'd

Medication (trade name)	Indication	Usual dosage and administration	Dosage forms, preparation, and storage	Contraindications, cautions, and comments	Monitoring
Metyrapone Metopirone	Diagnostic test of partial hypopituitarism (limited pituitary reserve) Diagnostic test for Cushing's syndrome (with adrenal hyperplasia)	Adults: 750 mg PO q.4h. for 6 doses Children: 15 mg/kg PO q.4h. for 6 doses Administration with food or milk may decrease GI distress	Tablet: 250 mg	Contraindicated in hypersensitivity and adrenal cortical insufficiency May cause GI distress IV administration may cause thrombophlebitis NOTE that several drugs, including carisoprodol, chlorpromazine, estrogens, meprobamate, and phenytoin, may cause decreased response to the metyrapone test and thus confound the interpretation of the results	Observe for GI distress
Mitotane Lysodren	Inoperable adrenocortical carcinoma (functional and nonfunctional)	Adults: 2-6 gm/24 hr PO in 3-4 divided doses and increase dose as tolerated to 8-10 gm/24 hr, or 9-10 gm/24 hr PO in 3-4 divided doses, and decrease dose if necessary Children: 1-2 gm/24 hr PO in 3-4 divided doses, and increase dose as tolerated to 5-7 gm/24 hr Administration with food or milk may decrease GI distress Decrease dose in severe liver impairment	Tablet: 500 mg	Contraindicated in known hypersensitivity Commonly causes GI distress, CNS depression, and skin toxicity Use with caution in patients with liver impairment May induce drug metabolizing enzymes and require dosage modification of concomitantly administered medications Long-term, high-dose therapy may cause impaired neurologic function and brain damage	Observe for GI distress Observe for signs of skin toxicity Monitor behavior and neurologic activity Assessments of behavioral and neurologic function should be performed at regular intervals for patients on long-term therapy (more than 2 years)

| ★ **Parametha-sone**
Alondra
Dilar
Haldrate
Haldrona
Haldrone
Monocortin
Stemex | Conditions responsive to corticosteroid therapy (see box, p. 1487) | Use minimum effective dose, particularly in chronic conditions (see box, p. 1488, top left)
Adults: 2-24 mg/24 hr PO as single or divided doses
Children: 0.06-0.08 mg/kg/24 hr PO as single or divided doses | Tablets: 1, 2 mg | *Contraindicated* in active or untreated tuberculosis; untreated or severe bacterial, fungal, or viral infections; acute psychoses; Cushing's syndrome; and active peptic ulcers
May mask signs of infection
May delay wound healing
May suppress pituitary adrenal function
Use with caution in patients with CHF, diabetes mellitus, hypertension, osteoporosis, infectious disease, and pregnancy
May cause fluid and electrolyte disturbances, such as sodium retention, potassium loss, calcium loss, fluid retention, and alkalosis
Use with caution in patients with cirrhosis or hypothyroidism
Do not administer smallpox vaccination while patient is receiving corticosteroid therapy
May cause or aggravate neurotic or psychotic behavior
Prolonged administration may result in posterior subcapsular cataract formation
Approximately 2½ times as potent as prednisone | Observe for cushingoid symptoms (moon-face, buffalo hump, muscle wasting, fluid retention, hirsutism, and mental changes)
Observe children for growth suppression
Monitor fluid and electrolyte status, particularly in elderly patients
Observe for signs of GI ulcers
Monitor for changes in mood, personality, or mentation
Monitor vision for cataract formation, particularly with prolonged administration |

Continued.

NURSING DRUG DIGEST—cont'd

Medication (trade name)	Indication	Usual dosage and administration	Dosage forms, preparation, and storage	Contraindications, cautions, and comments	Monitoring
Prednisolone Ataraxoid* Blephamide Liquifilm* Blephamide Ointment* Blephamide Ophthalmic* Blephamide S.O.P.* Cetapred* Delta-Cortef Econopred Fermisolone-P Hydeltra Hydeltrasol Hydeltra-T.B.A. Inflamase Isopto Cetapred* Meticortelone Meti-Derm Metimyd* Metreton Neo-Delta-Cortef*	Conditions responsive to corticosteroid therapy (see box, p. 1487)	Use minimum effective dose, particularly in chronic conditions (see box, p. 1488, top left)	Tablets: 1, 2.5, 5 mg Injectable: 25, 40, 50, 80, 100 mg/ml (prednisolone acetate and prednisolone tebutate are for IM, intralesional, or intraarticular use only—do not administer IV; prednisolone sodium phosphate can be administered by the IM, intralesional, intraarticular, and IV routes) *Shake* injectable suspension forms well before withdrawing dose	*Contraindicated* in active or untreated tuberculosis; untreated or severe bacterial, fungal, or viral infections; acute psychoses; Cushing's syndrome; and active peptic ulcers May mask signs of infection May delay wound healing	Observe for cushingoid symptoms (moonface, buffalo hump, muscle wasting, fluid retention, hirsutism, and mental changes) Observe children for growth suppression Monitor fluid and electrolyte status, particularly in elderly patients Observe for signs of GI ulcers Monitor for changes in mood, personality, or mentation Monitor vision for cataract formation, particularly with prolonged administration
	Acute, nonfatal conditions (e.g., acute rheumatic disorders)	*Adults:* 20-30 mg/24 hr PO, *or* (for acute inflamed joint *not* caused by infection) for small joints (e.g., interphalangeal): 10-15 mg intraarticularly and may be repeated in 3-5 days; for large joints (e.g., knee): 25-37.5 mg intraarticularly and may be repeated in 3-5 days			
	Chronic, nonfatal conditions (e.g., bronchial asthma, chronic rheumatoid arthritis)	*Adults:* 5-20 mg/24 hr PO in 3-4 divided doses	Injectable: 20 mg/ml (prednisolone sodium phosphate for IM, IV, intraarticular, and intralesional administration), 20 mg/ml (prednisolone tebutate for intraarticular and intralesional administration) NOTE: Because of its greater solubility, prednisolone is	May suppress pituitary adrenal function Use with caution in patients with CHF, diabetes mellitus, hypertension, infectious disease, osteoporosis, and pregnancy May cause fluid and electrolyte disturbances, such as sodium retention, potassium loss, calcium loss, fluid retention, and alkalosis	
	Acute, potentially fatal conditions (e.g., acute rheumatic carditis, systemic lupus erythematosus crisis)	*Adults:* 30-60 mg/24 hr PO or IV in 4 divided doses			

Neo-Hydeltra-
sol*
Nova-Pred
Optimyd*
Paracortol
Predate-
L.A.S.A.
Predate-100
Pred Forte
Pred Mild
Predne-Dome
Prednicon
Prednis
Predoxine
Predulose
PSI-IV
Sodasone
Sterane
Sterolone
Ulacort

Chronic, poten-
tially fatal con-
ditions (e.g., ne-
phrotic syn-
drome)
Congenital adre-
nal hyperplasia
Postoperative den-
tal inflammation
Can also be used
to treat derma-
tologic condi-
tions responsive
to intralesional
corticosteroid
therapy
See also Chapter
57, "Topical
Corticosteroids"

Adults: 30-40 mg/24 hr PO in 4
divided doses

Children: 2.5-10 mg/24 hr PO

Adults: 5 mg PO t.i.d. for 1-3
days
Adults: 2-60 mg intralesional
(dosage is highly variable
and must be individualized)
NOTE: For patients who are either seriously ill and cannot
take oral medications or
who are undergoing surgery,
IM prednisolone can generally be substituted for PO
therapy; IM administration
with a 20-gauge 3.9 cm (1.5
inch) needle is usually associated with little or no irritation
NOTE: If parenteral administration is planned, note which
salt form of prednisolone is
being used (see Dosage
Forms, Preparation, and
Storage); only the sodium
phosphate form should be
administered IV
Maximum oral adult dose: 250
mg/24 hr

less irritating to tissues
than prednisone and is
thus more suitable for IM,
intralesional, and intraarticular administration

Use with caution in pa-
tients with cirrhosis or
hypothyroidism
Do not administer
smallpox vaccination
while patient is receiv-
ing corticosteroid
therapy
May cause or aggravate
neurotic or psychotic
behavior
Prolonged administra-
tion may result in
posterior subcapsular
cataract formation

Continued.

NURSING DRUG DIGEST—cont'd

Medication (trade name)	Indication	Usual dosage and administration	Dosage forms, preparation, and storage	Contraindications, cautions, and comments	Monitoring
Prednisone Colisone Decortancyl Delta-Dome Deltasone Listacort Meticorten Orasone Paracort Servisone SK-Prednisone Steapred Uni-Pak Winpred Zenadrin	Conditions responsive to corticosteroid therapy (see box, p. 1487)	Use minimum effective dose, particularly in chronic conditions (see box, p. 1488, top left)	Tablets: 1, 2.5, 5, 10, 20, 50 mg	*Contraindicated* in active or untreated tuberculosis; untreated or severe bacterial, fungal, or viral infections; acute psychoses; Cushing's syndrome; and active peptic ulcers	Observe for cushingoid symptoms (moon-face, buffalo hump, muscle wasting, fluid retention, hirsutism, and mental changes)
	Acute, nonfatal conditions (e.g., acute rheumatic disorders)	*Adults:* 20-30 mg/24 hr PO		May mask signs of infection	Observe children for growth suppression
	Chronic, nonfatal conditions (e.g., chronic bronchial asthma, chronic rheumatoid arthritis)	*Adults:* 5-20 mg/24 hr PO in 3-4 divided doses		May delay wound healing	Monitor fluid and electrolyte status, particularly in elderly patients
	Acute, potentially fatal conditions (e.g., acute rheumatic carditis, systemic lupus erythematosus crisis)	*Adults:* 30-60 mg/24 hr PO in 4 divided doses		May suppress pituitary adrenal function	Observe for signs of GI ulcers
	Chronic, potentially fatal conditions (e.g., nephrotic syndrome)	*Adults:* 30-40 mg/24 hr PO in 4 divided doses		Use with caution in patients with CHF, diabetes mellitus, hypertension, infectious disease, osteoporosis, and pregnancy	Monitor for changes in mood, personality, or mentation
	Congenital adrenal hyperplasia	*Children:* 2.5-10 mg/24 hr PO		May cause fluid and electrolyte disturbances, such as sodium retention, potassium loss, calcium loss, fluid retention, and alkalosis	Monitor vision for cataract formation, particularly with prolonged administration
	Postoperative dental inflammation	*Adults:* 5 mg PO t.i.d. for 1-3 days		Use with caution in patients with cirrhosis or hypothyroidism	
				Do *not* administer smallpox vaccination while patient is receiving corticosteroid therapy	
				May cause or aggravate neurotic or psychotic behavior	
				Prolonged administration may result in posterior subcapsular cataract formation	
				Metabolized to prednisolone, the physiologically active form in the body	

Drug	Uses	Dosage	Preparations	Contraindications/Cautions	Nursing Considerations
Triamcinolone Aristform* Aristform D* Aristform R* Aristocort Aristoderm Aristogel Aristosol Aristospan Cinalone 40 Cinolone-T Flutone Kenacomb* Kenacort Kenalog Kenalog in orabase Kenalog-E Myco Triacet Cream & Ointment* Mycolog* Mytrex* Mysolone* Spencort SK-Triamcinolone Tramacin Triaderm Triamalone Tricilone NNG* Trimacort Trymex Viaderm-TA	Conditions responsive to corticosteroid therapy (see box, p. 1487) Corticosteroid-responsive dermatoses (see box, p. 1488 right) Dermal lesions responsive to intradermal administration (e.g., discoid lupus erythematosus, keloids) See also Chapter 57, "Topical Corticosteroids" Acute inflamed joint *not* caused by infection	Use minimum effective dose, particularly in chronic conditions (see box, p. 1488, top left) *Adults:* 4-48 mg/24 hr PO in 1-4 divided doses *Children:* (under 27 kg) 4-12 mg/24 hr PO in 1-4 divided doses; (27 kg and over) same as adult dose *Adults:* Apply a small amount of cream, ointment, lotion, spray, or paste to affected area b.i.d. to q.i.d. *Children:* Same as adults *Adults:* 0.25-1 mg intradermally per dermal lesion (each lesion so treated should be 1 cm or more distant from other treated lesions); use of a tuberculin syringe with a 23-25 gauge needle is recommended; for multiple injections ethyl chloride spray may be used to alleviate local discomfort *Adults:* small joints (e.g., interphalangeal): 2.5-5 mg intraarticularly; large joints (e.g., knee): 5-15 mg intraarticularly NOTE: For patients who are either seriously ill and cannot take oral medications or who are undergoing surgery, IM triamcinolone (33%-50% of dose administered q.12h.) can be substituted for PO therapy; for some patients and conditions, the weekly PO dose administered as a single IM dose may be effective for 4-30 days; administer IM doses deeply into the gluteal muscle IM injections of triamcinolone cause less tissue atrophy when injected into the gluteal as opposed to the deltoid site (see Chapter 2, "Preparation, Administration, and Monitoring of Medications") Do *not* administer IV	Cream: 0.025, 0.1% Ointment: 0.025, 0.1% Lotion: 0.1% Topical spray: 0.2% Dental paste: 0.1% Tablets: 1, 2, 4, 8, 16 mg Syrup: 2, 4 mg/5 ml Injectable: 10, 40 mg/ml (suspension for IM, intradermal, and intraarticular use) Generally, the 10 mg/ml injectable is administered either intradermally or intraarticularly, and the 40 mg/ml by the IM route *Shake* vial well before withdrawing dose	*Contraindicated* in active or untreated tuberculosis; untreated or severe bacterial, fungal, or viral infections; acute psychoses; Cushing's syndrome; and active peptic ulcers May mask signs of infection May delay wound healing May suppress pituitary adrenal function Use with caution in patients with CHF, diabetes mellitus, hypertension, infectious disease, osteoporosis, and pregnancy May cause fluid and electrolyte disturbances, such as sodium retention, potassium loss, calcium loss, fluid retention, and alkalosis Use with caution in patients with cirrhosis or hypothyroidism Do *not* administer smallpox vaccination while patient is receiving corticosteroid therapy May cause or aggravate neurotic or psychotic behavior Prolonged administration may result in posterior subcapsular cataract formation	Observe for cushingoid symptoms (moon-face, buffalo hump, muscle wasting, fluid retention, hirsutism, and mental changes) Observe children for growth suppression Monitor fluid and electrolyte status, particularly in elderly patients Observe for signs of GI ulcers Monitor for changes in mood, personality, or mentation Monitor vision for cataract formation, particularly with prolonged administration

BIBLIOGRAPHY

Dixon, R., & Christy, N. On the various forms of corticosteroid withdrawal syndrome. *The American Journal of Medicine,* 1980, *68,* 224-230.

Gotch, P.M. Teaching patients about adrenal corticosteroids. *American Journal of Nursing,* 1981, *81*(1), 78-81.

Johnson, L.K. If your patient has increased intracranial pressure, your goal should be: no surprises. *Nursing 83,* 1983, *13*(6), 58-63.

LaMont, J.T. Recommendations for inflammatory bowel disease. *Geriatrics,* 1982, *37*(3), 93-96, 102-105.

Self, T.H., Smith, S.L., Boswell, R.L., & Miller, W.A. Medical education provided by a clinical pharmacist: impact on the use and cost of corticosteroid therapy in chronic obstructive pulmonary disease. *Drug Intelligence and Clinical Pharmacy,* 1984, *18,* 241-244.

Sharfstein, S., Sack, D., & Fauci, A. Relationship between alternate-day corticosteroid therapy and behavioral abnormalities. *Journal of the American Medical Association,* 1982, *248,* 2987-2989.

Spiro, H.M. Is the steroid ulcer a myth? *The New England Journal of Medicine,* 1983, *309*(1), 45-47.

Spunt, A.L. Drug therapy for multiple sclerosis. *Drug Store News Continuing Education Program,* No. 679-401-16, December 12, 1983.

Subrt, P., & Raimer, S.S. Corticosteroids in the elderly. *Geriatrics,* 1983, *38*(2), 135-37, 141-2, 147, 151.

MISCELLANEOUS THERAPEUTIC AND DIAGNOSTIC AGENTS

Medications discussed in this section

CHAPTER 66

Ascorbic acid
Calcium
Cobalt
Copper
Cyanocobalamin
Fluorine
Folic acid
Iodine
Iron
Magnesium
Niacin
Phytonadione
Potassium
Pyridoxine
Riboflavin
Sodium
Sulfur
Thiamine
Vitamin A
Vitamin D
Vitamin E
Zinc

CHAPTER 67

Bicarbonate
Calcium
Magnesium
Potassium
Sodium

CHAPTER 68

Antirabies serum equine
BCG (Bacillus Calmette-Guerin vaccine
Cholera vaccine
Diphtheria toxoid
Hepatitis B immune globulin
Hepatitis B vaccine

CHAPTER 68—cont'd

Human diploid cell rabies vaccine
Human serum immune globulin
Influenza vaccine
Measles vaccine
Meningococcal polysaccharide vaccines
Mumps vaccine
Pertussis vaccine
Plague vaccine
Polyvalent pneumococcal vaccine
Poliomyelitis vaccine
Poliovirus vaccine
Rabies immune globulin, human
Rabies vaccine
Rubella vaccine
Smallpox vaccine
Tetanus immune globulin, human
Tetanus toxoid
Typhoid vaccine
Typhus vaccine
Varicella-zoster immune globulin
Yellow fever vaccine

CHAPTER 69

Black widow spider (*Lactrodectus mactans*) antivenin
Botulism antitoxin
Diphtheria antitoxin
Hymenoptera venom allergenic extracts (bee venom, yellow jacket, yellow hornet, white faced hornet, wasp)
North American coral snake (*Micrurus fulvius*) antivenin
Polyvalent Crotalidae antivenin
Tetanus antitoxin

CHAPTER 70

^{198}Au-Colloidal gold
^{57}Co-Cyanocobalamin
^{51}Cr-Sodium chromate
^{67}Ga-Gallium citrate
^{125}I-Fibrinogen
^{125}I-Human serum albumin
^{131}I-Human serum albumin
^{123}I-Orthoiodohippurate
^{131}I-Orthoiodohippurate
^{131}I-Rose bengal
^{123}I-Sodium iodide
^{131}I-Sodium iodide
^{111}In-Chloride
^{113m}In-Chloride
^{75}Se-Selenomethionine
^{99m}Tc-Antimony sulfide
^{99m}Tc-Calcium phytate
^{99m}Tc-Diphosphonates
^{99m}Tc-DTPA
^{99m}Tc-Human serum albumin
^{99m}Tc-HIDA
^{99m}Tc-Glucoheptonate
^{99m}Tc-Labeled RBC
^{99m}Tc-Pyrophosphate
^{99m}Tc-Sodium pertechnetate
^{99m}Tc-Sulfur colloid
^{201}Tl-Thallous chloride
^{133}Xe
^{169}Yb-Ytterbium DTPA

CHAPTER 71

Acetohydroxamic acid
Alprostadil
Aminobenzoic acid
Aminocaproic acid
Amrinone
Antihemophilic factor
Bromocriptine
Carbamide peroxide

CHAPTER 71—cont'd

Carbazochrome salicylate
Charcoal, activated
Chenodiol
Chymopapain
Chymotrypsin
Collagenase
Cyclosporine
Cyproheptadine
Dexpanthenol
Dicyclomine
Dihydroergotamine
Dimercaprol
Dipivefrin
Doxylamine
Edetate calcium disodium
Ergoloid mesylates
Ergonovine
Ergotamine
Factor IX complex
Fibrinolysin and desoxyribonuclease
Gonadotropin, chorionic
Hemin
Hyaluronidase
Lactase
Menotropins
Methysergide
Metyrosine
Oxytocin
Papain and urea
Pentoxifylline
Quinine
Ritodrine
Sodium cellulose phosphate
Sodium fluoride
Sodium polystyrene sulfonate
Somatropin
Streptokinase
Urokinase
Vasopressin

CHAPTER 66

Vitamins, Minerals, and Trace Elements

Ronald T. Coutts

Medications discussed in this chapter

Vitamins	Minerals
Ascorbic acid	Calcium
Cyanocobalamin	Iron
Folic acid	Magnesium
Niacin	Potassium
Phytonadione	Sodium
Pyridoxine	Sulfur
Riboflavin	*Trace elements*
Thiamine	Cobalt
Vitamin A	Copper
Vitamin D	Fluorine
Vitamin E	Iodine
	Zinc

Vitamins are organic compounds that in minute amounts are essential for normal body growth and metabolic function. Since the body cannot synthesize most vitamins (vitamins D and K are exceptions), they must be ingested. Vitamins are found in numerous plants and animal tissues. A balanced diet that includes dairy products, meat or fish, vegetables, fruits, and cereals will normally supply sufficient amounts of all vitamins, but if the diet is not an adequate source, vitamin supplements are necessary.

Vitamins are involved in biochemical reactions. All such reactions require catalysts, called enzymes, and the body contains hundreds of them. Some are specific in their action; others are nonspecific and capable of catalyzing many different biochemical reactions. Enzymes have two major component parts, the *apoenzyme* (a protein portion) and the *coenzyme* (a nonprotein prosthetic group), which play an important role in the interaction between the enzyme and substrate or target molecule on which it acts. Vitamins are components of the coenzyme portions of enzymes. Nicotinamide (vitamin B_3), for example, is a component of the important coenzymes nicotinamide adenine dinucleotide (NAD) and the corresponding phosphate (NADP). Numerous enzymes contain NAD or NADP as coenzymes. Metabolic oxidations, for example, require NADP.

It follows that enzyme deficiencies will seriously affect many biochemical reactions in the body and that a deficiency of even one vitamin can adversely affect diverse biochemical reactions and result in what first appears to be a considerable number of unrelated symptoms. When biochemical reactions are adversely affected by enzyme deficiencies, chemicals that are normally further metabolized can build up in the body's cells. This accumulation can lead to loss of cell function or even death of the cell. Symptoms of abnormal cellular behavior can be extremely variable. Severe mental disturbances, for example, may be particularly symptomatic.

Vitamins in common usage (i.e., A, B, C, D, E, and K) are classified according to their solubility characteristics. Vitamins A, D, E, and K are *fat-soluble vitamins;* vitamins B_1, B_2, B_6, nicotinic acid, nicotinamide, pantothenic acid, and vitamin C are the *water-soluble vitamins;* folic acid (i.e., vitamin B_c) and vitamin B_{12} are generally not assigned to either group. The former is water insoluble, whereas the latter is poorly soluble in water. Folic acid and vitamin B_{12} are separately classified as hemopoietic vitamins.

VITAMIN A

Vitamin A is one of the fat-soluble vitamins. It exists in a variety of forms (i.e., retinol, retinal, and retinoic acid); vitamin A is a collective name for these forms. Retinol (vitamin A_1) is present as a mixture of geometric isomers in the tissues of saltwater fishes, mainly in the liver. *Trans*-retinol and its oxidized product, retinal, have the greatest biologic potency.

Occurrence

The main sources of vitamin A are dietary. The carotenes are present in higher plants (e.g., green vege-

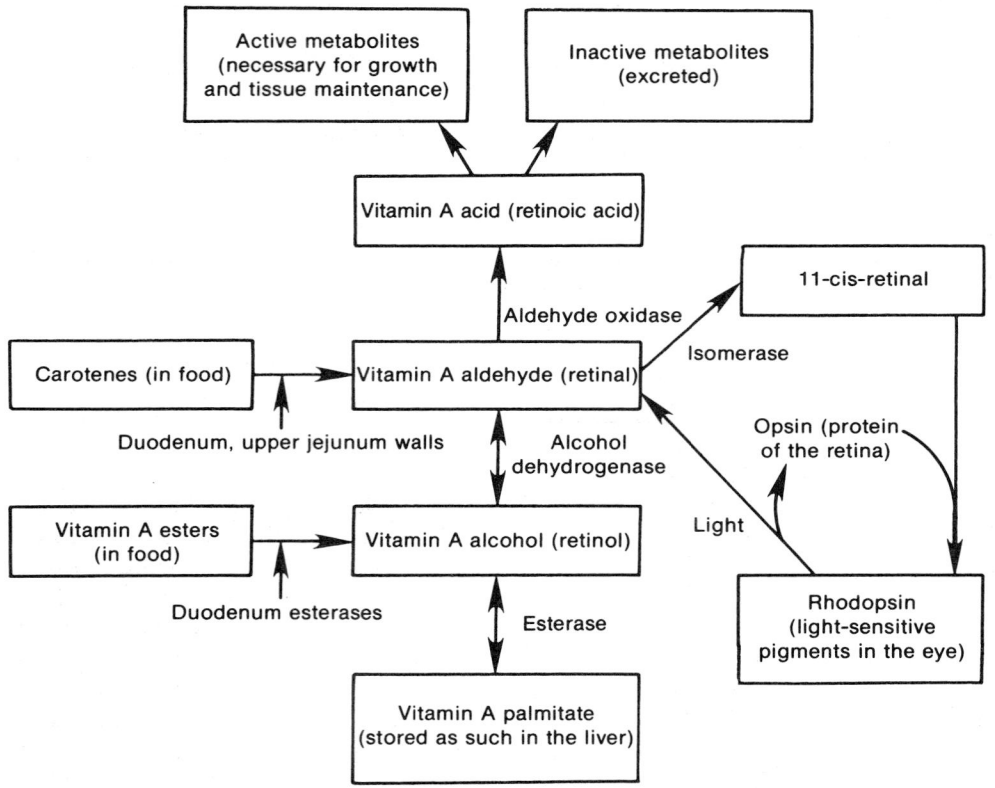

FIGURE 66-1. **Vitamin A. Carotenes are oxidized in the duodenum or upper jejunum to vitamin A aldehyde and subsequently reduced to vitamin A alcohol. Vitamin A is stored in the liver as the palmitate ester.**

tables and carrots) and algae, and are synthesized by photosynthetic bacteria. The carotenes are classified as *provitamins.* They are oxidized in humans in the duodenum or upper jejunum to vitamin A aldehyde and subsequently reduced to vitamin A alcohol. The process is illustrated in Figure 66-1.

Vitamin A is present in a large number of foods, especially fish liver oils, butter, and egg yolk. Cod, herring, halibut, and liver oils contain approximately 1000, 5000, and 50,000 to 100,000 international units (IU)* per gram respectively. Polar bear whole liver contains 20,000 IU of vitamin A per gram—a very rich source; acute vitamin A toxicity has been observed following its consumption.

Function

Vitamin A has a number of important roles in normal body function. It is required for the maintenance of health and life, for normal growth and reproduc-

tivity, and for the visual process (functioning of the retina).

It is vitamin A alcohol (retinol) that is essential for normal reproduction in both sexes, although its actual involvement in the biochemical process for this purpose is not known. Vitamin A aldehyde (retinal) is the derivative that is involved in the visual process. Vitamin A acid (retinoic acid) is known to be active in maintaining growth but has been shown to be incapable of maintaining reproductivity. Retinoic acid is also involved in some way in the synthesis of corticosterone from desoxycorticosterone.

Vitamin A is also believed to play a part in the synthesis of other corticosteroids, especially in the conversion of pregnenolone to progesterone and dehydroepiandrosterone to androstenedione.

Vitamin A requirement

A normal North American daily diet contains about 7500 to 10,000 IU (2.3 to 3 mg) of vitamin A, half of which is ingested in the form of provitamin (caro-

_____
*One IU Vitamin A = 0.30 μg of *all trans*-vitamin A alcohol.

tenes). The generally accepted daily requirement is 1400 to 2000 IU for infants, 2000 to 3300 IU for children, 4000 IU for adult women, and 5000 IU for adult men. Pregnant and lactating women require 5000 to 6000 IU per day. Vitamin A is stored in the liver mainly as the palmitate ester (Figure 66-1).

Vitamin A deficiency

Vitamin A deficiency retards normal growth and development. Usually tissue reserves are sufficiently large that a dietary lack of vitamin A is slow to manifest itself. However, reserves can be quickly used up in infections, hyperthermia, poisoning, and in other instances in which tissue maintenance is required.

Vitamin A deficiency is often associated with diseases that affect fat absorption, such as biliary tract or pancreatic disease, cirrhosis of the liver, and colitis. Deficiency is also associated with general malnutrition and is widespread in many developing countries. Because of their eating habits, a considerable number of North American youths have a low vitamin A intake, bordering on deficiency. Vitamin A deficiency can also be the result of disturbances in the conversion of carotene into the vitamin.

Typical results of vitamin A deficiency are nightblindness (nyctalopia), xerosis (dryness, for example, of the eye or skin), or keratinization of various membranes, especially xerophthalmia (conjunctivitis with atrophy and no liquid discharge in the eye), skin roughness, and the formation of defective bony tissue (thick spongy bone instead of thinner compact bone) and dentine.

Hypervitaminosis A

An intake of large excesses of vitamin A (i.e., 100,000 IU or more daily over a protracted period) is toxic. It has been observed in children whose parents have been overzealous in the prophylactic administration of vitamin preparations that include vitamin A, in children with minimal brain dysfunction who have been treated with large doses of vitamin A, in patients given megavitamin treatment, and in health food faddists. The symptoms of chronic overdoses of vitamin A include a dry, thickening skin with itching; some fissuring and peeling; erythematous eruptions; alopecia; tender, hard swellings on the back of the head; pain and swelling in all four extremities, especially tender, painful ankles; impairment and perhaps transient loss of vision; fatigue; anorexia; and headache. Acute poisoning results in irritability, severe headache, increased intracranial pressure, vomiting, and sometimes a great desire to sleep. Peeling of skin can result after 24 hours. Enlargement of the liver and spleen also occurs.

The toxic symptoms described are reversible and disappear rapidly on cessation of the vitamin A ingestion. Because of the danger of possible intoxication, it is best to restrict prophylactic doses to 2500 IU per day in the adult.

Vitamin A and calcium metabolism

Excessive vitamin A ingestion can have a harmful effect on the skeleton and on calcium metabolism. Three persons, ages 7, 16, and 46 years, experienced skeletal discomfort and elevated blood calcium levels after taking excessive doses of vitamin A. When ingestion of vitamin A was discontinued, these harmful effects were no longer observed. It is concluded that both vitamins A and D, if ingested in excess, may cause hypercalcemia and skeletal changes.

Vitamin A, oral contraceptives, and pregnancy

Women taking oral contraceptives show a significant increase in vitamin A levels. This increase is attributed to the profound influence that exogenous corticosteroids have on vitamin A metabolism. Administration of large doses of vitamin A to pregnant animals may be associated with an increased incidence of congenital malformations. It seems unlikely, however, that women who conceive soon after discontinuing oral contraceptives run any teratogenic risk from increased body vitamin A levels. A high vitamin A level during the first trimester of pregnancy has no detrimental effect on the outcome of pregnancy.

Vitamin A in the treatment of acne

Acne vulgaris is a psychologically distressing cutaneous condition, occurring especially during adolescence, and any agent more effective than present remedies in the treatment of acne would be most welcome. In 1971, a new remedy, tretinoin (retinoic acid; vitamin A acid; Retin-A), came into use. It is available for external use only in swabs (containing 0.05% alcohol solution of retinoic acid), as a 0.05% cream, and a 0.01% gel. The cream and gel are well tolerated even by sensitive patients, especially if they are applied every other day. If the skin accommodates to the drug (usually within 3 to 4 weeks), more frequent applications can be made with less adverse reaction. Once improvement is noted, the frequency of application may be reduced.

Mechanism of action. Retinoic acid causes peeling of the skin. In some instances the formation of comedones (i.e., blackheads) is suppressed; in many instances comedones become less firmly attached to the skin and are easily sloughed off. Initially a temporary worsening of the acne condition may be observed, since retinoic acid is known to stimulate proliferation of the follicular epithelium. Small comedones may enlarge and pustule formation may occur 2 to 3 weeks after starting treatment.

Adverse effects. The drug causes redness and peeling usually after 7 to 10 days of treatment. This reaction can be severe in persons with light complexions or in young adolescents. The skin of sensitive patients can become edematous, blistered, or crusted, whereas those with dark complexions can experience a mild loss of skin pigment.

Severe skin reactions may occur if retinoic acid is used in combination with other topical peeling agents; frequent washings with soap while retinoic acid is being used should be avoided, since irritation can occur. Also, since photosensitivity reactions may occur, persons applying retinoic acid to treat acne should avoid sunshine or should use sunscreens. When retinoic acid is used, the patient should be warned about possible inflammatory changes and the photosensitivity reaction.

Vitamin A and cancer

Vitamin A deficiency causes histologic changes in the mouth's mucous membranes that are reminiscent of some premalignant lesions. When animals were fed a vitamin A–deficient diet together with a known carcinogen (e.g., benzpyrene or dimethylbenzanthracene), the rate of cancer production was increased. In contrast, an excess of vitamin A in the diet inhibited the development of cancer in hamsters treated with these two carcinogens. Both retinol and retinoic acid are claimed to have this effect, and three possible mechanisms of action have been suggested: (1) vitamin A affects binding of carcinogens to tissues; (2) retinol inhibits the oxidation of benzpyrene to its carcinogenic epoxide; and (3) vitamin A may stimulate the body's immune system.

Vitamin A is too toxic for the systemic treatment of cancers, since large quantities of the vitamin would have to be ingested. However, preliminary studies suggest that retinoic acid ointments are of value in the treatment of skin carcinomas.

Vitamin A and the lungs

Vitamin A is crucial for the healthy metabolism and growth of epithelial cells. It has been shown, for example, that vitamin A influences the biochemistry of glycoprotein synthesis in lung tissue, and an absence of the vitamin from the diet of experimental animals results in subtle differences in the composition of glycoproteins. This difference in turn may result in the formation of thick layers of keratinizing squamous

cells in the bronchial mucus instead of normal mucus-secreting cells. Vitamin A, therefore, may promote the formation of healthy cells in the lining of the lung.

VITAMIN B COMPLEX

What was originally thought to be a single vitamin present in yeast, liver, whole-grain cereals, and in other sources has since proved to be a mixture of a large number of chemically unrelated substances, now designated the vitamin B complex. Different references assign a different number of substances to this group, but generally eight compounds are recognized as being members: thiamine (vitamin B_1), riboflavin (vitamin B_2), pyridoxine and related compounds (vitamin B_6), nicotinic acid (niacin) and nicotinamide (niacinamide), pantothenic acid, biotin, folic acid (vitamin B_c), and cyanocobalamin (vitamin B_{12}). Each is discussed briefly in Table 66-1.

In general, all these compounds are essential for certain biochemical reactions in which they often act as *coenzymes*. The effect of deficiency, therefore, can be extremely varied and can influence the nervous systems, the cardiovascular system, and metabolic processes. None of the eight compounds can be considered toxic. It appears that the body stores a proportion of an excess intake and excretes the remainder.

In the current literature few new references have been made to the majority of the eight compounds just described. Most attention has been focused on vitamin B_{12} and on folic acid. Three other compounds are considered by some as members of the vitamin B complex. They are *para*-aminobenzoic acid, choline, and inositol. Because none of the three can be truly considered to be a vitamin, comments on these compounds are brief.

Para-aminobenzoic acid (PABA)

Para-aminobenzoic acid is sometimes included as a member of the vitamin B complex because it is a constituent of folic acid. In microorganisms it is an essential nutrient for the synthesis of folic acid. Mammals, including humans, do not synthesize folic acid and therefore do not require dietary PABA for this purpose. Its main use today is as a chemical sunscreen agent.

Choline

Choline is classified by some as a B vitamin. However, three reasons exist as to why it should not be so classified: (1) it is present in animal tissues in relatively large quantities and not in "vitamin proportions"; (2)

it can be synthesized in the body from serine; and (3) it is not involved in enzymatic reactions.

It plays a role in human nutrition, being involved in the prevention of fatty infiltration and cirrhosis of the liver.

Inositol

Like choline, inositol has been assigned to the group of B vitamins, since it promoted growth of certain strains of yeast. However, it is now known that the body can synthesize inositol, that relatively high concentrations occur in animal tissues, and that no enzymatic reactions require inositol as a cofactor. Therefore it should not be classified as a B vitamin.

VITAMIN C

Vitamin C (ascorbic acid) is the vitamin that prevents or cures scurvy (Latin: *scorbutus*). Although it was known as early as 1720 that the ingestion of green vegetables or orange or lemon juice cured scurvy, it was not until 1932 that the chemical structure of vitamin C was determined. It was named ascorbic acid because of its ascorbutic properties. Ascorbic acid is synthesized by higher plants and by all animals except primates (including humans), guinea pigs, and a few others. It is not synthesized by microorganisms and is presumably not necessary for their growth.

Sources of vitamin C

In North Americans the normal daily intake of vitamin C is about 120 mg, half of which is in the form of citrus fruits or tomatoes. It is widely distributed in the body; tissue levels are highest at birth and greatly reduced in old age. Other good sources of the vitamin are cows' milk, cabbage, potatoes, spinach, paprikas, strawberries, red currants, and liver.

The minimum intake of ascorbic acid that will prevent scurvy is about 10 mg/day in humans. A daily intake of 30 to 40 mg results in moderate saturation of the tissues, and an intake of 60 to 100 mg results in complete tissue saturation.

Different countries have different recommended daily doses, ranging as follows: infants, 15 to 35 mg; children, 20 to 90 mg; and adults, 30 to 75 mg. The recommended daily dietary allowances in the United States are infants (to 1 year), 35 mg; children (1 to 10 years), 40 mg; adults, 45 mg; pregnant women, 60 mg; and lactating women, 80 mg.

Function

Ascorbic acid and its oxidized form, dehydroascorbic acid, form a redox system (i.e., a reversible oxidation-reduction system). It is believed that such a system plays an important role in biologic oxidations and reductions and in cellular respiration. It may also be involved in maintaining some enzyme systems in their reduced forms. It is therefore an important compound in body metabolism and in the metabolism of drugs. It is involved in carbohydrate metabolism and the hydroxylation of dopamine to noradrenaline and is probably involved in steroid synthesis.

Ascorbic acid is essential for the formation and the maintenance of intercellular ground substance and collagen. In deficiency, collagen levels decrease as a result of failure of the ascorbic acid–dependent hydroxylation of proline to hydroxyproline, a component of collagen. (Collagen is the chief component of connective tissue; it binds together all cells in the body.) Ascorbic acid is also necessary for the incorporation of iron into ferritin. Ferritin, a protein-iron complex, is the form in which iron is absorbed and stored in the body.

Vitamin C deficiency

The most important symptom of vitamin C deficiency is a marked tendency to bleeding; extensive patches of hemorrhage may appear in the gums and under the skin, in muscles, in fatty tissues, and in some internal organs. The patient will also suffer a marked impairment of connective tissue formation in addition to changes in bone structure and growth. Other symptoms are defective tooth formation and fissuring and roughening of the skin. Because vitamin C is involved in iron transportation, a deficiency of the vitamin can lead to disturbances in iron absorption and cause anemia.

The first signs of vitamin C deficiency is a fall in plasma levels to less than 1 mg/L. This sign may take up to 40 days to occur after ascorbic acid is removed from the diet. The leukocyte vitamin C content then slowly falls—within 3 to 4 months it will be almost zero. During this stage enlargement and keratosis of the hair follicles occur; hemorrhaging develops, gradually followed by changes in gingiva—characteristic signs of scurvy. Loss of teeth, hemorrhages in tissues, and acute diarrhea follow, then finally death.

Vitamin C and viral diseases, including the common cold

In 1942 a patient suffering from viral pneumonia was treated successfully with intramuscular vitamin C. In subsequent years reports have been made of many dramatic successful treatments of various viral infections with large amounts of vitamin C. Some au-

Text continued on p. 1532.

TABLE 66-1

Properties of compounds of the vitamin B complex

Name	Function	Daily requirement		Adult daily intake	Sources
Biotin	Coenzyme involved in the biosynthesis of fatty acids, in protein synthesis, and in carbohydrate metabolism. It may be involved in maintaining a steady blood sugar level.	Not known.		Uncertain. Formed by intestinal bacteria in relatively large quantities.	Liver, kidney, yeast, egg yolk, vegetables, nuts, and cereals
Pantothenic acid	Present in coenzyme A, which is involved in many oxidative biochemical reactions, including synthesis and oxidation of fatty acids. Involved in synthesis of cholesterol and acetylation of amines.	Not known. Normal dietary intake is adequate.		Around 5-10 mg. Also synthesized in human intestine.	Widely distributed in foods, including yeast, liver, kidney, and heart; royal jelly (food of queen bees) is rich source ($\sim$250 μg/gm)
Vitamin B$_1$ (thiamine, aneurin)	Required in many biochemical reactions, including metabolism of carbohydrates; involved in the stimulation of peripheral nerves.	*Adults:* *Children:* *Infants:*	1.0-1.3 mg 0.6-1.1 mg 0.2-0.5 mg	Around 2.2 mg.	Yeast, pork, liver, kidney, and whole-grain cereals
Vitamin B$_2$ (riboflavin, lactoflavin)	Required in many biochemical oxidation reactions, including amino acid metabolism.	*Adults:* *Children:* *Infants:*	1.3-2.0 mg 0.6-1.2 mg 0.4-0.6 mg	Around 2.6 mg.	Milk, liver, kidney, heart, and green vegetables
Vitamin B$_3$ (nicotinic acid [niacin] and nicotinamide [niacinamide])	Coenzymes of numerous dehydrogenases; involved in many biochemical reactions including oxidations, fermentation, and glycolysis.	*Adults:* *Children:* *Infants:*	13-20 mg 8-15 mg 5-8 mg	Around 8 to 17 mg; vitamin B$_3$ is also synthesized from tryptophan by intestinal bacteria.	Yeast, liver, lean meat, ground nuts, and leguminous plants
Vitamin B$_6$ (pyridoxine, pyridoxamine, and related compounds)	Coenzyme involved in many enzymatic reactions.	*Adults:* *Children:* *Infants:*	1.4-2.5 mg 0.5-1.2 mg 0.2-0.4 mg	Around 2 mg; also formed by intestinal bacteria.	Yeast, liver, whole-grain cereals (present in virtually all animal and vegetable foodstuffs)

Results of deficient intake	Results of excessive intake	Additional comments
Seborrheic dermatitis is the major deficiency symptom in humans. Lethargy, loss of appetite, nausea, and muscular pain are observed in experimentally produced deficiency. Diets rich in raw eggs and the presence of liver cirrhosis have been associated with biotin deficiency.	Not toxic. Excesses are excreted.	*Crib death:* The sudden death of apparently healthy babies in the third or fourth month of life ("crib death") may be partly the result of a deficiency of biotin. Such a deficiency would result in a lowering of blood sugar levels. Normally this would be of little significance, but under stress the body's extra demand for sugar cannot be met. Fatal hypoglycemia may be the result. Typical examples of mild stress are infection, a missed meal, excessive heat or cold, or a changed environment. Liver samples of infants who died of unexplained causes have been analyzed. Low levels of biotin were detected. "Crib deaths" are more common among bottle-fed babies. It may be significant that some infant formulas are deficient in biotin.
Virtually unknown in humans. Experimentally produced deficiency results in neuromuscular disturbances, reduced acetylating capacity of blood, and increased sensitivity to insulin.	Not known. Presumably any excess is excreted.	
Beriberi, a disease affecting the nervous system, accompanied by general fatigue and pain, extreme anorexia, nausea, vomiting, emotional disturbances, edema, and muscular paralysis.	Not toxic; urinary excretion increases when excess is ingested.	
Lesions of mucosa (e.g., corners of the mouth), skin lesions (especially of the anogenital region), bone marrow injury.	Not toxic; urinary excretion increases when excess is ingested.	
Pellagra—skin develops red pigmentation and lesions. Emotional and neurologic disturbances occur.	Intravenous doses in excess of 25 mg may cause anaphylactic shock. Oral doses in excess of 3 gm of nicotinic acid cause dilation of blood vessels, especially capillaries. Flushing and itching are commonly observed. Dermatoses, elevations in serum glucose levels, hyperuricemia, gouty arthritis, peptic ulceration, and hyperbilirubinemia (sometimes with liver damage) may occur. An advantageous result of ingesting high doses (3 gm daily) of nicotinic acid is a significant fall in serum cholesterol levels.	*Treatment of schizophrenia:* Nicotinic acid and nicotinamide have been recommended in the treatment of schizophrenia, and it is claimed that the earlier the treatment is begun in the course of the illness, the better are the results. Such treatment is said to be apparently without toxic effects. Controlled clinical trials have not confirmed these claims in acute or chronic schizophrenia; the recommended daily dose of nicotinic acid (3 gm) has no therapeutic effect in schizophrenia.
Varies greatly, depending on enzyme system affected. CNS disturbances and anemia are typical results. A syndrome of pyridoxine deficiency has been well defined only in infancy.	Not known; excesses that cannot be stored are excreted in urine.	

TABLE 66-1

Properties of compounds of the vitamin B complex—cont'd

Name	Function	Daily requirement		Adult daily intake	Sources
Vitamin B$_{12}$ (cyanoco-balamin)	Coenzyme involved in various biologic reactions, including DNA formation, protein metabolism, and probably lipid and carbohydrate metabolism, although its exact role is unknown. Vitamin B$_{12}$ plays an important role in hemopoiesis; with folic acid it is involved in the synthesis of nucleoprotein. Vitamin B$_{12}$ is required for the regeneration and functioning of cells (e.g., epithelial cells) and tissues (e.g., bone marrow). It is required for normal growth and reproduction, although its actual role in these processes is obscure.	*Adults:* *Children:* *Infants:*	5-8 µg 2-5 µg 1-2 µg	In North America the average daily diet contains about 15-30 µg vitamin B$_{12}$, of which approximately 25% is absorbed. Some is also synthesized by bacteria in the large intestine. Vitamin B$_{12}$ is destroyed by heating.	Liver, kidney, meat, and milk; plants contain very little

Results of deficient intake	**Results of excessive intake**	**Additional comments**
Strict vegetarians may have an inadequate dietary intake of vitamin B_{12} (see Additional comments). Other reasons for deficiency are (1) failure to form vitamin B_{12}–intrinsic factor complex (see Additional comments), (2) malabsorption in the ileum, (3) interference with absorption by bacteria or by the fish tapeworm in the small intestine. Deficiency symptoms are similar to those enumerated for folic acid deficiency and, in addition, progressive degeneration of the axis cylinders of the spinal cord neurons occurs.	Vitamin B_{12} is stored in many tissues, especially the liver. When sufficient reserves have accumulated, excess vitamin B_{12} is rapidly excreted in the urine.	*Absorption:* Vitamin B_{12} requires the *gastric intinsic factor of Castle* before it can be absorbed from the ileum. This factor is a glycoprotein that is secreted by the normal gastric mucosa. The dietary vitamin B_{12} then attaches itself to the intrinsic factor and the vitamin B_{12}–intrinsic factor complex is carried to the ileum where absorption occurs provided the Ca^{++} ion is present and the pH is >6—a complex absorption procedure. Adults with *pernicious anemia* are thought, because of absence of acid secretion in the stomach, to be unable to release vitamin B_{12} from the protein-bound form in which the vitamin is present in foodstuffs. Thus they cannot form a vitamin B_{12}–intrinsic factor complex. In children with pernicious anemia the intrinsic factor itself may be absent—a genetic defect. *Vitamin B_{12} deficiency in vegetarians:* Complete vegetarian diets that exclude milk products provide virtually no vitamin B_{12}. The consequences are megaloblastic anemia and degeneration of the spinal cord; some examples are occasionally reported. Unfortunately for diagnostic purposes, vegetarian diets are usually rich in folic acid, which masks the anemia of B_{12} deficiency so that irreparable nerve damage may be the first signs of vitamin B_{12} deficiency. Fortunately cases of this are rare. Indeed, some lifelong vegetarians show no evidence of B_{12} deficiency. This is thought to be because the body reabsorbs with high efficiency the B_{12} excreted daily into the bile stores accumulated earlier in life. Nevertheless, complete vegetarians are advised to take B_{12} supplements (i.e., 5 µg daily).

Continued.

TABLE 66-1

Properties of compounds of the vitamin B complex—cont'd

Name	Function	Daily requirement	Adult daily intake	Sources
Vitamin B$_c$ (folic acid, pteroylglutamic acid)	Folic acid in reduced form (tetrahydrofolic acid) plays an essential part in purine, nucleic acid, and DNA synthesis and thus is involved in all processes of cell division, particularly hemopoiesis. It plays a role in maintaining normal pregnancy. This role is not certain, but it is possible that it alters the action of the ovarian hormones on the uterus.	Not accurately known. Some authorities suggest 50 µg for adults increased in pregnancy up to 200-400 µg in the third trimester. Other authorities suggest a higher daily requirement. *Adults:* 400 µg *Pregnant women:* 500 µg *Lactating women:* 800 µg *Children:* 100-200 µg	Uncertain. May be only 100-200 µg, which is considered insufficient in pregnancy. Folic acid is heat sensitive; up to 90% of activity can be destroyed by heating.	Liver, yeast, kidney, dark green, leafy vegetables; the folic acid content of mother's and fresh cows' milk is usually sufficient to meet the requirements in infants

Results of deficient intake	Results of excessive intake	Additional comments
Inadequate nucleic acid synthesis resulting in megaloblastic anemia (especially in pregnancy). Clinical symptoms are megaloblastosis of bone marrow, macrocytic anemia, leukopenia, excessive segmentation of leukocytes, thrombocytopenia, and gastrointestinal disturbances. Functional damage to the small intestine may result. Deficiency in children may cause a loss of appetite and slow growth rather than megaloblastic anemia. (See Additional comments.)	Not known except when vitamin B_{12} is involved. Some of the excess is stored in various tissues including the liver; the remainder is excreted in the urine.	*Folic acid deficiency:* The hematologic symptoms of folic acid deficiency are indistinguishable from those of vitamin B_{12} deficiency. For this reason folic acid treatment can be dangerous in instances of B_{12} deficiency, since it will mask a deficiency of the latter vitamin by partially and temporarily correcting the hematologic damage while the more serious neurologic manifestations of B_{12} deficiency progress untreated. Multivitamin preparations do not contain more than 0.1 mg of folic acid because a daily dose of folic acid in excess of this amount will disguise a B_{12} deficiency. Folic acid deficiency is observed in instances of malnutrition often associated with alcoholism, in instances of malabsorption (sometimes drug induced), in sickle cell and other anemias, and in pregnancy. Some drugs (primidone, phenytoin, phenobarbital, and oral contraceptives) can contribute to folic acid deficiency because they interfere with its absorption. In the synthesis of nucleic acids folic acid must be converted to a reduced form, *folinic* acid. Some drugs can block this reduction step and therefore can contribute to folic acid deficiency. Examples are methotrexate, pyrimethamine, and triamterene. As well as in pregnancy, increased daily requirements of folic acid are necessary in malignant conditions and in severe infections. Daily doses up to 1 gm are recommended in those conditions. Folic acid deficiency is also a well-known side effect of anticonvulsant therapy. If steps are taken to correct folic acid deficiency during anticonvulsant therapy, a deterioration in seizure control can result. It would seem wise, therefore, to start giving folic acid supplements to all patients at the time anticonvulsant therapy is started.

thorities believe that the body functions best when its cells are saturated with vitamin C, but dietary sources of the vitamin are insufficient to produce the necessary cellular saturation.

Some respected scientists support the belief that cell saturation with ascorbic acid is essential for prolonged good health. It has been observed that the cells of the unborn fetus contain more vitamin C than cells of the newborn and that cellular ascorbic acid concentrations gradually decrease with increasing age. Many of the symptoms of aging have been likened to the symptoms of scurvy protracted over a long period of time. However, despite the enthusiastic support of an important minority of the medical profession, the majority is unconvinced of the role of vitamin C in preventing or curing the common cold and other viral infections. Evidence from various controlled clinical trials has not been encouraging. The administration of large doses of vitamin C did not prevent colds, and little or no reduction in their severity or duration was observed.

Vitamin C toxicity

Those who advocate the ingestion of large doses of vitamin C to prevent or cure a cold contend that the side effects produced by these high doses are minimal and of little concern. Those most commonly observed are flatulence, a tendency toward more frequent urination, and a laxative action of the vitamin. The latter can be minimized if vitamin C is taken after meals. Ascorbic acid in large doses produces an acidic urine, which could have an adverse effect on patients with a tendency toward gout or crystaluria or the formation of urate stones.

Other undesirable effects may result from the ingestion of large doses of vitamin C. It is reported to affect adversely the anticoagulant properties of warfarin and to interfere with some diagnostic biochemical tests on urine. The acidic urine that results from the ingestion of large amounts of vitamin C will promote an increase in the rate of excretion of weak basic drugs and a decrease, by promoting tubular reabsorption, in the rate of excretion of weakly acidic drugs. Alteration in drug excretion patterns will affect blood concentrations of drugs, which could have some clinical significance.

Vitamin C and smoking

The median level of vitamin C in the blood of cigarette smokers is at least 30% lower than that of non-smokers. Cigarette smoking must therefore be considered as a stress to the body. In some instances vitamin supplement may be required.

Vitamin C and decubiti

It has been claimed that vitamin C may be of value in the treatment of pressure sores. Surgical patients who received 250 mg to 1 gm ascorbic acid daily for a month showed significant reduction in the area of the pressure sore compared with patients who received a placebo.

Vitamin C and cancer

A study on 100 patients with terminal cancer who were treated with 10 gm per day of vitamin C showed that these patients survived longer (average 210 days) than a control sample of 1000 terminal patients (average survival 50 days). The quality of life of the treated patients also improved. A possible implication from these studies is that the ingestion of large doses of vitamin C over a lifetime may prevent or cure certain cancers. However, further controlled clinical studies on this subject are required.

VITAMIN D

Vitamin D is the name given to a group of chemically related compounds. The D vitamins are fat-soluble, water-insoluble solids, related in structure to the corticosteroids, ergosterol and cholesterol. The clinically useful D vitamins possess *antirachitic* properties (i.e., they prevent or cure *rickets*) and are named vitamin D_2 (ergocalciferol), vitamin D_3 (cholecalciferol, or activated 7-dehydrocholesterol), and vitamin D_4.

Sources of vitamin D

Vitamin D_2. Vitamin D_2 is an ultraviolet *irradiation* product of the sterol ergosterol. During this irradiation procedure the C_9—C_{10} bond of ergosterol cleaves and yields the antirachitic derivative ergocalciferol (vitamin D_2). Ergosterol itself has no antirachitic properties; it is sometimes referred to as provitamin D_2 and is mainly found in plants, yeast, ergot, and hens' eggs.

Vitamin D_3. In a similar manner ultraviolet irradiation of 7-dehydrocholesterol (provitamin D_3) yields vitamin D_3 as a result of cleavage of the C_9—C_{10} bond of 7-dehydrocholesterol. 7-Dehydrocholesterol is present in the tissues of higher animals including humans, having been formed from cholesterol by a reaction that takes place in the intestine. 7-Dehydrocholesterol has no antirachitic properties. It is transported in the body to the skin where, under the effect of ultraviolet irradiation by normal sunlight, it is converted to vitamin D_3. Once formed in this way, it is rapidly transported to the site where it is required in the body. Vitamin D_3 is the form of the vitamin present in fish liver oils or in irradiated milk.

The antirachitic properties of vitamin D_2 and D_3 differ greatly in some species, but in humans they have similar activities.

Vitamin D₄. Vitamin D_4 is a synthetic product that is formed by irradiation of 22-dihydroergosterol. The latter compound (provitamin D_4) has no antirachitic properties, whereas vitamin D_4 is appreciably active but less so than vitamin D_3.

The chemical structures of vitamins D_2, D_3, and D_4 are closely related. Irradiation of the provitamin precursors (ergosterol, 7-dehydrocholesterol, and 22-dihydroergosterol) causes ring opening of the corticosteroids, a structural feature that is essential for vitamin D activity.

Function

The activity of vitamin D is interrelated with the actions of the parathyroid hormone and of thyrocalcitonin, all three factors being necessary for the maintenance of calcium balance and a normal serum calcium level (see Chapter 62, "Parathyroid Hormone, Calcitonin, and Related Medications"). Although it is difficult to assign specific functions to each of these factors, it seems accepted that vitamin D is responsible for calcium transport in bone cells and that the vitamin causes, when required, an increase in intestinal absorption of dietary calcium. Vitamin D is necessary for the development of normal bone and for the calcification of rachitic bone. Vitamin D is also involved in the tubular reabsorption of phosphate.

Vitamin D requirements

In adults the body's needs are usually met by its own synthesis except in persons who spend limited periods in daylight. Additional quantities are normally obtained from fortified foodstuffs (e.g., milk, milk products, cereals, margarine, baby foods). During the period of active skeletal growth and in pregnancy and lactation the requirement is increased for both calcium and vitamin D, and vitamin supplements are recommended. In such cases oral administration of 400 IU* vitamin D per day is adequate in the vast majority of cases. It must be emphasized that serious toxicity may result from excessive ingestion of vitamin D. Supplements of as little as 1800 IU per day have proved to be toxic to some infants. In view of this danger supplementation in excess of 400 IU daily should only be carried out under medical supervision. The most commonly administered supplements are pure vitamin D_2 or D_3, especially the latter, or cod liver oil.

---

*One IU = 0.025 μg crystalline vitamin D_3.

Vitamin D deficiency

Deficiency of vitamin D results in an inadequate absorption of calcium and phosphate and causes rickets in children and *osteomalacia* in adults. In both diseases the failure of mineralization in bone leads to progressive demineralization and weakening of the skeleton. In children bone growth is particularly rapid in the epiphyses, vitamin D deficiency first shows there. In adults breakdown of bone occurs slowly and throughout the skeleton.

Hypervitaminosis D

All the D vitamins are toxic in large quantities. High dosages mobilize the bound calcium of the skeleton; plasma calcium levels rise (hypercalcemia); and urinary excretion of calcium and phosphate increases. The mobilized calcium is also taken up in the soft tissues, especially the kidneys. Clinical symptoms of *hypervitaminosis D* include headache, pain in the joints, and muscular weakness. Tremor of the limbs, loose skin, muscle spasm, and arterial hypertension are also observed, especially in children. Death is often the result of renal failure. The symptoms of vitamin D poisoning are reversible by stopping the ingestion of the vitamin.

Toxic effects of an excess of vitamin D appear, especially in children, when daily doses exceed 3000 to 4000 IU over a period of several months. Adults can normally ingest much larger daily doses of vitamin D before toxic symptoms become apparent, although some adults show profound toxic symptoms after receiving only slightly above the daily recommended dose. Since milk and baby foods are often enriched with vitamin D, the intake of the vitamin by children is bordering on the excessive in many countries including the United States and Canada.

Long-term anticonvulsant therapy

A considerable amount of evidence has now accumulated that patients on long-term anticonvulsant therapy, especially with phenytoin, are liable to develop rickets or osteomalacia. Controlled studies have been conducted. In one such study of 91 adult epileptic patients on long-term anticonvulsant therapy these patients were shown to have reduced serum calcium and phosphate levels and elevated alkaline phosphatase values compared with controls. Besides disturbances in calcium metabolism, radiologic changes in the femur of these patients were also observed. Similar observations have been made with other epileptic patients. Treatment with calcium and vitamin D generally results in steady improvement.

One instance of a 2-year-old epileptic child developing rickets has been reported. This child was receiving phenytoin (200 mg) and primidone (530 mg) daily, and severe rickets resulted. When phenytoin was replaced with methsuximide, 150 mg daily, and supplemental vitamin D (400 IU/day) was given, a steady improvement was noted.

It has been suggested that some anticonvulsant drugs accelerate the metabolic breakdown of vitamin D by liver enzyme induction, and this adversely affects calcium and phosphorus metabolism.

Metabolism of vitamin D

Initially it was generally accepted that vitamins D_2, D_3, and D_4 produced their antirachitic effects directly. It is now clear that this belief is incorrect, and that metabolic conversion to hydroxylated products is necessary for activity. Most studies have been conducted on cholecalciferol (vitamin D_3). It is metabolized in the liver to 25-hydroxycholecalciferol (25-OHD$_3$), and this compound stimulates bone *reabsorption* of calcium and the active transport of calcium from gut lumen to serum. 25-OHD$_3$ is further metabolized in the kidney to 1,25-dihydroxycholecalciferol (1,25-[OH]$_2$D$_3$), which is a still more active form of vitamin D. In a similar manner ergocalciferol (vitamin D_2) is metabolized to an active metabolite, 25-hydroxyergocalciferol (25-OHD$_2$).

Classic nutritional deficiency rickets of infants is now rare in the United States and Canada, especially since milk is fortified with vitamin D. However, the condition of pseudo–vitamin D–deficient rickets (Prader's syndrome) is not alleviated with vitamin D because it is caused by a deficiency of the enzyme that converts 25-OHD$_3$ to 1,25-[OH]$_2$D$_3$. Use of 1 μg per day of 1,25-[OH]$_2$D$_3$ intravenously has proved effective in healing rachitic lesions in a child, but this derivative is generally not available for routine clinical use.

A related synthetic vitamin D analog has been shown to be effective in the treatment of metabolic bone disease resulting from chronic renal failure. The compound is 1-hydroxycholecalciferol (1-OHD$_3$), which when administered at a dose of 2 μg orally per day caused a significant increase in both calcium absorption from the gastrointestinal tract and calcium content of bone in three patients suffering from renal bone disease.

VITAMIN E

Vitamin E is one of the fat-soluble vitamins. It is a collective name for various tocopherols that possess similar chemical structures. Eight tocopherols are known, but the most important of these is α-tocopherol, which comprises about 90% of the tocopherols

in animal tissues and has the greatest biologic activity. α-Tocopherol is found largely in plant materials. Among the richest sources are seed germ oils (especially corn and wheat), alfalfa, lettuce, eggs, and cereals. Animal tissues contain little tocopherol.

Function

The tocopherols are antioxidants, a property that has been demonstrated both in vivo and in vitro. For example, they prevent the oxidation of unsaturated fatty acids such as linoleic acid to toxic peroxides; they prevent the oxidation of vitamin A and the carotenes; and they prevent the oxidation of the thiol group (—SH), particularly in enzyme systems. In general, vitamin E appears to prevent undesired oxidation of essential cellular constituents and to prevent the formation of toxic oxidation products such as peroxides from dietary constitutents. Vitamin E may play a part in nucleic acid metabolism, in erythropoiesis, and in adenosine triphosphate (ATP) formation. The tocopherols seem to have an effect on the transport and metabolism of vitamin B_{12}.

To function as an antioxidant, α-tocopherol must itself be readily and preferentially oxidized. An oxidation product of α-tocopherol has been isolated and identified as α-tocopherolquinone, and a reversible oxidation-reduction system has been demonstrated.

Although extravagant claims of diverse pharmacologic actions attributable to vitamin E have been made (discussed later), numerous clinical trials have shown that apart from relieving symptoms of deficiency, which occur rarely, vitamin E displays no extraordinary pharmacologic properties. In fact, it has been called "the vitamin in search of a disease."

Vitamin E deficiency has not been demonstrated in humans except in some premature infants, some children with severe protein-calorie malnutrition, and rarely in adults with malabsorption syndromes. Severe protein-calorie malnutrition in children has produced a form of anemia that was successfully reversed with large doses of vitamin E. Some premature infants may develop hemolytic anemia associated with a low plasma vitamin E level. This condition can also be reversed with large doses of vitamin E. A rare genetic disease, the acanthocytosis syndrome, results in the formation of erythrocytes that spontaneously hemolyze in vitro. Sufferers have little or no circulating α-tocopherol; they have impaired intestinal absorption of the vitamin. Parenteral administration of vitamin E relieves the situation.

Other malabsorption syndromes exist, which are characterized by *steatorrhea*. Examples are cystic fibrosis, chronic pancreatitis, and biliary cirrhosis. In these conditions decreased erythrocyte lifetimes are also observed, and because fats are poorly absorbed, fat-soluble materials such as vitamin E are also poorly absorbed. These syndromes are alleviated only to some extent by administering vitamin E parenterally.

It must be emphasized that these human vitamin E deficiency conditions are rarely encountered. It has proved virtually impossible to completely deprive humans of vitamin E. A group of adult male mental patients were maintained on low vitamin E diets for protracted periods, in some instances as long as 8 years! Eventually their blood levels of α-tocopherol declined to about 20% of the original level. These patients remained in satisfactory health, although their red blood cells had a shorter survival time (110 days) than those of a control group of patients (123 days), but the cells performed their normal function. It was concluded from this study that humans require vitamin E, but the requirement is a modest one.

Recent claims that vitamin E is effective in treating intermittent claudication (a blood vessel disorder that results from arteriosclerosis of the legs and afflicts about 5% to 10% of elderly men, causing severe cramps) and benign breasts cysts in women await further clinical confirmation.

Many medical consultants believe that except for the vitamin E deficiency state associated with a hemolytic type of anemia that may occasionally occur in small or premature infants, supplements of vitamin E have no established value in preventing or treating any common human disorder.

Adverse effects of vitamin E

Vitamin E is essentially nontoxic. The likelihood of serious adverse effects from self-medication is low, although diarrhea and intestinal cramps have resulted with daily doses of 3200 IU. An isolated instance of vitamin E interfering with the action of warfarin has been reported. Some persons have experienced an allergic reaction to a deodorant (Mennen E deodorant) that contained vitamin E. Surprisingly this dermatologic reaction was attributed to the vitamin.

Daily requirement of vitamin E

The required daily intake of vitamin E is not known, since vitamin E deficiency has not been demonstrated in humans except in some premature infants. A daily intake of 10 IU* is probably more than sufficient and such a quantity is readily obtained in normal diets. The recommended daily allowance of vitamin E according to the US National Research Council is 25 to 30 IU. This higher figure is to accommodate those adults who eat large quantities of polyunsaturated

*One IU = 1 mg (±)-α-tocopheryl acetate or 0.73 mg (+)-α-tocopheryl acetate.

fats—such as in vegetable oils, margarine, and fish—to keep down blood cholesterol levels. Compared with saturated fats—such as in animal fats and butter—polyunsaturated fats are more susceptible to oxidation in the body, and therefore larger amounts of vitamin E (an antioxidant) are required to prevent this oxidation.

It is wrong, however, to argue that margarine eaters require more dietary vitamin E than butter eaters and should take vitamin E supplements daily, since polyunsaturated fats already contain more vitamin E than saturated fats. Margarine, for example, contains 10 to 15 times the amount of vitamin E present in butter; fish steaks are at least 10 times as rich in vitamin E as beef steaks. Thus regardless of whether a person's diet is rich in vegetable oils or animal oils, supplemental vitamin E is virtually unnecessary.

Vitamin E—a panacea?

Despite the assertion that vitamin E is of no value in the prevention or treatment of any common human disorders, large sums of money are spent on preparations containing vitamin E. It is suggested in the popular press that millions of people suffer pain or are crippled because of insufficient vitamin E in their diets, and children are destined to suffer and die prematurely unless vitamin E supplements are given to them. Vitamin E is claimed to prevent or cure literally dozens of human ailments. It is said to retard the aging process; to be beneficial in instances of sexual impotence, low sperm count, and sterility; to benefit the cardiovascular system including coronary, cerebral, and peripheral vascular disease, arteriosclerosis, heart attacks, angina pectoris, blood clots, congenital heart disease, phlebitis, varicose veins, and hemophilia; to improve or cure skin disorders such as skin aging, burns, sunburn, radiation burns, skin cancer, scarring, warts, acne, diaper rash, scleroderma, and brown pigmentation in older people; to improve or cure muscle weakness, muscle inflammation, muscular dystrophy, myasthenia gravis, poor posture, nocturnal leg cramps, and Dupuytren's contracture; to be beneficial in the treatment of allergies, asthma, and bee stings; to be helpful in pregnancy conditions (habitual spontaneous abortion, miscarriage, premature birth, and prolonged labor); and to be beneficial in diabetes, thyroid diseases, liver diseases, jaundice, kidney disease, bursitis, arthritis, emphysema, and ulcers. In most instances no direct evidence exists to support any of these claims.

Often reports in the scientific and medical literature describe how vitamin E benefits laboratory animals that are maintained on diets deficient in vitamin E. In some monkeys a lack of vitamin E results in a muscular condition resembling a type of human muscular dystrophy. Other animals develop brain abnormalities, degeneration of the liver, or damage to the heart. The rat's testicles degenerate and with this, of course, the sperm-producing cells. Many other observations have been made on other animals whose diets lacked vitamin E. All these studies served to prove that vitamin E was essential if animals were to enjoy normal health, but these studies did *not* show that additional vitamin E was of any benefit to the control animals (i.e., those maintained on diets containing sufficient vitamin E for normal development).

Unfortunately, the observations made on animals lacking vitamin E in their diets led to speculation that lack of vitamin E might also profoundly damage the human organism. The effects of administering vitamin E to humans with conditions resembling those produced in experimental animals (heart disease, muscular dystrophy, repeated miscarriage, infertility, and others) have proved over the years to be extremely disappointing. Extensive clinical studies have been conducted to determine whether vitamin E was of value in the treatment of heart ailments (arteriosclerotic, hypertensive, rheumatic, and coronary heart disease and angina pectoris). Some medical groups have reported exciting successful treatments. However, it soon became apparent that the claims made for vitamin E were unfounded. From all over the world reports were received that vitamin E had no therapeutic value in heart disease. Many controlled studies were made to prove this point conclusively. Often the conclusion was that no significant difference existed between a group of patients given vitamin E and another group receiving a placebo.

Most clinicians now conclude that reports of the efficacy of vitamin E in treating heart disease are essentially the uncontrolled personal impressions of clinicians who have faith in their remedy and transmit that faith to their patients. The claims of successful treatments have no scientific validity. Despite this conclusion enormous quantities of vitamin E are produced each year in North America for human use, and since no adverse side effects of large doses of the vitamin are known, most vitamin E advocates see no reason to curb their intake of the vitamin. It has been described as a modern "security blanket." I have received many unsolicited reports from the public of the vitamin's apparent utility in healing burns without scarring when applied topically.

VITAMIN K

Vitamin K occurs in a number of forms, all of which are derivatives of 2-methyl-1,4-naphthaquinone. Nat-urally occurring vitamin K is a fat-soluble substance found in green plants, tomatoes, alfalfa, vegetable oils, and hog liver fat. It is designated vitamin K_1; it is also known as phylloquinone, phytonadione, and 2-methyl-3-phytyl-1,4-naphthaquinone. Vitamin K_2 is a mixture of compounds (termed menaquinones) that are synthesized by various gram-positive bacteria. The vitamins K_2 possess various long-chain substituents in the 3-position of the 2-methyl-1,4-naphthaquinone nucleus. Vitamin K_1 is the only natural vitamin used therapeutically.

Synthetic compounds with vitamin K activity are known. The most potent, vitamin K_3 (menadione; 2-methyl-1,4-naphthaquinone), is available in water-soluble form as its sodium bisulfite derivative. Menadiol, sometimes referred to as vitamin K_4, is a reduced form of vitamin K_3 that is available in water-soluble form as its sodium diphosphate salt. Menadiol, menadiol sodium diphosphate, and menadione sodium bisulfite are all converted in vivo to vitamin K_3.

The water-soluble vitamins K are readily absorbed when administered orally. In contrast, vitamins K_1 and K_2 require adequate quantities of bile salts and pancreatic lipase to be absorbed from the gastrointestinal tract. If excess vitamin K is ingested, a little is stored in the liver and other tissues; however, most of an excess intake is excreted.

Function

Vitamin K is essential for normal blood clotting. It is involved in the hepatic biosynthesis of prothrombin (factor II), proconvertin (factor VII), thromboplastin (factor IX) and the Stuart factor (factor X), proteinous factors involved in the blood clotting process.

Vitamin K requirement

The requirement for vitamin K is not known accurately, but is probably low. Human requirements are generally satisfied with a balanced diet and with the vitamin synthesized by intestinal bacteria. The minimum daily requirement in adults is less than 0.1 μg/kg of body weight. In neonates hypoprothrombinemia is prevented by administering vitamin K_1 (10 μg/kg of body weight).

Vitamin K deficiency

Vitamin K deficiency is usually associated with a disease-induced fat absorption defect (e.g., enteritis, ulcerative colitis, or dysentery), bowel surgery (extensive resection), biliary tract obstruction or fistula, liver disease (e.g., hepatitis or advanced cirrhosis), or loss of gut flora such as could occur with the use of poorly absorbed sulfonamides or broad-spectrum antibiotics.

Newborn infants and premature babies may display

a hypoprothrombinemia because of vitamin K deficiency. Their diets lack sufficient vitamin K (human milk contains low vitamin K concentrations), and normal intestinal bacterial flora are not established. The resulting hemorrhagic disease of the newborn responds to vitamin K treatment.

Vitamin K toxicity

Naturally occurring vitamins K_1 and K_2 are believed to be nontoxic to humans even in large doses; occasionally reports are made of idiosyncratic reactions occurring when vitamin K_1 is administered. In contrast, the synthetic vitamins K (menadione and its water-soluble derivatives) are irritant to the skin and respiratory tract in humans and may induce hemolysis in individuals who have a glucose-6-phosphate dehydrogenase (G-6-PD) deficiency in their erythrocytes. In patients with severe hepatic disease the administration of large doses of vitamins K_1 or K_3 may aggravate the already depressed function of the liver.

Anticoagulant antidotal activity of vitamin K

With increasing use of coumarin drugs hemorrhage can result if the anticoagulant effect of these drugs is excessive. Reversal of this effect is a common indication for vitamin K therapy. It is important to restore a normal prothrombin time in patients who are receiving anticoagulants and are bleeding. Menadione (vitamin K_3) and its water-soluble salts are *not* effective for this purpose. It has been established that the 3-phytyl side chain in vitamin K_1 is an essential feature of that molecule's structure, which imparts on it the ability to reverse the coagulation defect induced by coumarin and its congeners. In the emergency treatment of drug-induced hypoprothrombinemia, therefore, vitamin K_1 (phytonadione) is the drug of choice.

Vitamin K in pregnancy

Excessive quantities of synthetic vitamin K may harm the fetus. If given in large doses near term, menadione and its water-soluble salts can raise serum bilirubin concentrations and increase the possibility of kernicterus.

MULTIVITAMIN PREPARATIONS

Parenteral multivitamins for the surgical patient

Most multivitamin preparations contain some of the B vitamins and large amounts of ascorbic acid. Beminol with C Fortis Injectable (Ayerst), Folbesyn (Lederle), Solu-B Sterile with Ascorbic Acid (Upjohn), and Solu-Zyme with Ascorbic Acid (Upjohn) are examples; the latter contains 10 mg of vitamin B_1, 10 mg of vitamin B_2, 250 mg of niacinamide, 45 mg of pantothenic acid, 5 mg of vitamin B_6, 25 μg of vitamin B_{12}, 5 mg of folic acid, and 500 mg of vitamin C in each daily dose. The products are available for intravenous administration before, during, and after surgery. The philosophy behind their use is to meet an increased vitamin requirement thought to be induced by surgery or trauma and to hasten the repair of tissues. The quantities of vitamins in these products are in considerable excess of recommended daily doses to prevent deficiency. The ascorbic acid content, for example, is in the dose range normally administered to treat fully developed scurvy. The ascorbic acid is present for its ability to accelerate tissue repair and wound healing. However, this ability has only been demonstrated in patients with a vitamin C deficiency, and this is rarely seen.

Multivitamin parenteral preparations are of value for patients who have undergone stomach or small intestine surgery and can no longer absorb adequate dietary sources of vitamins or for patients who will be fed intravenously for some time after surgery. They are also of value when rapid tissue saturation is necessary, as in beriberi. However, some clinicians consider that the routine use of parenteral multivitamin preparations, before, during, or after surgery is not warranted. Little evidence exists that such large doses of vitamin C or the B complex speed convalescence postoperatively. Fortunately such large doses are generally harmless, although they are expensive. Vitamins should be prescribed only when impaired absorption, increased need, or a dietary deficiency leading to a specific vitamin deficiency can be demonstrated.

Drug incompatibilities are possible when vitamins are added to intravenous solutions. B-complex vitamin preparations are incompatible with the antibiotics chloramphenicol and nafcillin and also with aminophylline and hydrocortisone. Ascorbic acid is not compatible with pencillin G.

Vitamins in pregnancy

Clinical studies indicate that routine multivitamin supplementation in pregnancy is generally not necessary. Nevertheless, over 30 prenatal multiple vitamin products are currently marketed. Most contain calcium (50 to 600 mg), although no evidence exists that calcium supplementation is required in pregnancy. Most also contain vitamin A (1500 to 15,000 IU) and vitamin D (133 to 1,000 IU). The pregnant woman can obtain enough vitamin A from an average of one green and one yellow vegetable daily and enough vitamin D from seasonal exposure to sunlight or by drinking three cups of vitamin D fortified milk daily.

Pregnant women should be aware of some claims

that vitamin A in excessive dosage may be teratogenic and that hypercalcemia or aortic stenosis may occur in infants born to mothers with hypervitaminosis D. Large doses of vitamin C (in excess of 1 gm daily) should be avoided as a cautionary measure, since the effects of large doses on the fetus are not known.

Some of the multivitamin preparations also contain 0.1 to 1.0 mg folic acid, and all contain iron (6.6 to 66 mg). Iron and folic acid supplements are recommended during normal pregnancy. Folic acid is essential to DNA synthesis and is necessary if cells are to replicate. The fetus uses maternal folic acid stores to such a degree that the mother may experience deficiency and consequently a severe megaloblastic anemia if her folic acid stores are marginal. It has been estimated that up to 50% of pregnant women may have a folic acid deficiency, especially since prolonged cooking of food sources in water destroys folic acid.

Folic acid is generally nontoxic, so a strong case can be made for the administration of folic acid prophylactically to pregnant women at a dose level of 0.3 to 0.4 mg daily throughout pregnancy. However, vitamin B_{12} blood levels should be determined before folic acid administration, since a vitamin B_{12} deficiency could be masked with such doses of folic acid.

Vitamin-mineral supplements for women taking oral contraceptives

Some multivitamin preparations are claimed by manufacturers to be of special value to patients who are taking oral contraceptives. Typically these preparations contain about 10 vitamins and two minerals. Claims such as this are misleading, since they imply that the use of oral contraceptives creates a special requirement for certain vitamins or minerals, but little evidence can be found to support this suggestion. Although some arguments are presented for supplements of vitamins B_6 and B_{12}, folic acid, and vitamin C and of zinc and iron, the conclusion of numerous clinicians is that women who are using oral contraceptives and who normally eat a well-balanced diet need no vitamin supplementation. Such a diet should include some of the following items: uncooked fruits, green and yellow vegetables, meat, milk, and whole-grain or enriched cereals. Iron deficiency is not expected in women taking oral contraceptives.

MINERALS AND TRACE ELEMENTS

The tissues of humans contain many elements that may be essential for normal body growth. Some are

Trace elements of living matter			
Aluminum	Chromium	Lithium	Silicon
Antimony	Cobalt	Manganese	Silver
Arsenic	Copper	Mercury	Strontium
Barium	Fluorine	Molybdenum	Tin
Boron	Gallium	Nickel	Vanadium
Bromine	Iodine	Rubidium	Zinc
Cadmium	Lead	Selenium	

present in trace quantities (picograms to micrograms per gram of wet tissue), whereas others are more abundant. Trace elements of living matter are identified in the box above, but not all can be said to be essential to animal life. Those that probably are essential are described in Table 66-2. This list is composed of elements that are known to cause deficiency syndromes in animals, and it is assumed from these animal studies that they are also necessary to prevent clinical abnormalities in humans. Four trace elements (cobalt, copper, iodine, and zinc) are of particular importance, since they have been proved to cause disease in humans. Trace elements are widely distributed in foods, and balanced diets easily supply human minimum daily requirements.

Some essential elements in nutrition are present in larger quantities in human tissues. These include calcium, chlorine, iron, magnesium, phosphorus, potassium, sodium, and sulfur, and many foodstuffs contain minerals that possess these elements. Sources and functions of these more abundant essential elements are summarized in Table 66-3.

SUMMARY

The various vitamins and minerals used to maintain normal growth and development and metabolic function have been presented. With an understanding of the indication for vitamin therapy, daily requirements, and toxicities associated with vitamins as well as signs of deficiencies, the nurse will be better able to help patients maintain adequate nutrition and use vitamins and minerals rationally with fewer adverse effects.

TABLE 66-2

Properties of essential trace elements

Trace element	Function	Effects of deficiency
Chromium	Glucose metabolism; may mediate insulin effect on membranes	Impaired glucose clearance; probably adversely affects growth, reproduction, and life span
Cobalt	Component of vitamin B_{12}; involved in biologic methylation (e.g., synthesis of methionine)	Pernicious anemia and methylmalonic aciduria
Copper	Essential for the action of many enzymes (e.g., cytochrome oxidase, lysine oxidase, and tyrosinase); required for mitochondrial function (e.g., drug metabolism), collagen metabolism, melanin formation, and oxygen transport	Anemia, leukopenia, neutropenia, Menke's syndrome, impaired mitochondrial function
Fluorine	Component of dental enamel; may be involved in iron absorption and required for normal growth of bones	Anemia and impaired growth and reproduction has been observed in rodents; defective bone growth; mottled tooth enamel
Iodine	Component of the thyroid hormones (i.e., thyroglobulin, thyroxine, and iodothyronines); involved in cellular oxidation processes	Thyroid diseases and impaired cellular function
Manganese	Essential for the action of pyruvate carboxylase and many intracellular enzymes; involved in oxidative phosphorylation and fatty acid metabolism; synthesis of mucopolysaccharides, proteins, and cholesterol	Defective body growth, bone growth, reproduction and central nervous system function
Molybdenum	Essential for the action of flavoenzymes (e.g., xanthine oxidase); involved in the metabolism of xanthine, hypoxanthine, and other substrates	Impaired growth; may cause impaired urate clearance
Nickel	Essential for normal ribonucleic acid metabolism; may be involved in membrane function	Unknown in humans; results in impaired reproduction in rats and defective lipid metabolism in chicks
Selenium	Involved in the action of some enzymes (e.g., erythrocyte glutathione peroxidase) and the degradation of intracellular peroxides; may play a role in the metabolism of tocopherol and sulfur-contained amino acids	Unknown in humans; liver necrosis and muscle disease have been observed in animals
Silicon	Involved in mucopolysaccharide metabolism and may be necessary for maintenance of connective tissue	Unknown in humans; causes impaired growth and impaired formation of connective tissue in chicks
Tin	Located in fatty tissue; may be involved in redox reactions	Unknown in humans; growth and dentition abnormalities are observed in rats
Vanadium	May be involved in lipid metabolism and oxygen transport	Unknown in humans; impaired growth, reproduction, lipid and bone metabolism have been observed in animals
Zinc	Essential component of more than 70 enzymes (e.g., alcohol dehydrogenase, DNA polymerase, carboxypeptidase) involved in the metabolism of carbohydrates, lipids, proteins, and nucleic acids; essential for normal growth and development The zinc content of breast milk falls during lactation and may be inadequate to meet the infant's zinc requirement	Acrodermatitis enteropathica—an autosomal recessive inherited disorder (chronic diarrhea, wasting, alopecia, thickened ulcerated skin at body orifices); probably implicated in hypogonadal dwarfism

TABLE 66-3

Properties of more abundant essential elements in nutrition

Element	Sources	Function
Calcium	Present in virtually all foodstuffs in varying amounts (0.5-1300 mg/100 gm); milk products, figs, oranges, kidney beans, kale, parsley, spinach, almonds, hazelnuts, soybean, and chocolate are rich sources	Calcium ion activates phospholipase C; required in the release of catecholamines from body stores; required in bone formation; essential for coagulation of blood; decreases permeability of blood and lymph vessels
Chlorine	Chloride is present in virtually all foodstuffs (0.4-3750 mg/100 gm); olives, bananas, dates, bread, dried coconut, cheese, and milk are rich sources	Chloride ion is important in electrolyte balance and in erythrocyte function; activates α-amylase
Iron	Present in relatively small quantities (0.2-19 mg/100 gm) in virtually all foodstuffs; liver, cocoa, wheat germ, yeast, spinach, soybeans, lentils are rich sources; also present in iron-fortified cereals	Iron is a component of cytochrome oxidase enzymes, which are essential in biologic oxidation reactions; essential for the production of hemoglobin and its metabolites and for myoglobin production
Magnesium	Present in virtually all foodstuffs (1-420 mg/100 gm); kidney beans, soybeans, spinach, brewer's yeast, various nuts, wheat germ, cocoa, and peanut butter are rich sources	Magnesium ion activates numerous enzymes (leucine aminopeptidase, hexosediphosphatase, alkaline phosphatase, inorganic pyrophosphatase, glycerophosphorylcholine diesterase, deoxyribonuclease, and others); essential for the formation of basic cell constituents from amino acids and the formation of purines
Phosphorus	Present in most foodstuffs (4-1753 mg/100 gm); yeast, nuts, meat, flour, egg yolk, and kidney beans are rich sources	Phosphorus is a component of the body's phosphatase and phospholipase enzymes, which are involved in numerous biochemical reactions; essential in the synthesis of cell constituents from glucose and in the derivation of energy from the degradation of foodstuffs, which involves adenosine triphosphate, diphosphate, and monophosphate
Potassium	Present in virtually all foodstuffs (0.2-3200 mg/100 gm); yeast, spinach, soybeans, most vegetables, molasses, fish, meat, milk products, egg powder, peanut butter, cocoa, and flour are rich sources	Potassium ion is important in water and electrolyte balance; necessary in the synthesis of cell constituents from amino acids and formation of purines; required for cellular maintenance and growth and in nervous system function; important in digestion and in muscle control; essential in recovery from severe diarrhea and diabetic acidosis
Sodium	Present in virtually all foodstuffs (0.3-2400 mg/100 gm); olives, fennel, canned vegetables, potato chips, sauerkraut, tomato ketchup, bread, pretzels, mayonnaise, mustard, dairy products, bacon, meat, and fish are excellent sources	Sodium ion is important in water and electrolyte balance; necessary in cellular maintenance and growth and in nervous system function; sodium deficiency is rarely encountered
Sulfur	Present in virtually all foodstuffs (1-630 mg/100 gm); eggs, meat, cocoa, nuts, vegetables, dried peaches, and dried apricots are rich sources	Sulfur is a component of some transferase enzymes (e.g., coenzyme A transferases, sulfotransferases); involved in drug detoxification (sulfate ester formation)

ADVERSE/SIDE EFFECTS OF VITAMINS, MINERALS, AND TRACE ELEMENTS*

The water-soluble vitamins (e.g., B complex, C) have relatively few adverse side effects when administered in therapeutic dosages. The fat-soluble vitamins, particularly A and D, have specific syndromes of adverse side effects associated with overdose or hypervitaminosis. (See the body of the chapter and the Nursing Drug Digest for adverse side effects associated with individual vitamins.)

Minerals and trace elements also possess relatively few adverse side effects when administered in therapeutic dosages. Effects are predominantly limited to the GI tract (i.e., nausea, diarrhea, and constipation).

*See Chapter 11, "Drug Toxicity," for an overview of drug toxicity.

CLINICALLY SIGNIFICANT DRUG INTERACTIONS*

Primary drug	Interacting drug	Possible effect(s)	Probable mechanism(s)
Calcium	Tetracyclines (except doxycycline)	Decreased tetracycline blood levels	Decreased GI absorption
Calcium	Thiazide diuretics	Hypercalcemia	Decreased calcium excretion
Iron	Tetracyclines	Decreased tetracycline blood levels	Decreased GI absorption
Phytonadione (vitamin K_1)	Oral anticoagulants	Decreased anticoagulant effect	Pharmacologic antagonism
Potassium	Potassium-sparing diuretics	Hyperkalemia	Decreased potassium excretion
Pyridoxine (vitamin B_6)	Levodopa	Decreased levodopa effect	Increased peripheral metabolism
Zinc	Tetracyclines (except doxycycline)	Decreased tetracycline blood levels	Decreased GI absorption

*See Chapter 10, "Drug Interactions" for an overview of drug interactions.

GENERAL NURSING IMPLICATIONS

Nursing of patients requiring vitamins, minerals, and trace elements

ASSESSMENT

Patients manifesting symptoms of nutritional deficiencies require a thorough history and physical examination including laboratory evaluation of blood and urine. The initial data base should include a detailed nutritional assessment including height, weight, other anthropometric measurements as indicated, and a detailed diet history. The patient's general appearance especially as related to the presenting problem should be documented. A history of alcohol, tobacco, or drug use should also be ascertained as well as a social history to identify problems related to diet and nutrition that may require referral for social service assistance. In addition, the patient's knowledge of food and nutrition as well as activity and exercise pattern should be assessed carefully. A detailed drug history should be completed identifying the use or misuse of vitamins, minerals, and trace elements. The drug history should also identify potential drug sensitivity, contraindications, cautions, potential drug interactions, and drug-taking patterns before therapy is initiated.

SENSITIVITY

Allergic reactions to vitamins, minerals, and trace elements are rare; however, any drug has the potential to cause a hypersensitivity reaction in a susceptible individual. Hypersensitivity reactions have been reported with topical vitamin A preparations and deodorants containing vitamin E.

CONTRAINDICATIONS

The specific vitamins, minerals, and trace elements are contraindicated in patients with known hypersensitivity to a particular agent or in the presence of toxicity. See the Nursing Drug Digest.

CAUTIONS

The vitamins, minerals, and trace elements should be used with caution in certain patients. See the Nursing Drug Digest.

DRUG INTERACTIONS

The various vitamins, minerals, and trace elements have been associated with interactions involving other drugs. See Clinically Significant Drug Interactions.

ADMINISTRATION

Vitamins, minerals, and trace elements are available in various dosage forms for oral use, including tablets, chewable tablets, drops, elixirs, and solutions. Other multivitamin preparations are available for intravenous administration after being diluted in appropriate intravenous solutions.

See the Nursing Drug Digest for specific information regarding the administration of these agents.

MONITORING PATIENT RESPONSE
Therapeutic response

The onset and duration of therapeutic effect vary with the particular agent. Patients should be monitored for changes in presenting symptoms and a general improvement in energy level, normal growth and development, improved appearance of affected tissues, and improvement in mood or well-being.

Adverse effects

The adverse affects associated with the use of vitamins, minerals, and trace elements are generally associated with excesses in amounts administered. Nurses should be aware of the signs of toxicity for these agents (See Table 66-1 and the Nursing Drug Digest) as well as signs that indicate the patient may have a nutritional deficit.

Many foods contain vitamin supplements, which can increase the risk of toxicity with certain agents.

PATIENT EDUCATION

The patient and family should be fully informed about the use and misuse of vitamins, minerals, and trace elements. They should understand the importance of eating a well-balanced diet and may require assistance with meal planning and preparation. The patient and family should understand the general action and adverse effects of vitamins, minerals, and trace elements and understand the correct administration of these agents, their storage, and how common adverse side effects (e.g., stomach upset with multivitamins or constipation with iron) can be minimized or prevented.

Misconceptions and fallacies should be clarified honestly after exploration with the patient and family. Both patients and families should be encouraged to discuss lay nutritional information and uses of vitamins, minerals, and trace elements so that they can make informed choices regarding medication use.

GENERAL INSTRUCTIONS FOR DISCHARGE/OUTPATIENTS

VITAMINS, MINERALS, AND TRACE ELEMENTS

This is a vitamin preparation used to prevent or treat vitamin deficiencies.

Take this medication exactly as prescribed. Do not take more than the recommended amount because unwanted or toxic effects can occur, especially if you are taking vitamin A, D, or K.

Vitamin preparations can interact with some other medications and cause unwanted effects. Do not take any other medications when you are taking vitamins unless told to do so by your health care provider. Let other health care providers know you are taking vitamin preparations.

Even though you are taking a vitamin preparation, it is still important that you eat a well-balanced diet including foods from all four of the basic food groups daily. If you have any questions about meal planning, contact your health care provider.

Do not take mineral oil when you are on vitamin therapy. This can affect the amount of vitamin absorbed. If you require a laxative, contact your health care provider.

Read the label on any vitamin preparation you are taking to be sure of the contents. Some vitamin preparations include iron.

Take tablet forms of this medication with meals and a full glass of water. Enteric-coated tablet, or tablets with a special coating to decrease stomach upset, should not be taken within 1 hour of milk or antacids. They should be swallowed whole, without chewing or breaking them up, with a full glass of water.

Liquid vitamin preparations should be carefully measured and taken with a small amount of water or fruit juice or taken directly on the tongue. If the vitamin is mixed in liquid, be sure to drink the entire amount of the liquid to ensure you take the correct amount of medication. Liquid vitamins should *not* be put in infant formula. They should be placed directly on the infant's tongue and followed with juice or formula as indicated.

Store this medication in a cool, dark, dry place. Refrigeration is not necessary.

Keep this medication and all other medications out of the reach of children.

In addition to the general instructions, following are instructions for specific vitamins.

Vitamin A

If you are pregnant or considering pregnancy, notify your health care provider before taking this medication. This medication could cause unwanted effects.

Be especially careful taking this medication. Too much vitamin A can cause unwanted toxic effects.

Unwanted effects associated with the use of this medication are not common; however, notify your health care provider if you develop a skin rash, nausea or vomiting, cracking of the lips or skin, or a loss of appetite.

Vitamin A-D preparations

If you are pregnant, considering pregnancy, or breastfeeding an infant, notify your health care provider before taking this medication. This medication could cause unwanted effects in unborn babies or nursing infants.

Unwanted effects associated with the use of this medication are not common; however, notify your health care provider if you develop loss of appetite, nausea, vomiting, diarrhea, weakness, a skin rash, or cracking of the lips and skin.

Vitamin B complex

Notify your health care provider if you develop flulike symptoms while taking this medication.

Vitamin B_1

Unwanted effects associated with the use of this medication are not common; however, notify your health care provider if you notice a skin rash, difficult breathing, or tightness of the throat while taking this medication.

Vitamin B_{12}

Follow the instructions on the prescription exactly. Do not inject any more or any less medication than prescribed. If you have any questions about how this medication should be administered, contact your health care provider.

It is important that you take this medication at regular intervals as indicated by your health care provider to prevent damage to nerve cells in your body.

Unwanted effects associated with the use of this medication are not common; however, notify your health care provider if you notice a skin rash, difficult breathing, or tightness of the throat.

Vitamin D

Always take this medication with milk as directed.

Unwanted effects associated with the use of this medication are not common; however, notify your health care provider if you notice any nausea, vomiting, drowsiness, or diarrhea while using this medication.

Vitamin E

Chew chewable tablets well before swallowing.

Vitamin C

Check the type of vitamin C preparation you have. Chew chewable tablets well before swallowing. Swallow regular tablets with a full glass of water. Effervescent tablets should be dissolved in a glass of water and taken immediately.

Unwanted effects associated with the use of this medication are not common; however, notify your health care provider if you notice low back pain or pain when urinating.

NURSING DRUG DIGEST

Medication (trade name*)	Indication	Usual dosage and administration	Dosage forms, preparation, and storage	Contraindications, cautions, and comments	Monitoring
Ascorbic acid (vitamin C) Erivit C Ferosorb-C* Megacin* Mol-Iron with Vitamin C* Natrascorb Niarb Super* Palmiron-C* Peridin-C* Tri-Tinic Capsules* Tri-Vi-Flor* Tri-Vi-Flor with Iron Drops* Tri-Vi-Sol* Trinsicon M Trihemic 600* Vita-C Vitacee Viterra-C Vitron C* Vi-Zac Capsules* Zentrol Chewables*	Prophylaxis and treatment of vitamin C deficiency; scurvy	*Adults:* 30-150 mg/day PO, SC, IM, or IV Minimum protective dosage against scurvy: 10 mg/day *Infants and Children:* 5 mg/kg/day PO, SC, IM or IV	Tablets: 25, 50, 100, 200, 250, 500, 1000 mg Chewable tablets: 100, 250, 500, 1000 mg Injectable: 50, 100, 200, 250, 500 mg/ml Syrup: 20 mg/ml Drops: 50, 100 mg/ml Protect solution from light	*Contraindicated* in renal failure Use large doses with caution in G-6-PD deficiency May cause kidney stones, particularly with dosages over 2 gm/day May cause pain and swelling at site of injection Ascorbic acid requirement is increased in smokers Rapid IV administration may cause syncope Sudden withdrawal of megadose therapy may result in scurvy	Monitor injection site Observe for diarrhea

Continued.

NOTE: For additional details regarding the individual agents listed in this table, see the text and other tables in this chapter.
*Indicates a multiple active ingredient product. For a complete listing of all active ingredients see the *Drug Reference Guide to Brand Names and Active Ingredients.*

NURSING DRUG DIGEST—cont'd

Medication (trade name)	Indication	Usual dosage and administration	Dosage forms, preparation, and storage	Contraindications, cautions, and comments	Monitoring
Calcium *Calcium carbonate* BioCal Cal-Sup Caltrate Os-Cal 500 *Calcium glubionate* Neo-Calglucon *Calcium gluconate* Calcet* Kalcinate* Supac* *Calcium lactate* Calcet* Calphosan* Calphosan B-12*	Prevention and treatment of calcium deficiency See also Chapter 62, "Parathyroid Hormone, Calcitonin, and Related Medications," and Chapter 67, "Fluids and Electrolytes"	*Adults*: 10-25 mEq PO q.d. to q.i.d. Dissolve effervescent tablets in a glassful of water *before* administration Administration with meals may decrease GI distress Parenteral: Administer by slow IV injection or infusion by slow IV drip Dosage *must* be individualized based on the patient's condition and serum calcium concentration Do *not* administer the gluconate salt by IM injection to children	Tablets: 1, 2, 4, 10 mEq Effervescent tablet: 25 mEq Syrup: 5.5 mEq/5 ml Injectable: 0.5 mEq/ml	*Contraindicated* in hypercalcemia, hypercalciuria, renal calculi, and severe renal disease Parenteral calcium is *contraindicated* in digitalized patients Use with caution in patients receiving high dosage of vitamin D NOTE: The calcium salts contain varying amounts of calcium (i.e., calcium chloride, 14 mEq/gm; calcium gluconate, 4.7 mEq/gm; calcium glucep-tate 4.5 mEq/gm; calcium glubionate, 4.5 mEq/gm; calcium lactate, 6 mEq/gm; calcium carbonate, 20 mEq/gm)	Monitor serum calcium Observe for signs of hypercalcemia (see Chapter 67, "Fluids and Electrolytes") Monitor injection site for irritation Monitor vital signs during parenteral administration
Cyanocobalamin (vitamin B₁₂) Bay Bee-12 Berubigen Betalin 12 Cabadon-M Cobex Cyanoject Cyomin Kaybovite-1000 Pernavit Redisol Rubesol-1000 Rubramin PC Ruvite 1000 Sytobex Vibal Vi-Twel	Pernicious anemia	*Adults*: 30μg/day IM or SC for 5-10 days, followed by monthly maintenance doses of 100 μg IM or SC; or 1000 μg/day PO, followed by weekly maintenance doses of 1000-3000 μg PO Do *not* administer IV	Capsule: 25 μg Tablets: 25, 50, 100, 250, 500, 1000 μg Timed-release tablet: 1200 μg Injectable: 30, 100, 1000 μg/ml Store injectable protected from light	*Contraindicated* in hypersensitivity to vitamin B₁₂ or cobalt May cause mild transient diarrhea, itching, or hypersensitivity reactions	Monitor hematology results

Generic names	Uses	Dosage	Dosage Forms	Remarks
Folic acid Berocca C* En-Cebrin F* Folbal Foldine Folvite Folvron* Hemocyte-F* Hemocyte Injection* Mission Prenatal* Niferex-150 Forte* Novofolacid Perihemin* Pronemia* Trinsicon* TriHemic 500* Tri-Tinic Capsules* Vitron-C-Plus* Zentinic* Zintinic*	Prophylaxis and treatment of folic acid deficiency; megaloblastic anemia	*Adults:* 0.4-1 mg/day PO, IM, IV, or SC *Children:* 0.1-0.4 mg/day PO, IM, IV, or SC	Tablets: 0.1, 0.25, 0.4, 0.8, 1, 5 mg Injectable: 5, 10 mg/ml	May rarely cause allergic reactions NOTE: The administration of folic acid in pernicious anemia without the concurrent administration of vitamin B_{12} may result in hematologic improvement, but with *continuing* neurologic progression of the condition — Monitor hematology results
Iron *Ferrous fumarate* Cefera* C-Ron* Feco-T Femiron Feostat Ircon Irolong* Hemocyte Toleron TriHemic 600* Trinsicon* Tri-Tinic*	Prevention and treatment of iron-deficiency anemia	*Adults:* 50-100 mg (elemental iron) PO t.i.d. *Children:* 15-45 mg (elemental iron) PO t.i.d. Administration with food or milk may decrease GI distress Oral liquid dosage forms should be administered in water or fruit juice (do *not* use milk) Parenteral: Individual dosages based on body weight and degree of iron-deficiency anemia; may be administered IM using a Z-track technique or IV	Tablets: 35, 60, 65 mg (elemental iron) Syrup: 30-40 mg (elemental iron)/5 ml Drops: 15 mg (elemental iron)/0.6 ml Oral solution: 25 mg (elemental iron)/ml Injectable: 50 mg (elemental iron)/ml	*Contraindicated* in hypersensitivity to iron, hemochromatosis, and hemosiderosis NOTE: The administration of iron in hemolytic anemia *without* iron deficiency may result in hemosiderosis Use with caution in infants Use with caution in patients with ulcer disorders Oral administration commonly causes nausea, constipation, or diarrhea — Monitor hematology results

Continued.

NURSING DRUG DIGEST—cont'd

Medication (trade name)	Indication	Usual dosage and administration	Dosage forms, preparation, and storage	Contraindications, cautions, and comments	Monitoring
Iron—cont'd *Ferrous gluconate* Fergon Ferralet Ferroid Fertinic Ironate Novofer-rogluc Simron *Ferrous sulfate* Feosol Fer-In-Sol Fer-Iron Fero-Grad Ferospace F. Iron* Fumaral* Ironized Yeast* Mol-Iron Vi-Daylin Plus Iron ADC Drops* Vi-Daylin/ F + Iron*		Administer IV doses slowly at a rate of 20-50 mg/min Do *not* use iron-dextran from multidose vials that contain a preservative (i.e., phenol) for IV administration Do *not* administer enteric-coated tablets with milk or antacids Protect teeth from staining by administering solutions and drops diluted in water or juice and drink from straw; follow with oral care Dosage must be individualized based on the patient's condition and serum iron concentration		Oral iron preparations may stain teeth IM administration may cause pain and discoloration at the injection site IV administration may cause headache, hypotension, nausea, and allergic-like reactions Iron usually darkens the stools Oral iron salts contain 15% to 35% elemental iron (i.e., ferrous fumarate, 34%; ferrous gluconate, 12%; ferrous lactate, 19%; ferrous succinate, 35%; ferrous sulfate, 20%)	
Niacin Nicamin Niconacid Nico-Span Novoniacin	Pellagra Hypercholesterolemia	*Adults:* 50-500 mg/day PO, SC, IM, or IV *Adults:* 250-1000 mg PO t.i.d. Maximum: 6 gm/day Administration with food or milk may decrease GI distress	Tablets: 25, 50, 100, 250, 500 mg Injectable: 50, 100 mg/ml	*Contraindicated* in hypersensitivity, active ulcer disease, hepatic dysfunction, and diabetes mellitus Use with caution in pregnancy and lactation May cause nausea, vomiting, severe flushing, pruritus, activation of peptic ulcers, and hypotension	Observe for activation of ulcers Monitor hepatic function Monitor blood glucose levels in diabetics

Drug	Uses	Dosage	Preparations	Cautions	Assessments
Phytonadione (vitamin K₁) Aquamephyton Konakion Mephyton Mono-Kay	Anticoagulant-induced prothrombin deficiency Hypoprothrombinemia secondary to antibacterial therapy Prevention of hemorrhagic disease in neonates	*Adults:* 2.5–50 mg/day PO, SC, IM, or IV When administered IV, inject slowly—*not exceeding 1 mg/min* *Children:* Prevention of hemorrhagic disease in neonates—0.5–1 mg IM or SC at birth and repeated in 6–8 hr if necessary	Tablet: 5 mg Injectable: 2, 10 mg/ml NOTE: Konakion injection is *for IM use only*	Large doses used to treat hypercholesterolemia commonly cause diarrhea, headache, dry skin, and rashes in addition to the other previously noted effects *Contraindicated* in hypersensitivity to vitamin K May cause pain and tenderness at the site of injection Rapid IV injection may cause flushing and hypotension Overdose in neonates may increase bilirubin levels Maximum dosages in adults may cause increased BSP retention and prolongation of prothrombin time Use with caution in patients with hepatic dysfunction or with G-6-PD deficiency	Observe for hypersensitivity Monitor neonate for signs of hyperbilirubinemia
Potassium *Potassium chloride* Apo-K K-10 Kaochlor Kato Powder Kay-Ciel K-Long Klor Klor-Con Kolyum Liquid/Powder* KEFF* Pan Chloride Slo-Pot Slow-K	Prevention and treatment of potassium deficiency See also Chapter 67, "Fluids and Electrolytes"	*Adults:* 20–100 mEq/day NOTE: For potassium, 1 mEq = 1 mmol Dilute *unflavored* liquid potassium preparation with fruit or vegetable juice to increase palatability Oral solid dosage forms should be taken with a full glass of water or liquid in an upright or high-Fowler's position, unless contraindicated, to prevent possible esophageal obstruction or ulceration that has been reported with the use of these agents Administration with food or milk may decrease GI distress; do *not* administer enteric-coated tablets with milk	Enteric-coated tablets: 10, 12 mEq Slow-release wax matrix tablets: 6.7, 8, 10 mEq Solution: 10%–20% (i.e., 20, 40 mEq/15 ml) Capsule: 8 mEq Elixir: 20 mEq/15 ml (generally with 1%–5% alcohol) Injectable: 2, 2.5 mEq/ml NOTE: Injectable must be further diluted in appropriate IV solution before use Injectable potassium may be diluted in normal saline or dextrose solutions. (NOTE: Administration of dextrose may decrease serum potassium concentration.)	*Contraindicated* in hyperkalemia, ventricular fibrillation, severe renal impairment, acute dehydration, and Addison's disease Use with caution in renal failure, ulcer disease, and heart block May cause nausea, vomiting, cramping, GI irritation, and diarrhea Slow-release wax matrix tablets (e.g., K-Long, Klotrix, K-Tab, Slo-Pot, Slow K) may cause GI ulcerations and strictures, although the incidence tends to be lower than with enteric-coated tablets	Monitor serum potassium Observe for symptoms of hyperkalemia (i.e., weakness, flaccid muscles, hypotension, confusion, ECG changes—see Chapter 67, "Fluids and Electrolytes") Monitor injection site for signs of pain or irritation Monitor vital signs during parenteral administration Observe for GI distress

Continued.

NURSING DRUG DIGEST—cont'd

Medication (trade name)	Indication	Usual dosage and administration	Dosage forms, preparation, and storage	Contraindications, cautions, and comments	Monitoring
Potassium— cont'd *Potassium citrate* Polycitra Syrup* Polycitra-K Syrup* Polycitra-LC-Sugar-Free* Potassium Triplex* Twin-K* *Potassium gluconate* Kao-Nor Kaon Kaylixir Kolyum Liquid/Powder* Potassium Rougier Royonate Twin-K*		Parenteral use: Administer IV *only* at a rate of 10-20 mEq/ hr; dilute to at least 30 mEq/L before infusion Dosage *must* be individualized based on the patient's condition and serum potassium concentration Ensure adequate renal function *before* administration		Oral solution has an unpleasant salty taste Oral solution may not be acceptable because of GI intolerance; however, it is generally the least toxic and least expensive of the various potassium preparations Other potassium salts (e.g., potassium aminobenzoate, potassium citrate, potassium gluconate) are available, but potassium chloride is generally preferred, particularly for the treatment of diuretic-induced hypokalemia, because it can treat (prevent) the possible resultant hypochloremic alkalosis at the same time as the potassium deficit	
Pyridoxine (vitamin B₆) Alba-Lybe* AVP Natal* Beelith* Beesix Doxine* Gravidox Hepp-Iron Drops* Hexa-Betalin Hexavibex Hydoxin Thera-Combex H-P* Vita-Metrazol*	Prophylaxis and treatment of pyridoxine deficiency	*Adults:* 10-20 mg/day PO, IM, or IV	Tablets: 5, 10, 25, 100, 500 mg Injectable: 50, 100 mg/ml Protect solution from light Discard solutions containing a precipitate	*Contraindicated* in hypersensitivity to pyridoxine May cause burning, stinging, or pain at the site of injection Pyridoxine may significantly decrease the effectiveness of levodopa	

Name	Uses	Dosage	Preparations	Remarks
Riboflavin (vitamin B₂) Alba-Lybe* Cerebro-Nicin* Geravite Elixir* Riobin-50 Thera-Combex H-P* Vita-Metrazol*	Prophylaxis and treatment of riboflavin deficiency	*Adults:* 2-20 mg/day PO, SC, IM, or IV	Tablets: 5, 10, 25, 50, 100 mg Injectable: 50 mg/ml Protect solution from light	High dosage may color the urine bright yellow
Thiamine (vitamin B₁) Alba-Lybe* Becrinol Betalin S Betaxin Bewon Biamine Cal-M* Cerebro-Nicin* Garavite Elixir* Glukor Injection* Hepp-Iron Drops* Ironized Yeast* Neuro B-12 Forte Injectable* Troph-Iron* Trophite*	Prophylaxis and treatment of thiamine deficiency Beriberi	*Adults:* 5-100 mg/day PO *Adults:* 10-20 mg IM or IV for 2 weeks, followed by 5-10 mg/day PO	Tablets: 5, 10, 25, 50, 100, 250, 500 mg Injectable: 100 mg/ml Elixir: 2.25 mg/5 ml (contains 10%-15% alcohol)	*Contraindicated* in hypersensitivity to thiamine IV administration has resulted in death from hypersensitivity An intradermal test dose is recommended to screen individuals with a greater probability of hypersensitivity (i.e., individuals with past or family history of allergy) May cause weakness, nausea, sweating, or hypersensitivity reactions Observe for signs of hypersensitivity

Continued.

NURSING DRUG DIGEST—cont'd

Medication (trade name)	Indication	Usual dosage and administration	Dosage forms, preparation, and storage	Contraindications, cautions, and comments	Monitoring
Vitamin A Anatola Andoin* Aquasol A Aquasol A & D* AVP Natal* Hyalex* Proctodon* Scott's Emulsion* Super A Testavol S Tri-Vi-Flor* Tri-Vi-Sol* Vi-Alpha Vi-Daylin ADC Drops* Vi-Daylin Plus Iron ADC Drops*	Prophylaxis and treatment of vitamin A deficiency	*Adults:* 5000-200,000 IU/day PO *Children:* 5000-30,000 IU/day PO	Capsules: 5000, 10,000, 25,000, 50,000 IU Injectable: 50,000 IU/ml	*Contraindicated* in hypervitaminosis A and hypersensitivity to vitamin A Overdose can result in hypervitaminosis A	Observe for hypervitaminosis A (fatigue, anorexia, gingivitis, headache, malaise, irritability, dry and cracking skin)
Vitamin D Alphamettes* Andoin* Aquasol A & D* Calciferol Cal-M* Deltalin Drisdol Hyalex* Scott's Emulsion* Tri-Vi-Flor* Tri-Vi-Flor w/ Iron Drops* Tri-Vi-Sol* Vi-Daylin ADC Drops* Vi-Daylin Plus Iron ADC Drops*	Refractory rickets Familial phosphatemia and hypoparathyroidism See also Chapter 62, "Parathyroid Hormone, Calcitonin, and Related Medications"	*Adults:* 12,000-500,000 IU/day PO or IM *Adults:* 50,000-200,000 IU/day PO or IM, *plus* 24 gm/day of calcium lactate in 6 divided doses Dose must be highly individualized depending on calcium intake, parathyroid function, and type of vitamin D used; see Chapter 62, "Parathyroid Hormone, Calcitonin, and Related Medications"	Capsules: 10,000, 25,000, 50,000 IU	*Contraindicated* in hypercalcemia, severe renal impairment, and hypervitaminosis D Maintain appropriate calcium intake Overdose may cause hypervitaminosis D	Observe for hypervitaminosis D (nausea, anorexia, weakness, thirst, impaired renal function) Monitor blood levels of calcium, phosphorus, and urea Monitor renal function

Vitamin E Aquasol E Dalfatol Ephynal Eprolin Epsilan-M Esorb Kell-E Lan-E Maxi-E Natopherol Novo-E Phytoferol Super Cardialine Tocopherex Tofaxin Vita-E Vi-Zac Capsules*	*No proved indication for use* Use may be indicated in the prevention of vitamin E deficiency	*Adults:* 60-75 IU/day PO or IM	Capsules: 30, 50, 100, 200, 400, 600, 800, 1000 IU Injectable: 100, 200 IU/ml Tablets: 100, 200, 400, 1000 IU Tablets, chewable: 200, 400 IU Drops: 50 IU/ml	Large dosages may cause diarrhea and skin reactions	Observe for diarrhea Monitor for untoward reactions when large doses are administered

BIBLIOGRAPHY

Aaron, H. (Ed.). Vitamin E. *The Medical Letter,* 1975, *17,* 69-70.

Abramovicz, M. (Ed.). Vitamin A toxicity. *The Medical Letter,* 1980, *22,* 19-20.

Abramovicz, M. (Ed.). Drugs for acne. *The Medical Letter,* 1980, *22,* 31-32.

Bacon, E. Vitamin and mineral supplementation, *Canadian Pharmaceutical Journal,* 1980, *113,* 88-91.

Cameron, E., & Pauling, L. Supplemental Ascorbate in the supportive treatment of cancer: prolongation of survival times in terminal human cancer. *Proceedings of the National Academy of Sciences of the United States of America,* 1976, *73,* 3685-3689.

Catto, G.R.D., MacLeod, M., Pelc, B., & Kodicek, E. 1α-hydroxycholecalciferol: a treatment for renal bone disease. *British Medical Journal,* 1975, *1,* 12-14.

Coulehan, J.L., Eberhard, S., Kapner, L., Taylor, F., Rogers, K., & Garry, P. Vitamin C and acute illnesses in Navajo schoolchildren. *New England Journal of Medicine,* 1976, *295,* 973-977.

DiFazio, C.L. Folic acid reviewed. *Hospital Pharmacy,* 1976, *11,* 124.

Dykes, M.H.M., & Meier, P. Ascorbic acid and the common cold: evaluation of its efficacy and toxicity. *Journal of the American Medical Association,* 1975, *231,* 1073-1079.

Eaton, M.L. Chronic hypervitaminosis A. *American Journal of Hospital Pharmacy,* 1978, *35,* 1099-1102.

Goodman, L.S. & Gilman, A. (Eds.). *The pharmacological basis of therapeutics* (5th ed.). New York: MacMillan, Inc., 1975.

Johnson, A.R., Hood, R.L., & Emery, J.L. Biotin and the sudden infant death syndrome. *Nature,* 1980, *285,* 159-160.

Juan, D. Vitamin D metabolism—update for the clinician. *Postgraduate Medicine,* 1980, *68*(5), 210-218.

Karlowski, T.R., Chalmers, T.C., Frenkel, L.D., Kapikian, A.Z., Lewis, T.L., & Lynch, J.M. Ascorbic acid for the common cold. *Journal of the American Medical Association,* 1975, *231,* 1038-1042.

King, G.G., & Burns, J.J., (Eds.). Second conference on vitamin C. *Annals of the New York Academy of Sciences,* 1975, *258,* 1-552.

Levander, O.A., & Cheng, L. Micronutrient interactions: vitamins, minerals and hazardous elements. *Annals of the New York Academy of Sciences,* 1980, *355,* 1-372.

Reidenberg, M. An idea on the way: vitamin A analogs and protection from carcinogens. *Hospital Pharmacy,* 1976, *11,* 120-121.

Schnoes, H.K., & DeLuca, H.F. Recent progress in vitamin D metabolism and the chemistry of vitamin D metabolites Federation Proceedings. *Federation of the American Society of Experimental Biologists,* 1980, *39,* 2723-2729.

Smith, F.R., & Goodman, D.S. Vitamin A transport in human vitamin A toxicity. *New England Journal of Medicine,* 1976, *294,* 805-808.

Ulmer, D.D. Trace elements. *New England Journal of Medicine,* 1977, *297,* 318-321.

CHAPTER 67

Fluids and Electrolytes

William D. Snively
Donna R. Helmer

Medications discussed in this chapter

Electrolytes
 Bicarbonate
 Calcium
 Magnesium
 Potassium
 Sodium

From the biologic standpoint it is useful to regard human body fluid as the lineal descendant of seawater—seawater that has been converted through eons of evolutionary development to serve the purposes of human physiology. Indeed, this concept helps explain the striking differences in the composition of extracellular fluid (ECF), which lies outside the body cells, and cellular fluid (CF), which resides inside the cells. These disparities are far from inconsequential, since about 20% of the body's energy output is devoted to maintaining contrasts such as high potassium (K^+) and high phosphate (PO_4^{--}) in the CF and high sodium (Na^+) and high chloride (Cl^-) in the ECF. The origin of CF apparently is the precambrian seas of approximately 2 billion years ago. The origin of ECF, on the other hand, goes back a mere 300 million years, when it was brought ashore by our remote aquatic ancestors in their epochal and courageous landfall. Geologists and paleontologists assure us that the composition of our CF closely resembles that of the precambrian seas, whereas the composition of our ECF resembles that of the cambrian seas.

Tough and durable, the human being has managed to inhabit almost every corner of the globe—desert, mountains, teeming towns, ocean depths, even outer space. Both hunted and hunter, we have survived countless struggles with infecting organisms. To do all this, humans must constantly make enormous adjustments of a chemical and physical nature. In ac-complishing these changes, we are concerned with three environments, first described in 1857 by the great Claude Bernard at the Sorbonne in Paris.

The first environment, Bernard pointed out, is the essentially hostile world that surrounds us. Bernard's second environment is that within the skin, not including the contents of the cells. The third environment is within the cells themselves. Bernard stated, "All the vital mechanisms, however varied they may be, have always but one end, that of preserving the constancy of the conditions of life, in the internal environment."

In this amazing statement Bernard meant by the *vital mechanisms* the body's mechanisms for maintaining homeostasis. In reality, he knew little about these mechanisms except that they *must* exist. By the *internal environment* he was referring quite clearly to the division of ECF known as *interstitial fluid*, the fluid that surrounds and bathes the body cells, supplying them with nutrients and carrying off their wastes. Bernard realized that what is essential from the standpoint of cellular health is the maintenance of healthy interstitial fluid. The interstitial fluid, of course, maintains its healthy state through intimate contact with the plasma, another portion of ECF, via the arterial and venous capillary beds of the microcirculation. In the area of the capillary beds essential nutrients and other chemicals are passed out of the bloodstream and are then ferried to the trillions of body cells by the interstitial fluid. Waste materials pass from cells to interstitial fluid to be carried to the bloodstream for disposal.

Thus when we talk of homeostasis, we are really referring to certain constants within the ECF that must be maintained if the ECF is to preserve the environment of life within the cells in a constant state. Claude Bernard first presented the gigantic concept just outlined, but he gave it no name. Walter Cannon, a great American physiologist, did name it in 1929. He called it *homeostasis,* which refers to the processes that tend to restore the internal environment to a steady state.

STEADY STATE

Let us define the constant, or steady, state. By this term we mean constant volume of ECF: a normal ratio between the volume of plasma and that of interstitial fluid, usually about 1:3.5, and normal levels of certain essential ingredients of ECF, including the electrolytes sodium (Na^+), potassium (K^+), calcium (Ca^{++}), phosphorus (P), magnesium (Mg^{++}), proteinate, carbonic acid (H_2CO_3), and bicarbonate (HCO_3^-). (These are called electrolytes because they develop electrical charges when placed in water.) However, other substances can be found in the ECF—oxygen (O_2), carbon dioxide (CO_2), urea, creatinine, amino acids, glucose, and many others. In addition, the temperature of ECF must be maintained within normal limits.

MECHANISMS OF HOMEOSTASIS

Homeostasis depends on a cluster of devices. Some of these are natural devices such as osmosis and diffusion. Some are really bloodborne messengers, or hormones, produced for the most part by the ductless, or endocrine, glands. The autonomic nervous system, both sympathetic and parasympathetic, also plays a gigantic role in maintaining homeostasis. Let us examine the natural processes more closely. Oxygen and carbon dioxide both diffuse from areas of greater concentration to areas of lesser concentration (i.e., they flow down the concentration gradient). Reduced hemoglobin gives off carbon dioxide in the pulmonary capillaries and picks up oxygen to become oxyhemoglobin for transport to the cells. Numerous natural processes are involved in exchanges between the tubular urine and the peritubular capillaries.

Hormones influence the cells. The cells they influence depend on the specific hormone in question. However, whether the hormone comes from the thyroid gland, the anterior pituitary gland, or the adrenal gland, it has to have a mediator to produce the desired result on the cells. That mediator is cyclic adenosine monophosphate (cAMP).

The autonomic nervous system, controlled largely by the hypothalamus, also plays an enormous role in body homeostasis. The hypothalamus not only exerts control over the autonomic nervous system, but also controls the pituitary gland and hence many of the body's endocrine glands. Numerous complex relationships exist between the endocrine glands and the autonomic nervous system. We refer to specific hook-ups as neuroendocrine transducers. One of these is represented by the relationship between the hypothalamus and the pituitary (anterior and posterior); the other consists of the connection between the endings of the sympathetic nervous system and the adrenal medulla.

The kidney is the key organ in the renocardiovascular homeostatic mechanism. Its role in maintaining body homeostasis is incalculable. For example, it is of primary importance in adjusting the concentration of electrolytes in the ECF as well as the total volume. It converts an unusable form of vitamin D to one that the body can use. It excretes the breakdown products of protein metabolism and of drugs as well as a multiplicity of toxins. It also rids the body of fixed acids such as phosphoric acid and sulfuric acid. It produces the hormone erythropoietin, essential for red blood cell production. Finally, as part of its role in maintaining the normal pH of body fluids it regenerates bicarbonate when the need arises.

How are the specific aspects of the steady state maintained? To begin with, the body defends ECF volume as its primary duty, maintaining its constancy even at the expense of other elements of composition such as the hydrogen ion (H^+) concentration. Primary hormonal controls of ECF volume include antidiuretic hormone (ADH) and aldosterone. Sodium and water intake are also involved. The portions of ECF that exist as plasma and as interstitial fluid are kept in their respective positions largely by natural processes such as the filtration pressure created by the pumping action of the heart and the colloidal osmotic pressure of albumin.

Control of the composition of ECF is enormously important. Sodium concentration is controlled by aldosterone and the water intake—which, strangely enough, is more important than the sodium intake. Potassium concentration is regulated by aldosterone, by potassium intake, and by sodium intake. Potassium conservation is far from perfect, being much inferior to that of sodium. Calcium concentration of the ECF is controlled by the hormone parathyroid hormone (PTH) and to a much lesser extent by the hormone calcitonin, by calcium intake and output, by vitamin D intake, and by the hydrogen ion concentration of the ECF. Regulation of the concentration of phosphorus, which is usually reciprocal with calcium, is carried out largely by the kidneys. Magnesium concentration is controlled in part by aldosterone. The prime factor in determining the concentration of proteinate is dietary intake, although any type of trauma tends to deplete the body of proteinate. The concentration of carbonic acid and base bicarbonate (sodium, potassium, calcium, and magnesium bicarbonate) is the prime determinant of acid-base balance. In turn, acid-base balance controls the level of hydrogen ion concentration, which will be normal when the ratio of carbonic acid to bicarbonate lies within normal. The level of carbonic acid in the ECF is adjusted by the lungs, that of bicarbonate by the kidneys. Oxygen concentration is controlled by diffusion, with the element always flowing down the concentration gradient. Carbon dioxide moves by the same principle as do amino acids, glucose, urea, and creatinine.

Factors that challenge homeostasis

Many factors challenge homeostasis. These factors include strains and stresses, changes in temperature, antigen-antibody reactions, genetic disorders, infection, endocrine disorders, psychosomatic disturbances—indeed, any factor that exerts an influence on the constant state of the internal environment.

ANATOMY OF BODY FLUIDS

Turning our attention to what we might call the anatomy of body fluids, let us examine the fluid and solid components of body weight in the adult. The average adult is about 40% solids and 60% fluids. In the adult ECF constitutes about 15% of body weight and cellular fluid 45%. (Interestingly enough, the more obese an individual is, the less is the percentage of body water, since fat does not contain important amounts of water.) The newborn is only some 23% solids and 77% fluids. In the neonate ECF constitutes 42% of body weight and cellular fluid, 35%. Why does the newborn have such a large percentage of body weight in the form of fluid? Several answers can be given: First of all, the neonate needs to have body fluid in an accessible form, and the most accessible form in which body fluid can exist is as ECF. The neonate is growing rapidly, and body homeostatic mechanisms are immature. Finally, the neonate has several times as much body surface area in relation to mass as does the adult. This means that the neonate loses considerably more water and electrolytes through the skin (in proportion to body weight) than does the adult.

If we were to take a cross section—as through the forearm or calf, for example—we would be able to see the microscopic anatomy of the body fluids. We would note the two types of ECF—namely, plasma and interstitial fluid. Both are ECF, but one is within the blood vessels and the other (about three and a half times as voluminous) is outside the blood vessels, surrounding the trillions of extravascular cells of the body. The CF is revealed as lying within the cells, both the cells in blood vessels and those outside the blood vessels. Obviously, CF is not a continuous fluid; it is divided into trillions of tiny compartments. The fluids of body cells are by no means constant in their composition, although they do have certain characteristics in common (such as a high level of potassium, magnesium, phosphate, and proteinate).

It might be useful to consider a topographic analogy of body fluid, with the CF as a great reservoir, the somewhat smaller ECF as a lake quite different in composition from CF but nevertheless in communication with it (over the cell membrane, of course). From the ECF stem water and electrolytes for important secretions and excretions, including those of the stomach, intestines, pancreas, liver, kidneys (urine), bowel (feces), and sweat glands (perspiration). Although most of the secretions and excretions have a fairly constant composition in health, they can vary greatly from the norm in disease. They all originate in the ECF, which means that if any of these fluids is depleted (e.g., by vomiting, diarrhea, excessive urination, or perspiration) the ECF can also be depleted as water and electrolytes flow from it to replenish those of secretions or excretions that have been lost abnormally. If the ECF is sufficiently drained, then additional water and electrolytes must be supplied by the oral or tube route if possible or by the parenteral route (preferably intravenously) if enteral feedings are not possible.

GAINS AND LOSSES

Gains and losses of body water and electrolytes are extremely important, since perhaps 90% of body fluid disturbances occur because of disparities between gains and losses. First, let us examine the gains: we can gain water alone through ingestion and through oxidation of foodstuffs and body tissues. When we ingest food, we gain both water and electrolytes as well as other essential nutrients. The same holds for tube feedings and parenteral feedings.

Now let us look at the routes of loss: water and electrolytes are lost through vomiting, through diarrhea and even normal stools, and through discharge of fluids from the lungs such as the bronchorrhea of bronchitis. Carbon dioxide and water vapor flow from the lungs in the normal process of respiration. Water and electrolytes are lost through perspiration; urine; and in exudate from burns, ulcers, bedsores, wounds, colitis, or fistulas. Via insensible loss through the skin, water alone is lost. Internal losses can also occur (e.g., in an obstructed intestine the water and electrolytes that accumulate are just as lost to the body as if they were outside the body). The same holds for losses to an injured area such as occurs in edema of an injured part or in massive urticaria. In various infections—notably hemorrhagic pancreatitis—large amounts of calcium are lost. Therapeutic measures such as paracentesis and gastric or intestinal suction can cause loss of water and electrolytes.

Significantly, the list of routes of gain is short, whereas the list of routes of loss is long (see box above). One of the first events that occurs when a person becomes seriously ill is that gains decrease and losses increase as part of the disease condition. Most seriously ill patients stand a great risk of developing a body fluid disturbance.

BASIC BODY FLUID DISTURBANCES

Body fluid disturbances consist of changes in *volume* of ECF, changes in *concentration* of electrolytes in ECF expressed as units of electrolyte per unit volume (bear in mind that we are speaking of concentration of electrolyte per unit of ECF, not of the total quantity in the body), or *shifts* of water and electrolytes from plasma to interstitial space or from interstitial space to plasma.

To review the basic body fluid disturbances, we are going to need some numbers that will give us at least a rough idea of the quantity of the body fluids and of the electrolytes. First let us consider the ECF. We can quantitate it in pounds or kilograms. A mild deficit represents a loss of about 2% of the body weight in ECF; a moderate deficit, 5%; and a severe deficit, 8%. We can, of course, have an ECF volume excess. We quantitate this condition by an acute weight gain in pounds or kilograms, and almost no limit can be placed on the gain until the lungs fill with fluid and patients can literally drown in their own secretions.

In speaking of the components of ECF we use different types of measuring units depending on the element concerned. For many we use milliequivalents (mEq) per liter (L). For example, the normal sodium content of ECF ranges from 137 to 147 mEq/L. Normal average values for most of these substances are shown in the box above. Recall that in discussing electrolytes, we are referring not to the total quantity of a given electrolyte in the body, but rather to its concentration, usually expressed as milliequivalents per liter. However, exceptions are made: the normal value for calcium, for example, is 4.5 mEq/L, or a little over 10 mg/

dl. (Laboratories have been measuring calcium so long in mg/dl that they have not yet gotten out of the habit.) Various authorities believe that the normal value for calcium is 10.2, 10.4, or 10.8 mg/dl. Values for albumin, that important protein of the plasma responsible largely for maintaining the plasma in the blood vessels, are expressed in grams rather than in milligrams or milliequivalents, since we have such a relatively large quantity of albumin. The normal is 4.5 gm/dl. Carbonic acid is measured in millimeters of mercury, the normal being 40. We have no ready measure for either of the two shifts of ECF that can occur; their detection depends on clinical assessment.

Thus, the basic unit of measurement for an electrolyte may vary depending on the equipment available and the agreed on standard for the area of practice. Values may be reported in milligrams per deciliter (mg/dl, mg/100 ml),* milliequivalents per liter (mEq/L), or millimoles per liter (mmol/L).

Regardless of how the values are presented, the nurse can easily convert from one measurement system to another by using the following two simple formulas and their variations.

1. Conversion of milligrams to milliequivalents.

$$mg \times \left(\frac{Valence}{Molecular\ (or\ atomic)\ weight} \right) = mEq$$

EXAMPLE: 100 mg of calcium = ? mEq of calcium

Valence of calcium = 2
Atomic weight of calcium = 40

$$100\ mg \times \left(\frac{2}{40} \right) = 5\ mEq$$

2. Conversion of milliequivalents to millimoles.

$$mmol = \frac{mEq}{Valence}$$

EXAMPLE: 5 mEq of calcium = ? mmol of calcium

Valence of calcium = 2

$$\frac{5\ mEq}{2} = 2.5\ mmol$$

All that then remains is to standardize the volume. For example, if one started with milligrams per deciliter and wished to convert to milliequivalents per liter, one would use the equation presented to convert milligrams to milliequivalents and then multiply the result by 10 to adjust for the reported volume (i.e., deciliter to liter).

In discussing the basic body fluid disturbances, which constitute the overwhelming preponderance of

_____
*Note that mg/dl = mg/100 ml = mg%.

body fluid problems, we will first cover the events preceding the disturbance. Obviously, the clinical history is invaluable in providing this information. Rather than listing the preceding events in precise terms, we will employ generalities, thus avoiding endless lists. Clinical observations, so essential for correct diagnosis, are listed specifically and include all the major symptoms and findings. Under the heading Laboratory Help we have included those findings usually indicative of the imbalance. Aspects of the disturbance of particular importance are included under the heading Of Special Significance.

In outlining the various modes of therapy under each imbalance, we would emphasize that the therapy chosen depends on a host of variables. Attention should always be focused on the condition bringing about the imbalance. (Emergency situations may necessarily delay this aspect of therapy.) Because the cause of the various imbalances varies so much from patient to patient, so must the mode of therapy chosen vary. The principles of therapy of body fluid disturbances in infants and children closely resemble those of therapy in the adult. Quantities will naturally be smaller for the young. Body surface area provides an excellent gauge for quantities regardless of age, with the possible exception of premature infants. A few general principles of therapy follow.

1. Give enough of whatever substance you are giving.
2. Logically, repair solutions should contain cellular as well as extracellular electrolytes.
3. In quantitating the amount of fluids to be given, consider repair of existing deficits, provision for maintenance, and replacement of concurrent losses (ongoing losses that are occurring from vomiting, diarrhea, heavy perspiration, tube drainage, fistulas, or insensible perspiration).
4. In correcting imbalances, never attempt to correct the entire deficit at one time. Rather, part—perhaps half—of the deficit should be corrected and electrolytes reassessed, then the rest of the deficit can be treated.
5. For internal or external losses of blood give whole blood.
6. Albumin should be administered if the serum albumin is below 3 gm/dl.
7. In urgent or emergency therapy do not use hyperalimentation (also referred to as high-caloric amino acid mixtures, complete parenteral alimentation, or total parenteral nutrition).
8. Hemodialysis or peritoneal dialysis—often used as a sort of court of last resort in severe poisoning—can be employed in certain extreme instances of body fluid disturbances.

Volume imbalances

Extracellular fluid volume deficit

Preceding events. A host of events can lead to this disturbance, all of which can be divided under two headings: (1) loss of water and electrolytes such as in gastroenteritis and (2) decreased intake of water and electrolytes such as in advanced debility. *Potential pharmacologic causes* are cathartics and emetics (see box, top right.)

Clinical observations. The clinical observations in ECF volume deficit are precise: the fontanel is depressed in an infant and the tongue of an adult has longitudinal furrows—both highly reliable signs. Inelastic skin gives us the clue in young and middle-aged persons. Other clinical observations include decreased tearing and salivation; slow filling of the veins of the hand when the arm is raised and lowered; and absence of moisture in the axilla and the groin, indicating a deficit of at least 1.5 L. We also observe a systolic blood pressure that is 10 mm Hg less when the person is standing than when he is supine. We see weight loss, not counting fluid that might be trapped in the intestines, in the peritoneal cavity, or as edema: 2% weight loss = mild deficit; 5% = moderate deficit; and 8% = severe deficit. Other clinical observations are decreased central venous pressure, subnormal temperature, urine flow rate under 40 ml/hr*, increased pulse rate, and increased respiratory rate. We see flat neck veins when the patient is supine, an increase in the urinary specific gravity, and a pinched facial expression.

Laboratory help. The laboratory gives us little help in diagnosing this deficit. However, in severe ECF volume deficit both sodium and chloride will be absent from the urine. The hemoglobin, hematocrit, and packed cell volume will be increased in proportion to the severity of the deficit, since they are in a lesser volume of plasma (i.e., hemoconcentration). This finding is of limited value unless the values before the onset of the ECF volume deficit are known (and they seldom are).

Of special significance. When this imbalance occurs, the kidney tubules deteriorate rapidly (for reasons not entirely clear). Moreover, ECF volume deficit quickly leads to other deficits. For both of these reasons ECF volume deficits should be corrected as rapidly as possible.

Modes of therapy. Deficits of ECF should be replaced either with a hypotonic or isotonic solution containing both extracellular and cellular electrolytes. Hypotonic solutions are often preferred, since they provide extra water for metabolic needs and kidney

---

*Adult rate.

Pharmacologic agents important in ECF volume deficit

As potential causes

Cathartics
Diuretics
Enemas

As modes of therapy

Replace ECF with hypotonic or isotonic balanced electrolyte solution by oral, tube, or parenteral route

---

Pharmacologic agents important in ECF volume excess

As potential causes

Corticosteroids (excessive administration)
Chlorpropamide
Isotonic (or stronger) solutions of sodium chloride
Sodium (excessive ingestion)

As modes of therapy

Withhold fluids temporarily
Start low-sodium diet
Administer potent diuretic (furosemide, thiazide, or ethacrynic acid)
Hemodialysis or peritoneal dialysis in extreme situation

---

function. Either the oral route, including nasogastric or gastrostomy tube, the rectal route via rectal tube, or the parenteral route may be employed (see box, above top).

Extracellular fluid volume excess

Preceding events. The events preceding ECF volume excess encompass any cause of retention of excessive sodium and water be it congestive heart disease, cirrhosis of the liver, or the nephrotic syndrome.

Potential pharmacologic causes are excessive ingestion of sodium or administration of isotonic (or stronger) solutions of sodium chloride (see box, above).

Clinical observations. In ECF volume excess the clinical observations are definite and usually obvious.

We see puffy eyelids and peripheral edema, which may be of the pitting variety. The patient may have ascites: pleural effusion; pulmonary edema (which can be detected by radiographic examination before being heard with a stethoscope); moist rales in the lungs (indicating an excess of 1.5 L or more of ECF); acute weight gain; a full, bounding pulse; slow emptying of the hand veins when the arm is raised; elevated central venous pressure; and distended neck veins. If the kidneys are normal, urinary volume will increase. If kidney disease is present, the blood urea nitrogen (BUN) and possibly the serum potassium levels may be elevated.

Laboratory help. The hemoglobin, hematocrit, and packed cell volume will be decreased in proportion to the severity of the excess, since they are in a greater volume of plasma (i.e., hemodilution). Unless the values before the onset of the imbalance are known, these findings are of limited value.

Of special significance. The patient may succumb from pulmonary edema. This imbalance may occur with the remobilization of edema fluid on the third day following a severe burn if the patient's fluid intake has not been carefully restricted during the first 2 days.

Modes of therapy. Fluids should be withheld temporarily. In most instances a low-sodium diet is indicated. One of the potent diuretics (e.g., furosemide, thiazides, or ethacrynic acid) may prove useful. In extreme situations hemodialysis or peritoneal dialysis can be lifesaving.

Concentration imbalances

In studying the concentration imbalances, remember: *concentration means units of electrolyte per unit volume of ECF—not total electrolyte in the body.*

Sodium deficit

Preceding events. Sodium, as the chief cation of ECF, is primarily responsible for maintaining its osmolality, or osmolarity.* A wide variety of events can lead to sodium deficit. First are those events resulting from loss of sodium, as exemplified by the losses in gastrointestinal secretions via vomiting or nasogastric

tube drainage. Second is sodium deficit caused by an excess of water, which dilutes the serum sodium; this is often referred to as water intoxication. Such excessive water gain could result, for example, from decreased renal blood flow or from a prolonged intravenous infusion of dextrose in water. The third type of preceding event is a combination of loss of sodium and excess of water resulting from inappropriate secretion of antidiuretic hormone (SIADH). Really an imbalance in its own right, SIADH is considered separately because of its enormous importance and the high current interest in the syndrome. The fourth cause of sodium deficit has been referred to as osmotic hyponatremia—really pseudohyponatremia caused by hyperglycemia, hyperlipidemia, or the hyperproteinemia of multiple myeloma. Pseudohyponatremia,

---

*The terms *osmolality* and *osmolarity* are not quite the same. Whereas a molar solution contains 1 gm molecular weight of a substance dissolved in a solvent to make 1 L, a 1 molal solution contains 1 gm molecular weight of the substance dissolved in 1 kg of the solvent. Osmolality is the more precise term. Measurement of the osmolality of the plasma or serum and of the ECF derives its importance from the fact that osmolality measures the concentration of free particles, be they molecules or ions, in a solution. Hence an increase or decrease of sodium and chloride ions, glucose, or urea molecules will increase or decrease the osmolality of the extracellular water. Serum osmolality normally amounts to 275 to 290 mOsm/kg of serum.

Pharmacologic agents important in sodium deficit

As potential causes

Ammonium chloride
Antidepressants (e.g., amitriptyline)
Antidiuretic hormone (excessive therapy)
Barbiturates
Chlorpropamide
Carbamazepine
Clofibrate
Diuretics (e.g., furosemide, thiazides, chlorthalidone, mercurial diuretics, amiloride, ethacrynic acid, mannitol, and dextrose)
Excessive water intake
Lithium
Low-sodium diet (carried to extremes)
Narcotics (e.g., morphine)
Oxytocin
Replacing fluid losses with water only
Tolbutamide
Vasopressin
Vincristine

As modes of therapy

Diuresis plus restriction of water
Replace salt and water (3% or 5% sodium chloride in water in extreme situations)
Restrict salt and water (when *total* body sodium and water are excessive)
Simply restrict water
Varies with pathogenesis of deficit

which actually involves no deficit of the concentration of sodium in the plasma water, does not require therapy from the standpoint of sodium concentration.

Potential pharmacologic causes (excluding SIADH) are excessive water intake, diuretics (e.g., furosemide, thiazides, chlorthalidone, mercurial diuretics, ethacrynic acid, mannitol, dextrose), replacing fluid losses with water only, low-sodium diet, chlorpropamide, narcotics, barbiturates, vincristine, antidepressants, clofibrate, and vasopressin (see box, p. 1558).

Clinical observations. The clinical observations in sodium deficit vary greatly but may include the following: apprehension; abdominal cramps; diarrhea; postural hypotension; dizziness with changes of position; vasomotor collapse; rapid, thready pulse; cold, clammy skin; and in extreme circumstances convulsions.

Laboratory help. The laboratory is of enormous help in detecting sodium deficit. The plasma sodium level will be below 137 mEq/L, and it may be far below this, sometimes as low as 100 mEq/L. The specific gravity of the urine is below 1.010 (except in the case of SIADH, when it will usually be above 1.012 and possibly much higher).

Of special significance. Intake-output records, which can predict possible hyponatremia by revealing a fluid intake greatly in excess of fluid output, should be carefully maintained.

Modes of therapy. The therapy will vary widely with the pathogenesis. In nonemergency situations oral replacement of salt and water will suffice. In severe deficits 3% or 5% sodium chloride in water may be required parenterally. When a great excess of water is producing the sodium deficit (i.e., dilutional hyponatremia), diuresis plus restriction of water should be employed. Sometimes simple restriction of water suffices. When the total sodium of the body and the body water are both excessive, although a *concentration* deficit of sodium exists, both sodium and water should be restricted (see box, p. 1558).

Sodium deficit (SIADH)

Preceding events. SIADH stems from a wide variety of circumstances that appear to bear little relation to one another. These circumstances are listed in the box at right.

Potential pharmacologic causes are hypoglycemic agents, antitumor agents, diuretics, analgesics, tranquilizers, and other agents (see the boxes, p. 1560).

Clinical observations. In the early stages the clinical observations in sodium deficit from SIADH resemble those from non–SIADH sodium deficit, but as the imbalance progresses, a sudden change is seen in the patient's condition, which had previously not been particularly alarming. This change consists of alterations in personality with the patient becoming uncooperative, antagonistic, even violent. The serum sodium level gives the clue to SIADH before the onset of these ominous symptoms. Following the psychiatric changes the patient goes on to convulsions, undoubtedly related to cerebral edema; coma; and if immediate

---

Conditions favoring or causing SIADH

CNS disorders

Aneurysm
Brain abscess
Cerebral hemorrhage
Guillain-Barré syndrome
Herpes simplex encephalitis
Limbic stimulation (pain, fear, or major trauma)
Tuberculous meningitis

Endocrine disturbances

Adrenal insufficiency
Hypopituitarism
Myxedema
Porphyria

Pulmonary disorders

Aspergillosis with cavitation
Chronic lung infection
Pneumonia
Status asthmaticus
Tuberculosis

Trauma or therapeutic procedures

Head injury, including facial injury
Heart valve operation
Major surgery
Prolonged mechanical pulmonary ventilation

Tumors

Adenocarcinoma of lung
Carcinoma of duodenum
Carcinoma of pancreas
Oat cell tumor of lung
Thymoma

Unexplained SIADH

Pharmacologic agents important in sodium deficit (SIADH)

As potential causes

Analgesics
Antitumor agents
CNS agents
Diuretics
Hypoglycemic agents
Miscellaneous agents (refer to box at right
    for generic names of agents.)

As modes of therapy

Discontinuation of pharmacologic agents
    prone to causing SIADH
Infusion of 3% or 5% hypertonic solution of
    sodium chloride
Intravenous infusion of potent diuretic
Restriction of water to 500 to 700 ml/day
    (simplest therapy, often sufficient)
Use of lithium carbonate
Use of demeclocycline

Pharmacologic agents causing SIADH

Analgesics

Acetaminophen
Morphine

Antitumor agents

Cyclophosphamide
Vincristine

CNS agents

Amitriptyline
Barbiturates
Carbamazepine
Fluphenazine
Nicotine
Thioridazine
Thiothixene

Diuretics

Chlorothiazide

Hypoglycemic agents

Chlorpropamide
Metformin
Tolbutamide

Miscellaneous agents

Clofibrate (stimulates release of ADH)
Isoproterenol

---

steps are not taken, death—often caused, it would appear, by herniation of the brain through the foramen magnum.

Laboratory help. The laboratory is of considerable help in SIADH; indeed, it is essential for early diagnosis. Symptoms indicative of SIADH can appear when the serum sodium level has dropped to 120 mEq/L, but may not appear until it has dropped to 115 or even 110. Both the serum osmolality and serum chloride concentration will be below normal. The BUN is normal; tests of renal function are normal; and if plasma levels of ADH are determined by bioassay, these will be elevated. Urine concentration of sodium is usually more than 20 mEq/L unless the patient is on a low-sodium diet. Specific gravity of the urine will be elevated—1.012 or more. SIADH, alone among the sodium deficit syndromes, pours out sodium in the urine (because the conserving effect of aldosterone has been shut off by the volume increase caused by water retention). In addition, the urine in SIADH usually will have more than 20 mOsm/dl and a higher osmolality than the serum. Normal amounts of adrenocortical hormones will be found in the urine.

Of special significance. Primary in prevention of SIADH is its early detection, to be accomplished only by repeated laboratory determinations on patients with an SIADH-prone condition (e.g., severe head in-

jury, including facial injury); oat-cell carcinoma of the lung; or limbic stimulation caused by pain, fear, or major trauma (see boxes, above and above left). The most important of these determinations are the serum sodium level and the osmolality of both serum and urine. In addition, intake-output records should be carefully maintained. Correctly, SIADH has been called the "nemesis for the unwary."

Modes of therapy. The simplest treatment of SIADH consists of restricting water intake to 500 to 700 ml/day. This therapy usually will be all that is required if the SIADH is detected early. On the other hand, when the imbalance is advanced, intravenous infusion of a potent diuretic may be indicated, or an intravenous infusion of a 3% or 5% solution of sodium chloride may be required. Some investigators have employed lithium carbonate with success. Others have used de-

---

Pharmacologic agents important in sodium excess

As potential causes

Corticosteroid therapy
Excessive intake of any electrolyte by any route
Hyperalimentation
Hypertonic sodium bicarbonate (as used in treating cardiac arrest or lactic acidosis from other causes)
Inadequate water intake
Intraamniotic injection of hypertonic sodium chloride (as used to induce abortion)
Renal toxin (e.g., mercuric bichloride)
Sodium-containing medications (e.g., sodium penicillin, sodium phosphate, and sodium bicarbonate)

As modes of therapy

Diuretic with replacement of water only
Hypotonic solution of water and electrolytes (*not* just dextrose in water)
Spironolactone (aldosterone antagonist)
Water orally

---

meclocycline. Nursing measures are extremely important. Intake-output records should be meticulously maintained. Such records may predict SIADH by revealing a fluid intake greatly in excess of output. Accurate daily weights also help. The cooperation of the patient in restricting fluid intake should be solicited by carefully explaining reasons for restrictions and involving the patient in care planning. Signs should be posted on the door of the room and on the bed stating that fluid restriction is mandatory, especially when patients are confused. In addition, the water pitcher should be removed from the bedside, and visitors should be instructed not to give the patient fluids. The head of the bed should be tilted down about 10 degrees to reduce stimulation of ADH by atrial receptors (see box, p. 1560, left).

Sodium excess

Preceding events. Sodium excess can be caused by an intake of sodium in excess of water intake. A classic case in an Eastern hospital was the mistaken preparation of infant formulas using salt instead of sugar, with tragic results. Sodium excess can also be caused by loss of water in excess of sodium loss.

This might occur in watery diarrhea; with the rapid respiration of acute laryngotracheobronchitis blowing off moisture through the lungs; with a hypothalamic tumor; with concussion; or in advanced debility, in which the individual is too aged or worn out to care to drink, unable to realize that drinking is necessary, or unable to obtain water independently.

Potential pharmacologic causes are inadequate water intake, excessive oral or parenteral intake of any electrolyte, renal toxins such as mercuric bichloride, hyperalimentation, corticosteroid therapy, sodium-containing medications such as sodium penicillin, hypertonic sodium bicarbonate (such as used in treating cardiac arrest or lactic acidosis from other causes), and intraamniotic injection of hypertonic sodium chloride (see box, left).

Clinical observations. Early in the process agitation is seen, which later may progress to mania or convulsions. In one child seen by the authors, an excess of undiluted evaporated milk had been given. The mother's presenting complaint was that the baby had not slept for several days and nights. The patient will have dry, sticky mucous membranes; the tongue will look as if one could strike a match on it. Oliguria will be present. The integument gives a misleadingly healthy appearance with firm, rubbery tissue turgor— which in reality is anything but healthy.

Laboratory help. The serum sodium level will be above 147 mEq/L; indeed, it may rise to the vicinity of 200 mEq/L. The specific gravity of the urine is unduly high, perhaps above 1.030.

Of special significance. The individual who has aspirated ocean water will have a sodium excess of the ECF. The imbalance often occurs on the fifth or sixth day after the onset of untreated diarrhea. It must be kept in mind that we are talking about sodium concentration per liter of ECF, not the total sodium in the body. Thus an infant may well die of sodium excess of the ECF even though his total body sodium is less than normal.

Modes of therapy. In simple sodium excess merely giving water by mouth as desired by the patient is adequate therapy. In advanced imbalances intravenous infusion of a hypotonic solution of water and electrolytes is mandatory. Tonicity might range from 50 to 75 mEq/L. Simple dextrose in water should *not* be given, since some electrolyte appears to be required. Other modes of therapy include use of a diuretic with water alone being replaced. Spironolactone, combating as it does the conserving action of aldosterone, may prove useful (see box, above left).

Potassium deficit

Preceding events. The events preceding potassium deficit may include prolonged inadequate intake such as in starvation. However, it requires a strikingly in-

TABLE 67-1

Potassium content of common foods: 100 gm, edible portion

Food	Potassium (mg)
Apple, raw, pared	110
Asparagus, boiled, drained	183
Avocado, raw	604
Banana, raw	370
Beans, white, cooked	416
Beef, hamburger	174
Bread, cracked wheat	134
Broccoli, spears, boiled, drained	267
Buttermilk (made from skim milk)	140
Cabbage, common varieties, raw	233
Catfish, freshwater, raw	330
Celery, raw	239
Cherries, sweet, raw	191
Chicken, light meat without skin, roasted	411
Chocolate, bitter or baking	830
Coffee, instant, beverage	36
Cucumber, raw, pared	160
Goose, flesh only, roasted	605
Grapefruit, raw, pulp, all varieties	135
Halibut, broiled	525
Ice milk	195
Lamb	290
Lemon juice, canned or bottled, unsweetened	140
Liver, beef, fried	380
Milk, cow, fluid, whole or skim	144
Molasses, cane, blackstrap	2927
Mushrooms, raw	414
Mussels, raw, meat only	315
Oatmeal, cooked	61
Ocean perch, Pacific, raw	390
Okra, boiled	249
Orange juice, frozen concentrate, diluted with three parts water	186
Parsnips, boiled	379
Peanuts, roasted	701
Peanut butter	670
Plums, raw	299
Pork, fresh cooked	390
Potatoes, boiled	407
Radishes, raw	322
Raisins, cooked	355
Rhubarb, cooked	203
Rice, brown, cooked	70
Rye wafers, whole-grain	600
Salmon, silver	339
Scallops, steamed	476
Spinach, boiled	324
Sturgeon, steamed	235
Sweet potatoes, baked	300
Tomato catsup	363
Tomatoes, ripe, raw	244
Turkey, dark meat, roasted	398
Turkey, white meat, roasted	411
Turnip greens, boiled	149
Watermelon, raw	100
Yeast, baker's	610
Yogurt (made from whole milk)	132

Potassium conversion equations and daily requirement

Conversion of mg of potassium to mEq
$$mg \times 0.0256 = mEq$$
Conversion of mEq of potassium to mg
$$\frac{mEq}{0.0256} = mg$$
Conversion of mEq of potassium to mmol
$$\frac{mEq}{Valence^*} = mmol$$
Daily potassium requirement of adult (*not* on medication):
$$2929.69 \ mg = 75 \ mEq$$

*The valence of potassium = 1; thus for potassium
1 mEq = 1 mmol

---

adequate diet to produce the deficit, since most foods have generous quantities of potassium (see Table 67-1 and box, above). Excessive loss of potassium from the body such as occurs in prolonged diarrhea is a common cause of the imbalance. A still more common cause is diuresis produced by potent diuretics. In the individual who is acclimated to heat and whose sweat, therefore, contains an unduly large quantity of potassium, excessive perspiration can produce a deficit of the electrolyte. Indeed, this condition has occurred in healthy young people receiving a usually adequate diet but working in a temperature of 130° F.

Potential pharmacologic causes are non–potassium-sparing diuretics (by all odds the most important), cathartics (used chronically), oral contraceptives, corticosteroids, licorice ingestion, absorbable alkalis (e.g., sodium bicarbonate), nonreabsorbable anion loads (e.g., penicillin and carbenicillin), thyroid preparations, magnesium deficit, calcium excess, and dextrose and insulin administration (see box, p. 1563).

Clinical observations. The clinical observations in potassium deficit relate almost entirely to muscle weakness—weakness of skeletal muscle, intestinal muscle, heart muscle, and respiratory muscle. Typically the individual with moderately severe potassium deficit will complain of the inability to walk any distance or climb stairs without becoming extremely fatigued. The patient will complain of constipation, perhaps of bloating. The patient will notice extra heartbeats and may have difficulty in breathing. The cause of death in severe potassium deficit is apnea.

Laboratory help. The laboratory is of great help in

Pharmacologic agents important in potassium deficit

As potential causes

Absorbable alkalis (e.g., sodium bicarbonate)
Acetazolamide
Albuterol (overdose)
Calcium excess
Cathartics (used chronically)
Corticosteroids
Corticotropin
Dextrose and insulin administration
Diuretics (by all odds most important cause, but does *not* include potassium-sparing diuretics—e.g., spironolactone and triamterene)
Epianhydrotetracycline (outdated tetracycline)
Insulin
Licorice ingestion
Magnesium deficit
Nafcillin
Nonreabsorbable anion loads (penicillin and carbenicillin)
Oral contraceptives
Potassium-free IV fluids (prolonged administration)
Thyroid preparations

As modes of therapy

Potassium orally or parenterally over two to three days
Various salts can be used; the chloride should be given if alkalosis is present. (*Always* assess for adequate renal function and urine output before IV administration of potassium.)

---

diagnosing potassium deficit. Repeated plasma potassium determinations below 3.5 to 4 mEq/L indicate a probable potassium deficit. Plasma pH is increased, and the chloride level is often below 98 mEq/L. The imbalance is also indicated by specific electrocardiographic (ECG) findings including low voltage, flattening or inversion of the T waves, depression of the ST segment, prolonged PR interval, widened QRS complex, exaggeration of the U wave, and merger of the T and U waves (often erroneously interpreted as a prolonged QT interval).

Of special significance. Recall that after the potassium of the blood is filtered through the glomerulus into the proximal convoluted tubules, virtually all is reabsorbed into the peritubular arterioles. Then in the distal tubules it is exchanged for the sodium of the tubular urine under the influence of the hormone aldosterone. CF contains 3500 mEq of potassium, whereas only 54 mEq is found in the ECF.

For various reasons metabolic alkalosis is commonly associated with potassium deficit. Indeed, a metabolic alkalosis permitted to go uncorrected will ultimately develop into potassium deficit. Conversely, an uncorrected potassium deficit will develop into metabolic alkalosis.

Modes of therapy. Potassium should be given orally if tolerated. If not, parenteral administration is indicated. Various potassium salts can be used, but the chloride should be employed if alkalosis is present. The infusion rate for parenteral administration should not exceed 20 to 25 mEq/hr for an adult. Infants and children should be given less, in proportion to body surface area. Potassium should not be infused intravenously until renal function is established. The commonly available food sources of potassium are bananas and oranges, but it takes enormous quantities to correct a potassium deficit (see box, left and Table 67-1).

Potassium excess

Preceding events. Preceding events of potassium excess include end-stage renal disease, crushing injuries and severe tissue trauma, excessive ingestion of a potassium salt (e.g., as in a suicide attempt), and excessive parenteral administration of potassium. The latter could occur through too-rapid administration of a standard solution containing potassium, or it could result—as has happened—through an error in making up a potassium-containing solution. It could also occur if the potassium was infused before renal function was established. Leakage from the body cells into the ECF can cause potassium excess. This can occur in metabolic acidosis, in hypoxia, or in familial hyperkalemia. Since aldosterone is in a sense an antagonist of potassium, administration of an antialdosterone preparation (such as spironolactone) can result in potassium excess. Addison's disease or other pathologic conditions of the adrenal glands in which aldosterone or the similarly acting desoxycorticosterone is no longer secreted in significant amounts can also cause potassium excess.

Potential pharmacologic causes are renal toxins such as mercuric bichloride, too rapid oral or parenteral administration of potassium-containing solutions (800 mEq by mouth has been fatal), potassium-sparing diuretics, succinylcholine, arginine hydrochloride, sea salt taken in great excess by food faddists, potassium-containing salt substitutes (especially if kidneys are impaired), and error in preparing potas-

---

Pharmacologic agents important in potassium excess

As potential causes

Arginine hydrochloride
Blood transfusions (multiple)
Captopril
Error in preparing potassium-containing
    parenteral solutions (e.g., decimal point
    in wrong place)
Heparin
Indomethacin
Mannitol (hyperosmotic infusion)
Potassium-containing salt substitutes if
    kidneys are impaired
Potassium-sparing diuretics (e.g.,
    spironolactone, triamterene), especially if
    a potassium supplement is given
Renal toxins (e.g., mercuric bichloride)
Sea salt taken in excess by food faddists
Succinylcholine
Testosterone
Too rapid oral or parenteral administration
    of potassium

As modes of therapy

Calcium gluconate intravenously to
    antagonize the cardiac toxicity of
    hyperkalemia
Hemodialysis or peritoneal dialysis (in
    end-stage renal disease)
Hypertonic dextrose solution intravenously
    plus insulin
Hypertonic sodium bicarbonate solution
    intravenously
Hypertonic sodium chloride solution
    intravenously
Low-potassium, high-carbohydrate diet
Sodium polystyrene sulfonate resin (to
    remove potassium from colon)

---

sium-containing parenteral solutions (e.g., decimal point in wrong place) (see box, above).

Clinical observations. Clinical observations in potassium excess include irritability combined with anxiety and gastrointestinal hyperactivity manifested by nausea, colic, and diarrhea. Auscultation over the abdomen reveals decreased bowel sounds. Chronic fatigue and drowsiness are often observed, as are depression and hypoactive tendon reflexes. The skeletal muscles feel soft and flabby, and the pulse may be weak and irregular. Cardiac dysrhythmias also occur. Thus bradycardia may be seen when the potassium reaches 7 mEq/L, heartblock at 9 mEq/L. Increased sensitivity to digitalis can be noted. Weakness is observed, and paresthesias can occur at only 6 mEq/L. These signs are particularly noticeable in the lips. With a severe deficit paralysis can occur. Death from failure of the cardiac muscle occurs at levels of approximately 10 mEq/L.

Laboratory help. Laboratory help consists of repeated serum potassium levels recorded at above 5.6 mEq/L. The ECG is helpful; at first decreased amplitude or disappearance of the P wave, prolongation of the PR interval, high T waves (tent-shaped), and depressed ST segments are observed. Later the T waves disappear, and heart block occurs.

Of special significance. Probably the most common cause of potassium excess is renal failure. Metabolic acidosis is commonly associated with potassium excess, just as metabolic alkalosis is associated with potassium deficit. Neglected potassium excess ultimately results in metabolic acidosis; conversely, neglected metabolic acidosis results in potassium excess.

Modes of therapy. One of the most effective means of treating potassium excess is by giving insulin plus a hypertonic solution of dextrose. In nonemergency situations a low-potassium, high-carbohydrate diet can be used. A sodium polystyrene sulfonate resin can be employed to remove potassium from the colon. Various intravenous solutions are employed, including calcium gluconate, hypertonic sodium bicarbonate solution, and hypertonic sodium chloride solution. In end-stage renal disease hemodialysis or peritoneal dialysis provides temporary relief (see box, left).

Calcium deficit

Preceding events. The events leading up to calcium deficit include loss of calcium-rich intestinal secretions such as occurs in chronic diarrhea, or immobilization of calcium can occur, which effectively removes it from the ECF. This immobilization can be seen in pancreatic infections such as acute hemorrhagic pancreatitis. In this case the immobilization of calcium is probably caused by a combination of calcium with necrotic fat. Excessive infusion of sodium citrate with citrated blood can remove calcium from the ECF, since the sodium citrate reacts with the calcium salts to form calcium citrate. A deficit of parathyroid hormone (PTH) such as can occur with inadvertent surgical removal of the parathyroid glands can bring about calcium deficit. Early in renal failure the level of phosphate in the ECF commonly rises because of the inability of the failing kidneys to excrete phosphate. When this happens, the level of calcium

---

Pharmacologic agents important in calcium deficit

As potential causes

Cytotoxic agents used for treatment of lymphoma and leukemia
Depletion of magnesium
Excessive use of cathartics
Fluoride poisoning
Low calcium intake
Low-fat diet
Magnesium sulfate
Oxalate poisoning
Phosphate-containing enemas
Sodium bicarbonate (alkalosis reduces ionized calcium)
Sodium citrate (administered with transfused blood)
Treatment with anticonvulsant drugs
Vitamin D deficit

As modes of therapy

Activated vitamin D (when renal problem exists)
Calcium gluconate intravenously
Calcium lactate (the chloride, gluconate, levulinate, or carbonate salt can be used)
Magnesium (when hypocalcemia is caused by magnesium depletion)
Vitamin D

---

drops, prompting additional secretion of PTH. As a result the level of calcium in the ECF rises. However, because of mechanisms not entirely clear, calcium does not perform its usual function; rather, it leaves the ECF as metastatic calcification of the tissues. Such metastatic calcification is also a problem in hemodialysis and peritoneal dialysis.

Potential pharmacologic causes are sodium citrate (administered with transfused blood), sodium bicarbonate (inducing reduction in ionized calcium), vitamin D deficit, excessive use of cathartics, depletion of magnesium, low-fat diet, phosphate-containing enemas, cytotoxic agents used for treatment of lymphoma and leukemia, and treatment with anticonvulsant drugs (see box, above).

Clinical observations. Clinical observations of calcium deficit include numbness with tingling of the fingers and circumoral region. Reflexes are hyperactive, and muscle cramps may occur. Trousseau's sign

is positive. (This consists of carpopedal spasm of the hand when the blood supply is decreased or when the nerve is stimulated by pressure.) Chvostek's sign is positive; thus tapping the facial nerve causes a spasm of the lip and cheek. Tetany occurs, as may laryngeal stridor, a sign of great danger, since it may cause obstruction to respiration. Fractures may occur because of the porosity of the bones. In severe calcium deficit convulsions sometimes occur.

Laboratory help. How does the laboratory help us? If the total plasma calcium level is below 4.5 mEq/L or 10 mg/dl, we have a calcium deficit. However, we must bear in mind that what really matters from the physiologic standpoint is not the total serum calcium, but the ionized calcium. Normally about half of the calcium in the serum is in the ionized form, while half is bound to the plasma protein albumin. Although it is the ionized calcium that is physiologically active, determination of this portion of the calcium is so difficult as to be impractical in most laboratories. Fortunately, in most instances the total calcium gives us an accurate idea of the concentration of the ionized calcium. This is not the case, however, if an albumin deficit is present. In such instances the total calcium gives a misleadingly low estimate of the ionized calcium. A simple correction is possible.

1. Measure the serum albumin (normal = 4.5 gm/dl).
2. Measure the total serum calcium (normal = 10 mg/dl).
3. For every gram per deciliter deficit in albumin, add 0.8 mg/dl to the serum calcium value.

EXAMPLE: A patient's serum albumin is 3.5 gm/dl. This represents a deficit of 1 gm/dl. The serum calcium is 10 mg/dl. Since the albumin deficit is 1 gm/dl, add 0.8 mg/dl to the calcium figure. This gives a "corrected" serum calcium value of 10.8 mg/dl, accurately reflecting the ionized calcium concentration. In the example cited, the patient's calcium value appeared normal, but was really elevated.

Additional tests are possible in the evaluation of calcium. One of these tests is immunoassay of PTH, which in many instances is far from reliable. A simple test on the urine is the urinary Sulkowitch test. Using this test, no precipitation occurs in the case of calcium deficit. The ECG helps us inasmuch as a prolonged QT interval is seen (as a result of lengthening of the ST segment) in calcium deficit.

Of special significance. Calcium deficit results from vitamin D deficiency regardless of the calcium intake.

Modes of therapy. Among the modes of therapy in calcium deficit is administration of vitamin D or, when a renal problem exists, of activated vitamin D. When the hypocalcemia is caused by magnesium depletion, magnesium should be given by mouth or parenterally. Oral administration of calcium can be carried out by giving lactate, chloride, gluconate, levulinate, or carbonate salts of calcium. Calcium gluconate can be given intravenously in emergency situations (see box, p. 1565).

Calcium excess

Preceding events. Among the main preceding events is excessive PTH, usually resulting from a parathyroid tumor. Another major cause is malignant disease. Excessive administration of vitamin D can also cause it. A dozen less common causes can be cited, such as idiopathic hypercalcemia of infancy and von Recklinghausen's disease.

Potential pharmacologic causes are excessive administration of vitamin D, milk alkali syndrome, use of thiazide diuretics, vitamin D sensitivity, vitamin A overdosage, calcium exchange resins, chronic alcoholism, and use of phosphate-binding antacids (see box, below).

Pharmacologic agents important in calcium excess

As potential causes

Alcohol (chronic excessive use)
Calcium exchange resins
Estrogens
Milk-alkali syndrome
Tamoxifen
Testosterone
Thiazides
Vitamin A (overdosage)
Vitamin D (sensitivity, idiopathic hypercalcemia, or excessive dosage)

As modes of therapy

Corticosteroids
Dextrose in water intravenously
Inorganic phosphates by mouth (danger of extraskeletal precipitation if the IV route is used)
Normal saline solution intravenously
Plicamycin (if hypercalcemia is secondary to malignancy)
Potent diuretics, notably furosemide
Propranolol
Salmon calcitonin (not consistently effective)
Sodium sulfate intravenously

Clinical observations. The clinical observations in excessive concentration of calcium in the ECF include hypotonic skeletal muscles; general symptoms such as anorexia, nausea, and vomiting; lethargy; polydipsia; and polyuria. Patients may complain of deep bony pain caused by osteoporosis or of pain in the lateral lumbar regions caused by the formation of kidney stones. More ominously symptoms of kidney failure caused by damage done by the kidney stones may be seen. As calcium excess becomes more severe, stupor, coma, and finally cardiac arrest may occur. In hypercalcemic crisis intractable nausea and vomiting, ECF volume deficit, stupor, and azotemia are observed.

Laboratory help. The laboratory is of considerable help. A plasma calcium level above 10.4 to 10.8 mg/dl indicates calcium excess. The correction referred to on p. 1565 should be made if the patient's serum albumin is below 4.5 gm/dl. Early in calcium excess a clue to the diagnosis is provided by rarefaction under the periostea of long bones as seen by radiographic examination. Later radiographic examination reveals generalized osteoporosis, widespread bone cavitation, or radiopaque urinary stones. Should kidney damage have occurred, the BUN will be elevated. Elevated PTH as determined by immunoassay is not always present in calcium excess, but certainly corroborates the diagnosis when it is present. Characteristic ECG changes include prolonged PR interval, absence of ST segment, and shortening of the QT interval (similar to the effect of digitalis). In hypercalcemia more than one determination of the serum calcium is advisable. Spurious elevations of calcium are sometimes seen following prolonged venous stasis or if the sample is exposed to a cork stopper. Once a diagnosis of hypercalcemia is confirmed, additional determinations are useful, such as the serum phosphorus, chloride, bicarbonate, and alkaline phosphatase levels and urinary calcium level. If the serum phosphorus level is depressed with hypercalcemia, then hyperparathyroidism, myeloma, or sarcoidosis is probably present. The serum chloride level is often elevated in primary hyperparathyroidism, but may be normal or depressed in patients with hypercalcemia plus adrenal crisis. Depression of the bicarbonate level will elevate the ionized fraction of the serum calcium; elevated bicarbonate level will depress it. The serum alkaline phosphatase level may be normal in hypercalcemia; if the enzyme is elevated, bone disease of hyperparathyroidism or malignancy of any type may be indicated. Determination of the urinary calcium level on a 24-hour urine collection with the patient on a normal phosphate intake will commonly reveal hypercalciuria in either primary or secondary hyperparathyroidism.

Of special significance. When kidney damage becomes manifest in calcium excess, it is probable that renal calculi have seriously damaged the kidneys; this is why early diagnosis is so important.

Modes of therapy. A wide variety of therapies are employed in calcium excess. Naturally, removal of a parathyroid tumor is primary. Parenteral administration of normal saline solution or of sodium sulfate is employed. A potent diuretic—most notably furosemide—may be given. Salmon calcitonin, although not consistently effective, is sometimes administered. Other measures include inorganic phosphates by mouth, plicamycin, dextrose in water infusion, corticosteroids, and propranolol (see box, p. 1566).

Magnesium deficit

Preceding events. The events preceding magnesium deficit usually represent a combination of liver malfunction and loss of intestinal contents. Chronic alcoholics appear especially prone to develop magnesium deficit because the alcoholic patient excretes excessive quantities of magnesium. This deficit may occur even though the magnesium content of the diet would have been adequate normally. Magnesium deficit can also occur in protein-calorie malnutrition (known in Africa as kwashiorkor and in Central and South America as pluricarencial syndrome). Until magnesium is added to the restorative program the child with this disease will likely not improve.

Potential pharmacologic causes are parenteral alimentation with magnesium-free fluid, alcohol in excess (especially as in chronic alcoholism), laxative abuse, use of diuretics, high intake of calcium salts when diet is low in magnesium, and the use of vitamin D in large doses (see box, top right).

Clinical observations. The clinical observations of magnesium deficit may take several weeks to develop, then neuromuscular irritability with tremor and hyperactive deep reflexes are seen. A positive Chvostek sign is observed. Disorientation, confusion, and visual or auditory hallucinations occur. Carphologia, or picking at the bedclothes, may be observed. Abnormal sensitivity to sounds, leg and foot cramps, and tachycardia are seen. Later hypertension and finally convulsions occur. Dramatic improvement may be seen with oral or parenteral administration of magnesium sulfate.

Laboratory help. The laboratory is helpful in that magnesium deficit is indicated by a plasma magnesium level below 1.4 mEq/L.

Of special significance. The preceding events of magnesium deficit are in many respects identical to those of potassium deficit. If improvement fails to occur with correction of a potassium deficit, then magnesium deficit should be suspected. Chronic alcoholics may develop magnesium deficit on a well-balanced diet. The symptoms of delirium tremens are strikingly similar to those of magnesium deficit. This is an easy imbalance to miss. One should thus keep it in mind and think of it if preceding events suggest its possibility.

Modes of therapy. Repair of magnesium deficit can be carried out by giving magnesium salts orally, intramuscularly, or intravenously. Hydrated magnesium sulfate is used most commonly (see box, below).

Pharmacologic agents important in magnesium deficit

As potential causes

   Alcohol (chronic overuse)
   Diuretics
   High intake of calcium salts when diet is low in magnesium
   Laxative abuse
   Parenteral alimentation with magnesium-free fluid
   Sodium sulfate
   Vitamin D in large doses

As modes of therapy

   Magnesium salts by oral or parenteral route, depending on urgency

---

Pharmacologic agents important in magnesium excess

As potential causes

   Hard water use in hemodialysis
   Magnesium infusion (excess)
   Magnesium-containing antacids (in renal impairment)
   Magnesium-containing laxatives (in renal impairment)

As modes of therapy

   Administer calcium gluconate parenterally (10% solution as a magnesium antagonist)
   Correct water deficit if present
   Discontinue medications containing magnesium

Magnesium excess

Preceding events. The most important preceding event of magnesium excess, a relatively unusual imbalance, is chronic renal disease, usually involving uremia. It is compounded by the administration of antacids containing magnesium salts to patients with renal impairment. Other events that tend to produce magnesium excess include untreated diabetic acidosis, parenteral administration of magnesium, Addison's disease with its lack of aldosterone and related corticosteroids, and hyperparathyroidism.

Potential pharmacologic causes are antacids or laxatives containing magnesium (see box, p. 1567, bottom).

Clinical observations. The clinical observations in magnesium excess include flushing and sweating, hypotension, and drowsiness. The deep tendon reflexes are weak to absent. Lethargy is seen. Ventricular premature contractions may occur, and bradycardia is observed. Respiration is impaired. If the imbalance progresses, coma supervenes.

Laboratory help. The laboratory is of assistance, with the normal plasma magnesium being 1.4 mEq/L. Magnesium excess involves considerably higher levels of magnesium—5 to 7 mEq/L. The ECG shows a prolonged PR interval, broadened QRS complex, elevated T waves, AV block, and evidence of premature ventricular contractions.

Of special significance. Hypermagnesemia is rarely seen except in patients who have impaired renal function or who are on hemodialysis or peritoneal dialysis.

Modes of therapy. In therapy of magnesium excess one first discontinues medications containing magnesium. Any water deficit present should be corrected. Calcium gluconate can be given intravenously as a magnesium antagonist in emergency situations (see box, p. 1567, bottom).

Protein deficit

Preceding events. The preceding events for protein deficit include a protein-poor diet, chronic disease of any kind, repeated surgical operations, severe trauma, and serious burns. Not only is the ingestion of protein reduced in trauma and burns, but also the excretion of protein is greatly increased because of the so-called toxic destruction of protein.

Potential pharmacologic causes are corticosteroids, thyroid preparations, and amphetamines (see box, above right).

Clinical observations. Clinical observations include striking mental and emotional depression; anorexia, which can be both a cause and a result of protein deficit; loss of muscle mass and tone contributing to the poor posture often seen in protein-deficient patients; weight loss; and a plasma-to–interstitial fluid

---

> ### Pharmacologic agents important in protein deficit
>
> **As potential causes**
>
> Amphetamines
> Corticosteroids
> Thyroid preparations
>
> **As modes of therapy**
>
> High-caloric, high-protein diet
> Amino acid mixtures
> High-protein tube feedings
> Anabolic hormones
> Parenteral hyperalimentation

---

shift of water and electrolytes caused by depressed serum albumin, permitting water and electrolytes to leave the microcirculation in abnormally great quantities. Reduced resistance to infection is another hallmark of protein deficit.

Laboratory help. The laboratory helps us chiefly with the serum albumin level determination. If this is below 4.5 gm/dl, a protein deficit can be assumed to be present. If the figure is 3 gm/dl or less, the deficit is severe indeed. Bear in mind that the chief osmotic protein of the circulating blood is albumin; hence it is albumin, not the total protein or serum proteins other than albumin, in which we are primarily interested.

Of special significance. It is extremely easy to fail to think of protein deficit, since it develops so slowly. Some individuals on fad diets can develop the imbalance. A pure vegetarian diet without milk products or eggs may produce protein deficit over a period of time, particularly if the vegetable proteins consumed are not chosen so that their amino acid contents are complementary. Decreased serum albumin is also observed as a natural consequence of aging.

Modes of therapy. Usually gradual in its development, protein deficit cannot be quickly repaired. The obvious—and certainly the most pleasant—method is the administration of a high-caloric, high-protein diet. Some patients, of course, are not able to take food by mouth. For these patients high-protein tube feedings offer an alternative. Anabolic hormones are sometimes employed in the repair of protein deficits but are generally not recommended.

A dramatic development in the restoration of body proteins is parenteral hyperalimentation. Patients whose gastrointestinal tracts for one reason or another are nonfunctional can have their protein nutrition restored and then maintained by hyperalimentation. Hyperalimentation causes tissue synthesis and growth by infusing intravenously large quantities of basic nutrients. Various mixtures of protein hydrolysates, amino acids, and hypertonic dextrose solutions are given. The large quantities of calories infused spare protein for tissue synthesis. The infusion is usually given via an indwelling catheter located in a large vein such as the superior vena cava. However, peripheral sites have also been used. The requirements for proper hyperalimentation are demanding; both the administration and preparation of the solutions require appropriate facilities (e.g., a laminar airflow hood) and personnel with appropriate qualifications and experience. As with so many lifesaving measures, hazards are many, particularly infections, but the results achieved are truly remarkable and unquestionably worth the travail (see box, p. 1568).

Since provision of parenteral hyperalimentation as administered in the hospital is expensive, interest has developed in providing it in the home. In one hospital the cost of maintaining the program for a full year for one patient was $73,720 (United States). However, when it was carried out at home the cost was reduced to 27% of this figure, or $19,700. The recent establishment of private companies that provide equipment, supplies, delivery, insurance, and services of pharmacists and nurses should have a major impact in further reducing the cost of home parenteral nutrition.

Acid-base disturbances

We will now discuss the four acid-base disturbances, each of which represents a special type of concentration imbalance. Before describing these individually, we will discuss some general principles concerning the maintenance of acid-base balance by the body.

Maintenance of acid-base balance. Among the most important laboratory values of use in evaluating the acid-base status of the body are the so-called blood gases. The first of the blood gases is oxygen, expressed as Po_2, or oxygen tension, measured in mm Hg. Its value in alveolar air and in arterial blood is normally—and ideally—about 100 mm Hg. In reality, we don't use the Po_2 in most acid-base disturbances, although sometimes it is essential. We also have the tension of carbon dioxide, the Pco_2, again measured in mm Hg. Its normal value in the alveolar air and in the arterial blood is 40 mm Hg. It is of enormous use in acid-base disturbances. Sometimes referred to as one of the blood gases is pH, the measurement of the hydrogen ion (H^+) concentration of the blood. Its normal value is 7.4 in either arterial or venous blood. Finally, also

referred to as a blood gas, although it isn't a gas at all, is bicarbonate (HCO_3^-), the anion of base bicarbonate, with the cation being either sodium, potassium, calcium, or magnesium. Its value is measured in milliequivalents per liter, and it normally is about 24 mEq/L in either arterial or venous blood. As already implied, we measure the Po_2 and the Pco_2 in arterial (or arterialized) blood, the pH and bicarbonate in venous blood. Of course, nothing is wrong with measuring pH and bicarbonate in arterial blood.

Now let us consider acid-base disturbances, using a sort of programmed learning approach to understanding them. First, acid-base disturbances make up four of the basic body fluid disturbances. They originate in deficit or excess of carbonic acid (H_2CO_3) or bicarbonate. Whatever the circumstantial or clinical cause of an acid-base disturbance, it does not occur unless it produces a deficit or excess of carbonic acid or of bicarbonate or of various combinations of these.

Remember that carbonic acid is in equilibrium in the ECF with the Pco_2 and water. If the Pco_2 is decreased, the carbonic acid is decreased; if it is increased, the carbonic acid is increased. This means that if we blow off carbon dioxide through the lungs, the body must convert carbonic acid to carbon dioxide and water. This mechanism has the effect of decreasing the hydrogen ion concentration of the ECF, since carbonic acid (H_2CO_3) is to a limited extent ionized into hydrogen (H^+) and bicarbonate (HCO_3^-) ions. Acid-base balance depends on the hydrogen ion concentration of the ECF. How do we measure hydrogen ions? A logical way would be the same way that we measure most other electrolytes—in units per liter, specifically in nanomoles (nmol) of hydrogen ions per liter (a nanomole, incidentally, is a billionth of a mole or a millionth of a millimole). However, except in certain academic hospitals, because of tradition and usage, we still measure hydrogen ions by the use of pH, the normal pH being 7.35 to 7.45.

The definition of pH is the reciprocal of the logarithm of the hydrogen ion concentration. It is not necessary to remember or to understand that mathematical definition; but it is necessary to remember that as the pH value goes up, the hydrogen ion concentration goes down; as the pH value goes down, the hydrogen ion concentration goes up. It is also interesting to note that changes in pH go in jumps of 10; thus, pH 8 is only one-tenth as acidic as pH 7. Conversely, pH 7 is ten times as acidic as pH 8. We wouldn't have to remember either of these peculiar facts if we used nanomoles per liter, since nanomoles is a simple arithmetic way of measuring. Thus in nanomoles per liter pH 7—extreme acidosis—has a value of 100 nmol/L; pH 7.4—approximate normality—has a nanomole figure of about 40 nmol/L; pH 8—extreme alkalosis—has a nanomole value of 10 nmol/L.

The hydrogen ion concentration of the ECF, on which acid-base balance depends, in turn depends on the ratio of carbonic acid to bicarbonate. Recall that in the body fluids the bicarbonate molecule is paired off electrically with sodium, potassium, magnesium, or calcium and referred to as base bicarbonate, since it is base, or alkaline.

Now, how do we measure carbonic acid or carbon dioxide? As already stated, we measure carbonic acid by determining the P_{CO_2}, or carbon dioxide pressure, in mm Hg, with the normal being 40 mm Hg. The normal P_{CO_2} of 40 mm Hg equals the P_{CO_2} of the alveolar air. Hence it must be measured either on arterial blood or on venous blood that has been made to approach arterial blood in composition. Arterialized blood is obtained by collecting the blood specimen from an extremity (e.g., an arm) that has been warmed for several minutes to a temperature of 45°C just before the blood is drawn. This is accomplished by submerging the forearm, hand, and fingers in a water bath with a temperature of 45°C. Alternatively, a towel soaked in water at 45°C can be wrapped around the forearm. The resulting heating of the capillaries speeds up the rate of blood flow and thus decreases the changes in blood composition caused by tissue respiration. The reason for using "arterialized" venous blood is that in some institutions facilities are not available to perform the arterial punctures necessary to obtain arterial blood.

How do we measure bicarbonate? We measure bicarbonate by treating serum with strong acid. The result is correctly referred to as the bicarbonate level. It is sometimes called the carbon dioxide or the carbon dioxide combining power, which is inaccurate and misleading and refers to the chemical method by which the determination is done rather than to what the value represents. The normal value for bicarbonate is approximately 24 mEq/L. Tests for bicarbonate are performed on arterial or venous blood. In many institutions, rather than chemical determination of bicarbonate, the P_{CO_2} is determined by a blood gas meter and the pH by a pH meter; from these two values and a simple formula the bicarbonate level can be derived.

Now let us examine how the body controls hydrogen ion concentration.

The body controls hydrogen ion concentration by three interrelated mechanisms: (1) body fluid buffers, (2) the lungs, and (3) the kidneys. First, consider the buffers. Buffers tend to prevent changes in hydrogen ion concentration when an acid or alkali is added to the body or generated within the body. Buffers occur in pairs. Each pair consists of a weak acid plus the salt of that acid. Actually, we have four major buffer pairs: the bicarbonate pair, primarily active in the ECF; the hemoglobin pair, active in the blood; the plasma protein pair, active in the plasma; and the phosphate pair, active in the cells. We need only be concerned with the buffer pair of clinical importance, the bicarbonate pair, which consists of carbonic acid and base bicarbonate.

Next, how do the lungs control hydrogen ion concentration? When the hydrogen ion concentration of the ECF becomes excessively high, the lungs reduce it by automatically blowing off carbon dioxide. This causes the carbonic acid of the ECF to break down into water, which is virtually neutral, and carbon dioxide, which is blown off. The net result is a decrease in the hydrogen ion concentration of the ECF. When, on the other hand, the hydrogen ion concentration is inadequate, the lungs retain carbon dioxide. This carbon dioxide combines with water in the ECF to form carbonic acid, and the net gain is increased hydrogen ion concentration. The lungs respond rapidly. If one hyperventilates for a minute or two, the pH of the ECF will move deep into the area of alkalosis. If, on the other hand, one holds the breath for a minute, the pH of the ECF will move deeply into the area of acidosis (see box, below).

How do the kidneys maintain acid-base balance? When the hydrogen ion concentration of the ECF be-

---

Carbon dioxide alterations: compensatory or primary?

P_{CO_2} elevated

If elevation of P_{CO_2} is compensatory, it will not rise higher than 62 mm Hg. If it is higher than this level a complicating respiratory acidosis is present.

P_{CO_2} depressed

If depressed P_{CO_2} is compensatory, it will be lowered about 1 mm Hg for each milliequivalent depletion of bicarbonate.
If P_{CO_2} is higher than predicted, complicating respiratory acidosis is present.
If P_{CO_2} is lower than predicted, complicating respiratory alkalosis is present.

comes excessively high, the kidneys, through a complex and ingenious series of reactions, throw out hydrogen ions and reabsorb—and even regenerate—bicarbonate. When, on the other hand, the bicarbonate content of the ECF becomes excessive, it flows out in the urine because of the renal threshold for bicarbonate. Naturally, in this situation the various mechanisms active for acidosis are canceled.

It is important to remember that the kidneys adjust the level of bicarbonate in the ECF. The lungs, on the other hand, involuntarily adjust the level of carbon dioxide and hence of carbonic acid. A host of clinical conditions and pharmacologic agents affect the kidneys, the lungs, or both to produce acid-base disturbances.

Let us review briefly: acid-base balance can be upset in four ways. First, a decrease in the bicarbonate of the ECF can occur through loss of bicarbonate in intestinal secretions or by neutralization or titration of bicarbonate in the body fluids—as by ketone bodies of diabetic acidosis, for example. In such an imbalance an excess of hydrogen ions is seen. Acidosis—specifically, *metabolic acidosis*—is present. The second imbalance involves an increase in bicarbonate. This can occur either because bicarbonate is added to the body (e.g., from taking excessive quantities of sodium bicarbonate [baking soda] or because the individual has lost chloride through vomiting, which forces the bicarbonate of the body fluids to increase in compensation so that the anions equal the cations). In this imbalance we have a deficit of hydrogen ions. We call it *metabolic alkalosis.*

In the third imbalance we have a decrease in carbonic acid. This is invariably caused by overbreathing, or hyperventilation, which blows off excessive quantities of carbon dioxide. The result is a deficit of hydrogen ions in the body fluids. Since the origin of this imbalance is respiratory, we call it *respiratory alkalosis.* The fourth acid-base disturbance involves an increase in carbonic acid resulting from inadequate ventilation on the part of the lungs, which simply are not disposing of carbon dioxide normally. This may be caused by intrinsic lung disease, or it may be the result of various pharmacologic agents (e.g., morphine). An excess of hydrogen ions is found in the body fluids. Since it is caused by pulmonary action, we refer to this imbalance as *respiratory acidosis* (Table 67-2).

Before we consider these four acid-base disturbances in clinical terms, let us examine a useful calculation that will help us determine whether a given case of metabolic acidosis is caused by a simple inorganic acid or by a complex organic acid. This little calculation really tells us how many abnormal organic anions are present in the ECF. It is therefore sometimes referred to as the *anion gap.* We prefer the briefer term *delta.* To obtain delta, subtract the sum of the chloride and bicarbonate values in milliequivalents from the sodium value in milliequivalents. If acidosis is present and the delta is greater than 13, organic acids are responsible for the imbalance. If, on the other hand, delta is 13 or less, any acidosis present has resulted from inorganic acids. If delta is less than 11, check for laboratory errors, since such a low delta is impossible. Now, with the concept of delta fixed in our minds, let us examine the acid-base disturbances.

Primary base bicarbonate deficit (metabolic acidosis)

Preceding events. The events preceding metabolic acidosis include the flooding of ECF with acids, which may be either endogenous or exogenous in origin. In certain clinical situations in which the acidosis is caused by organic acids, you will find a high delta—above 13. Sometimes this type of acidosis is referred to as increased anion gap acidosis. The clinical conditions in which it is seen include diabetic ketoacidosis, uremic acidosis, lactic acidosis (such as occurs in coronary thrombosis), starvation ketoacidosis, alcoholic ketoacidosis, and lactic acid acidosis caused by extreme exertion. Certain poisons (e.g., methanol, salicylates) also can produce it.

Next, let us examine the clinical situations in which the acidosis is caused by an inorganic acid. The delta is 13 or less, and this type of acidosis is sometimes referred to as a normal anion gap acidosis. The preceding events include diarrhea, renal tubular acidosis, and infusion of an excessive quantity of normal saline solution that simply dilutes the bicarbonate in the ECF and thus produces bicarbonate deficit (dilutional acidosis). Hyperalimentation can produce this type of acidosis, and so can an acid-producing tumor, such as multiple myeloma.

Potential pharmacologic causes are ethylene glycol, dithiazanine, streptozocin, isoniazid, cyanide, nitroprusside, fructose, sorbitol, epinephrine, alcohol, methanol, phenformin, chloride anion in hyperalimentation solutions, dinitrophenol, salicylates, amphotericin B, lithium carbonate, ammonium chloride, acetazolamide, and arginine hydrochloride (see box, p. 1572).

Clinical observations. Clinical observations in metabolic acidosis include hyperventilation, or deep, rapid breathing. This is compensatory and represents the automatic activity of the lungs in excreting carbon dioxide from the body and thus reducing the hydrogen ion concentration of the ECF. Such compensatory hyperventilation is not observed in a young infant.

Pharmacologic agents important in primary base bicarbonate deficit (metabolic acidosis)

As potential causes

Acetazolamide
Alcohol
Ammonium chloride
Amphotericin B
Chloride anion in hyperalimentation
    solutions
Cyanide
Diathiazanine
Dinitrophenol
Epianhydrotetracycline (outdated
    tetracycline)
Epinephrine
Ethylene glycol
Fructose
General anesthetics
Isoniazid
Lithium carbonate
Methanol (poisoning)
Nitroprusside
Paraldehyde (intoxication)
Salicylates (poisoning)
Sorbitol
Streptozocin

As modes of therapy

Hemodialysis or peritoneal dialysis (if
    extreme severity)
Replace ECF volume deficit if present
Replenish bicarbonate with sodium
    bicarbonate
Replenish serum potassium as acidosis is
    corrected
If diabetic ketoacidosis present, give insulin
    plus fluid and electrolyte replacement
If serum phosphate elevated, give oral
    aluminum hydroxide preparations
Remove excess serum potassium in acute
    stage

Here a significant question arises: in primary base bicarbonate deficit, how can you tell whether P_{CO_2} depression is truly compensatory or whether it has been brought about by a secondary respiratory alkalosis grafted on the metabolic acidosis? If the depression of the P_{CO_2} is compensatory, then the P_{CO_2} will be lowered about 1 mm Hg for each 1 mEq/L depression of the bicarbonate. If the P_{CO_2} is higher than that

predicted by the formula, then respiratory acidosis is present. If the P_{CO_2} is lower than the formula predicts, respiratory alkalosis is present. Other clinical observations in metabolic acidosis include weakness, dizziness, disorientation, and—if the acidosis becomes sufficiently severe—coma. Ultimately, death may occur.

Laboratory help. What help does the laboratory give us? The urine pH is often below 6, but this is not necessarily true in metabolic acidosis. The plasma pH is invariably below 7.35, and the plasma bicarbonate is below 24 mEq/L (since the imbalance was caused primarily by bicarbonate deficit). The P_{CO_2} is below 40 mm Hg for the reasons stated above.

Of special significance. The body attempts physiologic correction of the acidosis, with the kidneys excreting acid and regenerating bicarbonate and the lungs blowing off carbon dioxide. Metabolic acidosis is often associated with potassium excess.

Modes of therapy. Any ECF volume deficit should be repaired, preferably by a hypotonic balanced solution. If acidosis is severe, it may be advisable to administer sodium bicarbonate, correcting the imbalance gradually and periodically checking the pH and the bicarbonate level. In acute bicarbonate deficit excessive potassium should be removed. As acidosis recedes, potassium should be replenished. In diabetic ketoacidosis insulin plus fluid and electrolytes should be given. If the serum phosphate level is elevated, aluminum hydroxide should be administered orally. In extremely severe bicarbonate deficit hemodialysis or peritoneal dialysis may be required (see box, left).

Primary base bicarbonate excess (metabolic alkalosis)

Preceding events. Preceding events include loss of chloride such as with vomiting. When the chloride is lost, a compensatory rise in the bicarbonate occurs so that electrical equality between cations and anions will be maintained. We also see metabolic alkalosis because of excessive intake of absorbable alkalis such as sodium bicarbonate (i.e., baking soda).

Potential pharmacologic causes are excessive diuresis causing potassium deficit, laxative abuse, use of emetics, use of ACTH or corticosteroids, prolonged intravenous alimentation with potassium-free solutions, alkali therapy of peptic ulcer, and gastric suction causing excessive loss of hydrochloric acid and potassium (see box, p. 1573).

Clinical observations. Clinical observations in metabolic alkalosis include numbness and tingling of the extremities. Hypertonicity of muscles is present. Respirations are slow and shallow, sometimes with periods of apnea. The purpose of this hypoventilation is to retain carbon dioxide in the body and thus increase

---

> ## Pharmacologic agents important in primary base bicarbonate excess (metabolic alkalosis)
>
> ### As potential causes
>
> ACTH or corticosteroids
> Alkali therapy of peptic ulcer
> Diuretics (causing potassium deficit)
> Emetics
> Excessive intake of absorbable alkalis (e.g., sodium bicarbonate)
> Gastric suction, causing excessive loss of hydrochloric acid and potassium
> Laxative abuse
> Prolonged intravenous alimentation with potassium-free solutions
>
> ### As modes of therapy
>
> Administer calcium salt if deficit of ionized calcium exists
> Administer potassium chloride or ammonium chloride (any route)
> Carbonic anhydrase inhibitor when patient refractory to diuretics
> Dilute hydrochloric acid intravenously (*rarely* used and *not* generally recommended)
> Repair ECF volume deficits

the concentration of hydrogen ions. The P_{CO_2} will thereby be elevated. But how can we tell whether an elevated P_{CO_2} in metabolic alkalosis is compensatory or whether a secondary respiratory acidosis is present? P_{CO_2} over 55 mm Hg is usually too high for simple compensatory action. P_{CO_2} over 62 mm Hg is surely too high for compensatory action; thus respiratory acidosis must be present in addition to the metabolic alkalosis. Additional symptoms seen in metabolic alkalosis include bradycardia and tetany. If the alkalosis is allowed to progress unchecked, death may occur.

Laboratory help. How does the laboratory help us? The urine pH may be above 7, although many circumstances exist in which it is not. The plasma pH, however, is invariably above 7.45. The plasma bicarbonate is above 24 mEq/L, since it was an excess of bicarbonate that caused the imbalance in the first place. The P_{CO_2} is above 40 mm Hg, but not, as pointed out above, over 62 mm Hg in uncomplicated metabolic alkalosis.

Of special significance. The body attempts physiologic correction of the alkalosis, with the kidneys excreting the excess bicarbonate and the lungs retaining carbon dioxide to elevate the hydrogen ion concentration of the ECF. As stated above, metabolic alkalosis is often associated with potassium deficit, and vice versa.

Modes of therapy. The chloride of potassium or of ammonium administered by mouth may correct the imbalance. Any ECF volume deficit should be corrected. If a deficit of ionized calcium exists, calcium should be given. Carbonic anhydrase inhibitor is useful in patients refractory to diuretics. Less commonly used are intravenous ammonium chloride or dilute hydrochloric acid (see box, left).

Primary carbonic acid deficit (respiratory alkalosis)

Preceding events. The preceding events include hyperventilation from any cause. A host of situations both organic and functional can produce hyperventilation (e.g., voluntary hyperventilation, oxygen lack, fever, psychosomatic problems).

Potential pharmacologic causes are salicylates, P_{O_2} deficit, P_{CO_2} excess, and general anesthetics (see box, p. 1574).

Clinical observations. The clinical observations include deep, rapid breathing, or hyperventilation. As alkalosis develops with the continued blowing off of excessive carbon dioxide, the ionization of calcium is decreased, and the patient may suffer a relative calcium imbalance with tetany, paresthesias, and tingling and numbness of the extremities and of the circumoral region. The patient is unable to concentrate. Tinnitus may be bothersome. The patient's vision blurs. The patient sweats, has a dry mouth, and may go into coma. Extremely vigorous hyperventilation can produce a period of apnea, which may be disturbingly long. In fact, cases have been recorded in which voluntary hyperventilation was followed by permanent apnea.

Laboratory help. The laboratory helps us: the urine pH is usually above 7, and the plasma pH is higher than 7.45. The plasma bicarbonate is below 24 mEq/L because of the action of the kidneys in ridding the body of bicarbonate to counteract the deficit of hydrogen ions. The P_{CO_2} is below 40 mm Hg. Indeed, it may get into the 20 to 25 mm Hg range.

Of special significance. Since compensatory action on the part of the body must depend on the kidneys alone, it is slow, requiring hours or even days. Voluntary hyperventilation carried out so that a swimmer can swim a long distance underwater is unquestionably deadly. The mechanism is this: hyperventilation carried out for ½ minute, 1 minute, or even 2 or more minutes reduces the level of carbon dioxide in the ECF. The P_{CO_2} is the chief stimulus to respiration; with this gone the individual can swim comfortably without an overly strong urge to breathe. Anoxia will begin to

---

Pharmacologic agents important in primary carbonic acid deficit (respiratory alkalosis)

As potential causes

General anesthetics (second stage)
P_{CO_2} excess
P_{O_2} deficit
Quinine toxicity
Respiratory stimulants (e.g., caffeine and sodium benzoate, nikethamide, and doxapram)
Salicylate intoxication (early—usually followed by metabolic acidosis)
Sulfanilamide toxicity (early)

As modes of therapy

Inhalation of 5% carbon dioxide plus 95% oxygen sometimes used; dangerous because carbon dioxide may increase hyperventilation
Replace bicarbonate lost because of renal compensatory action
Sedation

Pharmacologic agents important in primary carbonic acid excess (respiratory acidosis)

As potential causes

Alcohol
General anesthetics
Great loss of potassium (causing paresis of respiration)
Opiates
Prolonged inhalation of carbon dioxide (carbon dioxide narcosis)
Sedatives that depress respiration (e.g., barbiturates)

As modes of therapy

Naloxone (intravenously, for narcotic overdose)
Should hyperkalemia and ventricular fibrillation occur, consider intravenous sodium bicarbonate
NOTE: Some authors have recommended the use of salicylates to increase the sensitivity of the respiratory center to carbon dioxide; however, we believe that the use of salicylates in therapy of respiratory acidosis is *contraindicated* because the dose of salicylate sufficient to stimulate respiration might well produce metabolic acidosis, thereby complicating the clinical problem by adding another form of acidosis.

---

occur, but the urge to breathe produced by hypoxia is not nearly as strong as that produced by a high content of carbon dioxide. So the individual swims merrily along, but is using up the oxygen of the brain. Moreover, the alkalosis produced by hyperventilation causes some vasoconstriction. If cerebral anoxia supervenes, the individual becomes unconscious. In case after case it has been reported that the swimmer continued to swim while unconscious. As the carbon dioxide in the ECF gradually builds up, the individual receives an urge in the respiratory center to breathe, and does—unconsciously—inhaling water. Unless the person in this circumstance is rescued promptly, death will occur because the lungs are full of water and the brain is hypoxic or anoxic. (The Heimlich maneuver appears to be an ideal method for expelling water from the lungs of a patient in this circumstance.)

Modes of therapy. Indicated psychotherapy should be administered. Sedation (e.g., with phenobarbital) may prove useful. If excessive amounts of bicarbonate have been lost because of renal compensation, bicarbonate replacement is indicated. Inhalation of 5% carbon dioxide plus 95% oxygen has been used, but is dangerous, since the carbon dioxide may increase the hyperventilation (see box, above).

Primary carbonic acid excess (respiratory acidosis)

Preceding events. The preceding events include respiratory obstruction, usually caused by disease of the lungs such as infection, asthma, or emphysema.

Potential pharmacologic causes are opiates, general anesthetics, alcohol, sedatives that depress respiration (e.g., barbiturates), prolonged inhalation of carbon dioxide and extreme loss of potassium (see box, above).

Clinical observations. The clinical observations include impaired respiration, disorientation, weakness, headache, and, if the imbalance is severe, coma.

Laboratory help. The laboratory helps us by identifying urine pH below 6 and plasma pH below 7.35. The plasma bicarbonate, after a period of time, will rise above 24 mEq/L because of the action of the kidneys in saving bicarbonate to combat the excessive

TABLE 67-2

Effects of various acid-base disturbances on pH, bicarbonate, and carbonic acid

	Metabolic acidosis	Metabolic alkalosis	Respiratory acidosis	Respiratory alkalosis
pH	Decreased	Increased	Decreased	Increased
Bicarbonate	Decreased	Increased	Increased	Decreased
Carbonic acid	Decreased	Increased	Increased	Decreased

hydrogen ion concentration of the ECF caused by the retention of carbon dioxide. The P_{CO_2} is above 40 mm Hg and may exceed 65. Bear in mind that the total pressure in the alveoli does not exceed 140 mm Hg unless oxygen is being administered. Hence if the P_{CO_2} rises to 70, the P_{O_2} cannot be higher than 70. If the P_{CO_2} goes to 80, the P_{O_2} would be 60.

Of special significance. Body compensation must depend on the kidneys alone and therefore is extremely slow, often taking days to occur.

Modes of therapy. It may be necessary to assist respiration by a respirator, intubation, or emergency bronchoscopy. Therapy should include maintenance of a patent airway and aspiration of excessive secretions. Give oxygen as needed, and administer artificial respiration when required. If hyperkalemia and ventricular fibrillation occur, sodium bicarbonate, IV, is sometimes used. Naloxone may be administered when respiratory depression is caused by narcotics (see box p. 1574, right, and box p. 1576, left).

Imbalances caused by shifts of ECF

The final two major imbalances are caused by shifts of water and electrolytes from plasma to interstitial fluid or from interstitial fluid to plasma. Recall that both plasma and interstitial fluid are ECF. Recall also that the interstitial fluid is between three and four times as voluminous as the plasma.

As we examine these final imbalances, let us review a highly pertinent subject—namely, the delivery of water, electrolytes, and other nutrients to the cells and transport of urea, carbon dioxide, and other wastes away from the cells. The delivery of water, electrolytes, dextrose, amino acids, vitamins, and other substances occurs in the arterial capillary bed. Filtration pressure generated by the heart, which tends to push nutrients out of the arterial capillary, provides a force of 32 mm Hg; it is opposed by a force of 22 mm Hg provided by the oncotic pressure of plasma albumin, which tends to hold the nutrients within the capillary bed. Subtracting 22 from 32, we see that a force of 10 mm Hg of filtration pressure produces net movement out of the capillary bed toward the cell. With the venous and lymph capillary bed we have a different situation. The oncotic pressure of albumin tending to draw materials into the venous capillaries is still 22 mm Hg, but the filtration pressure from the heart has diminished to 12 mm Hg. Again, 12 from 22 leaves 10 mm Hg, producing a net movement away from the cells and into the venous capillaries and the blind-ended lymph capillaries, which aid the venous capillaries in returning waste materials from the cell to the circulation.

Plasma-to–interstitial fluid shift

Preceding events. The preceding events include severe trauma such as a burn or crushing injury, a critical abdominal event in the nature of intestinal obstruction or perforated peptic ulcer, any ailment that depresses the plasma albumin such as chronic illness resulting in protein depletion (e.g., a malignancy), liver disease (since the liver is the site of albumin synthesis), loss from hemorrhage, childhood nephrosis, nephrosis of renal disease, and malnutrition (as starvation edema).

Potential pharmacologic causes are shock-inducing poisons (see box, p. 1576, top right).

Clinical observations. Clinical findings in plasma-to–interstitial fluid shift include pallor, rapid pulse, low blood pressure, cold extremities, apprehension, disorientation, and coma. As you can see, virtually the same symptoms are observed in surgical shock, with which plasma-to–interstitial fluid shift is closely related.

Laboratory help. What help does the laboratory give us? Little, although if we did an erythrocyte count and determined the hemoglobin and hematocrit, we would find them to be elevated, since they are now in a lesser total volume of plasma.

Of special significance. This shift occurs during the first few days of a severe burn. It is important during this period that the patient *not* be given excessive quantities of fluids.

Modes of therapy. Replace shifted water and electrolytes by mouth or intravenously. Administer a high-protein diet plus protein supplements. Give (parenterally) plasma, dextran, or electrolyte solution with

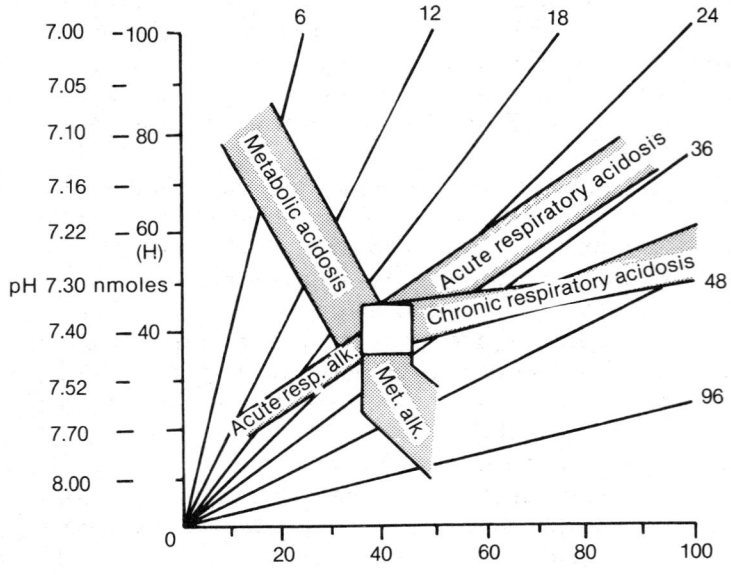

FIGURE 67-1. **Acid-base nomogram. The confidence bands describe the normal (i.e., with 95% confidence) steady-state response of humans to pure, uncomplicated respiratory or metabolic acid-base disorders. Because the respiratory adaptation to metabolic disorders occurs promptly, it is not necessary to segregate these disorders into acute or chronic components. Acid-base values (plotted as plasma pH on the ordinate and plasma Pco_2 on the abscissa) falling within a set of confidence bands are consistent with but not diagnostic of a pure disorder of that type. Values falling outside the confidence bands strongly suggest a mixed disorder of that type. The plasma bicarbonate isopleths are not required for analytic purposes. They simply reflect the bicarbonate concentration associated with a given set of pH and Pco_2 values. (Redrawn from *Audio-Digest Internal Medicine, Fluid and Electrolyte Alterations*, Dec. 17, 1980, 27 [24].)**

Signs and symptoms in infants and children with body fluid disturbances

General

Acute weight gain (in excess of 5%)
   ECF volume excess
Acute weight loss (in excess of 5%)
   ECF volume deficit
Anorexia
   ECF volume deficit
   Potassium deficit
   Protein deficit
   Primary bicarbonate deficit
Bounding pulse
   Interstitial fluid–to-plasma shift
Chronic weight loss
   Protein deficit
Chvostek's sign, positive
   Magnesium deficit
Coma
   Primary carbonic acid excess
Convulsions
   Calcium deficit
   Magnesium deficit
   Primary carbonic acid deficit
   Sodium deficit
Edema
   ECF volume excess
   Protein deficit
   Sodium deficit
Emotional depression
   Protein deficit
Engorgement of peripheral veins
   Interstitial fluid–to-plasma shift
Firm, rubbery integument
   Sodium excess
Flushed skin
   Sodium excess
Fontanel depressed
   ECF volume deficit
Hyperactive deep reflexes
   Calcium deficit
   Magnesium deficit
   Primary carbonic acid deficit
   Sodium deficit
Irritability
   Potassium excess
Nausea
   Potassium excess
Pallor
   ECF volume deficit
   Plasma-to–interstitial fluid shift
   Protein deficit
Ready fatigue
   Protein deficit
Skin dry and inelastic
   ECF volume deficit
Thirst
   Sodium excess
Weak to absent pulse
   Plasma-to–interstitial fluid shift

Upper body

Dry, sticky mucous membranes
   Sodium excess
Puffy eyelids
   ECF volume excess
Shortness of breath
   ECF volume excess
Tongue rough and dry
   Sodium excess

Middle body

Abdominal cramps
   Calcium deficit
   Sodium deficit
Cardiac dilatation
   Interstitial fluid–to-plasma shift
Carpopedal spasm
   Calcium deficit
Deep, rapid breathing
   Carbonic acid deficit
   Primary bicarbonate deficit (may be
      absent in young infants)
Depressed breathing
   Primary bicarbonate excess
Gaseous distention of intestines
   Potassium deficit
Intestinal colic
   Potassium excess
Moist rales in lungs
   ECF volume excess
   Interstitial fluid–to-plasma shift
Muscle cramps
   Calcium deficit
   Sodium deficit
Muscle hypertonicity
   Primary bicarbonate excess
Muscle hypotonicity
   Calcium excess
Respiratory distress
   Primary carbonic acid excess
Shortness of breath on exertion
   Potassium deficit
   Primary bicarbonate deficit
Silent intestinal ileus
   Potassium deficit
Soft, flabby muscles
   Potassium deficit
   Protein deficit

Lower body

Bone cavitation
   Calcium excess
Deep bony pain
   Calcium excess
Flank pain
   Calcium excess

electrolyte composition similar to that of plasma (Figure 67-1).

Interstitial fluid–to-plasma shift

Preceding events. This shift may occur during recovery from a plasma-to–interstitial fluid shift (e.g., on about day 3 following a severe burn). We also find that it may occur as a compensatory shift designed to shore up the volume of the plasma following hemorrhage.

Potential pharmacologic causes are salt-free albumin, dextran, or hypertonic dextrose solution intravenously (see box, p. 1576, bottom right).

Clinical observations. In many respects the clinical observations of this shift are the opposite of those seen in the preceding imbalance: bounding pulse; hypertension; abnormally large urinary volume; pulmonary edema (seen early by radiographic examination, later detected by auscultation); and finally, as the heart is overwhelmed, cardiac failure.

Laboratory help. We don't usually need help from the laboratory, but if we were to do an erythrocyte count and measure the hemoglobin and hematocrit, we would find that they are decreased.

Of special significance. This shift begins on the third day after a severe burn. It can be fatal if too much fluid is given the first 2 days.

Modes of therapy. If caused by hemorrhage, transfusion of whole blood is indicated. Following hemorrhage a balanced diet plus ferrous sulfate should be administered. In a severe shift tourniquets and phlebotomy may be required (see box, p. 1576, bottom right).

KEYS TO DIAGNOSIS

What are the keys to diagnosis of body fluid disturbances? As in all diagnostic problems medical and nursing histories are of enormous importance. In some respects this is more true of body fluid disturbances than of most other ailments. From these histories one will learn the preceding events that might have precipitated specific imbalances. Next, we are interested in weight changes, especially acute weight changes. (The patient commonly does not remember what he weighed a day or two before coming into the hospital.) Then we want to know the urine flow rate in milliliters per hour; catheterization usually will be necessary to obtain an accurate figure. The hemoglobin and hematocrit as well as the erythrocyte count should be carried out. We want to know the values for the serum protein, serum sodium, serum calcium, serum magnesium, serum potassium, serum pH, urine pH, osmolality of serum, osmolality of urine, Pco_2, and bicarbonate. These basic determinations are needed for a complete assessment of a suspected body fluid

disturbance. Many other tests may be required in special instances (see box, p. 1577, for signs and symptoms in infants and children with body fluid disturbances).

SUMMARY

This chapter has examined the physiologic role of body fluids and electrolytes, including acid-base balance. Homeostasis is maintained through a complex interaction of regulating factors and can be compromised by pathologic conditions and drug administration. Signs and symptoms of body excesses and deficits of various body fluids and electrolytes, as well as management or treatment, have also been discussed.

With a knowledge of the physiologic role of the body fluids and electrolytes and the causes, signs, symptoms, and treatment of excesses and deficits, the nurse should be able to provide optimum care to patients who require fluids and electrolytes.

BIBLIOGRAPHY

Auger, R., Zehr, J., Siekert, R., & Segar, W. Position effect on antidiuretic hormone. *Archives of Neurology*, 1970, *23*, 513-517.

Ballin, J. (Ed.). *AMA drug evaluations* (4th ed.). Chicago: AMA Department of Drugs, 1980.

Bernard, C. *Lecons sur les proprietes physiologiques en le alterations pathologiques des liquides de l'organisme.* Paris: Balliere, 1859 (2 vols.).

Bricker, N. (Ed.). *The sea within us.* New York: Science and Medicine Publishing Co., Inc., 1975.

Cannon, W. *The wisdom of the body.* New York: W.W. Norton and Co., Inc., 1932.

Cooke, C., Turin, M., & Walker, W. The syndrome of inappropriate antidiuretic hormone secretion (SIADH): pathophysiologic mechanisms in solute and volume regulation. *Medicine*, 1979, *58*, 240-251.

Daly, W., Papper, S., & Whang, R. (Eds.). *Clinical fluid and electrolyte management.* Washington, D.C.: U.S. Veterans Administration, 1976.

Duke, M. Thiazide-induced hypokalemia, association with acute myocardial infarction and ventricular fibrillation. *Journal of the American Medical Association*, 1978, *239*, 43-46.

Edelman, I., Leibman, J., O'Meara, M., & Birkenfeld, L. Interrelations between serum sodium concentration, serum osmolarity and total exchangeable sodium, total exchangeable potassium and total body. *Journal of Clinical Investigation*, 1958, *37*, 1236.

Felver, L. Understanding the electrolyte maze. *American Journal of Nursing*, 1980, *80*, 1591-1596.

Finberg, L., Kiley, J., & Luttrell, C. Mass accidental salt poisoning in infancy: a study of a hospital disaster. *Journal of the American Medical Association*, 1963, *184*, 187-190.

Goldberger, E. *A primer of water, electrolyte and acid-base syndromes* (5th ed.). Philadelphia: Lea & Febiger, 1975.

Goodhart, R., & Shils, M. *Modern nutrition in health and disease* (5th ed.). Philadelphia: Lea & Febiger, 1973.

Goodman, L., & Gilman, A. (Eds.). *The pharmacological basis of therapeutics* (6th ed.). New York: MacMillan Publishing Co., 1980.

Kubo, W., & Grant, M. The syndrome of inappropriate secretion of antidiuretic hormone. *Heart and Lung*, 1978, *7*, 469-475.

McCurdy, D. Mixed metabolic and respiratory acid-base disturbances: diagnosis and treatment. *Chest*, 1972, *62*, 35S-44S.

Metheny, N., & Snively, W. Perioperative fluids and electrolytes. *American Journal of Nursing*, 1978, *78*, 840-845.

Metheny, N., & Snively, W. *Nurses' handbook of fluid balance* (4th ed.). Philadelphia: J.B. Lippincott, 1983.

Myers, F., Jawetz, E., & Goldfien, A. *Review of medical pharmacology* (7th ed.). Los Altos, Calif.: Lange Medical Publications, 1980.

Newsome, H. Vasopressin: deficiency, excess and the syndrome of inappropriate antidiuretic hormone secretion. *Nephron*, 1979, *23*, 125-129.

Schwartz, W., Bennett, W., Curelop, S., & Bartter, F. A syndrome of renal sodium loss and hyponatremia probably resulting from inappropriate secretion of antidiuretic hormone. *American Journal of Medicine*, 1957, *23*, 529-542.

Snively, W., & Beshear, D. *Textbook of pathophysiology*. Philadelphia: J.B. Lippincott, 1972.

Snively, W., & Dick, R. Computer approach to diagnosis of body fluid disturbances. *Journal of the Indiana State Medical Association*, 1966, *59*, 233-246.

Snively, W., Leitch, G., & Beshear, D. Acid-base disturbances, a programmed text. *American Journal of Intravenous Therapy*, 1977, *4*, 22-40.

Snively, W., Leitch, G., & Beshear, D. Acid-base disturbances, a programmed text. *American Journal of Intravenous Therapy*, 1978, *5*, 26-41.

Snively, W., Leitch, G., & Beshear, D. Acid-base disturbances, a programmed text. *American Journal of Intravenous Therapy*, 1978, *5*, 36-56.

Snively, W., Leitch, G., & Beshear, D. Acid-base disturbances, a programmed text. *American Journal of Intravenous Therapy*, 1978, *5*, 26-34.

Snively, W., & Thuerbach, J. *Sea of life*. New York: David McKay, 1971.

Snively, W., & Thuerbach, J. Voluntary hyperventilation as a cause of needless drowning. *Journal of the Indiana State Medical Association*, 1972, *65*, 493-497.

Watseka, L., Sattler, L., & Steiger, E. Cost of a home parenteral nutrition program. *Journal of the American Medical Association*, 1980, *244*, 2303-2304.

Williams, S. *Nutrition and diet therapy* (5th ed.). St. Louis: The C.V. Mosby Co., 1985.

CHAPTER 68

Serums, Toxoids, and Vaccines

Karin E. Zenk

Medications discussed in this chapter

Serums
  Antirabies serum equine
  Hepatitis B immune glob-
    ulin
  Human serum immune
    globulin (HSIG)
  Rabies immune globulin,
    human
  Tetanus immune globu-
    lin, human
  Varicella-zoster immune
    globulin
Toxoids
  Diphtheria toxoid
  Tetanus toxoid
Vaccines
  Bacterial
    BCG (Bacillus Cal-
      mette-Guérin) vac-
      cine
    Cholera vaccine
    Meningococcal poly-
      saccharide vaccines

Vaccines—cont'd
  Bacterial—cont'd
    Pertussis vaccine
    Plague vaccine
    Polyvalent pneumococ-
      cal vaccine
    Typhoid vaccine
  Viral
    Hepatitis B vaccine
    Human diploid cell ra-
      bies vaccine
    Influenza vaccine
    Measles vaccine
    Mumps vaccine
    Poliomyelitis vaccine
    Poliovirus vaccine
    Rabies vaccine
    Rubella vaccine
    Smallpox vaccine
    Yellow fever vaccine
  Rickettsial
    Typhus vaccine

Serums, toxoids, and vaccines are used to prevent and treat various diseases. *Serums* are agents used to produce a passive immunity and to prevent the infectious disease from occurring or to relieve the symptoms of the disease after suspected or actual exposure. Passive immunity is immediate after administration, although the duration of the immunity is temporary, lasting only a few weeks. *Toxoids* (e.g., diphtheria toxoid) are prepared from formaldehyde-treated bacterial toxins. *Vaccines* are biologic agents. Both toxoids and vaccines are used to induce an active immunity against infectious diseases. Toxoids and vaccines initiate the formation of specific antibodies by stimulating the host's antigen-antibody mechanism. The onset of immunity takes from days to weeks; however, immunity is long term, lasting for years.

This chapter covers both agents that are required only in the occurrence of a special circumstance (e.g., animal bite, injury, or exposure to disease) and agents required for the routine immunization against common childhood communicable diseases and diseases encountered during travel. Requirements for childhood immunizations, adult immunizations, and immunization before travel change from time to time depending on the prevalence of disease. Local departments of health should be contacted for current immunization schedules and recommendations.

SERUMS

Various serums are obtained from animal or human sources in which antibodies have been formed against the respective pathogenic organism. Those derived from human sources cause fewer allergic reactions than those derived from animal sources. The serum is purified and standardized for injection. Serum sickness may occur with the use of serums in susceptible individuals and can occur several days to weeks after the administration of the serum. Some antiserums (e.g., diphtheria and tetanus), also called antitoxins (see Chapter 69, "Venom Allergenic Extracts, Antivenins, and Antitoxins"), can be used either therapeutically or prophylactically.

Antirabies serum, equine

Antirabies serum, equine (ARS) is made of the serum from hyperimmune horses. It is used only when rabies immune globulin, human (RIG) is not available and if the patient is not allergic to horses. The dosage is determined by the patient's weight. The serum is administered with one half of the dose usually infiltrated into the wound or bite (see RIG). Serum sickness is associated with the use of this serum, occurring more commonly in adults than in children.

Immune globulin

Immune globulin is indicated for the postexposure prophylaxis for all types of viral hepatitis, particularly hepatitis A, and non-A, non-B types and for varicella immunization. This preparation provides rapid immune protection lasting 2 months. The sterile solution of the globulins contains many antigens found in the adult human blood. Immune globulin is concentrated by alcohol fractionation from a plasma pool of approximately 1000 human donors, standardized to contain minimum levels of antibodies for diphtheria, poliomyelitis, measles, and hepatitis. Because of the availability of newer, more specific agents (i.e., hepatitis B immune globulin, varicella-zoster immune globulin) immune globulin is rarely used today in treatment or prevention of these conditions. However, the intravenous form (i.e., human serum immune globulin—Gamimune) is still used to treat IgG deficiency states (see the Nursing Drug Digest).

Hepatitis B immune globulin

Hepatitis B immune globulin is an antihepatitis B gamma globulin concentrated by cold alcohol fractionation from the plasma of human donors with high titers of antibody to hepatitis B surface antigens (HBsAg). Hepatitis B immune globulin is indicated for use *only* in the postexposure prophylaxis of hepatitis B caused by needle sticks or other inadvertent exposure (e.g., hemodialysis units, oncology units, or other areas where contraction of hepatitis B is of high risk resulting from percutaneous or mucosal exposure to blood, blood derivatives, or other body fluids from patients known to be positive for hepatitis B surface antigen).

Rabies immune globulin, human

Human rabies immune globulin (RIG) is produced from the plasma of hyperimmunized human donors. After a bite or wound from an infected animal, up to one half of the dose is infiltrated into the wound area and the rest is given as an intramuscular injection. Reactions to this preparation are rare.

Tetanus immune globulin, human

Tetanus immune globulin, human (TIGH) is effective in producing a passive immunity in patients with wounds that may be contaminated with *Clostridium tetani.* Because it is derived from human sources, there is less of a tendency for hypersensitivity. This preparation is used in individuals who have not had prior tetanus toxoid immunization.

Varicella-zoster immune globulin

Varicella-zoster immune globulin (VZIG) is prepared from human gamma globulin obtained from plasma with high titers of varicella-zoster antibodies. The vaccine is used for patients exposed to chickenpox or herpes zoster who are immunodeficient or immunosuppressed for whom varicella can be fatal, as well as for other selected patients. It is used to prevent or ameliorate varicella. VZIG is available from inventory centers in the United States and Canada.

Pain, redness, and swelling can occur at the site of injection. Allergic reactions, although rare, have been reported. The injection is made deep intramuscularly in the gluteal muscle. The dosage schedule is based on body weight, and the dose should be administered as soon as possible after exposure.

TOXOIDS

Diphtheria toxoid

Diphtheria toxoid is available in combination with tetanus toxoid, pertussis vaccine, and polio vaccine in various products (e.g., Diphtheria and Tetanus Toxoids Adsorbed, Diphtheria and Tetanus Toxoids and Pertussis Vaccine Adsorbed, Diphtheria-Pertussis-Tetanus-Polio vaccine) for immunization. Diphtheria toxoid is used for the primary immunization against diphtheria for infants 2 months of age or older and for preschool children. It is contraindicated in children older than 6 years of age and adults because of the danger of reactions to the diphtheria toxoid. Diphtheria toxoid is injected intramuscularly in different sites at an interval of 4 to 8 weeks. The primary series consists of three injections with another injection following 1 year later, and a reinforcing dose between 4 and 6 years of age (see the Nursing Drug Digest for specific information regarding various products containing diphtheria toxoid for immunization).

Tetanus toxoid

Tetanus is caused by the toxin-producing *Clostridium tetani*. Tetanus toxoid is given for prophylaxis. In the event of injury, the tetanus prophylaxis is individualized. A history of a previous immunization and a possible allergy to the tetanus toxoid should be ascertained. Tetanus boosters are indicated in the event of wounds. Wounds should be cleaned and debrided, as indicated, and all foreign material removed.

It is recommended that all individuals receive active immunization and booster injections when indicated. Basic immunization with adsorbed tetanus toxoid requires three injections, with the first two administered 4 to 6 weeks apart and a third injection given 6 to 12 months after the second injection. A booster of adsorbed tetanus toxoid is indicated 10 years after the third injection or 10 years after an intervening wound booster. Neonatal tetanus is preventable by the active immunization of the mother before or during the first 6 months of pregnancy with two intramuscular injections of adsorbed toxoid given 6 weeks apart.

Infants and young children usually receive the tetanus toxoid combined with pertussis vaccine and diphtheria toxoid between 2 months and 6 years of age. Combined tetanus and diphtheria toxoid, adult type (TD) is available for the basic immunization of children over 6 years of age and adults. With different preparations of the toxoid, the volume of a single booster dose should be modified as stated on the package label. Active immunization, not therapy after injury, is the best prevention of tetanus.

For protection against tetanus, adsorbed tetanus toxoid is usually given at the time of injury either as an immunization dose or as a booster for a previous immunization, unless the patient has received a booster or has completed initial immunization within the last 5 years.

The concentration of the tetanus toxoid varies in different products, so specific information on the volume of a single dose should be obtained from the package label. Different syringes, needles, and sites of injection are used for the tetanus toxoid, homologous tetanus immune globulin (human), or heterologous tetanus antitoxin (equine).

When the toxoid is to be given to patients actively immunized in the past with TD, TD toxoid is recommended for routine or wound boosters.

Patients actively immunized within the past 10 years should receive the adsorbed tetanus toxoid as a booster unless they have received boosters within the previous 5 years. Patients with severe neglected wounds older than 24 hours should be given adsorbed tetanus toxoid as indicated unless they have received a booster within the previous year.

VACCINES

There are generally three types of vaccines, bacterial vaccines, viral vaccines, and rickettsial vaccines. Bacterial vaccines, such as pneumococcal vaccine, are prepared from whole bacteria or from purified capsular polysaccharides of certain bacteria. Bacterial vaccines are usually composed of nonliving agents. Viral vaccines, such as measles vaccine, are composed of live attenuated viruses or, as in influenza vaccine, inactivated nonliving viruses.

Bacterial vaccines

BCG (Bacillus Calmette-Guérin) vaccine. BCG (Bacillus Calmette-Guérin) vaccinations are generally given to tuberculin-negative individuals who are at a high risk of contracting tuberculosis. These individuals include health workers who are exposed to patients with sputum-positive tuberculosis who will not or cannot take prophylactic isoniazid or patients who will be residing for a prolonged period in countries that have an increased prevalence of tuberculosis.

BCG vaccine is available in attenuated tubercle bacillus or in live bacillus Calmette-Guérin forms. The attenuated form is administered by the intradermal (intracutaneous) route. A small papule appears in 1 to 3 months. During this time contact with individuals with or suspected of having tuberculosis should be avoided. The vaccination should be repeated for patients with negative results to the Mantoux and Heaf tests more than 3 months after the initial vaccination.

The live forms of the vaccine are indicated for the active immunization against tuberculosis. One form is for intradermal administration and the other is for scarification. BCG should be injected intradermally over the insertion of the deltoid muscle, which lies midway between the acromion process and the lateral epicondyle process of the elbow. The tip of the shoulder should *not* be used because the use of this site has resulted in hypertrophic scar or keloid formation at the injection site. The tip of the shoulder had previously been used for the administration of BCG because it was felt that the clothing could conceal any scar resulting from the injection. This site is now *not* recommended (see the Nursing Drug Digest).

Cholera vaccine. Cholera vaccine is used for cholera prophylaxis. The vaccine is available in a saline suspension of killed *Cholera vibrios.* The vaccine is injected subcutaneously at the insertion of the deltoid muscle. The dosage varies with the patient's age. Three doses of varying amounts are required, and reinforcing doses may be indicated. Pain at the injection site for 1 to 2 days with fever, malaise, or headache may occur. As with other products, epinephrine should be available for the treatment of anaphylaxis or acute hypersensitivity reactions when this vaccine is administered.

Pertussis vaccine. Pertussis vaccine is used to prevent whooping cough. The use of this vaccine has rarely resulted in transient shocklike episodes, convulsions, or neurologic complications. The vaccine is administered subcutaneously in the upper arm at the site of the insertion of the deltoid. Three doses at 4-week intervals beginning at 3 months of age are recommended. Reinforcing doses 6 to 12 months after the third dose and at 5 years of age are indicated. Pertussis vaccine is also available in combination with other vaccines and tetanus toxoid (see the Nursing Drug Digest).

Pneumococcal vaccine. Pneumococcal vaccine is a mixture of 14 serologic subtypes of capsular polysaccharides of the *Pneumococcus* bacteria, chosen because they are responsible for over 80% of pneumococcal infections. The polyvalent pneumococcal vaccine is recommended for elderly patients, patients in nursing homes or other long-term care facilities, patients with chronic conditions (including diabetes mellitus, functional impairment, and cardiorespiratory, renal, or hepatic dysfunction). Use of the vaccine during pregnancy has not yet been established and thus use during pregnancy is not recommended. This vaccine is *not* recommended for use in children under 2 years of age because of the reported poor response.

The vaccine is administered by the deep intramuscular or subcutaneous route and should not be given to patients with any febrile or respiratory condition or any other active infection. The vaccine is not effective against pneumococcal disease caused by other types of organisms not present in the vaccine. Revaccination should not be completed at less than 5-year intervals because of the possible occurrence of more severe reactions at the site of the injection. Local reactions at the injection site within 24 to 72 hours occur after administration in some patients, along with a low-grade fever during the first 24 hours after the injection of the vaccine. Although rare, hypersensitivity reactions to the vaccine, or any component of the vaccine, can occur, and anaphylactic reactions have been reported rarely.

Typhoid vaccine. Typhoid vaccine against typhoid fever, spread by fecal-oral person-to-person contact may be required with travel to such areas as Mexico or India. Typhoid vaccine made from killed *S. typhi*, injected subcutaneously, enhances resistance to typhoid fever. Protection is short term and can be overcome by an increase in the number of ingested organisms. Typhoid fever can also occur in North America because of a spread by asymptomatic chronic intestinal carriers of the disease who are involved in food handling. A live, attenuated oral vaccine of an enzyme-deficient organism for immunization against typhoid fever is being studied and further testing is required.

Viral vaccines

Hepatitis B vaccine. Hepatitis B vaccine is indicated for preexposure protection or immunization against infections caused by the hepatitis B virus. Vaccination is recommended for individuals older than 3 months of age at risk for an infection, and particularly dentists, oral surgeons, dental hygienists, health care workers involved with an increased contact with blood

or blood products, or those involved with renal dialysis. Other high-risk individuals include homosexual men, drug abusers who use the intravenous route of administration, patients on hemodialysis and the sexual partners of chronic hepatitis B surface antigen (HBsAg) carriers.

Hepatitis A most commonly affects young adults and is transmitted via fecal contamination of food and water, with subsequent person-to-person contact. Hepatitis B is associated with complications of the GI tract, bleeding and clotting abnormalities, cirrhosis, ascites, chronic hepatitis, and primary hepatocellular cancer.

Hepatitis B vaccine is produced from chemically inactivated HBsAg particles obtained from the plasma of chronic HBsAg carriers and adsorbed onto aluminum hydroxide (alum). Because the vaccine can be produced from plasma obtained from homosexual men, concerns regarding the possibility of the transmission of acquired immune deficiency syndrome (AIDS) have been raised. However, these concerns appear to be unwarranted at this time. The transmission of AIDS seems to be prevented by the procedures used in the preparation of the vaccine and, to date, no cases have been reported.

Two initial doses are administered intramuscularly 1 month apart and a booster dose is administered 6 months after the initial dose. Hepatitis B vaccine is *not* to be administered intradermally or by the subcutaneous or intravenous routes. The dosage is individualized for children and adults, as well as for patients who are immunosuppressed or immunodeficient (see the Nursing Drug Digest). Vaccine-induced antibodies have persisted for years. Patients on dialysis or with an impaired immune response may not respond as well to the vaccine. The adverse effect associated with the use of hepatitis B vaccine appears to be temporary soreness at the injection site. No serious long-term effects have been reported.

The effectiveness of this vaccine for postexposure prophylaxis after accidental needle sticks, contact with patients with acute hepatitis B, or for neonates when mothers are infected has not been reported. In these situations, hepatitis immune globulin is recommended. Neonates born to mothers who are chronic HBsAg carriers probably should be vaccinated. In adults the antibody response to the vaccine is not inhibited by any previous or concurrent administration of hepatitis B globulin.

Influenza vaccine. Because of the recurrent shift of antigen components characterizing the influenza virus, influenza vaccine requires annual preparation to combat anticipated prevailing strains. Before the flu season, the USPHS Advisory Committee on Immunization Practices (ACIP) issues a yearly statement recommending which influenza vaccine is to be used, its dosage, and the selection of individuals recommended for vaccination.

Deaths related to influenza occur predominantly in chronically ill children and the elderly. Thus, an annual vaccination is recommended for these groups and for others at risk of developing adverse sequelae from lower respiratory tract infections, including patients with heart disease, chronic respiratory conditions, renal disease, diabetes mellitus, chronic severe anemic conditions, and compromised immune response. Influenza vaccine is also indicated for pregnant women who have underlying high-risk conditions.

Adverse effects associated with the use of the vaccine are usually minimal, including local reactions at the site of the injection (e.g., redness, induration) and systemic reactions (e.g., fever, malaise, myalgia), usually persisting for the first 24 to 48 hours. Allergic reactions have been reported, mainly associated with an allergy to egg protein. Thus, influenza vaccine is generally contraindicated in patients with a history of allergy to eggs.

In 1976, an increased risk of the development of Guillain-Barré syndrome (GBS) was associated with the use of the swine influenza vaccine, with an incidence 5 to 6 times greater in vaccinated as opposed to nonvaccinated persons. Before this time, there was no association between influenza vaccine and GBS. Continued surveillance will ultimately determine if this association was unique to the swine flu vaccine of 1976. Available evidence indicates that the risk of developing GBS from influenza vaccine is significantly lower than the risks associated with influenza in persons for whom the vaccine is recommended.

Measles, mumps, and rubella vaccines. Measles, mumps, and rubella vaccines are available in combination or separately for immunization against measles, mumps, and rubella, respectively.

Measles virus vaccine. Measles virus vaccine, live, attenuated is prepared with a more attenuated line of measles virus for the active immunization of children 12 months of age or older against measles (rubeola). The vaccine is prepared in the cell culture of the chick embryo. The vaccine should not be given to pregnant women. It is important to note that tuberculin skin sensitivity may be suppressed. The vaccine is administered subcutaneously in the outer aspect of the upper arm, and the vaccine is protected from light at all times. Moderate fever has been reported up to 1 month after the administration of the vaccine. Generally, fever

and rash in some individuals can occur between the fifth and twelfth days after the injection.

Mumps vaccine. Mumps vaccine is prepared from an attenuated strain of mumps virus grown in the cell cultures of chick embryos. The vaccine is indicated for use against mumps. The vaccine is used in children 15 months or older and in adults as indicated. The vaccine is contraindicated during pregnancy.

Mumps vaccine is administered subcutaneously and should not be given less than 1 month before or after an immunization with other live viruses. Monovalent or trivalent oral booster doses of poliomyelitis vaccine may be given simultaneously. However, tuberculin skin sensitivity tests may be affected (false negative response) by mumps vaccine for 4 or more weeks; thus, tuberculin skin testing should be completed concurrently or before the immunization with mumps vaccine. The injection is made into the outer aspect of the upper arm.

Rubella vaccine. Live, attenuated rubella vaccine is available for immunization of children between 15 months of age and puberty against rubella. The vaccine is contraindicated in pregnancy and in patients with a known hypersensitivity to neomycin. The vaccine is administered subcutaneously and has been associated with adverse effects consisting of local pain and induration at the injection site and other mild effects with children and arthralgia and arthritis in adult women.

It is important to note that approximately one fourth of the women who are immunized against rubella have reactions involving the joints (e.g., arthralgia, possible arthritis) beginning 2 to 4 weeks after the vaccination. Usually these effects are self-limiting; however, this vaccine should be used cautiously in adult women, particularly those of childbearing age. Women of childbearing age with a low titer should use contraception as indicated for 3 months after the immunization. It has not been substantiated that contact between pregnant women and newly vaccinated adults or children should be avoided.

To reduce the incidence of congenital rubella syndrome the National Advisory Committee on Immunizations in Canada (NAIC) recommends that rubella vaccine be given to all children of both sexes at 12 or more months of age. It also recommends that rubella vaccine be given at about 12 years of age to all girls who have no documented evidence of rubella vaccination to ensure that women entering childbearing age have been vaccinated. The committee also recommends that every effort be made to detect and vaccinate susceptible women of childbearing age.

Poliomyelitis and poliovirus vaccines. Both live,

attenuated oral vaccine (e.g., Sabin live oral vaccine) and inactivated preparations (e.g., Salk vaccine) for subcutaneous injection are available for immunization against poliomyelitis.

Poliomyelitis vaccine (Salk vaccine). The Salk vaccine is used for prophylaxis against poliomyelitis and is used primarily in childhood immunization. The vaccine should not be administered to patients with respiratory or other acute febrile conditions. The vaccine contains streptomycin, neomycin, and some animal proteins, and is thus contraindicated in patients with a known hypersensitivity to any of these components. The vaccine is injected subcutaneously into the area of insertion of the deltoid muscle. Three doses at 4-week intervals followed by a booster dose 6 to 12 months later are recommended. Recall doses should be given every 3 to 5 years.

Poliovirus vaccine (Sabin live oral vaccine). Oral poliovirus vaccine containing live, attenuated virus is used in preference to inactivated preparations (i.e., poliomyelitis vaccine) for immunization against polio. The virus multiplies in the host and provokes the production of serum antibodies. Live poliovirus is excreted by the host.

The Sabin live oral vaccine is used for prophylaxis against poliomyelitis primarily for childhood immunization, although the vaccine can be used for adults if a polio outbreak is suspected. Simultaneous administration of two or more live viruses should be avoided, and the vaccine should be administered only under the supervision of a physician. A period of 2 weeks should separate the administration of the preparations when indicated. It is important to note that the oral vaccine must *not* be administered parenterally. Two to three oral doses at intervals of 6 to 12 weeks between each dose is indicated, depending on age, with reinforcing doses.

The use of this vaccine has been associated with the risk of contracting poliomyelitis.

Rabies vaccines. Rabies is endemic in most parts of the world except in such countries as the United Kingdom, Japan, and Antarctica. The principal wild animal reservoir species vary from country to country.

Rabies is an acute, severe viral infection of the CNS caused by a bullet-shaped ribonucleic acid (RNA) virus belonging to the group rhabdovirus. It is transmitted in the saliva of infected animals, usually through a bite. In North America the domestic dog is usually associated with rabies, although other animals, including cats, skunks, raccoons, coyotes, bobcats, foxes, and insectivorous bats have been associated with this condition.

After the virus gains entry into the host, it incubates for 10 days to several months, averaging 20 to 60 days depending on the severity of the bite, its location, the size of the initial colony of rabies virus, the host's resistance, and the immediate treatment of the wound. The virus travels along the afferent sensory nerve pathways to the spinal cord on to the brain where it multiplies. The virus then follows the efferent motor nerve pathways to all body parts, especially the salivary glands. The treatment of choice is human diploid cell rabies vaccine.

Patients requiring rabies vaccine should be carefully assessed. It is important to ascertain what kind of animal was involved and if the exposure occurred in an endemic rabies area. The severity of the exposure should be identified (e.g., lick, scratch, bite with broken skin, or provoked or unprovoked attack). It should be identified if the patient knows the animal (e.g., a neighbor's pet) and the animal's appearance, behavior, and related circumstances. The animal's whereabouts should be documented, as well as whether the animal had been vaccinated. The involved area should be carefully assessed and cleansed. The patient should be calmed and the parents or the family should be allowed to remain with the patient as indicated. The location and extent of the wound should be determined, along with measures already used in treating the injury. The need for vigorous cleansing should be explained, because this can be painful. Analgesics or sedatives may be indicated.

Laboratory immunofluorescence of a skin biopsy, corneal impression smear, brain biopsy, and virus isolation from the saliva and other secretions may be indicated, although fluorescent antibodies and other antibodies are not usually detectable in the serum or the CSF before the eighth day.

It is important to be sure that the appropriate authorities have been notified.

For individuals at a high risk of being bitten by rabid animals (stock breeders, forest rangers, veterinarians), preexposure immunization may be indicated. Administration via the intradermal route into the lateral aspect of the upper arm is usually recommended. Serologic testing is usually not necessary after vaccination.

Human diploid cell rabies vaccine. Human diploid cell rabies vaccine (HDCRV) produced from human cells is associated with less hypersensitivity and fewer adverse effects than previous rabies vaccines. For complete protection, however, this vaccine must be administered with human rabies immunoglobulin (HRIG).

For the nonimmune patient, HDCRV is administered after exposure in five relatively painless intramuscular injections on days 0, 3, 7, 14, and 28. One half of the dose is infiltrated into the wound. HDCRV should not be administered with HRIG in the same syringe. A titer should be completed at the time of the last dose. Adverse effects include irritation at the site of the injection, headache, nausea, and fever.

For the immunized patient, the immediate dose of HDCRV is followed by a booster dose 3 days later. An HRIG injection should not be given.

Duck embryo vaccine. Duck embryo vaccine (DEV) is produced from infected duck embryos partially purified and inactivated with β-propiolactone. This vaccine is used to obtain an active immunity against rabies. A skin sensitivity test is indicated before administration to ensure that the patient is not allergic to duck protein. Epinephrine should be readily available for emergency use when this vaccine is given.

The vaccine is injected subcutaneously and the sites are rotated in the abdomen and the thigh of the patient. For bites below the waist, one injection is given daily for 21 days. For bites above the waist, injections are given twice daily for 7 days and then once daily for 7 days more. Either series is followed with a first booster in 10 days and a second booster in 20 days. Once immunity is established, it will continue for life.

Semple vaccine. Semple vaccine is obtained from the nervous tissue of rabbits and is *not* used today because of its increased association with allergic encephalitis.

Smallpox vaccine. Because the worldwide control of smallpox has been made possible, smallpox vaccination is no longer necessary, and the World Health Organization no longer requires it for international travel. The use of smallpox vaccine is limited to people directly involved in laboratory work with smallpox-related viruses (e.g., ariola, vaccinia, monkeypox).

CHILDHOOD AND ADULT IMMUNIZATION

For routine childhood immunizations, parents should be informed of the importance of completing the immunization series and of keeping records of the date and the type of immunization each child has received. The health care provider should record in the patient's chart the vaccine used, the date of administration, the manufacturer lot number, the volume injected, the site used, and any reactions. If the time sequence schedule is interrupted with a delay between doses it is not necessary to start the series over. This will not interfere with the final immunity achieved, no matter what length of time has elapsed.

Parents should be fully informed about childhood immunization schedules and the specific immuniza-

tion to be given—the name, purpose, and reactions that might occur. Advise parents to report any severe or unusual response. If severe, unusual reactions do occur they should be reported to local or state health officers, according to clinic or hospital policy, giving the product, manufacturer, and lot number. With bacterial vaccines, reactions usually occur within a few hours or days. However, with viral vaccines (live, attenuated) observation should be for a longer period—up to 30 days for vaccine-associated disorders. For rubella vaccine a 60-day surveillance period is maintained.

Active immunization is an important part of well-child care. The active immunization of infants and children when appropriately used can prevent disease and maintain health. Certain factors are considered when preparing a schedule for active vaccination. Changes occur from time to time in recommendations for routine immunization, and the nurse should be alert to these changes.

General ACIP Recommendations

In February, 1980, the USPHS Advisory Committee on Immunization Practices (ACIP) published revised recommendations for mumps vaccine. The changes include a clearer definition of individuals to be vaccinated, a definition of susceptible persons, and a statement regarding the possible association of mumps and diabetes.

Susceptible children, adolescents, and adults should be vaccinated against mumps unless contraindicated. Persons are susceptible unless they have had physician-diagnosed mumps in the past or laboratory evidence of immunity. They are not susceptible if they have had an adequate immunization with live mumps virus vaccine when 12 months of age or older. Persons born before 1957 are likely to have been infected naturally and generally may be considered immune. Live mumps vaccine should not be administered to infants younger than 12 months of age because persisting maternal antibodies may interfere with the development of the immunity. The ACIP states there is no proved association between mumps vaccination and pancreatic damage or the subsequent development of diabetes mellitus.

The ACIP also published new general recommendations on immunization in 1980. These changes clarify the recommendations on the simultaneous administration of vaccines and emphasize the need to report adverse reactions to vaccines. Experimental and extensive clinical experience has shown that most of the widely used antigens can safely and effectively be given simultaneously. Previously it had been recommended that individual live virus vaccines be given at least 1 month apart whenever possible. This was because of the theoretical concern that side effects would be more severe and that there could be a decreased antibody response. Field observations, however, have not found this to occur.

Sabin live oral polio vaccine can be given simultaneously with licensed combination measles, mumps, or rubella vaccine. Diphtheria and tetanus toxoid and pertussis vaccine (DPT) and measles vaccine or DPT and Sabin vaccine may be given simultaneously. The side effects are not increased, and the protective response is satisfactory. Simultaneous administration of all these antigens is feasible, particularly if there is doubt that the recipient will return to receive further doses of the vaccine.

The simultaneous administration of individual measles, mumps, or rubella vaccines at different sites will yield no different results from the administration of the combined vaccine at a single site. In addition, the simultaneous administration of pneumococcal polysaccharide vaccine and whole virus influenza vaccine has been found to give a satisfactory antibody response without any increased side effects.

All vaccines have been reported to cause some adverse effects, ranging from mild local reactions to severe systemic reactions, such as paralysis with trivalent oral polio vaccine (TOPV). To improve knowledge about adverse effects, all severe reactions should be evaluated and reported in detail to local, state, or provincial health officials and to the manufacturer.

Another change in vaccination policy has occurred recently with smallpox vaccination. The World Health Organization recommended in 1980 the cessation of smallpox vaccination (except for investigators) and the discontinuation of international smallpox vaccination certificates for travelers. This change is the result of the global eradication of the disease and the absence of evidence that smallpox would return as an endemic disease.

When to begin active immunization. For healthy infants active immunization is started at 2 months of age with a DPT (diphtheria and tetanus toxoids combined with pertussis vaccine) and TOPV. Measles vaccine should be given after 1 year of age so that interference by maternal antibodies will not occur. If measles vaccine is given earlier, a repeat dose of measles vaccine should be given after 1 year of age (Tables 68-1 and 68-2).

Adults should likewise be encouraged to maintain accurate immunization records and to keep immunizations up to date. Elderly patients, especially those in nursing homes, should be monitored for accurate

TABLE 68-1

Recommended schedule for active immunization in healthy infants and children

Age	Preparation
2 mo	DPT, TOPV
4 mo	DPT, TOPV
6 mo	DPT
1 yr	Tuberculin test
15 mo	Measles, rubella, mumps*
1½ yr	DPT, TOPV
4-6 yr	DPT, TOPV
14-16 yr	TD—repeat every 10 years

DPT—Diphtheria-pertussis-tetanus toxoid, TOPV—Trivalent oral polio vaccine, TD—Tetanus–diphtheria toxoid, adult strength.

NOTE: Interruption or delay of a series does not require restarting the immunization.

*Not to be administered to infants younger than 1 year of age because of possible interference from persisting maternal antibodies.

TABLE 68-2

Recommended schedule for active immunization for children not immunized in early infancy

Age	Preparation
UNDER 6 YEARS OF AGE	
First visit	DPT, TOPV, tuberculin test
1 mo after first visit	Measles,* mumps, rubella
2 mo after first visit	DPT, TOPV
4 mo after first visit	DPT, TOPV (optional)
10-16 mo after first visit or preschool	DPT, TOPV
OVER 6 YEARS OF AGE	
First visit	TD, TOPV, tuberculin test
1 mo after first visit	Measles, mumps, rubella
2 mo after first visit	TD, TOPV
8-14 mo after first visit	TD, TOPV
Age 14-16 yr	TD (repeat every 10 years)

DPT—Diphtheria-pertussis-tetanus toxoid, TOPV—Trivalent oral polio vaccine, TD—Tetanus-diphtheria toxoid, adult strength.

NOTE: Interruption of delay of series does not require restarting the immunizations.

*Measles vaccine is *not* routinely given before 15 months of age.

follow-up of immunizations, particularly routine immunizations against tetanus, diphtheria, influenza, and pneumonia. Special epidemiologic situations may indicate a tuberculosis skin test or immunization against viral hepatitis. Attention to tetanus is particularly important because it has been reported that over 50% of cases occur in patients older than 50 years of age, with an overall mortality of 50%. Diphtheria also occurs in adults.

Elderly patients should be assessed for immunization, because the immunization history is often neglected. This is particularly important because infectious diseases associated with a high mortality and morbidity (e.g., influenza, pneumonia, tetanus) can be prevented with the appropriate immunization. A comprehensive immunization program is recommended to ensure adequate protection, with updating and documentation as indicated.

Plague, typhoid, yellow fever, typhus, hepatitis A, or rabies vaccine are usually not required except for foreign travel to endemic areas or in special circumstances. Several vaccines can be administered simultaneously at different sites of injection, although typhoid, plague, and cholera vaccines, which can cause uncomfortable effects, may best be given at different times.

Immune globulin should not be given for 3 months before or at least 2 weeks after a live viral vaccine, although it does not appear to interfere with the immune response to oral polio virus vaccine or to yellow fever vaccine.

Storage of vaccines. Vaccines should be stored according to the manufacturer's instructions and as shown in the Nursing Drug Digest. There are usually specific requirements for temperature and light. If these instructions are not followed, a significant inactivation and reduced potency may occur.

Vaccine efficacy is an important consideration in view of the declining immunization status of children in North America. Vaccine failure has sometimes been attributed to mishandling. One study in which live virus vaccine from clinics and private offices was tested directly showed that one specimen in five had become inactive during transport or storage in the community. Vaccine spoilage is a problem that is easily avoided with attention to the following guidelines:

I. General rules
   A. Store vaccines well within the refrigerator, never in the refrigerator door, because of its lowered temperature.
   B. Use a styrofoam container to transport vaccines; add ice packs to protect vaccines. For polio vaccines use dry ice *only.*

II. Rules for specific agents
   A. *Poliovirus vaccine*
      1. Unopened vials. When maintained continuously in the frozen state, the vaccine will retain its potency for 12 months as indicated by the expiration date. Unopened poliovirus vaccine may be refrozen if it thaws in storage or transit, provided the temperature does not exceed the refrigerator temperature during that period. A maximum 10 freeze-thaw cycles is permissible for unopened vaccine provided the cumulative duration of the thawing does not exceed 4 hours and the temperature never exceeds 46° F (8° C) or the refrigerator temperature. Unopened vials of vaccine in the liquid state may be used up to 30 days provided they have been stored at 35° F to 46° F (2° C to 8° C) during that period.
      2. Opened vials. Once opened, poliovirus vaccine must be kept refrigerated between doses and used within 7 days. If the vaccine is *not* returned to the refrigerator between doses, it must be discarded according to agency guidelines, at the end of the day. Do *not* refreeze poliovirus vaccine after opening. Poliovirus vaccine has a variable red to yellow tinge. Color change may occur on thawing or storage, but it is unimportant if the vaccine remains crystal clear. The possibility of bacterial contamination should be considered, however, whenever a thawed and entered vial shows color changes from red to pink to yellow during subsequent storage.
   B. *Measles, rubella, mumps vaccines.* The measles, rubella, and mumps vaccines are extremely light and heat sensitive. Exposure of these vaccines to *light* either before or after reconstitution kills the live virus. Store reconstituted vaccine in a dark place (in its carton, within a towel, or wrapped with aluminum foil) in the refrigerator. Use only the diluent supplied to reconstitute the vaccine. After mixing, use the vaccine as soon as possible. Discard mixed vaccine if not used within 8 hours.
   C. *DPT* (diphtheria and tetanus toxoids and pertussis vaccine). Store DPT in the refrigerator. It should *not* be frozen because this reduces its potency. Shake the vial vigorously before withdrawing each dose.

D. *Influenza vaccine.* Store influenza vaccine in the refrigerator. Do *not* freeze this vaccine because this destroys its potency.

E. *Smallpox vaccine.* Smallpox vaccine should be stored below 32° F (0° C). Heat destroys its potency.

F. *Typhoid and cholera vaccines.* Store typhoid and cholera vaccines at a uniform temperature in the refrigerator.

Dosage. The dosage of vaccines in some instances differs from children to adults. The standard type of combined diphtheria-tetanus toxoids (DT) contains 7 to 25 Lf (flocculating units) of diphtheria toxoid per dose and may cause severe reactions in older children and adults. The adult tetanus-diphtheria toxoid (TD) contains not more than 2 Lf of diphtheria toxoid and is the recommended product for children over 6 years of age and adults. Always be sure to doublecheck the vaccine and the dosage before administration.

SUMMARY

Various serums, toxoids, and vaccines have been discussed. The importance of ensuring immunizations for the prevention of common childhood diseases, as well as for the prevention of diseases associated with travel cannot be overemphasized. The nurse has a role in promoting public safety in prevention and case finding in relation to the control of communicable diseases. With an understanding of the use, administration, and adverse effects associated with the various agents, the nurse can better help patients understand the importance of immunization and the completion of the immunization series. The nurse can also better educate patients regarding community safety and the importance of seeking health care in the case of injury, animal bite, or exposure to various contagious diseases that may require prophylactic or therapeutic treatment with serums, toxoids, or vaccines.

ADVERSE/SIDE EFFECTS OF THE SERUMS, TOXOIDS, AND VACCINES*

ALLERGIC REACTIONS

Anaphylaxis
Angioedema
Dyspnea
Hoarseness
Lacrimation
Pruritus
Sneezing
Urticaria
Wheezing

CENTRAL NERVOUS SYSTEM

Alteration of consciousness
Convulsions

Fever
Focal neurologic signs
Malaise

CUTANEOUS SYSTEM

Induration at injection site
Redness at injection site
Tenderness at injection site

GASTROINTESTINAL SYSTEM

Abdominal pain
Nausea
Vomiting

HEMATOLOGIC SYSTEM

Thrombocytopenia

NEUROMUSCULAR SYSTEM

Arthralgia
Arthritis-like symptoms
Myalgia
Polyneuralgia
Polyneuritis

*See Chapter 11, "Drug Toxicity," for an overview of drug toxicity.

CLINICALLY SIGNIFICANT DRUG INTERACTIONS*

Primary drug	Interacting drug	Possible effect(s)	Probable mechanism(s)
Influenza virus vaccine	Theophylline	Increased theophylline plasma levels	Inhibition of hepatic metabolism
Live virus vaccines	Immunosuppressive drugs (corticosteroids, irradiation, anticancer drugs)	Systemic infection from immunizing agent	Suppression of host defense mechanism
Measles vaccine	Tuberculin skin test	Depression of tuberculin skin test temporarily	Not established

*See Chapter 10, "Drug Interactions," for an overview of drug interactions.

GENERAL NURSING IMPLICATIONS

Nursing of patients requiring serums, toxoids, and vaccines

ASSESSMENT

Patients requiring serums, toxoids, or vaccines should have a general health assessment, with attention to the need for a specific serum, toxoid, or vaccine (e.g., childhood immunization, travel, injury). The patient's or parent's knowledge, as indicated, regarding the immunization should be assessed. Religious feelings should also be identified because some religious groups do not believe in immunization. It is not unusual for patients to be hesitant about immunizations, and this needs to be identified so that nursing assistance can be provided as indicated. Fears regarding the adverse effects associated with some immunizations (e.g., pertussis) need to be explored and the risks discussed carefully in relation to the benefits of the immunization so that the patient or the family can make an informed decision and an informed consent can be obtained. The initial assessment should include a detailed drug history to identify potential drug interactions, possible contraindications, cautions, and sensitivity. The patient's and family's use of the health care system, especially as related to follow-up immunization for children should be explored as indicated, and assistance with the completion of immunization schedules and other health care needs planned.

Patients requiring immunizations should be questioned regarding recent blood transfusions or injections of immune serum globulin. The vaccination should generally be delayed for 6 weeks because the presence of a passive immunity can prevent the formation of antibodies to the vaccine if immune globulin had been recently received.

A neurologic assessment should be completed, particularly in patients receiving DPT vaccine, including the identification of a history of convulsions, fainting spells, or previous reactions to DPT vaccine. If identified, the vaccination with DPT should be delayed until this condition has been reported to the prescriber.

Except for polio vaccine, all live virus vaccines are contraindicated in pregnancy. Women of childbearing age should be questioned regarding the possibility of pregnancy, and an accurate menstrual history should be obtained. The use of contraception may be indicated for 3 months after some vaccinations (e.g., rubella).

SENSITIVITY

Generally, allergic reactions to serums, toxoids, and vaccines are rare; however, any drug has the potential to cause a hypersensitivity reaction in susceptible individuals. Allergic reactions have been less common with the use of human diploid cell vaccines. It is important to note that allergic reactions are usually associated with the substance or protein used in the production of the serum, vaccine or toxoid rather than to the virus or active component itself. Thus, a careful history identifying any allergy to horses, ducks, eggs, chickens, or neomycin should be completed as indicated.

If a child or an adult has had a minor reaction to the vaccine, the remaining dose may be generally cut in half or in thirds to decrease the possibility of a systemic reaction. It is important to note that DPT reactions occur within hours of the administration of the vaccine and subside in 24 to 48 hours, whereas other vaccines, such as the viral antigens, may not cause symptoms for 10 to 28 days, and these reactions may not resolve as readily.

Although sensitivity to chickens, chicken eggs, and feathers is listed as a contraindication to the use of a vaccine, a history of egg sensitivity alone should not preclude the use of certain vaccines, including influenza, measles, mumps, typhus, or yellow fever that are grown in chick embryos or in chick embryo tissue. However, severe reactions following egg ingestion should serve as a warning for serious vaccine reactions. Intradermal testing with 1:1000 dilution of the vaccine is reliable in predicting reactions.

CONTRAINDICATIONS

The use of serums and vaccines is generally contraindicated in patients with the following conditions: acute febrile illness, immunologic deficiency, malignancy, immunosuppressive therapy, pregnancy, skin irritation or dermatitis (smallpox vaccine), or the administration of gamma globulin, plasma, or a blood transfusion in the previous 1 to 2 months (which postpones the immunization until the passively received antibodies decrease). See the Nursing Drug Digest for specific contraindications to each agent.

CAUTIONS

The various serums, toxoids, and vaccines should be used with caution in certain individuals. See the Nursing Drug Digest for cautions associated with specific preparations.

DRUG INTERACTIONS

Drug interactions can occur among certain serums, toxoids, and vaccines; however, these are rare. Interacting vaccines should generally be administered at different sites and at different times.

It is important to note that influenza vaccine can interfere with the hepatic metabolism of drugs and thus can dramatically prolong their half-lives by as much as 50%. Significant drug interactions have been reported with warfarin, phenytoin, oxtriphylline, and theophylline. A dose reduction may be necessary when influenza vaccine is administered to patients concurrently taking any of these drugs.

See Clinically Significant Drug Interactions for specific interactions.

ADMINISTRATION

Before any immunization is administered, it is important to note the age of the adult or the child for whom the serum, toxoid, or vaccine is indicated, and any contraindications, cautions, sensitivity, or possible drug interactions. It is important to ensure that a consent has been obtained and that the parent or the adult understands the benefits and risks associated with the administration of the specific agent. The nurse should doublecheck for allergies or a history of any reaction to a previous vaccination or to the constituents of the vaccine.

GENERAL NURSING IMPLICATIONS—cont'd

Nursing of patients requiring serums, toxoids, and vaccines—cont'd

ADMINISTRATION—cont'd

Inquire about any allergy to eggs, ducks, or chicken protein. If a positive history of an allergy exists, consult the Nursing Drug Digest of this chapter.

When administering live virus vaccines, make sure that the patient is not immunodeficient or on immunosuppressive agents (corticosteroids, irradiation, antineoplastics) (see Clinically Significant Drug Interactions). Be certain that the patient does not have a malignant neoplasm, leukemia, or lymphomas affecting the bone marrow or the lymphatic system. If the patient has any of these conditions, withhold the vaccination and contact the prescriber, because the administration of a live virus vaccine to these patients may cause a severe, disseminated disease associated with the virus administered.

The serum, toxoid, or vaccine should be carefully inspected for the expiration date and color changes. The nurse should be aware of the correct route of administration, dosage, and storage requirements. Observe the dilution and storage conditions carefully so that the active product is administered. Be sure to read all directions *each* time a preparation is given. Attention to these details is important before administering each preparation because drug companies and supplies can differ.

Have epinephrine ready when administering serums.

The various serums, toxoids, and vaccines are administered by various routes, including the oral, subcutaneous, intradermal, and intramuscular routes. Various sites are indicated for specific parenteral administration (e.g., insertion of deltoid muscle, outer aspect of upper arm). Be sure to identify the correct administration route and if the vaccine is live, attenuated, or killed, or inactivated. The correct recommended site of administration, the composition of the antigen and of the specific preparation prevents disease or the severity of it. Large doses of serums should generally be divided into smaller injections so that no more than 3 ml is administered per site in an adult. Be sure not to mix preparations in the same syringe that should *not* be mixed (e.g., rabies vaccine and antirabies serum).

See the Nursing Drug Digest for the dosage and administration of specific serums, toxoids, and vaccines.

MONITORING PATIENT RESPONSE

Therapeutic response

Generally monitor patients receiving serums, toxoids, or vaccines for the absence of the specific disease, hematologic response, or diminished signs and symptoms of disease.

Hepatitis B vaccine

A specific antibody develops in 75% to 90% of healthy patients after the first two doses of hepatitis B vaccine, and in 85% to 95% of patients after the third dose of the vaccine. Vaccine-induced antibodies have persisted for at least 3 years; booster shots may be indicated. Patients on dialysis or others with an impaired immune response may not respond as well. Serologic testing is not indicated except in patients whose subsequent management depends on a knowledge of their immune status.

Rabies

Monitor for the absence of the development of rabies encephalitis: fever (40° C, 104° F), flaccid paralysis of the extremities, and abnormal movements of the face and neck.

Monitor for signs of the *prodromal stage* (nonspecific symptoms): headache, fever, nausea, malaise, myalgia, sore throat or paresthesia, pain at the wound site, hyperesthesia, irritability, pupil dilation, and increased salivation.

NOTE: Depending on whether the spinal cord or brain is predominantly infected, symptoms progress to furious or paralytic rabies.

Monitor for signs of the *excitation stage* (furious rabies): increased agitation, marked restlessness, aimless pacing, hallucinations, excessive salivation, fever (103° F, 39.4° C), periods of excitement alternating with periods of calm, and severe painful contractions of the pharyngeal muscles when the patient tries to drink or sees water (hydrophobia).

Monitor for signs of the *paralytic stage:* progressive generalized paralysis, and death from respiratory failure after a generalized seizure, 2 to 3 days after entry into this stage or weeks later. Paralytic rabies is a form seen in about one fifth of cases, especially patients bitten by vampire bats, with flaccid paralysis usually beginning in the bitten limb and ascending symmetrically or asymmetrically until the muscles of deglutition and respiration are involved with death occurring within 2 to 3 weeks. Hydrophobia is unusual, but can occur in the late stage of illness.

Adverse side effects

Serums

Serum sickness may occur following the use of a serum within several days to weeks after administration. Patients should be monitored for fever, enlarged lymph nodes, splenomegaly, rash, or painful joints. The treatment of serum sickness is symptomatic, although corticosteroid therapy may be indicated in some patients.

Toxoids and vaccines

Generally, monitor patients for local redness, inflammation, or pain at the injection site. In addition, observe and report any allergic-like symptoms, such as wheezing, dyspnea, sneezing, hoarseness, tachycardia, GI discomfort, nausea, neck or chest pain, cyanosis, sweating, lacrimation, urticaria, angioedema, or pruritus. Observe and report any fever lasting longer than 2 to 3 days or any CNS signs and symptoms.

Points for monitoring and managing common and mild adverse side effects

For *diphtheria toxoid*, monitor for fever occurring during the first 24 to 48 hours, and soreness, redness, and swelling at the injection site.

Encourage the patient or parent to use aspirin or acetaminophen if a fever occurs, and to notify the health care provider if any unusual effects are noted.

For *hepatitis B vaccine*, monitor patients for temporary soreness and redness at the injection site, fever, rash, headache, fatigue, nausea, joint pain, myalgia, and arthralgia.

Continued.

GENERAL NURSING IMPLICATIONS—cont'd

Nursing of patients requiring serums, toxoids, and vaccines—cont'd

Points for monitoring and managing common and mild adverse side effects—cont'd

For *influenza vaccine*, monitor patients for local redness and swelling at the injection site 24 to 48 hours after the injection and fever, malaise, and myalgia occurring 6 to 12 hours after the vaccination and persisting for 1 to 2 days, especially in children.

Monitor patients for an allergic reaction, which is immediate: flare or wheal and a hypersensitivity reaction. Use is contraindicated in patients with an allergic response to eggs, including such signs as swelling of the lips or tongue or acute respiratory distress or collapse.

GBS has been associated with the swine flu vaccine 10 weeks following the injection. Monitor patients for other untoward effects.

For *measles vaccine*, monitor patients for anorexia or loss of appetite, malaise or weakness, rash, fever occurring 7 to 10 days after the immunization, and encephalitis (rarely).

Encourage the patient to use acetaminophen for a mild fever or discomfort, and to notify the health care provider if a high fever is noted.

For *mumps vaccine*, monitor the patient for mild fever.

For *pertussis vaccine*, monitor the patient for fever occurring during the first 24 to 48 hours, soreness, redness, or swelling at the injection site, a loss of consciousness, or convulsions (these effects require immediate reporting to the health care provider), or unusual bruising or bleeding (thrombocytopenia).

For *pneumococcal vaccine*, monitor the patient for local irritation at the injection site occuring 1 to 3 days after the vaccination, a low-grade fever for 24 hours after the vaccination, or anaphylaxis (rare), which can be caused by any component of the vaccine. Note and report any other untoward effect. (Epinephrine injection [1:1000] must be readily available for emergency use for an anaphylactic reaction when this vaccine is given.)

For *inactivated polio vaccine (IPV)* (Salk), monitor the patient for fever or restlessness.

For *live oral polio vaccine (TOPV)* (Sabin), although there are essentially no adverse side effects associated with this vaccine, paralysis can occur up to 2 months after the immunization.

Monitor the patient for tiredness, weakness, headache, sore throat, or other nonspecific complaints followed with vomiting, neck stiffness, personality change in children, followed with flaccid paralysis or sluggish tendon reflexes progressing over 48 to 72 hours and affecting any muscle or muscle group.

For *rabies vaccine*, monitor the patient for irritation at the injection site, headache, nausea, and fever.

Monitor patients requiring rabies vaccine for signs of wound infection, increased pain at the wound site, purulent drainage, or continued swelling of the area after 12 hours.

For *rubella vaccine*, monitor the patient for a mild rash lasting 24 to 48 hours within a few days of the immunization, painful or swollen joints (arthralgia, arthritis), or a loss of sensation of the hands and fingers (paresthesia).

For *tetanus vaccine*, monitor the patient for a fever occurring during the first 24 to 48 hours, soreness, redness, or swelling at the injection site, urticaria or hives, and malaise or general weakness. The onset may be delayed and may last for several days. A firm lump may be felt at the injection site, lasting for weeks or months, but will gradually disappear. Encourage the patient or parent to notify the health care provider if any unusual effects are noted.

See Adverse/Side Effects for an outline of the common adverse side effects associated with serums, toxoids, and vaccines.

PATIENT EDUCATION

The patient and the family, as indicated, should understand that immunizations for measles, mumps, rubella, diphtheria, pertussis, tetanus, and polio are still required because the antigens for these diseases cannot be totally eliminated from the environment.

Parents in North America have generally become lax in protecting their children from communicable diseases. This is probably because they have not experienced the impact of the contagious diseases of childhood. In addition, many lower socioeconomic groups do not have the needed health care resources.

The patient and the family, as indicated, should have a clear understanding of the anticipated schedule for the vaccination or treatment, its general action, purpose, and common associated adverse side effects. They should know how to monitor for the therapeutic response and the adverse effects, be able to manage the less severe effects, and

GENERAL NURSING IMPLICATIONS—cont'd

Nursing of patients requiring serums, toxoids, and vaccines—cont'd

PATIENT EDUCATION—cont'd

should be able to identify when the health care provider should be notified.

The lack of documentation of immunizations is a commonly encountered problem for nurses providing care to both children and adults, including elderly patients. Parents often cannot recall the exact immunizations their child has had, nor can adults usually give an accurate immunization history for themselves. Parents should be taught the importance of immunization records and be encouraged to keep immunization records for themselves and their family members. These records should be taken to the health care facility. Parents and adults should be taught to request and expect to receive records from health care providers regarding immunization.

Patients traveling to other countries should be referred to legal require- ments for entry and epidemiologic conditions that vary from country to country over time. Immunizations schedules should be planned carefully because they can take 2 to 3 months to complete, depending on the area of travel. Because several of the vaccines that are indicated require multiple doses at intervals of 4 weeks or at a specific time before entry into the country (e.g., cholera, 6 months), this is particularly important. Other vaccines can be administered simultaneously or at different sites (e.g., cholera, plague, typhoid).

Update information is available from local, state, or provincial health departments.

Rabies

It is important that nurses be aware of the prevalence of rabies in wild and domestic animals in their areas of practice, and they should encourage fami- lies and community members to pro- tect domestic pets with yearly vaccinations and stray control. People should be discouraged from keeping skunks, raccoons, and other wild car- nivorous pets. They should be encour- aged to avoid any unnecessary contact with animals such as playing with or petting stray dogs or exploring bat- infested caves. Education of the public regarding rabies is indicated. Travelers in particular should be encouraged to report bites before returning home.

Patients should be taught the imme- diate care for treating animal bites, scratches, and licks: scrub with soap under a running tap for at least 5 min- utes, removing any foreign material or debris, rinse with plain water, irrigate with 70% alcohol, tincture of iodine, or 0.01% aqueous iodine, and immediate- ly seek health care advice.

GENERAL INSTRUCTIONS FOR DISCHARGE/OUTPATIENTS

SERUMS, TOXOIDS, AND VACCINES

The immunization may cause redness or tenderness at the injection site. A fever may occur for 2 to 3 days. Report any unusually high fever or any fever that lasts longer than 2 to 3 days.

Keep a careful record of the date and type of each immunization received.

Bring this record card with you when- ever you visit your health care provider.

Report immediately any unusual signs such as a change in behavior or sei- zures.

Report any allergic symptoms such as difficulty breathing, rash, itching, swell- ing, excessive sneezing, chest pain, or nausea.

Do not use aspirin if you have received a viral vaccine. Acetaminophen can be used to control fever or mild discom- fort. If you have any questions, contact your health care provider.

NURSING DRUG DIGEST

Medication (trade name*)	Indication	Usual dosage and administration	Dosage forms, preparation, and storage	Contraindications, cautions, and comments	Monitoring
★ **Antirabies serum equine (ARS)**	A hyperimmune serum used to prevent rabies and used with rabies vaccine for postexposure treatment (generally *only* used if rabies immune globulin is *not* available)	*Adults and children:* 50 IU/kg of body weight; give up to one half of total dose infiltrated around the wound; give rest of dose IM; begin full 21-dose course of rabies vaccine immediately	Injectable: 1,000 unit/vial	*Contraindicated* in hypersensitivity Immediate shocklike reactions or delayed (7-14 days) serum sickness may occur (up to 40% in adults, less in children) because of sensitivity to horse serum. Take careful history from patient regarding allergy to horses. Skin test for sensitivity (intradermal) Wound should be thoroughly cleansed with soapy water and flushed with 70% isopropyl alcohol before infiltration of ARS	Observe for immediate sensitivity reactions and have epinephrine available for treatment
BCG vaccine	Prophylaxis against tuberculosis Recommended for persons exposed to environments in which risk of TB is increased, including newborn infants of mothers with TB	*Adults:* 0.1 ml intradermal multipuncture technique *Newborn infants:* 0.05 ml intradermal multipuncture technique *Older infants, children:* 0.1 ml intradermal multipuncture technique	Injectable: 1 ml ampule Reconstitution: add 1 ml sterile water for injection to 1 ml ampule of vaccine Each 1 ml of reconstituted vaccine contains 8 to 26 million colony-forming units	*Contraindicated* in patients who have not had a TB skin test within the previous 2 weeks, if acutely ill, with dysgammaglobulinemia, with extensive skin infections, allergic dermatitis, or burns	A papule will appear, which scales, ulcerates, and dries, leaving a smooth pink or blue scar after about 3 months

Agent	Use	Dosage	Storage/How Supplied	Comments
			Material not immediately used (within 2 hr) should be discarded Refrigerate at 4°-8° C Protect from light	There is lack of agreement concerning the importance of this vaccine for use in the United States and Canada Converts negative TB skin testers to positive reactors Active TB must be ruled out before the vaccine is administered Repeat vaccination may be considered in the absence of scarification Vaccination is generally ineffective if patient is receiving isoniazid	Check age of patient and which booster to verify dosage amount
Cholera vaccine	Prophylaxis against cholera Used only for persons traveling to endemic areas	*Adults and children over 10 years of age:* Two doses of 0.5 ml 1 week to 1 month apart; booster at 6-month interval 0.5 ml IM, SC, or intradermal *Children 5-10 years:* 0.3 ml, second dose 0.3 ml, booster dose 0.3 ml, IM, SC *Children 6 months-5 years:* 0.2 ml, second dose 0.2 ml, booster dose 0.2 ml, IM, SC	Injectable: 1, 1.5, 2.5, 10, 20 ml Refrigerate at 2°-8° C	*Contraindicated* in patients who have had serious reactions to this vaccine previously *Contraindicated* during acute illness or infection *Contraindicated* in infants younger than 6 months of age Side effects include malaise, fever, induration, and erythema at the site of the injection.

Continued.

NOTE: For additional details regarding the individual agents listed in this table, see the text and other tables in this chapter.
*Indicates a multiple active ingredient product. For a complete listing of all active ingredients see the *Drug Reference Guide to Brand Names and Active Ingredients*.
♦Indicates that the drug is generally available only in Canada.
★Indicates that the drug is generally available only in the United States.

NURSING DRUG DIGEST—cont'd

Medication (trade name)	Indication	Usual dosage and administration	Dosage forms, preparation, and storage	Contraindications, cautions, and comments	Monitoring
Diphtheria toxoid (DT) adsorbed Tri-Immunol* Triogen*	Prophylaxis for diphtheria	*Adults and children over 7 years:* 0.5 ml of TD (less potent, adult-strength tetanus diphtheria toxoids) IM at 4-6 week intervals and a booster dose at 6 months to 1 year after second dose *Primary immunization in children 6 weeks-7 years:* 0.5 ml of DPT (diphtheria and tetanus toxoids, and pertussis vaccine) at 4-8 week intervals for 3 doses; begin at 2 months of age; give fourth dose 1 year later (18 mo) and a booster before entering school (4-6 years of age)	Injectable: 5 ml vials and 0.5 ml Tubex sterile cartridge-needle units Keep refrigerated at 2°-8° C Shake vial vigorously before administering each dose	*Contraindicated* in active infection and immunosuppressive states Usually given in combination with tetanus toxoid and pertussis vaccine (DPT); also as DT in pediatric preparations; or in reduced amounts in adult preparation (TD) Advise patient that local reactions are usually self-limited and require no therapy *Common* tenderness at the injection site *Rare* fever, malaise, myalgia, or sterile abscess Fever much more common in preparations containing pertussis vaccine Acetaminophen may be used to control fever TD (tetanus, diphtheria toxoids in strength for adults and children over 7 years) contains the same amount of tetanus toxoid but only 10%-25% of diphtheria toxoid Mild to moderate temperature elevation (especially in products containing pertussis) accompanied by malaise occurring within several hours of administration and persisting for 1-2 days occur commonly	Observe for fever and malaise

Drug	Uses	Dosage	Dosage forms	Comments
Hepatitis B immune globulin H-BIG Hep-B-Gammagee Hyperhep	For postexposure prophylaxis following either parenteral exposure (e.g., accidental needlestick), direct mucous membrane contact (accidental splash) or oral ingestion (pipetting accident) of HBsAg-positive materials such as blood, plasma, or serum	*Adults:* Usual dose is 3 to 5 ml administered as soon as possible IM (not later than 7 days) after exposure and repeated 25 to 30 days after the first dose. *Children:* 0.06 ml/kg IM. For use in infants born to mothers who had hepatitis B infection during the last trimester, a dose of 3 ml given in divided volumes in four sites IM has been recommended. Administer in the gluteal or deltoid muscles (adults)	Injectable: 1, 5 ml	*Do not give IV.* May cause local pain and tenderness at the injection site, urticaria, and angioedema. Rarely causes allergic reactions. Use care in the disposal of used needles and syringes. Hospital workers should use care in working with patients with hepatitis to avoid inadvertent needlesticks; if this occurs, hepatitis B immune globulin should be administered as soon as possible (not later than 7 days)
Hepatitis B vaccine Heptavax-B	Prophylaxis for hepatitis B, preexposure	*Adults:* 1 ml IM initially, followed by 1 ml IM at 1 and 6 months. *Children:* 3 months to 10 years of age, 0.5 ml IM initially, followed by 0.5 ml IM at 1 and 6 months. For IM use only	Injectable: 3 ml/vial (20 µg/ml). Store at 2°-8° C. *Do not* freeze. Shake well before use	*Contraindicated* in hypersensitivity. May cause rash, nausea, fatigue, soreness at the injection site, and fever. Acetaminophen can be used to treat the fever. Use with caution in patients with severe cardiovascular disorders
★ **Human diploid cell rabies vaccine (HDCV)** Imovax Wyvac	Prophylaxis against rabies, preexposure and postexposure (Rabies vaccine of choice—note that a single dose of rabies immune globulin should be concurrently administered at the start of therapy)	*Adults:* Preexposure, 1 ml IM or intradermal, and repeated on days 7 and 21 or 28; a 1 ml IM booster is recommended at least once every 2 years. Postexposure, 1 ml IM, and repeated on days 3, 7, 14, and 28 after first dose; an additional dose on day 90 is considered optional. *Children:* Same as adults	Injectable: 1 ml single-dose vial of lyophilized vaccine and diluent (sterile water for injection). Store at 2°-8° C. *Do not* freeze. Use immediately after reconstitution	Recommended in preference to the rabies virus vaccine (duck embryo) because it requires fewer injections, is more effective, and has fewer adverse effects. Preexposure treatment is recommended for individuals at a high risk of exposure to rabies (e.g., veterinarians). Used in conjunction with rabies immune globulin. May cause some mild local reactions (e.g., itching, pain, redness) at the injection site

Continued.

NURSING DRUG DIGEST—cont'd

Medication (trade name)	Indication	Usual dosage and administration	Dosage forms, preparation, and storage	Contraindications, cautions, and comments	Monitoring
Human serum immune globulin (HSIG) Gamimune	IgG deficiency states	*Adults:* 100 mg/kg IV infusion once a month Infuse IV at a rate of 0.01-0.04 ml/kg/min (usually over 30 min) For IV use *only*	Injectable: 500 mg/ml Store at 2°-8° C Do *not* freeze May be diluted with D₅W Discard outdated, frozen, or turbid preparations	*Contraindicated* in hypersensitivity and patients with IgA deficiencies	Observe for allergic reactions
Influenza virus vaccine Fluogen Fluzone	Prophylaxis against influenza (used most commonly in elderly patients)	*Adults:* Inject in single dose, 0.5 ml IM into deltoid or thigh muscle (e.g., vastus lateralis) *Children:* 6 months-3 years of age, 0.25 ml IM; 3-12 years of age, 0.5 ml IM Do *not* administer IV	Injectable: 5 ml vials; 0.5 ml sterile cartridge-needle units	*Contraindicated* in patients highly sensitive to chicken eggs Influenza virus vaccine is usually reviewed annually to include strains that are anticipated to cause problems that year Common side effects are fever, malaise, erythema, myalgia, and pain at the injection site Encephalitis is rare Acetaminophen can be used to treat fever Have epinephrine injection (1:1000) available Consider annual injection in patients at risk: elderly patients, patients in nursing homes or extended care homes, patients with chronic cardiovascular, pulmonary, or renal disease, diabetes mellitus, adrenocortical insufficiency, and chronic metabolic disorders	

Measles virus vaccine, live Attenuvax

Prophylaxis against measles

Children 15 months or older:
0.5 ml SC
Do *not* administer IV

Injectable: Single-dose vial of lyophilized powder with diluent-containing syringe

Also available in combination with live mumps and rubella vaccines

Use *only* the diluent supplied for reconstitution

Use as soon as possible after reconstitution (discard after 8 hr)

Protect from light

Keep refrigerated at 2°-8° C

Contraindicated in severe febrile illness, during pregnancy, in leukemia or lymphoma, and in patients on drugs that interfere with immune mechanisms (corticosteroids, irradiation, anticancer drugs)

If given before 1 year of age, repeat after 15 months of age because maternal antibodies may interfere with the development of active immunity

If tuberculin skin testing is necessary, administer tuberculin skin test either before or simultaneously with measles vaccine because it depresses TB skin test temporarily

Measles vaccination may be neutralized by the antibody content of immune globulin, whole blood, or plasma; postpone vaccination 3 months after administration of any of these agents

Side effects include fever, convulsions with fever, thrombocytopenia with CNS effects

Acetaminophen may be used to treat fever

Use with caution in patients allergic to eggs or chickens

Centers for Disease Control state that vaccine may safely be given to patient allergic to eggs

Continued.

NURSING DRUG DIGEST—cont'd

Medication (trade name)	Indication	Usual dosage and administration	Dosage forms, preparation, and storage	Contraindications, cautions, and comments	Monitoring
Meningococcal polysaccharide vaccines Meningovax-AC Menomune-A Menomune-C Menomune-A/C Menomune-A/C/Y/ W-135	Prophylaxis against *Meningococcus* organisms	*Children over 2 years and adults:* 0.5 ml (50 µg) SC (not effective in children under 2 years of age)	Injectable: Monovalent serogroup A, monovalent serogroup C, and bivalent serogroups A-C, available in 10- and 50-dose vials with supplied diluent Reconstitute *only* with diluent supplied Store at 2°-8° C Discard unused reconstituted vaccine after 4 days	*Contraindicated* in active infection, immunosuppression, and pregnancy Side effects include localized erythema, headache, and low-grade fever Have epinephrine (1:1000) available for use	
Mumps virus vaccine, live Mumpsvax	Given for prophylaxis against mumps	*Adults and children:* 0.5 ml SC (same dose is used for all ages) Do *not* administer IV	Injectable: Single-dose vial of lyophilized vaccine with disposable syringe containing diluent The usual color of the vaccine is pink to red May exhibit some color change if shipped in dry ice When reconstituted, Mumpsvax's color is generally yellow Acceptable to administer if crystal clear and pink, red, or yellow in color Use *only* the diluent supplied for reconstitution; use as soon as possible after reconstitution (discard after 8 hr) Protect from light at all times Keep refrigerated at 2°-8° C	*Contraindicated* during pregnancy, in patients with dysgammaglobulinemia or hypogammaglobulinemia, in patients receiving immunosuppressive agents (corticosteroids, irradiation, antineoplastic agents), in patients with acute active infection, or in patients with blood dyscrasias, leukemia, lymphomas, or malignant neoplasms affecting bone marrow or lymphoid system Provides continuing protection against mumps for at least 10 years after immunization Warn patient that there may be pain at the site of injection and fever	

					May cause temporary depression of TB skin test Administer TB skin test either before or simultaneously with mumps vaccine The vaccine is of particular value in susceptible patients approaching puberty and in adolescents and adults Side effects include tenderness at the injection site, fever, and parotitis (rare) Acetaminophen can be used to treat the fever Defer vaccination for at least 3 months following blood or plasma transfusion or administration of immune serum globulin (human)	*Contraindicated* in children over 6 years of age and in adults *Contraindicated* in patients with brain damage or in children with fever or acute infections Convulsions after DPT are thought to be caused by the pertussis component; no further pertussis should be given in this instance May cause severe alteration of consciousness, focal neurologic signs, screaming episodes, cardiovascular collapse, and thrombocytopenia purpura (rare) May cause fever Fever may be treated with acetaminophen	Observe for signs of seizures, or altered state of consciousness Have parents report any unusual behavior immediately
Pertussis vaccine	Used prophylactically to immunize against pertussis (whooping cough)	*2 months to 6 years:* 1 ml at 4-8 week intervals SC in upper arm near insertion of the deltoid muscle for 3 doses; a reinforcing fourth dose should be given 1 year after completion of initial course and a booster on entering school (5 to 6 years of age) Pertussis vaccine is *not* administered to anyone over 6 years of age	Injectable: 1 ml ampule Also available as combination in DPT Keep refrigerated 2°-8° C Shake vial vigorously before administering each dose		

Continued.

NURSING DRUG DIGEST—cont'd

Medication (trade name)	Indication	Usual dosage and administration	Dosage forms, preparation, and storage	Contraindications, cautions, and comments	Monitoring
★ **Plague vaccine**	Prophylaxis against plague Administer only when patient has definite knowledge of potential contact with rodents and fleas in infested areas	*Adults and children over 10 years:* For primary immunization give two 0.5 ml doses 4 or more weeks apart Give a third dose of 0.2 ml 4 to 12 weeks after the second injection *Children under 10 years:* Give reduced dosage as follows: infants younger than 1 year give 0.1 ml, 1-4 years give 0.2 ml, 5-10 years give 0.3 ml with booster doses of 0.1 to 0.2 ml All doses are given IM	Injectable: 20 ml vials with 2 billion killed plague bacilli per ml Keep refrigerated	*Contraindicated* in acute infections and in patients receiving immunosuppressives Side effects include fever, myalgia, pain at the injection site, and lymphadenopathy	Monitor for hypersensitivity
Poliomyelitis vaccine, inactivated (IPV, Salk)	Prophylaxis against poliomyelitis (polio vaccine of choice for individuals with immunodeficiency and their household contacts)	*Adults and children:* Initial series, 3 doses of 1 ml each SC near the insertion of the deltoid muscle at 4-6 week intervals; a fourth dose is given 6-12 months after the third dose; booster series, 1 ml SC every 5 years	Injectable: 1, 10 ml Solution should be clear and cherry-red Store between 2-8° C Do *not* freeze	*Contraindicated* in acute infections, including respiratory infections Use with caution in patients hypersensitive to neomycin or streptomycin, and in pregnant patients Side effects are rare May cause erythema and tenderness at injection site Have epinephrine injection (1:1000) available Efficacy of boosters has not been clearly established	
Poliovirus vaccine, live oral (TOPv, Sabin) Orimune	Prophylaxis against poliomyelitis	*Infants:* First dose given PO at 2 months of age, and second and third at 8-week intervals thereafter (three doses total); a fourth dose is given at 15-18 months of age; *oral use only*	0.5 ml single-dose disposable pipette Must be stored in freezer compartment Thaw before use May be thawed and refrozen a maximum of 10 times Keep at refrigerated temperature during periods of thaw	*Contraindicated* in patients with impaired immunity (e.g., patients receiving corticosteroids or anticancer drugs or on irradiation); patients with dysgammaglobulinemias, lymphomas, or leukemia	

	Action	Dosage	Supply/Storage	Remarks
		Children and adolescents: Give first two doses PO at 6-8-week intervals; give the third 8-12 months after second dose; all children who completed the series should receive a booster dose at 4-6 years of age. *Not for parenteral use*	Cumulative periods of thaw should not exceed 24 hr; if exceeds 24 hr, must use within 30 days. Once opened must be used within 7 days	Usually used as the trivalent (Sabin strains types 1, 2, and 3) form; also available in monovalent form for use in epidemics of a particular strain. Advise parent (patient) to keep record of immunizations received. Ask patient if has diarrheal illness; if so, do not administer. Side effects are rare. Paralytic disease has been reported in patients receiving the vaccine and in some instances in persons who were in close contact with the patient who had been immunized (risk is about one chance per million doses)
Polyvalent pneumococcal vaccine Pneumovax 23 Pnu-Imune 23	Prophylaxis against *Pneumococcus* infection	*Children over 2 years and adults:* 0.5 ml SC or IM (deltoid or thigh muscle); detectable antibody levels remain for approximately 5 to 8 yr. *Do not administer IV*	Injectable: 0.5, 2.5 ml vial. Store vials in refrigerator at 2°-8° C	*Contraindicated* in febrile respiratory illnesses, hypersensitivity, active infection, pregnancy, children under 2 years of age. Side effects include local erythema and soreness at the injection site. Have epinephrine injection (1:1000) available

Continued.

NURSING DRUG DIGEST—cont'd

Medication (trade name)	Indication	Usual dosage and administration	Dosage forms, preparation, and storage	Contraindications, cautions, and comments	Monitoring
Rabies immune globulin, human (RIG) Hyperab Imogam	Postexposure rabies prophylaxis	*Children and adults:* 20 IU/kg IM administered *once* at the beginning of rabies treatment Infiltrate one half of this around the wound Do *not* administer IV	Injectable: 300 units/2 ml, 1500 units/10 ml vials Store at 2°–8° C	*Contraindicated in* hypersensitivity Use as soon as possible after rabies exposure Use with the usual 21 or 14 doses of rabies vaccine, *or* with the usual 5 doses of human diploid cell rabies vaccine This preparation is preferred over equine antirabies serum Wound should be thoroughly cleansed with soapy water and rinsed with 70% isopropyl alcohol before infiltration with RIG	
Rabies vaccine (duck embryo)	Prophylaxis against rabies, preexposure and postexposure (*not* recommended if human diploid cell rabies vaccine is available)	*Adults and children:* For immunoprophylaxis give two 1 ml doses SC; give a booster in 6 or 7 months Postexposure immunoprophylaxis, give 14 daily injections IM; when given with rabies immune globulin or antiserum, give 21 doses; two extra doses should be given 10 and 20 days after completion of 21-day course Rotate SC injection sites so each new injection is in a different site	Injectable: Single-dose vial of vaccine (dry powder) with one ampule of sterile water for injection as diluent per package Keep refrigerated between 2° and 8° C	*Contraindicated in* hypersensitivity Side effects include local reactions, especially tenderness at the injection site, regional lymphadenopathy, allergic reactions including urticaria and (rare) anaphylaxis Have epinephrine ready in case of allergic reaction Use caution in patients with a history of allergy, especially to chicken, duck eggs, or protein Severe abdominal distress with nausea and vomiting may occur within a few minutes of injection If CNS side effects occur, discontinue vaccine injections	Observe for neurologic side effects of the vaccine

Drug	Uses	Dosage and route	Administration	Contraindications/side effects
Rubella virus vaccine, live Meruvax II	Prophylaxis against rubella	*Adults and children:* (same dose for all ages) 0.5 ml SC; Do *not* inject IV	Injectable: Single-dose vial of lyophilized vaccine with disposable syringe containing diluent; Protect from light at all times; Refrigerate at 2°-8° C; Use only diluent supplied for reconstitution; Discard if not used within 8 hr of reconstitution; Color: may administer if crystal clear and pink, red, or yellow; Combinations of rubella virus vaccine with live measles and mumps virus vaccines are available	*Contraindicated* in hypersensitivity to neomycin; *Contraindicated* in pregnancy; In postpubertal females pregnancy must be ruled out before administration, and pregnancy prevented for 3 months after vaccination; *Contraindicated* in patients receiving immunosuppressive agents (corticosteroids, irradiation, antineoplastics), in patients with active, acute infections, or in patients with blood dyscrasias, malignant neoplasms, leukemia, lymphomas affecting bone marrow or lymphatic systems, and patients with immunodeficiencies; Side effects include fever, rash induration, erythema, and tenderness at the injection site; transient arthritis-like symptoms, arthralgia, polyneuralgia, and polyneuritis may occur within 2 months after immunization; incidence of adverse effects increases with age and may be higher in women; Ask patient if pregnant or receiving any corticosteroids, irradiation, or antineoplastics before administering vaccine

Continued.

NURSING DRUG DIGEST—cont'd

Medication (trade name)	Indication	Usual dosage and administration	Dosage forms, preparation, and storage	Contraindications, cautions, and comments	Monitoring
★ **Smallpox vaccine** Dryvax	Smallpox vaccination is justified only for investigators who are at special risk The World Health Organization has recommended cessation of smallpox vaccination (except for investigators) and discontinuation of international vaccination certificates for travelers	*Adults:* 0.01 ml with multiple puncture technique Inspect the site 6 to 8 days after vaccination A primary vaccination that is successful should show the typical smallpox lesion appearance	Injectable: Combination package (for 25 vaccinations) 1 vial dried vaccine, 1 container diluent, and 25 bifurcated needles Available from Centers for Disease Control, Atlanta, Georgia (403-329-3356)	*Contraindicated* in: patients with eczema or other skin conditions, wounds, or burns (and for siblings or other household contacts of such patients), patients receiving immunosuppressive drugs such as corticosteroids or antimetabolites, patients with leukemia, lymphomas, or other malignant neoplasms, and in pregnancy Rarely encephalomyelitis or generalized vaccinia occurs Patient should be cautioned not to touch the site because accidental spread may occur	Examine patient carefully for signs of skin conditions such as eczema (should never be given to these patients) Inspect vaccination site in 6 to 8 days for presence of a jennerian vesicle (if present, indicates successful vaccination)
Tetanus immune globulin, human (TIGH) Homo-Tet Hu-Tet Hyper-Tet Tet-Conn-G	For prophylaxis of patients with wounds contaminated with *Clostridium tetani* A passive immunization; use if patient has received less than two immunizing doses of tetanus toxoid, if the wound is unattended for more than 24 hr, or if the history of immunization is uncertain	*Adults and children:* Prophylaxis: 250 units as a single dose IM	Injectable: 250 unit vials or prefilled syringes	A gamma globulin preparation, so may cause pain and erythema at injection site Active immunization with tetanus toxoid should be used concomitantly in a different site and syringe Use if patient has received fewer than two immunizing doses of tetanus toxoid, if the wound was unattended for more than 24 hr, or if the history of immunization is uncertain	

	Dose	Form / Storage	Precautions / Contraindications
	Adults: Treatment: usual dose 3000-5000 units IM. *Do not* administer IV		The wound should be thoroughly cleansed with soapy water and rinsed with 70% iso-propyl alcohol
Tetanus toxoid Tri-Immunol* Triogen* — Prophylaxis for tetanus (*Clostridium tetani*). Used prophylactically for wound management in patients not completely immunized	*Adults and children not previously immunized:* 0.5 ml for 3 injections, IM or SC. The second injection is given 4-6 weeks after the first, and the third injection is given 6 months to 1 year after the second; give booster every 10 years	Injectable: Fluid and adsorbed forms: 0.5 ml pre-filled disposable syringes and 5 ml vial. Keep in refrigerator	*Contraindicated* in fever or acute infections. Generally given in combination with diphtheria toxoid and pertussis vaccine for primary immunization in infants and children. For primary immunization in adults TD (tetanus and diphtheria toxoids adsorbed for adult use) or tetanus toxoid alone may be used. Side effects are rare. Only some redness, induration, tenderness at the injection site (more common in persons over 25 years of age). Anaphylaxis may occur when multiple injections have inadvertently been administered within a few years
Typhoid vaccine — Prophylaxis against typhoid. Recommended for patients exposed to a carrier in the household or subject to unusual exposure because of occupation or travel	*Children 6 months to 10 years:* Two 0.25 ml doses 4 or more weeks apart, or 3 doses at weekly intervals SC. *Adults and children over 10 years:* Two 0.5 ml doses SC 4 or more weeks apart, or 3 doses at weekly intervals	Injectable: 5, 10, 20 ml vials with 8 units/ml. Store at 2°-8° C	*Contraindicated* if patient is acutely ill or has a chronic debilitating disease. Side effects include erythema and tenderness at the injection site, malaise, myalgia, headache, and fever

Continued.

NURSING DRUG DIGEST—cont'd

Medication (trade name)	Indication	Usual dosage and administration	Dosage forms, preparation, and storage	Contraindications, cautions, and comments	Monitoring
★ **Typhus vaccine**	For prophylaxis of louse-borne (epidemic) typhus	*Adults and children over 10 years:* Given in two doses SC at 4-week intervals Booster SC if needed at 6- to 12-month intervals NOTE: Because of the different methods of preparation, the adult dose for the Lederle product is 0.5 ml, and the adult dose for the Lilly product is 1.0 ml Children under 10 years receive one half of the adult dose	Injectable: 1 ml vial (Lederle) and 2 ml vial (Lilly)	*Contraindicated* in patients highly allergic to eggs Sensitivity testing required *before* use Do not use this vaccine if patient is acutely ill or has a chronic debilitating disease May cause stinging sensation at site of injection Take a careful allergy history from patient before administration Keep epinephrine ready in case of anaphylaxis Doublecheck brand and dosage use (see NOTE in Usual Dosage and Administration)	
Varicella-zoster immune globulin (VZIG)	Prevention or amelioration of varicella in susceptible immunocompromised children exposed to varicella and in neonates whose mothers develop a chickenpox rash within 5 days prepartum or postpartum	*Children:* 0-10 kg, 125 units deep IM; 10-20 kg, 250 units IM; 20-30 kg, 375 units IM; 30-40 kg, 500 units IM; 40+ kg, 625 units IM Administer *first* dose as soon as possible after exposure (after 4 days, the value of VZIG is uncertain) A *second* dose is recommended after 4 weeks for patients with continued or repeated exposure Administer by deep IM injection in the gluteal muscle, or in another large healthy muscle (e.g., vastus lateralis) when the gluteal site is contraindicated No more than 1.25 ml may be given at a single site to patients less than 10 kg; no more than 2.5 ml may be given at a single site to patients more than 10 kg For *IM injection only*	Injectable: 125 units/2.5 ml vial Available from various Red Cross Blood Service Centers in both the United States (617-449-0773) and Canada (416-923-6692) Store between 2° and 8° C	*Contraindicated* in severe thrombocytopenia and hypersensitivity to human serum immune globulin Adverse side effects are generally mild and transient Pain and irritation may occur at the injection site	Observe for allergic response (rare)

★ Yellow fever vaccine YF-Vax	Prophylaxis against yellow fever. Used for individuals 6 months of age or older who are traveling to or living in countries in which yellow fever is endemic. Also used for laboratory personnel exposed to yellow fever virus	*Adults and children over 6 mo:* 0.5 ml SC of reconstituted vaccine. Revaccinate every 10 years if necessary. Do *not* administer within 1 month of other live virus vaccines	Injectable: 1-, 5-, 20-, 100-, and 200-*dose* vials. Keep refrigerated below 5° C (frozen if possible) until reconstituted. Use only supplied diluent. Shake vial well *before* withdrawing dose. Once reconstituted use within 1 hr	*Contraindicated* in individuals allergic to eggs. Side effects include headache, myalgia, or low-grade fever. Symptoms are usually mild. Question patient carefully about possible allergy to eggs. Keep epinephrine ready in case of anaphylaxis. Because this is a live virus vaccine it should *not* be used in patients with dysgammaglobulinemia, or those receiving corticosteroids, antineoplastic, or immunosuppressive drugs

BIBLIOGRAPHY

A Guide to Immunization for Canadians. (2nd ed.). Health Protection Branch, Laboratory Centre for Disease Control, Ottawa: Minister of Supply and Services Canada, 1984.

Austrian, R. A reassessment of pneumococcal vaccine. *The New England Journal of Medicine,* 1984, *310*(10), 651-653.

Breman, J.G., & Arita, I. The confirmation and maintenance of smallpox eradication. *The New England Journal of Medicine,* 1980, *303,* 1263-1273.

Committee on Infectious Diseases. Expanded guidelines for use of varicella-zoster immune globulin. *Pediatrics,* 1983, *72*(6), 886-889.

Conner, C.S. Literature analysis influenza vaccine for 1981-1982. *Drug Intelligence and Clinical Pharmacy,* 1981, *15,* 913.

Devriendt, J., et al. Fatal encephalitis apparently due to rabies: occurrence after treatment with human diploid cell vaccine but not rabies immune globulin. *Journal of the American Medical Association,* 1982, *248,* 2304-2306.

Feng, C.S. An immunization program for the geriatric patient. *Geriatrics,* 1982, *37*(10), 78-84.

Furste, W., & Aguirre, A. Preventing tetanus. *American Journal of Nursing,* 1978, *78*(5), 834-837.

Gurevich, I. Viral hepatitis. *American Journal of Nursing,* 1983, *83*(4), 571-586.

Hayman, L.L. Varicella. *Nursing 83,* 1983, *13*(4), 41.

Hepatitis B vaccine. *The Medical Letter on Drugs and Therapeutics,* 1982, *24*(616), 75.

Hook, E.W. Typhoid fever today. *The New England Journal of Medicine,* 1984, *310*(2), 116-118.

Lawrence, C., & Summerly, M. Keloid formation after BCG vaccination. *Practitioner,* 1982, *226,* 326-328.

Levine, M., & Jones, M. Toxic reaction to phenytoin following a viral infection. *Canadian Medical Association Journal,* 1983, *128,* 1270-1271.

Morbidity and Mortality Weekly Report, 29 February 1980, 87.

Morbidity and Mortality Weekly Report, 22 February 1980, 76.

Nichols, A.O. Taking the fear out of rabies treatment. *Nursing 83,* 1983, *13*(6), 42-43.

Varicella-zoster immune globulin. *The Medical Letter on Drugs and Therapeutics,* 1982, *24*(610), 51-52.

White, M.J. Rabies update. *Nursing 80,* 1980, *10*(8), 53.

CHAPTER 69

Venom Allergenic Extracts, Antivenins, and Antitoxins

Karin E. Zenk

Medications discussed in this chapter

Venom allergic extracts	**Antivenins—cont'd**
Hymenoptera venom allergenic extracts (bee venom, yellow jacket, yellow hornet, white faced hornet, wasp)	North American coral snake *(Micrurus fulvius)* antivenin
	Polyvalent Crotalidae antivenin
Antivenins	**Antitoxins**
Black widow spider *(Lactrodectus mactans)* antivenin	Botulism antitoxin
	Diphtheria antitoxin
	Tetanus antitoxin

This chapter discusses a variety of miscellaneous agents that are physiologically and therapeutically related to the serums, toxoids, and vaccines discussed in Chapter 68. Specifically, *venom allergenic extracts, antivenins,* and *antitoxins* are discussed in this chapter. Venom allergenic extracts (e.g., *Hymenoptera* venom allergenic extracts) are an extract of the protein of any substance to which a human may be sensitive. They are used for the diagnosis or the desensitization therapy *(immunotherapy)* in conditions caused by hypersensitivity. Antivenins are proteinaceous materials used to treat venom poisoning. Like antitoxins, some antivenins such as black widow spider antivenin, polyvalent crotaline antivenin, and North American coral snake antivenin, contain antibodies and are used only therapeutically to treat envenomation. Antitoxins are serums given to neutralize certain toxins (e.g., diphtheria toxin). Antitoxic serums are formed in the bodies of animals (usually horses) that have been actively immunized by a specific toxin.

VENOM ALLERGENIC EXTRACTS

Hymenoptera is an order of insects having four membranous wings (e.g., bees, wasps, and ants). Stings or bites from these insects cause approximately 50 deaths annually in North America. Venom allergens are contained in the antivenin product Hymenoptera venom allergenic extracts, specifically Hymenoptera venom protein allergens of the honeybee, yellow jacket, yellow hornet, white-faced hornet, and wasp. This product is used either prophylactically to desensitize highly susceptible patients or to diagnose hypersensitivity. In the event of a positive sensitivity test, a great risk of anaphylaxis exists if further doses of the agent are used. With desensitization, small, incrementally increased doses of the agent (allergen) are injected, allowing the patient to build up an immunity. With one therapeutic regimen, serial injections of diluted agent (antitoxin or antivenin) are made at 15-minute intervals, provided no reaction occurs. If a reaction occurs after an injection, no dose is administered for 1 hour and then the last dose that failed to cause a reaction is repeated. This is then followed by maintenance doses.

The allergenic extracts should be used *only* by a clinician who is experienced in administering allergens after an allergy consultation because of the possibility of severe anaphylactic reactions. Use these preparations only where full emergency resuscitative equipment is available. Epinephrine should be available and drawn up in the appropriate dose. The patient should be observed for a period of time (usually 1 hour) in the office or clinical area after receiving these treatments, the length of time depending on the time the patient has been on the current dose and on the increase in dosage the patient has just received.

When receiving these treatments, the patient should be advised of the risk in taking these injections (i.e., that severe allergic reactions may occur, such as anaphylaxis). Patients on venom immunotherapy should be instructed how to self-administer epinephrine subcutaneously and to carry an emergency epinephrine kit during the Hymenoptera season, even while receiving venom immunotherapy. One such commercially available kit, Ana-Kit, contains two

0.3 ml doses of epinephrine in a preloaded syringe.

Even after reaching the maintenance dose, the patient may have some reaction when being stung. Because patients differ in their sensitivity to injections and treatment schedules, increases in doses must be individualized. If the patient has a local swelling or local reaction to an injection, the subsequent dose should be reduced.

Allergic response

Manifestations of allergic response to the allergenic extracts may occur in up to 30% of treated patients and include the following: large, painful swelling at the site of the injection; urticaria; itching; edema; flushing of the face, neck, or upper chest; bronchospasm; laryngeal edema; hypotension; GI complaints; fever; chills; lightheadedness; headache; persistent sneezing; dyspnea; cyanosis; tachycardia; perspiration; and wheezing. If a reaction occurs, a tourniquet should be applied to the extremity above the site of administration. The tourniquet should be removed every 10 to 15 minutes. Epinephrine should be administered. Severe shock reactions may require volume expansion, pressor agents, oxygen, and other resuscitative measures.

ANTIVENINS

An antivenin is a proteinaceous material used to treat venom poisoning. Black widow spider, polyvalent crotaline, and North American coral snake antivenins are used only therapeutically. They should be administered as soon as possible after the envenomation occurs. Hospitals located in areas where envenomation poses a hazard should carry an adequate supply of these products so that they may be immediately available, with expiration dates checked, when a patient is admitted. An antivenin is generally administered intravenously. Epinephrine injection should be on hand while sensitivity tests are performed or when the antivenin is administered.

Snake antivenins

The two major families of venomous snakes in North America are the pit vipers (Crotalidae) and the coral snakes (Elapidae). Of these the pit vipers are responsible for the vast majority of poisonous snakebites.

The pit viper group includes the rattlesnake, the copperhead, and the cottonmouth, or water moccasin. These snakes have a pit between the eye and the nostril, from which the pit viper derives its name. This pit is a heat receptor organ.

The coral snake *(Micrurus fulvius)* is found in the southeastern part of the United States.

Not all persons bitten by snakes are poisoned. The bite may have been by a nonpoisonous snake or the bite may have been by a poisonous snake, but the venom may not have been injected, or it may have been injected in too small an amount to cause poisoning symptoms. Therefore, an antivenin need not be given in all cases of snakebite. The term *envenomation* refers to cases in which the injection of the venom has occurred, and the term *snakebite* refers to bites by snakes, whether venomous or not.

Signs of envenomation

Persons who have been envenomated typically show signs of hemotoxicity and neurotoxicity. The symptoms depend on which of the two types of toxin predominates in the venom. All snake venoms may produce deleterious changes in several organ systems because they may contain 5 to 15 enzymes, 3 to 12 nonenzymatic proteins, plus various peptides and other substances.

Hemotoxicity. The pit viper venom contains hemotoxins (cytolysins) that cause the enzymatic destruction of cell walls and tissues. Hemolysis results, producing hemorrhage into vital organs. Thus, a person envenomated by a rattlesnake may have blood in the urine or bleeding from the mouth, nose, and gastrointestinal tract. These hemotoxins cause marked local swelling with pain, necrosis, discoloration, and hemorrhage at the site of the bite. In addition, tissue changes, which are caused by certain cytolytic proteins, chiefly enzymes, are the most dramatic manifestation of North American Crotalid venoms.

Neurotoxicity. Neurotoxicity, as produced by the coral snake, produces symptoms such as weakness and paralysis of the muscles of the mouth and the throat, and then paralysis of the muscles of respiration. The patient may be drowsy, have difficulty in breathing and swallowing, have a slow, weak pulse, ptosis (drooping of the eyelids), muscular pain, and weakness. Symptoms may progress to trismus (lockjaw), nausea, vomiting, coma, and eventually respiratory and cardiac failure. Convulsions may occur. In contrast to the pit viper poisoning, coral snake poisoning is *not* characterized by severe local pain, swelling, or local necrosis, and the onset of symptoms may be delayed for up to 10 to 12 hours following the bite. Neurotoxic symptoms resulting from pit viper envenomation include a tingling or numbness over the tongue, mouth, scalp, fingers, and toes, and around the wound. Vertigo, neuropathic muscle cramping, or paralysis with generalized weakness may occur.

Snakebites have occurred during pregnancy and may result in teratogenesis or abortion. The pathophysiologic mechanisms that account for the toxicity to the fetus include: (1) anoxia associated with shock following envenomation, (2) hemorrhages into the placenta and vascular uterine wall, and (3) uterine contractions caused by the venom. Delay in treatment, early gestation, and severe envenomation suggest an unfavorable outcome of the pregnancy. The administration of an antivenin neutralizes the venom and stops venom-induced uterine contractions.

Treatment of envenomation

The treatment of envenomation consists of emergency first aid followed by the use of an antivenin. Other medical and nursing treatments include using antibiotics (if signs of an infection appear); caring for the wound; supporting the patient's respiratory, circulatory, and hematologic systems; relieving the patient's pain and anxiety; treating serum sickness; and rehabilitating the patient using physical therapy to prevent contractures and deformities. Treatments *not* recommended are placing ice on the extremity, or packing it with ice, and fasciotomies. Freezing exacerbates the vascular and tissue damage. Several patients whose injured limbs had been packed in ice for 6 to 9 days had to have these limbs amputated because of cryotherapy, *not* because of venom poisoning. Fasciotomy, or making a deep cut in the edematous tissue, is not recommended because the damage done to the tissue in this way does not repair well and often leaves the patient with restricted movement of the extremity and severe scarring. The use of an antivenin alone usually results in a reduction of the edema and a much better outcome.

Antivenin therapy is the most important agent responsible for the decrease in fatalities from snake envenomation. First aid does *not* take the place of antivenin therapy. The purpose of the antivenin is to neutralize the venom at the local wound site before it can be absorbed into the general circulation. Local tissue reaction and survival are functions of the time between envenomation and antivenin administration. The antivenin should be diluted and administered intravenously by drip infusion under the supervision of a skilled clinician because an anaphylactic reaction to the horse serum or serum sickness may occur. Serum sickness is a delayed adverse reaction to horse serum manifested by lymphadenopathy, polyarthritis, and fever. This systemic reaction occurs several days after administration and is largely related to the amount of the horse serum administered, the hypersensitivity of

the patient, and the history of previous serum injection. The incidence of serum sickness with modern enzyme-treated serum is about 5% to 10%, and the syndrome occurs more commonly after the largest dose.

The antivenin may also be administered intramuscularly if it is necessary to use it in the field. Injecting antivenin into the wound site is generally *not* beneficial.

Polyvalent Crotalidae antivenin. Crotalidae antivenin is called polyvalent because it is used for treating several types of snake venoms: *Crotalus atrox, C. adamanteus, C. d. terrificus,* and *Bothrops atrox.* Because pit viper venoms share common *antigens,* it is possible to manufacture an antivenin that protects against the venoms of most species of pit vipers.

This mixture of four venoms is modified with formalin and mixed with aluminum hydroxide gel to prolong its adsorption into tissues. It is then injected into horses over a period of several weeks in gradually increasing doses as an immunity is built up. Blood is then withdrawn from the horses, and the cells are separated from the serum. The serum contains the horse's antibodies to the snake venoms and can be used to protect humans by passive immunity. The serum is refined, purified, standardized, freeze dried, and stored in vials. It is standardized by its ability to neutralize the toxic action of a standard venom tested by intravenous injection into mice.

The unreconstituted powder should be stored at a temperature not exceeding 37° C and kept from freezing. Properly reconstituted under sterile conditions, it should be stable for several hours providing it is stored in a refrigerator at 2° to 8° C.

Severity of viper poisoning. The grades of poisoning depend on the degree of the severity of the pit viper poisoning.

Grade 0. This is from the bite of a known venomous snake but no symptoms have occurred.

Grade I. In grade I, minimal envenomation has occurred. The patient has moderate pain, no systemic symptoms, and not more than a few centimeters or inches of swelling from edema.

Grade II. Grade II is moderate envenomation. It has the early signs of Grade I poisoning, but soon has more severe and widely dispersed pain, with progressing edema involving about half the distance between the bite site and the trunk; the regional lymph nodes are palpable and tender. Nausea, vomiting, and giddiness are usually present. Petechiae and ecchymoses are restricted to the area of the edema. There may be a fall in the hematocrit.

Grade III. Grade III is severe envenomation. On admission the patient's symptoms may resemble grades I or II, but intoxication is progressive. These patients may exhibit shock within a few minutes of the time of the injury. The edematous area extends to or involves part of the trunk. Petechiae and ecchymoses are commonly generalized in distribution. During the first 12 hours of therapy the pulse becomes rapid and thready, the temperature becomes subnormal, and the patient approaches a state of shock.

Grade IV. Grade IV is very severe. Sudden pain and rapidly spreading edema, marked local reaction with blister formation, and severe edema occur, which if obstructive to venous or arterial blood flow may result in gangrene or function loss. Systemic symptoms occur in a few minutes with signs of shock. There may be blood-tinged excretions, renal shutdown, hepatic or cardiovascular damage, and convulsions (especially in children). Coma and death may ensue within 30 minutes of the bite.

Dosage. The dose of antivenin depends on the severity of symptoms (Table 69-1).

In addition to the use of first aid, antivenin, antibiotics and analgesics, tetanus prophylaxis (see Chapter 68, "Serums, Toxoids, and Vaccines") is important in snakebite. Tetanus is a preventable disease. Prophylaxis should be ensured in all persons bitten by snakes. If the patient's immunization status is not known, generally administer human tetanus immune globulin 250 units intramuscularly immediately. Give tetanus toxoid in a separate syringe in a separate site.

TABLE 69-1

Antivenin dosing

Grade of poisoning	Envenomation	Dosage
Grade 0	No envenomation	No antivenin is given
Grade I	Minimal envenomation	1 to 5 vials (10 to 50 ml)
Grade II	Moderate envenomation	5 to 9 vials (50 to 90 ml)
Grade III	Severe envenomation	At least 9 vials and up to 15 vials (90 to 150 ml)

NOTE: Children require relatively larger doses of antivenin than adults because they receive more milligrams of toxin per kilogram of body weight

Patients who have had a basic series of tetanus immunizations and have had a booster in the past 5 years do *not* need an injection. Those who have had their basic immunization series but who have not had a booster in the last 5 years should be given 0.5 ml of fluid tetanus toxoid. Snake's mouths do not harbor *Clostridium tetani*, the organism that causes tetanus; however, the organism is carried into the wound by the fang puncture from dirt on the skin or from nonsterile first aid techniques.

ANTITOXINS

Antitoxins are serums (see Chapter 68) that are administered to neutralize certain toxins (e.g., diphtheria toxin). Antitoxic serums are formed in the bodies of animals, usually horses, that have been actively immunized by a specific toxin. Because these products are derived from animal serum, the possibility of both acute anaphylaxis and delayed serum sickness must be monitored for in patients receiving these medications. The nurse should also see that epinephrine (1:1000) is immediately available and should be able to intervene appropriately in any anticipated emergency.

The antitoxins commonly used in clinical practice are botulism antitoxin, diphtheria antitoxin, and tetanus antitoxin. These agents provide a passive immunity to the recipient against the specific toxin. Botulism antitoxin is administered to patients who have ingested contaminated or suspected food for both the prevention and treatment of botulism. Likewise, diphtheria antitoxin is administered for the prevention and treatment of diphtheria. Tetanus antitoxin also is used for prevention and treatment; however, it should *only* be used if tetanus immune globulin (human) is not available because of the significantly greater risk of anaphylaxis and serum sickness associated with its use.

SUMMARY

This chapter has discussed the venom allergenic extracts, antivenins, and antitoxins. These agents are used to desensitize patients and to treat poisoning caused by venoms and toxins. The major danger of therapy is associated with allergic or hypersensitivity reactions.

With an understanding of the use, action, administration, adverse side effects, and monitoring of these agents, the nurse will be better able to provide optimum therapy to patients who require venom allergenic extracts, antivenins, or antitoxins.

ADVERSE/SIDE EFFECTS OF VENOM ALLERGENIC EXTRACTS, ANTIVENINS AND ANTITOXINS*

ALLERGIC REACTIONS

Anaphylaxis
Angioedema
Dyspnea
Hoarseness
Lacrimation
Pruritus
Sneezing
Urticaria
Wheezing

CENTRAL NERVOUS SYSTEM

Malaise

CUTANEOUS SYSTEM

Induration at injection site
Redness at injection site
Tenderness at injection site

GASTROINTESTINAL SYSTEM

Abdominal pain

MUSCULOSKELETAL SYSTEM

Arthralgia
Arthritis-like symptoms
Myalgia

*See Chapter 11, "Drug Toxicity," for an overview of drug toxicity.

CLINICALLY SIGNIFICANT DRUG INTERACTIONS*

Primary drug	*Interacting drug*	*Possible effect(s)*	*Probable mechanism(s)*
Antivenins and antitoxins, horse serum (sensitivity test)	Antihistamines	Masking of allergic response	Reduction or blocking of allergic response by antihistamine

*Clinically significant drug interactions involving these agents have not been reported, except for the interaction noted above. However, the nurse should monitor for other possible drug interactions, particularly in relation to patients receiving immunosuppressives. See Chapter 10, "Drug Interactions," for an overview of drug interactions.

GENERAL NURSING IMPLICATIONS

Nursing of patients requiring venom allergenic extracts, antivenins, or antitoxins

ASSESSMENT

Patients requiring venom allergenic extracts, antivenins, or antitoxins should have a general health assessment, including an assessment aimed directly at the need for the specific preparation. The general assessment should include a history of an allergy, especially to horse serum, and a history of immunotherapy or previous horse serum injection. Patients requiring venom allergenic extracts or antivenins should be assessed for an immediate reaction associated with the sting or bite, and emergency measures that have been obtained or given should be identified. For snakebites, a history of the bite and a description of the snake should be included, as well as an identification of the geographic area where the bite occurred. The site of the snakebite should be carefully inspected and the patient should be assessed for hemotoxic or neurotoxic signs as indicated. Patients bitten by pit vipers should be assessed

for signs indicating the class of envenomation (e.g., grade of poisoning: 0, I, II, III, or IV). This information is important in dose selection and monitoring.

Women of childbearing age should be questioned regarding the possibility of pregnancy because some snakebites resulting in envenomation can cause adverse teratogenic effects. An immunization history for tetanus should also be obtained.

Patients requiring antitoxins should likewise be carefully assessed for signs of toxin effects. Patients admitted for botulism should be assessed for GI and other complaints, as well as for the onset of symptoms and their severity. The fluid and electrolyte status should be assessed. The source of the food contamination, as well as other individuals exposed to the source, should be identified. For other patients requiring selected antitoxins, recent travel or injury

should be identified especially when diphtheria or tetanus is suspected.

The nursing history should include a detailed drug history to identify possible drug interactions, contraindications, cautions, and sensitivity to the use of venom allergenic extracts, antivenins, or antitoxins. Allergic reactions to insect bites or stings, snakebites, injury, or food poisoning can be frightening, and patients and their families often require much support and understanding.

SENSITIVITY

Generally, allergic reactions to venom allergenic extracts, antivenins, and antitoxins are associated with an allergy to the animal source of the preparation (e.g., antivenin, allergy to horses). Because of the great risk of anaphylaxis associated with the use of these agents, epinephrine and emergency equipment should be readily available for use as necessary.

Nursing of patients requiring venom allergenic extracts, antivenins, or antitoxins—cont'd

CONTRAINDICATIONS AND CAUTIONS

These preparations are contraindicated in patients with a known hypersensitivity to a specific agent or any of its components.

DRUG INTERACTIONS

Drug interactions involving these agents have not been reported except for the interaction noted in Clinically Significant Drug Interactions. The nurse should monitor for other possible drug interactions, particularly in relation to patients receiving immunosuppressives.

ADMINISTRATION

Patients requiring *Hymenoptera* venom allergenic extract should have a scratch test or intradermal test before the administration of the preparation. This agent is administered subcutaneously for immunotherapy. With allergenic extracts, doublecheck the dilution before administration. Administering a stronger dilution than ordered may result in a severe allergic reaction.

Antivenins should be administered as soon as possible after envenomation. They are usually administered by intravenous infusion; however, depending on the specific agent, they can also be administered intramuscularly or subcutaneously.

North American coral snake antivenin is administered intravenously, whereas polyvalent crotaline antivenin can be administered subcutaneously, intramuscularly, or intravenously, depending on the severity of the patient's signs and symptoms. The injection of this preparation is usually above the swelling caused by the bite. Black widow spider antivenin is administered intramuscularly or, in severe cases, intravenously, diluted with saline.

Antitoxins, such as diphtheria antitoxin, can be administered either intramuscularly or intravenously. Botulism antitoxin can be administered subcutaneously or intramuscularly. A test for a sensitivity to horse serum should be done before administration.

Antivenins and antitoxins should be administered as soon as possible after the exposure to the toxin. Have the products listed in this chapter on hand at all times and check their expiration dates to be sure a potent antivenin or antitoxin is given.

Observe storage conditions carefully so that an active product is administered.

Inquire about any allergy to horse serum or a history of the previous administration of horse serum.

Have epinephrine ready when administering these agents. The dose of epinephrine in a child is 0.01 ml/kg/dose of the 1:1000 concentration. This is given subcutaneously. If the 1:10,000 concentration is used, the dose is 0.1 ml/kg/dose. The 1:10,000 concentration is available in a prefilled syringe and is given intravenously.

See the Nursing Drug Digest for specific information regarding the administration and storage of these agents.

MONITORING PATIENT RESPONSE
Therapeutic response

Monitor patients for decreased local reactions to the bite, injury, or effect of the toxin, as well as for diminished or absent generalized effects of the bite, sting, injury, or effect of the toxin.

Monitor patients requiring immunotherapy for a decreased sensitivity to the extract.

Adverse side effects

Monitor patients requiring antivenins for major adverse effects associated with the use of these agents, including an allergic reaction (observe and report any allergic-like symptoms such as wheezing, dyspnea, sneezing, hoarseness, tachycardia, GI discomfort, nausea, neck or chest pain, cyanosis, sweating, lacrimation, urticaria, angioedema, or pruritus) or serum sickness.

It is important to note that although a sensitivity can be readily observed, serum sickness may not be observed for 1 to 2 weeks after the injection.

See Adverse/Side Effects of Venom Allergenic Extracts, Antivenins, and Antitoxins for an outline of adverse effects associated with these agents.

PATIENT EDUCATION

The patient and the family, as indicated, should have a clear understanding of the anticipated therapy and the associated risks (e.g., allergic reactions, anaphylaxis) involved with the use of venom allergenic extracts, antivenins, or antitoxins. Patients requiring immunotherapy should understand the importance of following desensitization regimens and should be able to administer epinephrine subcutaneously at home in the event of an emergency associated with a hypersensitivity response to insect stings or bites. These patients should be encouraged to carry an epinephrine kit (e.g., ANA-Kit) during the *Hymenoptera* season. A family member should likewise be taught to recognize the signs of a hypersensitivity reaction and know how to administer epinephrine in an emergency, as well as how to seek appropriate emergency help.

Patients requiring antitoxins for inappropriate food preparation or handling should receive information as indicated to prevent a recurrence of botulism. Patients with an injury may require health education in relation to the prevention of accidents.

GENERAL INSTRUCTIONS FOR DISCHARGE/OUTPATIENTS

VENOM ALLERGENIC EXTRACTS, ANTIVENINS, AND ANTITOXINS

Report any allergic symptoms such as difficulty breathing, rash, itching, swelling, excessive sneezing, chest pain, or nausea.

You may experience fever, tiredness, and pain in your joints in about 7 to 12 days. This is called serum sickness and is a normal reaction that occurs in patients who have received treatment for snakebites; however, you should report these symptoms to your health care provider as soon as they are noted.

The treatment you received for your snakebite (or spiderbite) contained horse serum. If you need to receive a horse serum product in the future, you should advise the health care provider that you have received horse serum in the past and report any reactions you had.

Keep emergency epinephrine kits out of children's reach.

NURSING DRUG DIGEST

Medication (trade name*)	Indication	Usual dosage and administration	Dosage forms, preparation, and storage	Contraindications, cautions, and comments	Monitoring
Botulism antitoxin	Treatment of botulism caused by ingestion of infected food	*Adults:* Prophylactic, not less than 10,000 units types A and B and 1000 units type E, SC or IM Therapeutic, not less than 50,000 units each of types A and B and 5000 units of type E, IM or IV Repeat therapeutic dose q4-12h. IM prn *Persons who have consumed suspected food* and in whom symptoms have not developed should be given not less than 10,000 units each of types A and B and 1000 units of E IM or SC prophylactically	Injectable: Literature supplied with the antitoxin contains this information when obtained from the Centers for Disease Control, Atlanta, Georgia, 30333 Product is not commercially available in the United States, but must be obtained from the CDC Available in types A, B, or E, and as a trivalent ABE combination Store in refrigerator (2°-8° C) Avoid freezing	The antitoxin should be given early in the course of the disease Test for sensitivity to horse serum Have epinephrine available during sensitivity testing to this product, and during administration of the dose because severe allergic reactions may occur, including anaphylaxis Serum sickness may be delayed for 5 to 13 days Until the specific type of botulinus toxin has been identified, it is wise to use the trivalent ABE antitoxin	Monitor patient for hypersensitivity reaction Monitor over 5 to 13 days for signs of serum sickness
Black widow spider (*Lactrodectus mactans*) antivenin	Used to treat envenomation by black widow spider (*Lactrodectus mactans*)	*Adults and children:* Entire contents of one vial (2.5 ml serum) IM (usually the deltoid); may need to repeat in 1-3 hr The volume of injection may be divided into two injections for patients with small deltoid muscle mass, as indicated Dilute in 10-50 ml saline and administer IV over 15 min (use IV *only* in severe cases) *Elderly:* Same as adults Do *not* administer IV in other than severe cases	Injectable: 6000 antivenin units/vial with 2.5 ml sterile water for injection Shake vial to dissolve contents	Earliest possible use of the antivenin is recommended Test for horse serum sensitivity *before* use Have epinephrine ready for allergic reactions	Observe for signs and symptoms of possible anaphylaxis, such as dyspnea, sneezing, hoarseness, tachycardia, GI discomfort, nausea, neck or chest pain, cyanosis, sweating, lacrimation, urticaria, angioedema, and pruritus

Drug	Use	Dosage and Administration	Preparations	Remarks
Diphtheria antitoxin	To treat diphtheria or for prophylaxis in exposed, non-immunized susceptible individuals who are not under close surveillance	*Adults and children:* Prophylaxis, 1000 to 10,000 units IM; repeat in 2 weeks if necessary Treatment, dosage is empiric; 20,000 to 80,000 units or more by slow IV depending on duration of illness, degree of toxicity, and site and size of membrane Active diphtheria immunization with the toxoid should be given at the same time that the diphtheria antitoxin is given Administer diphtheria vaccine in a different site than the antitoxin The entire dose required should be given at one time if possible	Injectable: 10,000, 20,000 units/vial Store between 2°-8° C Do *not* freeze	Appropriate antibiotics, such as penicillin, help eliminate bacteria from the infected sites but are of no value against the toxin Serum sickness (urticaria, fever, pruritus, malaise, arthralgia) may occur in 7 to 12 days This is a product from horse serum; sensitivity testing must be done *before* use Have the appropriate dose of epinephrine drawn up in case of an allergic reaction during the sensitivity testing or during the administration of the antitoxin Monitor for hypersensitivity reactions Monitor for serum sickness
Hymenoptera venom allergenic extracts (bee, yellow jacket, yellow hornet, white-faced hornet, wasp) Pharmalgen Venomil	Used prophylactically to immunize highly susceptible individuals Also used to diagnose hypersensitivity to the stings of these insects	*Immunotherapy:* Administer SC as tolerated Maintenance: 100 µg IM or SC *Diagnostic skin testing:* Scratch test followed by an intradermal test Do *not* administer IV	Injectable: After reconstitution: *Single venom preparation:* 100 µg/ml *Mixed vespid preparation:* 300 µg/ml	*Contraindicated* in acute infections, immune deficiency, bleeding tendencies, and skin test–negative patients May cause systemic anaphylactic reaction Always keep tourniquet, epinephrine, and agents to treat shock and bronchospasm available when using these agents Should include a negative control with diluent and a positive control with histamine to properly interpret wheal and flare reaction if it occurs Anyone receiving these allergens should possess an emergency insect sting treatment kit (ANA-Kit) Observe patient 60 min after injection Observe for signs of possible anaphylaxis, such as dyspnea, sneezing, hoarseness, tachycardia, GI discomfort, chest pain, cyanosis, sweating, urticaria, angioedema, and pruritus

Continued.

NOTE: For additional details regarding the individual agents listed in this table, see the text and other tables in this chapter.
*These products are generally available from manufacturers under their *generic* names.
♦ Indicates that the drug is generally available only in Canada.
★ Indicates that the drug is generally available only in the United States.

NURSING DRUG DIGEST—cont'd

Medication (trade name)	Indication	Usual dosage and administration	Dosage forms, preparation, and storage	Contraindications, cautions, and comments	Monitoring
★ **North American coral snake antivenin (*Micrurus fulvius*)**	To treat bite of North American coral snake	*Adults and children:* 30 to 50 ml antivenin IV. The first 1 or 2 ml should be injected over a 3- to 5-min period with careful observation for allergic reactions. Some patients require 100 ml (10 vials). Rate of infusion is regulated by the severity of the envenomation and the tolerance to the antivenin. Until 30 to 50 ml has been given, administer at the maximum safe rate for IV fluids, based on body weight and the general condition of the patient	Injectable: 10 ml vials. Supplied as one vial of antivenin and one vial of diluent (10 ml bacteriostatic water for injection)	Tetanus prophylaxis is indicated because of a potential for a contaminated puncture wound. This is a horse serum product; therefore, severe allergic reactions, such as an anaphylaxis, may occur. Have the appropriate dose of epinephrine drawn up in case of an allergic reaction during the sensitivity testing or during the administration of the antivenin. Respiratory paralysis can occur; be prepared to assist the patient's ventilation. Serum sickness may occur 7 to 12 days after the dose is administered. The coral snake bite is a neurotoxin	Monitor patients carefully for hypersensitivity reactions. Monitor patients over 1 to 2 weeks for signs of serum sickness
Polyvalent Crotalidae antivenin	Used to treat envenomation by the North American rattlesnake, water moccasin, and copperhead	*Adults:* 1 to 15 or more vials IM, SC, or preferably IV, depending on the severity of the signs and symptoms. *Children:* May require more than adults. *Elderly:* Same dose as adults. If the bite is in an extremity, may inject part of the initial dose into the limb above the swelling—do *not* inject into a finger or a toe	Injectable: Lyophilized powder with diluent (10 ml bacteriostatic water for injection). Reconstitute immediately before administration. Discard unused reconstituted drug	Test for horse serum sensitivity *before* use. Have epinephrine ready for allergic reactions. May cause anaphylaxis. Often causes serum sickness. If the patient is allergic to horse serum, must desensitize the patient before treating with the antivenin	Observe for wheezing dyspnea, sneezing, hoarseness, tachycardia, GI discomfort, nausea, neck or chest pain, cyanosis, sweating, lacrimation, urticaria, angioedema, and pruritus, because these may be the signs and symptoms of anaphylaxis

| ★ Tetanus antitoxin (equine) | Prophylaxis in nonimmunized patients with tetanus-prone wounds, and as part of the therapy in patients with active tetanus

Use *only* if tetanus immune globulin (human) is not available (see Chapter 68, "Serums, Toxoids, and Vaccines") | *Adults and children:* 3000-5000 units within 24 hr after injury, IM
If 48 hr has elapsed give 10,000-20,000 units, IM
IV (preferred for therapy): 40,000-200,000 units or more
Initiate active tetanus immunization at the same time with the tetanus toxoid
Use different syringe and different site for tetanus antitoxin and toxoid | Injectable: 1500, 20,000 unit vial
Store between 2°-8° C | May cause anaphylaxis
Keep epinephrine 1:1000 ready for prompt treatment of any severe reaction
Other side effects are serum sickness (arthralgia, urticaria, fever, malaise) and pain at the injection site | Monitor for hypersensitivity reaction
Monitor for signs of serum sickness |

BIBLIOGRAPHY

Antivenom therapy and reactions. *Reactions*, 1980, 10-11.

Insect venom extracts. *The Medical Letter*, 1980, *22*, 37-38.

Insect venoms. *The Medical Letter*, 1983, *25*, 53-54.

Russell, F.E., Ruzic, N., & Gonzalez, H. Effectiveness of antivenin (Crotalidae) polyvalent following injection of crotalus venom. *Toxicon*, 1973, *11*, 461-464.

Zenk, K.E. Snake envenomation: what the pharmacist should know about successful therapy. *California Pharmacist*, 1976, *24*, 22-26.

Radiopharmaceuticals

Alec Shysh
Leonard I. Wiebe

Medications discussed in this chapter

Radiopharmaceuticals
^{198}Au-Colloidal gold
^{57}Co-Cyanocobolamin
^{51}Cr-Sodium chromate
^{67}Ga-Gallium citrate
^{125}I-Fibrinogen
^{125}I-Human serum albumin
^{131}I-Human serum albumin
^{123}I-Orthoiodohippurate
^{131}I-Orthoiodohippurate
^{131}I-Rose bengal
^{123}I-Sodium iodide
^{131}I-Sodium iodide
^{111}In-Chloride
^{113}In^m-Chloride
^{75}Se-Selenomethionine

Radiopharmaceuticals—cont'd
^{99}Tc^m-Antimony sulfide
^{99}Tc^m-Calcium phytate
^{99}Tc^m-Diphosphonates
^{99}Tc^m-DTPA
^{99}Tc^m-Human serum albumin
^{99}Tc^m-HIDA
^{99}Tc^m-Glucoheptonate
^{99}Tc^m-Labeled RBC
^{99}Tc^{m}Tc-Pyrophosphate
^{99}Tc^m-Sodium pertechnetate
^{99}Tc^m-Sulfur colloid
^{201}Tl-Thallous chloride
^{133}Xe
^{169}Yb-Ytterbium DTPA

This chapter discusses both the diagnostic and therapeutic uses of the radiopharmaceuticals. An overview of the physical structure of radioactive materials, radiation dosimetry, and biology is presented, as well as a discussion of the handling of radioactive materials and devices used with the diagnostic radiopharmaceuticals. Adverse reactions to these agents are described along with the prevention of *radioactive contamination*. The nurse's role in relation to preparing patients for the use of the radiopharmaceuticals and care after or during their use is also described.

RADIOPHARMACEUTICALS

A radiopharmaceutical is a compound containing a radionuclide designed for use in the diagnosis or therapy of various human diseases. A radiopharmaceutical has two main components: (1) the radionuclide, as an integral part of the formula, coupled to (2) the other pharmaceutical ingredients. Because the majority of the radiopharmaceuticals are administered parenterally, usually IV, they must meet the same stringent criteria of quality that are required for conventional medications. In nuclear medicine, the vast majority of these radioactive drugs are used for diagnostic purposes—only about 5% of them are used therapeutically. In diagnostic radiopharmaceuticals, the radioactive label is used as a tracer to provide information about organ structure, physiologic function, or metabolism. Therapeutic radioactive drugs are administered for the purpose of delivering large amounts of radiation to selected body tissues internally, so that the radiations emitted may selectively elicit an effect on living cells.

The diagnostic radiopharmaceuticals differ from conventional pharmaceutical agents in that the radioactive drugs usually have no pharmacologic effect because they are used in tracer quantities such that the amounts of the main ingredient are far below the minimum therapeutic dose. In these cases, the radiopharmaceuticals do not exhibit any conventional dose-response relationships.

The clinical use of a radioactive drug is determined by the characteristics of its two components: (1) the radioactive atoms themselves must possess certain physical properties so that the radiations emitted are compatible with the intended use, and (2) the carrier chemical form that influences the preferential localization in a particular organ or its participation in the physiologic function or metabolism of that organ or tissue.

In a hospital, the radiopharmaceuticals are prepared by a person who has specific training in the field, usually a radiopharmacist. The administration of the radioactive drug and the accompanying test procedures are carried out by specially trained nuclear medicine technologists and physicians or nurses who have expertise in this area. A radiation health officer is responsible for the proper handling and disposal of radioactive material and wastes.

It is important for nurses who are caring for "radioactive" patients to have a general understanding of various radiation parameters. Such specialized knowledge will allay the nurse's own concern about the safety of working with a patient who has received radioactive drugs and will also help the nurse converse intelligently and knowledgeably with the patient, who is often quite apprehensive about radiation. The nurse should understand the rationale for the various procedures and conditions, such as the restriction of visitors and the special collection of urine, that may be set forth by the radiation health officer, and should be aware of the possibility of radioactive contamination from the patient's clothing, bedding, or excreta. An understanding of the clinical radioactive procedures will also help the nurse assure that patients are properly prepared for specific tests (e.g., voiding just before a bone scan, administration of ancilliary medication and a recognition of the possible interaction between a patient's medication and the radioactive test), and assist them with questions and concerns they may have.

PHYSICAL ASPECTS OF RADIOACTIVE MATERIALS

Structure of matter

The concept of the existence of atoms as structural subunits of matter was advanced by Democritos in the fifth century BC. At that time, and until late in the eighteenth century when Lavasier proposed that there were 33 elements, the scientifically recognized elements were earth, water, air, and fire. Today, largely because of the pioneering efforts of scientists such as Dalton, Mendelof, Curie, Rutherford, and Thompson, we acknowledge the existence of over 100 naturally occurring and synthetic atomic elements. All matter is now believed to consist of atoms of these elements, usually found to occur in aggregations that are called molecules.

The structure of the atom has not been entirely resolved, with more than 30 subatomic particles and antiparticles being identified to date. The major subatomic particles are the *proton,* the *neutron,* and the *electron.* These particles are used as the basic structures to identify the elements and to rationalize the many chemical and physical characteristics of the elements (Table 70-1).

The spatial arrangement of these particles within the atom is such that the protons and neutrons inhabit a central region or nucleus (hence they are called nu-

TABLE 70-1

Mass and charge characteristics of the major subatomic particles

Subatomic particle	Symbol	A (mass in AMU*)	Charge (in units†)
Neutron	n	1.0089	0
Proton	p	1.0076	+1
Electron	e	0.00055	−1

*1 AMU = 1.66×10^{-24} gm.
†1 unit = 1.6×10^{-19} coulombs.

TABLE 70-2

Basic structure of some biologically important elements

Element name	Element symbol (X)	Atomic mass (A)	Atomic number (Z)
Hydrogen	H	1	1
Carbon	C	12	6
Nitrogen	N	14	7
Oxygen	O	16	8
Sodium	Na	23	11
Phosphorus	P	31	15
Sulfur	S	32	16
Chlorine	Cl	35	17
Potassium	K	41	19
Calcium	Ca	44	20

cleons), and electrons occupy the space around the nucleus at distances that are defined in terms of their energy. Atomic nuclei are designated according to their mass number A, their elemental symbol X, and their atomic number Z, in the following manner.

$$^A_Z X, \text{ where } A = n + p, \text{ and } Z = p$$
$$(n = \text{neutron}; p = \text{proton})$$

As the number of neutrons and protons in the nucleus increases, or as the ratio of protons to neutrons changes for a given element, the possibility of nuclear instability increases. In those cases where such nuclear instability exists, the atom will eventually undergo a nuclear rearrangement to attain a more stable state. During these rearrangements, nuclear energy is emitted in the form of radiation, and the element is said to have undergone radioactive decay.

The terms *nuclide* or *isotope* are applied to atoms of the same element (i.e., have the same Z number) that have a given atomic mass; a stable nuclide (or isotope) is one in which no spontaneous nuclear rearrangement is necessary, and no radioactive decay will occur. A radionuclide or radioisotope is an atom of a particular element that possesses a degree of nuclear instability and will emit radiation when it decays to a more stable nuclear configuration (Table 70-2).

Radioactive decay mechanisms

A nucleus may, as stated previously, be sufficiently unstable so as to emit energy as part of a rearrangement process toward a more stable state. The energy emitted (i.e., the radiation energy emitted) will assume one or more forms. In the simplest terms, this radiation will be either particulate or electromagnetic. In the electromagnetic case the radiations are called *gamma rays* or *x-rays*, depending on their exact origin. Particulate radiation will be in the form of negative electrons (beta particles), positive electrons (positrons), neutrons, or alpha particles.

The alpha particle, designated α, is a doubly charged helium ion (e.g., the helium nucleus). The emission of alpha radiation is accompanied by a nuclear transformation according to the general equation

$$_Z^A X \rightarrow _{Z-2}^{A-4} Y + \alpha + \text{energy};$$

where Y is the new element formed, and

$$\alpha \text{ is } _2^4He^{++}.$$

For example,

$$_{88}^{226}Ra \rightarrow _{86}^{222}Rn + \alpha + 4.79 \text{ MeV}$$

where Ra is radium, Rn is radon, and MeV is the emitted energy given in millions of electron volts, in this case, the energy belongs to the α particle.

Beta particles' emission is described by the general equation

$$_Z^A X \rightarrow _{z+1}^{A} Y + \beta^- + \text{energy}.$$

For example,

$$_6^{14}C \rightarrow _7^{14}N + \beta^- + 0.156 \text{ MeV}.$$

Positron emission results in a nuclear transformation according to the general equation

$$_Z^A X \rightarrow _{z-1}^{A} Y + \beta^+ + \text{energy}.$$

For example,

$$_6^{11}C \rightarrow _5^{11}B + \beta^+ + 0.97 \text{ MeV}.$$

In each instance, the energy is released in part as kinetic energy to the beta particle or positron. In many cases, gamma radiation also occurs during α, β, or β^+ emission. However, gamma radiation may also occur

alone, particularly as a result of a decay process called isomeric transition (IT). This does not result in a nuclear transformation, as is shown in the general equation

$$_Z^A X^m \rightarrow _Z^A X + \gamma + \text{energy}$$

where m designates the metastable state (the unstable or radioactive form) and, γ is the electromagnetic radiation (gamma ray).

For example,

$$_{43}^{99}Tc^m \rightarrow _{43}^{99}Tc + \gamma \text{ (0.14 MeV)}.$$

Other mechanisms by which radionuclides decay include internal conversion (IC) and electron capture (EC), both of which involve an interaction between the nucleus and the orbital electrons.

Mathematics of radioactive decay

The occurrence of radioactive decay is described as a probability, and consequently not all unstable (radioactive) nuclides decay at the same time, nor do different radionuclides decay at the same rate. The decay rate is usually referred to in terms of the number of atoms disintegrating per second or per minute, or in terms of the time required for one half of a given number of radioactive atoms to decay. The concept of *half-life* ($T_{1/2}$; the time required for one half of the atoms to decay) is used because of the exponential nature of the decay process. Linear and semilogarithmic plots of the radioactivity decay rate versus elapsed time illustrate these relationships (Figure 70-1).

The amount of radioactivity remaining can be easily calculated using a small scientific calculator or mathematical tables, or by referring to decay tables for a specific radionuclide. The calculation method requires one to solve the equation $A = A_o e^{-\lambda t}$, where A is the new value for the radioactivity (remaining activity), A_o is the calibrated amount of radioactivity, λ is the decay constant for the radionuclide (the fractional decay per unit time), t is the elapsed time (since calibration), and e is Euler's number (2.7183), an exponential quantity. The value of $e^{-\lambda t}$ may be determined using a hand calculator that has the e^x function, or alternately may be read out of mathematical tables that list e^{-x} values. Values of λ can similarly be obtained from tabulations of nuclear data, or can be calculated using the equation

$$\lambda = \frac{0.693}{T_{1/2}}$$

where $T_{1/2}$ is the known half-life of the radionuclide. Consider the following examples: Given a sample de-

FIGURE 70-1. *A,* Linear plot of radioactivity as a function of elapsed time in half-lives. *B,* Semilogarithmic plot of radioactivity as a function of decay time in half-lives.

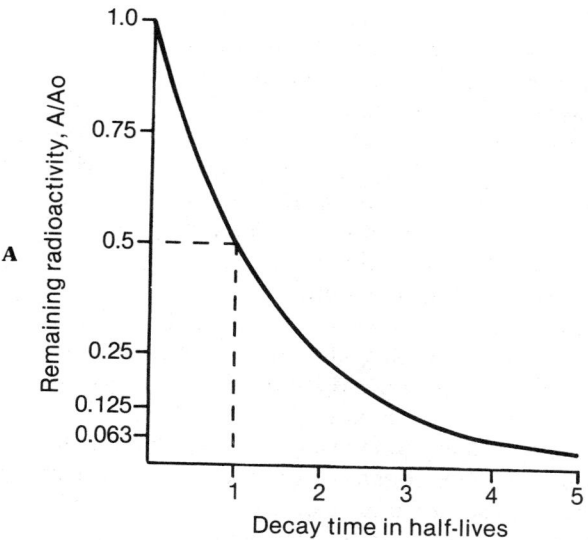

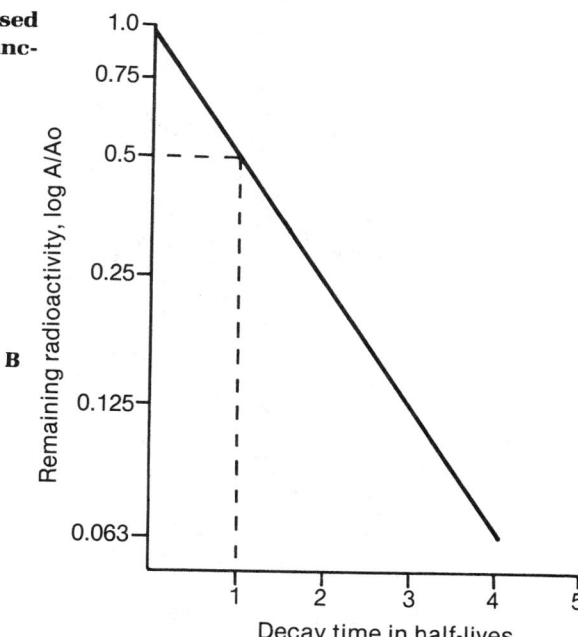

caying at a rate of 100 disintegrations per second, calculate the decay rate constant (λ) and determine the decay rate 6 hours after calibration.

1. Technetium 99m ($^{99}\text{Tc}^m$)

$$T_{1/2} \text{ (from tables)} = 6 \text{ hours}$$

$$\lambda = \frac{0.693}{6 \text{ hr}} = 0.1155 \text{ hr}^{-1}$$

and $A = 100 \times e^{-0.1155 \times 6}$
  $= 50$ disintegrations per second.

That is, after one half-life, 50% is remaining.
2. Iodine 131 (^{131}I)

$$T_{1/2} \text{ (from tables)} = 8.7 \text{ days} \ (= 208.8 \text{ hr}),$$

$$\lambda = \frac{0.693}{208.8 \text{ hr}} = 0.003314 \text{ hr}^{-1}$$

and $A = 100 \times e^{-0.003314 \times 6}$
  $= 98$ disintegrations per second.

That is, after 6 hours, 98% of the radioactive iodine remains.

Units of radioactive decay

Traditionally the units of radioactivity (i.e., the units for the rate of radioactive decay) were based on the *curie* (Ci). The curie was defined as the disintegration (decay) of 3.7×10^{10} atoms per second (dps). Subunits

TABLE 70-3

Conversion of curie units of radiation measurement to International System (SI) units

Curie unit (Ci)	SI unit (Bq)	Disintegrations per second (dps)
1 Picocurie (pCi)	37 mBq	0.037
1 Nanocurie (nCi)	37 Bq	37
1 Microcurie (μCi)	37 kBq	37,000
1 Millicurie (mCi)	37 MBq	37,000,000
1 Curie (Ci)	37 GBq	37,000,000,000

commonly used today include the kilocurie (3.7×10^{13} dps) for radiation sterilization, the millicurie (mCi; 3.7×10^7 dps) for internally administered radionuclides for radiotherapy and in vivo diagnostics, and the microcurie (μCi; 3.7×10^4 dps) and the nanocurie (nCi; 3.7×10 dps) for in vitro diagnostic tests. The introduction of the metric system has led to formulation of new units called the International System (SI) units.

The basic SI unit for radioactive decay is the *becquerel* (Bq), which is defined as one disintegration per second (1 dps). The relationship between curie units and SI units is shown in Table 70-3.

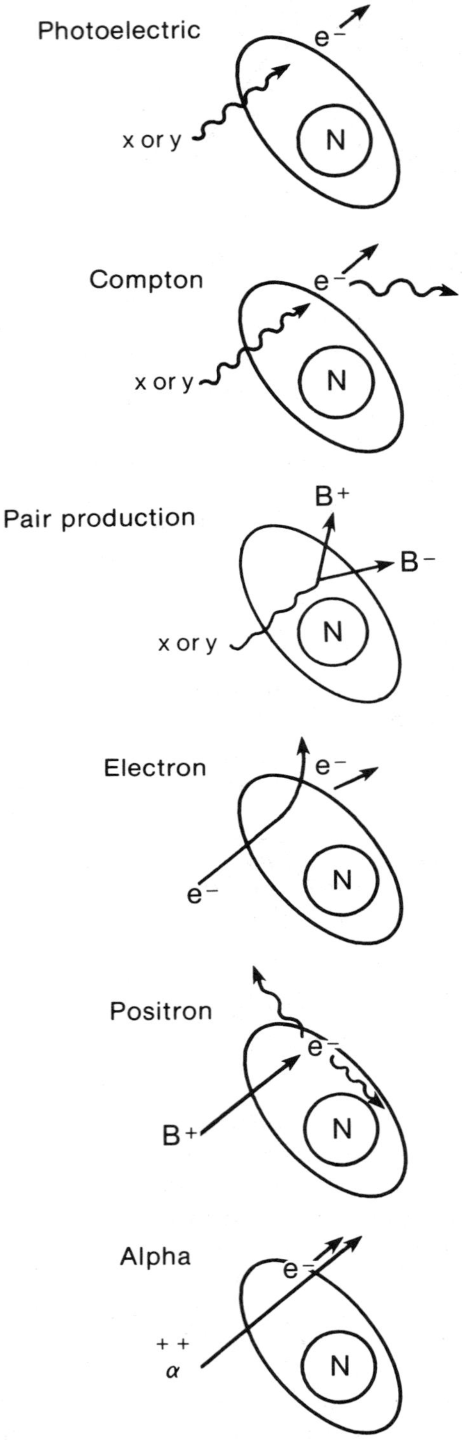

Photoelectric

Compton

x or y

Pair production

B+

B-

x or y

Electron

e-

e-

Positron

e-

B+

Alpha

e-

+ +
α

Mechanisms of interaction of radiation with matter

Radiation interacts with matter in a number of ways, depending on the energy associated with that radiation. Radiations emitted from atoms as a result of nuclear rearrangements (radioactive decay) and from x-ray machines are highly energetic. They interact primarily with orbital electrons of the atoms of the matter through which they are passing, removing these electrons from many of the atoms. This separation of electrons from atoms is called *ionization,* and consequently the radiation capable of causing this effect is called ionizing radiation.

Gamma rays and x-rays cause ionization in two ways, either by imparting all (photoelectric interaction) or part (Compton interaction) of their energy to an orbital electron, or by being converted directly to an ion pair by interaction with the nuclear force field. Electrons with considerable kinetic energy result in both cases; these are then capable of causing additional ionizations. Beta particles (electrons), positrons, and alpha particles with kinetic energy interact with orbital electrons of atoms that form the material through which they are passing. These interactions result from electrostatic repulsion and attraction of (−) or (+) charges of the particle with the (−) charge of the orbital electrons; the orbital electrons are deflected out of orbit (ionization), and the nuclear particle loses some of its kinetic energy in the process. This process of ionization continues until all of the kinetic energy of the ionizing radiation is dissipated. The positron combines with an electron when its kinetic energy has been dissipated; this combination of matter (electron) and antimatter (positron) results in annihilation (conversion of mass to energy) and the production of two new gamma rays; the combined energy of the latter $(2 \times 511 \text{ keV})$ is the energy equivalent of the rest of the mass of the electron and the positron combined.

These interactions can be depicted in the manner illustrated at left.

RADIATION DOSIMETRY

Historically, many methods were used quantitatively to measure the interaction of ionizing radiations with the matter through which they are passing.

This quantitative measurement is particularly important for living matter in two ways.

1. The amount of energy deposited in the biologic system is critical to the survival or well-being of that system.

TABLE 70-4

A comparison of SI and traditional units used for radiation dosimetry

Radiation quantity	Traditional unit (symbol)	SI unit (symbol)	Name for SI units (symbol)	Conversion factor
Absorbed dose	Rad	Joule per kilogram (J/kg)	Gray (Gy)	1 Gy = 100 rad
Exposure	Roentgen (R)	Coulomb per kilogram (C/kg)	—	1 rad = 0.01 Gy 1 C/kg = 3876 R
Dose equivalent	Rem	Joule per kilogram (J/kg)	Sievert (Sv)	1 R = 2.58 × 10⁻⁴ C/kg 1 Sv = 100 rem 1 rem = 0.01 Sv

2. The spatial distribution of the deposited energy will define the response of the biologic system, because of the heterogenous dispersion of vital subsystems (e.g., DNA) within the matrix (e.g., water).

The amount of radiation energy absorbed has been termed the *radiation absorbed dose,* which is known by the acronym *rad.* The rad is defined as being equal to 0.01 joule of absorbed energy per kg of absorbing material (or 100 ergs per gm); the SI unit, the gray (Gy), is 100 times larger, equivalent to 1 joule of energy per kg of absorbing material.

Different types of ionizing radiation (e.g., x-rays, alpha particles) are known to elicit unequal responses per unit of energy deposited (rad or Gy) in a biologic system, an effect attributed in large part to the spatial distribution (the linear energy transfer [LET]) of ionization or ion density along the path of the radiation. Consequently, the concept of *relative biologic effectiveness (RBE)* was introduced, where

$$RBE = \frac{\text{dose (rad or Gy) to produce an effect with x- or γ-rays}}{\text{dose (rad or Gy) to produce the same effect with another radiation.}}$$

The term *quality factor* (QF), usually determined through animal experiments, now largely replaces the RBE; in most cases the QF is numerically equal to the RBE. QF values for alpha particles and energetic beta particles (electrons) are 10 and 1.7, respectively, indicating that a given radiation absorbed dose (rad or Gy) from x-rays would elicit a biologic response that would be equaled by a much smaller radiation absorbed dose from alpha particles (10%) or beta particles (58%). The RBE dose was expressed in *roentgen equivalent* man (rem) units, where

$$rem = \text{Dose in rad} \times RBE.$$

The SI unit, the sievert (Sv), is derived in a similar manner, where

$$Sv = \text{Dose in Gy} \times QF.$$

The sievert is equivalent to 100 rem.

The relationship between SI and traditional units is given in Table 70-4.

The *absorption* of radiation energy by tissues is complex, consisting of variable factors such as tissue density (e.g., bone versus muscle), type of radiation (e.g., α versus γ) and energy of the radiation beam (e.g., 100 keV versus 1 MeV). For radiations most commonly encountered during medical applications, bone will absorb more x-ray and gamma ray energy than other soft tissues.

The radiation dose delivered by a radioisotope source may be measured using appropriate, precalibrated instruments, or calculated taking into account the radiation energy, the rate of decay, and the distance from the source. These calculations, although simple for the calculation of exposure dose rates for pure gamma sources, become more complex when calculating the radiation absorbed dose.

RADIATION BIOLOGY

The response of a biologic system to an exposure to ionizing radiation will depend on the total dose (rad or Gy) and the biologic effectiveness of the radiation (rem or Sv). In any case, the response (damage) will increase as the total dose increases and as the body fraction irradiated increases. The actual symptoms observed will depend directly on the amount of damage done in a given volume of tissue, and the overall amount of tissue damaged. In any case, the damage is virtually irreversible once the energy has been deposited (i.e., once the radiation has interacted with the system). The delayed response to a dose of ionizing radiation is the result of a progression of events beginning with energy deposition, proceeding through a chain of atomic, molecular, subcellular, and cellular reactions that may end in cell death, the destruction of organ function, and even the death of the organism (animal or human). Radioprotective drugs (e.g., histamine) must be present before or at the time of the radiation exposure to be effective at the atomic or molecular level. Thereafter, the treatment is limited to functional replacement therapy (e.g., electrolytes, platelets) and symptomatic treatment (e.g., antinauseants, antibiotics). Recovery from a radiation injury will depend entirely on the ability of the body to repair and regenerate the damaged tissue.

In mammals (including humans), radiobiologic effects can be conveniently divided into two major categories: the acute effects and the long-term effects. The acute effects include responses such as burns, nausea and vomiting, loss of hair, and the acute radiation syndromes. The acute radiation syndromes result from large, whole-body exposures, and depict damage to the hemopoietic system (up to 10 Gy), the gastrointestinal system (up to 100 Gy) and the central nervous system (over 50 Gy). Exposures that give rise to an acute syndrome can be expected to result in fatality in humans at doses above 4 Gy (400 rad). The mean survival times to be expected, expressed as a function of radiation absorbed dose, can be estimated from Figure 70-2.

The acute radiation syndromes in humans are encountered only infrequently. This is because of the relatively large dose required and of the nonuniformity of exposure experienced in most accidents involving humans or other large animals. Other acute effects, such as local burns and localized epilation, occur much

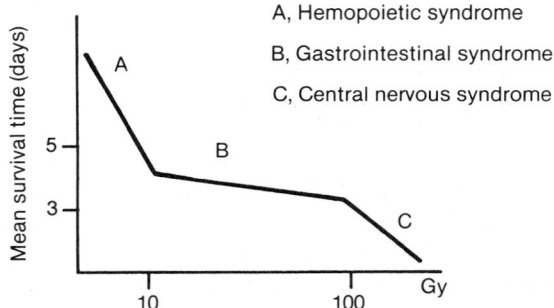

FIGURE 70-2. **The occurrence of predominant acute radiation syndromes with respect to mean survival time and radiation absorbed dose.**

more commonly; symptoms of gastrointestinal distress may be seen with real or imagined exposures.

The long-term effects of ionizing radiation are those that become manifest months, years, or even generations after the exposure to the ionizing radiation. The somatic long-term effects involve only the individual exposed, whereas the genetic long-term effects will not be evident in the individual exposed, but rather in a future generation. Somatic effects include lifespan shortening, sterility, cataract formation, and carcinogenesis; the relationship between dose and long-term lifespan shortening is not clear. Sterility and cataract formation are important considerations for localized exposures of the gonads and the eyes, respectively, because relatively large doses (large enough to cause death if the dose were delivered to the whole body) are required. A large variety of human cancers are known to be related to exposures to ionizing radiation; the latent period between exposure and disease generally ranges from 10 to 20 years. Genetic effects are extremely difficult to trace to one or more exposures to ionizing radiation. This is especially true in humans because there may be point mutations that are repaired or eliminated and that may result in recessive characteristics not expressed for several generations. Nonetheless, it is conceivable that genetic effects could occur, and individuals should attempt to minimize the dose to the gonads to the lowest level compatible with reason and benefit to those involved.

Tissues of various types respond differently to a given absorbed dose of radiation. Cells with high mitotic rates, long mitotic futures, and low degrees of differentiation are most radiosensitive. A radiation dose of 5 Gy will destroy stem cells in the bone marrow and epithelial cells in the lumen of the small intestine, but will not greatly affect cells of the central nervous system or mature bone cells.

It should be pointed out that the developing embryo and fetus represent a special case of a high sensitivity to ionizing radiation. In the embryo, all three conditions for high radiosensitivity are present. The result of in utero exposure is likely to result in death if the exposure occurs early after implantation, whereas exposure later during the first trimester (the period of organogenesis) will result in a high incidence of developmental abnormalities. Exposure of the fetus during the last trimester will have less severe effects unless relatively large doses are delivered, in which case the response will be similar to the response observed in an adult. For this reason, pregnant women should not handle radioactive materials or work in areas where such materials are being handled. The medical application of radiologic or nuclear medicine procedures to pregnant patients should be undertaken only after a careful assessment of the risk against the potential benefit to the patient.

HANDLING RADIOACTIVE MATERIALS

The safe handling of radioactive substances is directed toward minimizing direct personal exposure and reducing or eliminating laboratory and personal contamination. This requires the use of adequate shielding (e.g., lead, leaded-glass) to absorb radiation emitted by the radiation source, and protective clothing to avoid superficial contamination. The exposure (handling) time must be kept to a minimum, and the distance between the radiation source and personnel should be as great as practical.

Shielding against alpha and beta radiation can usually be adequately attained by the use of glass-walled containers, plastic barriers, or several centimeters of air. Shielding against gamma rays requires relatively large thicknesses of low-density material, or low to moderate thicknesses of materials such as lead or high-density concrete (Table 70-5). The attenuation of gamma and x-rays can be expressed mathematically by the equation

$$I = I_o e^{-\mu x},$$

where I = attenuated radiation intensity
I_o = radiation intensity before shielding
e = the base of the natural logarithm
μ = linear attenuation coefficient
x = thickness of the shield.

The thickness of the shielding required to reduce the radiation to half, *the half-value layer* (HVL), can be derived from this equation, and can be mathematically defined as

$$HVL = \frac{0.693}{\mu}$$

For example, the HVL for 140 keV photons from $^{99}Tc^m$ is 0.0256 cm for lead, 1.796 cm for aluminum, and 4.53 cm for water.

The distance from the radiation source can also be used to great advantage for radiation protection, because radiation intensity from a point (small) source is governed by the inverse square law, which states that the amount of radiation at a given distance is inversely proportional to the square of the distance. Calculations can be handled by application of the equation

$$\frac{I_1}{I_2} = \frac{D_2^2}{D_1^2}$$

where I_1 is the intensity at distance D_1 and I_2 is the intensity at distance D_2.

A source that delivers a dose rate (intensity) of 2 Gy per hour at 1 cm will deliver only 0.02 Gy per hour at a distance of 10 cm.

In all cases, the radiation dose to associated personnel can be kept well below the prescribed maximum permissible dose by a suitable combination of exposure time, distance, and shielding. Smoking and eating are not allowed in areas where open (unsealed) radioactive materials are being handled.

To reduce exposure to a minimum, handling and working procedures must be established so that atmospheric contamination is avoided. Extreme care must be taken when working with radioactive materials. Caution signs and labels must be displayed, appropriate monitoring devices must be employed, and

TABLE 70-5

Approximate penetration depth of nuclear radiations in air, soft tissue, and lead, expressed as maximum range for alpha and beta radiation and as half-value layer (HVL) for gamma radiation

Type of radiation	Energy (keV)	Penetration depth (mm)			Relative hazard	
		Air	Soft tissue	Lead	Internal	External
Alpha	1000	5	Low	Very low	High	Low
	5000	10	Low	Very low	High	Low
Beta	100	150	2	<0.2	High	Low
	1000	3200	4	0.3	High	Moderate
Gamma and x-ray	10	1250	1.5	<0.1	Moderate	Low
	100	33000	52	0.1	Moderate	Moderate
	1000	90000	80	9	High	High

personnel monitoring procedures must be established and adhered to. Waste disposal into sanitary sewage systems, by burial in soil, or by incineration is regulated by law for the protection of the general public. Records of the acquisition and disposal of radioactive materials, of personnel surveys, and of other radiation monitoring must be maintained. Licensing of individuals and facilities for radioisotope use and handling is governed by federal regulations that vary somewhat from country to country but comply with internationally accepted standards.

DIAGNOSTIC RADIOPHARMACEUTICALS
Clinically used radiation detection devices

Radiopharmaceuticals offer a noninvasive technique for assessing the morphologic structure or the physiologic function of an organ through the measurement, with a suitable detector, of the radiations emitted at the surface of the body. A variety of radiation detection instruments are currently used in nuclear medicine laboratories. The detector most commonly employed clinically is a thallium-activated sodium iodide crystal NaI(Tl) coupled to a photomultiplier tube and a *pulse height analyzer* (gamma spectrometer). Basically, in this type of detector, the gamma photon energy is absorbed within the NaI(Tl) crystal with the production of light flashes (scintillations). These light photons strike the photocathode of an adjacent photomultiplier tube that converts the scintillations into electronic pulses, the voltages of which are proportional to the amount of gamma ray energy absorbed by the NaI(Tl) crystal. The electronic pulse is amplified and the pulse height analyzer is used to sort out the electronic signals according to the gamma photon energy. The number of pulses produced in this system is proportional to the number of scintillations (photoelectric absorptions) in the NaI(Tl) crystal. Finally, the output is fed to some type of recording device: a scaler, rate meter, digital printer, magnetic tape, computer memory, photographic film, or a cathode ray tube oscilloscope screen.

Several types of gamma spectrometers are often used clinically: (1) nonimaging devices such as (a) collimated uptake scintillation probes and (b) well-type multisample gamma counters; and (2) imaging devices such as (a) rectilinear scanners and (b) gamma cameras.

Nonimaging devices

External scintillation probes. A scintillation crystal positioned over any region of the body can detect and quantitate the gamma ray–emitting radiophar-

maceutical that is contained in the underlying tissues. The crystal and photomultiplier tube are heavily shielded to minimize background and scatter radiation, and a *collimator* is used to restrict the field of view of the detector to the area under study. Basically, collimators consist of a hole or mosaic of holes separated by septa in a lead block. External scintillation probes are commonly used for thyroid uptake studies, radiorenograms, and circulation studies.

Gamma spectrometer well counters. A gamma spectrometer well counter consists of a NaI(Tl) crystal that is heavily shielded to eliminate most of the background radiation and permits the accurate detection of very low levels of radioactivity. Often, a hole or well is provided in the crystal so that the radioactive sample may be positioned into the crystal, thus enhancing detector geometry and efficiency. Automatic sample changers allow analysis, counting, and data processing for many radioactive samples. Recent models have the capability of counting gamma rays of different energies simultaneously in separate channels, and associated computers can be used for extensive data manipulation. Such well counters are routinely used for counting large numbers of samples, as in radioimmunoassay and numerous in vitro procedures.

Imaging devices

Rectilinear scanner. The development of the focusing collimators has led to the use of scanning devices for depicting or mapping the distribution of a radioactive compound within the underlying tissues, thus permitting the visualization of that organ. A typical rectilinear photoscanner consists of a shielded NaI(Tl) scintillation crystal (usually 3×2 inches or 5×2 inches) focused with a collimator to accumulate the gamma rays from a small, discrete area directly beneath it as it automatically moves back and forth over the portion of the body under study. The recording section may display the variations in counting rates by various means: (1) a light source moving parallel with the detector and exposing photographic film creates a photoscan where the intensity of the darkening of the film reflects the abundance of gamma ray emissions, (2) a mechanical tapper that burns dots on a special teledeltos paper when a gamma ray is detected by the crystal thus forming a dot scan, or (3) a direct color-coded typewriter ribbon system whereby various colored dots are imprinted on paper to reflect the intensity of gamma radiation seen by the crystal, resulting in a color-coded image.

In addition to these basic types of rectilinear scanners, many new sophisticated approaches are commercially available, using several detector heads and various collimators to enhance the sensitivity, spatial resolution, and focus at different depths of field. The advent of tomographic scanners permits the study of the distribution of radioactivity at different planes within the same organ.

Gamma scintillation camera. A gamma scintillation camera is a large detector that views all parts of the radiation field continually rather than by scanning the patient point by point. Gamma cameras commonly employ a single flat NaI(Tl) crystal (measuring from about 25 to 50 cm [11 to 21 inches] in diameter and about 1 cm [¼ to ½ inch] thick), which is viewed by an array of 19 to 91 photomultiplier tubes. As a scintillation is produced in the detector crystal by a gamma ray interaction, a computing circuit in combination with the array of photomultiplier tubes detects the position of the gamma ray and relays the signals to an oscilloscope screen where each detected gamma ray is reproduced as a dot of light. Multihole collimators (parallel or diverging) are used to restrict the field of view to the tissues directly beneath the detector. The output on the oscilloscope consists of an accumulation of dots of light, each one representing a gamma-ray interaction. These dots of light that produce an image of the biodistribution of the gamma ray–emitting radiopharmaceutical may be recorded on film or stored directly on tape for later replay or further data manipulation.

Gamma cameras may be used for static images (e.g., to portray the anatomic or functional structures by the accumulation of the radionuclide) or for dynamic studies whereby serial views are collected repeatedly over a period of time. Dynamic studies are commonly used to follow tagged tracer molecules through their physiologic pathways, thus yielding data on the functional integrity of various organs (e.g., blood flow through the various chambers of the heart may be visualized following a bolus injection of radiolabeled human serum albumin).

Various adaptations of the gamma camera are seen with different commercial manufacturers, including image magnification or minification, computer data storage and manipulation, analog-to-digital converters, and tomographic display. Whole-body imaging is possible by moving the patient or detector on specially designed platforms. Recent refinements in gamma imaging instrumentation have led to the use of tomographic techniques for displaying the distribution of radioactivity in a section or slice of the body at a given depth. The adaptation of gamma cameras to single photon emission tomographic (SPECT) procedures permits the depiction of the three-dimensional distribution of radiopharmaceuticals within the body and

allows for a more accurate localization of the radioactive tracer. The advent of the small compact cyclotron has permitted the availability of short-lived positron emitters; carbon-11 ($T_{1/2}$, 20 minutes), nitrogen-13 ($T_{1/2}$, 10 minutes), oxygen-15 ($T_{1/2}$, 2 minutes) and fluorine-18 ($T_{1/2}$, 110 minutes). These radionuclides are often referred to as *physiologic radionuclides* because they can be incorporated into naturally occurring biomolecules or drugs, allowing for precise tracer localization and measurements of physiologic function and local metabolism by application of computer-assisted tracer kinetics with positron emission tomography (PET). Such PET applications have produced exciting clinical advances in the study of local cerebral and myocardial function; however, the short half-lives of the radiotracers require an on-site cyclotron within the hospital.

Prerequisites for a diagnostic radiopharmaceutical

The ideal diagnostic radiopharmaceutical would provide data on a particular biologic function or structure while keeping the radiation dose to the patient at an acceptable low level. To conform with these criteria requires certain characteristics of both the pharmaceutical and radionuclidic moiety of the compound.

Biologic behavior. The radionuclide visualization of an organ requires that the administered labeled substance concentrate selectively in that organ. For example, to image a lesion such as an abscess or a tumor, the radiopharmaceutical must either be taken up in that lesion to a greater extent than in the surrounding tissue or blood, or be excluded from that lesion. In the former case an area of increased radioactivity or a hot lesion is detected, whereas in the latter case an area of decreased radioactivity or cold lesion is seen. A particular radiopharmaceutical is chosen for a specific diagnostic purpose because of its chemical or physical properties that result in the selective accumulation in a certain organ or region of the body.

Some common mechanisms for in vivo localization of radiopharmaceuticals. *Active transport* involves uptake caused by the metabolic activity of individual organs or tissues. The ability of the thyroid gland to concentrate radioiodine is a classic example of this type of localization. Other examples include renal scanning with radioiodinated orthoiodohippurate; and hepatobiliary imaging with radioiodinated rose bengal or with $^{99}Tc^{m}$-labeled iminodiacetic acids or pyridoxylidene glutamate.

Phagocytosis involves the engulfment or ingestion of small foreign particles primarily by the reticuloendothelial cells of the liver, spleen, and bone marrow. Radiolabeled colloidal particles of the size range of 50 to 5000 nm are readily removed from the central circulation by the liver, spleen, and bone marrow, thus allowing the visualization of these systems.

Cell sequestration is a technique commonly used to evaluate spleen function by its ability to sequester or remove from the blood circulation damaged radioactively tagged red blood cells.

Capillary blockade is a technique for the localization of radioactivity labeled particles (size 10 to 90 μm in diameter) in capillary beds (mean diameter 8 to 10 μm).

Simple or exchange diffusion mechanisms account for localization either on an ionic level or because of changes in tissue permeability. For example, myocardial uptake of radioactive thallium-201 (Tl) ions is the result of the similarity of Tl^+ to K^+ ions; bone scanning procedures with fluorine-18 or with technetium-99m phosphates are based on the exchange of the radiotracer with ions on bone hydroxyapatite crystal, whereas brain tumor scanning is usually based on changes in the permeability of the blood-brain barrier at the site of the tumor.

In *compartmental localization*, the radioactive tracer is introduced into a body compartment that can then be studied by scintiscanning or by kinetic analysis of the redistribution of that tracer. Some well-defined body compartments are the blood circulatory system, the renal system, the gastrointestinal tract, cerebrospinal fluid (CSF space), and the lung airway system. An example of this mechanism is the measurement of plasma volume following the injection of radiolabeled human serum albumin, which is initially confined to the vascular compartment and diffuses slowly into the extravascular space.

Other mechanisms. The preceding six mechanisms merely provide a basic outline to illustrate some common, well-established modes of radiopharmaceutical localization. However, several of these mechanisms, as well as other less understood modes, are often involved simultaneously. For example, ^{67}Ga citrate localizes in certain tumors and inflammatory sites presumably because of variations in blood perfusion, cell membrane permeability, cell growth rates, local pH changes, and via binding and transport mediated by plasma proteins or other substances. Newly developed, specialized radiopharmaceuticals are aimed at selected tissues by complex mechanisms, including binding to specific receptor sites, antigen-antibody reactions, unique metabolic transformations, or by other undetermined means. Recent developments in hybridoma technology have resulted in the availability of many specific monoclonal antibodies that can be radiolabeled for use as diagnostic or therapeutic pharmaceuticals.

Radionuclide characteristics

The principal characteristics of the radioactive element portion of the radiopharmaceutical that influence its use are the type of radiation emitted, energy, abundance, half-life, and availability. For diagnostic imaging and external detection, only X-rays and gamma rays provide detectable photons at the surface of the body. Beta particles and other particulate radiations, and even very low energy photons are absorbed within the tissues and only contribute to the radiation dose without yielding any useful information. High-energy beta particles are of particular internal hazard. Alpha particles, because of their high linear energy transfer, are not permitted in radiopharmaceuticals at all. Alternately, high-energy (hard) gamma rays necessitate the use of large amounts of shielding and heavy collimation. Even then these energetic gamma rays may pass through the detector crystal with only a few interactions and thus with a poor efficiency of detection. Most current scanning techniques rely on gamma radiation of about 80 to 500 keV of energy with photons of about 150 keV being almost ideal. For scanning, the yield of gamma ray photons from a particular nuclide should be of high abundance (high photon flux). For example, ^{51}Cr emits only about 9 photons per 100 disintegrations and is thus of limited use for imaging procedures.

Of natural concern in the use of diagnostic radiopharmaceuticals is the radiologic exposure of the patient. From a clinical viewpoint, it is desirable to retain the radiolabeled molecules in vivo no longer than absolutely necessary for the test. The physical half-life (Tp) is a definite value for each particular radionuclide, as discussed earlier. In addition, the administered radiopharmaceutical will undergo excretion from the body at a certain rate (Tb = biologic half-life, or time required for the elimination of one half of the initial radioactivity). Thus in a living system there is a loss of radioactivity following the administration both because of the physical decay of the radioisotope and because of the simultaneous biologic excretion. The net effective half-life (Te) may be expressed as

$$Te = \frac{Tp \times Tb}{Tp + Tb}.$$

For example, if [131]I (physical $T_{1/2}$ 8.1 days) labeled rose bengal were used in a liver function study where the biologic $T_{1/2}$ was 2 days, then the effective half-life of the radiopharmaceutical in the liver would be

$$Te = \frac{8.1 \times 2}{8.1 + 2} = 1.60 \text{ days.}$$

A commonly used guideline is that the physical half-life should be about 0.693 times the time at which the study is performed after the injection. The time interval between the administration and the start of the diagnostic test varies with different procedures, depending on the accumulation and the excretion kinetics of the tracer.

Finally, the radionuclide should be readily available to the various hospitals for routine clinical use.

Thus the desirable characteristics of a diagnostic radiopharmaceutical should include: (1) specificity of localization or metabolic reaction; (2) radioactive decay by emission of gamma rays of about 150 keV of energy in a high-photon flux with no beta particles or other particulate radiation; (3) a relatively short effective half-life, not much longer than the time required to complete the test; and (4) favorable production, formulation, and manufacture.

Although there is currently no ideal radionuclide or radiopharmaceutical, the most recent trend in the field of nuclear medicine is toward using short-lived low-energy radionuclides. Table 70-6 presents data on some commonly used diagnostic radiopharmaceuticals and allows a comparison of the properties of these radioactive drugs with the desirable characteristics just described. The physical half-life is important for such considerations as the expiration time of a radiopharmaceutical and for the length of the decay time required for the decontamination or disposal of radioactivity contaminated material. The physical $T_{1/2}$ value also provides for nursing personnel an insight into the length of time a patient remains radioactive after a diagnostic test, bearing in mind that both biologic excretion and radioactive decay reduce the patient's radioactivity simultaneously. The principle radiations, energies, and abundance are important in selecting the type of radiation detector and in adjusting the detection instruments to corresponding photopeak energies. The presence of beta particle radiation in diagnostic radiopharmaceuticals greatly increases the radiation absorbed dose and limits the amount of radioactive material that may be injected. The gamma ray intensity (Γ) and the half-value layer values are useful in estimating the thickness of the shielding required to maintain the exposure from a quantity of radioactive drug at an occupationally acceptable dose level under 2.5 mR/hour, as described earlier in this chapter under Handling Radioactive Material. The section on radiopharmaceutical application illustrating the main clinical use is meant to be used as a general guideline because many clinical variations of each test exist. The administered dosage, as determined by the nuclear medicine specialist, may vary depending on the particular instrument used and on the age, size, and clinical status of the patient. The estimated radiation absorbed dose serves as a guideline to indicate the approximate amount of radiation (rad) received by a patient from each procedure.

Referring to the previous portion of this chapter dealing with the radiation effects on tissues, it is evident from Table 70-6 that the diagnostic tests with radiopharmaceuticals deliver relatively small doses of radiation to target organs and to the whole body. Such information should provide the nurse with a relevant basis for allaying the patient's concerns about the radiation received from diagnostic radionuclide procedures.

Preparation of radiopharmaceuticals with short-lived radionuclides

The routine clinical use of short-lived radionuclides is impractical unless they can be readily provided to the nuclear medicine unit of a hospital. Generally, it is not practical to ship radioisotopes with half-lives of less than 10 to 15 hours any great distance from the site of production. Some hospitals with a direct access to a nuclear reactor or cyclotron facility may use short-lived isotopes such as ^{13}N ($T_{1/2} = 10$ minutes), ^{15}0 ($T_{1/2} = 2$ minutes), or ^{11}C ($T_{1/2} = 20$ minutes) for incorporation into biologically important compounds. I 123, with a physical half-life of 13 hours, a 159 keV gamma, and no β^- component, is an excellent radionuclide for diagnostic radiopharmaceuticals if it can be obtained in a pure form routinely and reliably. A great proportion of diagnostic imaging nuclear medicine procedures are based on radionuclides obtained from a radionuclide generator. A radionuclide generator system consists of one longer-lived radioactive isotope (a parent) that decays to a short-lived radioisotope (a daughter). The short-lived radioisotope may be removed by chemical means repeatedly as the parent nuclide decays. Such separation is often by chromatographic means where the parent is adsorbed onto a chromatographic column and the daughter is eluted or milked by passing a suitable solvent through the chromatographic media. Table 70-7 illustrates some medically useful radionuclide generating systems.

The clinical applications of the ^{99}Mo–^{99}Tc^m generating system are based on the favorable radiation characteristics of its components. The 67-hour half-life of the parent allows a practical use of these generators of about 1 week with a maximum amount of ^{99}Tc^m being generated every 23 hours. During manufacture, the chromatographic type generators are sterilized and the subsequent elution of the ^{99}Tc^m is achieved with sterile pyrogen-free isotonic saline. Several other

Text continued on p. 1636.

TABLE 70-6

Data on routinely used diagnostic radiopharmaceuticals

Radionuclide	$T_{1/2}$	Principle radiations energy (MeV) and abundance (%)	Γ*	HVL mm Pb	Radiopharmaceutical
Chromium-51 (^{51}Cr)	27.8 days	γ0.321 (9%)	0.18	2.0	^{51}Cr Sodium chromate
Fluorine-18 (^{18}F)	1.83 hr	γ0.510 (194%) β$^+$0.633	4.4	4.0	^{18}F Sodium fluoride
Gallium-67 (^{67}Ga)	3.3 days	γ0.093 (38%) γ0.185 (21%) γ0.300 (16%) γ0.393 (4%)	1.0	1.6	^{67}Ga Gallium citrate
Gold-198 (^{198}Au)	2.7 days	γ0.41 (95%) β$^-$0.97 (99%)	2.3	3.0	^{198}Au Colloidal gold (diagnostic)
Indium-111 (^{111}In)	2.8 days	γ0.17 (89%) γ0.25 (94%)	2.2	2.0	^{111}In DTPA ^{111}In Chloride
Cobalt-57 (^{57}Co)	270 days	γ0.122 (88%) γ0.014 (9%) γ0.136 (11%)	1.0	0.2	^{57}Co Cyanocobolamin capsule
Iodine-123 (^{123}I)	13 hr	γ0.159 (83%)	1.5	0.05	^{123}I Sodium iodide ^{123}I Orthoiodohippurate
Iodine-125 (^{125}I)	60.2 days	γ0.035 (67%) X-ray 0.027 (115%)	0.6	0.04	^{125}I Human serum albumin ^{125}I Fibrinogen
Iodine-131 (^{131}I)	8.04 days	γ0.364 (81%) γ0.637 (9%) γ0.284 (6%) γ0.722 (3%) β$^-$0.61 (87%) β$^-$0.34 (9%) β$^-$0.25 (3%)	2.2	3.1	^{131}I Sodium iodide ^{131}I Human serum albumin ^{131}I Macroaggregated human serum albumin ^{131}I Rose bengal ^{131}I Orthoiodohippurate

*Γ—Roentgens per hour from 1 mCi at 1 cm distance, HVL—Half value layer.

Radiopharmaceutical application				
Main clinical use	Usual adult dose	Time of test after administration	Radiation absorbed dose (rad)	
			Critical organ	Whole body
Spleen scanning with heat damaged ^{51}Cr tagged RBC	100-300 μCi IV	3-24 hr	Spleen 4-10	0.05-0.12
Determination of RBC mass; total blood volume; RBC survival time	20-200 μCi IV	Blood volumes, 15-20 min; RBC survival periodically up to 30 days	Lung <.02	<.04
Bone scanning to define altered osteogenic activity	1-2 mCi IV	2-3 hr	Bone 0.15-0.3	0.04-0.08
Tumor scanning; imaging and detection of abscesses and inflammatory lesions	3 mCi IV	48-72 hr	Bone marrow 4	0.78
Liver imaging	150-300 μCi IV	1-20 hr	Liver 6-12	0.4-0.8
Radionuclide cisternography	250-500 μCi intrathecally	2, 6, and 24 hr	Spinal cord 3-6	0.15-0.3
Hemopoietic marrow imaging	1-2 mCi IV	24-72 hr	Bone marrow 2.5-5	0.5-1.0
Cardiovascular imaging; circulation studies	1-3 mCi IV	5-15 min	Blood 0.15-0.3	0.01-0.03
Placental blood pool imaging	1 mCi IV	15 min	Blood 0.15	0.01
Diagnosis of pernicious anemia and diagnostic in defects of intestinal absorption	0.5 μCi oral	24 hr	Liver 0.05	0.005
Thyroid imaging; detection of metabolic thyroid tissue	200 μCi oral or IV	6-24 hr	Thyroid 2.0	0.002
Kidney scan and renal function radiorenogram	1-2 mCi IV	Immediately	Kidneys 0.7-1.4	
Determination of plasma and blood volume	2-5 μCi IV	15-20 min	Blood <0.05	<0.01
Detection of deep venous thrombosis	100 μCi IV	Daily counts for 5-7 days	Thyroid 0.02 (when blocked with Lugol's solution)	0.02
Thyroid uptake studies, thyroid imaging; detection of metastatic thyroid tissue	50 μCi oral or IV	24 hr	Thyroid 60-100 (depending on % uptake)	0.001-0.2 (depending on % uptake)
Determination of plasma and blood volume and blood circulation	2-5 μCi IV	15-20 min	Blood 0.04-0.08	0.02
Perfusion lung scanning, coronary perfusion scanning	300 μCi IV	5-20 min	Lungs 2.0	0.008
Liver imaging and liver function studies	0.15-0.3 mCi IV	Blood clearance studies 5-30 min Liver scan 15 min to 24 hr	Liver 0.2-1.4	0.2-0.4
Renal function studies	0.2-0.4 mCi IV	Immediately-30 min	Kidneys 0.2-0.4	0.006-0.012

Continued.

TABLE 70-6

Data on routinely used diagnostic radiopharmaceuticals—cont'd

	Physical characteristics of radionuclide				
Radionuclide	$T_{1/2}$	Principle radiations energy (MeV) and abundance (%)	Γ	HVL mm Pb	Radiopharmaceutical
Selenium-75 (75Se)	120 days	γ0.265 (60%) γ0.136 (57%) γ0.280 (25%) γ0.401 (12%)	2.0	2.2	75Se Selenomethionine
Technetium-99m (99Tcm)	6.03 hr	γ0.140 (98.4%) γ0.142 (1.6%)	0.72	0.3	99Tcm Sodium pertechnetate
					99Tcm Sulfur colloid
					99Tcm Antimony sulfide colloid
					99Tcm Calcium phytate colloid
					99Tcm HIDA
					99Tcm Pyridoxylidene glutamate
					99Tcm Macroaggregated human serum albumin
					99Tcm Human serum albumin solution
					99Tcm Pyrophosphate
					99Tcm Diphosphonates
					99Tcm Pyrophosphate
					99Tcm DTPA
					99Tcm Glucoheptonate
					99Tcm-labeled RBC (in vivo labeling or in vitro tagging with reinjection)
Thallium-201 201Tl	74 hr	X-rays 0.07-0.08 (90%) γ0.167 (10%) γ0.135 (3%)	0.47	0.23	201Tl Thallous chloride
Xenon-133 133Xe	5.3 days	γ0.081 (37%) β0.35 (100%)	0.73	0.1	133Xe gas for inhalation or 133Xe gas dissolved in saline for IV use
Ytterbium-169 169Yb	32 days	γ0.063 (45%) γ0.198 (35%) γ0.177 (22%)	2.0	0.1	169Yb Ytterbium DTPA

Main clinical use	Usual adult dose	Time of test after administration	Radiation absorbed dose (rad)	
			Critical organ	Whole body
Pancreatic scanning	250 μCi IV	15-20 min	Pancreas 3.5	1-2.5
Parathyroid scanning			Liver 7.0 Kidney 11	
Brain imaging	10-15 mCi IV	0.5-3 hr	Colon 1-2	0.1-0.2
Cerebral blood flow	5-15 mCi IV	Immediately; 2-4 sec intervals for 1 min		
Radionuclide angiography; relative blood flow	5-10 mCi IV	Immediately on bolus injection		
Thyroid imaging, salivary gland imaging	1-2 mCi IV	15 min-1 hr	Thyroid 0.2-0.4	0.01-0.02
Imaging RES cells of liver and spleen	1-3 mCi IV	15-30 min	Liver 0.3-1	0.02-0.06
Imaging RES of bone marrow	1-3 mCi IV	1-2 hr		
Lymphoscintigraphy	0.5-5 mCi SC			
Imaging areas of functional RES cells in liver, spleen, and bone marrow	1-8 mCi IV	15-30 min	Liver 0.3-2.4	0.02-0.16
Hepatobiliary imaging	3-5 mCi IV	Serial images up to 30 min-1 hr followed by static imaging	Small intestine 0.9-1.5	0.06-0.1
Perfusion lung scanning	1-3 mCi IV	15-30 min	Lungs 0.3-1	<0.01
Blood pool, cardiac function studies	1-20 mCi IV	Immediately on injection	Blood 0.04-0.8	0.01-0.2
Bone scanning	10 mCi IV	2-3 hr	Bone 0.5	0.1
Myocardial infarction detection and imaging	10-15 mCi IV	1-2 hr and at 24 hr	Bone 0.5-0.75	0.1-0.15
Renal imaging and renal function studies	10-15 mCi IV	Dynamic uptake up to 1 min then static image 30 min-1 hr	Bladder 5-7	0.2-0.3
Brain scanning	10-20 mCi IV	1 hr	Bladder 5-10	0.2-0.4
Renal imaging	10-15 mCi IV	Serial images up to 30 min then static image at 30 min-1 hr	Bladder 5-7	0.2-0.3
Brain scanning	10-20 mCi IV	1 hr	Bladder 5-10	0.2-0.4
Blood pool imaging, cardiac function studies	10-20 mCi IV	Immediately	Spleen	0.2-0.4
Myocardial imaging, evaluation of coronary artery disease	1-1.5 mCi IV	Several images 5-10 min after stress test then 2-6 hr later	Kidneys 1.5-2.2	0.24-0.36
Pulmonary ventilation studies, assessment of cerebral blood flow	5-10 mCi	Immediately	Lung 0.25-0.5	0.001-0.002
Radionuclide cisternography	0.5-2 mCi IV	4 hr and 24 hr	Spinal cord 12-48	0.1-0.4

TABLE 70-7

Some medically useful radionuclide generating systems

Radioactive parent nuclide	$T_{1/2}$	Radioactive daughter nuclide	$T_{1/2}$	Main radiations of daughter nuclide
^{99}Mo	67 hr	$^{99}Tc^m$	6 hr	γ140 keV, no β^-
^{113}Sn	118 days	$^{113}I^m$	100 min	γ392 keV, no β^-
^{81}Rb	4.7 hr	$^{81}Kr^m$	13 sec	γ190 keV, no β^-
^{82}Sr	25 days	^{82}Rb	75 sec	β^+
^{68}Ge	275 days	^{68}Ga	68 min	β^+
^{87}Y	80 hr	$^{87}Sr^m$	2.9 hr	γ388 keV, no β^-

types of Tc-generating systems are available, including solvent extraction and sublimation devices. Although the Tc 99m itself does not participate in any important biologic functions, because of its desireable radiation properties it is used extensively when incorporated into various chemical formulations.

$^{99}Tc^m$ radiopharmaceuticals

Because of the 6-hour half-life of $^{99}Tc^m$, radiopharmaceuticals containing this nuclide must be prepared freshly each day. The preparation of various radiopharmaceuticals involves a series of chemical manipulations such as reduction of the $^{99}Tc^{m7+}$ to lower valence states, chelation or incorporation into the required compound, pH adjustments, and stabilization. To facilitate such preparation, radiopharmaceutical kits, containing premeasured and prepackaged quantities of all the required ingredients except the radioactive $^{99}Tc^m$, are usually prepared. Before clinical use, the $^{99}Tc^m$ obtained from the nuclide generator is added or incorporated into the kit. These radiopharmaceutical kits may be purchased from commercial suppliers or manufactured by radiopharmacists in the hospital or in specialized radiopharmaceutical laboratories.

Quality control of radiopharmaceuticals

Because most of the diagnostic radiopharmaceuticals are administered by intravenous injection, strict quality control is essential. The various quality control procedures such as tests for stability, pyrogenicity, potency, toxicity, isotonicity, and product identity that are required for parenteral products are all applicable to the radiopharmaceuticals. In addition, the incorporation of the radioactive component also necessitates tests for radioactive assay, as well as radionuclide

and radiochemical purity, which must be carried out by the radiopharmacy department.

Radionuclidic purity is defined as the fraction or proportion of the total radioactivity present as the stated radionuclide. Some illustrations of radionuclidic impurities would be traces of ^{203}Hg in ^{197}Hg-labeled pharmaceuticals, various other iodine radioisotopes in ^{131}I-labeled products, and parent radionuclides in eluates from radionuclide generators (e.g., ^{99}Mo in products and ^{113}Sn in $^{113}In^m$ compounds). The presence of radionuclides other than the desired one may unduly increase the radiation dose to the patient and may degrade the quality of the scintigraphic images.

Radiochemical purity is defined as the proportion of the total radioactivity present as the stated chemical form. Examples of such impurities include free ionic $^{99}Tc^mO_4^-$ or hydrolyzed (colloidal) $^{99}Tc^m$ in technetium radiopharmaceuticals and free ^{131}I ions in ^{131}I-labeled organic compounds. Radiochemical impurities may often invalidate a diagnostic test (e.g., the presence of free $^{99}Tc^mO_4^-$ ions in a $^{99}Tc^m$-pyrophosphate preparation for bone scanning would indicate radioactivity in the thyroid, salivary glands, choroid plexus, stomach, and the skeleton, thus complicating or obscuring the diagnostic use of the scan).

Where the localization of the radiopharmaceutical depends on physical characteristics such as particle size, adequate quality control must ascertain the particle size distribution. In perfusion lung scanning, particles should be in the range of 10 to 100 μm in diameter as determined microscopically. The presence of smaller radiolabeled colloidal particles would result in localization in the reticuloendothelial system, thus confusing the scintigraphic image of the lungs. Each radiopharmaceutical formulation must undergo strict quality control testing, including a variety of physicochemical testing and biologic testing before its routine clinical use.

BASIC RATIONALE FOR SOME CLINICAL PROCEDURES USING RADIOPHARMACEUTICALS

The applications of radionuclide tracer compounds to clinical diagnostic nuclear medicine are expanding rapidly with advances in new improved selective radiopharmaceuticals, along with refinements in detection instruments and data manipulation. Although it is beyond the scope of this chapter to deal with all of the various procedures in depth, the following descriptions outline the basic underlying rationale for some well-established procedures using common radiopharmaceuticals. Because scintiscans form a part of the patient's records file when radionuclide imaging procedures are used, several representative scans are included as examples in the following section. These will help nurses recognize gamma camera scans and to differentiate them from other diagnostic modalities such as roentgenograms or ultrasound. In addition, these are helpful in preparing the patient for the specific procedure to increase knowledge and understanding and to reduce anxiety.

Central nervous system

Brain scanning. Brain scanning is based on the fact that a normal, intact blood-brain barrier (BBB) excludes the entry of many substances into the brain. Thus, intracranial lesions that alter the BBB will permit the penetration of radiopharmaceuticals and their localization at or around the site of the lesions. The process is nonspecific in that a variety of conditions that damage the BBB may result in the increased uptake of radiotracers. Clinical indications for brain scanning include the detection and localization of intracerebral space-occupying lesions such as neoplasms or abscesses, as well as evaluation of intracranial injury. The vascularization of the brain may be studied by taking rapid sequential scintigraphs (dynamic uptake) of the brain following an intravenous bolus injection of high radioactivity.

Radionuclide brain scanning procedures have employed a variety of radiopharmaceuticals, with Tc 99m sodium pertechnetate being one of the most common. When this agent is used, an oral dose of potassium perchlorate, 200 mg ½ hour before the scan is administered to block the uptake of the radiotracer by the choroid plexus. The chelates $^{99}Tc^m$ DTPA and $^{99}Tc^m$ glucoheptonate do not require the perchlorate block. Other radiopharmaceuticals for brain scanning in-

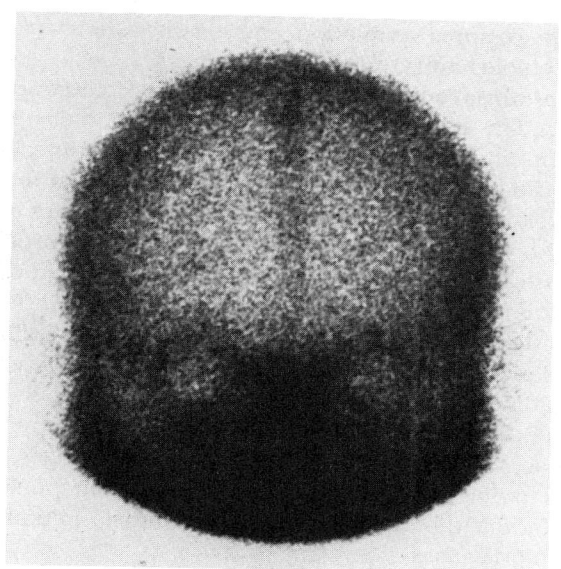

FIGURE 70-3. **Normal brain scan, anterior view, after a 20 mCi dose of $^{99}Tc^m$ glucoheptonate injected intravenously.**

clude ^{131}I human serum albumin, ^{197}Hg chlormerodrin, $^{113}In^m$ DTPA and ^{169}Yb DTPA. Recently the advent of positron computed tomography has made possible studies of local brain metabolism with ^{18}F-labeled glucose, and cerebral blood flow studies with short-lived ^{15}O or ^{11}C compounds.

Figure 70-3 is an example of a normal brain scan, anterior view, taken with a gamma camera following the intravenous injection of $^{99}Tc^m$ glucoheptonate. The dark portions of the image correspond to larger concentrations of radioactivity, whereas the lighter areas indicate the lesser uptake of the radiopharmaceutical. Normally the radiotracer distribution is symmetric and confined to the vascular component without crossing the intact BBB.

Radionuclide cisternography. Following the intrathecal injection of radiopharmaceuticals such as ^{111}In DTPA, ^{169}Yb DTPA, $^{99}Tc^m$ human serum albumin, or ^{131}I human serum albumin, the radiotracers diffuse to the basal cisterns and the subarachnoid space around the brain and then are absorbed into the bloodstream. Imaging with a gamma camera may be used to study the formation, resorption, and occlusion or flow of cerebrospinal fluid and to locate any CSF leaks.

Pulmonary system

Several components of the pulmonary system may be studied with radionuclides, including regional perfusion, regional ventilation, and airway patency of the bronchioles and lungs.

Pulmonary arterial perfusion. The scintigraphic evaluation of pulmonary arterial perfusion is most commonly accomplished by the intravenous injection of radioactively labeled particles (10 to 90 μm in diameter), which become lodged in the pulmonary capillary bed in the first pass of the circulation through the lungs. Adequate lung scans may be obtained with the injection of about 500,000 particles that will temporarily occlude less than 0.004% of the total capillary segments. Later these particles are broken down enzymatically and mechanically and are eventually removed from the circulation by phagocytes in the reticuloendothelial system. Perfusion scintimages are used to diagnose pulmonary embolism, bronchogenic carcinoma, tuberculosis, infections, fibrosis, and other related diseases.

The radiopharmaceuticals usually employed for the assessment of pulmonary arterial perfusion are macroaggregated human serum albumin (MAA) or human albumin microspheres (HAM) labeled with $^{99}Tc^m$, ^{131}I, or $^{131}In^m$. To assure a uniform distribution of the particles within the lungs and to avoid the effects of gravity on the particle distribution, the patient is injected with the scanning dose while in a supine position.

Figure 70-4, *A*, illustrates a normal lung perfusion scintigram, anterior view, following the intravenous injection of $^{99}Tc^m$ macroaggregated human serum albumin particles. In Figure 70-4, *B*, a similar study shows an obvious perfusion defect in the left lung associated with pulmonary thromboembolism.

Ventilation studies. Ventilation studies with radioactive gases are used to indicate the presence of any obstruction to the airflow or the trapping of air within the lungs. This test is usually done with ^{133}Xe gas whereby the patient inhales a ^{133}Xe air mixture in a closed system and holds the breath for 15 to 20 seconds for scintimaging with a gamma camera (single breath). The patient then rebreathes the ^{133}Xe-air mixture and additional scans are taken (equilibrium studies). This is followed by the inhalation of fresh air and the exhalation of the ^{133}Xe into a collecting bag while serial scintiscans are taken (washout studies). Normal lungs indicate the symmetric filling and emptying of all portions of the lungs without the regional trapping or exclusion of the radioactive gas. ^{133}Xe dissolved in saline may be injected intravenously so that the initial breathholding scan can also depict regional arterial perfusion. ^{127}Xe gas and $^{15}O_2$ gas, when available, are useful alternate choices for ventilation studies.

Radioactive aerosols. Radioactively labeled particles in a nebulized aerosol ($^{99}Tc^m$ human serum al-

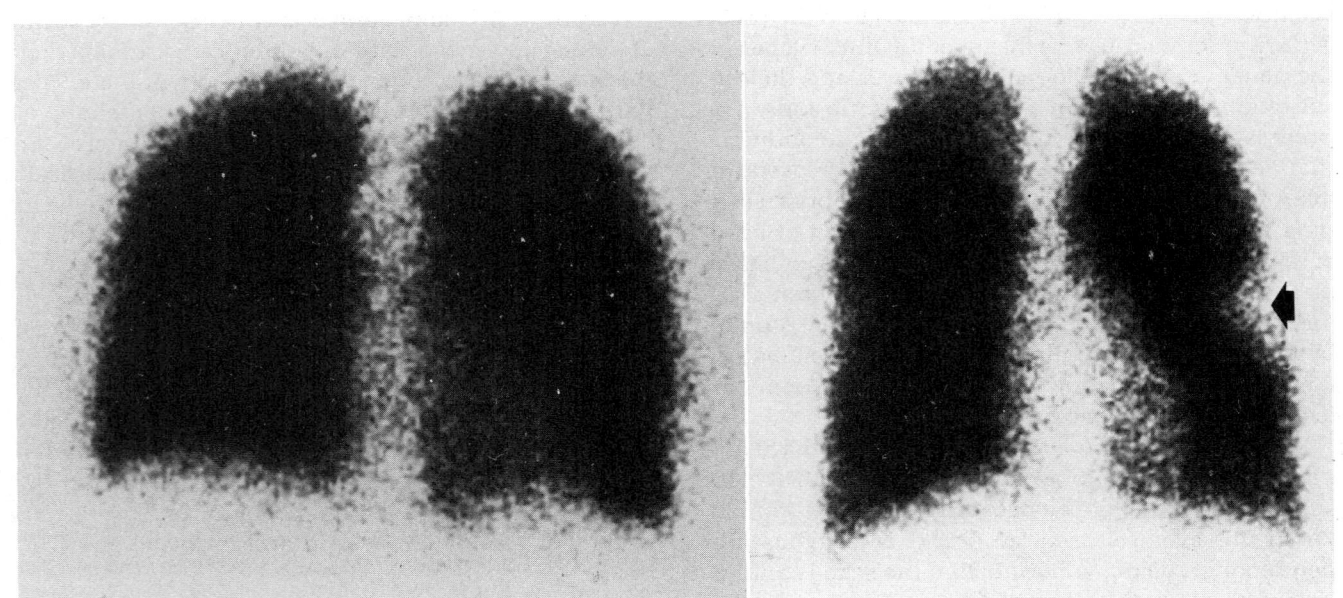

A   B

FIGURE 70-4. **Lung scans, anterior view, following intravenous injection of $^{99}Tc^m$ MAA.**
A, **Normal lung perfusion image.** *B,* **Lung scan in patient with pulmonary thromboembolism. A perfusion defect in the left lung is obvious.**

bumin, $^{99}Tc^m$ sulfur colloid, $^{99}Tc^m$ phytate, or other compounds) on inhalation will deposit in various portions of the tracheobronchial tree according to particle size (10 to 50 μm in the trachea and the bronchi, 2 to 6 μm in the terminal bronchioles and the alveolar ducts, and under 2 μm in the alveoli). Gamma camera scintimaging following inhalation can assess the bronchial space and the patency of the respiratory branching airways.

Skeletal system

Bone-seeking radiopharmaceuticals such as the $^{99}Tc^m$ phosphates and phosphonates, as well as the inorganic salts of ^{18}F and $^{87}Sr^m$, readily localize in a variety of osseous lesions, including neoplasms, osteomyelitis, healing fractures, and other bone conditions and diseases. The $^{87}Sr^{m++}$ ions exchange with Ca^{++} and the $^{18}F^+$ ions exchange with OH^- in bone hydroxyapatite, whereas the $^{99}Tc^m$ phosphates and

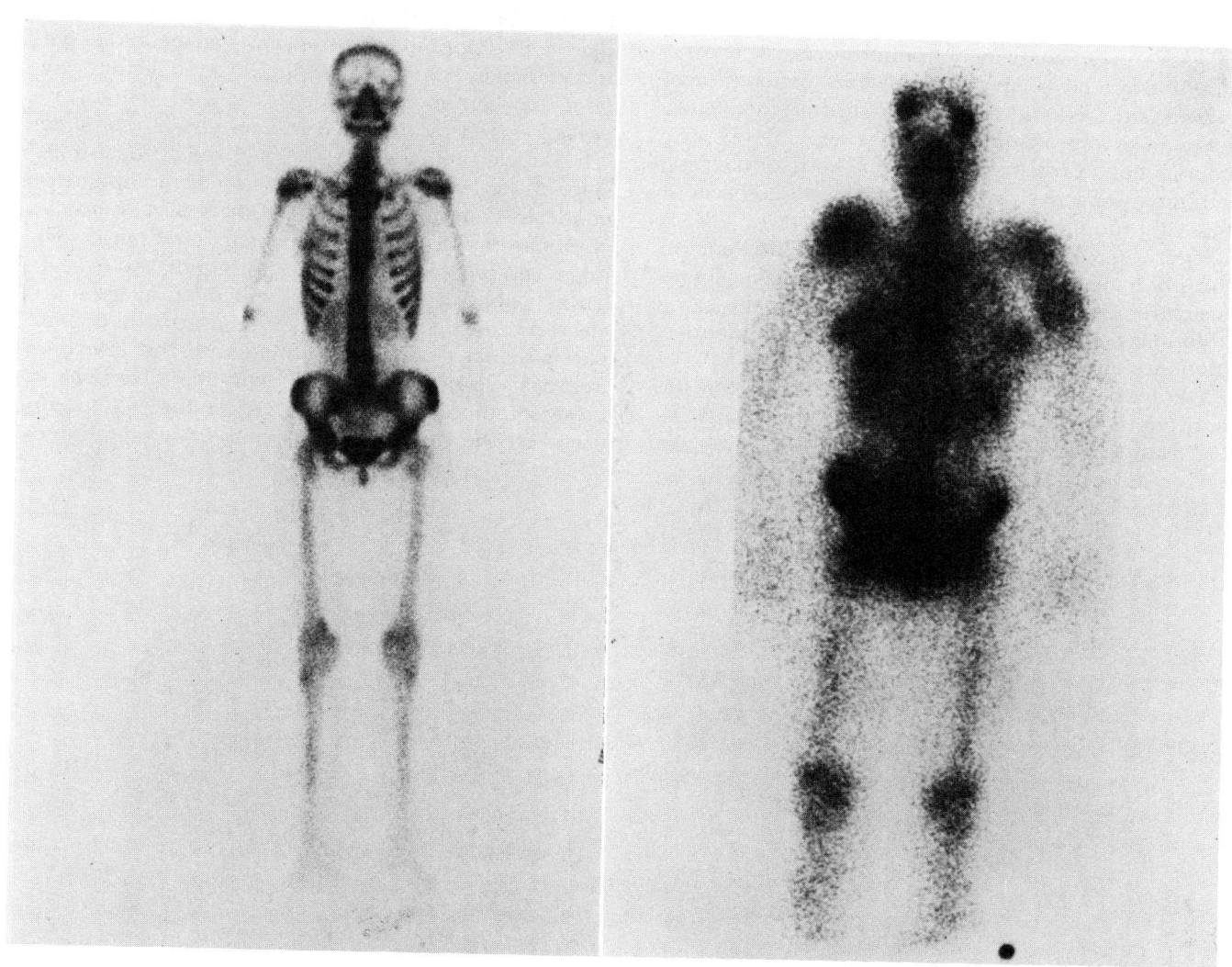

A

B

FIGURE 70-5. **Whole-body $^{99}Tc^m$ methylene diphosphonate bone scans, anterior view. A, Normal image in young patient. Normal, increased concentration of the radiopharmaceutical is seen at sites of active bone growth. Because the radiotracer is excreted in the urine, the bladder is readily visualized. B, Abnormal bone scan in patient with multiple metastatic spread showing abnormal uptake in the calvarium, sternum, scapula, left humerus, ribs, and pelvic bone.**

phosphonates localize mainly by chemiabsorption onto bone crystal and by affinity for immature collagen. The $^{99}Tc^m$ compounds are the most common radiopharmaceuticals for bone scanning procedures that find a particular application, because bone lesions can usually be detected much earlier by the scintigraphic technique than by conventional radiographic means. These radionuclide bone surveys are often employed for the detection, location, and evaluation of primary and metastatic bone tumors, osteomyelitis, arthritis, fractures, and a variety of metabolic bone diseases. The radiopharmaceuticals localize in the bone rapidly, but blood and soft tissue radioactivity must decrease to low levels to allow for useful bone images. The radioactivity not bound to the skeleton is rapidly excreted by the kidneys; thus patients must be well hydrated and are required to void just before the bone scan procedure (usually 1½ to 3 hours after the injection). Contamination of the body or clothing with the radioactive urine should be avoided because this will produce artifacts on the scan.

Figure 70-5, A, shows a normal $^{99}Tc^m$ methylene diphosphonate whole-body scan (anterior view), whereas Figure 70-5, B, illustrates a study with the same radiopharmaceutical in a patient with multiple metastatic lesions spread to the skeleton.

The active bone marrow may be visualized following intravenous injection of radioactive colloids such as $^{99}Tc^m$ sulfur colloid, which is taken up by RES cells (however, only about 5% of the total dose localizes in the bone marrow while the remainder accumulates in the liver and spleen). Radionuclides that participate in erythropoiesis may also be used for bone marrow imaging (e.g., ^{52}Fe citrate or ^{111}In indium chloride), where the radioindium is transported to bone marrow complexed to transferrin.

Liver

Radiopharmaceuticals may be used as aids in assessing liver function, morphology, or hemodynamic flow. Depending on the particular physiologic functions studied, the radiopharmaceuticals are either colloidal radiolabeled particles or radioactive soluble dyes and lipophilic substances. The colloidal particles (usually $^{99}Tc^m$ sulfur colloid, $^{99}Tc^m$ calcium phytate, $^{99}Tc^m$ antimony sulfide, ^{198}Au gold colloid, microaggregated radiolabeled serum albumin, or other $^{113}In^m$ labeled colloids) are phagocytized by the Kupffer cells of the liver. The second group of radiopharmaceuticals consisting of soluble dyes and lipophilic compounds (^{131}I or ^{123}I rose bengal, $^{99}Tc^m$ pyridoxylidene glutamate [PYG], $^{99}Tc^m$ iminodiacetic acids [HIDA], and other chemically similar agents) are cleared from the systemic circulation by the hepatic parenchymal cells and excreted into the intestinal tract via the hepatobiliary system. Static liver scans, most commonly done with $^{99}Tc^m$ sulfur colloid, are useful for the study of liver morphology, evaluation of

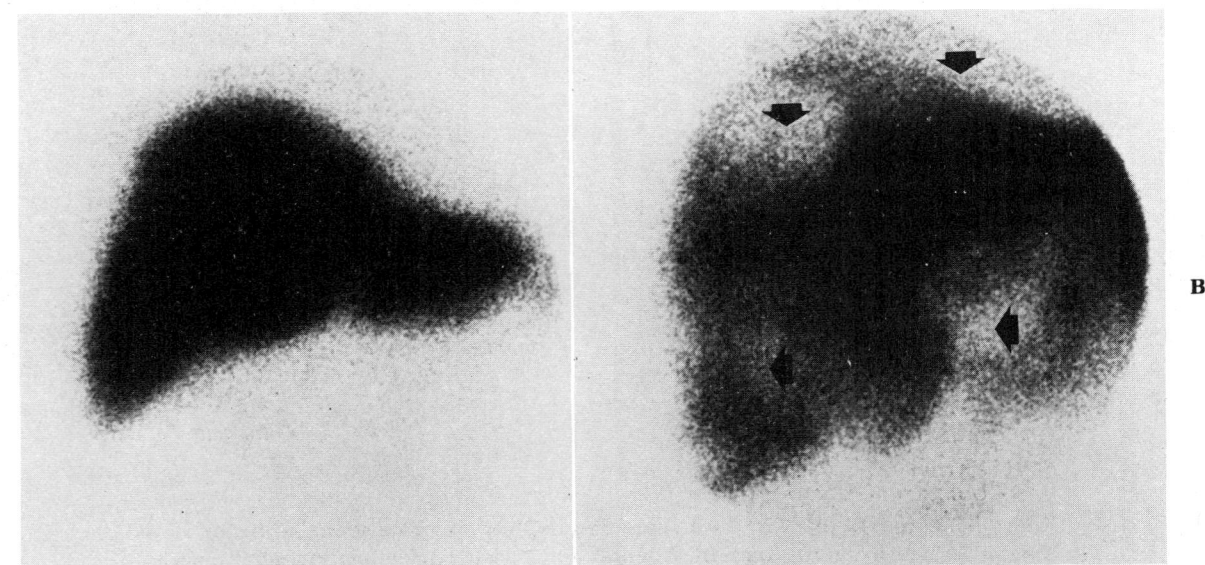

FIGURE 70-6. **Liver scans, anterior view, after intravenous $^{99}Tc^m$ sulfur colloid administration. A, Normal liver image. B, Liver scan in patient with widespread metastatic disease, showing liver enlargement and multiple space-occupying lesions.**

liver size, configuration, position, and for the detection of focal defects or space-occupying lesions such as metastases, abscesses, cysts, and fibrotic areas.

A normal liver scan (anterior view) following the injection of ^{99}Tc^m sulfur colloid is illustrated in Figure 70-6, *A*. In contrast, Figure 70-6, *B*, shows a liver scan in a patient with widespread metastatic disease associated with an enlarged liver and multiple focal defects that appear as cold spots on the image.

The evaluation of hepatocellular function may be achieved by measuring the rate of clearance of substances such as radioiodinated rose bengal. This study may be in the form of gamma camera imaging or by individual shielded collimated probes placed over the lateral area of the head, liver, and intestinal tract and measuring the changes in radioactivity over a period of time, thus yielding information about the functional status of the hepatic polygonal cells, liver blood flow, and integrity of the biliary system.

Radiopharmaceuticals such as ^{99}Tc^m–labeled PYG, HIDA, and other related compounds appear in the gallbladder within minutes of injection and are used for dynamic studies and static scans to identify and evaluate disease states and the patency of the hepatobiliary system.

Renal system

The radionuclide assessment of renal function is accomplished mainly by three types of tests: (1) the radionuclide renogram or radioactivity-versus-time graph; (2) dynamic studies to depict renal vascularization, renal plasma flow, and the excretory ability of the kidney; and (3) static scans with a gamma camera or rectilinear scanner to detect structural defects such as tumors, cysts, abscesses, or other lesions.

Renograms are usually performed by injecting tracer doses of ^{131}I orthoiodohippurate and recording the radioactivity for 20 to 30 minutes with collimated scintillation probes placed over each kidney. Alternately, a gamma camera may be used, viewing both kidneys simultaneously, obtaining sequential scintigrams along with the computer capability of data storage, replay, and analysis. The shape of the renogram depicts rates of renal blood flow, renal excretion, and urine outflow, whereas other parameters such as effective renal plasma flow may be calculated from related studies.

Renal vascularization may be studied with rapid sequential scintigraphs after an intravenous bolus injection of ^{99}Tc^m sodium pertechnetate. Often, radionuclide studies of kidney function include dynamic studies performed immediately after the injection of the radiopharmaceutical (initially providing data on renal blood perfusion) followed by additional scans (illustrating functional renal status such as glomerular filtration and tubular secretion with subsequent kidney drainage), and then finally by a static scan that demonstrates the morphologic structure of the kidney.

Routinely used radiopharmaceuticals include radioiodinated orthoiodohippurate (excreted primarily by renal tubular secretion with only 10% to 15% by filtration) ^{99}Tc^m DTPA (excreted by glomerular filtration) and ^{99}Tc^m glucoheptonate (excreted by both glomerular filtration and tubular secretion).

Thyroid

The affinity of the thyroid gland for iodides forms the underlying basis for the use of ^{131}I, ^{123}I, or ^{125}I as sodium iodide (oral solution, capsules, or intravenous injection) in assessing the structural and functional status of the thyroid gland. In the radioiodine uptake test (RAI), a tracer dose of radioactive iodide is administered and the radioactivity over the thyroid gland is measured, usually 24 hours later. The thyroid uptake is calculated as a percent of the administered dose and this value is used to assess the functional thyroid status. Thyroid gland imaging by rectilinear scanning or gamma camera techniques provides data about the size, shape, and position of the gland, the presence of functional hot or cold nodules, thyroid metastases, and displaced thyroid tissue (e.g., lingual thyroid). Tc 99m as sodium pertechnetate is also useful as a thyroid imaging radiopharmaceutical because the TcO_4^- ion is readily trapped by the thyroid gland, although the pertechnetate ion is not organified like the iodide ions.

Cardiovascular system

The use of radioactive compounds as tracers has provided a noninvasive diagnostic modality for evaluating numerous parameters concerning the cardiovascular system, including blood and plasma volume, relative blood flow and radionuclide angiography, blood pool imaging, quantitative radionuclide cardioangiography, myocardial perfusion imaging, and myocardial infarction imaging. Measurements of circulating blood and plasma volumes, with radionuclide techniques, are well-established, widely documented procedures based on the dilution principle $V_1C_1 = V_2C_2$, where V_1 = quantity of injected dose, C_1 = concentration of injected dose, V_2 = volume after equilibration, and C_2 = concentration after uniform mixing equilibration. Two important prerequisites for such radiotracer use is that these compounds maintain their radiochemical integrity in vivo and remain in the body compartments under study for the duration of the test. Radioiodinated human serum albumin (usually ^{125}I HSA) is commonly used to measure plasma volumes whereby a known volume of determined radioactivity is injected intravenously, a blood sample is collected after a thorough mixing in vivo (about 20 minutes), and a measured sample of plasma assayed for radioactivity. The application of hematocrit values can yield calculations for estimating whole-blood volume. In vitro labeling of the red blood cells with ^{51}Cr sodium chromate followed by intravenous reinjection into the patient with the subsequent collection of blood samples and radioactive assay is a commonly used technique for determining the red cell mass. Serial blood sampling for about 40 days following the reinjection of a patient's own ^{51}Cr-labeled RBC, with a plot of ^{51}Cr radioactivity per ml of RBC versus time, affords the estimation of red blood cell survival time.

Radiopharmaceuticals, as tracers, have achieved diagnostic use in evaluating the blood flow to the limbs and organs, as well as regional perfusion at the level of the microcirculation. Radiopharmaceuticals such as ^{131}I HSA, $^{99}Tc^m$ HSA, $^{99}Tc^m$ RBC, or $^{113}In^m$ transferrin, which are retained within the vascular compartment, permit quantitation by scintillation uptake probes or visualization of the vasculature by gamma camera dynamic studies, and along with computer data systems can generate radioactivity-versus-time curves for further analyses. With freely diffusible radiotracers such as $^{99}Tc^m$ pertechnetate or saline solutions of inert gases such as ^{133}Xe or $^{81}Kr^m$, the radionuclide angiogram studies must be done immediately on injection. Particulate tracers such as human serum macroaggregates (MAA) or microspheres (HAM) labeled with ^{131}I, $^{99}Tc^m$, or $^{113}In^m$, when injected intravenously or intraarterially at specific sites, can be used to study the microcirculation (e.g., AV shunts) at the level of the capillary bed. Such clinical applications of the radiopharmaceuticals are extremely diverse, covering virtually any organ or tissue, but some common procedures include the study of the cerebral blood flow, the renal blood flow, the peripheral perfusion of limbs, myocardial perfusion, the integrity of the blood supply to fractured or diseased bones, and the viability of grafts.

Radiopharmaceuticals that do not diffuse rapidly from the vascular compartment (e.g., radiolabeled RBC, HSA, or transferrin) and serial gamma camera scintigraphy are useful for blood-pool imaging. Such studies include the detection and evaluation of pericardial effusions, intracardiac shunts, abnormalities of individual cardiac chambers, aneurysms, and alterations in the patency of major vascular pathways. Blood-pool imaging may be useful in placental localization and for the detection of placenta previa, al-

though such radionuclide procedures in this case are generally being replaced by ultrasound techniques.

In the rapidly expanding field of nuclear cardiology a diversity of radiopharmaceuticals are used to assess myocardial performance. Quantitative radionuclide angiocardiography employs two main techniques: (1) the first-transit method, and (2) the gated blood-pool method. In the first-pass method an intravenous bolus injection of high radioactivity, usually $^{99}Tc^m$ sodium pertechnetate, is monitored by the gamma camera as the activity passes through the chambers of the heart. Rapid serial scintiphotos (25 or more per second) are collected during the initial 40 to 60 seconds of the first pass through the heart and the data are stored and analyzed by computer. The data can be used to display volumes of the heart chambers and the count rates of radioactivity in the ventricles during stages in the cardiac cycle. Such data are useful for measuring several aspects of cardiac performance, especially the determination of left ventricular ejection fraction, the determination of ventricular volume curves, the evaluation of regional wall motion, and the detection of intracardiac shunts.

In the gated blood-pool technique, an electronic signal from an electrocardiograph is used to trigger the collection of serial gamma camera images and data repeatedly only during specific portions of each cardiac cycle. For this study it is important that a high photon flux is available and that the radiotracer remain within the vascular blood pool for the duration of the study. $^{99}Tc^m$ HSA is often used, but may have the drawback of in vivo degradation. More recently, the patient's own RBC labeled with $^{99}Tc^m$ are used. The RBC may be tagged in vivo by intravenous administration of stannous pyrophosphate followed later by intravenous $^{99}Tc^m$ sodium pertechnetate; however, with this procedure a bolus injection is not possible. An in vitro labeling procedure whereby a blood sample is collected and the RBC treated with stannous chloride and sodium pertechnetate, followed by washing and resuspension in sterile normal saline provides a suitable radiopharmaceutical for an intravenous bolus injection. Data are accumulated by the computer for about 40 msec segments in synchronization with the R wave (end-diastole) and the downslope of the T wave (end-systole) for several hundred cardiac cycles. Computer reconstructed time-activity curves for the ventricles and a movie-type cineangiographic presentation of the cardiac cycle, as well as end-systole and end-diastole images, are produced for diagnostic purposes.

The regional myocardial localization of cations such as ^{43}K, ^{81}Rb, ^{131}Cs, and ^{201}Tl after an intravenous injection is directly related to the regional myocardial blood perfusion. With the use of such tracers, gamma scintigraphy of the heart is clinically indicated in the early (within the first 24 hours) evaluation of acute myocardial infarction and in the assessment of ischemic and coronary artery heart diseases. One of the most commonly used radiopharmaceuticals for myocardial perfusion studies is thallium 201-chloride, which distributes rapidly in myocardial tissue allowing for gamma scintigraphic imaging to indicate the size and shape of each ventricle, as well as myocardial and interventricular septum thickness and integrity. Perfusion defects or cold areas on the scan denote damaged myocardium such as an acute infarction or ischemia. To differentiate between an infarction and ischemic areas, imaging is performed under resting and stress conditions (e.g., exercise) where the patient is injected with ^{201}Tl at peak exercise and cardiac images are collected immediately and after several hours (redistribution studies). A perfusion defect or cold spot present at rest and at stress would indicate an infarction, whereas a cold area present at stress that later disappears at rest would suggest transient myocardial ischemia.

Another class of radiopharmaceuticals that has recently been introduced for myocardial imaging is radiolabeled substrates such as ^{13}N ammonia (participates in the synthesis of glutamine via the glutamine synthetase pathway) and ^{123}I-labeled fatty acids such as hexadecanoic acid (these are rapidly metabolized by the cardiac muscle). These substances can be used to study two aspects of myocardial physiology: (1) to monitor regional myocardial perfusion, and (2) to serve as sensitive indicators of the viability and metabolic function of the heart muscle. Ischemic, infarcted, or diseased areas are displayed as cold spots on the scan with these agents.

Infarction-avid radiopharmaceuticals represent another means of detecting, localizing, and assessing the extent of acute myocardial lesions. The ^{99}Tc^{m} phosphates, particularly the ^{99}Tc^{m} pyrophosphate, localize at sites of the damaged myocardium producing a hot spot on the scan. The infarction uptake of ^{99}Tc^{m} pyrophosphate is most predominant after 24 hours or more following the myocardial damage, and this radiopharmaceutical along with the ^{201}Tl study may be used to differentiate between recent and old infarctions.

ADVERSE REACTIONS TO DIAGNOSTIC RADIOPHARMACEUTICALS

In recognition that rapidly growing cells are especially sensitive to ionizing radiation, as explained in the section on radiation biology in this chapter, ra-

diopharmaceuticals should *not* generally be administered to pregnant or lactating women or to patients under 18 years of age unless the expected benefits to be gained from the diagnostic study outweigh the risks involved.

Diagnostic nuclear medicine techniques are based on the use of radioactive tracers that contain extremely small quantities of chemical substances, far below the threshold for pharmacologic activity. Furthermore, diagnostic radiopharmaceuticals differ from conventional therapeutic agents in that they are usually used only once per diagnostic routine, although repeat studies may be performed. Therefore it follows that the problems of drug toxicity and adverse side effects that often become apparent after chronic administration do not appear with diagnostic radioactive drugs.

Adverse reactions to the radiopharmaceuticals generally involve an unanticipated physiologic response of the patient to the vehicle carrying the radionuclide rather than to the radiation itself. Most of these types of reactions consist of a vaso-vagal reflex reaction with syncope, transient hypotension, flushing, bronchospasm, fever, hives, anaphylactic reactions, and nausea. The Society of Nuclear Medicine, together with the United States Pharmacopoeia and the United States Food and Drug Administration operate a data registry of adverse reactions to the radiopharmaceuticals. In 1978, the total incidence of reported adverse reactions was only 47 per 8 million diagnostic administrations. The vast majority of these reactions were allergic or pyrogen-like, with symptoms that resolved quickly. Such reactions were encountered more often with protein-containing products such as human serum albumin, whereas simple carrier-free solutions such as radioactive sodium pertechnetate, thallium chloride, and gallium citrate had a low incidence of reactions. Whenever radiolabeled protein-containing materials such as ^{99}Tc^{m} HSA or MAA are administered, especially in repeat studies, the possibility of hypersensitivity reactions should be considered, and drugs such as epinephrine, antihistamines, and corticosteroids should be readily available. In the presence of large right-to-left cardiovascular shunts, great caution should be used in the intravenous administration of radiolabeled macroaggregated particles because, under these circumstances, the particles enter the systemic circulation.

An estimated range for the incidence of severe reactions to the radiopharmaceuticals in the years 1976 to 1979 was only 0.02 to 0.09 per 10,000 examinations. Table 70-8 presents some of the adverse reactions seen following diagnostic radiopharmaceutical administration.

TABLE 70-8

Adverse reactions to diagnostic radiopharmaceuticals

Radiopharmaceutical	*Adverse reactions (in approximate order of incidence)*
$^{99}Tc^m$ HSA	Flushing, aseptic meningitis on intrathecal injection, fever, rash, allergic reactions
^{131}I or ^{125}I RISA	Allergic reactions, fever, aseptic meningitis following intrathecal injection
$^{99}Tc^m$ MAA and HAM	Allergic reactions, hives, itching, respiratory difficulty, cyanosis, pyrogen reaction, broncho-spasm, metallic taste
^{131}I MAA	Allergic reactions, dyspnea and cyanosis, bronchospasm, hypotensive response
$^{99}Tc^m$ Sulfur colloid	Allergic response, hives, rash, pruritus, pyrogen reaction, flushing, cyanosis
$^{99}Tc^m$ Glucoheptonate	Rash, nausea, chills, dizziness
$^{99}Tc^m$ DTPA	Allergic response, hives, itching, flushing
$^{113}In^m$ DTPA	Pyrogen response, aseptic meningitis following intrathecal injection
^{111}In DTPA	Pyrogen response, aseptic meningitis following intrathecal injection
^{169}Yb DTPA	Fixation to meningoencephalic structures
$^{99}Tc^m$ Phosphates	Allergic reactions, flushing, pyrogen reactions, headache
^{131}I Orthoiodohippurate	Anaphylactic shock, vaso-vagal reaction
^{131}I NaI	Allergic reactions, pruritus, rash, hives, nausea, vomiting, tachycardia

THERAPEUTICALLY USED RADIOPHARMACEUTICALS

The therapeutic radiopharmaceuticals are employed to deliver relatively large doses of radiation specifically to selected tissues or organs. Unlike the diagnostic radioactive drugs, the design of the therapeutic radiopharmaceuticals is based on the tissue destructive and ablative properties of the radiation. The generally desirable characteristics include the following.

1. Pure beta particle emission with energies in the range of 0.5 to 1 MeV Emax to provide energetic but limited irradiation
2. A relatively long physical half-life of about 2 to 14 days to allow for prolonged continuous biologic irradiation
3. Localization or uptake selectively by the organ or lesion to be irradiated with little or no deposition in other tissues
4. Pharmacologic safety and nontoxicity
5. Practical availability and feasibility of radiopharmaceutical formulation

Many radionuclides have physical properties that would render them suitable for therapy if an appropriate chemical form or vehicle were available to provide high localization in the tumor or tissue of interest with virtually no uptake in the surrounding organs or tissue. The recent advent of monoclonal antibody technology has created a novel approach for the targeting of radioactivity to specific tumor antigens. Although many therapeutic applications of various radioactive drugs have been reported and employed in

the last four decades, only several radiopharmaceuticals are currently used routinely, with the major radionuclides being ^{131}I, ^{32}P, ^{198}Au, and ^{90}Y. The decline in the application of radioactive drugs for routine therapy may be attributed to recent advances in the development of external beam therapy with high-energy photon beams and specialized ionizing particle beams together with computer-assisted accurate beam localization and radiation dose optimization, more precise techniques for positioning radioactive implants, and the expanding role of chemotherapy.

Radioiodine

Iodine-131, probably the most widely employed therapeutic radioactive drug, is used mainly for treating hyperthyroidism and thyroid cancer. In hyperthyroidism, the aim of ^{131}I therapy is to destroy a part of the thyroid gland that is producing too much thyroid hormone. A preliminary 24-hour radioiodine uptake test is used to determine the percent uptake by the thyroid gland, and the dosage of ^{131}I for the treatment of hyperthyroidism is then calculated on the basis of the estimated size of the thyroid gland and the percent of radioiodide uptake. The dosage regimen of ^{131}I for hyperthyroidism therapy varies; however, treatment with a single dose designed to deliver 80 to 100 μCi of ^{131}I per gram of thyroid tissue at 24 hours is effective in reducing hyperthyroidism in 60% to 80% of cases, whereas a subsequent smaller dose may be used in the remainder of patients. The local radiation dose to the thyroid from 80 μCi of ^{131}I per gram of tissue is about 7000 rad.

Data on certain therapeutic radiopharmaceuticals

	Physical characteristics of radionuclide				Radiopharmaceutical application			
Radionuclide	$T_{1/2}$	Principle radiations energy (MeV) and abundance (%)	Average β^- range in soft tissue	Chemical form	Main therapeutic application	Route of administration	Usual therapeutic dose range	Estimated radiation absorbed dose rad/mCi
^{198}Au	2.7 days	γ0.412 (95%) β^-0.97 (99%)	0.7-1 mm	Metallic colloidal gold	Malignant effusions in pleural or peritoneal cavity	Intracavity injection	Intrapleural 25-100 mCi; Intraperitoneal 35-150 mCi	Whole-body (from γ component only), 0.25 Intraperitoneal injection: liver, 6.5; spleen, 6.0; kidneys, 5.2; omentum, 45
^{131}I	8.04 days	γ0.364 (81%) γ0.637 (9%) β^-0.61 (87%) β0.34 (9%)	0.5 mm	Na^{131}I in solution or capsule	Persistent knee effusions	Intraarticular injection	4-8 mCi	
					Hyperactive thyroid conditions	Oral	1-10 mCi, various dosage regimens, depending on % uptake and on thyroid gland size; a single dose is often used to deliver 80-100 μCi/gm of thyroid tissue 80-200 mCi	Whole-body 0.45-0.5, thyroid (10% uptake) 600, thyroid (30% uptake) 1310
^{32}P	14.3 days	β^-1.71 (100%)	3.2 mm	^{32}P Sodium phosphate	Polycythemia vera, chronic leukemia	Intravenous preferably, may be given orally but about 20% is *not absorbed* by this route	1-5 mCi	Bone marrow, 13-15 Trabecular bone, 10 Cortical bone, 1
				NaH$_2$PO$_4$	Palliative in bone cancer		1-3 mCi	
				^{32}P Chromic phosphate colloid (insoluble)	Malignant effusions in pleural or peritoneal cavity	Intracavity injection	Intrapleural 5-10 mCi; Intraperitoneal 10-20 mCi	For IP injection, retroperitoneal lymph nodes, 517; omentum, 450; peritoneal serosa, 317; liver, 61; spleen, 60; kidneys, 52
^{90}Y	2.7 days	β^-2.26 (100%)	4 mm	Insoluble colloidal particles or microspheres	Irradiation of synovial membrane for chronic effusions associated with rheumatoid arthritis	Intraarticular injection	3-6 mCi	

β^- energies expressed as E (max)

The use of large therapeutic doses of ^{131}I in thyroid malignancy is aimed at destroying all of the thyroid tissue, including metastases. Such thyroid ablation doses are usually in the range of 80 to 200 mCi. Many variations are used in the management of thyroid malignancy, but a combination of the surgical removal of the thyroid cancer followed by ^{131}I ablation of the remaining thyroid tissue, including metastases, is a common procedure. The effectiveness of the radioiodine therapy depends on an adequate uptake (about 0.5% of the dose per gram of tumor) and the retention of the nuclide in the thyroid cancer (a biologic half-life of about 4 days). Administration of 150 mCi of ^{131}I deposits about 25,000 rad directly to the thyroid tumor. Such radiation levels may also be delivered to functional metastases of varying size and location, whereas whole-body radiation from therapeutic radioiodine is estimated at about 20 to 50 rad. Thus the whole-body radiation dose does not generally present any major complication. Follow-up procedures (6-month to 5-year intervals) often include a scan with a diagnostic dose of ^{131}I to delineate any residual thyroid tissue, followed by additional therapeutic ^{131}I treatments if necessary.

Phosphorus P-32

Phosphorus P-32 as the soluble phosphate is used most commonly for treating polycythemia vera. This application of ^{32}P was first reported in 1938 and the efficacy of this treatment because of the myelosuppressive properties of ^{32}P has been well documented. Several variations of treatment regimens have been reported, including phlebotomy alone or in combination with ^{32}P or alkylating agents. The Polycythemia Vera Study Group (PVSG) suggests an initial dose of ^{32}P of 2.3 mCi per square meter of body surface administered intravenously, not exceeding 5 mCi, followed 12 weeks later by reevaluation and further ^{32}P, if necessary, to a limit of 7 mCi. Careful blood monitoring is important during treatment, and the ^{32}P should be discontinued if serious hemopoietic depression occurs (platelet count below 100,000/μl or leukocytes below 3000/μl).

The short-range tissue destructive property of the ^{32}P particles is also used as a palliative in painful metastatic bone diseases. The ^{32}P is usually administered intravenously in a split schedule, such as 1.5-2 mCi daily for a total dose up to 15 to 20 mCi (less if hemopoietic depression occurs). Alleviation of intractable bone pain generally occurs within 2 to 3 weeks after therapy. The uptake of ^{32}P in bone tumors may be enhanced by the administration of vitamin D, calcium gluconate, or androgenic steroids such as testosterone.

Radioactive colloids

Radioactive colloids, in the form of insoluble ^{32}P chromic phosphate or inert colloidal gold-198 are often used to manage ascites or pleural effusions associated with malignancies. Following the instillation of a radioactive colloid into the peritoneal or pleural cavity, the colloidal particles plate out on the mesothelial membranes and free-floating malignant cells, providing selective local irradiations resulting in a reduction of fluid production and causing a palliative effect. Phosphorus-32, because of its higher beta energy and longer half-life, delivers about 885 rad/μCi/gm of tissue, compared with about 76 rad/μCi/gm for ^{198}Au. Because the penetrating gamma radiation from ^{198}Au also irradiates the whole body and presents a health hazard to attending health care personnel, treatment by the ^{32}P colloid is usually preferred.

Since the early 1960s a considerable interest has been generated in using radioactive nuclides for treating persistent synovitis, particularly of the knee joint. It appears that radiation levels of about 10,000 rad to the synovial surface are required for adequate therapeutic effects, and that insoluble colloidal particles are retained adequately within the synovia. The radiopharmaceuticals usually employed for medical synovectomy are colloidal gold ^{198}Au, colloidal or resin particles of ^{90}Y, or insoluble colloidal ^{32}P. Gold 198 has the disadvantage of an abundant, penetrating gamma ray that does little damage to the synovial membrane but greatly increases the whole-body radiation to the patient and medical personnel. Yttrium 90, with a high energy β^- (2.26 MeV), providing an average penetration of 4 mm up to a maximum 10 mm in tissue, may be of benefit in large joints or thick synovia, but should be used cautiously in small joints to avoid overirradiation and *radionecrosis* of overlying skin. Colloidal ^{32}P, with a β^- tissue penetration between that of ^{198}Au and ^{90}Y and a longer physical half-life, allows for the injection of smaller amounts of radioactive material (about 1 mCi), which provides a gradual deposition of radiation energy at the synovial surface. Table 70-9 summarizes the pertinent data on some of these commonly employed therapeutic radiopharmaceuticals.

SPECIAL CONSIDERATIONS FOR ADMINISTRATION OF THERAPEUTIC RADIOPHARMACEUTICALS

Because the therapeutic radiopharmaceuticals involve large doses of radiation, special considerations must be met regarding their safety from the viewpoint of the patient, nursing personnel and others involved in patient care, visitors, and nearby patients. In rec-

TABLE 70-10

Adverse effects from some therapeutic radiopharmaceuticals

Radiopharmaceutical	Adverse effects
^{198}Au Colloid	Depression of hemopoietic system with large doses of Au 198; occasional anorexia, nausea, or vomiting; abdominal adhesions; small bowel obstruction; fever; chromosomal abnormalities
^{131}I	Bone marrow depression with large doses of ^{131}I; acute thyroiditis; thyroid swelling; tenderness of neck; swelling of parotid and submaxillary salivary glands; pulmonary fibrosis after repeated ^{131}I treatments in patients with pulmonary thyroid metastases; hypoparathyroidism; increased incidence of hypothyroidism 5 to 10 years after ^{131}I treatment for hyperthyroidism; possible increased incidence (?) of thyroid carcinoma or leukemia many years following ^{131}I radiotherapy
NaH$_2$^{32}PO$_4$ (soluble IV treatments for hematologic disorders)	Bone marrow depression with large doses; possible induction of leukemia following treatments
^{32}P Chromic phosphate colloid (intracavity)	Abdominal pain; fever; loculation within cavity resulting in uneven irradiation
^{90}Y and ^{198}Au (intraarticular injection)	Immediate but transient joint inflammation; fever; fibrosis of synovial membrane; radionecrosis of the cartilage; leakage of radiocolloid from the joint resulting in the irradiation of regional lymph nodes

ognition of the high radiosensitivity of rapidly growing and dividing cells, radioactive drugs for therapy should *not* be administered to pregnant or lactating women or to patients under 18 years of age unless the expected benefits outweigh the risks involved. Care must be taken during the injection of therapeutic radioactive drugs because any subcutaneous or interstitial infiltration can cause radionecrosis at the injection site. Radiocolloid intracavity instillation is generally contraindicated in the presence of open lesions or unhealed surgical wounds, because leakage of the radioactive substance may occur. To facilitate the even distribution of the radiocolloid after intracavity injection, the patient should be turned at intervals of several hours after the injection.

Even with large doses of radioactive material, the signs and symptoms of the acute radiation syndrome are seldom seen because the effects are confined largely to the tissue or organ in which the radioactivity is localized. In most instances, the side effects that are commonly experienced are those that are restricted to the region of the body in which the radioactivity is deposited. Because of the short range of β^- particles only local radiation effects are seen with pure beta-emitters. However, when gamma ray emission is also present, as in ^{131}I or ^{198}Au, these penetrating photons contribute to the radiation dose received by the whole body and may also present a radiation hazard to other personnel. Table 70-10 presents some adverse side effects observed from selected therapeutic radiopharmaceuticals.

NURSING ASPECTS OF RADIATION PROTECTION ASSOCIATED WITH RADIOPHARMACEUTICAL USE

One of the important aspects of caring for patients who require radiopharmaceuticals is to prepare them both physically and psychologically for the specific diagnostic test or therapeutic procedure. Patients and their families should have a clear understanding of the need for the procedure or treatment and what to expect. They should be prepared for possible adverse effects and be informed of measures that are required to minimize the risk of radiation exposure or contamination. Both patients and their families, whenever possible should be involved in planning postprocedure or treatment care, especially when radioactive precautions are indicated. This is important because it can prevent undue anxiety, fear, and environmental contamination.

Patients and family members can be alarmed regarding the use of radioactive material, and misconceptions and fears should be identified and clarified. The patient and the family, as indicated, should be encouraged to ventilate feelings about the treatments, and they should be supported and reassured.

The assessment should include a menstrual history for women of childbearing age, who should *not* be exposed to nuclear medicine tests unless the expected benefits outweigh the risks. Tests should be completed only during the first 10 days of their menstrual cycle (the first day of menstrual flow until day 10) when less chance of pregnancy exists. Pregnant women or women who may be pregnant or mothers who are breast-feeding infants should *not* have nuclear medicine tests unless absolutely necessary and then only when the radiologist has been informed about the condition so that procedures can be modified as indicated. Pregnant or breastfeeding women should be encouraged to remind physicians and radiologists that they are pregnant or lactating.

A history of a hypersensitivity to a specific agent should be identified, as well as a history of an allergy, because certain patients may have an adverse reaction to some of the radiopharmaceuticals. Assessment of the patient is important in relation to identifying previous tests or radiation therapy. A history of a recent exposure to radioisotopes should also be noted because this can interfere with the interpretation of some test results.

The nurse needs to understand radiation safety so that unnecessary radiation exposure to nurses and other health care workers, patients, and visitors can be prevented. Diagnostic tests should *not* be ordered without a careful consideration of the value of the test in relation to obtaining useful information. Patients should be carefully prepared so that tests will not have to be repeated because foods or fluids were not withheld as indicated for the test or because a pretest medication or preparation was not administered on time.

A failure to prepare the patient may result in a poor diagnostic screening necessitating the repeated exposure to the specific agent and to its adverse side effects. This is also time consuming, depending on the test, uncomfortable because the patient may have to remain immobile for a period of time as indicated by the type of test, and expensive. The nurse should also be alert to the patient's anxiety related to the test results.

Many tests require a waiting period between the time of the injection and actual scanning, which could not only be stressful but also demand precautions. Activity restriction and limitations might be necessary to confine the patient to the room and to prevent the displacement of an intracavity catheter, if used, especially if it is to remain in place for any length of time.

Diagnostic nuclear medicine scintiscanning procedures

The diagnostic applications of the radiopharmaceuticals do not pose any serious radiation hazard to routine nursing care because of the small doses injected. Generally, no special precautions are required for dishes, utensils, or instruments used by the pa-

tients. However, the patients do emit some radiation for a time (depending on the half-life of the isotope and the rate of biologic excretion); thus an awareness of radiocontamination should be maintained.

If a patient should vomit within 12 hours of the oral ingestion of the radioisotope, the responsible specialist and radiation safety officer should be notified. Disposable rubber gloves and paper towels should be used for cleaning up the vomitus, and the radiation safety officer should be consulted for monitoring the contamination and ruling on the disposal of the contaminated towels, clothing, and other articles.

Generally, no special precautions are required for toilet use. Outpatients should be told that they contain a small amount of radioactive material and that they should avoid close contact with pregnant women or young children for 24 hours after the test, after which time their radioactivity will be greatly reduced by physical radionuclide decay and biologic elimination processes.

Therapeutic radiopharmaceuticals

Radiation hazards associated with therapeutic doses of the radiopharmaceuticals vary with the amount and type of the radionuclide administered. Patients are hospitalized if they contain in excess of 25 mCi of ^{198}Au, 15 mCi of ^{131}I; 30 mCi of ^{32}P, or 10 mCi of ^{90}Y. Nurses caring for radioactive patients should wear *film badges* or personnel *dosimeters* while on duty. Phosphorus-32, ^{90}Y, and other beta emitters, because of the limited range of these radiations, do not generally constitute any external radiation hazards to health care personnel, other patients, or visitors. Following an intracavity injection, any suspicion of leakage should be monitored with an appropriate detector to avoid any undue contamination.

Patients treated with the gamma-emitting radiopharmaceuticals may pose a significant radiation hazard because of the penetration and long range of the gamma rays. Individual hospitals have set rules and specific regulations involving such cases. Generally, the following precautions are followed.

Patients with radioactive gold. Patients with radioactive gold are placed in individual rooms, clearly marked with radiation warning labels, preferably at the end of a hall or in an outside corner of the building, or alternately spaced such that the exposure rate in adjacent beds does not exceed 0.25 mR/hour as determined by the radiation safety officer. Nursing and medical personnel should spend no more time than is absolutely necessary caring for the radioactive patient, and lead-shielded barriers interposed between the patient and the nurse should be used wherever possible. Usually, bed baths are omitted for the first 48 hours unless specially ordered and indicated, but bedding may be changed as usual unless there has been drainage from the injection site, in which case the specialist in charge should be notified for radioactive monitoring. Visiting restrictions are aimed at limiting the radiation dose received to under 50 mrem; thus visitors are usually allowed for a maximum of 1 hour per day, remaining at least 2 M from the patient. Persons under 18 years of age or pregnant women are excluded from visitation. Because radioactive gold colloid is not excreted, no special precautions are required for handling excreta. Because the physical half-life of ^{198}Au is 2.7 days, the radiation exposure from such patients will decrease according to the radioactive decay process described earlier in the chapter.

Patients with ^{131}I therapy. Iodine-131 radioactive therapy doses, administered orally, are taken up largely by the thyroid tissue, and the main portion of the dose not retained by the thyroid is excreted in the urine. Radioiodine is also excreted by the sweat glands and the salivary system, so that virtually any article in contact with the patient is contaminated with radioactivity. The precautions that must be taken in caring for these patients depend on the amount of radioactivity administered. Each hospital has a set of specific instructions for patients and nursing personnel. Generally, with smaller doses (several mCi of ^{131}I) the patient presents more of a radiocontamination problem rather than a radiation health hazard, although these patients should be instructed to keep close contact with other persons, especially children, to a minimum during the first week following treatment.

Patients receiving large doses of ^{131}I (in excess of 15 mCi), as for the treatment of cancer, are required to be hospitalized and put under special instructions and precautions until the radiation dose is reduced to lower levels by the process of radioactive decay and biologic elimination. The following general rules apply.

1. The patient is placed in a radioactive-designated single room with a private toilet, and the radiation levels in adjacent areas are monitored by the radiation safety officer.
2. Visitors are limited (usually ½ to 1 hour per day per person) and no one under 18 years of age or who is pregnant is allowed.
3. Nursing personnel, while attending the patient for routine care, should spend the minimum possible amount of time in the room. The radiation exposure dose to nursing or medical personnel should be monitored by the radiation safety officer.

To avoid unnecessary radiation exposure and to minimize radiocontamination from patients who have had high-dose ^{131}I therapy, the following further special precautions are observed in handling patient-related material.

1. *Vomitus.* If a patient vomits during the first 6 hours following oral ^{131}I administration, the vomitus and sputum are markedly radioactive. A large watertight container must be kept beside the bed for this purpose. The radiation safety officer will determine whether the level of radioactivity will permit flushing down the toilet or whether storage for radioactive decay is needed. Spilled vomitus should be wiped with disposable paper towels, while wearing rubber gloves, and all soiled linen, gloves, and towels should be retained in a specially marked container or a plastic bag kept in the patient's room for monitoring and proper disposal.
2. *Excretions.* Following therapeutic doses of ^{131}I, the urine is quite radioactive, especially during the first few hours. The radioactive urine is collected into a lead-shielded container kept in the patient's bathroom for radioactive decay and subsequent collection and disposal. Any spillage should be thoroughly wiped up with paper towels that are then retained in the radioactive waste container. Rubber gloves should be worn. There is usually little radioactivity in the stools, and these may be flushed away in the usual manner. The sputum is radioactive, so disposable utensils, plates, and cups should be used. These, as well as tissues and drinking straws, should be placed in the radioactive waste storage container, and housekeeping personnel should not empty the trash from the patient's room.
3. *Linens and bedding.* These will be contaminated by perspiration or possibly by urine and must be placed in plastic bags and stored in the patient's room until they are monitored for levels of radioactivity. Rubber gloves must be worn when handling bedding or linen or any other items used by the patient.
4. After the level of radioactivity in the patient is reduced sufficiently for discharge or transfer, the room must be thoroughly monitored for radiocontamination by the radiation safety officer.

Nurses should foster radiation safety in the hospital and community. In the hospital, breaks in radiation safety technique should be readily reported to the radiation safety officer. Nurses should avoid exposure when possible, wear lead aprons when assisting with radiographs or fluoroscopy, and wear rubber gloves when handling bedpans, urine specimens, dressings, tubing, or continuous drainage bags of patients who have had radiopharmaceuticals that require these precautions within the past few hours or days. Nurses should be aware of the tests and the therapy that do not require strict radiation precautions to prevent undue alarm for both staff members and patients. Nurses should request personal radiation monitors when practicing in areas where radiation precautions are indicated, and have the monitors checked as indicated. Nurses should be actively involved in hospital radiation safety committees so that nursing concerns in relation to patient care and staff protection can be effected. Radiation nurse clinical specialists should be used to promote patient care and safe hospital or community environments. It is also essential that nurses work toward legislation for licensure and certification of radiation technicians and technologists, and for the maintenance of safety standards to promote radiation safety. This may be done individually or through the professional organization.

SUMMARY

An overview of the various radiopharmaceuticals used for diagnostic or therapeutic purposes has been presented. With an understanding of the physical structure of radioactive materials, radiation dosimetry, and biology, as well as the administration of these agents, their adverse effects, and procedures for special handling and precautions, the nurse will be able to better plan the nursing care for patients requiring the radiopharmaceuticals.

BIBLIOGRAPHY

Berger, M.E., & Hübner, K.F. Hospital hazards: diagnostic radiation. *American Journal of Nursing*, 1983, *83*(8), 1155-1159.

Burcheil, S.W., & Rhodes, B.A. *Radioimmunology and radiotherapy.* New York: Elsevier Science Publishing Co., 1983.

Calgary radiation protection policy manual. Calgary, Alberta: Alberta Occupational Health and Safety Division of Radiation Health Branch, 1980.

Cardiovascular nuclear medicine. I. *Seminars in Nuclear Medicine*, 1979, *9*(4).

Cardiovascular nuclear medicine. II. *Seminars in Nuclear Medicine*, 1980, *10*(1).

Cardiovascular nuclear medicine. III. *Seminars in Nuclear Medicine*, 1980, *10*(2).

Early, P.J., Razzak, A., & Sodee, D.B. *Textbook of nuclear medicine technology* (3rd ed.). St. Louis: The C.V. Mosby Co., 1979.

Hladik, W.B., Nigg, K.K., & Rhodes, B.A. Drug-induced changes in the biologic distribution of radiopharmaceuticals. *Seminars in Nuclear Medicine*, 1982, *12*.

Kereiakes, J.G., & Rosenstein, M.R. *Handbook of radiation doses in nuclear medicine and diagnostic x-ray.* Boca Raton: CRC Press, Inc., 1980.

Krishnamurthy, G.T., & Blahd, W.H. Radioiodine ^{131}I therapy in the management of thyroid cancer. *Cancer*, 1977, *40*, 195.

L'Annunziata, M.F. *Radiotracers in agricultural chemistry.* New York: Academic Press, 1979.

Leahy, I.M., St. Germain, J.M., & Varricchio, C.G. *The nurse and radiotherapy—a manual for daily care.* St. Louis: The C.V. Mosby Co., 1979.

Matin, P. *Handbook of clinical nuclear medicine.* New York: Medical Examination Publishing Co., 1977.

National Council on Radiation Protection and Measurements (NCRP). Radiation protection for medical and allied health personnel (Report No. 48). National Council on Radiation Protection and Measurements, 1976.

Rayudu, G.V.S. *Radiotracers for medical applications.* Boca Raton: CRC Press, Inc., 1983.

Rhodes, B.A. *Quality control in nuclear medicine.* St. Louis: The C.V. Mosby Co., 1977.

Rhodes, B.A. & Cordova, M.A. Adverse reactions to radiopharmaceuticals. *Journal of Nuclear Medicine*, 1980, *21*, 1107.

Rosenfeld, S.D. & White, S.A. *Nuclear medicine technology review.* Chicago: Year Book Medical Publishers, Inc., 1977.

Saha, G.B. *Fundamentals of nuclear pharmacy.* New York: Springer-Verlag, 1983.

Shani, J., Atkins, H.L., & Wolfe, W. Adverse reactions to radiopharmaceuticals. *Seminars in Nuclear Medicine*, 1976, *6*, 305.

Spencer, R.P. *Therapy in nuclear medicine.* New York: Grune & Stratton, Inc., 1978.

Therapeutic uses of radionuclides. *Seminars in Nuclear Medicine*, 1979, *9*(2), 72-121.

Tubis, M., & Wolf, W. *Radiopharmaceuticals.* New York: John Wiley & Sons, Inc., 1976.

Varricchio, C.G. The patient on radiation therapy. *American Journal of Nursing*, 1981, *81*(2), 334-337.

CHAPTER 71

Unclassified and Miscellaneous Agents

Louis A. Pagliaro

Ann M. Pagliaro

Medications discussed in this chapter

Miscellaneous agents
  Acetohydroxamic acid
  Alprostadil
  Aminobenzoic acid
  Aminocaproic acid
  Amrinone
  Antihemophilic factor
  Bromocriptine
  Carbamide peroxide
  Carbazochrome salicylate
  Charcoal, activated
  Chenodiol
  Chymopapain
  Chymotrypsin

Miscellaneous agents—cont'd
  Collagenase
  Cyclosporine
  Cyproheptadine
  Dexpanthenol
  Dicyclomine
  Dihydroergotamine
  Dimercaprol
  Dipivefrin
  Doxylamine
  Edetate calcium disodium
  Ergoloid mesylates
  Ergonovine

Miscellaneous agents—cont'd
  Ergotamine
  Factor IX complex
  Fibrinolysin and desoxyribonuclease
  Gonadotropin, chorionic
  Hemin
  Hyaluronidase
  Lactase
  Menotropins
  Methysergide
  Metyrosine
  Oxytocin
  Papain and Urea

Miscellaneous agents—cont'd
  Pentoxifylline
  Quinine
  Ritodrine
  Sodium cellulose phosphate
  Sodium fluoride
  Sodium polystyrene sulfonate
  Somatropin
  Streptokinase
  Urokinase
  Vasopressin

CLINICALLY SIGNIFICANT DRUG INTERACTIONS*

Primary drug	Interacting drug	Possible effect(s)	Probable mechanism(s)
Acetohydroxamic acid	Oral iron preparations (e.g., ferrous sulfate)	Decreased iron levels	Decreased absorption (binding of iron to acetohydroxamic acid)
Aminobenzoic acid	Sulfonamides (e.g., sulfamethoxazole)	Decreased sulfonamide effect	Direct pharmacologic antagonism
Aminocaproic acid	Estrogens	Hypercoagulable state	Increase in clotting factors
Aminocaproic acid	Oral contraceptives	Hypercoagulable state	Increase in clotting factors
Bromocriptine	Antihypertensive medications (e.g., guanethidine)	Hypotension	Additive effect
Carbazochrome salicylate	Antihistamines (e.g., chlorpheniramine)	Decreased carbazochrome salicylate effect	Not established
Charcoal, activated	Antacids (e.g., calcium carbonate)	Decreased effectiveness of both agents	Binding in GI tract
Charcoal, activated	Laxatives (e.g., magnesium hydroxide)	Decreased effectiveness of both agents	Binding in GI tract
Charcoal, activated	Syrup of ipecac	Decreased effectiveness of both agents	Binding in GI tract

*See Chapter 10, "Drug Interactions," for an overview of drug interactions.

Continued.

CLINICALLY SIGNIFICANT DRUG INTERACTIONS—cont'd

Primary drug	Interacting drug	Possible effect(s)	Probable mechanism(s)
Chymotrypsin (topical)	Alcohol, topical	Decreased chymotrypsin effect	Chemical inactivation
Chymotrypsin (topical)	Antiseptics, topical (e.g., iodine)	Decreased chymotrypsin effect	Chemical inactivation
Collagenase (topical)	Antiseptics, topical (e.g., hexachlorophene)	Decreased collagenase effect	Chemical inactivation
Cyclosporine	Ketoconazole	Increased cyclosporine level and effect	Not established
Cyproheptadine	Metyrapone	Decreased metyrapone effect	Not established
Dimercaprol	Iron preparations, parenteral	Decreased dimercaprol effect	Binding of iron to dimercaprol
Metyrosine	Antipsychotic tranquilizers (e.g., chlorpromazine, haloperidol)	Increased extrapyramidal effects	Inhibition of catecholamine biosynthesis
Oxytocin	Sympathomimetic amines (e.g., epinephrine)	Hypertension	Potentiation of sympatho-mimetic amine effect
Quinine	Digoxin	Increased digoxin level and effect	Decreased renal clearance and other mechanisms not yet clearly established
Quinine	Gallamine, succinylcholine, tubocurarine	Neuromuscular blocking effects increased; may result in respiratory depression or apnea	Additive effect
Quinine	Warfarin	Increased anticoagulant effect	Additive effect on vitamin K–dependent clotting factor synthesis
Ritodrine	β-adrenergic blockers (e.g., propranolol)	Decreased ritodrine effect	Direct pharmacologic antagonism
Ritodrine	Corticosteroids (e.g., prednisone)	Pulmonary edema	Not established
Ritodrine	Sympathomimetic amines (e.g., epinephrine)	Increased sympathomimetic amine effects	Additive effect
Sodium fluoride	Calcium preparations (oral)	Decreased fluoride effect	Decreased GI absorption
Sodium polystyrene sulfonate	Magnesium hydroxide	Systemic alkalosis; grand mal seizure	Not completely established
Sodium polystyrene sulfonate	Sodium bicarbonate	Hypokalemia	Additive effect
Sodium polystyrene sulfonate	Oral antacids (e.g., calcium carbonate, sodium bicarbonate)	Metabolic alkalosis; decreased sodium polystyrene sulfonate effect	Additive effect; increased bicarbonate absorption from the GI tract
Somatropin	Glucocorticoids (e.g., hydrocortisone)	Decreased somatotropin effect	Antagonistic effect
Vasopressin	Carbamazepine	Increased antidiuretic effect	Additive effect
Vasopressin	Clofibrate	Increased antidiuretic effect	Additive effect

NURSING DRUG DIGEST

Medication (trade name*)	Indication	Usual dosage and administration	Dosage forms, preparation, and storage	Contraindications, cautions, and comments	Monitoring
Acetohydroxamic acid Lithostat	Adjunctive therapy (together with appropriate antibiotic) in the treatment of UTIs associated with the formation of struvite (magnesium-ammonium phosphate) as well as calcium stones	*Adults:* 10-15 mg/kg/day PO in 3-4 divided doses on an empty stomach Maximum: 1.5 gm/day *Children:* 10 mg/kg/day PO in 2-3 divided doses *Decrease dose in renal impairment*	Tablet: 250 mg	*Contraindicated* in pregnancy and severe renal impairment (i.e., creatinine clearance less than 20 ml/min) May cause headaches (usually mild), GI distress, and psychic symptoms (e.g., anxiety, depression, nervousness) May be teratogenic in humans Causes hemolytic anemia in a small percentage of patients (approximately 3%)	CBC and reticulocyte counts are recommended at regular intervals (generally after the first 2 weeks and every 3 months thereafter for chronic therapy) Monitor for hemolytic anemia
Alprostadil Prostin VR Pediatric Sterile Solution Prostin VR Sterile Solution	For use in infants with congenital heart defects to maintain the patency of the ductus arteriosus until palliative or corrective surgery can be performed	*Infants:* Continuous IV infusion Initial dose: 0.1 µg/kg/min, can be adjusted downward; duration of treatment usually 24 hr Infused per intraarterial or intravenous catheter usually placed at cardiac catheterization; infusion rates higher than 0.1 µg/kg/min have usually *not* produced greater effects and are *not* generally recommended Effective doses range from 0.01 to 0.4 µg/kg/min	Injectable: 500 µg/ml Store refrigerated between 2° and 8° C May be diluted with sterile NS or dextrose solutions Discard unused solution after 24 hr	*Contraindicated* in cyanosis with persistent fetal circulation, polysplenia, and neonates with total anomalous pulmonary venous return Use with caution in infants with bleeding tendencies or respiratory depression Commonly causes apnea, bradycardia, edema, focal seizures, pyrexia, and respiratory depression May cause flushing, GI distress, hypoglycemia, hematologic abnormalities (e.g., hemorrhage, thrombus formation, thrombocytopenia), and sepsis	Monitor Po₂ for increase indicating improved pulmonary blood flow Assess cardiac status to ensure ductus remains open Monitor improvement in infant's cardiovascular status; and improvement of hypoxia, metabolic acidosis, poor systemic perfusion, and heart failure Monitor for improvement in oxygenation in infants with cyanotic CHD Monitor blood pressure by means of an umbilical artery catheter or a Doppler transducer

Continued.

NOTE: For additional details regarding the individual agents listed in this table, see the "Clinically Significant Drug Interactions" table in this chapter.
*Indicates a multiple active ingredient product. For a complete listing of all active ingredients see the *Drug Reference Guide to Brand Names and Active Ingredients.*
♣ Indicates that the drug is generally available only in Canada.
★ Indicates that the drug is generally available only in the United States.

NURSING DRUG DIGEST—cont'd

Medication (trade name)	Indication	Usual dosage and administration	Dosage forms, preparation, and storage	Contraindications, cautions, and comments	Monitoring
Alprostadil— cont'd				Metabolized extensively in the lungs Short half-life of 5-10 min Alprostadil is commonly known as prostaglandin E_1	Monitor respiratory status throughout treatment
Aminobenzoic Acid Hill-Shade Neocylate* PABA Pabagel Pabanol Pabaplus Pabirin* PreSun RV Paba Lip Stick Sunbrella Sunscreen*	Prevention of sunburn Reduction of exposure to ultraviolet light	Adults: Apply evenly and liberally to areas of clean, dry skin; do not rub in Repeat application after swimming, excessive perspiration, towel drying, and during prolonged exposure to the sun Children: Same as adults For external use only	Gel: 1%, 2%, 3%, 4%, 5%, 6%, 8%, 10% Lotion: 1%, 2%, 3%, 4%, 5%, 6%, 8%, 10% Shake well before use	Contraindicated in hypersensitivity to aminobenzoic acid or related compounds (i.e., benzocaine, sulfonamides) Discontinue use if rash or irritation occurs; wash affected area and dry; consult health care provider if rash or irritation persists Do not apply to eyes or mucous membranes Some formulations may stain clothing; avoid contact with clothing until dry	Observe for rash or irritation
Aminocaproic Acid Amicar Capramol Epsamon Epsikapron	Hemorrhage caused by hyperfibrinolysis (NOTE: In lifethreatening conditions whole blood and fibrinogen may be required)	Adults: Initially, 5 gm PO: followed by 1 gm PO q.1h. to attain a plasma level of 0.13 mg/ml; or 5 gm by slow IV in 250 ml diluent over 1 hr, followed by 1 gm/hr administered by slow IV in 50 ml diluent Maximum: 30 gm/24 hr May need to decrease dose in renal impairment Rapid IV infusion may cause bradycardia, dysrhythmias, hypotension	Tablet: 500 mg Syrup: 250 mg/ml Injectable: 250 mg/ml Store between 15° and 30° C Injectable may be diluted in D_5W, NS, Ringer's solution, or sterile water for injection	Contraindicated during active intravascular clotting processes (e.g., disseminated intravascular coagulation and in hematuria) Use with caution in patients with cardiac, hepatic or renal dysfunction Use during the first and second trimesters of pregnancy only when need outweighs possible risks	Monitor adverse side effects: GI distress, myopathy (e.g., muscle weakness), and tinnitus Monitor therapeutic effects

Drug	Indication	Dosage	Preparation/Administration	Nursing considerations	Monitoring
	Subarachnoid hemorrhage (NOTE: *Not* an FDA-approved indication)	36 gm/24 hr IV by continuous infusion, administered as 18 gm in 400 ml D₅W q.12h. (or 1.5 gm/hr) for 10 days followed with 3 gm PO q.2h. until surgery. If surgery is not performed, therapy can be continued for 21 days; reduce dosage to 2 gm q.2h. for 3 days, followed by 1 gm q.2h. for 3 days, and discontinue	Treatment generally lasts for approximately 8 hr. Ensure proper insertion of needle to prevent possible thrombophlebitis	May cause GI distress, headache, myopathy, and tinnitus	
	Hemophiliacs undergoing dental extractions (NOTE: *Not* an FDA-approved indication)	6 gm PO immediately postoperatively followed by 6 gm PO q.6h. (i.e., 24 gm/24 hr) for 9-10 days (preoperative loading dose of factor VIII or IX to obtain at least 30%-50% factor levels should be done)			
Amrinone Inocor IV	Severe congestive heart failure that is refractory to conventional therapy	*Adults:* Initially 0.75 mg/kg by slow IV bolus over 2-3 min; may be repeated after 30 min. Maintenance: 5-10 μg/kg/min by continuous IV infusion for up to 24 hr; withdraw dosage gradually. Maximum: 10 mg/kg/day. NOTE: Dosages greater than 10 mg/kg/day or for longer than 24 hr are associated with an increased incidence of adverse effects. May need to decrease dosage in renal impairment	Injectable: 5 mg/ml. Store at room temperature. Protect from light. Discard solutions that are discolored or contain particulate matter. May be diluted before administration with NS. Do *not* dilute with dextrose solutions. Diluted solutions should be used within 24 hr	*Contraindicated* in hypersensitivity. Produces positive inotropic effects without increasing myocardial oxygen demand. Therapeutic plasma levels are between 1-2.5 μg/ml. Inotropic effects are independent of those of the digitalis glycosides and thus may be of additional benefit even in fully digitalized patients. May cause GI distress, fever, hypotension, and thrombocytopenia. Use with caution in hepatic impairment. Oral form is well absorbed (over 90%) from the GI tract	Monitor heart rate. Monitor hepatic function. Monitor fluid and electrolyte status. Monitor platelet count. Observe for fever, GI distress, and hypotension

Continued.

NURSING DRUG DIGEST—cont'd

Medication (trade name)	Indication	Usual dosage and administration	Dosage forms, preparation, and storage	Contraindications, cautions, and comments	Monitoring
★ **Antihemophilic factor** Factorate Hemofil	Hemophilia (factor VIII deficiency)	*Adults:* 10-20 units/kg IV push or slow infusion over 3 min q.8-24h. Dosage *highly* individualized *Children:* Same as adults Administer with plastic syringe because drug may bind to glass surface	Injectable: 250 units/vial supplied with sterile water for injection Store under refrigeration (2°-8° C) *until* reconstituted Reconstitute with supplied diluent *Discard* unused solution 3 hr after reconstitution	Use with caution in patients with A, B, or AB type blood because hemolysis may occur May cause backache, chills, or fever Half-life in plasma is approximately 12 hr	Monitor coagulation study results Observe for allergic reactions Monitor vital signs Monitor A, B, and AB blood type patients for hemolysis Monitor antihemophilic factor plasma levels
Bromocriptine Parlodel	Suppression of postpartum lactation Acromegaly Amenorrhea Galactorrhea, male hypogonadism Prolactin-secreting adenomas Prolactin-dependent menstrual disorders and infertility Parkinson's disease, idiopathic or postencephalitic	*Adults:* 2.5 mg PO b.i.d. for 14-21 days with meals *Adults:* Initially 1.25-2.5 mg PO q.h.s.; gradually increase to 2.5 mg PO b.i.d. to t.i.d. with meals For the treatment of acromegaly and prolactin-secreting adenomas a maximum of 20 mg/day can be administered in 4 equally divided doses *Adults:* Initially 1.25 mg PO b.i.d. with meals; gradually increase by 2.5 mg PO q.14-28 days as indicated Maximum for treatment of parkinsonism is 100 mg/day PO Administration with food or milk may decrease GI distress	Tablet: 2.5 mg Capsule: 5 mg	*Contraindicated* in hypersensitivity to ergot derivatives Commonly causes dizziness, GI distress and headache May cause fatigue, hypotension, lethargy, nervousness, and nightmares Highly bound to plasma proteins (approximately 96%) and metabolized primarily in the liver Acts as a dopamine agonist Semisynthetic derivative of ergot; however, bromocriptine is largely devoid of ergot-related pharmacologic activity	Gynecologic examination for women receiving long-term therapy is recommended every 6-12 months Monitor blood pressure for hypotension
Carbamide peroxide Cank-Aid Debrox Gly-Oxide Murine Ear Drops* Proxigel	Aid in debridement of minor oral lesions (e.g., canker sores, gingivitis) Aid in the removal of cerumen from the ear	*Adults:* Apply to affected area q.d. to q.i.d. or as indicated *Children:* Same as adults *Adults:* Place 5 drops in affected ear b.i.d. for 3-4 days *Children:* Same as adults For topical use only	Gel: 11% Solution: 6.5%	Do *not* apply to closed areas or wounds because liberation of oxygen may cause damage Discontinue use if redness or irritation occurs See also hydrogen peroxide in Chapter 55, "Antiseptics and Local Anesthetics"	Observe for local irritation

Drug	Uses	Dosage Forms	Dosage	Remarks	Nursing Implications
★ **Carbazo-chrome sa-licylate** Adrenosem Salicylate Adrenoxyl Adrestat F Statimo	Excessive capillary bleeding associated with surgery	Injectable: 5 mg/ml Tablet: 2.5 mg Syrup: 2.5 mg/5 ml	*Adults:* 10 mg IM h.s. preoperatively and repeated with "on-call" or preoperative medication on day of surgery; following surgery 5 mg PO or IM may be administered q.2-4h. as indicated *Children:* Half the adult dose Parenteral form is for *IM administration only* IV administration is *contraindicated*	*Contraindicated* in patients allergic to salicylates May cause pain or stinging at IM injection site Safety for use during pregnancy has not been established Effect may be inhibited by concurrent administration of antihistamines Repeated use may lead to the development of sensitivity to salicylates	Observe for sensitivity
Charcoal, activated Charcolanti-Dote Liquid-Antidose Medicoal	Adjunctive therapy in poisoning caused by substances that are effectively adsorbed by activated charcoal (see Appendix V, "Poisoning," for a list of substances effectively adsorbed by activated charcoal)	Suspension: 12.5 gm/60 ml, 40 gm/200 ml Powder: 15, 30, 120, 240 gm Powder must be mixed well with water *before* use	*Adults:* 25-100 gm (5-10 times the weight of poison ingested) PO as soon as possible after poisoning Dose has been repeated at 1, 3, 6, 9, 12, 18, 24, 30, and 36 hr when used to facilitate "gastric dialysis" of toxin *Children:* Same as adults Do *not* administer with milk or ice cream because this will decrease the effectiveness of the activated charcoal	Adsorbs toxic compounds Will color stools black A saline cathartic (e.g., magnesium sulfate) is often given concurrently to prevent constipation and speed the movement of the charcoal-toxin through the GI tract (to prevent possible dissociation and reabsorption of the toxin)	Monitor for signs of toxicity from ingested poison Monitor for signs of improvement
★ **Chenodiol** Chendol Chenix Cheno	Dissolution of gallstones in situ for patients at surgical risk	Tablet: 250 mg	*Adults:* Initially, 250 mg PO b.i.d. for 14 days Increase every 7 days by 250 mg/day until therapeutic response or toxicity occurs A lower total daily dose can sometimes be used with a once-a-day (q.h.s.) dosing regimen General dosage range is 13-16 mg/kg/day Therapy generally lasts for 6-24 months	*Contraindicated* in pregnancy May cause diarrhea, elevated hepatic function tests, and increased serum cholesterol For patients who can generally tolerate surgery well, cholecystectomy still appears to be the treatment of choice for gallstones Chenodiol is a natural bile acid that acts by reducing biliary cholesterol, thereby causing cholesterol-rich gallstones to gradually dissolve Gallstones generally recur within 5 years in approximately 50% of patients Often causes diarrhea (mild)	Monitor response with oral cholecystograms or ultrasonograms (partial response at least should be noted within 9 months) Monitor serum cholesterol levels every 6 months Monitor liver function tests Observe for diarrhea or other GI distress

Continued.

NURSING DRUG DIGEST—cont'd

Medication (trade name)	Indication	Usual dosage and administration	Dosage forms, preparation, and storage	Contraindications, cautions, and comments	Monitoring
Chymopapain Chymodiactin Disease	Treatment of herniated lumbar intervertebral disks in patients whose pain has not been relieved by conservative therapy, bed rest, and traction NOTE: Recommended for use only by specialists in the field of lumbar disk disease	*Adults:* 3000 units per disk; maximum dose for a patient with multiple disk herniation—10,000 units *Children: Not* recommended Injected intradiscally *only* by physicians who have completed a special course on the use of the drug Be sure epinephrine and emergency equipment are readily available in the case of an anaphylactic reaction Patient is usually under general anesthetic when drug is administered	Injectable: 10,000 units/vial Supplied as a sterile lyophilized powder in vials Refrigerate vials Reconstitute the vial's contents with 5 ml sterile water for injection Do *not* reconstitute with "bacteriostatic water for injection" because this may inactivate the chymopapain Use reconstituted solution *within* 60 min, and discard any unused portion	*Contraindicated* in patients allergic to papaya or papaya derivatives and in patients previously injected with chymopapain *Contraindicated* in patients with severe, progressive paralysis or a spinal cord tumor After injected intradiscally, this proteolytic enzyme breaks down herniated disk tissue that is pressing on tissues causing pain *Major adverse effect* is anaphylaxis (e.g., itching, urticaria, angioedema), which occurs in approximately 1% of patients Because it is a foreign protein, chymopapain can generate an immunologic response and should *not* be given to any patient more than once Patient should remain in the hospital 24-48 hr after the procedure Has not been fully tested in children or during pregnancy Paresis, paresthesias, hypalgesia and numbness of legs and toes, decreased reflexes, temporary loss of bowel and bladder control, and paralytic ileus have been reported	Monitor patients over 1-3 months for relief of severe back, hip and leg pain or other symptoms caused by herniated disk Monitor patients for adverse reactions: anaphylaxis (which can occur immediately or within an hour after the injection and last several days), hypotension, bronchospasm, back pain, stiffness, soreness, involuntary muscle spasm that may persist for days to months (residual stiffness or soreness of the lower back may persist several months) Monitor injection site for swelling and pain Monitor circulatory, motor, and neurologic function of the patient's legs

Drug	Use	Dosage	Preparations		
Chymotrypsin Alpha Chymar Alpha Chymolean Avazyme Biozyme* Catarase Chymar Chymase Chymetin Chymolase Chymoral Chymotest Enzeon Orenzyme* Quimotrase Zolyse Zonulyn	Relief of episiotomy symptoms	Adults: 4000-40,000 units PO q.i.d.	Capsules: 10,000 units	Transverse myelitis has been reported 21 days after administration as well as paraplegia and disk space infection Not recommended for patients who have had operative treatment of lumbar or lumbosacral disorders	Observe for signs of hypersensitivity Monitor for GI distress
	Enzymatic zonulysis for intracapsular lens extraction	Adults: Following dilation of the pupils with a suitable mydriatic and incision, the posterior chamber of the eye (under the iris) is irrigated with 1-2 ml of chymotrypsin solution; after 2-4 min irrigate with 2-3 ml of unused diluent or sodium chloride solution; if necessary, repeat procedure Following extraction of the lens, the pupil may be contracted with a suitable miotic *Not* to be used in patients under 20 years of age	Ophthalmic solution: 150, 300, 750 units/vial (with sodium chloride diluent) Store between 8° and 15° C Reconstitute *immediately* before use with supplied diluent Discard solutions that are cloudy or contain a precipitate Discard unused solution following procedure	*Contraindicated* in hypersensitivity and severe systemic infections May cause GI distress or hypersensitivity reactions *Contraindicated* in congenital cataracts, endothelial dystrophy, and high vitreous pressure May cause transient increase in intraocular pressure May cause corneal edema and striation Alcohol, antiseptics, blood, and serum can inactivate chymotrypsin	Observe eye for irritation or infection Monitor vision
★ **Collagenase** Nucleolycin Santyl	Enzyme used to help debride wounds (e.g., chronic dermal ulcers, severe	Adults: Apply to debrided and cleansed wound once daily For *topical use only*	Ointment: 250 units/gm	*Contraindicated* in hypersensitivity Acts by digesting collagen in necrotic tissue	Observe wound for signs of healing (i.e., formation of granulation tissue and reepithelization)

Continued.

NURSING DRUG DIGEST—cont'd

Medication (trade name)	Indication	Usual dosage and administration	Dosage forms, preparation, and storage	Contraindications, cautions, and comments	Monitoring
Cyclosporine Sandimmune	Prevention of organ (heart, kidney, liver) transplant rejection (*must* be used in conjunction with corticosteroids) NOTE: Recommended for use *only* by clinicians experienced in the management of organ transplants	*Adults:* 15 mg/kg PO (*or* 5 mg/kg/IV) as a single dose 4–12 hours before transplant surgery This daily dosage is continued for 2 weeks following surgery and then gradually reduced by one-third to one-half for long-term maintenance The oral solution may be diluted with milk or orange juice to increase palatability	Oral solution: 100 mg/ml Injectable: 50 mg/ml May dilute 1 ml of the injectable with 20–100 ml NS or D₅W	*Contraindicated* in hypersensitivity Use with caution in pregnancy Excreted in human breast milk May cause gum hyperplasia, hirsutism, hypertension, renal dysfunction, and tremors Concomitant use of other nephtotoxic drugs or other immunosuppressants (except the corticosteroids) should be avoided Cyclosporine acts primarily by inhibiting the proliferative response of T helper-cells; thus it generally does *not* significantly depress either white blood cell count or bone marrow Cyclosporine is highly protein bound (approximately 90%) and is metabolized primarily by the liver The dose-dependent nephrotoxicity of cyclosporine may be difficult to distinguish from kidney transplant rejection and may thus limit usefulness with renal transplants	Monitor cyclosporine blood levels in patients receiving the oral form to ensure adequate dosage and minimal toxicity (24 hour trough plasma levels of 50–300 ng/ml determined by RIA appear to minimize side effects and organ rejection) NOTE: Cyclosporine assay techniques and methodology may vary *greatly* from laboratory to laboratory Monitor for infection or lymphoma associated with immunosuppression Monitor renal function Monitor hepatic function Monitor for signs of organ transplant rejection Monitor for signs of neurotoxicity (e.g., amnesia, ataxia, confusion, paraparesis), particularly in cancer patients receiving other chemotherapy (e.g., cyclophosphamide, methotrexate)
Cyproheptadine Nuran Periactin Vimicon	Allergies Pruritus Rhinitis Stimulation of appetite	*Adults:* 4 mg PO t.i.d. to q.i.d. Maximum: 0.5 mg/kg/day	Tablet: 4 mg Syrup: 2 mg/5 ml	*Contraindicated* in newborn infants, hypersensitivity, mothers of nursing infants, asthma, COPD, and narrow-angle glaucoma	Monitor for drowsiness, GI distress, dry mouth, and decreased mental alertness

Drug	Uses	Dosage	Supplied/Side effects	Nursing considerations
		Children: 2-6 years, 2 mg PO b.i.d. to t.i.d.; 7-14 years, 4 mg PO b.i.d. to t.i.d. (NOTE: Children's dose can also be calculated on the basis of 0.25 mg/kg/day PO) Elderly: Start with small doses; increase dosage gradually. Administration with food or milk may decrease GI distress	May cause drowsiness, dry mouth, GI distress, increased appetite, and decreased mental alertness. May cause additive effects when administered with CNS depressants	Monitor for increased appetite
★ **Dexpanthenol** Dexol 300 Ilopan Rovite*	Adynamic (paralytic) ileus Postoperative abdominal distention	Adults: 250-500 mg IM, repeat in 2 hr, and then q,6-12h. prn. Dose may be *diluted* in bulk IV solutions (e.g., glucose, Ringer's lactate) and administered by *slow* IV infusion, but this route is *not* recommended. Children: 10 mg/kg IM, repeat in 2 hr, and then q,6-12h. prn	Injectable: 250 mg/ml. Do *not* freeze. Discard solutions that are discolored or that contain particulate matter. *Contraindicated* in hypersensitivity and hemophilia. Do *not* administer within 1 hr of succinylcholine	Monitor bowel sounds and abdominal distention
Dicyclomine Bentyl Bentyl with Phenobarb* Bentylol Cyclobec Dibent-PB* Dyspas Formulex Menospasm Merbentyl Pasmin Protylol Rocycle-10 Rocycle-20 Spasmoban Spasmoban-PH* Viscephen* Viscerol Wyovin	Irritable bowel syndrome Acute enterocolitis Infant colic	Adults: 10-20 mg PO t.i.d. to q.i.d.; or 20 mg IM q,4-6h. Children: (1-12 months) 5 mg (diluted with 5 ml of water) PO (syrup) t.i.d. to q.i.d.; (1-12 yr) 10 mg PO t.i.d. to q.i.d. Elderly: Start with lower doses and increase dosage gradually. Do *not* administer IV	Capsule: 10 mg. Tablet: 20 mg. Syrup: 10 mg/5 ml. Injectable: 10 mg/ml. Store at room temperature below 30° C. *Contraindicated* in GI obstruction, hypersensitivity, obstructive uropathy, severe ulcerative colitis, and myasthenia gravis. Use with caution in patients with narrow-angle glaucoma. Use with caution in presence of high environmental temperatures because heat prostration may occur. May cause blurred vision, drowsiness, dizziness, headache, palpitations, mental confusion, and urinary retention. Acts primarily by relaxing smooth muscles of the GI tract. Headache, GI distress, dilated pupils, dizziness, dry skin, CNS stimulation, and difficulty swallowing are signs of overdose	Monitor infants for signs of respiratory distress. Observe for signs of overdose

Continued.

NURSING DRUG DIGEST—cont'd

Medication (trade name)	Indication	Usual dosage and administration	Dosage forms, preparation, and storage	Contraindications, cautions, and comments	Monitoring
Dihydroergotamine D.H.E. 45 Plexonal*	Prevention or treatment of migraine headache	*Adults:* Immediately after the first symptoms of a migraine 1 mg IM or IV May repeat dose 1-2 additional times if necessary at 1-hr intervals Maximum: Do *not* exceed 6 mg per week	Injectable: 1 mg/ml Protect from heat Discard discolored solutions	*Contraindicated* in coronary artery disease, hypersensitivity, hypertension, infections (severe), hepatic dysfunction, peripheral vascular disease, pregnancy, and renal impairment May cause GI distress, muscle weakness, paresthesia, and transient bradycardia or tachycardia	Observe for signs of ergotism (e.g., acute GI distress, anuria, dilated pupils, slow weak pulse, thirst, twitching of extremities)
Dimercaprol BAL in Oil Sulfactin	Treatment of arsenic, gold, or mercury poisoning (together with appropriate supportive therapy)	Arsenic or gold poisoning *Adults:* 2.5-3 mg/kg IM q.4-6h. for 2 days, followed by 2.5-3 mg/kg IM b.i.d. to q.i.d. on day 3, and 2.5-3 mg/kg IM q.d. to b.i.d. for the next 10 days Mercury poisoning *Adults:* 5 mg/kg/day IM initially, followed by 2.5 mg/kg IM q.d. to b.i.d. for 10 days *Children:* Same as adults Administer by deep IM May cause pain at IM injection site IM use *only*	Injectable: 100 mg/ml	*Contraindicated* in renal or hepatic insufficiency Do *not* use for the treatment of cadmium, iron, or selenium poisoning because the resultant complex is *more* toxic, especially to the kidneys, than the heavy metals themselves Commonly causes fever in children Commonly causes tachycardia and increased blood pressure Alkalinization of the urine will help minimize possible dissociation of the dimercaprol–heavy metal complex and resultant nephrotoxicity Nausea, vomiting, and stupor are signs of dimercaprol overdose (i.e., doses greater than 5 mg/kg)	Monitor renal function Monitor heart rate and blood pressure Observe patient for pain or discomfort at injection site Monitor patients for signs of overdose, particularly those patients receiving greater than 5 mg/kg

Drug	Use	Dosage	How Supplied	Contraindications/Precautions	Nursing Implications
Dipivefrin Propine	Open (wide) angle glaucoma	*Adults:* 1 drop in affected eye(s) q.12h. Occlusion of the lacrimal duct during instillation and for 2 min after will decrease systemic absorption. For *ophthalmic use only*	Ophthalmic solution: 0.1% Keep container tightly closed. Store at room temperature	*Contraindicated* in narrow-angle glaucoma and hypersensitivity. Dipivefrin is actually a prodrug that is converted to epinephrine (see Chapter 24, "Sympathomimetics and Sympatholytics") in the eye. May cause local reactions such as burning, stinging, and photophobia. Effectively lowers intraocular pressure at a much lower concentration than epinephrine because it is much more effectively absorbed across the eye's surface into the anterior chamber	May be used *concomitantly* with edetate calcium disodium in the treatment of lead poisoning (3-4 mg/kg q.4h. for 2-7 days). Monitor for local irritation. Observe for systemic effects (e.g., increased heart rate, perspiration, trembling). See also Epinephrine, Chapter 24, "Sympathomimetics and Sympatholytics"
Doxylamine Consotuss* Decapryn Formula 44* Mercodol with Decapryn* NyQuil* Nyquil Nighttime Colds Medicine* Unisom	Insomnia; Antihistamine *component of* various cough and cold preparations (to treat allergy symptoms and rhinitis)	*Adults:* 25 mg PO 30 minutes before bedtime. *Children:* Use is *not* recommended. *Adults:* 5-15 mg PO q.d. to q.i.d. *Children:* 6-12 years, 5-7.5 mg PO q.d. to q.i.d. prn. *Elderly:* Start with low doses and increase gradually	Tablet: 25 mg. Syrup: in various strengths in combination with other cough and cold medications	*Contraindicated* in asthma, narrow-angle glaucoma, and hypertrophy of the prostate. May cause dry mouth, blurred vision, urinary retention, dizziness, and mental confusion. May potentiate the effects of other CNS depressants (e.g., alcohol, diazepam). May cause drowsiness and impair mental or motor ability when used as an antihistamine	Monitor for sedative effect as indicated. Observe for antihistamine effects as indicated. Monitor for adverse side effects, particularly in the elderly

Continued.

NURSING DRUG DIGEST—cont'd

Medication (trade name)	Indication	Usual dosage and administration	Dosage forms, preparation, and storage	Contraindications, cautions, and comments	Monitoring
Edetate calcium disodium Calcium Disodium Versenate Versenate	Treatment of lead poisoning	*Adults:* Dilute 1 gm with 250-500 ml NS or D₅W and administer by *slow* IV over 1 hr (or longer) q.d. to b.i.d. for 1-5 days. If additional therapy is required, it can be continued for an additional 5 days *following* a 2-day "rest period" *Children:* 50-70 mg/kg/day IM in 2-3 equally divided doses for 3-5 days (1 ml of procaine 1% is added to each 1 ml of undiluted edetate calcium disodium solution to keep volume to a minimum and to reduce pain at injection site). If additional therapy is required, it can be administered *following* a 4-day "rest period"	Injectable: 200 mg/ml	*Contraindicated* in severe renal impairment Do *not* administer IV in treatment of lead encephalopathy May cause renal tubular necrosis May cause pain at IM injection site Do *not* confuse edetate calcium disodium *with edetate disodium* (which is used to treat hypercalcemia)	Monitor BUN, fluid intake and output, and urinalysis for signs of renal impairment
Ergoloid mesylates Circanol H.E.A. Hydergine Trigot	Cerebral insufficiency Idiopathic decline in mental capacity	*Adults:* 1 mg PO q.i.d. with meals for 1 month; followed by 1 mg PO t.i.d. with meals for 2 months or longer as required If necessary, may be administered for short-term use parenterally: 0.3 mg IM, IV drip; *or* SC q.i.d. for 1 day, followed by 0.3 mg IM, IV drip; *or* SC t.i.d. *Adults:* 1 mg PO t.i.d. with meals Administration with food or milk may decrease GI distress	Injectable: 0.3 mg/ml Tablet: 1 mg Capsule: 1 mg Sublingual tablets: 0.5, 1 mg Oral solution: 1 mg/ml	*Contraindicated* in bradycardia, hypersensitivity, psychosis, and severe hypotension Ergoloid mesylates consist of a mixture in equal proportions of the following alkaloids: dihydroergocornine mesylate, dihydroergocristine mesylate, and dihydroergocryptine mesylate The ergoloid mesylates do *not* cause the vasoconstriction associated with the natural ergot alkaloids May cause GI distress and headache	Monitor patient for therapeutic effect Observe for adverse side effects including GI distress and headache

Drug	Uses	Dosage	Availability	Contraindications/Precautions	Nursing Considerations
Ergonovine Ergobasine* Ergotrate	Prevention and treatment of postpartum hemorrhage associated with uterine atony and puerperal morbidity	*Adults:* 0.2 mg IM (or IV in cases of excessive uterine bleeding) Dose may be repeated once in 2-4 hr if necessary To minimize late postpartum bleeding 0.2 mg PO may be administered q,6-12h. for an additional 48 hr NOTE: Administration before delivery of the placenta is generally *not* recommended	Injectable: 0.2 mg/ml Tablet: 0.2 mg Store protected from heat	*Contraindicated* in hypersensitivity, severe hypertension, threatened spontaneous abortion, toxemia, and use for the induction of labor Use with caution in patients with heart disease, hypertension, hepatic dysfunction, or renal dysfunction Generally, ergonovine produces a firm contraction of the uterus within a few minutes of parenteral administration May cause hypertension (generally immediately reversible by the administration of 15 mg IV chlorpromazine) Overdose may result in convulsions and gangrene	Observe for symptoms of ergotism (e.g., acute GI distress, anuria, dilated pupils, slow weak pulse, thirst, twitching of the extremities) Monitor blood pressure and ensure that chlorpromazine is readily available to treat hypertension
Ergotamine Bellergal* Bellergal-S* Bellermine-O.D.* Cafergot* Cafermine* Cafertrate* Ergocaf* Ergoklinine Ergomar Ergostat Femergin Gynergen Lingraine Medihaler-Ergotamine Migrastat* Wigraine* Wigrettes	Prevention or treatment of migraine headache	*Adults:* Immediately after the first symptoms of a migraine 2 mg PO, PR, or SL; *if necessary,* 4 additional 1 mg PO doses may be taken at ½-hr intervals; *or* 2 additional 2 mg SL doses may be taken at ½-hr intervals; *or* 1 additional 2 mg PR dose may be taken after 1 hr NOTE: Dosage must *not* exceed 6 mg in any 24-hr period or 10 mg in any 7-day period Oral inhalation: 1 spray at start of attack; repeat q 5 min prn (maximum: 6 metered sprays/24 hr; 15 metered sprays/week)	Tablets: 1, 2 mg Sublingual tablet: 2 mg Capsule: 1 mg Rectal suppository: 2 mg Metered aerosol: 0.36 mg/dose Shake metered aerosol well *before* use Store at room temperature below 30° C NOTE: The oral tablets are often found in combination with caffeine, which also possesses a cranial vaso-constricting effect	*Contraindicated* in angina pectoris, coronary artery disease, hypersensitivity, hypertension, infections (severe), lactation, peptic ulcer, pregnancy, renal impairment (severe), Raynaud's disease, thrombophlebitis, and thromboangitis obliterans Ergotamine apparently works by constricting cranial blood vessels May cause GI distress, muscle weakness, paresthesia, and transient bradycardia or tachycardia Discontinuation of long-term therapy with ergotamine may cause rebound migraine headaches and dysphoric mood	Monitor for signs of ergotism (e.g., acute GI distress, anuria, dilated pupils, slow weak pulse, thirst, twitching of the extremities)

Continued.

NURSING DRUG DIGEST—cont'd

Medication (trade name)	Indication	Usual dosage and administration	Dosage forms, preparation, and storage	Contraindications, cautions, and comments	Monitoring
★ **Factor IX complex (human, dried)** Konyne Proplex	Prevention or control of uncontrolled bleeding associated with deficiency of coagulation factors II, VII, IX, or X (often associated with Christmas disease)	*Adults:* Administer sufficient factor IX complex to raise factor IX concentration to at least 0.3 units of factor IX/ml of plasma Dosage is *highly* individualized based on patient response For IV infusion *only*	Injectable: 500 units factor IX/vial (also contains factors II, VII, and X) Store between 2° and 8° C until reconstituted Reconstitute with sterile water for injection Use immediately after reconstitution, although can be used within 3 hr *Discard* any unused solution	*Contraindicated* in severe liver dysfunction, intravascular coagulation, or fibrinolysis, and in neonates with vitamin K, deficiencies Discontinue treatment if evidence of intravascular coagulation is noted Infusion in patients with liver disease should be done cautiously because of possibility of transmission of HB₅Ag Rapid IV infusion may cause transient fever, chills, headache, flushing, tingling, hypertension, or irritation at injection site	Monitor for hypersensitivity Monitor blood coagulation factors
Fibrinolysin and desoxyribonuclease Elase Elase-Chloromycetin Ointment*	Enzymatic debriding agent	*Adults:* Apply in thin layer to local lesion daily until enzyme action is no longer desired; cover with petrolatum or other nonadhering dressing NOTE: Apply to clean wound; change dressing at least q.d. preferably b.i.d. to t.i.d. to obtain maximal effects of medication	Powder: 25 units fibrinolysin and 15,000 units desoxyribonuclease from bovine pancreas/vial Ointment: 1 unit fibrinolysin and 666 units of desoxyribonuclease per gram Disposable vaginal applicators available for use with 30 gm tube	*Contraindicated* in hypersensitivity Use cautiously in patients with history of allergic reactions to materials of bovine origin or mercury compounds	Monitor for adverse side effects, including local hyperemia particularly with higher concentrations After 2-4 days, monitor for healing of clean lesion and filling with granulation tissue

	Aseptic technique is indicated Remove necrotic debris and fibrinous exudates with saline peroxide or warm water so that newly applied drug (ointment) is in direct contact with lesion Solution may be applied topically as a liquid, spray, or wet dressing Spray: Spray solution using conventional atomizer Wet dressing: Mix vial of powder with 10-50 ml of normal saline; saturate sterile gauze with solution; pack ulcerated area with gauze ensuring contact with necrotic areas; surgical removal of heavy dry eschar at lesion is indicated before treatment with drug Allow gauze to dry in contact with lesion 6-8 hr so that necrotic tissue can slough and adhere to dressing; remove dried gauze to mechanically debride lesion; repeat wet-to-dry procedure t.i.d. to q.i.d. for 2-4 days For external use only	Solutions should be freshly prepared before use; loss of activity is reduced by refrigeration Discard any unused solution after 24 hr	After application, these products become rapidly and progressively less active, and insignificant activity remains after 24 hr
Vaginitis Cervicitis	Adults: Apply 5 ml of ointment deep into vagina with disposable vaginal applicator q.h.s. for 5 applications		Monitor for abnormal vaginal discharge, abdominal discomfort

Continued.

NURSING DRUG DIGEST—cont'd

Medication (trade name)	Indication	Usual dosage and administration	Dosage forms, preparation, and storage	Contraindications, cautions, and comments	Monitoring
Gonadotropin, chorionic A.P.L. Antuitrin-S Choranid Choron Entromone Follutein Glukor Injection* Pranturen Pregnesin Pregnyl Profas	Hypogonadotropic hypogonadism in males Induction of ovulation (used as an adjunct, with either clomiphene or menotropins) Prepubertal cryptorchidism	*Adults*: 1000-4000 units IM 3 times weekly for 2-28 weeks *Adults*: 5000-10,000 units IM 1 day following treatment with menotropins or 5-7 days following last dose of clomiphene *Children*: 500-1000 units IM 3 times weekly for 4-6 weeks; discontinue when desired response is observed Treatment for longer than 8 weeks is *not* recommended if progressive descent of testes does not occur Dosage is *highly* variable depending on patient response For IM use *only* May cause pain at injection site	Injectable: 2000, 5000, 10,000, 20,000 units/vial in powdered form supplied with 10 ml sodium chloride diluent Store between 15° and 30° C Stable in refrigerator for up to 90 days after reconstitution	*Contraindicated* (for treatment of cryptorchidism) in pituitary hypertrophy or tumor; precocious puberty *Contraindicated* (for male hypogonadism) in prostatic carcinoma or other androgen-dependent neoplasm *Contraindicated* (for induction of ovulation) in abnormal vaginal bleeding of undetermined origin, fibroid tumors of the uterus, ovarian cyst or enlargement, and thrombophlebitis (use associated with increased risk of thromboembolism) NOTE: Chorionic gonadotropin with menotropins is *not* the treatment of choice for induction of ovulation, but is used in patients who do not respond to less expensive or less hazardous treatment such as clomiphene Use with caution in patients with asthma, cardiac disease, epilepsy, migraine headaches, renal dysfunction	*For male hypogonadism:* Monitor serum testosterone concentrations, sperm count, and motility For determination of testicular function in delayed puberty, monitor serum testosterone concentrations before and 1 day following the course of treatment (should double if testes are normal) *For induction of ovulation:* Ovulation occurs within 18 hours after administration; pelvic examination should be completed daily for evaluation of ovarian size after the first sign of improvement until at least 2 weeks after chorionic gonadotropin administration Monitor basal body temperature daily to assist in determining occurrence of ovulation, and monitor changes in cervical mucus

Monitor estrogen determinations daily 1 week after beginning each course of menotropins; chorionic gonadotropin should *only* be given after estrogen production has been measured for the previous 24 hr following ovulation

Monitor for adverse side effects: bloating, stomach or pelvic pain associated with ovarian enlargement, or rupture of ovarian cysts and possible hemoperitoneum

Monitor for enlargement of breasts, headache, irritability, mental depression, edema of the lower extremities, tiredness

For prepubertal cryptorchidism: Monitor for stimulation of androgen production by testes resulting in development of secondary sex characteristics; descent of testes

NOTE: Effect may be permanent or temporary

Monitor males for acne, enlargement of penis and testes, growth of pubic hair, or rapid increase in height

Use cautiously in pregnancy; risk-benefit requires consideration; fetal death and congenital malformation have been reported in offspring of mothers treated with chorionic gonadotropin

False pregnancy tests may be obtained

Use associated with increased incidence of multiple births and possible prematurity

Continued.

NURSING DRUG DIGEST—cont'd

Medication (trade name)	Indication	Usual dosage and administration	Dosage forms, preparation, and storage	Contraindications, cautions, and comments	Monitoring
★ **Hemin** Panhematin	Amelioration of recurrent attacks of acute intermittent porphyria temporally related to the menstrual cycle in susceptible women	*Adults:* Initially, 1-4 mg/kg/day by slow IV over 10-15 min for 3-14 days based on clinical signs. If symptoms are not alleviated, the daily dose may be repeated *after* at least 12 hr. Maximum: Total daily amount of hemin *not* to exceed 6 mg/kg. Infuse into large arm or hand vein or through a central venous catheter. Phlebitis has occurred from injections into small veins. For IV use *only*	Injectable: 7 mg/ml available as a sterile lyophilized black powder in single-dose vials containing 313 mg hemin. Store lyophilized powder frozen until time of use. Reconstitute with 43 ml sterile water for injection, and shake well to aid dissolution *immediately* before administration	*Contraindicated* in hypersensitivity. Follow dosage guidelines carefully to prevent overdosage, which has led to renal shutdown. Because this drug is thought to act by reducing the rate of porphyrin/heme biosynthesis by inhibiting delta-aminolevulinic acid synthetase, drugs known to stimulate enzyme activity should be avoided; thus barbiturates, estrogens, sulfonamides, and anticoagulant drugs should *not* be given during hemin therapy. Improvement of neurologic signs may not be observed for weeks or months. Attacks tend to recur after prolonged remissions	Monitor for relief of symptoms: severe abdominal pain, hypertension, tachycardia, abnormal mental status or personality changes, psychotic behavior, control of mild to moderate progressive neurologic signs ranging from slight muscle weakness to flaccid paralysis or epileptiform convulsions. Observe for any untoward effects
Hyaluronidase Alidase Diffusin Enzodase Hyalase Hyazyme Infiltrase Wydase	Hemorrhoids. Increase absorption of other drugs administered SC. Adjunct to hypodermoclycis	*Adults:* 5000-10000 IU PR q.d. *Adults:* Add 150 IU to solvent of other drug being injected SC. *Adults:* 150 IU SC at injection site before clycis	Injectable: 60, 75, 150 IU/ml (for SC use *only*). Rectal suppository: 5000 IU. Once injectable is diluted, it is stable for 24 hr under refrigeration	*Contraindicated* in hypersensitivity. Do *not* inject into cancerous or infected areas	Monitor injection site for pain, irritation, abscess

Drug	Uses	Dosage	Remarks	Nursing Considerations
			May cause hypersensitivity (to test for hypersensitivity, inject 0.02 ml intradermally and observe in 5 min for wheal formation and pruritus) Used primarily to increase SC absorption of some drugs	Monitor patients receiving hypodermoclycis with dextrose solutions (e.g., D₅W) for hypovolemia, which may occur because of the lack of inorganic electrolytes in the solution
Lactase LactAid Lact-Ion Lactrose	Lactase insufficiency, milk intolerance	Capsule: 125 mg Oral drops: 200 units/drop *Adults*: 125-250 mg PO t.i.d. to q.i.d. with meals to aid in the digestion of dairy products Alternately, the capsules can be opened and the dosage can be sprinkled on dairy products *or* 800-2000 units (4-10 drops) added to each liter of milk	Toxicity appears to be minimal When added to milk, it takes approximately 2 hr to hydrolyze 70% of the lactose in 1 L at 30° C and approximately 24 hr at 6° C	Monitor for proper digestion of lactose Observe for any untoward effects
Menotropins Humegon Pergonal Pregova	Induction of ovulation (used as an adjunct with chorionic gonadotropin) Hypogonadotropic hypogonadism in males (used as an adjunct with chorionic gonadotropin)	Injectable: 75 IU of FSH and 75 IU of LH/vial Store between 15° and 30° C *Adults*: 75 IU each of FSH and LH IM q.d. for 9-12 days (followed by 5000-10,000 units of chorionic gonadotropin) May be repeated for 2 additional courses if necessary *Adults*: Following 5000 units of chorionic gonadotropin 3 times per week for 4-6 months; 75 IU each of FSH and LH IM 3 times per week (plus 2000 units of chorionic gonadotropin 2 times per week) for 4 months Dosage is *highly variable*, depending on patient response *For IM use only*	*Contraindicated* in elevated gonadotropin levels, thyroid dysfunction, pituitary tumor, and pregnancy Menotropins are a purified preparation of gonadotropins standardized for follicle stimulating hormone (FSH) and luteinizing hormone (LH) May result in multiple pregnancy, primarily twins May cause ovarian enlargement, hemoperitoneum, and arterial thromboembolism in females Occasionally causes gynecomastia in males	*For induction of ovulation*: Monitor serum estrogen levels, daily basal temperature, and complete pelvic examination *For treatment of hypogonadism in males*: Monitor serum testosterone levels, sperm count and motility

Continued.

NURSING DRUG DIGEST—cont'd

Medication (trade name)	Indication	Usual dosage and administration	Dosage forms, preparation, and storage	Contraindications, cautions, and comments	Monitoring
Methysergide Deseril Deseril Sansert	Prophylactic treatment and prevention of migraine and other severe recurring vascular headaches NOTE: It is *not* recommended for use to treat a migraine headache that has already started	*Adults:* Initially, 2 mg po q.h.s.; gradually increase to 2 mg t.i.d. with meals; average maintenance dose 4-8 mg/day Maximum: 12 mg/day *Children: Not* recommended for use in children under 12 years of age NOTE: A 1-month drug holiday is recommended following each 6-month course of treatment Decrease dose in renal failure	Tablet: 2 mg	*Contraindicated* in coronary artery disease, peripheral vascular disease, pregnancy, severe infection, impaired liver or renal function, and urinary tract diseases Approximately 50% of dose is excreted in unchanged form in urine May cause retroperitoneal fibrosis in patients receiving long-term maintenance therapy May cause edema, facial flush, GI distress, insomnia, weakness, and weight gain	Monitor patients for absence or decreased occurrence of migraine headache Observe for adverse effects, including coldness, numbness or tingling in the hands or feet, leg cramps, edema of the lower extremities, chest pain, shortness of breath, and girdle or flank pain Observe for signs of retroperitoneal fibrosis usually manifested as urinary tract obstruction
★ **Metyrosine** Demser	Pheochromocytoma (in preoperative patients and patients in whom surgery is contraindicated)	*Adults:* Initially, 250 mg PO q.i.d. Maintenance: may increase by 250-500 mg/day to a maximum of 4000 mg/day in divided doses *Children:* Use in children under 12 years of age is *not* recommended	Capsule: 250 mg	*Contraindicated* in hypersensitivity Commonly causes sedation, diarrhea, and extrapyramidal reactions (e.g., drooling, speech difficulty, tremor) May cause anxiety, depression, confusion, disorientation, and hallucinations May cause crystalluria Encourage fluid intake	Observe for psychic disturbance Monitor urinary output (should be maintained at 2000 ml or more per day)

Drug	Uses	Dosage/Preparation	Contraindications	Nursing considerations
Oxytocin Pitocin Syntocinon Uteracon	Induction or stimulation of labor in patients with a medical necessity (e.g., mild preeclampsia, premature rupture of membranes, uterine inertia) Control of postpartum uterine bleeding Initiate milk letdown	*Adults:* Initially 1-2 mUnits/minute by IV infusion (drip method); gradually increase dose, as necessary, in 1-2 mUnits/min increments at 15-30 min intervals until a uterine contraction pattern similar to normal labor is achieved *Adults:* 10-40 units (diluted in 1000 ml NS or D₅W) and administered by IV infusion (drip method) at a rate sufficient to control uterine atony; *or* 5-10 units IM after delivery of the placenta *Adults:* 1 spray into one or both nostrils 2-3 min before nursing or pumping the breasts Injectable: 10 units/ml, Store under refrigeration, Do *not* freeze, Dilute injectable with 1000 ml NS or D₅W *before* administration, Nasal spray: 40 units/ml	*Contraindicated* in fetal distress, hypertonic uterine patterns, hypersensitivity, significant cephalopelvic disproportion, severe toxemia, transverse lies, total placenta previa, unfavorable fetal presentation, and vasa previa In addition, the nasal spray formulation is *contraindicated* during pregnancy and labor May cause hypersensitivity, severe water intoxication, and fetal bradycardia	Monitor uterine tone Monitor uterine frequency, duration, and force of uterine contractions Monitor fluid status for signs of water intoxication Monitor blood pressure Monitor fetal heart rate for fetal bradycardia
★ **Papain and urea** Panafil Panafil-White	Enzymatic debridement and promotion of normal healing of surface lesions	*Adults:* Apply directly to lesion once or twice daily and cover with gauze Irrigate lesion with mild cleansing solution before each application of papain to remove liquefied necrotic material NOTE: Hydrogen peroxide solution may inactivate papain and should *not* be used to cleanse or irrigate lesion between application of papain or dressing changes For *external* use *only*	Ointment: 10% papain, 10% urea	*Contraindicated* in hypersensitivity *Contraindicated* for use in eyes	Monitor for adverse effects including itching or stinging associated with first application Monitor for normal healing of surface lesions, particularly those in which healing is slowed because of local infection, fibrinous or purulent debris, necrotic tissue, or eschar

Continued.

NURSING DRUG DIGEST—cont'd

Medication (trade name)	Indication	Usual dosage and administration	Dosage forms, preparation, and storage	Contraindications, cautions, and comments	Monitoring
Pentoxifylline Trental	Symptomatic treatment of chronic occlusive arterial disease	*Adults:* Initially, 400 mg PO b.i.d. Maintenance: 400 mg PO b.i.d. to t.i.d. Maximum dose: 1200 mg/day *Children:* Use is *not* recommended *Elderly:* Start with lower doses and increase gradually Tablets must be swallowed whole Administration with food or milk may decrease GI distress Dosage may need to be decreased in renal or hepatic impairment	Sustained release tablet: 400 mg	*Contraindicated* in patients with acute myocardial infarction, severe coronary artery disease, hemorrhage, intolerance to pentoxifylline or other xanthines (e.g., coffee, theophylline, theobromine), and peptic ulcer disease Metabolized extensively in the liver and eliminated through kidneys—use with caution in patients with liver or renal dysfunction; patients should be carefully monitored and dosage may need to be reduced Use cautiously in patients with labile blood pressure; any dose increase should be made gradually in the elderly, because peak plasma levels and metabolites are generally higher in this group Use with caution in pregnancy or nursing mothers because safety under these conditions has not been established Full effects may not be apparent for 2 months Commonly causes GI distress May cause dizziness, flushing, headache, and malaise	Monitor for relief of symptoms Monitor for improved peripheral blood flow, improved peripheral tissue oxygenation, and relief of intermittent claudication Monitor patients for adverse effects: nausea, flushing, abdominal discomfort, bloating, diarrhea, dizziness, dyspepsia, headache, and malaise Monitor for *overdose:* flushing, hematemesis, absent reflexes, tonic-clonic convulsions, loss of consciousness Monitor blood pressure carefully; dosage reduction may be indicated

Drug	Use	Dosage	Preparations/Notes	Cautions/Side Effects	Nursing Considerations
Quinine Novoquinine Quinamm	Nocturnal leg muscle cramps (prevention and treatment)	*Adults:* 250 mg PO q.h.s. If necessary, an additional 250 mg PO may be administered after the evening meal	Tablets: 250, 300 mg	May potentiate action of antihypertensive agents. Administration with other xanthines or with sympathomimetics may cause increased CNS stimulation. Dosage reduction of hypoglycemic agents may be required with concurrent administration. *Contraindicated* in pregnancy, G-6-PD deficiency, hypersensitivity, and optic neuritis. Use with caution in patients with tinnitus. May cause birth defects, including deafness and stillbirth, if administered during pregnancy. May cause nausea, vomiting, headache, blurred vision, and rashes. May cause cinchonism (i.e., GI disturbances, headache, nausea, tinnitus, visual disturbances)	Monitor for decreased occurrence or absence of nocturnal leg cramps. Observe for hypersensitivity (i.e., cutaneous flushing, dyspnea, gastric distress, fever, pruritus, skin rash, tinnitus)
★ **Ritodrine** Yutopar	To prolong pregnancy. To halt preterm labor. Reduction of recurrent attacks of premature labor	*Adults:* Initial dose: 0.1 mg/min IV gradually increasing to 0.15–0.35 mg/min; continue infusion for at least 12 hr after uterine contractions cease. NOTE: Patients require one-to-one nursing care and monitoring with IV administration. Oral maintenance: 10 mg PO 30 min *before* end of IV administration; then 10 mg q.2h. for first 24 hours followed by 10–20 mg q.4-6h. Maximum: 120 mg/day PO	Injectable: 10 mg/ml. Tablet: 10 mg. Dilute 150 mg in 500 ml of NS, D₅W, or Ringers solution. Discard unused solution after 48 hr. Discard discolored solutions of ritodrine	*Contraindicated* before the twentieth week of gestation and in active vaginal bleeding, severe preeclampsia, intrauterine infection, maternal cardiac disease, cervical dilation greater than 3-4 cm, advanced labor, cardiovascular disorders, fetal death, uncontrolled diabetes, and hypersensitivity. To minimize risk of hypertension, patients should maintain the lateral recumbent position	Monitor for decrease or cessation of uterine activity. During IV infusion maternal heart rate and blood pressure, uterine activity, and fetal heart rate should be monitored every 10-15 minutes. Monitor for: tachycardia (maternal heart rate should not exceed 135 beats/minute); nausea; tremors; light-headedness; and feeling of warmth over body

Continued.

NURSING DRUG DIGEST—cont'd

Medication (trade name)	Indication	Usual dosage and administration	Dosage forms, preparation, and storage	Contraindications, cautions, and comments	Monitoring
Ritodrine—cont'd				Patients receiving oral maintenance therapy require instruction regarding home care, including modified bed rest, refraining from preparing the breasts for nursing until 2 weeks before due date, avoiding sexual intercourse and orgasm, and notifying health care provider of signs of preterm labor: low back pain, cramping, increased vaginal discharge, uterine contractions Patients should be able to monitor pulse rate and know to notify health care provider, because medication is held if pulse is greater than 130 beats/min Use cautiously with corticosteroids because maternal pulmonary edema has been reported A persistent tachycardia (greater than 140 beats/min) may precede development of pulmonary edema Use cautiously in patients receiving potassium-depleting diuretics Commonly causes increased heart rate, headache, nausea, tremor, and vomiting.	Blood glucose of diabetics should be monitored closely since increases in insulin infusion doses may be required Observe for maternal pulmonary edema (even after delivery) Monitor maternal pulse rate and blood pressure and fetal heart rate, particularly during IV administration Monitor for adverse effects associated with β-sympathomimetic activity (e.g., increased heart rate, increased blood pressure, tremors, nausea, vomiting, headache)

Drug	Use	Dosage form	Dosing	Precautions/Contraindications	Monitoring
Sodium cellulose phosphate Calcibind Calcisorb	Treatment of recurrent calcium-containing stones caused by type I absorptive hypercalciuria in which both intestinal calcium absorption and urinary calcium remain abnormally high even with a low calcium intake	Powder: 2.5 gm/packet	*Adults:* 15 gm/day (5 gm with each meal) for patients with urinary calcium concentrations greater than 300 mg/day on a moderately calcium-restricted diet (e.g., avoidance of dairy products) 10 gm/day (5 gm with supper; 2.5 gm with other 2 meals) when urinary calcium falls to less than 150 mg/day 10 gm/day for patients with baseline urinary calcium concentrations below 300 mg/day on a moderately calcium-restricted diet *Children:* Use *not* recommended NOTE: Sodium cellulose phosphate should be taken *with* meals Powder form should be mixed in fruit juice, water, or a soft drink NOTE: Some patients find sodium cellulose phosphate unpalatable NOTE: Supplemental magnesium should be administered 1 hr before or 2 hr after the sodium cellulose phosphate dose to avoid binding of magnesium with the sodium cellulose phosphate	*Contraindicated* in bone disease (e.g., osteoporosis), enteric hyperoxaluria, hyperparathyroidism, hypocalcemia, hypomagnesemia, and renal hypercalciuria Sodium cellulose phosphate is an insoluble synthetic compound that exchanges sodium for calcium and other cations in the GI tract Sodium cellulose phosphate binds calcium in the intestinal tract, decreasing the amount in the urine without altering calcium balance May cause GI distress Patients taking sodium cellulose phosphate may develop hyperoxaluria and hypomagnesuria, which predispose to stone formation; they should take magnesium gluconate supplements (500 mg magnesium supplement per 5 gm sodium cellulose phosphate dose) and restrict dietary intake of oxalate and vitamin C	Monitor dietary calcium Patients should avoid dairy products, sardines, spinach, excess salt, and vitamin C Monitor for hyperoxaluria and hypomagnesuria Monitor patients for restriction of dietary intake of oxalate (found in spinach, rhubarb, chocolate, tea) and vitamin C, which can increase urinary oxalate Monitor fluid intake and output to maintain urine output of at least 2 L/day Monitor patients for decrease in frequency of passage of renal stones Monitor patients for adverse effects: GI discomfort, acute arthralgias Monitor parathyroid hormone concentrations and function

Continued.

NURSING DRUG DIGEST—cont'd

Medication (trade name)	Indication	Usual dosage and administration	Dosage forms, preparation, and storage	Contraindications, cautions, and comments	Monitoring
Sodium cellulose phosphate—cont'd				Use with caution in patients with congestive heart failure or hypertension A low calcium diet, high fluid intake and thiazides when necessary are generally recommended as adjunct therapy Every 15 gm of sodium cellulose phosphate contains 25-50 mEq of sodium, which may be excessive in some patients Sodium cellulose phosphate could cause hyperparathyroidism if the dosage is too high or if the drug is given to unsuitable patients Depletion of magnesium and trace metals may occur during long-term treatment	Monitor patients for depletion of magnesium and trace metals (copper, iron, zinc) especially during long-term therapy
Sodium Fluoride Flo-Tabs Flozenges Fluor-A-Day Flura-Drops Fluoretyl Fluorident Fluorinse Fluoritab Karidium Les-Cav	Prevention of dental caries	Topical use (oral rinse) *Adults:* Rinse mouth each day after brushing for 60 seconds with 5-10 ml *and* expectorate *Children:* Same as adults Do *not* swallow rinse Systemic use (tablets, drops) *Children:* infants, 0.55 mg PO q.d.; 2-5 years of age, 1.1 mg PO q.d.; over 5 years of age, 2.21 mg PO q.d.	Oral rinse: 0.05%, 0.2% Tablets: 0.55, 1.1, 2.21 mg Drops: 0.275, 0.55 mg	Systemic use is *contraindicated* in sodium-restricted diets and in communities where water with 0.7 ppm of fluoride is used May cause GI distress, headache, and skin rashes	Monitor for reduction in frequency of dental caries Monitor for hypersensitivity particularly to additives in commercial products

Drug	Indications	Dosage	Administration	Contraindications, Cautions, and Comments	Monitor
Luride Pedi-Dent Pediaflur Phos-Flur Primadent Solu-Flur Thera-Flur Vi-Daylin/F ADC Drops* Vi-Penta F Chewables*				NOTE: *Not* to be used in communities with fluoridated water (see Contraindications, Cautions, and Comments)	
Sodium polystyrene sulfonate Kayexalate	Hyperkalemia (in severe cases of hyperkalemia [e.g., >7.5 mEq/L] IV glucose and insulin may be indicated)	*Adults:* 15 gm (approximately 4 *level* teaspoonsful) PO q.d. to q.i.d. NOTE: 1 level teaspoon contains approximately 3.5 gm *Children:* Infants and small children, dose administered is based on an exchange rate of 1 mEq K$^+$/gm of powdered resin	Powdered resin: Protect from heat Reconstitute in drinking water or syrup before administration Suspensions should be freshly prepared *Discard* unused suspension after 24 hr	*Contraindicated* in *hypokalemia* Use with caution in patients on sodium restriction or in whom excess sodium may be problematic (e.g., those with CHF, edema, hypertension) Each gram of Kayexalate contains approximately 100 mg (4.1 mEq) of sodium May cause GI distress Constipation can be treated with 10-20 ml sorbitol syrup (70%) q.2h. prn	Monitor serum electrolytes Observe for signs of hypokalemia, hypocalcemia, and hypernatremia
Somatropin Asellacrin Crescormon	Growth failure resulting from decreased or failed pituitary growth hormone	*Children:* 0.5 IU/kg/week IM in 2-3 divided doses Dose is *highly* individualized based on patient response For IM use *only*	Injectable: 4 IU/vial with 2 ml sodium chloride injection as a diluent Keep refrigerated Solution should be reconstituted on day of use *Discard* unused solution after 24 hr	*Contraindicated* in diabetes mellitus, active intracranial lesions, and patients with closed epiphyses Adverse and side effects are reportedly minimal May cause hyperglycemia and ketosis	Monitor body growth Monitor urine for glycosuria

Continued.

NURSING DRUG DIGEST—cont'd

Medication (trade name)	Indication	Usual dosage and administration	Dosage forms, preparation, and storage	Contraindications, cautions, and comments	Monitoring
Streptokinase Bistreptase* Dornokinase* Kabikinase Streptase Varidase*	Lysis of intracoronary artery thrombi

Treatment of deep vein thrombosis, pulmonary embolism, arterial embolism, arterial thrombosis | *Adults:* Initially, (administered within 6 hr of symptoms of acute MI) 20,000 IU bolus into the thrombosed coronary artery via *coronary catheter;* followed by a maintenance dose of 2000 IU/min for 60 min administered via a volumetric infusion pump

Adults: Initially, (administered within 7 days of onset) 250,000 IU infused into a peripheral vein over 30 min, followed by a maintenance dose of 100,000 IU/hr for 24-72 hr

Children: Use is *not* recommended | Injectable: 250,000, 500,000 IU/vial
Store between 15° and 30° C
To reconstitute, add 5 ml of D₅W or sodium chloride for injection; gently mix by rolling and tilting the vial
Do *not* shake or agitate (shaking causes flocculation)
Discard solutions that contain a large amount of flocculation
May be slowly diluted with 45 ml sodium chloride injection or D₅W
If necessary, the total volume may be increased in multiples of 45 ml to a maximum of 500 ml
Store solution between 2° and 4° C
Discard any unused solution after 24 hr
The solution may be filtered through a 0.22-0.45 μ filter before administration; however, slight flocculation does *not* appear to interfere with the safe use of the solution
Do *not* add any other medication to streptokinase injection | *Contraindicated* in intracranial neoplasm, active internal bleeding, recent (within 2 months) intracranial or spinal surgery, and recent (within 2 months) cerebrovascular accident
May cause bleeding, hypersensitivity, and fever
Mild allergic reactions can be treated with an antihistamine or corticosteroid
Fever can be treated with acetaminophen (use of aspirin increases risk of hemorrhage)
Avoid IM injections and nonessential handling of patient
IV injections should be performed with caution | Monitor coagulation studies (i.e., thrombin time, activated partial thromboplastin time, prothrombin time)
Monitor hematocrit and platelet count
Observe for signs of hemorrhage (e.g., easy bruising, bleeding around the gums)
Monitor all injection sites |

CO_2

Drug	Use	Dosage	Preparation/Administration	Precautions/Contraindications	Nursing Considerations
Urokinase Abbokinase Breokinase Win-Kinase	Lysis of pulmonary emboli	*Adults:* Initially, 4400 IU/kg by IV infusion over 10 min, followed by 4400 IU/kg/hr at a rate of 15 ml/hr for 12 hr	Injectable: 250,000 IU/vial Store between 2° and 8° C Reconstitute *immediately* before use To reconstitute, add 5.2 ml of sterile water for injection *without* preservatives; rotate vial gently—do *not* shake Discard solutions that are discolored or contain a precipitate The solution may be filtered through a 0.22-0.45 μ filter May be diluted with up to 150 ml NS or D_5W Do *not* add any other medication to urokinase injection	*Contraindicated* in intracranial neoplasm, active internal bleeding, recent (within 2 months) intracranial or spinal surgery, and recent (within 2 months) cerebrovascular accident May cause bleeding, hypersensitivity, and fever Mild allergic reactions can be treated with an antihistamine or corticosteroid Fever can be treated with acetaminophen (use of aspirin increases risk of hemorrhage) Avoid IM injections and nonessential handling of patient IV injections should be performed with caution	Monitor coagulation studies (i.e., thrombin time, activated thromboplastin time, prothrombin time) Monitor hematocrit and platelet count Observe for signs of hemorrhage (e.g., easy bruising, bleeding around gums) Monitor all injection sites
Vasopressin Insipidin Pitressin Pitressin Tannate in Oil	Prevention and treatment of postoperative abdominal distention See also Chapter 36, "Diuretics and Antidiuretics"	*Adults:* Initially, 5 units IM after surgery, followed by 5-10 units IM q.3-4h. prn *Children:* Decrease dosage appropriately	Injectable: 20 units/ml; 5 units/ml in peanut oil (tannate salt)	*Contraindicated* in hypersensitivity and vascular disease Injectable in peanut oil is *contraindicated* in patients allergic to peanuts May cause water intoxication Use with caution in patients with asthma, congestive heart failure, hypertension, migraine, or renal failure May cause anaphylaxis, GI distress, pounding sensation in head, sweating, tremor, and urticaria	Observe for signs of water intoxication (i.e., drowsiness, headache, listlessness, convulsions, and coma) Observe for anginal pain and signs of myocardial infarction in patients with coronary artery disease (use in these patients is *not* recommended)

BIBLIOGRAPHY

Amiodarone HCl (Cordarone by Ives)—an investigational antiarrhythmic agent. Keeping up. *Hospital Pharmacy*, 1984, *19*, 384-385.

Atkinson, K., Biggs, J., & Darveniza, P. Cyclosporine-associated central nervous system toxicity after allogeneic bone-marrow transplantation. *New England Journal of Medicine*, 1984, *310*, 527.

Benotti, J., Grossman, W., Braunwald, E., & Carabellow, B.A. Effects of amrinone on myocardial energy metabolism and hemodynamics in patients with severe congestive heart failure due to coronary artery disease. *Circulation*, 1980, *62*(1), 28-34.

Brengman, S.L., & Burns, M. Ritodrine hydrochloride and preterm labor. *American Journal of Nursing*, 1983, *83*(4), 537-539.

Burckart, G.J. Editorial—Monitoring cyclosporine therapy. *Clinical Pharmacy*, 1983, *2*, 568.

Canafax, D.M., & Ascher, N.L. Cyclosporine immunosuppression. *Clinical Pharmacy*, 1983, *2*, 515-524.

Chymopapain for herniated lumbar discs. *The Medical Letter on Drugs and Therapeutics*, 1983, *25*(634), 41-42.

Conner, C.S. Intravenous streptokinase in acute myocardial infarction. *Drug Intelligence and Clinical Pharmacy*, 1983, *17*, 367-368.

Cyclosporine Neurotoxicity. *Drug Newsletter*, 1984, (April), 28.

Cyclosporine—a new immunosuppressive agent. *The Medical Letter On Drugs and Therapeutics*, 1983, *25*(642), 77-78.

Edwards, S., & Wing, D. Combination Drugs. *Drug Newsletter*, 1982, December.

Finkelstein, B.W. Ritodrine. *Drug Intelligence and Clinical Pharmacy*, 1981, *15*, 425-433.

Formulary Review of analgesics. Part III. Drug therapy of migraine. *Formulary Committee Bulletin*, Saskatchewan Health, 1980, *22*.

Fromm, H., Roat, J.W., & Gonzalez, V. Comparative efficacy and side effects of ursodeoxycholic and chenodeoxycholic acids in dissolving gallstones. *Gastroenterology*, 1983, *85*, 1257-1264.

Klein, N.A., Siskind, S.J., Frishman, W.H., Sonnenblick, E.H., & LeJemtel, T.H. Hemodynamic comparison of intravenous amrinone and dobutamine in patients with chronic congestive heart failure. *The American Journal of Cardiology*, 1981, *48*, 170-175.

Masson, E. Prostaglandins—a brief overview. *On Continuing Practice*, 1983, *10*(2), 13-14.

Phillipson, J.D., & Anderson, L.A. Pharmacologically active compounds in herbal remedies. *The Pharmaceutical Journal*, 1984, January, 41-44.

Plein, E.M. Sunscreens. *Nurse Practitioner*, 1981, May-June, 35, 39, 41, and 51.

Reichlin, S. Neural control of the pituitary gland: normal physiology and pathophysiologic implications. In *Current Concepts*, New York: The Upjohn Company, 1978.

Roehl, S.L., & Townsend, R.J. Alprostadil (Prostin VR Pediatric Sterile Solution, The Upjohn Company). *Drug Intelligence and Clinical Pharmacy*, 1982, *16*, 823-832.

Rosenberg, J.M. New Drugs Introduced in 1983. *Drug Store News Continuing Education Program*, 1984, Lesson no. 679-401-84-06.

Sodium Cellulose Phosphate (Calcibind). *The Medical Letter On Drugs and Therapeutics*, 1983, *25*(639), 67-68.

Ward, A., Brogden, R.N., & Heel R.C. Ursodeoxycholic acid: a review of its pharmacological properties and therapeutic efficacy. *Drugs*, 1984, *27*, 95-131.

Whall, C.W. Daily rinsing with fluoride: an effective anti-cavity procedure. *Pharmacy Times*, 1983, July, 26-29.

APPENDICES

Glossary

A

absence seizure (petit mal seizure) an epileptic seizure in which the patient has a brief lapse in awareness usually lasting less than 10 seconds; electroencephalograph shows 3 spike wave activity per second

absorption coefficient the fractional decrease in the intensity of a radioactive beam as it interacts with the absorbing material; usually described per unit thickness or per unit mass

acetonide grouping a chemical acetonelike combination

acid rebound consists of gastric hypersecretion of stomach acid after the initial buffering effect of the drug, occurs most noticeably with calcium carbonate

acid mucopolysaccharide major chemical constituent of ground substance of dermis

acidosis a pathologic condition resulting from accumulation of acid or loss of base from the body; characterized by an increase in hydrogen ion concentration (decrease in pH)

acinar cells a group of secretory cells surrounding a cavity

acini a collection of cells around a saclike dilatation, particularly one found in various glands

acne rosacea a common skin condition characterized by inflammatory papules, telangiectasia, or both of the central face

actin a protein that is contained in the thin filaments of the microfilamental structure of skeletal muscle and together with myosin is responsible for muscle contraction

actinic keratoses the superficial skin lesions on sun-exposed sites such as the face with microscopic atypical epidermal changes considered precancerous; grows slowly and tends to remain localized

action potential the electric activity developed in excitable tissue, such as cardiac tissue; subdivided into five phases (0 to 4); in muscle precedes and initiates events leading to contraction

active acquired immunity an immunity resulting from antibodies that the individual developed himself or herself; may be present after an infectious disease or may be artificially induced by injection of antigens such as with the injection of measles vaccine; these replicate in the recipient, who then develops antibodies in response

acute abdomen a sudden onset of abdominal pain, tenderness, and guarding, signifying an intraabdominal catastrophe

acute tubular necrosis damage to renal tubular function with a clinical picture of acute renal failure and necrosis of tubular cells

Addison's disease the partial or complete failure of the adrenocortex to secrete adrenocortical hormones

adenocarcinoma a cancer arising from gland-forming cells

adipocyte a fat cell

adjuvant chemotherapy the use of anticancer drugs after surgery in patients whose cancer is likely to recur

adrenal crisis an acute, life-threatening state arising from profound adrenal insufficiency; characterized by extracellular fluid volume deficit and hyperkalemia

adsorbent a substance that takes up another substance by adsorption (i.e., the attachment of one substance to the surface of another)

aerobe a microorganism that can live and grow in the presence of free oxygen

afterload (of the left ventricle) those factors, usually downstream from the ventricle, that determine impedance to outflow of blood from the ventricle and thus influence the forward cardiac output; in the absence of outflow obstruction, systemic vascular resistance is the primary factor

agonist a chemical substance that selectively "excites or activates" a receptor molecule; in turn triggers a sequence of events leading to an observable response

agranulocytosis a condition of decreased white blood cells; characterized by high fever and mucous membrane lesions

airways, large commonly defined as airways with a diameter greater than 2 mm; also called central or conducting airways

airways, small commonly defined as airways with a diameter less than 2 mm; also called peripheral airways

akinesia the inability to initiate movement

albuminuria the presence of detectable amounts of albumin in the urine; usually associated with kidney damage

aliphatic alcohols the alcohols containing open chain or fatty series of hydrocarbons

alkalosis a pathologic condition resulting from accumulation of base or loss of acid in the body; characterized by a decrease in hydrogen ion concentration (increase in pH)

alkylating agent a compound capable of introducing an alkyl (hydrocarbon radical) group onto other molecules by forming covalent bonds

allergenic extracts an extract of the protein of any substance to which a person may be sensitive; used for diagnosis or desensitization therapy in conditions caused by hypersensitivity; prepared from a great variety of substances from food to fungi

allergic rhinitis hay fever

allergic vasculitis the inflammation of blood vessels as a result of an allergic reaction; marked by such cutaneous lesions as papules, macules, vesicles, purpura, and small ulcers; accompanied by itching and usually by a slight fever and malaise

alopecia the loss of scalp hair

alpha particle a particle with a nucleus consisting of two protons and two neutrons carrying a double positive charge; a helium ion

alpha (redistribution) phase the period immediately following intravenous administration of a drug when the peak blood level begins to fall; primarily caused by redistribution of the drug throughout the body

amebic dysentery a disorder caused by *Entamoeba hystolytica*; associated with inflammation of the intestines, especially the colon, and symptoms of diarrhea and sometimes prostration

amebicide an agent destructive to amebas

amnesia the loss of memory (anterograde amnesia is loss of memory after the situation occurs)

amphoteric capable of acting either as a positively charged or negatively charged compound

amylase an enzyme that catalyzes the hydrolysis of starch into smaller molecules

anabolism any process of constructive metabolism

analgesia the loss of pain sensation

analgesic relieving pain; an agent that alleviates pain without causing unconsciousness

analogue a drug whose structure is very similar to another drug or compound

anaphylactic reactions a group of symptoms that represent a sometimes overwhelming and dangerous allergic reaction as a result of an extreme hypersensitivity to a drug; can result from a small dose of a drug, can develop suddenly, usually within a few minutes after taking the drug, can be rapidly progressive, and can lead to fatal collapse (anaphylactic shock) in a short time; symptoms can be mild (e.g., itching, hives, nasal congestion, nausea, abdominal cramps, and diarrhea) or severe (e.g., choking, shortness of breath, and cardiovascular collapse)

anasarca a generalized massive swelling caused by extensive accumulation of fluid

anergy a condition in which there is no response to the injection of an antigen

anesthesia the loss of all sensation

angioneurotic edema the swelling of the skin or mucous membranes; often associated with red, splotchy areas

anhedonia lacking interest or pleasure in acts or events that are normally pleasurable

anicteric without jaundice

anion a compound carrying a net negative charge; may include nonmetals, acid radicals, and hydroxyl ion (OH^-)

antagonist a substance that tends to nullify the action or effect of another

antianabolic the inhibition or slowing of the process of creating new tissue by protein synthesis and cell division; replaces damaged or aged tissues and is responsible for growth; antianabolic medications slow or inhibit anabolism

antibiotic anticancer agents those anticancer drugs that are produced by microorganisms (usually molds or fungi) that can kill other microorganisms and cancer cells

anticholinergic the process of blocking the passage of impulses through the parasympathetic nerves; parasympatholytic

antidiarrheal an agent that is effective in combating diarrhea

antigen a substance that on gaining access to animal tissues, stimulates the formation of antibody

antigenicity the ability to cause antibody formation

antihistamine a drug used to prevent actions of histamine

antileprotic a therapeutic agent effective in the treatment of leprosy

antimetabolite a drug that resembles normal compounds (usually vitamins or nucleotides) essential for cell growth but interferes with the function of these compounds and therefore inhibits cell growth and division

antimitotic inhibitor of cell division

antineoplastic anticancer

antiprotoplasmatic agents a general term for agents that are damaging to cell substance

antirachitic an agent used for treating rickets

antiseborrheic agents the topical compounds effective against seborrhea or seborrheic dermatitis

antiseptic a chemical agent that will arrest the growth of certain microorganisms

antisialagogue a drug that reduces secretion of saliva

antithyroid an agent or drug that inhibits normal thyroid activity

antitoxin the serums given to neutralize the toxins of certain diseases such as diphtheria; formed in the bodies of animals that have been actively immunized by a specific toxin

antitubercular a therapeutic agent effective in the treatment of tuberculosis

antitussive a cough suppressant

antivenin the proteinaceous material used to treat venom poisoning; some such as the black widow spider, polyvalent Crotalidae, and North American coral snake antivenins contain antibodies and are used only therapeutically

anuria no urine output

anxiolytic a pharmacologic agent that reduces anxiety

apical the upper part of a cell (nearest the follicular lumen for epithelial cells of the thyroid); pertaining to the apex

aplastic anemia a reduction in the number of red blood cells or hemoglobin concentration caused by failure of the bone marrow to produce new red blood cells

apnea cessation of breathing

appendicitis an inflammation of the vermiform appendix

argyria a generalized slate-gray coloration of skin and mucous membranes from excessive absorption and tissue deposition of silver salts

aspiration the act of breathing or drawing in of fluids, food, or foreign bodies into the respiratory passages

aspiration pneumonitis an inflammation of the lungs caused by aspiration of fluid, usually gastric contents

astringent causing contraction; usually associated with a drying effect on topical application; styptic

ataxia a lack of muscular coordination

atelectasis collapse of the lung

atom the smallest particle of an element that can react chemically; general symbol represented by X; the specific symbol derived from the name of the element

atomic mass unit (amu) the mass of a neutral atom of an element; expressed as $\frac{1}{12}$ of the mass of carbon, which carries an arbitrarily assigned value of 12; the energy equivalent of 1 amu equivalent to 931.2 MeV, the mass equivalent to 1.6604×10^{-24} gm

atomic number the number of protons in a nucleus; the general symbol represented by Z

atony a lack of muscle tone or strength

atopic dermatitis a common pattern of pruritic dermatitis tending to be familial; commonly associated with family background of asthma and hay fever

atopic patients those with a state of altered reactivity commonly comprising asthma, hay fever, and atopic dermatitis

atrioventricular (AV) node that portion of the specialized conduction system of the heart located low in the right atrium that provides an electric connection between the atria and the His-Purkinje system

atrophy a diminution of size or wasting away of tissues

autoantibodies the antibodies directed against antigens that are normal constituents of the same organism

autoimmune pertaining to the production of autoantibodies with associated dysfunction of the involved organ system

automaticity that property of specialized excitable tissue that permits self-activation through spontaneous development of an action potential

autonomous an activity that is not under the control of any external factors

azotemia the retention of urea and other nitrogenous waste products in the blood

B

bacillary dysentery a catarrhal, membranous, or necrotic inflammation of the mucous membrane of the large intestine as a result of the presence of bacteria of the genus *Shigella*; marked by symptoms of diarrhea, abdominal pain, and tenesmus

bacillus (pl. **bacilli**) in general any rod-shaped bacterium

bacterial resistance a measure of the tolerance that bacteria can develop toward specific antibiotic agents

bactericidal destructive to bacteria

bacteriostatic capable of inhibiting bacterial growth

barium enema a radiologic examination of the colon using barium sulfate as intracolonic contrast material

basal the lower part of a cell (nearest the basement membrane and blood supply for epithelial cells of the thyroid); pertaining to the base

becquerel a unit of radioactive decay equaling 1 disintegration per second (1 millicurie is equivalent to 37 megabecquerels)

benign not cancerous; a tumor that does not spread and destroy normal tissues

beta particle a particle emitted from the nucleus during radioactive decay; it has a single negative charge and the mass of an electron

beta (elimination) phase the period immediately following the alpha (redistribution) phase when the blood level of a drug falls more slowly primarily because of metabolism and excretion from the body

bloating the distention of the stomach or intestines with air or gases

blood-brain barrier a potential barrier to the free passage of substances from the bloodstream into the extracellular fluid of brain tissue; blood vessels subserving the brain have no gaps or pores, therefore substances must usually be reasonably lipid-soluble to pass through the capillary walls into brain tissue

blood urea nitrogen (BUN) the concentration of urea nitrogen in the blood; impairment of renal function is able to produce an increase in BUN

bronchiectasis a chronic dilation of the bronchi or bronchioles marked by fetid breath and paroxysmal coughing with the expectoration of mucopurulent matter

bruxism grinding teeth usually during sleep

buffalo hump the fat deposition at the back of the neck associated with prolonged use of large doses of glucocorticoids or the hypersecretion of cortisol occurring with Cushing's syndrome

buffer any substance in a fluid that tends to lessen the change in hydrogen ion concentration (reaction) that otherwise would be produced by adding acids or alkalis

C

capacitance vessels those blood vessels that hold the major proportion of the intravascular volume; the veins downstream from microvasculature (i.e., downstream from arterioles, capillaries, and venules)

carbamates a class of anticholinesterases used as insecticides and in medicine causing reversible inhibition of cholinesterase

carbon dioxide narcosis the stupor induced by toxic blood levels of carbon dioxide (i.e., 70 to 80 mm Hg carbon dioxide)

carcinogenic capable of causing cancer

carcinoid a yellow circumscribed tumor occurring in the small intestine, appendix, stomach, or colon

cardiac decompensation the inability of the heart to maintain adequate blood circulation

casts in urine the protein or cellular aggregates outlining the shape of renal tubules in which they are formed; presence indicates some forms of renal dysfunction

catabolic breaking down substances into more simple compounds

catabolism any process of destructive metabolism

catechol-o-methyltransferase (COMT) the enzyme responsible for methylation of the hydroxyl group in position 3 of the benzene ring of catecholamines such as norepinephrine, epinephrine, and isoproterenol; this inactivates these substances

catecholamines biogenic amines containing a catechol nucleus (3,4-dihydroxyphenylalanine); the most important examples include neurohumors dopamine and norepinephrine (noradrenaline) and the hormone epinephrine (adrenaline)

cathartic an agent that quickens and increases the evacuation from the bowels and produces purgation

cationic a compound carrying a net positive charge

cell cycle the sequence of events during the growth and division of cells

cephalic pertaining to the head or to the head end of the body

cercaria the final free-swimming larval stage of a trematode parasite, consisting of a body and tail

chelation a type of binding of two chemicals

chemotherapy a treatment with chemicals or drugs that can kill cancer cells

Chlamydia obligate intracellular infectious microorganisms that subvert the cell's metabolic processes for replication; now classified as bacteria

cholestasis a stop in bile flow

cholinesterases the enzymes catalyzing hydrolysis of choline esters

choreiform movements the involuntary irregular jerking movements of the arms and legs

chromatopsia a visual defect in which colorless objects appear to be tinged with color

chrysarobin a crystalline powdered reduction product of chrysophanic acid used formerly in topical therapy of psoriasis and other skin diseases

chyle the milky fluid taken up by the lacteal gland from the food in the intestine after digestion; it consists of lymph and emulsified fat; it passes into the veins by the thoracic duct, becoming mixed with the blood

chrysotherapy therapy with gold salts

chylomicrons a particle of emulsified fat, about 1 μm in diameter, found in the blood during digestion and absorption of fat

chyluria the presence of chyle in the urine, giving it a milky appearance

chyme the semifluid, homogeneous, creamy, or gruellike material produced by gastric digestion of food

ciliary muscle a muscle in the eye that regulates the shape of the lens and hence plays an important role in visual acuity for near and distant objects

cinchonism a drug toxicity syndrome characterized by tinnitus, headache, nausea, abdominal pain, and visual disturbances

coagulation the solidification of protein into a gelatinous mass

coccus (pl. **cocci**) a spherical bacterium

cochlear toxicity the toxic effects to the cochlea of the ear resulting in hearing dysfunction

coenzyme a low molecular weight substance that can combine with an inactive protein (apoenzyme) to form an active enzyme (holoenzyme)

collagen synthesis the production of the main tissue cellular and fiber component of the dermis

collimator a device of high absorption coefficient material (usually lead) to restrict the field of view of a detector to a given discrete area and to align rays in a parallel manner

colloid the homogeneous viscous fluid rich in thyroglobulin that is stored in the center of thyroid follicles

colloidal sulfur sulfur in a state of extremely fine division

colonoscopy an examination of the mucosa of the colon using a flexible instrument called the colonoscope

combination chemotherapy concomitant treatment with two or more anticancer drugs

combined modality treatment the use of chemotherapy in combination with surgery, radiation therapy, or both

comedogenicity potentially capable of producing acne comedones; adherent and sticky plugs in pilosebaceous follicles associated with acne

comedonal acne acne associated mainly with open or closed comedones (blackheads or whiteheads)

competitive inhibition a form of inhibition wherein the inhibitor competes for a receptor with other molecules; may be displaced from the receptor by increasing the numbers of other molecules through the principles of mass action

conduction velocity the speed with which an electrical impulse can be transmitted through excitable tissue

constipation infrequent or difficult evacuation of feces

constitutive resistance the bacterial resistance to antibiotics that reside in the chromosomal DNA; expressed in daughter cells after cell division but cannot be passed to other species

contact dermatitis the sensitization of the skin by direct contact to irritating substances; pruritus seen as early distressing symptom; skin may be edematous, have vesicles, and erythema; may be treated with 1:20 aluminum acetate (Burow's) solution used as a cool, wet compress for 15 minutes every 1 to 2 hours to relieve itching and loosen crusts; without oozing and crusting, calamine lotion with 0.25% phenol used to relieve pruritus; corticosteroid cream helpful also

contact urticaria a hivelike reaction at the site of contact with a topically applied compound or material

contractility inherent contractile capability of any muscle

Coombs' positive hemolytic anemia a form of anemia following premature destruction (hemolysis) of circulating red blood cells; serum antibodies reacting with circulating red blood cells able to lead to hemolysis and result in a positive Coombs' test

Coombs' test a test to detect the presence of antibodies on the surface of a patient's red blood cells; main indication for the direct Coombs' test to diagnose hemolytic anemia; since presence of small number of antibodies on the surface of red blood cells may not result in hemolytic anemia, a positive Coombs' test does not always signify hemolytic anemia

coronary artery disease (ischemic heart disease) a term used to encompass the breadth of disease (e.g., angina, myocardial infarction, dysrhythmias, and heart failure) that results from lack of an adequate oxygen supply to heart muscle; in the vast majority of cases in North America caused by fixed obstruction of the coronary arteries as a result of atherosclerosis

corticosteroid the hormones produced by (or synthetic derivatives of) the adrenal cortex affecting carbohydrate, fat, and protein metabolism and fluid and electrolyte balance; the hormones can be either natural or synthetic and include the glucocorticoids and mineralocorticoids

coryza a condition of the nasal mucosa characterized by profuse nasal discharge

count a single detected radioactive decay event

Crohn's disease regional ileitis; inflammatory bowel disease that may affect the GI tract from mouth to anus; cause unknown

cross resistance the resistance to a particular antibiotic that also provides resistance against a different antibiotic to which the bacteria may never have been exposed

cross sensitivity the sensitivity to one substance that predisposes an individual to sensitivity with other substances that are closely related in chemical structure

cross tolerance a tolerance to related drugs when tolerance develops after exposure to only one agent

crystalluria the excretion of crystals in the urine, producing renal irritation

curie a unit of radioactive decay rate, equalling 3.7×10^{10} decay events per second (see becquerel)

Cushing's syndrome a syndrome resulting from hypersecretion of glucocorticoids from the adrenal cortex or prolonged administration of corticosteroids, causing a cluster of symptoms including acne, amenorrhea, moon-face, buffalo hump, edema, hirsutism, glucose intolerance (diabetes mellitus), osteoporosis, thinning of skin, redistribution of subcutaneous fat, and muscle wasting

cycloplegia the paralysis of the ciliary muscle resulting in blurred vision for near objects

cysticercus a larval form of tapeworm, consisting of a single scolex enclosed in a bladderlike cyst

cystitis an inflammation of the urinary bladder associated with infections of the kidney, prostate, or urethra

D

dandruff the dry, scaly, or flaky material desquamated from scalp; may be mild variant of seborrheic dermatitis

debridement the removal of devitalized or contaminated tissue and foreign material

decay (radioactive) the disintegration of the nucleus of an unstable radionuclide

decay constant (disintegration constant) the fractional decay rate; in the equation $N = N_o e^{-\lambda\tau}$ where N_o equalling original number of atoms, N equalling final number after a given time, and $\lambda\ \tau = 0.693/T_{1/2}$

decongestant a drug used to reduce congestion and swelling of the nasal mucosa

defecation the evacuation of fecal material from the rectum

definitive host the animal in which a parasite passes its adult and sexual existence

dementia intellectual deterioration, particularly defective memory

demulcents a soothing oily or mucilaginous compound

denaturation the alteration of the basic nature or structure of a compound

dermatophytosis a chronic fungal infection that may involve skin, hair, or nails; also known as ringworm or tinea

desiccant an agent that causes drying

desquamation a peeling action usually causing separation of the epidermis in layers of scales

detrusor muscle a muscle in the urinary bladder that contracts and pushes down the bladder's contents, thereby facilitating urination

diabetes insipidus a disorder of the posterior pituitary gland characterized by passage of large amounts of dilute urine and great thirst

diapedesis the outward passage or migration through intact blood vessel walls of blood corpuscles during inflammatory reactions

diaphoretic a drug that causes increased perspiration

diarrhea an abnormal increase in frequency and fluid of fecal discharge

diathesis a predisposition to a certain condition or disease

diffusion constant a mathematical constant relating to ability to spread widely

digitalized the state of having a therapeutic total body level of a cardiac glycoside

digitalizing dose the amount of cardiac glycoside necessary to digitalize a patient

diplopia double vision

dissociative anesthesia quiescence; removal of environment

diuresis an increased excretion of urine

diverticular disease a disease of the colon, especially the sigmoid colon; characterized by the presence of herniation of mucosa through a defect in the muscle coat; associated with hypertrophy of the muscle coats

diverticulum a circumscribed pouch or sac of variable size created by herniation of the living mucous membrane through a defect in the muscular coat of a tubular organ

DNA deoxyribonucleic acid; the chemical within chromosomes that contains the genetic message of cells

dosimeter an instrument used to measure the dose resulting from an exposure to ionizing radiation

dropsy an old term for abnormal accumulation of fluid in the interstitial spaces and body cavities (i.e., edema)

drug fever the elevation of body temperature that occurs as an unwanted manifestation of drug action

dumping syndrome a syndrome caused by sudden, massive emptying of the stomach; characterized by nausea, vomiting, sweating, weakness, and diarrhea

dV/dt the rate of change of voltage in development of the action potential; most commonly used to describe phase 0

dysarthria the disturbance of speech as a result of emotional stress or paralysis; incoordination or spasticity of the muscles used for speaking

dysentery disorder(s) marked by inflammation of the intestines, especially the colon; attended by abdominal pain and frequent stools containing blood and mucus

dyskinesia the impairment of voluntary muscle movement

dysphoria a disorder of mood characterized by depression and anguish

dysrhythmia an abnormal rhythm (usually pertaining to the heart)

dystonia the impairment of muscular tonus

dystonic an abnormal increase in muscular tone causing unusual posturing

dysuria a pain and burning with urination

E

ecchymosis an extravasation of blood under the skin

eccrine sweat orifices the skin openings or pores of the terminal sweat duct

echolalia the automatic and meaningless repetition of another's words or phrases; also called ecophrasia

effective half-life the time required for the amount of radioactive compound in the body to be reduced by 50% as a result of both physical decay and simultaneous biologic elimination

efferent nerve a nerve that carries impulses from the CNS to a peripheral organ or tissue

effervescent the process of giving off gas bubbles

electron a negatively charged particle; has a mass of 0.000549 amu

electron volt (eV) the energy unit that is equivalent to the energy gained by an electron when it is passed through a potential difference of 1 volt; ionizing radiations usually have energies of thousands (KeV) or millions (MeV) of electron volts

electrophilic having an affinity for electrons, a property of the alkylating agents

emollients the topical agents that soften and soothe the skin

emulsion a preparation of one liquid dispersed in small globules throughout the body of a second liquid, usually an oil and water phase—creams or ointments commonly

encyst to become enclosed in a sac, bladder, or cyst

endemic common to one geographic region

endocarditis the inflammation of the endocardium, which can result from bacterial or fungal infection

endocrine the process of secreting internally; applies to organs whose function is to secrete into the blood or lymph a substance that has a specific effect on another organ or part

endocrine gland a specialized organ that secretes hormones directly into the bloodstream or lymphatic system

endocytosis the process by which droplets of colloid are surrounded by portions of apical membrane for transport into thyroid cells

endorphin literally an endogenous morphinelike substance; a pain-relieving substance produced within the body

endoscope an instrument for the examination of the interior of a hollow viscus

endoscopic retrograde cholangiopancreatography (ERCP) endoscopic cannulation through the duodenum of the common bile and pancreatic ducts for purposes of radiographic visualization

endoscopy the inspection of any cavity of the body by means of an endoscope

endothelium the innermost lining cell layer of blood and lymphatic vessels

enkephalin a long-chain protein produced in the brain and having an endorphin form as a part

enteric coating a special coating applied to tablets or capsules that prevents release and absorption of their contents until they reach the intestines

enterohepatic circulation the part of the bile that enters the gut to be reabsorbed, reexcreted through the liver into the gut, and recycled; remainder excreted in stool

enterotoxin a toxin specific for the cells of intestinal mucosa

enzyme an organic compound, commonly a protein; capable of accelerating or producing by catalytic action some change in a substrate for which it is often specific

eosinophilia an increased number of eosinophils in the blood

epidermis outer layer of skin

epigastric pertaining to the epigastrium (upper middle region of the abdomen)

epigastrium pertaining to the upper middle region of the abdomen located above the umbilicus

epistaxis a nose bleed

epithelium the general name given to all those tissues that cover the body surfaces, both externally and internally

erythema a redness caused by vascular dilatation

erythema multiforme an acute inflammatory skin disease characterized by the symmetrical eruption of a variety of lesions of various shapes

erythema nodosum a skin disease characterized by red, tender nodules on the anterior surface of the legs and may involve the face and arms

erythematous characterized by redness of skin as a result of vascular dilatation

eschar a thick, coagulated crust that forms after a thermal burn

esophageal manometric studies the pressure studies of the lower esophageal sphincter area to see if sphincter tone is normal, increased, or decreased

esophagitis the inflammation of the esophagus

essential (primary) hypertension an elevated blood pressure that is not a result of any known cause such as drugs, renovascular disease, or excess hormone production

esterification the chemical process of converting an acid into an ester

euglycemic having a normal blood glucose level

euphoria an exaggerated feeling of physical and emotional well-being not consonant with apparent stimuli or events; usually of psychologic origin but also seen in organic brain disease and toxic and drug-induced states

euthyroid a normal thyroid function

excitability an essential property of excitable tissue, which is the ability to develop an action potential, either spontaneously or after stimulation

excitation-contraction coupling the incompletely understood molecular mechanisms by which electrical or hormonal stimuli produce muscle contraction

excoriation the loss of skin produced by scratching

exercise hypotension an excessive fall in blood pressure induced by exercise

exfoliative dermatitis an inflammatory condition of the skin; characterized by redness and extensive scaling of dead epithelial cells

exocrine the external secretion of the gland through a duct

exocrine gland a specialized organ that secretes specific substances into the GI tract or "outwardly" from the body

exocytosis the process involved in the extrusion of vesicle contents from cells

exophthalmos an abnormal protrusion of the eyes

expectorant a drug used to decrease viscosity of airway secretions and to aid the elimination of secretions from the airways

extrapyramidal dysfunction the symptoms associated with nervous system dysfunction; include agitation, restlessness, tremor, rigidity, and spasm of certain muscle groups (i.e., face and hands)

extrapyramidal reactions akathisia, dyskinesia, muscle rigidity, oculogyric crisis, parkinsonism, salivation, and tremors

extrapyramidal syndrome a variety of signs and symptoms including muscular rigidity, tremors, drooling, restlessness, peculiar involuntary movements and postures, shuffling gait, protrusion of the tongue, chewing movements, blurred vision, and many other neurologic disturbances

extravasation the leakage or accidental injection of a drug outside of a vein into nearby tissues

exudation the accumulation and deposition of inflammatory cells, fluid, and cellular debris on tissue surfaces

F

fasciculations the disorganized twitching of groups of fibers in a muscle

festinating gait abnormal increased speed of walking as an attempt to "catch up" with a displaced center of gravity

fibroblast the main and "master" cell of the dermis; produces collagen, elastic tissue, and ground substance

filariform threadlike

filling pressure the pressure in the left ventricle at the end of diastole (i.e., end of filling)

film badge a dosimeter consisting of photographic film

fissure-in-ano a painful linear ulcer at the margin of the anus

fissures the abnormal clefts or grooves usually associated with loss of surface-covering tissue

flatulence the distention of the stomach or the intestines with air or gases

fluorination the addition of a fluorine group to a compound common to the majority of topical corticosteroids

follicle the smallest functional unit of the thyroid gland; a hollow spherical secretory structure lined by epithelial cells

folliculitis the inflammation of any portion of the hair follicle; may be caused by contact irritation, infection, or other causes

fomite an object such as a book, wooden object, or an article of clothing that is not in itself corrupted but is able to harbor pathogenic microorganisms that may be transmitted to others

formaldehyde a chemical disinfectant that results from degradation of methenamine in acid media; also used as a preservative

free radical a compound with an extra electron or proton, which is therefore unstable and reacts readily with other molecules

functional antagonism a pharmacologic term that describes the situation in which two agonists interact with different receptors and produce opposing effects

functional bowel syndrome see irritable bowel syndrome

fungicidal having a destructive (killing) action on fungi

fungistatic having an inhibiting action on the growth of fungi

G

gag reflex to retch or strive to vomit because of irritation to the fauces (i.e., the back of the throat)

gamma ray a short wavelength, high energy electromagnetic radiation originating from a decaying nucleus; energy range between 10 keV and 9 MeV

gastrectomy the cutting out or removal of the whole or part of the stomach

gastric lavage to wash out or remove gastric contents by means of a tube

gastrin a hormone obtained from the pyloric mucosa that when injected increases the flow of gastric juice

gastroscope an instrument to inspect the interior of the stomach and duodenum

gastroscopy inspection of the interior of the stomach by means of a gastroscope

gel chromatography a chemical analysis procedure that fractionally separates various drugs (or their metabolites)

gels the special topical formulations of colloids in gelatinous form; relatively firm in consistency though containing abundant liquid; often cosmetically elegant vehicles; particularly suitable on hairy sites

generalized tonic-clonic seizure (grand mal) an epileptic seizure sometimes preceded by a warning (aura); characterized by loss of consciousness, generalized stiffening (tonus), followed by generalized jerking (clonus) and sometimes with associated tongue biting and incontinence

gingival hypertrophy a spongy overgrowth of gum tissue peculiar to hydantoin toxicity

glabrous skin smooth or nonhairy skin

glomerular filtration the process of fluid in the blood being filtered across the capillaries of the glomerulus into the urinary space of Bowman's capsule

glossitis the inflammation of the tongue

glucocorticoid a natural or synthetic hormone related to the adrenal cortex that possesses major metabolic, antiinflammatory, and immunosuppressive effects

gluconeogenesis the formation of glycogen from fats and proteins

glucose-6-phosphate dehydrogenase (G-6-PD) an enzyme deficiency in the red blood cells of an individual; administration of certain drugs may cause hemolysis; most common in black, Oriental, and Mediterranean people

glycogenesis the formation of glycogen from glucose; glycogen usually stored in the liver until it is needed later by the body to replenish diminished glucose levels

glycogenolysis the process involved in the breakdown of glycogen to glucose

glycoprotein a protein containing carbohydrate

goiter an enlarged thyroid gland

gout the condition of hyperuricemia; characterized by acute arthritis and inflammation of the joints; usually affects the knee or foot

grand mal seizure see generalized tonic-clonic seizure

granular layer the usually relatively thin layer of epidermis containing microscopic basophilic-staining granules underlying the top keratin layer

granulocytopenia a decreased number of granulocytes in the blood

granulomatous the infiltration of tissue by granulocytes

gynecomastia an abnormal enlargement of the breasts in men

H

half-life (radioactive) the time required for one half of a given number of radioactive nuclides to decay

half-value layer (HVL) the thickness of an absorber, which when in the path of a beam of radiation will reduce the beam intensity to half

hematuria the condition of having blood in the urine

hemeralopia diminished vision in bright lighting

hemoglobinuria the presence of hemoglobin in the urine

hemolytic anemia an anemia resulting from the destruction of red blood cells

hemoptysis coughing up of blood or blood-stained sputum

hemorrhoid a varicose dilation of veins in the anal canal

hepatic porphyria an increase of porphyrins in the blood because of impaired liver function

Herxheimer's reaction an increase in symptoms after drug treatment; originally applied to the treatment of syphilis but now applies to other diseases as well

hirsutism abnormal hair growth, particularly facial hair in women

His-Purkinje system that portion of the specialized conduction system consisting of the bundle of His, right and left bundle branches, and terminal Purkinje fibers that provide an electric connection between the atrioventricular node and ventricular muscle

homeostatic pertaining to processes that tend to maintain a constancy of the body's internal milieu (e.g., to keep the blood pressure in the normal range)

homeostatic reflexes those reflexes that tend to maintain a constancy of the body's internal milieu (e.g., to keep blood pressure in the normal range)

hormonal pertaining to or of the nature of a hormone

hormone a chemical substance produced in the body that has a specific effect on the activity of a certain organ

hydrophilic readily absorbing moisture

hydrophobic not readily absorbing water or adversely affected by water

hydroscopic water attracting or binding

hydroxyapatite the main inorganic constituent of bone and teeth

hydroxyl group the chemical univalent hydroxyl (OH^-) radical

hypercapnia increased levels of carbon dioxide in the blood

hyperemia an increase in blood flow in an organ or tissue as a result of dilation of arterioles

hyperesthesia excessive sensitivity of the skin or of a special sense

hyperglycemia an elevated blood glucose level above normal

hyperhydrosis excessive perspiration

hyperkalemia condition of having a serum potassium level elevated above normal

hyperkeratotic the condition associated with excessive amounts of surface keratin on skin or mucous membrane

hyperlipidemia type I an elevated level of lipid in the blood; characterized by an increase in both cholesterol and triglycerides caused by the presence of chylomicrons

hyperlipidemia type IIA an elevated level of lipid in the blood; characterized by an elevation of cholesterol only and its normal carrier protein, low-density lipoprotein (LDL)

hyperlipidemia type IIB an elevated level of lipid in the blood; characterized by an elevation of cholesterol, a slight elevation of triglycerides, and elevation of the normal carrier proteins, low-density lipoprotein and very low density lipoprotein (VLDL)

hyperlipidemia type III an elevated level of lipid in the blood; characterized by an elevation of cholesterol, a mild to moderate elevation of triglycerides, and presence of elevated levels of abnormal carrier proteins LDL and VLDL

hyperlipidemia type IV an elevated level of lipid in the blood; characterized by a slight elevation of cholesterol, a moderate elevation of triglycerides and elevation of the normal triglyceride carrier protein VLDL

hyperlipidemia type V an elevated level of lipid in the blood; characterized by an elevation of cholesterol, marked elevation of triglyceride, elevation of the triglyceride carrier protein VLDL, and the presence of chylomicrons

hyperosmolarity a higher than normal concentration of osmotically active components

hyperosmotic containing a higher concentration of osmotically active components

hyperplasia an increase in the number of cells in a tissue

hyperreactivity the state of airways; associated with lung disease in which responses to various spasmogens are exaggerated

hypersensitivity a state of altered reactivity in which the body reacts with an exaggerated response to a foreign agent

hyperthyroidism an abnormally elevated thyroid function

hypertrophic subaortic stenosis an abnormal enlargement of the ventricular septum of the heart producing a functional obstruction of blood flow out of the ventricles

hypertrophy an abnormal enlargement or overgrowth of an organ or tissue, usually caused by an increase in size of cells

hyperuricemia an abnormally elevated level of uric acid in the blood

hyperventilation the rate of ventilation that eliminates greater than normal levels of carbon dioxide

hypervitaminosis a vitamin overdose

hypnosis the state of sleep induced by a hypnotic

hypnotic a pharmacologic agent used for the induction of sleep

hypoadrenocorticism (Addison's disease) the partial or complete failure of the adrenocortex to secrete adrenocortical hormones

hypocalcemia the reduction of the blood calcium below normal levels

hypochloremia the condition of having a low serum chloride

hypoglycemia a decreased blood glucose level (below normal)

hypokalemia a decreased blood potassium level (below normal)

hypokinesia abnormally diminished motor activity

hypomania a psychopathologic state and abnormality of mood falling somewhere between normal euphoria and mania

hyponatremia the condition of having a low serum sodium

hyposensitization desensitization therapy

hypothalamic-pituitary-adrenal axis the major neuroendocrine components of hormonal regulation in the body

hypothermia a body temperature that is below normal

hypothrombinemia a decreased level of the clotting factor thrombin in the blood

hypothyroidism an abnormally decreased thyroid function

hypovolemia an abnormally low volume of circulating blood

hypoxemia decreased levels of arterial oxygen

hypoxia decreased levels of oxygen in tissues

I

iatrogenic pertaining to adverse conditions or complications in a patient occurring as a result of treatment

ichthyotic skin conditions a group of hyperkeratotic skin conditions often hereditary and producing a fish-scale-like appearance

idiopathic hypertrophic subaortic stenosis (IHSS) a myopathic (muscular) disorder of the heart, usually of the left ventricle, that obstructs emptying; also called hypertrophic obstructive cardiomyopathy (HOCM) and muscular subaortic stenosis (MSS)

idiosyncratic pertaining to an abnormal susceptibility or tendency to develop a toxic reaction to a drug

ileostomy the surgical creation of an opening into the ileum; may be permanently placed on the surface of the skin of the abdominal wall

immune serum a serum that contains antibodies obtained from patients who have recovered from a disease and retain immune bodies in their blood serum

immunosuppression the impairment of the body's normal immunologic system

immunotherapy treatment by the production of immunity as is done with *Hymenoptera* venom extracts; results in a rise in serum levels of specific IgG

impetigo surface skin infection; usually staphylococcal, streptococcal, or a combination of these; often secondary infection to previous skin lesions

induration an area of tissue that becomes hard as a result of loss of normal pliability and elasticity

inflammatory bowel disease usually refers to intestinal disease associated with inflammatory changes in which the cause is unknown such as Crohn's disease or ulcerative colitis

insulin-dependent diabetes mellitus type I diabetes, formerly known as juvenile diabetes

intermediary host an animal in which a parasite passes in its larval or nonsexual existence

intermittent claudication pain of the lower limbs that is intermittent, occurs with exertion, and is caused by ischemia from inadequate blood flow usually secondary to atherosclerosis of the arteries to the lower body

interstitial between cells such as tissue spaces or cellular or chemical materials

interstitial nephritis the inflammatory changes usually confined to the interstitial tissue of the kidney resulting from toxic drug exposure and other factors

intertriginous pertaining to the sites of opposed surfaces of skin such as body folds or skin creases

intestinal (luminal) amebiasis *Entamoeba histolytica* organisms present in the intestinal lumen, on the mucosal surface of the bowel, and in the walls of the intestine

intraepidermal vesicle a fluid-filled blister cavity within the epidermis, usually less than 1 cm in diameter

intrarenal hemodynamics the pattern of blood flow or distribution in the various parts of the kidney; normally the renal cortex and outer medulla receive the major portion of the renal blood flow

intrathecal injection an injection of a drug directly into the lumbar space L4-5 and into the cerebrospinal fluid

intrinsic factor a component produced by parietal cells of the stomach that is necessary for the absorption of vitamin B_{12} and the prevention of pernicious anemia

iodination the incorporation and chemical reaction of iodine in a compound

ionization the process of changing a neutral atom to a positively or negatively charged species

irradiation the application of radiation to a substance to change it

irritable bowel syndrome a syndrome of unknown cause characterized by abdominal pain and constipation or less commonly diarrhea

isotopes the nuclides of the same atomic number (protons) but with varying numbers of neutrons and, hence, varying atomic weights

isotonic equal in tonicity or osmotic pressure to that of the blood, being about 300 mOsm/L

J

jaundice a yellowing of the skin and eyes; produced by liver damage or obstruction, with buildup of bile pigment

K

keratinization the process of forming keratin in skin

keratin layer the top layer of epidermis, varying considerably in thickness in different sites and composed of the tough, fibrous protein keratin

keratoconjunctivitis a disorder marked by inflammation of the conjunctiva at the border of the cornea

keratolytic pertaining to the dissolution or destruction of keratin

keratoplastic capable of producing keratin

kernicterus a neurologic complication of unconjugated hyperbilirubinemia in the infant; characterized by bile pigment in the cerebrospinal fluid and brain tissue

ketoacidosis acidosis associated with high ketone levels

ketone group the chemical carbonyl group with attached hydrocarbons

Kussmaul respiration a deep, gasping type of labored breathing usually associated with diabetic acidosis

L

lacrimation the secretion and discharge of tears

lactase an intestinal enzyme that splits lactose into glucose and galactose

larva an immature stage in the life history of an animal in which it is unlike the parent

laxative an agent that acts to promote the evacuation of the bowel

leukemia cancer of blood-forming cells

leukopenia a disorder marked by a decrease in the number of white blood cells

lipase any one of a family of enzymes that catalyzes the hydrolysis of fats

lipoatrophy the breakdown of subcutaneous fat tissue at the site of insulin injection

lipohypertrophy the buildup of subcutaneous fat tissue at the site of insulin injection

lipolysis the breakdown of fat

lipoprotein lipase a membrane-associated enzyme that catalyzes lipolysis, particularly of the lipid contained in chylomicrons

livedo reticularis a bluish discoloration of the legs with a "fishnet" appearance

loop of Henle part of the nephron adjoining the proximal and distal renal tubules forming a loop, where 25% to 30% of water and sodium chloride are reabsorbed (respectively in the descending limb and ascending limb)

lotions common topical formulations of liquid suspensions and dispersions

low-density lipoprotein (LDL) the carrier protein in the blood for cholesterol; so called because of its position after ultracentrifugation of serum

lupus erythematosus a morbid condition, ranging from mild to fulminant, with multisystem involvement; characterized by skin eruptions, fever, and a multitude of other constitutional symptoms

lymphadenopathy any disorder of lymph nodes or lymph vessels

lymphocytic leukemia a cancer of lymphocytes in the bone marrow and blood; also termed lymphoblastic leukemia

lymphokines chemical mediators concerned with regulation of immune function and released from lymphocytes in blood or tissues

lymphoma a cancer arising from lymphocytes

lysis dissolution or decomposition

lysosome a cytoplasmic cell structure or organelle containing enzymes important to cell catabolism or digestion and of potential importance in many disease states and inflammatory processes

M

malanosis coli a condition in which the mucous membrane of the colon is pigmented with melanin

malar pertaining to the cheek or cheek bone

malignancy cancer; an abnormal growth of cells that can spread and destroy normal tissues and result in death

mania a mood disorder characterized by excessive elation, hyperactivity, agitation, and accelerated thinking and speaking; sometimes manifested as flight of ideas

mass number the number of protons plus neutrons in a nucleus; the general symbol is A

mastication chewing

meconium first feces of a newborn infant

medullary interstitium the space between tubules in the renal medulla where normally hypertonicity is maintained by slow blood flow, allowing removal of sodium and chloride from the ascending limb, water from the descending limb of Henle, and urinary concentration in the collecting ducts in the presence of antidiuretic hormone

melena black, tarry stools or vomitus

Ménière's disease deafness, tinnitus, and dizziness occurring in association with nonsuppurative disease of the labyrinth

meningitis inflammation of the meninges that can result from bacterial, viral, or fungal infection

menorrhagia excessive bleeding during the menstrual period

messenger RNA a ribonucleic acid fraction that transmits genetic coded information from DNA to the protein synthesizing systems of the cell

metabolic alkalosis the state of bicarbonate retention resulting in a high blood pH because of an increased intake of bicarbonate or increased threshold of bicarbonate excretion

metacercaria the encysted resting or maturing stage of a trematode parasite in the tissues of an intermediate host (aquatic arthropods or fishes); may be the infective or transfer stage to man and other animals

metaphase the second phase of cell division

metastasis the spread of cancer cells from one part of the body to another

methemoglobin a form of hemoglobin in which the ferrous ion of heme has been oxidized to a ferric ion

methemoglobinemia the presence of methemoglobin in the blood, causing cyanosis because of the blood's inability to carry oxygen

microsomal enzymes a group of enzymes associated with a certain particulate fraction of liver homogenate that plays a prominent role in the metabolism of many drugs

miliaria a skin eruption involving the sweat gland apparatus; usually associated with obstruction, sweat retention, and inflammation; one form called prickly heat

miliary tuberculosis an acute form of tuberculosis in which tubercles the size of millet seeds develop in a number of organs of the body as a result of widespread dissemination of bacilli via the blood and lymph vessels

mineralocorticoid a natural or synthetic hormone related to the adrenal cortex; has several major effects, including sodium and water balance in the body

miosis constriction of the pupil as a result of the contraction of the sphincter muscles of the iris or paralysis of the radial (dilator) muscles of the iris

miotic a substance or drug that causes miosis (i.e., constriction of the pupil)

miscible capable of being mixed with another compound

mitosis the division of one cell into two cells, resulting in the growth of normal tissues and tumors; M-phase (metaphase)

mitral valve prolapse a common etiologic cause of mitral regurgitation caused by a myxomatous redundancy of the valve cusps and chordae tendineae, which permits prolapse during systole

moieties portions

monoamine oxidase the enzyme responsible for oxidatively removing the amine group from epinephrine, norepinephrine, tyramine, and related compounds, thus inactivating these substances

monoamine oxidase inhibitors (MAOIs) a group of antidepressant drugs that inhibit monoamine oxidase and raise the level of many monoamines

moon-face the development of a full, round face in response to excess secretion of adrenocortical hormone or prolonged corticosteroid therapy

morbilliform rash a measleslike rash

motor endplate the area of skeletal muscle cell directly adjacent to a motor nerve ending; is sensitive to acetylcholine

mucositis inflammation or damage to a mucous membrane, such as the lining of the mouth and throat

mutagenic producing changes in genetic material

mycoplasma bacteria without rigid cell walls; includes mycoplasma and ureaplasma species

mycosis any disease caused by the presence of a fungus

mycotoxicosis a systemic poisoning caused by toxins produced by fungal organisms

mydriasis dilation of the pupil because of contraction of the radial (dilator) muscles of the iris or paralysis of the sphincter (constrictor) muscles of the iris

mydriatic a substance or drug that causes mydriasis (i.e., dilation of the pupil)

myelocytic leukemia also called myelogenous leukemia; a cancer developing from the granulocytic white blood cells

myelosuppression damage to blood-forming cells in the bone marrow, resulting in anemia, leukopenia, or thrombocytopenia

myocarditis inflammation of the heart muscle

myosin a protein contained in the thick filaments of the microfilamental structure of skeletal muscle that interacts with actin in muscle contraction

myositis inflammation of a voluntary muscle

myxedema peculiar, nonpitting edema of skin, subcutaneous tissues, and other tissues; associated with thyroid dysfunction and caused by infiltration by mucopolysaccharides; severe hypothyroidism

N

nadir the lowest point; usually refers to blood count depression from chemotherapy

narcoanalysis an interview conducted while the patient is deeply sedated with medication so that the patient will lose inhibition and respond more truthfully

narcosis anesthesia

narcotherapy a therapeutic modality used in psychiatry in which the patient is kept asleep for long periods of time, usually many days

narcotic an agent chemically related to opium that produces decreased awareness of pain

nascent referring to the state of a chemical element just liberated from a chemical combination; is usually more reactive

nascent oxygen referring to oxygen just liberated from a chemical combination

natriuresis increased urinary sodium excretion

necrosis cell or tissue death

neoplasm any new and abnormal growth (e.g., a tumor)

nephrotic syndrome a condition caused by excessive loss of protein in the urine (more than 3.5 gm/24 hr), resulting in low serum protein, high serum cholesterol, and edema

nephrotoxicity the state of being toxic to the kidneys

neurodermatitis a chronic, itching, lichenoid (thickened) eruption on the axillary and pubic regions as a result of a nervous disorder

neurohumor a chemical substance that transduces an action potential across a synapse but can also overflow into the circulation and have more widespread effects (e.g., norepinephrine)

neuroleptanalgesia a state produced by a combination of a neuroleptic and analgesic

neuroleptanesthetic neuroleptanalgesic plus nitrous oxide

neuromodulator a substance that alters transmission of nervous information (messages)

neuromuscular blockade the inhibition of the muscular contraction activated by the nervous system, possibly resulting in muscle weakness or paralysis

neuromuscular junction the synapse between the motor nerve ending and the skeletal muscle cell

neutron an electrically neutral nuclear particle; has a mass of 1.00898 AMU

neutropenia a marked decrease in the number of neutrophilic leukocytes in the blood

nidus a point of origin, focus, or nucleus of a disease process

night terrors a sudden, apparent arousal out of stage 4 sleep (non-REM) in which the individual is not awake and is very difficult to arouse; characterized by intense fear and emotion

nitrazine paper absorbent strips of paper that turn specific colors when exposed to solutions of various acidity or alkalinity; also known as pH paper

nitritoid reaction a reaction similar to that seen following the administration of nitrites; caused by the administration of arsenicals or gold; characterized by hypotension, lightheadedness, fainting, and flushing

nociception the receiving of noxious sensations

nociceptive referring to a receptive neuron for painful sensations

noncompetitive inhibition a form of inhibition wherein the inhibitor occupies a receptor in an irreversible fashion and cannot be displaced from the receptor by increasing the numbers of other molecules through the principles of mass action

non-insulin-dependent diabetes mellitus type II diabetes; formerly known as adult- or maturity-onset diabetes

nonionic compounds without net negative or positive charge

nonrapid eye movement (non-REM) a stage of sleep characterized by cerebral "deactivation" and postural immobility

nonthrombocytopenic purpura a disorder characterized by purplish or red areas of the skin; does not involve a decrease in the number of platelets

normoglycemia normal blood glucose level

nucleophilic a property of molecules (e.g., nucleic acids and proteins) having electrons that can be shared with and thus form bonds with alkylating agents

nucleotides the compounds that form the nucleic acids DNA and RNA

nuclide an atom of an element characterized by its nuclear constitution

nystagmus involuntary, rapid movement of the eyeball in horizontal, vertical, or mixed directions

O

obstructive cardiomyopathy a myopathic (muscular) disorder of the heart that obstructs emptying, usually of the left ventricle; also called idiopathic hypertrophic subaortic stenosis (IHSS), hypertrophic obstructive cardiomyopathy (HOCM), and muscular subaortic stenosis (MSS)

occlusion air-tight coverage of the skin by natural body folds or aids, such as polyethylene wrap

occlusive conditions pertaining to air-tight coverage of the skin by natural body skin folds or aids, such as polyethylene wrap

oculogyric crisis prolonged fixation of eyeballs in one position, usually to the side or upward

ointments common topical formulations of water in oil emulsions; usually not readily water washable

oliguria diminished urine output

onycholysis separation of the nail from the nail bed

oogenesis the process of formation of ova in the ovaries before ovulation and fertilization

opiate a drug product containing or derived from opium

opportunistic infection an infection resulting from an organism that has been allowed access to the body by medical manipulation, physical debilitation, or a lack of normal bacterial flora because of antibiotic use

organophosphates a class of anticholinesterases used as insecticides and in medicine, causing irreversible inhibition of cholinesterase

orthostatic hypotension a significant drop of blood pressure resulting from change from recumbency to erect position

osmosis the passage of pure solvent from the lesser to the greater concentration when two solutions are separated by a membrane that selectively prevents the passage of solute molecules but is permeable to the solvent

osmotic pertaining to or of the nature of osmosis

osmotic effect effect of water and electrolytes in the renal tubule that are prevented from reabsorption because of the presence of a substance that exerts a high osmotic pressure in the tubule

osteoblasts a cell arising from a fibroblast and associated with the production of bone matrix

osteoclast a large multinucleated cell associated with the absorption of bone

osteolysis dissolution of bone; especially the removal or loss of the calcium of bone

osteomalacia softening of the bones

osteoporosis increased porosity of the bones

ototoxicity the state of being toxic to the organ of hearing

P

pain the conscious awareness of nociperception; a sensation of discomfort, distress, or agony, resulting from stimulation of specialized nerve endings

palatable having an acceptable taste

palilalia an abnormal condition characterized by increasingly rapid repetition of the same word or phrase

palliation a therapy that relieves symptoms and may prolong life but does not achieve a complete cure

pancytopenia a marked reduction in the cellular elements of the blood

papular urticaria a common condition in temperate parts of the world, usually occurring in children; caused by the bites of fleas, bedbugs, and other insects and representing a stage in the development of sensitization to them

papule a small, solid elevation on the skin

papulopustular lesions skin lesions characterized by raised, circumscribed elevations of skin, usually less than 1 cm in diameter and containing central loculations or cavities with pus

paradoxical bronchospasm constriction of the airways, occurring after treatment with a sympathomimetic bronchodilator

paralytic ileus paralysis of the smooth muscles of the intestines

paranoia delusion of persecution with marked suspiciousness

parkinsonism a group of neurologic disorders marked by hypokinesia, tremor, and muscle rigidity

paroxysmal a periodic, sudden recurrence or intensification of symptoms

partial complex seizure (psychomotor and temporal lobe) an epileptic seizure originating in the temporal lobe; characterized by confusion and olfactory, gustatory, psychic, visual, or auditory hallucinations; associated with directed but inappropriate motor activity (automatism); sometimes culminates in generalized tonic-clonic seizure

partial seizure (focal) an epileptic seizure in which symptoms are restricted to one part of the body (e.g., jerking of the right arm)

partition coefficient a mathematic expression relating the solubility relationship of a formulation or suspension in two different physical phases or between solute and solvent

passive acquired immunity acquired immunity to a disease produced by the administration of preformed antibody; done by transferring to a person via placenta or via the serum of an animal that has been actively immunized by injections with the specific toxins or organisms of those diseases

paste topical semisolid formulation composed usually of the active ingredient incorporated in a fatty base, a viscous or mucilaginous base, or a mixture of starch and petrolatum

patient compliance the degree of adherence to prescribed therapy

pemphigus a condition characterized by the sudden appearance of successive groups of bullae on apparently normal skin and the residual skin pigmentation that occurs as the bullae resolve

peptones a derived protein, a mixture of split products, produced by the hydrolysis of a native protein either by an acid or by an enzyme

percutaneous absorption the process of absorption through the skin from topical application

percutaneous transhepatic cholangiography the introduction of a small cannula through the skin into a liver bile duct to introduce radiopaque dye for radiologic visualization of ducts

periarteritis nodosa an inflammation of the arteries, giving a nodular appearance

peristalsis a wavelike movement by which the alimentary tract, or other tubular organs provided with both longitudinal and circular muscle fibers propel their contents

periungual situated near the nail

permeability the ability of certain substances to penetrate in solution a biologic or synthetic membrane

petechia a small, pinpoint, round, purplish-red spot caused by intradermal or submucous hemorrhage

petrolatum a purified mixture of semisolid hydrocarbons obtained from petroleum and commonly used as an ointment base or skin emollient

Peyronie's disease an induration and fibrosis of the corpora cavernosa of the penis, producing a fibrous chordae and deformity of the penis

phase 0 (depolarization) the phase of the cardiac action potential during which the potential difference rapidly loses negativity

phase 1 (repolarization) the phase of the cardiac action potential in which there is an initial period of rapid repolarization from approximately 20 mV to near 0

phase 2 (plateau phase) the phase of the cardiac action potential that is horizontal and near 0 potential difference

phase 3 (repolarization) the phase of the cardiac action potential during which the potential difference returns toward the nadir of negativity of the resting membrane potential

phase 4 (resting) the phase of the cardiac action potential between full depolarizations (i.e., from the nadir of negativity to phase 0); membrane resting potential

pheochromocytoma a vascular tumor of chromaffin tissue of adrenal medulla or sympathetic paraganglia that is only rarely malignant but produces excessive amounts of catecholamines; results in hypertension, tachycardia, and hyperglycemia (episodic or sustained) and the symptoms thereof

phlebitis inflammation of a vein

photon a discrete quantity of electromagnetic energy; in nuclear medicine usually refers to x-rays or gamma rays

photophobia an abnormal intolerance to light; can be a result of excessive dilation of the pupil

photoprotective protective against the potential adverse effects of ultraviolet light exposure

photosensitizers agents that can sensitize or prepare the skin for an allergic reaction to sun exposure

phototoxicity extreme sensitivity of skin to sunlight in which brief exposure may cause sunburn

physiologic dependence the need to continue ingestion of a pharmacologic agent to prevent the occurrence of withdrawal

pigmentary retinopathy a disorder of the retina, marked by pigmentary deposits and increasing loss of vision

pilosebaceous follicles the most common type of hair follicle; usually has sebaceous glands attached to the lumen via a duct (see Chapter 54, "Review of the Anatomy, Physiology, and Assessment of the Cutaneous System")

plasmapheresis the separation of plasma from red blood cells by centrifugation

plasmid extrachromosomal (cytoplasmic) DNA that can code for protein production and antibiotic resistance; can be transferred from species to species of bacteria

plasters tape or fabric coated on one side with an adhesive mixture with high tensile strength

platelets blood components that aid in clotting and control of bleeding

pleural effusion the presence of body fluid in the pleural or chest cavity

polar groups chemical groups of spatial orientation and charge, usually impeding water solubility but often aiding lipid solubility

polymerization the process of forming a larger and more complex compound by the combination of simpler molecules

polyuria the passage of a large amount of urine in a given period of time

positive inotropic effect an increase in inherent contractile capability

postprandial occurring after a meal

postsynaptic referring to the region on an organ or another nerve that receives innervation (i.e., the structure immediately adjacent to a nerve ending)

postural hypotension an excessive fall in blood pressure, induced by change from supine to upright position

preload (of the left ventricle) those factors, usually upstream from the left ventricle, that determine the amount of stretch of the left ventricular muscle at the end of diastole and thus influence the force of contraction of the ventricle and the forward cardiac output; commonly measured as the left ventricular end-diastolic volume or pressure

priapism persistent penile erection

primary pulmonary hypertension an elevated pressure in the pulmonary artery that is not a result of any known cause such as pulmonary embolus or elevated left heart pressure

prodrome a sign or symptom that serves as a warning or indication of an approaching disease, condition, or attack

prodrug an inactive or partially active drug that is metabolically changed in the body to an active drug

progesterone a hormone produced by the corpus luteum to prepare the uterus for the reception and development of the fertilized ovum by the glandular proliferation of the endometrium

prophylaxis preventive treatment

Propionibacterium acnes a common non-pathogenic gram-positive bacilli resident in the depths of pilosebaceous follicles

proptosis a synonym for exophthalmos

prostatism a condition resulting in the obstruction of urination; caused by hypertrophy (enlargement) of the prostate gland

prostatitis an inflammation of the prostate usually with pain or difficulty in urination; often caused by infection

proteinuria the presence of protein in the urine; indicates some forms of renal dysfunction

proton a positively charged nuclear particle; has a mass of 1.007277 AMU

Protozoa one-celled animal parasites

provitamin an inactive substance that is changed in the body to an active vitamin

pruritus the symptom of itch, associated with the desire to scratch

pseudomembranous colitis a severe colitis; possibly caused by an overgrowth of opportunistic organisms; usually occurs in debilitated individuals taking broad-spectrum antibiotics

psoriasis a common hereditary skin condition characterized by scaling inflammatory papules and plaques often in distinctive pattern and distribution

psychogenic having an emotional or psychologic origin as opposed to an organic basis

psychomotor seizure see partial complex seizure

psychoses a group of major mental disorders in which normal ability to function and contact with reality are severely impaired

ptosis a drooping, often of the upper eyelid, as a result of paralysis

pulse height analyzer a circuit designed to accept or reject electronic pulses according to their amplitude or energy; commonly used in gamma detection instrumentation to select certain gamma ray energies

purpura pinpoint purple-red spots under the skin or mucous membranes because of localized bleeding

purpuric rash a hemorrhagic skin rash

pyelonephritis an inflammation of the kidney, usually of bacterial origin, with symptoms of flank pain, chill, and fever

pylorus the distal aperture of the stomach through which the stomach contents pass into the duodenum

pyoderma a purulent skin disease

Q

quality factor (QF) an energy transfer dependent factor used to normalize the absorbed radiation dose of various radiations for biologic effectiveness

quaternary ammonium derivative a chemical structure characterized by having four organic (carbon) groups attached to a nitrogen atom; is a fairly strong base, highly water soluble, but relatively insoluble in lipids

QT interval the interval in the ECG from the beginning of the QRS complex to the end of the T-wave

R

radiation energy propagated through space as electromagnetic waves or corpuscular emissions

radiation absorbed dose (rad) an absorbed dose unit equivalent to 100 ergs/gm of irradiated material

radiation enteritis an inflammation of the intestines usually caused by radiation for some adjacent malignancy

radical a small chemical structure that, when attached to a larger compound, changes its properties to varying extents

radioactive contamination the deposition of radioactive material in any area where it is not desirable or intended; important from the viewpoint of possible interference with diagnostic procedures and from a radiation hazard to personnel

radioactivity the property of a nucleus to undergo spontaneous emission of particulate or gamma radiation

radioimmunoassay a precise laboratory method used for the specific measurement of hormones and other compounds; based on competition between unlabeled hormone and hormone labeled with a radioisotope for sites on a specific antibody

radionecrosis tissue death caused by radiation

radionuclide radioactive atoms of an element; characterized by specific nuclear constitution

radionuclide angiography visualization of blood vessels; requires the use of a gamma camera after a rapid bolus intravenous injection of a radiopharmaceutical

radiopharmaceutical a pharmaceutical compound containing a radioactive nuclide component

rapid eye movement (REM) sleep a stage of sleep characterized by dreaming and postural changes

rapid eye movement (REM) rebound the occurrence of greater than normal REM activity; may follow cessation of a REM-suppressant drug

Raynaud's phenomenon intermittent attacks of pallor followed by cyanosis of the extremities, usually the fingers; brought on by cold or emotion and associated with a number of conditions, particularly the collagen vascular diseases

reabsorption the removal (mobilization) of calcium from bone into the blood

rebound congestion congestion and swelling of the nasal mucosa that results from the late, vasodilator effects of decongestants

reflux a backward or return flow

reflux esophagitis esophageal irritation and inflammation that results from reflux of gastric contents into the esophagus

refractoriness the property of excitable tissue that determines how closely together two action potentials can occur

refractory resistant to conventional treatment

relative biological effectiveness (RBE) a factor used to compare the biological effectiveness of ionizing radiations of differing linear energy transfer characteristics

rem a dose unit obtained by multiplying the rad by the quality factor (QF)

remission clinical improvement associated with disappearance of the signs and symptoms of a disease

renogram a plot of radioactivity versus time by an external radiation detector placed over the kidneys; used for assessment of renal function following the injection of a radiopharmaceutical

renovascular hypertension an excessive elevation of the blood pressure resulting from ischemia of one or both kidneys caused by an obstruction of arterial blood flow to these organs

resistance the ability of an organism to remain unaffected by noxious agents and chemicals in its surrounding environment

resistance vessels those blood vessels (small muscular arteries, arterioles, and metarterioles) that form the major portion of the total peripheral resistance to blood flow

resting membrane potential the nadir of negativity during phase 4 of the cardiac action potential; for those cells that do not display automaticity, the cell remains at this potential difference throughout phase 4

reticulocytopenia a decrease in the number of reticulocytes

retinopathy any disorder of the retina

reverse triiodothyronine (rT₃) an inactive isomer of T_3; 3′,5,3-triiodothyronine

rhinitis an inflammation of the nasal mucosa, causing congestion and an increase in mucus secretion

rhinorrhea an increased nasal discharge, usually of a serous, watery character

ribonucleic acid (RNA) the chemical that translates the genetic message of DNA into production of proteins by cells

ribosomes intracellular structures at which protein synthesis occurs by the attachment of transfer RNA that provides the code for the amino acid sequence of the protein

rickets a form of osteomalacia in children

Rickettsia a group of similar intracellular infectious agents usually transmitted by an insect bite

rigidity stiffness in muscle movement

rods in general, any rod-shaped bacteria

roentgen a unit of radiation exposure to x-rays or gamma rays based on ionization of air

rosaniline dye a basic dye derived from triphenylmethane; often used in preparation of other dyes

rubefacient a topical agent that reddens the skin by producing blood vessel dilation

S

salicylism the syndrome of salicylate toxicity

saponified chemically hydrolyzed into soaps or acid salts and glycerol by heating with alkali

sarcoma a cancer of fibrous or supportive tissues, including bones and muscles

scintigraphy a photographic recording (taken by a gamma camera or other imaging device) of the distribution and intensity of radioactivity in various tissues and organs following the administration of a radiopharmaceutical

scintiscan (scintiphoto) a photographic display of the distribution of a radiopharmaceutical within the body

scolex the head of a tapeworm; the attachment end of the tapeworm

seborrhea a term commonly denoting excessive oiliness or dry or greasy scaling of the face or scalp

seborrheic dermatitis a common constitutional pattern of dermatitis, associated with scaling and erythema in a distinctive pattern and distribution such as face, scalp, and ear regions, and body folds or creases

serum creatinine level concentration of creatinine in the serum; impairment of renal function can produce an increase in serum creatinine level

serum sickness a hypersensitivity reaction characterized by urticarial rashes, edema, adenitis, joint pain, high fever, and prostration

sialorrhea increased salivation

sigmoidoscopy the inspection of the rectum and sigmoid colon by the aid of a long speculum (sigmoidoscope)

sinoatrial (SA) node the portion of the specialized conduction system located at the junction of the superior vena cava and right atrium that contains the normal dominant cardiac pacemaker

slow diastolic depolarization the slow loss of negativity that occurs during phase 4 of the action potential in cardiac cells having automaticity

somatic pertaining to or affecting the body

somatostatin the hormone that inhibits the release of insulin, gastrin, and growth hormone

specific activity the amount of radioactive material per unit weight or mass of a compound

spermatogenesis the process of formation in the testicles of spermatozoa

S-phase the phase of the cell cycle in which DNA is synthesized before mitosis (M-phase)

sphincter muscle a circular muscle surrounding an opening of an organ; closes off this opening or passage by contraction

spirochete several distinct species of bacteria that have a coil-like shape

sprue, celiac celiac sprue is a disease of the small intestine; associated with malabsorption; improves when gluten is withdrawn from the diet

status epilepticus recurrent, generalized tonic-clonic seizures without regaining consciousness

status spongiosus toxic and degenerative brain alteration usually associated with dissolution of brain substance

steatorrhea the passage of large amounts of fats in the feces

steroid any of a large group of substances chemically related to sterols and including vitamin D, certain hormones, and glycosides of digitalis

Stevens-Johnson syndrome a severe drug reaction characterized by multiform skin lesions, involvement of the mouth and anogenital membranes, and constitutional symptoms

Stokes-Adams syndrome loss of consciousness as a result of heart conduction block

stomatitis inflammation of the oral mucosa

striae linear, usually depressed, grooves or streaks in the skin; associated with atrophy or weakening of dermal elastic tissue; often assumes a silvery or purplish-pink discoloration

subacute myelo-optic neuropathy (SMON) characterized by muscular pain and weakness (usually below T12 vertebra), painful dysesthesia (especially of the limbs, often associated with significant alteration of gait), in some instances, optic atrophy

substantivity the property of continuing therapeutic action despite removal of the vehicle as applied to certain shampoos

sulfhemoglobinemia the production of an abnormal sulfur containing circulating hemoglobin in the blood

sulfhydryl groups the SH chemical groups or radicals

sulfonates a class of anticholinesterases used as insecticides

superinfection the development of a second infection that is superimposed on an initial infection currently under treatment; caused by organisms (bacteria or fungi) that are not susceptible to the drug(s) used to treat the original infection

suppository an easily fusible, medicated mass to be introduced into an orifice of the body

suppression the inhibition of glandular function by blocking normal stimulation

surface tension the resistance or tension force that acts to preserve the integrity of a surface

susceptibility the condition or quality of being sensitive or predisposed

syncope a sudden loss of consciousness

synergism the enhanced joint action of two or more agents that produces a greater effect than the sum of their individual actions

synergy a condition whereby the activity of two drugs is greater than the sum of their individual activity

systemic lupus erythematosus (SLE) a chronic disease of unknown cause marked by an erythematous rash on the face and other areas exposed to sunlight; involves the vascular and connective tissue of many organs, resulting in a wide variety of manifestations

T

tachyphylaxis the development of acute tolerance or a rapid diminution of pharmacologic response with repeated administration of a drug

tardive dyskinesia a late-occurring neurologic syndrome characterized by involuntary sucking and smacking of the lips, jaw movements, and darting of the tongue

telangiectasia a vascular lesion formed by dilation of small blood vessels such as capillaries

teratogenic causing malformations or damage to an embryo or fetus

therapeutic index the magnitude of difference between minimum therapeutic and minimum toxic concentration of a drug

threshold the level of potential difference at which a stimulus will produce a propagated action potential

thrombocytopenia a marked decrease in the number of platelets in the blood; can lead to easy bruising and bleeding

thrombopenia see thrombocytopenia

thrombocytopenic purpura large confluent areas of intradermal or subcutaneous hemorrhage as a result of thrombocytopenia

thyroglobulin a large glycoprotein containing the thyroid hormones in peptide linkage; synthesized and stored by the thyroid gland

thyroidectomy a procedure for the surgical removal of the thyroid gland

thyroiditis acute, subacute, or chronic disease of the thyroid gland; associated with inflammatory or infiltrative changes

thyrotoxicosis a synonym for hyperthyroidism

thyrotropin thyroid-stimulating hormone (TSH) secreted by specific cells of the anterior pituitary

thyroxine (T_4) 3,3′,5,5′-tetraiodothyronine, the principal thyroid hormone secreted by the thyroid gland (levothyroxine)

tincture an alcoholic solution

tinea infection a superficial fungus infection by dermatophytic fungi

tinea unguium a superficial fungus infection of the nail(s)

tinea versicolor a common, distinctive, asymptomatic superficial fungus infection of upper trunk and limbs; caused by *Pityrosporum obiculare*; produces pigment alterations

tinnitus a ringing or buzzing in the ears

tolerance the reduction of clinical effect in spite of continued similar dosing of a pharmacologic agent

tonometry the use of an instrument to measure intraocular pressure

tophaceous gout gout accompanied by tophi

tophus (pl., **tophi**) a deposit of sodium biurate in tissues near a joint or in bone

torticollis stiff contraction of the neck muscles with the head drawing to one side and the chin to the opposite side

toxic epidermal necrolysis a skin disease characterized by painful, large patches of necrotic epidermis; extensive raw areas form as the slightest pressure removes the epidermis from the underlying skin, making the patient appear scalded

toxic epidermal necrosis a severe form of exfoliative dermatitis, caused by staphylococci infection

toxic megacolon extreme dilation of the colon associated with toxic symptoms; occurs as a complication of inflammatory bowel disease

toxoid a toxin that has lost toxicity but retains the properties of combining with or stimulating the formation of antitoxin; adsorbed toxoids are bacterial toxoids adsorbed on aluminum hydroxide or alum providing prolonged antigenic stimulus

transcription the cellular process by which genetic information contained in DNA produces a complementary base sequence in an RNA chain to direct cellular protein synthesis

transduction a method of genetic recombination in bacteria, in which DNA from a lysed bacterium is transferred to another bacterium by a bacteriophage (a virus that can infect bacteria), thereby changing the genetic constitution of the second organism

transfer RNA a form of RNA that carries the code for protein synthesis to ribosomes where proteins are formed

translocation the shifting of a cellular or chemical segment or fragment from cytoplasm to nuclear receptors

transport, active movement of a substance across a barrier, involving an active process

transport, passive movement of a substance across a barrier by following the movement of another substance

tremor rhythmic shaking of a limb or muscle

trigone muscle a triangular-shaped muscle in the urinary bladder; when contracted impedes the flow of urine from the bladder

triiodothyronine (T_3) 3,5,3′-triiodothyronine, the principal and most active thyroid hormone at the cellular level (liothyronine)

trismus clenching or spasm of the jaw muscles

trophozoite the active, motile, feeding stage of a protozoon organism as contrasted with the nonmotile encysted stage

truncal obesity obesity preferentially affecting or located in the trunk of the body as opposed to the extremities

truncal vagotomy a procedure that surgically divides the trunk of the vagus nerve, usually in the region of the lower esophagus

tubercle bacilli the bacteria causing tuberculosis

tumor a lump, usually caused by abnormal growth of cells, that can be benign or malignant

U

ulcerative colitis an inflammatory bowel disease of unknown cause affecting the large bowel and rectum

universal antidote an antidote "supposedly for all toxins" made of one part magnesium oxide, one part tannic acid, and two parts activated charcoal

uremia a toxic condition resulting from renal insufficiency and accumulation of urea in the blood and manifesting symptoms of confusion, nausea, urinous odor of breath, and elevated blood pressure

urethritis an inflammation of the urethra; often associated with infection or trauma

uricosuric agent an agent that increases the urinary excretion of uric acid

urolithiasis formation of urinary calculi and the resultant clinical condition

urticaria a vascular reaction of the skin marked by transient appearance of smooth, slightly elevated patches that are redder or paler than the surrounding skin and often attended by severe itching; hives

V

vaccine a suspension of attenuated or killed microorganisms (bacteria, viruses, or rickettsiae); administered for the prevention, amelioration, or treatment of infectious disease

vagal pertaining to the vagus nerve

vagotomy a surgical interruption of the vagus nerve

vasoactive intestinal peptide a peptide that, in addition to causing vasodilation, has gastrointestinal effects such as inhibition of gastric secretion and stimulation of bile and pancreatic juice flow

vasoconstriction the diminution of the caliber or constricted size of a blood vessel; usually caused by autonomic nerve or chemical compound influences

vasomotor center a collection of cell bodies in the medulla oblongata of the brain that regulates or modulates blood pressure and cardiac function primarily via the autonomic nervous system

vasospastic angina an ischemic myocardial chest pain caused by spasm of the coronary arteries; has features different from classical exertional angina; also called Prinzmetal's angina

vehicle the medium or excipient in which the active therapeutic agent is carried or applied

vertigo a sensation as if the external world were revolving around the patient or as if the patient were revolving in space

very low density lipoprotein (VLDL) the carrier protein in the blood for triglycerides; so called because of its position after ultracentrifugation of serum

vesical sphincter the circular muscle surrounding the opening of the urinary bladder; when contracted, prevents urine from leaking from the bladder

vesicant a drug that is irritating to the skin on direct contact or to tissues on direct injection or extravasation

vestibular apparatus the portion of the ear that is associated with balance and position sense

vestibular toxicity toxic effects to the vestibule of the ear, resulting in dizziness, vertigo, and loss of balance

villous adenoma a polypoid or fungating type of lesion, usually occurring in the colon; composed of multiple, slender, fingerlike projections

viral gastroenteritis an inflammation of the intestine; caused by a virus and usually characterized by diarrhea, nausea and vomiting, and abdominal cramps

virucidal having a destructive (killing) action on viruses

virustatic having an inhibiting action on the growth of viruses

viscid glutinous or sticky

W

withdrawal the physiologic effects seen following the discontinuation of an agent that produces physiologic dependence; characterized by varying degrees of vomiting, sweating, diarrhea, anxiety, insomnia, hallucinations, chills, irritability, weakness, cramps, and spasms

Wolff-Parkinson-White syndrome the ECG pattern of a short PR interval with a widened QRS because of a delta wave that is commonly associated with supraventricular tachycardias; usually a result of an accessory electrical connection from atria to ventricles that lies outside the normal specialized conduction system and may be classified as a Kent bundle, Mahaim fibers, or a James fiber

wool fat the substance of which lanolin is a common chemical component

X

xanthoma small, flat plaques in the skin with a yellowish color; caused by deposits of lipids

x-ray a short wavelength, high-energy electromagnetic radiation resulting from the interaction of high-energy electrons with matter, especially metals

Z

Zollinger-Ellison syndrome a syndrome characterized by severe acid-peptic symptoms and complications; caused by hypersecretion of gastrin by an islet-cell tumor of the pancreas

Abbreviations Used in Text

A

AA	alcoholics anonymous
ACh	acetylcholine
AChE	acetylcholinesterase
ACIP	advisory committee on immunization practices
ACTH	corticotropin (formerly known as adrenocorticotrophic hormone)
ADA	American Diabetic Association
ADH	antidiuretic hormone
ADME	absorption, distribution, metabolism, and excretion
AHF	antihemophilic factor
AHG	antihemophilic globulin
AIDS	acquired immune deficiency syndrome
AM	ante meridiem; morning
AMP	adenosine monophosphate
AMU	atomic mass unit(s)
ANA	antinuclear antibody
ANS	autonomic nervous system
AP	action potential
APB	atrial premature beat(s)
ARDS	adult respiratory distress syndrome
ARS	antirabies serum, equine
ATP	adenosine triphosphate
ATPase	adenosine triphosphatase
AUC	area under the curve
AUC$_{o \to \infty}$	total area under the plasma concentration time curve
AV	atrioventricular
AVP	arginine-vasopressin

B

BAC	benzalkonium chloride
BAL	dimercaprol
BCG	bacillus Calmette-Guerin
BHI	biosynthetic human insulin
b.i.d.	twice daily
BM	bowel movement
BMR	basal metabolic rate
BP	blood pressure
Bq	becqueral
BUN	blood urea nitrogen

C

C	carbon
°C	degrees centigrade
Ca^{++}	calcium ion
CAC	cardioaccelerator center
CaCO$_3$	calcium carbonate
cAMP	cyclic adenosine monophosphate
Ca(OH)$_2$	calcium hydroxide
C$_b$	concentration in blood; blood level
CBC	complete blood count
CDC	Centers for Disease Control
CF	cellular fluid
cf.	compare
cGMP	cyclic guanosine monophosphate
CH$_3^+$	methyl group
ChA	choline acetyltransferase
CHD	congenital heart defect(s)
ChE	cholinesterase
CHF	congestive heart failure
CHO	carbohydrate
Ci	curie(s)
CIC	cardioinhibitory center
Cl$^-$	chloride ion
CL$_R$	renal clearance
CL$_T$	total clearance
cm	centimeter; one hundredth of a meter
CNS	central nervous system
CO	cardiac output
CO$_2$	carbon dioxide
COMT	catechol-O-methyltransferase
COOH$^-$	carboxyl group
COPD	chronic obstructive pulmonary disease
C$_p$	average plasma concentration
C$_p$	plasma concentration
Cp$_1$	plasma concentration at time 1
Cp$_2$	plasma concentration at time 2
CPAP	continuous positive airway pressure
Cp$_{mid}$	midpoint plasma concentration
Cp$^{ss}_{max}$	maximum steady state plasma concentration
Cp$^{ss}_{min}$	minimum steady state plasma concentration
CrCl	creatinine clearance
CSF	cerebrospinal fluid
CTZ	chemoreceptor trigger zone
C$_u$	concentration of drug in urine

D

DAWN	Drug Abuse Warning Network
DC	direct current
DDAVP	desmopressin
DDT	chlorophenothane
DET	diethyltryptamine
DEV	duck embryo vaccine
DIT	diiodotyrosine
DJD	degenerative joint disease
DKA	diabetic ketoacidosis
dl	deciliter; 100 ml; one tenth of a liter
Dm	diffusion constant
DMSO	dimethyl sulfoxide
DMT	dimethyltryptamine
DN	dibucaine number
DNA	deoxyribonucleic acid
DOM	2,5-dimethoxy-4-methylamphetamine
dps	disintegration (decay) per second
DPT	diphtheria and tetanus toxoid and pertussis vaccine
DS	double strength
DT	diphtheria toxoid
D_5W	five percent dextrose in water
$D_{10}W$	ten percent dextrose in water
$D_{40}W$	forty percent dextrose in water
dV/dt	rate of depolarization
DVT	deep vein thrombosis

E

E	epinephrine
ECF	extracellular fluid
ECG	electrocardiogram
ECT	electroconvulsive therapy
ED_{50}	minimum dose effective for 50% of the population
EDTA	edetate disodium (formerly known as ethylenediamine-tetraacetate)
EEG	electroencephalogram
e.g.	for example
E_i^j	allele
EMG	electromyelogram
EMU	epidermal-melanin unit
EPSP	excitatory postsynaptic potential
ERCP	endoscopic retrograde cholangiopancreatography
ERV	expiratory reserve volume
ESF	erythropoietic stimulating factor
EW	Edinger-Westphal

F

F	fraction of dose available to systemic circulation
°F	degrees Fahrenheit
FAS	fetal alcohol syndrome
FBS	fasting blood sugar
FDA	Food and Drug Administration
FDC	food, drug, and cosmetic
FEV_1	forced expiratory volume in the first second
FFA	free fatty acids
FIF	forced inspiratory flow
F_{IV}	fraction available from intravenous administration

FRV	functional residual volume
FSH	follicle-stimulating hormone
FT_3I	free triiodothyronine index
FT_4I	free thyroxine index
FVC	forced vital capacity

G

GABA	gamma-aminobutyric acid
GBS	Guillain-Barré syndrome
GFR	glomerular filtration rate
GGT	gamma glutamyl transpeptidase
GI	gastrointestinal
gm	gram
G-6-PD	glucose-6-phosphate dehydrogenase
Gy	gray

H

h.	hours
H^+	hydrogen ion
H_1	histamine one
HA	acidic drug
HBsAg	hepatitis B surface antigen
HCG	human chorionic gonadotrophin
HCl	hydrochloric acid; hydrochloride
HCO_3^-	bicarbonate ion
H_2CO_3	carbonic acid
HDCRV	human diploid cell rabies vaccine
HDL	high density lipoprotein(s)
Hg	mercury
HHNK	hyperglycemic hyperosmolar nonketotic coma
hr^-	reciprocal of hour; per hour
H_2O	water
HOCM	hypertrophic obstructive cardiomyopathy
HP	His-Purkinje
HPA	hypothalamic-pituitary-adrenal
HPB	Health Protection Branch
HPV	hypoxic pulmonary vasoconstriction
hr	hour
HSIG	human serum immune globulin
H_2SO_4	sulfuric acid
HT	hydroxytryptamine
HTP	hydroxytryptophan
HTSI	human thyroid-stimulating immunoglobulin
HVL	half-value layer

I

IA	intraarterial
IC	inspiratory capacity
ICF	intracellular fluid
ICU	intensive care unit
IDDM	insulin-dependent diabetes mellitus
IDL	intermediate density lipoprotein(s)
i.e.	that is
IgE	immune globulin E
IgG	immune globulin G
IHSS	idiopathic hypertrophic subaortic stenosis
IM	intramuscular
in	inch
INH	isoniazid

IPPB	intermittent positive pressure breathing		**mOsm**	milliosmole(s); one thousandth of an osmole
IPSP	inhibitory postsynaptic potential		**mRNA**	messenger ribonucleic acid
IPV	poliomyelitis vaccine, inactivated; Salk vaccine		**msec**	millisecond; one thousandth of a second
IQ	intelligence quotient		**MSS**	muscular subaortic stenosis
IU	International Unit(s)		**MTC**	minimum toxic concentration
IV	intravenous		**mV**	millivolt; one thousandth of a volt

J

J	flux; flow; joule
JPB	junctional premature beats

K

K⁺	potassium ion
KCl	potassium chloride
keV	thousand electron volt(s)
kg	kilogram; 1000 gm
KI	potassium iodide
Km	permeability constant
k$_m$	rate constant of metabolism
k$_m$C	rate of metabolism

L

L	liter
LATS	long-acting thyroid stimulator
lb	pound
LD$_{50}$	minimal dose lethal for 50% of test animals
LDL	low density lipoprotein(s)
LES	lower esophageal sphincter
LET	linear energy transfer
Lf	flocculating units
LH	luteinizing hormone
LNMP	last normal menstrual period
LSD	lysergic acid diethylamide
LTM	long-term memory

M

m	meter(s); mole(s)
m²	square meters
MAC	minimum alveolar concentration
MAO	monoamine oxidase
MAOI	monoamine oxidase inhibitor
MAOIs	monoamine oxidase inhibitors
MAT	multifocal atrial tachycardia
mCi	millicurie(s)
MEC	minimum effective concentration
mEq	milliequivalent(s)
MeV	million electron volt(s)
mg	milligram; one thousandth of a gram
mg/dl	milligrams per deciliter; milligrams per 100 milliliters
Mg⁺⁺	magnesium ion
MHPG	3-methoxy,4-hydroxyphenylglycol
MI	myocardial infarction
min	minute(s)
MIT	monoiodotyrosine
ml	milliliter(s); one thousandth of a liter
mm	millimeter(s); one thousandth of a meter
mmol	millimole(s); one thousandth of a mole

N

N	nitrogen
Na⁺	sodium ion
NaCl	sodium chloride
Na$_2$CO$_3$	sodium carbonate
NaI(Tl)	thallium-activated sodium iodide
NAD	nicotinamide adenine dinucleotide
NADP	nicotinamide adenine dinucleotide phosphate
NaHCO$_3$	sodium bicarbonate
NAIC	National Advisory Committee on Immunizations in Canada
NaOH	sodium hydroxide
NAP	nerve action potential
nCi	nanocurie; one billionth of a curie
NE	norepinephrine
nEq	nanoequivalents; one billionth of an equivalent
NF	National Formulary
ng	nanogram; one billionth of a gram
NG	nasogastric
NIAAA	National Institute on Alcoholism and Alcohol Abuse
NIDA	National Institutes of Drug Abuse
NL	normal
nm	nanometer(s); one billionth of a meter
nmol	nanomole(s); one billionth of a mole
nonIV	route of administration other than intravenous
non-REM	nonrapid eye movement
NPH	neutral protamine Hagedorn
NS	normal saline; 0.9% sodium chloride
NSAIDs	nonsteroidal antiinflammatory drugs

O

O⁼	oxygen ion
O$_2$	oxygen
OH⁻	hydroxyl group

P

p	para
P	phosphorus
PABA	aminobenzoic acid (formerly known as para-aminobenzoic acid)
Paco$_2$	partial pressure of carbon dioxide in the alveoli; carbon dioxide tension
PAH	para-amino-hippurate
Pao$_2$	partial pressure of oxygen in the arteries
PAO$_2$	partial pressure of oxygen in the alveoli
Pap	Papanicolaou
PAPS	3'-phosphoadenosine-5'-phosphosulfate

PAS	aminosalicylic acid (formerly known as para-aminosalicylic acid)
PAT	paroxysmal atrial tachycardia
PAWP	pulmonary artery wedge pressure
PCBs	polychlorinated biphenyls
pCi	picocurie; one trillionth of a Curie
P$_{CO_2}$	partial pressure of carbon dioxide
PCP	phencyclidine
PEEP	positive end-expiratory pressure
pg	picogram; one trillionth of a gram
PGE$_1$	prostaglandin E$_1$
PGE$_{2\alpha}$	prostaglandin E$_{2\alpha}$
PGE$_2$	prostaglandin E$_2$
pH	potential of hydrogen; measurement of the degree of acidity or alkalinity of a solution
pK$_a$	acid dissociation constant
PKU	phenylketonuria
PM	post meridiem; night
PMN	polymorphonuclear
pmol	picomole; one trillionth of a mole
PNS	peripheral nervous system
PO	by mouth; orally
P$_{O_2}$	partial pressure of oxygen
PO$_4^{--}$	phosphate ion
PPD	purified protein derivative
PPHP	5-phenyl-5′-para-hydroxyphenylhydantoin
PPI	patient package insert
PR	by rectum; rectally
prn	as needed
pro-PTH	proparathyroid hormone
PSP	phenolsulfonphthalein
PSVT	paroxysmal supraventricular tachycardia
PT	prothrombin time; parathyroid
PTA	plasma thromboplastin antecedent
PTC	phenylthiocarbamide
PTH	parathyroid hormone
PTT	partial thromboplastin time
PZI	insulin protamine zinc suspension (formerly known as protamine zinc insulin)

Q

q.	every
q.a.m.	every morning
q.d.	every day; daily
QF	quality factor
q.h.s.	every evening at bedtime; at bedtime
q.i.d.	four times daily
q.o.d.	every other day

R

R	Roentgen
RA	rheumatoid arthritis
rad	radiation absorbed dose
RAS	reticular activating system
RBC	red blood cell
RBE	relative biologic effectiveness
rem	roentgen equivalent man
REM	rapid eye movement
RIG	rabies immune globulin, human
RNA	ribonucleic acid
RUQ	right upper quadrant
RV	residual volume

S

S	sulfur
SA	sustained-action; sinoatrial
S&A	sugar and acetone
SAR	structure-activity relationship
SC	subcutaneous
SD	standard deviation of measurement
SE	standard error of measurement
sec	second(s)
SGOT	serum oxaloacetic transaminase
SGPT	serum glutamic pyruvic transaminase
SH	sulfhydryl
SI	international system
SIADH	syndrome of inappropriate antidiuretic hormone secretion
SL	sublingual
SMON	subacute myelo-optic neuropathy
SO$_4^{--}$	sulfate ion
SPCA	serum prothrombin conversion accelerator
SRS-A	slow-reacting substances of anaphylaxis
SSKI	saturated solution of potassium iodide
STM	short-term memory

T

t	time
T$_{1/2}$	half-life
t$_1$	time 1
t$_2$	time 2
T$_3$	liothyronine
T$_4$	levothyroxine; thyroxine
TB	tuberculosis
TBG	thyroxine-binding globulin
TD	combined tetanus and diphtheria toxoid, adult type
THC	tetrahydrocannabinol
TI	therapeutic index; ratio of minimum toxic to minimum effective dose
t.i.d.	three times daily
TIGH	tetanus immune globulin, human
TLC	total lung capacity
TOPV	poliovirus vaccine, live oral (formerly known as trivalent oral polio vaccine); Sabin vaccine
t$_{peak}$	time to reach peak concentration
TRH	thyrotropin-releasing hormone
TSH	thyrotropin (formerly known as thyroid stimulating hormone)
TU	tuberculin unit
T$_3$U	liothyronine-uptake

U

u	unit(s)
U$_\infty$	total amount of drug eliminated unchanged in the urine
UDPGA	uridine diphosphate α-D-glucuronic acid
UGDP	University Group Diabetes Program
URT	upper respiratory tract
USAN	United States Adopted Names
USP	*United States Pharmacopeia*
USPHS	United States Public Health Services
UTIs	urinary tract infections
UVA	ultraviolet light A

V

V	volume of urine excreted
VC	vital capacity
V_d	volume of distribution
vitamin B_1	thiamine
vitamin B_2	riboflavin
vitamin B_6	pyridoxine
vitamin B_{12}	cyanocobalamin
vitamin B_c	folic acid
vitamin C	ascorbic acid
vitamin D_2	ergocalciferol
vitamin D_3	cholecalciferol
vitamin K_1	phytonadione
vitamin K_3	menadione
vitamin K_4	menadiol
VLDL	very low density lipoprotein(s)
V_{max}	maximum rate of metabolism
VPB	ventricular premature beat(s)
V_T	tidal volume
v/v	volume-volume ratio
VZIG	varicella-zoster immune globulin

W

WBC	white blood cell
WHO	World Health Organization
wk	week
W-P-W	Wolff-Parkinson-White
w/v	weight-volume ratio

Y

| yr | year(s) |

Miscellaneous Symbols

μg	microgram; one millionth of a gram
μ	mu; micro
β	beta
Γ	gamma
α	alpha
λ	lambda; radionuclide decay constant
%	percent
=	equals; equal to
$\approx$	approximately equals
τ	tau; dosing interval
Δt	change in time; time interval
ΔU	amount excreted unchanged in the urine
<	less than
>	greater than
$\uparrow$	increase
$\downarrow$	decrease
$\propto$	proportional to
$\star$	indicates that the drug is generally available only in the United States
$\maltese$	indicates that the drug is generally available only in Canada
$\pm$	plus or minus; with or without
+	plus; with
$m\mu$	millimicron
ΔCs	concentration gradient
−	minus; without
β_1	beta one
β_2	beta two
μCi	microcurie; one millionth of a curie
μm	micrometer

Drug Names that Look or Sound Alike

Ann M. Pagliaro
Louis A. Pagliaro

A

Acetazolamide	Acetohexamide
Acetohexamide	Acetazolamide
Achromycin	Aureomycin
Actidil	Actifed
Actifed	Actidil
Aerolone	Aralen, Arlidin
Afrin	Aspirin
Agoral	Argyrol
Aldactazide	Aldactone
Aldactone	Aldactazide
Aldomet	Aldoril
Aldoril	Aldomet, Elavil, Equanil, Mellaril
Allerest	Sinarest
Ambenyl	Ambodyrl, Aventyl
Ambodryl	Ambenyl
Amcil	Amoxil
Amitriptyline	Nortriptyline
Amoxil	Amcil
Antuitrin	Anturan
Anturan	Antuitrin, Artane
Anusol	Aquasol
Aquasol	Anusol
Aralen	Aerolone, Arlidin
Argyrol	Agoral
Arlidin	Aerolone, Aralen
Arthralgen	Auralgan, Ophthalgan
Aspirin	Afrin
Atarax	Enarax, Marax
Auralgan	Arthralgen, Ophthalgan
Aureomycin	Achromycin
Avazyme	Orenzyme
Aventyl	Ambenyl, Ambodryl, Bentyl
Azathioprine	Azulfidine
Azlin	Mezlin
Azulfidine	Azathioprine

B

Bacitracin	Bactrim
Bactocill	Pathocil
Bactrim	Bacitracin, Zactirin
Banthine	Brethine
Belladenal	Belladonna, Bentyl
Belladonna	Belladenal
Beminal	Benemid
Benadryl	Belladenal, Bentyl, Benylin, Caladryl
Benemid	Beminal

Benoxyl	PanOxyl
Bentyl	Aventyl, Bontril
Bentylol	Aventyl
Benylin	Benadryl
Betalin	Benylin
Bicillin	V-cillin, Wycillin
Bontril	Bentyl
Brethine	Banthine
Butabarbital	Butalbital
Butalbital	Butabarbital
Butazolidin	Sterazolidin

C

Caladryl	Benadryl
Calamine	Calomel
Calomel	Calamine
Camalox	Maalox
Catapres	Combipres, Diupres, Hydropres
Cheracol	Geritol
Clinistix	Clinitest
Clinitest	Clinistix
Clofibrate	Clorazepate
Clomiphene	Clonidine
Clonidine	Clomiphene
Clorazepate	Clofibrate
Clotrimazole	Co-trimoxazole
Codeine	Coldene
Colace	Orinase
Coldene	Codeine
Combex	Combid
Combid	Combex
Combipres	Catapres, Diupres
Cort-dome	Cortone
Cortone	Cort-dome
Co-trimoxazole	Clotrimazole
Coumadin	Kemadrin
Cytarabine	Vidarabine

D

Dacarbazine	Procarbazine
Dalmane	Demulen
Danthron	Dantrium
Dantrium	Danthron
Darvon-N	Darvocet-N
Daunorubicin	Doxorubicin

Demerol	Demulen, Deprol, Dicumarol
Demulen	Demerol, Dicumarol
Deprol	Demerol
Desoxyn	Digoxin
Diamox	Trimox
Diazepam	Diazoxide
Diazoxide	Diazepam
Digitoxin	Desoxyn, Digoxin
Digoxin	Desoxyn, Digitoxin
Dilantin	Delautin, Phelantin
Dilaudid	Dilantin
Dilone	Dolene, Dyclone
Dimentabs	Dimetapp, Dimetane
Dimetane	Dimetapp
Dimetapp	Dimetane, Dimentabs
Diupres	Catapres
Diuril	Doriden
Diutensin	Salutensin, Unitensin
Dolene	Dilone
Donnagel	Donnatal
Donnatal	Dianabol, Donnagel
Donnazyme	Entozyme
Doriden	Doxidan, Loridine
Doxidan	Doriden
Doxorubicin	Daunorubicin
Drisdol	Drysol
Drysol	Drisol
Dyclone	Dilone
Dymelor	Demerol, Pamelor
Dyrenium	Pyridium

E

Ecotrin	Edecrin
Edecrin	Ecotrin
Elavil	Aldoril, Equanil, Mellaril
Emetine	Emetrol
Emetrol	Emetine
Enarax	Atarax, Marax
Enduron	Imferon
Enduronyl	Inderal
Entozyme	Donnazyme
Equanil	Aldoril, Elavil
Esidrix	Lasix
Esimil	Estinyl, Ismelin
Estinyl	Esimil
Ethamide	Ethionamide

Ethionamide	Ethamide, Ethinamate
Eurax	Urex
Euthroid	Synthroid, Thyroid

F

Feosol	Fer-in-sol, Festal
Fer-in-sol	Feosol
Festal	Feosol
Flagyl	Flexical
Flexical	Flagyl
Fostex	pHisoHex
Fulvicin	Furacin
Furacin	Fulvicin

G

Ganatrex	Kantrex
Gantanol	Gantrisin
Gantrisin	Gantanol
Garamycin	Terramycin
Gelfoam	Ger-o-foam
Geritol	Cheracol
Ger-o-foam	Gelfoam
Glaucon	Glucagon
Glucagon	Glaucon
Guanethidine	Guanidine
Guanidine	Guanethidine

H

Haldol	Halog, Winstrol
Halog	Haldol
Haloperidol	Haloprogin
Haloprogin	Haloperidol
Hexadrol	Hexalol
Hexalol	Hexadrol
Herplex	Hiprex
Hiprex	Herplex, Histex
Histex	Hiprex
Hycodan	Hycomine
Hycomine	Hycodan
Hydropres	Catapres, Diupres
Hygroton	Regroton
HyperHep	Hyper-Tet
Hyperstat	Hyper-Tet, Nitrostat

Hyper-Tet   HyperHep, Hyperstat
Hytone   Vytone

I

Imferon   Enduron, Imuran
Imuran   Imferon
Inderal   Enduronyl, Imuran, Isordil
Indocin   Ismelin, Lincocin
Ismelin   Estinyl, Indocin, Ritalin
Isordil   Inderal, Isuprel

K

Kafocin   Keflin
Kantrex   Ganatrex
Kaochlor   K-Lor
Kaon   Kaolin
Keflex   Keflin
Keflin   Kafocin, Keflex
Kemadrin   Coumadin
K-Lor   Kaochlor

L

Lasix   Esidrix, Lidex
Leritine   Loridine
Levodopa   Methyldopa
Levorphanol   Levallorphan
Lidaform   Vioform
Lidex   Lasix
Lincocin   Indocin
Loridine   Leritine
Luminal   Tuinal

M

Maalox   Camalox
Marax   Atarax, Enarax
Mebaral   Medrol, Mellaril
Mebendazole   Metronidazole
Medrol   Mebaral
Mellaril   Aldoril, Elavil, Mebaral
Mephenytoin   Mesantoin, Mephyton
Mephyton   Mephenytoin
Mesantoin   Mephenytoin
Methadone   Mephyton
Metronidazole   Mebendazole
Methyldopa   Levodopa
Mezlin   Azlin
Milontin   Miltown, Minocin
Miltown   Milontin
Minocin   Milontin
Myambutol   Nembutal

N

Nardil   Norinyl
Nembutal   Myambutol
Nicobid   Nitro-bid

Nilstat   Nitrostat, Nystatin
Nitro-bid   Nicobid
Nitrostat   Hyperstat, Nystatin
Norinyl   Nardil
Norlutate   Norlutin
Norlutin   Norlutate
Nortriptyline   Amitriptyline

O

Omnipen   Unipen
Ophthalgan   Arthralgen, Auralgan
Orenzyme   Avazyme
Orexin   Ornex
Orinase   Colace, Ornade, Tolinase
Ornade   Orinase, Ornex
Ornex   Orexin, Ornade
Otobione   Otobiotic
Otobiotic   Otobione, Urobiotic
Ovral   Ovulen
Ovulen   Ovral

P

Pabalate   Robalate
Pabanol   Panadol
Pamelor   Dymelor
Panadol   Pabanol, Valadol
PanOxyl   Benoxyl
Pantopon   Protopam
Parest   Trest
Pathocil   Bactocill, Placidyl
Penicillin   Polycillin
Pentacine   Pentazocine
Pentazocine   Pentacine
Pentobarbital   Phenobarbital
Pentothal   Pentritol
Pentritol   Pentothal
Percodan   Percobarb, Percorten
Percorten   Percodan
Periactin   Peritrate, Persantine, Taractan
Peritrate   Periactin
Persantine   Persistin, Trasentine
Persistin   Persantine
Pertofrane   Persantine
Phelantin   Dilantin
Phenaphen   Phenergan
Phenergan   Phenaphen, Theragran
Phenobarbital   Pentobarbital
pHisoHex   Fostex
Physostigmine   Pyridostigmine
Piperacetazine   Piperazine
Piperazine   Piperacetazine
Pitocin   Pitressin
Pitressin   Pitocin
Placidyl   Pathocil
Polycillin   Penicillin
Ponstel   Pronestyl
Pralidoxime   Pyridoxine
Prednisolone   Prednisone
Prednisone   Prednisolone

Procaine	Procan
Procarbazine	Dacarbazine
Procan	Procaine
Pronestyl	Ponstel
Propadrine	Propoxyphene
Propoxyphene	Propadrine
Protopam	Pantopon
Psorex	Serax
Pyridium	Pyridoxine
Pyridostigmine	Physostigmine
Pyridoxine	Pralidoxime, Pyridium

Q

Quarzan	Questran
Questran	Quarzan
Quinidine	Quinine
Quinine	Quinidine

R

Regonol	Regroton
Regroton	Hygroton, Regonol
Rifadin	Ritalin
Ritalin	Ismelin, Rifadin
Robalate	Pabalate

S

Salutensin	Unitensin
Sebical	Sebulex
Sebulex	Sebical, Sebutone
Sebutone	Sebulex
Senokap	Senokot
Senokot	Senokap
Serax	Eurax, Psorex, Xanax, Xerac
Sinarest	Allerest
Slo-Phyllin	Somophyllin
Somophyllin	Slo-Phyllin
Sparine	Sterine
Sporicidin	Sporostacin
Sporostacin	Sporicidin
Sterazolidin	Butazolidin
Sterine	Sparine
Sulfamerazine	Sulfamethazine
Sulfamethazine	Sulfamethizole, sulfamerazine
Surbex	Surfak
Surfak	Surbex
Synalar	Syntar
Syntar	Synalar
Synthroid	Euthroid, Thyroid

T

Tace	Tao
Tao	Tace
Taractin	Tinactin
Tedral	Teldrin
Tegopen	Tegretol, Tegrin
Tegretol	Tegrin

Tegrin	Tegopen, Tegretol
Teldrin	Tedral
Temaril	Tepanil
Tepanil	Temaril, Terfonyl, Tofranil
Terfonyl	Tofranil
Terramycin	Garamycin
Theolair	Thyrolar
Thyrar	Thyrolar
Thyroid	Euthroid
Thyrolar	Theolair, Thyrar
Tinactin	Taractin
Tobramycin	Trobicin
Tofranil	Terfonyl
Tolectin	Tolinase
Tolinase	Orinase, Tolectin
Trasentine	Persantine
Trest	Parest
Triaminic	TriHemic
TriHemic	Triaminic
Trimox	Diamox, Wymox
Trobicin	Tobramycin
Tuinal	Luminal, Tylenol
Tylenol	Tuinal
Tylox	Wymox
Tyzine	Visine

U

Unicap	Unipen
Unipen	Omnipen, Unicap
Unitensen	Salutensin
Uracel	Uracid, Uracil
Uracid	Uracel, Uracil, Urised, Uristix
Uracil	Uracel
Urex	Eurax
Urised	Uracid, Uristat, Uristix
Uristat	Uristix
Uristix	Urised, Uristat
Urobiotic	Otobiotic

V

Valadol	Panadol
Valmid	Vanobid
Valpin	Velban
Vanobid	Valmid
Vasocidin	Vasodilan
Vasodilan	Vasocidin
Vasosulf	Velosef
V-Cillin	Bicillin, Wycillin
Velban	Valpin
Velosef	Vasosulf
Verstran	Vesprin
Vesprin	Verstran
Vibramycin	Viomycin
Vicon-C	Vitron-C
Vidarabine	Cytarabine
Vigran	Wigraine
Vioform	Lidaform
Viomycin	Vibramycin

Visine   Tyzine
Vitron-C   Vicon-C
Vontrol   Vosol
Vosol   Vontrol
Vytone   Hytone

W

Wigraine   Vigran
Winstrol   Haldol
Wycillin   Bicillin, V-Cillin
Wymox   Tylox

X

Xanax   Xerax, Zantac, Zomax
Xerac   Eurax, Serax, Xanax, Zomax

Z

Zactirin   Bactrim, Zarontin, Zaroxolyn
Zantac   Xanax
Zarontin   Zactirin, Zaroxolyn
Zaroxolyn   Zarontin
Zentron   Zarontin
Zomax   Xanax

Compatibility Guide for Combining IV Medications

Philip K. Ng

<table>
<tr><td colspan="2">Key to table on pp. 1708-1711</td></tr>
<tr><td>C</td><td>Compatible in dextrose and dextrose-saline solution</td></tr>
<tr><td>☐</td><td>No information available</td></tr>
<tr><td>C*</td><td>Compatible initially; unstable, use immediately since potency may be lost after prolonged exposure</td></tr>
<tr><td>C?</td><td>Compatibility studies showed conflicting results</td></tr>
<tr><td>C^a</td><td>Compatible in dextrose solution</td></tr>
<tr><td>C^b</td><td>Compatible in saline solution</td></tr>
<tr><td>±X</td><td>Stable for X hours after mixing</td></tr>
<tr><td>±X^a</td><td>Stable for X hours after mixing in dextrose solution</td></tr>
<tr><td>☐ I</td><td>Incompatible</td></tr>
</table>

NOTE: Compatibility (physical and/or chemical) sometimes depends on the relative concentrations of the drugs in the same solution. Hence, certain drugs may be compatible in one concentration but incompatible in another concentration.

Reproduced with permission from: Ng, P. Compatibility guide for combining I.V. medications. *American Journal of Nursing,* 1979, *79,* 1292-1295.

Compatibility here means that the drugs in the same IV solution are at least *physically* compatible (cloudiness, precipitation, or gas formation will not occur). Although the drugs may be physically compatible, possible pharmacologic chemical incompatibility (inactivation or degradation of one drug in the presence of the other) may occur. Whenever in doubt, do *not* mix the two drugs together. For additional information regarding pharmacologic interactions see Chapter 10, "Drug Interactions."

Generic names are used in the chart and are supplemented by trade names, in parentheses, when the information applies *only* to that product.

For additional information regarding stability after reconstitution and dilution see the Nursing Drug Digest for each specific drug.

	Amikacin SO4	Aminophylline	Amphotericin B	Ampicillin Na	Atropine SO4	Calcium gluconate	Carbenicillin Na2	Cefazolin Na	Cephalothin Na	Chloramphenicol Na succinate	Clindamycin PO4	Dexamethasone Na PO4	Diazepam	Digoxin	Dopamine HCl	Epinephrine HCl	Erythromycin gluceptate	Erythromycin lactobionate
Amikacin SO4	C	±8	I	I		C	±8	±8	I	C	C	C				C	I	
Aminophylline	±8	C		C*		C		C?	I	Ca	I	C	C	C			I	C
Amphotericin B	I		C	I		I	I								I			
Ampicillin Na	I	C*	I	C	I	I	Ca	Cb		C	I				±1a	I	I	
Atropine SO4				I	C						I					I		
Calcium gluconate	C	C	I	I		C		I	I	C	I						I	C
Carbenicillin Na2	±8		I	Ca			C	Cb		I	Ca				Ca	I	I	I
Cefazolin Na	±8	C?		Cb		I	Cb	C		Cb	Cb	Cb	C				I	
Cephalothin Na	I	I				I				C	Ca	Ca			±6a	I	I	I
Chloramphenicol Na succinate	C	Ca		C	I	C	I	Cb	Ca	C		C			Ca	I	I	I
Clindamycin PO4	C	I		I		I	Ca	Cb	Ca		C							
Dexamethasone Na PO4	C	C						Cb		C		C	I				C	
Diazepam		C						C					I	C	C	I		
Digoxin		C												C	C			
Dopamine HCl			I	±1a			Ca		±6a	Ca					C			
Epinephrine HCl	C		I	I	I	I			I		I				I	C	I	
Erythromycin gluceptate	I	I		I		C	I	I	I	I		C				I	C	
Erythromycin lactobionate		C					I		I	I								C
Furosemide (Lasix)		±8											I					
Gentamicin SO4			I	I			I	I	I		Ca				±6a			
Heparin Na	I	C?	C	C	I	Ca		Cb	C	Ca	Ca	C	I	C	Ca		C?	I

Furosemide (Lasix)	Gentamicin SO₄	Heparin Na	Insulin injection (Regular)	Isoproterenol HCl	Levarterenol bitartrate (Levophed)	Lidocaine HCl	Meperidine HCl (Demerol)	Metaraminol bitartrate (Aramine)	Methicillin Na	Morphine SO₄	M.V.I. (Multi-Vitamin Infusion)	Nafcillin Na	Penicillin G potassium	Potassium chloride	Procainamide HCl	Solu-Cortef (hydrocortisone Na succinate)	Solu-Medrol (methylprednisolone Na succinate)	Sodium bicarbonate	Tobramycin SO₄	Vitamin B complex with C (Berocca-C)	Vitamin C
		I		C				C	±8				C	C		C		C		±8	C
±8		C?	I	I	I	C	I	C	Cᵃ	I	I	C*	C*	C	C	C	±6	±8ᵃ		I	I
	I	C						I					I	I		±12ᵃ	±7ᵃ				
	I	C		I		C?		I					C?	Cᵃ		C?				I	
		I			I		C	I		C								I		I	
		Cᵃ			Cᵃ		C	C					C	C	C	C	I	I		C	±8ᵃ
	I			I		C								C		Cᵃ	C	Cᵃ	I	C*	
	I	Cᵇ											Cᵇ	Cᵃ		C	Cᵃ		I	C	
	I	C	±8ᵃ	C	C?	I		I	C				Cᵃ	C		C	I	I	I	I	±6
		Cᵃ			C?	C	C	C	Cᵃ		Cᵃ	C	C	C	C	C*	Cᵃ	C		C	Cᵃ
	Cᵃ	Cᵃ											Cᵃ	C		C	C	C	Cᵇ	I	Cᵃ
		C				C		I	C		Cᵃ	C	C	C		C				±8	
I		I		I	I	I	I						I					I		I	
		C												C		C				C	
	±6ᵃ	Cᵃ			C	Cᵃ						±6ᵃ	Cᵃ			Cᵃ	Cᵃ	I			
			I	I	C*	C	I	I		Cᵃ			I					I		I	
		C?					I	Cᵃ				Cᵃ	C	C	C	C	C				C
		I			C		I	C				C	C		C		C			I	C?
C						I	I											I			
	C	I						I		I											
	I	C	C	C	C	C	I		C?	I		C	C?	C	C	C?			I	C	Cᵃ

	Amikacin SO₄	Aminophylline	Amphotericin B	Ampicillin Na	Atropine SO₄	Calcium gluconate	Carbenicillin Na2	Cefazolin Na	Cephalothin Na	Chloramphenicol Na succinate	Clindamycin PO₄	Dexamethasone Na PO₄	Diazepam	Digoxin	Dopamine HCl	Epinephrine HCl	Erythromycin gluceptate	Erythromycin lactobionate
Insulin injection (Regular)		I							±8ᵃ									
Isoproterenol HCl		I					I		C				I			I		
Levarterenol bitartrate (Levophed)	C	I		I	I	Cᵃ			C?	C?			I		C	I		
Lidocaine HCl		C		C?				C	I	C		C	I		Cᵃ	C*		C
Meperidine HCl (Demerol)		I			C				C				I			C		
Metaraminol bitartrate (Aramine)	C	C	I	I	I	C			I	C		I				I	I	I
Methicillin Na	±8	Cᵃ				C			C	Cᵃ		C				I	Cᵃ	C
Morphine SO₄		I		C														
M.V.I. (Multi-Vitamin Infusion)		I								Cᵃ		Cᵃ				Cᵃ		
Nafcillin Na		C*								C		C						
Penicillin G potassium	C	C*	I	C?		C		Cᵇ	Cᵃ	C	Cᵃ	C			±6ᵃ		Cᵃ	C
Potassium chloride	C	C	I	Cᵃ		C	C	Cᵃ	C	C	C	C	I	C	Cᵃ	I	C	C
Procainamide HCl		C				C				C						C		
Solu-Cortef (hydrocortisone Na succinate)	C	C	+12ᵃ	C?		C	Cᵃ	C	C	C*	C	C			C	Cᵃ	C	C
Solu-Medrol (methylprednisolone Na succinate)		±6	±7ᵃ			I	C	Cᵃ	I	Cᵃ	C				Cᵃ		C	
Sodium bicarbonate	C	±8ᵃ			I	I	Cᵃ		I	C	C		I		I	I		C
Tobramycin SO₄							I	I	I		Cᵇ							
Vitamin B complex with C (Berocca-C)	±8	I		I	I	C	C*	C	I	C	I	±8	I	C		I		I
Vitamin C	C	I				±8ᵃ			±6	Cᵃ	Cᵃ						C	C?

Furosemide (Lasix)	Gentamicin SO₄	Heparin Na	Insulin injection (Regular)	Isoproterenol HCl	Levarterenol bitartrate (Levophed)	Lidocaine HCl	Meperidine HCl (Demerol)	Metaraminol bitartrate (Aramine)	Methicillin Na	Morphine SO₄	M.V.I. (Multi-Vitamin Infusion)	Nafcillin Na	Penicillin G potassium	Potassium chloride	Procainamide HCl	Solu-Cortef (hydrocortisone Na succinate)	Solu-Medrol (methylprednisolone Na succinate)	Sodium bicarbonate	Tobramycin SO₄	Vitamin B complex with C (Berocca-C)	Vitamin C
		C	C										I	C				I			C
		C		C		C*					C			C				I			C
		C			C	C*			I		C	C*		C		C		I			C
		C		C*	C*	C		C	C				C	C		C		C?			C
I		I					C		I	I						C?	I	I			
I						C		C	I				I	C	C	C?	I	C			
	I	C?			I	C	I	I	C	I		Cᵃ		C		I		I		I	Cᵃ
		I				I	C		I	C								I			
			C	C						C			C*								
	I	C		C*					C					C		I		C		I	I
		C?	I			C		I	Cᵃ		C*		C	C	C	C	C	I		C	±8ᵃ
		C	C	C	C	C	C	C				C	C	C		C*	C	C		C	C
		C					C						C		C	C				C	
		C?		C	C	C?	C?	I				I	C	C*	C	C	C	±8ᵃ		I	C*
							I	I					C	C		C	C	±8ᵃ		I	
	I	I	I	I		C?	I	C	I	I		C	I	C		±8ᵃ	±8ᵃ	C		I	I
		I																	C		
I		C	C	C	C	C			I			I	C	C	C	I	I	I		C	C
		Cᵃ					Cᵃ		I			±8ᵃ	C			C*		I		C	C

Poisoning

ANTIDOTES

Antidote	Trade name	Indication	Dosage	Comments
Amyl nitrite inhaler, sodium thiosulfate, sodium nitrite	Cyanide Antidote Kit	Cyanide poisoning	*Adults or children over 25 kg:* give entire ampule of sodium nitrite IV *Children under 25 kg:* adjust the doses according to hemoglobin: Hemoglobin / Initial dose 3% sodium nitrite (ml/kg) 8 gm — 0.22 ml (6.6 mg) 10 gm — 0.27 ml (8.7 mg) 12 gm — 0.33 ml (10.0 mg) 14 gm — 0.39 ml (11.6 mg) Hemoglobin / Initial dose 25% sodium thiosulfate (ml/kg) 8 gm — 1.10 ml 10 gm — 1.35 ml 12 gm — 1.65 ml 14 gm — 1.95 ml	Follow instructions in the kit (see dosage column)
Atropine	Various	Control of symptoms of organophosphate poisoning	Initial dose: *adults,* 2 mg IV; *children,* 0.05 mg/kg	Drug should be given until symptoms, i.e., bradycardia, excessive pulmonary secretion, are effectively controlled
Calcium disodium edetate (EDTA)	Calcium Disodium Versenate	Used for severe lead poisoning in conjunction with dimercaprol; may be useful for other types of heavy metal poisoning	50 mg/kg/day IV or IM divided into 3 doses for 5 days; allow 2 days off and repeat course if necessary	*IV use:* dosage should be diluted in 250 ml of D_5W or NS and infused over 1 to 2 hr *IM use:* procaine 1% (1 ml for each ml of EDTA) should be added to decrease pain at injection site
Deferoxamine	Desferal	Severe iron poisoning	90 mg/kg IM (up to 1 gm) q.8h. *or* 15 mg/kg/hr IV up to 90 mg/kg q.8h.	IV use is indicated when the patient is hypotensive and blood flow to IM injection sites is expected to be poor

Reprinted with permission from Manoguerra, T. Pediatric poisoning. In L. Pagliaro & R. Levin (Eds.). *Problems in Pediatric Drug Therapy.* Hamilton: Drug Intelligence Publications, Inc., 1979.

ANTIDOTES—cont'd

Antidote	Trade name	Indication	Dosage	Comments
Dimercaprol	BAL in Oil	Arsenic, gold, and mercury poisoning; for severe lead poisoning in conjunction with EDTA	Variable according to indication; generally 4 mg/kg IM q.4h.	
Methylene blue	None	Methemoglobinemia	0.2 ml/kg IV injected over 5 min	
Naloxone	Narcan	Poisoning with narcotics or narcotic derivatives	*Adults:* 0.4 mg IV, repeat prn *Children:* 0.01 mg/kg IV, repeat prn	Effect may be short lived; repeated doses usually necessary; patients should be monitored closely
Penicillamine	Cuprimine	Oral therapy of copper, lead, mercury and arsenic poisoning	*Children:* 100 mg/kg/day PO for 5 days, maximum of 1 gm/day *Adults:* 500 mg q.6h. for 1 day, 250 mg q.6h. for 1 day, 250 mg q.8h. until chelation complete	
Physostigmine	Antilirium	Severe anticholinergic poisoning *Indications for physostigmine use:* seizures, severe hypertension, dysrhythmias, hallucinations and delirium when injury to patient likely	*Adults:* 2 mg IV slowly; repeat prn *Children:* 0.5 mg IV slowly; repeat prn	Should be administered until desired effect achieved or excess cholinergic symptoms develop
Pralidoxime (2-PAM)	Protopam	Organophosphate poisoning	*Adults:* 1 gm IV over 2 min; repeat q.8-12h. prn *Children:* 250 mg IV over 2 min; repeated q.8-12h prn	Should be used after severe symptoms have been controlled by atropine

SUMMARY OF EMERGENCY TREATMENT
OF POISONING

State of patient or nature of poison	Emergency treatment
Syrup of ipecac *can be used to induce vomiting in all poisonings* **except** *in the following instances, which should be treated as indicated.*	
Alcohol	Be prepared to administer artificial respiration
Corrosive acids or alkalis	Dilutional therapy with up to 2 glassfuls of water or milk. Do *not* induce vomiting
Household detergents	Administer liberal quantities of milk or water
Liquid bleaches	Give milk of magnesia or aluminum hydroxide gel
Methanol	Give 30 ml (1 fl oz) of an alcohol containing beverage (e.g., gin, vodka, whiskey) every 3 or 4 hours
Petroleum products	Give several ounces of mineral oil (medicinal grade) or give activated charcoal
Pregnancy or cardiac disease	Administer activated charcoal if appropriate
Strychnine	Give activated charcoal; keep patient warm, quiet, and in subdued lighting. (Emesis may be induced [syrup of ipecac] provided the emetic is administered *immediately* after the ingestion of the strychnine.)
Tricyclic antidepressants, Phenothiazines	Induction of emesis is probably contraindicated; the safest emergency treatment is to administer activated charcoal
Turpentine	Administer a demulcent, milk, or several egg whites mixed with water
Unconscious, drowsy, agitated, or convulsing patient	Keep the patient warm and provide supportive care
Activated charcoal *can be given in all poisonings* **except** *in the following instances, which should be treated as indicated.*	
Alcohol	Administer artificial respiration if necessary
Boric acid	Give syrup of ipecac
Corrosive acids and alkalis	Dilutional therapy with up to 2 glassfuls of water or milk. Do *not* induce vomiting
Cyanide	Give syrup of ipecac
Iron preparations	Give syrup of ipecac
Methanol	Administer 30 ml (1 fl oz) of an alcohol-containing beverage (e.g., gin, vodka, whiskey) every 3 or 4 hours
Turpentine	Give milk or several egg whites beaten with water
Unconscious, drowsy, agitated, or convulsing patient	Keep the patient warm and provide supportive care

Reprinted with permission from Coutts, R. Geriatric poisoning. In L. Pagliaro & A. Pagliaro (Eds.). *Pharmacologic aspects of aging.* St. Louis: The C.V. Mosby Co., 1983.

SUBSTANCES ADSORBED BY
ACTIVATED CHARCOAL

ORGANIC SUBSTANCES EFFECTIVELY ADSORBED BY ACTIVATED CHARCOAL

Acetaminophen
Amphetamines
Antipyrine
Aspirin
Atropine
Barbiturates
Benzodiazepines
Camphor
Chlorinated hydrocarbons (e.g., DDT)
Chloroquine
Chlorpheniramine
Chlorpromazine

Cocaine
Digitalis
Digoxin
Glutethimide
Ipecac
Malathion
Meprobamate
Morphine
Nicotine
Opium
Oxalates
Parathion
Penicillin

Phenobarbital
Phenol
Phenol-
    phthalein
Phenothia-
    zines
Phenytoin
Propoxy-
    phene
Quinine
Salicylates
Strychnine
Sulfonamides
Tricyclic anti-
    depressants

INORGANIC SUBSTANCES EFFECTIVELY ADSORBED BY ACTIVATED CHARCOAL

Antimony salts
Arsenic
Iodine

Lead
Mercury
Phosphorus

Potassium
    permanga-
    nate
Selenium
Silver

Reprinted with permission from Coutts, R. Geriatric poisoning. In L. Pagliaro & A. Pagliaro (Eds.). *Pharmacologic aspects of aging.* St. Louis: The C.V. Mosby Co., 1983.

Products Lacking Adequate Evidence
of Effectiveness

January 1981

Dear Health Professional:

I am writing to furnish you with a list of prescription drug products currently classified by the Food and Drug Administration (FDA) as lacking adequate evidence of effectiveness. You may wish to consider this list in your professional practice.

All of the products on this list were marketed prior to the 1962 amendments to the Federal Food, Drug, and Cosmetic Act and were originally approved by the FDA only for safety. As a result of these amendments, the FDA initiated a review of the effectiveness of all prescription drug products approved between 1938 (when the new drug law was first enacted) and 1962. This review considered more than 3400 products and is now almost 90 percent complete.

The drug products on the accompanying list are listed alphabetically by trade name. These products are in various stages of administrative review and remain on the market pending final resolution of the issues in each case. This means in some cases that the FDA considers the active ingredient not to have been shown to be effective by appropriate clinical trials, in other cases that not all ingredients in a combination contribute to the claimed effect, in yet other cases that a purported controlled release effect is not proven, or in other cases that not all of the claimed indications are supported by adequate clinical trials.

There are numerous other drug products that have active ingredients which are identical or similar to those on the list but which are marketed by other firms under different product names. The same effectiveness issues apply to these other products, and their fate is tied directly to their counterparts on the list. Because the list identifies the ingredients in each product, it is possible to recognize these other drug products by comparing the ingredients.

Under the terms of a settlement agreement to a lawsuit over the FDA's implementation of this drug efficacy review, the agency is accelerating its review of the drug products on this list. Nevertheless, this review could still take up to four more years to complete. In the meantime, I hope this list will be helpful to you in explaining the status of these products and in your selection of drugs for your patients.

Sincerely yours,

Mark Novitch,
Acting Commissioner
of Food and Drugs

**PRESCRIPTION DRUG PRODUCTS CURRENTLY
CLASSIFIED BY THE FOOD AND DRUG
ADMINISTRATION AS LACKING ADEQUATE EVIDENCE
OF EFFECTIVENESS**

January 1981
(Revised February 1984)

Unresolved issues for drug products on this list:

1. For products containing only a single active ingredient, the issue in most cases is whether the effectiveness of that entity for any indication is supported by adequate and well-controlled trials.

2. For combination drugs, the issue in most cases is whether *all* of the ingredients contribute to the claimed effect (i.e., whether one or more of the ingredients is superfluous).

3. For controlled release dosage forms, the issue in most cases is whether the controlled release product in fact produces the desired blood level of active ingredient(s) for a longer period of time than that produced by the conventional dosage form of the drug product.

4. For products marked with an asterisk (*), the issue is whether the product is effective for *all* of its claimed indications; such products are judged effective for at least one indication. The less-than-effective indications at issue are identified.

Trade name	Active ingredient(s)	Dosage form/route of administration	Firm	Remarks
Actifed-C Expectorant	Codeine Guaifenesin Pseudoephedrine Triprolidine	Syrup/oral	Burroughs Wellcome	Drug is included on list of 200-most prescribed drugs (National Prescription Audit, IMS America, Ltd., as reported in *Pharmacy Times*, April, 1983)
Ambenyl Expectorant	Ammonium chloride Bromodiphenhydramine Codeine sulfate Diphenhydramine Guaiacolsulfonate potassium Menthol	Syrup/oral	Marion	
Amesec	Aminophylline Amobarbital Ephedrine	Capsule/oral Enteric-coated tablet/oral	Lilly	
Aminophylline and Amytal	Aminophylline Amobarbital	Capsule/oral	Lilly	
Ananase	Bromelains	Enteric-coated tablet/oral	Rorer	
Anaspaz-PB	L-Hyoscyamine Phenobarbital	Tablet/oral	B.F. Ascher	
Antora-B.T.D.	Pentaerythritol tetranitrate Secobarbital	Capsule/oral	Mayrand	
Arlidin	Nylidrin	Tablet/oral	USV	
Atropine sulfate, Hyoscyamine sulfate, Scopolamine hydrobromide, and Phenobarbital	Atropine Hyoscyamine Phenobarbital Scopolamine	Tablet/oral	National Alliance	
Atropine sulfate, and Phenobarbital	Atropine Phenobarbital	Tablet/oral	Numerous manufacturers	
Avazyme	Chymotrypsin	Enteric-coated tablet/oral	Wallace	
Barbidonna	Atropine Hyoscine Hyoscyamine Phenobarbital	Tablet/oral Elixir/oral	Mallinckrodt Wallace	
Barophen	Atropine Hyoscyamine Phenobarbital Scopolamine	Elixir/oral	National	
Bay-Ase	Atropine Hyoscine hydrobromide Phenobarbital Scopolamine	Elixir/oral	Bay Labs	
Belabarb	Atropine Hyoscine Hyoscyamine Phenobarbital	Tablet/oral	Arnar-Stone	
Belladenal	Bellafoline levorotatory alkaloids of belladonna as the maleates Phenobarbital	Tablet/oral	Sandoz	

Trade name	Active ingredient(s)	Dosage form/route of administration	Firm	Remarks
Belladenal-S	Bellafoline levorotatory alkaloids of belladonna as the maleates Phenobarbital	Tablet/oral	Sandoz	
Belladonna alkaloids and phenobarbital	Atropine Hyoscyamine Phenobarbital Scopolamine	Tablet/oral	Lemmon	
Bellastal	Atropine Hyoscyamine Phenobarbital Scopolamine	Capsule/oral	Warton	
Bentyl/Phenobarbital	Dicyclomine Phenobarbital	Capsule/oral Tablet/oral Syrup/oral	Merrell Dow	
Brophed	Ephedrine Hydroxyzine Theophylline	Tablet/oral	Cord	
Butabar Belladonna	Belladonna alkaloids Butabarbital	Elixir/oral	National	
Butibel	Belladonna extract Butabarbital	Tablet/oral Elixir/oral	McNeil	
Cantil with Phenobarbital	Mepenzolate Phenobarbital	Tablet/oral	Merrell Dow	
Cartrax	Hydroxyzine Pentaerythritol tetranitrate	Tablet/oral	Roerig	
Cetacaine	Benzocaine Tetracaine	Aerosol/topical Jelly/topical Liquid/topical Ointment/topical	Cetylite	
Chardonna-2	Belladonna extract Phenobarbital	Tablet/oral	Rorer	
Chymoral	Chymotrypsin Trypsin	Enteric-coated tablet/oral	Armour	
Combid	Isopropamide iodide Prochlorperazine maleate	Sustained release capsule/oral	Smith Kline & French	Drug is included on list of 200-most prescribed drugs (National Prescription Audit, IMS America, Ltd., as reported in *Pharmacy Times*, April, 1983)
Corovas	Pentaerythritol tetranitrate Secobarbital	Sustained release capsule/oral	Amfre-Grant	
Cordran-N	Flurandrenolide Neomycin	Cream and ointment/topical	Lilly	
Cortisporin-G	Gramicidin Hydrocortisone Neomycin Polymyxin B	Cream/topical	Burroughs Wellcome	
Cyclandelate	Cyclandelate	Tablet/oral	Cord Premo	
Cyclospasmol	Cyclandelate	Capsule and tablet/oral	Ives	
Dainite	Aluminum hydroxide gel (dried) Aminophylline Benzocaine Ephedrine Phenobarbital	Tablet/oral	Wallace	

Continued.

Trade name	Active ingredient(s)	Dosage form/route of administration	Firm	Remarks
Dainite-KI	Aluminum hydroxide gel (dried) Aminophylline Benzocaine Ephedrine Phenobarbital Potassium iodide	Tablet/oral	Wallace	
Daricon PB	Oxyphencyclimine Phenobarbital	Tablet/oral	Beecham	
Deprol	Benactyzine Meprobamate	Tablet/oral	Wallace	
Di-Ademil-K	Hydroflumethiazide Potassium chloride	Tablet/oral	E.R. Squibb	
Dimetane Expectorant	Brompheniramine maleate Guaifenesin Phenylephrine Phenylpropanolamine	Syrup/oral	A.H. Robins	
Dimetane-DC Expectorant	Brompheniramine maleate Codeine phosphate Guaifenesin Phenylephrine Phenylpropanolamine	Syrup/oral	A.H. Robins	
Dimetapp	Brompheniramine Phenylephrine Phenylpropanolamine	Elixir and sustained release tablet/oral	A.H. Robins	
Diutensin	Cryptenamine tannates Methyclothiazide	Tablet/oral	Wallace	
Donnatal	Atropine Hyoscyamine Phenobarbital Scopolamine	Elixir/oral Capsule/oral Tablet/oral	Robins	
Donnatal Extentabs	Atropine Hyoscine Hyoscyamine Phenobarbital	Sustained release tablet/oral	Robins	
Enarax	Hydroxyzine Oxyphencyclimine	Tablet/oral	Pfizer	
Gantrisin*	Sulfisoxazole	Cream/vaginal	Hoffmann- La Roche	Less than effective indications: for the treatment of *Haemophilis vaginalis*, for the treatment of trichomoniasis, for the treatment of vulvovaginal candiasis
Homapin-PB	Homatropine methylbromide Phenobarbital	Tablet/oral	Mission	
Hybephen	Atropine Hyoscyamine Phenobarbital Scopolamine	Tablet/oral	Beecham	
Ilotycin No. 90	Erythromycin	Ointment/topical	Lilly	
Iodochlorhydroxyquin with Hydrocortisone	Hydrocortisone Iodochlorhydroxyquin	Cream/topical	Byk-Gulden	
Isoxsuprine	Isoxsuprine	Tablet/oral	Cord Premo	

Trade name	Active ingredient(s)	Dosage form/route of administration	Firm	Remarks
Kinesed	Atropine Hyoscine Hyoscyamine Phenobarbital	Tablet/oral	ICI	
Koro-sulf	Sulfisoxazole	Cream/vaginal	Holland-Rantos	
Levsin with Phenobarbital	Hyoscyamine Phenobarbital	Elixir/oral Drops/oral Tablet/oral	Kremers-Urban	
Librax	Chlordiazepoxide Clidinium	Capsule/oral	Roche	Drug is included on list of 200-most prescribed drugs (National Prescription Audit, IMS America, Ltd., as reported in *Pharmacy Times*, April, 1983)
Lufyllin-EPG	Dyphylline Ephedrine Guaifenesin Phenobarbital	Elixir/oral Tablet/oral	Wallace	
Luftodil	Ephedrine Guaifenesin Phenobarbital Theophylline	Tablet/oral	Wallace	
Marax	Ephedrine Hydroxyzine Theophylline	Tablet/oral Syrup/oral	Roerig	
Mepergan Fortis	Meperidine Promethazine	Capsule/oral	Wyeth	
Methan-drosteno-lone	Methandrostenolone	Tablet/oral	Bolar Par	
Midrin	Acetaminophen Dichloralphenazone Isometheptene	Capsule/oral	Carnrick	
Milpath	Meprobamate Tridihexethyl chloride	Tablet/oral	Wallace	
Miltrate	Meprobamate Pentaerythritol tetranitrate	Tablet/oral	Wallace	
Mycolog	Gramicidin Neomycin Nystatin Triamcinolone acetonide	Cream and ointment/topical	E.R. Squibb	Drug is included on list of 200-most prescribed drugs (National Prescription Audit, IMS America, Ltd., as reported in *Pharmacy Times*, April, 1983)
Myco Triacet	Gramicidin Neomycin Nystatin Triamcinolone	Ointment/topical	Premo	
Naturetin with K	Bendroflumethiazide Potassium chloride	Tablet/oral	E.R. Squibb	
Neo-Aristo-cort	Neomycin Triamcinolone acetonide	Cream and ointment/topical	Lederle	
Neo-Aristo-derm	Neomycin Triamcinolone acetonide	Aerosol foam/topical	Lederle	
Neo-Deca-dron	Dexamethasone sodium phosphate Neomycin	Cream/topical	Merck Sharp & Dohme	
Neo-Delta-Cortef	Neomycin Prednisolone	Ointment/topical	Upjohn	
Neo-Cort-Dome	Hydrocortisone Neomycin	Cream/topical	Dome	

Continued.

Trade name	Active ingredient(s)	Dosage form/route of administration	Firm	Remarks
Neo-Cortef	Hydrocortisone Neomycin	Cream/topical Lotion/topical Ointment/topical	Upjohn	
Neo-Medrol Acetate	Methylprednisolone Neomycin	Cream/topical	Upjohn	
Neo-Oxylone	Fluorometholone Neomycin	Ointment/topical	Upjohn	
Neosporin-G	Gramicidin Neomycin Polymyxin B	Cream/topical	Burroughs Wellcome	
Neo-Synalar	Fluocinolone acetonide Neomycin	Cream/topical	Syntex	
Neoquess	Atropine Hyoscyamine Phenobarbital Scopolamine	Tablet/oral	O'Neal, Jones & Feldman	
Neomycin-Hydrocortisone	Neomycin Hydrocortisone	Ointment/topical	Ambix	
Nylidrin	Nylidrin	Tablet/oral	Cord	
Nystatin-Neomycin-Gramicidin-Triamcinolone	Gramicidin Neomycin Nystatin Triamcinolone	Cream/topical	Premo Byk-Gulden	
Nystatin-Neomycin-Gramicidin-Triamcinolone	Gramicidin Neomycin Nystatin Triamcinolone	Ointment/topical	Byk-Gulden Clay-Park	
Orenzyme	Chymotrypsin Trypsin	Enteric-coated tablets/oral	Merrell Dow	
Papase	Proteolytic enzymes from carica papaya	Chewable tablet/oral or buccal	Warner-Lambert Parke-Davis	
Parafon Forte	Acetaminophen Chlorzoxazone	Tablet/oral	McNeil	
Pathibamate	Meprobamate Tridihexethyl chloride	Tablet/oral	Lederle	
Peritrate with Phenobarbital	Pentaerythritol tetranitrate Phenobarbital	Sustained release tablet/oral	Warner-Lambert Parke-Davis	
Phenergan Pediatric Expectorant with Dextromethorphan	Citric acid Dextromethorphan Ipecac fluid extract Potassium guaiacolsulfonate Promethazine Sodium citrate	Syrup/oral	Wyeth	
Phenergan Expectorant Plain	Citric acid Ipecac fluid extract Potassium guaiacolsulfonate Promethazine Sodium citrate	Syrup/oral	Wyeth	Drug is included on list of 200-most prescribed drugs (National Prescription Audit, IMS America, Ltd., as reported in *Pharmacy Times*, April, 1983)
Phenergan Expectorant with Codeine	Citric acid Codeine Ipecac fluid extract Potassium guaiacolsulfonate Promethazine Sodium citrate	Syrup/oral	Wyeth	Drug is included on list of 200-most prescribed drugs (National Prescription Audit, IMS America, Ltd., as reported in *Pharmacy Times*, April, 1983)

Trade name	Active ingredient(s)	Dosage form/route of administration	Firm	Remarks
Phenergan VC Expectorant Plain	Citric acid Ipecac fluid extract Phenylephrine Potassium guaiacolsulfonate Promethazine Sodium citrate	Syrup/oral	Wyeth	
Phenergan VC Expectorant with Codeine	Citric acid Codeine phosphate Ipecac fluid extract Phenylephrine Potassium guaiacolsulfonate Promethazine Sodium citrate	Syrup/oral	Wyeth	Drug is included on list of 200-most prescribed drugs (National Prescription Audit, IMS America, Ltd., as reported in *Pharmacy Times*, April, 1983)
Phenobarbital and Belladonna	Atropine Hyoscyamine Phenobarbital Scopolamine	Elixir/oral	Pharmaceutical Assoc.	
Potaba	Aminobenzoate Potassium	Tablet, capsule, and powder/oral	Glenwood	
Priscoline	Tolazoline	Injectable/injection	Ciba	
Pro-Banthine with Phenobarbital	Phenobarbital Propantheline bromide	Tablet/oral	Searle	
Propazine	Isopropamide iodide Prochlorperazine	Capsule/oral	Cord	
Quadrinal	Ephedrine Phenobarbital Potassium iodide Theophylline calcium salicylate	Tablet/oral	Knoll	
Quibron Plus	Butabarbital Ephedrine Guaifenesin Theophylline	Capsule/oral Elixir/oral	Mead Johnson	
Racet	Hydrocortisone Iodochlorhydroxyquin	Cream/topical	Lemmon Pharmacal	
Rautrax	Flumethiazide Potassium chloride Rauwolfia serpentina	Tablet/oral	E.R. Squibb	
Rautrax Improved	Hydroflumethiazide Potassium chloride Rauwolfia serpentina	Tablet/oral	E.R. Squibb	
Rautrax-N	Bendroflumethiazide Potassium chloride Rauwolfia serpentina	Tablet/oral	E.R. Squibb	
Rautrax-N Modified	Bendroflumethiazide Potassium chloride Rauwolfia serpentina	Tablet/oral	E.R. Squibb	
Roniacol	Nicotinyl alcohol tartrate	Tablet/oral Sustained release tablet/oral	Roche	
Roniacol	Nicotinyl alcohol	Elixir/oral	Roche	
Ruhexatal Pb	Mannitol hexanitrate Phenobarbital	Tablet/oral	Lemmon	
Ruhexatal & Reserpine	Mannitol hexanitrate Reserpine	Tablet/oral	Lemmon	

Continued.

Trade name	Active ingredient(s)	Dosage form/route of administration	Firm	Remarks
Saplix	Atropine Hyoscyamine Phenobarbital Scopolamine	Elixir/oral Tablet/oral	Reid-Provident	
Spasmatol	Atropine Hyoscyamine Phenobarbital Scopolamine	Elixir/oral	Pharmaceutical Assoc.	
Susano	Atropine Hyoscyamine Phenobarbital Scopolamine	Elixir/oral	Halsey Drug	
T.C.M.	Meprobamate Tridihexethylchloride	Tablet/oral	Zenith	
Terra-Cortril	Hydrocortisone Oxytetracycline	Ointment/topical	Pfizer	
Tigan*	Trimethobenzamide	Capsule/oral	Beecham	Less than effective indications: vomiting secondary to gastroenteritis, nausea and vomiting associated with radiation therapy, travel sickness, nausea and vomiting caused by infections, underlying disease processes or drug administration, emesis associated with operative procedures or Ménière's syndrome
Tigan	Trimethobenzamide	Suppository/rectal	Beecham	
Tri-Statin	Gramicidin Neomycin Nystatin Triamcinolone	Cream/topical	Clay-Park	
Trocinate	Thiphenamil	Tablet/oral	Poythress	

Trade name	Active ingredient(s)	Dosage form/route of administration	Firm	Remarks
Tuss-Ornade	Caramiphen edisylate Chlorpheniramine maleate Isopropamide iodide Phenylpropanolamine	Sustained release capsule and liquid/oral	Smith Kline & French	Drug is included on list of 200-most prescribed drugs (National Prescription Audit, IMS America, Ltd., as reported in *Pharmacy Times*, April, 1983)
Tussionex	Hydrocodone Phenyltoloxamine	Tablet and suspension/oral	Pennwalt	
Valpin PB	Anisotropine methylbromide Phenobarbital	Tablet/oral	Endo	
Vasocon-A	Antazoline Naphazoline	Solution/ophthalmic	Cooper	
Vasodilan	Isoxsuprine	Solution/intramuscular Tablet/oral	Mead Johnson	Drug is included on list of 200-most prescribed drugs (National Prescription Audit, IMS America, Ltd., as reported in *Pharmacy Times*, April, 1983)
Vioform-Hydrocortisone	Hydrocortisone Iodochlorhydroxyquin	Cream/topical Ointment/topical	Ciba	
Vistrax	Oxyphencyclimine Hydroxyzine	Tablet/oral	Pfizer	
Vytone	Diiodohydroxyquin Hydrocortisone	Cream/topical	Dermik	
Westhiazole	Sulfathiazole	Jelly/vaginal	Westwood	
Wyanoids HC	Belladonna extract Bismuth subcarbonate Bismuth oxyiodide Boric acid Ephedrine sulfate Hydrocortisone acetate Peruvian balsam Zinc oxide	Suppository/rectal	Wyeth	

Therapeutic and Toxic Concentrations of Selected Drugs

Louis A. Pagliaro
Ann M. Pagliaro

Drug	Plasma (P) or serum (S)	Usual therapeutic concentration range	Usual toxic concentration range
Acetaminophen	P	5-20 µg/ml	150+ µg/ml (4 hr after injection)
Carbamazepine	P	4-11 µg/ml	10+ µg/ml
Digitoxin	P	10-22 ng/ml	30+ ng/ml
Digoxin*	P	0.5-2.0 ng/ml	2.4+ ng/ml
Disopyramide	P	2-5 µg/ml	8+ µg/ml
Ethosuximide	S	40-100 µg/ml	100+ µg/ml
Lidocaine	P	1.5-6 µg/ml	6+ µg/ml
Lithium	S	0.5-1.5 mEq/L	1.5+ mEq/L
Phenobarbital	P	1-5 mg/100 ml	5+ mg/100 ml
Phenytoin	S	10-20 µg/ml	25+ µg/ml
Primidone	P	5-10 µg/ml	12+ µg/ml
Procainamide	P	4-8 µg/ml	10+ µg/ml
(N-acetylprocainamide)	P	10-20 µg/ml	30+ µg/ml
Quinidine	P	3-6 µg/ml	7+ µg/ml
Salicylates (salicylic acid)	P	100-250 µg/ml (antiinflammatory effect)	300+ µg/ml
Theophylline	S	10-20 µg/ml	20+ µg/ml
Valproic acid	P	50-100 µg/ml	

Note that these values may vary depending on which analytic laboratory methods are used in measuring the drug concentration. In addition, it should be emphasized that these values are presented as a general guide and that because of individual variability, the patient's status must *always* be used in conjunction with laboratory test results to determine the optimum therapy. The values presented are for adults and may not necessarily apply to children or to elderly patients.

*Note that the measurement of endogenous digoxin-like material, particularly in neonates, can result in spuriously high digoxin values. This laboratory test interference occurs predominantly, and to varying degrees, with the various immunoassays used to determine plasma digoxin concentrations.

Adverse Drug Effects Index

*Adverse Drug Effects Index**

A

Abdominal cramps; *see* Abdominal pain
Abdominal pain; *see also* Epigastric distress
  alclofenac and, 1328
  anticholinesterases and, 509
  benoxaprofen and, 1329
  bisacodyl and, 883, 898
  cascara sagrada and, 899
  castor oil and, 899
  clomiphene and, 1454
  dichlorophen and, 965
  diflunisal and, 1330
  docusates and, 900
  glycerin and, 901
  laxatives and, 894
  loperamide and, 890
  mebendazole and, 967
  melarsonyl and, 936
  melarsoprol and, 936
  phenolphthalein and, 883
  probenecid and, 1355
  senna and, 906
Acid rebound
  antacids and, 840
  calcium carbonate and, 834
  sodium bicarbonate and, 835
Acid-base disturbances; *see* Electrolyte imbalance;
    Metabolic acidosis; Metabolic alkalosis
Acne
  anabolic steroids and, 1474-1475
  androgens and, 1474
  corticosteroids and, 1356
    topical, 1282-1283, 1284
  progestins and, 1459
Acneform rash; *see* Rashes
Addiction; *see* Drug abuse
Adrenal failure
  corticosteroids and, 1284
Agranulocytosis; *see also* Blood dyscrasias
  antipsychotics and, 181, 329, 334
  aprinidine and, 669
  chlorpromazine and, 181
  cimetidine and, 841
  co-trimoxazole and, 1076
  doxepin and, 371
  furazolidone and, 934
  indomethacin and, 1323
  levamisole and, 1351
  nonsteroidal antiinflammatory drugs and, 1334
  phenylbutazone and, 1322, 1334
  sulfasalazine and, 1076
  sulfonamides and, 1075-1076, 1081
Air embolism
  hydrogen peroxide and, 1215, 1224

Airway resistance increase
  beta-adrenergic blockers and, 693
Akathisia
  antipsychotics and, 329, 335
Albuminuria
  ipecac and, 591
  melarsonyl and, 936
  melarsoprol and, 936
  methenamine and, 790
Alkalosis; *see also* Metabolic alkalosis
  antacids and, 840
  calcium carbonate and, 834
  sodium bicarbonate and, 835
Allergic dermatitis; *see also* Allergic reactions
  clomiphene and, 1454
  neomycin and, 1027
  topical corticosteroids and, 1283, 1284-1285
Allergic reactions; *see also* Allergic dermatitis; Ana-
    phylaxis; Hypersensitivity
  aminoglycosides and, 1023
  antipsychotics and, 329, 331
  asparaginase and, 1170, 1173
  cephalosporins and, 981
  dacarbazine and, 1173
  dermatitis in; *see* Allergic dermatitis
  epinephrine and, 1170
  epipodophyllotoxins and, 1171
  formalin and, 1224
  general anesthetics and, 241
  haloprogin and, 1129
  influenza vaccine and, 1584
  insulin and, 1380
  iodine compounds and, 1212, 1224
  local anesthetics and, 1222, 1224
  mechlorethamine and, 1173
  neomycin and, 793, 1023, 1027, 1284
  pancreatic enzymes and, 837
  parabens and, 1217
  penicillin and, 981
  phenolphthalein and, 883
  rabies vaccine and, 1586
  radiopharmaceuticals and, 1644
  sedative-hypnotics and, 259
  sulfamethoxazole and, 1077
  sulfonamides and, 1076, 1081
  tetracycline and, 1042
  venom allergenic extracts and, 1611, 1614
  zomepirac and, 1330
Alopecia
  anticancer drugs and, 1140, 1146, 1152
  asparaginase and, 1173
  azathioprine and, 1356, 1360
  chlorambucil and, 1173
  cisplatin and, 1171
  colchicine and, 1353, 1356
  cyclophosphamide and, 1167, 1179, 1350, 1356,
    1360
  dactinomycin and, 1145, 1146, 1160
  daunorubicin and, 1161
  doxorubicin and, 1161

Alopecia—cont'd
  epipodophyllotoxins and, 1171
  ifosfamide and, 1168
  interferon and, 1173
  mechlorethamine and, 1166, 1173
  melphalan and, 1173
  mitomycin and, 1163
  nitrosoureas and, 1168, 1173
  phensuximide and, 424
  primidone and, 426
  progestins and, 1459
  remittive agents and, 1360
  valproic acid and, 429
  vincristine and, 1169, 1173
Amenorrhea; *see also* Sexual dysfunction
  cyclophosphamide and, 1167, 1350, 1351, 1357
  mechlorethamine and, 1166, 1173, 1176-1183
Amnesia
  general anesthetics and, 241
  muscarinic blockers and, 457
Anaphylaxis, 181; *see also* Allergic reactions; Hy-
    persensitivity
  amphotericin B and, 1109, 1118, 1120, 1126
  antitoxins and, 1613, 1614
  asparaginase and, 1185
  bleomycin and, 1146, 1159
  cholera vaccine and, 1582
  chymopapain and, 1658
  doxorubicin and, 1146
  epinephrine and, 181, 1147
  local anesthetics and, 1222, 1224
  methocarbamol and, 288
  muscle relaxants and, 288
  phenolphthalein and, 883
  pneumococcal vaccine and, 1583
  radiopharmaceuticals and, 1643
  serums and, 1589, 1590
  tetracyclines and, 1042, 1044
  thyrotropin and, 1431
  toxoids and, 1589, 1590
  vaccines and, 1589, 1590
  vasopressin and, 1681
Anemia; *see also* Blood dyscrasias
  acetohydroxamic acid and, 1653
  amphotericin B and, 1109, 1118, 1120, 1126
  aplastic
    chloramphenicol and, 1053
    indomethacin and, 1323
    mephenytoin and, 419
    nonsteroidal antiinflammatory drugs and,
      1334
    phenylbutazone and, 1322, 1334
    sulfonamides and, 1075-1076, 1081
  cisplatin and, 1171
  colchicine and, 1353
  flucytosine and, 1112
  general anesthetics and, 241
  hemolytic
    acetohydroxamic acid and, 1653
    cephalosporins and, 989

Anemia—cont'd
    hemolytic—cont'd
        indomethacin and, 1323
        mefenamic acid and, 1328
        methyldopa and, 694
        methylene blue and, 796
        nitrofurantoin and, 792, 796
        penicillins and, 989
        primaquine and, 939
        stibophen and, 973
        sulfonamides and, 1075-1076, 1081
        urinary tract drugs and, 796
    megaloblastic, 1353
        nitrofurantoin and, 792
    nitrofurantoin and, 792
    oxyphenbutazone and, 1342
    phenylbutazone and, 1343
    piroxicam and, 1343
    quinidine and, 669
    remittive agents and, 1359
Angina
    sympathomimetics and, 477
Angioneurotic edema
    barbiturates and, 259
    cinoxacin and, 795
    methenamine and, 795
    muscle relaxants and, 288
    nalidixic acid and, 795
    neomycin and, 795
    nitrofurantoin and, 795
    sedative-hypnotics and, 259
    sulfonamides and, 1076
    urinary tract drugs and, 795
Anhedonia
    indomethacin and, 1323
    nonsteroidal antiinflammatory drugs and, 1335
Anorexia
    aminosalicylic acid and, 1096
    amphetamines and, 387
    cardiac glycosides and, 652, 653
    central nervous system stimulants and, 387
    cyclophosphamide and, 1350
    dextroamphetamine and, 394
    ethionamide and, 1096
    pemoline and, 402
    propranolol and, 709
    pyrazinamide and, 1096
    vitamin A and, 1523
    vitamin D and, 1442
Anovulation; see also Sexual dysfunction
    cyclophosphamide and, 1350, 1357
Anticholinergic effects
    acetophenazine and, 340
    amoxapine and, 368
    antidysrhythmics and, 670
    antipsychotics and, 329, 331, 333
    atropine and, 456
    butaperazine and, 340
    chlorpromazine and, 341
    chlorprothixene and, 328, 342
    cyclobenzaprine and, 293
    diphenhydramine and, 867
    diphenidol and, 867
    disopyramide and, 675
    fluphenazine and, 343
    loxapine and, 327
    mesoridazine and, 344
    molindone and, 327, 345
    parasympatholytics and, 456
    phenothiazines and, 327
    promazine and, 348

Anticholinergic effects—cont'd
    thioridazine and, 349
    thiothixene and, 328
    trazodone and, 379
    triflupromazine and, 350
Anuria
    sulfonamides and, 1077
Anxiety
    tricyclic antidepressants and, 360
Aplastic anemia; see Anemia
Apnea
    alprostadil and, 1653
    diazepam and, 417
    muscarinic blockers and, 522
    narcotics and, 304
    oxygen and, 557
Apnea neonatorum
    halothane and, 247
Arterial hypertension; see also Hypertension
    vitamin D and, 1533
Arterial thromboembolism
    menotropins and, 1671
Arthralgia
    gold salts and, 1357
    rubella vaccine and, 1584
Arthritis
    rubella vaccine and, 1584
Aseptic bone necrosis
    corticosteroids and, 1357
Aseptic meningitis; see also Meningitis
    sulindac and, 1324
Asthma; see also Respiratory dysfunction
    aspirin and, 1321
    beta-adrenergic blocking agents and, 693
    iodine and, 1224
    mercury compounds and, 1224
    muscle relaxants and, 288
    sedative-hypnotics and, 259
    sodium salicylate and, 1321
Ataxia
    fluorouracil and, 1146
    muscle relaxants and, 286
    nabilone and, 870
    phenytoin and, 425
Atrial fibrillation; see also Cardiac dysrhythmias
    syrup of ipecac and, 856
Atropine-like side effects; see Anticholinergic effects
Auditory dysfunction; see Hearing loss
Azoospermia; see also Sexual dysfunction
    cyclophosphamide and, 1350, 1357
Azotemia
    sulfonamides and, 1077

B

Behavioral disturbances
    alcohol and, 140
    corticosteroids and, 1356, 1491, 1495
    cyclopentolate and, 467
Bell's palsy
    methyldopa and, 693
Bleeding; see also Blood dyscrasias
    alprostadil and, 1653
    anticoagulants and, 724, 729
    carbenicillin and, 989
    cyclophosphamide and, 1350, 1357
    dicumarol and, 750
    epinephrine and, 1224
    ethacrynic acid and, 772
    heparin and, 750
    moxalactam and, 989

Bleeding—cont'd
    phenylbutazone and, 1343
    platelet aggregation inhibitors and, 727
    streptokinase and, 1680
    urokinase and, 1681
Bloating
    hydroxychloroquine and, 1349
    plantago seed and, 905
Blood dyscrasias; see also Bleeding; specific dyscrasia
    alprostadil and, 1653
    anticancer drugs and, 1140
    anticonvulsants and, 409
    antidysrhythmics and, 670
    antihistamines and, 590
    antiparkinsonian drugs and, 386
    antipsychotics and, 329
    antithyroid medications and, 1424
    aurothioglucose and, 1363
    butyrophenones and, 326
    captopril and, 695
    chloramphenicol and, 1053
    co-trimoxazole and, 931
    general anesthetics and, 259
    indomethacin and, 1323
    mephenytoin and, 419
    nonsteroidal antiinflammatory drugs and, 1331, 1334
    novobiocin and, 1057, 1068
    oxyphenbutazone and, 1342
    penicillamine and, 1368
    pentamidine and, 939
    perphenazine and, 859
    phenacemide and, 422
    platelet aggregation inhibitors and, 729
    plicamycin and, 1145, 1146
    primaquine and, 939
    pyrimethamine and, 940
    quinacrine and, 940
    quinine and, 941
    sulfonamides and, 1075
    suramin and, 942
    tricyclic antidepressants and, 360
    valproic acid and, 429
Blurred vision; see Visual disturbances
Bone; see also Bone marrow depression; Fractures
    corticosteroids and, 132
    tetracyclines and, 1042
Bone marrow depression; see also Myelosuppression
    anticancer drugs and, 1140-1141, 1146, 1150-1151
    chloramphenicol and, 1053, 1060, 1062
    cytarabine and, 1160
    daunorubicin and, 1161
    doxorubicin and, 1161
    flucytosine and, 1127
    nonsteroidal antiinflammatory drugs and, 1334
    phenylbutazone and, 1322, 1334
    procarbazine and, 1190
    radiopharmaceuticals and, 1647
    remittive agents and, 1359
    sulfonamides and, 1075-1076, 1081
    thioguanine and, 1164
    vidarabine and, 1118
Bone pain; see also Fractures
    tamoxifen and, 1454, 1471
Bradycardia; see also Cardiac dysrhythmias
    alprostadil and, 1653
    atenolol and, 701
    beta-adrenergic blockers and, 693
    bethanechol and, 465

Drug Interaction Index

Drug Interaction Index*

A

Acetaminophen
oral anticoagulants and, 730
Acetazolamide, 108
aspirin and, 305
lithium and, 361
methenamine compounds and, 796
probenecid and, 1355
quinidine and, 178, 671
Acetohexamide, 1392; see also Oral hypoglycemics
aspirin and, 1332
choline salicylate and, 1332
magnesium salicylate and, 1332
oxyphenbutazone and, 1332
phenylbutazone and, 1332
quinidine and, 178
salicylates and, 1332
salsalate and, 1332
Acetohydroxamic acid
iron and, 1651
Activated charcoal, 171, 890, 895
antacids and, 1651
laxatives and, 1651
syrup of ipecac and, 1651
Acyclovir
probenecid and, 1118
Adrenaline, 235, 236; see also Epinephrine
α-Adrenergic agonists; see Alpha-adrenergic agonists
β-Adrenergic agonists; see Beta-adrenergic agonists
β-Adrenergic blockers; see Beta-adrenergic blockers
Albuterol, 479; see also Beta-adrenergic agonists
Alclofenac
warfarin and, 1328
Alcohol, 85, 173-174, 1225
acetohexamide and, 1392
amebicides and, 923, 924
anticancer drugs and, 1173, 1351
antidepressants and, 362
antihistamines and, 594
antiprotozoals and, 923, 924
antitussives and, 594
aspirin and, 305, 731, 1321, 1332
barbiturates and, 260, 410
benzodiazepines and, 260
bishydroxycoumarin and, 114, 115
bronchodilators and, 561
cefamandole and, 990
cefoperazone and, 990
central nervous system depressants and, 174
cephalosporins and, 990
chloral hydrate and, 174, 260
chlorpromazine and, 859
chlorpropamide and, 174, 1392

Alcohol—cont'd
chymotrypsin and, 1652
codeine and, 592
cyclizine and, 858
cyclobenzaprine and, 288
cyclophosphamide and, 1351
desipramine and, 370
diazepam and, 288
disulfiram and, 115, 174, 1225
fenoprofen and, 1326
furazolidone and, 923
general anesthetics and, 242
glipizide and, 1392
glutethimide and, 260
glyburide and, 1392
guanethidine and, 697
hypnotics and, 260, 262
insulin and, 1392
meclizine and, 858
meprobamate and, 114, 260
metronidazole and, 115, 174, 922, 926, 937
moxalactam and, 990
muscle relaxants and, 286, 288
naproxen and, 1336
narcotic analgesics and, 305
nitrofurantoin and, 798
oral anticoagulants and, 114, 115, 730
oral hypoglycemics and, 177, 182, 260, 1392
phenothiazines and, 330, 857, 858, 859, 861
phenytoin and, 114
procarbazine and, 1171, 1174
salicylates and, 178, 305, 1321, 1332
sedatives and, 260, 262
sulfonylureas and, 1392
tetrachloroethylene and, 961
thiazide diuretics and, 774
tolazamide and, 1392
tolbutamide and, 114, 182, 1392
vasodilators and, 730
Alkylating agents, 1174, 1175; see also specific agent
Allopurinol, 1350, 1354
ampicillin and, 1355
azathioprine and, 1350, 1354, 1357, 1359
mercaptopurine and, 1143, 1147, 1148, 1354, 1357
oral anticoagulants and, 730, 1354, 1357
prazosin and, 695
probenecid and, 1355
thiazide diuretics and, 1354
Alpha-adrenergic agonists; see also specific agent
atropine and, 458
bethanechol and, 458
bethanidine and, 479
debrisoquine and, 479
diazoxide and, 695
guanethidine-like drugs and, 479
monoamine oxidase inhibitors and, 479
muscarinic agonists and, 458
muscarinic blockers and, 458
phenelzine and, 479

Alpha-adrenergic agonists—cont'd
pilocarpine and, 458
scopolamine and, 458
tranylcypromine and, 479
Alpha- and beta-adrenergic agonists; see also Alpha- adrenergic agonists
amitriptyline and, 479
beta-adrenergic blockers and, 479
bethanidine and, 479
debrisoquine and, 479
guanethidine-like drugs and, 479
imipramine and, 479
monoamine oxidase inhibitors and, 479
phenelzine and, 479
propranolol and, 479
timolol and, 479
tranylcypromine and, 479
Aluminum hydroxide, 890
tetracyclines and, 838, 1045
Ambenonium
mecamylamine and, 528
Amebicides, 922, 923, 924; see also specific agent
Amikacin, 1029; see also Aminoglycosides
general anesthetics and, 242
intravenous compatibility and, 1708, 1709
ticarcillin and, 1029
Amiloride
hydrochlorothiazide and, 773
lithium and, 773
Aminobenzoic acid
aspirin and, 305
sulfonamides and, 1651
Aminocaproic acid
estrogens and, 1651
oral contraceptives and, 1651
Aminoglycosides, 1028, 1029; see also specific agent
anticholinesterases and, 510
cephaloridine and, 990
cephalosporins and, 990
cephalothin and, 990, 1028
cisplatin and, 1174
ethacrynic acid and, 773, 1028
furosemide and, 773, 1028
loop diuretics and, 773
methoxyflurane and, 1028
muscle relaxants and, 1028
neomycin and, 1285
neuromuscular blockers and, 523
oral anticoagulants and, 1028
penicillins and, 991, 1028
polymyxin B and, 1057
succinylcholine and, 1028
ticarcillin and, 1029
tubocurarine and, 1028
Aminophylline
B-complex vitamins and, 1537
ethylenediamine and, 1284, 1287
intravenous compatibility and, 1708, 1709

*This index provides a comprehensive cross-reference of all drug-drug interactions that are discussed in this text. See also the General Index.

General Index

A

A chain, 1377, 1378
A-200 Pyrinate (Pyrethrins), 952
AA; *see* Alcoholics Anonymous
Aarane (Cromolyn sodium), 574
Abbocin (Oxytetracycline), 938, 1050
Abbokinase (Urokinase), 1681
Abbreviations, 1697-1701
Abdomen
  aminoglycoside and infection in, 1024
  fluid in, 758
  kidney assessment and, 758
Abdominal cramps; *see* Abdominal pain
Abdominal pain; *see* Adverse Drug Effects Index
Abdominal surgery
  kanamycin and, 1026
  neomycin and, 1026
Abducens nerve, 219
Aberel (Tretinoin), 1274
Abortive cold, 586
Abscess
  abdominal, aminoglycoside and, 1024
  brain, bacitracin and, 1052
  liver, 918, 919
Absence seizure, 405-406
Absorbable moiety, 825
Absorption
  drug interaction and, 171
  food and, 83-87
  across membrane, 83-92
  of oral medication, 32
  physiologic factor and, 85-86
  of radiation, 1625
  across skin, 92
    corticosteroid and, 1279
  subcutaneous, 45
  of suppository, 37
Abuse, drug; *see* Drug abuse
Acanthocytosis, 1534
Acatalasia, 159, 161-162
Accelerase (Pancrelipase), 851
Accessory nerve, 220
Accidental pediatric poisoning, 132; *see also* Poisoning
Accountability, 26-28
Accumulative effect, strychnine and, 12
Accurbron (Theophylline), 582
Acebutolol, 686
Aceclidine, 456
Acecoline (Acetylcholine), 463
Acenocoumarol, 750
  pharmacokinetics of, 724
Acephen (Acetaminophen), 321
Acetal (Aspirin), 322
Acetaldehyde, 96
Acet-Am (Theophylline), 582
Acet-Am Expectorant (Theophylline), 582
Acetamin (Acetaminophen), 321
Acetaminophen, 303, 321-322, 1355
  activated charcoal and, 1715
  and chlorzoxazone, 1722
  dichloralphenazone and isometheptene, 1721
  elderly and, 135
  food and, 84
  hepatotoxicity of, 112

Acetaminophen—cont'd
  inflammation and, 1319, 1321
  metabolism and, 97, 116
  nephrotoxicity of, 112
  oral anticoagulants and, 730
  probenecid and, 1355
  saliva and, 109
  syndrome of inappropriate secretion of antidiuretic hormone and, 1560
  therapeutic concentration of, 1726
  toxic concentration of, 1726
  toxigenesis and, 116-117
  vaccine reaction and, 1593
Acetanilid, 9
Acetate formation, 102
Acetazolam (Acetazolamide), 414
Acetazolamide, 414
  angle-closure glaucoma and, 414
  aspirin and, 305
  excretion of, 95
  lithium and, 361
  metabolic acidosis and, 1571, 1572
  methenamine compounds and, 796
  potassium deficit and, 1563
  probenecid and, 1355
  quinidine and, 178, 671
  urinary pH and, 108
Acetest, 1383, 1384
Acetexa (Nortriptyline), 375
Acetic acid, 805
  as antiseptic, 1218
  metabolic pathway and, 96
  paraldehyde and, 258
  as urinary tract irrigant, 792
Acetic acid derivative, 1323-1324
  indomethacin as, 1323, 1333, 1334, 1336
  sulindac as, 1323-1324, 1333
  tolmetin as, 1324
Acetoacetic acid, 1380, 1384
Acetohexamide, 1400; *see also* Oral hypoglycemics
  diabetes and, 1373, 1374
  drug interactions and; *see* Drug Interaction Index
  enzyme inhibition and, 115
  metabolic activation and, 116
  phenylbutazone and, 178, 1332
Acetohydroxamic acid, 1653
  iron and, 1651
Acetone, 1380, 1384
Acetonide grouping, 1278
Acetophen (Aspirin), 752, 1337
Acetophenazine, 340
  enzyme induction and, 114
Acetoxyl (Benzoyl peroxide), 1266
Acetyl coenzyme A, 102
Acetyl hydrazine, 1092
Acetylation
  slow inactivation and, 159, 162
  sulfonamides and, 1074
Acetylcholine, 383, 463
  airway smooth muscle and, 545
  anticholinergic and, 857
  anticholinesterase and, 506
  atropine and, 446
  autonomic nervous system and, 439, 444
  cholinergic nerve and, 453
  depolarizing agent and, 520
  gastric secretion and, 817
  histamine and, 545
  muscle fiber and, 212
  nondepolarizing agent and, 521

Acetylcholine—cont'd
  phenoxybenzamine and, 685
  receptor site and, 73
  synapse and, 212
  as transmitter, 213-214, 443, 519, 520
Acetylcholinesterase, 214, 505
Acetylcysteine, 591, 626
Acetylisoniazid, 1091
  metabolic pathway and, 102
N-Acetylprocainamide, 664, 665
  metabolic activation and, 116
  therapeutic concentration of, 1726
  toxic concentration of, 1726
Acetyl-Sal (Aspirin), 752
Acetylsalicylic acid; *see* Aspirin
Acetylstrophanthidin, 648
N-Acetyltransferase
  metabolic pathway and, 102
  procainamide and, 181
ACh; *see* Acetylcholine
AChE; *see* Acetylcholinesterase
Achromycin (Tetracycline), 1050
Achrostatin V (Nystatin), 1132
Acid; *see also* specific acid
  aldehyde oxidized to, 96
  as antiseptic, 1218
  corrosive, poisoning and, 1714
  as keratolytic, 1251-1253
  lipid solubility of, 89
  organic, secretion of, 765
  renal excretion of, 764
  timing of drug administration and, 13
α-Acid glycoprotein, 665
Acid peptic disorder, 830-832
Acid rebound, 834, 835, 840
Acid urine, drug excretion and; *see* Acidifier, urinary
Acid-base balance, 1569-1571
  disturbance of, 1569-1575; *see also* Electrolyte imbalance; Fluid and electrolyte disturbance
    bicarbonate deficit in, 1571-1572
    bicarbonate excess in, 1572-1573
    carbonic acid deficit in, 1573-1574
    carbonic acid excess in, 1574-1575
    clinical conditions with mixed, 1576
    maintenance of balance and, 1569-1571
  homeostasis and, 1554
  hydrogen ion excretion and, 759
Acid-base nomogram, 1576
Acid-fast bacilli, 1090
Acidification
  drug absorption and, 85, 172
  gastric, 817
  urinary; *see* Acidifier, urinary
Acidifier
  chemical reaction and, 75
  urinary, 172, 787-789
    discharge instructions and, 798
    methenamine and, 740
    nursing implications for, 797
Acidity, titratable, 764
Acidogen (Glutamic acid hydrohloride), 852
Acidoride (Glutamic acid hydrochloride), 852
Acidosis
  metabolic, 1571-1572
    ketoacidosis and, 1384
  respiratory, 1571, 1574-1575
Acid-stable penicillin, 982
Acidulin (Glutamic acid hydrochloride), 852
Acillin (Ampicillin), 998

*For information regarding drug interactions or adverse effects consult the Drug Interaction Index (p. 1747) or the Adverse Drug Effects Index (p. 1727) *before* consulting the General Index.

Acinar cell, 836
Acinetobacter
  aminoglycosides and, 1021
  chloramphenicol and, 1053
Acini, 822
ACIP; *see* Advisory Committee on Immunization
    Practice
A.C.N. (Niacin), 744, 749
Acnaveen (Salicylic acid), 1272
Acne
  anabolic steroids and, 1474-1475
  androgens and, 1474
  benzoyl peroxide in, 1255-1256
  corticosteroids and, 1356
    topical, 1282-1283, 1284
  progestins and, 1459
  resorcinol in, 1256
  sulfur in, 1256
  tetracycline and, 1043
  tretinoin in, 1255
  vitamin A and, 1523-1524
Acne-Dome Medicated Cleanser (Salicylic acid),
    1272
Acneiform eruption, 184
  muscle relaxant and, 288
  tar preparation for, 1258
  topical corticosteroid and, 1282, 1284
Acneiform rash; *see* Rash
Acnesarb (Salicylic acid), 1272
Acnomel (Resorcinol and sulfur combination),
    1271
Acoustic nerve, 219-220
Acquired immune deficiency syndrome, 1583
Acridil (Triprolidine), 610
Acrisorcin, 1114-1115, 1124
Acrynic acid, 1030
Actamer, 964; *see* Bithionol
Actazine (Piperacetazine), 347
Actest (Corticotropin), 416, 1501
ACTH (Corticotropin), 416, 1501
Acthar (Corticotropin), 416, 1501
Actidil (Triprolidine), 610
Actidilon (Triprolidine), 610
Actifed (Guaifenesin; Pseudoephedrine; Triproli-
    dine), 500, 610, 625, 629
Actifed Expectorant (Triprolidine), 610
Actifed-C (Codeine; Guaifenesin; Triprolidine), 610,
    612, 629
Actifed-C Expectorant (Codeine; Guaifenesin;
    Pseudoephedrine; Triprolidine), 1718
Actin, 1434-1437
Actinomyces, 891, 980, 1072
Actinomyces israelii
  penicillin and, 891, 980
  sulfonamide and, 1072
  tetracycline and, 891
Action of drug
  duration of, 80-81
  mechanism of, 71-77
  onset of, 80-81
Action potential, 211-212, 639
Acti-Prem (Triprolidine), 610
Activated charcoal, 171, 1651, 1657, 1714, 1715
  antacids and, 1651
  as antidiarrheal, 890, 895
  laxatives and, 1651
  syrup of ipecac and, 1651
Active metabolite, 95
Active transport, 108
  radiopharmaceutical and, 1629
Active tubular secretion, 172

Actol Expectorant (Noscapine), 618
Acupuncture, 198
Acute gout; *see also* Gout
  colchicine and, 1352, 1355
  hyperuricemia and, 1352
  ibuprofen and, 1352
  indomethacin and, 1352
  naproxen and, 1325, 1352
  phenylbutazone and, 1352
  sulindac and, 1352
Acutuss Expectorant with Codeine (Codeine; Guai-
    fenesin), 612
Acyclovir, 1117, 1118, 1124
  probenecid and, 1118
A/D (Aspirin), 752
Adalat (Nifedipine), 744
Adalin (Carbromal), 268
Adanon (Methadone), 315
Adapin (Doxepin), 371
Adatuss D.C. Expectorant (Guaifenesin; Hydroco-
    done), 312, 629
Addiction, 13, 188-203: *see also* Drug abuse
  definition of, 188
  narcotic, 191-194, 302
  substances of abuse and, 191-201
    alcohol in, 196-198
    amphetamine in, 199-200
    barbiturate in, 200
    cocaine in, 199-200
    hallucinogen in, 200-201
    marijuana in, 198-199
    nonmedical use of prescription drug in, 200
    opiate in, 191-194
    phencyclidine in, 198
    tobacco in, 194-195
  theory of, 189-191
    conditioning, 190-191
    intrapsychic, 190
    somatic, 189-190
Adenosine diphosphate, 725
Adenosine triphosphatase, 648
Adenosine triphosphate
  affective disorder and, 355
  metabolic pathways and, 102
S-Adenosylmethionine, 102
Adenyl cyclase, 546, 547
ADH; *see* Antidiuretic hormone
Adipex (Phentermine), 403
Adipex-P (Phentermine), 403
Adipocyte, 1380
Adipose tissue, insulin and, 1380
Adjuvant chemotherapy, 1139-1140
Adlerika (Magnesium sulfate), 418, 903
Administration, drug; *see* Drug administration
Admixture, 9
Adphen (Phendimetrazine), 402
A-D-R (Racemethionine), 800
Adrenal failure, 1284
Adrenal medulla, 453
Adrenal cortical carcinoma, 1171, 1491-1492
Adrenal gland, 453
  carcinoma of, 1171, 1491-1492
  corticosteroid and, 1486-1518; *see also* Cortico-
    steroid
  failure of, 1284
  levamisole and, 1351
  steroid inhibitor and, 1491-1492
Adrenalcorticosteroid; *see* Corticosteroid
Adrenalin (Epinephrine), 235, 236, 487, 576
Adrenalin In Oil (Epinephrine), 576
Adrenatrate (Epinephrine), 487, 576

α-Adrenergic agonist; *see* Alpha-adrenergic ago-
    nist
β-Adrenergic agonist; *see* Beta-adrenergic agonist
α-Adrenergic blocker; *see* Alpha-adrenergic block-
    er
β-Adrenergic blocker; *see* Beta-adrenergic blocker
Adrenergic bronchodilator, 547
Adrenergic nerve, 453
Adrenergic neuron blocking agent, 474
Adrenergic receptor, 453-456
Adrenergic synapse, 214
Adrenocortical hormone
  metabolic alkalosis and, 1572, 1573
Adrenocorticosteroid, 1486-1491; *see also* Corti-
    costeroids
  children and, 132
  metabolic acidosis and, 1572, 1573
Adrenosem Salicylate (Carbazochrome salicylate),
    1657
Adrenoxyl (Carbazochrome salicylate), 1657
Adrestat F (Carbazochrome salicylate), 1657
Adriamycin (Doxorubicin), 1161
Adroyd (Oxymetholone), 1483
Adrucil (Fluorouracil), 1162
Adsorbent, 890-891
  general, 890
  ion-exchange resin as, 890-891
Adsorbocarpine (Pilocarpine), 470
Adult immunization, 1587-1588
Adumbran (Oxazepam), 277
Adverse drug reactions, 27, 180-187; *see also* Tox-
    icity; Adverse Drug Effects Index; specific
    agent
  child and, 132
  clinical consideration in, 182
  definition of, 180
  drug toxicity and, 180
  elderly and, 135, 137
  frequency of, 158
  incidence of, 180
Advil (Ibuprofen), 1339
Advisory Committee on Immunization Practice,
    1584, 1586-1587
Aerolate Liquid (Theophylline), 582
Aerolate Sr & Jr & III (Theophylline), 582
Aerolone (Isoproterenol; Propylene glycol), 490,
    579, 1270
Aerophylline (Dyphylline), 574
Aeroseb-Dex (Dexamethasone), 1301, 1504
Aeroseb-HC (Hydrocortisone), 1307
Aerosol
  administration of, 1261
  metered-dose, 551
  radioactive, 1638-1639
Aerosporin (Polymyxin B), 1069
Affective disorder, 352-381
  antidepressant side effect and, 360
  depressed patient and, 356-360
    depressive syndrome in, 352-353
    theory of, 353-356
  discharge and, 366-367
  drug digest and, 368-380
  drug interactions and, 361
  nursing implications and, 362-365
Afferent fiber system, 207
Afferent nerve, 433-434
African trypansomiasis, 917
Afrin (Oxymetazoline), 494, 620
Afrin Pediatric (Oxymetazoline), 494
Afrinol (Pseudoephedrine), 625
Afrinol Repetabs (Pseudoephedrine), 500

Asmatane Mist (Epinephrine), 487, 576
Asminyl (Dyphylline; Dyphylline), 574, 582
Asmolin (Epinephrine), 487, 576
Asparaginase, 1170, 1173, 1185
Aspergillus, 1112
 amphotericin B and, 1109
Aspergum (Aspirin), 322
Aspiration, emetics and, 855
Aspirin, 303, 322-323, 752-753, 1319-1322, 1333, 1334, 1336, 1337; *see also* Salicylates
 accidental poisoning and, 132
 action of, 725
 activated charcoal and, 890, 895, 1715
 adverse effect of, 180, 1321, 1337
  child and, 132
 as analgesic, 1319
 antacid and, 834
 as antiinflammatory drug, 1319-1322
 as antipyretic, 1319
 cyclooxygenase and, 1319
 diarrhea and, 890
 discharge instruction and, 740
 dosage regimen and, 1321-1322
 drug digest and, 1337
 drug interactions and, 1321; *see also* Drug Interaction Index
 duodenal ulcer and, 830
 duodenum and, 830, 1321
 food and, 84
 gastric erosion and, 832
 gastric mucus and, 820
 gastritis and, 820, 1321
 and law of conservation of dose, 71
 malaria and, 921
 metabolic activation and, 116
 nerve cell membrane permeability and, 212
 pharmacodynamics of, 1319-1321
 pharmacokinetics of, 726, 1321, 1321
 prostaglandin and, 725
 prosthetic heart valve and, 727
 renal excretion and, 1321
 transient ischemic attack and, 727
 in trichinosis, 956
 urinary pH and, 173, 305, 1321, 1332
Aspirin Free Anacin-3 (Acetaminophen), 321
Aspirin Free Dristan (Chlorpheniramine; Phenylephrine), 604, 620
Aspogen (Dihydroxyaluminum aminoacetate), 844
Assertiveness training, 198
Assessment
 of gastrointestinal system, 813-829; *see also* Gastrointestinal system, assessment of
 of renal system, 757-758
 of skin, 1195-1209; *see also* Skin
Association area, 216
Astasol (Acetaminophen), 321
Asthma; *see also* Respiratory dysfunction; Adverse Drug Effects Index
 antihistamine and, 586
 benoxaprofen and, 1329
 diclofenac and, 1328
 expiratory work and, 538
 hyperventilation and, 589
 sleep laboratory finding and, 253
Asthmagyl (Ephedrine), 487, 575
AsthmaHaler (Epinephrine), 487, 576
AsthmaNefrin (Epinephrine), 487, 576
Asthmophylline (Theophylline), 582
Astrin (Aspirin), 752
Astrocyte, 207
AT 10 (Dihydrotachysterol), 1447
Atabrine (Quinacrine), 940, 972

Atarax (Hydroxyzine), 274, 868
Ataraxoid (Hydroxyzine; Prednisolone), 274, 1514
Atarzine (Promazine), 348
Atasol (Acetaminophen), 321
Ataxia, 286, 425, 870
Atelectasis, 557
 intubation and, 556
Atenol, 686
Atenolol, 693, 701
 pharmacokinetics of, 688
Atensine (Diazepam), 270, 294
Athlete's foot, 1113
Athose (Methadone), 315
Athrombin-K (Warfarin), 752
Ativan (Lorazepam), 274
Atlachlor (Chlorpheniramine), 604
Atom, 1621
Atomic mass, 1621
Atomic number, 1621
Atomizer, 11
Atonic seizure, 406
Atony
Atony of detrusor muscles of bladder, 794-795
Atosil (Promethazine), 871
ATP; *see* Adenosine triphosphate
Atracurium, 529
Atrial fibrillation, 652, 856; *see also* Cardiac dysrhythmias
Atrial flutter, 652; *see also* Cardiac dysrhythmias
Atrioventricular block, 654
Atrioventricular node, 640
 antidysrhythmic drug and, 662
 cardiac glycoside and, 649
Atrobarb (Atropine; Phenobarbital), 278, 464
Atromidin (Clofibrate), 748, 753
Atromid-S (Clofibrate), 748, 753
Atrophy of adipose tissue, 1380
Atropine, 85, 86, 446, 449, 464, 517; *see also* Anticholinergics
 activated charcoal and, 1715
 adrenergic agonists and, 458
 anticholinesterase and, 507
  poisoning and, 507
 as antidote, 1712
 bethanechol and, 794-795
 as bronchodilator, 550
 central nervous system effect of, 456
 chloroform and, 234
 clindamycin-associated colitis and, 1053
 in diarrhea, 890
  with diphenoxylate, 889-890
 drug receptor in child and, 133
 gastric secretion and, 817
 general anesthetic and, 224
 halothane and, 235
 hyoscine, hyoscyamine, and phenobarbital, 1718, 1720, 1721
  and scopolamine, 1718, 1719, 1720, 1722, 1723
 hyoscine hydrobromide, phenobarbital, and scopolamine, 1718
 hyoscyamine, phenobarbital and scopolamine, 1724
 in inhibitory postsynaptic potential, 443
 intravenous, 64
  compatibility and, 1708, 1709
 metoclopramide and, 859
 as muscarinic blocker, 453, 454
 neostigmine and, 795, 808
 and phenobarbital, 1718
 propranolol and, 499
 psychosis and, 331
 salivary secretion and, 815

Atropine—cont'd
 temperature regulation and, 184
Atropine-like drugs, 456-457; *see also* Anticholinergics
 poisoning and, 456
Atropine-like effects, 849; *see also* Anticholinergic effects
 of disopyramide, 668
 of quinidine, 668
Atropisol (Atropine), 464
Atrovent (Ipratropium), 578
A.T.S. (Coal tar), 1267
Attapulgite, 890
 absorption interactions and, 171
Attention deficit disorder, 385
Attenuvax (Measles virus vaccine, live), 1599
A.T.V. (Diethylstilbestrol), 1462
Atypical pseudocholinesterase, 163, 531
Au 198; *see* Gold 198
Aubason (Desoximetasone), 1300
Auditory dysfunction; *see* Hearing loss
Auditory nerve, 219
Augmentin (Nortriptyline), 375
Augustinian Sisters, 4, 5
Auranofin; *see also* Gold salts
 adverse effect of, 1347
 dosage regimen and, 1347-1348
 drug interaction and, 1347
 elimination of, 1347
 immunoglobulin and, 1347
 lysosome and, 1347
 penicillamine and, 1347
 pharmacokinetics and, 1347
 rheumatic disease and, 1347-1348
Aureomycin (Chlortetracycline), 1040, 1048
Aurothioglucose, 1363; *see also* Gold salts
 rheumatic disease and, 1346-1347
Ausabel theory of addiction, 190
Autoantibody, thyroid, 1413
Autoimmune thyroiditis, 1413, 1420-1421
Automaticity of heart, 661
Autonomic nervous system, 207, 435, 453-456
 cholinergic and adrenergic nerve in, 453
 cholinergic and adrenergic receptor in, 453-456
 homeostasis and, 1553
 parasympathetic division of, 446-449
 sympathetic division of, 439-446
 trimethaphan and, 685
 type of control by, 449
Autorhythmicity of heart, 639
Autosomal dominant disorder, 161
Autosomal recessive disorder, 161
AV node; *see* Atrioventricular node
Availability of drug, 78-82
Avantyl (Nortriptyline), 375
Avazyme (Chymotrypsin), 1659, 1718
AVC cream (Aminacrine; Sulfanilamide; Allantoin), 918
AVC with Dienestrol (Dienestrol), 1462
Aventyl (Nortriptyline), 375
Average dose, 73
Avercillin (Penicillin G), 1012
Aversive conditioning
 alcoholism and, 197
 tobacco smoking and, 195
Avlocardyl (Propranolol), 498, 709
Avlochlor (Chloroquine), 929
Avlosulfon (Dapsone), 1103
AVP Natal (Pyridoxine; Vitamin A), 1548, 1550
Axon, 207-210
Ayds Weight Suppressant (Phenylpropanolamine), 498
Ayercillin (Penicillin G procaine), 1014

Bone marrow imaging, 1640

Bone pain, 1454, 1471; see also Fractures

Bonine (Meclizine), 869

Bontril PDM (Phendimetrazine), 402

Bontril slow release (Phendimetrazine), 402

Borax, 1218

Borborygmi, 828

Boric acid, 1130, 1218

   in belladonna extract, bismuth subcarbonate, bismuth oxyiodide, boric acid, ephedrine sulfate, hydrocortisone acetate, peruvian balsam, and zinc oxide, 1725

   poisoning from, 1714

Boron, sweat and, 110

Boston Collaborative Drug Surveillance Program, 180

Bothrops atrox, 1612

Botulism antitoxin, 1613, 1616

Boutons, 209, 212

Bovine insulin, 1379

Bowel, fluid in, 758

Bowel preparation, prophylactic

   kanamycin and, 1026

   neomycin and, 1026

Bowel sounds, 827-828

B-Pam (Diazepam), 417

BPN Ointment, 1062

Bq; see Becquerel

Bradycardia; see also Adverse Drug Effects Index

Bradykinesia, 382

Brain, 214-218

   abscess of, 1052

   cerebrum in, 214-217

   diencephalon in, 217

   hindbrain in, 218

   midbrain in, 217-218, 217-218

   peptide of, 144

   scanning of, 1637

   tumor of, 1168

Brainstem

   enkephalin in, 302

   opiate receptor in, 302

   pain modulation and, 300

   pain transmission and, 300

Bran, 879, 898

Breacol (Chlorpheniramine; Phenylpropanolamine), 605, 622

Breast cancer, 1170

   androgens and, 1473

   cyclophosphamide and, 1167

   estrogens and, 1454, 1457

   hexamethylmelamine and, 1171

   ifosfamide and, 1168

   melphalan and, 1168

   methotrexate and, 1142

   reserpine and, 692, 709

   tamoxifen and, 1170

   thiotepa and, 1169

   vinblastine and, 1169

   vincristine and, 1169

   vindesine and, 1170

Breast milk

   clindamycin and, 1060

   drugs in, 131-132

   nicotine and, 520

Breatheasy (Epinephrine), 487, 576

Breathing, 535; see also Respiration

   reflex and, 545

Breathing circuit, 230-231

Breokinase (Urokinase), 1681

Brethine (Terbutaline), 501, 581

Bretylate (Bretylium; Bretylium tosylate; Terbutaline), 485, 501, 581, 674

Bretylin (Bretylium; Bretylium tosylate), 485, 674

Bretylium, 485

   adverse effect of, 669

   catecholamines and, 669

   digitalis glycosides and, 671

   mechanism of action and pharmacologic effect of, 663-664

   norepinephrine and, 474

   pharmacokinetics and, 666

   use of, 668

Bretylium tosylate, 674

Bretylol (Bretylium; Bretylium tosylate), 485, 674

Brevicon (Norethindrone), 1466, 1469

Brevimytal (Methohexital), 248

Brevital (Methohexital), 248

Bricanyl (Terbutaline), 501, 581

Bridine (Povidone-iodine), 1240

Brietal (Methohexital), 248

Brioschi (Sodium bicarbonate), 848

Bristagen (Gentamicin), 1033

Bristopen (Oxacillin), 1011

Bristuron (Bendroflumethiazide), 778

Broad beta disease, 719

Brocasipal (Orphenadrine), 297, 401

Brocon C.R. (Brompheniramine), 603

Brocon Chewable (Brompheniramine; Phenylpropanolamine), 603, 623

Bromazepam, 267

   properties of, 255

Bromelains, 1718

Bromide, 25, 530

   in breast milk, 132

   first use of, 252

   by rectal route, 10

Bromine, sweat and, 110

Bromisovalum, 267

Bromocriptine, 393, 1651, 1656

   antihypertensives and, 1651

Bromodiphenhydramine, 603

   ineffectiveness of, 1718

Brompheniramine, 603-604

   with phenylephrine and phenylpropanolamine, 1720

Brompheniramine maleate, guaifenesin, phenylephrine, and phenylpropanolamine, 1720

   with codeine phosphate, 1720

Bromo-Seltzer (Acetaminophen; Sodium bicarbonate), 321, 848

Bromphen (Brompheniramine), 603

Brompton's cocktail, 310

Bromural (Bromisovalum), 267

Bronchi, 544

Bronchial artery, 547

Bronchial asthma; see Asthma

Bronchial gland goblet cell, 546

Bronchicide (Guaifenesin), 629

Bronchiole, 544

   respiratory, 535-536

   terminal, 535-536, 544

    velocity of air flow through, 537

Bronchoconstriction, reflex and, 545-546

Bronchodilators, 544-585; see also specific agent

   action of, 546, 547

   administration of, 561-564

   adverse effect of, 558, 564, 566

   alpha-receptor antagonist in, 548

   anticholinergic in, 550

   beta-receptor selective, 547-548

   caution for, 561

Bronchodilators—cont'd

   central nervous system stimulation and, 548

   cilia effect and, 546

   contraindication to, 560-561

   corticosteroid in, 550, 551

   discharge/outpatient instruction and, 569

   drug digest for, 571-583

   drug interaction and, 559, 561

   emergency therapy with, 551

   histamine release and, 545

   intestinal metabolism and, 106

   mediator release and, 550-551

   monitoring response and, 564

   nonselective, 547

   nursing implications and, 559-560

   oxygen with, 554, 555

   parasympatholytic in, 550

   patient education and, 566-561, 566-568

   phosphodiesterase inhibitor in, 548-550

   respiratory gas in, 551-558

    carbon dioxide in, 552-554

    oxygen in, 551-552, 554-558

   selection of, 551

   sensitivity of, 560

   sympathomimetic, 547

   target effect and, 124

Broncho-Grippex (Guaifenesin), 629

Bronchospasms; see also Adverse Drug Effects Index

Broncho-Tussin (Codeine; Terpin hydrate), 612, 633

Brondecon (Guaifenesin; Oxtriphylline), 581, 629

Bronicolixir (Ephedrine), 575

Bronitin (Ephedrine; Guaifenesin; Theophylline), 575, 582, 629

Bronitin Mist (Epinephrine; Pyrilamine), 487, 576, 608

Bronkaid (Ephedrine; Theophylline), 487, 575, 582

Bronkaid Mist (Epinephrine), 487, 576

Bronkaid Mistometer (Epinephrine), 576

Bronkephrine (Ethylnorepinephrine), 489, 577

Bronkodyl (Theophylline), 582

Bronkodyl S-R (Theophylline), 582

Bronkolixir (Phenobarbital; Theophylline), 279, 582

Bronkometer (Isoetharine), 578

Bronkosol (Isoetharine), 578

Bronkotabs (Ephedrine; Theophylline), 487, 575, 582

Brophed (Ephedrine; Hydroxyzine; Theophylline), 1719

Bro-T's (Carbromal), 268

Brucellosis

   aminoglycosides and, 1024

   tetracyclines and, 1043

Brugia malayia, 955

Bruit, hypertension and, 758

Bryrel (Piperazine), 969

Bubartal (Butabarbital), 267

Buccal route, 90

Bucladine (Buclizine), 865

Buclizine, 864, 865

   discharge/outpatient instruction and, 864

Buf Foot-Care Lotion (Propylene glycol), 1270

Buf-Acne Cleansing Bar (Salicylic acid and sulfur combination), 1273

Buff-A Comp (Butalbital), 268

Buffer, 759

Bufferin (Aspirin), 322, 753, 1337

   with Codeine No.3 (Aspirin), 311, 322

Buffinol (Magnesium oxide), 846

Bukozide (Bendroflumethiazide), 778

Bu-Lax (Docusate potassium), 901
Bulk-forming laxatives, 879-880, 897; see also Lax-
    atives
    action of, 879
    discharge/outpatient instruction for, 897
    vincristine and, 1169
Bullae, 795
Bumetanide, 770, 779
Bumex (Bumetanide), 779
Bupivacaine, 1242
    local anesthetic and, 1220, 1221, 1222
Burdeo (Hexachlorophene), 1235
Bureau of Human Prescription Drugs, 916
Buretrol, 63
Burkitt's lymphoma, 1142
Burn therapy
    silver compound and, 1213
    sulfonamide and, 1080
    ulcer and, 832
Burns, 1215, 1224
Burow's solution (Aluminum acetate), 1214
Busulfan, 1168, 1173, 1185
Butabar Belladonna (Belladonna alkaloids; Buta-
    barbital), 1719
Buta-Barb (Butabarbital), 267
Butabarbital, 267
    with belladonna alkaloid, 1719
    with belladonna extract, 1719
    with ephedrine, guaifenesin and theophylline,
    1723
    properties of, 256
Butabell HMB (Atropine; Butabarbital), 267,
    464
Butagesic (Phenylbutazone), 1343
Butalbital, 268
    properties of, 256
Butaperazine, 340
    enzyme induction and, 114
    as piperazine, 327
Butazolidin (Phenylbutazone), 1343
Butazolidin-Alka (Antacid; Phenylbutazone),
    1322
Butibel (Belladonna extract; Butabarbital),
    1719
Butibel (Belladonna extract; Butabarbital), 1719
Buticaps (Butabarbital), 267
Butigetic (Butabarbital), 267
Butiserpazide (Butabarbital; Reserpine), 267, 500,
    710
Butisol (Butabarbital), 267
Butone (Phenylbutazone), 1343
Butorphanol, 317-318
Butterfly needle, 61
Butyl aminobenzoate, 1055
Butylone (Pentobarbital), 278, 422
Butylparaben, 1216
Butyrophenones, 326; see also specific agent
    as antiemetic, 860
    droperidol and, 238
    metyrosine and, 1652
    narcotic analgesics and, 305
    parkinsonism and, 383
Byrol (Piperazine), 969

C

C3 (Codeine), 311, 613
C4 (Codeine), 311, 613
C3 Cold Cough (Chlorpheniramine), 605
C3 Cold Cough Capsules (Dextromethorphan;
    Phenylpropanolamine), 614, 623
C cells, 1439
Cabadon-M (Cyanocobalamin), 1544

Cafergot (Ergotamine), 1665
Cafermine (Ergotamine), 1665
Cafertrate (Ergotamine), 1665
Caffedrine (Caffeine), 393
Caffeine, 393
    behavior change and, 140
    beverage and, 393
    bronchodilation and, 550
    diethylpropion and, 395
    diphenhydramine and, 395
    intramuscular injection of, 15
    methamphetamine and, 400
    methylphenidate and, 401
    respiratory alkalosis and, 1574
    saliva and, 109
    sleep and, 261, 263
    and sodium benzoate, 1574
Calamine lotion
    phenol and, 1216
    zinc salts and, 1213
Calan (Verapamil), 679, 747
Calcarine sulcus, 215
Calcet (Calcium carbonate; Calcium gluconate;
    Calcium lactate), 215, 844, 1544, 1677
Calcibind (Sodium cellulose phosphate),
    1677
Calciferol (Vitamin D), 1448, 1550
Calcification
    extraskeletal, 882
    of pancreas, 836
    vitamin D and, 1442
Calcimar (Calcitonin, salmon), 1447
Calciparine (Heparin), 751
Calcisorb (Sodium cellulose phosphate),
    1677
Calcitonin, 1439-1441, 1442, 1443
    calcium and, 1440
    salmon, 1447
Calcitriol, 1442, 1443, 1444, 1447
    cholestyramine and, 1443
Calcium, 546, 1544, 1621; see also specific agent
    aminoglycoside-induced neuromuscular block-
    ade and, 1023
    bone and, 1437
    calcitonin and, 1440
    cardiac glycosides and, 652, 654
    concentration of
        homeostasis and, 1553
        parathyroid hormone and, 1553
    deficit of, 1564-1566
        pharmacologic agent in, 1565
    excess of, 1566-1567
        pharmacologic agent in, 1566
        potassium deficit and, 1562, 1563
    extracellular fluid and, 1555-1556
    heart rate and, 645
    ion metabolism and, 1434-1437
    low intake of, 1565
    metabolic alkalosis and, 1573
    metabolism of, vitamin A and, 1523
    in nutrition, 1540
    regulation of, 1434
    sodium fluoride and, 1652
    tetracyclines and, 1045, 1541
    thiazide diuretic and, 1541
Calcium antacid, 878
Calcium carbonate, 75, 834, 840, 844, 1544; see also
    Antacids; Calcium
    activated charcoal and, 1651
    constipation and, 878
    pepsin and, 833

Calcium carbonate—cont'd
    sodium polystyrene sulfonate and, 1652
    urinary pH and, 108
Calcium channel blocker
    absorption of, 715
    action of, 714
    bioavailability of, 715
    vasodilation and, 713, 716
Calcium chloride, 1565, 1566
Calcium current antagonist, 667
Calcium disodium edetate, 75, 1664, 1712
Calcium Disodium Versenate (Calcium disodium
    edetate), 1664
Calcium entry blocker, 664
Calcium exchange resin, 1566
Calcium glubionate, 1544
Calcium gluconate, 1544
    calcium deficit and, 1565, 1566
    intravenous compatibility and, 1708
    magnesium excess and, 1567, 1568
    phosphorus 32 uptake and, 1646
    potassium excess and, 1564
Calcium lactate, 1544
    calcium deficit and, 1565, 1566
Calcium levulinate, 1565, 1566
Calcium salts, 1027; see also specific agent
    magnesium deficit and, 1567
Calcium undecylenate, 1133
Calculation
    of body surface area, 134
    of dose for child, 12
    of rate of infusion, 58-61
Calculi
    of pancreatic duct, 836
    salivary duct and, 815
Caldesene (Undecylenic acid; Zinc undecylenate),
    1133
Caliber of arterial system, 643
Cal-M (Niacin; Thiamine; Vitamin A), 749, 1448,
    1550, 1549
Calmurid (Urea), 1275
Calomel, 9, 18, 1225
    children and, 12
Calphosan (Calcium lactate), 1544
Calphosan B-12 (Calcium lactate), 1544
Cal-Sup (Calcium carbonate), 1544
Caltrate (Calcium carbonate), 1544
Camalox (Calcium carbonate; Magnesium oxide),
    844, 846
Camcolit (Lithium), 373
Camoqiun (Amodiaquine), 928
cAMP; see Cyclic adenosine-3',5'-monophosphate
Camphor
    activated charcoal and, 1715
    intramuscular injection of, 15
    local anesthetic and, 1222
    lung excretion and, 110
Camphorated tincture of opium, 889, 910
Canadian nursing, early, 5
Cancer; see also Carcinoma
    breast, melphalan and, 1168
    cervical, 1169
    chemotherapy for, 1350; see also Anticancer
    drug
    head, 1171
    invasion of, 1139, 1646
    kidney, 1170
    lung; see Lung cancer
    neck, 1171
    ovary; see Ovarian cancer
    pain in, 308

Cholinergic—cont'd
  long-term memory and, 144
  urinary, 794-795
    discharge instruction and, 798
    nursing implication for, 797
Cholinergic agonist, 546
Cholinergic antagonist, 546
Cholinergic nerve, 453
Cholinergic receptor, 453-456
Cholinergic synapse, 214
Cholinesterase, 456, 505
Cholinesterase inhibitor, 456
  aminoglycoside-induced neuromuscular block-
    ade and, 1023
  recovery period and, 225
Cholinesterase reactivators, 505-518; see also specific agent
  acetylcholinesterase in, 505
  adverse effect of, 509
  anticholinesterase and, 505-507
  carbamate poisoning and, 508
  cholinesterase in, 505
  description of, 507-508
  discharge/outpatient instruction for, 512
  drug digest of, 513-517
  drug interaction and, 510
  insecticide and, 508
  organophosphate poisoning and, 508
  sulfonate poisoning and, 508
Choloxin (Dextrothyroxine), 748
Chomphyl (Aminophylline), 572
Chondrus, 879-880
Chooz (Calcium carbonate; Magnesium trisilicate),
  844, 847
Chophylline (Oxtriphylline), 581
Choranid (Gonadotropin, chorionic), 1668
Choreiform movements, 409
Choriocarcinoma, gestational, 1142
Chorionic gonadotropin; see Gonadotropin, cho-
  rionic
Choron (Gonadotropin, chorionic), 1668
Christian Church, first centuries of, 3
Chromatography, 1379
Chromium, trace element and, 1539
Chromium-51, 1630, 1632
Chromium-51 sodium chromate, 1632
  cardiovascular system and, 1642
Chromium-51-labeled red blood cell, 1642
Chromosomal mediated resistance to tetracycline,
  1041
Chronic benign pain, 302, 308
Chronic cancer pain, 308
Chronic gout; see Gout, chronic
Chronic obstructive pulmonary disease, 557, 559-
  560
Chronic pain, 151, 302, 308
  cancer, 308
Chronulac (Lactulose), 902
Chrysarobin compound, 1258
Chrysomysin (Chlortetracycline), 1048
Chrysotherapy, 1346-1348
Church of England, 4
Chyluria in filariasis, 956
Chymar (Chymotrypsin), 1659
Chymase (Chymotrypsin), 1659
Chyme, 825
Chymetin (Chymotrypsin), 1659
Chymodiactin (Chymopapain), 1658
Chymolase (Chymotrypsin), 1659
Chymopapain, 1658-1659
Chymoral (Chymotrypsin; Trypsin), 1659, 1719

Chymotest (Chymotrypsin), 1659
Chymotrypsin, 822, 825, 1659
  alcohol and, 1652
  antiseptics and, 1652
  ineffectiveness of, 1718
  iodine and, 1652
  and trypsin, 1719, 1722
Chymotrypsinogen, 822
Ci; see Curie unit
CIC; see Cardioinhibitory center
Ciclopirox, 1127
Cidomycin (Gentamicin), 1033
Cilia
  activity of, 546-547
  factor inhibiting, 546
Cillimycin (Lincomycin), 1068
Cimetidine, 260, 835, 842, 849
  drug interactions and, 175; see also Drug Inter-
    action Index
  enzyme inhibition and, 115, 172
  food and, 84
  gastric erosion and, 832
  nursing implication for, 840-841
  pancreatic enzyme and, 837
  reflux esophagitis and, 832
  ulcer and gastritis and, 820
    duodenal, 830
    stress, 832
Cinalone 40 (Triamcinolone), 1517
Cinchona alkaloid, 669
Cinchonism, 669, 925, 941, 1675
Cinchophen, 164
Cingulate sulcus, 215
Cinobac (Cinoxacin), 802
Cinolone-T (Triamcinolone), 1517
Cinoxacin, 789-790, 797, 802
  administration of, 789-790, 798
  dosage and, 789-790
  excretion of, 790
  nalidixic acid and, 741
  nursing implication for, 797
  sensitive organism to, 789
  toxicity of, 790
Cin-Quin (Quinidine), 678
Circanol (Ergoloid mesylates), 1664
Circlidrin (Nylidrin), 494, 745
Circulation
  general, oral medication and, 89-90
  overload of, 65
  percutaneous absorption and, 1207
  radiopharmaceutical and, 1641
  systemic, injection into, 83
Circulatory failure; see Cardiopulmonary arrest
Cirrhosis, alcoholic, 112, 125-127, 128
Cisplatin, 1171, 1172, 1173, 1186
  aminoglycosides and, 1174
  functional disruption and, 76
  vinblastine and bleomycin, regimen of, 1144,
    1169
Cisternography, radionuclide, 1637
Citanest (Prilocaine), 1249
Citra (Chlorpheniramine; Pheniramine; Phenyl-
    ephrine), 496, 605, 608, 620
Citra Forte (Hydrocodone; Pheniramine; Phenyl-
    ephrine; Pyrilamine), 312, 496, 608, 617, 620
Citra Forte Syrup (Hydrocodone), 617
Citrate of Magnesia (Magnesium citrate), 902
Citric acid
  codeine, ipecac fluid extract, potassium guaia-
    colate, promethazine and sodium citrate,
    1722
  and phenylephrine, 1723

Citric acid—cont'd
  dextromethorphan, ipecac fluid extract, potas-
    sium guaiacolsulfonate, promethazine, and
    sodium citrate, 1722
  ipecac fluid extract, phenylephrine, potassium
    guaiacolsulfonate, promethazine, and so-
    dium citrate, 1723
Citrobacter
  aminoglycoside and, 1021
  mecillinam and, 984
Citrocarbonate (Sodium bicarbonate), 848
Citro-Mag (Magnesium citrate), 902
Civalin (Ascorbic acid), 799
Claforan (Cefotaxime), 1003
Claripex (Clofibrate), 748, 753
Claudication, intermittent, 716
Claviton (Tridihexethyl), 471
Cleanser as antiseborrheic, 1257-1258
Clear Eyes (Naphazoline), 493
Clearance of drug, 120-122
Clearasil Medicated Cleanser (Salicylic acid), 1272
Clemastine, 606
Cleocin (Clindamycin), 1063
Clidinium, 466
  with chlordiazepoxide, 1721
Climestrone (Estrogens, esterified), 1464
Clinazine (Trifluoperazine), 349
Clindamycin, 1053-1054, 1059-1061, 1063
  aminoglycoside and, 1024
  breast milk and, 1060
  crossing of placenta and, 1060
  cross-resistance and, 1054, 1060
  drug interactions and; see Drug Interaction In-
    dex
  excretion of, 759
  intravenous compatibility and, 1708, 1709
  local irritation from, 36
Clindamycin phosphate, 1708, 1710
Clinical nurse specialist, 26; see also Nurse
Clinicydin (Bacitracin; Neomycin; Polymyxin B),
    1035, 1062, 1069
Clinitest, 1077, 1082
  cephalothin and, 183
  color change and, 1384
  false positive reading and, 1383, 1384
Clinoril (Sulindac), 1344
Clipoxide (Chlordiazepoxide; Clidinium), 269,466
Clistin (Carbinoxamine), 604
Clistin-D (Carbinoxamine; Phenylephrine), 496,
    604
Clitoral enlargement, 1474, 1475
Clobetasol, 1297, 1500
  potency of, 1278
Clobetasol butyrate, 1278, 1284
Clobetasone, 1298, 1500
  potency of, 1278
Clobetasone butyrate, 1278
Clocortolone, 1298-1299, 1500
Cloderm (Clocortolone), 1298
Clofazimine, 1095, 1103
Clofibrate, 748, 753
  action of, 720, 725
  angina pectoris and, 727
  oral anticoagulants and, 176
  oral hypoglycemic and, 177
  pharmacokinetics of, 720, 725-726
  platelet aggregation inhibitors and, 730
  sodium deficit and, 1558, 1559
  syndrome of inappropriate secretion of antidi-
    uretic hormone and, 1560
  vasopressin and, 1652

Gallamine triethiodide, 529

Gallium-67, 1632

Gallium-68, 1636

Gallium citrate, 1632
  in breast milk, 132
  localization of, 1630

Gamene (Lindane), 951

Gametocyte, 920

Gamimune (Human serum immune globulin), 1598

Gamma benzene hexachloride (Lindane), 944

Gamma ray, 1622
  characteristic of, 1630-1631
  penetration depth of, 1627

Gamma scintillation camera, 1629

Gamma spectrometer, 1628

Gamma spectrometer well counter, 1628

Gamma-aminobutyric acid, 214
  benzodiazepine and, 254

Gammacorten (Dexamethasone), 1504

Gammahydroxybutyrate, 385

Gamophen (Hexachlorophene), 1235

Ganal (Fenfluramine), 396

Ganglia, 435-439
  basal, 216
  motor, 436-439
  sensory, 435-436

Ganglionic blockers, 523, 795; see also specific
    agent
  adverse effect of, 521-522
  drug digest of, 528-531
  drug interaction and, 523
  nursing implication of, 524-526
  trimethaphan and, 685

Ganglionic stimulants, 519-532; see also specific
    agent
  adverse effect of, 621-622
  drug digest of, 528-531
  drug interaction and, 523
  lobeline as, 520
  nicotine as, 519-520
  nursing implication of, 524-526

Ganglionic synapse
  in parasympathetic division, 449
  in sympathetic division, 443-444

Ganglionic transmission, 519

Gangrene; see Adverse Drug Effects Index

Ganphen (Promethazine), 871

Gantanol (Sulfamethoxazole), 1086

Gantrisin (Sulfisoxazole), 1087, 1720

Gantrisin Cream (Sulfisoxazole), 1087

Gantrisin Ophthalmic (Sulfisoxazole), 1087

Gap junction, 1377

Garamycin (Gentamicin), 1033

Garamycin Ophthalmic (Gentamicin), 1033

Garamycin Otic (Gentamicin), 1033

Garavite Elixir (Thiamine), 1549

Gardenal (Phenobarbital), 423

Gas
  blood, 539-542
  lung excretion of drug and, 110
  respiratory, 535
  therapeutic, 18

Gas exchange
  in lung, 535
  problem of, 539-542

Gaseous anesthetic, 232-233
  cyclopropane in, 233
  ethylene in, 233
  nitrous oxide in, 232-233
  second gas effect and, 228

Gastrectomy, 820
  stress ulcer and, 832

Gastric acid hypersecretion, 820, 830; see also Gas-
    tric secretion
  diarrhea and, 887

Gastric content; see also Gastric secretion
  average volume of, 826
  reflux of, 816
  pH of, 833

Gastric inhibitory polypeptide
  insulin and, 1378

Gastric emptying change, 795

Gastric inhibitory polypeptide, 1378

Gastric motility, 820

Gastric mucus, 820

Gastric secretion; see also Gastric content
  cephalic phase of, 817
  diarrhea and, 887
  hormonal phase of, 817
  vagal phase of, 817

Gastric ulcer, 820, 831-832

Gastrin, 816, 817
  esophageal function and, 816
  pancreatic, 822

Gastrin-secreting tumor of pancreas, 836

Gastritis, 820, 832

Gastrix (Oxyphencyclimine), 469

Gastrocolic reflex, 827, 878

Gastroenteritis, 421, 828

Gastroesophageal junction, 815

Gastrointestinal bleeding; see also Bleeding
  nonsteroidal antiinflammatory drug and, 1334
  oxyphenbutazone and, 1342
  phenylbutazone and, 1343

Gastrointestinal cancer, 1168

Gastrointestinal effect; see Adverse Drug Effects In-
    dex

Gastrointestinal hormone, 1377-1378

Gastrointestinal infection, tetracycline and, 1043

Gastrointestinal medications, 811-913; see also
    specific agent
  anatomy and physiology in, 813-829
  antacid, ulcer medication, and digestant in, 830-
    853; see also Antacids; Digestants; Ulcer
    medications
  emetics and antiemetics in, 854-876; see also
    Emetics and antiemetics
  laxatives and antidiarrheals in, 877-912; see also
    Laxatives and antidiarrheals

Gastrointestinal organism
  kanamycin and, 1024
  metabolism and, 95, 106
  neomycin and, 1024
  tetracycline and, 1043

Gastrointestinal secretion; see Gastric secretion

Gastrointestinal system; see also Gastrointestinal
    effect
  anatomy and physiology of, 813-829
    esophagus in, 815-816
    large intestine in, 826-828
    liver and biliary tree in, 820-822
    mouth in, 813-815
    pancreas in, 822-825
    small intestine in, 825-826
    stomach in, 816-820
  autonomic nerve stimulation and, 455
  organism of; see Gastrointestinal organism
  postpurgation of, 916
  prepurgation of, 915
  somatostatin and, 1378
  tetracycline toxicity and, 1042

Gastroscopy, 831

Gas-X (Simethicone), 850

Gated blood-pool method, 1642

Gaviscon Antacid (Magnesium trisilicate), 847

Gaysal (Phenobarbital), 278

gBh (Lindane), 951

Ge 68; see Germanium-68

Gel chromatography, 1379

Gelatin capsule, 33

Gelumina (Magnesium trisilicate), 847

Gelusil (Aluminum hydroxide gel; Magnesium ox-
    ide; Simethicone), 843, 847, 850

Gelusil II (Simethicone), 850

Gelusil Extra Strength Liquid (Magnesium hydrox-
    ide), 846

Gelusil M (Simethicone), 850

Gemfibrozil, 720, 721

Gemonil (Metharbital), 420

Genapex (Gentian violet), 1128, 1235

Genecillin VK-500 (Penicillin V), 1015

General anesthetics, 223-251; see also Anesthetics;
    specific agent
  adverse effect of, 241
  antihypertensive and, 697
  balanced anesthesia in, 225
  barbiturate and, 256
  class of, 224
  clinical, 238-239
    course of, 225
  definition in, 224-225
  discharge/outpatient instruction in, 244
  drug digest of, 245-250
  drug interactions with, 242
  effective concentration of, 232
  gaseous, 232-233
  halogenated, epinephrine and, 487, 559
  history of, 223-224
  ideal drug in, 225-226
  inhalation, 228-232
    administration of, 228-231
    effective dose in, 231
    effect of, 231-232
    potency of, 231
  intravenous agent in, 236-238
  malignant hyperpyrexia and, 239
  mechanism of action of, 239-240
  medication with, 224
  metabolic acidosis and, 1572
  nursing implications of, 242-244
  preanesthetic medication in, 238
  properties of, 226, 230
  respiratory acidosis and, 1572
  sign and stage of anesthesia in, 226, 227
  uptake and distribution of, 226-228
  volatile liquid in, 233-236

Generalized seizure, 405-406
  anticonvulsant choice and, 406; see also Anti-
    convulsant; specific agent

Geneserine (Physostigmine), 516

Geneserp (Reserpine), 500, 710

Genetics, 157-169
  addiction and, 189-190
  drug metabolism and elimination and, 111
  drug response and, 157-169
    category and associated condition in, 161-167
    disposition of drug in, 167-168
    monogenic condition affecting, 158-167
    pharmacogenetic condition affecting, 158-167
    single factor altering body action on drug in,
      161-165
    single factor altering drug action on body in,
      165-167
    terminology in, 161
    transmission of trait in, 161

Herpes keratoconjunctivitis, 1116
Herpes simiae, 1117
Herpes simplex, 1122-1123, 1284
  acyclovir and, 1117
  encephalitis and, 1115, 1116
  trifluridine and, 1115, 1116
  vidarabine and, 1115, 1116
Herpes zoster
  immune globulin and, 1581
  interferon and, 1117
  vidarabine and, 1116
Herpesvirus; see also Herpes simplex; Herpes zoster
  acyclovir and, 1117
  idoxuridine and, 1116
  ribavirin and, 1117
Herplex (Idoxuridine), 1130
Herplex-D (Idoxuridine), 1130
Hetacillin, 983, 1009; see also Ampicillin
  food and, 84
Hetastarch, 545
Heterozygous, 161
Hetrazan (Diethylcarbamazine), 965
Hexa-Betalin (Pyridoxine), 378, 1548
Hexachlorophene, 1215, 1216-1217, 1224, 1235, 1652
  adverse drug reaction in child and, 132
Hexadecanoic acid, 1643
Hexadrol (Dexamethasone), 1365, 1504
Hexafluorenium bromide, 530
Hexamead-PH (Hexachlorophene), 1235
Hexamethonium, 443, 449, 520
  excretion of, 95, 765
Hexamethylmelamine, 1171, 1173, 1187
Hexaphenyl (Hexachlorophene), 1235
Hexavibex (Pyridoxine), 378, 1548
Hexobarbital, 273; see also Barbiturates
  history of use of, 224
  liver function and, 112
  metabolism induction and, 113
  properties of, 256
Hexocyclium methysulfate, 467
Hexyphen (Trihexyphenidyl), 403
Hibanil (Chlorpromazine), 341, 866
Hibicare (Chlorhexidine gluconate), 806, 1234
Hibiclens (Chlorhexidine gluconate), 806, 1234
Hibitane (Chlorhexidine gluconate), 806, 1234
Hibitane Tincture (Chlorhexidine gluconate), 806, 1234
Hiccups, intractable, 859
Hi-Fibran (Plantago seed), 905, 911
High blood pressure; see Hypertension
High-surface-area drug, 171
Hill-Shade (Aminobenzoic acid), 1654
Hindgut, 817
Hindus, ancient, 3
Hi-Pen (Penicillin V), 1015
Hippuric acid, 95
  metabolic pathway and, 102
Hirschsprung's disease, 877
Hirsutism, 288, 425, 706, 1203
Hiserpia (Reserpine), 500
Hispril (Diphenylpyraline), 607
Histadyl EC (Ammonium chloride; Ephedrine), 575, 628
Histalet DM Syrup (Dextromethorphan), 615
Histalet Forte (Pyrilamine), 609
Histalet Syrup (Pseudoephedrine), 625
Histalet X Guaifenesin), 630
Histalon (Chlorpheniramine), 605
Histamine
  agents producing release of, 545

Histamine—cont'd
  airway smooth muscle and, 545
  excretion and, 765
  gastric secretion and, 817
  general anesthetic and, 241
  metabolic pathway and, 102, 103
  phenoxybenzamine and, 685
  teratogenesis and, 593
Histamine 2 blocker, 830
Histan (Pyrilamine), 609
Hista-Nil (Diphenylpyraline), 607
Histantil (Promethazine), 871
Histaspan (Chlorpheniramine), 605
Histaspan-D (Methscopolamine; Phenylephrine), 469, 621
Histatapp Elixir (Brompheniramine), 603
Histiocyte, 1198
Histoplasma
  amphotericin B and, 891, 1109
  miconazole and, 1112
Historal (Chlorpheniramine; Methscopolamine; Pseudoephedrine), 469, 605, 625
History
  of allergic responses, 31
  of drug, 31
  drug therapy, 3-29
    accountability and, 26-28
    administration and, 16-17
    advance in delivery system and, 25-26
    care of medicine and, 15-16
    drug form and, 14
    inhalation and, 17-18
    measurement and, 16
    normal saline injection and, 11, 15
    oral route of, 8-10
    parenteral route of, 10-13, 15
    rectal route of, 10
    right patient, right drug, and right time and, 18-19
  nursing
    American and Canadian, 5
    dark age of, 5-6
    early practice and, 3-5
    early schools of nursing and, 8
    1800s, 6
    80s, 26-28
    expanding role and, 25-26
    50s, 24-25
    Florence Nightingale and, 6-8
    40s, 19-24
    1914 to 1918, 13-15
    postwar years and, 15-18
    60s and 70s, 25-26
    research and, 24-25
    teaching in 50s, 24-25
    30s, 18-19
    turn of century, 8-13
    war years and, 13-15, 23-24
  of general anesthetic use, 223-224
Histostab (Antazoline), 603
HMS Liquifilm (Medrysone), 1510
H2O2; see Hydrogen peroxide
Hodgkin's disease, 1171
  dacarbazine and, 1169
  MOPP regimen for, 1166
  procarbazine and, 1171
  vinblastine and, 1169
  vincristine and, 1169
Hold (Dextromethorphan), 615
Hold 4-Hour Cough Suppressant (Dextromethorphan), 615

Hold Liquid Cough Suppressant (Dextromethorphan), 615
Homapin (Homatropine hydrobromide), 467
Homapin-PB (Homatropine methylbromide; Phenobarbital), 1720
Homatrisol (Homatropine hydrobromide), 467
Homatrocel (Homatropine hydrobromide), 467
Homatropine hydrobromide, 467
Homatropine methylbromide and phenobarbital, 1720
Homeostasis, 1553-1554
Homeostatic temperature, 1199
Homo-Tet (Tetanus immune globulin), 1606
Homozygous, 161
Honvol (Diethylstilbestrol), 1462
Hookworm, 957-958
Hormestrin (Estrone), 1465
Hormones; see also specific hormone
  antineoplastic, 1170
  drug metabolism and elimination and, 112-113
  esophageal function and, 816
  female sex; see Estrogen
  gastric secretion and, 817
  growth, 1378
  laxative and, 893
  male sex; see Testosterone
  parathyroid, 1437-1438
  polypeptide, somatostatin and, 1378
  thyroid, 1407, 1408
Hormonin (Estradiol; Estrone), 1463, 1465
Hot Lemon (Chlorpheniramine), 605
Hotel Dieu
  in Montreal, 5
  in Paris, 4, 7
  in Quebec, 5
Household bleach, 1211
Household detergent, poisoning from, 1714
HPA; see Hypothalamus-pituitary-adrenal axis
H.P. Acthar (Corticotropin), 416
H.P. Acthar Gel (Corticotropin), 1501
HSIG (Human serum immune globulin), 1598
H-Stadur (Chlorpheniramine), 605
5-HTP (5-Hydroxytryptophan), 354
HTSI; see Human thyroid-stimulating immunoglobulin
Hub of needle, 47
Humagel (Paromomycin), 938, 1036
Human albumin microsphere, 1638
  labeled with technetium 99m, 1638
Human chorionic gonadotrophin, 1668
  vomiting in pregnancy and, 860
Human diploid cell rabies vaccine, 1585-1586, 1597
Human insulin, biosynthetic, 1391; see also Insulin
Human rabies immunoglobulin, 1585-1586
Human serum albumin, radiolabeled; see Radiolabeled human serum albumin
Human serum immune globulin, 1581, 1598
Human serum macroaggregate, 1632, 1643, 1644
  cardiovascular system and, 1642
  pulmonary system and, 1638
Human serum macroaggregated albumin, 1640
Human serum microsphere, labeled
  with indium 113m, 1642
  with iodine 131, 1642
  with technetium 99m, 1642
Human teratogenesis; see Teratogenicity
Human thyroid-stimulating immunoglobulin, 1413
Humatin (Paromomycin), 938, 1036
Humegon (Menotropins), 1671
Humidity, oxygen and, 555
Humorsol (Demecarium bromide), 513

Multiple disease states, elderly and, 136
Multiple drop therapy, 40, 182
Multiple myeloma, 1168
Multipolar neuron, 209, 210
Multi-Symptom (Pseudoephedrine), 500
Multivitamins, 1537-1538; see also Vitamins
  infusion of, 63
    intravenous compatibility and, 1709, 1710,
      1711
  oral contraceptive and, 1538
  pregnancy and, 1537-1538
  surgical patient and, 1537
Mumps vaccine, 1584, 1600
  administration of, and schedule, 1587
  diabetes and, 1586
  storage of, 1588
Mumps virus vaccine, live, 1600
Mumpsvax (Mumps virus vaccine, live), 1600
Muracine (Tetracycline), 1050
Muriamic (Glutamic acid hydrochloride), 852
Murine 2 (Tetrahydrozoline), 502
Murine Ear Drops (Carbamide peroxide), 1656
Murine Plus (Tetrahydrozoline), 502
Muripsin (Glutamic acid hydrochloride), 852
Murocoll (Epinephrine), 487, 576
Muscarinic agonists, 456, 458, 459; see also specific
      agent
  adverse effect of, 457-458
Muscarinic blockers, 456, 458, 459; see also specific
      agent
  adverse effect of, 457-458
  drug interactions and, 458
Muscarinic cholinergic receptor, 453
Muscle; see also specific muscle
  airway smooth, 545
  agonist, 284, 285
  cardiac, 637
  of eye, 219
  insulin and, 1380
  pain in, 836, 841
  respiratory, 535
  rigidity of, 328
  spasms of, 284-285
  weakness of, 856, 1357; see also Adverse Drug
      Effects Index
Muscle relaxants, 284-298, 305 see also specific
      agent
  adverse effect of, 286-287, 288
  centrally acting, 285-287
  discharge instruction and, 290
  drug interactions and, 288; see also Drug Inter-
      action Index
  drug therapy and, 285
  halothane and, 235
  laxative and, 893
  nursing digest of, 291-297
  nursing implications of, 289-290
  peripherally acting, 287
  physiology and, 284-285
Muscle spindle, 284, 285
Mustargen (Mechlorethamine), 1189
Mutamycin (Mitomycin), 1163
Myambutol (Ethambutol), 1104
Myasthenia gravis, 212; see also Adverse Drug Ef-
      fects Index
  anticholinesterase and, 506
Mybephen (Atropine), 464
Mycelex (Clotrimazole), 1127
Mycetism, 1108; see also Antifungal and antiviral
Mychel (Chloramphenicol), 1063

Mycifradin (Neomycin), 1035
Myciguent (Neomycin), 1035
Mycin (Chloramphenicol), 1063
Mycinettes Sugar Free (Terpin hydrate), 633
Mycitracin (Bacitracin), 1062
Mycivin (Lincomycin), 1068
Myco Triacet (Gramicidin; Neomycin; Nystatin;
      Triamcinolone), 1721
Myco Triacet Cream & Ointment (Gramicidin; Nys-
      tatin; Triamcinolone), 1067, 1132, 1517
Mycobacterial antigen, 1091
Mycobacterium leprae, 1094
Mycobacterium tuberculosis, 891, 1090; see also
      Tuberculosis
Mycolog (Gramicidin; Neomycin; Nystatin; Tri-
      amcinolone), 1067, 1132, 1315, 1517, 1721
Mycoplasma, 1041
Mycosis, 1108; see also Antifungal and antiviral;
      Fungus
  superficial, 1113
    agent for, 1113-1115
  systemic, 1108
    agent for, 1108-1113
Mycostatin (Nystatin), 891, 1132
Mycotoxicoses, 1108; see also Antifungals and an-
      tivirals
Mydfrin (Phenylephrine), 621
Mydplegic (Cyclopentolate), 467
Mydrap-ES (Hydralazine), 704
Mydriacyl (Tropicamide), 471
Mydriatic, precaution with, 41
Mydrilate (Cyclopentolate), 467
Myelin sheath, 207-210
Myelocytic leukemia, 1170
Myelogenous leukemia, acute, 1143
Myelomas, multiple, 1168
Myelosuppression; see Adverse Drug Effects Index
Mylanta (Aluminum hydroxide gel; Magnesium
      hydroxide), 843, 846
Mylanta II (Simethicone), 850
Mylanta-2 Extra Strength (Simethicone), 850
Mylaxen (Hexafluorenium bromide), 530
Mylepsine (Primidone), 426
Myleran (Busulfan), 1185
Mylicon (Simethicone), 850
Myocardial infarction, 418, 528, 667, 692, 694; see
      also Adverse Drug Effects Index
  beta-adrenergic blocker and, 692
  imaging and, 1641
  sulfinpyrazone and, 727
Myocardial ischemia, 667
Myocardial perfusion imaging, 1641
Myocarditis, 694
  trypanosomiasis and, 917
Myocardol (Pentaerythritol tetranitrate), 746
Myochrysine (Gold sodium thiomalate), 1366
Myoclonus seizure, 406
Myocon (Nitroglycerin), 745
Myoquin (Iodochlorhydroxyquin), 1238
Myoforte (Chlorzoxazone), 292
Myoplegine (Succinylcholine), 531
Myosin, 1434-1437
Myotatic reflex, 212
Myotenlis (Succinylcholine), 531
Myotonachol (Bethanechol), 465, 808
Myotrol (Orphenadrine), 297, 401
Myser Plus (Hydralazine), 704
Mysoline (Primidone), 426
Mysolone (Triamcinolone), 1517
Mystaform Ointment (Iodochlorhydroxyquin),
      1238

Mystaform-HC (Iodochlorhydroxyquin), 1238
Mysuran (Ambenonium), 513
Mytelase (Ambenonium), 513
Mytrate (Epinephrine), 487, 576
Mytrex (Gramicidin; Nystatin; Triamcinolone),
      1067, 1132, 1517
Mytrox (Gramicidin), 1067
Myxedema
  hypothyroidism and, 1420
  pretibial, 1413
Myxedema coma, 1407, 1423
  hypothyroidism and, 1421

N

Nabilone, 870
Nack (Chlordiazepoxide), 269
Naclex (Benzthiazide), 779
NAD; see Nicotinamide adenine dinucleotide
Nadolol, 686, 706
  pharmacokinetics of, 688
Nadopen-V (Penicillin V), 1015
Nadostine (Nystatin), 1132
NADP; see Nicotinamide adenine dinucleotide
      phosphate
Nafcil (Nafcillin), 1010
Nafcillin, 982-983, 1010, 1537; see also Penicillins
  excretion of, 759
  food and, 84
  intravenous compatibility and, 1710, 1711
  oral, 983
  potassium deficit and, 1563
  staphylococcal infection and, 980
Nafrine (Oxymetazoline), 494, 620
Nail plate changes, 1204, 1204-1205
Nailbed discoloration, 1146
NaI(Tl); see Thallium-activated sodium iodide
      crystal
Nalbuphine, 318-319
Nalcrom (Cromolyn sodium), 574
Naldecon (Chlorpheniramine; Phenylephrine;
      Phenylpropanolamine), 496, 605, 621, 623
Naldecon-CX (Guaifenesin), 630
Naldegesic (Pseudoephedrine), 625
Naldetuss (Dextromethorphan), 615
Nalfon (Fenoprofen), 1339
Nalgesic (Fenoprofen), 1339
Nalidixic acid, 791, 795, 796, 797, 800, 804, 805
  administration of, 791, 798
  adverse effect of, 791
  dosage and, 791
  excretion of, 791
  neonate and, 133
  nursing implications for, 797
  sensitive organism to, 791
  urinary pH and, 108
Nallpen (Nafcillin), 1010
Nalorphine, 74
Naloxone, 237, 321
  as antagonist, 74
  as antidote, 1713
  apomorphine and, 856
  dissociation and, 148
  fentanyl and, 237
  mood and, 144
  narcotic overdose and, 303
  paregoric and, 910
  respiratory acidosis and, 1575
  sensitivity to stimuli and, 142
Naltrexone, 191
Nalutron (Progesterone), 1470
Nandrobolic LA (Nandrolone), 1482

Nyquil (Doxylamine; Ephedrine), 487, 575, 1663
Nyquil Nightime Colds Medicine (Dextromethorphan; Doxylamine; Ephedrine), 487, 575, 615, 1663
Nysolone (Gramicidin; Nystatin; Triamcinolone), 1067, 1132, 1315
Nystaform Ointment (Nystatin), 1132
Nystaform-HC (Hydrocortisone; Iodohydroxyquin; Nystatin), 1309
Nystatin, 1113-1114, 1119, 1132
  Candida albicans and, 891
  in gramicidin, neomycin, nystatin, and triamcinolone, 1285, 1721, 1722, 1724
  in ice cups, 1151
  with iodochlorhydroxyquin and hydrocortisone, 1285
Nytilax (Senna), 907

O

O & B Suppository (Belladonna), 465
Obedrin-LA (Methamphetamine), 400
Obepar (Phendimetrazine), 402
Obesamead (Phentermine), 403
Obesity
  blood pressure and, 643
  central nervous system stimulant and, 384
  diet and, 1375
  hyperglycemia and, 1375
  insulin and, 1375
  insulin resistance and, 1375
  non insulin-dependent diabetes and, 1373
  oral hypoglycemic and, 1375, 1376
Obetrol (Dextroamphetamine), 395
Obeval (Phendimetrazine), 402
Obidoxime, 507
Objective
  evaluation and, 31
  planning and, 31
Obligatory parasite, 915
Obotan (Dextroamphetamine)
Obstruction
  airway, 537-539
  of common bile duct, 822
  intestinal, 879
  of pancreatic drainage, 837
Obstructive cardiomyopathy, 651, 654
Obstructive lung disease, 538
Occlusive dressing, 1262
  topical corticosteroid and, 1280-1281
Octocaine (Lidocaine), 1245
Ocuclear (Oxymetazoline), 494
Ocular complication, 185, 1131
Ocular infection
  natamycin and, 1114
  sulfonamide and, 1080
Oculogyric crisis, 328
Oculomotor nerve, 219
Ocusert (Pilocarpine), 92, 470
Ocusert Pilo (Pilocarpine), 470
Ocusol Drops (Tetrahydrozoline), 502
Oestrilin (Estrogens, conjugated), 1464
  with Methyltestosterone (Estrogens, conjugated; Methyltestosterone), 1464
Ogen (Estropipate), 1465
25-OHD$_2$; *see* 25-Hydroxyergocalciferol
25-OHD$_3$; *see* 25-Hydroxycholecalciferol
1,25-(OH)$_2$D$_3$; *see* 1,25-Dihydroxycholecalciferol
Oil, 32
Oil of wintergreen; *see* Methyl salicylate
Oil enema, 885
Oil preparation, 8-9

Ointment
  administration of, 1261
  ophthalmic, 39
  topical, 44
    corticosteroid and, 1281
  vaginal, 38
Oleandomycin, 1057
  Streptomyces antibioticus and, 1057
Olfactory nerve, 218
Olicin (Troleandomycin), 1070
Oligodendroglia, 207
Olive oil enema, 904
Olivopontocerebellar degeneration, 383
Omazine (Chlorpromazine), 341
Omnipen (Ampicillin), 998
Onchocerca volvulus, 956
Onchocerciasis, 956
Oncovin (Vincristine), 1191
On-off autonomic control, 449
Onset (Isosorbide dinitrate), 743
Onset of action, 80-81
Open drop method for anesthetic, 228
Ophthaine (Proparacaine), 1249
Ophthalmia neonatorum, 1055, 1213
Ophthalmic medications, 39-41; *see also* specific agent
  absorption and, 91-92
  administration of, 39-41
  monitoring of, 41
  preparation of, 39-40
Ophthalmic nerve, 219
Ophthalmic reactions; *see* Adverse Drug Effect Index
Ophthel-S (Sulfacetamide), 1085
Ophthetic (Proparacaine), 1249
Ophthochlor (Chloramphenicol), 1063
Opiate, 303, 827, 858, 895; *see also* Narcotics; specific agent
  activated charcoal and, 1715
  addiction to, 13, 191-194
  colonic motility and, 828
  constipation and, 878
  diarrhea and, 888, 889
  health consequence of, 192
  in patent medication, 13
  respiratory acidosis and, 1574
  in suppository, 10
  tincture of opium in, 889, 911
Opiate antagonist, 142
Opiate receptor
  brainstem and, 302
  medulla and, 302
  spinal cord and, 301
  thalamus and, 301
Opium alkaloid, 316
Opium derivative, laxative and, 893
Opium tincture, 889, 911
Opponent process theory, 191
Op-Sulfa30 (Sulfacetamide), 1085
Optic nerve, 218-219
Optic tract, 218
Opticrom (Cromolyn sodium), 574
Optimyd (Prednisolone), 1515
Optinoxan (Methaqualone), 276
Optomethasone (Dexamethasone), 1504
Optopentolate (Cyclopentolate), 467
Optopilo (Pilocarpine), 470
Optosulfex (Sulfacetamide), 1085
Optozoline (Naphazoline), 493, 619
Oradrate (Chloral hydrate), 269
Oraflex (Benoxaprofen), 1337

Oragest (Medroxyprogesterone), 1466
Oral antacid; *see* Antacid
Oral anticoagulant, 260; *see also* Anticoagulant; specific agent
  action of, 723
  administration of, 735-736
  chemistry of, 723
  discovery of, 721-722
  drug interactions and; *see* Drug Interaction Index
  enzyme induction and, 113, 114
  enzyme inhibition and, 115
  monitoring and, 736
  pharmacokinetics of, 723-724
  use of, 724
Oral cavity, 815
Oral contraceptives, 260, 1451-1454; *see also* specific agent
  biphasic, 1452
  breakthrough bleeding and, 261
  combination, 1452
  drug interactions and, 176; *see also* Drug Interaction Index
  enzyme induction and, 114
  hepatotoxicity of, 112
  menstrual cycle and, 1451-1452
  mini pill progestin only, 1453
  monophasic, 1452
  multivitamins and, 1538
  postcoital estrogen only, 1453
  potassium deficit and, 1562, 1563
  thromboembolic disorder and, 1453-1454
  triphasic, 1452-1453
  types of, 1452
Oral hypoglycemics, 1373-1375, 1400-1401; *see also* specific agent
  biguanide, 1375
  characteristics of, 1374
  drug interactions and, 176-177; *see also* Drug Interaction Index
  enzyme inhibition and, 115
  history of, 1373
  mechanism of action of, 1373-1374
  non insulin-dependent diabetes and, 1373
  obesity and, 1375, 1376
  primary failure and, 1374
  secondary failure and, 1374
  sodium deficit and, 1560
  sulfonylurea and; *see* Sulfonylurea
  syndrome of inappropriate secretion of antidiuretic hormone and, 1560
  University Group Diabetes Program and, 1375
Oral medication, 31-37; *see also* specific agent
  absorption of, 32, 83-90, 981
  cephalosporin and, 986
  administration of, 35-37
  amoxicillin and, 983
  capsule in, 33
  contraindication for, 33
  corticosteroid and, 172; *see also* Corticosteroid
  cyclacillin and, 983
  early drugs and, 8-10
  liquid, 32
  monitoring of, 37
  penicillin G in, 981-982
  penicillin V in, 982
  preparation of, 33-34
  tablet in, 32-33
Oramide (Tolbutamide), 1401
Oranixon (Mephenesin), 296
Orap (Pimozide), 346

Sandimmune (Cyclosporine), 1660
Sandoptal (Butalbital), 268
Sandril (Reserpine), 501, 710
Sanoma (Carisoprodol), 292
Sanorex (Mazindol), 400
Sansert (Methysergide), 1672
Santyl (Collagenase), 1659
Saplix (Atropine; Hyoscyamine; Phenobarbital; Scopolamine), 1724
S-Aqua (Benzthiazide), 779
SAR; see Structure-activity relationship
Saralasin, 687
Sarcoma
    cyclophosphamide and, 1167
    dacarbazine and, 1169
    doxorubicin and, 1144
    Ewing's
        dactinomycin and, 1145
        vincristine and, 1169
    methotrexate and, 1142
    vincristine and, 1169
Sarcoptes scabiei, 945
Sarin as irreversible anticholinesterase, 506
Sarodant (Nitrofurantoin), 805
Saroflex (Chlorzoxazone), 292
Saronil (Meprobamate), 276
Saroten (Amitryptyline), 368
SAS-500 (Sulfasalazine), 1087
Satric (Metronidazole), 937
Saturated solution
    of potassium iodide, 1416, 1427
    of sodium iodide, 1427
Saventrine (Isoproterenol), 490, 579
Savlon (Cetrimide), 1232, 1233
Savlon Hospital Concentrate (Cetrimide with chlorhexidine), 1233
Scabanca (Benzyl benzoate), 950
Scabane (Lindane), 951
Scabicides; see Pediculicides and scabicides
Scabies, 945-946
    canine, 946
    secondary infection of, 946
    topical corticosteroid and, 1283-1284
Scabiol (Benzyl benzoate), 950
Scalp lesions, 1262
Scan
    bone, 1639-1640
    brain, 1637
    liver, 1640-1641
Scanner, rectilinear, 1628-1629
Scarlet red, 1219
Schistosoma hematobium, 959
Schistosoma japonicum, 891, 959
Schistosoma mansoni, 891, 959
Schistosomiasis, 891, 959
    diarrhea and, 888
Schizont, 920
Schools of nursing, early, 8
Schwann cell, 210
Sciatic nerve, 52, 53
Scintillation, 1628
Scintillation camera, gamma, 1629
Scintillation probe, 1628
Sclerosing agent, hemorrhoid and, 1216
Scolex, 954
Scoline (Succinylcholine), 531
Scopolamine, 457, 458, 471, 857, 873
    with atropine, hyoscyamine, and phenobarbital, 1718, 1719, 1720, 1722, 1723, 1724
    central nervous system effect of, 456
    general anesthetic and, 224
    and memory for stimulus, 142

Scopolamine—cont'd
    nausea and vomiting and, 857
    to reverse poisoning from anticholinergic, 510
    sustained release of, 93
Scott's Emulsion (Vitamin A; Vitamin D), 1448, 1550
Scratch, animal, 1585
Scurvy, 1525
SDM No. 22 (Pentaerythritol tetranitrate), 746
SDM No. 23 (Pentaerythritol tetranitrate), 746
SDM No. 35 (Pentaerythritol tetranitrate), 746
[75]Se; see also Selenium-75
Sea salt, 1564
Seatworm, 957
Sebaceous gland, 1200
Seborrheic dermatitis, 1256-1258
Sebucare (Salicylic acid), 1272
Sebulex (Salicylic acid; Ssulfur), 1273
Sebusan (Selenium sulfide), 1273
Sebutone (Coal tar; Salicylic acid), 1267
Secobarbital, 280; see also Barbiturates
    athletic person and, 150
    general anesthetic and, 224
    hazard of, in pregnancy, 131
    intake of information and, 141
    intellectual person and, 150
    with pentaerythritol tetranitrate, 1718, 1719
    properties of, 256
Secogen (Secobarbital), 280
Second cranial nerve, 218-219
Second gas effect of anesthetic, 228
Secotabs (Secobarbital), 280
Secretin, 822
    gastric secretion and, 817
    volume of food to duodenum and, 820
Secular hospital, 4
Sedalone (Methaqualone), 276
Sedaril (Hydroxyzine), 868
Sedation, 457, 588, 859; see also Adverse Drug Effects Index
    stimulant and, 384
Sedative-hypnotics, 252-283; see also specific agent
    accidental poisoning and, 132
    adverse effects of, 253-254, 259
    animal bite and, 1585
    barbiturates in, 256-257; see also Barbiturates
    behavior change and, 140
    benzodiazepines in, 254-256; see also Benzodiazepines
    chloral hydrate in, 257-258
    chlormezanone in, 258
    constipation and, 878
    difference between, 252
    discharge/outpatient instruction and, 264
    drug digest of, 265-282
    drug interactions and, 260; see also Drug Interaction Index
    duodenal ulcer and, 830
    elderly and, 136
    ephedrine and, 547, 550
    ethchlorvynol in, 258
    eye-hand coordination and, 142
    general anesthetic and, 224
    glutethimide in, 258
    hydroxyzine in, 258
    liver function and, 112
    and memory for stimulus, 142
    meprobamate in, 258
    methaqualone in, 258
    methyprylon in, 258
    nonmedical use of, 200
    nursing implications of, 261-263

Sedative-hypnotics—cont'd
    paraldehyde in, 258
    physiology of sleep in, 252-253
    preanesthetic medication and, 225, 238
    psychomotor task and, 142
    rectal, 10
    withdrawal syndrome and, 200
Sedatuss (Dextromethorphan), 615
Sedatuss Expectorant (Guaifenesin), 631
Sedolatan (Prenylamine), 746
Sedonal Natrium (Secobarbital), 280
Sedralex (Hyoscyamine), 468
Sedural (Phenazopyridine), 801
Seebrine (Methyldopa), 705
Seffin (Cephalothin), 1006
Segmentation, 887
    of colon, 878
Segontin (Prenylamine), 746
Seguril (Furosemide), 781
Seizures; see also Convulsions
    alcohol withdrawal and, 408
    alprostadil and, 1653
    anticonvulsant choice and, 406
    classification of, 405-406
    generalized, 405-406
    infantile, 408
    partial, 405
    penicillin G and, 981
    pregnancy and, 407
    psychomotor, 405
    in status epilepticus, 407-408
    unclassified, 406
    unilateral, 406
Seldane (Terfenadine), 610
Selective bronchodilator, 547-548
Selenium, 1257, 1273
    activated charcoal and, 1715
    as antiseborrheic, 1256-1257
    trace element and, 1539
Selenium-75, 1634
Selenium-75 selenomethionine, 1634
Self-induced vomiting, 860
Self-medication program, 30
Selium (Chlordiazepoxide), 269
Sellymin (Sodium bicarbonate), 848
Seloken (Metoprolol), 492, 706
Selsun (Selenium), 1273
Selsun Blue (Selenium), 1273
Semilente (Insulin zinc, prompt), 1403
Semilente Iletin (Insulin zinc, prompt), 1403
Semilumar valve, 637
Semitard (Insulin zinc, prompt), 1403
Semoxydrine (Methamphetamine), 400
Semple vaccine, 1586
Semustine, 1168
Senna, 882, 906-907
Senna fluid extract, 882
Senna glyoside, 882
Senna laxative, 897
    discharge/outpatient instruction for, 897
Senna leaf, 882
Sennoside A and B, 882
Senokap DSS (Senna), 907
Senokot (Senna), 907
    with plantago (Plantago seed; Senna), 905, 907
Senokot-S (Senna), 907
Senolax (Senna), 907
Sensitivity; see also Allergy reaction; Hypersensitivity
    aminoglycoside and, 1019-1020
    antibiotic and, 1059
    intravenous medication and, 65

Tonelax (Danthron), 900

Tonic, 13

Tonic seizure, 406

Tonic-clonic seizure, 406

Tonilen (Demecarium bromide), 513

Tonoftal (Tolnaftate), 1132

Tooth discoloration; see Adverse Drug Effects Index

Topex Acne Clearing Medication (Benzoyl peroxide), 1266

Tophaceous gout, 1354
  allopurinol and, 1354
  probenecid and, 1354
  sulfinpyrazone and, 1354

Topical corticosteroids, 1197, 1277-1316; see also Corticosteroids
  adverse effect of, 1281-1285, 1286, 1288, 1290, 1490- 1491
  amount of, 1279-1280
  antibiotic and, 1285
  antiinflammation and, 1278-1279
  antiproliferation and, 1279
  basic action of, 1277
  concentration of, 1280
  cosmetic appearance and, 1381
  cost of, 1281
  discharge/outpatient instruction for, 1291
  drug digest of, 1292-1315
  drug interactions and, 1284, 1287, 1288
  formulation of, 1281
  frequency of application of, 1280
  metabolism and, 1281
  nursing implication for, 1288-1290
  occlusion and, 1280-1281
  percutaneous absorption of, 1279
  potency of, 1278
  precaution for, 1285
  reservoir and, 1281
  site of, 1280
  structure-activity relationship and, 1277-1278
  tachyphylaxis and, 1280
  tolerance and, 1280
  type of disease and, 1280
  vehicle and, 1281

Topical medication, 44-45, 1208; see also specific agent
  drug absorption and, 92

Topicort (Desoximetasone), 1300

Topisolon (Desoximetasone), 1300

Topitracin (Bacitracin), 1062

Topsyn Gel (Fluocinomide), 1304

TOPV (Poliovirus vaccine, live oral), 1602

Torecan (Triethylperazine) 872

Toresten (Triethylperazine) 872

Toronto insulin (Insulin injection), 1403

Torticollis, 328

Tosmilen (Demecarium bromide), 513

Totacillin (Ampicillin), 999

Total body fluid of elderly, 135

Total intestinal preparation, 884, 885, 907

Total lung capacity, 536

Total parenteral nutrition, 64; see also Parenteral alimentation

Total plasma clearance, 121

Toxic concentration, 1726

Toxic epidermal necrolysis, 184, 1076, 1354

Toxic nodular goiter, 1414

Toxicity, 180-187
  adverse drug reaction and, 180-182; see also Adverse drug reaction; Adverse Drug Effects Index

Toxicity—cont'd
  of aminoglycosides, 1022-1023
  of anesthetics, 239
  of barbiturates, 200
  cutaneous, 183-184
  of digitalis, 176, 652, 653
  drug interactions in, 182-183; see also Drug interactions; Drug interaction index
  drug metabolism and elimination and, 116-117
  laboratory test interference in, 183
  organ, 183-186
  cutaneous, 183-184
  fever and, 184-185
  hematologic complication and, 185
  hepatotoxicity and, 185
  ocular complication and, 185
  ototoxicity and, 185
  pulmonary complication and, 186
  renal complication and, 185-186
  sexual dysfunction and, 186
  overdosage in, 182
  parkinsonism and, 383; see also Extrapyramidal effect
  side effect and, 180-182
  specific organ, 183-186
    cutaneous toxicity in, 183-184
    fever and, 184-185
    hematologic complication and, 185
    hepatotoxicity and, 185
    ocular complication and, 185
    ototoxicity and, 185
    pulmonary complication and, 186
    renal complication and, 185-186
    sexual dysfunction and, 186

Toxocara canis, 959

Toxocara cati, 959

Toxocariasis, 959

Toxoid, 1580, 1581-1582, 1589, 1591-1592
  adverse effect of, 1589, 1591-1592
  diphtheria, 1581, 1596
  discharge/outpatient instruction and, 1593
  drug digest and, 1594-1609
  drug interaction and, 1589, 1590
  nursing implication for, 1590-1593
  recommended schedule for, 1587
  tetanus, 1581-1582, 1607

Toxoplasma gondii, 1079

Toxoplasmosis, 1079

TPN; see Total parenteral nutrition

Trac Tabs (Atropine; Hyoscyamine; Methenamine; Methylene blue), 464, 468, 802, 803

Trace elements, 1521, 1538, 1539-1540
  adverse effect of, 1540
  drug interaction and, 1541
  nursing implication and, 1541

Trachea, 544
  velocity of air flow through, 537

Tracheostomy, 538

Trachoma, 1043
  sulfonamide and, 1078

Tracrium (Atracurium), 529

Training, alcoholism treatment and, 198

Training schools, early, 8

Trait, transmission of, 161; see also Genetics

Tral Filmtab (Hexocyclium methylsulfate), 467

Tral Gradumet (Hexocyclium methylsulfate), 467

Tramacin (Triamcinolone), 1314, 1517

Trancin (Fluphenazine), 343

Trancopal (Chlormezanone), 269

Trandate (Labetalol), 704

Tranimul (Diazepam), 270, 295

Tranquil (Acetaminophen), 321

Tranquiline (Meprobamate), 276

Tranquilizer
  antipsychotic; see Antipsychotics

Transact (Sulfur), 1274

Transcellular path, 1206-1207

Transdermal delivery system, scopolamine and, 857

Transderm-Nitro (Nitroglycerin), 733, 745

Transderm-SCOP (Scopolamine), 471, 873

Transderm-V (Scopolamine), 471, 873

Transepidermal transport, 1206-1208

Transference, placebo and, 148

Transferrin, radiolabeled, 1642

Transfusion reaction, 181

Transient ischemic attack
  aspirin and, 727, 1319
  dipyridamole and, 1355
  probenecid and, 1355

Transmitter compound, 299
  central nervous system and, 213-214; see also Neurotransmitter agent

Transport, 108
  alteration of, 1207
  membrane, oral medication and, 89
  radiopharmaceutical and, 1629
  transepidermal, 1206-1208

Trans-retinol, 1521

Transverse colon, 827

Tranxene (Clorazepate), 269

Tranxilene (Clorazepate), 269

Tranylcypromine, 378, 479; see also Monoamine oxidase inhibitors
  drug interactions and; see Drug Interaction Index
  enzyme inhibition and, 115

Tranzine (Chlorpromazine), 341, 866

Trasicor (Oxprenolol), 707

Trates (Nitroglycerin), 745

Trauma
  extrathoracic airway obstruction and, 538
  head, 217
    anticonvulsant and, 408
  nerve, 210
  ulcer and, 832

Travamine (Dimenhydrinate), 867

Tray, medication, 20, 21

Trazodone, 379

Treatment plan
  diabetes and, 1373
  rheumatoid arthritis and, 1319, 1320

Trecator (Ethionamide), 1104

Trecator-SC (Ethionamide), 1104

Trelmar (Meprobamate), 276

Trematode, 959-960
  clonorchiasis and, 960
  fascioliasis and, 959
  paragonimiasis and, 959-960
  schistosomiasis and, 959

Tremin (Trihexyphenidyl), 403

Tremor, 328, 360, 382, 579, 1424

Trental (Pentoxifylline), 1674

Treponema pallidum, 980, 1041, 1043

Trescatyl (Ethionamide), 1104

Tresortil (Methocarbamol), 297

Tretinoin, 1255, 1274-1275, 1523

TRH; see Thyrotropin-releasing hormone

Triacetin, 1133

Triaderm (Triamcinolone), 1517

Triador (Methaqualone), 276

Triamalone (Triamcinolone), 1517

Virosterone (Testosterone), 1485
Virus, 1115, 1284; *see also* Antifungal and antiviral
    diarrhea and, 891
    formalin and, 1219
    hepatitis and; *see* Viral hepatitis
    iodine compound and, 1211, 1212
    replication of, 1117
    slow, 382
    vaccine for, 1583-1586
    vitamin C and, 1525-1532
Viscephen (Dicyclomine), 1661
Visceral innervation, 440-441
Visceral larva migrans, 959
Visceral leishmaniasis, 917
Viscerol (Dicyclomine), 1661
Viscous lidocaine, 1221
Visine Eye Drops (Tetrahydrozoline), 502
Visken (Pindolol), 708
Vistaril (Hydroxyzine), 274, 868
Vistrax (Oxyphencyclimine; Hydroxyzine), 469, 868,
    1725
Visual disturbances; *see* Adverse Drug Effects In-
    dex
Visudrisone (Medrysone), 1510
Visumiotic (Demecarium bromide), 513
Visutensil (Guanethidine), 489, 703
Vita-C (Ascorbic acid), 1543
Vitacee (Ascorbic acid), 799, 1543
Vita-E (Vitamin E), 1551
Vital capacity, 536
Vitalone (Methaqualone), 276
Vita-Metrazol (Pyridoxine; Riboflavin), 1548, 1549
Vitamin, 1521-1551; *see also* specific vitamin
    adverse effect of, 1524, 1540, 1541, 1542
    chemical reaction and, 75
    constipation and, 878
    cystic fibrosis and, 837
    discharge/outpatient instruction and, 1542
    drug digest and, 1543-1551
    drug interactions and, 1541
    enzyme and, 1521
    fat-soluble, 1521
    intravenous antibiotic and, 64
    lung and, 1524
    mineral and trace element and, 1538, 1539-1540
    mineral oil and, 892, 1443
    multivitamin preparation and, 1537-1538
    nursing implications for, 1541
    water-soluble, 1521
Vitamin A, 1521-1525, 1550
    in acne, 1255, 1523-1524
    adverse effect of, 1524, 1540, 1541
    calcium metabolism and, 1523
    cancer and, 1524
    cholestyramine and, 739
    cystic fibrosis and, 837
    deficiency of, 1523
    function of, 1522
    hypervitaminosis and, 1523
      calcium excess and, 1566
    mineral oil and, 880
    occurrence of, 1521-1522
    oral contraceptive and, 1523
    pregnancy and, 1523
    requirement for 1522-1523
Vitamin A Acid Gel (Tretinoin), 1274, 1523
Vitamin B$_1$, 1526-1527; *see also* Thiamine
Vitamin B$_2$, 1526-1527, 1549
    food and, 84
Vitamin B$_3$, 1526-1527; *see also* Niacin
Vitamin B$_6$, 1526-1527; *see also* Pyridoxine
    affective disorder and, 354

Vitamin B$_6$—cont'd
    isoniazid and, 162, 1092
    levodopa and, 397
    levodopa-carbidopa and, 399
    penicillamine and, 1359
Vitamin B$_{12}$, 243, 1353, 1528-1529; *see also* Cyano-
    cobalamin
    adverse effect of, 1442, 1444
    nitrous oxide and, 243
Vitamin B$_c$, 1530-1531; *see also* Folic acid
Vitamin B complex, 1524-1525, 1526-1531, 1537
    inositol and, 1525
    para-aminobenzoic acid and, 1524
    with vitamin C, intravenous incompatibility and,
      1710, 1711
Vitamin C, 799, 1521-1532, 1542; *see also* Ascorbic
    acid
    aspirin and, 1321
    cancer and, 1532
    common cold and, 1525-1532
    decubiti and, 1532
    deficiency of, 1525
    function of, 1525
    intestinal drug sulfation and, 106
    intravenous compatibility and, 1710, 1711
    penicillin G and, 1537
    smoking and, 1532
    source of, 1525
    toxicity of, 1532
    viral disease and, 1525-1532
Vitamin D, 1441-1442, 1444, 1524, 1532-1533, 1550
    anticonvulsant and, 1533-1534
    calcium deficit and, 1565
    cholestyramine and, 739
    cystic fibrosis and, 837
    deficiency of, 1533
    elderly and, 138
    function of, 1533
    hypervitaminosis and, 1533
      calcium excess and and, 1566
    magnesium deficit and, 1567
    metabolism and, 116, 1534
    mineral oil and, 880, 1443
    osteomalacia and, 1533
    phosphorus-32 uptake and, 1646
    requirement for, 1533
    rickets and, 1532, 1533
    rifampin and, 1443
    source of, 1532-1533
    thiazide diuretic and, 1443
Vitamin D$_2$, 1532
Vitamin D$_3$, 1532-1533
Vitamin D$_4$, 1533
Vitamin E, 1537, 1541, 1551
    adverse effect of, 1535
    assertions about, 1535-1536
    cystic fibrosis and, 837
    function of, 1534-1535
    mineral oil and, 880
    requirement for, 1535
Vitamin K, 1536-1537, 1547; *see also* Phytonadione
    anticoagulant and, 164, 737, 738, 1537, 1541
    cholestyramine and, 739
    cystic fibrosis and, 837
    deficiency and, 164, 1536-1537
    function of, 1536
    mineral oil and, 880
    pregnancy and, 1537
    requirement for, 1536
    toxicity of, 1537
Viterra-C (Ascorbic acid), 1543

Vitron C (Ascorbic acid), 1543
Vitron-C-Plus (Folic acid), 1545
Vi-Twel (Cyanocobalamin), 1544
Vivactil (Protriptyline), 377
Vivarin (Caffeine), 393
Vividyl (Nortriptyline), 375
Vivol (Diazepam), 270, 295, 417
Vi-Zac Capsules (Ascorbic acid; Vitamin E), 1543,
    1551
VLDL; *see* Very low density lipoprotein
Volatile anesthetics, 233-236, 242; *see also* Anes-
    thetics; specific agent
    chloroform in, 234
    divinyl ether in, 234
    enflurane in, 235-236
    ether in, 233-234
    ethyl chloride in, 234
    halothane in, 234-235
    isoflurane in, 236
    methoxyflurane in, 235
Volital (Pemoline), 402
Voltaren (Diclofenac), 1338
Volume
    of distribution, 119, 120
      child and, 133
      elderly and, 135
      infant and, 133
    fluid, imbalance of, 1557; *see also* Fluid and elec-
      trolyte disturbance
    lung, 536
    stroke, 645
Volume-control device, 62, 63
Vol-U-Trol, 63
Vomiting, 854, 858-860; *see also* Antiemetic; Emetic
    cause of, 855
    oral medication and, 37
    during pregnancy, 860
    psychologic component of, 860
Vomiting center, 854, 855
von Economo's disease, 382
Von Liebig, 223
Vontrol (Diphenidol), 867
Vumon (Teniposide), 1190
Vytone (Diiodohydroxyquin and hydrocortisone),
    1725
VZIG (Varicella-zoster immune globulin), 1608

W

W-135 (Meningococcal polysaccharide vaccine),
    1600
Wafer, 9
Wampocap (Niacin), 744, 749
WANS (Pentobarbital), 278, 422
War years
    World War I and, 13-15
    World War II and, 23-24
Warcoumin (Warfarin), 752
Warfarin, 752; *see also* Oral onticoagulants
    dicumarol sensitivity and, 164
    drug interactions and, 262; *see also* Drug Inter-
      action Index
    elderly and, 135
    enzyme induction and, 113, 114
    genetics and, 160, 165-166
    hazard of, 45
      in pregnancy, 131
    intramuscular injection and, 57
    metabolic pathway and, 99
    pharmacokinetics of, 724
    prolonged bleeding and, 182
    resistance to, 160, 165-166